Occupational Therapy *for* Physical Dysfunction

Seventh Edition

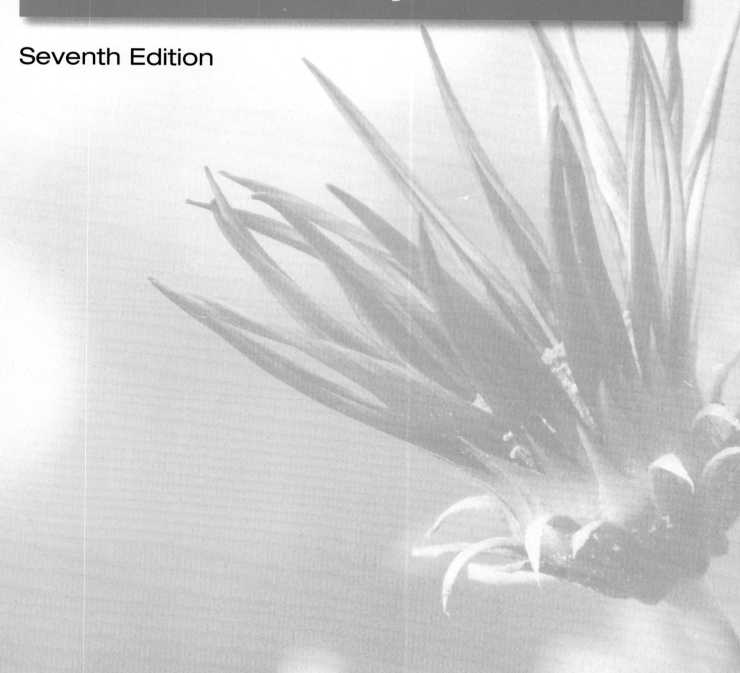

Occupational Therapy *for* Physical Dysfunction

Seventh Edition

EDITORS

Mary Vining Radomski, PhD, OTR/ L, FAOTA

Clinical Scientist, Occupational Therapist
Courage Kenny Research Center
Occupational Therapist
Courage Kenny Rehabilitation Institute
Minneapolis, Minnesota

Catherine A. Trombly Latham, ScD, OTR/L, FAOTA

Professor Emerita
Department of Occupational Therapy
College of Health and Rehabilitation Sciences: Sargent College
Boston University
Boston, Massachusetts

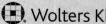 **Wolters Kluwer** | Lippincott Williams & Wilkins
Health

Philadelphia · Baltimore · New York · London
Buenos Aires · Hong Kong · Sydney · Tokyo

Senior Editor: Michael Noble
Product Manager: John Larkin, Heather Rybacki
Development Editor: Kelly Horvath
Marketing Manager: Shauna Kelley
Designer: Teresa Mallon
Compositor: Absolute Service, Inc.

Seventh Edition
Copyright © 2014 Lippincott Williams & Wilkins, a Wolters Kluwer business

351 West Camden Street
Baltimore, MD 21201

Two Commerce Square
2001 Market Street
Philadelphia, PA 19103

Printed in China

9 8 7 6 5 4 3 2 1

Library of Congress Cataloging-in-Publication Data

Occupational therapy for physical dysfunction / editors, Mary Vining Radomski, Catherine A. Trombly Latham. -- Seventh edition.
  p.; cm.
Includes bibliographical references and index.
  ISBN 978-1-4511-8921-6 (hardback : alk. paper)
  I. Radomski, Mary Vining, editor of compilation. II. Latham, Catherine A. Trombly editor of compilation.
  [DNLM: 1. Occupational Therapy. 2. Disabled Persons--rehabilitation. WB 555]
  RM735
  615.8'515--dc23

2013029668

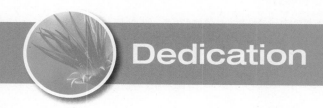

Dedication

To the profession's authors—past, present, and future.

Preface

The seventh edition of *Occupational Therapy for Physical Dysfunction* emphasizes four key themes that are essential to the best possible occupational therapy for adults with physical disabilities and to the future of the profession:

- Reliance on evidence/research to inform occupational therapy assessment and intervention
- Occupation as the central intervention and outcome of occupational therapy services
- Importance of expert activity analysis that synthesizes theoretical knowledge, clinical skills, and awareness of person and contextual factors to occupational therapy practice
- Appreciation for the individuality, unique circumstances, and priorities of each patient/client.

These themes are evident in the book's organization, features, ancillaries, terminology, and authorship.

ORGANIZATION

Similar to the previous edition, the seventh edition is composed of six sections with 45 chapters.

Section I lays the foundation for the rest of the textbook. Chapter 1 addresses theoretical foundations (with emphasis on the Model of Occupational Functioning), and Chapter 2 addresses practical foundations of occupational therapy for adults with physical dysfunction.

Section II presents the areas of assessment in which an occupational therapist working in acute medical, inpatient/outpatient rehabilitation, and community-based rehabilitation settings should be competent. The chapter sequence generally represents the order in which occupational therapists might conduct assessment, beginning with appraisal of the specific context and evaluating the person's occupational roles and competence, followed by assessment of the person's abilities and capacities that support role performance and finally assessment of the relevant environmental constraints and enablers of performance.

Section III presents three mechanisms of therapeutic change: occupation and occupation as therapy, learning, and therapeutic rapport.

Section IV presents therapeutic technologies that enable and support occupational functioning: splinting, wheelchairs, adapted or assistive devices, and physical agent modalities.

Section V elucidates intervention principles and practices for persons with physical dysfunction. As in earlier editions, this section does not provide recipes for the treatment of people with particular diagnoses but rather descriptions of best practice. The professional occupational therapist can choose from these for a particular patient who has his or her own particular goals and manifestation of a diagnosis.

Section VI includes discussions of the practice of occupational therapy for particular major diagnostic categories, each written by a specialist in that area. These experts alert therapists who are beginning to practice with one of these populations to various commonly encountered impairments that affect occupational functioning and to the specialized assessments and treatments that have been developed for persons carrying the diagnosis.

In addition to the textbook, the following three chapters from the sixth edition are now available to readers on thePoint, the book's website (thepoint.lww.com): Optimizing Motor Behavior Using the Bobath Approach, Optimizing Motor Behavior Using the Brunnstrom Movement Therapy Approach, and Managing Deficit of First-Level Motor Control Capacities Using Rood and Proprioceptive Neuromuscular Facilitation Techniques. The intervention techniques described in these chapters are not adequately supported by current evidence, and to remain consistent with the key themes described above, we did not include them in the book. However, because many practitioners continue to refer to these approaches and related concepts, these chapters are preserved to serve as important resources.

FEATURES

This edition also has a number of features that emphasize the scientific and reflective foundations of clinical practice.

The chapters in Section II (Assessment of Occupational Function) include **Assessment Tables** that summarize the psychometric properties, strengths, and weaknesses of the assessment methods described in the chapter.

Evidence Tables (where evidence exists) are included in chapters in Section III (Therapeutic Mechanisms), Section IV (Therapeutic Technologies), Section V (Intervention for Occupational Function), and Section VI (Rehabilitation to Promote Occupational Function for Selected

Diagnostic Categories). These tables summarize research studies that address the interventions mentioned in the chapters and/or Case Examples. They are not exhaustive compendia of all research but represent the current best evidence for the effectiveness of the interventions and serve as examples of culling critical information from research articles. Readers will find information pertaining to these tables and other features in this volume's **User's Guide**.

The **Case Examples** in this edition continue to highlight the "whys" of the assessment and intervention process. In general, Case Examples are designed to help students appreciate how various topics described in the chapter relate to and inform occupational therapy practice. Readers will find that the Case Example format in this edition describes the actions of therapy ("Occupational Therapy Process") along with the therapist's internal dialogue to explain why he or she approached occupational therapy assessment and/or intervention as he or she did ("Clinical Reasoning Process").

New to this edition are three **Activity Analysis Case Examples**, the goal of which is to explicate the clinical reasoning that occupational therapists use in selecting and modifying activities to meet patients' therapeutic goals. Three types of activity analyses are introduced in Chapter 12 by Catherine Verrier Piersol, PhD, OTR/L, and modeled in later chapters by other authors. In Chapter 27 (Restoring Competence for Homemaker and Parent Roles), Susan Fasoli, ScD, OTR/L, developed an **Activity-Focused Analysis Case Example**. This is a deconstruction of the activity itself outside of the client-specific application or context. This type of activity analysis is intended to provide a schema that readers may use to build a repertoire of therapeutic occupations and emphasizes occupation-as-means. In Chapter 37 (Hand Impairments), Cynthia Cooper, MFA, MA, OTR/L, CHT, developed a **Client-Focused Activity Analysis Case Example**. This is a description of the reasoning involved in the therapeutic use of occupation-as-means for a particular therapeutic goal for a specific person. In Chapter 25 (Restoring the Role of Independent Person), Anne Birge James, PhD, OTR/L, developed an **Environment-Client Focused Activity Analysis Case Example**. This is a deconstruction of the specific activity-environment-person fit to determine and/or optimize the likelihood of successful performance of occupation-as-end. Activity Analysis Case Example templates are also available on thePoint (thepoint.lww.com) should readers choose to use them to develop activity analyses on their own.

As in the previous edition, a **Glossary** and boxes highlighting **Clinical Reasoning** (opportunities to develop clinical reasoning skills that go beyond the material that can be looked up in the chapter), **Procedures for Practice** (how to do a particular assessment or treatment), **Definitions**, **Research Notes** (examples of application of research, including that from other disciplines, to practice), **Safety Notes** (precautions to be observed), and **Resources** (where to find information and equipment) are included throughout the chapters to showcase and emphasize key concepts.

ANCILLARIES

As indicated above, a website is available at thepoint.lww .com. Students can go to the site to see how an expert would answer the questions posed in Clinical Reasoning Boxes throughout the text. Clinical Reasoning Boxes (questions and answers) from the sixth edition are also available on the site. Instructors' Resources have been posted, including PowerPoint slides that provide lecture outlines for each chapter and an image bank containing all images and tables from the book.

Also at thePoint, students can access audiovisual content in which core techniques are demonstrated. Brief video clips help learners visualize and review key aspects of practice, including the measurement of upper extremity range of motion and hand strength, upper and lower extremity dressing techniques for individuals with hemiplegia and paraplegia (new to this edition), how to fabricate a splint, and how to assist clients as they transfer into and out of a wheelchair.

TERMINOLOGY

Throughout this book, readers will note an amalgam of occupational therapy terminology, derived from the *Occupational Therapy Practice Framework: Domain & Process, Second Edition* (American Occupational Therapy Association, 2008), *International Classification of Functioning* (World Health Organization, 2001), *Occupational Functioning Model*, and generic "OT speak." This supports our aim to develop multilingual practitioners. The use of various terms and frameworks in the textbook reflects the different ways in which practicing occupational therapists and occupational therapy scholars talk about the work we do each day. If you find yourself needing to think twice to do some translation, get used to it. In practice, we must be proficient at adapting our language based on the needs of those with whom we communicate, understanding that most of us spend our day with people who have never heard of occupational therapy, much less our professional vocabulary. Similarly, some authors elected to refer to recipients of occupational therapy services as clients, others as patients. This too reflects ways in which appropriate terminology varies based on the context of the situation. In general, the term "patient" is most often used in acute medical and inpatient rehabilitation settings; it reflects a more passive role of the person receiving care and is the term used by other professionals on the health care team. The term "client" is used in reference to a person living in the community who is receiving outpatient, home-based, or community-based services. It reflects the assumption that the person receiving services is ready to assume a more directive role in organizing his or her care.

AUTHORS

Sixty-eight outstanding clinical and academic occupational therapists and experienced lay persons contributed to this edition. They each did so with the desire to contribute to the profession of occupational therapy by

sharing their knowledge and skills with occupational therapists preparing to enter the field.

Mary Vining Radomski
Catherine A. Trombly Latham

REFERENCES

American Occupational Therapy Association. (2008). Occupational therapy practice framework: Domain & process (2nd ed.). *American Journal of Occupational Therapy, 62,* 625–683.
World Health Organization. (2001). *International Classification of Functioning, Disability and Health–Short version.* Geneva, Switzerland: World Health Organization.

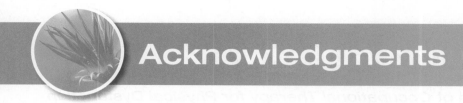

Acknowledgments

We gratefully acknowledge the many individuals who have helped us with the seventh edition of *Occupational Therapy for Physical Dysfunction*. As always, we relied on the accommodation, practical assistance, and occasional indulgence of our friends and loved ones, most notably our husbands, Jim Radomski and John Latham; we thank them for their help with this work. Heather Rybacki, Managing Editor at Lippincott Williams & Wilkins, worked with us throughout the planning and editing of the seventh edition. John Larkin, Product Manager, and Russ Hall (Absolute Service, Inc.) orchestrated and prepared the production of the book. We appreciate their expertise, professionalism, and the continuity that they brought to this project.

Many others were quick to agree to our requests for assistance with photographs, videography, and ancillaries. Emily Eastman, occupational therapy student at St. Catherine University, was an exceptional model for the new range of motion and manual muscle testing photographs. We appreciate Jennifer Theis, MS, OTR/L, who developed the storyboards for the new video on car transfers and dressing techniques, and Kelly Tollefson (and her sister/driver, Amy) and Susan Hagel, MS CTRS, who demonstrated these techniques in the videos. Thanks too to the Courage Kenny Rehabilitation Institute for providing space for our photography and videography sessions and to Cheryl Smith and Matthew White, OTR/L of the Courage Kenny Research Center. We are especially grateful to Elizabeth Plummer, who allowed us to use her beautiful photograph on the cover of the book.

As mentioned in the Preface, we recognize the contribution, commitment, and hard work of this edition's authors. In this edition, we are particularly grateful to the authors who are also members of the U.S. Army Medical Specialists Corps including MAJ Charles Quick, MAJ Priscillia Bejarano, LTC Andrew Fabrizio, MAJ Jose Rafols, MAJ Sarah Mitsch, MAJ(P) Kathleen Yancosek, and those with recent military service (Valerie Rice, Lisa Smurr Walters, and Lynsay Whelan). We recognize the historically important ways that military clinicians have influenced our profession and their service to our country. All of these authors stand on the shoulders of 51 previous authors who have shaped the textbook's content since the first edition was published in 1977 (see the list that follows). Past and present authors have taken on this work with a desire to advance the profession by sharing their expertise with you and for that, we are most grateful.

Mary Vining Radomski
Catherine Trombly Latham

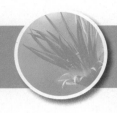

Contributing Authors

of Past Editions of *Occupational Therapy for Physical Dysfunction*

First Edition
Anna Deane Scott, MEd, OTR
Catherine Anne Trombly, MA, OTR
Hilda Versluys, MEd, OTR

Second Edition
Anne G. Fisher, MS, OTR
Beverly J. Myers, BS, OTR
Lillian Hoyle Parent, MA, OTR
Cynthia A. Philips, MA, OTR
Anna Deane Scott, MEd, OTR
Catherine Anne Trombly, MA, OTR
Hilda P. Versluys, MEd, OTR
Patricia L. Weber, MS, OTR

Third Edition
Patricia Weber Dow, MS, OTR
Anne G. Fisher, ScD, OTR
Beverly J. Myers, MHPE, OTR/L
Lillian Hoyle Parent, MA, OTR
Cynthia A. Philips, MA, OTR/L, ASHT
Lee Ann Quintana, MS, OTR
Anna Deane Scott, MEd, OTR
Catherine Anne Trombly, MA, OTR
Hilda Powers Versluys, MEd, OTR

Fourth Edition
M. Irma Alvarado, MA, OTR
Ben Atchinson, MEd, OTR
Julie Bass Haugen, PhD, OTR
Jane Bear-Lehman, MS, OTR
Karen Bentzel, MS, OTR
Bette R. Bonder, PhD, OTR/L
Felice Celikyol, MA, OTR
Barbara Cooper, PhD (abd), OT(C)
Wendy Coster, PhD, OTR
Jean Deitz, PhD, OTR/L
Glenn Digman, MSW, MA, OTR/L
Patricia Weber Dow, MS, OTR
Brian Dudgeon, MS, OTR/L
Maria Elena Echevarria, BS, OTR/L
Marilyn Ernest-Conibear, MA, OT(C)
Judy R. Feinberg, PhD, OTR
Glenn Goodman, MOT, OTR/L
Laura Devore Hollar, MSOT, OTR
Karen Jacobs, EdD, OTR/L, CPE
Lyn Jongbloed, PhD, OT(C)
Katherine A. Konosky, MS, OTR
Mary Law, PhD, OT(C)
Susan L. Lee, BS, OTR/L

Lori Letts, MA, OT(C)
Kathryn Levit, BS, OTR
Cheryl Linden, MS, OTR
Jaclyn Faglie Low, PhD, OTR
Colleen T. Lowe, M.P.H., OTR/L, CHT
Virgil Mathiowetz, PhD, OTR
Beverly J. Myers, MHPE, OTR
Elizabeth M. Newman, BS, OTR/L
Cynthia A. Philips, MA, OTR/L, ASHT
Janet L. Poole, MA, OTR
Robert E. Post, PhD, PT
Lee Ann Quintana, MS, OTR
Nancy Pearson Rees, MOT, OTR
Patricia Rigby, MHSc, OT(C)
Joyce Shapero Sabari, PhD, OTR
Anna Deane Scott, MEd, OTR
Cara Stewart, BS, OTR
Debra Stewart, BSc, OT(C)
Susan Strong, BSc, OT(C)
Dorie B. Syen, OTR, CHT
Linda Tickle-Degnen, PhD, OTR/L
Jeannette Tries, MS, OTR/L
Catherine A. Trombly, ScD, OTR/L
Hilda Powers Versluys, MEd, OTR/L
Anne M. Woodson, BS, OTR
Ruth Zemke, PhD, OTR

Fifth Edition
Jennifer Angelo, PhD, OTR, ATP
Michal S. Atkins, MA, OTR
Wendy Avery-Smith, MS, OTR/L
Julie Bass Haugen, PhD, OTR
Jane Bear-Lehman, PhD, OTR
Karen Bentzel, MS, OTR
Bette R. Bonder, PhD, OTR/L
Alfred G. Bracciano, EdD., OTR
Mary Ellen Buning, MS, OTR, ATP
Nancy Callinan, MA, OTR, CHT
Felice Gadaleta Celikyol, MA, OTR
Barbara Acheson Cooper, MHSc, Ph.,D., OT(C)
Cynthia Cooper, MFA, MA, OTR/L, CHT
Lois F. Copperman, PhD, OTR/L
Elin Schold Davis, OTR/L, CDRS
Jean C. Deitz, PhD, OTR/L
Lisa Deshaies, OTR, CHT
Brian Dudgeon, PhD, OTR/L
Donald Earley, MA, OTR
Susan E. Fasoli, ScD, OTR/L
Nancy A. Flinn, MA, OTR, BCN
Susan Jane Forwell, MA, OT(C)

Glenn Goodman, PhD, OTR/L
Julie McLaughlin Gray, MA, OTR
Carolyn Schmidt Hanson, PhD, OTR
Lucinda L. Hugos, MS, PT
Nancy Huntley, OTR, CES
Jeanne Jackson, PhD, OTR
Douglas D. Jones, J.D., MEd
Theodore I King II, PhD, OT
Mary Law, PhD, OT(C)
Lori Letts, PhD (abd), OT(C)
Kathryn Levit, MA, OTR
Jaclyn Faglie Low, PhD, OTR
LTC Stephen Luster, MS, OTR/L, CHT
Virgil Mathiowetz, PhD, OTR
Amy C. Orroth, OTR/L, CHT
Monica Pessina, MEd, OTR
Susan L.Pierce, OTR, CDRS
Carolyn Robinson Podolski, MS, OTR/L
Lee Ann Quintana, MS, OTR
Mary Vining Radomski, MA, OTR
COL Valerie Rice, PhD, OTR/L, CPE
Patricia Rigby, MHSc, OT(C)
Joyce Shapero Sabari, PhD, OTR, BCN
Shoshana Shamberg, MSEd, OTR/L
Jo M. Solet, EdM., PhD, OTR/L
Debra Stewart, MSc, OT(C)
Susan Strong, MSc, OT(C)
Linda Tickle-Degnen, PhD, OTR/L
Catherine A. Trombly, ScD, OTR/L
Anne M. Woodson, BS, OTR
Y. Lynn Yasuda, MSEd, OTR
Ruth Zemke, PhD, OTR

Sixth Edition

Anne Armstrong, MA, OTR/L
Michal S. Atkins, MA, OTR/L
Wendy Avery, MS, OTR/L
Julie Bass-Haugen, PhD, OTR
Jane Bear-Lehman, PhD, OTR
Karen Bentzel, MS, OTR/L
Bette R. Bonder, PhD, OTR/L
Alfred G. Bracciano, EdD, OTR
Mary Ellen Buning, PhD, OTR, ATP
Nancy Callinan, MA, OTR/L, CHT
Cynthia Cooper, MFA, MA, OTR/L, CHT
Lois Copperman, PhD, OTR(L)
Elin Schold Davis, OTR/L, CDRS

Jean C. Deitz, PhD, OTR/L
Lisa Deshaies, OTR/L, CHT
Brian J. Dudgeon, PhD, OTR/L
Susan E. Fasoli, ScD, OTR/L
Nancy A. Flinn, PhD, OTR/L, BCN
Susan Forwell, PhD, OT(C)
Glenn Goodman, PhD, OTR/L
Julie McLaughlin Gray, PhD (candidate), OTR/L
Carolyn Schmidt Hanson, PhD, OTR/L
Lucinda L. Hugos, MS, PT
Nancy Huntley, OTR/L, CES
Jeanne Jackson, PhD, OTR
Anne Birge James, PhD, OTR/L
Sharon Kurfuerst, EdD, OTR/L
Catherine A. Trombly Latham, ScD, OTR/L
Lori Letts, PhD (abd), OT Reg (Ont)
Kathryn Levit, PhD, OTR/L
Joanna Bertness Lipoma, MOT, OTR
Jaclyn Faglie Low, PhD, OTR
Mandy Lowe MSc, OT Reg (Ont)
Stephen Luster, MS, OTR/L, CHT
Colleen Maher, MS, OTR/L CHT, MLD
Virgil Mathiowetz, PhD, OTR/L
E. Stuart Oertli, MS, OTR
Karin J. Opacich, PhD, MHPE, OTR/L
Amy C. Orroth, OTR/L, CHT
Monica Pessina, PhD, MEd, OTR
Susan Lanier Pierce, OTR, CDRS, SCDCM
Carolyn Robinson Podolski, MA, OTR, SCDCM
Lee Ann Quintana, MS, OTR/L
Mary Vining Radomski, MA, OTR/L
Valerie Rice, PhD, OTR/L, CPE
Patricia Rigby, MHSc, OT Reg (Ont)
Pamela Roberts, MSHA., OTR/L, CPHQ
Kathy Longenecker Rust, MS, OT
Dory Sabata, OTD, OTR/L
Joyce Shapero Sabari, PhD, OTR, BCN
Shoshana Shamberg, MSEd, OTR/L
Margarette L. Shelton, PhD, OTR
Jo M. Solet, Ed.M., PhD, OTR/L
Debra Stewart, MSc, OT Reg (Ont)
Kathy Stubblefield, OTR/L
Linda Tickle-Degnen, PhD, OTR/L
Michael Williams, PhD
Anne M. Woodson, BS, OTR
Y. Lynn Yasuda, MSEd, OTR
Ruth Zemke, PhD, OTR

Contributing Authors

Khader A. Almhdawi, PhD, OT
Assistant Professor
Department of Rehabilitation Sciences,
Faculty of Applied Medical Sciences
Jordan University of Science & Technology
Irbid, Jordan

Mattie Anheluk, MOT, OTR/L
Occupational Therapist
Courage Kenny Comprehensive Outpatient Rehabilitation
Instructor Scientist
Courage Kenny Research Center
Minneapolis, Minnesota

Michal S. Atkins, MA, OTR/L
Occupational Therapy Clinical Instructor
Department of Occupational and Recreational Therapy
Rancho Los Amigos National Rehabilitation Center
Downey, California

Wendy W. Avery, MS, OTR/L
Occupational Therapist
Amedisys Home Health
Bluffton, South Carolina

Julie D. Bass, PhD, OTR/L, FAOTA
Professor
St. Catherine University
St. Paul, Minnesota
Associate Director
Institute for the Study of Occupation and Health
American Occupational Therapy Foundation
Bethesda, Maryland

MAJ Priscillia D. Bejarano, MA, OTR/L, CHT
Assistant Chief
Occupational Therapy Services
Landstuhl Regional Medical Center
United States Army
Landstuhl, Germany

Karen Bentzel, M.S., OTR/L
Occupational Therapist
Lancaster General Hospital
Lancaster, Pennsylvania
Heartland Home Care
York, Pennsylvania

Bette R. Bonder, PhD, OTR/L, FAOTA
Professor
Master of Occupational Therapy Program
College of Science and Health Professions
Department of Psychology
Cleveland State University
Cleveland, Ohio

F. D. Blade Branham, PT, DPT, CHT
Eisenhower Medical Center
Rancho Mirage, California

Mary Ellen Buning, PhD, OTR/L, ATP/SMS
Assistant Professor
Department of Neurological Surgery
School of Medicine
University of Louisville
Louisville, Kentucky
Director
Assistive Technology Resource Center
Frazier Rehabilitation & Neuroscience Institute
Louisville, Kentucky

Nettie Capasso, MA, OTR/L
Supervisor
Inpatient Adult Occupational Therapy
Rusk Institute of Rehabilitation Medicine at NYU Langone
    Medical Center
New York, New York

Cynthia Cooper, MFA, MA, OTR/L, CHT
Owner
Cooper Hand Therapy
Scottsdale, Arizona
Adjunct Faculty
Occupational Therapy Department
A.T. Still University
Mesa, Arizona

Lois F. Copperman, PhD, OTR
Clinical Associate Professor
Department of Neurology
Oregon Health and Science University
Portland, Oregon

Oana Craciunoiu, M.Sc., OT Reg. (Ont.)
Occupational Therapist
Bridgepoint Health Hospital
Toronto, Ontario
Canada

Jean C. Deitz, PhD, OTR, FAOTA
Professor Emeritus
Division of Occupational Therapy
Department of Rehabilitation Medicine
University of Washington
Seattle, Washington

Lisa D. Deshaies, OTR/L, CHT
Clinical Specialist
Occupational Therapy Department
Rancho Los Amigos National Rehabilitation Center
Downey, California
Adjunct Clinical Faculty
Division of Occupational Science and Occupational Therapy
University of Southern California
Los Angeles, California

Margaret R. Dimpfel, MOT, OTR/L, ATP
Occupational Therapist, Clinical Specialist
Department of Veterans Affairs
VA Puget Sound Health Care System- Seattle Division
Seattle, Washington

Claire-Jehanne Dubouloz, PhD, OT Reg. (Ont.), FCAOT
Professor
School of Rehabilitation Sciences
University of Ottawa
Ottawa, Ontario
Canada

Brian J. Dudgeon, PhD, OTR, FAOTA
Professor and Director Occupational Therapy
University of Alabama at Birmingham
Birmingham, Alabama

Mary Y. Egan, PhD, OT Reg. (Ont.), FCAOT
Professor
School of Rehabilitation Sciences
University of Ottawa
Ottawa, Ontario
Canada

LTC Andrew J. Fabrizio, MS, OTR/L, CHT
Chief, Occupational Therapy
Southern Region Medical Command Occupational Therapy
    Consultant
Dwight David Eisenhower Army Medical Center
Fort Gordon, Georgia

Susan E. Fasoli, ScD OTR/L
Research Health Science Specialist
Providence VA Medical Center
Providence, Rhode Island

Rachel Feld-Glazman, MS, OTR/L
Neuro-Rehabilitation Clinical Specialist
Occupational Therapy Department
Rusk Institute of Rehabilitation Medicine at NYU Langone
    Medical Center
New York, New York

Nancy A. Flinn, PhD, OTR/L
Senior Scientific Adviser
Public Affairs
Allina Health
Minneapolis, Minnesota

Susan J. Forwell, PhD, OT(C), FCAOT
Associate Professor
Department of Occupational Science and Occupational Therapy
University of British Columbia
Vancouver, British Columbia
Canada

Setareh Ghahari, PhD, MSc, BSc (OT)
Post Doctoral Fellow
University of British Columbia
Vancouver, British Columbia
Canada

Gordon Muir Giles, PhD, OTR/L, FAOTA
Professor
Samuel Merritt University
Oakland, California
Director of Neurobehavioral Services
Crestwood Behavioral Health, Inc.
Sacramento, California

Glenn D. Goodman, PhD, OTR/L
Professor and Director
Master of Occupational Therapy Program
College of Science and Health Professions
Cleveland State University
Cleveland, Ohio

Kim Grabe, MA, OTR/L
Acute care occupational therapist
Courage Kenny Rehabilitation Institute/Abbott Northwestern
    Hospital
Instructor Scientist
Courage Kenny Research Center
Minneapolis, Minnesota

Alison Hammond, PhD, OT
Professor in Rheumatology Rehabilitation
Centre for Health Sciences Research
University of Salford
Greater Manchester
United Kingdom

Carolyn Schmidt Hanson, PhD, OTR
Research Occupational Therapist
Brain Rehabilitation Research Center
North Florida/South Georgia Veterans Administration
    Healthcare System
Gainesville, Florida

Shayne E. Hopkins, OTR/L
Occupational Therapist
Inpatient Rehabilitation
Courage Kenny Rehabilitation Institute
Minneapolis, Minnesota

Lucinda L. Hugos, MS, PT
Assistant Professor and Physical Therapist
Oregon Health & Science University
Oregon Research Health Science Specialist
Portland VA Medical Center
Portland, Oregon

Nancy Huntley OTR/L, CES
Cardiac Rehabilitation Therapist
Fairview Southdale Hospital
Edina, Minnesota

Anne Birge James, PhD, OTR/L
Professor
Occupational Therapy Program
University of Puget Sound
Tacoma, Washington

Jennifer Kaldenberg, MSA, OTR/L, SCLV, FAOTA
Director of Occupational Therapy Services &
Adjunct, Assistant Professor of Vision Rehabilitation
New England Eye Institute & New
England College of Optometry
Boston, Massachusetts

Catherine A. Trombly Latham, ScD, OT(retired), FAOTA
Professor Emerita, Clinical Assistant Professor & Fieldwork
    Coordinator
Department of Occupational Therapy
College of Health & Rehabilitation Sciences: Sargent College
Boston University
Boston, Massachusetts

Kathryn Levit, PhD, OTR/L
Assistant Professor and Academic Fieldwork Coordinator
Shenandoah University
Winchester, Virginia

Colleen Maher, OTD, OTR/L, CHT
Assistant Professor
Department of Occupational Therapy
University of the Sciences
Philadelphia, Pennsylvania

Virgil G. Mathiowetz, PhD, OTR/L, FAOTA
Associate Professor and Assistant Director,
Program in Occupational Therapy
University of Minnesota
Minneapolis, Minnesota

MAJ Sarah Mitsch, OTR/L
Chief, Occupational Therapy Amputee Section
Military Advanced Training Center
Walter Reed National Military Medical Center
Washington, District of Columbia

M. Tracy Morrison, OTD, OTR/L
Clinical Scientist
Courage Kenny Research Center and Courage Kenny
    Rehabilitation Institute
Minneapolis, Minnesota
Adjunct Assistant Professor
University of Kansas Medical Center
Department of Occupational Therapy Education
Kansas City, Kansas

Karin J. Opacich, PhD, MHPE, OTR/L, FAOTA
Director, Undergraduate Public Health and
Clinical Associate Professor, Health Policy & Administration
School of Public Health
University of Illinois at Chicago
Chicago, Illinois

Amy Clara Orroth OTR/L, CHT
Senior Occupational Therapist
Massachusetts General Hospital
Boston, Massachusetts

Monica Ann Pessina, OTR, MEd, PhD
Assistant Professor
Department of Anatomy and Neurobiology
Boston University School of Medicine
Lecturer
Department of Occupational Therapy
College of Health & Rehabilitation Sciences: Sargent College
Boston University
Boston, Massachusetts

Susan Pierce, OTR, SCDCM, CDRS
President and CEO
Adaptive Mobility Services, Inc.
Orlando, Florida

Catherine Verrier Piersol, PhD, OTR/L
Assistant Professor
Department of Occupational Therapy
Clinical Director
Jefferson Elder Care
Jefferson School of Health Professions
Thomas Jefferson University
Philadelphia, Pennsylvania

Janet M. Powell, PhD, OTR/L, FAOTA
Associate Professor and Head
Division of Occupational Therapy
University of Washington
Seattle, Washington

MAJ Charles D. Quick, MS, OTR/L, CHT
Chief
Occupational Therapy Services
Landstuhl Regional Medical Center
United States Army
Landstuhl, Germany

Mary Vining Radomski, PhD, OTR/L, FAOTA
Clinical Scientist
Courage Kenny Research Center
Occupational Therapist
Courage Kenny Rehabilitation Institute
Minneapolis, Minnesota

MAJ Jose Rafols, OTD, MHSA, OTR/L
Assistant Chief, Occupational Therapy
Dwight David Eisenhower Army Medical Center
Fort Gordon, Georgia

Valerie J. Berg Rice, PhD, MHA, MS, CPE, OTR/L, FAOTA
Chief, Army Research Laboratory - Human Research &
    Engineering Directorate - Cognitive Sciences Branch
Army Medical Department Field Element
Ft. Sam Houston
San Antonio, Texas
Consultant
General Ergonomics
Selma, Texas

Patricia Rigby, PhD, MSc
Associate Professor
Department of Occupational Science and Occupational
    Therapy
Faculty of Medicine
University of Toronto
Occupational Therapist
Bridgepoint Health Hospital
Toronto, Ontario
Canada

Pamela Roberts, PhD, OTR/L, SCFES, FAOTA, CPHQ
Manager – Rehabilitation and Neuropsychology
Cedars-Sinai Medical Center
Los Angeles, California

Kathy Longenecker Rust, MS, OT
Tactile Communication & Neurorehabilitation Laboratory
Department of Biomedical Engineering
University of Wisconsin
Madison, Wisconsin

Joyce Shapero Sabari, PhD, OTR, FAOTA
Associate Professor and Chair
Occupational Therapy Program
SUNY Downstate Medical Center
Brooklyn, New York

Dory Sabata, OTD, OTR/L, SCEM
Clinical Assistant Professor
University of Kansas Medical Center
Occupational Therapy Education
Kansas City, Kansas

Lisa Smurr Walters, MS, OTR/L, CHT
Supervisor, Occupational Therapy
Center for the Intrepid
Department of Orthopedics and Rehabilitation
San Antonio Military Medical Center
Ft. Sam Houston, Texas

Jo M. Solet, MS EdM PhD OTR/L
Clinical Instructor in Medicine
Harvard Medical School
Cambridge, Massachusetts
Cambridge Health Alliance
Cambridge, Massachusetts

Jennifer L. Theis, MS, OTR/L
Staff Occupational Therapist
Program Coordinator for Spinal Cord System of Care
Department of Rehabilitation Services
Courage Kenny Rehabilitation Institute
Minneapolis, Minnesota

Linda Tickle-Degnen, PhD, OTR/L, FAOTA
Professor and Chair
Department of Occupational Therapy
Tufts University
Medford, Massachusetts

Orli M. Weisser-Pike, OTR/L, CLVT, SCLV
Assistant Director
Low Vision Service, Hamilton Eye Institute
University of Tennessee Health Science Center
Memphis, Tennessee

Lynsay R. Whelan, OTR/L
Occupational Therapist
Touch Bionics, Inc.
Hilliard, Ohio

Christine M. Wietlisbach, OTD, OTR/L, CHT, MPA
Eisenhower Medical Center
Rancho Mirage, California
Clinical Instructor
Department of Occupational Therapy
School of Allied Health Professions
Loma Linda University
Loma Linda, California

Anne M. Woodson, OTR
Adjunct Faculty
Department of Occupational Therapy
School of Health Professions
University of Texas Medical Branch
Galveston, Texas

MAJ(P) Kathleen E. Yancosek, PhD, OTR/L, CHT
Research Director
Baylor University
U.S. Army Occupational Therapy Program
Fort San Houston, Texas
Assistant Chief, Occupational Therapy
San Antonio Military Medical Center
Fort San Houston, Texas
Deputy Division Chief, Military Performance Division
U.S. Army Research Institute of Environmental Medicine
Natick, Massachusetts

Joette Zola, OTR/L, STAR-C
Occupational Therapist
Outpatient Brain Injury Program
Lead Therapist, Cognitive Impairment Group – Allina Health
    STAR Program
Courage Kenny Rehabilitation Institute
Minneapolis, Minnesota

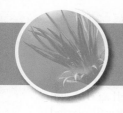

About the Cover Artist

Cover and Interior Art: **Transition**
Artist: **Elizabeth Plummer**

The cover and thematic image for this volume, "Transition," is a photograph taken by Elizabeth Plummer (St. Paul, MN), so named by the artist because the flower is blossoming rather than fading as it may appear at first glance. Elizabeth was struck by a car in 1994, resulting in a traumatic brain injury. Because of her physical limitations, she finds that shooting photography helps her express her creative self, and she endorses the helpfulness of long lenses!

This User's Guide introduces you to the many features of *Occupational Therapy for Physical Dysfunction*, Seventh Edition. By taking full advantage of these features as well as the text, you will develop the ability to practice using sound measurement, theoretically based interventions, and reflective reasoning.

Each chapter includes features that help you focus on the key points, deepen your knowledge, and guide you to select correct assessment and intervention tools.

LEARNING OBJECTIVES AND DIAGRAMS set forth each chapter's learning goals and how the information in the chapter fits within the Occupational Functioning Model.

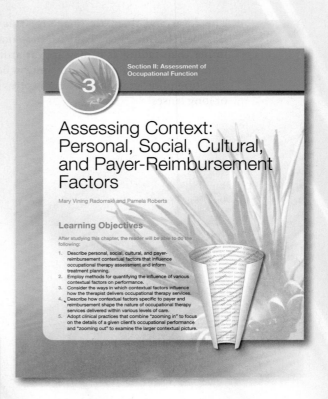

Section II: Assessment of Occupational Function

3

Assessing Context: Personal, Social, Cultural, and Payer-Reimbursement Factors

Mary Vining Radomski and Pamela Roberts

Learning Objectives

After studying this chapter, the reader will be able to do the following:

1. Describe personal, social, cultural, and payer-reimbursement contextual factors that influence occupational therapy assessment and inform treatment planning.
2. Employ methods for quantifying the influence of various contextual factors on performance.
3. Consider the ways in which contextual factors influence how the therapist delivers occupational therapy services.
4. Describe how contextual factors specific to payer and reimbursement shape the nature of occupational therapy services delivered within various levels of care.
5. Adopt clinical practices that combine "zooming in" to focus on the details of a given client's occupational performance and "zooming out" to examine the larger contextual picture.

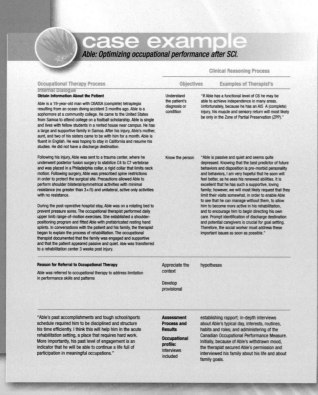

case example
Able: Optimizing occupational performance after SCI.

Occupational Therapy Process Internal Dialogue	Clinical Reasoning Process	
	Objectives	Examples of Therapist's
Obtain Information About the Patient	Understand the patient's diagnosis or condition	"If Able has a functional level of C6 he may be able to achieve independence in many areas. Unfortunately, because he has an AIS A (complete) injury, his muscle and sensory return will most likely be only in the Zone of Partial Preservation (ZPP)."
Able is a 19-year-old man with C6AISA (complete) tetraplegia resulting from an ocean diving accident 3 months ago. Able is a sophomore at a community college. He came to the United States from Samoa to attend college on a football scholarship. Able is single and lives with fellow students in a rented house near campus. He has a large and supportive family in Samoa. After his injury, Able's mother, aunt, and two of his sisters came to be with him for a month. Able is fluent in English. He was hoping to stay in California and resume his studies. He did not have a discharge destination.		
Following his injury, Able was sent to a trauma center, where he underwent posterior fusion surgery to stabilize C4 to C7 vertebrae and was placed in a Philadelphia collar, a rigid collar that limits neck motion. Following surgery, Able was prescribed spine restrictions in order to protect the surgical site. Precautions allowed Able to perform shoulder bilateral/symmetrical activities with minimal resistance (no greater than 3+/5) and unilateral, active only activities with no resistance.	Know the person	"Able is passive and quiet and seems quite depressed. Knowing that the best predictor of future behaviors and disposition is pre-morbid personality and behaviors, I am very hopeful that he soon will feel better, as he sees his renewed abilities. It is excellent that he has a supportive, loving family; however, we will most likely request that they limit their visits somewhat, in order to enable Able to see that he can manage without them, to allow him to become more active in his rehabilitation, and to encourage him to begin directing his own care. Prompt identification of discharge destination and potential caregivers is crucial for goal setting. Therefore, the social worker must address these important issues as soon as possible."
During the post-operative hospital stay, Able was on a rotating bed to prevent pressure sores. The occupational therapist performed daily upper limb range-of-motion exercises. She established a shoulder-positioning program and fitted Able with prefabricated resting hand splints. In conversations with the patient and his family, the therapist began to explain the process of rehabilitation. The occupational therapist documented that the family was engaged and supportive and that the patient appeared passive and quiet. Able was transferred to a rehabilitation center 3 weeks post injury.		
Reason for Referral to Occupational Therapy	Appreciate the context	hypotheses
Able was referred to occupational therapy to address limitation in performance skills and patterns	Develop provisional	
"Able's past accomplishments and tough school/sports schedule required him to be disciplined and structure his time efficiently. I think this will help him in the acute rehabilitation setting, a place that requires hard work. More importantly, his past level of engagement is an indicator that he will be able to continue a life full of participation in meaningful occupations."	**Assessment Process and Results** **Occupational profile:** Interviews included	establishing rapport; in-depth interviews about Able's typical day, interests, routines, habits and roles; and administering of the Canadian Occupational Performance Measure. Initially, because of Able's withdrawn mood, the therapist secured Able's permission and interviewed his family about his life and about family goals.

CASE EXAMPLES stress the underlying rationales for assessments, interventions, and activity analyses and help students apply what they learn in practice.

DYNAMIC VIDEO CLIPS on thePoint demonstrate range of motion, manual muscle testing, construction of hand splints, adapted dressing techniques, and transferring patients.

FEATURES TO HELP YOU BE A SUCCESSFUL OCCUPATIONAL THERAPIST

Occupational therapists who practice competently and ethically do so from a background of evidence that assessments are valid and reliable and treatments are efficacious. Two table features of *Occupational Therapy for Physical Dysfunction* support evidence-based practice.

ASSESSMENT TABLES, located at the end of each assessment chapter, help the therapist select an appropriate measure and interpret the results. Terms used in these tables include the following:

- **Reliability** is a measure of an instrument's stability. Interobserver or interrater reliability refers to the outcome when two different individuals administer the instrument to a particular person and achieve similar results. Test–retest reliability, or intrarater reliability, refers to the constancy of results over repeated use of the instrument by the same tester in the absence of change in the person being tested. This type of reliability applies most directly to practice in which the same therapist measures the patient's abilities before and after treatment.
- **Sensitivity** is the ability of an instrument to detect clinically important changes. The more sensitive the instrument, the greater likelihood that small changes will be detected.
- **Validity** is the ability of an instrument to measure what it is intended or presumed to measure. Criterion validity is determined by comparing the examined test to an agreed-on *gold standard* (accepted test). Predictive validity is its ability to predict future outcomes.

Assessment Table 38-1		Comparing interventions and their outcomes					
Intervention	Description of Intervention Tested	Participants	Dosage	Type of Best Evidence and Level of Evidence	Benefit	Statistical Probability	Reference
Intervention to improve voluntary hand function in incomplete individuals with C4-C7 spinal cord injury	Comparison of 2 treatment groups: Conventional occupational therapy and functional electrical stimulation therapy	22 individuals with incomplete C4-C7 tetraplegia. Single-site.	1 dose defined as 60 min per day, 5 days per week for 8 weeks). Conventional OT group: 2 units of conventional OT FES group: I unit of conventional OT and 1 unit of FES	Randomized control; small groups (10 and 12) No control who did not receive treatment. Level: IIB	Group that received FES and conventional OT showed greater improvement than group that had 2 hours of conventional OT.	FIM P=0.015; SCIM UE sub-scale < 0.0001; Hand test TRI-HFT: 10 objects=0.054; Rectangular blocks= 0.124; Able to hold wooden bar= 0.065	Kapadia, Zivanovic, Furlan, Craven, McGillivray, & Popovic, 2011
Intervention to improve self-efficacy, ability to set/achieve goals, and perceived independent-living status	Occupational therapists and other health care providers conducted health promotional seminars, group discussions, physical and recreational activities.	SCI=16 MS=12	10 full day sessions, twice a month for 5 months.	Small group, quasi-experimental repeated-measures; non-randomized Level: IIIC	Yes. Self-efficacy and ability to formulate and achieve goals in the areas of independent-living skills improved for intervention participants.	Statistically significant difference in the change in self-efficacy scores t(38)=2.855 p=0.007	Block,Vanner, Keys, Rimmer, &Skeels, 2010

EVIDENCE TABLES, located at the end of each chapter which is devoted to a treatment or a diagnosis, list some of the best evidence concerning the treatments mentioned in the chapter. Terms used in the evidence tables include the following:

- **Effect size** is a unitless indication of the strength of the relationship between the treatment and the outcome (Rosenthal, 1984). There are several representations of effect size, including r, Hedges's g, Cohen's d, and η^2 (eta squared). Effect size, "r," is interpreted like a correlation coefficient: 1.0 equals a perfect, strong, relationship, and 0 equals no relationship (Rosenthal, 1984). An effect size of $r = 0.10$ is considered small; of 0.30, medium; and of 0.50, large (Cohen, 1988) (η^2, eta squared, is interpreted similarly to "r").
- **Level of evidence** rating scale used in this textbook is the American Occupational Therapy Association's Evidence-Based Project Scale (Trombly & Ma, 2002): Level I (highest) to Level IV (lowest). The higher the level, the better the evidence that the intervention was the cause of the change reported. The scale also presents grades relating to sample size, internal validity (how well the study controlled for alternate explanations of outcome), and external validity (how well the study generalizes to persons other than the study participants or to settings other than the study setting). For example, a rating of IC2c means that the study was a randomized controlled trial (I), with 20 or fewer participants in each group (C), that had no strong alternative explanation for outcome but had one or two threats to validity (2), and that the participants do not necessarily represent the population of patients of that diagnosis AND the treatment does not represent current practice OR it was carried out in an unnatural (laboratory) setting (c).
- **Statistical probability** indicates the likelihood that the outcome was due to chance. A probability level of 0.05 indicates that there are only five chances out of a hundred that the outcome occurred by chance (Rosenthal & Rosnow, 1991).

Evidence Table 38-1   Comparing interventions and their outcomes

Intervention	Description of Intervention Tested	Participants	Dosage	Type of Best Evidence and Level of Evidence	Benefit	Statistical Probability	Reference
Intervention to improve voluntary hand function in incomplete individuals with C4-C7 spinal cord injury	Comparison of 2 treatment groups: Conventional occupational therapy and functional electrical stimulation therapy	22 individuals with incomplete C4-C7 tetraplegia. Single-site.	1 dose defined as 60 min per day, 5 days per week for 8 weeks). Conventional OT group: 2 units of conventional OT FES group: I unit of conventional OT and 1 unit of FES	Randomized control; small groups (10 and 12) No control who did not receive treatment. Level: IIB	Group that received FES and conventional OT showed greater improvement than group that had 2 hours of conventional OT.	FIM P=0.015; SCIM UE sub-scale < 0.0001; Hand test TRI-HFT: 10 objects=0.054; Rectangular blocks= 0.124; Able to hold wooden bar= 0.065	Kapadia, Zivanovic, Furlan, Craven, McGillivray, & Popovic, 2011
Intervention to improve self-efficacy, ability to set/achieve goals, and perceived independent-living status	Occupational therapists and other health care providers conducted health promotional seminars, group discussions, physical and recreational activities.	SCI=16 MS=12	10 full day sessions, twice a month for 5 months.	Small group, quasi-experimental repeated-measures; non-randomized Level: IIIC	Yes. Self-efficacy and ability to formulate and achieve goals in the areas of independent-living skills improved for intervention participants.	Statistically significant difference in the change in self-efficacy scores t(38)=2.855 p=0.007	Block, Vanner, Keys, Rimmer, & Skeels, 2010

REFERENCES

Cohen, J. (1988). *Statistical power analysis for the behavioral sciences* (2nd ed.). Hillsdale, NJ: Erlbaum.

Rosenthal, R. (1984). *Meta-analytic procedures for social research.* Beverly Hills: Sage Publications.

Rosenthal, R., & Rosnow, R. L. (1991). *Essentials of behavioral research: Methods and data analysis* (2nd ed.). New York: McGraw-Hill, Inc.

Trombly, C. A., & Ma, H.-I. (2002). A synthesis of effects of occupational therapy for persons with stroke. Part I: Restoration of roles, tasks, and activities. *American Journal of Occupational Therapy, 56,* 250–259.

SUMMARY REVIEW QUESTIONS let you assess your ability to recall the information presented in each chapter. The answers are found in the chapter.

Summary Review Questions

1. List three key epidemiological factors of the SCI population and describe how these factors influence evaluation and treatment.
2. List three precautions the therapist must consider in planning for an outing with a patient with C5 injury.
3. What is a tenodesis grasp? Why is it important, and how can the occupational therapist facilitate it?
4. List five parts of the initial occupational therapy evaluation of a patient with SCI.
5. Describe a typical feeding setup for person with C5 tetraplegia.
6. What are the functional expectations for the patient with a C7 injury?
7. You read in the medical chart that a patient lost consciousness at the time of injury. How do you modify your evaluation? Describe how concomitant brain injury may alter your treatment goals and interventions.
8. What are the roles of the occupational therapist in the transition phase?

Nurses are the primary trainers of bowel and bladder routines, and occupational therapists have a vital role in supporting the acquisition of these new skills and habits. A typical bowel program for a person with paraplegia includes taking oral medications to allow for optimal feces consistency and establishing a daily routine of transferring to the toilet, managing clothing, inserting a suppository, and, after waiting for some time, inserting a finger in the anus (called digital stimulation), which causes reflexive defecation. The occupational therapist may assist in facilitating skill acquisition in a person with poor vision and/or cognitive deficits. A magnifying mirror and a lamp may be placed on the floor to help the person see and further break down the activity to better reinforce each step. Persons with low tetraplegia have added challenges in becoming independent in bowel care. They may achieve independence or assist in managing their bowel care only after much practice. To compensate for poor trunk control, individuals perform the bowel program on a commode; to compensate for finger paralysis, they require a tool called the dill stick to stimulate the anal reflex to defecate (Figure 38-4); and to compensate for lack of sensation in the anus and/or parts of the hand, they require a mirror. For safe task performance, occupational therapists may practice commode mobility and dill stick insertion focusing on effective visual compensation. When patients become skillful at bowel evacuation practices, they decrease the

risk of complications. Most individuals, after discharge, opt to carry out their bowel program in the morning every other day and can complete the procedure within 45 minutes (Kirshblum, Gulati, O'Conner, & Voorman, 1998).

As with the bowel program, the goal of the bladder program is to achieve a simple routine with minimal risk of complications. Recurring urinary tract infection is a frequent complication and the most frequent cause of rehospitalization after spinal cord injury (Cardenas, Hoffman, Kirshblum, & McKinley, 2004). To avoid complications, patients must empty their bladder routinely. An indwelling catheter, which is a catheter that stays in the urethra and is changed only periodically, is commonly inserted soon after the person is admitted to the acute care hospital (Consortium for Spinal Cord Injury, 2008 [Early Acute Management]).Although some patients continue to use an indwelling catheter, an effort is made

Clinical Reasoning in Occupational Therapy

Helping the Client Hire a Caregiver

Able is hiring his first caregiver. A. What activities will the caregiver need to perform? B. What important precautions does the caregiver need to exercise? C. As Able's therapist how would you facilitate the caregiver's learning?

PROCEDURES FOR PRACTICE BOXES provide step-by-step directions for carrying out particular assessment or intervention practices.

to rest between sessions?")
• Facilitate solving problems ("What do you think is the best way for you to hold your pen?" "What do you think will make you sleep better at night?")
• Engage the person in activities that are personally relevant and meaningful.

Later in the continuum of care, therapists can facilitate positive coping by helping the patient identify optimal transportation, reduce environmental barriers and facilitate the return to gainful employment.

To understand the complexity of the psychosocial adjustment to SCI, we must also examine the reactions of the patient's relevant others. Family members and friends may also experience distress, sadness, anger or a myriad of other emotions. Concurrently, they may have to reassess their future commitment to the injured person. A mother, for example, may grieve and be sad while having to decide whether to take her fully dependent son home after a turbulent adolescence.

We must also examine our own emotional reactions and the influence of these emotions on the patient and therapeutic process. For example, sometimes upon interviewing a newly injured person, I become especially sad as I strongly identify with something in the patient's life narrative (e.g., the struggles of a mother with two young children). I am reminded of my projection, as the patient may be more accepting and positive. As occupational therapists, we contribute to psychosocial adaptation after SCI by incorporating the following considerations into evaluation and treatment.

• Set aside all preconceived biases about who the patient is and how he or she should feel or behave. Instead,

CLINICAL REASONING BOXES give opportunities to solve clinical problems by applying the knowledge gained in each chapter to real-life situations. The answers supplied by experienced therapists are located on the website, thePoint (thepoint.lww.com).

concentrate on learning to know patients' factors, their unique life contexts, and their individual reactions to their trauma or illness.
• Provide psychological support. At times when the patient is overwhelmed with sadness, it is okay just to be present and available to the person. It is okay to stop an

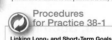
Procedures for Practice 38-1

Linking Long- and Short-Term Goals to Anticipated Rehabilitation Outcomes

P.B. is a 20-year-old man with C8 tetraplegia beginning multidisciplinary inpatient rehabilitation. The following examples of outcome and long- and short-term goals are not meant to be exhaustive lists of intervention plans but rather to illustrate the linkage between global outcome projections and therapy plans.

• Projected outcome of rehabilitation stay: In 8 weeks, P.B. will resume self-maintenance roles, requiring no more than occasional physical assistance from family members to manage in the home environment.
• Examples of long-term occupational therapy goals (to be achieved in 8 weeks):
  1. P.B. will perform upper body dressing independently and require no more than moderate assistance for lower body dressing.
  2. P.B. will use adaptive equipment to feed himself independently.
• Examples of short-term occupational therapy goals (to be achieved in 2 weeks):
  1. P.B. will don a pullover shirt with no more than general verbal cues.
  2. P.B. will participate in the evaluation of various types of adaptive equipment for self-feeding and use selected aids to feed himself independently after set up by therapist.

thePoint, the website associated with this textbook, has, in addition to the answers to the Clinical Reasoning Boxes, the clinical reasoning boxes with answers from the sixth edition as well as an image bank and learning objectives. To access and log onto thePoint, go to www. thepoint.lww.com and register.

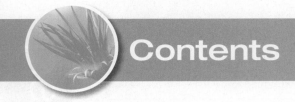

Contents

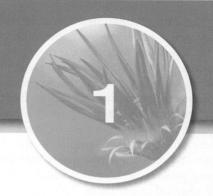

Conceptual Foundations for Practice

Catherine A. Trombly Latham

Learning Objectives

After studying this chapter, the reader will be able to do the following:

1. Describe the Occupational Functioning Model (OFM).
2. Relate the American Occupational Therapy Association's Occupational Therapy Practice Framework (OTPF) to the OFM.
3. Use the language of the Occupational Functioning Model, the American Occupational Therapy Association's OTPF, and the World Health Organization's International Classification of Functioning (ICF) interchangeably.
4. Organize assessment and treatment planning according to the Occupational Functioning Model.

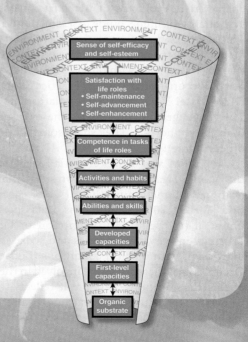

How do occupational therapists know what to do when a person with occupational dysfunction secondary to a disease or injury that results in physical impairment is referred to them? First, they have *specific knowledge* about what the diagnosis means in terms of limitations of bodily structure or function and subsequent probable limitation of occupational performance, and they know the outcome of research on the effectiveness of interventions available—the evidence base of practice. Second, they have *specific skills* for assessing and treating persons with occupational dysfunction secondary to physical impairment. Third, they know *how therapy is organized*—the conceptual foundation for practice. The organization or process of occupational therapy is found in various conceptual models of practice. A conceptual model is a representation of an object or process that indicates how various parts fit into a whole or work together for a particular purpose.

Conceptual models of practice are meant to be used in conjunction with the American Occupational Therapy Association's Occupational Therapy Practice Framework (OTPF). That framework describes the domain and process of the entire practice of occupational therapy (American Occupational Therapy Association [AOTA], 2008). The framework aims to standardize the language of the domain and process of occupational therapy. Because the framework is not a conceptual model (AOTA, 2008), it is expected that occupational therapists will apply pertinent aspects of the framework through the particular conceptual model they choose to guide their practice. Therapists may choose from among many different conceptual models of practice in order to put the framework into practice. An occupational therapy model of practice is a way of conceptualizing the interrelatedness of the person's characteristics and his or her environment, occupation, and quality of life to guide assessment and intervention. This textbook has chosen the Occupational Functioning Model (OFM) to conceptualize the process of occupational therapy for persons with physical dysfunction. How, then, do the Occupational Therapy Practice Framework and the OFM relate? What are their similarities and differences? The language and process of the two are comparable (Tables 1-1 and 1-2). They share some ideas and differ on others (Table 1-3).

The OFM also shares some language and ideas with the World Health Organization's International Classification of Functioning (ICF) (World Health Organization [WHO], 2001). The ICF is a classification tool for universal (transcultural) description of functioning and disability in everyday activities and social involvement of individuals with medical conditions (Bilbao et al., 2003). Occupational therapists were involved in the development of this classification; therefore it reflects the philosophy of occupational therapy regarding health being a state enabling full participation in life's activities (Mahaffey &

Colaianni, 2012). Both occupational therapy (here represented by the OFM) and the ICF believe that recovery goes beyond remediating impairments, and both focus on the interaction between the person and the environment (Mahaffey & Colaianni, 2012). However, the ICF is neither detailed nor focused enough to guide occupational therapy practice. The ICF is used frequently in epidemiological research and public policy making because its language is discipline free and because it has been adopted internationally. See Table 1-4, which relates the ICF language to that of the OFM.

THE OCCUPATIONAL FUNCTIONING MODEL

The OFM guides assessment and treatment of persons with physical dysfunction leading to competence in occupational performance and subsequent feelings of self-empowerment. In this textbook, the diagrams on the title pages of each of the chapters (except chapter 2 and chapters on diagnostic categories) indicate how the pieces of the various aspects of the OFM fit together and where the contents of each chapter fits in the overall model.

The OFM was derived from clinical practice with persons with physical impairments. The primary belief is that people who are competent in their life roles experience a sense of self-efficacy, self-esteem, and life satisfaction. Research indirectly supports the idea that competency is related to satisfaction or a positive quality of life (Elavsky et al., 2005; Eriksson et al., 2009; Korpershoek, van der Bijl, & Hafsteinsdóttir, 2011; Robinson-Smith, Johnston, & Allen, 2000). Successful performance strengthens personal efficacy beliefs (Bandura, 1977, 1997, 2001; Brock et al., 2009; Resnick, 1998). The goal of treatment, according to the OFM, is to enable competent engagement in valued roles whether by restored self-performance (personal agency) or by directing others (proxy agency) (Bandura, 2001).

Another assumption of the OFM is that the ability to carry out one's roles, tasks, and activities of life depends on basic abilities and capacities (e.g., strength, perception, and ability to sequence information). As do other systems (WHO, 2001), this hierarchical organization assumes that lower level capacities and abilities are related to higher level performance of everyday tasks and activities. This organization has been tangentially supported by research (Dijkers, 1997, 1999; Geertzen et al., 1998; Michielsen et al., 2009; Pollard, Johnston, & Dieppe, 2011; Sveen et al., 1999). However, the relationship is not linear (Michielsen et al., 2009). Only part of the variance associated with function is accounted for by any one ability. For example, Lynch and Bridle (1989) found a moderately strong ($r = -0.65$; $p < 0.01$) negative relationship between the scores of the Jebsen-Taylor Hand Function Test (Jebsen et al., 1969) and the scores of the Klein-Bell Activities of Daily Living (ADL) Scale (Klein & Bell, 1982).

Table 1-1   **The Domains of the Occupational Functioning Model and the Occupational Therapy Practice Framework**

Occupational Functioning Model	Occupational Therapy Practice Framework (AOTA, 2008)
Competence and Satisfaction with Life Roles and Competence in the Performance of Tasks of Life Roles	*Areas of Occupation*
Life roles and the tasks that comprise them are defined by the patient or client. Generally, roles fall into one of the following three categories: *Self-maintenance roles*—These roles maintain self, family, pets, and home, including all basic activities of daily living (BADL) and instrumental activities of daily living (IADL) associated with self-care; all IADL associated with care of family; and all IADL associated with care of home, and other possessions. *Self-advancement roles*—These roles add to the person's skills, possessions, or other betterment. *Self-enhancement roles*—These roles contribute to personal accomplishment and enjoyment or sense of well-being and happiness.	*ADL*—Care of one's body including bathing and showering, bowel and bladder management, dressing, eating, self-feeding, functional mobility, personal device care, personal hygiene and grooming, sexual activity, and toilet hygiene *IADL*—Activities to support daily life in the home and community including, care of others, child rearing, care of pets, communication management, community mobility, financial management, health management and maintenance, home establishment and management, meal preparation and cleanup, religious observance, safety and emergency maintenance, and shopping *Rest and sleep*—Rest, sleep, sleep preparation, and sleep participation *Education*—Participation in formal or informal education; exploration of informal educational needs or interests *Work*—Employment interests and pursuits, employment seeking and acquisition, job performance, retirement preparation and adjustment, and volunteer exploration and participation *Play*—Play exploration and participation *Leisure*—Leisure exploration and participation *Social participation*—Engaging in activities that result in successful interaction at the community, family or peer/friend levels
Competence in the Performance of Activities and Habits of the Tasks of Life Roles	*Performance Patterns—Person*
Activities—Smaller units of goal-directed behavior that comprise tasks *Habits*—Chains of action sequences acquired by frequent repetition that can be carried out with minimal attention. Therapy aims to sustain useful habits, release useless habits, and develop new habits.	*Habits*—Automatic behavior integrated into more complex patterns of daily behavior; can be useful, dominating, or impoverished and either support or interfere with performance in areas of occupation *Routines*—Patterns of behavior that provide structure for daily life *Rituals*—Symbolic actions that contribute to the client's identity and reinforce values and beliefs *Roles*—A set of behaviors expected by society, shaped by culture, and defined by the client
Abilities and Skills	*Performance Skills*
Abilities and skills that are basic to interaction with objects and physical and social environments include: *Motor*—Adequate strength, coordination, range of motion, dexterity, and muscular endurance *Sensory*—Abilities to adequately receive and interpret sensory stimuli to enable occupational performance *Cardiorespiratory*—Adequate cardiac and pulmonary function to sustain performance *Visual-perception*—Adequate visual acuity and ability to perceive and interpret sensory stimuli and to perceive self and objects in space to enable occupational performance *Cognitive*—Abilities and skills that are basic to interaction with the environment, to organizing life tasks, and to solving occupational problems; abilities include attention, memory, problem solving *Socioemotional*—Abilities and skills that enable occupational performance in a social context or environment	Abilities that clients demonstrate in the actions they perform. *Motor and praxis skills*—Actions or behaviors used to move and physically interact with tasks, objects, contexts, and environments; includes planning, sequencing, and executing novel movements *Sensory-perceptual skills*—Actions or behaviors used to locate, identify, respond and interpret sensory events *Emotional regulation skills*—Actions or behaviors used to identify, manage, or express feelings while engaging in activities alone or with others *Cognitive skills*—Actions or behaviors used to plan and manage the performance of an activity *Communication and social skills*—Actions or behaviors used to communicate and interact with others in an interactive environment

(continued)

| Table 1-1 | The Domains of the Occupational Functioning Model and the Occupational Therapy Practice Framework *(continued)* |

Occupational Functioning Model	Occupational Therapy Practice Framework (AOTA, 2008)
Developed Capacities	*Client Factors*
Voluntary responses that have developed from first-level capacities	Values, beliefs, and spirituality. Body functions, including mental functions; sensory functions and pain; neuromusculoskeletal and movement-related functions; cardiovascular, hematological, immunological, and respiratory functions; voice and speech functions; digestive, metabolic, and endocrine functions; genitourinary and reproductive functions; and skin and related structure functions
First-Level Capacities	*Client Factors*
The reflexive subroutines of voluntary movement and behavior. These functional foundations for movement and behavior include sensorimotor, cognitive-perceptual, and socioemotional capacities.	(as above)
Organic Substrate	*Body Structures*
Structural and physiological foundation for movement, cognition, perception and emotions. The substrate includes central nervous system organization and the integrity of skeleton, muscles, peripheral nerves, heart, lungs, and skin.	Those anatomical parts of the body that correspond to the functions mentioned above.
Environment and Context	*Contexts and Environments*
Physical—Including the natural and built environments, objects and utensils, and the requirements that tools and utensils pose for use\n\n*Personal*—Including age, gender, activity history, sense of competency, and spirituality\n\n*Cultural*—Including norms, values, beliefs, and routines or rituals of the family, ethnic group, community, or religious group\n\n*Social*—Including therapeutic interaction and relationships with family members, peers and friends, and community\n\n*Temporal*—Including temporal demands of role tasks, activities and habits; balance of activity types; and balance of activity and rest\n\n*Situational*—Including circumstances related to the setting or surroundings at a given moment	*Cultural*—Including ethnicity, beliefs, activity patterns, and behavior standards\n\n*Personal*—Including age, gender, socioeconomic status, and educational status\n\n*Temporal*—Including stage of life, time of year or day, duration, rhythm of activity, and history\n\n*Virtual*—Defined as the communication that occurs via air waves or computers with an absence of physical contact\n\n*Physical*—Including built and natural nonhuman environments and objects in them\n\n*Social*—including relationships with individuals, groups, organizations, and systems
	Activity Demands
The OFM has no comparable concept within the hierarchical model. Activity analysis is, however, a basic therapeutic process within the OFM. Three analyses are described in Chapter 12.\n\n1. Task-focused activity analysis—Deconstruction of activity itself outside of the client-specific application to build student's or clinician's repertoire of therapeutic occupations\n\n2. Client-focused activity analysis—Description of the reasoning used in the therapeutic use of occupation-as-means for a particular therapeutic goal for a particular person\n\n3. Client-environment fit analysis—Deconstruction of the specific activity-environment-person fit to determine and/or optimize the likelihood of successful performance of occupation-as-end	*Objects used and their properties*—Tools, materials, equipment\n\n*Space demands*—Size, arrangement, temperature, etc.\n\n*Social demands*—Social environment and cultural contexts\n\n*Sequence and timing*—Rules, sequences\n\n*Required actions and performance skills*—Sensory, perceptual, motor, praxis, emotional, cognitive, communication and social performance skills\n\n*Required body functions*—Those physiological functions required to support the actions required of the activity\n\n*Required body structures*—Anatomical parts of the body that are required to perform the activity

Table 1-2   The Process of Occupational Therapy

Process	Occupational Functioning Model	Occupational Therapy Practice Framework (AOTA, 2008)
Goal of therapy	Satisfactorily engage in self-identified, important life roles through which the person gains a sense of self-efficacy and self-esteem	Support health and participation in life through engagement in occupation
Evaluate to identify the problem(s)	• Identify roles, tasks, and activities the person wants to do or needs to do • Observe and analyze the person's performance, preferably within usual context • Identify inadequate performance • Identify impaired abilities or capacities that contribute to inadequate performance and assess level of impairment using valid, reliable assessment tools administered according to the standardized protocol • Identify environmental or contextual enablers or hindrances • Interpret assessment data to the patient and family and document in the patient's record	• Develop an occupational profile to understand the client's occupational history, patterns of daily living, interests, values, needs, problems with performance, and priorities • Do an analysis of occupational performance by observation within personally relevant context to specifically identify effectiveness of client's performance skills • Measure performance skills • Interpret assessment data to identify facilitators and barriers to performance • Develop hypotheses about what strengths and weaknesses the client brings to occupation
Plan intervention	• Plan in collaboration with the person or family, after presenting the current evidence, to determine whether the person wants to engage in either remediation of impaired abilities or capacities to enhance overall performance or restoration of occupational performance through relearning and/or adaptation of method or environment • With the patient, establish short-term goals that directly relate to the long-term goal of successful role functioning identified by the patient and that can be objectively and reliably measured • Select interventions that have evidence for effectiveness for the immediate goal	• With the client, develop a plan with objective, measurable goals and a time frame to guide action • Plan occupational therapy intervention based on theory and evidence • Consider discharge needs and plan • Select outcome measures • Refer to other professionals as needed
Implement the intervention	Use therapeutic mechanisms, as appropriate: *Occupation* • Occupation-as-end to restore occupational functioning • Occupation-as-means to optimize abilities or capacities *Therapeutic rapport* *Education*—Learning or relearning *Adjunctive therapies*—Therapies such as orthoses, technological aids, physical agent modalities, mobility aids used to facilitate performance *Contextual and environmental modification*—To facilitate performance	Determine the types of occupational therapy interventions to be used and carry them out • Therapeutic use of self • Occupation-based intervention • Purposeful activity • Preparatory methods • Consultation • Education • Advocacy Monitor and document client's response
Evaluate the result	• Assess patient outcomes • Determine whether the short-term goals were achieved • Determine whether achievement of the short-term goals resulted in desired occupational performance • If not, reevaluate and modify the plan relative to achieving targeted outcomes • If yes, determine whether the person was satisfied with his or her achievement • Plan for the next level of therapy or plan for discharge and referral as appropriate	• Determine success in achieving targeted outcomes • Modify the plan as needed • Determine need for continuation, discontinuation or referral
Types of outcomes	• Satisfactory occupational performance to allow expected discharge success • Voiced, or otherwise indicated, sense of self-efficacy and self-esteem • Prevention of further disability through education and follow-up, if necessary	• Occupational performance • Adaptation • Health and wellness • Participation • Prevention • Quality of life • Role competence • Self-advocacy • Occupational justice

Table 1-3 The Similarities and Differences between the Occupational Functioning Model and the AOTA Occupational Therapy Practice Framework

	Occupational Therapy Practice Framework (AOTA, 2008)	Occupational Functioning Model
Central focus	Occupation to achieve health (Gutman et al., 2007)	Self-fulfillment through role competence
A conceptual model	No	Yes
Describes the relationships (dynamic interaction) among the terms and categories in the classification system	No (Nelson, 2006)	Yes
Domain	Incorporates all aspects of occupational therapy practice	Limited to practice for those with physical dysfunction
Hierarchical	No (Smith Roley & Delany, 2009)	Yes; successful performance of higher occupations depends on lower abilities, skills, and capacities
Clients include person, organization, society	Yes	No; limited to practice with individuals
End goal	Support health and participation in life through engagement in occupation	Satisfactorily engage in self-identified, important life roles through which the person gains a sense of self-efficacy and self-esteem
Process	Evaluation, planning, intervention, outcome monitoring	Evaluation, planning, treatment, reevaluation
Evaluation	Occupational profile and occupational performance; factors that influence performance skills and patterns	Role performance; task and activity performance; skills, abilities; developed capacities; first-level capacities; and organic substrate, as needed Environmental and contextual influences on performance
Top-down evaluation process	Yes	Yes
Process of evaluating, planning, treating, and monitoring outcome is iterative, not sequenced	Yes	Yes
Process is collaborative, i.e., client centered	Yes (Gutman et al., 2007)	Yes
Key skill of occupational therapist	Analysis of occupational performance: observe, analyze, and interpret performance and detect the client, contextual, or environmental factors that enable successful performance or that impede that performance	Activity analysis: observe, analyze, and interpret performance and detect the clinically relevant impairment and/or the contextual-environmental enablers or barriers to performance
Interventions	Therapeutic use of self Therapeutic use of occupation and purposeful activities Preparatory methods Education Consultation Advocacy	Therapeutic rapport Therapeutic use of occupation as occupation-as-means and/or occupation-as-end Learning (education) Therapeutic technologies

Table 1-3 The Similarities and Differences between the Occupational Functioning Model and the AOTA Occupational Therapy Practice Framework *(continued)*

	Occupational Therapy Practice Framework (AOTA, 2008)	Occupational Functioning Model
Occupational therapy intervention approaches	Create, promote (health promotion)	Collaborate
	Establish, restore (remediation, restoration)	Remediate skills and abilities
	Maintain	Restore activities, tasks, and role performance by relearning or adaptation
	Modify (compensation, adaptation)	
	Prevent (disability prevention)	
Evidential support	None offered (Smith et al., 2009)	Tangential supporting evidence, that is, incidental evidence of the various assumptions, but not direct evidence for the model
Practical usefulness (usable and clinically relevant; use of everyday language)	No (Gutman et al., 2007; Nelson, 2006)	Yes

The correlation is negative because better performance on the Jebsen-Taylor is indicated by less time (lower score), whereas better performance on the Klein-Bell is indicated by a higher score. Filiatrault et al. (1991) found a similar relationship ($r = 0.6$) between the Fugl-Meyer Motor Function Test (upper extremity subtest) (Fugl-Meyer et al., 1975) and the Barthel Index (ADL) (Mahoney & Barthel, 1965).

Rudhe and van Hedel (2009) found relationships within a similar range between manual muscle testing and self-care activities, although they found higher relationships ($r > .82; R2 > .67$) between finger and thumb strength and grooming. These outcomes do indicate that sensorimotor control of the upper extremities is related to self-care, but because the variance (r^2) is only approximately 40%

Table 1-4 Occupational Functioning Model Related to the World Health Organization International Classification of Functioning

Occupational Functioning Model	World Health Organization International Classification of Functioning Classification (WHO, 2001)
Self-efficacy and self-esteem as a by-product of successful role performance	No corresponding concept
Satisfaction with life roles • Self-maintenance • Self-advancement • Self-enhancement	**Participation:** involvement in a life situation; the nature and extent of a person's societal functioning; the interaction between the person having a disability and/or impairment with contextual factors
Competence in **tasks of life roles** Mastery of **activities and habits** Having **abilities and skills** that underlie mastery and competence	**Activity:** the execution of a task or action by an individual; the nature and extent of functioning at the level of the individual; all that a person does at any level of complexity
Developed capacities **First-level capacities** **Organic substrate**	Bodily **structures** and psychological and physiological **functions**
Environment and context: the milieu in which occupation occurs, including natural and built physical environments, tools and utensils, social relationships, cultural situations, and time	**Contextual factors:** the complete background to a person's life and living, including both external environmental factors[a] and internal personal factors.[b] Environmental factors include all aspects of the physical, social, and attitudinal world.

[a]Natural environment (weather or terrain), human-made environment (tools, furnishings, and the built environment), social attitudes, customs, rules, practices and institutions, and other individuals.
[b]Age, race, gender, educational background, experiences, personality and character style, aptitudes, fitness, lifestyle, habits, upbringing, coping styles, social background, profession, and experience.

$(0.65^2$ or $0.60^2)$, other unidentified variables must account for the remaining approximately 60% variance associated with ADL. This makes sense because, in addition to upper extremity function, ADL independence requires such skills as sitting and standing balance, perception of positions of objects in space, ability to sequence steps of a procedure, environmental support, and so forth.

It appears that the relationship between two adjacent levels of performance (e.g., capacities and abilities) is stronger than between two nonadjacent levels (e.g., capacities and roles) (Dijkers, 1999; Pollard, Johnston, & Dieppe, 2011). The relationship between levels is strong both at the low end of the model (Pendlebury et al., 1999; Pollard, Johnston, & Dieppe, 2011) and at the high end (Dijkers, 1997, 1999; Pollard, Johnston, & Dieppe, 2011). Pendlebury et al. (1999) found a strong ($r = 0.90$) relationship between deficits in organic substrate and deficits of motor capacities and abilities. In a large sample of persons with spinal cord injury, Dijkers (1999) found a moderately strong relationship ($r = 0.24$–0.42) between life satisfaction and roles related to social integration and occupation (work) but not between impairments and life satisfaction ($r = 0.04$–0.07). He concluded that "these relationships suggest a causal chain [i.e., one link leading to the next]. . . . The impact of impairment on quality of life is almost entirely through its impact on disability, and the effect of disability is largely through its impact on handicap" (Dijkers, 1999, p. 874). This suggests that the relationship between low-level capacities and abilities and higher level tasks and roles is not direct. That is, having a particular ability, such as strength, does not ensure that a person can accomplish a given activity or task (Dagfinrud et al., 2005). Likewise, the ability to accomplish a single activity does not account for role performance. Many capacities contribute to the development of one ability, and many abilities are needed to engage successfully in an activity. When one capacity or ability is impaired, occupational dysfunction does not automatically occur. A person may adaptively use other capacities and abilities to allow accomplishment of the activity (Foroud & Whislaw, 2010).

Research is needed to clarify the multivariate relationships among lower level abilities and capacities and higher level activities, tasks, and roles. Researchers also must verify whether remediation of impaired capacities and abilities results in more complete and more versatile participation in the activities and tasks of importance in people's lives than would learning specific routines of activities in an adapted way. This is a key question for the practice of occupational therapy with persons having physical dysfunction.

Another assumption of the OFM is that satisfactory occupational functioning occurs only within enabling environments and contexts particular to the individual. True occupational functioning does not occur in a vacuum nor in a controlled situation such as the clinic; occupational functioning is the successful interaction of the person with the objects, situations, and surroundings of his or her home, family, and community. Although the contexts of particular actions and occupations used to regain lost abilities and capacities may be controlled at first, therapy is not complete until generalization to the person's particular environment has occurred (Raina, Rogers, & Holm, 2007).

Achievement of occupational functioning after injury or disease is accomplished through occupation as well as adjunctive therapies described in this textbook. In the OFM, occupation has two natures: occupation-as-end and occupation-as-means (Trombly, 1995). Occupation-as-end equates to the higher levels of the OFM, at which the person tries to accomplish a functional goal (an activity or task) by using whatever skills, abilities, habits, and capacities he or she has. Occupation-as-means, on the other hand, is *the therapy* used to bring about changes in impaired capacities and performance skills. Occupation-as-means is therapeutic because the goal presents challenges to impaired capacities and abilities, and the successful achievement of that goal results in improved organic or behavioral impairments. Both occupation-as-end and occupation-as-means derive their therapeutic impact from the qualities of purposefulness and meaningfulness (see Chapter 11 for discussion of these concepts).

The constructs of the occupational functioning model shown in the diagram on the title page are described next.

Sense of Self-Efficacy and Self-Esteem

The goal of occupational therapy is the development of competence in the activities and tasks of one's cherished roles, which promotes a sense of self-efficacy and self-esteem. *Competence* refers to effective interaction with the physical and social environments (Fig. 1-1). To be competent means to have the skills that are sufficient or adequate to meet the demands of a situation or task (Gage et al., 1994; White, 1959). It does not equate to excellence, normality, or the ability to do everything, and it recognizes that there are degrees of sufficiency and adequacy in people (Gage et al., 1994; Mocellin, 1992; White, 1971).

Competence develops by enabling a person to engage in graduated, goal-directed activity that is accomplishable by that person and that produces a feeling of satisfaction (White, 1959). Occupational therapists help people achieve competence through graded engagement in occupation, vicarious engagement in occupation (watching others), virtual engagement in occupation, developmental and instrumental learning with immediate and precise feedback, and therapeutic interaction with the therapist (Radomski, 2000; Robinson-Smith, Johnston, & Allen, 2000).

When people feel competent, they have a sense of self-efficacy. The most powerful source of personal efficacy expectations is past accomplishments in similar situations

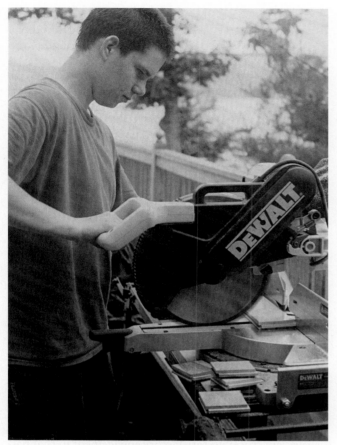

Figure 1-1 Competency in self-advancement role of contractor's helper.

(Fig. 1-2). They have perceived their capability to perform a behavior (Williams, 2010). Self-efficacy is concerned not with the skills one possesses but with the judgments of what one can do with those skills. Perceived self-efficacy is influenced through an ongoing evaluation of success

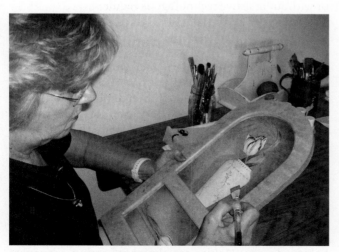

Figure 1-2 For this accomplished artist, painting a picture is a task of one of her self-advancement roles (worker). For another person for whom painting is a hobby, it would be classified as a task of a self-enhancement role (hobbyist).

and failure with each task people participate in over the course of their lives (Gage & Polatajko, 1994). Self-efficacy is likely to lead people to esteem themselves (Hughes, Galbraith, & White, 2011).

Satisfaction with Life Roles [Areas of Occupation][1]

Being in control of one's life means being able to engage satisfyingly in one's life roles or to voluntarily reassign a role to another. Role performance is a vital component of productive, independent living (Hallett et al., 1994). Various occupational therapy scholars have proposed taxonomies of roles. The OTPF categorizes a role as a subunit of the performance patterns of the person (see Table 1-1). The framework's equivalent to the OFM's category of role performance is called "areas of occupation," which includes activities of daily living (ADL), instrumental activities of daily living (IADL), rest and sleep, education, work, play, leisure, and social participation.

The OFM sorts roles into three domains related to aspects of self-definition: self-maintenance, self-advancement, and self-enhancement (Rogers, 1984; Trombly, 1993, 1995), but recognizes that the assignment of roles to a particular category is not absolute. Some roles may be classified in one domain by one person but in another domain by another person, depending on the motivation or context. For example, volunteering may be classified by one person as a self-advancement role because volunteering promotes skills that will be useful in a worker role. Another person may classify volunteering as self-enhancement because it promotes a sense of satisfaction without expectation of gain. The individuality of motivation underscores the importance of assessing each person from his or her own point of view, letting each define his or her roles and their meaning. That is a major aspect of client-centered therapy.

Self-Maintenance Roles [Activities of Daily Living and Instrumental Activities of Daily Living]

Self-maintenance roles are associated with maintenance of the self and care of the family, pets, and home. Examples of roles in this domain are independent person, grandparent, parent, son, daughter, homemaker (Fig. 1-3), home maintainer (Fig. 1-4), exerciser, cat owner, and caregiver.

Self-Advancement Roles [Work and Education]

Self-advancement roles are those that draw the person into productive activities that add to the person's skills, possessions, or other betterment. Self-advancement roles

---

[1]The comparable Occupational Therapy Practice Framework language is added in brackets to assist the student in using the language interchangeably.

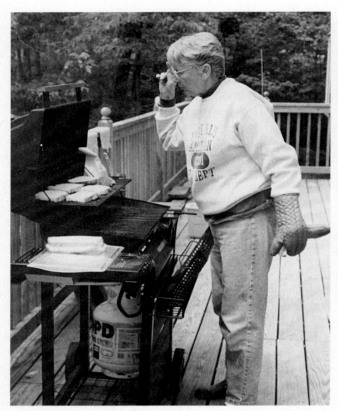

Figure 1-3 Self-maintenance role: homemaker; task: meal preparation; activity: grilling fish.

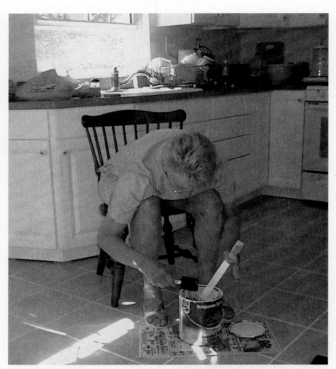

Figure 1-4 Self-maintenance role: home maintainer; task: painting the walls; activity: preparing the paint.

correspond to the participation category of the ICF (Table 1-4). Examples of roles in the self-advancement role domain include worker (Figs. 1-1 and 1-5), student, intern, commuter, shopper, investor, manager, and voter.

Self-Enhancement Roles [Play, Leisure, Social Participation]

Self-enhancement roles contribute to the person's sense of accomplishment and enjoyment or sense of well-being and happiness (Figs. 1-2 and 1-6). Examples of roles in this domain include hobbyist, friend, club member, religious participant, vacationer, golfer, moviegoer, and violinist.

Competency in Tasks of Life Roles [Areas of Occupation]

Roles consist of constellations of tasks. For example, the role of homemaker may include the tasks of food preparation (Fig. 1-3) and service, housecleaning, laundry, and decorating (Fig. 1-4). The tasks identified for the same role by different people may be different (Nelson & Payton, 1991; Trombly, 1993, 1995). The value ascribed to tasks varies among people of similar situations and may vary from what therapists consider important for patients. Because people have different values, each person must

define his or her role by identifying the tasks that he or she believes are crucial to satisfactory engagement in that particular role. The therapist cannot assume that particular tasks are or are not important to a person's interpretation of a role.

Tasks consist of constellations of related activities and are therapeutically developed using occupation-as-end, that is, practicing the activities constituting the task in normal temporal order and environmental demand, with or without assistive technology as required.

Activities and Habits [Performance Patterns]

Activities, in the OFM, are smaller units of goal-directed behavior that, taken together, comprise tasks (Figs. 1-1 to 1-6). Activities bring together abilities and skills within a functional context. For example, one task of the gardener is pest control. Activities that make up this task may include hanging lures, spreading granular insect killer, mixing and spraying liquids, and picking insects off plants. Furthermore, each of these activities consists of even smaller units of behavior, such as opening the package and pouring granular insect killer into a garden spreader. Some activities, such as picking insects off plants, require full attention. Others, called habits, do not. Habits are chains of action sequences that are so well learned that the person does not have to pay attention to do them under ordinary circumstances

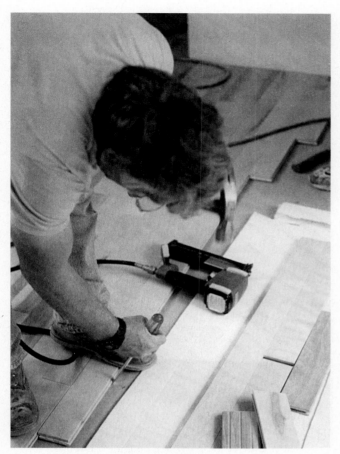

Figure 1-5 Self-advancement role: contractor; task: installing floor; activity: moving the wood into place.

and in familiar contexts. Physical dysfunction disrupts habits, requiring attention to be paid to the simplest of ADL. This adds to the fatigue experienced by many persons (Wallenbert & Jonsson, 2005). Using the OFM, occupational therapists seek to help the person sustain or relearn adaptive habits, let go of habits that are no longer adaptive, and develop new habits, given the person's changed abilities and capacities.

Activities and habits are learned using occupation-as-end, that is, "task-specific training." In task-specific training, functional and meaningful activities are practiced over and over using assistive technology, adaptive methods, or adapted environment to enable performance, if necessary. See Chapter 11 for a more complete discussion of the therapeutic use of occupation-as-end.

Abilities and Skills [Performance Skills]

Activities depend on more basic abilities (Clark, Czaja, & Weber, 1990; Fleishman, 1972; Fleishman & Quaintance, 1984; Kielhofner, 2008). A person with a great number

of highly developed abilities can become proficient at a greater variety of activities. An ability is a general trait, such as muscle strength or memory, that individuals bring with them to a new task (Fleishman, 1972). In the OFM, abilities are seen as a combination of endowed talents and acquired skills. A skill is the ability to use one's knowledge to effectively and readily execute performance (Merriam-Webster Online, 2011). Skill enables goal achievement under a wide variety of conditions with a degree of consistency and economy. Abilities and skills develop from one or more developed capacities. They are more voluntary and organized and evidence smoother execution than do developed capacities. The OFM identifies six categories of abilities and skills: motor, sensory, cognitive, perceptual, socioemotional, and cardiorespiratory.

To accomplish the activity of hanging lures in the previous example of the gardener, the person needs certain abilities, such as coordination, dexterity, and ability to follow directions. The person also needs to be able to translate these endowed talents into the skilled actions required to hang the lures. Carefully analyzed occupation-as-means is used to develop deficient abilities and skills. In the process of repeatedly accomplishing occupations that demand greater levels of the deficient ability or skill, in varying contexts, the patient gains greater levels of that ability or skill. By varying the context, the therapist encourages more robust learning. See Chapter 11 for a more complete discussion of the therapeutic use of occupation-as-means.

Developed Capacities [Client Factors]

Developed capacities reflect the organization of first-level capacities into more mature, less reflexive, and more voluntary responses. For example, to support dexterity, an ability, a person needs independent use of fingers, graded release, and pinch, which are developed capacities that derive from reflexive grasp and automatic release (first-level capacities). This organization is normally acquired through maturation. In therapy, occupation-as-means is used to develop these capacities. Therapeutic demands for gradually more mature and varied responses are made through repeated opportunities to engage in selected occupations.

First-Level Capacities [Client Factors]

First-level capacities are the functional foundation for movement, cognition, perception, and emotional life based on the integrity of the organic substrate. In the motor domain, first-level capacities are reflex-based motor responses that reflect the organization of primary visual, sensory, and motor systems. Examples include reflexive grasp, reflexive release, primitive

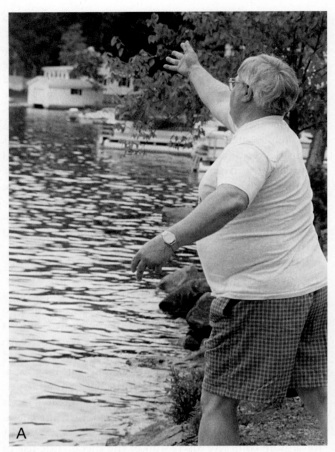
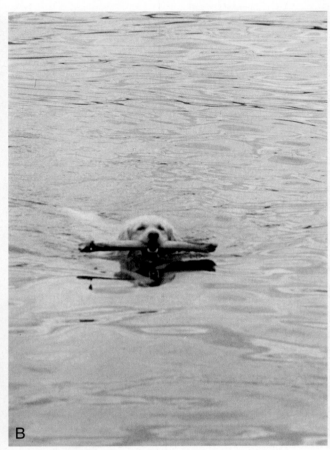

Figure 1-6   A. Self-enhancement role: pet owner; task: exercise dog; activity: throw the stick. **B.** Molly with stick.

Clinical Reasoning in Occupational Therapy Practice

Occupational Self-Analysis

Occupational therapists evaluate a patient's occupational profile. Practice this skill by analyzing your own occupational profile. The following directions are one way to determine the profile.

1. Make an occupational diary by listing awake hours along the left side of a piece of 11 × 8.5-inch paper and listing the days of the week across the top.
2. Fill in activities or tasks you do hour by hour in a typical week.
3. Classify these into role categories: self-maintenance, self-advancement, or self-enhancement.
4. Calculate what percentage of time you engaged in these role categories (hours spent in one role category/total awake hours × 100%).
5. Do these percentages align with your values and goals? To what extent does performance of these roles contribute to your self-esteem or role satisfaction?

6. Do you feel occupationally balanced, that is, physically, mentally, socially, emotionally, and spiritually healthy? Or are you stressed because of occupational imbalance? How have you gauged your balance—using time distribution, degree of challenge of the occupations in your life, type of occupations (physical, mental, etc.), or degree of self- or other-centeredness?
7. Make another chart. Choose a favorite role. What tasks make up this role for you? Are the tasks the same as those of your classmates who chose the same role?
8. Choose the key task from your answer to Question 7. What activities comprise this task?
9. Choose one activity from your answer to Question 8. What abilities are needed to do this activity?
10. What type of impairments would prevent you from doing the activity as you usually do it?
11. What type of environmental or contextual barriers would prevent or hamper you from doing the activity? Enable or facilitate your performance?

reaching, kicking, and stepping. They are the subroutines that Bruner (1973) described as underlying the development of all voluntary movement. The ability to recognize a connection between an instrumental, nonreflexive response given consistently within a particular perceptual situation is a first-level capacity of cognition and perception. The fascination of babies with human faces is a first-level capacity of the socioemotional domain.

Organic Substrate [Client Factors]

Organic substrate is the structural and physiological foundation for movement, cognition, perception, and emotions, including the primordial central nervous system (CNS) organization in the neonate; the CNS organization that is spared or recovers spontaneously after injury or illness; and the integrity of the skeleton, muscles, sensory and motor nerves, heart, lungs, and skin. If the organic substrate is not present, therapy cannot generate it. If it exists at all, therapy attempts to develop it into first-level capacities through techniques classified as augmented maturation (see Web Chapters A through C).

Environment and Context [Contexts and Environments]

The words *environment* and *context* are often used interchangeably. In current health care literature, the term *context* is used to encompass all that influences any aspect of human functioning, including physical, social, personal, temporal, and situational influences, as well as familial and cultural beliefs and practices that influence the life of an individual. Context is the interpretive dimension of the circumstances surrounding occupational engagement. Seemingly similar circumstances may result in different occupational behavior depending on the person's interpretation of the circumstances. It is this interpretive dimension of context that is important to the occupational therapist.

Environment is defined as the complex of external factors, circumstances, objects, structures, and social surround that inhibit or facilitate occupational functioning. Research has shown that familiarity of environment positively affects daily functioning (Geusgens et al., 2010). Successful and satisfactory performance of complex, cognitive IADL, which involve equipment and planning, has been found to be more affected by the environment than physical ADL, such as basic self-care (Raina, Rogers, & Holm, 2007).

Context in the OTPF refers to cultural, physical, social, personal, temporal, and virtual aspects of living. Similar to the OTPF, the OFM assumes that context and

environment surround and permeate all levels of the occupational functioning hierarchy. However, the OFM distinguishes between the greater influence of context and environment at the higher levels of the hierarchy and the lesser influence at the lower levels. At the lower levels, the immediate physical and personal context and environment influence the actions. For example, organization of a reaching movement was shown to differ when actual, natural objects and utensils were used versus when simulated objects were used (Ma, Trombly, & Robinson-Podolski, 1999; Wu et al., 1998). Cultural and social contexts pertain less to this level. At the higher levels of activities, tasks, and roles, however, all aspects of context and environment—personal, social, cultural, temporal, situational, and physical—interact with the person's abilities to yield occupational functioning for the particular person. The diagram of the OFM on the title page depicts these ideas about context and environment within the limitations of two-dimensional representation. Chapters 3 and 30 discuss the influence of personal, social, cultural and situational contexts on occupational functioning, and Chapters 10 and 31 discuss the influence of physical context.

When the challenges of the environment exceed the capabilities of a person, that person is said to be disabled (Bilbao et al., 2003; Institute of Medicine, 2007). A person with impaired abilities and capacities, however, may be able to accomplish activities and tasks of his or her roles if the environment is adapted to enable that (Geusgens et al., 2010). Therefore, occupational therapy treatment may focus on changing the environment or context rather than on remediating the person's impaired abilities or capacities.

THE PROCESS OF OCCUPATIONAL THERAPY FOR PERSONS WITH PHYSICAL DYSFUNCTION

The process of occupational therapy follows the universal plan for problem solving: identify the problem, determine possible solutions, intervene, and evaluate the result. The occupational therapist, however, focuses only on problems related to the person's occupational life, including occupational balance. What a person needs to do, wants to do, and can do are identified. Discrepancy between what the person needs or wants to do and what he or she can do identifies the problem. The occupational therapist then uses various occupational, adaptive, and adjunctive therapies to intervene, or the occupational therapist may detect the person's dissatisfaction or stress caused by an occupational imbalance and intervene using educational therapies. The processes of the OFM and the OTPF are similar (Table 1-2). A discussion of the OFM process follows.

Assessment [Evaluation]

The hierarchical organization of the OFM indicates that higher level occupational functioning is established on a foundation of abilities and capacities. Assessment *always* follows a top-down approach. That is, the therapist determines what roles and tasks the person was responsible for in life before the accident or disease and what the person is expected to be, and wants to be, responsible for in post-rehabilitation life, including the context and environment in which the person typically engaged in these valued roles and tasks (Mathiowetz, 1993; Mayer, Keating, & Rapp, 1986; Trombly, 1993, 1995). The Role Checklist (Barris, Oakley, & Kielhofner, 1988; Colon & Haertlein, 2002; Cordeiro et al., 2007; Oakley et al., 1986), the Canadian Occupational Performance Measure (COPM) (Carswell et al., 2004; Eyssen et al., 2011; Law et al., 2005), and the Client-Oriented Role Evaluation (Toal-Sullivan & Henderson, 2004) are examples of assessments the therapist may use to gather this information. The therapist may also measure the patient's sense of self-efficacy concerning the ability to do the tasks required to fulfill particular roles by having the patient assign a number on a visual analog scale that ranges from 0 (not at all confident) to 10 (absolutely certain) for each major task that defines a specific role (Gill et al., 1994). For example, "on this scale from 0 to 10, how confident are you that you can prepare your own lunch without help?" Other assessments of self-efficacy are the Self-Efficacy for Functional Activities Scale (Resnick, 1999) and the Self-Efficacy Gauge designed especially for occupational therapists to measure the patient's current level of perceived self-efficacy and the change in perceived self-efficacy over time (Gage et al., 1994).

Wilcock et al. (1997), focusing on the importance of occupational balance, developed an assessment that can be used to gauge balance. It asks subjects to rate their current and ideal involvement in physical, mental, social, and rest occupations. A therapist can also determine whether the person feels that his or her life is in balance, and what the imbalance may be, through careful interviewing or the use of the Life Balance Inventory, which determines a person's satisfaction with time use in four dimensions: health (self-care), relationships, identity (e. g. vocational or social activities) and challenge (e. g. hobbies) (Matuska, 2012).

When evaluating a patient's competence to accomplish the roles he or she identifies as important, the therapist observes the patient attempting to do the tasks and activities, also identified by the person, of those roles in the most familiar context. The Assessment of Motor and Process Skills (AMPS) (Fisher, 2003), the Klein-Bell ADL Scale (Klein & Bell, 1982), the Barthel Index (Della Pietra et al., 2011; Mahoney & Barthel, 1965; Tennant, Geddes, & Chamberlain, 1996), and the Performance Assessment of Self-Care Skills (PASS) (Holm & Rogers, 1999; Skidmore et al., 2006) are examples of observational assessments

of tasks and activities. Using an assessment that structures observation of performance and having knowledge of the probabilities established by the diagnosis and age of the person, the therapist detects which of the myriad abilities and capacities assumed to be related to accomplishment of these activities are impaired (the process of activity analysis applied to assessment; see Chapter 12 for client-centered activity analysis procedure and example). The therapist then assesses these abilities and capacities more directly using assessments that have been validated and found reliable for the type of patient being evaluated. For example, if the patient's goal is to shave with an electric razor, but he appears to lack the grasp strength and endurance to do so, strength and endurance are assessed according to the procedures described in Chapter 7. A person whose abilities and capacities are found deficient may be treated to optimize them, allowing not only shaving but other occupations.

Some therapists prefer to use a bottom-up evaluation procedure in which capacities, abilities, and skills are assessed before occupational performance (Gutman et al., 2007; Weinstock-Zlotnick & Hinojosa, 2004). However, this practice often results in emphasizing these lower level factors without translation of the regained abilities to occupational performance. Furthermore, when this approach is used, the patient often fails to see the connection between therapy to optimize skills and abilities and achievement of his or her occupational goals.

The environment in which the patient will live, work, or play is assessed to determine whether it enables or hinders occupational functioning. Assessments of the home environment have been developed (e.g., Safety Assessment of Function and the Environment for Rehabilitation [SAFER] [Chui et al., 2002] and Home Occupational-Environmental Assessment [Baum & Edwards, 1998]), but assessments of other environments have not yet been developed (Letts, Baum, & Perlmutter, 2003). To assess the effects on occupational performance of other physical and social environments typical for the patient, the occupational therapist needs to observe performance under those conditions, using the process of client-environment fit activity analysis (see Chapter 12). In practice, this assessment usually occurs immediately before or after discharge from an inpatient rehabilitation setting.

Treatment [Intervention]

Treatment may focus on changing the environment (Raina, Rogers, & Holm, 2007), changing the impaired skills and abilities of the person (Lum et al., 2009), teaching specific tasks or activities using goal-directed training (Mastos et al., 2007), or teaching compensatory ways to accomplish activities and tasks. Treatment to improve occupational functioning, then, may start toward the bottom of the OFM hierarchy, focusing on optimizing abilities and capacities; or it may start higher, at the activity level of the hierarchy, focusing on restoring competence in doing the activities and tasks of valued roles that the patient has identified as concerns; or it may start peripheral to the person, focusing on modifying the context or environment. The starting point should acknowledge the problem that the patient has identified as an immediate concern, although treatment may not actually start there. For example, if the patient identified resuming fishing as the goal, the therapist may choose to teach adaptive methods to enable that. If, however, the evidence and the experience of the therapist indicated that it would be more effective to start treatment by regaining finger dexterity to enable various activities related to fishing (e.g., baiting the hook and removing the fish from the line), the therapist must help the patient understand how treatment of this lower level ability addresses the stated concern at the task level. In addition, the therapist must ensure carryover of any gained dexterity to the fishing task. Optimizing impaired abilities and capacities is accomplished through remedial therapy in which a change in physiological structure, function, or organization is sought through occupation-as-means. If remediation of deficit abilities or capacities does not restore occupational functioning, if economic constraints prevent such thorough treatment, or if the patient is not committed to the extensive work required to recover abilities and capacities, a degree of competence can be restored using goal-specific training and/or adaptive therapy. Adaptive therapy seeks to find and promote a balance among the person's goals and environmental demands and his or her current capacities and abilities (Thoren-Jonsson, Moller, & Grimby, 1999). In this type of therapy, the method of doing an activity may be modified, assistive technology may be used to enable completion of the activity, and/or the physical or social environments may be modified. The person may be counseled to reassess the need to accomplish a particularly difficult activity alone and opt to employ another to do it.

Optimizing Abilities and Capacities [Intervention]

It is believed that remediating impaired sensorimotor, cognitive, perceptual, and emotional capacities and abilities to as high a level as a person's organic substrate allows will enable versatile performance of activities. Versatile performance allows the person to adjust to changes in the social and physical environments, whereas if a person learns only one compensatory response, adaptation to new situations is less likely. As in the typical development of these capacities and abilities, therapy engages the patient in circumscribed encounters with the environment using occupation-as-means. Using the example of the man who wanted to shave, the therapist might start treatment by providing a cuff to hold the razor to eliminate the need for grasp (adaptive therapy) and let the patient shave as

much as he could. Then the occupational therapist would finish the activity. Day by day, the patient's endurance for shaving would increase, and he would do more of the task on his own (occupation used as a means of remediation). Concurrently, the therapist would engage the patient in other activities that require grasp strength until the patient was able to hold the razor.

Occupation-as-means, that is, activities that provide stretch of soft tissues, active or passive movement to preserve and restore full range of motion, resistance and other stress to strengthen weak muscles, or graduated, increasing levels of aerobic exercise to improve endurance, is used to optimize motor abilities and capacities. The intervention techniques for optimizing abilities and capacities are described in Chapter 20; adjunctive therapies that support this approach are discussed in Chapters 15, 18, and 19; and the application of the approach, in combination with complementary approaches, is illustrated in Chapters 36–42.

When impairment of the CNS results in the inability to move voluntarily to effect a desired change in the environment, a therapist may use occupation-as-means in conjunction with controlled sensory input and ontogenetic or recovery-based developmental postures or patterns (augmented maturation) to facilitate change in first-level and developed capacities of sensorimotor organization. Whereas some therapists have anecdotally reported success using controlled sensory stimulation and developmental movements or postures to develop motor control, as described in the Bobath (1990), Brunnstrom (1970), Rood (1956), and proprioceptive neuromuscular facilitation (PNF) (Knott & Voss, 1968) approaches, there is little to no evidence in the literature to support these approaches. However, because some therapists do find aspects of these approaches clinically helpful, especially when there is a need to optimize first-level capacities, chapters describing these approaches have been preserved online (see pages 675, 677, 679 for access), but they have been removed from this textbook because we subscribe to the AOTA Centennial Vision: We envision that occupational therapy is a . . . science-driven and evidence-based profession. . . . (AOTA, 2008).

Alternatively, because of the preponderance of research that documents that neural reorganization occurs secondary to practice of goal-directed movements, the therapist may use motor learning principles in conjunction with occupation-as-end to bring about change in voluntary movement behavior (Mastos et al., 2007). The application of motor learning principles and methods of treatment for persons with CNS impairment is described in Chapters 13 and 21. This approach emphasizes motor performance using functional tasks, includes modification of the environment to improve task performance, and stresses practice that fits the nature of the task. The approach further heeds the research findings on the effect of context on the organization of movement, which indicates that practicing a skill under simplified, non–context-specific conditions is different from practicing with an actual object in a context-specific situation (Mathiowetz & Wade, 1995; Trombly & Wu, 1999; Wu et al., 1998).

Restoring Competence [Intervention]

Restoration of occupational functioning depends on developing competence in the valued tasks and activities of the patient's life roles. Competence in tasks and activities is synthesized through successful engagement with the environment. Occupational therapists are skilled in developing graduated encounters with objects and the surrounding physical and social environments to promote successful performance. They are also expert in teaching compensatory methods to accomplish activities. Some therapists use this approach exclusively (Mayer, Keating, & Rapp, 1986). Others believe that first optimizing the impaired abilities and capacities requires less compensation and produces more versatility of performance. There is no research to support one point of view over the other.

When activity, task, and role levels of the OFM are dysfunctional, treatment may aim at making people as independent as possible in spite of any residual impairment. The occupational therapist will concentrate on helping a person find ways to compensate by reorganizing activity patterns or adapting techniques, equipment, or the environment. The goal is independence. People are considered independent when they perform tasks for themselves using assistive equipment, alternative methods, or adapted environments, as required, or when they appropriately oversee completion of activities by others on their own behalf (Moyers & Dale, 2007). The therapist teaches the patient to recognize and use remaining abilities in adapted ways and teaches the principles and concepts of adapted methods so that the person can become an independent problem solver. For example, Chapter 24 explains how to help develop habits as a means of addressing cognitive-related performance problems that interfere with previously automated tasks. Therapeutic mechanisms of change include occupation-as-end, teaching-learning, and therapeutic rapport. The treatment procedures for restoring or preventing loss of role performance are described in Chapters 25–32.

SUMMARY

This chapter describes one model, the OFM, to guide the process of occupational therapy for persons with occupational dysfunction secondary to physical impairments and relates that model to the Occupational Therapy Practice Framework, which is an official document of the American Occupational Therapy Association concerning domain and process of the entire practice of occupational therapy. The framework needs an organizational model to guide assessment and intervention. That model can be the OFM, the Model for Human Occupation (MOHO) (Kielhofner, 2008), the Occupational Adaptation Model (Jack & Estes, 2010) or any number of other models (see Table 3-1) that complement your way of thinking and analyzing problems and that facilitate clinical reasoning. Furthermore, this chapter relates the OFM to the WHO ICF, an international classification of the effects of impairment and the process of rehabilitation.

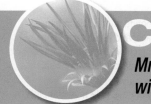

case example

Mr. J.: Application of the Occupational Functioning Method to a Patient with Spinal Cord Injury

Occupational Therapy Process		Clinical Reasoning—Examples of Therapist's Internal Dialogue
Obtain Information About the Patient	Mr. J. is a patient with a spinal cord injury (SCI) (see Chapter 38 for a description of this condition, including special circumstances such as tenodesis grasp).	He can become independent in self-care and other tasks and activities important to him if he is willing to work hard. Even though he may choose, in the future, to employ a personal care attendant to help with dressing and personal care to conserve his energy, as many others with his level of SCI do, he needs to learn the adapted techniques so he can be independent if he needs to be.
	Diagnosis: fracture/dislocation of C6–7 of his spine in a diving accident. Status: post cervical laminectomy and fusion; medically stable. He exhibits C6 functional level.	
	Interview: Mr. J. is 24 years old, a college graduate, who lives with his parents in a second-floor apartment in a small city. He has four older siblings who are all married. He has many friends.	He will have to relocate to a first-floor apartment or to a building with an elevator. This needs to be discussed soon and a referral made to Social Services.

His sociability should make developing rapport with him easy. |
Evaluate to Identify Problem(s)	Interview: In addition to his role as independent person, Mr. J. identified self-advancement and self-enhancement roles of worker and sportsman.	Mr. J. values his roles as independent person, worker, friend, and sportsman. He appears ready to work to regain those roles.
	Mr. J's worker role was that of computer programmer. The company is holding his job for him. He identifies keyboarding as a major physical task of this role.	Although he cannot do keyboarding now because of paralysis of his fingers, he should be able to resume his job with adaptations and reasonable accommodations. However, he also needs to regain activities of daily living (ADL) independence, functional mobility, and commuter activities and skills in order to do so.
	Swimmer, basketball player, camper, and friend are his major self-enhancement roles.	
	The family is supportive, but they expect Mr. J. to be independent in self-care, with the prospect of resuming work, at discharge.	Because of the paralysis, he will need to learn adaptive methods of resuming his sports interests.
	Assessment: *Observation*: Mr. J. was unable to accomplish any tasks or activities associated with the independent person role; he is dependent in all basic self care.	There is no need to evaluate any other activities until he can do basic self-care activities. It will be frustrating for him.
	He is unable to move his lower limbs; movements of the upper limbs are weak and incomplete; unable to grasp. His sitting balance is poor.	I am going to introduce him to Mr. L. who has a similar disability and who is nearing discharge after gaining many skills and resuming several of his roles. It will let Mr. J. see the possibilities for recovery of his own roles.
	Measurement: Manual muscle testing revealed that Mr. J.'s proximal upper extremity musculature rated 4 to 5, with the exception of the triceps, which graded 2 (see Table 7-1, which describes muscle strength grading). Wrist extensors graded 3+ on the left and 4− on the right; wrist flexors and finger and thumb muscles graded 0 bilaterally.	He will need to learn adaptive ischial pressure relief methods and how to use tenodesis grasp.
Plan Intervention	During our planning conversation, Mr. J. agreed that treatment to increase the strength of his arms and to promote sitting balance would enable him to do the activities and tasks that he needs and wants to do. Again, he mentioned sports activities being important to him.	Weakness of the proximal upper extremity musculature, wrist extensors, and sitting balance can be improved through occupation-as-means that uses activities that provide Mr. J.'s current strength with a just-right challenge, one that is within his capability but also requires effort. The activity needs to be repetitious enough to build muscular endurance. Strength and endurance training will be done in tandem.

Implement Intervention

During occupational therapy, Mr. J. engaged in *occupation-as-means* to remediate the weakness of his upper arms and wrists and to improve his balance. He also engaged in *occupation-as-end* to learn adapted ways to accomplish important tasks and activities of his independent person and worker roles and to overcome environmental barriers.

Because of paralysis of his trunk and lower extremities, Mr. J. is required to use a wheelchair, which needs to be adapted to allow propulsion without requiring grasp.

The physical therapist and I collaborated on developing his permanent wheelchair order, teaching him to use it and teaching and supervising his ischial pressure relief maneuvers.

Mr. J. and I enjoyed a beneficial *therapeutic relationship* in which he knew that I would not make demands for action that were beyond his capabilities and that I was available to help him work through his feelings of loss.

He participated in group *educational sessions* for social, emotional, and practical problem solving; members are other persons with similar activity limitations.

I used simulated basketball shooting games (bean bag shoot, etc.) among other activities, and he enjoyed them enough to work hard while in the clinic. His enthusiasm is spurring on others and making his family less stressed.

Because of his returning strength, he is able to accomplish more ADL each day. I determined his openness to using adaptive devices, and he was willing as long as the devices increased abilities. I must continue to organize those practice sessions to keep the physical and emotional demands within his capabilities.

Relearning basic ADL can be distressing; I am paying close attention to his emotional responses and make the opportunity to discuss these with him.

Mr. J has "down" periods but seems able to work through them with the help of the other group members and his own optimistic life outlook. He enjoys sharing new ideas and "tricks" with the others, as well as learning "tricks" of wheelchair usage from them.

Evaluate the Result

Mr. J. is able to wheel himself 50 feet on flat carpeting and is able to mount one step or curb with the wheelchair. He is happy with his progress and expects to develop more advanced wheelchair skills on his own.

Mr. J. uses gravity, momentum, and leverage to move his body in the wheelchair and bed.

His proximal upper extremity musculature recovered to normal strength, but because the triceps remained at less than functional strength, he cannot elevate himself off the wheelchair cushion. Therefore, he learned an adaptive method of relieving ischial pressure to maintain skin integrity. Mr. J. was glad to take control and responsibility for regular pressure relief so I expect that he will be faithful to this procedure to prevent decubiti.

Mr. J.'s wrist extensor strength improved to 4+ bilaterally, which allowed a functional tenodesis grasp. This enabled showering, dressing, and bowel and bladder management. He showers using a bath bench and handheld showerhead, and he dresses independently using adaptive methods and devices.

He keyboards using universal cuffs with typing sticks tipped with rubber ends. His computer is adapted to allow one-key depression for all operations. He feels ready to return to work; he plans on resuming work part time (noon to 4 pm).

He plans on joining the local wheelchair basketball team.

Acknowledging his loss caused by the accident, he has worked hard in therapy and feels ready to resume his previous roles.

The people he will be playing wheelchair basketball with after discharge are expert wheelchair users and will teach him their "tricks." He has the initiative and desire to become expert.

The problem-solving skills he probably developed while camping and playing sports, and those he learned in therapy, have served him well in learning adapted techniques for self-care so he should be able to solve any new activity problem that presents itself after discharge.

Ischial pressure relief is so important, I am sending a work sheet reminder and a programmed reminder alarm home with him to help him remember during the exciting transition time from hospital to home.

His time to do self-care will improve with practice, but I will remind him that for purposes of energy conservation, he may prefer to receive assistance with these activities.

His speed will increase with practice, but at some point he may be interested in returning to occupational therapy to evaluate strategies to boost his speed, such as speech recognition software.

This schedule will allow enough time for morning care.

Go, Mr. J.!

Mr. J. successfully completed this first phase of his rehabilitation. He will likely need intermittent rehabilitation "tune-ups" for many years as his interests, needs, and capacities change. For example, he may soon want to return to outpatient therapy to review technologies to assist him with his job and to resume driving.

Clinical Reasoning in Occupational Therapy Practice

Treatment Planning for Mr. J.

When Mr. J. began occupational therapy, he had extensive impairments that prevented him from engaging in the activities and tasks of his valued roles. The occupational therapist, in collaboration with Mr. J., must decide what approach to take in treatment. What are the pros and cons of concentrating therapeutic intervention on restoration of activities, tasks, and roles (occupation-as-end) versus remediation of capacities and abilities using occupation-as-means?

Summary Review Questions

1. Describe the OFM.
2. In what ways are the OFM and the OTPF similar? Dissimilar?
3. What is the overall goal of occupational therapy for persons with occupational dysfunction caused by physical impairments according to the OFM? According to the OTPF?
4. Using the OFM as your model of practice, what would you assess first in a patient with stroke: level of spasticity of the upper extremity, ADL, or role history and expectations?

5. Define *ability* and *developed capacity*. Give an example of each. To what levels of the OTPF and the ICF do these terms correspond?
6. Define *task* and *activity*. Give an example of each. To what levels of the OTPF and the ICF do these terms correspond?
7. What distinguishes occupation-as-means from occupation-as-end?

Glossary

Ability—Competence in doing; natural aptitude or acquired proficiency (Merriam-Webster Online, 2011). A general trait an individual brings to learning a new task (Fleishman, 1972).

Activity, activities—In the Occupational Functioning Model (OFM), activities are considered small units of goal-directed behavior that make up tasks. The Occupational Therapy Practice Framework defines activity as a class of human actions that are goal directed; the term *occupation* encompasses activity (AOTA, 2008, pp. 629, 669). In the International Classification of Functioning (ICF), activity is defined as the "execution of a task or action by an individual" and includes everything a person does at any level of complexity from basic physical and mental functions of the person as a whole (e.g., acquisition of knowledge or grasp) to complex skills and behavior (e.g., driving a car or interacting with persons in formal settings) (WHO, 2001).

Activity analysis—A process used to identify the properties inherent in a given occupation, task, or activity, as well as the skills, abilities, and capacities required to complete it. Activity analysis is used to analyze and assess performance, to select occupations to remediate deficient capacities and abilities, or, knowing the person's skills, abilities, and capacities, to modify an activity or environment to ensure successful completion of the activity.

Adaptive therapy—Therapy that promotes a balance among a person's goals, capabilities, and environmental demands by use of assistive technology, adaptation of the environment or methods of accomplishing an activity, and/or redefinition of goals.

Augmented maturation—Therapeutic techniques that challenge further development of first-level capacities or developed capacities, such as controlled sensory stimulation and activities that promote responses in developmental postures or patterns.

Capacities—Potential attributes that, once developed into abilities and skills, will contribute to occupational functioning. Capacities are the basis of performance.

Context—Interrelated conditions in which something exists or occurs (Merriam-Webster Online, 2011). In health care, context has personal, social, cultural, physical, temporal, and situational dimensions, which together qualify a person's experience. In the OFM, context is considered the circumstantial milieu in which occupation occurs and may be fully understood.

Environment—The tangible objects, structures, or conditions by which one is surrounded and in which one's daily occupations occur. The aggregate of physical, social, and cultural conditions that influence the life of an individual (Merriam-Webster Online, 2011). In the OFM, environment is considered the encompassing surround in which the person accomplishes the activities and tasks of his or her life.

Functioning—An umbrella term encompassing all body functions, activities, and participation (WHO, 2001).

Impairment—Any significant deviation or loss of body structure or physiological or psychological function (WHO, 2001).

Occupation—The breadth and meaning of everyday activity (AOTA, 2008, p. 628).

Occupation-as-end—Occupation is the functional goal (activity, task) to be learned or accomplished. Its therapeutic impact comes from its characteristics of purpose and meaning (Trombly, 1995). Through repeated carrying out of an occupation ("task-specific training"), the patient will relearn the actions and routine of an activity, or through adaptation, the activity will be made possible for the person, given his or her current capacities and abilities.

Occupation-as-means—Occupation that is used as the therapeutic change agent to remediate impaired abilities or capacities. Its therapeutic effect derives from characteristics of purpose and meaning (Trombly, 1995).

Occupational balance—The distribution of occupations within a person's life. When the occupations are balanced, the person perceives him- or herself to be healthy or stress free; too much or too little of an occupation or type of occupation is unhealthy. The dimension through which satisfactory balance may be achieved differs for different people and at different times in one person's life. Dimensions identified to date are time (hours spent in self-care, play, work, and rest for example), degree of difficulty (challenging occupation versus relaxing occupation),

degree of self-focus (occupation is meaningful for the person versus being meaningful for others; care of one's self versus care of others) (Rogers, 1984; Stamm et al., 2009; Wilcock et al., 1997).

Occupational dysfunction—Inability to accomplish a necessary or desired occupational goal, for example, maintain one's self (i.e., care for self, dependents, and home); advance oneself through work, learning, and financial management; or enhance the self by engaging in self-actualizing activities that add enjoyment to life, because of either impairment of abilities and skills or environmental barriers. Occupational dysfunction is the focus of occupational therapy (Rogers, 1984).

Occupational Functioning Model—A conceptual model that guides occupational therapy evaluation and treatment of persons with occupational dysfunction secondary to physical dysfunction. The particulars of the model are as follows: (1) To engage satisfactorily in a life role, a person must be able to do the tasks that, in his or her opinion, make up that role. (2) Tasks are composed of activities, which are small units of behavior. (3) To be able to do a given activity, one must have certain sensorimotor, cognitive, perceptual, emotional, and social abilities. (4) Abilities are developed from capacities that the person has gained through learning or maturation. (5) These developed capacities depend on first-level capacities that derive from a person's genetic endowment or spared organic substrate (Trombly, 1993, 1995).

Participation—Ability to engage in all areas or aspects of human life, including the full experience of being involved in a practice, custom, or social behavior (WHO, 2001); involvement in a life situation (AOTA, 2008, p. 673).

Performance patterns—Patterns of behavior related to daily life activities that are habitual or routine, including habits, routines, rituals, and roles (AOTA, 2008, p. 673).

Performance skills—The abilities clients demonstrate in actions they perform, including motor and praxis, sensory-perceptual, emotional regulation, cognitive, and communication and social skills (AOTA, 2008, pp. 639, 673).

Self-efficacy—Perceived capability to perform a behavior (Williams, 2010). Belief in personal competence (Brock et al., 2009).

Skill—Competence in doing (Merriam-Webster Online, 2011).

References

American Occupational Therapy Association. (2008). *Occupational therapy practice framework: Domain and process* (2nd ed.). Bethesda, MD: AOTA Press and American Occupational Therapy Association. (2008). Occupational therapy practice framework: Domain and process (2nd ed.). *American Journal of Occupational Therapy, 62,* 625–683.

Bandura, A. (1977). Self-efficacy: Toward a unifying theory of behavior change. *Psychological Review, 84,* 191–215.

Bandura, A. (1997). *Self-efficacy.* New York: W. H. Freeman.

Bandura, A. (2001). Social cognitive theory: An agentic perspective. *Annual Review of Psychology, 52,* 1–26.

Barris, R., Oakley, F., & Kielhofner, G. (1988). The role checklist. In B. J. Hemphill (Ed.), *Mental health assessment in occupational therapy* (pp. 73–91). Thorofare, NJ: Slack, Inc.

Baum, C. M., & Edwards, D. F. (1998). *Guide for the home occupational-environmental assessment.* St. Louis, MO: Washington University Program in Occupational Therapy.

Bilbao, A., Kennedy, C., Chatterji, S., Üstün, B., Vasquez Barquero, J. L., & Barth, J. T. (2003). The ICF: Applications of the WHO model of functioning, disability and health to brain injury rehabilitation. *NeuroRehabilitation, 18,* 239–250.

Bobath, B. (1990). *Adult hemiplegia: Evaluation and treatment* (3rd ed.). London: Heinemann.

Brock, K., Black, S., Cotton, S., Kennedy, G., Wilson, S., & Sutton, E. (2009). Goal achievement in the six months after inpatient rehabilitation for stroke. *Disability and Rehabilitation, 31,* 880–886.

Bruner, J. (1973). Organization of early skilled action. *Child Development, 44,* 1–11.

Brunnstrom, S. (1970). *Movement therapy in hemiplegia.* New York: Harper & Row.

Carswell, A., McColl, M. A., Baptiste, S., Law, M., Polatajko, H., & Pollock, N. (2004). The Canadian Occupational Performance Measure: A research and clinical literature review. *Canadian Journal of Occupational Therapy, 71,* 210–222.

Chui, T., Oliver, R., Marshall, L., & Letts, L. (2002). *Safety assessment of function and the environment for rehabilitation tool manual.* Toronto, Canada: COTA Comprehensive Rehabilitation and Mental Health Services.

Clark, M. C., Czaja, S. J., & Weber, R. A. (1990). Older adults and daily living task profiles. *Human Factors, 32,* 537–549.

Colon, H., & Haertlein, C. (2002). Spanish translation of the Role Checklist. *American Journal of Occupational Therapy, 56,* 586–589.

Cordeiro, J. R., Camelier, A., Oakley, F., & Jardim, J. R. (2007). Cross-cultural reproducibility of the Brazilian Portuguese version of the Role Checklist for persons with chronic obstructive pulmonary disease. *American Journal of Occupational Therapy, 61,* 33–40.

Dagfinrud, H., Kjeken, I., Mowinckel, P., Hagen, K. B., & Kvien, T. K. (2005). Impact of functional impairment in ankylosing spondylitis: Impairment, activity limitation, and participation restrictions. *Journal of Rheumatology, 32,* 516–523.

Della Pietra, G. L., Savio, K., Oddone, F., Reggiani, M., Monaco, F., & Leone, M. A. (2011). Validity and reliability of the Barthel Index administered by telephone. *Stroke, 42,* 2077–2079.

Dijkers, M. (1997). Quality of life after spinal cord injury: A meta-analysis of the effects of disablement components. *Spinal Cord, 35,* 829–840.

Dijkers, M. P. J. M. (1999). Correlates of life satisfaction among persons with spinal cord injury. *Archives of Physical Medicine and Rehabilitation, 80,* 867–876.

Elavsky, S., McAuley, E., Motl, R. W., Konopack, J. F., Marquez, D. X., Hu, L., Jerome, G. J., & Diener, E. (2005). Physical activity enhances long-term quality of life in older adults: Efficacy, esteem, and affective influences. *Annals of Behavioral Medicine, 30,* 138–145.

Eriksson, G., Kottorp, A., Borg, J., & Tham, K. (2009). Relationship between occupational gaps in everyday life, depressive mood and life satisfaction after acquired brain injury. *Journal of Rehabilitation Medicine, 41,* 187–194.

Eyssen, I. C. J. M, Steultjens, M. P. M., Oud, T. A. M., Bolt, E. M., Maasdam, A., & Dekker, J. (2011). Responsiveness of the Canadian Occupational Performance Measure. *Journal of Rehabilitation Research & Development, 48,* 517–528.

Filiatrault, J., Arsenault, A. B., Dutil, E. M., & Bourbonnais, D. (1991). Motor function and activities of daily living assessments: A study of three tests for persons with hemiplegia. *American Journal of Occupational Therapy, 45,* 806–810.

Fisher, A. G. (2003). *Assessment of motor and process skills: Development, standardization, and administration manual* (5th ed.). Fort Collins, CO: Three Star Press.

Fleishman, E. A. (1972). On the relation between ability, learning, and human performance. *American Psychologist, 27,* 1017–1032.

Fleishman, E. A., & Quaintance, M. K. (1984). *Taxonomies of human performance.* New York: Academic Press.

Foroud, A., & Whislaw, I. Q. (2010). Reaching-to-eat in humans post stroke: Fluctuating components within a constant pattern. *Behavioral Neurosciences, 124,* 851–867.

Fugl-Meyer, A. R., Jaasko, L., Leyman, I., Olsson, S., & Steglind, S. (1975). The post stroke hemiplegic patient: 1. A method for evaluation of physical performance. *Scandinavian Journal of Rehabilitation Medicine, 7,* 13–31.

Gage, M., Noh, S., Polatajko, H. J., & Kaspar, V. (1994). Measuring perceived self-efficacy in occupational therapy. *American Journal of Occupational Therapy, 48,* 783–790.

Gage, M., & Polatajko, H. (1994). Enhancing occupational performance through an understanding of perceived self-efficacy. *American Journal of Occupational Therapy, 48,* 452–461.

Geertzen, J. H. B., Dijkstra, P. U., van Sonderen, E. L. P., Groothoff, J. W., ten Duis, H. J., & Eisma, W. H. (1998). Relationship between impairments, disability and handicap in reflex sympathetic dystrophy patients: A long-term follow-up study. *Clinical Rehabilitation, 12,* 402–412.

Geusgens, C. A., van Heugten, C. M., Hagedoren, E., Jolles, J., & van den Heuvel, W. J. (2010). Environmental effects in the performance of daily tasks in healthy adults. *American Journal of Occupational Therapy, 64,* 935–940.

Gill, D. L., Kelley, B. C., Williams, K., & Martin, J. J. (1994). The relationship of self-efficacy and perceived well-being to physical activity and stair climbing in older adults. *Research Quarterly for Exercise and Sport, 65,* 367–371.

Gutman, S., Mortera, M. H., Hinojosa, J., & Kramer, P. (2007). The issue is: Revision of the occupational therapy practice framework. *American Journal of Occupational Therapy, 61,* 119–126.

Hallett, J. D., Zasler, N. D., Maurer, P., & Cash, S. (1994). Role change after traumatic brain injury in adults. *American Journal of Occupational Therapy, 48,* 241–246.

Holm, M. B., & Rogers, J. C. (1999). Functional assessment: The Performance Assessment of Self-Care Skills (PASS). In B. J. Hemphill (Ed.), *Assessments in occupational therapy mental health: An integrative approach* (pp. 117–124). Thorofare, NJ: Slack, Inc.

Hughes, A., Galbraith, D., & White, D. (2011). Perceived competence: A common core for self-efficacy and self-concept? *Journal of Personality Assessment, 93,* 278–289.

Institute of Medicine (US) Committee on Disability in America; Field, M. J., & Jette, A. M. (Eds.). (2007). *The future of disability in America.* Washington, DC: National Academy Press.

Jack, J., & Estes, R. I. (2010). Documenting progress: Hand therapy treatment shift from biomechanical to occupational adaptation. *American Journal of Occupational Therapy, 64,* 82–87.

Jebsen, R. H., Taylor, N., Trieschmann, R., Trotter, M., & Howard, L. (1969). An objective and standardized test of hand function. *Archives of Physical Medicine & Rehabilitation, 50,* 311–319.

Kielhofner, G. (2008). *Model of human occupation: Theory and application* (4th ed.). Philadelphia: Lippincott Williams & Wilkins.

Klein, R. M., & Bell, B. (1982). Self-care skills: Behavioral measurement with Klein-Bell ADL Scale. *Archives of Physical Medicine & Rehabilitation, 63,* 335–338.

Knott, M., & Voss, D. E. (1968). *Proprioceptive neuromuscular facilitation techniques.* New York: Harper & Row.

Korpershoek, C., van der Bijl, J., & Hafsteinsdóttir, T. B. (2011). Self-efficacy and its influence on recovery of patients with stroke: A systematic review. *Journal of Advanced Nursing, 67,* 1876–1894.

Law, M., Baptiste, S., Carswell, A., McColl, M., Polatajko, H., & Pollack, N. (2005). *Canadian occupational performance measure* (3rd ed.). Ottawa, Canada: Canadian Association of Occupational Therapists.

Letts, L., Baum, C., & Perlmutter, M. (2003). Person-environment-occupation assessment with older adults. *OT Practice, 8,* 27–34.

Lum, P. S., Mulroy, S., Amdur, R. L., Requejo, P., Prilutsky, B. I., & Dromerick, A. W. (2009). Gains in upper extremity function after stroke via recovery or compensation: Potential differential effects on amount of real-world limb use. *Topics in Stroke Rehabilitation, 16,* 237–253.

Lynch, K. B., & Bridle, M. J. (1989). Validity of the Jebsen-Taylor Hand Function Test in predicting activities of daily living. *Occupational Therapy Journal of Research, 9,* 316–318.

Ma, H.-I., Trombly, C. A., & Robinson-Podolski, C. (1999). The effect of context on skill acquisition and transfer. *American Journal of Occupational Therapy, 53,* 138–144.

Mahaffey, L., & Colaianni, D. (2012). Understanding ICF's connection to occupational therapy services. *OT Practice, 17,* 7–8.

Mahoney, F. I., & Barthel, D. W. (1965). Functional evaluation: The Barthel Index. *Maryland State Medical Journal, 14,* 61–65.

Mastos, M., Miller, A. C., Eliasson, A. C., & Imms, C. (2007). Goal-directed training: Linking theories of treatment to clinical practice for improved functional activities in daily life. *Clinical Rehabilitation, 21,* 47–55.

Mathiowetz, V. (1993). Role of physical performance component evaluations in occupational therapy functional assessment. *American Journal of Occupational Therapy, 47,* 225–230.

Mathiowetz, V., & Wade, M. G. (1995). Task constraints and functional motor performance of individuals with and without multiple sclerosis. *Ecological Psychology, 7,* 99–123.

Matuska, K. (2012). Description and development of the Life Balance Inventory. *OTJR: Occupation, Participation and Health, 32*(1), 220–228.

Mayer, N. H., Keating, D. J., & Rapp, D. (1986). Skills, routines, and activity patterns of daily living: A functional nested approach. In B. Uzzell & Y. Gross (Eds.), *Clinical neuropsychology of intervention* (pp. 205–222). Boston: Martinus Nijhoff.

Merriam-Webster Online (2011). Merriam-Webster, Inc. Retrieved July 28, 2011 from http://www.merriam-webster.com/dictionary.

Michielsen, M. E., de Niet, M., Ribbers, G. M., Stam, H. J., & Bussmann, J. B. (2009). Evidence of a logarithmic relationship between motor capacity and actual performance in daily life of the paretic arm following stroke. *Journal of Rehabilitation Medicine, 41,* 327–331.

Mocellin, G. (1992). An overview of occupational therapy in the context of the American influence on the profession: Part 2. *British Journal of Occupational Therapy, 55,* 55–60.

Moyers, P. A., & Dale, L. M. (2007). *The guide to occupational therapy practice* (2nd ed.). Bethesda, MD: AOTA Press.

Nelson, C. E., & Payton, O. D. (1991). The issue is: A system for involving patients in program planning. *American Journal of Occupational Therapy, 45,* 753–755.

Nelson, D. L. (2006). Critiquing the logic of the *Domain* section of the occupational therapy practice framework: Domain and process. *American Journal of Occupational Therapy, 60,* 511–523.

Oakley, F., Kielhofner, G., Barris, R., & Reichler, R. (1986). The Role Checklist: Development and empirical assessment of reliability. *Occupational Therapy Journal of Research, 6,* 157–170.

Pendlebury, S. T., Blamire, A. M., Lee, M. A., Styles, P., & Matthews, P. M. (1999). Axonal injury in the internal capsule correlates with motor impairment after stroke. *Stroke, 30,* 956–962.

Pollard, B., Johnston, M., & Dieppe, P. (2011). Exploring the relationships between International Classification of Functioning, Disability and Health (ICF) constructs of impairment, activity limitation and participation restriction in people with osteoarthritis prior to joint replacement. *BMC Musculoskeletal Disorders, 12,* 97–104.

Radomski, M. V. (2000). Self-efficacy: Improving occupational therapy outcomes by helping patients say "I can." [American Occupational Therapy Association] *Physical Disabilities Special Interest Section Quarterly, 23,* 1–3.

Raina, K. D., Rogers, J. C., & Holm, M. B. (2007). Influence of the environment on activity performance in older women with heart failure. *Disability and Rehabilitation, 29,* 545–557.

Resnick, B. (1998). Efficacy beliefs in geriatric rehabilitation. *Journal of Gerontological Nursing, 24,* 34–44.

Resnick, B. (1999). Reliability and validity testing of the Self-Efficacy for Functional Activities Scale. *Journal of Nursing Measurement, 7,* 5–20.

Robinson-Smith, G., Johnston, M. V., & Allen, J. (2000). Self-care self-efficacy, quality of life, and depression. *Archives of Physical Medicine and Rehabilitation, 81,* 460–464.

Rogers, J. C. (1984). The Foundation: Why study human occupation? *The American Journal of Occupational Therapy, 38,* 47–49.

Rood, M. S. (1956). Neurophysiological mechanisms utilized in the treatment of neuromuscular dysfunction. *American Journal of Occupational Therapy, 10,* 220–225.

Rudhe, C., & van Hedel, H. J. A. (2009). Upper extremity function in persons with tetraplegia: Relationships between strength, capacity, and the spinal cord independence measure. *Neurorehabilitation and Neural Repair, 23*(5), 413–421.

Skidmore, E. R., Rogers, J. C., Chandler, L. S., & Holm, M. B. (2006). Developing empirical models to enhance stroke rehabilitation. *Disability and Rehabilitation, 28,* 1027–1034.

Smith Roley, S., & Delany, J. (2009). Improving the occupational therapy practice framework: Domain & process. *OT Practice, 14,* 9–12.

Sveen, U., Bautz-Holter, E., Sødring, K. M., Wyller, T. B., & Laake, K. (1999). Association between impairments, self-care ability and social activities 1 year after stroke. *Disability and Rehabilitation, 21,* 372–377.

Tennant, A., Geddes, J. M. L., & Chamberlain, M. A. (1996). The Barthel Index: An ordinal or interval measure? *Clinical Rehabilitation, 10,* 301–308.

Thoren-Jonsson, A.-L., Moller, A., & Grimby, G. (1999). Managing occupations in everyday life to achieve adaptation. *American Journal of Occupational Therapy, 53,* 353–362.

Toal-Sullivan, D., & Henderson, P. R. (2004). Client-Oriented Role Evaluation (CORE): The development of a clinical rehabilitation instrument to assess role change associated with disability. *American Journal of Occupational Therapy, 58,* 211–220.

Trombly, C. (1993). Anticipating the future: Assessment of occupational function. *American Journal of Occupational Therapy, 47,* 253–257.

Trombly, C. A. (1995). Occupation: Purposefulness and meaningfulness as therapeutic mechanisms. *American Journal of Occupational Therapy, 49,* 960–972. Reprinted in R. Padilla & Y. Griffiths (Eds.). (2011). *A professional legacy: The Eleanor Clarke Slagle lectures in occupational therapy 1955–2010* (3rd ed.). Bethesda, MD: AOTA Press.

Trombly, C. A., & Wu, C.-Y. (1999). Effect of rehabilitation tasks on organization of movement after stroke. *American Journal of Occupational Therapy, 53,* 333–344.

Wallenbert, I., & Jonsson, H. (2005). Waiting to get better: A dilemma regarding habits in daily occupations after stroke. *American Journal of Occupational Therapy, 59,* 218–224.

Weinstock-Zlotnick, G., & Hinojosa, J. (2004). The issue is: Bottom-up or top-down evaluation: Is one better than the other? *American Journal of Occupational Therapy, 58,* 594–599.

White, R. W. (1959). Motivation reconsidered: The concept of competence. *Psychological Reviews, 66,* 297–333.

White, R. W. (1971). The urge towards competence. *American Journal of Occupational Therapy, 25,* 271–274.

Wilcock, A. A., Chelin, M., Hall, M., Hamley, N., Morrison, B., Scrivener, L., Townsend, M., & Treen, K. (1997). The relationship between occupational balance and health: A pilot study. *Occupational Therapy International, 4,* 17–30.

Williams, D. M. (2010). Outcome expectancy and self-efficacy: Theoretical implications of an unresolved contradiction. *Personality and Social Psychology Review, 14,* 417–425.

World Health Organization. (2001). *International classification of functioning, disability and health (ICF).* Geneva, Switzerland: World Health Organization.

Wu, C.-Y., Trombly, C., Lin, K.-C., & Tickle-Degnen, L. (1998). Effects of object affordances on reaching performance in person with and without cerebrovascular accident. *American Journal of Occupational Therapy, 52,* 447–456.

ACKNOWLEDGMENT

I am indebted to my coeditor, Mary Vining Radomski, for her contributions to this chapter and to my family and friends for posing for the photographs.

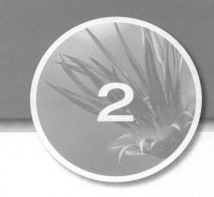

2

Practical Foundations for Practice: Planning, Guiding, Documenting, and Reflecting

Mary Egan and Claire-Jehanne Dubouloz

Learning Objectives

After studying this chapter, the reader will begin to be able to do the following:

1. Describe aspects of clinical reasoning that shape provision of occupational therapy services.
2. Identify how different types of research and expert and patient evidence can inform practice.
3. Discuss issues related to determining the objective of therapy and identifying long- and short-term goals.
4. Describe the purpose of documentation and documentation requirements for occupational therapy services.
5. Commit to professional development plans based on continuous reflection on practice.

Occupational therapists, like all health professionals, use a process to plan, guide, document, and learn from their work with each patient. Throughout this process, there are many decisions to make. This process can seem overwhelming at first, but it does get easier over time. In some ways, implementing this process is like planning a trip.

To plan a trip, you need to decide where you want to go and the best way to get there. You also have to consider your resources, particularly how much time and money you have. Most importantly, if you are traveling with a partner, you have to be in agreement about where you are heading and how you are going to get there.

To help with your planning, you consult with maps, guidebooks, websites, and friends and family who have taken similar trips. You determine what information is the most trustworthy. For example, you are likely to be more confident about a glowing hotel recommendation from a trusted guidebook than about one from the website of that hotel.

Clinical reasoning in occupational therapy is a lot like going on a trip with a partner. First, you must determine whether you should be "traveling" together. This is *screening* to determine whether there are good reasons to enter into a therapeutic relationship with the patient. Next, you have to be sure that you are both in agreement about where you are going. This is the *overall objective of therapy*. You need to know how much time, money, and other means you have for the trip. These are the *resources* that you and the patient have at hand. You also must have a map to your destination. This is your *practice model*. You look for travel tips from people who have been there before. This is *research* and *expert clinical and patient evidence*.

Next, you sketch out your itinerary, including stops along the way, as best you can by combining all this evidence. These are your *intervention plan* and *short-term goals*. As you travel, you and your partner may change your plans a bit to respond to new challenges or opportunities. This is your *intervention implementation*. Often, at the end of the trip, you adjust plans toward a new travel goal. This is your *discharge plan*. An additional feature of occupational therapy is the creation of an official record of the trip. This is your *documentation*. Finally, because travel is such a big part of your life, you consider your experience and put plans in place to ensure that you continue to develop as a traveler. This is your *reflection and development plan*.

This chapter is structured around these basic considerations for practice. Note that these considerations inform the reflection involved in the major decision points regarding a particular patient's care and are summarized in Table 2-1. This table provides the outline for the case example format used throughout the textbook. Table 2-2 outlines the various ways in which this journey is documented. The chapter concludes with a discussion of the ways therapists reflect to improve their clinical competence.

SCREENING: SHOULD WE TAKE THIS TRIP?

Screening is defined as reviewing information relevant to a prospective patient to determine the need for further evaluation and intervention (Moyers, 1999). Therapists gather this information through chart review and a brief interview.

Occupational therapists review relevant documents in the patient's medical record before beginning assessment or treatment. Other team members' assessments (e.g., the physician's history and physical, social service or psychology intake notes, and nursing assessments) help the therapist create a preliminary clinical image related to disease, severity of illness or disorder, comorbidities, age, sex, and personal and social background (Rogers & Holm, 1991). After the chart review, the occupational therapist typically introduces him- or herself to the patient and/or significant other, informs them of the referral, and briefly describes the nature of occupational therapy and the anticipated services. The purpose of this conversation is to ensure the appropriateness of the referral and obtain preliminary consent for occupational therapy intervention. The conversation may take place during the first few minutes of the initial assessment session, such as with outpatients or patients receiving home care, or as a brief encounter in the patient's hospital room, with the assessment scheduled to take place later.

Required Documentation: Screening Note

If the screening suggests that the referral to occupational therapy is inappropriate or the patient does not wish to have occupational therapy, the therapist records that orders were received and a screen was performed and explains why further assessment and treatment appear unwarranted. If the screening suggests that occupational therapy is appropriate and the patient wishes to receive this service, the therapist documents this and, with the patient's input, proceeds to determine the overall objective of therapy. Table 2-2 shows the purpose of typical documentation throughout the occupational therapy process and what must be included.

OVERALL OBJECTIVE: WHERE ARE WE HEADED?

All health care intervention is focused on arriving at a particular goal. A key component of our profession is the ability and commitment of occupational therapists to consider the unique experiences and desires of each patient in determining the goal of our work. Using a structured interview, the clinician identifies the client's needs and goals in the context of his or her life (Fisher, 1998). Fisher extolled the value of this aspect of the assessment process: "This step is critical, and it must occur, even under the pressures of cost containment, reduced duration of care, staff cuts, and increased accountability. In fact,

Table 2-1	**Clinical Reasoning Underlying the Process of Delivering Occupational Therapy Services**

Service Delivery	Clinical Reasoning Objectives	What the Therapist . . .		Documents
		Does	Thinks (Examples of Internal Questions and Self-reflections)	
Screen	Understand the patient's diagnosis or condition	Obtain and review background information	What do I know about the patient's medical diagnosis?	Informal note-taking and record keeping
			What impairments, activity limitations, and participation restrictions are typical for individuals with this diagnosis or condition?	
			Do the patient's records and information from referral sources suggest that occupational therapy services would be appropriate for this patient at this time?	
Assess occupational functioning	Know the person	Interview, listen, write	What do I need to know about this patient's current and past occupational functioning?	Daily contact notes
			What does the patient's past tell me about his or her priorities, strategies, and resources under the present circumstances?	
			Which of the patient's current concerns relate to his or her occupational functioning?	
			What seem to be the patient's main priorities regarding his or her occupational functioning?	
	Appreciate the context		Are there social, cultural, personal contextual factors that may affect the evaluation or intervention process?	
			Who should I talk with to better understand the patient's situation, occupational functioning, and/or needs?	
			Where is the patient in his or her recovery relative to onset of the condition?	
			What is the projected duration of this episode of care?	
			What sorts of resources are available to support the occupational therapy process?	
			What other medical, rehabilitation, and therapy services have been or are involved in the patient's care?	
			What have been the outcomes of past or current services?	
	Reflect on competence	Consult others (as needed)	Do I have adequate experience, education, and training to provide occupational therapy services to this patient?	
			If not, should I share responsibility with someone who can provide coaching or assistance?	
			Should this patient be referred elsewhere for services?	
	Develop provisional hypotheses		What physical, cognitive, or contextual barriers may be interfering with the patient's occupational function?	
	Consider the evaluation approach	Select evaluation tools and methods	Do I want to observe function to make inferences about impairment?	Evaluation note
			Do I want to assess specific impairments to make inferences about function?	
			How can I use existing information from other disciplines to inform questions about barriers to occupational functioning?	

Table 2-1 **Clinical Reasoning Underlying the Process of Delivering Occupational Therapy Services** *(continued)*

Service Delivery	Clinical Reasoning Objectives	What the Therapist . . . Does	Thinks (Examples of Internal Questions and Self-reflections)	Documents
	Consider the evaluation tools		Are there standardized assessments that will help specify the nature of the barriers to occupational functioning? What are the psychometric properties of these assessments (e.g., reliability and validity)? On what diagnostic groups have this assessment been tested? What forms of evaluation or specific tools will put the patient most at ease, given what I know about his or her background?	
	Interpret observations	Administer evaluation; observe; take notes on performance	How closely am I adhering to administration instructions for standardized assessments? Does the patient seem to understand the instructions? What physical, cognitive, sensory processing capacities are challenged by this assessment? What strategies or approaches does the patient use to perform the assessment?	
	Synthesize results	Write up evaluation findings	How does the patient's performance compare to that of others? To what extent could the patient's performance have been affected by unrelated factors (e.g., fatigue, medication, pain, distraction, etc.)? Do patterns emerge in the patient's performance across task or assessment?	
Plan intervention	Develop intervention hypotheses		What seem to be the most salient barriers (i.e., physical, cognitive, emotional, or contextual) to the patient's occupational functioning?	Intervention plan
	Consider the evidence		What type of intervention is supported by the best scientific evidence? If limited evidence is available, what type of intervention approach do experts recommend? What kind of outcomes have I observed with past patients?	
	Select an intervention approach or model		What intervention approach or model has the strongest evidence of effectiveness in the rehabilitation research literature for patients similar to my current patient?	
	Reflect on competence	Consult others (as needed)	Do I have adequate experience, education, and training to provide occupational therapy services to this patient? If not, should I share responsibility with someone who can provide coaching or assistance? Should this patient be referred elsewhere for services?	
	Consider the patient's appraisal of performance	Discuss evaluation impressions and findings with patient and possible course of intervention	To what extent does the patient understand and/or agree with my hypotheses regarding barriers to his or her occupational functioning? Given what I suspect are underlying barriers to occupational functioning, what does the patient seem to want to achieve in therapy at this time? Are there any constraints on the length of time that I am able to provide services to this patient?	

(continued)

Table 2-1	Clinical Reasoning Underlying the Process of Delivering Occupational Therapy Services *(continued)*

Service Delivery	Clinical Reasoning Objectives	What the Therapist . . .		Documents
		Does	**Thinks (Examples of Internal Questions and Self-reflections)**	
	Consider what will occur in therapy, how often, and for how long	Specify treatment activities, time frame, and intensity	What specific techniques or activities should be used in therapy, given the approach I have selected and what I know about the person? What does the literature suggest about the optimal time frame, intensity, and duration of therapy needed to achieve results? If there is no scientific evidence in this area, what do experienced clinicians recommend about time frame, intensity, and duration?	
	Ascertain patient's endorsement of intervention plan	Discuss with patient and modify as necessary	What are the indicators that this patient understands the intervention plan that I've proposed? What are the indicators that this patient (and/or significant others) endorse the plan as proposed?	
Provide intervention and monitor progress	Assess the patient's comprehension	Provide instructions for therapy exercises, tasks, and activities	Does the patient seem to understand what I am saying? Am I using language or expressions that likely make sense to this person?	Daily contact notes
	Understand what the patient is doing	Observe patient's performance	What specific actions is the patient taking? What do the actions infer about how the patient is thinking or processing? Why does the patient appear to be performing in this manner?	Weekly and/or monthly progress notes Home programs
	Compare actual performance to expected performance	Discuss with patient; readminister selected assessments; modify the treatment plan as needed	To what extent does this patient's performance support my hypotheses regarding the nature of his or her barriers to occupational functioning? Is the patient's performance improving at the rate I anticipated? If not, why? To what extent is the patient adhering to home recommendations, exercises, and activities?	
	Know the person		What does the patient's performance tell me about who this patient is? How should these insights further shape the intervention plan?	
	Appreciate the context		Are there other possible factors that are interfering with his or her occupational functioning? If so, what might they be? Does the patient seem to understand what I am saying? Am I using language or expressions that likely make sense to this person?	
	Consider alternatives to current services		Is the patient making enough progress toward his or her occupational therapy goals to warrant continuation? Are the goals still appropriate? Would services from other providers be beneficial?	

Table 2-1 **Clinical Reasoning Underlying the Process of Delivering Occupational Therapy Services** *(continued)*

Service Delivery	Clinical Reasoning Objectives	What the Therapist . . . Does	Thinks (Examples of Internal Questions and Self-reflections)	Documents
Discontinue occupational therapy services	Anticipate present and future patient concerns	Write and discuss recommendations; together, develop an adherence plan	Given what I know about the diagnosis or condition, who he or she is, and his or her progress to date, what should this patient continue to do (or discontinue) to optimize his or her occupational functioning? What does the patient think needs to be in place to help him/her to adhere to the discharge recommendations?	Home program
	Analyze the patient's comprehension		Does the patient seem to understand what I am saying? Am I using language or expressions that likely make sense to this person? What other people in the patient's life also need to understand this information?	Referral
	Decide whether or when the patient should return for therapy	Plan for follow-up	Do I expect the patient's occupational functioning to change at some point in such a way that therapy should then be resumed? If so, when would it make sense to reevaluate the patient's need for occupational therapy services? Are there resources to pay for follow-up occupational therapy services? Does the patient seem to understand under what circumstances to contact me again, or should we schedule a time at which he or she will return? Are there other services in the community that this patient should be accessing at this point?	Discharge summary

there is some evidence that taking more time, initially, to establish client-centered performance will result in overall outcomes being enhanced and overall costs reduced" (Fisher, 1998, pp. 515–516).

Many patients value the possibility of helping inform the goals of therapy (Holliday, Ballinger, & Playford, 2007). In fact, evidence supports the idea that intervention that considers patients' goals is more effective and efficient (Jack & Estes, 2010). Getting to know patients and their hopes for therapy is an important part of beginning the process (Holliday, Ballinger, & Playford, 2007). Learning about their preferences and needs regarding goal setting (for example, what information they might need to be able to participate in goal setting) is also important (Levinson et al., 2005).

There will be times when patients are not able to express their goals for therapy. For example, they may be overwhelmed by their personal situation, too ill, or simply unaware of what occupational therapy can offer. When working with such individuals, we have a responsibility to provide the support they need to participate as much as they can and to actively listen for their valued goals

(Hobson, 1996), rather than substituting them with ideas about what we think is best (Levack et al., 2011).

Once the overall goal is set, we can begin to use clinical reasoning to move toward achieving these goals.

CLINICAL REASONING: HOW ARE WE GOING TO GET THERE?

Clinical reasoning is the thinking process by which therapists collect and use information to make decisions about the care of an individual client (Rogers, 1983). Clinical reasoning is ongoing. It begins as the therapist first reads a patient's referral; extends through assessment, intervention, and discharge; and continues as the clinician reflects on the process and results of intervention with a patient as he or she plans therapy for another patient. Clinical reasoning in practice typically does not occur as a tidy progression of thoughts. It may appear cyclic or even chaotic as therapists dance back and forth between hypothesis testing and storytelling throughout each patient's care (Hagedorn, 1996). Note how the same internal questions and self-reflections in Table 2-1 are repeated at various junctures in the delivery of services.

| Table 2-2 | **Overview: Types of Occupational Therapy Documentation** | | | |

Documentation	Purpose	Typical Formats	Contents	When to Document
Contact, treatment or visit note	Brief account of an individual session	Short narrative note, checklist, or flow sheet	• Amount of time spent evaluating or treating the client • Brief characterization of intervention (e.g., activities of daily living instruction, strengthening, compensatory strategy training) • Description of client response relative to short-term goals	After each evaluation or treatment session
Evaluation report	Detailing of assessment findings, interpretation of results, estimated outcomes of intervention, goals, time frame, and treatment plan	• Therapist's observations and findings written or typed into a fill-in-the-blank form or template (as in an electronic medical record) • Handwritten or dictated and typed report	• Background information on the client (age, sex, and diagnosis); summary of medical history, secondary problems, and comorbidities; and precautions and contraindications • Referral source, services requested, date of referral • Date(s) of evaluation sessions and amount of time • Premorbid or prior level of functioning in occupational function; self-report of problems and priorities (Occupational Profile [AOTA 2002]) • Assessment results: scores, observations, summary, and analysis of assessment findings (Analysis of Occupational Performance [AOTA, 2002]) • Intervention plan: projected outcomes of therapy, goals, and time frame; statement of client participation in goal setting for therapy; general description of treatment plan (including treatment approach and recommended frequency of treatment sessions)	After completing the assessment, synthesizing the results, and collaborating with client about therapy goals
Progress report	Summary of progress toward functional goals, interventions employed, updated goals, and treatment plan	• Fill-in-the-blank form or template or checklist with section for handwritten comments • Flow sheet (as used with clinical pathways) • Handwritten or dictated and typed report	• Dates of service and dates of progress period • Number of treatment sessions during progress period • Overview of activities, techniques, and modalities used • Summary of instruction provided to client or family • Description of adaptive equipment issued or recommended • Client's response to intervention specific to therapy goals • Recommendations regarding continuation of therapy • Revised goals and time frame for achievement • Revised treatment plan (treatment approach and recommended frequency of sessions) • Statement of client participation in goal setting for therapy	Daily, weekly, or monthly, depending on setting
Discharge report	Review of occupational therapy assessment, intervention, and outcome	• Fill-in-the-blank form or template or checklist with section for handwritten comments • Flow sheet (as used with critical pathways) • Handwritten or dictated and typed report	• Dates of referral, service initiation, and discontinuation • Total number of evaluation and treatment sessions • Summary of client's progress toward each therapy goal • Overview of interventions employed specific to each goal • Description of maintenance program and discharge instructions • Recommendations for follow-up, maintenance programs, referrals to other services or agencies	After the last session in an episode of care

From Allen, C. A. (1997). Clinical reasoning for documentation. In J. D. Acquaviva (Ed.), *Effective documentation for occupational therapy* (2nd ed., pp. 53–62). Bethesda, MD: American Occupational Therapy Association.
American Occupational Therapy Association [AOTA]. (2008). Occupational therapy practice framework: Domain & process (2nd ed.). *American Journal of Occupational Therapy, 62,* 625–683.
American Occupational Therapy Association [AOTA]. (2008). Guidelines for the documentation of occupational therapy. *American Journal of Occupational Therapy, 62,* 684–690.
Wilson, D. (1997). Clinical reasoning for documentation. In J. D. Acquaviva (Ed.), *Effective documentation for occupational therapy* (2nd ed., pp. 1–3). Bethesda, MD: American Occupational Therapy Association.

The Three-Track Mind

In their classic study of clinical reasoning among American occupational therapists, Mattingly and Fleming (1994) observed that therapists reasoned with a "three-track mind," using procedural, narrative, and conditional forms of reasoning.

- *Procedural reasoning* refers to rational, linear thinking about the nature of the client's problems and the optimal course of action in treatment (Mattingly, 1991; Rogers, 1983). This thinking is generally based on logical ideas of "if, then" that therapists have learned in their courses and clinical training (Unsworth, 2004). For example, a therapist may think, "If my activities of daily living (ADL) assessment shows that the patient has trouble rising from the bath, then he needs some type of tub seat."
- *Narrative reasoning* refers to thinking in story form to place the client's functioning in the context of his or her background and broader experience (Schell & Cervero, 1993). Therapists employ narrative reasoning when they try to understand the meaning of disability in the patient's life in order to link the patient's goals and values to the therapy process (Mattingly, 1991). For example, a therapist may think, "This patient prides herself on her beautiful home. I should ask how she would feel about installing tub equipment, and if she has any ideas that could help minimize the impact of environmental adaptations on the appearance of her bathroom." Unsworth (2004) refers to this type of reasoning as "interactive" because it "is concerned with understanding the client as a person and his or her perception of events that have led him or her to see the therapist" (p. 11).
- *Conditional reasoning* uses therapist's understanding of the unique patient and his or her specific condition and life situation to predict what might happen if different therapeutic plans are carried out. For example, a therapist may think, "This patient will likely eventually need a roll-in shower. It may be distressing to think about disease progression. However, she has raised this issue of disease progression with me once. She would probably appreciate planning for the long term when considering any home adaptations right now."

Two Additional Tracks of Reasoning: Pragmatic Reasoning and Generalization Reasoning

Schell and Cervero (1993) added *pragmatic reasoning* to this classic list of types of occupational therapy reasoning. Pragmatic, or management, reasoning (Lyons & Crepeau, 2001) considers the logistics and practical aspects of delivering services to clients within a given setting or organization. Therapists employ pragmatic reasoning when they consider norms of the department or expectations related to accreditation, personnel, or reimbursement factors as they provide occupational therapy services (Schell & Cervero, 1993). In many ways, pragmatic reasoning places limits around what can currently be offered by the therapist. For example, a therapist might reason, "I think I understand the layout of this patient's bathroom, but I know that in a small space like this you really need to see and measure to determine the best equipment to recommend. Therapists do not normally do home visits from my facility. I need to ask if there are rules against this or whether I might be allowed to go. If I cannot see the patient's bathroom, I need to find a way to get more precise information."

Generalization reasoning is a subcategory in which a therapist's previous experience with patients judged to be similar to the specific patient whom they are treating adds to their knowledge about the situation (Unsworth, 2004). For example, a therapist might think, "I have had a lot of patients who never used bath seats that were recommended for them. I wonder what might keep this patient from using a bath seat, and whether there's anything we can do about this, or whether we need to find another plan?"

The Lenses through Which We See: Worldview

Overarching all these forms of reasoning are the therapist's preferences and skills and his or her worldview (Hooper, 1997). Worldview includes the therapist's values, beliefs, ethics, faith/spirituality, personal style, and motivation (Unsworth, 2004). Our worldviews serve as the lenses through which we see the world. These lenses affect *all* of our reasoning but are incredibly difficult to reflect on because we tend to take for granted that everyone sees things through similar invisible lenses. (Chapter 3 expands upon this topic in the discussion regarding personal context.)

Reflecting on one's worldview is an essential concurrent subprocess of reflection during the clinical reasoning process. Such reflection is particularly important when patients seem hesitant or even hostile regarding our recommendations. In these situations we must identify our own preconceived ideas regarding the patient's situation through critical reflection (Kinsella, 2000). For example, a therapist might think, "This patient gets help from her husband to take a bath. I think she could bathe alone if she had a bath seat. When I suggest this, she keeps telling me it will not work. Why is it so important for me that she be independent in this activity? Maybe there are other aspects of the situation, such as maintaining autonomy (that is, being able to carry out the activity in the way she wishes) or enjoying the intimacy that this shared activity involves, that are more important to her than my professional idea of independence."

The interactive nature of the different forms of reasoning is illustrated in Figure 2-1. The reasoning of novice

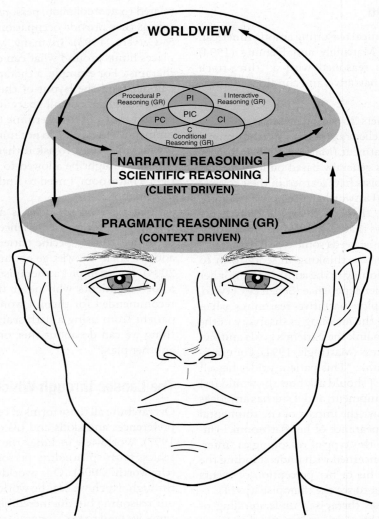

WORLDVIEW

Procedural P
Reasoning (GR)

PI

I Interactive
Reasoning (GR)

PC

PIC

CI

C
Conditional
Reasoning (GR)

NARRATIVE REASONING
SCIENTIFIC REASONING
(CLIENT DRIVEN)

PRAGMATIC REASONING (GR)
(CONTEXT DRIVEN)

Figure 2-1 Clinical reasoning in client-centered occupational therapy. (Reprinted with permission from Unsworth, C. A. [2004]. Clinical reasoning: How do pragmatic reasoning, worldview and client-centeredness fit? *British Journal of Occupational Therapy, 67*, 17. Note: Generalization reasoning (GR) is a subcategory of each type of reasoning in the model.

therapists tends to be dominated by procedural reasoning, a tendency to rely on formulas for practice and a reluctance to discuss potentially painful issues with patients (Mitchell & Unsworth, 2005). This seems to be part of beginning to practice. With experience, therapists more easily move between different forms of reasoning (i.e., procedural, interactive, conditional, and pragmatic forms of reasoning). Their thinking also flows more fluidly between the steps of assessment and decision making, and they more easily find ways to address difficult issues with patients (Mitchell & Unsworth, 2005).

Recently, Unsworth (2011) added another related consideration in clinical reasoning: the patient's reasoning. Patients have both theoretical information about their health and functioning (Krefting, 1991) and practical knowledge about living in their own bodies and in their

own communities, particularly after many years with a particular condition. This information is a valuable resource for clinical reasoning.

Evidence-Based Practice: Adding Knowledge from Research

We have just discussed five aspects or tracks of thinking that run through an occupational therapist's mind as he or she reasons about what to do. We have also considered how these tracks of reasoning may interact with the patient's reasoning to influence the intervention plan. There is one additional important track: the evidence-based practice (EBP) track. In this track, the therapist considers evidence from research literature, the patient, and clinical experts regarding the potential benefits of specific therapy decisions.

In everyday life, we rarely make a decision without consulting some form of evidence. Should we take the bus, plane, or train to visit family at Thanksgiving? Any form of transportation that will not get us there should be ruled out immediately. Our final decision will likely rest on the relative cost (in dollars) and benefit (in time) of each of the remaining transportation methods. In occupational therapy, evidence helps us rule out ineffective actions and make the best choices from among the remaining options.

Evidence-based medicine has provided the starting point for evidence-based occupational therapy. In evidence-based medicine, intervention decisions are based on the "integration of best research evidence with clinical expertise and patient values" (Sackett et al., 1997, p. 1).

Which evaluations and which treatments to use are two of these important decisions. Information in Section II of this textbook will help you make evidence-based evaluation choices. An understanding of the different levels of evidence for the effectiveness of treatment, provided below, will help you make evidence-based intervention choices, which are further discussed in Sections V and VI. In this chapter, we examine how occupational therapists use experimental research, clinical practice guidelines, and qualitative research to guide intervention planning.

Guidance from Experimental Research

When properly designed and interpreted, intervention studies answer the question, "What is the benefit of this intervention?" This benefit is called the "treatment effect." Well implemented randomized controlled trials (RCTs) are the most trustworthy of intervention studies. To understand this, imagine a researcher trying to determine the level of effectiveness of an ADL retraining program for patients after a stroke. Using a pretest/posttest study design, the researcher measures ADL before the treatment starts, using the 100-point Barthel Index. After the intervention, the researcher reassesses the patients using the same test. She finds that the patients have improved, on average, by 15 points, which is judged an important difference. Can the researcher conclude that this occupational therapy intervention was effective? Unfortunately not. It is possible that these patients developed better skills on their own or with the help of other interventions they received in rehabilitation.

To control for these possibilities, the researcher carries out another study. Here she examines the average change in ADL for a group who receives the intervention (intervention group) and a group who does not receive the intervention (control group). She subtracts the change in the control group (which provides an idea of how much patients change over time without occupational therapy) from the change in the intervention group to determine the treatment effect of occupational therapy. She finds a treatment effect of 12 points, which is still considered an important change.

Although this is clearly a better estimate of the effect of occupational therapy on ADL, one serious problem remains. That is, were the patients who were put into the intervention group simply the patients in the study who were more likely to get better on their own? To control for this possibility, the researcher conducts a third study in which patients are randomly assigned to either the intervention group or the control group. This study is an RCT.

As stated previously, the treatment effect is calculated by subtracting the change in the control group from the change in the treatment group. The treatment effect represents an estimate of the average benefit of treatment experienced by the patients in the study. Researchers also generally provide an estimate of the confidence interval (CI) around this estimate. The CI provides an estimate of the average benefit of treatment that would likely be observed had the study been done repeatedly with different samples. In our example RCT, the researcher found a treatment effect of 10 with a 95% CI of 7–13, meaning that through statistical calculations, she estimates an average change somewhere between 7 and 13 in 95 out of 100 such studies of the intervention.

This estimate of effect is often presented as a standardized effect size. A standardized effect size is calculated by dividing the treatment effect by the standard deviation of the outcome variable in the population from which the study sample originated. Because this information is usually not available, it is estimated by the standard deviation of the control group or both groups (Coe, 2002).

For example, the researcher who carried out the RCT of interventions to improve ADL post stroke might calculate a standardized effect size so that she could compare her findings with those of another RCT in which a different test with a different scale was used. To do this, she divides the effect size she found (10 points) by the standard deviation in Barthel Index scores at baseline (15 points), giving her a standardized effect size of 0.67.

Some evaluations come with indications of what an important or clinically significant difference in the measure is. In other situations, the therapist estimates this number by looking at the scale and determining how much change would represent an important difference for a patient. Of course, this is something that can be done in consultation with the patient. For example, a 10° increase in fifth digit distal interphalangeal joint finger flexion for a violinist may be enormously important, whereas the same change for a professor may be virtually unnoticeable.

Although RCTs provide very strong evidence of the effectiveness of an intervention, systematic reviews provide even more robust evidence. In a systematic review, the researcher uses an established process to locate as many studies as possible regarding a particular intervention with a particular type of patient. This provides an overview of the results of many related studies. If these RCTs examined similar outcomes, a meta-analysis can be performed by statistically combining the results. The result is a more precise estimate of the treatment effect.

Guidance from Clinical Practice Guidelines

Although a systematic review will provide a comprehensive summary of the anticipated effects of a particular treatment, clinical practice guidelines (CPGs), "statements used to assist practitioners to make decisions about appropriate health care for specific clinical circumstances" (Field & Lohr, 1990), generally focus on which types of care are most helpful for a particular condition. Therefore, they are generally broader in nature and particularly helpful to the practitioner.

A search for broad CPGs specific to a health problem of interest can provide helpful information for occupational therapy. For instance, evidence-based clinical practice guidelines for interdisciplinary rehabilitation of chronic nonmalignant pain syndrome patients (Sanders, Harden, & Vincente, 2007) provide guidelines for pharmaceutical and nonpharmaceutical interventions for people with chronic pain. Among the recommendations are "helping clients learn awareness of body mechanics and dynamic posture, initiation and activation of a long-term exercise program to

gradually increase general fitness, strength, coordination, and a range of flexibility and motion, postural and muscle balance, as well as specific physical coping strategies" (p. 308). Additional recommendations include assisting clients to modify work and other activities and enabling clients to develop exercise routines they can incorporate into their daily routines.

It is important to know that not all CPGs are created equal. To considered high quality and trustworthy, a CPG must have been rigorously developed, using proper EBP principles and submitted for thorough, independent review. The AGREE II (an acronym for Appraisal of Guidelines for Research and Evaluation II) instrument can be applied to evaluate these and four other essential domains critical to a CPG that can be relied on to provide proper clinical advice (AGREE Next Steps Consortium, 2009). Applying this instrument to eight stroke-rehabilitation CPGs, Hurdowar et al. (2007) found widely varying quality. Therefore, it is helpful to be aware of the AGREE criteria when determining whether a particular CPG should be applied (Procedures for Practice 2-1).

To ensure that your interventions are informed by "integration of best research evidence with clinical expertise and patient values" (Sackett et al., 1997, p. 1), it is

 Procedures for Practice 2-1

Criteria for Evaluating a Clinical Practice Guideline (AGREE II Instrument)

Domain 1: Scope and purpose

1. The overall objective(s) of the guideline is(are) specifically described.
2. The health question(s) covered by the guideline is(are) specifically described.
3. The population (patients, public, etc.) to whom the guideline is meant to apply is specifically described.

Domain 2: Stakeholder involvement

4. The guideline development group includes individuals from all the relevant professional groups.
5. The views and preferences of the target population (patients, public, etc.) have been sought.
6. The target users of the guideline are clearly defined.

Domain 3: Rigor of development

7. Systematic methods were used to search for evidence.
8. The criteria for selecting the evidence are clearly described.
9. The strength and limitations of the body of evidence are clearly described.
10. The methods used for formulating the recommendations are clearly described.
11. The health benefits, side effects, and risks have been considered in formulating the recommendations.

12. There is an explicit link between the recommendations and the supporting evidence.
13. The guideline has been externally reviewed by experts prior to its publication.
14. A procedure for updating the guideline is provided.

Domain 4: Clarity and presentation

15. The recommendations are specific and unambiguous.
16. The different options for management of the condition or health issue are clearly presented.
17. Key recommendations are easily identifiable.
18. The guideline describes facilitators and barriers to its application.

Domain 5: Applicability

19. The guideline provides advice and/or tools on how the recommendations can be put into practice.
20. The potential resource implications of applying the recommendations have been considered.
21. The guideline presents monitoring and/or auditing criteria.

Domain 6: Editorial independence

22. The views of the funding body have not influenced the content of the guideline.
23. Competing interests of guideline development members have been recorded and addressed.

important to abandon interventions that, although popular, have excellent evidence of *ineffectiveness*. That is, repeated well-designed studies have demonstrated that the interventions do not produce the intended effects. Also, you may wish to keep an open mind regarding new therapies with emerging research evidence. These interventions may not have been tested using RCT methods but may have some demonstrated evidence of effectiveness in studies such as single-case studies, which are often used to demonstrate potential effectiveness of an intervention before a full RCT is mounted.

Guidance from Qualitative Research

There is increasing interest in making use of the results of qualitative research in EBP. We return to our trip analogy to illustrate how this type of research can provide useful information for treatment planning.

Suppose that you and your partner have chosen to visit Nepal, a place you have never been before. In planning for the trip, you wish to learn a bit about the cultural aspects of Nepalese daily life, either from someone who has studied the culture (an ethnographer), gathered the stories of the people (a historian), or, better yet, from the Nepalese themselves. There may be specific aspects of life that most interest you. You may wish, for example, to better understand the experience of young children living at a very high elevation in the mountains of the Himalayas, the evolution of friendships in that context, or their family organization with regards to daily living. Qualitative research will be the best source for exploring these questions.

Qualitative research approaches are used to understand a phenomenon, provide an understanding of a historical and cultural view of a phenomenon (ethnography), a lived experience of people (phenomenology), a systematization of a social process (grounded theory), or the story of an individual living through a particular experience (biographical approach) (Creswell, 2013). Although quantitative evidence is often helpful in narrowing the choices so that intervention decisions can be made, qualitative evidence can help expand your understanding of issues related to developing a holistic view of a client. This might include issues related to practicing in a client-centered manner or interacting effectively with families and appreciating the experience of patients before, during, and after their treatments in rehabilitation—in short, multiple important aspects critical to the values and approach of occupational therapy.

Qualitative research reports can make you aware of a phenomenon, such as the lived experience of your client during occupational therapy, or provide you with a better understanding of a process, such as a patient's process of change during physical rehabilitation. For example, a metasynthesis of qualitative research done by an interdisciplinary team (Dubouloz et al., 2010) led to the construction of a model of personal change that patients may go through during rehabilitation.

Qualitative research uses three main tools to collect data: interviews, observations, and written and/or audiovisual documents. Semi-directed interviews are the most popular tool; they allow an open-ended style of interaction between researcher and participant in order to explore in-depth perceptions, values, and so on. Often, in the research report, key quotations from participants are used to express the essence of a phenomenon studied. Such quotations can enhance your ability to listen for the essence of your patients' experiences.

Just as with quantitative research, the results of some qualitative studies are more trustworthy than others. Those that can be most highly trusted clearly name the research process selected and plainly document the procedures used. In addition, four main criteria of rigor must be addressed: credibility, transferability, dependability, and confirmability (Lincoln & Guba, 1985).

The strategy of triangulation is well known as a way to assure credibility of the research process at the level of data sources (through use of multiple sources of data), data analysis (through the examination of data by more than one researcher), and data collection methods (through different ways of collecting data) (Creswell, 2013).

Practical Considerations for Using Evidence to Guide Practice

Sharing your findings with the patient regarding the best evidence available for decision making is an essential part of therapy. However, you must make sure that this evidence is understandable to the patient. Present it briefly and in plain language, with consideration of the strength of the evidence (Tickle-Degnen, 2008), providing details as requested. Finally, put the information in perspective. That is, the results of current research are the best estimates of average treatment effect for patients with similar characteristics rather than an exact prediction of what may happen with one particular patient.

It is very easy to become overwhelmed at the thought of having to review the evidence for every clinical situation. It is important to know that this is not possible or expected. Instead, we suggest four strategies to keep practice more evidence based (Straus et al., 2005). First, have a good idea of the major systematic reviews and CPGs available for patients with conditions you often see. Important EBP resources include the Cochrane Library, OTseeker, and American Occupational Therapy Association (AOTA) EBP resources. Second, if you work for an organization with a librarian, ask him or her to help you set up alerts for topics of particular importance to your patients. These regular e-mail notifications of relevant, new articles will help you remain aware of new and important research in your area. Third, set up a buddy system to share your information.

Fourth, keep a list of your clinical questions and review this list for themes. Do not hesitate to assign one of these questions to a student trainee (Phillips & Glasziou, 2008).

We see from the above discussion that EBP encompasses knowledge of quantitative and qualitative evidence, with consideration of the trustworthiness of this evidence. Tonelli (2006) points out that good clinical reasoning should take into consideration not only this research evidence but also experiential evidence, understanding of current theories of pathology and their relationship to function, patient goals and values, and aspects of the context in which one is working. These ideas are supported in discussions of client-centered, occupation-focused practice (Canadian Association of Occupational Therapists et al., 1999; Egan et al., 1998). Resources 2-1 provides evidence-based occupational therapy websites.

PLANNING INTERVENTION: YOUR JOURNEY WITH YOUR PATIENT PARTNER

Once the overall objective of occupational therapy is determined and the evidence has been considered, you begin to plan the specifics of your journey. The occupational therapist uses a practice model to begin to form a hypothesis regarding how best to understand the journey to the goal (i.e., what is causing current problems, what needs to be done to get to the overall objective, etc.). To do this, the occupational therapist carries out specific assessments and begins to estimate how the patient will journey toward this objective, reflecting on relevant research evidence. The occupational therapist shares these ideas with the patient. Together they plot the *short- and long-term goals*, or milestones along the way to the objective, which interventions will be used, and how long it is likely to take to get to each step. Also, the occupational therapist and patient will discuss the anticipated outcomes of the current intervention (i.e., how far along the way to the overall objective the therapist will be able to accompany the patient and which resources the patient may use to continue this journey on his or her own).

Estimate Outcomes and Set Collaborative Goals

An outcome of therapy is an anticipated end result, given a specific set of parameters (Bryant, 1995). Outcomes are chosen, in part, according to expected length of stay, or anticipated number of outpatient or home-based sessions, and the type of funding available. The contemporary rehabilitation environment often requires clinicians to identify key expected outcomes for and with persons served, to measure these outcomes, and to determine how outcomes can be achieved in a resource-wise or cost-effective manner (Cope & Sundance, 1995). Interdisciplinary rehabilitation teams typically establish a plan of care for a given episode of care that delineates the overall patient-specific outcomes, with each discipline setting goals that contribute to these core outcomes.

The Occupational Therapy Practice Framework (OTPF) (AOTA, 2002, 2008b) suggests that the overarching outcome of occupational therapy intervention is to enable recipients to engage in occupations that allow them to participate in valued roles within their homes,

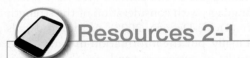 **Resources 2-1**

Evidence-Based Practice

The AGREE Collaboration (Appraisal of Guidelines Research and Evaluation) is an instrument for assessing the quality of clinical practice guidelines (www.agreecolla boration.org).

AOTA's Evidence Brief Series is a site available to members of AOTA that includes summaries of research related to occupational intervention related to various diagnostic groups (www.aota.org).

The Centre for Evidence Based Medicine is a site at University of Toronto that offers resources for understanding the steps for using evidence in practice and teaching others about this process (www.cebm.utoronto.ca).

The Cochrane Collaboration is the international organization that produces and disseminates hundreds of systematic reviews of health care interventions (www.cochrane.org).

Occupational Therapy Critically Appraised Topics contains critically appraised topics (short summaries of evidence on a topic of interest focused around a clinical question) usually developed from several critically appraised papers (summaries of single studies) (www.otcats.com).

The Centre for Evidence-Based Rehabilitation is a site created by McMaster Occupational Therapy Evidence-Based Practice Group with results of systematic reviews of research evidence in interventions used by occupational therapists and forms and guidelines to critically review qualitative and quantitative research articles (www.srs-mcmaster.ca/ResearchResourcesnbsp/ResearchGroups/CentreforEvidenceBasedRehabilitation/tabid/543/Default. aspx).

OTseeker (Occupational Therapy Systematic Evaluation of Evidence) is a site created by a team of occupational therapists at the Universities of Queensland and Western Sydney with abstracts of systematic reviews and quality ratings of randomized controlled trials relevant to occupational therapy (www.otseeker.com)

schools, workplaces, and/or communities (AOTA, 2002, 2008b). This may be achieved through improvements related to (1) function (remediation of impairments); (2) occupational performance (independence in ADL, work, and play); (3) health and well-being (symptom status improvement and prevention of disability); and (4) quality of life (purposeful participation in community life, emotional well-being, balance of activity and rest, and life satisfaction) (Moyers, 1999). Global outcomes of occupational therapy intervention can also be identified according to resumption of self-maintenance, self-advancement, and self-enhancement roles (Trombly, 1993, 1995). In selecting and projecting treatment outcomes, occupational therapists are urged to look beyond functional independence or relearning of physical skills as the highest aims of occupational therapy (Radomski, 1995) and rather help patients attain wholeness, autonomy, meaning, and purpose in their daily lives (Crabtree, 2000).

Predicting therapy outcomes forces clinicians to answer two key questions in intervention planning: (1) In what broad ways will this client's life, health, and functioning improve as a result of therapy at this point in the recovery or adaptation process? and (2) How long will it take to realize these benefits? The answers require an appreciation for the continuum of care and a realization that not every dysfunction, impairment, or inefficiency can or should be addressed within a given episode of care. For example, resumption of self-maintenance roles may be an appropriate outcome for a patient who had a stroke and is expected to receive inpatient rehabilitation for 2–3 weeks. On the other hand, resumption of self-advancement roles would probably not be an appropriate outcome of inpatient rehabilitation. Occupational therapy services to promote work readiness can likely be provided more cost effectively when the individual is an outpatient. Treatment planning based on anticipated therapy outcomes not only reflects good stewardship but it is also required by accreditation bodies, such as The Joint Commission (TJC) and the Commission on Accreditation of Rehabilitation Facilities (CARF International).

Long- and Short-Term Goals

Once the occupational therapist and patient/family member conceptualize global therapy outcomes, they work backward to establish a sequence of long- and short-term goals to get there (Cope & Sundance, 1995). A goal is a measurable, narrowly defined end result of therapy to be achieved in a specified time (Bryant, 1995). Long-term goals reflect what will be achieved by the time the patient is discharged from treatment or discharged to the next level of care on the continuum (Moorhead & Kannenberg, 1997). In occupational therapy, long-term goals always relate to expectations of the patient's functional skills and/or resumption of roles. This is a tricky area insofar as attainment of

occupation-related goals among patients with very similar levels of disability varies widely. Therapists should always frame these expectations with the knowledge that individual patients may do better than expected. Because occupational performance is produced by a combination of person, environment, and occupation factors, there are many ways to reengage in valued occupations.

Short-term goals are the small steps that cumulatively result in long-term goal achievement. Short-term goals are based either on expected improvements specific to client factors (AOTA, 2002) or impairments that ultimately contribute to improved function or on the patient's improved ability to perform portions of the functional task (McGuire, 1997). A patient's occupational therapy goals are always linked to a predicted outcome and typically complement the work of other rehabilitation disciplines. Procedures for Practice 2-2 illustrates how long- and short-term goals support outcome realization. Definition 2-1 describes how to use goal-attainment scaling to measure progress.

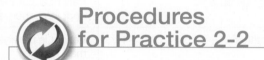

Procedures for Practice 2-2

Linking Long- and Short-Term Goals to Anticipated Rehabilitation Outcomes

P. B. is a 20-year-old man with C8 tetraplegia beginning multidisciplinary inpatient rehabilitation. The following examples of outcome and long- and short-term goals are not meant to be exhaustive lists of intervention plans but rather to illustrate the linkage between global outcome projections and therapy plans.

- Projected outcome of rehabilitation stay: In 8 weeks, P. B. will resume self-maintenance roles, requiring no more than occasional physical assistance from family members to manage in the home environment.
- Examples of long-term occupational therapy goals (to be achieved in 8 weeks):

  1. P. B. will perform upper body dressing independently and require no more than moderate assistance for lower body dressing.
  2. P. B. will use adaptive equipment to feed himself independently.

- Examples of short-term occupational therapy goals (to be achieved in 2 weeks):

  1. P. B. will don a pullover shirt with no more than general verbal cues.
  2. P. B. will participate in the evaluation of various types of adaptive equipment for self-feeding and use selected aids to feed himself independently after set up by therapist.

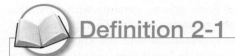

Definition 2-1

Goal-Attainment Scaling

Goal-attainment scaling is a method for evaluating the effectiveness of therapy that produces a quantitative index of patient progress over time and a means by which one patient's progress can be compared with other patients in the same program (Ottenbacher & Cusick, 1990). Goal-attainment scaling was developed for use in the mental health field (Kiresuk & Sherman, 1968) and has been used to measure change as a result of cognitive rehabilitation (Rockwood, Joyce, & Stolee, 1997) and brain injury rehabilitation (Joyce, Rockwood, & Mate-Kole, 1994; Trombly, Radomski, & Davis, 1998; Trombly et al., 2002).

For each goal, a five-point behaviorally defined scale is constructed as exemplified below. Ottenbacher and Cusick (1990) provided an excellent summary regarding how quantitative outcome data can then be calculated and interpreted.

Problem area: Patient relies on other people to make transportation arrangements for her.

Predicted Attainment	Score	Goals
Most favorable outcome	+2	Patient accurately makes her own transportation arrangements without supervision or assistance.
Greater than expected outcome	+1	Patient accurately makes her own transportation arrangements with occasional cueing.
Expected outcome	0	Patient accurately makes her own transportation arrangements with ongoing supervision.
Current status	−1	Patient is provided with information about transportation arrangements made for her.
Least favorable outcome	−2	Patient is unable to successfully use transportation information provided for her.

Collaborating with Clients to Set Goals

Collaborative goal setting between clients and therapists, an accreditation requirement of CARF International (2011) and TJC (2011), presents benefits and challenges to both patients and therapists. Ponte-Allan and Giles (1999) suggest that the nature of goal setting may be linked with actual therapy outcomes. They compared patients whose goals were functional, independence-oriented statements with patients whose goals were general, less functional statements or who made no goal statements at all. Although there were no differences in age, sex, side of stroke, or levels of disability at admission, patients who had functional goals had higher discharge scores on the Functional Independence Measure™ for grooming, upper and lower extremity dressing, and toilet and tub transfers.

Collaborating with patients in goal setting is a critical counterbalance to therapist-biased expectations and priorities in treatment planning (Procedures for Practice 2-3); it reflects a philosophy of care rather than simply a periodic conversation between therapist and patient (Sumsion & Law, 2006). This practice philosophy requires that therapists tolerate the stress that can occur during goal setting (Foye et al., 2002) and remain attentive and flexible as patients' goals change throughout the recovery and adaptation process (Donnelly et al., 2004). Therapists appreciate that many patients must be coached on how to participate in goal setting (Nelson & Payton, 1997), probing for concerns, goals, and ideas. Asking a patient, "What are your occupational therapy goals?" is likely to be met with a perplexed look and a vague response. As one patient put it, "Asking one question about goals on an initial evaluation is probably not adequate" (Nelson & Payton, 1997, p. 582). Clearly, the time and energy invested in collaborative goal setting not only benefits patients but also contributes to the empathic partnership that holds so much reward and satisfaction for therapists (Gahnstrom-Strandqvist et al., 2000).

Select Treatment Approaches and Methods

In Chapter 1, Trombly Latham outlines that intervention might focus on changes to the person, the environment, or the occupation to promote function. Intervention is also often discussed as focusing on remediation, adaptation, or metacognitive strategies.

Remediation

Remediation aims to restore an impaired capacity or ability with the expectation that this improvement will bring about

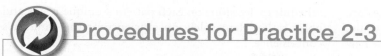

Procedures for Practice 2-3

Suggestions for Collaborating with Clients to Set Meaningful Occupational Therapy Goals

- Incorporate life history information into the assessment process so that you are able to get a glimpse of what the patient has found meaningful and important during the course of his or her life events (Spencer, Davidson, & White, 1997). Awareness of the patient's personal context enables the clinician to discuss, frame, or propose possible therapy outcomes and goals in ways that the patient will understand.
- Appreciate that patients' ability to identify and advance their goals for therapy will be influenced by where they are in the recovery and adaptation process. Individuals who are acutely ill or whose hospitalization has insulated them from the real-world impact of newly acquired disabilities will often be unable to anticipate the challenges that await them in the community. Outpatients or home-based clients are typically more able to articulate needs and hopes for therapy because of their experiences with performance gaps.
- Consider the broad continuum of care (inpatient to home health to outpatient to work reentry) as you aim to match the "right" goals with the "right" time frame by asking, "What does the person both value and need from occupational therapy at this point in his or her recovery?"

- Appreciate that many patients are unfamiliar with occupational therapy services and what we have to offer them and therefore are unable to independently generate goals for therapy. The therapist sometimes facilitates collaborative goal setting by proposing a menu of possible goals to address in therapy and modifying that list with the patient.
- Acknowledge the influence of cognitive function on a person's capacity to set meaningful goals. For a person to establish a meaningful goal, he or she must first accurately appraise his or her current status and compare it with past, or premorbid, performance. The individual must be able to imagine what is both possible and likely (given present condition and status) and how much time and effort is required to attain what is envisioned. Solicit input from family if the patient seems unable to independently determine or communicate his or her goals for therapy.
- If you are unable to arrive at consensus of broad therapy outcomes, try to agree on short-term goals. For example, a patient who is starting therapy 3 months after brain injury and wants only to work toward resuming his career as an air-traffic controller hopes for a broad outcome the clinician views as unrealistic. Instead of haggling over what the future may or may not hold for this individual (which dampens energy, hope, and motivation), the patient and therapist agree that, to return to work, he needs to be able to independently get ready each morning, so they can begin their work there.

---

general change in the patient's activities, tasks, and roles. Remedial approaches typically address body structures and functions (World Health Organization, 2001), which comprise client factors in the OTPF (AOTA, 2002, 2008b). Because it aims to fix underlying impairments, remediation may be somewhat slow to affect occupational function. Moreover, our current understanding of motor learning points to the importance of task-specific practice for improvement of particular tasks (Mastos et al., 2007; Mathiowetz & Haugen, 1995). A remedial approach is often emphasized when patients are in the early stages of recovery and rehabilitation.

Adaptation

An adaptive approach is used when the patient wants to optimize his or her level of independence while continuing to work toward restoration of fundamental capacities and abilities. Adaptive therapy entails three possible therapy actions: changing the context (e.g., modifying the environment or task demands), helping the patient reestablish habits and routines, and acquiring compensatory skills and metacognitive strategies.

Learning new skills and strategies generally takes longer to affect occupational function than, for example, does

changing elements of the physical context. Acquiring the skills to transfer in and out of a wheelchair, however, may have benefits that carry over to other activities also requiring such transfers, thus enabling performance of a number of occupational roles. To benefit from this approach, patients must value the new skills and strategies, wish to participate in training, and be capable of recognizing opportunities in which the new skills and strategies can be used.

Metacognitive Strategies

A promising new approach to adaptive therapy is the use of metacognitive strategies. Metacognition refers to the higher order thinking that allows individuals to set a goal, plan action(s) to meet the goal, monitor progress toward the goal, and adjust action plans accordingly. The approach was first applied in occupational therapy in child health, in programs such as the Co-op Approach (goal, plan, do, check) (Polatajko & Mandich, 2004). Using this approach, the occupational therapist acts as a coach, helping patients to move through the stages toward a self-identified goal. In later stages, the therapist helps the patient develop the ability to apply the strategy whenever he or she encounters a problem in occupational performance.

Early evidence strongly suggests that such strategies are also effective in improving performance in activities adults identify that they need and want to do and that these new problem-solving abilities may transfer to additional valued activities (McEwen et al., 2009; Skidmore et al., 2011; Toglia et al., 2010) (see further discussion in Chapter 24).

Determining the Optimal Treatment Approaches

As noted previously, wise treatment decisions are based on patient goals and values, research evidence, experiential evidence, understanding of current theories of pathology and their relationship to function, and aspects of the context in which one is working. Although the research literature and your own experience will often point you in the direction of a particular intervention, it is important to note that all interventions must be tailored to the specific patient.

For example, systematic review evidence demonstrates that occupational therapy is effective in improving ADL, such as dressing, following stroke (Steultjens et al., 2003). However, the patient you are working with, Jean, a 40-year-old woman who is the single parent of an 18-month-old girl, may be extremely concerned about how she will continue caring for her young daughter (see Case Example). You know, from your understanding of function, that she is probably quite capable of relearning to dress independently. However, she has told you that resuming child care is her only current goal. You use what evidence you can find on parenting and stroke (Rogers & Kirshbaum, 2010), what Jean tells you about her daughter, the tasks she needs to perform, her concerns, your knowledge of the stroke, and the common functional difficulties experienced by people who have similar stroke-related deficits (in this case, apraxia and fatigue). Working with Jean, you tailor an intervention that includes environmental adaptation, energy conservation, repetitive practice, and metacognitive techniques.

Required Documentation: Evaluation Note

An occupational therapy evaluation note is added to the medical record when assessment and treatment planning are complete.

Implementing Intervention

Once therapists collaboratively determine therapy outcomes, goals, and approaches, treatment begins. Clinicians continue to make decisions regarding how the treatment is best delivered (i.e., one-on-one or group treatment) and by whom.

How Treatment Is Delivered: Individual or Group Sessions

Occupational therapy occurs during one-on-one sessions with the patient or in pairs or small groups. Although clinicians must be sensitive to associated costs, they base scheduling decisions on each patient's unique needs and goals rather than solely on efficiency or the clinician's convenience.

Individual Treatment. Clinicians typically schedule individual sessions for assessment and reassessment. Individual sessions are also appropriate when patient privacy must be protected, such as during dressing training and when the patient seems particularly vulnerable or in need of emotional support. Patients who are easily distracted, such as those in early phases of recovery from brain injury, are also best treated individually.

Group Treatment. Groups typically consist of patients engaged in parallel activities, such as performing individualized exercise regimens at the same time and place, or in collaborative activity, such as preparing a meal together. Patients tend to be grouped according to similar goals, treatment, or education needs or to similar diagnoses, conditions, or limitations. Beyond its value from an economic standpoint, group treatment offers many benefits to patients. Group therapy can provide social support to patients as well as encouragement as they observe others mastering challenges similar to those they face.

Who Delivers Treatment

Economic trends in health care require that the most appropriate person perform therapeutic tasks to optimize efficiency (Russell & Kanny, 1998). Occupational therapists make decisions about who will carry out the treatment plan (occupational therapist and/or occupational therapy assistant. Occupational therapists orchestrate the treatment plan and are ultimately responsible for service delivery (AOTA, 2008a). They typically spend their time conducting evaluations, identifying problems, planning solutions, and supervising implementation (Dunn & Cada, 1998; Glantz & Richman, 1997). Occupational therapy assistants spend most of their time delivering direct service and documenting results (Dunn & Cada, 1998; Glantz & Richman, 1997).

Required Documentation: Daily Contact Notes

Each time the patient is seen for assessment and treatment, the clinician documents the contact (see Table 2-2).

Monitoring Progress

Clinicians continuously monitor client responses to intervention and their progress toward goals. At regular intervals, typically weekly for inpatients and at least monthly for outpatients, clinicians formally reassess status relative to goals, analyze barriers to and enablers of progress, evaluate effectiveness of the treatment approach, and make decisions about continuing, modifying, or discontinuing treatment. If short-term goals are met but long-term goals are not, the short-term goals are upgraded (Moyers, 1999). If short-term goals are not met or performance has leveled off, the therapist examines and possibly modifies the treatment approach, reflects on the caliber of his or her skills with the treatment methods, looks for transient explanatory factors, consults with experts, and/or considers discontinuing therapy.

Required Documentation: Weekly and/or Monthly Progress Notes

Progress notes document the formal examination of the patient's progress toward treatment goals (Allen, 1997). For outpatients with Medicare, therapists also must complete monthly recertification forms detailing the patient's progress toward goals, which must be signed by the patient's physician every 30 days.

Discontinuing Therapy

Therapy is discontinued when goals have been met, the patient's performance has leveled off or deteriorated in such a way that he or she is not benefiting from services, or the individual chooses to stop. Ideally, the patient and family participate in discharge planning, which entails setting up a maintenance program, referring to other services, and/or planning for follow-up.

- Set up the maintenance program. Patients and families receive instructions that allow them to extend the benefits of treatment after discharge. Therapists typically provide written and oral information regarding continued exercise, recommended equipment, and strategies or techniques that optimize function. The plan must fit well with the patient's daily routine, incorporate the patient's goals, and be feasible given the patient's environment and resources. It is also essential that the patient has a clear idea of the goals of the program and how it works (Radomski, 2011).
- Help the patient establish an adherence plan. People with chronic health problems may have particular difficulty adhering to recommended maintenance plans for many reasons. It can be helpful to talk about this early on, normalizing the situation and allowing for later discussions of difficulties with adherence. The adherence plan can include ways to work the recommendations into daily routines, use of reminder systems, and provisions for monitoring outcomes, so that even slow progress or maintenance is recognized and provides reinforcement for adhering to the program (Radomski, 2011).
- Refer to other services. Many patients who discontinue occupational therapy at one site continue treatment at another level of care. For example, often persons receiving inpatient rehabilitation receive additional occupational therapy in long-term care facilities, through home health agencies, or as outpatients. To continue intervention seamlessly, therapists pass information along to the next tier of intervention. Therapists may also identify areas of need that are outside their scope of practice or competence and refer patients to appropriate disciplines or specialists.
- Plan for follow-up. Implicit in intervention plans geared to addressing the right issues at the right time in a patient's recovery and adaptation is the expectation that the therapist will not treat all possible problems during a given episode of care. A scheduled occupational therapy follow-up session is a mechanism by which the clinician can screen for the need for more services. A follow-up session is necessary when the patient improves, gets worse, or anticipates changed needs or goals or when the social or environmental context changes (Moyers, 1999). Some clients are ambivalent about discontinuing occupational therapy, recognizing lack of progress but fearing abandonment and stalled recovery or deterioration. Planned follow-up assures patients that occupational therapy services will be available to them if needed in the future.

Required Documentation: Home Program, Referrals, and Discharge Summary

Not only are written home programs and referrals provided to the patient and referral source, but these reports are also added to the medical record. The discharge summary provides an overview of services provided, outcomes, and recommendations. Allen (1997) suggested that creating this document can be a reflective process for the clinician, who considers whether goals were met and which factors contributed to or interfered with the patient's progress.

DOCUMENTATION: THE OFFICIAL RECORD OF THE TRIP

As a traveler, keeping detailed notes of your trip is a personal choice. However, occupational therapists are professionally and legally required to document their work with each patient in the medical record. This record is "a confidential, patient-identifiable, document or compilation of documents that chronicles the medical history of a patient throughout the course of his or her treatment at that facility or from that provider" (Iyer, Levin, & Shea, 2006, p. 3). This information will include therapy goals, assessment details, interventions provided, intervention outcomes, the patient's status at the end of therapy, and plans for discharge. Such plans may include further therapy or instructions to the patient regarding when he or she should contact the therapist again.

The AOTA (2008a) outlines several purposes of occupational therapy documentation. These purposes are to

- articulate the rationale for provision of occupational therapy services and the relationship of this service to the client's outcomes
- reflect the occupational therapy therapist's clinical reasoning and professional judgment
- communicate information about the client from the occupational therapy perspective
- create a chronological record of client status, occupational therapy services provided to the client, and client outcomes

In the course of their daily work, occupational therapists produce a number of reports, including daily contact notes, evaluation summaries, weekly or monthly progress notes, and discharge summaries (see Table 2-2). Documentation formats include computerized records, checklists, forms, and narrative notes. Regardless of format, to communicate in these documents, therapists must be clear about their target audience (McGuire, 1997; Robertson, 1997). That is, who will read this note and what do they need or want to know about the occupational therapy that was provided to this patient? Clinicians aim to provide succinct descriptions of functional status, anticipated outcome, and progress to date, so that a single document meets a number of stakeholders' information needs (McGuire, 1997). The reading audience may include members of the treatment team, who want to know how best to collaborate; the third-party payer, who wants to decide whether to pay for services; the accrediting agency, such as TJC or CARF International, which wants to determine whether quality services are provided at the institution; the legal system, which wants evidence in malpractice litigation; and the patient and significant others, who want to understand the care (Robertson, 1997).

McGuire (1997) outlined six principles that reflect excellent standards for occupational therapy documentation and meet the requirements of Medicare, the largest third-party payer in the United States.

1. Focus on function. Clinicians describe the patient's previous or premorbid level of function in key areas, review current status, and/or provide estimates of potential improvements or outcomes as a result of therapy.
2. Focus on underlying causes. Clinicians combine their understanding of the patient's medical condition with their assessment results to identify specific impairments that restrict or limit occupational performance.
3. Focus on progress. Clinicians describe the patient's progress toward goals according to objective measures, detailed observation, and/or standardized levels of independence.
4. Focus on safety. Many stakeholders look to the occupational therapist to provide information about the patient's safety and competence in self-management, self-advancement, and self-enhancement roles.
5. State expectations for progress or explain slow progress or lack of progress. Occupational therapists must "document a continued expectation that the patient's condition will continue to improve significantly in a reasonable and generally predictable amount of time" (McGuire, 1997, p. 441). Therapists should document setbacks that delay progress, such as medication changes, medical complications, and social disruptions.
6. Summarize needed skilled services. Occupational therapists avoid detailing the specific therapeutic interventions used during a given treatment session or period but emphasize the provision of skilled services. Skilled services include evaluations, direct intervention, such as training in techniques or strategies, task modification, selection or construction of equipment or orthotics, and instructions to the patient or caregiver about maintenance programs.

Because, as noted above, many of your readers will not be occupational therapists, ensure that the information is relatively jargon free. The greatest considerations for documentation, however, are accuracy and completeness.

Accuracy and completeness are essential because the document serves as a record of what you have done and found that others will refer to as they make their own treatment decisions. Importantly, in the event of legal action, the medical record will be called into evidence to act as a witness to the event. For this reason, all entries must be dated and signed, and any corrections made in such a way that the original entry can still be seen. Further charting guidelines and regulations may be obtained from TJC, your state department of health, and your employer (Iyer, Levin, & Shea, 2006).

The Health Insurance Portability and Accountability Act and Personal Health Information

The Health Insurance Portability and Accountability Act, 1996 (HIPAA) is a complex federal law designed, in part, to ensure the protection of personal health information (PHI). The "privacy standards" within this law present guidelines for the transfer of PHI (also known as *individually identifiable health information*) to another person or agency.

Individually identifiable health information refers to data that could be used to identify someone who has received health services. Any information that would allow another person to know that a particular patient has received health care services or to become aware of that patient's medical condition is individually identifiable health information. In addition to diagnosis, such information may include the treating physician, the patient's date of birth, the patient's social security number, and information regarding therapy.

Before transmitting PHI to another person or agency, therapists must explain to the patient where they plan to transmit the information and for what purposes. They must then obtain the patient's permission to do so. With the exception of emergency circumstances or when the information has been properly ordered as part of a judicial process, information cannot be transmitted without the patient's permission. Importantly, specific state legislation may have even stricter requirements for PHI transmission, and in these cases, state legislation determines the rules for such transmission (White & Hoffman, 2003–2004).

REFLECTION: BECOMING A BETTER TRAVELER

When a therapist considers what he or she has done, why it has worked or not worked, and what can be learned to strengthen work with future patients, the therapist is engaging in reflective practice (Crist, 2007).

Using Practice Experience to Improve Competence

You, as an occupational therapy professional, are ultimately responsible for assessing, improving, maintaining, and documenting your own competence to practice (AOTA, 2010; Youngstrom, 1998). As Holm (2000) reminded us, high standards of competence are inextricably linked to high ethical standards. Competence has many dimensions, including knowledge, critical reasoning, interpersonal abilities, performance skills, and ethical reasoning (AOTA, 2010). Like occupational therapy services, continuing competence entails assessment, goal-directed action, and documentation.

Self-Assessment

The cornerstone of continuing growth of competence is reflection on yourself and your practice. Therapists deliberately and regularly take stock of their status and determine where they can grow. Clinicians interested in growth ask for feedback from peers and formally review their own performance. Schell (1992) recommended that clinicians annually outline their strengths, areas needing improvement, accomplishments of the past year, and goals for the coming year (see Procedures for Practice 2-3 for suggestions).

Goal-Directed Action

Having assessed your professional strengths and weaknesses, you have many ways to improve your competence, including the following:

- Participate in your professional national and state occupational therapy associations. During such volunteer service, you will encounter other occupational therapists who are committed to the profession and their own growth.
- Become a research-sensitive practitioner (Cusick & McCluskey, 2000). Make research evidence a vital part of the way that you provide services.
- Because even the most dedicated therapists make them (Scheirton, Mu, & Lohman, 2003), commit to learning from your mistakes. Reflect on your errors or inefficiencies, and consider what you would do differently should you face similar circumstances in the future. Be willing to discuss what you learn in this process with others.
- Establish a mentoring relationship. Mentors benefit from the relationship as they expand into new areas of practice, and protégés benefit from coaching and intellectual stimulation (Smith, 1992).
- Keep a journal to document information and questions; to reflect on ideas, concerns, and beliefs; and, ultimately, to identify learning needs (Tryssenaar, 1995).
- Start a journal club at work in which clinicians regularly read and discuss research articles relevant to their occupational therapy practice.
- Volunteer for medical record reviews and audits. By reviewing the documentation of others and submitting your documentation to the same scrutiny, you will learn how you can make your documentation clearer and more useful.

Documentation of Professional Continuing Education

Crist, Wilcox, and McCarron (1998) recommended that occupational therapists use "transitional portfolios" (p. 729) to plan and document their professional competence. More than a résumé or a curriculum vitae, the transitional portfolio features completed and exemplary work (e.g., certificates of attendance, awards, and articles), in-process projects and plans for professional development, and a reflective journal with ideas, goals, and feelings about one's reading, research, and work experiences. Resources available to clinicians include the professional development tool (which includes self-assessments, professional development plans, and portfolio template) developed for members of AOTA (AOTA, 2003). By systematically collecting and organizing information and artifacts specific to accomplishments, progress, and goals, occupational therapists take responsibility for their present and future professional competence.

In summary, occupational therapists feel competent when clients achieve results that translate into meaningful improvements in their daily lives (Gahnstrom-Strandqvist et al., 2000). Such results can be achieved as clinicians combine their knowledge of evidence with their insights regarding patients' values and goals to plan and implement intervention that is not only effective but also rewarding for patient and therapist alike.

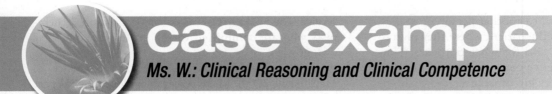

case example
Ms. W.: Clinical Reasoning and Clinical Competence

Occupational Therapy Intervention Process	Clinical Reasoning Process	
	Objectives	Examples of Therapist's Internal Dialogue
Patient Information Jean W. is a 40-year-old woman who was admitted to a stroke rehabilitation unit 3 weeks after experiencing a stroke. She was referred to the unit for general rehabilitation.	Appreciate the context	"Why has Jean been referred to occupational therapy? How long will she likely be a patient on the unit? What does she want to achieve while she is here?"
In conversation with the therapist, Jean tearfully states that her only goal is to be able to care for her 18-month-old daughter, Annabel, who is currently staying with her sister. On the Canadian Occupational Performance Measure, Jean states that her only goal is child care and rates her current performance and satisfaction as 0. The occupational therapy discharge note from acute care mentions probable perceptual problems, possible memory problems, and lack of motivation for therapy.	Know the person	"I wonder if Jean's worry about being able to care for her child is sapping her energy to participate in therapy. I wonder about the current extent of her perceptual problems and how they might interfere with child care activities. I wonder if fatigue may also be a part of the picture."
The therapist and Jean agree that resuming her child care responsibilities will be the primary objective of her work in occupational therapy. The therapist explains what perceptual and cognitive problems are and how learning more about them can help the therapist suggest ways to work around their impact on daily functioning. The therapist consults Stroke Engine (strokengine.ca) for evidence-based advice regarding evaluation and carries out the recommended assessments. She also asks Jean to carry out a number of simulated child care tasks to get a preliminary idea of the probable impact of any perceptual problems on daily tasks.	Select evaluation tools and methods	"I wonder how the apraxia I'm seeing on evaluation will affect child care in real life? I wonder what the effect of fatigue is on these evaluations?"
The therapist tries to develop a deeper understanding of how the goal could be achieved, including environmental resources.	Consult others as needed	"Is there any literature about parenting and stroke? Or about parenting and other neurological conditions with similar impacts? Are there any experts in this area? Where does their knowledge come from? (This area seems to call for a combination of knowledge from research and personal experiences of other patients.) How can Jean's sister be a resource for her rehabilitation in this area? Does Jean consent to have me speak with her?"
The therapist explains to Jean that she has observed a mild apraxia on testing and some possible short-term memory problems that are worsened by fatigue. She states that she believes that within the 3 weeks of treatment available, Jean could likely get to the point of safely carrying out basic child care tasks with supervision. Further progression could be worked out through home-care occupational therapy.	Discuss evaluation impressions and findings with patient and possible course of intervention	"Jean's sister will be a key player in ensuring that Jean has the opportunity to progress after her work here (that is, through providing opportunities to gradually resume independent care of Annabel). I should include her as much as possible in planning and treatment, with Jean's continued consent."

Jean and the therapist work on daily sessions of graded activity and metacognitive strategies to solve problems related to child care tasks. In the second week of treatment, Jean's sister brings in Annabel so that she can practice these tasks in a more real-life situation. In the week prior to discharge, Jean tries these activities at home.

Specify treatment activities, time frame, and intensity; provide instructions for therapy exercises, tasks, and activities; and observe patient's performance	

On a reevaluation with the Canadian Occupational Performance Measure, Jean scores an 8 for performance and satisfaction with child care activities.

Discuss with patient; readminister selected assessments; and modify the treatment plan as needed	"Has the intervention led to the desired changes?"

Jean had no further financial resources for occupational therapy and was very concerned that she might not be able to continue moving forward in her ability to care for Annabel. During the last two sessions, the therapist provided Jean with general guidelines for grading her child care activities and provided a written copy of this document. Jean's sister attended the final occupational therapy session so that she could provide Jean with help and encouragement with future activity grading. The therapist also helped Jean find an online group for young stroke survivors.

Plan for follow-up	"What kind of support would help Jean continue to progress toward her objective? What resources are available (e.g., home care, support groups, etc.)? What kind of support would be acceptable to her?"

 # Clinical Reasoning in Occupational Therapy Practice

Going Home but Feeling Sad

After 3 weeks of occupational therapy intervention, you observe that Jean seems to have decreased interest and a slightly depressed mood during the intervention, especially when thinking about the near future of being home alone. What might be causing these feelings? How might these feelings be addressed during the occupational therapy sessions?

Summary Review Questions

1. You have just taken a position in small rural hospital where you, as the sole occupational therapist, see both inpatients and outpatients. You receive a referral to see Barbara Khouzam, a 63-year-old woman with osteoarthritis of the carpometacarpal joint of her dominant hand. Using the resources described in this chapter, find research evidence related to appropriate occupational therapy intervention.

2. Working in the role described in Question 1, you receive a referral to see George Lee, an 85-year-old man who has fractured a hip. He is being discharged tomorrow, and the referring physician is asking you to see him to recommend equipment to maximize his independence in toileting and bathing. In your interview with George, you learn that he is adamant that he does not need or want equipment. Write down your thoughts about this using at least three of the five clinical reasoning tracks described in the chapter.

3. You are working in a large rehabilitation center that employs 20 occupational therapists. You have been

assigned to a new unit for people who are experiencing disability as a result of lifesaving cancer treatment. List the types of information that Tonelli (2006) recommends should be included for best practice, and describe at least one specific source for each type as you take on your new responsibilities.

4. Draft two long-term and two short-term occupational therapy goals for a hypothetical client with multiple sclerosis who wishes to return to clerical work.

5. Write a brief statement (fewer than 25 words) that you could use to describe occupational therapy to a new client as a prelude to collaborative goal setting. Compare descriptions with classmates, and then share with family and friends who know little about occupational therapy.

6. Note which of the following pieces of information you can communicate under HIPAA provisions without the patient's consent:
   - The results of an assessment of ADL functioning to the patient's physiotherapist
   - The times and dates of occupational therapy sessions to the patient's employer
   - The results of cognitive testing to the patient's spouse

   For information that you are not allowed to communicate, state whether there are special conditions under which you would be allowed to communicate this information.

7. Knowing that the patient's file may be called into evidence as a "witness to the event" should legal action be taken, list everything that should be included in documentation and how corrections should be made if errors occur.

8. Describe what competence looks like in action regarding knowledge, critical reasoning, interpersonal abilities, performance skills, and ethical reasoning. Describe what incompetence looks like for each area.

Glossary

Accreditation—The process in which a health care agency is assessed by an outside body to determine whether it meets specific standards of quality and safe patient care (Nicklin, 2011).

CARF International—Founded in 1966 as the Commission on Accreditation of Rehabilitation Facilities, CARF International is an accrediting organization of health and human service agencies (CARF International, 2011).

Comorbidities—Medical problems additional to the diagnosis with which a person is referred to occupational therapy that may affect the anticipated outcome and/or treatment approach.

Continuum of care—A system of services of varying intensity that address the ongoing or intermittent needs of persons with disabilities, ranging from acute medical interventions to rehabilitation to subacute rehabilitation to home health services to outpatient treatment to community wellness opportunities (CARF, 2004).

Episode of care—A discrete interval of service provision related to the achievement of specific therapeutic goals. Patients typically participate in many episodes of care during the recovery and rehabilitation process.

Evidence-based practice (EBP)—The use of the current literature, client choice, expertise, and clinical judgment to best serve clients (Law & MacDermid, 2008).

Goal—Specific statements regarding key priority areas for intervention and specific performance levels to be attained by the patient for defined activities within a specified period (Holliday, Ballinger, & Playford, 2007).

Health Insurance Portability and Accountability Act, 1996 (HIPAA)—A U.S. Federal law that includes provisions to protect personal health information. The privacy standards within this law present guidelines for the transfer of personal health information to another person or agency (White & Hoffman, 2003–2004).

The Joint Commission (TJC)—A not-for-profit organization that is the oldest and largest health care facility accrediting body in the United States (TJC, 2011).

Outcome—The level of performance attained by the patient at the end of therapy.

Qualitative research—A type of inquiry carried out using inductive logic and an emergent design to describe, understand or explain a human phenomenon in depth and in relation to its context.

Randomized controlled trials (RCTs)—A type of study used to provide high quality evidence regarding the effectiveness of a particular intervention. Study participants are assigned by chance to either receive the treatment being studied or not. The average outcome of each group is compared to determine the effect of treatment.

References

The AGREE Collaboration. (2001). Appraisal of Guidelines for Research & Evaluation (AGREE) Instrument. Retrieved July 3, 2013 from http://www.agreecollaboration.org/pdf/agreeinstrumentfinal.pdf.

The AGREE Next Steps Consortium (2009). Appraisal of Guidelines for Research & Evaluation. Retrieved July 8, 2013 from http://www.agreetrust.org/wp-content/uploads/2013/06/AGREE_II_Users_Manual_and_23-item_Instrument_ENGLISH.pdf.

Allen, C. (1997). Clinical reasoning documentation. In J. D. Acquaviva (Ed.), *Effective documentation for occupational therapy* (2nd ed., pp. 53–66). Bethesda, MD: American Occupational Therapy Association.

American Occupational Therapy Association. (2002). Occupational therapy practice framework: Domain and process. *American Journal of Occupational Therapy, 56,* 609–639.

American Occupational Therapy Association. (2008a). Guidelines for documentation of occupational therapy. *American Journal of Occupational Therapy, 62,* 684–690.

American Occupational Therapy Association. (2008b). Occupational therapy practice framework: Domain and process (2nd ed.). *American Journal of Occupational Therapy, 62,* 625–683.

American Occupational Therapy Association. (2010). Standards for continuing competence. *American Journal of Occupational Therapy, 64,* S103–S105.

Bryant, E. T. (1995). Acute rehabilitation in an outcome-oriented model. In P. K. Landrum, N. D. Schmidt, & A. McLean (Eds.), *Outcome-oriented rehabilitation* (pp. 69–93). Gaithersburg, MD: Aspen.

Canadian Association of Occupational Therapists, Association of Canadian Occupational Therapy University Programs, Association of Canadian Occupational Therapy Regulatory Organizations & President's Advisory Council. (1999). Joint position paper on evidence-based occupational therapy. *Canadian Journal of Occupational Therapy, 66,* 267–269.

Commission on Accreditation of Rehabilitation Facilities. (2004). *2004 medical rehabilitation standards manual.* Tucson, AZ: Commission on Accreditation of Rehabilitation Facilities.

CARF International. (2011). About us. Retrieved from http://www.carf.org/About/.

Coe, R. (2002). It's the effect size, stupid: What the effect size is and why it is important. *Education-line.* Retrieved August 15, 2013 from http://www.leeds.ac.uk/educol/documents/00002182.htm

Cope, D. N., & Sundance, P. (1995). Conceptualizing clinical outcomes. In P. K. Landrum, N. D. Schmidt, & A. McLean (Eds.), *Outcome-oriented rehabilitation* (pp. 43–56). Gaithersburg, MD: Aspen.

Crabtree, J. (2000). What is a worthy goal of occupational therapy? *Occupational Therapy in Health Care, 12,* 111–126.

Creswell, J. W. (2013). *Qualitative inquiry and research design: Choosing among five approaches - 3rd edition.* Thousand Oaks, CA: Sage.

Crist, P. (2007). Clinical reasoning and reflective practice. *ADVANCE for Occupational Therapy Practitioners.* Retrieved from http://occupational-therapy.advanceweb.com/Article/Clinical-Reasoning-and-Reflective-Practice.aspx.

Crist, P., Wilcox, B. L., & McCarron, K. (1998). Transitional portfolios: Orchestrating our professional competence. *American Journal of Occupational Therapy, 52,* 729–736.

Cusick, A., & McCluskey, A. (2000). Becoming an evidence-based practitioner through professional development. *Australian Occupational Therapy Journal, 47,* 159–170.

Donnelly, C., Eng, J. J., Hall, J., Alford, L., Giachino, R., Norton, K., & Kerr, D. S. (2004). Client-centred assessment and the identification of meaningful treatment goals for individuals with spinal cord injury. *Spinal Cord, 42,* 302–307.

Dubouloz, C. J, King, J., Ashe, B., Paterson, B., Chevrier, J., & Moldoveanu, M. (2010). The process of transformation in rehabilitation: What does it look like? *International Journal of Therapy and Rehabilitation, 17,* 604–615.

Dunn, W., & Cada, E. (1998). The national occupational therapy practice analysis: Findings and implication for competence. *American Journal of Occupational Therapy, 52,* 721–728.

Egan, M., Dubouloz, C. J., von Zweck, C., & Vallerand, J. (1998). The client-centred evidence-based practice of occupational therapy. *Canadian Journal of Occupational Therapy, 65,* 136–143.

Field, M. J., & Lohr, L. K. (1990). *Clinical practice guidelines: Directions for a new program.* Washington, DC: National Academy Press.

Fisher, A. G. (1998). Uniting practice and theory in an occupational framework. *American Journal of Occupational Therapy, 52,* 509–521.

Foye, S. J., Kirschner, K. L., Brady Wagner, L. C., Stocking, C., & Siegler, M. (2002). Ethical issues in rehabilitation: A qualitative analysis of dilemmas identified by occupational therapists. *Topics in Stroke Rehabilitation, 9,* 89–101.

Gahnstrom-Strandqvist, K., Tham, K., Josephsson, S., & Borrell, L. (2000). Actions of competence in occupational therapy practice. *Scandinavian Journal of Occupational Therapy, 7,* 15–25.

Glantz, C. H., & Richman, N. (1997). OTR-COTA collaboration in home health: Roles and supervisory issues. *American Journal of Occupational Therapy, 51,* 446–452.

Hagedorn, R. (1996). Clinical decision-making in familiar cases: A model of the process and implications for practice. *British Journal of Occupational Therapy, 59,* 217–222.

Hobson, S. (1996). Being client-centred when the client is cognitively impaired. *Canadian Journal of Occupational Therapy, 63,* 133–137.

Holliday, R. C., Ballinger, C., & Playford, E. D. (2007). Goal setting in neurological rehabilitation: Patients' perspectives. *Disability and Rehabilitation, 29,* 389–394.

Holm, M. B. (2000). Our mandate for the new millennium: Evidence-based practice. *American Journal of Occupational Therapy, 54,* 575–585.

Hooper, B. (1997). The relationship between pretheoretical assumptions and clinical reasoning. *American Journal of Occupational Therapy, 51,* 328–338.

Hurdowar, A., Graham, I. D., Bayley, M., Harrison, M., Wood-Dauphinee, S., & Bhogal, S. (2007). Quality of stroke rehabilitation clinical practice guidelines. *Journal of Evaluation in Clinical Practice, 13,* 657–664.

Iyer, P., Levin, B. J., & Shea, M. A. (2006). *Medical legal aspects of medical records.* Tuscon, AZ: Lawyers & Judges Publishing Company.

Jack, J., & Estes, R. I. (2010). Documenting progress: Hand therapy treatment shift from biomechanical to occupational adaptation. *American Journal of Occupational Therapy, 64,* 82–87.

The Joint Commission. (2011). About the Joint Commission. Retrieved from http://www.jointcommission.org/about_us/about_the_joint_commission_main.aspx.

Joyce, B. M., Rockwood, K. J., & Mate-Kole, C. C. (1994). Use of goal attainment scaling in brain injury in a rehabilitation hospital. *American Journal of Physical Medicine and Rehabilitation, 73,* 10–14.

Kinsella, E. A. (2000). *Professional development and reflective practice: Strategies for learning through professional experience.* Ottawa, Canada: CAOT Publications.

Kiresuk, T. J., & Sherman, R. E. (1968). Goal attainment scaling: A general method for evaluating comprehensive community mental health programs. *Community Mental Health Journal, 4,* 443–453.

Krefting, L. (1991). The culture concept in everyday practice of occupational and physical therapy. *Physical and Occupational Therapy in Paediatrics, 11,* 1–16.

Law, M., & MacDermid, J. (2008). *Evidence-based rehabilitation.* Thorofare NJ: Slack Inc.

Levack, W. M. M., Dean, S. G., Siegert, R. J., & McPherson, K. M. (2011). Navigating patient-centered goal setting in inpatient stroke rehabilitation: How clinicians control the process to meet perceived professional responsibilities. *Patient Education and Counseling, 85,* 206–213.

Levinson, W., Kao, A., Kuby, A., & Thisted, R. A. (2005). Not all patients want to participate in goal setting: A national study of patient preferences. *Journal of General Internal Medicine, 20,* 531–355.

Lincoln, Y. S., & Guba, E. G. (1985). *Naturalistic inquiry.* Beverly Hills, CA: Sage.

Lyons, K. D., & Crepeau, E. B. (2001). The clinical reasoning of an occupational therapy assistant. *American Journal of Occupational Therapy, 55,* 577–581.

Mastos, M., Miller, K., Eliasson, A. C., & Imms, C. (2007). Goal-directed training: Linking theories of treatment to clinical practice for improved functional activities in daily life. *Clinical Rehabilitation, 21,* 47–55.

Mathiowetz, V., & Haugen, J. B. (1995). Motor behavior research: Implications for therapeutic approaches to central nervous dysfunction. *American Journal of Occupational Therapy, 48,* 733–745.

Mattingly, C. (1991). What is clinical reasoning? *American Journal of Occupational Therapy, 45,* 979–986.

Mattingly, C., & Fleming, M. H. (1994). *Clinical reasoning: Forms of inquiry in a therapeutic practice.* Philadelphia: FA Davis.

McEwen, S. E., Polatajko, H. J., Huijbregts, M. P. J., & Ryan, J. D. (2009). Exploring a cognitive-based treatment approach to improve motor-based skill performance in chronic stroke: Results of three singe case experiments. *Brain Injury, 23,* 1041–1053.

McGuire, M. J. (1997). Documenting progress in home care. *American Journal of Occupational Therapy, 51,* 436–445.

Mitchell, R., & Unsworth, C. A. (2005). Clinical reasoning during community home visits: Expert and novice visits. *British Journal of Occupational Therapy, 68,* 215–223.

Moorhead, P., & Kannenberg, K. (1997). Writing functional goals. In J. D. Acquaviva (Ed.), *Effective documentation for occupational therapy* (2nd ed., pp. 75–82). Bethesda, MD: American Occupational Therapy Association.

Moyers, P. A. (1999). A guide to occupational therapy practice. *American Journal of Occupational Therapy, 53,* 247–322.

Nelson, C. E., & Payton, O. D. (1997). The planning process in occupational therapy: Perceptions of adult rehabilitation patients. *American Journal of Occupational Therapy, 51,* 576–583.

Nicklin, W. (2011). *The value and impact of health care accreditation: A literature review.* Ottawa, Canada: Accreditation Canada.

Ottenbacher, K. J., & Cusick, A. (1990). Goal attainment scaling as a method of clinical service evaluation. *American Journal of Occupational Therapy, 44,* 519–525.

Ponte-Allan, M., & Giles, G. M. (1999). Goal setting and functional outcomes in rehabilitation. *American Journal of Occupational Therapy, 53,* 646–649.

Phillips, R., & Glasziou, P. (2008). Evidence based practice: The practicalities of keeping abreast of clinical evidence while in training. *Postgraduate Medicine Journal, 84,* 450–453.

Polatajko, H. J., & Mandich, A. (2004). *Enabling occupation in children: The Cognitive Orientation to Daily Living (CO-OP) Approach.* Ottawa, Canada: CAOT Publications.

Radomksi, M. V. (1995). There is more to life that putting on your pants. *American Journal of Occupational Therapy, 49,* 487–490.

Radomski, M. V. (2011). More than good intentions: Advancing adherence to therapy recommendations. *American Journal of Occupational Therapy, 65,* 471–477.

Robertson, S. C. (1997). Why we document. In J. D. Acquaviva (Ed.), *Effective documentation for occupational therapy* (2nd ed., pp. 29–38). Bethesda, MD: American Occupational Therapy Association.

Rockwood, K., Joyce, B., & Stolee, P. (1997). The use of goal attainment scaling in measuring clinically important change in cognitive rehabilitation patients. *Journal of Clinical Epidemiology, 50,* 581–588.

Rogers, J. (1983). Eleanor Clarke Slagle Lectureship-1983: Clinical reasoning: The ethics, science and art. *American Journal of Occupational Therapy, 37,* 601–616.

Rogers, J. C., & Holm, M. B. (1991). Occupational therapy diagnostic reasoning: A component of clinical reasoning. *American Journal of Occupational Therapy, 45,* 1045–1053.

Rogers, J., & Kirshbaum, M. (2010). Parenting after stroke. In G. Gillen (Ed.), *Stroke rehabilitation: A function-based approach* (pp. 583–597). St. Louis: Mosby.

Russell, K. V., & Kanny, E. M. (1998). Use of aides in occupational therapy practice. *American Journal of Occupational Therapy, 52,* 118–124.

Sackett, D. L., Richardson, W. S., Rosenberg, W., & Haynes, R. B. (1997). *Evidence-based medicine: How to practice and teach EBM.* New York: Churchill Livingstone.

Sanders, S. H., Harden, R. N., & Vicente, P. J. (2005). Evidence-based practice guidelines for the interdisciplinary rehabilitation of chronic nonmalignant pain syndrome patients. *Pain Practice, 5,* 303–315.

Scheirton, L., Mu, K., & Lohman, H. (2003). Occupational therapists' responses to practice errors in physical rehabilitation settings. *American Journal of Occupational Therapy, 57,* 307–314.

Schell, B. B. (1992). Setting realistic career goals. *Occupational Therapy Practice, 3,* 11–20.

Schell, B. A., & Cervero, R. M. (1993). Clinical reasoning in occupational therapy: An integrative review. *American Journal of Occupational Therapy, 47,* 605–610.

Skidmore, E. R., Holm, M. B., Whyte, E. M., Dew, M. A., Dawson, D., & Becker, J. T. (2011). The feasibility of metacognitive strategy training in acute inpatient stroke rehabilitation: Case report. *Neuropsychological Rehabilitation, 21,* 208–223.

Smith, B. C. (1992). Mentoring: The key to professional growth. *Occupational Therapy Practice, 3,* 21–28.

Spencer, J., Davidson, H., & White, V. (1997). Helping clients develop hopes for the future. *American Journal of Occupational Therapy, 51,* 191–198.

Steultjens, E. M. J., Dekker, J., Bouter, L. M., van de Nes, J. C. M., Cup, E. H. C., & van den Ende, C. H. M. (2003). Occupational therapy for stroke patients: A systematic review. *Stroke, 34,* 676–687.

Straus, S. E., Richardson, W. S., Glasziou, P., & Haynes, R. B. (2005). *Evidence-based medicine: How to practice and teach EBM* (3rd ed.). Edinburgh: Churchill Livingstone.

Sumsion, T., & Law, M. (2006). A review of evidence on the conceptual elements informing client-centred practice. *Canadian Journal of Occupational Therapy, 73,* 153–162.

Tickle-Degnen, L. (2008). Communicating evidence to clients, managers and funders. M. Law & J. MacDermid (Eds.), *Evidence-based rehabilitation* (pp. 263–295). Thorofare, NJ: Slack, Inc.

Toglia, J., Johnston, M. V., Goverover, Y., & Dinn, B. (2010). A multicontext approach to promoting transfer of strategy use and self regulation after brain injury: An exploratory study. *Brain Injury, 24,* 664–677.

Tonelli, M. R. (2006). Integrating evidence into clinical practice: an alternative to evidence-based approaches. *Journal of Evaluation in Clinical Practice, 12,* 248–256.

Trombly, C. A. (1993). Anticipating the future: Assessment of occupational therapy function. *American Journal of Occupational Therapy, 47,* 253–357.

Trombly, C. A. (1995). Occupation: Purposefulness and meaningfulness as therapeutic mechanisms. *American Journal of Occupational Therapy, 49,* 960–9672.

Trombly, C. A., Radomski, M. V., & Davis, E. S. (1998). Achievement of self-identified goals by adults with traumatic brain injury: Phase I. *American Journal of Occupational Therapy, 52,* 810–818.

Trombly, C. A., Radomski, M. V., Trexel, C., & Burnett-Smith, S. E. (2002). Achievement of self-identified goals by adults with traumatic brain injury: Phase II. *American Journal of Occupational Therapy, 56,* 489–498.

Tryssenaar, J. (1995). Interactive journals: An educational strategy to promote reflection. *American Journal of Occupational Therapy, 49,* 695–702.

Unsworth, C. A. (2004). Clinical reasoning: How do pragmatic reasoning, worldview and client-centredness fit? *British Journal of Occupational Therapy, 67,* 10–19.

Unsworth, C. A. (2011). The evolving theory of clinical reasoning. In E. A. S. Duncan (Ed.), *Foundations of occupational therapy* (3rd ed., pp. 209–231). Edinburgh: Elsevier.

White, T. J., & Hoffman, C. A. (2003–2004). Privacy standards under the Health Insurance Portability and Accountability Act: A practical guide to promote order and avoid potential chaos. *West Virginia Law Review, 106.* Retrieved from http://heinonline.org/HOL/Page?handle=hein.journals/wvb106&div=25&g_sent=1&collectio==journals.

World Health Organization. (2001). *International Classification of Function, Disability and Health (ICF).* Geneva, Switzerland: World Health Organization.

Youngstrom, M. J. (1998). Evolving competence in the practitioner role. *American Journal of Occupational Therapy, 52,* 716–720.

3

Assessing Context: Personal, Social, Cultural, and Payer-Reimbursement Factors

Mary Vining Radomski and Pamela Roberts

Learning Objectives

After studying this chapter, the reader will be able to do the following:

1. Describe personal, social, cultural, and payer-reimbursement contextual factors that influence occupational therapy assessment and inform treatment planning.
2. Employ methods for quantifying the influence of various contextual factors on performance.
3. Consider the ways in which contextual factors influence how the therapist delivers occupational therapy services.
4. Describe how contextual factors specific to payer and reimbursement shape the nature of occupational therapy services delivered within various levels of care.
5. Adopt clinical practices that combine "zooming in" to focus on the details of a given client's occupational performance and "zooming out" to examine the larger contextual picture.

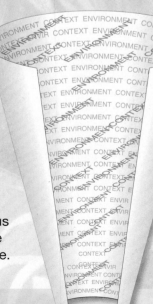

Much as a phrase, punch line, or couplet can be understood only in the larger context of a story, joke, or poem, a client's performance during occupational therapy assessment can be interpreted only in light of the broader context of his or her life, background, and/or circumstances. For example, lack of eye contact during an initial interview may easily be misinterpreted as lack of interest or motivation unless the therapist appreciates the contribution of cultural background—that avoiding eye contact is a way of showing respect in some cultures, including the Vietnamese culture (Farrales, 1996). Difficulty selecting clothing during a dressing assessment may be erroneously attributed to a patient's poor decision-making skills unless the therapist appreciates the contribution of social role experiences— that for 50 years, the patient's wife set out his clothing each morning.

The term *context* refers to the whole situation, background, or environment that is relevant to a particular event or personality. Contextual factors serve to characterize a situation and throw light on its meaning (*Webster's Third New International Dictionary*, 1993); together they provide the complete picture of an individual's life (World Health Organization, 2001). During the assessment process, occupational therapists try to obtain a complete picture of the patient's functioning, appreciating that a person's function at any moment is shaped by a dynamic array of contextual factors and not solely by his or her capacities, acquired skills, and abilities.

Occupational therapists are likely to best understand a client's occupational performance if viewed through a telephoto lens that zooms in and out. Borrowing from Kanter (2011), effective therapists are able to zoom in to bring details regarding a client's capacities, skills, and roles into focus and zoom out to see the bigger picture, including the influence of contextual factors on performance. Chapters 4–9 have to do with zooming in during the occupational therapy assessment process, and this chapter focuses on zooming out by describing examples of influential personal, social, cultural, and payer-reimbursement factors.

The role of context in occupational function cannot be exhaustively explored in one chapter; whole texts and careers have been devoted to each of these complex constructs. Clinicians need not obsess about correctly labeling or pigeonholing each and every contextual factor, but using these examples, readers are encouraged to reflect on other contextual factors not discussed herein. This overview, however, has one superordinate aim: to describe the potential contextual influences on occupational performance so that therapists may thoughtfully plan, conduct, and interpret the results of occupational therapy assessment.

CONTEXT AND OCCUPATIONAL FUNCTION

Occupational function is always embedded in context, with physical, cultural, social, and personal factors shaping its form (Nelson, 1988). Consider how contextual factors change the picture: a middle-aged homemaker preparing eggs and toast for her children before they leave for school versus a middle-aged homemaker preparing the same breakfast in an unfamiliar rehabilitation setting as part of an occupational therapy assessment to determine readiness for discharge after a mild stroke.

The important role of context in occupational function is described by a number of models and frameworks from occupational therapy, rehabilitation, and health fields. Each of the models or frameworks summarized in Table 3-1 emphasizes the dynamic relationship between a person; his or her cultural, social, and physical contexts; and the continuum of function to disability relative to chosen roles and tasks. The aforementioned models universally downplay the contribution of physical impairments and elevate the role of context in the explanation of human functioning and disablement but use slightly different terminology. Assessment Table 3-1 provides examples of measures that assess personal, social, and cultural context. In the occupational functioning model (OFM), occupation is presumed to occur and be understood within a unique contextual milieu that, while peripheral to a client's primary diagnosis, influences his or her occupational functioning (see Chapter 1).

- Personal context reflects an individual's internal environment derived from his or her gender, values, beliefs, cultural background, or state of mind.
- Social context refers to factors in the human environment (roles, resources, and structure) that enable or deter the person's occupational function.
- Cultural context has to do with the norms, values, and behaviors related to the community or society in which the occupational function occurs.
- Payer-reimbursement context refers to policies and regulations that determine availability and reimbursement of occupational therapy services in various settings.

The convenience of describing personal, social, cultural, and payer-reimbursement contextual factors as separate and distinct entities belies their complexity, interrelatedness, interactive, and dynamic influences. For example, one's culture may influence family structure, norms for coping, and such individual matters as food preferences, humor, and definition of personal space (that is, aspects of personal context). Likewise, personal context may influence social and cultural context in that a person's spiritual beliefs often shape his or her social network, preferred roles, and definitions of acceptable behavior. The relatively stable factors, such as age, generational

Table 3-1 | **Selected Models or Frameworks That Specifically Include Context as an Element in Human Function**

Models and Frameworks	Synopsis of Role of Context in Occupation and/or Human Function
Ecology of Human Performance (Dunn, Brown, & McGuigan, 1994)	The interaction between a person and the environment affects his or her behavior and performance. Human performance can be understood only through the "lens" of context, which includes temporal (age, development, and health status), physical, cultural, and social features that operate external to a person. In essence, the interrelationship between person and context determines which tasks fall within the individual's performance range.
Person-Environment-Occupation Model of Occupational Performance (Law et al., 1996)	Occupational function is the result of the transactive relationship "between people, their occupations and roles, and the environments in which they live, work, and play" (p. 9). This model emphasizes the interdependence of person and environment (defined as those contexts and situations that occur outside the individual such as cultural, socioeconomic, institutional, and social considerations). It also recognizes the temporal or changing nature of person, environment, occupation characteristics, and their interrelationships.
Occupational Therapy Intervention Process Model (Fisher, 1998)	Occupational performance occurs as a "transaction between the person and the environment as he or she enacts a task" (p. 514). Therapists must be aware of the client's performance context (composed of temporal, environmental, cultural, societal, social, role, motivational, capacity, and task dimensions) in order to understand, evaluate, and interpret a person's occupational performance.
International Classification of Functioning, Disability, and Health (World Health Organization, 2001)	"A person's functioning and disability are conceived as a dynamic interaction between health conditions and contextual factors" (p. 10). Contextual factors include personal and environmental factors. Personal factors are internal influences of functioning that are not part of a health condition or functional state such as gender, age, social background, fitness, lifestyle, and habits. Environmental factors, external influences on functioning, include features of the physical, social, and attitudinal world.
Occupational Therapy Practice Framework (American Occupational Therapy Association, 2008)	The overarching outcome of occupational therapy is to advance clients' engagement in occupation to support life participation in the context of their unique situations. Defined as "a variety of interrelated conditions within and surrounding the client that influence performance" (p. 670), context (cultural, personal, temporal, and virtual) is included in the domain of occupational therapy.

cohort, and gender identity, may pervade most tasks and situations and are not easily changed in occupational therapy. For example, a patient's educational background may affect how the therapist provides home instruction but is unlikely to be a focus of intervention (Procedures for Practice 3-1). On the other hand, the more dynamic contextual factors, such as pain, stress level, and social dynamics, are transient, circumstantial, and potentially more responsive to environment, task, and therapy than stable contextual factors. For example, upper extremity pain that interferes with an individual's concentration likely varies with time of day and activity. Therefore, the therapist considers its effect on performance during all aspects of occupational therapy assessment and likely addresses the issue in the intervention plan.

Importance of Personal, Social, Cultural, and Payer-Reimbursement Context to Assessment

Paying attention to contextual factors is central to occupational therapy assessment for three key reasons. First, doing so provides the therapist with a more complete picture of the client, which in turn guides selection of assessments

and the interpretation of results. Scholar/researcher Mary Egan (2007) described an experience early in her career that illustrates the importance of considering contextual factors in planning the occupational therapy assessment. She reportedly started a cognitive-perceptual evaluation on a professor who was receiving rehabilitation after a stroke when 10 minutes into the session, he became enraged and demanded to return to his room. In hindsight, Dr. Egan realized how threatening her assessments must have been to a person whose livelihood and self-definition depended upon thinking, writing, and speaking. She speculated that the process would have been more effective had she begun by acknowledging his loss and suffering, educating him about the process and rationale, and then conducting the assessment with his approval.

Dr. Egan's experience highlights the importance of considering contextual factors when planning assessment. It is equally important to consider the influence of contextual factors when interpreting assessment findings as exemplified in the following scenario. Mr. S. appears to have difficulty attending to instructions during an occupational therapy homemaking assessment. The therapist might solely attribute the problem to cognitive

Assessment Table 3-1	Summary of Measures for Assessing Personal, Social, and Cultural Context

Instrument and Reference	Description	Time to Administer	Validity	Reliability	Sensitivity	Strengths and Weaknesses
Rapid Estimate of Adult Literacy in Medicine (REALM) (Murphy et al., 1993)	Reading recognition test composed of a 66-item reading list that allows clinicians to estimate patients' reading skills	2–3 minutes	Concurrent validity: significant correlation ($p < 0.0001$) between REALM and standardized measures of reading including the Peabody Individual Achievement Test-Revised ($r = 0.97$), Wide Range Achievement Test-Revised ($r = 0.88$), and Slosson Oral Reading Test-Revised ($r = 0.96$) (Davis et al., 1993)	Excellent test–retest reliability ($r = 0.99$, $p < 0.001$)	No information	Strengths: Brief Minimal training needed Spanish version available The REALM-SF has only seven items on the reading list and has strong correlation with the REALM ($r = 0.94$, $p < 0.001$) (Arozullah et al., 2007).
CAGE Questionnaire (Ewing, 1984)	Involves asking four questions to persons seeking medical services to identify possible alcohol abuse	5–10 minutes	Convergent validity for four CAGE questions with alcohol-related items of the Army's Health Risk Appraisal ranged from (Φ coefficient) 0.1713–0.3496, moderately weak Criterion validity: persons with cutoff score of 2 were at 3.5 times greater risk for military discharge because of alcoholism (Bell et al., 2003).	Good test–retest reliability (2–30 days) for four questions (r ranged from 0.73 to 0.83) (Bell et al., 2003)	In a study of individuals with traumatic brain injury, specificity and sensitivity of CAGE were high (86% and 91%, respectively) (Ashman et al., 2004).	Strength: Appropriate for use with clinical populations Weaknesses: Poor sensitivity when modified to detect drug abuse or when used to determine preinjury substance abuse (Ashman et al., 2004) CAGE was shown to be unable to discriminate between those who were heavy drinkers and those who were not heavy drinkers in the general population (Bisson, Nadeau, & Demers, 1999).

(continued)

Assessment Table 3-1 · Summary of Measures for Assessing Personal, Social, and Cultural Context (continued)

Instrument and Reference	Description	Time to Administer	Validity	Reliability	Sensitivity	Strengths and Weaknesses
Numeric Pain Rating Scale (NPRS) (Jensen, Karoly, & Braver, 1986)	Presented as a vertical column of numbers (from 10 to 0), with 10 referring to "pain as bad as it can be" and 0 labeled as "no pain." The patient identifies the number (by pointing or circling) that best reflects pain intensity over the past 24 hours.	Approximately 2 minutes	Demonstrated construct validity in its ability to discriminate between patients with cervical radiculopathy (CR) who had made clinical improvements and those who did not (Young et al., 2010)	Moderate test–retest reliability, with an Intraclass correlation coefficient (ICC) of 0.76 (95% confidence interval of 0.51–0.87) for patients with mechanical neck pain (Cleland, Childs, & Whitman, 2008)	Minimal detectable change (MDC) (amount of change needed to exceed measurement error) of the NPRS varies by clinical population: 2.1 points for patients with mechanical neck pain (Cleland, Childs, & Whitman, 2008) and 4.1 points for patients with CR (Young et al., 2010). The threshold for minimal clinically important difference (MCID) (the smallest difference that patients perceive as beneficial) also varies by diagnosis: 1.3 points for those with neck pain (Cleland, Childs, & Whitman, 2008) and 2.2 points for those with CR (Young et al., 2010).	Strengths: Brief screening tool Widely used and understood by patients and professionals Involves interval data that can be analyzed using parametric statistics (Williamson & Hoggart, 2005) Weakness: Limited research regarding reliability and validity with neurorehabilitation populations
Fatigue Severity Scale (FSS) (Krupp et al., 1989)	Self-report questionnaire designed to evaluate the impact fatigue has on a patient. The patient rates the severity of his or her fatigue symptoms by reading each of the nine statements and circling a number from 1 to 7 (1 reflects strong disagreement with the statement, and 7 reflects strong agreement with the statement) based on how accurately it reflects his or her condition during the past week.	Relatively brief (approximately 3–5 minutes)	Convergent validity: FSS scores with other measures of fatigue including the Multidimensional Assessment of Fatigue and Rhoten Fatigue Scale (as summarized in Whitehead, 2009).	Test–retest reliability: Eleven subjects with fatigue-related conditions were retested after an average of 10 weeks in which no change in fatigue was clinically anticipated. Paired t-test differences were not significant; correlation coefficient was 0.84 (Krupp et al., 1989).	Based on test–retest values (Krupp et al., 1989), the minimal detectable change is 1.44 points.	Strengths: The FSS is brief and relates fatigue to daily functioning; it has been used on rehabilitation populations including multiple sclerosis, stroke, Parkinson's disease (Whitehead, 2009), and mild to moderate traumatic brain injury (Merritta et al., 2010). Weakness: Requires ability to read

Instrument	Description	Time to Complete	Validity	Reliability	Sensitivity/Specificity	Strengths/Weaknesses
The Hospital Anxiety and Depression Scale (HADS) (Zigmond & Snaith, 1983)	Self-administered questionnaire designed to detect depression and anxiety in a medical outpatient clinical setting; composed of 16 questions related to psychological rather than somatic complaints	Less than 20 minutes	Moderate correlation between patient self-ratings on HADS and psychiatric interview assessment for anxiety ($r = 0.54$, $p < 0.05$); moderately strong for depression ($r = 0.79$, $p < 0.01$)	Good internal consistency (Cronbach alpha value of 0.83 for anxiety subscale and 0.84 for depression subscale) (Pallant & Bailey, 2005).	Good sensitivity and specificity for separate subscales with cutoff score of ≥ 8 (HADS anxiety: sensitivity 0.89, specificity 0.88; HADS depression: sensitivity 0.80; specificity 0.88) (Olsson, Mykletun, & Dahl, 2005).	Strengths: Brief screen such that patient could complete while waiting for appointment; Has been translated into Arabic, Dutch, French, German, Hebrew, Swedish, Italian, and Spanish; Appropriate for wide range of medical diagnoses. Weaknesses: Patients must be able to read in order to complete the HADS; Use of total score not adequately sensitive in identifying cases of psychiatric illness (Poole & Morgan, 2006)
Beck Depression Index (BDI) – FastScreen for Medical Patients (Beck, Steer, & Brown, 2000).	Self-report tool that screens for depression in adults and adolescents; composed of seven items extracted from the 21-item Beck Depression Inventory II.	Less than 5 minutes to complete	Construct validity: moderately strong correlation between BDI-FastScreen and HADS ($r = 0.62$, $p < 0.001$)	Good internal consistency (alpha values of the BDI-FastScreen for family practice, internal medicine, and pediatric patients were 0.85, 0.85, and 0.88, respectively) (Beck, Steer, & Brown, 2000)	BDI-FastScreen cutoff score of ≥ 4 had 100% sensitivity and 84% specificity rates (Scheinthal et al., 2001).	Strengths: Very brief with good psychometric properties; Responses to BDI-FastScreen not related to sex, ethnicity, age, or total number of medical conditions (Beck, Steer, & Brown, 2000). Weakness: Does not specifically inform occupational therapy intervention planning; serves only to identify persons in need of referral for more in-depth psychiatric assessment
Norbeck Social Support Questionnaire (NSSQ) (Norbeck, Lindsey, & Carrieri 1981)	Self-administered questionnaire consisting of nine items; patients list individuals in their personal network and specify the nature of their relationship; measures three functional types of social support (affect, affirmation, and aid)	Approximately 10 minutes	Concurrent validity: statistically significant correlation with the Personal Resources Questionnaire, another measure of social support ($r = 0.35$–0.41, $p < 0.05$) (Norbeck, Lindsey, & Carrieri, 1983)	High degree of test-retest reliability (0.85–0.92); High internal consistency within three types of support (0.89–0.97) (Norbeck, Lindsey, & Carrieri, 1981)	No information	Strength: Instrument may provide useful structure for interviewing clients about the nature of their social support. Weakness: Specific subscale scores may be more relevant to research than practice.

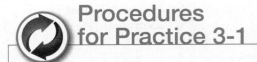

Procedures for Practice 3-1

Assessing Literacy

Health literacy pertains to a person's ability to process and comprehend basic health information necessary to make decisions (Institute of Medicine, 2009); a person's ability to read is part of this basic competency. Clients with low literacy may try to hide their difficulties with reading, compromising the assessment and the value of written home instructions (Parikh et al., 1996). Occupational therapists use written materials in assessment and treatment. Use of a reading screen allows the clinician to identify patients who need simplified, audiotaped, or pictorial education materials.

The Rapid Estimate of Adult Literacy in Medicine (REALM) (Murphy et al., 1993) is a widely used reading recognition test that takes 2–3 minutes to administer and score. It contains three columns of health-related words of increasing difficulty, 66 words in all. The client is asked to start at the top of list 1 and read the words aloud until he or she completes the three lists or is unable to read additional words. He or she is allowed 5 seconds to pronounce each word. The clinician takes note of all words pronounced correctly; this number becomes the raw score that is converted to grade range estimates.

Recently, researchers developed a seven-item version of the REALM, called the Rapid Estimate of Adult Literacy in Medicine–Short Form (REALM-SF) (Arozullah et al., 2007). The REALM-SF has excellent agreement with the original instrument. Online access to the REALM-SF word list, scoring instructions and interpretation, and a Spanish version is available from the Agency for Healthcare Research and Quality (2009).

impairment related to his right cerebrovascular accident if she did not know that Mr. S. was awake much of the previous night, as nurses addressed his roommate's deteriorating medical condition.

Second, paying attention to contextual factors may impact the outcome of occupational therapy services by informing the focus of intervention. A qualitative study involving rural women with HIV/AIDS underscores that sometimes patients care more about contextual factors (such as paying the bills and interacting with family) than the illness or condition itself (Phillips et al., 2011). The following example illustrates how the therapist may need to address issues related to social context in order to help the patient achieve his or her goals. Even with adequate strength and mobility, Mrs. P. remained dependent in lower extremity dressing after her total hip replacement because her husband, fearful that she may overexert, insisted on assisting with dressing. Because independence was important to Mrs. P., the therapist taught Mrs. P. lower extremity

dressing techniques and taught Mr. P. how to support the process without providing physical assistance.

Finally, therapists employ what they learn about the context of patients' lives (past and present) during assessment to improve engagement in the occupational therapy intervention process itself. For example, "knowing what makes them tick" can improve participation for persons with dementia (Galik, Resnick, & Pretzer-Aboff, 2009), and simple awareness of nursing home residents' life story appeared to help staff form empathetic relationships, which in turn appear to help reduce agitation (Egan et al., 2007).

Looking in the Mirror: Therapist as Contextually Influenced Being

Appreciating the influence of context on function requires that therapists acquire a complex combination of knowledge, attitudes, and skills. Rather than focusing on how a client fits into the therapist's world (via assumptions, schedule, and conventions), the therapist examines how he or she can understand and fit into the client's world (St. Clair & McKenry, 1999). To accomplish this shift, therapists must acknowledge and inventory the contextual factors that influence their own function. As I become aware of my own beliefs and biases, social background, and culturally based expectations, I will be able to appreciate their influence on collaborations with patients and coworkers (Odawara, 2005).

PERSONAL CONTEXT

"Life is suddenly reduced to a one dimension picture, known as physical function, and continually referred to as 'outcome.' The typical outcome process ignores . . . emotional and interpersonal needs and skills. Within those parameters lies the answer to true recovery . . . I refuse to have an 'outcome.' I do have a *life*!" (Cannon, 1994, p. 3)

Personal context refers to the intrapersonal environment that shapes an individual's experience. These factors play a role in determining the client's unique response to the onset of illness or impairment and contribute to his or her ability to adapt (National Center for Medical Rehabilitation and Research, 1993). Some aspects of a person's internal environment, such as age and long-standing beliefs, are stable; others, such as pain, mood, and adaptation to illness or injury (see Chapter 30), may be constantly in flux.

Age and Generational Cohort

A person's age or age at onset of disability appears to have implications for length of stay and outcome of rehabilitation, with elders generally having longer lengths of stay and poorer outcomes (Graham et al., 2010; Sendroy-Terrill, Whiteneck, & Brooks, 2010). A person's age may influence rehabilitation outcomes and his or her occupational functioning in three primary ways: (1) age-related changes in capacities and abilities; (2) developmental shifts in goals, values, and priorities; and (3) the individual's generation-based worldview.

In tandem with age-related changes in capacities (which are discussed in Chapter 32), Royeen (1995) hypothesized that people undergo "occupational shifts" (p. 11) during the life cycle that lead to major changes in patterns of activity. She posited that early adulthood is characterized by establishing worker roles while realigning social roles to adjust to marriage and parenthood. In middle adulthood, people maintain work and leisure roles but may undergo sudden occupational shifts related to caregiving roles of parents, children, and grandchildren. During maturity (age 45 years to retirement), people continue their work and leisure roles, but occupational shifts arise from death of family members, loss of provider status, and adjustments in life goals. An increased awareness of the limits of time appears to shape people's priorities and occupations as they age (Carstensen, Fung, & Charles, 2003). Older people tend to seek activities that create or develop emotional bonds and that contribute to life meaning more so than young adults, and these motivations actually have a positive impact on well-being for many elders (Carstensen, Fung, & Charles, 2003).

A person's generational cohort (group who share the same birth years and specific defining experiences) may also impact occupational performance through his or her attitudes and beliefs (Kramer, 2010). Consider the ways in which generational identity may influence participation in occupational therapy and interactions among intergenerational occupational therapy colleagues from four contemporary generational groups in the United States:

- The Veterans (born 1925–1945) respect authority, hierarchy, and believe that sacrifice and hard work pay off (Kramer, 2010).
- Baby Boomers (born 1946–1964) value independence, creativity, and prefer work that offers both personal reward and public recognition (Kramer, 2010).
- Generation Xers (born 1963–1980) tend to prioritize work-life balance and self-reliance and may need clarification regarding how tasks perceived as menial relate to larger goals (Kramer, 2010).
- Millennials (born 1980–2000), who tend to be practical and techno-savvy, have a unique appreciation for diversity—variety in people, environments, and activities. They are accustomed to participant-oriented decision making and expect to work in collaboration with others in their endeavors (Lancaster & Stillman, 2002).

Of course, generalizations about patterns of aging may or may not apply to specific individuals, and therapists are cautioned against age-related patient biases (Rybarczyk et al., 2001). Catastrophic loss of function, as with illness or disability, is an individual experience that takes place against a backdrop of other age-related changes, developmental tasks, and worldviews. For example, a person's adaptation to a spinal cord injury (SCI) may occur as he or she is also adapting to a new marriage or career. An elderly patient's efforts to relearn motor skills and standing balance may be complicated by declines in capacities associated with age and beliefs that if a person works hard enough, he or she will always achieve goals. A client who has lived and aged with a long-standing disability will likely have different health concerns and vulnerabilities than a young person with a new injury (Amsters et al., 2005).

Symptoms: Pain and Fatigue

A patient's intrapersonal environment is also shaped by his or her ongoing experience with symptoms such as pain and fatigue that influence both assessment and functioning. Occupational therapists try to understand the extent to which these symptoms contribute to the patient's performance during assessment.

Pain

Pain, acute and chronic, interferes with occupational function and quality of life for many people receiving occupational therapy services (Ehde et al., 2003). People with spinal cord injury who use manual wheelchairs report upper extremity pain, with the most severe pain occurring while pushing the wheelchair up an incline and during sleep (Curtis et al., 1999). Dalyan, Cardenas, and Gerard (1999) found that upper extremity pain was associated with lower employment rates and greater disability for outpatients with spinal cord injury. Many stroke patients have upper extremity pain as well, typically beginning 2 weeks after the onset of stroke (Chantraine et al., 1999). In addition to its contribution to disability and to decreased quality of life, pain is linked to depression (Dalyan, Cardenas, & Gerard, 1999), inefficiencies in information processing (Luoto et al., 1999), and coping strategies (Molton et al., 2009).

Many people with disabilities are used to living with pain and differentiating between usual pain and unexpected pain (Dudgeon et al., 2006). Because many recipients of occupational therapy services may be reluctant to mention their concerns about pain to therapists (Dudgeon et al., 2002), therapists take responsibility to routinely ask and/or assess. One commonly used subjective measure of pain is the Numeric Pain Rating Scale (NPRS) (Jensen, Karoly, & Braver, 1986).

Numeric Pain Rating Scale. The NPRS is a brief self-report questionnaire in which patients rate their pain intensity using an 11-point scale (Jensen, Karoly, & Braver, 1986).

Patients are asked to circle or point to one of the numbers that are listed vertically on the page (where 10 indicates pain as bad as it can be and 0 indicates no pain). If administered by interview, the therapist describes the scale and reference points and asks the patient to describe his or her level of pain by specifying a numeric rating. The NPRS may be used to better understand the patient's overall pain experience or how pain changes during an activity.

Fatigue

Fatigue is the subjective experience of lacking the physical or mental energy necessary to do usual and desired activities (Besharat et al., 2011). Many people with disability or chronic health conditions appear to experience fatigue, including those with stroke (Lerdahl et al., 2009), multiple sclerosis (Besharat et al., 2011), and brain injury (Gordon, 2008). Fatigue appears to be associated with personality characteristics (Besharat et al., 2011), depression (Merritta et al., 2010), and the nature of the neurological impairment itself (Cantor et al., 2008). If significant fatigue is suggested, clinicians try to quantify or characterize the patient's level of fatigue using a fatigue visual analog scale or a standardized questionnaire such as the Fatigue Severity Scale (Krupp et al., 1989)—information that is used during assessment and to inform referrals to other professionals.

In summary, because people who are fatigued or in pain generally do not perform at their best, occupational therapists often try to understand patients' status and experience in order to plan the assessment process, interpret findings, and determine the focus of occupational therapy intervention. If pain or fatigue management becomes the focus of intervention, therapists use assessments with good psychometric properties and known responsiveness to change (such as the NPRS and Fatigue Severity Scale), so that these measures can be readministered to ascertain progress. During assessment, questionnaires and numerical or visual analog scales should be the catalysts for, rather than replacements of, more in-depth conversations with clients about their experience with pain and fatigue. Conversations to explore the extent to which pain and fatigue levels are manageable or tolerable will be a prelude to problem solving about the kinds of strategies that might help (Zelman et al., 2004).

Coping and Beliefs

People's coping strategies, mental health, and spirituality may impact the ways in which they deal with sudden-onset disability and the experience of loss and ambiguity. During the assessment process, occupational therapists try to understand these aspects of personal context in order to understand their possible influence on performance; make referrals to specialists, if needed; and lay the groundwork for engaging with the patient in ways that advance adaptation and wholeness.

There is no question that persons with disabilities are at risk for anxiety and depression during the acute and chronic stages of injury (Hart et al., 2011; Kennedy & Rogers, 2000). Even so, most people with disability find that they are able to adjust to physical changes and live a happy, relatively normal life (Quale & Schanke, 2010); that is, most people are resilient.

Resilience in a rehabilitation setting is defined as "the ability of adults who are facing a severe and potentially disabling physical injury to maintain relatively stable, healthy levels of psychological and social functioning and to maintain positive emotions and a positive perception of self and the future" (Quale & Schanke, 2010, p. 13). A person's mood and coping strategies contribute to resilience, and both have far-reaching consequences (Pollard & Kennedy, 2007) and can be modifiable (Kennedy et al., 2011). In a study in which mood, coping, independence, and social support were assessed at 12 weeks post-SCI and 10 years later, Pollard and Kennedy (2007) found that rates of anxiety and depression and coping strategies changed little over the 10-year period. This underscores the importance of identifying problems with emotional distress and maladaptive coping early in the recovery period, because left untreated, they are unlikely to resolve over time (Pollard & Kennedy, 2007).

Identifying Emotional Distress

Early identification and treatment of mood disorders is important, as depression and anxiety appear to interfere with attention and concentration during assessment (Eysenck & Keane, 1990) and negatively influence outcome of intervention (Lai et al., 2002). Although occupational therapists do not diagnose mood disorders, they have numerous opportunities to observe behavior. According to Scherer and Cushman (1997), certain patterns of behavior may indicate psychological distress and warrant referral to a psychologist or psychiatrist for further assessment and treatment.

Depression. People feeling transitory sadness and discouragement or normal grief may display signs that are similar to those of depression but will differ in terms of persistence of symptoms and their effect on self-esteem (Gorman, Sultman, & Luna-Raines, 1989). That is, sadness and normal grief resolve with time and generally do not lead to lowered self-esteem, as suggested by the following signs of possible clinical depression (Gorman, Sultman, & Luna-Raines, 1989; Scherer & Cushman, 1997):

- Significant declines in functioning lasting 2 weeks or more
- Feelings of worthlessness, inadequacy, or self-doubt
- Diminished interest in virtually all activities, even formerly enjoyable activities

- Depressed or irritable mood most of the time
- Vegetative disturbances: lethargy, insomnia or excessive sleep, change of appetite with weight change of more than 5%, or periods of excessive activity or slowness almost every day
- Very poor concentration·
- Withdrawal from social interaction
- Recurrent thoughts of death or suicide

Anxiety. Anxiety is defined as a "subjectively painful warning of impending danger, real or imagined, that motivates the individual to take corrective action to relieve the unpleasant feelings and is experienced both psychologically and physiologically" (Gorman, Sultman, & Luna-Raines, 1989, p. 51). Anxiety is different from fear. Anxiety is characterized by a diffuse feeling of dread, whereas fear is a reaction to a specific temporary external danger (Gorman, Sultman, & Luna-Raines, 1989). Here are some signs of possible anxiety disorder (Gorman, Sultman, & Luna-Raines, 1989; Scherer & Cushman, 1997) that may prompt referral to a psychiatrist or psychologist:

- Panic attack (choking feeling, nausea, dizziness, palpitations or chest pain, fear of dying, or losing control)
- Distorted, unrealistic fears or perceptions of a situation or object
- Disruption of normal routines or daily activities associated with irrational fears

Despite their best intentions, occupational therapists often have difficulty recognizing these disorders. Therefore, occupational therapists are advised to use standardized screens to identify patients in need of psychological or psychiatric services (Ruchinskas, 2002). The Hospital Anxiety and Depression Scale (Zigmond & Snaith, 1983) and the Beck Depression Index-FastScreen for Medical Patients (Beck, Steer, & Brown, 2000) are good examples.

Identifying Coping Strategies

Coping strategies are things people do to maintain psychosocial adaptation during stressful periods (Holahan & Moos, 1987). Like mood disorders, how a person copes with stress impacts the outcome of rehabilitation efforts (Kennedy et al., 2011). In general, active coping strategies are oriented toward confronting, addressing, and/or cognitively reinterpreting the problem, and avoidance strategies are oriented toward reducing tension by avoiding the problem (Holahan & Moos, 1987). Active coping strategies such as accepting an intractable situation, trying to see the positive side, and learning more about the problem are associated with adaptation and improved rehabilitation outcomes (Kennedy et al., 2011). Avoidance strategies, such as trying to reduce tension by drinking (see Procedures for Practice 3-2) and avoiding people in general, are associated with distress and compromised effort in rehabilitation (Kennedy et al., 2011).

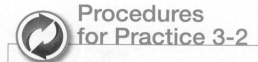

Procedures for Practice 3-2

Assessing Possible Substance Abuse

Alcohol use is a risk factor for traumatic onset of injury and disability such as spinal cord and brain injury (Andelic et al., 2010) and may be a factor in long-term adjustment to disability (Koponen et al., 2011; Tate et al., 2004). Kolakowsky-Hayner et al. (1999) found alarmingly high rates of preinjury heavy drinking among patients who were treated in a level I trauma center and subsequently in rehabilitation (57% of patients admitted with spinal cord injury and 42% of patients admitted with traumatic brain injury). Preinjury substance abuse has been associated with worse rehabilitation outcomes (Bogner et al., 2001) and predicts postinjury substance abuse (Kolakowsky-Hayner et al., 1999). Despite the implications for rehabilitation, health care providers are often reluctant to ask patients about substance use because of time constraints, lack of knowledge, and reluctance to intervene (Taj, Devera-Sales, & Vinson, 1998).

An occupational therapist who suspects that a patient is a substance abuser has an ethical obligation (Moyers & Stoffel, 1999) to perform a screening test and, if indicated, refer the patient for further assessment and intervention. Here are two screening methods.

- Ask a pointed question. Taj, Devera-Sales, and Vinson (1998) were able to identify 74% of at-risk or problem drinkers when physicians incorporated a simple question into their routine examinations ("On any single occasion during the past 3 months, have you had more than five drinks containing alcohol?"). They presented the alcohol screening question between two other general health questions ("In the past 3 months, have you used tobacco?" and "Do you regularly wear your seat belt when riding in the car?"; p. 329).
- Use a mnemonic when interviewing clients about suspected alcohol abuse. The CAGE Questionnaire (Ewing, 1984) asks four questions related to patients' perceptions of need to **cut** down, **annoyance** with criticism, **guilt** about drinking, and need for a drink as an **eye-opener** first thing in the morning.

The good news is that anyone can learn active coping strategies, thoughts, and actions (Quale & Schanke, 2010). Experts recommend trying to identify maladaptive coping strategies early on in the rehabilitation process and then promoting active coping strategies in rehabilitation to maximize treatment efficacy (Hall et al., 2011). Throughout the episode of care, occupational therapists informally take notice of patients' coping patterns and talk with patients about how they have coped with other stressful events, reinforcing past episodes of resilience when possible.

Spirituality

Spirituality refers to the beliefs and practices about the world and one's place in it that give a person transcendent meaning in life (Egan & Swedersky, 2003; Pulchaski & Romer, 2000). These beliefs may be expressed as a religious faith or directed toward nature, family, or community. It reflects a person's overriding system of meaning that influences use of time, choice of actions, and perceptions of purpose. As such, spirituality is central to a person's coping and occupational function (Christiansen, 1997). Therapists who incorporate spirituality into their practice do so by dealing with clients' religious concerns, encouraging patients' core sense of self, and addressing or confronting patients' experience of suffering (Egan & Swedersky, 2003). These connections with clients become opportunities for the therapist's development as well (Egan & Swedersky, 2003). Procedures for Practice 3-3 describes ways to discuss coping, spiritual beliefs, and meaning systems with patients.

Cultural Background and Identity

Because of the increasingly diverse populations in most communities, occupational therapists consider the influence of culture on occupational therapy assessment and occupational functioning (Suarez-Balcazar et al., 2009). Culture is broadly defined as a system of learned and shared guidelines for perceiving, interpreting, and interacting with others and the environment that informs values, beliefs, and behavior (Jezewski & Sotnik, 2001).

Culture is not biologically inherited or determined by geography or ethnicity (Krefting, 1991). Ethnicity has to do with group norms and practices associated with a person's culture of origin (Breland & Ellis, 2012). It may

 Procedures for Practice 3-3

Assessing Patients' Coping, Spiritual Beliefs, and Meaning Systems

People typically share personal information with those they trust. Therefore, to explore patients' beliefs and meaning systems, therapists invest in establishing therapeutic rapport (see Chapter 14). Without the rapport that comes with time and consistency of care providers, patients may perceive questions about their spirituality, for example, as intrusive or offensive. Therapists who are aware of their own coping strategies and belief systems will be best able to comfortably discuss these issues with their patients.

In general, discussions of these very personal and potentially sensitive matters begin at a superficial level and progress to deeper, more personal levels as dictated by the patient and therapist's comfort with each other and the subject matter. Here are examples of this progression.

- Ask the client to provide an hour-by-hour account of a typical day prior to the injury or onset of illness (Radomski, 1995). How a person is used to spending his or her time richly defines his or her valued activities and priorities.
- Take a brief life history, asking the patient to give you an overview of his or her life course, including past goals and obstacles (Kleinman, 1988). People often use stories or narratives to make connections and meaning attributions between a series of life events (Mattingly, 1991).
- Ask the patient about his or her explanatory model of the illness or disability. Kleinman (1988) suggested that faced with illness, disability, or suffering, people attempt to construct models to explain the whys of their experiences. They make attributions about causation and outcome that are more likely to be based on personal beliefs and culture than on facts or medical information. For example,

patients may feel responsible for permanent impairments because they did not try hard enough in rehabilitation to overcome them (Luborsky, 1997). If the person views onset of illness or disability as God's punishment for a past sin or mistake, he or she may not feel empowered to invest in rehabilitation efforts. Only as patients' explanatory models are acknowledged may they be negotiated with the therapist or health care team (Kleinman, 1988).

- To begin to understand the role of spirituality in patients' lives, ask them questions about meaning and past experiences in which their coping skills were taxed, such as the following (Cox & Waller, 1991; Mattison, 2006):
  1. What gives your life meaning? What is your greatest hope?
  2. When you are discouraged and feeling despondent, what keeps you going?
  3. What comforts or encourages you? Where have you found strength in the past?
  4. What have you done in the past when you have lost someone or something important?
  5. What do you think the message in this is for you?
- Pulchaski and Romer (2000) recommended an acronym (FICA) for aspects of a spiritual assessment: *F*, faith; *I*, importance and influence; *C*, community; and *A*, address.
  F. What things do you believe in that give meaning to your life?
  I. How have your beliefs influenced your behavior during this illness? What roles do your beliefs play in regaining your health?
  C. Are you a part of a spiritual or religious community? Is this a support to you and how?
  A. How would you like me, your health care provider, to address these issues in your health care?

have implications in economic, social, and political realms but contributes little to a therapist's appreciation of a patient's personal context. Furthermore, clinicians are cautioned about the reliability and accuracy of ethnic designations in hospital records (Stansbury et al., 2004). Because there is as much variation within ethnic groups as between them, a person's ethnic background is not a reliable gauge of his or her cultural identity.

The influence of culture on a person's experience is dynamic and individualized and may exert obvious or subtle influences on how people cope with disability. Consider the rehabilitation challenges of a recent immigrant from India with a right hemiplegia who refuses to feed herself with her left hand because in her culture, the left hand is always relegated for personal hygiene tasks (Pinto & Sahu, 2001). Although cultural rules are learned, they are also graded, flexible, task- and environment-specific, and often self-selected. For example, the degree to which immigrants have assimilated the customs and patterns of behavior of their new country or region is determined by how recently they emigrated, the primary language spoken at home, and the amount of contact with their homeland (Krefting, 1991). People adopt the culture of specific subgroups and environments; the expectations for behavior of a clinician in an occupational therapy clinic are different from expectations for a broker working at the New York Stock Exchange.

Culture and Occupational Performance

Cultural background and identity have implications for the ways in which occupational therapists understand social interactions, activities of daily living (ADL), and performance on standardized assessments. As illustrated earlier, occupational therapists consider the influence of various cultural aspects of communication, such as beliefs about communication based on social hierarchy, turn-taking in conversation, forms of address (using first or surnames), use of gestures, and concept of personal space (Hearnden, 2008). The cultural overtones of ADL are also particularly salient to occupational therapists. Because the nature of ADL routines (importance and frequency) is highly personal and differs between cultural groups and even between generations within the same ethnic group, Jezewski and Sotnik (2001) recommend considering three key questions when working with patients who are members of foreign-born groups:

- Are there differences in ADL activities in the person's country of origin in comparison to how they are performed in the United States?
- How do persons with disabilities perform ADL in the culture of origin?
- Given his or her cultural background, how might the individual respond to receiving assistance in these personal activities (p. 19)?

Culturally Aware Therapists

Although therapists' cultural awareness appears to be associated with more years of experience (Suarez-Balcazar et al., 2009), all occupational therapists take responsibility for providing culturally sensitive services. Clinicians can begin to understand potential cultural influences on performance by using resources such as those available through the Center for International Rehabilitation Research Information & Exchange (CIRRIE) (http://cirrie.buffalo.edu/). However, the dynamic influence of culture on human experience requires that clinicians resist attempts to characterize or stereotype clients based on ethnic or geographical background. Rather, occupational therapists attempt to recognize and then step outside of their own cultural backgrounds and biases to appreciate and accept the culturally based customs, values, and beliefs of each client (Procedures for Practice 3-4).

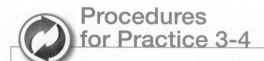

Procedures for Practice 3-4

Cultural Assessment

Experts advise against using cultural cookbooks to gain insights about culturally based habits and behaviors of various ethnic groups, as they can lead to stereotyping individual patients (Lipson, 1996). Instead, therapists consider the unique influence of culture on each individual's experience by carefully attending to nuances of body language, word choice, and gestures and adopting an attitude of curiosity about each client's situation and background (Bonder, Martin, & Miracle, 2004).

Lipson (1996, p. 3) suggested the following questions as key elements of a cultural assessment of any patient. Occupational therapists may get the answers to these questions in the medical record or talk directly with patients or loved ones.

- Where was the person born? If an immigrant, how long has the patient lived in this country?
- What is the patient's ethnic affiliation and how strong is the patient's ethnic identity?
- Who are the client's major support people, family members or friends? Does he or she live in an ethnic community?
- What are the primary and secondary languages and the speaking and reading ability?
- How would you characterize the nonverbal communication style?
- What is the person's religion, its importance in daily life, and current practices?
- What are his or her food preferences and prohibitions?
- What is the person's economic situation, and is the income adequate to meet the needs of the patient and family?
- What are the health and illness beliefs and practices?
- What are the customs and beliefs around such transitions as birth, illness, and death?

Finally, culturally aware occupational therapists understand that many evaluation tools are based on norms developed for a white middle-class population (Krefting, 1991; Paul, 1995). Culturally reflective clinicians assess the cultural validity of their standardized assessment tools (Krefting, 1991). While clinicians try to select criterion- and norm-referenced tests appropriate for the person's background, it is very difficult to devise culturally unbiased tests that include only items that reflect the knowledge, experience, and skills common to all cultures (Paul, 1995). Because it is nearly impossible to locate culture-specific tools for all of the diverse cultural groups in North America, therapists must make every effort to attempt to understand a client's individual cultural background before interpreting performance on the most appropriate standardized tests.

SOCIAL CONTEXT

"Every long winded well-meaning expression of sympathy was a giant highlighting marker over the fact that I was different. Our family's misfortune now set us apart. More than anything I wanted people to treat me like the old Lee" (Woodruff & Woodruff, 2007, p. 253).

Onset of disability occurs within the social context of the person's social resources, roles, and preferences that together influence occupational pursuits, satisfaction, health, and well-being (Helliwell & Putnam, 2004). For example, some people select tasks and activities that put them in contact with a social network; others select occupations that allow them to avoid social interaction, as in the case of individual preferences for hobbies or careers. Social networks may facilitate an individual's chosen occupations through emotional support, assistance, or instruction; unfortunately, some social relationships interfere with a person's optimal function. Only if occupational therapists are aware of the social context in which occupational function occurs can they orchestrate intervention that will outlive their own involvement in a client's recovery and adaptation.

Social Network and Support

The characteristics of a person's social network and support are relatively stable social contextual factors that influence his or her identity, opportunities, and function. Langford et al. (1997) suggested that a social network is an interactive web of people who provide each other with help and protection; that is, they give and receive social support. Social networks vary in terms of the following characteristics: reciprocity (extent to which resources and support are both given and received), intensity (extent to which social relationships offer emotional closeness), complexity (extent to which social relationships serve many functions), and density (extent to which network members know and interact with each other) (Heaney & Israel, 1997). Social support is defined as aid and assistance exchanged through social relationships and interactions (Heaney & Israel, 1997). This dynamic construct is composed of (1) social companionship and daily emotional support, (2) assistance (physical, informational, and emotional) during times of trouble, and (3) exchanges that contribute to self-esteem and approval (van Leeuwen et al., 2010).

Occupational therapists are fundamentally interested in patients' social networks because families and caregivers play a pivotal role in the patients' care and quality of life (McPherson et al., 2011). Additionally, the nature of a patient's social support appears to influence his or her life satisfaction over time, with functionally dependent persons who receive little social support at particular risk for poor adjustment (van Leeuwen et al., 2010). Therefore, during the assessment, occupational therapists first try to identify the composition and characteristics of the client's social network (i.e., who these individuals are and the nature of their relationships). Occupational therapists must step outside of their own possible biases and expectations to appreciate that patients' social networks take many forms, including traditional nuclear families, same-sex partners, friendships, and acquaintances. Any biases against nontraditional families are not aligned with the profession's stance on nondiscrimination and inclusion (American Occupational Therapy Association, 2009).

Therapists also attempt to determine the types of support that individuals in the social network are willing and able to provide. For example, long-standing intimate ties typically provide emotional support and long-term assistance, whereas neighbors and friends most often provide short-term instrumental and informational support (Heaney & Israel, 1997). Key players in the social network assume as much or as little responsibility as they are able, and the patient–family unit becomes the primary recipient of occupational therapy services (Brown, Humphry, & Taylor, 1997). Therapists can learn a lot about patients' social networks and resources by simply talking with them. An alternative method of assessing a patient's social network and resources is the Norbeck Social Support Questionnaire (Norbeck, Lindsey, & Carrieri, 1981). It is a standardized, self-administered questionnaire consisting of nine items and taking about 10 minutes to complete. Patients list individuals in their personal network and specify the nature of these relationships, the frequency of contact, and the extent to which they provide emotional and tangible support

Finally, occupational therapists appreciate that some social relationships are harmful to patients. Accredited hospitals and rehabilitation facilities are mandated to have policies in place to identify patients who may be victims of physical assault, sexual assault, and domestic or elder abuse or neglect (Joint Commission on Accreditation of Healthcare Organizations, 2010). Therapists must familiarize themselves with employers' policies and procedures that describe how to report, document, and respond to cases of suspected maltreatment. For example, at Mercy and Unity Hospitals in suburban Minneapolis, physical and occupational therapists are expected to screen all outpatients for family violence (J. L. Miller, personal communication, August 26, 2011).

Caregiver Adaptation: A Dynamic Social Factor

Long-standing intimate ties in the patient's social network (hereafter also referred to as family) are critical to the patient's ability to adapt to chronic illness and disability. Families influence outcome of services because they provide a context for individual change and because they represent continuity in patients' lives (Brown, Humphry, & Taylor, 1997). The ability of significant others to provide needed support, however, is shaped by their own emotional and physical health and place in the adaptation process (Grant et al., 2000). Many relatives of persons with traumatic brain injury (Webster, Daisley, & King, 1999), stroke (Epstein-Lubow et al., 2009), multiple sclerosis (Figved et al., 2007), and Alzheimer's disease (Pruchno & Potashnik, 1989), for example, experience significant levels of subjective burden and mood disorders as well as role changes in work, leisure, and social life (Frosch et al., 1997). To contribute to patients' long-term quality of life, occupational therapists assess family members' adaptation needs on an ongoing basis.

All of the personal, social, and cultural contextual factors described in this chapter can be applied to the significant other's occupational functioning as caregiver. That is, a spouse's ability to learn and reinforce new techniques and strategies is affected by his or her own health concerns and distractions, age and generation, sex, mood, cultural background, makeup of the social network, and culture of the community (Murray, Manktelow, & Clifford, 2000). Furthermore, caregivers' goals and perceptions of need from health providers change as they adapt to the patient's illness or injury.

In their pioneering study, Corbin and Strauss (1988) described the work of adapting to chronic disability over time as "a set of tasks performed by an individual or couple, alone or in conjunction with others, to carry out a plan of action designed to manage one or more aspects of the illness" (p. 9). This work consists of not only adjustments to self-maintenance tasks and roles but also the work involved in redefining one's identity. Corbin and Strauss used the term *illness trajectory* to refer to the sequence of physiological changes associated with an illness, injury, or disorder and the adaptive work demanded of a patient and family that accompanies each phase. They further suggested that most trajectories have five types of phases, distinctly ordered according to various diagnoses and individual courses: acute, comeback, stable, unstable, and downward.

- Acute phase. The patient requires immediate medical attention and focuses on physiological stabilization and recovery. Patient and family may wonder how life will change because of the illness, injury, or disorder.
- Comeback phase. The patient is in the midst of physical and emotional recovery and focuses on getting physically well and regaining functional abilities. Patient and family may ask questions such as these: Will I (he or she) come back? How long will it take before I (he or she) peak? Corbin & Strauss (1988) explain that "in the comeback trajectory, the present is seen as overbearing, and the future is put on hold while one awaits answers to the foregoing questions" (p. 46).
- Stable phase. The patient undergoes very few changes in the course of illness or functional abilities, as in the remission phase of multiple sclerosis or permanent spinal cord injury. Patient and family focus on maintaining stable health while wondering how long the phase will last and what can be done to extend it.
- Unstable phase. The patient has periodic but erratic downturns in function or exacerbations of illness (as might come, for example, with bladder infection). Unstable phases hamper normal living, and people in this phase ask questions like these: How long until we get this under control? How much longer can I (or we) go on like this?
- Downward phase. The patient slowly or rapidly loses health and function. With increasing incapacity, the patient and family view the present as temporary and the future as unknown. They are concerned with questions such as these: How fast and how far? When will it end? What can we do to slow it down?

Although there are no standardized methods for determining a person's phase in an illness trajectory, sensitivity to each person's changing path in this journey is prerequisite to creating a treatment plan that meshes with patient and family real-time needs and priorities. A family-centered approach allows the therapist to capitalize on the family's priorities and contributions to the patient's recovery and adaptation. This mindset, however, requires that therapists "follow the family's lead rather than impose professional decisions" (Brown, Humphry, & Taylor, 1997, p. 598).

Patient–Therapist Social Interactions

Occupational therapy assessment is not a neutral process (Luborsky, 1997). Gans (1998) suggests, "Part of the way the patient behaves with you is a function of the way you are with the patient. This effect may comprise 75%, 25%, or 2% of what goes on between you and the patient, but it is there" (p. 4). The therapist is endowed with power to shape the interaction by selecting certain questions and omitting others (Luborsky, 1995), to judge or evaluate the responses of the patient, and even to determine whose expectations and "reality" are correct (Abberley, 1995). Therapists' communication patterns set the tone for patient experience. For example, when providers are perceived as unfriendly, interrupt, or fail to encourage questions and dialogue about concerns, patients report less satisfaction with the services they receive (Abdulhadi et al., 2007).

Perhaps to meet self-imposed expectations around outcome, Abberley (1995) suggested that some occupational therapists unwittingly define the client as the problem and themselves as the solution, with failure of intervention always attributed to the patient and success always credited to the clinician's efforts. Gans (1998) believes that a primary source of clinician gratification should stem from "the privilege of participating intimately in another person's life" (p. 5). He further suggests that when the work no longer feels like a privilege, one should try to figure out why (e.g., volume of caseload, private life that is distracting or burdensome, burnt out, or ethically questionable employer expectations that corrode integrity). Effective occupational therapists take steps to manage the stresses associated with patients' overwhelming challenges (Stevenson, Phillips, & Anderson, 2011) so that their personal needs do not infiltrate into social interactions with patients.

Clinicians also examine their expectations of their own supportive roles in patients' lives. They recognize that professional helpers are typically not able to provide support over long periods. They realize that professional–lay relationships are not characterized by reciprocity typical of social networks and often entail invisible but palpable power differentials that interfere with the provision of genuine emotional support (Heaney & Israel, 1997). In essence, they realize that, as professionals, they should not attempt to assume a long-term role in the social network but rather work with the patient and family to create permanent social links that meet the patient's needs.

CULTURAL CONTEXT OF THE LARGER SOCIETY AND COMMUNITY

"I used to dream about being in a world where being disabled was no big deal, where no one considered it a tragedy. No one thought you were inspiring or felt sorry for you. . . . I imagined what a relief it would be to be seen every day as perfectly ordinary." (Tollifson, 1997, p. 105)

The dominant culture influences the ease with which a person with a disability feels accepted and integrated into the community. Luborsky (1994) suggested that culturally based requirements for the status of a full adult person

in Europe and North America, such as self-sufficiency, activity, and upright posture, are often at odds with full participation for persons with disabilities. Adapted equipment may be rejected because of its appearance and acceptability in public rather than its functional value (Luborsky, 1994, 1997). Patients and family may respond to embarrassment or guilt over disability by attempting to keep the disability private and refusing help from friends or neighbors (Armstrong & Fitzgerald, 1996). Loss of social status is further compounded when insidious cultural beliefs hold persons with disabilities responsible for their impairments or as having varying degrees of deservedness in terms of accommodation and assistance (Askew, 2011). "At a deep level there is a bias that either they are culpable for the cause of the impairment, or for not working harder at rehabilitation to be able to 'overcome' the odds regardless of how realistic that is" (Luborsky, 1994, p. 251). As abhorrent and illogical as such notions are, patients, families, and occupational therapists are not immune to the subtle but pervasive influences of the sociocultural context in which they live.

Occupational therapists are challenged to check many of their own assumptions about people with disabilities. For example, Kielhofner (2005) reminded us that the person-first terminology that therapists are urged to use is objectionable to some disability activists and scholars who suggest that the term "disabled person" more accurately reflects his or her true minority status. Many people resent the notion that their impairments reflect some sort of personal tragedy (Wakefield, 2005; Watson, 2002) and, instead, view their disability with pride as a part of their identity (Eddey & Robey, 2005). However, while some interpret rehabilitation and remediation of impairments as an effort to remove a flaw or a negative characteristic (Kielhofner, 2005), rehabilitation hospital settings may nurture growth, self-redefinition, and even personal transformation after sudden-onset disability (Devlieger, Albrecht, & Hertz, 2007).

PAYER-REIMBURSEMENT CONTEXT

Laws and health care policies influence the nature and intensity of occupational therapy services available to a given patient by dictating the services he or she is eligible to receive and the extent to which services are reimbursed. The payer-reimbursement context for various health care settings may drive the type and length of assessment, availability of tools and equipment, and methods used in practice.

Consider how the payer-reimbursement context influences the nature of occupational therapy assessment and intervention in the following scenario. Mrs. J. is a 60-year-old woman who experienced sudden-onset left hemiparesis. An ambulance transported Mrs. J. to a certified stroke center, at which she received evaluation by medical specialists, imaging, and tissue plasminogen activator (tPA). (If provided within an established time frame, tPA can significantly reduce the effects of stroke and permanent disability.) Mrs. J. was admitted to the neurointensive care unit and within 2 days was evaluated by an occupational therapist. The occupational therapy assessment suggested that Mrs. J. had a very active lifestyle before her stroke but now has left hemiparesis of the arm and leg and slight left facial droop. She required moderate assistance for eating, grooming, dressing, bathing, toileting, functional transfers, and mobility. Mrs. J.'s ability to perform instrumental activities of daily living was not assessed. Occupational therapy in the intensive care unit and on the acute stroke floor was provided at bedside because Mrs. J. had multiple IVs and was being monitored for cardiac arrhythmias. The goals were to improve participation in activities of daily living and functional mobility. Because her stroke diagnosis was included in the Centers for Medicare and Medicaid Services (CMS) 13 qualifying diagnoses for inpatient rehabilitation and she required multiple therapies (physical therapy, occupational therapy, and speech-language pathology), Mrs. J. was admitted to the inpatient rehabilitation unit 5 days after the onset of her stroke. Her therapy focus shifted from basic daily activities to restoration of function for eventual return home. Mrs. J. continued to demonstrate significant improvement and progressed to supervision for daily activities. She had hoped to stay in the inpatient rehabilitation setting until she reached an independent level; however, her insurance placed a limit on her length of stay. After discharge, Mrs. J. planned to transition to outpatient rehabilitation with the goals of increased independence for home and community reintegration, including eventual return to work and driving.

This scenario illustrates how occupational therapists need to understand payer-reimbursement aspects of the contextual picture so that they use patients' covered services in ways that yield the most benefit and value. To that end, occupational therapists understand governmental policies and laws and stay abreast of ongoing changes to the health care system.

Governmental Policies and Laws

Many Americans' health care services are paid for by government-funded programs such as Medicare and Medicaid. One of the largest payers of occupational therapy services is Medicare, a federally administered health insurance program for people age 65 years and older, those of all ages with end-stage renal disease, and those under age 65 years with certain qualifying disabilities. Divided into two parts, Medicare A and Medicare B, this program helps to cover inpatient care in hospitals and skilled nursing centers, as well as some aspects of hospice and home health care, and outpatient services, including physician

visits and those medically necessary services provided by occupational therapy practitioners (CMS, 2005b).

Another government-administered health insurance program is Medicaid. Medicaid is designed to assist low-income individuals and families who fit into specific eligibility groups that are established by federal and state law (CMS, 2005a). Although funded by the federal government, Medicaid is administered individually by states. Each state is permitted to establish its own guidelines for both Medicaid eligibility and the coverage of services (CMS, 2005a). Requirements can vary significantly from state to state for both recipients and service providers. Occupational therapy services may or may not be covered under Medicaid. When services are covered, the conditions warranting care are specifically identified, and there may be requirements regarding the frequency and duration of occupational therapy services for which Medicaid will pay.

According to the CMS (formerly the Health Care Financing Administration), private insurance funds approximately one-third of total health care service and primarily cover children and adults under the age of 65 years who are not disabled (Federal Interagency Forum on Aging-Related Statistics, 2004; Henry J. Kaiser Family Foundation, 2007). Public programs including Medicare, Medicaid, and the State Children's Health Insurance Program fund approximately 45% of health care spending for Americans (Federal Interagency Forum on Aging-Related Statistics, 2004; Henry J. Kaiser Family Foundation, 2007). Medicaid covered 7% of health care costs of Medicare enrollees age 65 years and older; out-of-pocket costs account for approximately 19%, with another 4% from other funds such as foundations (Federal Interagency Forum on Aging-Related Statistics, 2010).

Beyond Medicare and Medicaid, there are other government-sponsored health programs. Depending on state law, those who are injured on the job are frequently covered under workers' compensation. People who are under the age of 65 years and are disabled may be able to apply for state or federal assistance. Health care from the Veterans Administration is available for veterans of the U.S. military. Those who are uninsured may be eligible to apply for state assistance under the Medicaid system or may need to pay privately for health care services.

Consider how payer-reimbursement factors have influenced occupational therapy practice in the following brief history of Medicare. In 1966, Medicare was enacted as a means of providing health coverage for the elderly (age 65 years and older) and the disabled. In 1983, Congress implemented the Medicare Prospective Payment System (PPS) for acute care hospitals in an effort to contain costs and standardize care. Acute care hospital PPS is based on more than 490 diagnostic related groups (DRGs). Since the enactment of the DRGs, temporary exemption has been in effect for rehabilitation hospitals and units, children's hospitals and units, alcohol and drug programs, long-term care, cancer specialty hospitals, and psychiatric hospitals and units. The impact of the DRGs was significant. Hospital lengths of stay became shorter, and discharges to all types of postacute care providers rose (such as inpatient rehabilitation facilities, skilled nursing facilities, and long-term care hospitals). The Balanced Budget Act (Balanced Budget Act of 1997) enacted and mandated PPS for nursing facilities, rehabilitation hospitals and units, and home health agencies. Skilled nursing was included in the PPS in 1998 that based payment on a per diem allowance. Home health was included in 2000, and payment for that was based per episode of care. Inpatient rehabilitation was included in 2002, and payment was based per discharge.

Changes in Medicare policy over time have influenced occupational therapy practice in all of the aforementioned settings. Shorter acute care lengths resulted in fewer occupational therapy sessions, with a greater focus on discharge-readiness assessment than intervention. Similarly, the duration of inpatient rehabilitation services is shaped, in part, by condition-specific Medicare payment. As a result, occupational therapists often focus on helping patients meet self-care goals during inpatient rehabilitation and address issues associated with community and work reintegration during other phases of the continuum of care.

Standards of occupational therapy practice also reflect priorities of regulatory agencies such as the Joint Commission on Accreditation of Healthcare Organizations (TJC), the U.S. Department of Health and Human Services, fiscal intermediaries, and the Commission on Accreditation for Rehabilitation Facilities (CARF). For example, within hospital or institutional care settings, services must be prescribed by a physician and provided under a physician-approved plan of care; services must be performed by a qualified occupational therapist or an occupational therapy assistant under the supervision of an occupational therapist; and services provided must be reasonable and necessary for the individual's illness or injury. In addition to these requirements, regulations can also place limits on the amount of therapy intervention, including the amount of time services are provided and the overall length of service provision, requiring the therapist to outline and provide a plan of care within these guidelines.

Health Care Reform

There are continual changes to the health care delivery system that will shape the future payer-reimbursement context. The Patient Protection and Affordable Care Act of 2010 will bring the most significant changes to American health care since the prospective payment reform in 1983. Health reform law introduces important changes for health care providers that will unfold over the next decade. Between the years 2010 and 2013, we will see regulation and coverage changes. Major changes slated to occur in 2014 are expected to bend the cost curve by 2015–2020. The health care landscape will continue to evolve as providers experiment with new models and work to achieve integration through accountable care organizations, medical homes, value-based purchasing, and/or bundling.

Accountable Care Organizations

Many believe the key to health care reform is the development of an efficient, affordable primary care delivery system that is patient-centered, coordinated, team-based care and supported by health information technology. Accountable care organizations, or ACOs, are a proposed system design and payment reform solution to address rapidly rising health care costs, related inefficiencies within the current health care delivery system (duplication of services, for example), and poor health outcomes experienced by many Americans. The goal of an ACO is to create an integrated network of providers in order to improve individual and population level health outcomes and control costs. Services delivered across the continuum of care (in hospitals, outpatient clinics, primary care centers, community clinics, inpatient rehabilitation, skilled nursing facilities, etc.) and throughout the life span will be integrated and coordinated, and providers will be held jointly accountable for patients' outcomes (Lowell & Bertko, 2010; McClellan et al., 2010). Occupational therapy practitioners have roles to play in every facet of an ACO, including providing expert guidance on client-centered care and contributing to the governance structure that oversees the management of the ACO.

Medical Home

The medical home has emerged as a promising model for transforming organization and delivery of primary care to address care fragmentation and dismantling the silos in health care delivery. The medical home is also known as the primary care medical home, advanced primary care, and the health care home. However, the model is most commonly referred to as the patient-centered medical home (PCMH), emphasizing the central tenet that quality care is always patient centered. Under the PCMH, each patient is assigned to a personal physician practice that is held accountable for providing, coordinating, and evaluating care (Gulley et al., 2011). Many of the principles driving the efforts to transform primary care align with core occupational therapy beliefs and values and thus the opportunity exists for occupational therapy practitioners to engage in educating primary care providers on how to provide care that is truly patient centered and relevant to daily life across the life span.

Value-Based Purchasing

On May 6, 2011, the CMS released its hospital value-based purchasing final rule, which was required under the Patient Protection and Affordable Care Act (U.S. Department of Health and Human Services, 2011). This final rule relates specially to Medicare reimbursement; however, private payers may follow CMS's lead. Value-based purchasing means that Medicare reimbursement will be based on quality achievements that link payment to performance. Higher quality achievements will receive higher payment. Medicare value-based purchasing will likely include four components: reporting hospital quality data for annual payment update (RHQDAPU) based on specific quality indicators, a penalty/reward system based on metrics from the RHQDAPU, a payment penalty for certain negative conditions that are hospital acquired, and a payment penalty for high readmissions rate as compared to peers (Department of Health and Human Services, 2011). Value-based purchasing aims to transform Medicare from a passive payer of claims based on volume of care to an active purchaser of care that is based on quality of services.

Bundling

Bundling payment, especially bundling acute and post-acute payment into one payment is a potential way to make acute care hospitals accountable for hospital readmissions, as well as bring greater efficiencies and cost savings to an entire episode of care. Bundling across providers for services is designed to result in better coordination and continuity of care across settings. Better coordinated care may reduce unnecessary duplication of services and potentially decrease medical errors and cost. Bundling payment, which seems conceptually quite simple, is complex and will require testing and demonstrations that will allow health systems to experiment with various models (MedPAC, 2008). It is important for occupational therapy services to be involved in the testing of these models to ensure that occupational therapy remains an important and viable service.

Staying Engaged and Informed

Health care reform needs to equally and equitably distribute the costs and benefits of quality health care to all individuals. To that end, occupational therapy professionals must be aware of legislative and regulatory activities that may impact the practice of occupational therapy. For example, yearly in the *Federal Register*, revisions to payment policies under the physician fee schedule are published. These revisions impact reimbursement for health care services including the reimbursement and regulatory situations that impact the delivery of occupational therapy.

Ultimately, each practitioner needs to be accountable for the value of services provided and integrated with other practitioners to ensure optimal outcome. Measuring and improving the value of occupational therapy remains a central priority of the profession (Porter, 2010). **It is important for every occupational therapy practitioner to be a member of their national and state occupational therapy organizations in order to shape the future of occupational therapy for the clients we serve in the context of health care reform.**

GENERAL COMMENTS ON CONSIDERING PERSONAL, SOCIAL, CULTURAL, AND PAYER-REIMBURSEMENT CONTEXT

Zooming in to identify and quantify specific barriers to occupational functioning and zooming out to observe contextual factors that may influence assessment methods and a patient's performance promise to result in the client-centered services to which our profession aspires. Enacting such practices in real life requires clinician commitment and vigilance. If nothing else, the discussion of contextual factors underscores that occupational therapists ought to not get too comfortable with their findings, scores, or impressions and ought to learn to tolerate the ambiguity of "it just depends." The imposing influence of contextual variables serves to keep us humble and on-guard against jumping to the wrong conclusions about assessment findings and our clients.

Occupational therapists struggle to balance their preeminent concerns for service to patients with very real demands for efficiency and productivity. Clinicians typically devote 30 minutes to 3 hours assessing each patient; the short lengths of stay in acute settings allow less time; inpatient rehabilitation settings (with possibly longer stays) allow somewhat more. How does one have time to assess the web of personal, social, and cultural contextual factors on top of all pertinent areas of occupational function (roles, tasks, activities, abilities and skills, and capacities)? Here are some general guidelines:

- Review the assessments of other professionals. Many patients who are referred to occupational therapy are also assessed by social workers, psychologists, speech-language pathologists, physical therapists, physicians, therapeutic recreation specialists, chaplains, and/or nurses. Reviewing the assessments of team members greatly adds to the occupational therapist's ability to understand a patient's personal, social, and cultural context without using limited assessment time to do so.
- Take advantage of informal conversations with patients. Luborsky (1997) pointed out the value of attending to patients' informal remarks made during structured assessments. He described how a patient's

comments during transitions between various standardized tools provide insights not captured by the tools themselves. He further stated that patients' informal remarks "can be essential to gaining an understanding of the way subjects make sense of the assessment; to providing us with important information on the validity of the assessment tool; and to identifying important areas for clinical intervention" (p. 12).

- Keep in mind that contextual factors influence your clinician attitudes, habits, and practices as much as they are likely to impact the patient's occupational performance. Try to notice when you find yourself responding to situations and rushing to conclusions in ways that might be unduly influenced by contextual factors.

It is advisable to use each and every moment with patients to try to understand who they are, where they come from, and how they are interpreting their experience in therapy. Gans (1998) links this investment to patient outcome: "Our ongoing, relentless determination to understand the uniqueness of each patient is what the patient, to the degree he or she can, experiences as love . . . [and] patients who feel cared about and valued make the most gains in therapy" (p. 5). It is unrealistic to expect therapists to understand the full picture of all the factors that shape a patient's life and performance during an arbitrarily defined assessment period. The richness of conversations that relate to important contextual factors grows as the therapeutic relationship deepens and continues to inform the intervention process.

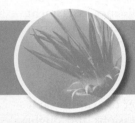

case example

Mrs. N.: Appreciating Context During Assessment

Occupational Therapy Assessment Process	Clinical Reasoning Process	
	Objectives	Examples of Therapist's Internal Dialogue
Patient Information Mrs. N., a 30-year-old wife and mother of three young children, was referred to outpatient occupational therapy for assessment and treatment approximately 6 months after a suspected brain injury. She was injured when a shelf at a convenience store broke and its contents fell on her head. After the accident, Mrs. N. frequently complained of headaches, fatigue, and dizziness accompanied by dramatic decrease in her activity level and was observed to be forgetful, even unsafe (e.g., leaving stove burners turned on, losing track of her children, forgetting to take medication). With a high school education, Mrs. N. worked full time as a teaching assistant at a day care center but was unable to return to work following her injury. As a recent immigrant from Saudi Arabia, Mrs. N. spoke very little English. (She spoke and wrote in Arabic.) The consulting neuropsychologist opted not to perform a battery of standardized cognitive assessments because of concerns about communication, cultural biases of the tests themselves, and possible religious discomfort associated with spending hours of assessment time with the neuropsychologist, a man. Therefore, assessment and observations in occupational therapy were particularly important in establishing her rehabilitation needs.	Understand the patient's diagnosis or condition	"Mrs. N.'s complaints and presentation are certainly consistent with a brain injury. It appears that she did not seek medical attention immediately after the accident and that she has never received any rehabilitation services. These symptoms must be frightening for her."
	Know the person	"It is going to be challenging for me to try to get to know Mrs. N. and to provide the kind of encouragement and support that I feel is so important to my approach with patients, given our language barriers."
	Appreciate the context	"I realize that I need an assessment strategy that is different from what I am used to. It would not make much sense for me to rely on scores from standardized tests. I will also be sensitive to the fact that it is possible that some of what Mrs. N. says to me may be lost in translation."
	Develop provisional hypotheses	"My guess is that some of Mrs. N.'s problems can be attributed to brain injury, but I wonder what effect anxiety and/or depression may have on her overall functioning."

Assessment Process

Mrs. N. appeared to doze in the waiting room prior to her initial occupational therapy session. She was cooperative and soft-spoken; she was able to respond in English to approximately 30% of the questions. She stayed awake for most of each of the three 1-hour assessment sessions. Mr. N., also a native of Saudi Arabia, served as translator but often dominated interactions with details of his own stress related to his wife's status. He appeared to be on the verge of tears on at least two occasions as he described his inability to work full time because of his wife's need for supervision, assistance, and transportation to medical appointments.

Consider evaluation approach and methods	"I think that I can learn the most about Mrs. N.'s functioning with a dynamic assessment approach—observing her response to various demands and challenges that I set up.

Patient's and Husband's Report of Abilities and Limitations

Through her husband, Mrs. N. indicated that she was primarily concerned about her memory and endurance and that her ultimate goals were to completely resume her roles as mother, homemaker, and worker. (At the time of her assessment, Mr. N. prepared all of the family meals, and their oldest daughter, age 9 years, did most of the household chores.) Through her husband, Mrs. N. indicated that she had very little activity or routine in her day. She woke anywhere between 8:00 am and noon. After rising, she sat for approximately half an hour, avoiding movement so as to avoid dizziness. She did not prepare meals for herself, eating only a cookie with tea instead of breakfast or lunch. She typically spent her afternoons napping, sitting alone at the window, or watching television. She fell asleep at approximately 9:00 pm, but her husband reported that he regularly found her crying in the middle of the night. Her inactivity contrasted dramatically with reports of her premorbid status: working full time, attending language and driving classes, managing all household tasks, caring for her children, and socializing with friends. With the patient's permission, the therapist also contacted Mrs. N.'s American-born, English-speaking sister-in-law, who confirmed the dramatic decline in Mrs. N.'s activity level and abilities, Mr. N.'s understandable stress given these changes, and her own willingness to serve as a resource.

Interpret observations	"Descriptions of Mrs. N.'s premorbid activities and her self-reports of long-term goals contradict my assumptions about Muslim women from the Middle East. Prior to meeting Mrs. N., I expected that Mrs. N. would have a narrow sphere of activities that centered exclusively on her home and children. Mrs. N.'s premorbid engagement in work outside of her home and language and driving lessons and her goals to return to these roles reminds me of the importance of trying to understand each patient as an individual rather than drawing conclusions based on cultural or ethnic stereotypes."

"It is helpful to get a snapshot of Mrs. N.'s functioning through her husband and her sister-in-law. I feel fairly confident that I am following all that Mr. N. is telling me, as his sister-in-law tells me much the same thing." |

Observations of Cognitive Function

Mrs. N. performed the Contextual Memory Test (CMT) (Toglia, 1993), a test of immediate and delayed recall of 20 pictures associated with morning hygiene. Her performance on this test suggested moderate memory deficits but adequate awareness of these limitations. Her husband translated instructions to a 10-step task to which she jotted notes. After a 25-minute delay and interference activities, she was able to use her own notes to carry out the task with 70% accuracy. She appeared to make errors because she did not carefully review her notes and approached two steps in what appeared to be a hasty and impulsive manner.

	"I know that I am supposed to follow the CMT's administration protocol, but under these circumstances, I just cannot. However, the picture format of this test might give me a sense of her ability to learn new information. I appreciate that the veracity of assessment findings are in question, as all responses were reported through her husband."

Observations of Performance of Functional Tasks

The therapist requested that Mrs. N. select a familiar stove-top meal to prepare in occupational therapy and asked her to bring necessary supplies and ingredients to one of her assessment sessions. Mr. N. reportedly reminded Mrs. N. to do so. As instructed by the therapist, Mrs. N. made an obvious effort to remember to turn off the stove burner once she finished preparing her dish. She sat next to the stove throughout the task, but having removed the pan from the stove to serve the food, she did not return to turn off the burner (which was left on for 5 minutes, until the therapist turned it off). She appeared well organized in her approach to the task, removing all ingredients and supplies from the cupboard ahead of time and cleaning up as she proceeded. Despite these efforts, she forgot to add one of the ingredients she had set out on the table and asked the therapist whether she had added another. Mrs. N. frequently requested rest during occupational therapy sessions that entailed physical activity. She generally tolerated approximately 5 minutes of standing or walking before requesting to sit and rest because of fatigue and dizziness. During one of the three sessions, Mrs. N. complained of headache and intermittently rested her head on the table.

	"I thought it would be a good idea to have Mrs. N. prepare a familiar dish so as to remove at least one novelty variable. I am impressed that she is willing to try every activity that I propose and that says a lot to me about her motivation to use therapy to improve her functioning."

Analysis of Results

Mrs. N.'s performance of functional tasks in occupational therapy seemed consistent with the kinds of problems reported at home by Mrs. N., her husband, and her sister-in-law. Specifically, Mrs. N.'s performance on pencil-and-paper and kitchen tasks were marked by forgetfulness, absent-mindedness, and poor endurance. Furthermore, given her dramatic decline in activity, reports of frequent crying and decreased appetite, the therapist was concerned about depression. Given his own stress, the therapist questioned whether Mr. N. would be able to maintain all of the roles he had assumed since his wife's injury.

The following recommendations were suggested as prerequisite to commencing occupational therapy treatment:

- Referral to a woman psychologist for further evaluation and treatment of possible mood disorder
- Referral to a neurologist specializing in balance disorders (she had never had this complaint exhaustively evaluated)
- Schedule of a family conference with Mrs. N.'s sister-in-law, brother-in-law, and attorney to make arrangements to assist Mr. N. at home, enabling him to put in more hours at work
- Work with the hospital patient representative to provide a translator for future occupational therapy sessions

Occupational Therapy Problem List

1. Decreased memory and concentration capabilities and inadequate strategies to compensate for these problems
2. Deconditioning associated with prolonged inactivity complicated by poor nutrition
3. Lack of structure or routine for daily activities and inability to judge independently which tasks were within her competence level

"I requested an interpreter from the patient representative, but it has taken a little longer than I would like to find someone. Our policies and procedures recommend against using a family member as an interpreter, and I can see that logic. Mr. N. has is own stresses and maybe his own agenda. He needs to be freed up to take care of his other responsibilities and I think it would be beneficial for Mrs. N. to participate in occupational therapy sessions on her own."

"I am concerned that Mrs. N. may not make substantive progress toward her goals if she is depressed, and so I recommended that she see a psychologist or psychiatrist before beginning occupational therapy intervention. Similarly, her complaints about dizziness have never been medically evaluated, and we need to find out what is going on. Given what Mr. and Mrs. N. have told me and what I have seen of Mrs. N.'s performance, I am very concerned about her safety at home. I am not confident in offering any definitive suggestions until I observe her in her own environment."

Synthesize results

"I have addressed similar issues with other clients, and I am confident I can help Mrs. N. address these problems as well."

Clinical Reasoning in Occupational Therapy Practice

Effects of Payer-Reimbursement Context on Occupational Therapy Service Provision

D.W. is a 58-year-old widowed man who was admitted to the hospital after a fall from a ladder during which he suffered a traumatic brain injury. D.W. underwent a craniotomy because of a subdural hematoma. Prior to the accident, he lived alone and worked full time as a construction worker. He does not have any family in the area but does have a son and daughter who live in another state. After the accident, he has both motor and cognitive deficits. D.W. has executive functioning cognitive deficits, is unable to utilize his dominant right upper extremity, requires maximal assistance with his activities of daily living (ADL), and is dependent with his instrumental activities of daily living (IADL). D.W.'s insurance is a health maintenance organization (HMO) that limits inpatient rehabilitation coverage and also limits outpatient occupational therapy coverage to 12 visits in a calendar year. Identify the contextual factors that affect occupational therapy service delivery. What considerations would need to be given for occupational therapy service provision?

Summary Review Questions

1. Consider your morning self-care routine—the activities you performed today to get ready to leave for school or work. List the personal, social, and contextual factors that influenced your performance. If someone who did not know you judged your performance, what aspects might they consider unusual? What aspects might he or she consider normal for someone of your age and background?
2. Write a paragraph describing the possible influences on occupational functioning of one of the contextual factors not discussed in this chapter. For example, how might geography, social class, or gender help or hinder performance?
3. Outline circumstances in which you would use standardized instruments to assess contextual factors and those in which you would use more informal methods.
4. Make a private list of your own biases. What assumptions do you have about people who are different from you in terms of age, sex, cultural and educational background, sexual orientation, and abilities (physical, cognitive, and emotional)? List the steps you can take to debunk these biases and measures to minimize their effects during interactions with patients.
5. Why is it important to identify maladaptive coping strategies during the occupational therapy assessment process?
6. If a patient reports low back pain during a homemaking assessment, what methods might you use to obtain more specific information about his or her complaints?
7. Summarize at least three ways in which social context may influence a stroke survivor's occupational performance.
8. Describe at least three ways in which a patient's cultural background might influence occupational therapy assessment.
9. What are at least two ways in which government and third-party reimbursement impact occupational therapy for patients with physical dysfunction?

Glossary

Context—The interrelated conditions or circumstances in which something occurs (*Webster's Third New International Dictionary*, 1993).

Cultural context—Stable and dynamic norms, values, and behaviors associated with the community or societal environments in which occupational functioning occurs.

Culture—A system of learned and shared guidelines for perceiving, interpreting, and interacting with others and the environment that informs values, beliefs, and behavior (Jezewski & Sotnik, 2001).

Ethnicity—Group norms and practices associated with one's culture of origin (Breland & Ellis, 2012). In and of itself, ethnicity does not predict cultural identity.

Payer-reimbursement context—Policies and regulations that determine availability and reimbursement of occupational therapy services in various settings.

Personal context—A person's internal environment, derived from stable and dynamic factors such as sex, age, mood, and cultural identity.

Social context—The social environment consisting of stable and dynamic factors such as premorbid roles, social network, and support resources.

Social network—An interactive web of people who provide each other with helpfulness and protection. Social networks typically vary in terms of reciprocity, complexity, intensity, and density (Heaney & Israel, 1997).

Social support—The aid and assistance (emotional, instrumental, information, and appraisal) exchanged through a social network (Heaney & Israel, 1997).

Spirituality—Beliefs and practices that give a person transcendent meaning in life (Pulchaski & Romer, 2000).

References

Abberley, P. (1995). Disabling ideology in health and welfare: The case of occupational therapy. *Disability and Society, 10,* 221–232.

Abdulhadi, N., Shafaee, M. A., Freudenthal, S., Östenson, C., & Wahlström, R. (2007). Patient-provider interaction from the perspectives of type 2 diabetes patients in Muscat, Oman: A qualitative study. *BMC Health Services Research, 7,* 162.

Agency for Healthcare Research and Quality. (2009). Rapid Estimate of Adult Literacy in Medicine–Short Form. *Health Literacy Measurement Tools.* Retrieved May 25, 2013 from http://www.ahrq.gov/professionals/quality-patient-safety/quality-resources/tools/literacy/index.html

American Occupational Therapy Association. (2008). Occupational Therapy Practice Framework: Domain and process (2nd ed.). *American Journal of Occupational Therapy, 62,* 625–683.

American Occupational Therapy Association. (2009). Occupational therapy's commitment to nondiscrimination and inclusion. *American Journal of Occupational Therapy, 63,* 819–820.

Amsters, D. I., Pershouse, K. J., Price, G. L., & Kendall, M. B. (2005). Long duration spinal cord injury: Perceptions of functional change over time. *Disability and Rehabilitation, 27,* 489–497.

Andelic, N., Jerstad, T., Sigurdardottir, S., Schanke, A. K., Sandvik, L., & Roe, C. (2010). Effects of acute substance use and pre-injury substance abuse on traumatic brain injury severity in adults admitted to a trauma centre. *Journal of Trauma Management Outcomes, 4,* 6.

Armstrong, M. J., & Fitzgerald, M. H. (1996). Culture and disability studies: An anthropological perspective. *Rehabilitation Education, 10,* 247–304.

Arozullah, A. M., Yarnold, P. R., Bennett, C. L., Soltysik, R. C., Wolf, M. S., Ferreira, R. M., Lee, S. Y., Costello, S., Shakir, A., Denwood, C., Bryant, F. B., & Davis, T. (2007). Development and validation of a short-form, rapid estimate of adult literacy in medicine. *Medical Care, 45,* 1027–1033.

Ashman, T. A., Schwartz, M. E., Cantor, J. B., Hibbard, M. R., & Gordon, W. A. (2004). Screening for substance abuse in individuals with traumatic brain injury. *Brain Injury, 18,* 191–202.

Askew, E. (2011). (Re)Creating world in seven days: Place, disability, and salvation in *Extreme Makeover: Home Edition. Disability Studies Quarterly 31.* Retrieved July 1, 2013 from http://www.dsq-sds.org/article/view/1590/1558.

Balanced Budget Act of 1997, Pub. L. No. 105–33, § 4421 (1997).

Beck, A. T., Steer, R. A., & Brown, G. K. (2000). *BDI-Fast Screen for Medical Patients.* San Antonio, TX: The Psychological Corporation.

Bell, N. S., Williams, J. O., Senier, L., Strowman, S. R., & Amoroso, P. J. (2003). The reliability and validity of the self-reported drinking measures in the Army's Health Risk Appraisal survey. *Alcoholism: Clinical and Experimental Research, 27,* 826–834.

Besharat, M. A., Pourhosein, R., Rostami, R., & Bazzazian, S. (2011). Perfectionism and fatigue in multiple sclerosis. *Psychology and Health, 26,* 419–432.

Bisson, J., Nadeau, L., & Demers, A. (1999). The validity of the CAGE scale to screen for heavy drinking and drinking problems in a general population survey. *Addiction, 94,* 715–722.

Bogner, J. A., Corrigan, J. D., Mysiw, J., Clinchot, D., & Fugate, L. (2001). Comparison of substance abuse and violence in the prediction of long-term rehabilitation outcomes after traumatic brain injury. *Archives of Physical Medicine and Rehabilitation, 82,* 571–577.

Bonder, B. R., Martin, L., & Miracle, A. W. (2004). Culture as emergent in occupation. *American Journal of Occupational Therapy, 58,* 159–168.

Breland, H. L., & Ellis, C. (2012). Is reporting race and ethnicity essential to occupational therapy evidence? *American Journal of Occupational Therapy, 66,* 115–119.

Brown, S. M., Humphry, R., & Taylor, E. (1997). A model of the nature of family-therapist relationships: Implications for education. *American Journal of Occupational Therapy, 51,* 597–603.

Cannon, P. (1994). If I live, does the injury take my life? *Viewpoints: Issues in Brain Injury Rehabilitation, 26,* 3–4.

Cantor, J. B., Ashman, T., Gordon, W., Ginsberg, A., Engmann, C., Egan, M., Spielman, L., Dijkers, M., & Flanagan, S. (2008). Fatigue after traumatic brain injury and its impact on participation and quality of life. *Journal of Head Trauma Rehabilitation, 23,* 41–51.

Carstensen, L. L., Fung, H. H., & Charles, S. T. (2003). Socioemotional selectivity theory and the regulation of emotion in the second half of life. *Motivation and Emotion, 27,* 103–123.

Centers for Medicare and Medicaid Services. (2005a). Medicaid program: General information. Retrieved December 20, 2005 from www.cms.hhs.gov/MedicaidGenInfo.

Centers for Medicare and Medicaid Services. (2005b). Medicare program: General information. Retrieved December 22, 2005 from www.cms.hhs.gov/MedicareGenInfo.

Chantraine, A., Baribeault, A., Uebelhart, D., & Gremion, G. (1999). Shoulder pain and dysfunction in hemiplegia: Effects of functional electrical stimulation. *Archives of Physical Medicine and Rehabilitation, 80,* 328–331.

Christiansen, C. (1997). Acknowledging a spiritual dimension in occupational therapy practice. *American Journal of Occupational Therapy, 51,* 169–172.

Cleland, J. A., Childs, J. D., & Whitman, J. M. (2008). Psychometric properties of the Neck Disability Index and numeric pain rating scale in patients with mechanical neck pain. *Archives of Physical Medicine and Rehabilitation, 89,* 69–74.

Corbin, J. M., & Strauss, A. (1988). *Unending work and care: Managing chronic illness at home.* San Francisco: Jossey-Bass.

Cox, B. J., & Waller, L. L. (1991). *Bridging the communication gap with the elderly.* Chicago: American Hospital.

Curtis, K. A., Drysdale, G. A., Lanza, D., Kolber, M., Vitolo, R. S., & West, R. (1999). Shoulder pain in wheelchair users with tetraplegia and paraplegia. *Archives of Physical Medicine and Rehabilitation, 80,* 453–457.

Dalyan, M., Cardenas, D. D., & Gerard, B. (1999). Upper extremity pain after spinal cord injury. *Spinal Cord, 37,* 191–195.

Davis, T. C., Long, S. W., Jackson, R. H., Mayeaux, E. J., George, R. B., Murphy, P. W., & Crouch, M. A. (1993). Rapid estimate of adult literacy in medicine: A shortened screening instrument. *Family Medicine, 25,* 391–395.

Devlieger, P. J., Albrecht, G. L., & Hertz, M. (2007). The production of disability culture among young African-American men. *Social Science & Medicine, 64,* 1948–1959.

Dudgeon, B. J., Gerrard, B. C., Jensen, M. P., Rhodes, L. A., & Tyler, E. J. (2002). Physical disability and the experience of chronic pain. *Archives of Physical Medicine and Rehabilitation, 83,* 229–235.

Dudgeon, B. J., Tyler, E. J., Rhondes, L. A., & Jensen, M. P. (2006). Managing usual and unexpected pain with physical disability: A qualitative analysis. *American Journal of Occupational Therapy, 60,* 92–103.

Dunn, W., Brown, C., & McGuigan, A. (1994). The ecology of human performance: A framework for considering the effect of context. *American Journal of Occupational Therapy, 48,* 595–607.

Eddey, G. E., & Robey, K. L. (2005). Considering the culture of disability in cultural competence education. *Academic Medicine, 80,* 706–712.

Egan, M. (2007). Speaking of suffering and occupational therapy. *Canadian Journal of Occupational Therapy, 74,* 293–301.

Egan, M. Y., Munroe, S., Hubert, C., Rossiter, T., Gauthier, A., Eisner, M., Fulford, N., Neilson, M., Daros, B., & Rodrigue, C. (2007). Caring for residents with dementia and impact of life history knowledge. *Journal of Gerontological Nursing, 33,* 24–30.

Egan, M., & Swedersky, J. (2003). Spirituality as experienced by occupational therapists in practice. *American Journal of Occupational Therapy, 57,* 525–533.

Ehde, D. M., Jensen, M. P., Engel, J. M., Turner, J. A., Hoffman, A. J., & Cardenas, D. D. (2003). Chronic pain secondary to disability: A review. *The Clinical Journal of Pain, 19,* 3–17.

Epstein-Lubow, G. P., Beevers, C. G., Bishop, D. S., & Miller, I. W. (2009). Family functioning is associated with depressive symptoms in caregivers of acute stroke survivors. *Archives of Physical Medicine and Rehabilitation, 90,* 947–955.

Ewing, J. A. (1984). Detecting alcoholism: The CAGE questionnaire. *Journal of the American Medical Association, 252,* 1905–1907.

Eysenck, M. W., & Keane, M. T. (1990). *Cognitive psychology: A student's handbook.* London: Lawrence Erlbaum.

Farrales, S. (1996). Vietnamese. In J. G. Lipson, S. L. Dibble, & P. A. Minarik (Eds.), *Culture & nursing care: A pocket guide* (pp. 280–290). San Francisco: UCSF Nursing.

Federal Interagency Forum on Aging-Related Statistics. (2004). *Key indicators of well-being.* Washington, DC: U.S. Government Printing Office.

Federal Interagency Forum on Aging-Related Statistics. (2010). *Older Americans 2010, Key indicators of well-being.* Washington, DC: U.S. Government Printing Office.

Figved, N., Myhr, K.-M., Larsen, J.-P., & Aarsland, D. (2007). Caregiver burden in multiple sclerosis: The impact of neuropsychiatric symptoms. *Journal of Neurology, Neurosurgery, and Psychiatry, 78,* 1097–1102.

Fisher, A. G. (1998). Uniting practice and theory in an occupational framework. *American Journal of Occupational Therapy, 52,* 509–521.

Frosch, S., Gruber, A., Jones, C., Myers, S., Noel, E., Westerlund, A., & Zavisin, T. (1997). The long term effects of traumatic brain injury on the roles of caregivers. *Brain Injury, 11,* 891–906.

Galik, E. M., Resnick, B., & Pretzer-Aboff, I. (2009). "Knowing what makes them tick": Motivating cognitively impaired older adults to participate in restorative care. *International Journal of Nursing Practice, 15,* 48–55.

Gans, J. S. (1998). Enhancing the therapeutic value of talking with patients in the rehabilitation setting. *Rehabilitation Outlook, Summer,* 4–5.

Gordon, W. A. (2008). Post TBI Fatigue. *Journal of Head Trauma Rehabilitation, 23,* 2.

Gorman, L. M., Sultman, D., & Luna-Raines, M. (1989). *Psychosocial nursing handbook for the nonpsychiatric nurse.* Baltimore: Williams & Wilkins.

Graham, J. E., Radice-Neumann, D. M., Reistetter, T. A., Hammond, F. M., Dijkers, M., & Granger, C. V. (2010). Influence of sex and age on inpatient rehabilitation outcomes among older adults with traumatic brain injury *Archives of Physical Medicine & Rehabilitation, 91,* 43–50.

Grant, J. S., Bartolucci, A. A., Elliot, T. R., & Giger, J. N. (2000). Sociodemographic, physical, and psychosocial characteristics of depressed and non-depressed family caregivers of stroke survivors. *Brain Injury, 14,* 1089–1100.

Gulley, S. P., Rasch, E. K., & Chan, L. (2011). If we build it, Who will come? Working-age adults with chronic health care needs and the medical home. *Medical Care, 49,* 149–155.

Hall, P. A., Marshall, J., Mercado, A., & Tkachuk, G. (2011). Changes in coping style and treatment outcome following motor vehicle accident. *Rehabilitation Psychology, 56,* 43–51.

Hart, T., Brenner, L., Clark, A. N., Bogner, J. A., Novack, T. A., Chervoneva, I., Nakase-Richardson, R., & Arango-Lasprilla, J. C. (2011). Major and minor depression after traumatic brain injury. *Archives of Physical Medicine and Rehabilitation, 92,* 1211–1219.

Henry J. Kaiser Family Foundation. (2007). Health care costs: A Primer. Retrieved September 10, 2011 from http://www.kff.org/insurance/upload/7670.pdf.

Heaney, C. A., & Israel, B. A. (1997). Social networks and social support. In K. Glanz, F. M. Lewis, & B. K. Rimer (Eds.), *Health behavior and health education* (pp. 179–205). San Francisco: Jossey-Bass.

Hearnden, M. (2008). Coping with differences in culture and communication in health care. *Nursing Standard, 23,* 49–57.

Helliwell, J. F., & Putnam, R. D. (2004). The social context of well-being. *Philosophical Transactions of the Royal Society B, 359,* 1435–1446.

Holahan, C. J., & Moos, R. H. (1987). Personal and contextual determinants of coping strategies. *Journal of Personality and Social Psychology, 52,* 946–955.

Institute of Medicine. (2009). *Measures of health literacy: Workshop summary.* Washington, DC: The National Academies Press.

Jensen, M. P., Karoly, P., & Braver, S. (1986). The measurement of clinical pain intensity: A comparison of six methods. *Pain, 27,* 117–126.

Jezewski, M. A., & Sotnik, P. (2001). Culture brokering: Providing culturally-competent rehabilitation services to foreign-born persons. In J. Stone (Ed.), CIRRIE Monograph Series. Buffalo, NY: CIRRIE, State University of New York.

Joint Commission on Accreditation of Healthcare Organizations. (2010). *Comprehensive accreditation manual for hospitals.* Oakbrook Terrace, IL: Joint Commission on Accreditation of Healthcare Organizations.

Kanter, R. M. (2011). Zoom in, zoom out. *Harvard Business Review, March,* 112–116.

Kennedy, P., & Rogers, B. A. (2000). Anxiety and depression after spinal cord injury: A longitudinal analysis. *Archives of Physical Medicine and Rehabilitation, 81,* 932–937.

Kennedy, P., Lude, P., Elfström, M. L., & Smithson, E. F. (2011). Psychological contributions to functional independence: A longitudinal investigation of spinal cord injury rehabilitation. *Archives of Physical Medicine and Rehabilitation, 92,* 597–602.

Kielhofner, G. (2005). Rethinking disability and what to do about it: Disability studies and its implication for occupational therapy. *American Journal of Occupational Therapy, 59,* 487–496.

Kleinman, A. (1988). *The illness narratives: Suffering, healing, and the human condition.* New York: Basic Books.

Kolakowsky-Hayner, S. A., Gourley, E. V., Kreutzer, J. S., Marwitz, J. H., Cifu, D. X., & McKinley, W. O. (1999). Pre-injury substance abuse among persons with brain injury and spinal cord injury. *Brain Injury, 13,* 571–581.

Koponen, S., Taiminen, T., Hiekkanen, H., & Tenovuo, O. (2011). Axis I and II psychiatric disorders in patients with traumatic brain injury: A 12-month follow-up study. *Brain Injury, 25,* 1029–1034.

Kramer, L. W. (2010). Generational diversity. *Dimensions of Critical Care Nursing, 29,* 125–128.

Krefting, L. (1991). The culture concept in the everyday practice of occupational and physical therapy. *Physical and Occupational Therapy in Practice, 11,* 1–16.

Krupp, L. B., LaRocca, N. G., Muir-Nash, J., & Steinberg, A. D. (1989). The Fatigue Severity Scale: Application to patients with multiple sclerosis and systemic lupus erythematosus. *Archives of Neurology, 46,* 1121–1123.

Lai, S. M., Duncan, P. W., Keighley, J., & Johnson, D. (2002). Depressive symptoms and independence in BADL and IADL. *Journal of Rehabilitation Research and Development, 39,* 589–596.

Lancaster, L. C., & Stillman, D. (2002). *When generations collide.* New York: Harper Collins Publishers, Inc.

Langford, C. P. H., Bowsher, J., Maloney, J. P., & Lillis, P. (1997). Social support: A conceptual analysis. *Journal of Advanced Nursing, 25,* 95–100.

Law, M., Cooper, B., Strong, S., Stewart, D., Rigby, P., & Letts, L. (1996). The person-environment-occupation model: A transactive approach to occupational performance. *Canadian Journal of Occupational Therapy, 63,* 9–23.

Lerdahl, A., Bakken, L. N., Kouwenhowven, S. E., Pedersen, G., Kirkevold, M., Finset, A., & Kim, H. S. (2009). Poststroke fatigue: A review. *Journal of Pain and Symptom Management, 38,* 928–949.

Lipson, J. G. (1996). Culturally competent nursing care. In J. G. Lipson, S. L. Dibble, & P. A. Minarik (Eds.), *Culture and nursing care: A pocket guide* (pp. 1–10). San Francisco: UCSF Nursing.

Lowell, K. H., & Bertko, J. (2010). The accountable care organization (ACO) model. Building blocks for success. *Journal of Ambulatory Care, 33,* 81–88.

Luborsky, M. R. (1994). The cultural adversity of physical disability: Erosion of full adult personhood. *Journal of Aging Studies, 8,* 239–253.

Luborsky, M. R. (1995). The process of self-report of impairment in clinical research. *Social Science Medicine, 40,* 1447–1459.

Luborsky, M. (1997). Attuning assessment to the client: Recent advances in theory and methodology. *Generations, 21,* 10–15.

Luoto, S., Taimela, S., Hurri, H., & Alaranta, H. (1999). Mechanisms explaining the association between low back trouble and deficits in information processing. *Spine, 24,* 255–261.

Mattingly, C. (1991). The narrative nature of clinical reasoning. *American Journal of Occupational Therapy, 45,* 998–1005.

Mattison, D. (2006). The forgotten spirit: Integration of spirituality in health care. *Nephrology News and Issues, 20,* 30–32.

McClellan, M., McKethan, A. N., Lewis, J. L., Roski, J., & Fisher, E. S. (2010). A national strategy to put accountable care into practice. *Health Affairs, 29,* 982–990.

McPherson, C. J., Wilson, K. G., Chyurlia, L., & Leclerc, C. (2011). The caregiving relationship and quality of life among partners of stroke survivors: A cross-sectional study. *Health and Quality of Life Outcomes, 9,* 29. Retrieved May 25, 2013 from http://www.hqlo.com/content/9/1/29.

MedPAC. (2008). A path to a bundled payment around a hospitalization. Retrieved September 10, 2011 from http://post-acute.org/bundling/index_files/Page885.htm.

Merritta, C., Cherian, B., Macaden, A. S., & John, J. A. (2010). Measurement of physical performance and objective fatigability in people with mild-to-moderate traumatic brain injury. *International Journal of Rehabilitation Research, 33,* 109–114.

Molton, I. R., Stoeb, B. L., Jensen, M. P., Ehde, D. M., Raichle, K. A., & Cardenas, D. D. (2009). Psychosocial factors and adjustment to chronic pain in spinal cord injury: Replication and cross-validation. *Journal of Rehabilitation Research & Development, 46,* 31–42.

Moyers, P. A., & Stoffel, V. C. (1999). Alcohol dependence in a client with a work-related injury. *American Journal of Occupational Therapy, 53,* 640–645.

Murphy, P. W., Davis, T. C., Long, S. W., Jackson, R. H., & Decker, B. C. (1993). Rapid Estimates of Adult Literacy in Medicine (REALM): A quick reading test for patients. *Journal of Reading, 37,* 124–130.

Murray, S. A., Manktelow, K., & Clifford, C. (2000). The interplay between social and cultural context and perceptions of cardiovascular disease. *Journal of Advanced Nursing, 32,* 1224–1233.

National Center for Medical Rehabilitation Research. (1993). *Research plan for the National Center for Medical Rehabilitation Research* (NIH Publication 93-3509). Bethesda, MD: National Center for Medical Rehabilitation Research.

Nelson, D. L. (1988). Occupation: Form and performance. *American Journal of Occupational Therapy, 42,* 633–641.

Norbeck, J. S., Lindsey, A. M., & Carrieri, V. L. (1981). The development of an instrument to measure social support. *Nursing Research, 30,* 262–269.

Norbeck, J. S., Lindsey, A. M., & Carrieri, V. L. (1983). Further development of the Norbeck Social Support Questionnaire. *Nursing Research, 32,* 4–9.

Odawara, E. (2005). Cultural competency in occupational therapy: Beyond a cross-cultural view of practice. *American Journal of Occupational Therapy, 59,* 325–334.

Olssøn, I., Mykletun, A., & Dahl, A. A. (2005). The hospital anxiety and depression rating scale: A cross-sectional study of psychometrics and case finding abilities in general practice. *BMC Psychiatry, 5,* 46.

Pallant, J. F., & Bailey, C. M. (2005). Assessment of the structure of the Hospital Anxiety and Depression Scale in musculoskeletal patients. *Health and Quality of Life Outcomes, 3,* 82.

Parikh, N. S., Parker, R. M., Nurss, J. R., Baker, D. W., & Williams, M. V. (1996). Shame and health literacy: The unspoken connection. *Patient Education and Counseling, 27,* 33–39.

Patient Protection and Affordable Care Act, Pub. L. No. 111–148 (2010). Retrieved September 3, 2011 from http://www.gpo.gov/fdys/pkg/PLAW-111publ148/content-detail.html.

Paul, S. (1995). Culture and its influence on occupational therapy evaluation. *Canadian Journal of Occupational Therapy, 62,* 154–161.

Phillips, K. D., Moneyham, L., Thomas, S. P., Gunther, M., & Vyavaharkar, M. (2011). Social context of rural women with HIV/AIDS. *Issues in Mental Health Nursing, 32,* 374–381.

Pinto, P. E., & Sahu, N. (2001). Working with people with disability: An Indian perspective. In. J. Stone (Ed.), CIRRIE Monograph Series. Buffalo, NY: CIRRIE, State University of New York.

Pollard, C., & Kennedy, P. (2007). A longitudinal analysis of emotional impact, coping strategies and post-traumatic psychological growth following spinal cord injury: A 10-year review. *British Journal of Health Psychology, 12,* 347–362.

Poole, N. A., & Morgan, J. F. (2006). Validity and reliability of the Hospital Anxiety and Depression Scale in a hypertrophic cardiomyopathy clinic: The HADS in a cardiomyopathy population. *General Hospital Psychiatry, 28,* 55–58.

Porter, M. E. (2010). What is the value in health care? *New England Journal of Medicine, 363,* 2477–2481.

Pruchno, R. A., & Potashnik, S. L. (1989). Caregiving spouses: Physical and mental health in perspective. *Journal of the American Geriatrics Society, 37,* 697–705.

Pulchaski, C., & Romer, A. L. (2000). Taking a spiritual history allows clinicians to understand patients more fully. *Journal of Palliative Medicine, 3,* 129–137.

Quale, A. J., & Schanke, A. K. (2010). Resilience in the face of coping with a severe physical injury: A study of trajectories of adjustment in a rehabilitation setting. *Rehabilitation Psychology, 55,* 12–22.

Radomski, M. V. (1995). There is more to life than putting on your pants. *American Journal of Occupational Therapy, 49,* 487–490.

Royeen, C. B. (1995). The human life cycle: Paradigmatic shifts in occupation. In C. B. Royeen (Ed.), *The practice of the future: Putting occupation back into therapy.* Bethesda, MD: American Occupational Therapy Association.

Ruchinskas, R. (2002). Rehabilitation therapists' recognition of cognitive and mood disorders in geriatric patients. *Archives of Physical Medicine and Rehabilitation, 83,* 609–612.

Rybarczyk, B., Haut, A., Lacey, R. F., Fogg, L. F., & Nicholas, J. J. (2001). A multifactorial study of age bias among rehabilitation professionals. *Archives of Physical Medicine and Rehabilitation, 82,* 625–632.

Scheinthal, S. M., Steer, R. A., Giffin, L., & Beck, A. T. (2001). Evaluating geriatric medical outpatients with the Beck Depression Inventory-Fastscreen for medical patients. *Aging and Mental Health, 5,* 143–148.

Scherer, M. J., & Cushman, L. A. (1997). A functional approach to psychological and psychosocial factors and their assessment in rehabilitation. In S. S. Dittmar & G. E. Gresham (Eds.), *Functional assessment and outcome measures for the rehabilitation health professional* (pp. 57–67). Gaithersburg, MD: Aspen.

Sendroy-Terrill, M., Whiteneck, G. G., & Brooks, C. A. (2010). Aging with traumatic brain injury: Cross-sectional follow-up of people receiving inpatient rehabilitation over more than 3 decades. *Archives of Physical Medicine & Rehabilitation, 91,* 489–497.

Stansbury, J. P., Reid, K. J., Reker, D. M., Duncan, P. W., Marshall, C. R., & Rittman, M. (2004). Why ethnic designation matters for stroke rehabilitation: Comparing VA administrative data and clinical records. *Journal of Rehabilitation Research and Development, 41,* 269–278.

St. Clair, A., & McKenry, L. (1999). Preparing culturally competent practitioners. *Journal of Nursing Education, 38,* 228–234.

Stevenson, A. D., Phillips, C. B., & Anderson, K. J. (2011). Resilience among doctors who work in challenging areas: A qualitative study. *British Journal of General Practice, 61,* e404–e410.

Suarez-Balcazar, Y., Rodawoski, J., Balcazar, F., Taylor-Ritzler, T., Portillo, N., Barwacz, D., & Willis, C. (2009). Perceived levels of cultural competence among occupational therapists. *American Journal of Occupational Therapy, 63,* 498–505.

Taj, N., Devera-Sales, A., & Vinson, D. C. (1998). Screening for problem drinking: Does a single question work? *Journal of Family Practice, 46,* 328–335.

Tate, D. G., Forchheimer, M. B., Krause, J. S., Meade, M. A., & Bombardier, C. H. (2004). Patterns of alcohol and substance use and abuse in persons with spinal cord injury: Risk factors and correlates. *Archives of Physical Medicine and Rehabilitation, 85,* 1837–1847.

Toglia, J. P. (1993). *The Contextual Memory Test*. Tucson, AZ: Therapy Skill Builders.

Tollifson, J. (1997). Imperfection is a beautiful thing: On disability and meditation. In K. Fries (Ed.), *Staring back: The disability experience from the inside out*. New York: Penguin Putnam.

U.S. Department of Health and Human Services. (2011). Medicare program: Hospital inpatient value-based purchasing program; final rule. *Federal Register, 76,* 26490–26547.

van Leeuwen, C. M. C., Post, M. W. M., van Asbeck, F. W. A., van der Woude, L. H. V., de Groot, S., & Lindeman, E. (2010). Social support and life satisfaction in spinal cord injury during and up to one year after inpatient rehabilitation. *Journal of Rehabilitation Medicine, 42,* 265–271.

Wakefield, D. (2005). *I remember running: The year I got everything I ever wanted–and ALS*. New York: Marlowe & Company.

Watson, N. (2002). Well, I know this is going to sound very strange to you, but I don't see myself as a disabled person: Identity and disability. *Disability and Society, 17,* 509–527.

Webster's Third New International Dictionary. (1993). Springfield, MA: Merriam-Webster Inc.

Webster, G., Daisley, A., & King, N. (1999). Relationship and family breakdown following acquired brain injury: The role of the rehabilitation team. *Brain Injury, 13,* 593–603.

Whitehead, L. (2009). The measurement of fatigue in chronic illness: A systematic review of unidimensional and multidimensional fatigue measures. *Journal of Pain and Symptom Management, 37,* 107–128.

Williamson, A., & Hoggart, B. (2005). Pain: A review of three commonly used pain rating scales. *Issues in Clinical Nursing, 14,* 798–804.

Woodruff, L., & Woodruff, B. (2007). *In an Instant*. New York: Random House.

World Health Organization. (2001). *International Classification of Functioning, Disability and Health: Short version*. Geneva, Switzerland: World Health Organization.

Young, I. A., Cleland, J. A., Michener, L. A., & Brown, C. (2010). Reliability, construct validity, and responsiveness of the Neck Disability Index, Patient-Specific Functional Scale, and Numeric Pain Rating Scale. *American Journal of Physical Medicine and Rehabilitation, 89,* 831–839.

Zelman, D. C., Smith, M. Y., Hoffman, D., Edwards, L., Reed, P., Levine, E., Siefeldin, R., & Dukes, E. (2004). Acceptable, manageable, and tolerable days: Patient daily goals for medication management of persistent pain. *Journal of Pain and Symptom Management, 28,* 474–487.

Zigmond, A. S., & Snaith, R. P. (1983). The Hospital Anxiety and Depression Scale. *Acta Psychiatrica Scandinavia, 67,* 361–370.

4

Assessing Roles and Competence

Susan E. Fasoli

Learning Objectives

After studying this chapter, the reader will be able to do the following:

1. Understand the nature and importance of assessment in occupational therapy.
2. Evaluate roles, competence, and occupational functioning, beginning with clients' perception of their occupational performance concerns.
3. Understand the measurement criteria necessary for reliable and valid assessments used in occupational therapy practice.
4. Describe and select appropriate validated assessments of occupational performance (roles, tasks, and activities) based on client needs.

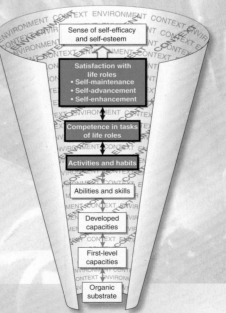

Participation in the occupations of everyday life is a vital part of human development and the lived experience (Law, 2002). Occupational therapists provide services to optimize the occupational performance of persons who have or are at risk for developing occupational dysfunction. This chapter describes many assessments of occupational performance and competence in valued life roles, tasks, and activities. Later chapters discuss assessment of the abilities and capacities (components of occupational function) required to carry out the tasks and activities involved in various life roles.

The goal of occupational therapy is to enable individuals to achieve competency and satisfaction in their chosen life roles and in the activities that support function and participation in these roles. Such competency and satisfaction can be achieved through personal independence or by directing others, such as a caregiver or attendant. Occupational performance is the ability to carry out basic activities of daily living (BADL) or activities of daily living (ADL), instrumental activities of daily living (IADL), education, work, play or leisure, and social participation (American Occupational Therapy Association [AOTA], 2008). Whenever a person has a health disorder, injury, or disease that results in a physical and/or cognitive impairment, independence in these areas of occupation may be jeopardized.

The evaluation of occupational performance often begins with a semistructured interview to assess the client's needs, problems, and concerns regarding role participation and competence in daily living tasks and activities (AOTA, 2008). During this interview, the therapist gathers valuable information from the client and family members about the tasks and roles that are most important to them and about activities that the client can and cannot do. After identifying the client's areas of difficulty in occupational performance, the therapist completes further assessments (either impairment-based or disease-specific) to clarify the factors that limit performance. If the limiting factors can be improved or eliminated by direct intervention, the therapist chooses an intervention approach that is appropriate for the problem. When the limiting factors are not amenable to change, the therapist teaches the individual to compensate for these limitations by adapting the task or by changing the environment in which it is performed.

It is important to recognize that occupational performance, or the ability to carry out activities during daily life, depends on the individual's culture, gender, roles that he or she wishes to undertake, and environment. Thus, occupational performance is a personal concept. The individuality of a person's roles and his or her day-to-day functioning make it both difficult and time consuming to assess all aspects of occupational performance. Therefore, it is important for the occupational therapist to carefully select evaluations that best measure a client's occupational performance needs. As outlined by Trombly Latham (see Chapter 1), assessments should be done using a top-down approach that begins with an evaluation of roles, tasks, and activities.

Life roles include self-maintenance (e.g., independent person, caregiver and home maintainer), self-enhancement (e.g., friend and moviegoer), and self-advancement (e.g., worker and student) (Trombly, 1995).

This top-down approach to assessment includes consideration of the environment in which a person lives (see Chapter 10) and incorporates considerations of personal, social, and cultural context (Chapter 3). Assessment does not ignore the more basic abilities, or performance skills, that enable occupational performance, such as strength, endurance, problem solving, or depth perception. Rather, it begins with a function-based assessment of the tasks and activities that the client needs, wants, or is expected to accomplish and is having difficulty performing (Law et al., 2005). Looking at this process from the perspective of the World Health Organization's International Classification of Functioning, Disability and Health (ICF) (World Health Organization [WHO], 2001), occupational therapists first assess activities and participation, evaluating impairments in body functions (i.e., performance skills) as needed to explain difficulties in performance. By beginning with a focus on clients' needs and considering their roles and the environment in which they live, therapists acknowledge the values and goals that these individuals bring to occupational therapy. This approach reflects a client-centered philosophy, recognizing that it is the person who is engaged in therapy who should articulate the goals of therapy and drive the rehabilitation process (Law, 1998).

TIMING, SEQUENCE, AND SETTINGS FOR EVALUATING OCCUPATIONAL PERFORMANCE

Competence in occupational performance areas (e.g., ADL, IADL, leisure, and work) is evaluated over time based on the client's identified needs and interests. Assessments of self-care and personal mobility are usually done early because they form the basis for planning restorative therapy and/or adaptations to optimize ADL. As recovery continues and discharge plans are considered, further evaluations are used to assess a client's ability to manage home and child care responsibilities, gain access to home and community, engage in leisure activities and family recreation, or return to valued education or work pursuits.

Assessment of roles and competence by occupational therapists can take place in many environments, such as a hospital, rehabilitation center, workplace, school, or community setting. It is important to note that the setting in which an assessment is performed can affect a client's performance. Research indicates that the results of an assessment performed at one location (e.g., rehabilitation center) do not necessarily predict performance in another location (e.g., home) (Rogers et al., 2003). For example, Park, Fisher, and Velozo (1994) reported that process skills were better when older adults completed IADL tasks in the familiar environment of their homes rather than the occupational therapy clinic, whereas motor skills remained stable across settings. This research supports evaluation of a client's performance in the environment in which tasks typically occur, whenever possible.

MEASUREMENT CONCEPTS

Several important measurement concepts must be considered when choosing evaluations to assess roles and competence in occupational therapy. These concepts include whether the assessment is a standardized measure with established reliability and validity, its responsiveness to change, its level of measurement and clinical utility, and whether it involves direct observation or self-report.

Properties of the Assessment

A standardized measure is a published assessment tool that provides detailed instructions on test administration and scoring and has published results of reliability and validity (Finch et al., 2002). A reliable assessment is one that consistently measures the attribute under study, no matter who is scoring (interrater reliability) or when the assessment occurs (test–retest reliability). A valid assessment is one that measures what it claims to measure. Most evaluations of occupational performance have content validity, meaning that the test items well represent the area being tested. Some items of a valid assessment, however, may be more important than others. For example, when assessing homemaker competence during meal preparation, "can use the stove safely" is more critical in many ways than "can stir batter."

The use of nonstandardized checklists commonly found in the clinic is not recommended because of their inherent lack of reliability and validity. Because the tasks listed in nonstandardized checklists are rarely operationally defined, the same methods are not necessarily used to evaluate task performance across clients and therapists. The Centers for Medicare and Medicaid Services (CMS) recommend the use of validated tests and measures when assessing a client's functional abilities and needs (Centers for Medicare & Medicaid Services, 2011). Because many private insurers follow CMS guidelines when establishing their own standards, it is critically important that occupational therapists use objective measures to reliably document occupational performance for all clients receiving services. When using standardized assessments, occupational therapists can more efficiently target client needs and goals and accurately measure changes in occupational performance that are both clinically significant and meaningful to their clients. In order to best meet patient needs, the therapist should select assessments based on the population for which it was validated and adhere to administration instructions exactly as directed (e.g., not adding or dropping items) so that reliability is not reduced across multiple testing sessions.

An assessment that includes a wide range of test items will be more responsive to detecting decrements in occupational performance. For a therapist working on a day-to-day basis with a client to improve her ability to dress, the assessment should be sensitive enough to allow progress to be noted when different areas of the body can be dressed or different articles of clothing are donned. Responsiveness is directly related to the number of items on an assessment and to the number of categories on the scoring scale. An assessment with 50 items is likely to be more responsive than one with 10 items. The level of measurement also contributes to the test's responsiveness or sensitivity in detecting clinical change. For most evaluations of roles, tasks, and activities, the level of measurement is ordinal; that is, the scores are rank ordered to indicate the client's performance. For example, scores might range from 1 (dependent, is unable) to 7 (independent, is able). The range of ordinal scores varies depending on the assessment scale. A scoring system that uses a 1 to 7 Likert-type scale is likely to be more responsive to changes in performance than one using a 1 to 3 scale.

Reevaluation

Periodic reevaluations are performed to monitor the client's response to therapy. At a minimum, it is important to record the level of performance at admission and discharge because these records may be used for program evaluation, to justify occupational therapy services to third-party payers, in legal actions, or when determining whether a patient will be discharged home or to an extended-care facility. Discharge evaluations can also aid transitions from one level of care to the next (e.g., rehabilitation hospital to home-based therapy) by providing valuable information about the client's abilities and occupational performance needs.

In order to interpret whether changes in test scores are meaningful, it is important to understand what constitutes a clinically significant difference. From a client's perspective, a clinically significant change could reflect greater independence in valued activities, such as transferring into the tub or completing lower body dressing. The therapist may use the concept of clinically significant change to determine whether her treatment methods are effective or whether the course of intervention needs to be altered to better impact performance. A clinically significant change score is one that exceeds the measurement error that typically occurs during routine test administration. One more commonly used index of change is the minimal clinically important difference (MCID) (Haley & Fragala-Pinkham, 2006). The MCID can be calculated for a standardized assessment and used to demonstrate that changes in occupational performance exceed measurement error and are clinically meaningful. An increasing number of standardized assessments used by occupational therapists, such as the Barthel Index and Functional Independence Measure™ (FIM™), have documented MCIDs to aid interpretation of patient outcomes. The concept of clinically significant change is gaining research attention and will be increasingly important as occupational therapists are required to better substantiate the effectiveness of their interventions.

Clinical Utility

The clinical utility of an assessment tool is another important consideration. Clinical utility refers to all of the practical factors of an instrument, such as its cost, the amount of training needed, availability of a manual with clear instructions, and ease of administration and interpretation. In most occupational therapy settings, managers prefer to use assessments that efficiently provide useful information for treatment planning and evaluating client outcomes.

Direct Observation versus Self-Report

Standardized assessments gather information about occupational performance from either direct observation or self-report by the client or family members. Observation of activities that are important to the client is the most direct method of assessing competence in occupational performance. This method is preferred for accuracy, detection of inefficient or unsafe methods, and determining the underlying reason(s) that a particular task cannot be performed. Direct observation of the wide range of occupational performance areas, however, can be time consuming and costly (Law & Letts, 1989). Self-report of one's competence in occupational tasks and roles through interview is often the easiest, fastest, and least expensive method of assessing functional abilities and may inform the direct observation of selected activities.

There is a concern that self-reports and interviews may not accurately reflect what the person can do. Studies that compared self-report ratings with direct observation of functional performance have yielded conflicting results. Some researchers reported high levels of agreement between these two methods, especially for daily self-care tasks (Collin et al., 1988); others found that clients consistently overrated their abilities (Edwards, 1990; Sagar et al., 1992). If a client reports questionable data and does not allow direct observation, the therapist should verify the report with others who have knowledge of his or her actual performance. False information may be related to the client's lack of insight and limited awareness of abilities and needs and is not necessarily a conscious intent to deceive. In these cases, proxy reports and interviews with family members or caregivers can provide additional information about client performance from the family's perspective. Although self-report and direct observation in the environment where the task ordinarily occurs are preferred, the assessment methods chosen for a particular client ultimately will depend on the nature of the disability, the supportiveness of the client's environment, and the time constraints encountered during rehabilitation.

Assessing Outcomes

As indicated earlier, occupational therapists administer various assessments to obtain information for the purpose of planning intervention. Some measures are administered in order to quantify the overall benefits of intervention (also referred to as outcomes of intervention). Recent studies have shown initial reliability and validity of the Australian Therapy Outcome Measures for Occupational Therapy (AusTOMS-OT) (Perry et al., 2004; Unsworth, 2005; Unsworth et al., 2004). The AusTOMS-OT was developed to be consistent with ICF terminology and provides a snapshot of the client's occupational performance across four domains of functioning: impairment, activity, participation, and distress/well-being. The AusTOMS-OT is suitable for clients of varied diagnoses and ages across treatment settings (hospital, outpatient clinics, and home or extended care) and consists of 12 function-focused scales, including learning and applying knowledge, upper limb use, self-care, and domestic life, among others. To use the AusTOMS-OT, the therapist administers standardized assessments as described below, works collaboratively with the client to select goals for therapy, and then chooses related AusTOMS-OT scales (e.g., self-care or functional walking and mobility) for scoring. Four scores are given for each of the selected scales to reflect the therapist's perception of performance impairments in relation to the four domains. This quick and easy-to-use measurement tool has strong potential to document change in patient status over the course of therapy and allows the therapist and client to examine the effectiveness of intervention. This unique approach, although focused on occupational performance, allows for a single assessment of the client's strengths and limitations across ICF domains. Although it is currently used extensively in the United Kingdom and Australia, more widespread use in the United States is expected.

The assessments discussed in this chapter are generic measures that can be used to evaluate occupational performance of clients with a variety of diagnoses and levels of disablement. Refer to the chapters that follow for specific measures that assess the effects of a particular disease or condition (e.g., orthopedic injuries and chronic obstructive pulmonary disease) on occupational performance.

ASSESSMENT METHODS AND TOOLS

A comprehensive top-down assessment of occupational performance begins with an overview and identification of a client's occupational needs, is followed by evaluation of his or her engagement and competence in life roles and tasks, and continues with an assessment of the abilities or performance skills (e.g., coordination, strength, and organization) needed to accomplish valued activities. See Assessment Table 4-1 for descriptions, reliability and validity data, and strengths/weaknesses of many of the evaluations discussed in this chapter. Resources 4-1 has contact information regarding purchase of these assessments.

(text continued on page 91)

Assessment Table 4-1 | Summary of Assessments of Occupational Function

Instrument & Reference	Description	Time to Administer	Validity	Reliability	Sensitivity	Strengths and Weaknesses
Occupational Performance Needs						
Canadian Occupational Performance Measure (COPM), 4th edition (Law et al., 2005)	Semistructured interview with ordinal scale to measure changes in client perception of performance and satisfaction with performance in self-care, productivity, and leisure occupations	30–40 minutes	Numerous studies support COPM as a valid measure of occupational performance. Combined COPM and Functional Independence Measure (FIM™) scores were 65% accurate in predicting discharge status (Simmons, Crepeau, & White, 2000).	Test-retest reliability at 1–2-week intervals ranges from 0.63 to 0.89 for performance; and 0.76 to 0.88 for satisfaction (AOTA, 2007).	Carswell et al. (2004) report COPM is more sensitive to perceived changes in client status than other disability measures, including Short Form 36 and FIM™. A 2-point change in score is clinically significant (AOTA, 2007).	Strengths: Psychometrics studied in wide range of diagnoses (Carswell et al., 2004). Translated into 20 languages and used in more than 35 countries around the world.
Australian Therapy Outcome Measure for Occupational Therapy (AusTOMs) (Unsworth, 2005)	Consists of 12 function-focused scales (e.g., self-care and domestic life) that are scored across four domains derived from International Classification of Functioning, Disability and Health (ICF). Occupational performance is rated by therapist after completion of other standardized assessments. Useful tool for documentation of progress, program evaluation, etc.	5–10 minutes (scores based on other standardized assessment outcomes)	Construct validity established with EuroQuol-5D (Unsworth et al., 2004).	Self-care scale: Moderate to high interrater reliability across three domains (Intraclass Correlation Coefficient (ICC) ≥ 0.79); somewhat lower for impairment domain (ICC = 0.70). Intrarater reliability also moderate to high (ICCs = 0.74–0.94) across domains (Scott et al., 2006).	Sensitivity to change is documented, particularly in clients at acute and subacute facilities and for those with neurological diagnoses.	Strengths: Scoring allows holistic assessment across levels of occupational performance (impairment through participation). Tests are quick to administer/complete. Weaknesses: Scores are based on therapist perception of client outcomes. Reliability studies ongoing.

Assessment	Administration Time	Description	Validity	Reliability	Strengths and Weaknesses
Occupational Performance History Interview-II (OPHI-II, version 2.1) (Kielhofner et al., 2004).	45–60 minutes	Semistructured interview intended to give a broad and detailed appreciation of a person's life history, the impact of disability, and the direction in which the person would like to take his or her life. Specific criteria are provided to rate performance on three scales: occupational performance, identity, and behavior. Rasch analysis has been used to calibrate and convert ordinal scores to interval data.	Validity for all three scales is excellent. More than 90% of subjects tested (with varied ages, nationalities, and diagnoses) were validly measured, and over 90% of raters used scales validly, with approximately the same degree of severity or leniency. (Kielhofner et al., 2001).	Test-retest reliability studies not available; manual provides detailed information on the rating process to improve observer reliability.	Adequate. Person separation statistic showed that the scale can distinguish meaningful differences among persons of approximately three different levels of competence, identity and environmental support (Kielhofner et al., 2001).	Strengths: Specific criteria assist with rating. Rasch analysis has been used to calibrate and convert ordinal scores to interval data. Weakness: Evidence of rater reliability not well reported in research literature.
Life Balance Inventory (LBI) (Matuska, 2012a, 2012b). Available online at http://minerva.stkate.edu/lbi.nsf	10–15 minutes	Self-report questionnaire used to rate satisfaction with amount of time spent on activities the client does or would like to do. Life balance ratings are provided for four dimensions: health, relationships, challenge/interests, and identity needs (Matuska, 2012a).	Acceptable content validity; combined congruence and equivalence model provided best fit with measures of stress and personal well-being (Matuska, 2012b)	Internal consistency was very good (Cronbach's α = 0.89–0.97).	Not established	Strengths: Theory-based assessment, low cost, and easily accessed; useful for treatment planning. Weaknesses: Its use with varied patient groups and sensitivity to change have not been examined.

(continued)

Assessment Table 4-1   Summary of Assessments of Occupational Function (continued)

Instrument & Reference	Description	Time to Administer	Validity	Reliability	Sensitivity	Strengths and Weaknesses
Roles and Community Integration						
Role Checklist (Oakley et al., 1986) Available from: Frances Oakley, MS, OTR, FAOTA Board Certification in Gerontology National Institutes of Health Building 10, CRC, Room 1-1469 10 Center Drive MSC 1604 Bethesda MD 20892-1604 E-mail: foakley@cc.nih.gov	Written inventory/ checklist that provides data on client perceptions of role participation and values throughout the life span	15 minutes	Content validity of role taxonomy is based on literature review and expert opinion; construct validity based on Model of Human Occupation (MOHO) (AOTA, 2007).	Test-retest reliability ranged from 73% to 97% agreement for three time categories (mean = 88%); agreement for roles was 77%–93% (mean = 87%) (AOTA, 2007).	Not established	Strengths: Appropriate across age groups. Translated into 10 languages. Can be adapted for verbal administration by therapist.
Reintegration to Normal Living Index (RNL) (Wood-Dauphinee et al., 1988).	Eleven declarative statements regarding how well clients perceive their return to normal living after a disabling event (e.g., "I am comfortable with how my self-care needs are met.") are rated by either a visual analog scale or 3- or 4-point categorical scale. A validation study (Stark et al., 2005) used a 10-point Likert-type scale to increase precision of scoring. Recently modified version (mRNL) rephrased questions to improve validity (Miller, Clemson, & Lannin, 2011).	Less than 10 minutes	Good construct validity of mRNL confirmed by Rasch analysis (Miller, Clemson, & Lannin, 2011).	Internal consistency (Cronbach's α = 0.80) and test-retest reliability (ICC (3,1) = 0.83, p = 0.0001) both acceptable (Miller, Clemson, & Lannin, 2011).	Not established	Strengths: Emphasis placed on client's perceptions of autonomy in life situations. Weakness: Initial problems in RNL domains were more likely reported by proxy than client scores; important to compare client and proxy reports.

Instrument	Description	Time to Administer	Validity	Reliability	Responsiveness	Strengths/Weaknesses
Community Integration Measure (CIM) (McColl et al., 2001). Primary author M. A. McColl may be contacted at mccollm@post.queensu.ca	Ten-item, qualitative measure based on client-centered model of community integration. Client agreement with test statements is measured by 5-point scale. Sample items include "I feel that I am accepted in this community" and "I know my way around this community."	Approximately 5 minutes	Criterion validity supported by comparisons with Community Integration Questionnaire and Satisfaction with Life Scale (Reistetter et al., 2005). Discriminates well between persons with brain injury and neurologically intact controls.	Cronbach's α for internal consistency originally reported at 0.87. Replication study reported slightly lower yet acceptable internal consistency (0.72–0.83).	Not established	Strengths: Quick and easy to administer and score and readily understood by clients and families. Weakness: Psychometrics to date have only been examined with clients diagnosed with traumatic brain injury (TBI), potentially limiting generalizability of this tool to other disability groups. Specific instructions to relate test results to treatment planning are not provided.

Activities of Daily Living

Instrument	Description	Time to Administer	Validity	Reliability	Responsiveness	Strengths/Weaknesses
Barthel Index (Mahoney & Barthel, 1965). Information available online at www.strokecenter.org/trials/scales/barthel.pdf	Self-report and direct observation used to evaluate 10 activities: feeding, bathing, grooming, dressing, bowel and bladder control, toilet use, transfers between chair and bed, mobility, and stair climbing. The total score ranges from 0 (total dependence) to 100 (total independence).	5–10 minutes if verbal report; 25 minutes or longer for direct observation	High correlations between Barthel Index and clinical judgment. Well correlated with index of motor ability (r = 0.73–0.77) (AOTA, 2007).	Internal consistency α coefficients 0.87–0.92 for original version; 0.90–0.93 for modified scoring (Shah, Vanclay, & Cooper, 1989). Test-retest reliability κ = 0.98 in clients with stroke (Wolfe et al., 1991).	Lacks sensitivity to amount of assistance needed. Initially high functioning clients can reach "ceiling" score and show no further improvement (Shah, Vanclay, & Cooper, 1989).	Strengths: Excellent reliability and validity. Widely used. Time to administer. Minimal clinically important difference (MCID) established for 20-point scale of Barthel Index (MCID = 1.85) (Hsieh et al., 2007). Weaknesses: "Ceiling" effect for higher level clients. Only fair sensitivity to change.

(continued)

Assessment Table 4-1   Summary of Assessments of Occupational Function (continued)

Instrument & Reference	Description	Time to Administer	Validity	Reliability	Sensitivity	Strengths and Weaknesses
Functional Independence Measure (Granger et al., 1993)	Eighteen items (13 motor and 5 cognition) in the areas of self-care, sphincter control, transfers, locomotion, communication, and social cognition. A 7-point ordinal scale rates level of independence in activities of daily living (ADL) (independent without equipment = 7). Scores are based on clinical observation. Follow up data can be gathered from phone interviews.	Approximately 45 minutes, depending on client abilities	Excellent validity reported. Motor FIM™ able to predict level of assistance required in 83% of TBI clients tested; cognitive FIM™ predicted 77% of those requiring supervision (Corrigan, Smith-Knapp, & Granger, 1997).	Numerous studies have reported excellent reliability in wide range of diagnostic groups. Chau et al. (1994) reported interrater ICC at 0.94, test–retest ICC at 0.93.	Greater sensitivity to change reported in motor than cognitive scales in persons with stroke (van der Putten et al., 1999) and multiple sclerosis (Sharrack et al., 1999).	Strengths: Extensive validation, widely recognized and used. Excellent reliability and validity in measuring disability. MCID established for stroke: Total FIM™ (MCID = 22); motor FIM™ (MCID = 17); cognitive FIM (MCID = 3) (Beninato et al., 2006). Weaknesses: FIM™ scores do not provide information regarding factors (e.g., body functions and environmental support) that influence occupational performance.
Klein-Bell Activities of Daily Living Scale (Klein & Bell, 1982)	Behavior rating scale consists of 170 specific items to rate performance in six ADL areas: dressing, elimination, mobility, bathing/hygiene, eating, and emergency phone communication. Performance is observed and scored as either able or unable; scores also are weighted from 1 to 3 points based on item difficulty.	30 minutes depending on client's level of ability and fatigue	Validity was established on 14 patients by comparing the total score at discharge against the hours of assistance required. A correlation of −0.86 ($p < 0.01$) was obtained, indicating that the amount of assistance decreases as the Klein-Bell score increases.	Interrater agreement = 0.92 even without extensive training (Klein & Bell, 1982).	Specificity of test items makes this test highly responsive to changes in client status.	Strengths: Highly responsive. Excellent reliability and validity. Appropriate for clinical purposes and research. Weaknesses: Higher level subjects may reach test "ceiling."

Instrumental Activities of Daily Living (IADL)

Nottingham Extended Activities of Daily Living (NEADL) Scale (Nouri & Lincoln, 1987). Available at http://www.nottingham.ac.uk/iwho/documents/neadl.pdf	Quick to administer self-report questionnaire consisting of 22 items in four sections: mobility, kitchen, domestic, and leisure tasks. Respondents rate amount of assistance needed to complete tasks on 4-point scale.	10–15 minutes	Validity was established when compared to Frenchay Activities Index and Stroke Impact Scale (Wu et al., 2011).	High interrater reliability reported with stroke (Schlote et al., 2004). Satisfactory test–retest reliability with multiple sclerosis clients ($r = 0.81–0.90$) (Nicholl, Lincoln, & Playford, 2002).	Contradictory reports may be due to comparison to different measures. More responsive than Frenchay Activities Index (Wu et al., 2011); insensitive to change when compared with components of SF-36 and London Handicap Scale (Harwood & Ebrahim, 2000).	Strengths: Quick to administer, easily understood by clients; appropriate for mail surveys. Weaknesses: Questionable responsiveness to change over time; not as specific as semistructured questionnaires (e.g., COPM) for guiding treatment planning.
The Assessment of Motor and Process Skills (AMPS) (Fisher, 1993, 1995)	The AMPS is an observational assessment that evaluates motor and process skills that directly impact occupational performance. Client chooses 2 or 3 ADL tasks for assessment from a list of more than 100. Computerized scoring and Rasch methods are used to generate adjusted instrumental activities of daily living (IADL) ability measures. These take into account severity of the rater who scored performance and the relative challenge of tasks performed.	30–60 minutes for administration and scoring	Many published studies have demonstrated the validity of the AMPS. Validity as a cross-cultural measure has been reported.	Extensive research documents reliability across cultural and diagnostic groups. Intrarater reliability is excellent ($r = 0.93$). Test–retest reliability reported to be $r = 0.88$ for motor skills, $r = 0.86$ for process skills. (Fisher, 1995).	Excellent responsiveness to client change has been reported.	Strengths: Excellent reliability and validity. Evaluation tasks are chosen by client and are meaningful and relevant to his daily life situation. Appropriate for use across ages (3 years to adult) and diagnostic groups. Weaknesses: Training requirements are extensive, which limits clinical utility.

(continued)

Assessment Table 4-1   Summary of Assessments of Occupational Function *(continued)*

Instrument & Reference	Description	Time to Administer	Validity	Reliability	Sensitivity	Strengths and Weaknesses
The Kohlman Evaluation of Living Skills (KELS) (Kohlman Thomson, 1993).	Self-report and observation assessment of 17 IADL tasks in five areas: self-care, safety and health, money management, transportation and telephone, and work and leisure. Items such as "use of money to purchase items" or "use of phone book and telephone" are scored as 0 (independent) or 1 (needs assistance). A score of 5.5 or less indicates that client is able to live independently.	30–45 minutes	Concurrent validity studies that compared KELS with Global Assessment Scale (0.78–0.89) and BaFPE (−0.84) indicate high agreement.	Interrater reliability in multiple studies is reported to be high (r = 0.84–1.00) (Kohlman Thomson, 1993).	Not established	Strengths: Easy to administer. Few materials are required. Can be used in many settings and with many diagnostic groups. Weaknesses: Tasks provide good screening of basic abilities, but higher level clients may reach test "ceiling."
Performance Assessment of Self-Care Skills (PASS) version 3.1. (Holm & Rogers, 2008; Rogers & Holm, 1989a, 1989b). Contact: mbholm@pitt.edu	Performance-based, criterion-referenced assessment of functional status and change consisting of 26 core tasks organized in four domains: functional mobility, personal self-care, and IADL tasks with either a cognitive emphasis or physical emphasis. Observed performance is rated for independence, safety, and adequacy.	Varies widely depending on number of items administered. Entire test requires 1.5–3 hours to complete.	Content and construct validity established (AOTA, 2007).	Interrater reliability percentage of agreement for PASS-C and PASS-H was 0.80–0.99. Test–retest reliability ranged from 0.82 to 0.97 with 3-day interval (Rogers & Holm, 1989a, 1989b).	Authors report sensitivity to change at discharge.	Strengths: Actual objects are used during performance of test items, increasing ecological validity. Clear instructions for administration and scoring. Criterion referenced. Low cost. Weaknesses: Time needed to assemble items. Materials for test kit.

Safety Assessment of Function and the Environment for Rehabilitation (SAFER-HOME) (Chiu et al., 2006; Oliver et al., 1993)	The SAFER-HOME tool consists of an easy-to-use checklist of 75 items grouped into 12 areas of concern including living situation, mobility, kitchen, household management, self-care, and recreation. A combination of observation, interview, and task performance is used to rate each item.	Approximately 1 hour, depending on administration method, client's functioning level, and home environment.	Construct validity has been supported in relation to cognitive impairment, but further research is needed. (Chiu & Oliver, 2006).	Interrater and test-retest reliability demonstrated via κ or percentage agreement was acceptable to excellent (Letts et al., 1998). Internal consistency of SAFER-HOME version 2 is good with Cronbach's α = 0.859 (AOTA, 2007).	Fair. The revised 4-point rating scale of *SAFER-HOME* version 2 may better measure changes postintervention than original tool.	Strengths: Clear assessment guidelines and recommendations. Revised 4-point scoring may increase sensitivity to change. Weaknesses: Lack of sensitivity to change. Reliability and validity of the revised scale (SAFER-HOME, version 3) are not established.
The Kitchen Task Assessment (KTA) (Baum & Edwards, 1993).	The KTA assesses six cognitive abilities during the task of making cooked pudding from a package: initiation, organization, inclusion of all steps, safety and judgment, and task completion. The level of support needed from the therapist is scored from 0 (independent) to 3 (not capable). Unlike the AMPS, this measure does not evaluate motor skills during task performance.	Less than 30 minutes	Construct validity was supported by highly significant correlations between KTA scores and other cognitive measures, including the Token Test, Clinical Dementia Rating, and Short Blessed Dementia Scale.	Internal consistency of the KTA ranges from 0.87 to 0.96, and interrater reliability for the total score is 0.85.	KTA scores significantly differentiated cognitive performance across all stages of dementia (Baum & Edwards, 1993). Sensitivity to client change over time has not been established.	Strengths: Good reliability and validity in lower functioning adults with dementia. Quick and easy to administer. Weaknesses: Little data to support KTA use with other rehabilitation populations (Duncombe, 2004). Higher functioning clients will easily reach test "ceiling."
Rabideau Kitchen Evaluation Revised (Neistadt, 1992, 1994)	Direct observation of meal preparation tasks that involve preparing a hot beverage and cold sandwich. Each task is broken down into component steps that are rated on a 0- (no assist needed) to 3-point scale (unable and requires direct intervention) (Neistadt, 1994). Six levels of task difficulty help guide the grading of tasks, based on client abilities (highest level involves preparation of fruit salad or baking frozen pastries).	20-30 minutes depending on tasks performed	Criterion validity reported with the Wechsler Adult Intelligence Scale-Revised (WAIS-R) block design test (r = 0.60, p = 0.0002), suggesting that both tests measure common skills.	Interrater reliability is r = 0.86. Test-retest reliability on a small sample yielded was r = 0.80 (Neistadt, 1992).	Not established	Strengths: Reliable kitchen assessment based on information-processing theory. Dynamic assessment approach indicates amount of cognitive support needed for task completion. Weaknesses: Primarily validated with persons with TBI, limiting generalizability to other diagnostic groups. Choice of tasks is limited by test design.

(continued)

Assessment Table 4-1	Summary of Assessments of Occupational Function *(continued)*

Instrument & Reference	Description	Time to Administer	Validity	Reliability	Sensitivity	Strengths and Weaknesses
Work Assessments						
VALPAR Component Work Sample Series & Dexterity Modules (Valpar Corp.)	Direct observation of work tasks selected to evaluate client's specific job requirements and needs. Each work sample consists of a scoring manual and standardized equipment ranging from common items to large equipment. Examples of dexterity module include small parts assembly, tool manipulation, and bimanual coordination.	Dependent on number of work samples tested. Samples range in time from 20 to 90 minutes.	The work samples have been criterion-referenced according to the Department of Labor's *Dictionary of Occupational Titles (DOT)*, yielding good face and content validity (AOTA, 2007).	Test-retest reliability for work samples 1-16 of the original series ranged from 0.70 to 0.99 for work rate and accuracy scores over a 1-week interval (AOTA, 2007).	Measures are highly sensitive to detecting changes in client performance over time.	Strengths: High face validity and reliability. Normative tables provide error and time percentiles for each sample. Weaknesses: Work samples emphasize physical components of work tasks and should be supplemented with assessments of worker interests, goals, and psychosocial/contextual factors influencing performance.
Worker Role Interview (WRI) version 10.0 (Braveman et al., 2005; Velozo, Kielhofner, & Fisher, 1998)	A semistructured interview that assesses psychosocial/ environmental factors of concern to the injured worker or client with a long-term disability and poor/limited work history. Complements observations made during other physical or behavioral work assessments: designed to identify specific variables influencing client's ability to return to work.	30–60 minutes and 15 minutes for scoring	Content areas were based on MOHO, and extensive literature review of factors that influence return to work.	Test-retest reliability for total score with a 6–12-day interval was 0.95. Interrater reliability was 0.81 with three raters (Biernacki, 1993).	Not established	Strengths: Test items reflect occupational therapists' interest in the meaning of work. Psychometrics of WRI (version 9.0) confirmed (Forsyth et al., 2006). Weaknesses: Time to administer can be lengthy.

Leisure Assessments

Assessment	Description	Time	Validity/Reliability	Sensitivity	Strengths/Weaknesses
Activity Card Sort (ACS), 2nd edition (Baum & Edwards, 2008)	Card sort consists of 89 photographs depicting instrumental, leisure, and social activities. Respondent is asked to sort cards into categories related to activity performance prior to injury/illness, current patterns, and most important. Comparison of previous to current scores for each area of occupation reflects change in activity participation that can be addressed in treatment planning. Three test versions allow use in multiple settings.	20–30 minutes	Content, construct, and predictive validity well established (Baum & Edwards, 2008). Test–retest reliability for 1-week interval was 0.89. Reliability also studied in Israeli and Hong Kong samples (Baum & Edwards, 2008).	Good sensitivity for clinical and research purposes	Strengths: Strong psychometrics. Easy to administer and use. Provides useful data for treatment planning. Weaknesses: Addresses activity participation of older adults; not appropriate for young clients.
Modified Interest Checklist (Kielhofner & Neville, 1983). Derived from Interest Checklist (Matsutsuyu, 1969; Rogers, Weinstein, & Figone, 1978)	Self-report questionnaire and 68-item interview checklist. Gathers data about a client's interest patterns over time (past, present, and future). Activities range from gardening and yard work, to bowling, watching television, and driving. Recommended for use MOHO.	10–15 minutes	Face validity evident. Rogers (1988) reported that Interest Checklist discriminates among diagnostic groups and normal control subjects. Good test–retest reliability (0.92) within 3-week interval for original version (Rogers, Weinstein, & Figone, 1978).	Not established	Strengths: Quick to administer. Participation in wide range of activities is assessed over time. Provides activity ideas for treatment planning (Klyczek, Bauer-Yox, & Fiedler, 1997). Weaknesses: Lack of strong validity and sensitivity data. Clients may misinterpret some items (e.g., level of participation is unclear: do clients perform versus watch activities such as auto racing or concerts?). Limited testing with clients who have physical versus psychosocial disabilities.

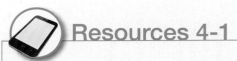

Resources 4-1

Assessments

The assessments discussed in this chapter may be obtained either from the resources listed below or from published articles on instrument development and psychometric properties that are included in the reference list. For additional information on assessments not discussed in this chapter, refer to *Occupational therapy assessment tools: An annotated index* (AOTA, 2007).

Activity Card Sort, 2nd edition

American Occupational
Therapy Association
4720 Montgomery Lane
P.O. Box 31220
Bethesda, MD 20824-1220
Phone: (877) 404-AOTA
Fax: (770) 238-0414
http://store.aota.org

Assessment of Motor and Process Skills (AMPS) (7th edition, revised 2012)

Center for Innovative
OT Solution
Email: info@innovativeOT
solutions.com
www.innovativeOT
solutions.com

Australian Therapy Outcome Measures for Occupational Therapy

(AusTOMs-OT, 2nd edition)
School of Occupational
Therapy
LaTrobe University
Victoria, 3086, Australia
Phone: 61-3-9479-5700
Fax: 61-3-9479-5737
E-mail: c.unsworth@
latrobe.edu.au

Canadian Occupational Performance Measure (COPM) (4th edition)

Canadian Association of
Occupational Therapists
CTTC Building, Suite 3400
1125 Colonel By Drive
Ottawa Ontario K1S 5R1,
Canada
Phone: 613-523-CAOT
(2268)
Toll-free in Canada and the
continental United States:
800-434-CAOT (2268)
www.caot.ca

Functional Independence Measure (FIM™)

Uniform Data System for
Medical Rehabilitation
270 Northpointe Parkway,
Suite 300
Amherst, New York 14228
Office Hours: Mon–Fri, 8:30
a.m.–5:30 p.m. EST
Phone: 716-817-7800
Fax: 716-568-0037
E-mail: info@udsmr.org

Idyll Arbor Leisure Battery (IALB) Leisure Assessment Inventory

Idyll Arbor
39129 264th Ave SE
Enumclaw, WA 98022
Phone: 360-825-7797
Fax: 360-825-5670
E-mail: sales@idyllarbor.com

Kohlman Evaluation of Living Skills (KELS) (3rd edition)

AOTA
4720 Montgomery Lane
P.O. Box 31220
Bethesda, MD 20824-1220
Phone: 877-404-AOTA
Fax: 770-238-0414
http://store.aota.org

Modified Interest Checklist

MOHO Clearinghouse
UIC Office of Publications
Services (MC 291)
828 S. Wolcott Ave.
Room B-4
Chicago, IL 60612
Phone: 312-996-4193
Fax: 312-996-0633
Free Download at: http://
www.uic.edu/depts/moho
/images/Modified%20
Interest%20Checklist.pdf

Occupational Performance History Interview-II (OPHI-II) (version 2.1, 2004)

MOHO Clearinghouse
UIC Office of Publications
Services (MC 291)
828 S. Wolcott Ave.
Room B-4
Chicago, IL 60612
Phone: 312-996-4193
Fax: 312-996-0633
http://www.uic.edu
/depts/moho/images
/OfflineOrderform.pdf

Safety Assessment of Function and the Environment for Rehabilitation – Health Outcome Measurement and Evaluation (SAFER-HOME, version 3)

VHA Rehab Solutions
477 Mount Pleasant Rd.,
Suite 500
Toronto, Ontario M4S 2L9,
Canada
Phone: 416-489-2500
Fax: 416-489-7533
www.vha.ca

Valpar Component Work Samples

Valpar International
Corporation
P.O. Box 5767
Tucson, AZ 85703
Phone: 800-633-3321
Fax: 262-797-8488
E-mail: sales@valparint.com

Worker Role Interview (WRI) (version 10.0, 2005)

MOHO Clearinghouse
UIC Office of Publications
Services (MC 291)
828 S. Wolcott Ave.
Room B-4
Chicago, IL 60612
Phone: 312-996-4193
Fax: 312-996-0633
http://www.uic.edu
/depts/moho/images
/OfflineOrderform.pdf

Identification of Occupational Performance Needs

A client-centered occupational therapy assessment recognizes that engagement in life roles and occupations of one's choice is a personal issue and that the client's perception is an important force that drives the occupational therapy process (Law et al., 2005). Information about a person's occupational roles and tasks, developmental stage, and the environment in which he or she lives is best obtained through interview. Although this can be done through informal narrative interviews, more structured interview-based assessments are recommended. Neistadt's (1994) research indicated that informal client interviews often lead to goals that are vague and not specifically related to occupation. The occupational therapist is advised to select a range of standardized assessments that incorporate semistructured interviews to identify occupational need areas, as well as direct measures of abilities and skills during observation of task performance.

Semistructured Interview Assessments

A semistructured interview assessment that is widely used to evaluate a client's perception of his or her occupational performance is the Canadian Occupational Performance Measure (COPM) (Law et al., 2005). The COPM helps clients to identify concerns with occupational performance, assists in goal setting, and measures changes in client perceptions of occupational performance over the course of therapy. The COPM is a generic measure that can be used with clients across all developmental stages who have a variety of disabilities. It is client centered and addresses roles, role expectations, and activity performance within the client's own environment.

The COPM is administered in a four-step process that includes problem definition, priority setting, scoring, and reassessment. During the initial COPM interview, clients or caregivers identify activities that are important to them and are in need of occupational therapy intervention in the areas of ADL, work, and leisure. After all of the occupational performance problems are identified, clients score them in terms of importance, their perception of current performance, and satisfaction with that performance. It is important to be aware that a client with a new illness may not recognize or be ready to identify these issues. The therapist and the client may begin treatment by working on identified concerns and can return to this semistructured interview process later to see whether other issues emerge. Reassessment is completed at discharge or when the client and the therapist consider it necessary for further treatment planning (Fig. 4-1).

Another semistructured interview assessment that is used to identify occupational performance needs is the Occupational Performance History Interview-II (OPHI-II),

Through an interview, clients identify occupational performance activities that are important to them and which they are having difficulties performing satisfactorily. These are scored on a 1–10 scale.

Activity Problems	Importance	Performance	Satisfaction
Doing up fasteners	9	3	1
Washing face and hands	10	1	1
Preparing sandwich	5	1	4
Holding a book	7	3	5
Visiting friends	9	2	4

Figure 4-1 Example of the scores for the Canadian Occupational Performance Measure.

version 2.1 (Kielhofner et al., 2004). OPHI-II is a broad assessment of occupational life history in work, leisure, and daily activities that was developed using the Model of Human Occupation (Kielhofner, 2008). The OPHI-II contains three valid scales that provide insight into the nature of occupational performance and adaptation (see Assessment Table 4-1). Test items explore a client's ability to organize time for responsibilities; identify interests, goals, and role expectations; recognize personal responsibilities and values; and participate in varied environments (e.g., leisure, home, and work settings). OPHI-II, version 2.1 includes paper key forms that can be used to easily obtain interval measures without computer analysis. These measures can identify when performance in one area (e.g., works toward goals) deviates from others, indicating needs for intervention. An accompanying Life History Narrative Form is used to document qualitative information from the interview. OPHI-II can be used with occupational therapy clients who are adolescents or older and who are seen in psychiatry, physical disability, or gerontology practices (Kielhofner et al., 2004).

Another concept related to occupational performance is that of life balance. The life balance model proposes that a person's activity configuration should meet important needs, which are "(1) basic instrumental needs necessary for sustained biological health and physical safety; (2) to have rewarding and self-affirming relationships with others; (3) to feel engaged, challenged and competent; and (4) to create meaning and a positive personal identity" (Matuska & Christiansen, 2008, p. 11). The Life Balance Inventory (LBI) is based on this model, in which the balance of one's everyday activities is measured in terms of activity configuration *congruence* and activity configuration *equivalence*. Congruence is high when there is a match between the *actual* activities a person engages in regularly and his or her *desired* activity configuration or engagement. Activity configuration equivalence is conceptualized as a satisfactory balance of activity engagement across four dimensions: health, relationships, challenge/interests, and identity needs (Matuska, 2012a).

The LBI is a reliable and valid online tool (Matuska, 2012b) in which respondents first identify daily activities they do or want to engage in (e.g., gardening and participating in professional organizations) and then rate their perceived satisfaction with the amount of time they spent doing those activities within the past month. A printout provides life balance scores for each of the four dimensions above. The LBI and this conceptualization of life balance can facilitate interview discussions about client-centered goals and help identify ways in which the client can improve satisfaction and reduce stress while engaged in occupational roles and routines.

Assessing Roles and Community Integration

Trombly (1995) sorts life roles into three domains that correspond well to the Occupational Therapy Practice Framework (OTPF) (AOTA, 2008): self-maintenance, self-advancement, and self-enhancement (see Chapter 1). Widely used role assessments in occupational therapy include the OPHI-II, discussed above, and the Role Checklist (Oakley et al., 1986). The Role Checklist is a two-part self-report assessment. Part I assesses participation in 10 major life roles: student, worker, volunteer, caregiver, home maintainer, friend, family member, religious participant, hobbyist/amateur, participant in organizations, and other. Test items address past, present, and future performance of these roles. Part II measures how valuable or important each role is to the client. This assessment has been used to evaluate perceptions of role participation in persons with mental illness, mothers with young children, persons with physical disabilities, and adolescents.

Community integration refers to the ability of a person to live, work, and enjoy his or her free time within the community setting. A client's competence and ability to engage in community tasks and roles after a disabling event or illness are related to intrinsic abilities or performance skills as well as characteristics of the environment in which he or she lives. Although most of the following assessments emphasize the client's perception of his or her competence in community or societal integration, others, such as the Craig Hospital Inventory of Environmental Factors (CHIEF) (Whiteneck et al., 2004), focus on environmental factors that limit community integration. For example, questions on the CHIEF address how the design and layout of the home or workplace, or features of natural or man-made environments (e.g., terrain, noise, and lighting) impact occupational performance and participation. Knowledge of the content and focus of these and other assessments will help the occupational therapist choose tools that best measure and identify occupational performance areas in need of intervention.

The Reintegration to Normal Living (RNL) Index (Wood-Dauphinee et al., 1988) is an easy-to-use 11-item assessment of how well individuals return to normal living patterns following incapacitating disease or injury. Client perceptions of reintegration are measured along several domains: mobility, self-care, daily activity, recreational activity, and family roles. This assessment has been tested with a wide variety of diagnostic groups including patients with arthritis, fractures, amputations, stroke, spinal cord injury, traumatic brain injury, and hip fracture. A validation study of community-dwelling persons with limited mobility (Stark et al., 2005) replaced the original visual analog scale with a 10-point Likert-type scale so clients could more accurately rate their performance. A recent study yielded good construct validity and internal consistency with a mixed sample of community dwelling individuals after rehabilitation (Miller, Clemson, & Lannin, 2011).

The Community Integration Measure (CIM) (McColl et al., 2001) uses 10 items to gather qualitative information about a person's experience with community integration and participation. It is based on a theoretical model that is client centered and differs from other community assessments because it makes no assumptions about the relative importance of particular activities or relationships (McColl et al., 2001). For example, the CIM does not assume that independent participation is a better measure of community integration than supported or mutual participation with others. Although this easy-to-use measure was developed for and tested primarily with persons diagnosed with traumatic brain injury, it has been used in practice with clients who have a wide range of disabilities (McColl et al., 2001). The CIM is able to differentiate persons with and without disabilities and correlates significantly with other measures of community integration and life satisfaction. A replication study (Reistetter et al., 2005) showed that the CIM correlated better with the Satisfaction with Life Scale than the Community Integration Questionnaire (CIQ) (Willer, Ottenbacher, & Coad et al., 1994).

Many assessments of health-related quality of life have been developed for use with persons with chronic illness. Examples of these assessments that have excellent reliability and validity include the Sickness Impact Profile (Bergner et al., 1981) and the Medical Outcomes Study Short Form 36 (SF-36) (Jenkinson, Wright, & Coulter, 1994).

Assessing Tasks and Activities

Occupational therapists use a variety of assessment tools to measure baseline and discharge performance in tasks and activities of importance to the client, including ADL, IADL, work, and leisure.

Activities of Daily Living

ADL generally include mobility at home, feeding, dressing, bathing, grooming, toileting, and personal hygiene (AOTA, 2008). Direct observation of problem activities identified by the client should be done at the time of day when they are normally performed and, if possible, in the place where they usually occur. Remember that many people may have strong feelings of modesty regarding personal care, and those feelings should be respected. The client's endurance and safety should be closely monitored, and ADL performance can be evaluated over several therapy sessions if slow performance or fatigue occurs. Items that would be unsafe or obviously unsuccessful (such as tub transfers) are postponed until the patient's physical status improves. When the patient is not independent in a required task at the time of discharge, plans are developed to ensure that others can assist with this task and that additional therapy is received if warranted.

Most standardized ADL evaluations were designed for program evaluation to document the level of independence achieved by patients as the result of a particular program. Several ADL assessments used by occupational therapists are briefly described in the following paragraphs. The Barthel Index (Mahoney & Barthel, 1965) is a reliable and valid assessment of 10 activities (see Assessment Table 4-1). The total score for these 10 activities can range from 0 to 100 (total independence), and the score for each activity is weighted according to its importance for independent functioning (Mahoney & Barthel, 1965). A score of 60 seems to be the transition point from dependency to assisted independence. Scores may be derived from client interview or direct observation. The reliability and validity of the Barthel Index also has been established when administered during telephone interviews (Della Pietra et al., 2011).

The Modified Barthel Index (Shah, Vanclay, & Cooper, 1989) was developed to increase sensitivity to changes observed when patients progressed from one level of assist to another during rehabilitation. A third 20-point Barthel Index includes the same test items with weighted, variable subscores ranging between 0 and 1 (e.g., bathing) or between 0 and 3 (e.g., transfers) (Collin et al., 1988). Differences in sensitivity were not found between these two modified versions of the Barthel in a sample of stroke survivors requiring rehabilitation (Hocking et al., 1999). The original 10-item version of the Barthel Index, scoring 0 to 100 with 5-point increments, continues to be most widely used and recommended for stroke research (Quinn, Langhorne, & Stott, 2011).

The FIM™ (Granger & Hamilton, 1992) uses a 7-point ordinal scale to evaluate occupational performance for 18 items (13 motor and 5 cognition) (see Assessment Table 4-1) and is a basic measure of the severity of disability based on burden of care, not impairment.

(Granger et al., 1993). The scale rates a client's performance by taking into account his or her need for assistance from another person or a device. The FIM™ instrument is intended to measure what the person with disability actually does, whatever the diagnosis or impairment, and is scored according to information gathered by members of the rehabilitation team during client observation. The FIM™ can be used during rehabilitation to track changes in ADL and provide data for program evaluation. It has been shown to predict functional status at discharge and length of rehabilitation stay (Heinemann et al., 1994). The FIM™ is part of a uniform data system that collects information about rehabilitation outcomes and effectiveness and is an integral part of the Inpatient Rehabilitation Facility–Patient Assessment Instrument (IRF-PAI) (University at Buffalo Foundation Activities, Inc., 2004) (see Fig. 10-6, Case Example: FIM™ assessment). Researchers have established MCID values for the modified 20-point Barthel Index (Hsieh et al., 2007) and FIM™ (Beninato et al., 2006) (see Assessment Table 4-1 for specifics).

The Klein-Bell Activities of Daily Living Scale (Klein & Bell, 1982) documents a client's ability to perform in six BADL (see Assessment Table 4-1). These ADL are broken down into 170 simple behavioral items, each of which is scored separately. The large number of items makes the Klein-Bell one of the most responsive ADL assessments. Each item is scored as achieved (no physical or verbal assistance) or unable (assistance needed), and raw scores are converted to percentage scores to make communication of results easier to understand. If the client can perform the test item with adapted equipment during the discharge evaluation, he or she is given credit for accomplishing that activity. Emphasis is placed on the person's ability to physically complete components of ADL tasks (e.g., inserting foot into pant leg, grasping waistband to pull up pants, and zipping). It does not well distinguish when a client is unable to complete the task because of other factors, such as impaired organization or safety awareness. When impairments become apparent during ADL assessment, the therapist will further evaluate performance skills (e.g., sequencing, coordination, and balance) as needed for comprehensive treatment planning.

Instrumental Activities of Daily Living

Although many IADL assessments include a few self-care items, their focus is primarily home management tasks such as meal planning, preparation, and cleanup; laundry; shopping for food and clothing; routine and seasonal care of the home; and yard work and other maintenance tasks that were the responsibility of the patient prior to therapy and may require assessment and intervention. Several standardized IADL assessments used by occupational therapists are described in the following paragraphs.

The Nottingham Extended ADL Scale (Nouri & Lincoln, 1987) is a self-report questionnaire that assesses occupational performance of 22 daily activities during the previous few weeks (see Fig. 4-2 and Assessment Table 4-1). Although originally developed for use with stroke survivors, its use has also been studied in clients after hip replacement surgery (Harwood & Ebrahim, 2000), with multiple sclerosis (Nicholl, Lincoln, & Playford, 2002), and with Parkinson's disease (Clarke et al., 2009). The Nottingham Extended ADL Scale is a reliable and valid

measure of functional independence; however, conflicting reports of its responsiveness to change have been published (Harwood & Ebrahim, 2000; Wu et al., 2011).

The Assessment of Motor and Process Skills (AMPS) (Fisher, 1993, 1995; Fisher & Bray Jones, 2010) is an innovative observational assessment. It uses a 4-point scale to rate 16 motor and 20 process skill items during performance of client-selected, challenging IADL tasks. The motor skills (e.g., stabilizes, reaches, and transports) are the actions observed during task performance that are thought to be related to underlying abilities in postural control, mobility, coordination, or strength. Process skills (e.g., sequences, initiates, and adjusts) are used to organize and adapt actions during actual performance and represent the underlying attentional, conceptual, organizational, and adaptive capacities of the client (Park, Fisher, & Velozo, 1994). It is important to note that the AMPS is a test of skill in occupational performance and is not designed to evaluate the presence of neuromuscular, biomechanical, or cognitive impairments (e.g., strength, range of motion, and memory) or underlying capacities. Unlike impairments and underlying capacities that often are evaluated separately from task performance, the motor and process skills of the AMPS are goal-directed actions that occur in the context of occupation. As a result, the AMPS is used to assess activities and participation, not body functions or contextual factors (WHO, 2001). A pilot study to develop a driving task for the AMPS provides an example of the range of test items used to evaluate occupational performance (Robertson & Carswell, 2011).

Occupational therapists must attend a training workshop and become calibrated as a reliable rater before using the AMPS. Once trained, scoring is done by computer. The AMPS has been shown to discriminate well between people without disabilities and those with cognitive or physical disabilities. A significant advantage of AMPS is its flexibility in allowing the client to choose which tasks are used for assessment.

The Kohlman Evaluation of Living Skills (KELS) is a short living skills assessment that is administered through interview and direct observation (Kohlman Thomson, 1993) (see Assessment Table 4-1). Individual items are scored as independent, needs assistance, or not applicable. Although originally created for use in short-term psychiatric units, it is also a good measure of IADL performance in elderly clients. When compared with standardized assessments for cognition, affect, and functional status of community living older adults, the KELS showed good convergent validity and strong correlations with executive function measures (Burnett, Dyer, & Naik, 2009). When combined with other assessments and client input, the KELS data can help determine the environment that will allow a person to live as independently and safely as possible.

Nottingham Extended ADL Scale

The following questions are about everyday activities. Please answer by ticking ONE box for each question. Please record what you have ACTUALLY done in the last few weeks.

DID YOU....	Not at all	with help	on your own with difficulty	on your own
1. Walk around outside?	☐	☐	☐	☐
2. Climb stairs?	☐	☐	☐	☐
3. Get in and out of a car?	☐	☐	☐	☐
4. Walk over uneven ground?	☐	☐	☐	☐
5. Cross roads?	☐	☐	☐	☐
6. Travel on public transport?	☐	☐	☐	☐
7. Manage to feed yourself?	☐	☐	☐	☐
8. Manage to make yourself a hot drink?	☐	☐	☐	☐
9. Take hot drinks from one room to another?	☐	☐	☐	☐
10. Do the washing up?	☐	☐	☐	☐
11. Make yourself a hot snack?	☐	☐	☐	☐
12. Manage your own money when out?	☐	☐	☐	☐
13. Wash small items of clothing?	☐	☐	☐	☐
14. Do your own housework?	☐	☐	☐	☐
15. Do your own shopping?	☐	☐	☐	☐
16. Do a full clothes wash?	☐	☐	☐	☐
17. Read newspaper or books?	☐	☐	☐	☐
18. Use the telephone?	☐	☐	☐	☐
19. Write letters?	☐	☐	☐	☐
20. Go out socially?	☐	☐	☐	☐
21. Manage your own garden?	☐	☐	☐	☐
22. Drive a car?	☐	☐	☐	☐

Figure 4-2 Nottingham Extended Activities of Daily Living Scale (NEADL), University of Nottingham, 2007. Used with permission.

The Performance Assessment of Self-Care Skills (PASS), version 3.1 (Rogers & Holm, 1989a, 1989b) is a performance-based observational tool to document functional status and change during rehabilitation (Fig. 4-3) (see Assessment Table 4-1). The PASS has both clinic and home versions and is designed to assess the types of assistance needed for home and community safety. Unlike the KELS, the PASS is criterion referenced, meaning that only selected items or the entire test can be administered depending on the client's needs and time availability. The PASS provides input regarding the client's level of independence in task completion, safety needs, and quality of task outcome. It is appropriate for use with adults of varied diagnoses (e.g., arthritis, cardiopulmonary disease, and dementia) and provides excellent data for treatment planning and documentation of patient outcomes (AOTA, 2007).

The Safety Assessment of Function and the Environment for Rehabilitation-Health Outcome Measurement and Evaluation (SAFER-HOME) was developed to provide occupational therapists with a comprehensive, consistent measure to simultaneously assess safety and occupational performance in the home (Chiu et al., 2006; Oliver et al., 1993). Test items assess both the environmental situation and functional ability of the client in 12 categories (see Assessment Table 4-1). For example, the living situation category addresses whether stairs are in good condition, the presence of scatter rugs and electric cords, and environmental clutter that might impact home safety. Level of safety risk is rated on a 4-point scale ranging from 0 (no problem) to 3 (severe problem) (AOTA, 2007). The instruction manual includes a list of recommendations to help the occupational therapist identify solutions to difficult problem areas.

Kitchen Tasks. Two assessments of performance during kitchen tasks have been developed for use in occupational therapy. The Kitchen Task Assessment (KTA) (Baum & Edwards, 1993) uses the task of making pudding to assess the cognitive support required by persons with dementia and Alzheimer's disease to complete a basic cooking task. Thus, the KTA provides information about performance as well as components of occupation, such as initiation, sequencing, organization, and problem solving. There is a significant relationship between scores on the KTA and other neuropsychological assessments but limited evidence of its use with clients who have physical versus psychosocial and cognitive disabilities.

The Rabideau Kitchen Evaluation Revised (RKE-R) (Neistadt, 1992, 1994) is an assessment of meal preparation that was primarily developed for adults with brain injury. All task components are scored according to the number of verbal cues or the amount of physical assistance required for safe completion. This quick assessment can help with discharge planning by providing information about a client's safety and independence during basic kitchen tasks. The RKE-R was found to differentiate among stroke survivors with/without unilateral spatial neglect (Katz et al., 1999) and was significantly related to neuropsychological measures of verbal memory, simple auditory attention, visuospatial skills, and overall cognitive performance (Yantz et al., 2010).

Child Care

Child care and parenting activities include but are not limited to the physical care and supervision of children and the use of age-appropriate activities, communication, and behaviors to facilitate child development (AOTA, 2008). Because no standard evaluations exist, the occupational therapist must work with the client to identify and assess performance needs during required and valued child care tasks, while taking into account the ages and personalities of the children involved. The COPM can be used to assess child care concerns and to determine what interventions and adaptations may be needed to enhance a client's competence and satisfaction in this area. The AusTOMS-OT provides a means to document the degree to which limitations in child care and parenting abilities are related to impairments in structure or function, activity limitations, participation restrictions, and level of distress/well-being (Unsworth, 2005) and how these change in response to intervention.

Work

Work assessments are used to determine whether an individual has the ability to perform necessary job skills and is otherwise prepared for employment in terms of work habits, work quality, ability to learn or acquire new skills, and ability to work with others as a team member, supervisor, or supervisee. Velozo (1993) described two categories of work evaluations: (1) standardized commercial evaluations such as those used in vocational rehabilitation and (2) highly technical evaluations of physical and work capacity. He questioned whether these work evaluations truly reflect occupational therapists' interest in the meaning of work and emphasized our unique role in linking work evaluations to the psychosocial and environmental factors that contribute to client performance.

Standardized vocational evaluation systems use job analysis or work samples to determine an individual's ability to perform tasks similar to those encountered at work. In the United States, the Dictionary of Occupational Titles (U.S. Department of Labor, 2011) provides a taxonomy for measurement of work performance that lists specific job requirements, including skills and equipment. One standardized work assessment system that

Task #H14: IADL: Medication Management

Assistive Technology Devices (ATDs) used during task:

1.

2.

3.

Total # of ATDs used: _____

	Assist level →															
		INDEPENDENCE DATA									**SAFETY DATA**		**ADEQUACY DATA**		**SUMMARY SCORES**	
Subtasks	MOBILITY/ADL/IADL SUBTASKS	Verbal Supportive (Encouragement) 1	Verbal Non-Directive 2	Verbal Directive 3	Gestures 4	Task or Environment Rearrangement 5	Demonstration 6	Physical Guidance 7	Physical Support 8	Total Assist 9		Unsafe Observations	QUALITY: Standards not met/ improvement needed	PROCESS: Imprecision, lack of economy, missing steps	INDEPENDENCE	SAFETY ADEQUACY
1 Med 1 C-P	Reports next time first medication is to be taken correctly (based on testing time, matches direction on label)															
2 Med 1 C-P	Opens first pill bottle with ease (by second try)															
3 Med 1 C-P	Distributes pills from first pill bottle into correct time slots for the next 2 days (all pills & all slots indicated; days indicated)															
4 Med2 N-C-P	Reports next time second medication is to be taken correctly (based on testing time, matches direction on label)															
5 Med2 N-C-P	Opens second pill bottle with ease (by second try)															
6 Med2 N-C-P	Distributes pills from second pill bottle into correct time slots for the next 2 days (all pills and all slots indicated; days indicated)															

Figure 4-3 Performance Assessment of Self-Care Skills (PASS), version 3.1. Score sheet to record type of assistance needed, safety, and adequacy of performance during assessment. Summary scores (0–3), based on the client's level of independence, safety awareness, and overall performance, are described in test manual. © Rogers & Holm, 1989, 1994. Used with permission.

is often used is the VALPAR Component Work Samples (see Resources 4-1). The VALPAR system consists of a wide range of work samples that evaluate specific occupational performance skills (e.g., range of motion, problem solving, physical capacities, and mobility) during simulated job tasks. Although evidence of the reliability and validity for this standardized evaluation system is extensive, a potential disadvantage of the VALPAR Component Work Samples is its expense.

Because a large proportion of work evaluations are administered to clients who have musculoskeletal or soft-tissue injuries, their primary focus is on the physical capacities required for work tasks. Many standardized functional capacity evaluations (FCE) are available to measure physical capacity (e.g., strength, endurance, and freedom from pain) during work-related tasks, such as lifting, sitting, and standing (AOTA, 2007). In addition to evaluating a client's physical performance, a comprehensive work assessment must also include contextual information regarding the client's work environment and history, his medical condition and contraindications, and the whole person context in which he lives (e.g., information about nonwork occupations such as homemaker, caregiver, or recreational roles) (Strong et al., 2004).

Semistructured interviews, such as the Worker Role Interview (WRI) (Braveman et al., 2005; Velozo, Kielhofner, & Fisher, 1998), can complement fce by providing important information regarding the psychosocial and environmental factors that influence return to work. This well established tool can be used to assess other behaviors considered important for work, such as punctuality, communication skills, ability to work with others, and grooming. The WRI is well suited to the needs of clients from varied cultures and diagnostic groups (Forsyth et al., 2006).

Leisure

Leisure involves engaging in self-chosen, motivating, and goal-directed activities for amusement, relaxation, spontaneous enjoyment, and/or self-expression. Hersch (1990) pointed out that "the concept of leisure encompasses a multitude of meanings: the leisure event itself, the amount and frequency of the activity, its meaningfulness to the participant, and the social context" in which it is performed (p. 55). Leisure serves many purposes in one's life by fulfilling physical, social, and intellectual needs, particularly for the older adult (Hersch, 1990). Participation in leisure is an important area of occupation that is closely related to life satisfaction (AOTA, 2007). The occupational therapist can facilitate leisure exploration with clients through use of checklists and semistructured interviews that focus on identifying interests, skills, opportunities, and leisure activities that are appropriate for the individual. Leisure participation

involves the planning and engagement in appropriate leisure activities, maintaining a balance of leisure activities with other areas of occupation, and obtaining needed supplies and adaptations to allow for successful engagement (AOTA, 2007).

Because participation in leisure is viewed as an integral component of occupational performance and functioning, many IADL assessments address the client's leisure interests and pursuits along with IADL (e.g., home management and community mobility), work/education, and social/participation needs. The LBI (Matuska, 2012a), the COPM (Law et al., 2005), the OPHI-II, version 2.1 (Kielhofner et al., 2004), the Nottingham Extended ADL Scale (Nouri & Lincoln, 1987), and the RNL Index (Wood-Dauphinee et al., 1988) all include items related to leisure activities. The Activity Card Sort (2nd edition) (Baum & Edwards, 2008) is another reliable and valid assessment of actual and desired activity engagement that crosses the domains of IADL, leisure and social activities. The Activity Card Sort (2nd edition) captures changes in activity patterns related to the impact of a disability or illness and provides the therapist with immediate feedback regarding valued activities for treatment planning. Any of these assessments can help the therapist identify the client's leisure interests within the context of other occupational performance needs.

Several assessments specific to evaluation of leisure interests and participation continue to be used by occupational therapists. For example, the Modified Interest Checklist (Kielhofner & Neville, 1983; Matsutsuyu, 1969) gathers information about a client's level of interest and participation in 68 different leisure activities. Activities are rated on a 3-point scale ranging from no interest to strong interest. This modified scale assesses current interests, how these have changed over time, and whether the client wishes to participate in these and other activities in the future. The Modified Interest Checklist is particularly useful for appreciating the impact of disability or illness on the client's experiences and engagement in meaningful leisure activities (Kielhofner, 2008). It can be used for treatment planning with clients throughout the life span, from adolescence through old age.

Other leisure assessments, such as the Nottingham Leisure Questionnaire (Drummond et al., 2001) and the Leisure Diagnostic Battery (Witt & Ellis, 1984), are reliable and valid tools that have been frequently used in research but are not readily available for clinic use. The Idyll Arbor Leisure Battery (IALB) (Hawkins et al., 2002) is composed of several scales to assess client attitudes, interests, motivation, and satisfaction with leisure pursuits. Although used primarily by recreational therapists, this battery has established reliability and validity and may be used by occupational therapists for program development and evaluation (AOTA, 2007). Please refer to Resources 4-1 for more information.

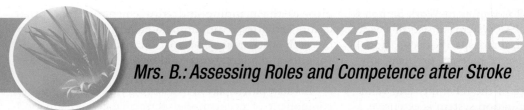

case example
Mrs. B.: Assessing Roles and Competence after Stroke

Occupational Therapy Assessment Process	Clinical Reasoning Process	
	Objectives	Examples of Internal Dialogue

Patient Information

Mrs. B. is a 53-year-old married woman who experienced a left ischemic cerebrovascular accident 1 month ago while at work. She received a thrombolytic medication within the first 3 hours of her stroke and is reported to have made excellent progress during 3 weeks of inpatient rehabilitation. She has recently been discharged home and is now being referred to outpatient rehabilitation for continued occupational, physical, and speech therapy. The occupational therapy discharge summary reports continued limitations in instrumental activities of daily living (IADL) tasks, with mild to moderate right-sided paresis and mild aphasia.

Mrs. B. lives with her husband and 15-year-old daughter. Her 19-year-old son is a college freshman, living 4 hours from home. Mrs. B. is an elementary school teacher who also coaches her daughter's skating team and volunteers at the town library. Her husband has a demanding full-time job and travels 1–2 weeks per month. The occupational therapist focuses the initial occupational assessment on Mrs. B.'s ability to resume self-maintenance roles and to engage in valued life roles and tasks now that she is home.

Understand the patient's diagnosis or condition

"Mrs. B. had a pretty significant stroke and would likely have had greater limitations in motor abilities and language if she had not received such good care from emergency services. She is probably having difficulty using her dominant hand for daily tasks, and I wonder how she is getting around and managing at home when her husband is at work."

Know the person

"It must have been terrible for her to have a stroke while she was at work—at least it happened during lunch and not while she was in the classroom with her students. It sounds like she was pretty busy managing multiple roles—as mother, teacher, coach, and volunteer—in addition to taking care of home responsibilities. I wonder how she is dealing with this sudden change in routine."

Appreciate the context

"It must be difficult for her husband and daughter to take on more home management tasks while Mrs. B. is recovering from her stroke. I wonder if they have friends or other family members who can help with shopping, driving, etc."

Develop provisional hypotheses

"Given her diagnosis and good rate of recovery, I think she will do well in therapy. I expect that her motor impairments will be the biggest barrier to regaining independence in home and leisure tasks. Her mild aphasia will likely limit her return to teaching, at least in the short term."

Assessment Process

The therapist selected the following evaluation tools: Canadian Occupational Performance Measure (COPM) to obtain information about the client's perceived problems and priorities and the Assessment of Motor and Process Skills (AMPS) to assess IADL motor and process skills.

Consider evaluation approach and methods

"Because of her mild aphasia, it might be difficult and a bit frustrating for her to verbally describe her priorities for therapy on the COPM. I will talk with the speech therapist to see whether she might benefit from using a written list of activities to report concerns during this evaluation. It might also be helpful to have her husband present during the COPM to help clarify issues, as needed. The AMPS will give me the chance to observe how her right-sided paresis affects IADL performance and whether other cognitive and process-related impairments are a concern."

Assessment Results

During an interview using the COPM, Mrs. B. reported that it was very important for her to resume responsibilities in managing household tasks and fulfilling her roles as wife and mother. Planning and preparing meals and grocery shopping were also very important to her. She expressed frustration with the clumsiness in her dominant right hand and with her low endurance and fatigue when walking a distance with a cane. She was very concerned about returning to her job as a teacher because of her mild aphasia and expressed a strong desire to help prepare her daughter's skating team for the state finals in 2 months.

Interpret observations

"Mrs. B. seems to have good awareness of her impairments and needs for therapy and is generally able to make her needs known despite her mild aphasia and word-finding problems."

"I wonder whether the problems Mrs. B. had with sequencing and organizing tasks during the AMPS are related to the fact that she performed these in the rehab clinic, not at home. As she begins to take on more challenging tasks, it will be important to see how she performs in familiar versus unfamiliar settings."

The AMPS revealed that process skills were mildly impaired in the sequencing and organizing of chosen tasks. Although she required additional cues/support to initiate tasks, she showed good pacing once engaged and was able to adjust and adapt her approach to tasks when difficulties arose. Motor skills were mildly to moderately impaired, as she had difficulty reaching for items at or above shoulder height, lifting a medium-sized sauce pan from the stove to sink and manipulating items with her right hand. However, she was able to use her paretic right hand to stabilize and transport items during bilateral tasks. Extra time was needed for task completion, because she needed frequent rest breaks when performing IADL from an ambulatory level.

Occupational Therapy Problem List

Decreased participation and independence in IADL.

Impaired endurance and functional mobility, contributing to decreased productivity during IADL.

Reduced organizing and sequencing skills during IADL in an unfamiliar environment.

Mild to moderate hemiparesis in right arm, impeding functional use of the limb during occupational tasks.

"It seems like Mrs. B.'s mild hemiparesis is having the greatest impact on her performance of IADL, and she shows great determination and desire to improve the functional use of her right arm and hand. I'll administer a couple of stroke-specific assessments to get a better handle on her motor strengths and weaknesses so we can decide on a therapy program to best address these concerns. She is a great candidate for outpatient therapy."

Synthesize results

"Mrs. B. has experienced significant changes in her daily routine and ability to engage in important life roles and tasks since her stroke. I will talk more with her family to see how they think she is coping with these changes. Although fatigue is common during early recovery from stroke, depression might also be affecting her initiation and reports of fatigue during IADL."

"It will be important to get a better handle on Mrs. B.'s ability to return to her coaching and teaching roles, but this will be a longer term process. First, I'll use the Modified Interest Checklist to help identify meaningful activities to use in therapy so we can begin to work on problem areas and help her to feel more productive as she continues to recover from her stroke."

 Clinical Reasoning in Occupational Therapy Practice

Relating assessment to intervention and outcomes in occupational performance

During her first outpatient treatment session, Mrs. B. described frequent difficulties when using her right hand to carry items from the fridge or trying to grasp and place laundry items into the washer. She described feeling "tired all the time" and was frustrated by the extra time and effort needed to do previously simple tasks, such as paying household bills.

How might the occupational therapist address Mrs. B.'s concerns? How might the results of occupational therapy assessments guide the use of occupation as both an intervention and outcome of occupational therapy services?

Summary Review Questions

1. Define self-report and direct observation methods of assessment. What are the advantages and disadvantages of these methods when evaluating a client's occupational performance?
2. Distinguish between IADL and BADL, and describe one standardized assessment for each.
3. What are three measurement concepts or psychometric properties of standardized evaluation instruments? Define each and provide an example of how these properties might affect the results of occupational therapy assessments administered in the clinic.
4. Describe how a semistructured assessment such as the COPM can be used to measure occupational performance and establish the client's treatment plan.
5. Compare two different IADL measures. Describe the assessment and its psychometric properties, strengths, and weaknesses. Based on this information, which measure would you choose to evaluate a client recently admitted for outpatient rehabilitation services following stroke? Why?
6. A client-centered approach has been emphasized when assessing occupational roles and competence. List three ways in which this approach might influence occupational therapy intervention.

Glossary

Activities of daily living (ADL)—Activities or tasks that a person does every day to maintain personal care. Also referred to as basic activities of daily living (BADL).

Instrumental activities of daily living (IADL)—Complex activities or tasks that a person does to maintain independence in the home and community.

Leisure—Activities or tasks that are not obligatory, are intrinsically motivating, and are done for enjoyment.

Life balance—A satisfying pattern of daily activity that is healthful, meaningful, and sustainable to an individual within the context of his or her current life circumstances (Matuska & Christiansen, 2008).

Life roles—Areas of occupation associated with self-maintenance (e.g., ADL and IADL), self-advancement (e.g., work and education), and self-enhancement (e.g., leisure) that involve specific tasks and activities (see Chapter 1).

Occupational performance—Ability of individuals to satisfactorily perform purposeful daily activities (occupations). This involves the dynamic transaction among the client, the context or environment, and the activity.

Reliability—The ability of an assessment to consistently measure performance and to differentiate among clients under various conditions (Finch et al., 2002).

Validity—The extent to which an instrument measures what it is intended to measure (Finch et al., 2002).

Work—An area of occupation that includes activities needed for engaging in remunerative employment or volunteer pursuits (AOTA, 2008).

References

American Occupational Therapy Association. (2007). *Occupational therapy assessment tools: An annotated index* (3rd ed.). Bethesda, MD: AOTA.

American Occupational Therapy Association. (2008). Occupational therapy practice framework: Domain and process (2nd ed.). *American Journal of Occupational Therapy, 62,* 625–683.

Baum, C., & Edwards, D. F. (1993). Cognitive performance in senile dementia of the Alzheimer's type: The Kitchen Task Assessment. *American Journal of Occupational Therapy, 47,* 431–436.

Baum, C., & Edwards, D. F. (2008). *Activity card sort (ACS)* (2nd ed.). Bethesda, MD: AOTA.

Beninato, M., Gill-Body, K. M., Salles, S., Stark, P. C., Black-Schaffer, R. M., & Stein, J. (2006). Determination of the minimal clinically important difference in the FIM instrument in patients with stroke. *Archives of Physical Medicine and Rehabilitation, 87,* 32–39.

Bergner, M., Bobbit, R. A., Carter, W. B., & Gilson, B. S. (1981). The Sickness Impact Profile: Development and final revision of health status measure. *Medical Care, 19,* 787–805.

Biernacki, S. (1993). Reliability of the worker role interview. *American Journal of Occupational Therapy, 47,* 797–803.

Braveman, B., Robson, M., Velozo, C., Kielhofner, G., Fisher, G., Forsyth, K., & Kerschbaum, J. (2005). *Worker role interview (WRI)* (version 10.0). Chicago: Model of Human Occupation Clearinghouse.

Burnett, J., Dyer, C. B., & Naik, A. D. (2009). Convergent validation of the Kohlman evaluation of living skills as a screening tool of older adults' ability to live safely and independently in the community. *Archives of Physical Medicine and Rehabilitation, 90,* 1948–1952.

Carswell, A., McColl, M. A., Baptiste, S., Law, M., Polatajko, H., & Pollock, N. (2004). The Canadian Occupational Performance Measure: A research and clinical literature review. *Canadian Journal of Occupational Therapy, 71,* 210–222.

Centers for Medicare & Medicaid Services. (2013). Covered medical and other health services (Chapter 15, Rev. 170, 5-10-13). Medicare benefit policy manual. Retrieved from http://www.cms.gov/manuals/Downloads/bp102c15.pdf on 07/14/13.

Chau, N., Daler, S., Andre, J. M., & Patris, A. (1994). Inter-rater agreement of two functional independence scales: The Functional Independence Measure (FIM) and a subjective uniform continuous scale. *Disability and Rehabilitation, 16,* 63–71.

Chiu, T., & Oliver, R. (2006). Factor analysis and construct validity of the SAFER-HOME. *OTJR: Occupation, Participation and Health, 80 (4),* 132–142.

Chiu, T., Oliver, R., Ascott, P., Choo, L. C., Davis, T., Gaya, A., Goldsilver, P., McWhirter, M., & Letts, L. (2006). Safety assessment of function and the environment for rehabilitation: Health outcome measurement and evaluation (SAFER-HOME), version 3 Manual. Toronto, Canada: COTAHealth.

Clarke, C. E., Furmston, A., Morgan, E., Patel, S., Sackley, C., Walker, M, Bryan, S., & Wheatley, K. (2009). Pilot randomised controlled trial of occupational therapy to optimise independence in Parkinson's disease: The PD OT trial. *Journal of Neurology, Neurosurgery & Psychiatry, 80,* 976–978.

Collin, C., Wade, D. T., Davies, S., & Horne, V. (1988). The Barthel ADL index: A reliability study. *International Disabilities Studies, 10,* 61–63.

Corrigan, J. D., Smith-Knapp, K., & Granger, C. V. (1997). Validity of the functional independence measure for persons with traumatic brain injury. *Archives of Physical Medicine and Rehabilitation, 78,* 828–834.

Della Pietra, G. L., Savio, K., Oddone, E., Reggiani, M., Monaco, F., & Leone, M. A. (2011). Validity and reliability of the Barthel Index administered by telephone. *Stroke, 42,* 2077–2079.

Drummond, A. E., Parker, C. J., Gladman, J. R., & Logan, P. A. (2001). Development and validation of the Nottingham leisure questionnaire (NLQ). *Clinical Rehabilitation, 15,* 647–656.

Duncombe, L. W. (2004). Comparing learning of cooking in home and clinic for people with schizophrenia. *American Journal of Occupational Therapy, 58,* 272–278.

Edwards, M. M. (1990). The reliability and validity of self-report activities of daily living scales. *Canadian Journal of Occupational Therapy, 57,* 273–278.

Finch, E., Brooks, D., Stratford, P. W., & Mayo, N. E. (2002). *Physical rehabilitation outcome measures: A guide to enhanced clinical decision making* (2nd ed.). Hamilton, Canada: B.C. Decker.

Fisher, A. G. (1993). The assessment of IADL motor skills: An application of many-faceted Rasch analysis. *American Journal of Occupational Therapy, 47,* 319–329.

Fisher, A. G. (1995). *Assessment of motor and process skills*. Fort Collins, CO: Three Star Press.

Fisher, A. G. & Bray Jones, K. (2010). *Assessment of Motor and Process Skills. Volume 2: User Manual* (7th ed.). Fort Collins, CO: Three Star Press.

Forsyth, K., Bravemen, B., Kielhofner, G., Ekbladh, E., Haglund, L., Fenger, K., Keller, J. (2006). Psychometric properties of the Worker Role Interview. *Work, 27,* 313–318.

Granger, C. V., & Hamilton, B. B. (1992). The Uniform Data System for medical rehabilitation report of first admissions for 1990. *American Journal of Physical Medicine and Rehabilitation, 71,* 108–113.

Granger, C. V., Hamilton, B. B., Linacre, J. M., Heinemann, A. W., & Wright, B. D. (1993). Performance profiles of the Functional Independence Measure. *American Journal of Physical Medicine and Rehabilitation, 72,* 84–89.

Harwood, R. H., & Ebrahim, S. (2000). A comparison of the responsiveness of the Nottingham extended activities of daily living scale, London handicap scale and SF-36. *Disability and Rehabilitation, 22,* 786–793.

Hawkins, B. H., Ardovino, P., Brattain Rogers, N., Foose, A. & Ohlsen, N. (2002). *Idyll Arbor Leisure Battery (IALB) Leisure Assessment Inventory.* Enumclaw, WA: Idyll Arbor.

Haley, S. M., & Fragala-Pinkham, M. A. (2006). Interpreting change scores of tests and measures used in physical therapy. *Physical Therapy, 86,* 735–743.

Heinemann, A. W., Linacre, J. M., Wright, B. D., Hamilton, B. B., & Granger, C. V. (1994). Prediction of rehabilitation outcomes with disability measures. *Archives of Physical Medicine and Rehabilitation, 75,* 133–143.

Hersch, G. (1990). Leisure and aging. *Physical and Occupational Therapy in Geriatrics, 9,* 55–78.

Hocking, C., Williams, M., Broad, J., & Baskett, J. (1999). Sensitivity of Shah, Vanclay and Cooper's modified Barthel Index. *Clinical Rehabilitation, 13,* 141–147.

Holm, M. B., & Rogers, J. C. (2008). Performance Assessment of Self-Care Skills (PASS). In B. Hemphill-Pearson (Ed.), *Assessments in Occupational Therapy Mental Health* (2nd ed., pp. 101–110). Thorofare, NJ: SLACK.

Hsieh, Y.-W., Wang, C.-H., Wu, S.-C., Chen, P.-C., Sheu, C.-F., & Hsieh, C.-L. (2007). Establishing the minimal clinically important difference of the Barthel Index in stroke patients. *Neurorehabilitation and Neural Repair, 21,* 233–238.

Jenkinson, C., Wright, L., & Coulter, A. (1994). Criterion validity and reliability of the SF-36 in a population sample. *Quality of Life Research, 3,* 7–12.

Katz, N., Hartman-Maeir, A., Ring, H., & Soroker, N. (1999). Functional disability and rehabilitation outcome in right hemisphere damaged patients with and without unilateral spatial neglect. *Archives of Physical Medicine and Rehabilitation, 80,* 379–384.

Kielhofner, G. (2008). *Model of human occupation: Theory and application* (4th ed.). Philadelphia: Lippincott Williams & Wilkins.

Kielhofner, G., Mallinson, T., Crawford, D., Nowak, M., Rigby, M., Henry, A., & Walens, D. (2004). *User's manual for the OPHI-II* (version 2.1). Chicago: Model of Human Occupation Clearinghouse, University of Illinois at Chicago.

Kielhofner, G., Mallinson, T., Forsyth, K., & Lai, J.-S. (2001). Psychometric properties of the second version of the Occupational Performance History Interview (OPHI-II). *American Journal of Occupational Therapy, 55,* 260–267.

Kielhofner, G. & Neville, A. (1983). *The modified interest checklist.* Unpublished manuscript.

Klein, R. M., & Bell, B. (1982). Self-care skills: Behavioral measurement with Klein-Bell ADL Scale. *Archives of Physical Medicine and Rehabilitation, 63,* 335–338.

Klyczek, J. P., Bauer-Yox, N., & Fiedler, R. C. (1997). The interest checklist: A factor analysis. *American Journal of Occupational Therapy, 51,* 815–823.

Kohlman Thomson, L. (1993). *The Kohlman evaluation of living skills* (3rd ed.). Rockville, MD: AOTA.

Law, M. (Ed.). (1998). *Client-centered occupational therapy.* Thorofare, NJ: Slack.

Law, M. (2002). Participation in the occupations of everyday life. *American Journal of Occupational Therapy, 56,* 640–649.

Law, M., Baptiste, S., Carswell, A., McColl, M., Polatajko, H., & Pollock, N. (2005). *Canadian occupational performance measure* (4th ed.). Ottawa, Canada: CAOT.

Law, M., & Letts, L. (1989). A critical review of scales of activities of daily living. *American Journal of Occupational Therapy, 43,* 522–528.

Letts, L., Scott, S., Burtney, J., Marshall, L., & McKean, M. (1998). The reliability and validity of the Safety Assessment of Function and the Environment for Rehabilitation (SAFER). *British Journal of Occupational Therapy, 61,* 127–132.

Mahoney, F. I., & Barthel, D. W. (1965). Functional evaluation: The Barthel Index. *Maryland State Medical Journal, 14,* 61–65.

Matsutsuyu, J. S. (1969). Interest checklist. *American Journal of Occupational Therapy, 23,* 23–328.

Matuska, K. (2012a). Development of the Life Balance Inventory. *Occupational Therapy Journal of Research, 32,* 220–228.

Matuska, K. (2012b). Validity evidence for a model and measure of life balance. *Occupational Therapy Journal of Research, 32,* 229–237.

Matuska, K., & Christiansen, C. (2008). A proposed model of lifestyle balance. *Journal of Occupational Science, 15,* 9–19.

McColl, M., Davies, D., Carlson, P., Johnston, J., & Minnes, P. (2001). The community integration measure: Development and preliminary validation. *Archives of Physical Medicine and Rehabilitation, 82,* 429–434.

Miller, A., Clemson, L., & Lannin, N. (2011) Measurement properties of a modified Reintegration to Normal Living Index in a community-dwelling adult rehabilitation population. *Disability and Rehabilitation, 33,* 1968–1978.

Neistadt, M. E. (1992). The Rabideau Kitchen Evaluation Revised: An assessment of meal preparation skill. *Occupational Therapy Journal of Research, 12,* 242–255.

Neistadt, M. E. (1994). A meal preparation treatment protocol for adults with brain injury. *American Journal of Occupational Therapy, 48,* 431–438.

Nicholl, C. R., Lincoln, N. B., & Playford, E. D. (2002). The reliability and validity of the Nottingham extended activities of daily living scale in patients with multiple sclerosis. *Multiple Sclerosis, 8,* 372–376.

Nouri, F. M., & Lincoln, N. B. (1987). An extended activities of daily living scale for stroke patients. *Clinical Rehabilitation, 1,* 301–305.

Oakley, F., Kielhofner, G., Barris, R., & Reichler, R. K. (1986). The Role Checklist: Development and empirical assessment of reliability. *Occupational Therapy Journal of Research, 6,* 157–170.

Oliver, R., Blathwayt, J., Brockley, C., & Tamaki, T. (1993). Development of the Safety Assessment of Function and the Environment for Rehabilitation (SAFER) tool. *Canadian Journal of Occupational Therapy, 60,* 78–82.

Park, S., Fisher, A. G., & Velozo, C. A. (1994). Using the assessment of motor and process skills to compare occupational performance between clinic and home settings. *American Journal of Occupational Therapy, 48,* 697–709.

Perry, A., Morris, M., Unsworth, C., Duckett, S., Skeat, J., Dodd, K., Taylor, N., & Riley, K. (2004). Therapy outcome measures for allied health practitioners in Australia: The AusTOMs. *International Journal for Quality in Health Care, 16,* 285–291.

Quinn, T. J., Langhorne, P., & Stott, D. J. (2011). Barthel Index for stroke trials: Development, properties and application. *Stroke, 42,* 1146–1151.

Reistetter, T. A., Spencer, J. C., Trujillo, L., & Abreu, B. C. (2005). Examining the Community Integration Measure (CIM): A replication study with life satisfaction. *Neurorehabilitation, 20,* 139–148.

Robertson, D. & Carswell, M. A. (2011). Adding a driving task to AMPS: A pilot study. *Canadian Journal of Occupational Therapy, 78,* 103–109.

Rogers, J. C. (1988). The NPI interest checklist. In B. Hemphill (Ed.), *Mental health assessments in occupational therapy* (pp. 93–114). Thorofare, NJ: Slack.

Rogers, J. C., & Holm, M. B. (1989a). Performance of Self-Care Skills-Clinic (PASS-Clinic, Version 3.1). Unpublished test. University of Pittsburgh, Pittsburgh, PA (Available from mbholm@pitt.edu).

Rogers, J. C., & Holm, M. B. (1989b). Performance of Self-Care Skills-Home (PASS-Home, Version 3.1). Unpublished test. University of Pittsburgh, Pittsburgh, PA (Available from mbholm@pitt.edu).

Rogers, J. C., Holm, M. B., Beach, S., Schulz, R., Cipriani, J., Fox, A., & Starz, T. W. (2003). Concordance of four methods of disability assessment using performance in the home as the criterion method. *Arthritis and Rheumatism, 49,* 640–647.

Rogers, J. C., Weinstein, J. M., & Figone, J. J. (1978). The interest checklist: An empirical assessment. *American Journal of Occupational Therapy, 32,* 628–630.

Sagar, M. A., Dunham, N. C., Schwartes, A., Mecum, L., Halverson, K., & Harlowe, D. (1992). Measurement of activities of daily living in hospitalized elderly: A comparison of self-report and performance-based methods. *Journal of the American Geriatrics Society, 40,* 457–462.

Schlote, A., Kruger, J., Topp, H., & Wallesch, C. W. (2004). [Interrater reliability of the Barthel Index, activity index, and the Nottingham extended activities of daily living: The use of ADL instruments in stroke rehabilitation by medical and nonmedical personnel]. [German]. *Rehabilitation (Stuttgart), 43,* 75–82.

Scott, F., Unsworth, C. A., Fricke, J., & Taylor, N. (2006). Reliability of the Australian therapy outcome measures for occupational therapy self care scale. *Australian Journal of Occupational Therapy, 53,* 265–276.

Shah, S., Vanclay, F., & Cooper, B. (1989). Improving the sensitivity of the Barthel Index for stroke rehabilitation. *Journal of Clinical Epidemiology, 42,* 703–709.

Sharrack, B., Hughes, R. A. C., Soudain, S., & Dunn, G. (1999). The psychometric properties of clinical rating scales used in multiple sclerosis. *Brain, 122,* 141–159.

Simmons, D. C., Crepeau, E. B., & White, B. P. (2000). The predictive power of narrative data in occupational therapy evaluation. *American Journal of Occupational Therapy, 54,* 471–476.

Stark, S. L., Edwards, D. F., Hollingsworth, H., & Gray, D. B. (2005). Validation of the Reintegration to Normal Living Index in a population of community-dwelling people with mobility limitations. *Archives of Physical Medicine and Rehabilitation, 86,* 344–345.

Strong, S., Baptiste, S., Cole, D., Clarke, J., Costa, M., Shannon, H., Reardon, R., & Sinclair, S. (2004). Functional assessment of injured workers: A profile of assessor practices. *Canadian Journal of Occupational Therapy, 71,* 13–23.

Trombly, C. A. (1995). Occupation: Purposefulness and meaningfulness as therapeutic mechanisms. 1995 Eleanor Clarke Slagle Lecture. *American Journal of Occupational Therapy, 49,* 960–972.

University at Buffalo Foundation Activities, Inc. (2004). *The Inpatient Rehabilitation Facility–Patient Assessment Instrument (IRF-PAI) training manual: Effective 4/01/04.* Buffalo, NY: University at Buffalo Foundation Activities, Inc.

Unsworth, C. A. (2005). Measuring outcomes using the Australian therapy outcome measures for occupational therapy (AusTOMS-OT): Data description and tool sensitivity. *British Journal of Occupational Therapy, 68,* 354–366.

Unsworth, C. A., Duckett, S., Duncombe, D., Perry, A., Morris, M., Taylor, N., & Skeat, J. (2004). Validity of the AusTOM scales: A comparison of the AusTOMs and EuroQol-5D. *Health and Quality of Life Outcomes, 2,* 1–17.

U.S. Department of Labor. (2011). *Dictionary of occupational titles.* (4th ed.). Washington, DC: United States Department of Labor. Retrieved from http://www.occupationalinfo.org/index.html on 7/14/13.

van der Putten, J. J., Hobart, J. C., Freeman, J. A., & Thompson, A. J. (1999). Measuring change in disability after inpatient rehabilitation: Comparison of the responsiveness of the Barthel Index and the Functional Independence Measure. *Journal of Neurology, Neurosurgery, and Psychiatry, 66,* 480–484.

Velozo, C. A. (1993). Work evaluations: Critique of the states of the art of functional assessment of work. *American Journal of Occupational Therapy, 47,* 203–209.

Velozo, C., Kielhofner, G., & Fisher, G. (1998). *Worker Role Interview (WRI).* Chicago: Model of Human Occupation Clearinghouse.

Whiteneck, G. G., Harrison-Felix, C. L., Mellick, D. C., Brooks, C. A., Charlifue, S. B., & Gerhart, K. A. (2004). Quantifying environmental factors: A measure of physical, attitudinal, service, productivity, and policy barriers. *Archives of Physical Medicine and Rehabilitation, 85,* 1324–1335.

Willer, B., Ottenbacher, K. J., & Coad, M. L. (1994). The community integration questionnaire: A comparative examination. *American Journal of Physical Medicine and Rehabilitation, 73,* 103–111.

Witt, P. A., & Ellis, G. D. (1984). The *Leisure Diagnostic Battery*: Measuring perceived freedom in leisure. *Society and Leisure, 7,* 109–124.

Wolfe, C. D., Taub, N. A., Woodrow, E. J., & Burney, P. G. (1991). Assessment of scales of disability and handicap for stroke patients. *Stroke, 22,* 1242–1244.

Wood-Dauphinee, S., Opzoomer, A., Williams, J. I., Marchand, B., & Spitzer, W. O. (1988). Assessment of global function: The Reintegration to Normal Living Index. *Archives of Physical Medicine and Rehabilitation, 69,* 583–590.

World Health Organization. (2001). *International Classification of Functioning, Disability and Health (ICF).* Geneva: World Health Organization.

Wu, C. Y., Chuang, L. L., Lin, K. C., & Horng, Y. S. (2011). Responsiveness and validity of two outcome measures of instrumental activities of daily living in stroke survivors receiving rehabilitative therapies. *Clinical Rehabilitation, 25,* 175–183.

Yantz, C. L., Johnson-Greene, D., Higginson, C., & Emmerson, L. (2010). Functional cooking skills and neuropsychological functioning in patients with stroke: An ecological validity study. *Neuropsychological Rehabilitation, 20,* 725–738.

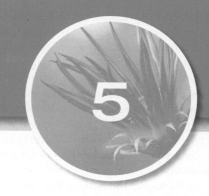

Assessing Abilities and Capacities: Vision and Visual Processing

Orli Weisser-Pike

Learning Objectives

After studying this chapter, the reader will be able to do the following:

1. Define and differentiate between visual functions and functional vision.
2. Identify some conditions in adults that cause vision-related problems.
3. Differentiate between correctable and uncorrectable vision impairments.
4. Describe screening techniques for visual acuity, visual fields, and oculomotor control.
5. Understand the impact of vision impairments on performance skills, patterns, and activity demands.
6. Become familiar with other vision-related professions.

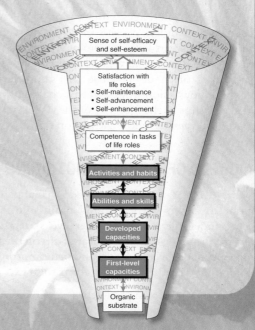

Eyes are remarkable organs that must shrink life-size images so that the reflected light from those images fits through a small aperture, the pupil, and lands perfectly in focus on the retina, the only place in the human body where nerve tissue—indeed the brain—can be seen by the naked eye. Upside down and inverted on the retina, light is converted into an electrical impulse that makes its way to the back of the head, the primary visual cortex, where the image is further processed and assigned meaning. *This is the sensory component of vision.* Additional features of the image are identified and recognized, compared with previously memorized images, and assigned meaning. *This is the cognitive component of vision* where interpretation occurs. Furthermore, the eyes have to point to the same target to produce a unified image. They must work together in a smooth and coordinated manner to follow a moving target. They also must be able to move as a team when searching for information in the environment, jumping from one target to the next, and be able to keep the target in focus regardless of whether it is near or far. *This is the motor component of vision.*

Occupational performance problems can occur when a deficit arises in any of these components. Take, for example, Mr. K., a 78-year-old man who was admitted to the hospital following a cardiac event. In the rush to get him to the hospital, his wife removed his spectacles so that he would not worry about keeping track of them while admitted for medical care. On the third day following his admission, the occupational therapist administered a cognitive screening test. Mr. K. scored poorly on the test not because he experienced a cognitive decline but because he could not see to read the instructions he was given. This example illustrates how important it is for occupational therapy practitioners to screen a client's vision in order to determine factors that hinder or support engagement in desired occupations.

Because occupational therapy practitioners are likely to see people of all ages who have problems with sensory, cognitive, or motor aspects of vision, it is useful to distinguish between key terminology, such as "visual functions" and "functional vision." Note, however, that vision specialists often do not use the same terminology to describe how vision works. In this chapter, the term *visual function* refers to the integrity of the visual system, whereas *functional vision* tells how the person operates.

MODELS OF VISUAL FUNCTIONING

Warren (1993a, 1993b) described a visual perceptual hierarchy in adults with acquired brain injuries (Fig. 5-1). This model suggests that higher level skills (such as visual attention and visual memory) are built on the foundations of visual acuity, visual fields, and oculomotor control. The components in the hierarchy are as follows:

1. Visual attention and alertness
2. Visual scanning

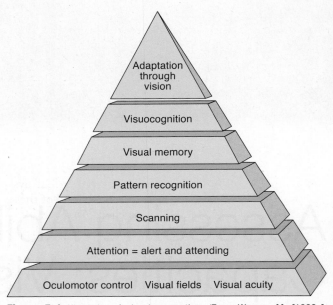

Figure 5-1 Hierarchy of visual perception. (From Warren, M. [1993a]. A hierarchical model for evaluation for evaluation and treatment of visual perceptual dysfunction in adult acquired brain injury, Part 1. *American Journal of Occupational Therapy, 47,* 43. Copyright 1993 by the American Occupational Therapy Association, Inc. Reprinted with permission.)

3. Pattern recognition
4. Visual memory
5. Visual cognition

The model illustrates that without good foundational sensory or motor components, faulty visual perception may occur, leading to faulty learning.

More recently, Colenbrander (2009) described three distinct stages of visual functioning: optical, retinal, and neural. In the optical stage, light enters the eyeball and lands onto the retina. Any abnormalities of the eyeball that might interfere with the path of the light reaching the retina will likely cause visual problems. Refractive errors are some examples of problems in the optical stage. If the eyeball is too long, for example, as in the case of shortsightedness, the light does not reach the retina at the right spot, leading to blurry vision.

In the retinal stage, light landing on the retina is translated into neural impulses. Retinal diseases, such as macular degeneration, can cause problems at this stage. A person with macular degeneration may not notice areas of missing information from the visual field and may only discover vision loss when shutting one eye.

In the third stage, neural impulses are processed by the inner retina and other centers in the brain. At this stage, the image is analyzed, interpreted, and translated into a mental picture, which Colenbrander (2009) terms as the "mental model of the environment" (p. 120). The mental model is one in which the environment appears to be stable in spite of a constantly changing retinal image.

Colenbrander (2009) proposed use of the term "cognitive visual dysfunction" (p. 122) to describe problems that exist in the presence of normal input to the brain, such as failure to recognize familiar faces (prosopagnosia), difficulty visually attending to one side, and difficulty naming colors.

POPULATIONS AND VISION PROBLEMS

Many recipients of occupational therapy services may have correctable vision impairments. However, some vision impairments are not correctable, and visual dysfunction can persist despite vision correction. All of these conditions may coexist in the same client. Because most visual impairments are "hidden" problems, the occupational therapist should not assume that a person's vision problem has been, or can be, corrected just because that person wears glasses.

Correctable Vision Impairments

The most common correctable vision impairments are refractive errors, which affect approximately 42.2 million (35.3%) of Americans age 40 years or older (National Eye Institute, 2006). Refractive errors include myopia (near-sightedness), hyperopia (farsightedness), astigmatism (asymmetrical or distorted vision at any distance), and presbyopia (loss of accommodation of the lens, which occurs around age 40 years). Occupational therapy practitioners are likely to encounter clients across the life span who wear glasses or contact lenses to help focus the incoming image on the retina. Lenses may be designed to correct for one particular distance, as in the case of single vision lenses, or for multiple distances, as in the case of bifocals, trifocals, or progressive lenses. Surgical procedures, such as LASIK and cataract extraction, can also improve refractive errors.

Uncorrectable Vision Impairments and Low Vision

Massof (2002) estimated that there are 1.5 million Americans older than age 45 years with uncorrectable vision impairments; there are approximately a quarter of a million new cases each year. Nearly 12% of individuals ages 55–64 years and 27% of individuals age 85 years and older report some form of visual impairment that impacts their ability to complete everyday activities such as walking outside, managing medications, or preparing a meal (Campbell et al., 1999; Schoehborn & Heyman, 2009). People with uncorrectable losses of visual acuity and visual field are considered to have low vision or blindness, a condition that supports medical necessity for rehabilitation by an occupational therapy practitioner (Centers for Medicare & Medicaid Services, 2002). Table 5-1 shows levels of visual impairment.

Table 5-1 **Levels of Vision Impairment**

Definition of Levels of Vision Impairment	
Moderate	Best corrected visual acuity is less than 20/60.
Severe	Best corrected visual acuity is less than 20/160, or visual field is 20° or less (legal blindness).
Profound	Best corrected visual acuity is less than 20/400, or visual field is 10° or less (moderate blindness).
Near-total	Best corrected visual acuity is less than 20/1000, or visual field is 5° or less (severe blindness).
Total	No light perception (total blindness).

From Centers for Medicare & Medicaid Services. (2002). *Transmittal AB-02-078*. Department of Health and Human Services. Retrieved from https://www.cms.gov /transmittals/downloads/AB02078.pdf.

Neurologically Based Visual Dysfunction

Beyond age-related vision loss and impairments, many clients experience vision problems because of neurologically based disability or illness. In a study of 328 patients who suffered a stroke, over 90% had visual problems in eye alignment, visual fields, and visual attention (Rowe et al., 2009). Many service members with blast-related brain injuries receive occupational therapy screening for vision problems (Brahm et al., 2009; Cockerham et al., 2009; Dougherty et al., 2010).

ASSESSING VISION

The purpose of assessing vision as part of the occupational therapy evaluation is to elucidate client factors—visual functions and functional vision—that hinder or support engagement in desired occupations (American Occupational Therapy Association, 2008; Warren, 2011). Insofar as observed behaviors are frequently attributed to cognitive changes rather than impaired vision, all neurologically impaired clients should receive an occupational therapy vision screen to rule out visual dysfunction (Warren, 2011). Screening is also considered for older clients whose vision may have been affected by age-related eye diseases. See Definition 5-1 for other professions involved in vision assessment and treatment.

The occupational therapy assessment of vision includes a basic eye history; interviews with the client and/or family about subjective complaints (e.g., difficulty concentrating, double vision, eye strain, and bumping into objects on one side); screening of visual acuity, visual fields, and ocular motility; screening for visual attention and visual search; observations of functional tasks (Table 5-2); and formal vision-related questionnaires. Assessment Table 5-1 describes and summarizes the psychometric properties of various occupational therapy vision assessments. Also see information about how to obtain some of these assessments in the Resources 5-1.

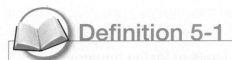

Definition 5-1

Vision-Related Professions

- Ophthalmologist—Medical doctor with an additional year of training in general medicine followed by a minimum of 3 years in organ-specific training. Ophthalmology is concerned with the anatomy and function of the eye, including prevention, diagnosis, and medical and surgical treatment of eye conditions and diseases. Additionally, there are numerous subspecialties in ophthalmology (such as glaucoma and neuro-ophthalmology), which necessitate additional years of training (American Academy of Ophthalmology, 2011).
- Optometrists—Primary eye care providers who receive a doctorate in optometry after 4 years of postgraduate training but are not medical physicians. Although they are educated in limited management of eye diseases (e.g., they cannot perform surgery), their focus is primarily on correcting refractive impairments. There are also subspecialties within optometry, such as behavioral optometry and developmental optometry, which are aimed at treating the functional impact of vision impairments (American Optometric Association, 2011).
- Orthoptist—Eye care specialist who works in ophthalmology and is trained in a 2-year fellowship at an accredited program following a baccalaureate degree. Emphasis is on evaluation and treatment of disorders of binocular vision, eye movements, and eye alignment in children and adults (American Association of Certified Orthoptists, 2011).
- Low-vision therapist—Practitioner who works with an ophthalmologist, optometrist, or orthoptist to provide the client training in use of optical devices and methods to compensate for vision loss (Academy for Certification of Vision Rehabilitation and Education Professions, 2011).
- Orientation and mobility specialist—Trains the client with low vision and blindness to independently and safely travel from one place to another (Academy for Certification of Vision Rehabilitation and Education Professions, 2011).
- Vision rehabilitation therapist—Teaches people with low vision and blindness to compensate for vision loss using nonvisual strategies and technologies, including braille (Academy for Certification of Vision Rehabilitation and Education Professions, 2011).
- Teachers of the visually impaired—Also known as itinerant teachers; work in the educational system and are trained in special education to provide specific instruction to students with visual impairments, their teachers, and their families (Olmstead, 2005).
- American Occupational Therapy Association specialty certification in low vision—Recognition of occupational therapy practitioners with specialized knowledge and skills in low vision (Warren et al., 2006).

Table 5-2 Observation of Functional Tasks

Impact of Client Factors on Performance Patterns, Performance Skills, and Activity Demands	Possible Visual Function Problem	Possible Functional Vision Problem
The client fails to visually identify a close family member entering the room. The client feels embarrassed and decides henceforth not to have any visitors.	**Reduced visual acuity** caused by opacity of the lens (e.g., cataract) leading to difficulty distinguishing facial features	**Prosopagnosia** caused by damage to face recognition centers in the brain.
The client has difficulty reading the daily menu to select meals. She is given her food tray last because staff does not know what she ordered. Client settles for undesired food and does not consume sufficient calories for healing.	**Blurry vision** up close when reading caused by lack of accommodation of the lens (presbyopia)	**Dyslexia** or **dysphasia** can lead to problems deciphering written language.
When playing a game of Bingo, client reads the number 25 on the card as a 5 and misses the first numeral. He misses opportunities to win. He also has trouble writing checks and leaves a large space at the left margin of the line. He gives up financial management and hands control of financial matters to his neighbor, because he has no relatives in the state.	**Reduced visual acuity** caused by a retinal disease (e.g., macular degeneration) leading to a central blind spot slightly displaced to the left of fixation A left homonymous **visual field defect** caused by damage to the optic pathways on the right side of the brain (e.g., stroke)	**Hemi-inattention** caused by dysfunction of the attentional system of the brain (may exist with or without a visual field defect) leading to missed information on the left side.
Client reaches for her beverage on the right side of the placemat but misses, despite looking at it. She knocks the drink over and spills red wine on her friend's white blouse. She is so embarrassed that she bursts out crying.	**Constricted visual fields** caused by damage of the optic nerve (e.g., glaucoma) leading to tunnel vision	**Eye–hand coordination deficits** caused by dysfunction of coordination centers in the brain
Client cannot find a grapefruit spoon in a drawer full of cutlery. She fumbles for the spoon and accidentally cuts herself on a knife that she did not notice.	**Reduced contrast sensitivity** from swelling of the retina caused by a systemic disease (e.g., diabetes)	**Figure-ground separation difficulties** caused by inability to inhibit competing or distracting visual information

Assessment Table 5-1 Summary of Assessments of Vision and Visual Processing

Instrument & Reference	Description	Time to Administer	Validity	Reliability	Sensitivity	Strengths & Weaknesses
Brain Injury Visual Assessment Battery for Adults (BiVABA) (Warren, 1998)	A collection of instruments to screen for visual processing impairments following brain injury. The intention of the battery is to find out whether and how visual processing impairments prevent or hinder participation in occupations; items are selected based on the visual perceptual hierarchy (Fig. 5-1). Norms and cutoff scores are not relevant because the intention is to identify deficiencies in primary visual functions.	Entire battery may take upward of 1 hour; some subtests may take as little as 3–5 minutes.	Not reported	Not reported	Not reported	Strength: Comprehensive assessment battery for foundational visual skills; detailed instructions for setup and testing; extensive interpretation guidelines. Weaknesses: No psychometric data available. Requires practice in administration and interpretation before working with clients.
The Self-Report Assessment of Functional Visual Performance (SRAFVP) (Warren et al., 2008). Available in Warren (2011). *Occupational Therapy Interventions for Adults with Low Vision*. Bethesda, MD: American Occupational Therapy Association.	A 45-item activities of daily living (ADL) performance measure that combines a self-report assessment of 38 items and optional observations of seven ADL tasks. Both sections are scored using a three-point ordinal scale. Tasks are ordered by level of visual difficulty with the most visually demanding items listed first; scores yield a "recovery profile" showing tasks that client is unable to complete, tasks that are difficult, and tasks for which client is mostly independent.	Self-report may take up to 40 minutes.	Differentiated between individuals with complete homonymous hemianopsia and those with macular sparing for reading tasks (*p* = 0.03) and eye coordination (*p* = 0.047) but not with navigation (*p* = 0.787)	Internal consistency: Cronbach's α for the 38 items = 0.96 (Mennem, Warren, & Yuen, 2012).	Not reported	Strength: Developed for clients with low vision. Weaknesses: May not be appropriate for clients with oculomotor dysfunction; no psychometric data available. Copyrighted; requires explicit permission by the authors.
National Eye Institute Visual Function Questionnaire, 25-item version (NEI VFQ-25) (Mangione, 2000).	This quality-of-life questionnaire can be administered by an interviewer or completed as a self-report. Twenty-five statements specific to the impact of vision loss on general health, well-being, and ADL are scored on a 5-point ordinal scale. Higher scores = higher quality of life	Interview may take up to 60 minutes.	Statistically significant correlation between the 25-item NEI VFQ and clinical indicators of visual function (Pearson correlations ranged from .11–.70, p<.05)	Good internal consistency among NEI VFQ-25 subscales (Cronbach's α = 0.73–0.87; driving α = 0.45; overall α = 0.93)	Not reported	Strengths: Available in the public domain for clients with low vision. May be self-administered or administered via interview by the practitioner.

(continued)

Assessment Table 5-1 Summary of Assessments of Vision and Visual Processing (continued)

Instrument & Reference	Description	Time to Administer	Validity	Reliability	Sensitivity	Strengths & Weaknesses
Melbourne Low-Vision Activities of Daily Living Index (MLVAI) (Haymes, Johnston, & Heyes, 2001b).	A 25-item ADL performance measure combining a questionnaire and observations of performance in structured, standardized tasks. Both sections are scored using 4-point ordinal scales. Higher scores = lower disability	May take up to 60 minutes	Moderately high correlation with vision impairment ($r = -0.68$, $p = 0.001$).	Good internal consistency (Cronbach's α = 0.96) Strong test-retest reliability (Spearman's correlation coefficient = 0.94; $p = 0.001$), and the interpractitioner reliability for five different pairs of practitioners was 0.90 or higher ($p = 0.001$).	Not reported	Strength: For clients with low vision; measure of functional performance related to visual functioning. Weaknesses: Observation portion is culturally specific (Australian). Available on request from the author.
Catherine Bergego Scale (CBS) (Azouvi et al., 2003)	Assesses behavioral neglect. Ten items from everyday life situations (e.g., grooming left side of face, collisions with people or objects on the left). Unilateral neglect (UN) scored on 4-point scale, where 0 indicates no neglect observed and 3 indicates severe neglect: Client only able to access right hemispace	Unknown, but would be observed during the occupational therapist's evaluation of ADL	CBS score correlated significantly with performance on five paper and pencil tests (Spearman's ρ = 0.50-0.74). Significant correlation between CBS and Barthel Index Spearman's ($\rho = -0.63$) Correlated with line-bisection subtest of the Behavioral Inattention Test (Spearman correlation = .56) (Luukkainen-Markkula et al., 2011).	Internal consistency: Spearman's rho ranged from 0.58 to 0.88. Strong inter-rater reliability (Spearman rank order correlation coefficient = .96, $p<.0001$)	Authors found it more sensitive than conventional paper and pencil tests.	Strengths: Direct observations of clients' function during everyday activities; provides the client with insight into their deficits. Several items of the CBS and the line-bisection test of Behavioral Inattention Test (BIT) were found to be especially sensitive in identifying the combination of visual neglect and visual field deficits in stroke patients (Luukkainen-Markkula et al., 2011). Weaknesses: Training recommended for inexperienced therapists unfamiliar with unilateral neglect (UN). Difficulty differentiating sensory and motor neglect.
Behavioral Inattention Test (Wilson et al., 1987)	Assesses visual neglect Fifteen-item standardized test battery: six pen and paper tests (such as line bisection, letter cancellation, and star cancellation) and nine behavioral tasks. Cutoff scores are used to indicate neglect.	Approximately 30 minutes	Correlation between BIT and Barthel Index: $r = 0.642$ (Cassidy et al., 1999) Correlation between BIT behavior subtests and items on an ADL checklist: $r = 0.77$ (Hartman-Maier & Katz, 1995)	Test-retest: $r = 0.99$ Interrater reliability: $r = 0.99$	Behavioral subtests were found to differentiate between groups: neglect and no neglect (Hartman-Maier & Katz, 1995)	Strength: Includes functional as well as conventional tests Weakness: Two subtests (map navigation and picture scanning) were found not to correlate with a functional ADL (Hartman-Maier & Katz, 1995). Measures neglect in peripersonal space only and cannot distinguish between sensory and motor neglect.

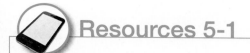

Resources 5-1

Evaluation Materials

Visual Acuity and Contrast Sensitivity Charts

Precision Vision (www.precisionvision.com)

Good-Lite Company (www.good-lite.com)

Minnesota Reading Acuity Charts
(www.shoplowvision.com)

Pepper Visual Skills for Reading Test and Morgan Low Vision Reading Comprehension Assessment provided by Fork in the Road Vision Rehabilitation Services, LLC (www.lowvisionsimulators.com)

Brain Injury Visual Assessment Battery for Adults provided by visABILITIES Rehab Services (www.visabilities.com)

Visually guided actions and interactions with one's surroundings are dependent on a mental model of the environment, discussed earlier in the chapter (Colenbrander, 2009). In the past, therapists often evaluated visual perception without a good understanding of the optical system and how it provides the foundation for vision (Cate & Richards, 2000; Hunt & Bassi, 2010; Warren, 1999;). What may be thought of as a deficit in visual perception, such as the ability to differentiate a figure from its background, may be the result of a problem in the sensory or motor components of vision. Warren (1993b) recommended that therapists' limited time was best spent evaluating the foundations for visual function rather than higher level visual cognitive skills.

Screening the Foundations of Visual Function

Visual acuity, visual fields, and oculomotor control form the foundations for visual function. Although deficits in any of these visual functions can affect client performance, clients may not complain of any problems, or they may make complaints that appear unrelated to vision. Therefore, it is important to screen the foundations of visual function even if the client denies visual difficulties. However, prior to screening visual functions, all clients should be screened for refractive errors.

Refractive Errors

Clients should use their best available vision when participating in visual screens. This is particularly true when screening visual acuity. Without adequate correction, clients may demonstrate greater visual acuity impairment, leading the occupational therapist to presume that visual acuity is hindering occupational performance. Refractive errors are easily correctable. Correctable vision impairments that go untreated are associated with poorer quality of life, reduced participation in daily occupations, and increased risk of injury (Vitale, Cotch, & Sperduto, 2006). If glasses are not available, the client can view the acuity chart through a small pinhole punched into an index card (Scheiman, Scheiman, & Whittaker, 2007). The pinhole method is a quick screen to determine whether visual acuity can be improved with eyeglasses or contact lenses, which can only be prescribed by an ophthalmologist or optometrist.

Visual Acuity

Visual acuity testing demonstrates the sharpness of vision at the part of the retina with which the person fixates on the target—the fovea. Visual acuity is not constant throughout the retina: it rapidly decreases from the fovea (the area of greatest acuity) outward to the periphery. Therefore, visual acuity describes only the small area of sharpest vision, known as central visual acuity, or central vision. There are many measurements of visual acuity. "Best-corrected visual acuity" reflects the client's potential visual acuity using prescriptive lenses. "Presenting visual acuity" denotes the client's visual acuity at initial testing. "Pin hole visual acuity" indicates that the measurement was taken with the client viewing the visual acuity chart through a tiny aperture.

Traditionally, visual acuity is measured for distance (e.g., driving) at 6 meters (20 feet) and for near tasks (e.g., reading) at 40 centimeters (16 inches). The notation of visual acuity as a fraction (e.g., 20/20) describes the magnification required by the observer. The numerator denotes the distance at which the client recognizes the stimulus (measured in meters or feet), and the denominator is the size of the letter or symbol on the chart (measured by a unit called an M-size). A person with 6/6 (20/20) vision requires no magnification, because the value of the fraction is 1. However, a person with 6/60 (20/200) requires 10× magnification; it also means that this person is only able to recognize at 6 meters (20 feet) a stimulus that a person with "standard" vision could recognize at 60 meters (200 feet) (see Procedures for Practice 5-1).

Visual acuity is screened using a standardized logarithmic letter or symbol chart, such as the Early Treatment of Diabetic Retinopathy Study (ETDRS) chart, which is considered the gold standard for visual acuity measurement (International Council of Ophthalmology, 2002). Other charts, such as LEA Symbols, LEA Numbers, or Sloan Letters are also appropriate for screening visual acuity (Chaplin & Bradford, 2011). Regardless of the chart being used, it is essential that the examiner position the client at the testing distance for which the chart is intended. Most charts are designed in the metric system but provide a corresponding measure in feet (Snellen equivalent). Visual acuity screening should be carried out with the best correction available; in other words, clients should wear their glasses or corrective lenses. If the glasses/lenses are not available, have the client look through a pinhole in a piece of paper, as described earlier (International Council of Ophthalmology, 2002).

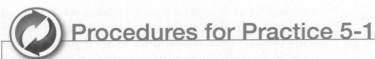

Procedures for Practice 5-1

Screening for Distance Visual Acuity

Equipment: ETDRS-type chart

Setup

- Client must wear contact lenses or glasses for distance (single vision for distance or multifocals) if typically worn. If the client wears bifocals, trifocals, or progressive multifocals, ensure that the client views the chart through the upper segment of the glasses.
- Client is seated directly opposite the chart, which is positioned at eye level. A common testing distance is 4 meters. Most ETDRS-type charts are calibrated to be used at distances of 4, 2, and 1 meters.
- The room should have standard illumination.

Procedure

- Patch the client's left eye.
- Instruct the client to name the letters on the chart, starting at the top row. If using a symbol chart, instruct the client to name the symbols or match them to a handheld symbol key. If using a "tumbling C" chart (e.g., for illiterate or dysphasic clients), instruct the client to point to the direction of the opening in the "C" (i.e., the direction of the gap in the letter).
- If the client is reluctant to name the letters, encourage guessing.

- If the client cannot name the letters, encourage the client to draw the letters in the air or on a piece of paper.
- If the client cannot identify any characters on the top line, bring the chart to a closer distance as specified in chart instructions. If the client cannot identify any characters at the shortest distance for which the chart is designed (e.g., 1 meter), note this in the client's record and proceed to screen the other eye.
- Record the last line in which the client was able to identify three or more characters on the line. The size of the characters is noted as an M-size (e.g., 16M). When noting visual acuity as a fraction, write the distance of the client from the chart in meters as the numerator (e.g., 4 meters) and the M-size of the characters on the last line in which 3 or more characters were read as the denominator (e.g., 4/16).
- Return the chart to the furthest testing distance and repeat with the left eye, followed by both eyes together.
- Record score separately in the following order: right eye, left eye, both eyes.
- Fractions can be converted from meters to feet using 20 as the numerator, e.g, 4/16 to 20/80.
- Visual acuity worse than 4/8 (20/40) with prescriptive lenses is an indication for a referral to an eye physician.

Adapted from International Council of Ophthalmology. (2002). Visual standards: Aspects and ranges of vision loss with emphasis on population surveys. Retrieved from http://www.icoph.org/downloads/visual-standardsreport.pdf.

Cataract is an example of a disease of the crystalline lens that can cause a disruption in the optical stage of image formation, leading to decreased visual acuity. Macular degeneration is an example of an age-related disease that causes a disruption in the retinal stage of image formation, in which the image is converted into neural impulses. People with loss of central visual acuity commonly refer to their vision as being blurry or veiled; common complaints include reading difficulties and inability to distinguish facial features. People with central vision loss may be observed tilting or shaking their heads or gazing in different directions when attempting to identify the target. Because visual targets are not distinct, clients may try to get closer to the target, enlarge the target, or view the target from an angle.

Contrast Sensitivity

Contrast sensitivity is the ability to detect a visual target against a background of similar tone or hue and more accurately reflects conditions of the visual environment, such as sidewalk curbs, or facial features. Contrast sensitivity is also referred to as "low contrast acuity" and is closely related to problems experienced in everyday activities, particularly falls (American Academy of Ophthalmology

Vision Rehabilitation Committee, 2007). Various charts are available to measure contrast sensitivity. The salient feature in all of them is that the size of the stimulus is constant, whereas the contrast of the stimulus fades.

Diabetes is a systemic disease that can damage the blood vessels of the eye and is the leading cause of new cases of blindness in American adults older than age 20 years (Centers for Disease Control and Prevention, 2011). Despite having good visual acuity, many people with diabetic retinopathy have reduced contrast sensitivity related to vascular damage (Arend et al., 1997).

Visual Field

The visual field is defined as the boundary of what is seen while looking straight ahead. It is commonly described monocularly as extending approximately 50° superiorly, 70° inferiorly, 90° temporally, and 60° nasally. However, the visual fields of both eyes overlap, and the horizontal binocular field is increased by 30° from 150° monocularly to 180° binocularly (Scheiman, Scheiman, & Whittaker, 2007) as shown in Figure 5-2. Defects can affect all areas of the peripheral visual fields, only one side of the visual field in each eye, only the center of the visual field, or only the upper or lower portion of the visual field.

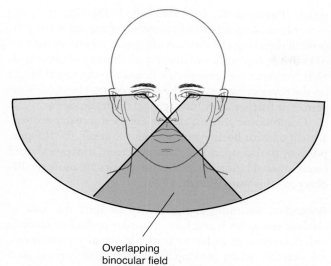

Overlapping
binocular field

Figure 5-2 Visual fields. The illustration shows the limits of the visual fields in each eye, including the area where the visual fields of each eye overlap. The overlapping field is the binocular visual field, where visual targets appear to have solidity and depth. In clients with double vision, objects within the overlapping area appear duplicated when both eyes are open.

Peripheral Visual Field. Confrontation testing is typically used to screen for gross visual field defects. Confrontation testing has been found to be relatively unreliable and should therefore be used in conjunction with functional observations (Warren, 1998). Typically, visual fields are measured in each eye separately, and the client's visual fields are compared to the examiner's visual fields when sitting juxtaposed to the client. More recently, Scheiman (2011) recommended testing both eyes together rather than one at a time, insofar as the purpose of the occupational therapy screen is to determine whether a bilateral visual field defect is hindering the client's occupational performance (see Procedures for Practice 5-2).

Damage to the optic nerves or the visual pathways may result in visual field losses. Glaucoma is a constellation of diseases that causes degeneration of the cells that form the optic nerve. Glaucoma is known as "the silent thief." Visual field loss often goes unnoticed by clients until it is too late, because, in general, they pay less attention to the edges of their sight. Glaucoma is the second leading cause of blindness in the United States, after macular degeneration (Prevent Blindness America, 2008). Damage to the optic nerve leads to contraction or constriction of the visual fields in one or both eyes, commonly referred to as "tunnel vision," yet central visual acuity may remain intact. A person with constricted visual fields may have difficulty finding his or her way in unfamiliar or dark areas, bump into people or obstacles, and have difficulty reaching for objects. Because they do not see the entire picture, clients commonly move away from visual targets in order to get a wider view of the scene.

Hemianopic Visual Field. Hemianopic visual field defects are caused by damage to the visual pathways beyond the

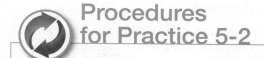

Procedures for Practice 5-2

Screening for Peripheral Visual Field Defect Using the Binocular Confrontation Method

Equipment: Interesting Target Mounted on a Wand

Setup

- Client should not wear glasses (as they may obscure the visual targets).
- Client is seated directly opposite examiner, approximately 20 inches away.
- Background behind examiner should be dark and distraction free.

Procedure

- Instruct client to look at your finger, which you hold between your own eyes. Let the client know you will be moving a target from the side, and the client should tell you when it is first seen while looking at your finger.
- Move target in from all angles, starting at 12 o'clock and moving clockwise to the 2, 4, 6, 8, 10 o'clock positions.
- Compare the client's response with yours.
- A problem is indicated if the client cannot see the target when you do.

From Scheiman, M. (2011). *Understanding and managing vision deficits: A guide for occupational therapists* (3rd ed.). Thorofare, NJ: Slack.

organ of the eye. The most common ones seen by occupational therapy practitioners are hemianopia and quadrantanopia: visual field defects on the same side in each eye. Clients frequently refer to a field loss in one eye and sometimes lack awareness that, in fact, the field loss is bilateral. Some clients with brain damage may not be aware of their visual field defects or may present with lack of attention to the affected side. Take care to differentiate between this (hemi-inattention) and a true visual field defect, keeping in mind that they can coexist in the same client.

Central Visual Field. A scotoma is an area of reduced central vision commonly described as a "blind spot," surrounded by intact visual fields. The client may or may not be aware of the presence of one or more scotomas because of "perceptual completion." Perceptual completion occurs when the mental model of the visual target or the environment is perceived as complete, despite missing visual input. Scotomas vary in amount, size, location, and density (Fletcher & Schuchard, 1997). Testing methods require a high degree of accuracy in order to detect the presence of small or relative blind spots; this is called "macular perimetry." Careful observations during reading tasks can also detect the presence of scotomas (see Reading Assessment).

Oculomotor Functions

Control of eye movements depends on a complex interaction at cortical and subcortical levels. Colenbrander (2009) suggested that eye movements used to search for or follow moving visual targets are made in direct response to the mental model of the environment. Because detailed vision is restricted to a small portion of the central retina—the fovea—eye movements are necessary in order to position and maintain the fovea on visual targets of interest, particularly during motion (Purves et al., 2004; Warren 1998). Foveation refers to positioning of the object of interest on the area of clearest vision. Gaze stabilizing movements are reflexive reactions to head and body motions. These compensatory eye movements are generated by the vestibular/ocular/cervical response system. The vestibular-ocular reflex is initiated when the vestibular system detects a change in head position during a visual task. Feedback is provided to the oculomotor system to produce compensatory eye movements in order to maintain a steady visual image (Purves et al., 2004; Warren, 1998). Gaze shifting movements, saccades and pursuits, are made for the purpose of directing the eyes toward visual targets of interest or maintaining targets of interest on the area of clearest vision. Vergence eye movements help keep the visual target on the fovea of each eye as the target moves closer (convergence) or further away (divergence) from the viewer.

Oculomotor control can be assessed in each eye separately or with both eyes together. However, for the purposes of the occupational therapy screen, the tests should be conducted binocularly because deficits are more readily observed this way (Warren, 1998).

Saccades. Scanning is the ability to shift the area of clearest vision back and forth in order to find or identify visual targets. In order to scan the visual environment, for example when looking for a particular person in a crowded room, the observer makes quick eye movements called saccades (see Procedures for Practice 5-3).

Smooth Pursuits. When tracking and following moving targets, the eyes must keep the object of regard in the area of clearest vision, the fovea. The eyes make smooth pursuits in order to maintain continued fixation on the moving target, as when watching an airplane take off (see Procedures for Practice 5-4).

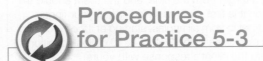

Procedures for Practice 5-3

Screening of Saccades

Equipment: Two interesting targets (e.g., two tongue depressors, one with a green circle on the end and the other with a red circle on the end)

Setup

- Client must wear contact lenses or glasses for distance (single vision for distance or multifocals) if typically worn. If the client wears bifocals, trifocals, or progressive multifocals, ensure that the client views through the upper segment of the glasses.
- Client is seated directly in front of and facing the examiner.

Procedure

- Hold wands approximately 16 inches from the face, separated by approximately 8 inches.
- Give no instructions regarding head movement.
- Tell the client, "Look at the red dot when I say red. Look at the green when I say green, and remember to wait until I say to look."
- Tell the client to look from one target to the other for a total of 10 fixations, five round trips.
- Observe
  - Ability to complete five round trips
  - Accuracy of eye movements (overshooting or undershooting target)
  - Movement of head or body

Adapted from Maples, W., Atchley, J., & Ficklin, T. (1992). Northeastern State University College of Optometry's oculomotor norms. *Journal of Behavioral Optometry, 3*, 143–150.

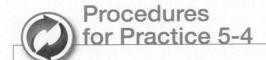

Procedures for Practice 5-4

Screening of Smooth Pursuits

Equipment: Interesting target mounted on a wand

Setup

- Client is seated directly in front of and facing the examiner.
- Client must wear contact lenses or glasses for distance (single vision for distance or multifocals) if typically worn.
- Hold target approximately 16 inches from the client's face.

Procedure

- Give no instructions regarding head movement.
- Tell the client, "Watch the target, and don't take your eyes off of it."
- Move target clockwise two rotations and counterclockwise for two rotations.
- Observe
  - Number of rotations the client is able to complete
  - Ability to maintain fixation, that is, the number of times the client has to refixate
  - Movement of the head or body

Adapted from Maples, W., Atchley, J., & Ficklin, T. (1992). Northeastern State University College of Optometry's oculomotor norms. *Journal of Behavioral Optometry, 3*, 143–150.

Convergence. Convergence is a reflexive response elicited when the viewer attends to a visual target moving closer to the viewer (see Procedures for Practice 5-5). A break in fixation normally occurs when the target is within 2–4 inches of the face, and recovery of a single image takes place at 4–6 inches. The client may not report seeing a double or blurry image because of suppression of vision from one eye. Therefore, it is important to observe the eyes and note when one eye drifts out or in during convergence and pulls back in or out with fusion.

Binocular Vision

Binocular vision allows us to blend the two slightly different images from each eye into a singular image containing volume and depth. Binocular vision depends on good eye alignment and the ability of the eyes to work as a team. In screening binocular vision, the therapist checks objective eye alignment and accommodation.

Eye Alignment. Eye alignment is objectively measured by observation of the light reflected off of the corneas with both eyes at the same time. The client should wear glasses or corrective lenses if typically worn. The therapist asks the seated client to gaze at a target at least

Normal

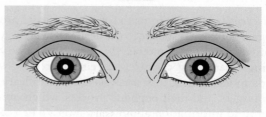

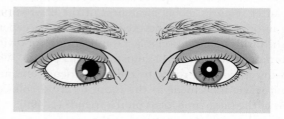

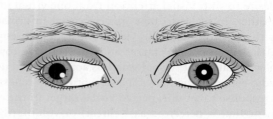

Figure 5-3 Eye alignment showing how a single light source reflects on both corneas in reference to the pupils. In normally aligned eyes, the reflections are located in the center of the pupil of each eye. In eyes that are out of alignment, the light reflections are different from each other.

20 feet away, so that the eyes are in the position of primary gaze. The therapist holds a penlight centered approximately 16 inches away from the client's eyes. The therapist observes the light reflection in each eye; the reflection should be in the same position in both eyes (Fig. 5-3). Discrepancies in positions of the reflections are noted (Warren, 1998).

Accommodation. Accommodation describes the ability of the lens to strengthen its optical power so that close objects are seen clearly. Decline in accommodation becomes functionally significant around age 40 years. If the client is older than age 40 years, expect accommodation to be decreased, necessitating reading glasses.

Visual Processing Deficit Screening

The ability to use vision for completing daily tasks depends not only on the solid foundations of acuity, field, and oculomotor control but also on the ability to engage vision with other sensory input as well as with motion and cognition (International Council of Ophthalmology, 2008). The client's ability to use vision to interact with the environment may be diminished if the information cannot adequately be processed.

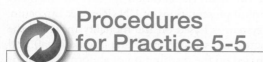

Procedures for Practice 5-5

Screening for Convergence Deficits

Equipment: Penlight or target; ruler

Setup

- Client is seated directly opposite the therapist.
- Client must wear contact lenses or glasses for distance (single vision for distance or multifocals) if typically worn.
- Client's head should be vertically erect.

Procedure

- Slowly move the penlight or target toward client at eye level (do not shine light directly into the client's eyes; direct it at the brow slightly above eye level).
- Ask the client to keep his or her eyes on the light and to report when the light appears blurred or when two lights are seen. Note the distance at which this occurs. Observe for a break in fusion.
- When the break in fusion occurs, move the target in another inch or so and begin to move it away from the client.
- Ask the client to let you know when he or she can see one light again. Note the distance at which fusion is reported.

Adapted from Warren, M. (1998). *Brain Injury Assessment Battery for adults: Test manual.* Birmingham, AL: visABILITIES Rehab Services, Inc.

Visual Attention and Visual Search

Visual attention is a prerequisite for higher visual processing; *visual search* is a response to the desire to selectively find and attend to targets of interest (Warren, 2011). Two visual processes seamlessly coexist: the central process, which attends to visual detail for analysis and identification of visual targets, and the peripheral process, which provides background information about the viewer's whereabouts in space. The former requires selective attention, whereas the latter requires global awareness of the environment. The amount of attention devoted to each process depends on the task, and attention may be apportioned or divided accordingly. Warren (2011) illustrates this point: "When crossing a crowded room to talk to a friend, one must monitor the movement in the room to avoid collisions while at the same time focus on the friend" (p. 409).

Visual search (or scanning) is the motor response to the desire to shift visual attention from one visual target to another. In order to take in new visual information from the environment, the viewer must first disengage from the current visual target and redirect gaze toward the new visual target. Visual search is accomplished using saccadic eye movements, which can originate reflexively (as a response to an unexpected visual target in the environment that is perceived as a threat) or voluntarily (as a response to the deliberate desire to search the environment for specific visual targets).

Screening for visual attention and visual search deficits occurs at the same time and cannot be separated into components, because visual search is the expression of the client's ability to selectively attend to, disengage from, and shift visual attention to find new targets (Warren, 2011). A good visual search includes the following features (Warren, 2011):

- Initiation of a horizontal or vertical pattern
- An organized and efficient strategy
- Symmetrical search of both sides of the scene
- Sustained engagement in the visual search without drifting off
- Successful identification of targets
- Ability to search increasingly complex environments

Hemi-Inattention. Hemi-inattention is a disorder characterized by the loss of ability to attend, respond, or react to sensory stimuli on the side contralateral to the brain lesion. Three main features of hemi-inattention are generalized difficulty with alertness and attention, spatial bias (preference for initiating and confining visual search to the ipsilateral side), and difficulty forming a mental representation of space that includes the involved side (Warren, 2011). The disorder occurs most commonly in lesions of the right hemisphere with hemi-inattention involving the left side. The severity of the disorder ranges from mild to severe, with the terms visual neglect and hemispatial neglect reserved to describe the most severe condition, which may be accompanied by a left hemianopsia (Warren, 2011). Unilateral neglect and visual neglect are terms often used interchangeably, but they are not the same (see below).

Unilateral Neglect. Unilateral neglect (UN) is a category of disorders that broadly refers to the failure to detect, report, or respond to stimuli (people or objects) presented to the side that is opposite of a brain lesion (Hillis, 2006; Plummer, Morris, & Dunai, 2003). UN can involve sensory, motor, and representational modalities that may not be detected in assessment of vision (Goff, 2010). In severe cases of neglect, evidence suggests that in addition to the features of hemi-inattention described above, attention to visual stimuli on the extreme ipsilateral side is diminished as well, leading to the characterization of neglect as "a bilateral, asymmetrical compression of experienced space" (Ellis, Jordan, & Sullivan, 2006, p. 861). For example, a client with a right-brain stroke may appear to not see a person sitting on the left side of his body or fail to shave the left side of his face. Clients with UN are often not aware that they are missing information and believe they are seeing things as complete (Toglia & Cermak, 2009). Although it is typically associated with right parietal lobe damage, UN can occur after unilateral lesion of a diverse range of brain structures (Cumming et al., 2009).

There are two main classification systems for the many types and clinical presentations of UN (Pierce & Buxbaum, 2002). One system is based on the modality in which the neglect is elicited (i.e., sensory, motor, representational), and the other is based on the distribution of abnormal behavior (i.e., personal or spatial) (Plummer, Morris, & Dunai, 2003) (see Definition 5-2). This chapter addresses aspects of sensory neglect (specifically visual neglect), personal neglect, and spatial neglect (motor neglect is described further in Chapter 8).

Although, to onlookers, it may appear that clients with UN do not see stimuli on the contralateral side of their brain lesion, UN is generally believed to be an attention-based processing impairment, not an impairment of the eyes or visual system (Gillen, 2009). Occupational therapists attempt to discern between possible symptoms of visual field deficits and UN during the assessment process (see Table 5-3) and administer specific assessments of UN if it is suspected (see options in Assessment Table 5-1) so that the most appropriate intervention plan may be developed.

When screening for visual attention and visual search deficits, the occupational therapist must consider the context in which the search occurs. A visual search of the area immediately surrounding the body—the peripersonal space—requires a different search strategy than a visual search of the larger environment—the extrapersonal space. (Also see Figure 24-4 for depiction of extrapersonal versus peripersonal space.)

Peripersonal Space Visual Search. A visual search of peripersonal space requires high amounts of selective attention, because visual targets at close range can be inspected

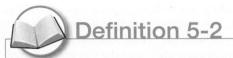

Definition 5-2

Categories of Unilateral Neglect

- **Sensory neglect** (also called "input neglect and perceptual neglect") refers to a condition in which the client is not aware of the visual, auditory, or tactile stimuli on the part of the body contralateral to the lesion.
- **Motor neglect** (also called "output neglect") presents as impaired initiation or execution of movement in response to a stimulus even when the person is aware of the stimulus that cannot be explained by a motor deficit or weakness.
- **Representational neglect** pertains to disregard of the contralesional half of mental visualizations of a task, action, or environment. For example, the client with right-brain stroke is asked to imagine and then describe her bedroom as if she were standing in the doorway, but she omits the left-sided details in her description.
- **Personal neglect** refers to lack of awareness of the side of the body opposite the brain damage, such as failing to comb one side of the head.
- **Spatial neglect** refers to the failure to respond to stimuli on the contralateral side of space, further characterized as peripersonal neglect (failure to eat food on half of the plate) or extrapersonal neglect (bumping into a doorway).

Adapted from Plummer, P., Morris, M. E., & Dunai, J. (2003). Assessment of unilateral neglect. *Physical Therapy, 83,* 732–740.

for greater detail than those in the distant environment. Assessments conducted at close range are commonly given in the form of pen-and-paper tests administered at a desk. Examples of tests include line bisection, single-letter cancellation, design copy, and draw a clock (Goff, 2010; Rengachary et al., 2009; Warren, 2011). A computerized

Table 5-3   Scanning: Visual Field Defect Versus Hemi-Inattention

Visual Field Defect	Hemi-Inattention
Abbreviated scanning pattern	Disorganized, random scanning pattern
Scanning pattern is organized	Asymmetrical search pattern in hemispace
Rescanning is observed	Scanning pattern is carried out with reduced effort and little or no rescanning
Length of time/effort are appropriate for the task	Task is completed swiftly, or if client is aware of deficit, will take an inordinate amount of time in an attempt to compensate

Reprinted with permission from Warren, M. (1998). *Brain Injury Assessment Battery for adults: Test manual.* Birmingham, AL: visABILITIES Rehab Services, Inc.

reaction time test—the Posner Cueing Paradigm—was shown to have the greatest sensitivity to detecting left-sided visual neglect when compared with some of the aforementioned tests in clients in the acute and chronic phases of stroke recovery (Rengachary et al., 2009).

Extrapersonal Space Visual Search. The area that extends beyond arm's reach is extrapersonal space and represents the larger environment through which an individual moves. Global awareness of the environment must be balanced with selective attention to the visual details of targets. Wider eye and head movements are required to effectively perform visual searches of the environment; searches can be conducted when the client/viewer is stationary or while the client performs a mobility task.

Three visual search strategies are used by people with normal visual attention: clockwise, counterclockwise, or rectilinear (Warren, 1998). The ScanBoard was developed to assess visual search of extrapersonal space when the client is stationary (Warren, 1998). The client is required to point out 10 numbers as he or she sees them without cueing. The therapist records the order of the numbers read. The ScanBoard tells if the client used an organized, sequential search strategy or whether the search was disorganized, random, or abbreviated (Warren, 1998). Visual search of extrapersonal space during ambulation can be observed by asking the client to identify features of the environment while walking through it. Warren (1998) recommended placing ten 1-inch letters or numbers along each side of a hallway at various heights and distances from one another and then asking the client to point out and read each letter or number during ambulation (Warren, 1998, 2011).

Reading Assessment

Reading difficulty is the most frequently cited complaint in clients with vision impairments (Watson, 1999). Reading is a complex task that involves many cognitive processes other than vision. Assessments were developed to examine the impact of central vision loss on particular aspects of reading: acuity, size, speed, accuracy, and comprehension. In low vision reading assessments, the size of print is calibrated using the same unit of measure, M-size, as the characters on visual acuity charts. Newsprint positioned at 40 centimeters (16 inches) from the reader roughly corresponds to a print size of 1.0M, also considered the size of standard print.

The Minnesota Reading Acuity Charts (MNRead) were designed to measure the effect of print size on reading speed. The client reads the sentences out loud while the examiner records the time taken to read each sentence. The smallest print size that is read fluently and without errors in the fastest time is called the "critical print size." The smallest print size read, regardless of reading speed, is termed "reading acuity" (Legge et al., 1989). The critical print size is used to determine the amount of magnification the client needs in order to read "standard" print.

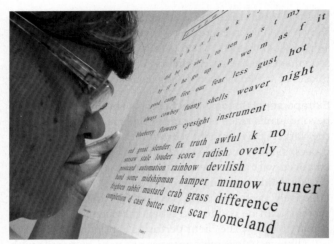

Figure 5-4 Client performing the Pepper Visual Skills for Reading test.

Visual recognition of words, eye movement control during reading, and the interference of central scotomas are measured using the Pepper Visual Skills for Reading Test (VSRT). The client is required to read aloud unrelated letters and words in rows with varied spacing while the examiner records errors and the time to complete the test (Fig. 5-4). The test reveals reading rate, line mastery, and prevalent errors in reading for the print size in which the test is presented (Watson, Baldesare, & Whittaker, 1990).

A client's reading grade level can be calculated using the Morgan Low Vision Reading Comprehension Assessment. The test uses the "cloze" method, in which a word is omitted from a sentence, and the client is required to provide the missing word after reading it only once (Watson et al., 1996).

Formal Vision-Related Questionnaires

The National Eye Institute 25-Item Visual Function Questionnaire (VFQ-25) Version 2000 (Mangione et al., 2001) is a standardized vision-specific quality of life outcome measure designed to evaluate the impact of visual symptoms on visual tasks (e.g., reading medication labels and driving) and general health (e.g., emotional well-being and social functioning). It has been extensively used in research and is available in the public domain.

The Melbourne Low-Vision Activities of Daily Living Index (MLVAI) is a standardized test of basic and instrumental activities of daily living (ADL) for clients with low vision. The therapist conducts an interview and observes structured tasks that are scored according to descriptive criteria (Haymes, Johnston, & Heyes, 2001b). The Weighted Melbourne Low-Vision ADL Index ($MLVAI_w$) uses the same criteria from the MLVAI but includes the client's rating of the importance of the ADL items. The ranking of importance allows the therapist to measure the impact of low vision on the client's perception of disability (Haymes, Johnston, & Heyes, 2001a).

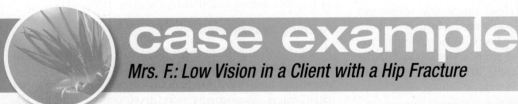

case example

Mrs. F.: Low Vision in a Client with a Hip Fracture

Occupational Therapy Assessment Process	Clinical Reasoning Process	
	Objectives	**Examples of Internal Dialogue**
Client Information	Understand the client's diagnosis or condition	"Mrs. F. broke her leg at the hip—I wonder if she tripped over something she did not see? The macular degeneration is likely to make it difficult for her to recognize the people on the unit and read postsurgical instructions. I wonder what her vision is like now compared to what it used to be before her eye disease. It is important for me to know her level of vision impairment so that I can modify instructions accordingly."
Mrs. F. is a 78-year-old woman who was admitted for inpatient rehabilitation following repair to the right femoral neck. Other chronic health conditions include osteoarthritis, hypertension, and macular degeneration. Her expected length of stay in the rehabilitation unit is 8 days.		
Mrs. F. was a homemaker who did not learn to drive until she turned age 55 years. Prior to getting her driver's license, her hobbies included cross-stitching and reading romance novels. Once she got her license, she and her husband would plan weekend excursions to visit family and friends across state borders.	Know the person	"She does not strike me as someone who takes care of herself—she seems like someone who always takes care of others. I wonder if she has been to see her eye doctor lately to get a dilated eye exam."

Mrs. F. lost her husband of 58 years 6 months ago. Of her four children, one lives locally, one lives several states away, and one lives overseas. Her second child committed suicide at age 30 years. Her relationships with her children are strained, and they rarely come to visit.

Appreciate the context	"I imagine it has been very difficult keeping up with housework, paying bills, cleaning, and driving—not only because of her vision loss but also coping with the recent loss of her husband."
Develop provisional hypotheses	"Even though Mrs. F. is here for a broken hip, I imagine that one of the greatest barriers to her successful rehabilitation will be her vision loss, particularly in tasks requiring appreciation of details. I am predicting that she has poor visual acuity, contrast sensitivity loss, and a scotoma that makes reading very difficult. She might also be depressed because she has suffered so many losses in such a short time. She is going to be spending a lot of time in one place, so she will likely desire to engage in activities within her peripersonal space—requiring greater attention to visual details."

Assessment Process

In addition to completing an occupational profile and observations of performance in activities of daily living (ADL), the therapist chose the Canadian Occupational Performance Measure (COPM) to obtain information about Mrs. F.'s perceived problems and priorities. The therapist also screened visual acuity using an Early Treatment of Diabetic Retinopathy Study (ETDRS) chart at 4 meters with glasses, the Minnesota Reading Acuity (MNRead) chart (to obtain information about reading acuity and critical print size), the Pepper Visual Skills for Reading Test (VSRT) (to obtain information on reading accuracy), and the Morgan Low Vision Reading Comprehension Assessment (LVRCA) (to estimate current grade-level reading ability).

Consider evaluation approach and methods	"I already know that she will not be able to do certain ADL tasks because of her postsurgical non–weight-bearing status. I need to evaluate her vision to give me a better understanding of how her loss of vision impacts her ability to engage in other daily activities."

Assessment Results

The COPM revealed that although her highest priority was to do everything possible to allow her hip to heal and be a "good patient," Mrs. F. was very concerned about her ability to cope with the demands of the therapists and nursing staff. She disclosed that she was more worried about potential embarrassing situations caused by her "hidden disability" (like difficulty recognizing faces or reading therapy instructions) than those caused by her temporary dependence on others for mobility assistance. She was dissatisfied with her ability to read instructions, sign her name on admission forms, and distinguish the faces of the therapists and nursing staff.

Best corrected visual acuity at 4 meters using both eyes was 4/16 (equivalent to 20/80), indicating moderate vision impairment displaced to the left of fixation.

The MNRead, which Mrs. F. held at 33 centimeters, revealed a reading acuity of 1.3M and a critical print size of 2.5M. Reading speed was not calculated.

The VSRT was administered at 3.2M. Mrs. F. demonstrated frequent misidentification of word beginnings, indicating a possible central scotoma. The LVRCA was administered at 3.0M, and Mrs. F.'s reading grade level was equivalent to that of a fifth grader.

Interpret observations	"Mrs. F. is highly motivated to participate in her own therapeutic process but is concerned about the disabling impact her vision loss has on her ability to meet the challenges that the clinical staff might present to her. She seems willing to accept help for limitations caused by her hip fracture—look at her bossing her visitor to go fetch her a box of tissues from the bathroom or a drink from the vending machine. Yet she is clearly concerned that she will embarrass herself when she is asked to read something, such as the breakfast menu, and it is revealed that she cannot see. She is worried that everyone will think she is illiterate.
	The reading tests were really difficult for her to complete and made a huge emotional impact on her. She broke down and cried. She said she felt like a complete idiot. I guess this was the first time that she could not "fudge" it—she is not used to being alone now, and when her husband was alive he did all of the reading."

Occupational Therapy Problem List

1. At risk for poor adherence to rehabilitation efforts related to hip fracture because of vision limitations. Difficulty acknowledging vision loss to others.
2. Decreased awareness of how her vision loss can potentially interfere with the therapy process.
3. Difficulty recognizing faces of staff on the unit.
4. Difficulty reading print size smaller than the equivalent of subheadings in a newspaper.
5. Decreased comprehension of reading materials.

Synthesize results

"She is putting up a good front and is managing to hold herself together for the most part. I would like to screen for depression in the following days, once we establish a good therapeutic relationship. I think that doing the reading tests really opened the floodgates and touched a deep sorrow for all the losses she has had to face in the past year and might be facing in the near future—losing her husband, her eyesight, her driver's license, and possibly her ability to take care of her house. She was not expecting me to address her vision loss, because she came here for her hip. I would also like to involve her eye-care provider and find out when she is due for an appointment and what tools might be available to help her. I wonder if since her husband's passing, her home has gotten so disorganized that she tripped and fell over something that was not put away, causing the hip fracture. She will benefit from a home assessment prior to discharge."

 # Clinical Reasoning in Occupational Therapy Practice

Effects of an Old Stroke on Visual Function

During her inpatient rehabilitation, Mrs. F. was observed to eat only the food on the right side of her plate. Her medical history revealed an old stroke on the right side of her brain.

What might you suspect to find in the occupational therapy vision screen?

Summary Review Questions

1. What is the difference between visual function and functional vision?
2. How do you understand the Occupational Therapy Practice Framework, 2nd edition, in the context of visual function and functional vision?
3. What are the foundations for visual function?
4. Your client with brain injury did poorly on a test of figure-ground administered by another therapist. List two possible reasons why.
5. Why is it important to assess contrast sensitivity?
6. Name four vision-related professions. Where would you be most likely to interact with workers in those professions? What information would you exchange?
7. What is the difference between low vision and visual dysfunction?
8. Name three age-related eye diseases and describe their impact on visual function.
9. What are three distinguishing features of hemi-inattention, and how does it differ from a visual field defect?
10. Why is it important to screen vision as early as possible?

Glossary

Contrast sensitivity—The ability to distinguish the edges of objects against backgrounds of similar color or hue.

Hemi-inattention—A disorder of attention resulting in decreased visual search to one side.

Pursuits—Slow movements of the eyes allowing the moving object of regard to remain in the area of clearest vision.

Saccades—Quick movements of the eyes from one target to another while positioning the visual targets in the area of clearest vision.

Scanning—The act of visually searching the environment.

Tracking—The act of visually following a moving target.

Unilateral neglect (UN)—A category of disorders that broadly refers to the failure to detect, report, or respond to stimuli (people or objects) presented to the side that is opposite of a brain lesion (Hillis, 2006; Plummer, Morris, & Dunai, 2003).

Visual acuity—Sharpness of vision.

Visual field—The span of vision; what one sees all around while looking straight ahead.

Visual perception—The visual and cognitive processes required to adapt to the environment.

References

Academy for Certification of Vision Rehabilitation and Education Professionals. (2011). *About ACVREP*. Retrieved March 11, 2012 from http://www.acvrep.org.

American Academy of Ophthalmology. (2011). *About ophthalmology & eye M.D.s*. Retrieved from http://www.aao.org/about/eyemds.cfm.

American Academy of Ophthalmology Vision Rehabilitation Committee. (2007). *Preferred Practice Pattern® Guidelines: Vision rehabilitation for adults*. San Francisco: American Academy of Ophthalmology.

American Association of Certified Orthoptists. (2011). *What is orthoptics*. Retrieved from http://www.orthoptics.org/index.htm.

American Occupational Therapy Association. (2008). Occupational therapy practice framework: Domain and process (2nd ed.). *American Journal of Occupational Therapy, 62*, 625–683.

American Optometric Association. (2011). *Doctors of optometry and their education*. Retrieved from http://www.aoa.org/x5879.xml.

Arend, O., Remky, A., Evans, D., Stüber, R., & Harris, A. (1997). Contrast sensitivity loss is coupled with capillary dropout in patients with diabetes. *Investigative Ophthalmology & Visual Science, 38*, 1819–1824.

Azouvi, P., Olivier, S., de Montety, G., Samuel, C., Louis-Dreyfus, A., & Tesio, L. (2003). Behavioral assessment of unilateral neglect: Study of the psychometric properties of the Catherine Bergego Scale. *Archives of Physical Medicine and Rehabilitation, 84*, 51–57.

Brahm, K., Wilgenburg, H., Kirby, J., Ingalla, S., Chang, C., & Goodrich, G. (2009). Visual impairment and dysfunction in combat-injured service members with traumatic brain injury. *Optometry and Vision Science, 86*, 817–825.

Campbell, V. A., Crews, J. E., Moriarty, D. G., Zack, M. M., & Blackman, D. K. (1999). *Surveillance for sensory impairment, activity limitation, and health-related quality of life among older adults – United States, 1993–1997*. Retrieved from http://www.cdc.gov/mmwr/preview/mmwrhtml/ss4808a6.htm.

Cassidy, T.P., Bruce, D.W., Lewis, S., & Gray, C.S. (1999). The association of visual field deficits and visuo-spatial neglect in acute right-hemisphere stroke patients. *Age and Ageing, 28*(3), 257–260.

Cate, Y., & Richards, L. (2000). Relationship between performance on tests of basic visual functions and visual-perceptual processing in persons after brain injury. *The American Journal of Occupational Therapy, 54*, 326–334.

Centers for Disease Control and Prevention. (2011). *National Diabetes Fact Sheet: National estimates and general information on diabetes and pre-diabetes in the United States*. Atlanta: U.S. Department of Health and Human Services.

Centers for Medicare & Medicaid Services. (2002). *Transmittal AB-02-078*. Department of Health and Human Services. Retrieved from https://www.cms.gov/transmittals/downloads/AB02078.pdf.

Chaplin, K., & Bradford, G. (2011). Eye charts 102: Challenges with current recommended eye charts. *Visibility, 5*, 1–6.

Cockerham, G., Goodrich, G., Weichel, E., Orcutt, J., Rizzo, J., Bower, K., & Schuchard, R. (2009). Eye and visual function in traumatic brain injury. *Journal of Rehabilitation Research & Development, 46*, 811–818.

Colenbrander, A. (2009). The functional classification of brain damage-related vision loss. *Journal of Vision Impairment and Blindness, 103*, 118–113.

Cumming, T. B., Plummer-D'Amato, P., Linden, T., & Bernardt, J. (2009). Hemispatial neglect and rehabilitation in acute stroke. *Archives of Physical Medicine and Rehabilitation, 90*, 1931–1936.

Dougherty, A., MacGregor, A., Han, P., Heltemes, K., & Galarneau, M. (2010). Visual dysfunction following blast-related traumatic brain injury from the battlefield. *Brain Injury, 25*, 8–13.

Ellis, A., Jordan, J., & Sullivan, C. (2006). Unilateral neglect is not unilateral: Evidence for additional neglect of extreme right space. *Cortex, 42*, 861–868.

Fletcher, D., & Schuchard, R. (1997). Preferred retinal loci relationship to macular scotomas in a low-vision population. *Ophthalmology, 104*, 632–638.

Gillen, G. (2009). *Cognitive and perceptual rehabilitation: Optimizing function*. St. Louis: Mosby.

Goff, J. (2010). Assessing unilateral neglect in acute care: Raising clinician awareness. *OT Practice, 15*, 14–17.

Hartman-Maier, A. & Katz, N. (1995). Validity of the Behavioral Inattention Test (BIT): Relationships With Functional Tasks. *American Journal of Occupational Therapy 49* (6), 507–516

Haymes, S., Johnston, A., & Heyes, A. (2001a). A weighted version of the Melbourne Low-Vision ADL Index: A measure of disability impact. *Optometry and Vision Science, 78*, 565–579.

Haymes, S., Johnston, A., & Heyes, A. (2001b). The development of the Melbourne Low-Vision ADL Index: A measure of vision disability. *Investigative Ophthalmology & Visual Science, 42*, 1215–1225.

Hillis, A. E. (2006). Neurobiology of unilateral spatial neglect. *Neuroscientist, 12*, 153–163.

Hunt, L., & Bassi, C. (2010). Near-vision acuity levels and performance on neuropsychological assessments used in occupational therapy. *American Journal of Occupational Therapy, 64*, 105–113.

International Council of Ophthalmology. (2002). *Visual standards: Aspects and ranges of vision loss with emphasis on population surveys*. Retrieved from http://www.icoph.org/downloads/visualstandardsreport.pdf.

International Council of Ophthalmology. (2008). *Assessment and rehabilitation of functional vision*. Retrieved from http://www.icoph.org/standards.

Legge, G., Ross, J., Luebker, A., & LaMay, J. (1989). Psychophysics of reading VIII: The Minnesota low-vision reading test. *Optometry and Vision Science, 66,* 843–853.

Luukkainen-Markkula, R., Tarkka, I. M., Pitkänen, Sivenius, J., & Hämäläinen, H. (2011). Comparison of the Behavioural Inattention Test and the Catherine Bergego Scale in assessment of hemispatial neglect. *Neuropsychological Rehabilitation, 21,* 103–116.

Mangione, C. (2000). *NEI VFQ-25 scoring algorithm*. Bethesda, MD: National Eye Institute.

Mangione, C., Lee, P., Gutierrez, P., Spritzer, K., Berry, S., & Hays, R. (2001). National Eye Institute Visual Function Questionnaire (VFQ-25). *Archives of Ophthalmology, 119,* 1050–1058.

Maples, W., Atchley, J., & Ficklin, T. (1992). Northeastern State University College of Optometry's oculomotor norms. *Journal of Behavioral Optometry, 3,* 143–150.

Massof, R. (2002). A model of the prevalence and incidence of low vision and blindness among adults in the U.S. *Optometry and Vision Science, 79,* 31–38.

Mennem, T. A., Warren, M., & Yuen, H. K. (2012). Preliminary validation of a vision-dependent activities of daily living instrument on adults with homonymous hemianopsia. *American Journal of Occupational Therapy, 66,* 478–482.

National Eye Institute. (2006). *Progress in eye and vision research 1999–2006*. U.S. Department of Health and Human Services. Retrieved from http://www.nei.nih.gov/strategicplanning/NEI_ProgressDoc.pdf.

Olmstead, J. (2005). *Itinerant teachers*. American Foundation for the Blind. Retrieved from http://www.afb.org/Section.asp?SectionID=44&TopicID=256.

Pierce, S. R., & Buxbaum, L. J. (2002). Treatments of unilateral neglect: A review. *Archives of Physical Medicine and Rehabilitation, 83,* 256–268.

Plummer, P., Morris, M. E., & Dunai, J. (2003). Assessment of unilateral neglect. *Physical Therapy, 83,* 732–740.

Prevent Blindness America. (2008). *Vision problems in the U.S.: 2008 Update to the fourth edition*. National Eye Institute, National Institutes of Health, and the U.S. Department of Health and Human Services. Retrieved September 8, 2011, from http://www.preventblindness.net/site/DocServer/VPUS_2008_update.pdf?docID=1561.

Purves, D., Augustine, G. J., Fitzpatrick, D., Hall, W. C., LaMantia, A., McNamara, J. O., & Williams, S. M. (Eds.). (2004). *Neuroscience* (3rd ed.). Sunderland, MA: Sinauer Associates.

Rengachary, J., d'Avossa, G., Sapir, A., Shulman, G., & Corbetta, M. (2009). Is the Posner Reaction Time Test more accurate than clinical tests in detecting left neglect in acute and chronic stroke? *Archives of Physical Medicine and Rehabilitation, 90,* 2081–2088.

Rowe F, Brand D, Jackson CA, Price A, Walker L, Harrison S, Eccleston C, Scott C, Akerman N, Dodridge C, Howard C, Shipman T, Sperring U, MacDiarmid S, Freeman C. (2009). Visual impairment following stroke: Do stroke patients require vision assessment? *Age and Ageing, 38,* 188–193.

Scheiman, M. (2011). *Understanding and managing vision deficits: A guide for occupational therapists* (3rd ed.). Thorofare, NJ: Slack.

Scheiman, M., Scheiman, M., & Whittaker, S. (2007). *Low vision rehabilitation: A practical guide for occupational therapists*. Thorofare, NJ: Slack.

Schoehborn, C., & Heyman, K. (2009). *Health characteristics of adults aged 55 years and over: United States, 2004–2007*. Centers for Disease Control and Prevention. Retrieved from http://www.cdc.gov/nchs/data/nhsr/nhsr016.pdf.

Toglia, J., & Cermak, S. A. (2009). Dynamic assessment and prediction of learning potential in clients with unilateral neglect. *American Journal of Occupational Therapy, 64,* 569–579.

Vitale, S., Cotch, M., & Sperduto, R. (2006). Prevalence of visual impairment in the United States. *Journal of the American Medical Association, 295,* 2158–2163.

Warren, M. (1993a). A hierarchical model for evaluation and treatment of visual perceptual dysfunction in adult acquired brain injury, part 1. *The American Journal of Occupational Therapy, 47,* 42–54.

Warren, M. (1993b). A hierarchical model for evaluation and treatment of visual perceptual dysfunction in adult acquired brain injury, part 2. *The American Journal of Occupational Therapy, 47,* 55–66.

Warren, M. (1998). *Brain Injury Assessment Battery for adults: Test manual*. Birmingham, AL: visABILITIES Rehab Services, Inc.

Warren, M. (1999). *Occupational therapy practice guidelines for adults with low vision*. Bethesda, MD: American Occupational Therapy Association.

Warren, M. (2011). Interventions for adults with vision impairment from acquired brain injury. In M. Warren & E. Barstow (Eds.), *Occupational therapy interventions for adults with low vision*. Bethesda, MD: American Occupational Therapy Association.

Warren, M., Bachelder, J., Velozo, C., & Hicks, E. (2008). The *self-report assessment of functional visual performance*. Birmingham, AL: Occupational Therapy Departments at University of Alabama at Birmingham and University of Florida at Gainesville.

Warren, M., Bettenhausen, D., Kaldenberg, J., Sokol-McKay, D., & Weisser-Pike, O. (2006). Occupational therapy in low-vision rehabilitation: A reflection on specialized practice. *OT Practice, 20,* 19–23.

Watson, G. (1999). Using low vision effectively. In D. Fletcher (Ed.), *Low vision rehabilitation: Caring for the whole person*. San Francisco: American Academy of Ophthalmology.

Watson, G., Baldesare, J., & Whittaker, S. (1990). The validity and clinical uses of the Pepper Visual Skills for Reading Test. *Journal of Visual Impairment and Blindness, 84,* 119–123.

Watson, G., Wright, V., Long, S., & De l'Aune, W. (1996). The development and evaluation of a low vision reading comprehension test. *Journal of Visual Impairment and Blindness, 90,* 486–494.

Wilson, B., Cockburn, J., & Halligan, P. (1987). Development of a behavioral test of visuospatial neglect. *Archives of Physical Medicine and Rehabilitation, 68(2),* 98–102.

Acknowledgments

Many thanks go to Luke Skilbeck, CO, COMT, for his assistance in thoroughly reviewing this chapter for accuracy. Thanks go to Lee Ann Quintana, MS, OTR/L, for her thoughtful work in developing and writing the previous edition of this chapter.

Assessing Abilities and Capacities: Cognition

Mary Vining Radomski and M. Tracy Morrison

Learning Objectives

After studying this chapter, the reader will be able to do the following:

1. Appreciate the role of cognition in occupational performance.
2. Describe specific cognitive capacities and abilities and analyze their influence on occupational function.
3. Select cognitive assessment methods and tools based on individual clients' characteristics, properties of various measures, and requirements of the setting or episode of care.
4. Anticipate and describe factors that should be considered in interpreting the results of cognitive assessment.
5. Distinguish occupational therapy's contribution to multidisciplinary cognitive assessment from that of other rehabilitation disciplines.

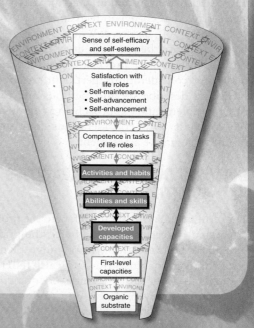

ognition refers to the integrated functions of the human mind that together result in thought and goal-directed action. Cognition underlies being and doing and is evidenced in how people interact with others and perform both simple and complex activities of daily life. Perhaps the central role of cognition in occupational performance is best illustrated as one imagines what it must be like to suddenly lose the ability to concentrate, remember, and problem solve. Survivors of traumatic brain injury (TBI) describe how their once-familiar routines and environments become chaotic, confusing, and frightening, which devastates their sense of identity and competence (Erikson et al., 2007).

Occupational therapists assess cognition because many people seeking occupational therapy services are likely to have some degree of cognitive impairment that influences their ability to participate in rehabilitation and achieve rehabilitation outcomes (Skidmore et al., 2010). Cognitive changes can be temporary, relatively static, or progressive. As above, many survivors of TBI experience deficits in information processing speed, attention, memory, and executive functions that persist for months or years postinjury (Skandsen et al., 2010). A significant number of persons who sustain a spinal cord injury also have a concurrent TBI with similar implications for cognition (Macciocchi et al., 2008). Individuals with chronic conditions may also experience cognitive changes including those with multiple sclerosis (Rogers & Panegyres, 2007), Parkinson's disease (Caviness et al., 2007), cancer (Boykoff, Moieni, & Subramanian, 2009), epilepsy (Helmstaedter et al., 2003), systemic lupus erythematosus (McLaurin et al., 2005), and human immunodeficiency virus/acquired immunodeficiency syndrome (Heaton et al., 2004). Even individuals with mild stroke who are independent in activities of daily living (ADL) may have executive dysfunction that impacts their ability to work, drive, and engage in recreational activities (Edwards et al., 2006; Wolf, Barbee, & White, 2011).

This chapter begins with descriptions of specific cognitive domains and processes. We then review clinical reasoning considerations pertinent to cognitive assessment and describe specific methods and tools based on three complementary approaches to cognitive assessment. We conclude with considerations for interpreting the results of cognitive assessment.

DEFINING COGNITIVE CAPACITIES AND ABILITIES

The term cognition generally refers to the product of many integrated processes carried out by the brain that allow humans to be aware, think, learn, judge, plan, and execute behavior (National Institutes of Health [NIH], n.d.). These domains and processes include orientation, perception, attention, memory and learning, judgment, reasoning, language, and executive functions (NIH, n.d.). How these processes and domains precisely interact to enable being,

| Table 6-1 | **Possible Observable Manifestations of Cognitive Dysfunction** |

Cognitive Domain	Examples of Patient Performance That Suggest Cognitive Dysfunction
Orientation	Mr. K. is asked to report the correct date, time, or location. Sometimes during morning sessions he responds correctly but later in the day provides illogical or far-fetched answers.
Attention	Mrs. G. sorts a basket of laundry into two piles based on color. She stops and looks around every time she hears an overhead page, requiring cues to restart the task.
Memory	Mr. B. takes his medication right before breakfast. Two hours later, Mr. B. reports that he cannot recall whether or not he took his morning pills (episodic memory failure).

thinking, and doing is unclear, but it appears that executive functions may control and coordinate the other cognitive operations in the service of goal-directed action (Salthouse, 2005). Consider the working definitions that follow and how dysfunction might be observed in everyday activities (see Table 6-1).

Primary Cognitive Operations

Primary cognitive operations such as orientation, attention, and memory are thought to be prerequisite to higher level thinking abilities such as executive functions and metacognition. That is, people must have a sense of place or time and some ability to focus their attention and remember information in order to reason, problem solve, plan, and execute complex activities.

Orientation

Orientation refers to the awareness of self in relation to person, place, time, and circumstance (Sohlberg & Mateer, 1989). Orientation deficits are typically symptoms of brain dysfunction, with disorientation to time and place being most common (Lezak, 1995).

Attention

The term attention was famously defined by William James as "the taking possession by the mind, in a clear and vivid form, of one out of what seem several simultaneously present objects or trains of thought" (James, 1890, pp. 403–404). Attentional abilities are dependent on multiple brain regions including the cingulate cortex, limbic system, prefrontal cortices, and sensorimotor regions (Posner, 1980). Each person is thought to have a limited capacity for consciously attending to information—a hard-wired upper limit that dictates how many inputs

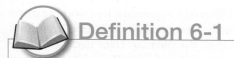

Definition 6-1

Components of Attention and Influence on Performance

Component of Attention	Definition	Implications: Performance during Meal Preparation
Focused attention	Basic response to stimuli as in turning head to sound of bell (Sohlberg & Mateer, 2001)	None. This level of attention is considered low level and often recovered as individuals emerge from coma and gain conscious awareness.
Sustained attention	Vigilance; maintaining attention over time during continuous activity (Sohlberg & Mateer, 2001)	To peel several potatoes, an individual must stay focused for the duration of the task.
Selective attention	Freedom from distractibility; occurs when an individual concentrates on one set of stimuli while ignoring competing stimuli (Sohlberg & Mateer, 2001)	The cook ignores the noise from the television while measuring or counting ingredients.
Alternating attention	Capacity for mental flexibility; occurs as one flexibly shifts attention between multiple operations (Sohlberg & Mateer, 2001)	The cook interrupts meal preparation to answer the telephone and then quickly resumes setting the table while monitoring the status of food simmering on the stove.
Divided attention	Ability to respond to two tasks simultaneously (Sohlberg & Mateer, 2001)	The cook browns the meat while talking with a family member.

can be simultaneously processed (Lezak, 1995). Deficits in attention are common following brain injury as numerous and diffuse neural regions work to support the individual's attentional abilities. Deficits can also be experienced because of a lack of sleep or decreased nutrition (Groeger et al., 2011).

Learning is dependent on attention as individuals cannot encode into memory stimuli or content they do not attend to. Definition 6-1 describes five components of attention (Sohlberg & Mateer, 2001) and their implications for task performance.

Memory

Memory broadly refers to information storage and retrieval (Lezak, 1995). Rather than a unitary process or construct, there are many types of neural processes that support an individual's memory capacity (Sohlberg & Turkstra, 2011). Experts still debate about what transpires during the process of remembering (Cowan, 2008). Atkinson and Shiffrin's (1971) Information-Processing Model, which highlights stages of acquiring and employing new knowledge and skills, is one of many conceptions as to how this process occurs (Fig. 6-1). We use this model to introduce

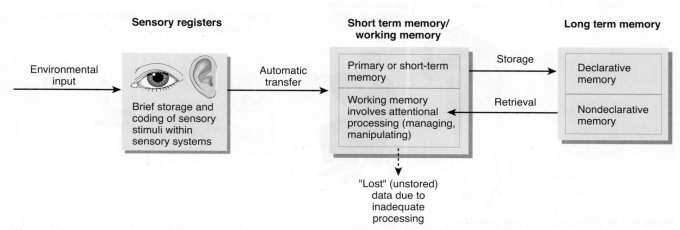

Figure 6-1 Human information-processing diagram that incorporates concepts proposed by Atkinson and Shiffrin (1971) and Levy (2011).

memory-related concepts, acknowledging the continued debate regarding precise terms and their meanings in this realm. (Also see Dubuc [2011] and Levy [2011] for more in-depth information on the following discussion.)

Sensory Registers. Information from the environment is briefly (milliseconds) held in registers (or stores) specific to the human senses (Lezak, 1995). This registration stage has been called the intake valve for determining what data from the environment are ultimately stored. This phase is influenced by acuity of the senses (such as hearing and vision), affective set, and perception.

Short-Term Memory/Working Memory. The short-term phase of information processing reflects "faculties of the human mind that can hold a limited amount of information in a very accessible state temporarily" (Cowan, 2008, p. 324). It has many labels: primary memory, immediate memory, short-term memory, and working memory. The term *primary memory* pertains to a pattern of neural firing associated with a given idea, about which the person may or may not be aware (Cowan, 2008). This includes data just transferred from the sensory registers related to one's focus of attention (Levy, 2011). The term *working memory* pertains to the attention-related processes that are involved in managing incoming information and manipulating stored information for planning and problem solving (Cowan, 2008). It can be thought of as the seat of conscious thought; it connotes the effortful deployment of cognitive resources during this stage as well as the manipulation of information involved in active thinking (Sohlberg & Turkstra, 2011). Many experts believe that for input from sensory registers to proceed to storage in long-term memory, the input must

be the subject of deliberate concentration in working memory for approximately 30 seconds (Lezak, 1995). Without this focused attention, the memory trace decays, and the memory is not retained (Lezak, 1995). Unlike long-term memory, which is thought to have an infinite capacity, working memory has a restricted holding capacity of seven plus or minus two chunks of information (Miller, 1956). In addition to its role in information processing, working memory is the foundation of concentration and problem solving (Baddeley, 1990). Based on electrochemical activity in the brain, working memory reflects the contribution of attention to the memory process (Lezak, 1995).

Long-Term Memory. Whereas data in working memory have a short shelf life, information in long-term memory can be stored for minutes to a lifetime (Lezak, 1995). When we remember information (an event that occurred an hour ago or a year ago), we have located and retrieved data from long-term memory and are holding it for conscious attention and thought in limited-capacity working memory. Storage in long-term memory is based on relatively permanent changes in brain cell structure (Glover, Ronning, & Bruning, 1990), although there does not appear to be a single local storage site for stored memories (Lezak, 1995).

Long-term memory is thought to consist of two subsystems, explicit (or declarative) memory and implicit (or nondeclarative) memory (Fig. 6-2). Declarative memory pertains to factual information and includes episodic memory (knowledge of personal information and events such as what you ate for breakfast) and semantic memory (knowledge of facts about the world such as that horses are big and ants are small) (Eysenck & Keane, 1990). Prospective memory is another form of declarative

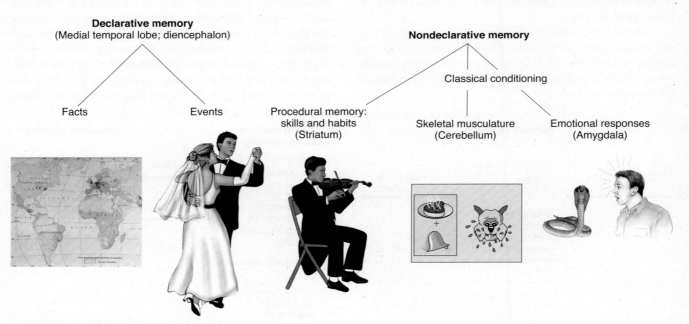

Figure 6-2 Two subsystems of long-term memory.

memory, having to do with remembering to do tasks that one intends (Fish, Wilson, & Manly, 2010). Implicit or nondeclarative memory differs from explicit memory because it does not involve conscious awareness of learning (Sohlberg & Turkstra, 2011). This includes procedural memory, which pertains to knowing how to do things; it allows us to learn and perform skilled motor actions (Eysenck & Keane, 1990).

Memory impairments are typically characterized as mild, moderate, or severe based on the results of cognitive assessment. The term *neurologic amnesia* is reserved to describe losses of broad categories or segments of memory resulting from brain trauma, stroke, or tumor (Dubuc, 2011) (see Definition 6-2).

Executive Abilities

The term *executive abilities* (also called executive functions) refers to a group of higher order thinking processes that enable individuals to achieve self-determined goals and engage independently and purposefully in complex everyday tasks, such as work and academic life (Lezak, 1995). As outlined in Table 6-2, the domains and functions that comprise executive processing underlie the personalized methods through which individuals begin, accomplish, and complete tasks. As such, executive abilities are critical to occupational performance.

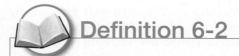

Definition 6-2

Types of Amnesia

Retrograde	Loss of ability to recall events that occurred before the trauma
Anterograde	Decreased memory of events occurring after trauma
Posttraumatic amnesia (PTA)	Period following trauma during which the patient is confused and disoriented and seems to lack the ability to store and retrieve new information

Executive Functions in Everyday Life

Executive abilities determine our ability to problem solve, plan, establish goals, monitor our work, and initiate and terminate tasks. Individuals with executive deficits commonly experience significant disability when they encounter novelty and complexity such as when discharged from clinical environments to return home (Baum et al., 2008).

Table 6-2   Possible Observable Manifestations of Problems with Executive Processing

Domain	Examples of Performance That Suggest Executive Dysfunction
Initiation	Mrs. M. wants to create a photo album for her son. She has an empty photo album and a large bag of photographs on a table and a free afternoon but cannot get herself to begin.
Inhibition	Mr. G. finds himself lost while driving in a new city. Two hours later he notices a shopping center he continually passes by and realizes he has circled the same one-half mile block the entire time.
Task persistence	Mr. J. selects a 60-piece model of an antique car to assemble for his nephew. He dumps the pieces on the table top and tries to fit together the two pieces that are within easiest reach. When that does not work, he quits the task.
Organization	Ms. C. has missed her therapy session again. The occupational therapist notices that Ms. C. showed up 4 hours late for her last therapy session and arrived on the wrong day for preceding session. When telephoned, Ms. C. exclaims, "I thought the appointment was tomorrow! I am so upset. I need this therapy to help me get my life back together!"
Generative thinking	Mr. F. is a member of a support group for individuals with brain injury. An occupational therapist leads the group and makes a suggestion to move a future meeting time to a new day because of upcoming holidays. Mr. F. rarely participates in group dialogue, but becomes very agitated by the change and states, "I cannot have any changes in my schedule! I want us to keep the meeting time the same!"
	As assigned, Ms. D. brings ingredients to her outpatient therapy session so that she can prepare a familiar, favorite recipe. The recipe involves making a graham cracker crust, to be prepared during the session. Ms. D. puts large graham crackers in a bowl and starts the electric mixer. After giving Ms. D. sufficient time to self-correct, the therapist stops the task as cracker pieces fly out of the bowl and around the kitchen.
Awareness	When Ms. S. arrives to her outpatient therapy, the therapist observes her disheveled appearance. She is wearing flip-flops despite the cold winter conditions, and she smells of body odor. When asked her about her plans for the day, she reports that she is going to a job interview immediately after the therapy session.

From Sohlberg, M. M., & Mateer, C. A. (2001). *Cognitive rehabilitation*. New York: Guilford Press.

Simple daily tasks (such as ADL) that were premorbidly performed through habit, or procedural memory, become novel and layered in complexity following a disabling injury or condition. Many individuals with executive deficits describe feelings of mental fatigue and a decreased mood when they return home from a hospital setting. They may experience deterioration in personal grooming and cleanliness, an inability to manage household tasks (such as managing personal finances), and/or difficulties returning to work. To help prevent excess disability, it is critically important that occupational therapists accurately assess patients' executive abilities before they have returned to their homes or at other significant transitions in recovery.

Executive Abilities and Brain Function

Neuroscientists use a variety of measurement methods to link brain functions to brain structures. One commonly used method is magnetic resonance imaging (MRI), which provides three-dimensional reconstructed images of the brain and skull. Advances from the field of cognitive neuroscience have enabled scientists to link executive abilities to prefrontal and subcortical brain regions (Alexander, Delong, & Strick, 1986). In addition, clinicians now realize that individuals with basal ganglia disorders associated with Parkinson's disease, for example, often experience executive dysfunction and cognitive impairment prior to experiencing severe motor impairments (Goldman & Litvan, 2011). Depending on what area of the brain is affected, people may have difficulties in some domains of executive functioning and not others. During the assessment process, clinicians try to determine which, if any, aspects of executive processing are impaired to focus intervention on specific areas of concern.

Self-Awareness and Metacognition

Self-awareness is an executive ability that pertains to the ability to process information about the self and compare it with a long-standing self-evaluation (Dougherty & Radomski, 1993). Some consider self-awareness to be the highest of all integrated activities of the brain (Prigatano & Schacter, 1991). It has two primary dimensions: (1) appreciation of personal attributes, such as physical and cognitive strengths and weaknesses, and (2) initiation of compensatory strategies in response to known personal attributes. In general, persons with TBI tend to be more aware of physical deficits than cognitive or emotional changes (Anderson & Tranel, 1989), and typically, the more severe the brain injury, the more problems the individual has with self-awareness (Sherer et al., 2005). Interestingly, some family members view unawareness as a blessing in persons with dementia (Fleming, Strong, & Ashton, 1996), whereas for other caregivers, it is associated with higher levels of subjective distress (Prigatano et al., 2005).

Crosson et al. (1989) proposed a three-level self-awareness hierarchy consisting of intellectual awareness, emergent awareness, and anticipatory awareness. This hierarchy helps clinicians specify awareness problems and is a useful structure for characterizing progress in this realm (e.g., a patient who previously endorses his wife's report of his memory failures [intellectual awareness] now writes himself an errand list before leaving the house [anticipatory awareness]).

1. Intellectual awareness is a person's ability to understand at some level that a particular function is impaired. Severe deficits in memory impede intellectual awareness because such awareness requires recall of the past.
2. Emergent awareness is the ability of a person to recognize a problem when it is actually happening.
3. Anticipatory awareness, which depends on the existence of intellectual and emergent awareness, is the ability to anticipate a challenge or problem resulting from physical or cognitive impairments.

Self-awareness is fundamental to metacognition, which is defined as "thinking about thinking" (Flavell, 1979, p. 906) and intimately linked to executive processing (Fernandez-Duque, Baird, & Posner, 2000). As in the previous example, to initiate note-taking in response to prospective memory demands (a metacognitive strategy), a person must appreciate vulnerability from memory deficits and anticipate the challenge the activity represents (intellectual and anticipatory awareness). Scientific evidence suggests executive processes work in a supervisory fashion over other cognitive domains, whereas metacognition involves both knowledge of one's cognitive abilities and regulation to coordinate cognitive processes through monitoring (e.g., error detection) and control (e.g., error correction or prevention) (Fernandez-Duque, Baird, & Posner, 2000). Although executive processing and metacognition are behaviorally interrelated, patients may have problems in one area but not the other. For example, patients can experience difficulty in organizing and planning tasks while maintaining good metacognitive knowledge about these deficits (Lysaker et al., 2011). This enables them to anticipate their cognitive vulnerabilities and initiate strategies to circumvent potential problems.

The importance of executive functions and metacognition to satisfying and productive role performance cannot be overstated. Impairments in executive functions are major factors associated with the loss of everyday competence (Goverover, 2004) and social autonomy and with the inability to return to work long after TBI (Mazaux et al., 1997). Decreased metacognition after TBI may prevent survivors from recognizing their deficits, which limits performance and diminishes motivation to participate in rehabilitation therapies. Executive functions reciprocally influence metacognition. Metacognition informs the selection of reasonable goals for a given undertaking as well as strategies that best facilitate performance. Ongoing monitoring of task performance with adjustment of strategies and incorporation of feedback can in turn affect self-awareness, altering percepts of personal strengths and weaknesses.

In summary, cognition is understood as an array of domains and processes. Occupational therapists must understand these constructs in order to assess cognition. For clarity and convenience, in this section we have described various cognitive domains and processes as separate and discrete entities. However, doing so belies the reality of their inseparability, as evidenced in the concept of dual-task performance. Based on an experimental dual-task paradigm from cognitive psychology, older adults and clinical populations demonstrate greater decrements in performance of a relatively simple primary task (such as walking) when a secondary (cognitive) task is added (McCulloch, 2007; McDowell, Whyte, & D'Esposito, 1997; Sosnoff et al., 2011) than do healthy controls. These dual-task conditions appear to be sensitive to frontal brain damage (McDowell, Whyte, & D'Esposito, 1997) and illustrate how attention, memory, and executive functions intersect in function. Dual-task performance involves divided attention, challenges the resource limitations of working memory, and requires flexible allocation of attention, which is thought to represent an executive ability (McCulloch, 2007; McDowell, Whyte, & D'Esposito, 1997). Although dual-task assessment methods have not yet been formalized in occupational therapy practice, dual-task performance is clearly relevant to the complexities of real-world occupational performance.

THE PROCESS OF COGNITIVE ASSESSMENT

Occupational therapists assess cognition for many reasons: (1) to measure baseline, progress, and/or outcome status; (2) to understand the patient's cognitive strengths, weaknesses, and capacity for strategy use in order to plan intervention; and (3) to estimate the patient's ability to safely perform every day activities (Baum & Katz, 2010). The purpose and methods will vary by patient, setting, competence of the therapist, roles of neuropsychology and/or speech language pathology personnel, and the point in the continuum of care at which the patient is assessed. However, one aspect of occupational therapy cognitive assessment is consistent: the focus on occupational performance. Occupational therapists have the potential to contribute a critical and unique perspective to the cognitive assessment process by combining their understanding of cognitive domains and operations and task analysis with keen observation and interpretation skills.

Procedures for Practice 6-1 describes the general process for assessing cognition, which represents a segment of a comprehensive occupational therapy evaluation. A cognitive assessment should incorporate patient/family self-report, measures of specific cognitive domains or processes, and observations of functional performance; occupational therapists may conduct part or all of the assessments, depending on setting. Examples of these assessment approaches are included in Assessment Table 6-1. In-depth and more extensive analyses of cognitive assessments can be found in the work of Katz (2011) and Gillen (2009).

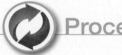 Procedures for Practice 6-1

Procedures for Assessing Cognition

Prepare	Review the patient's medical record to learn about diagnosis, background, results of procedures and other diagnostics, other disciplines involved in care. Look for information about possible language-communication problems, literacy, or medical issues (e.g., pain or fatigue) that may confound cognitive assessment.
	Obtain information from patient and/or family about perceptions of current status and priorities. Informally observe functional performance to establish hypotheses regarding possible areas of cognitive dysfunction.
	If information is not available in the medical record, perform a vision screen to assure that the patient has adequate visual skills to participate in a valid cognitive assessment.
	Coordinate with members of the interdisciplinary team so that elements of cognitive assessment are complementary and not duplicative.
Select	Decide what approach and/or measure(s) to use to assess cognition. Consider factors described above (e.g., diagnosis, patient priorities, and contributions of other team members), purpose of cognitive assessment, and psychometric properties of assessment options relative to patient characteristics.
Administer	If using standardized measures or methods, follow published setup and administration procedures. Observe and note behaviors during assessment; record assessment scores.
Interpret	Use scoring guidelines, if available, to interpret score. Consider the extent to which other variables (such as pain, fatigue, and stress) may have influenced performance.
Report	Document results in medical record; discuss results with patient, family, and/or team members.

| Assessment Table 6-1 | Summary of Assessments of Cognition |

Instrument and Reference	Description	Time to Administer	Validity	Reliability	Sensitivity	Strengths and Weaknesses
Selected Measures Involving Self-Report						
Self-Awareness of Deficits Interview (SADI) (Fleming, Strong, & Ashton, 1996)	Tool designed to obtain both qualitative and quantitative data on status of self-awareness. The patient is asked about self-awareness of deficits, self-awareness of functional limitations because of deficits, and ability to set realistic goals. A therapist familiar with the patient's level of functioning assigns a score in each realm (0–3, with 0 representing full awareness).	10 minutes	SADI moderately correlated with the Dysexecutive Questionnaire (DEX) ($r = 0.40$, $p < 0.05$). Regression analyses indicated that SADI scores were significantly predicted by a set of executive functioning measures ($p < 0.01$, $R^2 = 0.31$) (Bogod, Mateer, & MacDonald, 2003).	Strong interrater reliability (Intraclass correlation coefficient [ICC] = 0.82). Strong test-retest reliability (ICC = 0.94) (Simmond & Fleming, 2003)	No information	Strength: Brief semistructured interview with questions that are relevant to treatment planning Weakness: Potential for bias because clinician judges the extent to which patient responses reflect level of self-awareness disorder
Behavioral Rating Inventory of Executive Function-Adult version (BRIEF-A) (Roth, Isquith, & Gioia, 2005)	A standardized self-report and informant report questionnaire that measures an adult's appraisal of his or her executive functioning in everyday life. The BRIEF-A measures the following domains: inhibit, self-monitor, plan and organize, initiate, task monitor, emotional control, working memory, and organization of materials. The BRIEF-A is composed of 75 items with composite scores falling into two broad indexes: behavioral regulation and metacognition. An overall summary score results in a global executive composite. Higher values reflect greater difficulty experienced by the individual.	35 minutes	Convergent validity has been established through correlations with other self-reports and informant reports of frontal dysfunction. There appears to be a significant relationship between frontal lobe volumes and self-reported deficits measured by the BRIEF-A (Garlinghouse et al., 2010).	Moderate to high internal consistency ($\alpha = 0.73$–0.90 for clinical scales; 0.93–0.96 for index and global scores). High internal consistency for both the self-report ($\alpha = 0.80$–0.94 for clinical scales; 0.96–0.98 for index and global scores) and informant form (α range = 0.85–0.95 for clinical scales; 0.96–0.98 for index and global scales). Good test-retest reliability ($r = 0.82$–0.94) for self-report forms and high ($r = 0.91$–0.94) for informant reports (Roth, Isquith, & Gioia, 2005)	A study by Rabin et al. (2006) found the BRIEF-A to be sensitive to mild cognitive impairments among a group of 28 individuals with mild cognitive impairment and cognitive complaints when compared with controls.	Strengths: Good to excellent reliability; user-friendly; provides specific information on patient perceptions of executive functioning in daily life Weaknesses: The majority of validity studies have been conducted by the creators of the BRIEF-A; more studies are needed to further validate this tool.

Selected Measures of Functional Cognitive Performance

Measure	Description	Time	Validity	Reliability	Sensitivity	Strengths and Weaknesses
Observed Tasks of Daily Living–Revised (OTDL-R) (Diehl et al., 2005)	An assessment of everyday problem solving in which the patient performs nine tasks related to medication use, telephone use, and financial management.	25–30 minutes	OTDL-R scores were associated with measures of executive functioning (moderate correlation with the Toglia Category Assessment, $r = 0.506$, and moderately strong correlation with the Deductive Reasoning Test, $r = 0.796$) (Goverover & Hinojosa, 2002). OTDL-R scores were significantly different among four groups (community-dwelling older adults, older adults living in nursing homes, individuals with schizophrenia, and individuals with brain injury) ($p < 0.001$) (Goverover & Josman, 2004).	Internal consistency for the total measure (Cronbach's $\alpha = 0.82$)	Not established	Strength: Measure of everyday cognition that can be administered at bedside. Weakness: Does not provide a comprehensive picture of cognitive function, especially related to unstructured situations
Arnadottir OT-ADL Neurobehavioral Evaluation (A-ONE) (Arnadottir, 1990)	There are two parts to the instrument. Part 1 involves observing ADL performance and completing the (1) Functional Independence Scale and (2) Neurobehavioral Specific Impairment Subscale. Part 2 is optional, enabling the clinician to cross-link the neurobehavioral impairment to the most likely lesion site.	25 minutes	Content validity established through expert input. Discriminant validity: compared scores of 50 persons with stroke and 79 healthy controls. Significant Mann-Whitney U test suggests A-ONE discriminates between groups for all items of the Functional Independence Scale and all but six items of the Neurobehavioral Subscale.	Interrater reliability: Functional Independence Scale, $\kappa = 0.83$); Neurobehavioral Specific Impairment Subscale ($\kappa = 0.86$). Test-retest reliability within 1 week ($r_s = 0.85$)	No information	Strength: Standardized methods for combining assessment of ADL with assessment of some areas of cognition so that therapists can assess both areas at the same time. Weakness: Neurobehavioral subscale does not include assessment in key cognitive capacities such as memory and attention.
Executive Function Performance Test (EFPT) (Baum et al., 2003)	A standardized top-down performance-based measure of executive functioning. The EFPT examines the execution of four basic tasks associated with self-maintenance: simple cooking, telephone use, medication management, and bill paying. The EFPT uses an ordinal scoring system that highlights individuals' ability levels through measurement of the cues provided by the clinician.	60 minutes	Concurrent validity was established ($\rho = 0.61$) with the Assessment of Motor and Process Skills (AMPS) (Cederfeldt et al., 2011). Construct validity was established by Baum et al. (2008) with control EFPT total scores significantly ($p \leq 05$) lower (better) than mild stroke scores and moderate stroke scores ($p \leq 0.0001$). Mild stroke scores were also significantly lower than moderate stroke scores ($p \leq 0.0001$).	Excellent interrater reliability of the overall EFPT (ICC = 0.91). Internal consistency is excellent for total sample scores ($\alpha = .94$) (Baum et al., 2008). Test-retest reliability has not been evaluated.	Performance-based measures are not diagnostic tests and thus difficult to determine sensitivity or specificity. As such, sensitivity has not been investigated for the EFPT.	Strengths: One of few standardized performance-based measures and the only performance-based measure that provides clinicians with guidance on the level of cues needed to support clients' functional abilities; excellent reliability and validity. Weaknesses: Requires a full hour; cannot be used as an outcome tool without test-retest reliability established

(continued)

Assessment Table 6-1	Summary of Assessments of Cognition (*continued*)				
Instrument and Reference	Description	Time to Administer	Validity	Reliability	Sensitivity	Strengths and Weaknesses
The Multiple Errands Test (MET) (Shallice & Burgess, 1991)	A naturalistic performance-based measure of executive functioning deficits. The MET is set up much like a scavenger hunt. Participants are given a task list (typically 12 tasks); tasks with rules (typically 9 rules); and a map of the test environment. Participants are told to begin the test and to complete the test as they wish. Patients are successful only with careful planning with test goals and rules in mind.	60 minutes	Dawson et al. (2009) established ecological validity with good to strong correlations ($p \geq 0.51$) when the MET was compared to the Dysexecutive Questionnaire, AMPS and Stroke Impact Scale. Among participants with stroke, rule adherence and time to complete task showed the most robust correlations with measures of daily life function. Among the people with TBI, robust correlations were also seen between rule adherence and the process score of the AMPS, as well as between total errors and weighted errors with the DEX.	Moderate interrater reliability based on two studies: ICCs $\geq$ 0.70 (Alderman et al., 2003) and ICC $\geq$ 0.60 (Dawson et. al, 2009).	The MET has not been tested for sensitivity.	Strengths: Complex performance-based test that measures individuals' performance deficits as they navigate dynamic real-world environments, possibly sensitive to otherwise undetectable high-level problems Weaknesses: Site specific, requiring careful preparation prior to each test session; questionable clinical use given the complexity of the test for both participants during test execution and administrators during test setup and evaluation; does not have a standardized test manual or scoring system. The MET requires a significant amount of time for test setup and high rater skill. Morrison et al. (2005) suggested scoring focus only on quantifiable performance deficits versus behavioral lapses identified during the test session.

Selected Tools for Assessing Cognitive Capacities and Abilities

Tool	Description	Time	Validity	Reliability	Strengths/Weaknesses
Galveston Orientation and Amnesia Test (GOAT) (Levin, O'Donnell, & Grossman, 1979)	A widely used measure of orientation to person, place, time, and memory for events preceding and following injury. Ten questions with weighted error points deducted from a total of 100 points.	10–15 minutes	Performance on the GOAT strongly related to aspects of the Glasgow Coma Scale (for eye opening, $\chi^2 = 21.09$, $p < 0.00001$; for verbal responding, $\chi^2 = 19.53$, $p < 0.000001$).	Good interrater reliability (Kendall τ coefficient = 0.99, $p < 0.001$)	Well suited to track fluctuations in confusional period after traumatic brain injury	Strength: Brief test that evaluates PTA and RA (see Definition 6-1) Weakness: Designed for use after TBI; may be difficult to use with other populations of rehabilitation patients
Test of Everyday Attention (TEA) (Robertson et al., 1996)	Test of sustained, selective, and divided attention based on eight ecologically plausible subtests such as map and telephone search (selective attention), elevator counting and lottery (sustained attention), and telephone dual task (divided attention).	45–60 minutes	Concurrent validity: moderate to moderately strong correlation between TEA subtests and other measures of attention ($r = 0.42$–0.63). Discriminant validity: statistically significant differences between older healthy controls and older stroke patients on all subtests ($p < 0.001$) and on five of eight subtests with younger paired subjects.	Test–retest reliability (across parallel forms of the test) is strong across subtests of the parallel versions ($r = 0.66$–0.90).		Strengths: Development of TEA was based on investigations for functional-neuroanatomical specialization of attention. Subtests have ecological validity for clients. There are three parallel forms of the TEA to prevent patients from learning the test with repeated administration. Weaknesses: Not appropriate for patients with significant visual problems; rather lengthy assessment of one dimension of cognitive function
Rivermead Behavioral Memory Test (RBMT) (Wilson, Cockburn, & Baddeley, 1985)	Assesses memory skills necessary for everyday life including remembering names, faces, routes, and appointments.	30–45 minutes	Discriminant validity: Wilson et al. (1989) found statistically significant differences between persons with brain injury and healthy controls on all RBMT subtests ($p < 0.001$).	Interrater reliability: 100% agreement when 40 subjects with brain injury were scored separately but simultaneously by two raters (Wilson et al., 1989)		Strengths: Subtests are similar to everyday tasks; useful in the characterization of memory disorders for a wide range of diagnostic groups (Lezak et al., 2004). There are four parallel forms of the RBMT to prevent patients from learning the test with repeated administration. Weakness: Requires intact visual and verbal skills
Contextual Memory Test (Toglia, 1993)	Dynamic assessment of recall, awareness of memory capacity, and memory strategy use, in which client tries to remember 20 objects related to one of two themes (ADL routine or restaurant).	30–40 minutes	Concurrent validity: strongly correlated with the RBMT ($r = 0.80$–0.84).	Reliability for parallel forms of test ($r = 0.73$–0.81). Test–retest reliability for persons with brain injury ($r = 0.85$–0.94)	Not established	Strength: One assessment that provides information about memory and information about metamemory Weakness: Potential for cultural bias–associated pictures (Josman & Hartman-Maeir, 2000)

(continued)

Assessment Table 6-1 | Summary of Assessments of Cognition (*continued*)

Selected Cognitive Screens and Microbatteries

Instrument and Reference	Description	Time to Administer	Validity	Reliability	Sensitivity	Strengths and Weaknesses
Mini-Mental State Examination (MMSE) (Folstein, Folstein, & McHugh, 1975).	Screening tool involving a therapist-administered interview composed of 11 questions related to orientation, attention, learning, calculation, abstraction, information, construction, and delayed recall. Scores of 0–30, with scores of 24 or below suggestive of possible cognitive disorder (Tombaugh & McIntyre, 1992).	5–10 minutes	Concurrent validity: MMSE score is highly correlated with Weschler Adult Intelligence Scale (for verbal IQ, Pearson $r = 0.776$, $p < 0.0001$; for performance IQ, Pearson $r = 0.660$, $p < 0.001$).	24-hour test-retest reliability, Pearson $r = 0.887$. Interrater reliability, Pearson $r = 0.827$	Concerns about sensitivity of MMSE with scores <24 (Kukull et al., 1994). Improved sensitivity when the MMSE (Teng & Chui, 1987) is used in combination with draw a clock (Suhr & Grace, 1999; Watson, Arfken, & Birge, 1993).	Strengths: Widely used and understood by many rehabilitation and medical disciplines; brief screen that is helpful in determining need for more in-depth cognitive assessment (Zwecker et al., 2002) Weaknesses: Bias toward verbal items and, therefore, insensitive to damage in right hemisphere; poor sensitivity to mild cognitive deficits
The Montreal Cognitive Assessment (MoCA) (Nasreddine et al., 2005)	A screening tool developed to measure mild cognitive impairment. The MoCA screens attention and concentration, executive functions, memory, language, visuoconstructional skills, conceptual thinking, calculations, and orientation. The MoCA has been validated on a range of patients, including those with stroke, Parkinson's disease, and dementia (Dalrymple-Alford et al., 2010; Dong et al., 2010; Nasreddine et al., 2005) but can be used on any patient experiencing memory difficulties who scores within the normal ranges on the MMSE (Nasreddine et al., 2005).	10–15 minutes	Excellent concurrent validity among patients with mild Alzheimer's disease ($r = 0.87$) (Nasreddine et al., 2005). Also discriminant validity established on a variety of diagnostic groups with neurological impairments (see Nasreddine, 2013).	Excellent internal consistency ($\alpha = 0.83$); excellent test-retest reliability ($r = 0.92$) (Nasreddine et al., 2005)	Using a cutoff of a raw value of 26 to identify mild cognitive impairment; sensitivity is good (0.97) but specificity is poor (Nasreddine et al., 2003)	Strengths: Highly sensitive to mild cognitive impairment in many populations; user friendly with normative values; best used as a screening tool; found to be more sensitive to cognitive impairment after mild stroke than the MMSE and a better predictor of outcome of acute rehabilitation (Toglia et al., 2011) Weaknesses: May be overly sensitive with current published cutoff values (potentially suggesting impairment where this is none). Therapists should be cautious in determining mild cognitive impairment based only on the MoCA as an evaluation tool.

Loewenstein Occupational Therapy Cognitive Assessment (LOTCA) (Katz et al., 1989)	Microbattery consisting of 20 subtests in four areas: orientation, perception, visuomotor operations, and thinking operations.	30–45 minutes	Discriminant validity: All subtests, except identification of objects, differentiated between patients with craniocerebral injury and healthy controls and stroke patients and healthy controls using Wilcoxon two-sample tests (p < 0.0001).	Katz et al. (1989) observed improved test scores between test scores at admission and after 2 months for TBI and stroke patients.	Strength: Provides a snapshot of a number of cognitive capacities in a relatively short amount of time Weaknesses: Does not pick up subtle cognitive deficiencies on persons with mild injuries; does not include measure of memory
Cognistat (Neurobehavioral Cognitive Status Examination) (Kiernan et al., 1987)	Microbattery comprised of 10 subtests in the areas of orientation*, attention, comprehension*, repetition*, naming*, construction, memory, calculation, similarities, and judgment.	20–25 minutes	Discriminant analysis: Wilcoxon analysis suggested that four of the subtests (see areas marked with asterisks in column to the left) discriminated between elderly persons with stroke and healthy independent elderly (Katz, Elazar, & Itzkovich, 1996); statistically significant differences in mean scores for healthy controls, persons with Alzheimer's type dementia, and neurosurgical patients on 9 of 10 subtests (Katz et al., 1997).	No information	Found to be more sensitive than MMSE with neurosurgical patients (Schwamm et al., 1987) Strengths: Scores as average, mild, moderate, or severe impairment and presented in a profile of performance in each domain; normative data available for healthy elderly persons (Eisenstein et al., 2002). Weaknesses: Some test items (construction subtest) may be too difficult for both stroke patients and healthy elderly persons (Osmon et al., 1992); not appropriate for geriatric or psychiatric patients (Engelhart, Eisenstein, & Meininger, 1994).

Self-Report Measures

Self-reports measures consist of standardized interviews and questionnaires in which the patient rates his or her performance in various aspects of cognitive functioning. Keep in mind that individuals with impaired self-awareness may minimize problems on self-reports. Discrepancies between the patient's self-report and that of significant others may be used as indicators of inaccurate perceptions of competency (O'Keeffe et al., 2007).

Measures of Functional Cognitive Performance

Occupational therapists' education and expertise lend themselves especially well to this aspect of cognitive assessment. There are three themes in the realm of assessing cognitive functional performance: dynamic assessment, informal observations of function, and performance-based assessments.

Dynamic Assessment

Unlike static assessments, which identify and quantify impairment at a specific point in time, dynamic assessment refers to an approach in which the clinician uses cues and feedback to understand how to elicit the patient's best performance (Toglia & Cermak, 2009). Dynamic Interactional Assessment (DIA) (Toglia, 1998) is an example of a dynamic assessment approach. DIA consists of awareness questioning, cueing and task grading, and strategy investigation (Toglia, 1998). Patients predict their performance before beginning the assessment task. Graded verbal cues are offered as needed once the patient begins work, and parameters of the task are changed, if necessary, to buoy the patient's performance. The therapist also asks questions about what strategies or approaches the patient uses. Toglia (1993) incorporated DIA into a number of the standardized assessment tools she developed, including the Contextual Memory Test. In addition to these specific measures, therapists can convert any task (such as organizing the messy cupboard in Fig. 6-3) into a dynamic assessment by deliberately manipulating task and environment variables and offering strategies and cues to determine in what conditions the patient performs at his or her best (Dougherty & Radomski, 1993).

Informal Observation

Informal observation of task performance enables the therapist to make hypotheses about cognitive strengths and weaknesses and identify domains warranting further evaluation. For example, during an ADL or homemaking evaluation, occupational therapists observe attention to task by counting episodes of distraction in a specific

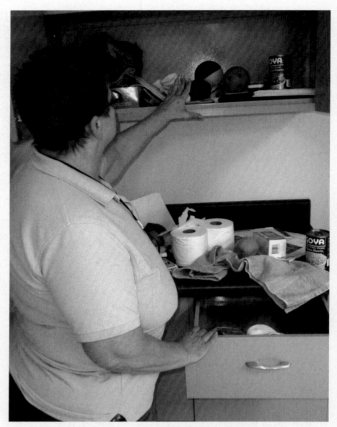

Figure 6-3 Example of informal observation of performance: the patient is asked to organize an array of items in a storage cupboard.

time period or environment, memory for instructions, performance accuracy, and evidence of organization and planning. Of course, informal observations are highly subjective and easily influenced by the clinician's definition of "normal" and his or her acumen in using the observable (behavior) to make inferences about internal cognitive processes. Informal observations may be preferable for patients who cannot understand verbal or written instructions, as with communication deficits or speaking another language.

Performance-Based Assessment

In general, performance-based assessment involves patient performance of a task (or tasks) that simulate an everyday activity, "under the observation of the examiner, who utilizes behaviorally based measures to quantify different aspects of functional capacity" (Loewenstein & Acevedo, 2010, p. 98). Many disciplines and fields (e.g., occupational therapy, educational psychology, and neuropsychology) use this approach to characterize what a person does under standardized, directed conditions (Moore et al., 2007). Performance-based assessments vary widely in their structure, complexity, and assessment objectives as exemplified by standardized functional assessments and measures of executive functioning.

Standardized Functional Assessment. Whereas informal observations yield hypotheses that inform continued evaluation and intervention, standardized, semistructured functional assessments provide information about what a patient can or cannot do in ADL or instrumental activities of daily living (IADL). As exemplified by the Arnadottir OT-ADL Neurobehavioral Evaluation (A-ONE) (Arnadottir, 1990), this approach allows the therapist to examine cognition in the context of functional tasks.

The A-ONE evaluates performance of ADL and examines the effect of neurobehavioral dysfunction on task performance. There are two parts to the instrument; part 2 is considered optional. During part 1, the occupational therapist observes the patient performing dressing, hygiene, transfer and mobility, feeding, and communication tasks and completes the Functional Independence Scale by assigning a numerical score (0–4) for each aspect of the various tasks. For example, a score is assigned to each of the activities of dressing (donning shirt, pants, socks, and shoes; fastening clothing). While observing the patient's performance of each component, the therapist also rates the patient in terms of presence of neurobehavioral impairments, again using a 0–4 scale. For example, the patient is scored on each of the following possible neurobehavioral impairments specified for the task of dressing: motor apraxia, ideational apraxia, unilateral body neglect, somatoagnosia, spatial relations, unilateral spatial neglect, abnormal tone, perseveration, and organization and sequencing. The scores on the Functional Independence Scale and Neurobehavioral Scale are not additive but used to establish patterns of performance and impairment. Occupational therapists may use the results of part 1 to localize cerebral dysfunction based on functional performance (part 2). Part 1 of the A-ONE, which takes approximately 25 minutes to administer, was standardized on patients with cortical central nervous system dysfunction. Its author recommends that therapists attend a training seminar before using the tool (Arnadottir, 1990).

Performance-Based Measures of Executive Functioning. Deficits in executive abilities can be difficult to assess in clinical environments (Baum et al., 2008). Formal, standardized measures of specific cognitive domains and function often fail to detect existing deficiencies in executive abilities and complex task performance (Tranel, Hathaway-Nepple, & Anderson, 2007). This is because the inherent structures of these assessments typically do not adequately challenge executive processes, commonly resulting in a false negative in the detection of executive impairments. To identify executive impairments,

Lezak (1995) suggested that clinicians ask "how" or "whether" patients perform complex tasks. Inefficiencies during task performance are common hallmarks among individuals with executive deficits (Levine et al., 2011). The valid assessment of executive abilities depends on adequate task complexity, novelty, and challenge (Alderman et al., 2003).

Performance-based assessments are designed to incorporate the cognitive complexity that people typically encounter in IADL, work, school, and community life. Performance-based assessments typically require the patient to problem solve, manage distractions, and incorporate some degree of multitasking—all elements of executive abilities. We describe two performance-based assessments as examples: the Executive Function Performance Test (EFPT) (Baum et al., 2008) and the Multiple Errands Test (MET) (Alderman et al., 2003; Shallice & Burgess, 1991).

The EFPT was developed by Baum et al. (2008) to measure individuals' functional abilities through the performance of four test tasks identified as supportive of independent everyday living: preparing a light meal, managing medications, using the telephone, and paying bills. The EFPT examines three primary executive abilities—task initiation, task execution, and task completion—and measures the level of therapist assistance required to support patients during each task performance. Examiners use a 0–5 ordinal scoring system based on the level of cue they provide. For example, the level of cue advances after two cues of each type have been administered. Advancement in cues is reflected through a scoring paradigm where a score of 0 equals complete independence, 1 equals verbal guidance, 2 equals gestural guidance, 3 equals direct verbal instruction, 4 equals physical assistance, and 5 equals total assistance from the therapist. The EFPT has a detailed administration manual that includes details of test setup, the examiner's script, and specific criteria for timing, circumstances of cue provision. On average, the test for the EFPT takes 30 minutes and can be reliably administered once therapists have studied the test manual. However, novice therapists should practice administering the EFPT on nonpatients with special attention to the cueing system. Following test completion, test scores result in executive function component scores ranging from 0 to 20; task scores ranging from 0 to 25, and the overall total score ranging from 0 to 100 with 0 equaling a perfect performance on all functional tasks. The EFPT is one of few performance-based measures with psychometric rigor (Baum et al., 2008; Cederfeldt et al., 2011). This tool has been used with multiple patient populations with several ongoing studies investigating the validity of separating EFPT tasks to shorten test time.

The MET was created to capture the everyday performance failures reported by patients with high-level executive dysfunction (Shallice & Burgess, 1991). The MET is a naturalistic measure of executive performance designed to present ongoing and dynamic challenges throughout test performance. Patients are presented with a list of 12 everyday tasks and 9 rules. Test initiation and task execution is left to the participant without interference or cueing from the examiner. The MET is site specific, which means the test tasks are dependent on the test location. To date, a standardized manual with scoring system that is site neutral does not exist. The MET does not have an easily replicated scoring system, which creates significant challenge to clinicians attempting to administer the test in clinical settings. Questions about the clinical utility of the MET remain as this test is extremely challenging for patients with TBI and requires significant skill and time to administer. Since the first publication, alternative versions of the MET have been published in effort to simplify the administration and to meet site-specific needs (Alderman et al., 2003; Dawson et al., 2009; Knight, Alderman, & Burgess, 2002; Morrison et al., 2005; Rand et al., 2009).

Measures of Specific Cognitive Domains and Processes

While performance-based assessments are designed to have relevance to performance in real-world contexts (Connor & Maier, 2011), tools and methods that assess specific cognitive capacities and abilities are generally composed of desktop activities with standardized administration and scoring procedures. Cognitive screens and microbatteries allow the clinician to assess a number of cognitive domains using a single tool. A cognitive screen takes less than 15 minutes to administer and provides the clinician with a general sense of a patient's cognitive status but little information about what specific areas may be impaired. A microbattery may take up to 45 minutes to administer and consists of a number of subtests, typically associated with an array of cognitive capacities and abilities. Many instruments have demonstrated reliability and validity and standardized scoring criteria that greatly reduce therapist bias.

INTERPRETING RESULTS OF PERFORMANCE ON COGNITIVE ASSESSMENT

An individual's cognitive performance at any point in time is determined by many interacting variables, including neurobiological, affective, cultural, task, and environmental influences. Changes in any of these domains improve or detract from a person's cognitive status and thereby his or her occupational functioning. Therefore, to effectively assess cognition and interpret findings, occupational therapists must appreciate how variables can affect performance during cognitive assessment. What follows is a brief summary of each influence, supported with specific examples from the literature.

Neurobiological Influence on Cognition

Throughout this chapter, we have alluded to the neurobiological influence on cognition; that is, the ways in which changes to the anatomy and physiology of the brain impact cognition. Persons with stroke have local damage to brain tissue that often results in predictable and specific cognitive deficits, such as frontal lobe damage leading to executive dysfunction and temporal lobe damage affecting memory. Neurobiological changes that accompany aging also seem to affect thinking abilities and memory. Crystallized intelligence (well practiced, overlearned skills and knowledge) is reportedly maintained or strengthened into the eighth decade of life, whereas fluid intelligence, which entails reasoning and problem solving for unfamiliar challenges, begins a slow decline in the sixth decade of life (Lezak, 1995). Normal age-related cognitive changes underscore the importance of using age-normed cognitive assessments whenever possible.

Changes or deterioration of other functions of the human body have secondary neurobiological influences on cognition. For example, visual-perceptual impairments alter the inputs into the memory process, limiting what a person can accurately remember. Diminished visual acuity in and of itself is associated with significantly reduced performance on neuropsychological evaluations (Hunt & Bassi, 2010). Dehydration and anemia may also negatively impact cognition (Denny, Kuchibhatla, & Cohen, 2006; Lieberman, 2007), as do some medications. Researchers suggest a link between adjuvant chemotherapy for operative primary breast cancer and cognition (Schilling et al., 2005).

Affective Influences on Cognition

A person's emotional state has a pervasive influence on cognition (Chepenik, Cornew, & Farah, 2007). For example, anxious people differ from others in several aspects of attentional functioning. Anxious people are more likely to attend to threat-related stimuli and use limited-capacity working memory for worry, self-concern, and other task-irrelevant distractions (Beaudreau & O'Hara, 2009). Persons with depression also frequently complain about poor memory but often do not demonstrate memory deficits on neuropsychological testing (Lezak, 1995). Depressed individuals are thought to show passive disengagement with the environment in that their attentional focus is on internal concerns rather than environmental events (Eysenck & Keane, 1990). Depressed people also demonstrate a negative recall bias (a tendency to recall more negative information about themselves than others do) (Baddeley, 1990). Memory problems associated with depression seem to have a secondary effect on executive processes, possibly because of distractions by dysfunctional negative thoughts that occupy limited-capacity working memory during problem solving and task performance (Channon & Green, 1999). As discussed in Chapter 3, patients who are anxious or depressed must be referred to specialized psychological or medical services.

Transient mental distractions can also impair cognition. Pain and fatigue (especially mental fatigue) are thought to be irrelevant inputs that interfere with memory trace formation and diminish the function of limited-capacity working memory by occupying attention that is therefore unavailable to incoming data (Denburg, Carbotte, & Denburg, 1997; Dick & Rashiq, 2007; Seminowicz & Davis, 2007). Therefore, clients who are tired or in pain may be unable to demonstrate their cognitive capabilities during assessment (Bryant, Chiaravalloti, & DeLuca, 2004). Under such circumstances, the occupational therapist may defer cognitive assessment to another time or, at a minimum, consider the influence of these factors when interpreting the assessment results.

Sociocultural Influences on Cognition

Experts suggest that basic processes of perception and cognition are influenced by cultural and social factors, such as education. Nisbett and Masuda (2003) summarized a series of studies that illustrate information-processing differences in East Asian and Western cultures. They suggested that Americans tended to focus their attention on objects and object attributes, but Japanese subjects tended to focus on the field, background, relationship, or context of the objects. Culture may also influence displays of self-awareness. Prigatano, Ogano, and Amakusa (1997) suggested that, because incompetence in personal care is a sign of disgrace in Japan, Japanese patients with TBI tended to overestimate their abilities in this realm. On the other hand, Japanese people generally believe it is impolite to report high estimations of social and interpersonal skills. Therefore, Japanese patients with TBI tended to underestimate their abilities in this realm. Beyond cultural background, performance on cognitive tests appears to be shaped by years of education. In a study involving a random sample of age stratified healthy older adults, younger age and higher education were associated with better performance on cognitive testing (Ganguli et al., 2010). This suggests a possible education-related bias in cognitive assessments: persons with higher education may score within normal limits on cognitive tests even with decrements in their functioning and/or persons with lower education who perform poorly on cognitive assessments may, in fact, be cognitively intact.

Task and Environment as Contextual Mediators of Cognition

People bring their neurobiological, emotional, and sociocultural predispositions to all information processing, but performance at a given moment is mediated by characteristics of the task and environmental contexts. Here is an example of task-cognition interplay. When a task is familiar, the thinker requires relatively little attention to recognize a problem type and determine a hypothesis and plan of action (Mayer, 1992). A familiar task or problem prompts the individual to retrieve a large number of interconnected units of knowledge, both related facts and previous solutions (Mayer, 1992). This suggests that patients who are expert cooks may outperform those who rarely cook on functional cognitive assessments that involve meal preparation. The environment similarly affects cognition. Contextual cues in the environment enhance recall of similar tasks or previously effective techniques or solutions. The stimulus-arousal properties of the environment also influence cognitive function. Lighting and noise can focus attention or, as is often the case for persons with brain injury, provide distractions that derail thinking.

In summary, cognition consists of specific but interrelated capacities and abilities that are influenced by neurobiological, affective, sociocultural variables, and task and environmental contexts. This discussion, although not exhaustive, highlights the complexity, if not the mystery, of cognitive function, which is an appreciation necessary for assessing cognitive capacities and abilities in occupational therapy. This discussion also evidences the importance of knowing something about the patient (i.e., diagnosis, education and cultural background, psychological and medical status, literacy, and communication abilities) before assessing his or her cognitive status. In judging the cognitive status of another person, teasing out performance confounders is as important as selecting and correctly administering the assessment tool. Whereas assigning and summing scores on standardized instruments requires the attentiveness of a trained technician, observing and interpreting performance during assessment requires the insight of a professional.

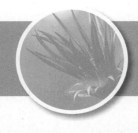

case example
D.B.: Assessing Cognitive Function

Occupational Therapy Assessment Process	Clinical Reasoning Process	
	Objectives	**Examples of Therapist's Internal Dialogue**

Patient Information

D.B. is a 26-year-old single male who sustained a TBI as a result of a pedestrian–auto accident. Upon admission to the emergency department, he had a Glasgow Coma Scale score of 6, and records indicate that he was in a coma for approximately 10 days. In addition to the brain injury, D.B. sustained fractures in both legs, a tibia-fibula fracture on the right and fracture of the femur on the left. D.B. participated in inpatient rehabilitation for 3 weeks. D.B. graduated from college with a degree in law enforcement and worked in a rural community as a police officer at the time of his injury. His former girlfriend broke off the relationship approximately 1 month ago. Unable to return to his own apartment because of concerns about safety, D.B. was discharged from the inpatient rehabilitation unit to his brother's home.

At approximately 3 months post-TBI, D.B. was referred to outpatient occupational therapy to assess readiness for independent living. The occupational therapist focuses the assessment on D.B.'s ability to assume self-maintenance roles and identification of cognitive deficits interfering with role and task performance.

	Objectives	Examples of Therapist's Internal Dialogue
	Understand the patient's diagnosis or condition	"D.B. had a severe brain injury and will likely have significant, long-term cognitive impairments. He sounds like someone who is used to being active, and mobility restrictions may be confusing and frustrating. I wonder how he is getting around now that he is 3 months post-injury."
	Know the person	"I know that I have certain stereotyped expectations of cops. I expect him to be sort of rigid and reluctant to take instructions from women. I wonder if D.B.'s girlfriend could not handle the changes related to the TBI or if there were long-standing issues that led to the recent breakup. Either way, D.B. must feel sad and isolated."
	Appreciate the context	"I wonder what transpired during the past 2 months at the brother's home. How much of a role is the brother willing to play in this transition?"
	Develop provisional hypotheses	"Given his diagnosis and history, I presume that D.B.'s cognitive impairments are the biggest barriers to independent living."

Assessment Process

The therapist selected the following evaluation tools: Canadian Occupational Performance Measure (COPM) to obtain information about the client's perceived problems and priorities, Executive Function Performance Test (EFPT) to evaluate D.B.'s executive functioning, Cognistat to obtain a general picture of cognitive capabilities, and systematic observation of the client's response to the presentation of homework.

| | Consider evaluation approach and methods | "Because he has not been assessed in occupational therapy for over 2 months and he has not had a neuropsychological evaluation, I want to get a full picture of his occupational functioning. The COPM will tell me about his priorities and give me a snapshot of his awareness of deficits. The EFPT will provide me with information about his ability to safely perform tasks at home. With this test, I can observe his ability to begin and complete activities of daily living. I will gain insight into his ability to sequence and problem solve through task steps, which will help identify the level of support he needs to live independently. Cognistat will give me a sense of his cognitive strengths and weaknesses and be useful in benchmarking cognitive change. His response to homework will help me observe his use of compensatory cognitive strategies." |

Assessment Results

COPM: D.B. indicated that his ability to function independently was limited because of lower extremity fractures. He was dissatisfied with his inability to drive, the slowness with which he donned lower extremity clothing, his low stamina when walking outside the home, and lack of avocational outlets because of mobility limitations. When queried about known dependence on family members to take medications and his lack of initiation of self-maintenance tasks, D.B. quickly dismissed these reports as awkwardness associated with being a guest in their home.

EFPT: When the therapist administered the EFPT, she noted D.B. answered all pretest questions as if he experienced no difficulties living independently, which conflicted with the information provided by his brother. When the therapist observed D.B.'s performance, she noted he experienced no difficulty with the hand-washing task, which indicated he would be able to perform the rest of the EFPT tasks. D.B. had the following scores for the rest of the EFPT tasks:

1 = hand washing
0 = telephone use
3 = taking medication
5 = paying bills

Cognistat: D.B.'s cognitive status profile indicated the following: performance within the average range for orientation, comprehension, naming, construction; and mild impairment in similarities, judgment, calculations, repetition; mild to moderate impairment in attention and memory.

  Informal observation: During each of his two outpatient evaluation sessions, the therapist gave D.B. oral instructions specific to three homework assignments to complete at home, all of which he agreed to do but did not make note of. He completed none of them. He seemed motivated throughout the assessment and did not appear distracted by pain or emotional distress during his sessions.

Occupational Therapy Problem List

1. Decreased initiation of ADL and IADL
2. Decreased productivity because of poor stamina and limited repertoire of appropriate avocational outlets
3. Memory inefficiency and inadequate repertoire of memory compensation strategies
4. Decreased awareness of cognitive deficits interfering with compensatory strategy use

Interpret observations

Synthesize results

"D.B. seems to be quite aware of concrete changes in his mobility but less aware of possible cognitive changes related to initiation and memory of medications. I wonder how much family members are helping to prevent any errors in daily life that might otherwise give him feedback about his cognitive changes."

"Based on D.B.'s performance on the EFPT tasks, I am concerned he is having difficulty performing tasks on his own because he is having problems with higher order thinking abilities, like problem solving and working memory. I noticed he had to be cued to remember to turn off the stove after cooking. He also needed specific verbal direction in figuring out when to take the medications. He could not do the mathematics required for bill paying and did not catch the balance difference in the available money and bill sums. If he has problems like this on the EFPT, it is likely he is going to have problems living alone and functioning independently without support."

"D.B.'s performance on the Cognistat does not surprise me all that much given the severity of his TBI. He seems to have a number of cognitive strengths that I think will really help him participate in the therapy process."

"I'm guessing that D.B. has not had to take responsibility for keeping track of information in recent months; no doubt his brother has done that for him. I bet D.B. has not had much experience with his memory changes and does not appreciate that he needs to compensate for these changes. He seems to be a really good candidate for outpatient rehabilitation at this point."

"Overall, D.B. seems to have rather superficial awareness of his limitations; he acknowledges physical but not cognitive changes. His brother's report of D.B.'s need for supervision with medications and prompts for ADL and IADL seem consistent with what I saw on his performance of the EFPT. I will want to incorporate opportunities for dynamic assessment into the treatment plan. I need to talk a little more with D.B.'s brother about the role he would like to play in the therapy program. Maybe he needs a break and wants the team to take a more dominant role for a while."

 Clinical Reasoning in Occupational Therapy Practice

Effects of Environment on Cognitive Function

During his inpatient rehabilitation, D.B. was observed to have decreased attentional capacities, especially with complex tasks. How might this problem be evident during the occupational therapy homemaking assessment? What factors in the environment might exaggerate these problems? What factors might minimize them?

Summary Review Questions

1. Analyze bill paying and grocery shopping in terms of the specific cognitive capacities and abilities required.
2. Compare the advantages and disadvantages of the three approaches to cognitive assessment described in this chapter.
3. Describe each variable that influences a person's ability to think. How would you expect these variables to affect cognitive assessment of an elderly illiterate client? How would you expect these variables to affect cognitive assessment of a college student?
4. Explain the occupational therapist's contribution to the rehabilitation team in the realm of cognitive assessment. Specifically, outline the ways in which occupational therapy complements the assessments of other professionals and the unique elements of occupational therapy.

Glossary

Attention—The ability to deploy limited mental resources for purposes of concentration. Human activities have various attentional demands, including sustained attention (length of time), selective attention (competing stimuli), divided attention (multiple simultaneous stimuli), and alternating attention (shifts back and forth between various stimuli).

Cognition—The general term that reflects the mental enterprises related to absorbing information, thinking, and goal-directed action.

Dual-task performance—Conditions in which performance of a single task is compared to performance of the single task performed simultaneously with a secondary task. *Dual-task cost* refers to the decrement in performance of a relatively simple primary task when a secondary (cognitive) task is added (McCulloch, 2007).

Executive function—Metaprocesses that enable a person to initiate, plan, self-monitor, and correct his or her approach to goal-directed tasks. Executive disorders often result from frontal lobe damage and are evidenced by problems with self-control, self-direction, and organization (Lezak, 1995).

Memory—The result of interactive cognitive systems that receive, code, store, and retrieve information.

Neuropsychological evaluation—A long battery of standardized tests for purposes of diagnosis, patient care and planning, rehabilitation evaluation, and research (Lezak, 1995). Typically, the examiner is a doctor of psychology with specialized training in cognitive processes and brain–behavior relationships.

Orientation—Awareness of self in relation to person, place, time, and circumstance (Sohlberg & Mateer, 1989).

Self-awareness—The capacity to objectively perceive the self (Prigatano & Schacter, 1991) and (with a reasonable degree of accuracy) to compare that conception to a premorbid standard.

References

Alderman, N., Burgess, P. W., Knight, C., & Henman, C. (2003). Ecological validity of a simplified version of the multiple errands shopping test. *Journal of the International Neuropsychological Society, 9,* 31–44.

Alexander, G. E., Delong, M. R., & Strick, P. L. (1986). Parallel organization of functionally segregated circuits linking basal ganglia and cortex. *Annual Review of Neuroscience, 9,* 357–381.

Anderson, S. W., & Tranel, D. (1989). Awareness of disease states following cerebral infarction, dementia, head trauma: A standardized assessment. *Clinical Neuropsychologist, 3,* 327–339.

Arnadottir, A. (1990). *The brain and behavior: Assessing cortical dysfunction through activities of daily living.* St. Louis: Mosby.

Atkinson, R. C., & Shiffrin, R. M. (1971). The control of short-term memory. *Scientific American, 225,* 82–90.

Baddeley, A. (1990). *Human memory: Theory and practice.* Boston: Allyn & Bacon.

Baum, C. M., Connor, L. T., Morrison, T., Hahn, M., Dromerick, A. W., & Edwards, D. F. (2008). Reliability, validity, and clinical utility of the Executive Function Performance Test: A measure of executive function in a sample of people with stroke. *American Journal of Occupational Therapy, 62,* 446–455.

Baum, C. M., & Katz, N. (2010). Occupational therapy approach to assessing the relationship between cognition and function. In T. D. Marcotte & I. Grant (Eds.), *Neuropsychology of everyday functioning* (pp. 62–90). New York: The Guilford Press.

Baum, C. M., Morrison, T., Hahn, M., & Edwards, D. F. (2003). *Test manual: Executive Function Performance Test.* St. Louis: Washington University.

Beaudreau, S. A., & O'Hara, R. (2009). The association of anxiety and depressive symptoms with cognitive performance in community-dwelling older adults. *Psychology and Aging, 24,* 507–512.

Bogod, N. M., Mateer, C. A., & MacDonald, S. W. S. (2003). Self-awareness after traumatic brain injury: A comparison of measures and their relationship to executive functions. *Journal of the International Neuropsychological Society, 9,* 450–458.

Boykoff, N., Moieni, M., & Subramanian, S. K. (2009). Confronting chemobrain: An in-depth look at survivors' reports of impact on work, social networks, and health care response. *Journal of Cancer Survivorship, 3,* 223–232.

Bryant, D., Chiaravalloti, N. D., & DeLuca, J. (2004). Objective measurement of cognitive fatigue in multiple sclerosis. *Rehabilitation Psychology, 49,* 114–122.

Caviness, J. N., Driver-Dunckley, E., Connor, D. J., Sabbagh, M. N., Hentz, J. G., Noble, B., Evidente V. G., Shill H. A., Adler C. H. (2007). Defining mild cognitive impairment in Parkinson's disease. *Movement Disorders, 22,* 1272–1277.

Cederfeldt, M., Widell, Y., Andersson, E. E., Dahlin-Ivanoff, S., & Gosman-Hedström, G. (2011). Concurrent validity of the Executive Function Performance Test in people with mild stroke. *British Journal of Occupational Therapy, 74,* 443–449.

Channon, S., & Green, P. S. (1999). Executive function in depression: The role of performance strategies in aiding depressed and non-depressed participants. *Journal Neurology Neurosurgery & Psychiatry, 66,* 162–171.

Chepenik, L. G., Cornew, L. A., & Farah, M. J. (2007). The influence of sad mood on cognition. *Emotion, 7,* 802–811.

Connor, L. T., & Maier, A. (2011). Putting executive performance in a theoretical context. *OTJR: Occupation, Participation and Health, 31,* S3–S7.

Cowan, N. (2008). What are the differences between long-term, short-term, and working memory? *Progress in Brain Research, 169,* 323–338.

Crosson, B., Barco, P. P., Velozo, C. A., Bolesta, M. M., Cooper, P. V., Werts, D., & Brobeck, T. C. (1989). Awareness and compensation in postacute head injury rehabilitation. *Journal of Head Trauma Rehabilitation, 4,* 46–54.

Dalrymple-Alford, J. C., MacAskill, M. R., Nakas, C. T., Livingston, L., Graham, C., Crucian, G. P., Melzer, T. R., Kirwan, J., Keenan, R., Wells, S., Porter, R. J., Watts, R., Anderson, T. J. (2010). The MoCA: Well-suited screen for cognitive impairment in Parkinson disease. *Neurology, 75,* 1717–1725.

Dawson, D. R., Anderson, N. D., Burgess, P. Cooper, E., Krpan, K. M., & Stuss, D. T. (2009). Further development of the Multiple Errands Test: Standardized scoring, reliability, and ecological validity for the Baycrest version. *Archives of Physical Medicine & Rehabilitation, 90,* S41–S51.

Denburg, S. D., Carbotte, R. M., & Denburg, J. A. (1997). Cognition and mood in systemic lupus erythematosus. *Annals of the New York Academy of Sciences, 823,* 44–59.

Denny, S. D., Kuchibhatla, M. N., & Cohen, H. J. (2006). Impact of anemia on mortality, cognition, and function in community-dwelling elderly. *The American Journal of Medicine, 119,* 327–334.

Dick, B. D., & Rashiq, S. (2007). Disruption of attention and working memory traces in individuals with chronic pain. *Anesthesia & Analgesia, 104,* 1223–1229.

Diehl, M., Marsieke, M., Horgas, A. L., Rosenberg, A., Saczynski, J. S., & Willis, S. L. (2005). The Revised Observed Tasks of Daily Living: A performance-based assessment of everyday problem solving in older adults. *Journal of Applied Gerontology, 24,* 211–230.

Dong, Y. H., Sharma, V. K., Chan, B. P. L., Venketasubramanian, N., Teoh, H. L., Seet, R. C. S., Tanicala, S., Chan, Y. H., & Chen, C. (2010). The Montreal Cognitive Assessment (MoCA) is superior to the Mini-Mental State Examination (MMSE) for the detection of vascular cognitive impairment after acute stroke. *Journal of Neurological Sciences, 299,* 15–18.

Dougherty, P. M., & Radomski, M. V. (1993). *The cognitive rehabilitation workbook.* Gaithersburg, MD: Aspen.

Dubuc, B (nd). Brain and mind: Memory and the brain. Retrieved May 24, 2013. http://thebrain.mcgill.ca/flash/d/d_07/d_07_p/d_07_p_tra/d_07_p_tra.html

Edwards, D. F., Hahn, M., Baum, C., & Dromerick, A. W. (2006). The impact of mild stroke on meaningful activity and life satisfaction. *Journal of Stroke and Cerebrovascular Diseases, 15,* 151–157.

Eisenstein, N., Engelhart, C. I., Johnson, V., Wolf, J., Williamsom, J., & Losonczy, M. B. (2002). Normative data for healthy elderly persons with the Neurobehavioral Cognitive Status Exam (Cognistat). *Applied Neuropsychology, 9,* 110–113.

Engelhart, C., Eisenstein, N., & Meininger, J. (1994). Psychometric properties of the Neurobehavioral Cognitive Status Exam. *The Clinical Neuropsychologist, 8,* 405–415.

Erikson, A., Karlsson, G., Borell, L., & Tham, K. (2007). The lived experience of memory impairment in daily occupation after acquired brain injury. *OTJR: Occupation, Participation and Health, 27,* 84–94.

Eysenck, M. W., & Keane, M. T. (1990). *Cognitive psychology: A student's handbook.* London: Lawrence Erlbaum.

Fernandez-Duque, D., Baird, J. A., & Posner, M. I. (2000). Executive attention and metacognitive regulation. *Consciousness and Cognition, 9,* 288–307.

Fish, J., Wilson, B. A., & Manly, T. (2010). The assessment and rehabilitation of prospective memory problems in people with neurological disorders: A review. *Neuropsychological Rehabilitation, 20,* 161–179.

Flavell, J. (1979). Metacognition and cognitive monitoring: A new area of cognitive-developmental enquiry. *American Psychologist, 34,* 906–911.

Fleming, J. M., Strong, J., & Ashton, R. (1996). Self-awareness of deficits in adults with traumatic brain injury: How best to measure? *Brain Injury, 10,* 1–15.

Folstein, M. F., Folstein, S. E., & McHugh, P. R. (1975). "Mini-Mental State": A practical method for grading cognitive state of patients for the clinician. *Journal of Psychiatric Research, 12,* 189–198.

Ganguli, M., Snitz, B. E., Lee, C. W., Vanderbilt, J., Saxton, J. A., & Chang, C. C. (2010). Age and education effects and norms on a cognitive test battery from a population-based cohort: The Monongahela-Youghiogheny Healthy Aging Team. *Aging & Mental Health, 14,* 100–107.

Garlinghouse, M. A., Roth, R. M., Isquith, P. K., Flashman, L. A., & Saykin, A. J. (2010). Subjective rating of working memory is associated with frontal lobe volume in schizophrenia. *Schizophrenia Research, 120,* 71–75.

Gillen, G. (2009). *Cognitive and perceptual rehabilitation: Optimizing function.* St. Louis: Mosby.

Glover, J. A., Ronning, R. R., & Bruning, R. H. (1990). *Cognitive psychology for teachers.* New York: Macmillan.

Goldman, J. G., & Litvan, I. (2011). Mild cognitive impairment in Parkinson's Disease. *Minerva Medica, 102,* 441–459.

Goverover, Y. (2004). Categorization, deductive reasoning, and self-awareness: Association with everyday competence in persons with acute brain injury. *Journal of Clinical and Experimental Neuropsychology, 26,* 737–749.

Goverover, Y., & Hinojosa, J. (2002). Categorization and deductive reasoning: Predictors of instrumental activities of daily living performance in adults with brain injury. *American Journal of Occupational Therapy, 55,* 509–516.

Goverover, Y., & Josman, N. (2004). Everyday problem solving among four groups of individuals with cognitive impairments: Examination of the discriminant validity of the Observed Tasks of Daily Living-Revised. *Occupational Therapy Journal of Research, 24,* 103–112.

Groeger, J. A., Lo, J. C., Burns, C. G., & Dijk, D. J. (2011). Effects of sleep inertia after daytime naps vary with executive load and time of day. *Behavioral Neuroscience, 125,* 252–260.

Heaton, R. K., Marcotte, T. D., Rivera Mindt, M., Sadek, J., Moore, D. J., Bentley, H., McCutchan, J. A., Reicks, C., Grant, I. & The HNRC Group (2004). The impact of HIV-associated neuropsychological impairment on everyday functioning. *Journal of the International Neuropsychological Society, 10,* 317–331.

Helmstaedter, C., Kurthen, M., Lux, S., Reuber, M., & Elger, C. E. (2003). Chronic epilepsy and cognition: A longitudinal study in temporal lobe epilepsy. *Annals of Neurology, 54,* 425–432.

Hunt, L. A., & Bassi, C. J. (2010). Near-vision acuity levels and performance on neuropsychological assessments used in occupational therapy. *American Journal Occupational Therapy, 64,* 105–113.

James, W. (1890). *The Principles of Psychology (Vol. 1).* New York: Henry Holt.

Josman, N., & Hartman-Maeir, A. (2000). Cross-cultural assessment of the Contextual Memory Test. *Occupational Therapy International, 7,* 246–258.

Katz, N. (2011). *Cognition, Occupation, and Participation Across the Life Span* (3rd ed.). Bethesda, MD: American Occupational Therapy Association.

Katz, N., Elazar, B., & Itzkovich, M. (1996). Validity of the Neurobehavioral Cognitive Status Examination (COGNISTAT) in assessing patients post CVA and healthy elderly in Israel. *Israel Journal of Occupational Therapy, 5,* E185–E198.

Katz, N., Hartman-Maeir, A., Weiss, P., & Armon, N. (1997). Comparison of cognitive status profiles of healthy elderly persons with dementia and neurosurgical patients using the Neurobehavioral Cognitive Status Examination. *NeuroRehabilitation, 9,* 179–186.

Katz, N., Itzkovich, M., Averbuch, S., & Elazar, B. (1989). Loewenstein Occupational Therapy Cognitive Assessment (LOTCA) battery for brain-injured patients: Reliability and validity. *American Journal of Occupational Therapy, 43,* 184–192.

Kiernan, R. J., Mueller, J., Langston, J. W., & Van Dyke, C. (1987). The Neurobehavioral Cognitive Status Examination: A brief but differentiated approach to cognitive assessment. *Annals of Internal Medicine, 107,* 481–485.

Knight, C., Alderman, N., & Burgess, P. W. (2002). Development of a simplified version of the Multiple Errands Test for use in hospital settings. *Neuropsychological Rehabilitation, 12,* 231–255.

Kukull, W. A., Larson, E. B., Teri, L., Bowen, J., McCormick, W., & Pfanschmidt, M. L. (1994). The Mini-Mental State Examination Score and the clinical diagnosis of dementia. *Journal of Clinical Epidemiology, 47,* 1061–1067.

Levin, H. S., O'Donnell, V. M., & Grossman, R. G. (1979). The Galveston Orientation and Amnesia Test. *Journal of Nervous and Mental Disease, 167,* 675–684.

Levine, B., Schweizer, T. A., O'Connor, C., Turner, G., Gillingham, S., Stuss, D. T., Manly, T., & Robertson, I. H. (2011). Rehabilitation of executive functioning in patients with frontal lobe brain damage with goal management training. *Frontiers in Human Neuroscience, 5,* 9.

Levy, L. L. (2011). Cognitive information processing. In N. Katz (Ed.), *Cognition, occupation, and participation across the life span* (3rd ed., pp. 93–115). Bethesda, MD: American Occupational Therapy Association.

Lezak, M. D. (1995). *Neuropsychological assessment* (3rd ed.). New York: Oxford University.

Lezak, M. D., Howieson, D. B., Loring, D. W., Hannay, H. J., & Fischer, J. S. (2004). *Neuropsychological assessment* (4th ed.). New York: Oxford University Press.

Lieberman, H. R. (2007). Hydration and cognition: A critical review and recommendations for future research. *Journal of the American College of Nutrition, 26,* 5555–5615.

Loewenstein, D., & Acevedo, A. (2010). The relationship between instrumental activities of daily living and neuropsychological performance. In T. D. Marcotte & I. Grant (Eds.), *Neuropsychology of Everyday Living* (pp. 93–112). New York: The Guildford Press.

Lysaker, P. H., Buck, K. D., Carcione, A., Proccacci, M., Giampaolo, S., Guiseppe, N., & Dimaggio, G. (2011). Addressing metacognitive capacity for self reflection in the psychotherapy for schizophrenia: A conceptual model of the key tasks and processes, *Psychology and Psychotherapy: Theory, Research and Practice, 84,* 58–59.

Macciocchi, S., Seel, R. T., Thompson, N., Byams, R., & Bowman, B. (2008). Spinal cord injury and co-occurring traumatic brain injury: Assessment and incidence. *Archives of Physical Medicine and Rehabilitation, 89,* 1350–1357.

Mayer, R. E. (1992). *Thinking, problem solving, cognition.* New York: Freeman.

Mazaux, J. M., Masson, F., Levin, H. S., Alaoui, P., Maurette, P., & Barat, M. (1997). Long-term neuropsychological outcome and loss of social autonomy after traumatic brain injury. *Archives of Physical Medicine and Rehabilitation, 78,* 1316–1320.

McCulloch, K. (2007). Attention and dual-task conditions: Physical therapy implications for individuals with acquired brain injury. *Journal of Neurologic Physical Therapy, 31,* 104–118.

McDowell, S., Whyte, J., & D'Esposito, M. (1997). Working memory impairments in traumatic brain injury: Evidence from a dual-task paradigm. *Neuropsychologia, 35,* 1341–1353.

McLaurin, E. Y., Holliday, S. L., Williams, P., & Brey, R. L. (2005). Predictors of cognitive dysfunction in patients with systemic lupus erythematosus. *Neurology, 64,* 297–303.

Miller, G. A. (1956). The magical number seven, plus or minus two: Some limits on our capacity for processing information. *Psychological Review, 63,* 81–97.

Moore, D. J., Palmer, B. W., Patterson, T. L., & Jeste, D. V. (2007). A review of performance-based measures of functional living skills. *Journal of Psychiatric Research, 41,* 97–118.

Morrison M. T., Ryan, J., Wolf, T., Savre, J., Dromerick, A., Hollingsworth, H., Connor, L., White, D., Baum, D., Polatajko, H., & Edwards, D. (2005). Assessment of executive dysfunction in individuals with mild stroke: The Multiple Errands Test–Revised. Paper presented at the Mild Stroke Symposium of the International Neuropsychological Society, Dublin, Ireland, July 2005.

Nasreddine, Z. S., Collin, I., Chertkow, H., Phillips, N., Bergman, H., & Whitehead, V. (2003). Sensitivity and Specificity of the Montreal Cognitive Assessment (MoCA) for detection of mild cognitive deficits. *Canadian Journal of Neurological Sciences, 30,* S2, 30. Presented at Canadian Congress of Neurological Sciences Meeting, Québec City, Québec, June 2003.

Nasreddine, Z. S., Phillips, N. A., Bédirian, V., Charbonneau, S., Whitehead, V., Collin, I., Cummings, J. L., & Chertkow, H. (2005). The Montreal Cognitive Assessment (MoCA): A brief screening tool for mild cognitive impairment. *Journal of the American Geriatric Society, 53,* 695–699.

Nasreddine, Z. (2013). The Montreal Cognitive Assessment (MoCA). Retrieved May 24,2013 from http://www.mocatest.org/default.asp

National Institutes of Health. (n.d.). NIH Toolbox: Assessment of Neurological and Behavioral Function. Retrieved May 24, 2013 from http://www.nihtoolbox.org/WhatAndWhy/Pages/default.aspx

Nisbett, R. E., & Masuda, T. (2003). Culture and point of view. *Proceedings of the National Academy of Sciences U.S.A., 100,* 11163–11170.

O'Keeffe, F., Dockree, P., Moloney, P., Carton, S., & Robertson, I. H. (2007). Awareness of deficits in traumatic brain injury: A multidimensional approach to assessing metacognitive knowledge and online-awareness. *Journal of the International Neuropsychology Society, 13,* 38–49.

Osmon, D. C., Smet, I. C., Winegarden, B., & Gandhavadi, B. (1992). Neurobehavioral Cognitive Status Examination: Its use with unilateral stroke patients in a rehabilitation setting. *Archives of Physical Medicine and Rehabilitation, 73,* 414–418.

Posner, M. I. (1980). Orienting of attention. *Quarterly Journal of Experimental Psychology, 32,* 3–25.

Prigatano, G. P., Borgaro, S., Baker, J., & Wethe, J. (2005). Awareness and distress after traumatic brain injury: A relative's perspective. *Journal of Head Trauma Rehabilitation, 20,* 359–367.

Prigatano, G. P., Ogano, M., & Amakusa, B. (1997). A cross-cultural study on impaired self-awareness in Japanese patients with brain dysfunction. *Neuropsychiatry, Neuropsychology, and Behavioral Neurology, 10,* 135–143.

Prigatano, G. P., & Schacter, D. L. (1991). *Awareness of deficit after brain injury: Clinical and theoretical issues.* New York: Oxford University.

Rabin, L. A., Roth, R. M., Isquith, P. K., Wishart, H. A., Nutter-Upham, K. E., Pare, N., Flashman, L. A., & Saykin, A. J. (2006). Self- and informant reports of executive function on the BRIEF-A in MCI and older adults with cognitive complaints. *Archives of Clinical Neuropsychology, 21,* 721–732.

Rand, D., Rukan, S. B., Weiss, P. L., & Katz, N. (2009). Validation of the Virtual MET as an assessment tool of executive functions. *Neuropsychological Rehabilitation, 19,* 583–602.

Robertson, I. H., Ward, T., Ridgeway, V., & Nimmo-Smith, I. (1996). The structure of normal human attention: The Test of Everyday Attention. *Journal of the International Neuropsychological Society, 2,* 525–534.

Rogers, J. M., & Panegyres, P. K. (2007). Cognitive impairment in multiple sclerosis: Evidence-based analysis and recommendations. *Journal of Clinical Neurosciences, 14,* 919–927.

Roth, R. M., Isquith, P. K., & Gioia, G. A. (2005). *Behavior Rating Inventory of Executive Function—Adult Version (BRIEF-A).* Psychological Assessment Resources, Lutz, FL.

Salthouse, T. A. (2005). Relations between cognitive abilities and measures of executive functioning. *Neuropsychology, 1,* 532–545.

Schilling, V., Jenkins, V., Morris, R., Deutsch, G., & Bloomfield, D. (2005). The effects of adjuvant chemotherapy on cognition in women with breast cancer: Preliminary results of an observational longitudinal study. *Breast, 14,* 142–150.

Schwamm, L. H., Van Dyke, C., Kiernan, R. J., Muerrin, E. L., & Mueller, J. (1987). The neurobehavioral cognitive status examination: Comparison with the cognitive capacity screening examination and the mini-mental status examination in a neurosurgical population. *Annals of Internal Medicine, 107,* 486–490.

Seminowicz, D. A., & Davis, K. D. (2007). Interactions of pain intensity and cognitive load: The brain stays on task. *Cerebral Cortex, 17,* 1412–1422.

Shallice, T., & Burgess, P. W. (1991). Deficits in strategy application following frontal lobe damage in man. *Brain, 114,* 727–741.

Sherer, M., Hart, T., Whyte, J., Nick, T. G., & Yablon, S. A. (2005). Neuroanatomic basis of impaired self-awareness after traumatic brain injury. *Journal of Head Trauma Rehabilitation, 20,* 287–300.

Simmond, M., & Fleming, J. (2003). Reliability of the self-awareness of deficits interview for adults with traumatic brain injury. *Brain Injury, 17,* 325–337.

Skandsen, T., Finnanger, T. G., Andersson, S., Lydersen, S., Brunner, J. F., & Vik, A. (2010). Cognitive impairment 3 months after moderate and severe traumatic brain injury: A prospective follow-up study. *Archives of Physical Medicine and Rehabilitation, 91,* 1904–1913.

Skidmore, E. R., Whyte, E. M., Holm, M. B., Becker, J. T., Butters, M. A., Dew, M. A., Munin, M. C., & Lenze, E. J. (2010). Cognitive and affective predictors of rehabilitation participation after stroke. *Archives of Physical Medicine and Rehabilitation, 91,* 203–207.

Sohlberg, M. M., & Mateer, C. A. (1989). *Introduction to cognitive rehabilitation theory and practice.* New York: Guilford Press.

Sohlberg, M. M:, & Mateer, C. A. (2001). *Cognitive rehabilitation.* New York: Guilford Press.

Sohlberg, M. M., & Turkstra, L. S. (2011). *Optimizing cognitive rehabilitation: Effective instructional methods.* New York: Guilford Press.

Sosnoff, J. J., Boes, M. K., Sandroff, B. M., Socie, M. J., Pula, J. H., & Motl, R. W. (2011). Walking and thinking in persons with multiple sclerosis who vary in disability. *Archives of Physical Medicine and Rehabilitation, 92,* 2028–2033.

Suhr, J. A., & Grace, J. (1999). Brief cognitive screening of right hemisphere stroke: Relation to functional outcome. *Archives of Physical Medicine and Rehabilitation, 80,* 773–776.

Teng, E. L., & Chui, H. (1987). The Modified Mini-Mental State (3MS) Examination. *Journal of Clinical Psychiatry, 48,* 314–318.

Toglia, J. P. (1993). *The Contextual Memory Test.* Tucson, AZ: Therapy Skill Builders.

Toglia, J. P. (1998). A dynamic interactional model to cognitive rehabilitation. In N. Katz (Ed.), *Cognition and occupation in rehabilitation.* Bethesda, MD: American Occupational Therapy Association.

Toglia, J., & Cermak, S. A. (2009). Dynamic assessment and prediction of learning potential in clients with unilateral neglect. *American Journal of Occupational Therapy, 63,* 569–579.

Toglia, J., Fitzgerald, K. A., O'Dell, M. W., Mastrogiovanni,, A. R., & Lin, C. D. (2011). The Mini-Mental State Examination and Montreal Cognitive Assessment in persons with mild subacute stroke: Relationship to functional outcome. *Archives of Physical Medicine and Rehabilitation, 92,* 792–798.

Tombaugh, T. N., & McIntyre, N. J. (1992). The Mini-Mental State Examination: A comprehensive review. *Journal of the American Geriatric Society, 40,* 922–935.

Tranel, D., Hathaway-Nepple, J., & Anderson, S. W. (2007). Impaired behavior on real-world tasks following damage to the ventromedial prefrontal cortex. *Journal of Clinical and Experimental Neuropsychology, 29,* 319–332.

Watson, Y. I., Arfken, C. L., & Birge, S. J. (1993). Clock completion: An objective screening test for dementia. *Journal of the American Geriatric Society, 41,* 1235–1240.

Wilson, B. A., Cockburn, J., & Baddeley, A. (1985). *The Rivermead Behavioral Memory Test.* Reading, UK: Thames Valley Test; Gaylord, MI: National Rehabilitation Services.

Wilson, B. A., Cockburn, J., Baddeley, A., & Hiorns, R. (1989). The development and validation of a test battery for detecting and monitoring everyday memory problems. *Journal of Clinical and Experimental Neuropsychology, 11,* 855–870.

Wolf, T. J., Barbee, A. R., & White, D. (2011). Executive dysfunction immediately after mild stroke. *OTJR: Occupation, Participation and Health, 31(Suppl. 1),* S23–S29.

Zwecker, M., Levenkrohn, S., Fleisig, Y., Zeilig, G., Ohry, A., & Adunsky, A. (2002). Mini-Mental State Examination, Cognitive FIM Instrument, and the Loewenstein Occupational Therapy Cognitive Assessment: Relation to functional outcome of stroke patients. *Archive of Physical Medicine and Rehabilitation, 83,* 342–345.

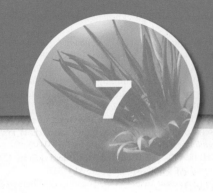

7

Assessing Abilities and Capacities: Range of Motion, Strength, and Endurance

Lynsay R. Whelan

Learning Objectives

After studying this chapter, the reader will be able to do the following:

1. Determine when evaluation of motion, strength, and endurance is appropriate and the best methods for obtaining such data.
2. Evaluate range of motion of the upper extremity using a goniometer.
3. Evaluate underlying causes of decreased motion and strength including edema, scar tissue, and pain.
4. Perform a manual muscle test to evaluate strength of the upper extremity.
5. Determine functional endurance level.
6. Interpret the findings of the evaluations in this chapter and incorporate the results into intervention planning in a functional manner.

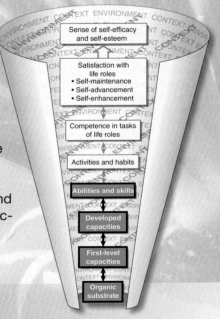

INTRODUCTION

The assessments presented in this chapter are appropriate for patients who are unable to do or are restricted in doing the occupational tasks and activities important to them because of range of joint motion, strength, or endurance impairments. Being able to move (mobility, or range of motion [ROM]) and use the extremities against resistance (strength) for an extended period (endurance) is essential for the completion of most occupational tasks. For example, a person who cannot fully flex the elbow, is too weak to lift a spoon to the mouth, or is too fatigued to lift the utensil repeatedly cannot eat a meal independently. Because deficits in these abilities and capacities may lead to impaired occupational functioning, it is within the realm of occupational therapy to assess them. Keep in mind that occupational therapy assessments of mobility, strength, and endurance focus on how deficits in these areas impact occupational functioning. Occupational therapists also consider other variables in the overall evaluation, including environmental and contextual constraints that contribute to performance ability. The majority of this chapter will focus on evaluating limitations that impact upper extremity (UE) function and occupational performance.

Use of the assessments described in this chapter allows for the establishment of the patient's baseline abilities. Reassessment produces documentation of progress or lack thereof as well as return to function within normal limits (WNL). With the demands for efficiency in health care delivery, it is essential that occupational therapists be skilled in their evaluations of patients to justify continuation or discharge of therapy services.

The Occupational Therapy Practice Framework (OTPF) (American Occupational Therapy Association [AOTA], 2008) recognizes that client factors impacting mobility, muscle power, and endurance (such as neuromusculoskeletal and movement-related body functions and structures) can impact occupational functioning. The OTPF also recognizes that activity demands and contextual factors contribute to an individual's success in performing various tasks (AOTA, 2008). Similarly, the Occupational Functioning Model recognizes the sensorimotor abilities, motor skills, cardiorespiratory (CR) skills, and contextual influences that impact function in life roles. Although this chapter will focus on the assessment of occupational performance and intervention planning portions of the occupational therapy process, it is important to also remember that the occupational profile or subjective portion of the evaluation influences the therapists' decisions regarding what objective measures to analyze in determining the factors impacting performance (AOTA, 2008).

FUNCTIONAL UPPER EXTREMITY ASSESSMENT

Depending on the reason for the referral to occupational therapy services, a screening (or preliminary assessment to determine whether more in-depth evaluation is needed) of motion and functional strength may be more appropriate than individual measurement of motion and strength at each joint and muscle. It is often appropriate to screen some areas while taking formal measurements of others, which is why therapists will often begin with the functional screen. For example, a patient may be referred to therapy following a distal radius fracture. When individuals have a cast on their wrist, they may lose motion at the shoulder and elbow as well because of nonuse and protective posturing. It would be appropriate to screen the shoulder and elbow and compare bilaterally to ensure motion there is WNL and then do specific ROM measurements at the wrist and hand. If deficits are noted on the screen at the shoulder or elbow, then it would also be appropriate to complete specific measurements where the limitation was noted.

Similarly, a gross screening of UE strength may be more appropriate than testing individual muscles. This screening is often appropriate in inpatient and rehabilitation settings in which the patient may be experiencing more gross weakness from debilitation. During the screening, if the therapist determines any patterns such as weakness in one specific nerve distribution, he or she may wish to then do more specific manual muscle testing (MMT) of muscles innervated by that nerve (for more information on functional screening of the UE, see Procedures for Practice 7-1). Note that, depending on the practice setting, the terms upper limb or upper quadrant may be used rather than upper extremity.

FUNCTIONAL LOWER EXTREMITY ASSESSMENT

Physical therapists typically complete any needed formal measurements of ROM and strength of the lower extremities (LE). However, there is a role for occupational therapists in the functional assessment of the lower extremities insofar as they are commonly consulted regarding return to independence in activities of daily living (ADL) and instrumental activities of daily living (IADL) for patients with, for example, various orthopedic, neurological, and other debilitating chronic conditions. In these cases, evaluation of LE function is typically done with the demonstration of ADL/IADL tasks and functional transfers. Occupational therapists are not interested in the exact degree of motion at the hip, knee, or ankle as much as they are interested in whether that motion, for example, allows

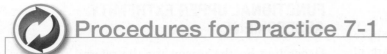

Procedures for Practice 7-1

Functional Active Range of Motion and Strength Screen

- The patient should be seated if possible.
- The patient should perform the motions bilaterally, if possible. If not, the unimpaired or least impaired side should move first to set a baseline for normal for this person.
- Observe for complete movements, symmetry of movements, and timing of movements.
- Demonstrate the movements if the patient has a language barrier or cognitive deficits.
- To estimate the amount of active movement in the following motions, give instructions such as these to the patient:

Motion/Resisted Motion	Examples of Instruction
Shoulder flexion	Lift your arms straight up in front of you and reach toward the ceiling. Now, with your arms straight in front of you, do not let me push you down.
Shoulder abduction	Move your arms out to the side. Now reach over your head. With your arms straight out, do not let me push you down.
Shoulder horizontal abduction and adduction	Raise your arms forward to shoulder height. Move each arm out to the side, then back again while keeping your arm level. Push against me this time.
External rotation	Touch the back of your head with your hand, like you are washing your hair. Now push against me, like you were going to throw a ball overhand.
Internal rotation	Touch the small of your back with your hand like you are tucking in your shirt. Now push against my hand.
Elbow flexion and extension	Start with your arms straight down by your sides. Now bend your elbows so your hands touch your shoulders. Push and pull against me starting with your arm flexed like you are making a muscle.
Forearm supination and pronation	With your arms at your side and your elbows flexed to 90°, rotate your forearms so the palms of your hands face the floor and then the ceiling. Now, like we are shaking hands, resist my motion.
Wrist flexion and extension	Move your wrists up and down. Now, resist my pressure.
Finger flexion and extension	Make a fist, then open your fingers. Squeeze my hands (ensure your hand is interlocked in the web space to avoid injury of your own hand).
Finger opposition	Touch your thumb to the tip of each finger one at a time. Now, try to hold your thumb to your index finger and small finger without letting me break the circle.

the individual to transfer to and from a toilet or complete dressing independently and safely.

For example, an occupational therapist is consulted to evaluate and treat a patient following a hip replacement. The therapist evaluates the patient's LE motion and strength as it relates to the patient's ability to perform bed mobility; functional transfers; and ADL/IADL tasks, such as dressing, bathing, and meal preparation, while following any precautions the surgeon has prescribed. Patients may be asked to demonstrate how they would put on their socks or retrieve an item from the bottom shelf of the refrigerator while following their hip precautions. The therapist may develop a treatment plan after evaluation that provides or recommends adaptive equipment

and educates the patient on compensatory techniques for completing ADL/IADL tasks with modified independence (see Procedures for Practice 7-2 and Figs. 7-1 to 7-3 for additional information regarding functional LE assessment).

If the physical therapy evaluation is not available for review prior to the occupational therapy evaluation, the occupational therapist should screen motion and strength to ensure safety when engaging in functional tasks as long as it is not contraindicated by the physician's orders, the condition, or the weight-bearing status of the patient. The therapist should have the client demonstrate ankle, knee, and hip motion either lying in bed or at the edge of the bed with resistance if it is not contraindicated.

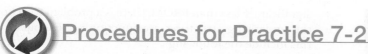

Procedures for Practice 7-2

Motion	Example Instructions
Hip	Show me how you would move from lying down to sitting on the edge of the bed.
	How would you get on and off the commode?
	Show me how you would get in and out of the tub.
	How would you get something from a bottom shelf?
Knee	Show me how you would put on your socks.
	How would you get on and off the commode?
	How would you get something from a bottom shelf?
Ankle	Show me how you will wash your feet.
	Show me how you would put on your socks.
Functional transfers	Show me how you would get in and out of bed (assess bed mobility, supine to sit, sit to stand, stand to sit, and sit to supine).
	Show me how you would sit on the commode (assess stand to sit and sit to stand with toilet or bedside commode transfers).
	Show me how you will get in and out of the shower (assess shower bench or transfer bench or safety in getting in and out of tub or walk-in shower as appropriate to patient).
	Show me how you will get in and out of the car (use real or simulated car).
	Show me how you will get up from this chair (cushioned seating versus solid chair).

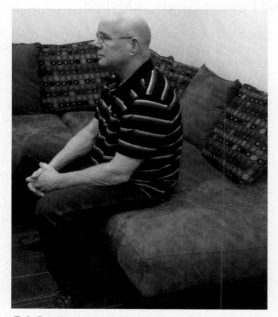

Figure 7-1 Functional lower extremity assessment with patient at edge of bed. Note the motion required to sit in this position.

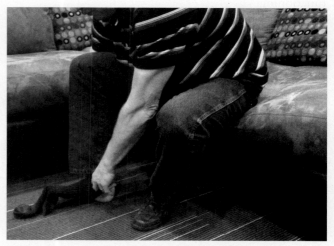

Figure 7-2 Functional lower extremity assessment with patient donning socks. Note the hip, knee, and ankle position. How could this task be modified?

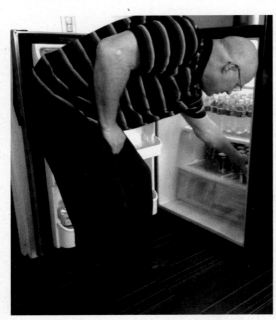

Figure 7-3 Functional lower extremity assessment with patient reaching for bottom shelf item. What adaptive equipment could assist in this task? How would you educate the patient?

If weakness is noted, the therapist should take extra precautions during the functional screening and ensure a gait belt is used. The occupational therapist should also ensure that the appropriate mobility device is being used during the functional screening.

RANGE OF MOTION MEASUREMENT

Normally, each joint can move in certain directions and to certain limits of motion based on the joint itself as well as the integrity of surrounding tissues. Trauma or disease that affects joint structures or the surrounding tissues can decrease motion at the joint and limit occupational functioning.

Measurement of joint range may be done actively or passively. Passive range of motion (PROM) is the amount of motion at a given joint when the joint is moved by an outside force. Typically, the outside force comes from the therapist or therapeutic equipment. Active range of motion (AROM) is the amount of motion at a given joint achieved when the patient contracts the muscles that control the desired motion. Additional types of ROM include self range of motion (SROM), where the client performs ROM on the affected side by using the nonaffected side, and active assistive range of motion (AAROM) where the therapist, the client, or another caregiver may provide support during active motion to allow the client to move beyond their current AROM limits. These are not typically measured in an evaluation but may be used in treatment to improve deficits in ROM. It is normal to have slightly more PROM than AROM; however, if AROM is

significantly less than PROM, there is a problem with how the underlying structures are functioning. Examples of this include the following:

- If the tendon is not intact, including lacerations or avulsions to the tendon, the result is that the tendon cannot pull along its anatomical path to produce AROM, but the joint can still be moved passively.
- Muscle weakness or loss of strength can prevent full contraction and, therefore, full motion.
- Pain may be caused by edema in or injury to surrounding tissue. The individual may be able to move further passively because he or she is not actively using the injured tissue and therefore has less pain.
- Scar tissue can adhere to underlying structures and impede motion.

If both AROM and PROM are limited, underlying causes could include a bony block to motion, capsular tightness around the joint, tightness of the muscle-tendon unit, edema, contractures, or more extensive scar tissue such as from burns.

If limitations in AROM are observed, they are formally measured and documented. If there are no contraindications (see Safety Note 7-1), the therapist then attempts to move the joint through its full PROM. If the joint is free to move to the end range, the problem is with active motion.

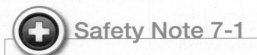

Safety Note 7-1

Precautions in the Evaluation of Active and Passive Range of Motion

- Carefully review consult/referral to therapy and note any contraindications to motion or restrictions in motion by the referring provider.
- Limited motion protocols may require that motion only be tested within the limits prescribed even if the patient feels they can move beyond these limits. For example, following tendon repair, the surgeon may prescribe a limited arc of motion to avoid overstressing the repair during the healing process.
- Avoid pushing passive range of motion when the underlying cause of the limitation is unknown, particularly with trauma.
- Avoid increasing edema or pain for the sake of a measurement. For example, immediately following casting the therapist would expect tightness of the tissues that have been immobilized, and active range of motion (AROM) measurements may be all that is needed to set baseline goals. It may be appropriate to try a heat modality (if edema does not contraindicate this) and then remeasure AROM to see whether increasing the extensibility of the soft tissues helps to improve ROM.

If the end range cannot be attained when the therapist moves the limb, the problem is with passive motion, and the PROM limitation is measured and recorded.

When recording PROM, the therapist should also note any abnormal end-feel. End-feel is the descriptive term used to describe what the therapist feels at the end range of passive limits of motion. Cyriax, Kaltenborn, and Paris are three different classification systems of end-feel (Petersen & Hayes, 2000). All three require more research into the interrater reliability of the classifications (Petersen & Hayes, 2000; van de Pol, van Trijffel, & Lucas, 2010). Commonly used terms for end-feel, mostly based on the Cyriax and Kaltenborn systems include:

- bony, hard, or bone-to-bone end-feel, where movement stops as the bony surfaces meet such as elbow extension
- capsular end-feel, which is somewhat firm or leathery but has some give, such as end range of shoulder external rotation
- soft end-feel or tissue approximation, which is when soft tissue stops the movement, such as elbow flexion
- spasm end-feel, where the tissue responds with a harsh movement in the opposite direction
- empty end-feel, where there is no "feel," but rather the patient asks to stop because of pain
- springy end-feel, where there is some rebound at the end range of motion (Petersen & Hayes, 2000; van de Pol, van Trijffel, & Lucas, 2010)

Although some of these may be a normal end-feel, it is important to note when they are abnormal. For example, a bony end-feel prior to full wrist extension may indicate underlying pathology or a capsular end-feel during elbow extension when the elbow is at 30° may be the result of capsular tightness from immobilization.

A goniometer is the most common tool used for measuring joint motion of the UE. Every goniometer has a protractor, an axis, and two arms. The stationary arm extends from the protractor, on which the degrees are marked. The movable arm has a center line or pointer to indicate angle measurement. The axis is the point at which these two arms are riveted together. A full-circle goniometer, which measures 360°, or 0°–180° in each direction, permits motion measurement in both directions, such as flexion and extension, without repositioning the tool. When using a half-circle goniometer, the protractor must be positioned opposite to the direction of motion so that the indicator remains on the face of the protractor. A finger goniometer is designed with a shorter movable arm and flat surfaces to fit comfortably over the finger joints. Figure 7-4 shows examples of these types of goniometers.

Some clinics use a manual or electronic inclinometer rather than a goniometer to measure ROM. These devices use gravity rather than the therapist's visual skills to determine the starting position for measurement and therefore can improve accuracy, particularly in more complex motions

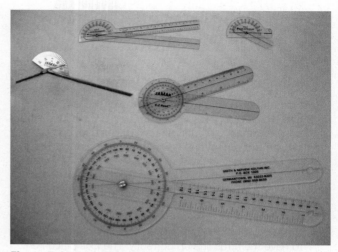

Figure 7-4 Types of goniometers. The small half-circle goniometer and modified half-circle (*top*) is used to measure small joints, such as the wrist. The small finger goniometer (*middle left*) has flat arms that fit over the fingers. The small and large full-circle goniometers (*middle right and bottom*) are used to measure with the 360° method and for larger joints.

such as compound spine motions (Gerhardt, Cocchiarella, & Lea, 2002). It is important to note that the position of the individual being measured may need to change with the use of an inclinometer because gravity is used to obtain the starting position. Another potential tool is the electrogoniometer. This tool can offer continuous measurement of ROM once positioned and calibrated (Yen & Radwin, 2000). This may be particularly helpful in work and industry type settings where repetitive work tasks and ergonomic impact are being assessed. When using the electrogoniometer, the therapist should calibrate the instrument for the task being performed to decrease errors often seen at angles greater than 45° (Yen & Radwin, 2000). Because the goniometer is most commonly used in occupational therapy practice and the general principles apply to the alignment of other instruments, the figures depicting ROM measurement in this chapter include standard goniometers.

Reliability

The therapist must place the axis and arms appropriately to ensure accuracy and reliability. See Procedures for Practice 7-3 for general principles to follow when using the goniometer. The specific placement of the goniometer for each joint is described and demonstrated in this chapter.

In addition to goniometer placement, multiple patient-related and environmental factors can affect accuracy and reliability of ROM measurements. Patient-related factors include pain, fear of pain, fatigue, and feelings of stress or tension. For the most accurate and reliable results, every effort should be made to make the patient physically and emotionally comfortable, including talking to the patient and describing the procedure that is to follow.

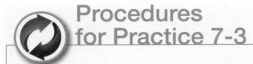

Procedures for Practice 7-3

Principles of Goniometer Placement

- Place the axis of the goniometer over the axis of motion. The axis of motion for some joints coincides with bony landmarks, but for others it must be found by observing movement and finding the point around which the movement occurs. In that case, the axis of motion can change position during movement, so it is acceptable for the goniometer to be repositioned at the end of range. When the two arms of the goniometer are placed correctly, they intersect at the axis of motion (Triffitt, Wildin, & Hajioff, 1999), so it is more important to have the arms line up correctly. The axis placement then automatically falls in line.
- Position the stationary arm parallel to the longitudinal axis of the body segment proximal to the joint being measured, although there are some exceptions.
- Position the movable arm parallel to the longitudinal axis of the body segment distal to the joint being measured, with some exceptions.

Environmental factors include time of day, temperature of the room, type of goniometer used, and training and experience of the tester. For the most reliable pretest–posttest information, the same tester should use the same goniometer at approximately the same time of day.

Intrarater reliability is consistently higher than interrater reliability for ROM testing using a universal goniometer. Intrarater reliability refers to *one* therapist consistently measuring the same joint angle over multiple trials, whereas interrater reliability concerns *multiple* therapists consistently measuring the same joint angle. In one study of shoulder internal and external rotation measured in the supine position, intrarater reliability was good ($r = 0.58$–0.71), and interrater reliability was fair to good ($r = 0.41$–0.66) (Awan, Smith, & Boon, 2002). A second study found that combined finger flexion measured with a ruler was a reliable measure when taken by different therapists, but that goniometric measures of the finger joints were more reliable when a single therapist was involved (Ellis & Bruton, 2002).

Active motion measurements are more reliable than passive ones. In one study by Sabari et al. (1998), 30 adults were measured for both active and passive ROM for shoulder flexion and abduction in two positions, sitting and supine. The AROM measurements were more reliable than the PROM measurements for both positions. Furthermore, the researchers found only a moderate range of agreement ($r = 0.64$–0.81) between goniometric measurements of shoulder movements with the patient sitting and supine. The authors concluded that the position of the patient can affect ROM. Therefore, therapists should record the testing

position, and the same position should be used each time the patient is retested (Sabari et al., 1998). This chapter demonstrates measurement of shoulder ROM in a sitting patient because it measures shoulder mobility in the position more frequently used for functional task performance.

A multicenter study looked at the reliability of three goniometric techniques for measuring passive wrist flexion and extension: radial, ulnar, and volar-dorsal approaches. The study found the volar-dorsal approach to be slightly more reliable. The interclass correlation coefficient (ICC) was 0.93 for flexion and 0.84 for extension with the volar-dorsal approach, whereas the corresponding values were 0.88 and 0.80 for the radial approach and 0.89 and 0.80 for the ulnar approach (LaStayo & Wheeler, 1994). All three approaches are reliable, but they are not interchangeable. The therapist must be sure to document which approach is being used and use the same approach consistently to document progress.

It is commonly believed that experience plays a major role in the reliability of ROM measurements. A study of how therapist experience influences reliability of goniometric measurements found no dramatic difference in reliability between experienced physical therapists and inexperienced therapy students measuring ankle joint angle. All of the inexperienced therapists were uniformly trained on specific testing procedures (Somers et al., 1997). Thus, interrater reliability may be more dependent on training than experience.

Recording Range of Motion

Depending on the facility, ROM may be documented electronically or on paper, making it a part of the medical record and a legal document. This form should include the date that the measurements were taken, whether the measurements represent AROM or PROM, the starting and ending position for each movement, whether the right versus the left side was tested, and the physical or electronic signature of the therapist performing the measurements. A sample form is provided in Figure 7-5. When reading the goniometer, always state your results as a range using two numbers. The first number is the starting position of the extremity, and the second number is the limit of motion at end range. At reevaluation, compare the initial evaluation measurements to evaluate progress.

The most common method of determining ROM is the Neutral Zero Method recommended by the Committee on Joint Motion of the American Academy of Orthopaedic Surgeons (AAOS) (Greene & Heckman, 1994). The ROM normative data presented in this chapter is also from the AAOS, although it is important to note that other sources, such as the American Medical Association (AMA), have documented these averages differently, and these sources may be seen in practice as well. In the Neutral Zero Method, the anatomical position is considered to be 0, or if a given starting position is different from anatomical position, it is defined

Patient's Name _____

Type of motion: AROM _____
  PROM _____

| LEFT | | | | RIGHT | |
Date	Date	Joint To Be Measured		Date	Date
		Shoulder			
		Flexion	0–180		
		Extension	0–60		
		Abduction	0–180		
		Horizontal abduction	0–45		
		Horizontal adduction	0–140		
		Internal rotation	0–70		
		External rotation	0–90		
		Internal rotation (alt)	0–90		
		External rotation (alt)	0–60		
		Elbow and Forearm			
		Flexion–extension	0–150		
		Supination	0–80		
		Pronation	0–80		
		Wrist			
		Flexion	0–80		
		Extension	0–70		
		Ulnar deviation	0–30		
		Radial deviation	0–20		
		Thumb			
		CM flexion	0–15		
		CM extension	0–20		
		MP flexion–extension	0–50		
		IP flexion–extension	0–80		
		Palmar Abduction	0–70		
		Radial Abduction	0–80		
		Opposition cm.			
		Index Finger			
		MP flexion	0–90		
		PIP flexion–extension	0–100		
		DIP flexion–extension	0–90		
		Abduction	no norm		
		Adduction	no norm		
		Middle Finger			
		MP flexion	0–90		
		PIP flexion–extension	0–100		
		DIP flexion–extension	0–90		
		Abduction	no norm		
		Adduction	no norm		
		Ring Finger			
		MP flexion	0–90		
		PIP flexion–extension	0–100		
		DIP flexion–extension	0–90		
		Abduction	no norm		
		Adduction	no norm		
		Little Finger			
		MP flexion	0–90		
		PIP flexion–extension	0–100		
		DIP flexion–extension	0–90		
		Abduction	no norm		
		Adduction	no norm		

Therapist's signature: _____

Figure 7-5 Sample range of motion recording form.

as 0. Measurement is taken from the stated starting position to the stated end position. If the patient cannot achieve the stated starting and end positions, the actual starting and end positions are recorded to indicate limitations in movement. An example using elbow flexion, is as follows:

0°–150°: No limitation
20°–150°: A limitation in extension (problem with the start position)
0°–120°: A limitation in flexion (problem with the end position)
20°–120°: Limitations in flexion and extension (problems with start and end positions)

To record hyperextension of a joint, which may be occasionally seen in metacarpophalangeal (MP) and elbow joints, the AAOS recommends a separate measurement to describe the available ROM without confusion. For example, if 20° of elbow hyperextension (an unnatural movement) is noted, it should be recorded as follows:

0°–150° of flexion
0° of extension
0°–20° of hyperextension

If a joint is fused, the starting and end positions are the same, with no ROM. This is recorded as "fused at X°." If a joint that normally moves in two directions cannot move in one direction, the ROM-limited motion is recorded. For example, if wrist flexion is 15°–80° with a 15° flexion contracture, the wrist cannot be positioned at zero or be moved into extension; therefore, wrist extension is −15° or a 15° extension lag.

Because there are various systems of notations, each having its own meaning, it is important to clarify the intended meaning to ensure consistency among therapists and physicians within the same facility.

RANGE OF MOTION MEASUREMENT OF THE UPPER EXTREMITY

This chapter addresses ROM of the UE, because most functional activities require UE use and manipulation skills. For the measurements given here, unless otherwise noted, the patient is seated with trunk erect against the back of an armless straight chair, although the measurements can be taken with the patient standing or supine, if necessary. This procedure can be done actively or passively. For active movement, take special care to ensure that there are no substitutions of movement.

A substitution or compensatory movement is the use of an alternate muscle or position to complete a motion, possibly preventing measurement of the true limits of motion. In order to avoid this error, the therapist should watch the individual as the motion is completed rather than focusing too intently on the goniometer. For PROM, the tester supports both the body part and the goniometer proximal and distal to the joint, leaving the joint free to move. Comfortable handling of the goniometer together with the movable body segment may require practice.

On the pages that follow, the reader will find narrative and pictorial descriptions to help in understanding and practicing measurement of UE ROM. The narrative descriptions frequently use the sagittal, transverse, and frontal planes of motion to describe the motion being measured (see Fig. 7-6 for pictorial clarification of these planes of motion).

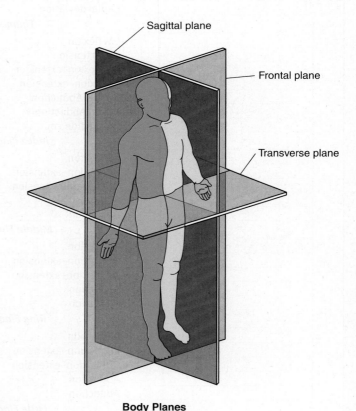

Body Planes

Figure 7-6 Planes of motion of the body.

Shoulder Flexion

Movement of the humerus anteriorly in the sagittal plane (0°–180°), which represents both glenohumeral and axioscapular motion (Figs. 7-7 and 7-8): starting position deviates from the anatomical position to allow the palm of the hand to face the body.

Goniometer Placement

Axis. A point around which motion occurs through the lateral aspect of the glenohumeral joint; at the start of motion, it lies approximately 1 inch below the acromion process with arm in neutral rotation. At the end position, the axis has moved, and the goniometer must be repositioned.

Stationary Arm. Parallel to the lateral midline of the trunk.

Movable Arm. Parallel to the longitudinal axis of the humerus on the lateral aspect.

Possible Substitutions

Trunk extension/rotation, shoulder abduction. Having the patient place the arm not actively being tested against a wall or chair in front of the patient may prevent excessive trunk motion used as a substitution method (Gerhardt, Cocchiarella, & Lea, 2002).

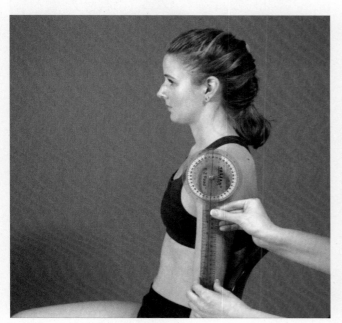

Figure 7-7 Shoulder flexion, start position.

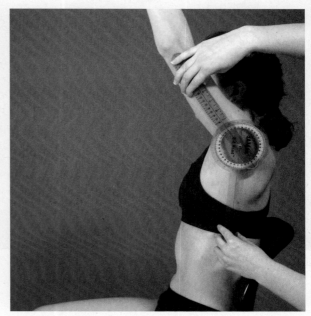

Figure 7-8 Shoulder flexion, end position.

Shoulder Extension

Movement of the humerus posteriorly in the sagittal plane with the arm in neutral rotation (0°–60°) (Figs. 7-9 and 7-10): some natural internal rotation occurs at the end range and is permitted (Greene & Heckman, 1994).

Goniometer Placement

Axis. A point around which motion occurs; it lies approximately 1 inch below the acromion process through the lateral aspect of the glenohumeral joint.

Stationary Arm. Parallel to the lateral midline of the trunk.

Movable Arm. Parallel to the longitudinal axis of the humerus on the lateral aspect.

Possible Substitutions

Trunk flexion/rotation, excessive scapular elevation and downward rotation, shoulder abduction.

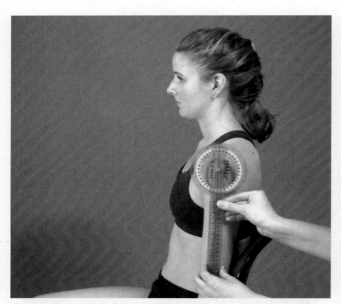

Figure 7-9 Shoulder extension, start position.

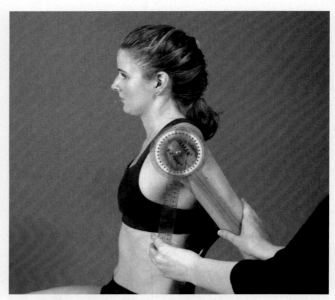

Figure 7-10 Shoulder extension, end position.

Shoulder Abduction

Movement of the humerus laterally in the frontal plane (0°–180°), which represents both glenohumeral and axioscapular motion (Figs. 7-11 and 7-12).

Goniometer Placement

Axis. A point through the anterior or posterior aspect of the glenohumeral joint.

Stationary Arm. Along the trunk, parallel to the spine.

Movable Arm. Parallel to the longitudinal axis of the humerus.

Possible Substitutions

Lateral flexion of trunk, scapular elevation, shoulder flexion or extension. If excessive lateral flexion of the trunk is noted, the arm not being actively tested may be stabilized at 90° of abduction against a wall or other stable object to prevent trunk motion (Gerhardt, Cocchiarella, & Lea, 2002).

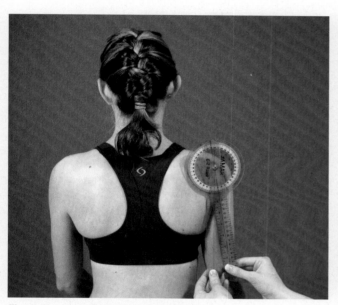

Figure 7-11 Shoulder abduction, start position.

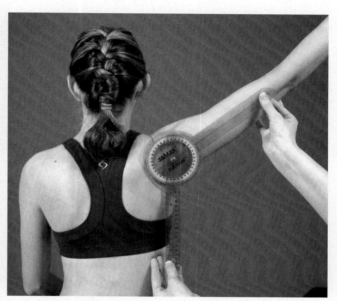

Figure 7-12 Shoulder abduction, end position.

Horizontal Abduction

Movement of the humerus on a horizontal (transverse) plane from 90° of shoulder abduction (0°–45°) (Figs. 7-13 and 7-14).

Goniometer Placement

Axis. On top of the acromion process.

Stationary Arm. Across the shoulder, anterior or posterior to the neck and in line with the opposite acromion process.

Movable Arm. Parallel to the longitudinal axis of the humerus on the superior aspect.

Possible Substitutions

Trunk rotation or trunk flexion, scapular motion, shoulder flexion (can be avoided by stabilizing the arm in 90° abduction).

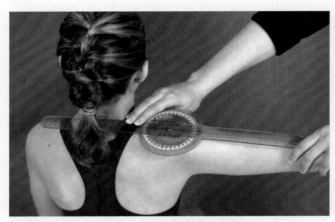

Figure 7-13 Shoulder horizontal abduction, start position.

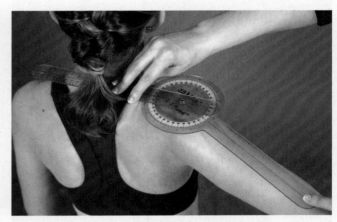

Figure 7-14 Shoulder horizontal abduction, end position.

Horizontal Adduction

Movement of the humerus on a horizontal (transverse) plane from 90° of shoulder abduction through 90° of shoulder flexion, across the trunk to the limit of motion (0°–140°) (Figs. 7-15 and 7-16).

Goniometer Placement

Axis. On top of the acromion process.

Stationary Arm. Across the shoulder, anterior to the neck and in line with the opposite acromion process.

Movable Arm. Parallel to the longitudinal axis of the humerus on the superior aspect.

Possible Substitution

Trunk rotation, scapular motion, shoulder flexion/extension (can be avoided by stabilizing the arm in 90° abduction).

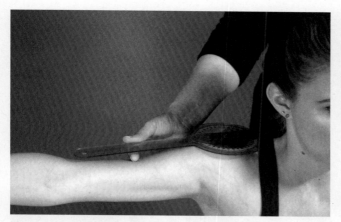

Figure 7-15 Shoulder horizontal adduction, start position.

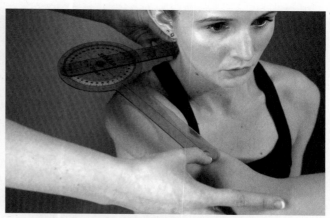

Figure 7-16 Shoulder horizontal adduction, end position.

Internal Rotation

Rotation of the humerus internally around the longitudinal axis of the humerus (0°–70°) (Figs. 7-17 and 7-18). Preferably the zero start position is with the arm abducted to 90° and elbow flexed at 90° with the forearm moving toward the floor from this starting position.

Goniometer Placement

Axis. Olecranon process of the ulna.

Stationary Arm. Perpendicular to the floor, which will be parallel to the lateral trunk if the patient is sitting up straight with hips at 90°. The goniometer reads 90° at the start, and this score must be adjusted from the final score when recording ROM. *Note:* If the patient is supine with the shoulder abducted to 90° and the elbow flexed to 90°, the stationary arm is perpendicular to the floor, with the movable arm along the ulna. The goniometer reads 0° at the start (Boone & Smith, 2000).

Movable Arm. Parallel to the longitudinal axis of the ulna.

Possible Substitutions

Scapular elevation and downward rotation, trunk flexion, elbow extension.

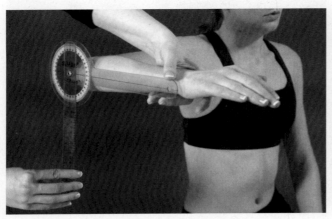

Figure 7-17 Shoulder internal rotation, start position.

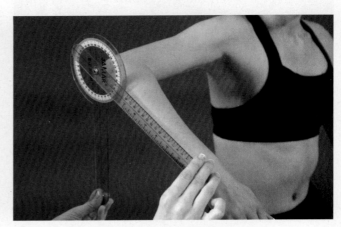

Figure 7-18 Shoulder internal rotation, end position.

External Rotation

Movement of the humerus laterally or upward from the ground in the 90° abducted start position around the longitudinal axis of the humerus (0°–90°) (Figs. 7-19 and 7-20).

Goniometer Placement

Axis. Olecranon process of the ulna.

Stationary Arm. Perpendicular to the floor. The goniometer will read 90° at the start, and this must be considered when recording the ROM score.

Movable Arm. Parallel to the longitudinal axis of the ulna.

Possible Substitutions

Scapular depression and upward rotation, trunk extension, elbow extension.

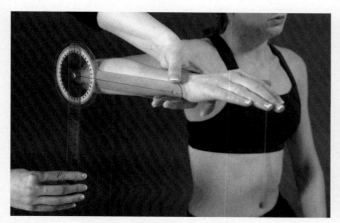

Figure 7-19 Shoulder external rotation, start position.

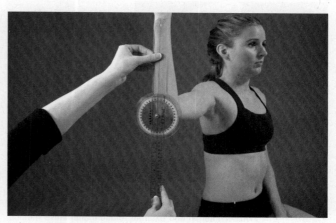

Figure 7-20 Shoulder external rotation, end position.

Internal and External Rotation: Alternative Method

If shoulder limitation prevents positioning for the previously described method, the patient may be seated with the humerus adducted to the side and elbow flexed to 90° with forearm in neutral (Figs. 7-21 and 7-22). This method is inaccurate in internal rotation if the patient has a large abdomen (internal rotation, 0°–90°; external rotation, 0°–60°).

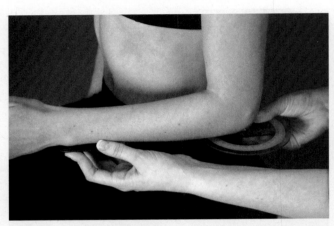

Figure 7-21 Shoulder internal and external rotation, alternative method, start position.

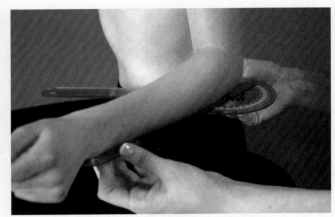

Figure 7-22 Shoulder external rotation, alternative method, end position.

Elbow Flexion–Extension

Movement of the supinated forearm anteriorly in the sagittal plane (0°–150°) (Figs. 7-23 and 7-24). Significant elbow extension is not typically seen in the adult population, but children and some hypermobile adults may demonstrate 10°–15° of hyperextension at the elbow, although most functional tasks are completed in the 30°–130° arc of flexion (Greene & Heckman, 1994).

Goniometer Placement

Axis. Lateral epicondyle of the humerus.

Stationary Arm. Parallel to the longitudinal axis of the humerus on the lateral aspect.

Movable Arm. Parallel to the longitudinal axis of the radius.

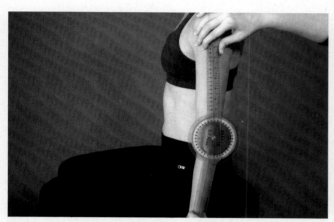

Figure 7-23 Elbow flexion, start position (elbow extension).

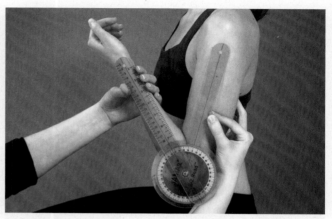

Figure 7-24 Elbow flexion, end position.

Forearm Supination

Rotation of the forearm laterally around its longitudinal axis from midposition so that the palm of the hand faces up (0°–80°) (Figs. 7-25 and 7-26). Starting position is with the forearm in neutral, and the humerus stabilized against the body.

Goniometer Placement

Axis. Longitudinal axis of the forearm displaced toward the ulnar side.

Stationary Arm. Perpendicular to the floor, which should also be parallel with the humerus if no substitution movements are allowed.

Movable Arm. Across the distal radius and ulna on the volar surface.

Possible Substitutions

Adduction and external rotation of the shoulder.

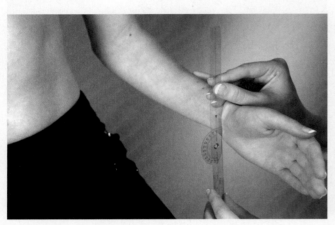

Figure 7-25 Supination, start position.

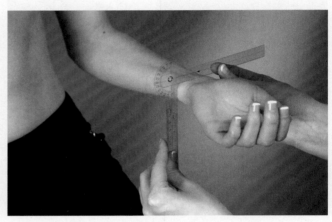

Figure 7-26 Supination, end position.

Forearm Pronation

Rotation of the forearm medially around its longitudinal axis from neutral so that the palm of the hand faces down (0°–80°) (Figs. 7-27 and 7-28). Functional forearm rotation is 50° of both pronation and supination (Greene & Heckman, 1994).

Goniometer Placement

Axis. Longitudinal axis of forearm displaced toward the ulnar side.

Stationary Arm. Perpendicular to the floor, which should also be parallel with the humerus if no substitution movements are allowed.

Movable Arm. Across the distal radius and ulna on the dorsal surface.

Possible Substitutions

Abduction and internal rotation of the shoulder.

Although the distal forearm method described here for supination and pronation has been the gold standard, two additional methods (the handheld pencil and plumbline goniometer methods) have shown high interrater and intrarater reliability in a more functional measure of supination and pronation. The handheld pencil method can be easily used in the clinic to determine functional forearm rotation. The standardized method is to have the client seated with hips and knees at 90°, feet flat on the ground, arms adducted to the sides with elbow flexed to 90°, forearm unsupported in neutral. The client holds a standard 15-cm pencil in a tight fist, with the pencil extending from the radial aspect of the hand. The goniometer is aligned with the axis at the head of the third metacarpal, stationary arm perpendicular to the floor, and moveable arm parallel to the pencil (Karagiannopoulos, Sitler, & Michlovitz, 2003).

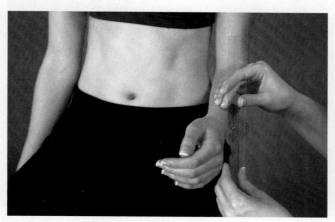

Figure 7-27 Pronation, start position.

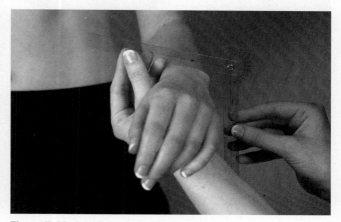

Figure 7-28 Pronation, end position.

Wrist Flexion (Volar Flexion)

Movement of the hand volarly in the sagittal plane (0°–80°) (Figs. 7-29 and 7-30). Starting with the forearm pronated and digits in a relaxed position will prevent any negative impact of the tenodesis effect on demonstrating the limits of motion.

Goniometer Placement

Axis. On the dorsal aspect of the wrist joint in line with the base of the third metacarpal in the proximal capitate region. (*Note:* The lunate protrudes as the wrist is flexed forward, and the capitate is located distal to the lunate and proximal to the base of the third metacarpal.)

Stationary Arm. Along the midline of the dorsal surface of the forearm.

Movable Arm. Parallel to the longitudinal axis of the third metacarpal.

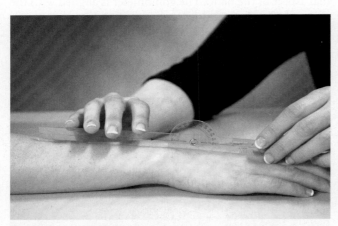

Figure 7-29 Wrist flexion, start position.

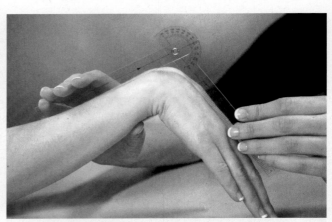

Figure 7-30 Wrist flexion, end position.

Wrist Extension (Dorsiflexion)

Movement of the hand dorsally in the sagittal plane (0°–70°) (Figs. 7-31 and 7-32). Again, prevent the tenodesis effect by reminding the patient to relax the fingers rather than trying to maintain them in full extension while measuring wrist motion.

Goniometer Placement

Axis. Same position as wrist flexion or, if the goniometer does not accommodate this position, on the volar surface of the wrist in line with the palmaris longus tendon in line with the third metacarpal at the level of the carpal bones.

Stationary Arm. Along the midline of the volar surface of the forearm.

Movable Arm. Parallel to the longitudinal axis of the third metacarpal. The movable arm may need to rest between the third and fourth digits if the digits prevent correct alignment.

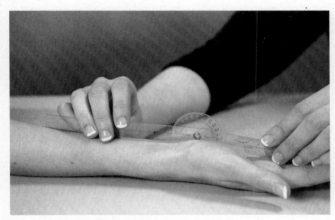

Figure 7-31 Wrist extension, start position.

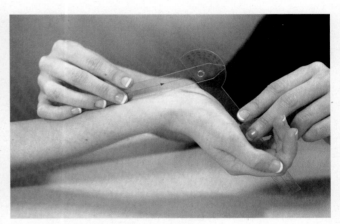

Figure 7-32 Wrist extension, end position.

Wrist Ulnar Deviation

Movement of the hand toward the ulnar side in a frontal plane (0°–30°) (Figs. 7-33 and 7-34). The AAOS recommends a starting position with the forearm pronated, whereas the AMA recommends neutral forearm rotation. Proper alignment of the goniometer is easier in pronation.

Goniometer Placement

Axis. On the dorsal aspect of the wrist joint in line with the base of the third metacarpal over the capitate where the motion is observed.

Stationary Arm. Along the midline of the forearm on the dorsal surface. After positioning the patient, stabilizing the forearm can assist in isolating motion to the wrist.

Movable Arm. Along the midline of the third metacarpal. (*Note:* Do not be distracted by additional abduction of the third digit, and palpate the third metacarpal to ensure alignment.)

Possible Substitutions

Wrist extension, wrist flexion.

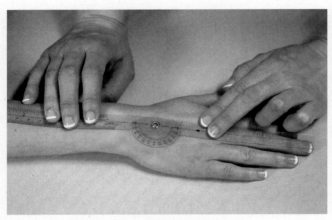

Figure 7-33 Wrist ulnar deviation, start position.

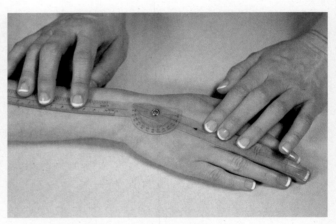

Figure 7-34 Wrist ulnar deviation, end position.

Wrist Radial Deviation

Movement of the hand toward the radial side in a frontal plane (0°–20°) (Figs. 7-35 and 7-36).

Goniometer Placement

Axis. On the dorsal aspect of the wrist joint in line with the base of the third metacarpal over the capitate.

Stationary Arm. Along the midline of the forearm on the dorsal surface. After positioning the patient, stabilizing the forearm can assist in isolating motion to the wrist.

Movable Arm. Along the midline of the third metacarpal.

Possible Substitution

Wrist extension.

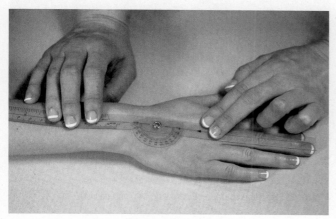

Figure 7-35 Wrist radial deviation, start position.

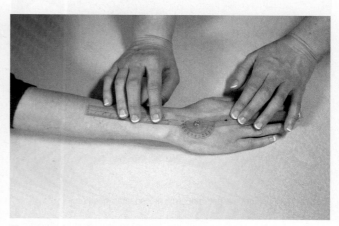

Figure 7-36 Wrist radial deviation, end position.

Thumb Carpometacarpal Flexion

Movement of the thumb across the palm in the frontal plane (0°–15°) (Figs. 7-37 and 7-38).

Goniometer Placement

Axis. On the radial side of the wrist at the junction of the base of the first metacarpal and the trapezium.

Stationary Arm. Parallel to the longitudinal axis of the radius.

Movable Arm. Parallel to the longitudinal axis of the first metacarpal. For accuracy, the arms of the goniometer must remain in full contact with skin surface over the bones. (*Note:* Avoid excessive pressure with the edge of a half-circle goniometer.) The axis of the goniometer may lift off the skin at greater degrees of motion in order to keep the arms in contact. These statements apply to all flexion–extension measurements of the thumb and fingers.

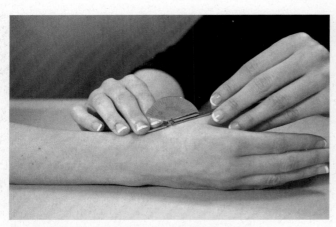

Figure 7-37 Thumb carpometacarpal flexion, start position.

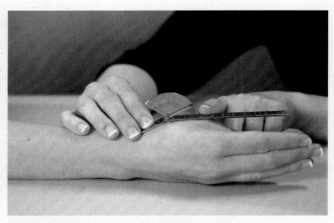

Figure 7-38 Thumb carpometacarpal flexion, end position.

Thumb Carpometacarpal Extension

Movement of the thumb away from the palm in the frontal plane (0°–20°) (Figs. 7-39 and 7-40).

Goniometer Placement

Axis. On the volar side of the wrist at the junction of the base of the first metacarpal and the trapezium.

Stationary Arm. Parallel to the longitudinal axis of the radius.

Moveable Arm. Parallel to the longitudinal axis of the first metacarpal.

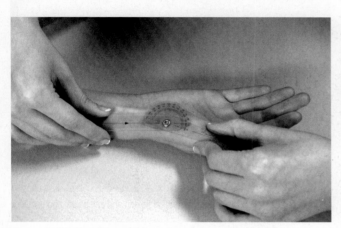

Figure 7-39 Thumb carpometacarpal extension, start position.

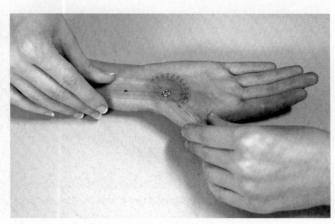

Figure 7-40 Thumb carpometacarpal extension, end position.

Thumb Metacarpophalangeal Flexion–Extension

Movement of the thumb across the palm in the frontal plane (0°–50°) (Figs. 7-41 and 7-42).

Goniometer Placement

Axis. On the dorsal aspect of the MP joint.

Stationary Arm. On the dorsal surface along the midline of the first metacarpal.

Movable Arm. On the dorsal surface along the midline of the proximal phalanx of the thumb.

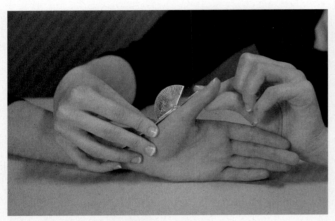

Figure 7-41 Thumb metacarpophalangeal flexion, start position (extension).

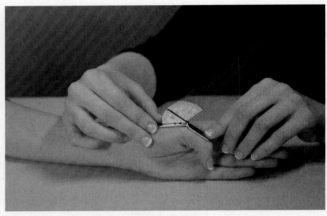

Figure 7-42 Thumb metacarpophalangeal flexion and extension, end position.

Thumb Interphalangeal Flexion–Extension

Movement of the distal phalanx of the thumb toward the volar surface of the proximal phalanx of the thumb (0°–80°) (Figs. 7-43 and 7-44).

Goniometer Placement

Axis. On the dorsal aspect of the interphalangeal (IP) joint.

Stationary Arm. On the dorsal surface along the proximal phalanx.

Movable Arm. On the dorsal surface along the distal phalanx. (*Note:* If the thumbnail prevents full goniometer contact, shift the movable arm laterally to increase accuracy. Also, thumb MP and IP flexion and extension can be measured on the lateral aspect of the thumb using lateral aspects of the same landmarks.)

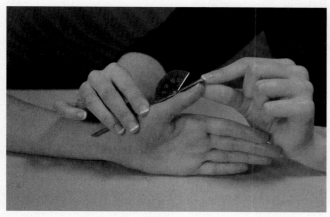

Figure 7-43 Thumb interphalangeal flexion, start position (extension).

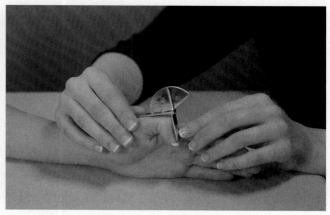

Figure 7-44 Thumb interphalangeal flexion, end position.

Thumb Palmar Abduction

Movement of the thumb perpendicular to the palm (0°–70°) (Figs. 7-45 and 7-46).

Goniometer Placement

Axis. Over the trapezium on the dorsal aspect of the hand.

Stationary Arm. On the dorsal surface parallel to the second metacarpal.

Movable Arm. Parallel to the first metacarpal.

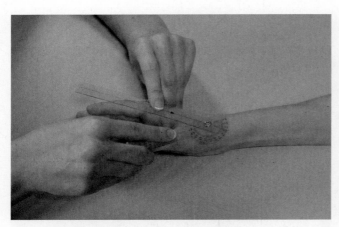

Figure 7-45 Thumb palmar abduction, start position.

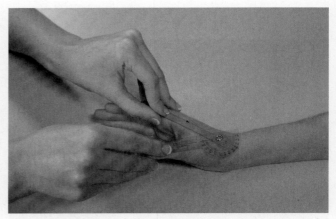

Figure 7-46 Thumb palmar abduction, end position.

Thumb Radial Abduction

Movement of the thumb radially and in line with the plane of the palm (0°–80°) (Figs. 7-47 and 7-48).

Goniometer Placement

Axis. Over the trapezium on the dorsal aspect of the hand.

Stationary Arm. On the dorsal surface parallel to the second metacarpal.

Movable Arm. Parallel to the first metacarpal.

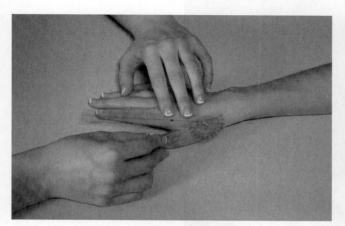

Figure 7-47 Thumb radial abduction, start position.

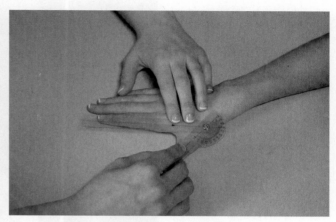

Figure 7-48 Thumb radial abduction, end position.

Opposition: Ruler Measurements

The pad of the thumb rotates to meet the pad of each finger. The little finger rotates to better meet the pad of the thumb. As a summary measure of opposition, record the distance from the tip of the thumb pad (not the thumbnail) to the tip end of the little finger or base of little finger (Fig. 7-49).

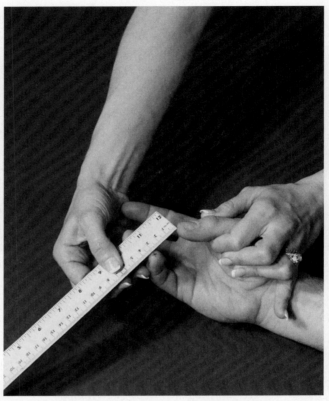

Figure 7-49 Measurement of opposition to the little finger using a centimeter ruler.

Finger Metacarpophalangeal Flexion–Extension

Movement of the finger at the MP joint (0°–90°) (Figs. 7-50 and 7-51). Hyperextension is normal at this joint.

Goniometer Placement

Axis. On the dorsal aspect of the MP joint of the finger being measured.

Stationary Arm. On the dorsal surface along the midline of the metacarpal of the finger being measured.

Movable Arm. On the dorsal surface along the midline of the proximal phalanx of the finger being measured.

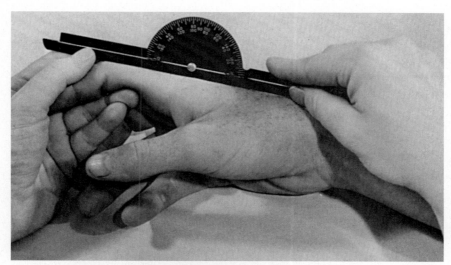

Figure 7-50   Finger metacarpophalangeal flexion, start position (extension).

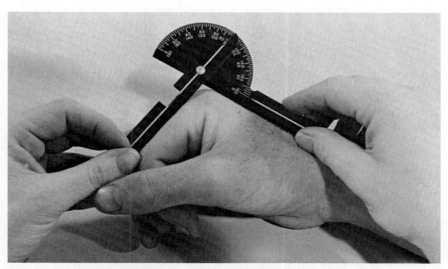

Figure 7-51   Finger metacarpophalangeal flexion, end position.

Finger Proximal Interphalangeal Flexion–Extension

Movement of the middle phalanx toward the palmar surface of the proximal phalanx (0°–100°) (Figs. 7-52 and 7-53).

Goniometer Placement

Axis. On the dorsal aspect of the proximal interphalangeal (PIP) joint of the finger being measured.

Stationary Arm. On the dorsal surface along the midline of the proximal phalanx of the finger being measured.

Movable Arm. On the dorsal surface along the midline of the middle phalanx of the finger being measured.

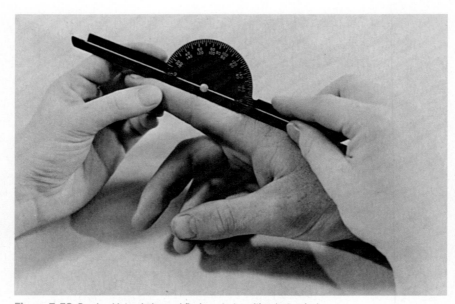

Figure 7-52   Proximal interphalangeal flexion, start position (extension).

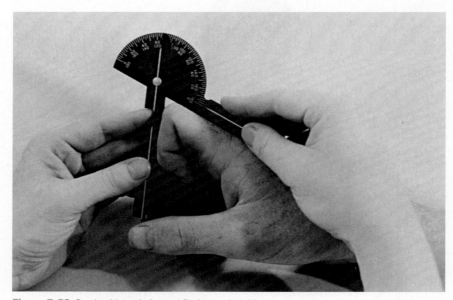

Figure 7-53   Proximal interphalangeal flexion, end position.

Finger Distal Interphalangeal Flexion–Extension

Movement of the distal phalanx toward the palmar surface of the middle phalanx (0°–90°) (Figs. 7-54 and 7-55).

Goniometer Placement

Axis. On the dorsal aspect of the distal interphalangeal (DIP) joint of the finger being measured.

Stationary Arm. On the dorsal surface along the midline of the middle phalanx of the finger being measured.

Movable Arm. On the dorsal surface along the midline of the distal phalanx of the finger being measured. (*Note:* If the fingernail prevents full goniometer contact, shift the arms laterally to increase accuracy. If contact with the palm impacts goniometer alignment, a hooked-fist position may improve accuracy of measurement. Also, finger PIP and DIP flexion and extension can be measured from the lateral aspect of each finger using the lateral aspect of the same landmarks. This method may be more accurate when joints are enlarged or when there is diffuse edema noted along the digit.)

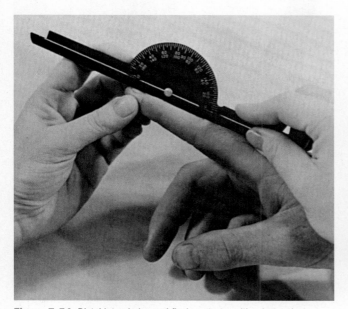

Figure 7-54   Distal interphalangeal flexion, start position (extension).

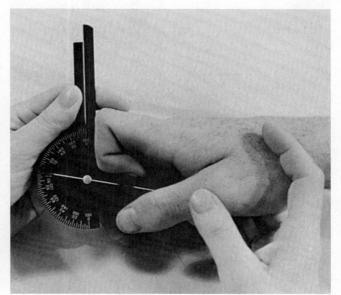

Figure 7-55   Distal interphalangeal flexion, end position.

Composite Measurement and Recording of Total Finger Flexion

A method of recording composite digital motion used by hand therapists is to sum the values for the degrees of flexion motion of the MP, PIP, and DIP joints, taking into consideration extension deficits (Ellis & Bruton, 2002). Total active motion (TAM) or total passive motion (TPM) can then be expressed by a single number. The formula for calculating these values is as follows: (MP + PIP + DIP flexion) − (MP + PIP + DIP extension deficits) = TAM or TPM.

Another method for measuring combined flexion of the PIP and DIP joints or combined flexion of the MP, PIP, and DIP joints using a centimeter ruler is illustrated in Figures 7-56 and 7-57.

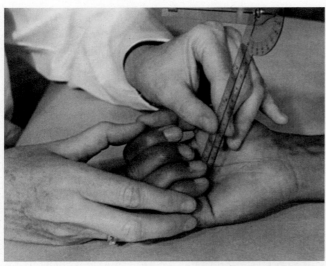

Figure 7-56 Proximal and distal interphalangeal combined finger flexion; ruler measurement.

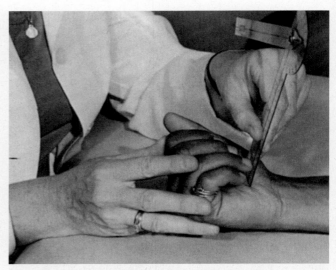

Figure 7-57 Metacarpophalangeal and proximal and distal interphalangeal combined finger flexion; ruler measurement.

Finger Abduction

Movement of the index, ring, and little fingers away from the midline of the hand in a frontal plane. The middle finger, which is the midline of the hand, abducts in both radial and ulnar directions (Figs. 7-58 and 7-59).

Goniometer Placement

Axis. On the dorsal aspect of the MP joint of the finger being measured.

Stationary Arm. Along the dorsal surface of the metacarpal of the finger being measured.

Movable Arm. Along the dorsal surface of the proximal phalanx of the finger being measured.

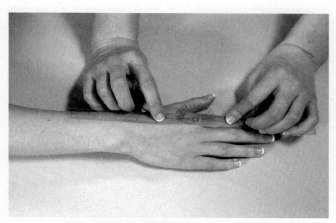

Figure 7-58 Finger abduction, start position.

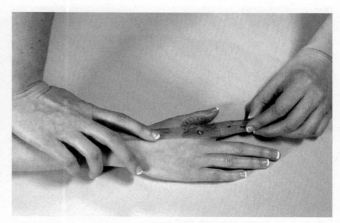

Figure 7-59 Finger abduction, end position.

Finger Adduction

Movement of the index, ring, and little fingers toward the midline of the hand in a frontal plane. Note that the middle finger cannot adduct as it is already in midline (Figs. 7-60 and 7-61).

Goniometer Placement

Axis. On the dorsal aspect of the MP joint of the finger being measured.

Stationary Arm. Along the dorsal surface of the metacarpal of the finger being measured. The middle finger is not measured.

Movable Arm. Along the dorsal surface of the proximal phalanx of the finger being measured.

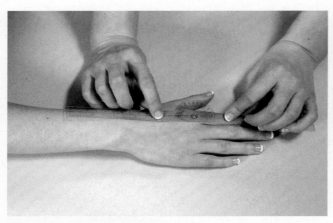

Figure 7-60 Finger adduction, start position.

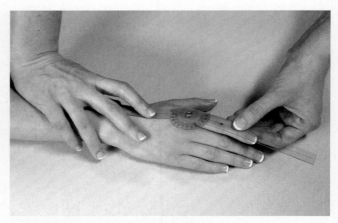

Figure 7-61 Finger adduction, end position.

Metacarpophalangeal Deviation Correction Measurement

When there is ulnar deviation deformity of the MP joints, often seen in rheumatoid arthritis, this additional measurement is taken (Figs. 7-62 and 7-63).

The active range is compared with the passive range to determine whether muscle weakness is present. PROM is compared with the norm of 0° deviation to determine whether a fixed deformity exists.

Goniometer Placement

Axis. Over the MP joint of the finger being measured.

Stationary Arm. Placed along the dorsal midline of the metacarpal.

Movable Arm. Placed along the dorsal midline of the proximal phalanx.

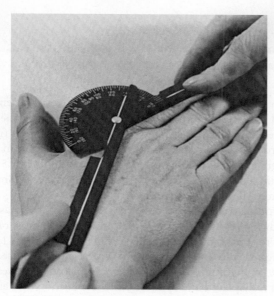

Figure 7-62 Metacarpophalangeal deviation correction, start position.

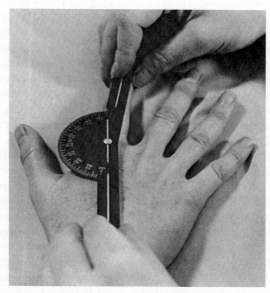

Figure 7-63 Metacarpophalangeal deviation correction, end position.

Interpreting the Results

The initial evaluation is interpreted by reviewing the recording form to identify which joints have significant limitation. A significant limitation is one that decreases occupational functioning or may lead to deformity. Limits of motion scores can be used in several ways. First, the therapist can compare the scores of the involved to the uninvolved extremity. A study of more than 1,000 healthy male subjects, however, found a significant difference in ROM between the dominant and nondominant sides. The nondominant side had greater range in many of the UE joints tested (Gunal et al., 1996). This information should be kept in mind when comparing the two sides. The patient's scores can be compared with the average limits (norms) expected for each motion. The average limits stated by the Committee on Joint Motion of the American Academy of Orthopaedic Surgeons (Greene & Heckman, 1994) are commonly used and are included here. However, patients may be functional with less ROM than is noted in the norms for particular joints. The emphasis in occupational therapy is to enable occupational functioning.

With the significant limitations and probable cause in mind, treatment goals that reflect the identified problem can be developed. For example, if skin, joint, and/or muscle tissues have shortened as a result of immobilization, the goal is to increase range by stretching these tissues. If the limitation is caused by edema, pain, spasticity, or muscle weakness, the primary goal is to reduce or correct the underlying problem, and the secondary goal is to prevent loss of ROM caused by the immobility imposed by the primary condition. If the cause is bony ankylosis or long-standing contracture, the goal is to teach the patient methods of compensation, because these conditions do not respond to nonsurgical treatment.

Comparing initial evaluation scores to mid- and post-treatment scores is important to assess the outcome and redirect treatment, if necessary. Interpretation of a re-evaluation that shows improvement following treatment must be tempered with the realization that changes may occur simply as a result of remeasurement. For ROM measurements to reflect actual change, the amount of change must exceed measurement error, which was found to be 5° for both the upper and lower extremities (Groth et al., 2001). For example, an increase of 10° in shoulder flexion is considered an improvement, but 5° may be accounted for by measurement error.

EDEMA

Edema, one cause of limited ROM, is quantified using circumferential or volumetric measurements. A millimeter tape is used to measure the circumference of a body part not easily submerged (as required by volumetric measurement) or when the edema is very localized (such

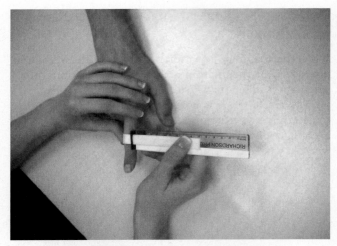

Figure 7-64 Measuring edema using circumferential method.

as to a single digit, making measurement of the entire hand unnecessary). With circumferential measurements, it is essential to measure at exactly the same place from test to test. Using anatomic landmarks can assist in the placement, such as over the third digit PIP joint or 5 cm proximal to the ulnar styloid (see Fig. 7-64 for an example of circumferential measurement).

Volumetric measures document changes in the mass of a body part by use of water displacement and is most often used to measure hand edema. A water vessel that is large enough to allow submersion of the whole hand is used as shown in Figure 7-65. When the hand is placed in the vessel, water is displaced and spills out into a collection beaker via the spout near the top and is then measured with a graduated cylinder. An edematous hand displaces more water

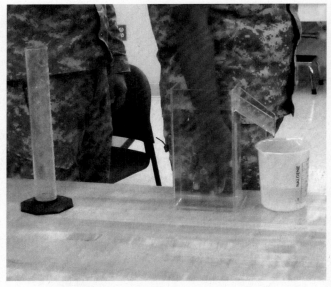

Figure 7-65 Measuring edema of the hand using a volumeter. Note the water being displaced into the graduated beaker as the hand is submerged.

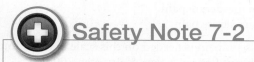

Safety Note 7-2

Precautions for Edema Measurements

Immersing the hand in water is sometimes contraindicated, such as with open wounds or skin conditions, immediately postoperatively, with percutaneous pinning and external fixation devices, healing skin grafts, and suspicion of infection. It is also inappropriate if having the extremity in the dependent position during testing significantly increases pain and edema or if spasticity or paralysis impacts the measurement (Dewey et al., 2007; Maihafer et al., 2003).

than does a nonswollen hand, so a lower reading is considered an improvement. The therapist should not expect the hand volume to be the same bilaterally, because the dominant hand typically has more muscle mass. Precautions with using this method are listed in Safety Note 7-2.

Dodds et al. (2004) examined therapists' ability to orient the extremity consistently within the volumeter and to measure the displaced water accurately. Following this protocol in the clinic setting, the therapist should follow the steps below:

1. An adjustable table should be set at a height that allows the client to keep the shoulder in neutral position when placing the hand in the volumeter on the tabletop. The therapist should ensure that the volumeter is stable, and the table is level.
2. The volumeter should be filled with room temperature water to the point of overflow. Any excess water should be wiped out of the collection beaker.
3. The client should be positioned parallel to the volumeter with the volar forearm and palm of the hand facing his or her body. The client should stand to the side of the table that will allow his or her thumb to face the spout of the volumeter.
4. The client should be instructed to note the dowel in the volumeter and slowly lower his or her hand into the volumeter at a rate that allows the water to collect in the beaker below the spout until the web space between the third and fourth digits rests on the dowel and the water stops dripping. Tell the client to avoid touching the sides of the volumeter during the test.
5. The therapist should stand behind the client to support the trunk and prevent any rotation or leaning and can provide verbal cues to the client to prevent excess motion and ensure the hand is properly positioned. Instruct the client to remain silent until the test is complete to avoid motion from talking.
6. After the client removes his or her hand from the volumeter and dries it (provide a towel), the therapist uses

the 500-mL graduated cylinder to measure the amount of displaced water to the nearest 5 mL. The use of a 10-mL micropipette allows the therapist to measure the displaced water to the nearest 1 mL, thereby increasing accuracy. Occasionally, more than 500 mL will be displaced, and multiple graduated cylinders will be needed, or the water will be measured to 500 mL and then discarded, the graduated cylinder dried out, and the remaining water measured and added to the 500 mL already measured.

This protocol showed high reliability over two repeated tests on 50 hands, showing a test–retest reliability of 0.99 (Dodds et al., 2004). To interpret findings, compare the measurement of the affected part with that of its contralateral counterpart. If edema is present, the short-term goal of treatment may be to decrease edema more than 10 mL, which is more than the standard error of measurement of less than 3 mL (Dodds et al., 2004). However, it is important to remember the reasoning behind wanting the decrease in edema. For example, the entire short-term goal may be written as, "The patient will demonstrate a 10-mL decrease in volumeter measurement of edema of the right hand in order to increase hand function with dressing tasks."

A second method of measuring edema of the whole hand is the figure-of-eight technique (Pellecchia, 2004). This method is based on the understanding that edema of the hand tends to collect more dorsally. Using a ¼-inch wide tape measure with the wrist in neutral and fingers adducted, the tape is started at the medial aspect of the wrist just distal to the ulnar styloid. The tape is then run across the volar surface of the wrist to the most distal point of the radial styloid and then run diagonally across the dorsum of the hand to the fifth MP joint. The tape is then run across the heads of the metacarpals to the second MP joint and then back across the dorsum of the hand to the starting point. The measurement recorded is the distance measured by the tape in centimeters (Fig. 7-66). The interrater and the intrarater reliabilities for this method are high ($r = 0.98$–0.99) (Leard et al., 2004; Pellecchia, 2004). When the figure-of-eight measurement was compared to the submersion method in a normal population, the two methods were highly correlated ($r = 0.94$–0.95) (Maihafer et al., 2003). The figure-of-eight measurement technique may be especially appropriate when volumetry is contraindicated.

In a study by Dewey et al. (2007), this method has also been shown to be reliable and valid in the measurement of edema in patients with burns to the hands. Intrarater reliability in this population was ICC = 0.96–0.97, and interrater reliability was ICC = 0.94. Correlation between the figure-of-eight method and volumetry was also good ($r = 0.83$–0.90). This study emphasized the time efficiency and cost savings of the figure-of-eight method and the preference for this method, particularly in the intensive care unit setting. They identified a standard error of

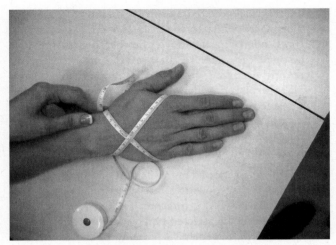

Figure 7-66 Measuring edema of the hand using the figure-of-eight method.

measurement in the 33 hands measured of 1.16 cm and recommended that changes in this measurement must exceed this number in order to be clinically significant (Dewey et al., 2007).

PAIN

Pain is another possible cause of ROM limitations. Pain or fear of pain may affect a person's willingness to move. Pain is very subjective, and although therapists often assign a numerical value to the intensity of pain, that number is very individual and cannot be compared to any normative value or with any other patient (Farrar, Berlin, & Strom, 2003). Pain is also multidimensional, and by discussing the different components with the patient, the therapist can elicit a better understanding of how pain is impacting function. Components of pain include intensity, duration, location, description of type of pain, and the emotional impact of pain (Williamson & Hoggart, 2005). Because pain is subjective, self-report measures provide the most valid measure of the experience. Several self-report measures include the Visual Analog Scale (VAS), the Wong-Baker FACES® Pain-Rating Scale, the Numerical Rating Scale (NRS), and the Verbal Rating Scale (VRS) (Hockenberry & Wilson, 2009; Williamson & Hoggart, 2005).

The VAS consists of a 100-mm line with ends of the line designated with descriptions such as "no pain at all" and "the worst pain possible." The patient marks on the line the point that represents the intensity of the pain he or she feels. The score is obtained by measuring the line from the zero point to the patient's mark in cm. A review of data from two randomized controlled trials using the VAS suggests the following:

- 0–4 mm: no pain
- 5–44 mm: mild pain

- 45–74 mm: moderate pain
- 75–100 mm: severe pain

A 33% decrease in pain is needed on this scale in order for it to be significant (Jensen, Chen, & Brugger, 2003).

The NRS also has good sensitivity and is frequently used when evaluating pain. The 0–10 range is typical for the NRS, but this scale has also been used with 0–20 and 0–100 ranges. With the NRS, it has been suggested that a difference of 2 points on the 0–10 scale indicates a clinically significant difference (Farrar, Berlin, & Strom, 2003). This knowledge can be helpful in goal writing. For example, a patient with osteoarthritis of the carpometacarpal (CMC) joint of the right dominant hand may report a pain level of 7 out of 10 on initial evaluation. The therapist should ask in the discussion of pain with the client, "What would you like to be able to do if you had less pain in your hand?" The client may list several activities, such as completing housework, gardening, and caring for his or her pets. A short-term goal written to reflect this information could be, "The patient will report a decrease in pain of the right hand to 5 out of 10 or less with the use of joint protection techniques and clinical treatment in order to increase function for household and leisure tasks."

The verbal rating scale asks patients to describe their pain such as "none," "mild," "moderate," or "severe." Some therapists will turn this description into a 4-point scale. All of the pain-rating tools described have been researched for their reliability and sensitivity in detecting change in pain levels. Examples of the various pain scales can be found in Figures 7-67 and 7-68.

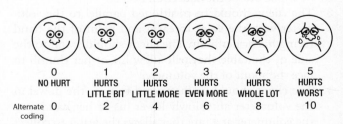

| 0 | 1 | 2 | 3 | 4 | 5 |
| NO HURT | HURTS LITTLE BIT | HURTS LITTLE MORE | HURTS EVEN MORE | HURTS WHOLE LOT | HURTS WORST |

Alternate coding: 0 2 4 6 8 10

Brief word instructions: Point to each face using the words to describe the pain intensity. Ask the child to choose face that best describes their own pain and record the appropriate number.

Original instructions: Explain to the person that each face is for a person who feels happy because he has no pain (hurt) or sad because he has some or a lot of pain. Face 0 is very happy because he doesn't hurt at all. Face 1 hurts just a little bit. Face 2 hurts a little more. Face 3 hurts even more. Face 4 hurts a whole lot. Face 5 hurts as much as you can imagine, although you don't have to be crying to feel this bad. Ask the person to choose the face that best describes how he is feeling.

Rating scale is recommended for persons age 3 years and older.

Figure 7-67 FACES Pain Scale.

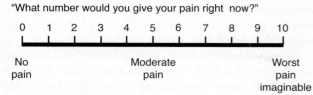

"What number would you give your pain right now?"

0   1   2   3   4   5   6   7   8   9   10

No   Moderate   Worst
pain   pain   pain
                                      imaginable

Figure 7-68 Example Pain Scales.

Often the therapist will ask the client about pain at the beginning of the evaluation, but it is also important to ask about increases in pain during the evaluation of ROM and strength. The report of pain should be documented along with the ROM limitations. By asking questions regarding where the pain is specifically located and the type and intensity of the pain, underlying conditions impacting motion and strength can sometimes be identified.

For example, a patient may present for evaluation following a distal radius fracture, but the pain he or she reports may be along the volar wrist and thenar aspect of the hand with a description of burning and pins and needles radiating into the radial digits. This pain may actually be from compression of the median nerve at the wrist level (i.e., carpal tunnel syndrome) from the initial injury or from the edema that resulted from the injury. The therapist may choose to do additional testing, and it may be appropriate to contact the referring orthopedic surgeon if this is a new finding.

It is important to know your patient population when selecting the most appropriate pain scale, and often one clinic will need more than one scale depending on the age, education, culture, and cognitive skills of the population being served. For example, the Wong-Baker FACES pain scale is more appropriate for the pediatric population than is asking children to rate their pain with the NRS (Hockenberry & Wilson, 2009). The clinician can also note any observations of pain, such as facial expressions (e.g., wincing) or physical motion (e.g., retraction of the extremity being tested).

SCAR TISSUE

Scar tissue, particularly scars that cross joints or run along tendons, can significantly impact motion. All wounds will heal with scar tissue, but not all scar tissue will impact motion. The size, color, and characteristics of any wounds or scars should be described during initial and subsequent evaluations. Typically, by manipulating the scar tissue with the fingers and pinching the skin around the scar, a therapist can determine whether any significant scar adhesions exist. Skin puckering around the scar with motion can also be a sign of adhesions (see additional information on wound healing and scar tissue in Chapters 19 and 37).

MUSCLE STRENGTH

Muscular strength, the "ability of the muscle to exert force," is a key component of muscular fitness (American College of Sports Medicine, 2010b, p. 86). Weakness is a lack or reduction of the power of a muscle or muscle group. When weakness limits or impairs the individual's occupational functioning, determining the degree and distribution of weakness to establish an appropriate intervention plan is necessary. Treatment can be focused on remediating the weakness, or it can focus on alternative ways of accomplishing the task. Weakness can manifest in several forms. It can be general, such as with Guillain-Barré syndrome, or it can be local, such as with a peripheral nerve lesion. In the former case, muscles throughout the body are assessed; in the latter case, just the muscles innervated by the involved nerve are tested. In both cases, the muscles to be tested are the ones contributing to the functional limitations on which treatment will focus.

A maximum voluntary contraction (MVC), the maximum amount of tension that can be produced under voluntary control, is commonly used to measure strength (Wilmore & Costill, 1999). Because muscle testing is a measurement of voluntary contraction of an isolated muscle or muscle group, strength testing is inappropriate for patients who lack the ability to contract a single muscle or a muscle group in isolation such as patients who exhibit patterned movement.

In this chapter, a technique called the "break test" is used. In the break test, the muscle to be tested is positioned at its greatest mechanical advantage. Once the extremity is positioned, the patient is asked to hold the position as the tester imparts external force (i.e., his or her hand and own strength) to overcome the contractile force of the muscle or muscle group. In other words, the therapist tries to break the patient's isometric contraction (Bohannon, 1988). *Safety Message: The therapist must ensure that providing resistance is not contraindicated by the diagnosis or the surgeon's orders for therapy. For example, putting resistance against a patient with a healing fracture, following various surgeries such as tendon or nerve repairs, after chest/heart/lung surgery, initially after myocardial infarction, where there is a history of bone metastasis, or after recent back/neck surgery is contraindicated. Precautions should also be taken with various neurodegenerative disorders so as not to stress fatigued or weakened muscles.*

The term *mechanical advantage* refers to the length–tension relationship of a muscle. The passive tension exerted by the elastic components in the lengthened muscle and surrounding tissue and the active tension generated by the contractile elements of the contracting muscle contribute to the total tension of a muscle (Hall & Brody, 1999). A muscle is able to generate its greatest total tension or sustain the heaviest load when positioned at a length that gives it optimal mechanical advantage. This is usually slightly (10%) longer than resting length. Developed (active) tension, which is the total tension minus the elastic contribution, is greatest at resting length but decreases as the muscle shortens or lengthens. The length–tension principle is used to elicit the best response from prime movers during muscle testing. Furthermore, this principle is used to reduce the contribution of synergist muscles when testing the prime mover. Synergist muscles are placed at a mechanical disadvantage (either lengthened or shortened), whereas the prime mover is asked to resist the applied force (Hall & Brody, 1999). For muscles or muscle groups too weak to resist an external force, muscle strength is evaluated by isotonic contraction, in which the muscle is required to move the mass of the body part against gravity without applied resistance or with the effect of gravity decreased (Hislop & Montgomery, 1995; Kendall et al., 2005).

Gravity as resistance is considered an important variable and is used to test all motions when practical. Standard procedures for evaluation against gravity and with gravity eliminated are described in this chapter. Tests of the UE described here for the most part are motion tests for the purpose of evaluating strength in terms of functional ability. Tests of individual muscles in the wrist and hand are included because of the responsibility of the occupational therapist in the rehabilitation of hand injuries. The movements of the face, head, neck, and trunk, although important in the assessment of some patients,

have not been included in the interest of conserving space; however, this information can be found in references listed at the end of this chapter.

Prior to the start of MMT, an ROM scan should be done to determine what ROM is available at each joint. Although the available range is considered to be full ROM for the purposes of muscle testing, notation should be made of any limitation. The muscle or muscle group is assigned a grade according to the amount of resistance it can take. Two grading systems are presented here: Table 7-1 equates the Medical Research Council (1976) Oxford system to the descriptive grading system (Clarkson, 2000).

Procedures for Practice 7-4 shows the sequence of steps for testing every muscle or muscle group to ensure reliability and accuracy. There are additional considerations when performing an MMT. First, although fatigue differs for each person and each muscle, a rest of 2 minutes between maximum effort contractions of the same muscle is considered adequate (Milner-Brown, Mellenthin, & Miller, 1986). Second, for the comfort and convenience of the patient, all testing in one position is done before the patient changes to another position. Also, the positions of head, neck, and proximal parts are usually kept the same from test to test, although preliminary study results indicated that this does not affect tension development (Anderson & Bohannon, 1991; Bohannon, Warren, & Cogman, 1991).

Other methods of muscle testing can provide more specific data regarding strength, such as isokinetic testing done mostly in research and handheld dynamometry,

Table 7-1 Muscle Testing Grading System

Numerical Grade	Descriptive Grade	Definition
5	Normal	The part moves through full ROM against gravity and takes maximal resistance.
4	Good	The part moves through full ROM against gravity and takes moderate resistance.
4−	Good minus	The part moves through full ROM against gravity and takes less than moderate resistance.
3+	Fair plus	The part moves through full ROM against gravity and takes minimal resistance before it breaks.
3	Fair	The part moves through full ROM against gravity and is unable to take any added resistance.
3−	Fair minus	The part moves less than full range of motion against gravity.
2+	Poor plus	The part moves through full ROM in a gravity-eliminated plane, takes minimal resistance, and then breaks.
2	Poor	The part moves through full ROM in a gravity-eliminated plane with no added resistance.
2−	Poor minus	The part moves less than full ROM in a gravity-eliminated plane, no resistance.
1	Trace	Tension is palpated in the muscle or tendon, but no motion occurs at the joint.
0	Zero	No tension is palpated in the muscle or tendon, and no motion occurs.

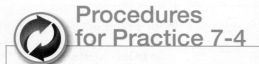

Procedures for Practice 7-4

Muscle Testing Procedures

1. Explain the procedure and demonstrate the desired movement.
2. Position the patient so that the direction of movement will be against gravity.
3. Stabilize proximal to the joint that will move to prevent substitutions.
4. Instruct the patient to move actively to the end position. If the patient cannot move actively against gravity, place the patient in a gravity-eliminated position, and ask him or her to move actively in this position.
5. If the patient can move actively against gravity, tell the patient to hold the contraction at the end position.
6. Apply resistance:
   - to the distal end of the segment into which the muscle inserts
   - in the direction the movement came from
   - by starting with light resistance and increasing to maximal resistance over a 2- to 3-second period
7. Palpate over the prime mover to determine whether the muscle is contracting or whether gravity and/or synergistic muscles are substituting.
8. Record the appropriate grade according to the resistance tolerated before the muscle broke or by the amount of movement achieved without resistance in an against-gravity or gravity-eliminated position.

which uses MMT set up with the dynamometer directly against the body part being tested to register specific muscle strength when resistance is applied. The majority of the research shows moderate to good reliability and validity with the use of the handheld dynamometer, and the limitations seem to be a lack of standardized testing procedures and the inability of the therapist to resist against the body part being tested (Stark et al., 2011). The joint is placed in a gravity-eliminated position, and the handheld dynamometer is placed perpendicular to the limb segment. The patient is asked to build a maximum contraction against the dynamometer for a 1- to 2-second period and then to hold that contraction against the dynamometer for 4–5 seconds. The recorded measure is the maximum isometric value that was achieved by the patient. This type of measurement is particularly helpful for quantifying antigravity strength, grades 3+ to 5 (Hayes et al., 2002).

Reliability

Reliability is essential for meaningful evaluation. Most important to the reliability of the scores of repeated tests is strict adherence to the exact procedures of testing. In addition, reliability of muscle testing scores is affected by the interest and cooperation of the patient and by the experience and tone of voice of the tester, with higher volume eliciting greater muscle contractions (Johannson, Kent, & Shepard, 1983). The most suitable environment is free of distractions, is at a comfortable temperature, and has proper lighting. Other factors known to affect outcome are posture, fatigue, the patient's ability to understand directions, the therapist's operational definitions of various grades, and test positions (Kendall et al., 2005). For reliability, these variables must be controlled from test to test and among therapists at the same facility. It is necessary for the inexperienced therapist to develop a kinesthetic sense of minimal, moderate, and maximal resistances by working with experienced therapists, each testing the same patient and discussing the grade to be assigned.

MMT is a valid and reliable procedure to measure muscle strength (Herbison et al., 1996; Schwartz et al., 1992). A study of reliability for testing intrinsic hand muscles found the correlation for intrarater reliability to range from 0.71 to 0.96 and from 0.72 to 0.93 for interrater reliability (Brandsma et al., 1995). Florence et al. (1992) performed MMT on patients with Duchenne muscular dystrophy and, using a standard method of testing and the modified Medical Research Council grading scale (Table 7-1), found that reliability for muscle grades 0–5 ranged from 0.80 to 0.99. The most reliable grades were 3 and below, with the least reliable grades being 3+ (0.80), 4− (0.83), and 5− (0.83), those that involve a developed kinesthetic sense of minimal, moderate, and maximal resistance.

Recording Muscle Strength Scores

Muscle strength must be accurately documented in the medical record, identifying muscle tested, grades assigned to the right and left sides, date of testing, and electronic or physical signature of the therapist performing the evaluation. A sample form is presented in Figure 7-69. On that form, the peripheral nerve and spinal segmental levels are listed beside each muscle to assist the therapist in interpreting the results of the muscle test.

On the pages that follow, the reader will find narrative and pictorial descriptions to help in understanding and practicing measurement of UE strength.

Patient's Name: _____ Age: _____

	LEFT			RIGHT	
Date	Date			Date	Date

Scapula

		ELEVATION			
		Upper trapezius (accessory) CN XI, C3-4			
		Levator scapulae (dorsal scapular) C5, C3-4			
		DEPRESSION			
		Lower trapezius (accessory) CN XI, C3-4			
		Latissimus dorsi (thoracodorsal) C6-8			
		ADDUCTION			
		Middle trapezius (accessory) CN XI, C3-4			
		Rhomboids (dorsal scapular) C5			
		ABDUCTION			
		Serratus anterior (long thoracic) C5-7			

Shoulder

		FLEXION			
		Anterior deltoid (axillary) C5-6			
		Coracobrachialis (musculocutaneous) C5-6			
		Pectoralis major-clavicular (pectoral) C5-6			
		Biceps (musculocutaneous) C5-6			
		EXTENSION			
		Latissimus dorsi (thoracodorsal) C6-8			
		Teres major (lower subscapular) C5-6			
		Posterior deltoid (axillary) C5-6			
		Triceps-long head (radial) C7-8			
		ABDUCTION			
		Supraspinatus (suprascapular) C5-6			
		Middle deltoid (axillary) C5-6			
		ADDUCTION			
		Latissimus dorsi (thoracodorsal) C6-8			
		Teres major (lower subscapular) C5-6			
		Pectoralis major (pectoral) C5-T1			
		HORIZONTAL ABDUCTION			
		Posterior deltoid (axillary) C5-6			
		Pectoralis major (pectoral) C5-T1			
		Anterior deltoid (axillary) C5-6			
		EXTERNAL ROTATION			
		Infraspinatus (suprascapular) C5-6			
		Teres minor (axillary) C5-6			
		Posterior deltoid (axillary) C5-6			
		INTERNAL ROTATION			
		Subscapularis (upper, lower subscapular) C5-7			
		Teres major (lower subscapular) C6-7			
		Latissimus dorsi (thoracodorsal) C6-8			
		Pectoralis major (pectoral) C5-T1			
		Anterior deltoid (axillary) C5-6			

Elbow

		FLEXION			
		Biceps (musculocutaneous) C5-6			
		Brachioradialis (radial) C5-7			
		Brachialis (musculocutaneous) C5-6 (radial) C7-8			
		EXTENSION			
		Triceps (radial) C6-8			

Figure 7-69 Sample form for recording manual muscle strength. (Reprinted with permission from Pansky, B. [1996]. *Review of gross anatomy* [6th ed.]. New York: McGraw-Hill.) *(continued)*

Patient's Name: _____   Age: _____
 LEFT   RIGHT

Date	Date		Date	Date
		Forearm		
		PRONATION		
		Pronator teres (median) C6-7		
		Pronator quadratus (median) C8-T1		
		SUPINATION		
		Supinator (radial) C5-6		
		Biceps (musculocutaneous) C5-6		
		Wrist		
		EXTENSION		
		Ext. carpi radialis longus (radial) C6-7		
		Ext. carpi radialis brevis (radial) C7-8		
		Ext. carpi ulnaris (radial) C7-8		
		FLEXION		
		Flexor carpi radialis (median) C6-7		
		Palmaris longus (median) C7-8		
		Flexor carpi ulnaris (ulnar) C8-T1		
		Fingers		
		DIP FLEXION		
		1st flexor profundus (median) C8-T1		
		2nd flexor profundus (median) C8-T1		
		3rd flexor profundus (ulnar) C8-T1		
		4th flexor profundus (ulnar) C8-T1		
		5TH MP FLEXION		
		Flexor digiti minimi (ulnar) C8-T1		
		PIP FLEXION		
		1st flexor superficialis (median) C7-T1		
		2nd flexor superficialis (median) C7-T1		
		3rd flexor superficialis (median) C7-T1		
		4th flexor superficialis (median) C7-T1		
		ABDUCTION		
		1st palmar interosseus (ulnar) C8-T1		
		2nd palmar interosseus (ulnar) C8-T1		
		3rd palmar interosseus (ulnar) C8-T1		
		1st dorsal interosseus (ulnar) C8-T1		
		2nd dorsal interosseus (ulnar) C8-T1		
		3rd dorsal interosseus (ulnar) C8-T1		
		4th dorsal interosseus (ulnar) C8-T1		
		MP EXTENSION		
		1st extensor digitorum (radial) C7-8		
		2nd extensor digitorum (radial) C7-8		
		3rd extensor digitorum (radial) C7-8		
		4th extensor digitorum (radial) C7-8		
		Extensor digiti minimi (radial) C7-8		
		IP EXTENSION		
		1st lumbrical (median) C8-T1		
		2nd lumbrical (median) C8-T1		
		3rd lumbrical (ulnar) C8-T1		
		4th lumbrical (ulnar) C8-T1		

Figure 7-69 *(continued)*

Patient's Name: _____ Age: _____

		LEFT	RIGHT	
Date	Date		Date	Date

		Thumb		
		EXTENSION		
		Extensor pollicis longus (radial) C7-8		
		Extensor pollicis brevis (radial) C7-8		
		FLEXION		
		Flexor pollicis longus (median) C8-T1		
		Flexor pollicis brevis (median) C8-T1		
		ABDUCTION		
		Abductor pollicis longus (radial) C7-8		
		Abductor pollicis brevis (median) C8-T1		
		ADDUCTOR		
		Adductor pollicis (ulnar) C8-T1		
		OPPOSITION		
		Opponens pollicis (median) C8-T1		
		Opponens digiti minimi (ulnar) C8-T1		
		Hip		
		FLEXION		
		Iliopsoas (femoral) L2-3		
		EXTENSION		
		Gluteus maximus (inf. gluteal) L5-S2		
		Knee		
		FLEXION		
		Hamstrings (tibial) L5-S2		
		EXTENSION		
		Quadriceps (femoral) L2-4		
		Ankle		
		DORSIFLEXION		
		Tibialis anterior (deep peroneal) L4-S1		
		Extensor digitorum longus (deep peroneal) L4-S1		
		Extensor hallucis longus (deep peroneal) L4-S1		
		PLANTARFLEXION		
		Gastrocnemius (tibial) S1-2		
		Soleus (tibial) S1-2		

Therapist's signature: _____ Date: _____

Figure 7-69 *(continued)*

PROXIMAL UPPER EXTREMITY MEASUREMENT

Scapular Elevation

Prime Movers

Upper trapezius and levator scapulae.

Against-Gravity Position (Fig. 7-70)

Start Position. Patient sitting erect with arms at side.

Stabilize. Trunk is stabilized against the chair back.

Instruction. "Lift your shoulders toward your ears like you are shrugging. Do not let me push them down."

Resistance. The therapist places his or her hands over each acromion and pushes down toward scapular depression. A normal adult trapezius cannot be broken.

Substitution. It could appear that the patient's shoulders elevated if he or she placed the hands on the legs to push the shoulders into elevation.

Gravity-Eliminated Position (Fig. 7-71)

Start Position. Prone with arms at side and therapist supporting under the shoulder.

Stabilize. The trunk is stabilized against the mat or plinth.

Instruction. "Lift your shoulder toward your ear."

Palpation. The upper trapezius is palpated on the shoulder at the curve of the neck. The levator scapulae is palpated posterior to the sternocleidomastoideus on the lateral side of the neck.

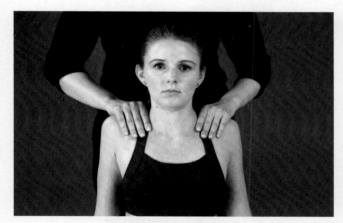

Figure 7-70 Scapular elevation against gravity.

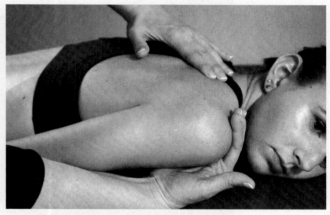

Figure 7-71 Scapular elevation, gravity eliminated.

Scapular Depression

Prime Movers

Lower trapezius and latissimus dorsi.

Resistance Test (Fig. 7-72)

Start Position. This movement is tested in a gravity-eliminated position because the patient cannot be positioned to move against gravity. The patient lies prone with arms by the sides.

Stabilize. The trunk is stabilized by the mat or plinth.

Instruction. "Reach your hand down toward your feet."

Resistance. The therapist's hand cups the inferior angle of the scapula; the therapist pushes up toward scapular elevation. When the inferior angle is not easily accessible because of tissue bulk, apply resistance at the distal humerus if the shoulder joint is stable and pain free.

Palpation. Palpate the lower trapezius lateral to the vertebral column as it passes diagonally from the lower thoracic vertebrae to the spine of the scapula. Palpate the latissimus dorsi along the posterior rib cage or in the posterior axilla as it attaches to the humerus.

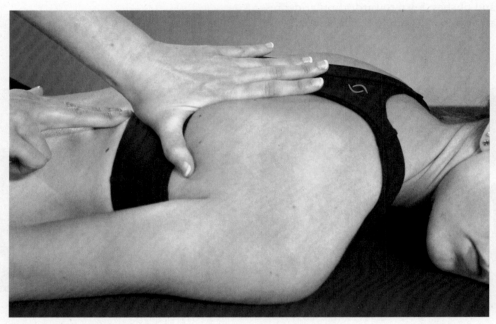

Figure 7-72 Scapular depression.

Scapular Adduction: Retraction

Prime Movers

Middle trapezius and rhomboids.

Against-Gravity Position for the Middle Trapezius (Fig. 7-73)

Start Position. Prone on a mat with the shoulder abducted to 90° and the elbow flexed to 90°.

Stabilize. The trunk is stabilized against the mat or plinth. Additional stabilization over the contralateral scapula provides counterpressure during action and resistance.

Instruction. "Raise your elbow toward the ceiling. Do not let me push it down."

Resistance. Apply resistance laterally at the vertebral border of the scapula or, if the shoulder is stable and pain free, downward at the distal humerus.

Palpation. With your hand over the vertebral border of the scapula, feel to determine whether the scapula stays adducted during resistance. Palpate the middle trapezius between the vertebral column and vertebral border of the scapula at the level of the spine of the scapula.

Against-Gravity Position for the Rhomboids (Fig. 7-74)

Start Position. Prone on the mat with the shoulder internally rotated and with the back of the hand resting on the lumbar region.

Stabilize. The trunk is stabilized against the mat or plinth. Additional stabilization over the contralateral scapula will provide counterpressure during action and resistance.

Instruction. "Lift your hand off of your back. Do not let me push it down."

Resistance. Apply downward resistance against the distal humerus or, if the shoulder is unstable or painful, against the vertebral border of the scapula in the direction of scapular abduction.

Palpation. Palpate the rhomboids along the vertebral border of the scapula near the inferior angle. The rhomboids are located deep to the trapezius, and the positioning of the hand in the small of the back allows the trapezius to remain relaxed so the rhomboids can be palpated.

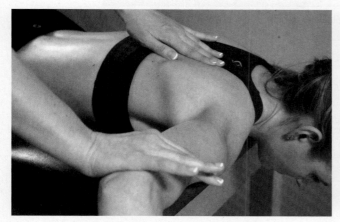

Figure 7-73 Scapular adduction, test for middle trapezius.

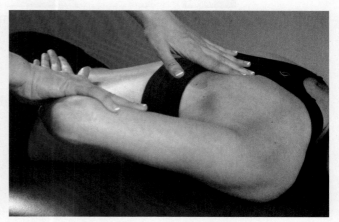

Figure 7-74 Scapular adduction, test for rhomboids.

Gravity-Eliminated Position for the Middle Trapezius and Rhomboids (Fig. 7-75)

Start Position. Sitting erect with the humerus abducted to 90° and supported.

Stabilize. The trunk is stabilized by the chair. Note a table or the therapist's arm can be used to support the arm of the individual being tested.

Instruction. "Try to move your arm backward."

Grading. If the scapula moves toward the spine, give a grade of 2. If no movement is noted, palpate the scapular adductors.

Palpation. Same as previously described.

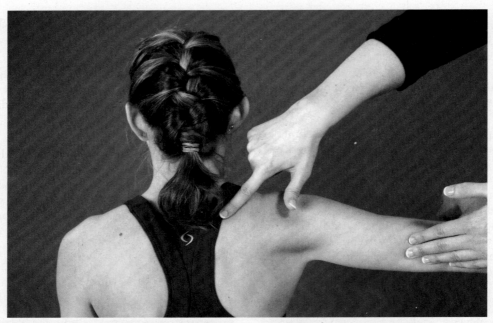

Figure 7-75 Scapular adduction, gravity eliminated. The therapist is pointing to the middle trapezius.

Scapular Abduction: Protraction

Prime Mover

Serratus anterior.

Against-Gravity Position (Fig. 7-76)

Start Position. Supine with the humerus flexed to 90°. The elbow may be flexed or extended.

Stabilize. The trunk is stabilized on the mat or plinth.

Instruction. "Reach your arm toward the ceiling."

Resistance. According to the rule, resistance should be applied along the axillary border of the scapula. Because it is difficult to apply resistance there, therapists often resist this motion either by grasping the distal humerus or by cupping the hand over the patient's elbow and pushing down or back toward scapular adduction. (*Note:* This method is not used if the glenohumeral joint is unstable or painful.)

Gravity-Eliminated Position (Fig. 7-77)

Start Position. Sitting erect with the humerus flexed to 90° and supported.

Stabilize. The trunk is stabilized against the chair.

Instruction. "Try to reach your arm forward."

Grading. Movement of the scapula into abduction receives a grade of 2. If no movement occurs, palpate the serratus anterior.

Palpation. Palpate the serratus anterior on the lateral ribs just lateral to the inferior angle of the scapula.

Substitution. In the gravity-eliminated position, this motion can be achieved by inching the arm forward on a supportive surface using the finger flexors.

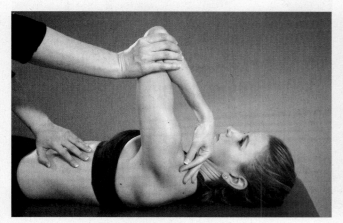

Figure 7-76 Scapular abduction against gravity.

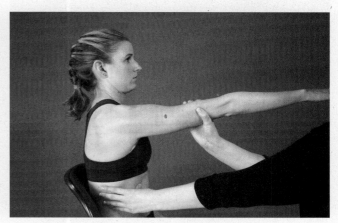

Figure 7-77 Scapular abduction, gravity eliminated.

Shoulder Flexion

Prime Movers

Anterior deltoid; coracobrachialis; and pectoralis major, clavicular head; biceps, both heads.

Against-Gravity Position (Fig. 7-78)

Start Position. Sitting in a chair with the arm down at the side in midposition.

Stabilize. Over the clavicle and the scapula.

Instruction. "Lift your arm in front of you to shoulder height. Do not let me push it down."

Resistance. The therapist's hand, placed over the distal end of the humerus, pushes down toward extension. Movement above 90° involves scapular rotation; these motions are separated for muscle testing, although they are not separated for ROM measurement.

Substitutions. Shoulder abductors, scapular elevation, or trunk extension.

Gravity-Eliminated Position (Fig. 7-79)

Start Position. Lying on the side with the arm along the side of the body in midposition; therapist supports the arm under the elbow.

Instruction. "Try to move your arm so your hand is at the level of your shoulder."

Palpation. Palpate the anterior deltoid immediately anterior to the glenohumeral joint. The coracobrachialis may be palpated medially to the tendon of the long head of the biceps, which is palpated on the anterior aspect of the humerus. The clavicular head of the pectoralis major may be palpated below the clavicle on its way to insert on the humerus below the anterior deltoid.

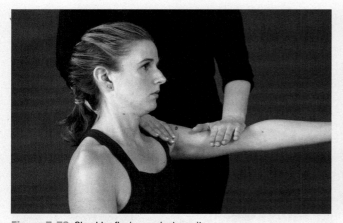

Figure 7-78 Shoulder flexion against gravity.

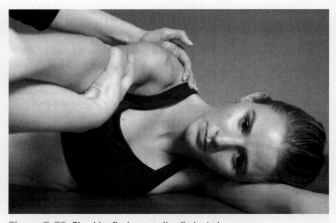

Figure 7-79 Shoulder flexion, gravity eliminated.

Shoulder Extension

Prime Movers

Latissimus dorsi; teres major; posterior deltoid; and triceps, long head.

Against-Gravity Position (Fig. 7-80)

Start Position. Sitting with the arm by the side and the humerus internally rotated.

Stabilize. Over the clavicle and scapula; make sure the patient remains upright.

Instruction. "Move your arm straight back as far as it will go. Keep your palm facing the back wall."

Resistance. The therapist's hand, placed over the distal end of the humerus, pushes forward toward flexion.

Substitutions. Shoulder abductors, tipping the shoulder forward, bending the trunk forward.

Gravity-Eliminated Position (Fig. 7-81)

Start Position. Lying on the side with the arm along the side of the body and in internal rotation. Therapist supports the elbow during the motion.

Instruction. "Try to move your arm backward."

Palpation. The latissimus dorsi and teres major form the posterior border of the axilla. The latissimus dorsi is inferior to the teres major. The posterior deltoid is immediately posterior to the glenohumeral joint. The triceps are palpated on the posterior aspect of the humerus.

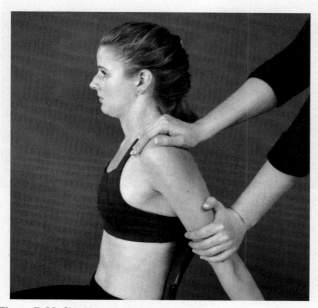

Figure 7-80 Shoulder extension against gravity.

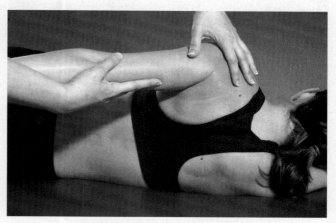

Figure 7-81 Shoulder extension, gravity eliminated.

Shoulder Abduction

Prime Movers

Supraspinatus and middle deltoid.

Against-Gravity Position (Fig. 7-82)

Start Position. Sitting erect with the arm down at the side and in midposition.

Stabilize. Over the clavicle and the scapula.

Instruction. "Raise your arm out to the side to shoulder level. Do not let me push it down."

Resistance. The therapist's hand, placed over the distal end of the humerus, pushes the humerus down toward the body. Movement above 90° involves scapular rotation and is not measured.

Substitutions. The long head of the biceps can substitute if the humerus is allowed to move into external rotation; trunk lateral flexion.

Gravity-Eliminated Position (Fig. 7-83)

Start Position. Supine with the arm supported at the side in midposition. The therapist supports the elbow during the motion.

Instruction. "Try to move your arm out to the side."

Palpation. The supraspinatus lies too deep for easy palpation. Palpate the middle deltoid below the acromion and lateral to the glenohumeral joint.

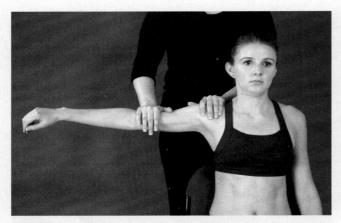

Figure 7-82 Shoulder abduction against gravity.

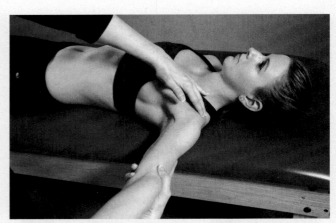

Figure 7-83 Shoulder abduction, gravity eliminated.

Shoulder Adduction

Prime Movers

Pectoralis major, teres major, and latissimus dorsi.

Gravity-Eliminated Position (Fig. 7-84)

The patient cannot be positioned for this motion against gravity.

Start Position. Supine with the humerus abducted to 90° and the forearm in midposition.

Stabilize. The trunk is stabilized by the mat.

Instruction. "Bring your arm down to your side, and do not let me pull it away."

Resistance. The therapist's hand, placed on the medial side of the distal end of the humerus, attempts to pull the humerus away from the patient's body.

Palpation. The pectoralis major forms the anterior border of the axilla, where it may be easily palpated. Palpation of the teres major and the latissimus dorsi is described earlier in the chapter.

Grading. Antigravity grades can only be estimated; a question mark should be entered beside the grade on the form. With experience, the therapist develops the skill to estimate reliably.

Substitutions. On a supporting surface, the arm can be inched down using the finger flexors.

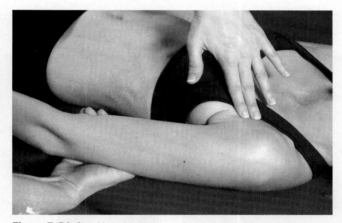

Figure 7-84 Shoulder adduction.

Shoulder Horizontal Abduction

Prime Mover

Posterior deltoid.

Against-Gravity Position (Fig. 7-85).

Start Position. Prone with the arm over the edge of the mat. The shoulder is abducted to 90°, and the elbow is flexed to 90°.

Stabilize. The scapula and trunk are stabilized by the mat. Counterpressure over the contralateral scapula is helpful during action and resistance.

Instruction. "Raise your elbow toward the ceiling."

Resistance. The therapist's hand, placed on the posterior surface of the distal end of the humerus, pushes the arm down toward horizontal adduction.

Gravity-Eliminated Position (Fig. 7-86)

Start Position. Sitting in a chair with the humerus supported in 90° of flexion and the elbow straight. The therapist supports the elbow.

Stabilize. The trunk is stabilized against the back of the chair.

Instruction. "Try to move your arm out to the side."

Palpation. Palpate the posterior deltoid immediately posterior to the glenohumeral joint.

Substitution. Trunk rotation.

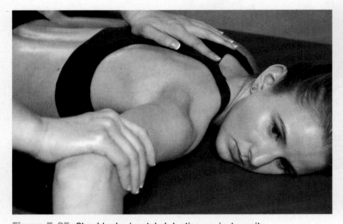

Figure 7-85 Shoulder horizontal abduction against gravity.

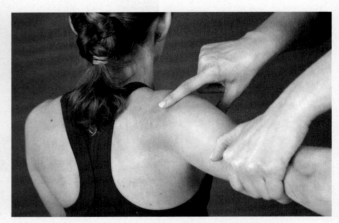

Figure 7-86 Shoulder horizontal abduction, gravity eliminated.

Shoulder Horizontal Adduction

Prime Movers

Pectoralis major and anterior deltoid.

Against-Gravity Position (Fig. 7-87)

Start Position. Supine with the humerus abducted to 90° in neutral rotation and the elbow extended.

Stabilize. The table stabilizes the scapula and trunk. If the elbow extensors are weak, be sure to support the distal end of the forearm so the hand does not fall into the patient's face during horizontal adduction.

Instruction. "Move your arm in front of you and across your chest."

Resistance. The therapist's hand, placed on the anterior surface of the distal end of the humerus, pulls the arm out toward horizontal abduction.

Gravity-Eliminated Position (Fig. 7-88)

Start Position. Sitting in a chair with the arm abducted to 90°.

Stabilize. The trunk is stabilized against the back of the chair. The therapist supports the arm under the elbow.

Instruction. "Try to bring your arm across your chest."

Palpation. Palpate the pectoralis major along the anterior border of the axilla. The anterior deltoid is immediately anterior to the glenohumeral joint below the acromion process and superior to the pectoralis major.

Substitutions. Trunk rotation can substitute. The arm can be inched across a supporting surface using the finger flexors.

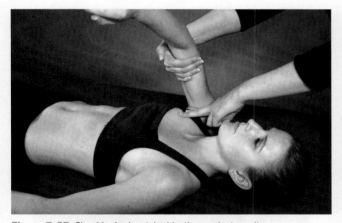

Figure 7-87 Shoulder horizontal adduction against gravity.

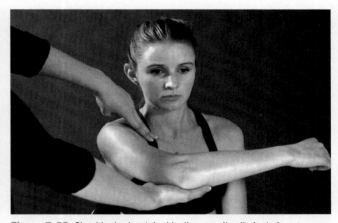

Figure 7-88 Shoulder horizontal adduction, gravity eliminated.

Shoulder External Rotation

Prime Movers

Infraspinatus, teres minor, and posterior deltoid.

Against-Gravity Position (Fig. 7-89)

Start Position. Prone with the humerus abducted to 90° and supported by the mat. The elbow is flexed to 90° and is hanging over the edge of the table.

Stabilize. The humerus is held just proximal to the elbow to allow only rotation.

Instruction. "Lift the back of your hand toward the ceiling."

Resistance. The therapist's hand, placed on the dorsal surface of the distal end of the forearm, pushes toward the floor. The therapist's other hand keeps the patient's elbow supported and flexed to 90° to prevent supination.

Substitutions. Scapula adduction combined with downward rotation can substitute. The triceps may substitute when resistance is applied.

Gravity-Eliminated Position (Fig. 7-90)

Start Position. Prone with the entire arm hanging over the edge of the mat. The arm is in internal rotation.

Stabilize. The trunk and scapula are stabilized on the mat.

Instruction. "Try to turn your palm outward."

Palpation. Palpate the infraspinatus inferior to the spine of the scapula. Palpate the teres minor between the posterior deltoid and the axillary border of the scapula; it is superior to the teres major. Palpation of the posterior deltoid was described earlier.

Substitution. Supination may be mistaken for external rotation in a gravity-eliminated position.

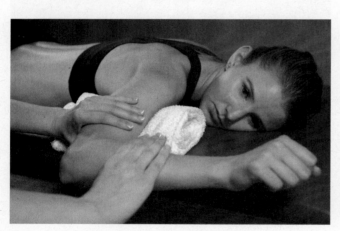

Figure 7-89 Shoulder external rotation against gravity.

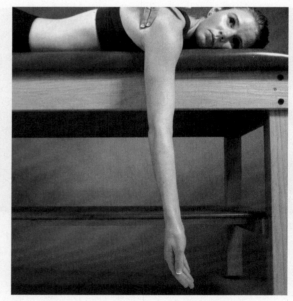

Figure 7-90 Shoulder external rotation, gravity eliminated.

Alternative Gravity-Eliminated Position (Fig. 7-91)

Start Position. Sitting in a chair with the humerus adducted to the side and the elbow flexed to 90°.

Stabilize. The distal end of the humerus is held against the body to allow only rotation.

Instruction. "Try to move the back of your hand out to the side."

Palpation. Same as previously described.

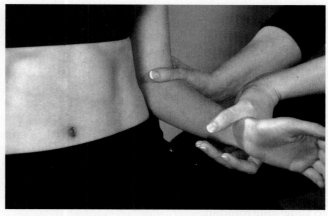

Figure 7-91 Shoulder external rotation, alternative position with gravity eliminated.

Shoulder Internal Rotation

Prime Movers

Subscapularis, teres major, latissimus dorsi, pectoralis major, and anterior deltoid.

Against-Gravity Position (Fig. 7-92)

Start Position. Prone with the humerus abducted to 90° and supported by the mat. The elbow is flexed to 90° and hangs over the edge of the mat.

Stabilize. The humerus is held just proximal to the elbow to allow only rotation.

Instruction. "Lift the palm of your hand toward the ceiling."

Resistance. The therapist's hand, placed on the volar surface of the distal end of the forearm, pushes toward the floor. The therapist's other hand keeps the patient's elbow supported and flexed to 90° to prevent supination.

Substitutions. Scapular abduction combined with upward rotation can substitute. The triceps can substitute as in external rotation.

Gravity-Eliminated Position (Fig. 7-93)

Start Position. Prone with the entire arm hanging over the edge of the mat. The arm is in external rotation.

Stabilize. The trunk and scapula are stabilized by the mat.

Instruction. "Try to turn your palm inward."

Palpation. The subscapularis is not easily palpated but may be found in the posterior axilla. Palpate the teres major, latissimus dorsi, pectoralis major, and anterior deltoid as previously described.

Substitutions. Scapular abduction combined with upward rotation can substitute. Pronation may be mistaken for internal rotation in a gravity-eliminated position.

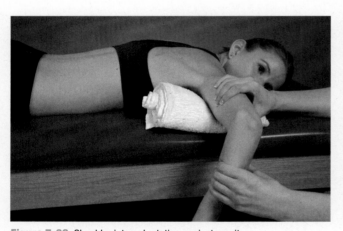

Figure 7-92 Shoulder internal rotation against gravity.

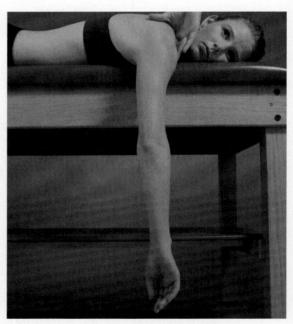

Figure 7-93 Shoulder internal rotation, gravity eliminated.

Alternative Gravity-Eliminated Position (Fig. 7-94)

Start Position. Sitting in a chair with the humerus adducted to the side and the elbow flexed to 90°.

Stabilize. The distal end of the humerus is held against the body to allow only rotation.

Instruction. "Try to move the palm of your hand in toward your stomach."

Palpation. Same as previously described.

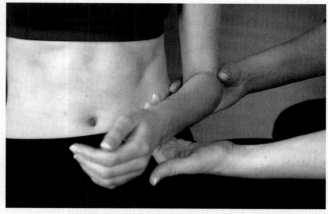

Figure 7-94 Shoulder internal rotation, alternative position with gravity eliminated.

Elbow Flexion

Prime Movers

Biceps, brachialis, and brachioradialis.

Against-Gravity Position (Fig. 7-95)

Start Position. Sitting in a chair with the arm at the side. The position of the forearm determines which muscle is working primarily: forearm in supination, biceps brachii; forearm in pronation, brachialis; forearm in midposition, brachioradialis.

Stabilize. Stabilize the distal end of the humerus during the action. While applying resistance, provide counter-pressure at the front of the shoulder.

Instruction. While the patient is in each of the three forearm positions, say, "Bend your elbow to touch your shoulder, and do not let me pull it back down."

Resistance. For each of the three positions, the therapist's hand is placed on the distal end of the forearm and pulls out toward extension.

Gravity-Eliminated Position (Fig. 7-96)

Start Position. Sitting with the arm supported by the therapist in 90° of abduction and elbow extension. The position of the forearm determines which muscle is working, as described earlier.

Stabilize. Distal humerus.

Instruction. "Try to move your hand toward your shoulder."

Palpation. The biceps is easily palpated on the anterior surface of the humerus. With the biceps relaxed and the forearm pronated, palpate the brachialis just medial to the distal biceps tendon. With the forearm in midposition, palpate the brachioradialis along the radial side of the proximal forearm.

Substitution. In a gravity-eliminated plane, the wrist flexors may substitute.

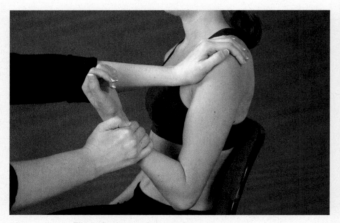

Figure 7-95 Elbow flexion against gravity.

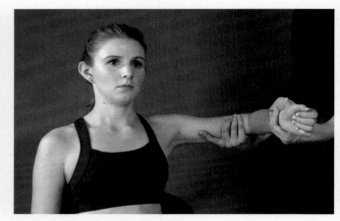

Figure 7-96 Elbow flexion, gravity eliminated.

Elbow Extension

Prime Mover

Triceps.

Against-Gravity Position (Fig. 7-97)

Start Position. Prone with humerus abducted to 90° and supported on the table. The elbow is flexed, and the forearm is hanging over the edge of the table.

Stabilize. Support the arm under the anterior surface of the distal humerus.

Instruction. "Straighten your arm, and do not let me push it back down."

Resistance. Apply resistance with the elbow at 10°–15° less than full extension so that the elbow does not lock into position, which may indicate greater strength than the patient actually has. The therapist's hand, placed on the dorsal surface of the patient's forearm, pushes toward flexion.

Gravity-Eliminated Position (Fig. 7-98)

Start Position. Sitting, with the humerus supported by the therapist in 90° of abduction. The elbow is fully flexed.

Stabilize. The humerus is supported and stabilized.

Instruction. "Try to straighten your elbow."

Palpation. The triceps are easily palpated on the posterior surface of the humerus.

Substitutions. In the gravity-eliminated position, no external rotation of the shoulder is permitted, so as to avoid letting the assistance of gravity produce extension. On a supporting surface, finger flexion may be used to inch the forearm across the surface.

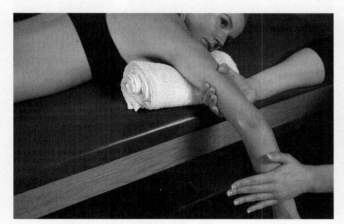

Figure 7-97 Elbow extension against gravity.

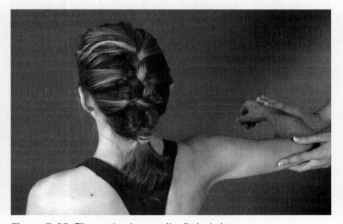

Figure 7-98 Elbow extension, gravity eliminated.

Pronation

Prime Movers

Pronator teres and pronator quadratus.

Against-Gravity Position (Fig. 7-99)

Start Position. Sitting with the humerus adducted, elbow flexed to 90°, and forearm supinated. The wrist and fingers are relaxed.

Stabilize. The distal humerus is stabilized to keep it adducted to the body.

Instruction. "Turn your palm to the floor, and do not let me turn it back over."

Resistance. The therapist's hand encircles the patient's volar wrist with the therapist's index finger extended along the forearm. The therapist applies resistance in the direction of supination.

Substitutions. Shoulder abduction or wrist and finger flexion may substitute.

Gravity-Eliminated Position (Fig. 7-100)

Start Position. Sitting with the humerus flexed to 90° and supported. The elbow is flexed to 90°, and the forearm is in full supination. The wrist and fingers are relaxed.

Stabilize. The humerus is stabilized.

Instruction. "Try to turn your palm away from your face."

Palpation. The pronator teres is palpated medial to the distal attachment of the biceps tendon on the volar surface of the proximal forearm. Pronator quadratus is too deep to palpate.

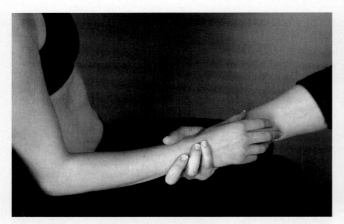

Figure 7-99 Pronation against gravity.

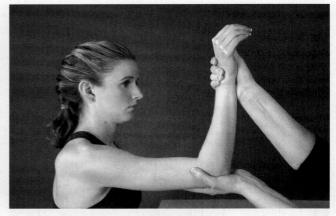

Figure 7-100 Pronation, gravity eliminated.

Supination

Prime Movers

Supinator and biceps.

Against-Gravity Position (Fig. 7-101)

Start Position. Sitting, with the humerus adducted, elbow flexed to 90°, and forearm pronated. The wrist and fingers are relaxed. To differentiate the supinator from the supination function of the biceps, isolate the supinator by extending the elbow. The biceps does not supinate the extended arm unless resisted (Kendall et al., 2005).

Stabilize. The distal humerus is stabilized.

Instruction. "Turn your palm up toward the ceiling, and do not let me turn it back over."

Resistance. Same as for pronation except that resistance is in the direction of pronation.

Substitutions. The wrist and finger extensors may substitute.

Gravity-Eliminated Position (Fig. 7-102)

Start Position. Sitting with the humerus flexed to 90° and supported. The elbow is flexed to 90°, and the forearm is in full pronation. The wrist and fingers are relaxed.

Stabilize. The humerus is stabilized and supported.

Instruction. "Try to turn your palm toward your face."

Palpation. The supinator is palpated on the dorsal surface of the proximal forearm just distal to the head of the radius. Palpation of the biceps was described earlier.

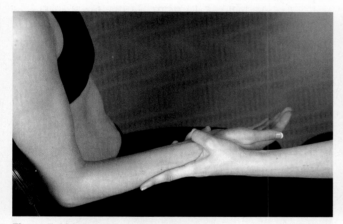

Figure 7-101 Supination against gravity.

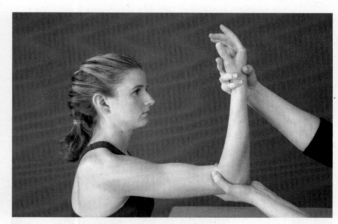

Figure 7-102 Supination, gravity eliminated.

WRIST AND HAND MEASUREMENT

Because many tendons of the wrist and hand cross more than one joint, test positions for individual muscles must include ways to minimize the effect of other muscles crossing the joint. As a general rule, to minimize the effect of a muscle, place it opposite the prime action. For example, to minimize the effect of the extensor pollicis longus (EPL) on extension of the proximal joint of the thumb, flex the distal joint.

Wrist Extension

Prime Movers

Extensor carpi radialis longus (ECRL), extensor carpi radialis brevis (ECRB), and extensor carpi ulnaris (ECU).

Against-Gravity Position (Figs. 7-103 and 7-104)

Start Position. The forearm is supported on a table in full pronation with fingers and thumb relaxed or slightly flexed.

Stabilize. The forearm is stabilized on the table.

Instruction. "Lift your wrist as far as you can, and do not let me push it down."

Resistance. To test the ECRL, which extends and radially deviates, apply resistance to the dorsum of the hand on the radial side in the direction of flexion and ulnar deviation (Fig. 7-103). To test the ECRB, apply resistance on the dorsum of the hand and push into flexion. To test the ECU, which extends and ulnarly deviates, apply resistance to the dorsum of the hand on the ulnar side and push in the direction of flexion and radial deviation (Fig. 7-104).

Substitutions. EPL and extensor digitorum (ED).

Gravity-Eliminated Position

Start Position. The forearm is supported on the table in midposition with the wrist in a slightly flexed position.

Instruction. "Try to bend your wrist backward."

Palpation. Palpate the tendon of the ECRL on the dorsal surface of the wrist at the base of the second metacarpal. The muscle belly is on the dorsal proximal forearm adjacent to the brachioradialis. Palpate the tendon of the ECRB on the dorsal surface of the wrist at the base of the third metacarpal adjacent to the ECRL. The muscle belly of the ECRB is distal to the belly of the ECRL on the dorsal surface of the proximal forearm. Palpate the ECU on the dorsal surface of the wrist between the head of the ulna and the base of the fifth metacarpal. The muscle belly is approximately 2 inches distal to the lateral epicondyle of the humerus (Rybski, 2004).

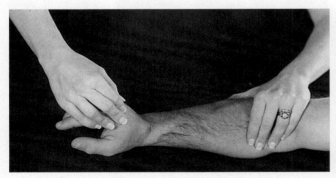

Figure 7-103 Wrist extension. Resistance is being given to the extensor carpi radialis.

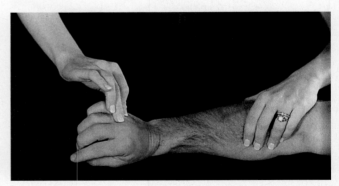

Figure 7-104 Wrist extension. Resistance is being given to the extensor carpi ulnaris.

Wrist Flexion

Prime Movers

Flexor carpi radialis (FCR), palmaris longus, and flexor carpi ulnaris (FCU).

Against-Gravity Position (Figs. 7-105 and 7-106)

Start Position. The forearm is supinated, the wrist is extended, and the fingers and thumb are relaxed.

Stabilize. The forearm is stabilized on the table with the back of the hand raised off the table to allow the wrist to go into slight extension.

Instruction. "Bend your wrist all the way forward, and do not let me push it back."

Resistance. To test the FCR and palmaris longus, the therapist applies resistance over the heads of the metacarpals on the volar surface of the hand toward extension. To test for the FCU, the therapist applies resistance over the head of the fifth metacarpal on the volar surface of the hand toward wrist extension and radial deviation.

Substitutions. Abductor pollicis longus, flexor pollicis longus, flexor digitorum superficialis (FDS), and flexor digitorum profundus (FDP).

Gravity-Eliminated Position

Start Position. Forearm in midposition, wrist extended, and fingers and thumb relaxed.

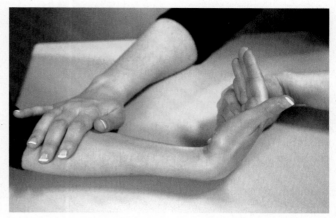

Figure 7-106 Wrist flexion. The therapist is resisting the flexor capri ulnaris.

Stabilize. The forearm rests on the table.

Instruction. "Try to bend your wrist forward."

Palpation. Palpate the FCR (Figure 7-105) on the volar surface of the wrist in line with the second metacarpal and radial to the palmaris longus (if present). Palpate the FCU (Figure 7-106) on the volar surface of the wrist just proximal to the pisiform bone. The palmaris longus is a weak wrist flexor. The tendon crosses the center of the volar surface of the wrist (Figure 7-107). It is not tested for strength and may not even be present; if it is present, it will stand out prominently in the middle of the wrist when wrist flexion is resisted or the palm is cupped with the thumb and fifth digit opposed to one another.

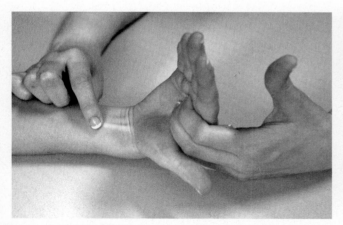

Figure 7-105 Wrist flexion. The therapist is pointing to the flexor carpi radialis longus tendon as she gives resistance.

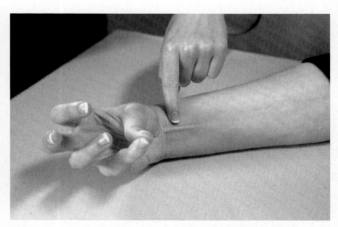

Figure 7-107 The therapist is pointing to the tendon of the palmaris longus as the patient cups her hand in an effort to make his tendon stand out.

Finger Metacarpophalangeal Extension

Prime Movers

ED, extensor indicis proprius, and extensor digiti minimi.

Against-Gravity Position (Fig. 7-108)

Start Position. The forearm is pronated and supported on the table. The wrist is supported in neutral position, and the finger MP and IP joints are in a relaxed flexed posture.

Stabilize. Wrist and metacarpals.

Instruction. "Lift this knuckle straight as far as it will go [touch the finger that is to be tested]. Keep the rest of your fingers bent. Do not let me push your knuckle down." (*Note:* Be sure to demonstrate this action.)

Resistance. Using one finger, the therapist pushes the head of each proximal phalanx toward flexion, one at a time.

Substitution. Apparent extension of the fingers can result from the rebound effect of relaxation following finger flexion. Flexion of the wrist can cause finger extension through tenodesis action.

Gravity-Eliminated Position

Start Position. Forearm supported in midposition, wrist in neutral position, and fingers flexed.

Stabilize. Wrist and metacarpals.

Instruction. "Try to move your knuckles back as far as they will go, one at a time. Keep the rest of your fingers bent."

Palpation. Palpate the muscle belly of the ED on the dorsal–ulnar surface of the proximal forearm. Often the separate muscle bellies are discernible. The tendons of this muscle are readily seen and palpated on the dorsum of the hand. The extensor indicis proprius tendon is ulnar to the ED tendon. Palpate the belly of this muscle on the mid- to distal dorsal forearm between the radius and ulna. Palpate the extensor digiti minimi tendon ulnar to the ED. Actually, it is the tendon that looks as if it were the ED tendon to the little finger because the ED to the little finger is only a slip from the ED tendon to the ring finger.

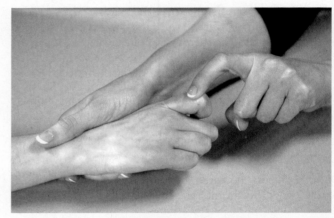

Figure 7-108 Finger metacarpophalangeal extension. The tendons of the extensor digitorum can be seen on the back of the patient's hand.

Finger Interphalangeal Extension

Prime Movers

Lumbricals, interossei, ED, extensor indicis proprius, and extensor digiti minimi.

According to electromyographic evidence, the intrinsics, especially the lumbricals, are the primary extensors of the IP joints (Long, 1968; Long & Brown, 1962). Except for the lumbricals and interossei, the other muscles have been discussed. The interossei are discussed under their alternative action of finger abduction and adduction. The lumbricals, arising as they do from the flexor profundus and inserting on the ED, have a unique action in regard to finger extension. Contracting against the noncontracting flexor profundus, the lumbricals pull the tendons of the profundus toward the fingertips. This slackens the profundus tendons distal to the insertion of the lumbricals, allowing the ED to extend the IP joints fully, regardless of the position of the MP joints (Long, 1968). The interossei flex the MP joints while extending the IP joints and, in fact, operate to extend only when the MP joints are flexed or flexing (Long, 1968).

Against-Gravity Position for the Lumbricals

There is no reliable test for lumbrical function. Test 1 is traditional. Test 2 is suggested in accordance with electromyographic evidence.

Start Position. The forearm is supinated and supported. The wrist is in neutral position. Test 1: MPs are extended with the IPs flexed. Test 2: MPs are flexed with the IPs extended.

Stabilize. Metacarpals and wrist.

Instruction. Test 1: "Bend your knuckles and straighten your fingers at the same time." (*Note:* Be sure to demonstrate this movement.) Test 2: "Straighten your knuckles and keep your fingers straight at the same time."

Resistance. Test 1: The therapist holds the tip of the finger being tested and pushes it toward the starting position. Test 2: The therapist places one finger on the patient's fingernail and pushes toward flexion (Fig. 7-109).

Substitution. Nothing substitutes for DIP extension in the event of the loss of lumbrical function when the MP joint is extended. Other muscles of the dorsal expansion can substitute for DIP extension when the MP joint is flexed.

Palpation. Lumbrical muscles lie too deep to be palpated.

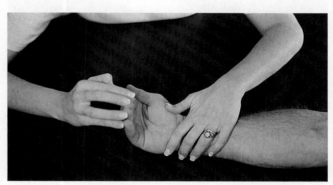

Figure 7-109 Finger interphalangeal extension. Resistance is given to the lumbricals as described for test 2.

Finger Distal Interphalangeal Flexion

Prime Mover

FDP.

Against-Gravity Position (Fig. 7-110)

Start Position. Forearm supinated and supported on a table; wrist and IP joints relaxed.

Stabilize. Firmly support the middle phalanx of each finger as it is tested to prevent flexion of the proximal IP joint; the wrist should remain in neutral position.

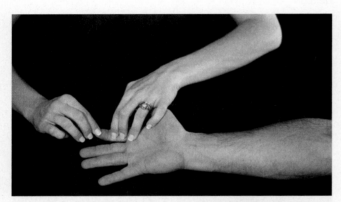

Figure 7-110 Finger distal interphalangeal flexion. The other joints of the finger are prevented from flexing.

Instruction. "Bend the last joint on your finger as far as you can."

Resistance. The therapist places one finger on the pad of the patient's finger and applies resistance toward extension.

Substitutions. Rebound effect of apparent flexion following contraction of extensors. Wrist extension causes tenodesis action.

Gravity-Eliminated Position

Start Position. The forearm is in midposition, resting on the ulnar border on a table. The wrist and IP joints are relaxed in neutral position.

Stabilize. Same as previously described.

Instruction. Same as previously described.

Palpation. Palpate the belly of the FDP just volar to the ulna in the proximal third of the forearm. The tendons are sometimes palpable on the volar surface of the middle phalanges.

Finger Proximal Interphalangeal Flexion

Prime Movers

FDS and FDP.

Against-Gravity Position for the Flexor Digitorum Superficialis (Fig. 7-111)

Start Position. Forearm supinated and supported on the table; wrist and MP joints relaxed and in zero position. To rule out the influence of the FDP when testing the FDS, hold all IP joints of the fingers not being tested in full extension to slight hyperextension. Because the FDP is essentially one muscle with four tendons, preventing its action in three of the four fingers prevents it from working in the tested finger. In fact, the patient cannot flex the distal joint of the tested finger at all. In some people, the FDP slip to the index finger is such that this method cannot rule out its influence on the PIP joint of the index finger. This should be noted on the test form.

Stabilize. All IP joints of the other digits of the hand.

Instruction. Point to the PIP joint and say, "Bend just this joint."

Resistance. Using one finger, the therapist applies resistance to the head of the middle phalanx toward extension.

Substitutions. FDP. Wrist extension causes tenodesis action.

Gravity-Eliminated Position

Start Position. Forearm supported in midposition, with the wrist and MP joints relaxed in neutral position. Again, rule out the influence of the FDP by holding all the joints of the untested fingers in extension.

Stabilize. Proximal phalanx of the finger being tested as well as all IP joints of the other digits of the hand.

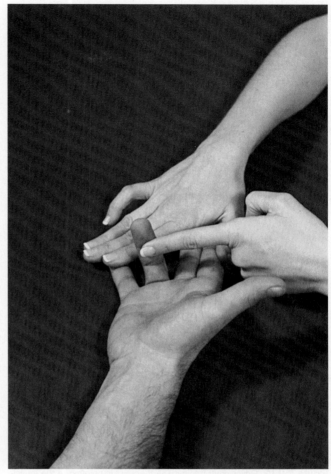

Figure 7-111 Finger proximal interphalangeal flexion. The flexor profundus is prevented from substituting because the therapist is holding in extension all fingers not being tested.

Instruction. Point to the PIP joint and say, "Try to bend just this joint."

Palpation. Palpate the FDS on the volar surface of the proximal forearm toward the ulnar side. Palpate the tendons at the wrist between the palmaris longus and the FCU.

Finger Metacarpophalangeal Flexion

Prime Movers

FDP, FDS, dorsal interossei (DI), volar (palmar) interossei, and flexor digiti minimi.

The tests for the first four muscles are discussed under their alternative actions. The flexor of the little finger has no other action and is described here.

Against-Gravity Position for the Flexor Digiti Minimi (Fig. 7-112)

Start Position. Forearm supported in supination.

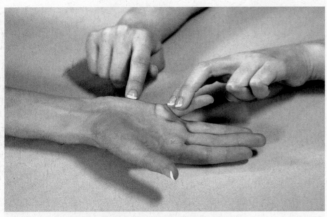

Figure 7-112 Flexor digiti minimi. The therapist is pointing to the muscle belly.

Stabilize. Other fingers in extension.

Instruction. "Bend the knuckle of your little finger toward your palm while you keep the rest of the finger straight."

Resistance. Using one finger, the therapist pushes the head of the proximal phalanx toward extension. The therapist must be sure the IP joints remain extended.

Substitutions. The FDP, FDS, or third volar interosseus may substitute.

Gravity-Eliminated Position

Start Position. Forearm supported in midposition.

Stabilize. Other fingers in extension.

Instruction. "Try to bend the knuckle of your little finger toward your palm while you keep the rest of the finger straight."

Palpation. The flexor digiti minimi is found on the volar surface of the hypothenar eminence.

Finger Abduction

Prime Movers

DI (4) and abductor digiti minimi.

Gravity-Eliminated Position (Fig. 7-113)

Start Position. The pronated forearm is supported with the wrist neutral. The fingers are extended and adducted. Be sure the MP joints are in neutral or slight flexion.

Stabilize. The wrist and metacarpals are gently supported.

Instruction. "Spread your fingers apart, and do not let me push them back together."

Action. Because the midline of the hand is the third finger and abduction is movement away from midline, the action of each finger is different. It is important to know which DI you are testing. The first DI abducts the index finger toward the thumb. The second DI abducts the middle finger toward the thumb. The third DI abducts the middle finger toward the little finger. The fourth DI abducts the ring finger toward the little finger. The abductor digiti minimi abducts the little finger ulnarly.

Resistance. Using the thumb and index finger to form a pincer, the therapist applies resistance at the radial or ulnar side of the head of the proximal phalanx in an attempt to push the finger toward midline. Applying resistance to the radial side of the heads of the index and middle fingers tests the first and second DI. Applying resistance to the ulnar side of the middle, ring, and little fingers tests the third and fourth DI and the abductor digiti minimi.

Substitutions. ED.

Grading. Normal finger abductors do not tolerate much resistance. If the fingers give way to resistance but spring back when the resistance is removed, the grade is 5. The grade is 4 if the muscle takes some resistance. The grade is 3 when there is full AROM. The grade is 2 if there is partial AROM. The grade is 1 when contraction is felt with palpation. The grade is 0 when no contractile activity is palpable.

Palpation. The first DI fills the dorsal web space and is easy to palpate there. Palpate the abductor digiti minimi on the ulnar border of the fifth metacarpal. The other interossei lie between the metacarpals on the dorsal aspect of the hand, where they may be palpated; on some people, the tendons can be palpated as they enter the dorsal expansion near the heads of the metacarpals. When the DI are atrophied, the spaces between the metacarpals on the dorsal surface appear sunken.

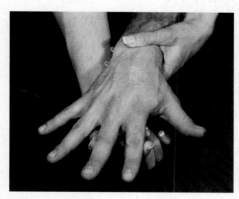

Figure 7-113 Finger abduction.

Finger Adduction

Prime Movers

Volar (palmar) interossei (3).

Gravity-Eliminated Position (Fig. 7-114)

Start Position. The forearm is pronated, and the MPs are abducted and in extension.

Stabilize. Both of the therapist's hands are needed for resistance. The forearm and wrist can be supported on a table.

Instruction. "Bring your fingers together and hold them. Do not let me pull them apart."

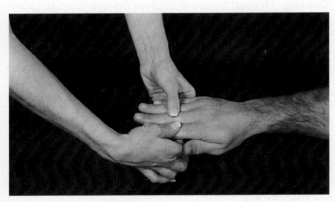

Figure 7-114 Finger adduction.

Action. Because the midline of the hand is the third finger and adduction is movement toward midline, the action of each finger is different. The first palmar interosseus (PI) adducts the index finger toward the middle finger. The second adducts the ring finger toward the middle finger, and the third adducts the little finger toward the middle finger.

Resistance. The therapist holds the heads of the proximal phalanx of two adjoining fingers and applies resistance in the direction of abduction to pull the fingers apart. For the index and middle finger pair, the first PI is tested. For the middle and ring finger pair, the second PI is tested. For the ring and little finger pair, the third PI is tested.

Substitutions. Extrinsic finger flexors.

Grading. Same as with the finger abductors.

Palpation. The PI are usually too deep to palpate with certainty. When these muscles are atrophied, the areas between the metacarpals on the volar surface appear sunken.

Thumb Interphalangeal Extension

Prime Mover

EPL.

Against-Gravity Position (Fig. 7-115)

Start Position. Forearm supported in midposition, wrist flexion of 10°–20°, and thumb MP and IP flexion.

Instruction. "Straighten the end of your thumb."

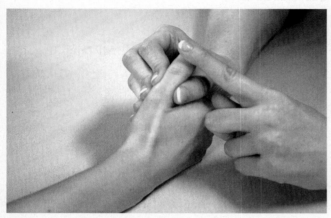

Figure 7-115 The therapist is resisting the extensor pollicis longus, whose tendon is prominent.

Stabilize. Proximal phalanx into MP flexion.

Resistance. The therapist places one finger over the dorsum of the distal phalanx (thumbnail) and pushes only the DIP toward flexion.

Substitutions. Relaxation of the flexor pollicis longus produces apparent extensor movement as a result of rebound effect. Because the abductor pollicis brevis, adductor pollicis, and flexor pollicis brevis insert into the lateral aspects of the dorsal expansion, they may produce thumb IP extension when the EPL is paralyzed. To prevent this, the position of maximal flexion of CMC and MP joints, wrist flexion of 10°–20°, and full forearm supination are used to put these synergists in a shortened, disadvantaged position while testing the EPL (Howell et al., 1989).

Gravity-Eliminated Position

Start Position. Forearm supinated, thumb flexed.

Instruction. "Try to straighten the end of your thumb."

Palpation. The tendon of the EPL may be palpated on the ulnar border of the anatomical snuffbox and on the dorsal surface of the proximal phalanx of the thumb.

Thumb Metacarpophalangeal Extension

Prime Movers

Extensor pollicis brevis (EPB) and EPL.

Against-Gravity Position for the Extensor Pollicis Brevis (Fig. 7-116)

Start Position. Forearm supported in midposition, MP and IP joints flexed.

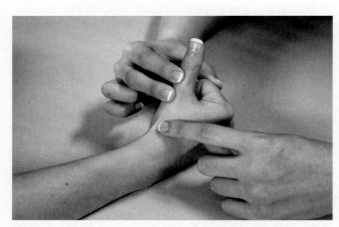

Figure 7-116 The therapist is resisting the extensor pollicis brevis, whose tendon can be seen.

Stabilize. Firmly support the first metacarpal in abduction.

Instruction. "Straighten the knuckle of your thumb while keeping the end joint bent." (*Note:* You may have to move the thumb passively a few times for the patient to get the kinesthetic input regarding the movement.)

Resistance. The therapist's index finger, placed on the dorsal surface of the head of the proximal phalanx, pushes toward flexion.

Substitution. EPL.

Gravity-Eliminated Position

Start Position. Forearm supinated, MP and IP joints flexed.

Stabilize. First metacarpal in abduction.

Instruction. "Try to straighten the knuckle of your thumb while keeping the end joint bent."

Palpation. Palpate the tendon of the EPB on the radial border of the anatomical snuffbox medial to the tendon of the abductor pollicis longus. The EPB may not be present.

Thumb Abduction

Prime Movers

Abductor pollicis longus and abductor pollicis brevis.

Against-Gravity Position for the Abductor Pollicis Longus (Fig. 7-117)

Start Position. Forearm supinated, wrist in neutral position, thumb adducted.

Stabilize. Support the wrist on the ulnar side and hold it in neutral position.

Instruction. "Bring your thumb away from your palm. Do not let me push it back in."

Action. Patient abducts the thumb halfway between thumb extension and palmar abduction. The therapist may have to demonstrate this action while giving the instructions.

Resistance. The therapist's finger presses the head of the first metacarpal toward adduction.

Substitutions. Abductor pollicis brevis and EPB.

Gravity-Eliminated Position

Start Position. Forearm in midposition, wrist in neutral position, thumb adducted.

Stabilize. Support the wrist on the ulnar side and hold it in neutral position.

Instruction. "Try to bring your thumb away from your palm."

Palpation. Palpate the tendon of the abductor pollicis longus at the wrist joint just distal to the radial styloid and lateral to the EPB.

Against-Gravity Position for the Abductor Pollicis Brevis (Fig. 7-118)

Start Position. Forearm is supported in supination, wrist in neutral position, and thumb adducted.

Stabilize. Support the wrist in neutral position by holding it on the dorsal and ulnar side.

Instruction. "Lift your thumb directly out of the palm of the hand. Do not let me push it back in."

Resistance. The therapist's finger presses the head of the first metacarpal toward adduction.

Substitution. Abductor pollicis longus.

Gravity-Eliminated Position

Start Position. Forearm is supported in midposition, wrist in neutral position, thumb adducted.

Stabilize. Support the wrist in neutral position by holding it on the dorsal and ulnar side.

Instruction. "Try to move your thumb away from the palm of your hand."

Palpation. Palpate the abductor pollicis brevis over the center of the thenar eminence.

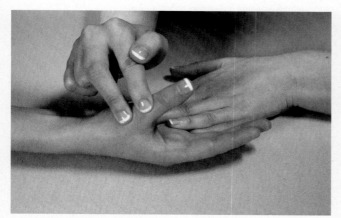

Figure 7-117 The therapist is resisting the abductor pollicis longus, which moves the thumb away from the palm halfway between extension and palmar abduction.

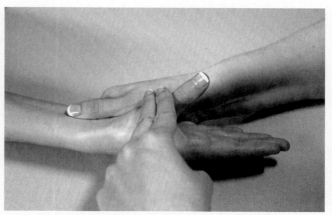

Figure 7-118 The therapist is resisting the abductor pollicis brevis, which moves the thumb directly up from the palm of the hand (palmar abduction).

Thumb Interphalangeal Flexion

Prime Mover

Flexor pollicis longus.

Against-Gravity Position (Fig. 7-119)

Start Position. Elbow flexed and supported on a table. Forearm supinated so that the palmar surface of the thumb faces the ceiling; thumb extended at the MP and IP joints.

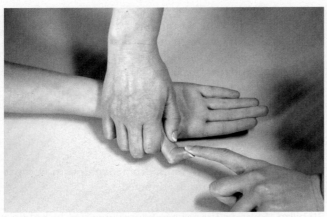

Figure 7-119 The therapist is resisting the flexor pollicis longus.

Stabilize. Proximal phalanx, holding MP joint in extension.

Instruction. "Bend the tip of your thumb as far as you can, and do not let me straighten it."

Resistance. The therapist's finger pushes the head of the distal phalanx toward extension.

Substitution. Relaxation of the EPL causes apparent rebound movement.

Gravity-Eliminated Position

Start Position. Forearm supinated to 90° so that the thumb can flex across the palm.

Stabilize. Proximal phalanx, holding MP joint in extension.

Instruction. "Try to bend the tip of your thumb as far as you can."

Palpation. Palpate the flexor pollicis longus on the palmar surface of the proximal phalanx.

Thumb Metacarpophalangeal Flexion

Prime Movers

Flexor pollicis brevis and flexor pollicis longus.

Against-Gravity Position for the Flexor Pollicis Brevis (Fig. 7-120)

Start Position. Elbow flexed and supported on the table. Forearm supinated so that the palmar surface of the thumb faces the ceiling; thumb is extended at both the MP and IP joints.

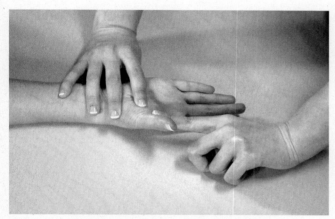

Figure 7-120 The therapist is resisting the flexor pollicis brevis.

Stabilize. Firmly support the first metacarpal.

Instruction. "Bend your thumb across your palm, keeping the end joint of your thumb straight. Do not let me pull it back out."

Resistance. The therapist's finger pushes the head of the proximal phalanx toward extension.

Substitution. Flexor pollicis longus; the abductor pollicis brevis and the adductor pollicis through insertion into the extensor hood. To rule out the effect of the flexor pollicis longus when testing the flexor pollicis brevis, a test position of maximal elbow flexion, maximal pronation, and maximal wrist flexion has been recommended (Howell et al., 1989).

Gravity-Eliminated Position

Start Position. Forearm supinated to 90° so that the thumb can flex across the palm.

Stabilize. First metacarpal.

Instruction. "Try to bend your thumb into your palm, keeping the end joint of your thumb straight."

Palpation. Palpate the flexor pollicis brevis on the thenar eminence just proximal to the MP joint and medial to the abductor pollicis brevis.

Thumb Adduction

Prime Mover

Adductor pollicis.

Against-Gravity Position (Fig. 7-121)

Start Position. Forearm pronated, wrist and fingers in neutral position, thumb abducted, and MP and IP joints of the thumb in extension.

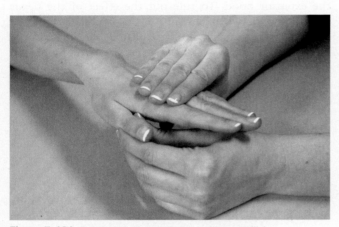

Figure 7-121 The therapist is resisting the adductor pollicis.

Stabilize. Metacarpals of fingers, keeping the MP joints in neutral.

Instruction. "Lift your thumb into the palm of your hand, and do not let me pull it out."

Resistance. The therapist grasps the head of the proximal phalanx and tries to pull it away from the palm toward abduction.

Substitutions. The EPL, flexor pollicis longus, or flexor pollicis brevis may substitute.

Gravity-Eliminated Position

Start Position. Same except forearm is in midposition.

Stabilize. Metacarpals of fingers, keeping the MP joints in neutral.

Instruction. "Try to bring your thumb into the palm of your hand."

Palpation. Palpate the adductor pollicis on the palmar surface of the thumb web space.

Opposition

Prime Movers

Opponens pollicis and opponens digiti minimi.

Against-Gravity Position (Fig. 7-122)

Start Position. Forearm supinated and supported, wrist in neutral position, thumb adducted and extended.

Stabilize. Hold the wrist in a neutral position.

Instruction. "Touch the pad of your thumb to the pad of your little finger. Do not let me pull them apart."

Resistance. The therapist holds along the first metacarpal and derotates the thumb or holds along the fifth metacarpal and derotates the little finger. These can be resisted simultaneously using both hands.

Substitutions. The abductor pollicis brevis, flexor pollicis brevis, or flexor pollicis longus may substitute.

Gravity-Eliminated Position

Start Position. Elbow resting on the table with forearm perpendicular to the table, wrist in neutral position, thumb adducted and extended.

Stabilize. Hold the wrist in a neutral position.

Instruction. "Try to touch the pad of your thumb to the pad of your little finger."

Palpation. Place fingertips along the lateral side of the shaft of the first metacarpal where the opponens pollicis may be palpated before it becomes deep to the abductor

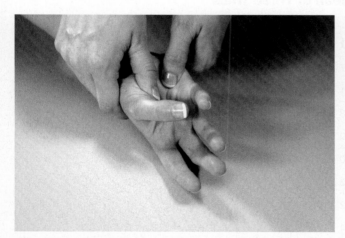

Figure 7-122 The therapist is resisting both the opponens pollicis and the opponens digiti minimi.

pollicis brevis. The opponens digiti minimi can be palpated volarly along the shaft of the fifth metacarpal.

Interpreting the Muscle Test

After recording all muscle test scores, the therapist reviews the scores and looks for the weak muscles and the distribution and significance of the weakness. Any muscle that grades "good minus" (4−) or below is considered weak. "Good plus" (4+) muscles are functional and usually require no therapy. "Good" (4) muscles may or may not be functionally adequate for the patient, depending on his or her occupational task requirements. The pattern of muscle weakness is important. The pattern may indicate general weakness caused by disuse secondary to immobilization, or it may reflect the level of spinal innervation in a patient after spinal cord injury or the distribution of a peripheral nerve in the case of peripheral nerve injury. A pattern of imbalance of forces in agonist and antagonist muscles may be deforming; therefore, counterpositioning or splinting should be considered along with strengthening of the weak muscles.

The pattern of significant strength is also important. For example, a muscle test of a patient with an injured spinal cord that indicates some strength in a muscle innervated by a segment below the diagnosed level of injury is hopeful for more recovery. Or, because muscles are reinnervated proximally to distally after peripheral nerve injury, findings showing beginning return of strength in particular muscles help to track the progress of nerve regeneration.

Short-term goals move the patient from the level of strength determined by testing to the next higher level. For example, if a muscle grades 3, the short-term goal is to improve strength to 3+; if it grades 3+, the goal is to increase strength to 4−, and so on. However, the goal should not purely reflect the numerical increase in the muscle strength. Improved strength should instead be reflected in some sort of functional task. For example, the short-term goal may state, "The patient will demonstrate an increase in left elbow muscle strength to 3+, as needed for independent hygiene tasks of brushing the teeth and washing the face." The required strength for occupational functioning must always be kept in mind when establishing goals.

If the muscle is being reevaluated, the scores are compared with those of the previous test. The frequency of reevaluation depends on the nature of expected recovery. Expected rapid recovery requires frequent reevaluation. For example in a young, healthy individual recovering from a fracture that has been cleared by the surgeon to begin strengthening, it may be appropriate to reevaluate every 2 weeks until full strength is returned. However, in an individual recovering from a peripheral nerve injury when nerve healing is slow and expected to only heal 1 inch every month, it may be more appropriate to wait 4 weeks between reevaluations. If significant gains are noted in therapy and the patient would benefit from a change in the treatment plan, then a reevaluation should be completed to document these gains and the change in treatment plan. If the repeated muscle test shows that the patient is making gains, the program is considered beneficial, and its demands are upgraded. If repeated muscle tests show no gains despite program adaptations, the patient is considered to have reached a plateau and to no longer benefit from remedial therapy. In that case, the focus of treatment shifts to teaching the patient compensatory strategies and the use of adaptive equipment to enable participation in desired tasks and activities.

There are, of course, exceptions to these standards. Patients with degenerative diseases are expected to get weaker; therefore, therapy is aimed at maintaining their strength and function for as long as possible, and efficacy is confirmed with repeat tests. A plateau for these patients is desirable; it indicates that the therapy is effective for maintaining strength and should be continued. Documentation of how this maintenance of strength impacts independence in ADL and IADL tasks should also be used to justify continued services. These patients often benefit from rehabilitation to maintain their current level of independence as well as compensatory techniques in order to conserve energy and maintain independence. For example, an individual may have the functional strength needed in order to shower standing and use basic techniques for all required steps including squeezing the shampoo bottle, lathering the body, bending and reaching to clean all body parts, and rotating in the shower to rinse. However, the person may be so tired following this routine that he or she does not have the energy to cook a meal or engage in

a favorite hobby. In this case, activity analysis would aid in determining compensation techniques and equipment to conserve energy so the individual can both shower and have enough energy to also engage in additional ADL and IADL tasks. The individual may benefit from a shower bench, long-handled sponge, removable shower head, and pump bottles to aid in completing this task with modified independence.

GRASP AND PINCH STRENGTH MEASUREMENT

More specific measurements beyond MMT grading can demonstrate more discrete changes in grip and pinch strength. In a review of 42 studies of hand-grip strength, the methods, equipment, and metrics were evaluated to determine standardization of procedures (Roberts et al., 2011). Normative data for both grip and pinch strength has long been established (Mathiowetz et al., 1985). Abbreviated versions of the norms are listed in Tables 7-2 and 7-3. When individual scores are outside of these established norms, an individual with unilateral injury may also be compared to him- or herself by using the 10% rule. In right-handed individuals, the dominant side is typically 10% stronger than the nondominant side, although left-handed individuals typically demonstrate equal strength bilaterally (Roberts et al., 2011).

Definitions of handedness vary widely in the literature. In a literature review on how handedness impacts grip strength, the difference between a definitive preference for the right versus left hand and degree of preference are discussed (Clerke & Clerke, 2001). In a discussion with a client, the individual may state that he or she writes with the left hand but completes most sports and

| Table 7-2 | **Dynamometer Norms in Pounds: Mean of Three Trials** |

	Norms at Age	20	25	30	35	40	45	50	55	60	65	70	75+
Men	Right	121	121	122	120	117	110	114	101	90	91	75	66
	SD	21	23	22	24	21	23	18	27	20	21	21	21
	Left	104	110	110	113	113	101	102	83	77	77	65	55
	SD	22	16	22	22	19	23	17	23	20	20	18	17
Women	Right	70	74	79	74	70	62	66	57	55	50	50	43
	SD	14	14	19	11	13	15	12	12	10	10	12	11
	Left	61	63	68	66	62	56	57	47	46	41	41	38
	SD	13	12	18	12	14	13	11	12	10	8	10	9

N = 628; age range = 20–94; SD = standard deviation. Reprinted with permission from Mathiowetz, V., Kashman, N., Volland, G., Weber, K., Dowe, M., & Rogers, S. (1985). Grip and pinch strength: Normative data for adults. *Archives of Physical Medicine and Rehabilitation, 66,* 69–74.

Table 7-3 **Pinch Meter Norms in Pounds: Mean of Three Trials**

		Norms at Age	20	30	40	50	60	70	75+
Tip	Men	Right	18	18	18	18	16	14	14
		Left	17	18	18	18	15	13	14
	Women	Right	11	13	11	12	10	10	10
		Left	10	12	11	11	10	10	9
Lateral	Men	Right	26	26	26	27	23	19	20
		Left	25	26	25	26	22	19	19
	Women	Right	18	19	17	17	15	14	13
		Left	16	18	16	16	14	14	11
Palmar	Men	Right	27	25	24	24	22	18	19
		Left	26	25	25	24	21	19	18
	Women	Right	17	19	17	17	15	14	12
		Left	16	18	17	16	14	14	12

Tip pinch average standard deviation (SD): men, 4.0; women, 2.5. Lateral pinch average SD: men, 4.6; women, 3.0. Palmar pinch average SD: men, 5.1; women, 3.7. $N = 628$; age range = 20–94. Reprinted with permission from Mathiowetz, V., Kashman, N., Volland, G., Weber, K., Dowe, M., & Rogers, S. (1985). Grip and pinch strength: Normative data for adults. *Archives of Physical Medicine and Rehabilitation, 66,* 69–74.

household tasks with the right hand. This individual may demonstrate better scores on dexterity testing on the left, while demonstrating higher grip scores on the right. Clerke and Clerke (2001) suggest that more research be done regarding the effect of handedness with greater specificity of how handedness is defined. The literature they reviewed included variations in grip strength up to 40% between an individual's hands (Clerke & Clerke, 2001). The therapist should consider each person's unique situation when evaluating this area. A mechanic may appear to have good return of strength following a carpal tunnel release but continue to complain of difficulty with work tasks compared preoperatively. Further activity analysis of his or her work tasks and occupation-based treatment and goals should be the focus rather than purely a numerical goal.

Grip-strength norms were originally established using the Jamar dynamometer, which is most commonly used in research. However, interinstrument reliability, or the ability of multiple instruments to be used interchangeably, has been established between devices with various levels of confidence (see Table 7-4 for a listing of instruments used to measure grip strength). Although these instruments can be used with various levels of confidence against the norms,

Table 7-4 **Dynamometer Equipment: Dynamometer Interinstrument Reliability Compared to the Jamar Dynamometer**

Excellent	Moderate to Excellent	Low	Unclear
• Dexter • Baseline • Rolyan Hydraulic	• Baltimore Therapeutic Equipment (BTE) work simulator • BTE Primus • Martin Vigorimeter • MicroFET 4 • DynEx	• Sphygmomanometer • Vigorimeter	• Grippit dynamometer

From Roberts, H. C., Denison, H. J., Martin, H. J., Patel, H. P., Syddall, H., Cooper, C., & Sayer, A. A. (2011). A review of the measurement of grip strength in clinical and epidemiological studies: Towards a standardised approach. *Age and Ageing, 40,* 423–429.

the selected instrument still must be calibrated every 4–12 months. It is recommended to use the same instrument at the same time of day using a standard protocol and instructions for body and instrument position when evaluating and reevaluating individual patients. In the use of the Jamar dynamometer, there are five grooves along the handle used to select the grip position. The second grip position from the gauge is the standard position used, although hand size and nail length may impact which position allows for maximum grip strength. It was also recommended that a change in score of at least 6 kg or 13 pounds is needed to be clinically significant (Roberts et al., 2011).

The pinch norms can be used with the B & L, JTech, and NK pinch meters because they have been found to be interchangeably reliable: for symptomatic subjects ($r > 0.90$) and for nonsymptomatic subjects ($r = 0.80$) (MacDermid, Evenhuis, & Louzon, 2001).

As with any tool of measurement, the instrument must be calibrated and set at 0 to start. Dynamometers and pinch meters can be calibrated by placing known weights on or suspending them from the compression part of the meter (Fess, 1987). With this procedure, the Jamar dynamometer was found to be accurate to within 7% (Shechtman, Gestewitz, & Kimble, 2005), and the B & L pinch meter was found to be accurate within 1% (Mathiowetz, Vizenor, & Melander, 2000).

The standard method of measurement used in the study from which the norms were established reflects the recommendations of the American Society of Hand Therapists (ASHT) (Fess, 1992). Test–retest reliability of this method using the Jamar hydraulic dynamometer was found to be 0.88; interrater reliability (two raters, same time) was 0.99. Interrater (two raters, same time) reliability of averaged B & L pinch meter scores was 0.98, and test–retest reliability was 0.81 (Mathiowetz et al., 1984).

A vigorimeter cannot be used interchangeably with a dynamometer. However, it is an acceptable alternative hand strength–measuring device for patients whose diagnoses contraindicate stress on joints and/or skin, because it requires the patient to squeeze a rubber bulb rather than a steel handle. The vigorimeter is a commercially available instrument for which norms have been published (Fike & Rousseau, 1982; Roberts et al., 2011).

Fong and Ng (2001) studied the effect of wrist position on grip strength in a normal population. Their review of the literature on this topic revealed many conflicting findings. However, the methods in many of these studies were highly varied as well. They followed the basic ASHT recommendations for test position but deviated by using a testing board to secure the wrist in the position they were testing and then rested this board on a table. They found the highest grip scores with the wrist in 15° or 30° of extension with no radial or ulnar deviation and did find significant differences in scores when the wrist was positioned in 15° of ulnar deviation. They did not test for positions with less ulnar deviation, and further research

is needed in this area, as well as with populations with UE conditions (Fong & Ng, 2001).

With occupational therapy practice moving into the community and home, the need for valid tools that are quick, portable, and easy to use is increasing. Grip strength has been studied as a method to evaluate overall strength and function. Various studies have revealed a range of correlation, with moderate correlation in individuals under the age 55 years. In a study of women over age 75 years, standardized grip-strength measurements were compared with computerized strength measurements using an isokinetic dynamometer and functional evaluations including the Barthel Index (BI) self-report of ADL function and the Timed Get-Up-and-Go Test (TUG) (Tietjen-Smith et al., 2006). Limitations of the study included that it was conducted in a busy assisted-living facility with high traffic and a lack of isolated, quiet areas for testing as well as their very specific patient population. Moderate correlation was found between grip and overall strength ($r = 0.583$). However, the authors caution against using grip alone to determine function because the grip measurements did not correlate with the BI. Although strength is important for completing ADL tasks, it is important to remember with this aging population that many other factors impact their independence (Tietjen-Smith et al., 2006).

Grasp

The patient should be seated in a chair without arms with his or her shoulder adducted and neutrally rotated, the elbow flexed at 90°, the forearm neutral and wrist between 0° and 30° of extension and up to 15° of ulnar deviation. Feet should be flat on the floor (Fess, 1992; Lindstrom-Hazel, Krat, & Bix, 2009). The handle of the dynamometer is set at the second position. The task is demonstrated to the patient. After the dynamometer is positioned in the patient's hand, the therapist says, "Ready? Squeeze as hard as you can," and urges the patient on throughout the attempt saying "Harder! . . . Harder! . . . Relax" (Mathiowetz et al., 1985). The patient squeezes the dynamometer with as much force as he or she can three times, with a 1-minute rest between trials. The score is the average of the three trials. Note that research has suggested that a single trial is as reliable as multiple trials (Coldham, Lewis, & Lee, 2006). This may be appropriate for cases in which multiple trials would cause undue pain or stress (see Fig. 7-123 and Table 7-2 for normative data and standardized position for grip-strength testing).

Pinch

Three types of pinch are typically evaluated because they are involved in accomplishing occupational tasks and activities efficiently. The seating and positioning of the arm should be the same as with grip testing, with the addition

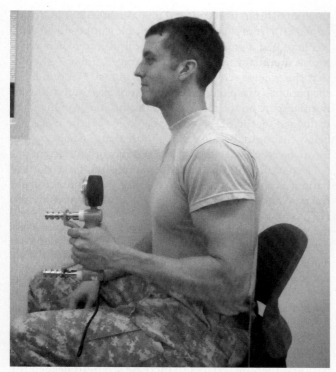

Figure 7-123 Measuring grasp using a dynamometer. The patient's upper arm is close to his body, and the elbow is flexed to 90°.

that the fingers should be allowed to flex. With both tip and three-jaw pinch, it is important to note that in order to keep the forearm in a neutral position, the pinch gauge must be held vertically, and the wrist will naturally extend to assume the best testing position (MacDermid, Evenhuis, & Louzon, 2001).

Tip Pinch (Fig. 7-124 and Table 7-3)

The patient pinches the ends of the pinch meter between the tips of the thumb and index finger (Mathiowetz et al.,

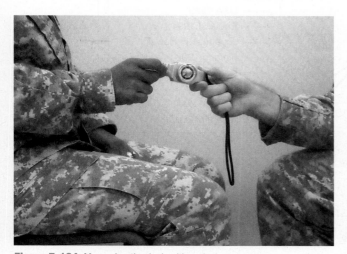

Figure 7-124 Measuring tip pinch with a pinch meter.

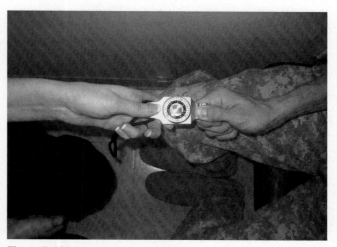

Figure 7-125 Measuring lateral pinch.

1985). The test is administered by first giving the patient instructions and a demonstration. Next, the therapist says, "Ready? Pinch as hard as you can." The patient is urged on as he or she attempts to pinch. Three trials, with a rest between each trial, are completed. The average of three trials is recorded. It is important to observe for any compensation techniques because some individuals will naturally try to use the middle finger to assist without recognizing their deviance from the instructed test position.

Lateral Pinch: Key Pinch (Fig. 7-125 and Table 7-3)

The patient pinches the meter between the pad of the thumb and the lateral surface of the index finger. The instructions and procedure are the same as for tip pinch, but the pinch gauge is held horizontally. Interestingly, in a study of key pinch in children ages 5–12 years, differences were found according to age, but no significant differences were found by hand or gender in this age range. Based on these findings, comparing the right to left side in this age range should be possible as long as the injury or condition is not bilateral (De Smet & Decramer, 2006).

Palmar Pinch: Three-Jaw Chuck (Fig. 7-126 and Table 7-3)

The patient pinches the meter between the pad of the thumb and the pads of the index and middle fingers. The instructions and procedure are the same as for tip pinch.

Interpretation of Grasp and Pinch Scores

The scores are compared with those of the other hand or to norms to ascertain whether the patient has a significant limitation. Lindstrom-Hazel, Krat, and Bix (2009) questioned the current normative data based on the fact that it is more than 20 years old, and the differences in individual's activities compared to when the data were

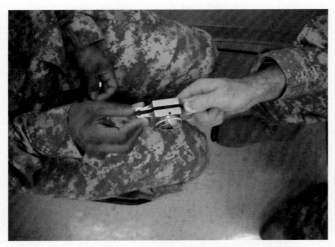

Figure 7-126 Measuring palmar pinch or three-jaw chuck pinch.

collected. They determined that students using standardized methods could demonstrate high levels of interrater reliability (ICC = 0.99 for grip strength; ICC = 0.95–0.99 for pinch strength), indicating that, with training, students could contribute to collecting new normative data (Lindstrom-Hazel, Krat, & Bix, 2009).

In a recent Australian study of grip strength, the researchers compared their normative data to other studies that have collected norms in various countries. The trends and variations in these data are interesting to acknowledge and have been included in Figures 7-127 and 7-128 (Massy-Westropp et al., 2011).

The accuracy of the Jamar dynamometer was found to be 7%, which means that, if the patient scored 50 pounds, the actual strength may range from 46.5 to 53.5 pounds (Shechtman, Gestewitz, & Kimble, 2005). Grasp and pinch scores are considered abnormal if they are associated with a

functional limitation and/or if they are three standard deviations (SD) from the mean. For example, suppose a 40-year-old man had a grasp score of 50 pounds after three trials for his dominant right hand are averaged. Table 7-2 shows that the average score for his age group is 117 pounds, so the patient's grasp score was 67 pounds less than the mean normal score on the table. When the difference in his score is divided by the SD given in the table (21), he is 3.2 SD below the mean. Because this is more than 3 SD below the mean, he is considered to have a significant limitation.

Expanding on this patient example, imagine that the patient is a carpenter and recovering from a metacarpal fracture and can now demonstrate a full composite fist. He has an average score of 50 pounds on the right dominant hand, and an average of 100 pounds on the left nondominant hand. Using the 10% rule, the therapist would anticipate that 110 pounds was the patient's right hand strength prior to injury. The therapist's assessment could be written as, "Patient is 7 weeks post–metacarpal fracture with good return of motion. He demonstrates 45.5% of right hand strength compared to the left and 42.7% compared to established norms for his age and gender. The patient would benefit from continued occupational therapy services to increase strength needed for work and daily tasks." Grasp and pinch measurements can be quickly and easily reevaluated over time to monitor the progress of the patient and the effectiveness of the treatment plan.

DEXTERITY MEASUREMENT

Dexterity requires hand ROM, hand strength, and sensation in order to manipulate objects. Individuals who lack full hand motion and function often complain about their inability to manipulate objects for writing, fastening clothing,

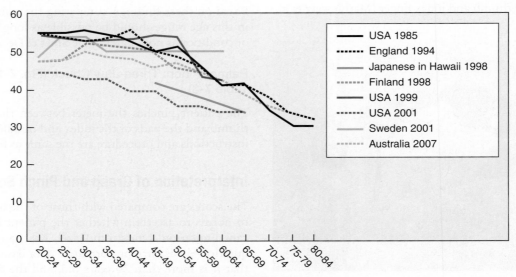

Figure 7-127 Comparison of male normative grip data across studies.

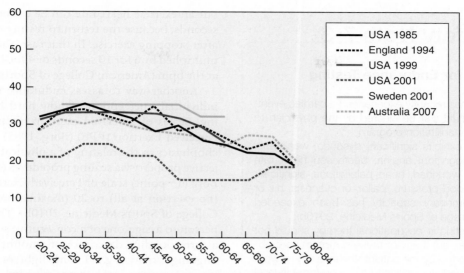

Figure 7-128 Comparison of female normative grip data across studies.

or turning a key in a car or door. The therapist may wish to further evaluate dexterity in these cases. Yancosek and Howell (2009) did a thorough review of common adult dexterity assessments and their psychometric properties. Further information on dexterity assessments can be found in Chapter 37.

ENDURANCE MEASUREMENT

Occupational therapists treat a variety of conditions that can impact an individual's endurance, including cardiac or pulmonary impairments, a major trauma or illness requiring bed rest, loss of significant muscle function, or the need to use a prosthesis or adaptive equipment. There are two components of endurance. The first is cardiovascular endurance, which is when during continuous physical activity both the circulatory and respiratory systems must supply adequate oxygen to continue the task (American College of Sports Medicine, 2010b). The second is muscular endurance, in which the muscles engaged during the task can continue to work without fatigue (American College of Sports Medicine, 2010b). Both of these aspects of endurance are vital to engagement in ADL and IADL tasks, which is why in some settings this is referred to as activity tolerance. The therapist may evaluate one aspect or both depending on the patient's symptoms.

Cardiovascular Aspects of Endurance

The role of the occupational therapist here is most clearly seen in the role of therapists in cardiac rehabilitation programs, although these same principles may apply to an individual receiving therapy after prolonged bed rest or to an individual in home health with decreased endurance. Once an individual is cleared to begin a cardiac rehabilitation program from his or her physician following

a cardiac event, the first activities that test CR fitness are typically self-care tasks (American College of Sports Medicine, 2010b). As the person progresses, household management tasks create a good challenge to the patient's endurance. Additionally, if the patient will be returning to work, the occupational therapist can assess the patient's workplace to gain a better understanding of the job demands and use task analysis to develop a program to return the patient to the endurance level needed to complete work tasks through a work-hardening program (American College of Sports Medicine, 2010b).

It is important for the therapist working with patients with decreased endurance to know the limitations and contraindications to pushing them in their progress to regain cardiovascular endurance. Additional information regarding safety during testing can be found in Safety Note 7-3. There are several measures of CR fitness that are beyond the scope of this chapter; however, the basic concepts will be explained to gain a better understanding of the contraindications. The criterion measure of CR fitness is maximal oxygen uptake (VO_{2max}) and is associated with heart functional capacity (American College of Sports Medicine, 2010b). It increases with physical training and decreases with bed rest and age. With physical training, the heart rate becomes lower for the same level of work, which is referred to as the "training effect." The training effect indicates improvement in circulatory system efficiency (American College of Sports Medicine, 2010a) (see further discussion of this topic in Chapter 42).

VO_{2max} is typically measured in a laboratory environment, which is not always available, but there is a linear relationship between oxygen uptake and heart rate for various intensities (i.e., light to moderately heavy exercise). Intensity of an activity is estimated in terms of light, moderate, or heavy work or metabolic equivalent (MET) level.

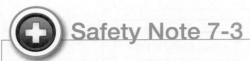

Safety Note 7-3

Precautions for Endurance Testing

- If the patient has recently experienced a cardiac event, he or she should first be cleared by the physician to engage in a rehabilitation program.
- If the patient exhibits significant dyspnea, weakness, changes in cognition, angina, decreased heart rate for increased workload, heart palpitations, significant changes in blood pressure, pallor, or cyanosis, his or her cardiopulmonary capacity has been exceeded (American College of Sports Medicine, 2010b).
- Endurance testing in occupational therapy should not reach this level, but if any of these symptoms are observed or reported by the patient, the intensity of work should be immediately reduced to a comfortable level or terminated, and the patient should be evaluated.

One MET equals basal metabolic rate (American College of Sports Medicine, 2010a). Basal metabolic rate is the amount of oxygen consumption necessary to maintain the metabolic processes (e.g., respiration, circulation, peristalsis, temperature regulation, and glandular function) of the body at rest and is quantified as 3.5 mL of oxygen per kilogram of body weight per minute. The energy cost of activities or exercise can be rated using multiples of METs. An exercise that is rated 4 METs requires four times the amount of oxygen per kilogram of body weight per minute than that of the basal rate. The oxygen consumption of daily living, recreational, and vocational tasks has been measured for normal subjects, and the METs required for each task have been calculated (see Table 42-1 for MET values of various activities). These costs are estimates that vary with environmental conditions, such as humidity and temperature, and personal conditions, such as anger or stress.

Because heart rate relates linearly to VO_{2max} except at the upper limits (80%–90%) of maximal capacity, if a person's heart rate is 70% of maximal heart rate (HR_{max}), he or she is using approximately 70% of VO_{2max} as long as there is no underlying pulmonary disorder. HR_{max} has traditionally been estimated by subtracting the person's age from 220; however, a more accurate formula is $HR_{max} = 206.9 - (0.67 \times age)$ (American College of Sports Medicine, 2010b). The pulse taken immediately after activity is then related to the person's HR_{max} as a percentage of maximum. A constant heart rate obtained during exercise indicates a steady state, that is, a balance of oxygen intake and consumption (Fletcher et al., 2001). Heart rate is measured by placing the index and middle fingers lightly but firmly over the radial artery at the wrist (lateral to the FCR) and counting the number of beats per minute (bpm). It is most accurate to count for a full minute, but an exercise heart rate can be counted for only 10–15 seconds, because the return to resting rate occurs quickly after stopping exercise. In that case, the obtained value is multiplied by 6 for 10 seconds or 4 for 15 seconds to arrive at the bpm (American College of Sports Medicine, 2010a).

Another way to assess endurance is to ascertain the individual's perception of how hard he or she is working. Scales of perceived exertion, such as the Rating of Perceived Exertion (RPE) (Borg, 1985), are based on psychophysics or the relating of a physical property to a subjective property via scaling procedures (Russell, 1997). The Borg (15-point) scale of Perceived Exertion ranges from 6 (no exertion at all) to 20 (maximal exertion) (American College of Sports Medicine, 2010b). This scale allows the person to assign one of a consecutive set of numbers with a corresponding descriptor of amount of exertion to the ongoing activity (e.g., 11, fairly light; or 17, very hard). For dynamic activities, the Borg scale has been found over the years to correlate validly with heart rate and oxygen uptake (Finucane, Fiddler, & Lindfield, 2005). Therapists should be aware that perceived exertion for a given level of oxygen uptake is higher for arm work than leg work (Russell, 1997). Lamb, Eston, and Corns (1999) looked at test–retest reliability and found it to differ by as much as 3 RPE when the level of agreement between trials was examined, and the scores of the two trials were not merely correlated. Nevertheless, these scales provide a good estimate when used repeatedly for the same patient and therefore may be used clinically during ongoing continuous activity, such as walking, bicycling, scrubbing floors, painting a wall, mowing the lawn, raking leaves, and calisthenic exercises. These scales do not apply to activities composed of sporadic variable movements.

The therapist should orient the person to the scale using the standardized instructions published by Borg (1985) prior to the start of the activity. The scale should be enlarged and posted so that it can be seen easily from where the person is engaging in activity. At appropriate intervals depending on the task, the therapist prompts the patient to rate exertion at that moment. The decision to continue depends on the goal and precautions for the particular patient.

Another measure easily used when engaging in functional tasks is the Talk Test. The client should be able to continue talking in full sentences during engagement in therapeutic tasks. This is correlated with the ventilator threshold, and when the client can no longer talk comfortably they have passed this threshold (American College of Sports Medicine, 2010a).

Muscular Aspects of Endurance

Muscular fitness is a combination of muscular strength and muscular endurance (American College of Sports Medicine, 2010b). This chapter has already explored the evaluation of muscular strength with MMT, grip, and pinch strength testing. Muscular endurance is the ability of the muscle to perform multiple repetitions of a contraction without fatigue (American College of Sports Medicine, 2010b). Endurance may be decreased because of local trauma or reduction of innervation. In normal muscle contraction against low resistance, only a few of the available motor units are needed at any one time. The active and resting units take turns. Fatigue rarely occurs in conditions required for ADL tasks. However, if the person sustains a contraction that exceeds 15%–20% MVC for the muscle group involved, blood flow to the working muscle decreases, causing a shift to anaerobic metabolism, which limits duration of contraction. The limitation is signaled by symptoms of muscle fatigue (cramping, burning, and tremor, which are secondary to the accumulation of lactic acid) and slowed nerve conduction velocity to the muscle fibers, which reduce tension and eventually result in inability to hold the contraction (American College of Sports Medicine, 2010a). Strength and endurance are closely related. As muscle gains strength, its endurance for a given level of work also increases.

For neurologically disadvantaged muscle, such as after a spinal cord injury, peripheral nerve injury, or stroke, fewer motor units or muscle fibers may be available than are required for daily activity. Such muscles work at as much as 50%–75% MVC to do otherwise low-intensity work (Trombly & Quintana, 1985).

Endurance can be measured dynamically or statically. Dynamic assessments include the number of repetitions per unit of time. When evaluating both cardiovascular and muscular endurance, the percentage of maximal heart rate generated by the task or MET level can also be documented. Static assessment is the amount of time a contraction can be held (American College of Sports Medicine, 2010b; Fletcher et al., 2001).

Intensity, duration, and frequency of the activity are considerations in evaluation of endurance. Intensity is related to both resistance and speed. The heavier the resistance or the faster the pace is, the higher the intensity. The intensity of the test activity must be kept constant from test to test to gauge improvement.

The decision to measure dynamically or statically depends on the functional goal of the patient and his or her cardiopulmonary status. If the patient's self-advancement and self-enhancement roles require mostly isotonic activity, endurance should be evaluated dynamically. To measure endurance in terms of number of repetitions, use a light repetitive activity such as the Box and Block Test, which is described in Chapter 37. It can be adapted to measure UE endurance for light work by counting the number of blocks the patient can transfer before becoming fatigued.

For some individuals, engaging in a task as light as the Box and Block Test will not demonstrate the decreased endurance that may be impairing their ability to return to work. In these cases, a functional capacity evaluation may be appropriate or a test of endurance, using equipment such as the Baltimore Therapeutic Equipment (BTE) work simulator. This equipment can be set up to simulate a variety of work and daily tasks. A static trial can be completed to gain a numeric value for the individual's MVC for that task, and then to test endurance, the therapist can set the resistance level at 20%–30% of that maximum. The therapist can see on the equipment if the patient is decreasing in speed and showing fatigue. The time, repetitions, and weight can be documented for later comparison to show progress in the area of endurance. Although these numbers can be used clinically to demonstrate progress, the therapist should use caution when relating them to work capacity. Research suggests that endurance time, VO_2, heart rate, and RPE were all significantly different in lifting endurance on the BTE when compared to actual lifting (Ting et al., 2001). The discussion in this research suggests that the differences could result from the decreased metabolic and cardiovascular demands when using the BTE and the difference in the lifting task based on the design of the BTE, which changes both the dynamic and static aspects of the lift and allows for additional compensation by the individual lifting (Ting et al., 2001).

If the patient expects to return to a job or hobby that requires maintaining grasp or holding loads (isometric contractions), static endurance should be tested. To measure statically, the amount of time a person can hold an object or position requiring a certain level MVC is noted. Normally, a person can hold 25% MVC for 5–6 minutes, 50% MVC for 1–2 minutes, and 100% MVC only momentarily (Dehn & Mullins, 1977).

Isometric holding increases blood pressure and stresses the cardiopulmonary system (Pollock et al., 2000). This is true especially if the person holds his or her breath (Valsalva maneuver) while holding the contraction. Therefore, persons being tested should talk (e.g., count or sing) while doing an isometric contraction to preclude breath holding. Isometric testing can produce arrhythmias and, therefore, electrocardiogram and blood pressure should be monitored during isometric testing of patients with heart disease or abnormalities. The results of isometric testing cannot be extrapolated to gauge isotonic aerobic exercise capacity (Pollock et al., 2000).

In a review of the literature in the care of individuals following stroke, Ma and Trombly (2002) discuss the importance of meaningful and purposeful tasks in the evaluation and treatment of endurance. The studies they reviewed found that the number of repetitions and length of time a person was willing to engage in a task both increased when the task was meaningful or preferred (Ma & Trombly, 2002). Assessment Table 7-1 lists many of the tests used to measure ROM, strength, and endurance.

Assessment Table 7-1 | Abilities and Capacities: Range of Motion, Strength, and Endurance

Instrument and Reference	Description	Time to Administer	Validity	Reliability	Sensitivity	Strengths and Weaknesses
Measurement of range of motion	Interval scale. Range varies with joint being measured	Full evaluation of all joints in the UE, 45 minutes to an hour	Gold standard	Intrarater reliability for shoulder external rotation, interclass correlation coefficient (ICC) = 0.58–0.67, internal rotation ICC = 0.63–0.71. Interrater reliability external rotation = 0.41–0.66, internal rotation ICC = 0.41–0.66 (Awan, Smith, & Boon, 2002)	In the upper and lower extremities, measurement error is estimated at 5° (Groth et al., 2001).	Strengths: Relatively fast and inexpensive measure. Measurements are consistently more accurate when done by the same therapist with the patient in the same position from test to test. Weaknesses: Interrater reliability is consistently lower than intrarater reliability. Accuracy of measurement is dependent on the consistent placement of the goniometer.
Hand Volumetry (Dodds et al., 2004)	Interval scale because it is a direct measure of the volume of water displaced	10–20 minutes	Gold standard. Direct measurement of hand volume	Test-retest reliability ($r = 0.99$) (Dodds et al., 2004)	Variation of measurement 3–5 mL (Dodds et al., 2004)	Strength: Gold standard for edema measurement. Weakness: Hand must be immersed in water, so therapist must be aware of any contraindications. Takes considerable time.
Figure-of-eight technique to measure hand edema (Dewey et al., 2007; Pellecchia, 2004)	Interval scale	1–4 minutes	Correlation coefficient between figure-of-eight technique and hand volumetry ICC = 0.83–0.95 (Dewey et al., 2007; Maihafer et al., 2003)	Intratester ICC for figure-of-eight ICC = 0.96-0.99; Intertester reliability ICC 0.94–0.99 (Dewey et al., 2007; Leard et al., 2004)	Recommend change of 1.16 cm to be clinically significant in patients with burns to the hands (Dewey et al., 2007)	Strengths: Fast measurement. Can be used with individuals with open wounds or skin conditions. Weakness: Larger studies of various patient populations needed.
Visual Analog Scale for pain measurement	Interval scale with scores measured along the 10-cm line	1 minute	Gold standard; however, still a subjective measure	Not established; in studies, a decrease in pain level resulted in less need for medication, showing clinical significance (Farrar, Berlin, & Strom, 2003).	Recommend 33% change for clinical significance (Farrar, Berlin, & Strom, 2003)	Strengths: Fast measurement. Can be used to monitor changes in pain in a single patient. Weakness: Cannot be used to compare pain levels between patients.

Assessment	Scale	Time	Validity	Reliability	Norms	Strengths/Weaknesses
Numerical pain-rating scale	0–10 scale of self-perceived pain level	1 minute	Subjective measure	In studies, a decrease in pain level resulted in less need for medication showing clinical significance (Farrar, Berlin, & Strom, 2003).	Recommend change in pain level by at least two levels to be significant (Farrar, Berlin, & Strom, 2003)	Strengths: Fast measurement. Can be used to monitor changes in pain in a single patient. Weakness: Cannot be used to compare pain levels between patients.
Manual muscle testing	Ordinal scale from 0 to 5	Depending on the number of muscles being tested, up to 1 hour	Gold standard	In a reliability test for intrinsic hand muscles, intrarater ($r = 0.71$–0.96) and interrater ($r = 0.72$–0.93) reliability (Brandsma et al., 1995). In an evaluation of reliability for the deltoid muscles, Pollard et al. (2005) found that two testers agreed exactly 82% of the time, ($\kappa = 0.62$).	Not established	Strength: No equipment needed. Weakness: Dependent on training and experience of the tester.
Handheld dynamometry	Interval scale; measurement is in kilograms	Depending on the number of muscles being tested, up to 1 hour	Direct measure of strength	Interrater reliability ICC = 0.79–0.96, and intrarater reliability ICC = 0.87–0.98 (Ottenbacher et al., 2002).	Norms established (Bohannon, 1988)	Strength: Reliable testing device. Weaknesses: Validity and sensitivity not established. Expense of device.
Grip strength test	Interval scale; measures resistance in pounds or kilograms	5 minutes	Recommended by American Society of Hand Therapists as a valid measure of hand strength (Fess, 1992)	Test–retest reliability Jamar dynamometer $r > 0.80$, and interrater reliability $r = 0.98$ (Roberts et al., 2011).	Norms established with gold standard Jamar dynamometer (Mathiowetz et al., 1985); recommend 13-pound change for clinical significance (Roberts et al., 2011)	Strengths: Quick and easy measure. Norms available. Weakness: Dynamometers need to be calibrated regularly in order to be accurate.
Pinch test	Interval scale; measures resistance in pounds or kilograms	5 minutes	Recommended by American Society of Hand Therapists as a valid measure of pinch strength (Fess, 1992)	Interrater reliability $r = 0.98$; test–retest reliability was $r = 0.81$ (Mathiowetz et al., 1984).	Norms established (Mathiowetz et al., 1985)	Strengths: Quick and easy measure. Norms available. Weakness: Pinch meters need to be calibrated regularly in order to be accurate.
Borg rating of perceived exertion scale	Ordinal scale, from 6 to 20	1 minute	Valid measure of exercise intensity (Chen, Fan, & Moe, 2002)	Not established	Not established	Strength: Good measure for individuals. Weakness: Not consistent between individuals.

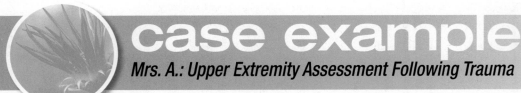

case example
Mrs. A.: Upper Extremity Assessment Following Trauma

Occupational Therapy Assessment Process	Clinical Reasoning Process	
	Objectives	Examples of Therapist's Internal Dialogue

Patient Information

Mrs. A. is a 42-year-old right-handed woman 8 weeks status post open reduction internal fixation (ORIF) of a right humerus fracture following a gunshot wound (GSW) during an assault in a parking lot in the city (about 45 minutes away). Her radial nerve (which is frequently injured during humerus fractures) was not lacerated, but she did have wrist drop for a week following the injury and surgery that has slowly been improving (neuropraxia). She complains of UE weakness, stiffness, and decreased motion. She also complains of pain and fatigue that are increasingly limiting her self-maintenance, self-advancement, and self-enhancement roles.

She is a married dental hygienist, although her husband frequently travels for work. They live in a one-story house. She has two grown children and enjoys gardening, working out at the gym, and shopping. She was previously seen at another facility recommended by the injury lawyer but has decided to transfer to a new facility because it is closer to her home. She recently had a follow-up with her surgeon, who referred her to occupational therapy for evaluation and to begin strengthening training.

Understand the patient's diagnosis or condition

"Mrs. A. is very active and has not been able to fully return to work following this trauma. I wonder if her weakness is impacting her ability to engage in her work tasks?"

Know the person

"Mrs. A. is frequently home alone during the week. I wonder if she is having any problems with the trauma being so recent, and if this is impacting her engagement in tasks? I wonder if she has been avoiding any home maintenance or self-care tasks because of her fatigue?"

Appreciate the context

"I bet being a dental hygienist requires good endurance of the muscles in both upper extremities to hold and manipulate the tools all day long. I wonder what she is currently doing at work?"

Develop provisional hypotheses

"She has been working in therapy to regain her motion, but now that she is able to work toward improving her strength and endurance, I bet she will be motivated by the potential to fully return to work. I wonder how the trauma itself is impacting her engagement in activities?"

Assessment Process

To determine Mrs. A.'s perception of her occupational dysfunction and her priorities, the therapist administered the Canadian Occupational Performance Measure (COPM). To determine to what extent motion, strength, and endurance problems affected Mrs. A.'s occupational functioning, a manual muscle test on selected muscle groups, grip- and pinch-strength assessments, numeric pain-rating scale, and engagement in 1 minute of wrist activity on the Baltimore Therapeutic Equipment (BTE) for endurance during work tasks were administered.

Consider evaluation approach and methods

"I need to get a picture of what occupations are important to her. I also need to know exactly how her arms are functioning in terms of motion, strength, and endurance. I would like to know how much pain she is having at rest and during activity."

Assessment Results

The results of the COPM are as follows:
Difficulty holding dental hygienist tools for prolonged periods (performance 3, satisfaction 2).

Difficulty with morning activities of daily living, including showering and dressing. She has problems squeezing bottles, bathing the left side of the body such as her armpit and back, and putting on jewelry (performance 6, satisfaction 5).

Difficulty engaging in shopping tasks because of the fear associated with it. She was on a shopping trip when the trauma occurred (performance 5, satisfaction 4).

Interpret observations

"Mrs. A. is involved in a number of gross and fine motor activities during the day and seems to be having problems with all of them."

Inability to do heavy meal preparation activities, including cutting vegetables and carrying dishes (performance 6, satisfaction 4).

Unable to garden as desired, specifically planting, digging with a trowel, and weeding (performance 3, satisfaction 2).

The results of Mrs. A.'s range of motion and manual muscle test are displayed below. Grip strength using a Jamar dynamometer was 18 pounds on the right and 58 pounds on the left. Tip pinch strength was 3 pounds on the right and 12 pounds on the left. Lateral pinch was 5 pounds on the right and 14 pounds on the left. Palmar pinch was 4 pounds on the right and 13 pounds on the left.

Active range of motion:
Shoulder, wrist, and hand AROM within normal limits.
Elbow extension–flexion right: 30°–120°
Elbow flexion left: 0°–150°
Elbow hyperextension left: 0°–5°
Supination right: 0°–60°
Supination left: 0°–90°
Pronation right: 0°–80°
Pronation left: 0°–90°

Mrs. A. has a 22-cm scar along the dorsal aspect of her arm that is red in appearance and flat. There is mild adhesion noted along the scar, and the scar does pucker with elbow motion.

Select manual muscle strength	Right	Left
Shoulder flexion	5	5
Shoulder abduction	4–	5
Elbow flexion	4	5
Elbow extension	4	5
Forearm supination	4	5
Forearm pronation	4	5
Wrist flexion	5	5
Wrist extension	3+	5
Digital extension	3+	5

Mrs. A. reported a 5 on the numeric pain-rating scale at rest and described it as burning pain, but stated that pain increases to 6 during morning activities of daily living, 6 during meal preparation, and 7 during work tasks. She describes this pain as sharp pain.

Using the BTE, Mrs. A. demonstrated only five repetitions of wrist motion during 1 minute when set at 70% of her maximum voluntary contraction, which was 3 pounds.

"Mrs. A. is weak in the muscles that have debilitated because of nonuse, as well as the muscles innervated by the radial nerve. The dynamometer test showed a significant decrease in grip strength for her right hand, which is her dominant hand, but grip strength was within normal limits for her left hand. Her right hand pinches were also significantly limited compared to the left or to the norms, whereas all three pinches of her left hand were within normal limits. The weakness in her right hand also contributes to her difficulty in many occupational tasks, such as work tasks, opening jars, and manipulating garden tools."

"Mrs. A.'s scores on the visual analog scale indicate increased pain in her hands and shoulders during many functional activities, with less, although still significant, pain at rest. She describes these pains differently, and burning pain can sometimes be attributed to the nerve trying to heal."

"The results of endurance testing on the BTE demonstrate decreased endurance with activities requiring wrist extension such as manipulating tools for work."

Occupational Therapy Problem List

Decreased ability to perform morning activities of daily living, including bathing and dressing, because of decreased motion, weakness, and low endurance.

Decreased ability to perform meal preparation tasks because of weak grasp and pinch on the dominant side.

Decreased ability to perform work-related tasks, including manipulating tools for prolonged periods of time because of weakness and decreased endurance of the muscles innervated by the radial nerve.

Decreased ability to garden because of weakness and pain.

Decreased engagement in shopping tasks based on psychosocial factors.

Synthesize results

"I wonder what adaptations she is already using in her activities of daily living and instrumental activities of daily living tasks and whether additional adaptations would be helpful until her strength and endurance are regained."

"Mrs. A. has problems with decreased motion, weakness, and endurance. She is motivated to return to work, and I should use activities for her therapy and goals to work on full return to work."

"I need to find out what all her works tasks involve and what sort of time she has between patients."

"I wonder if she is already seeking assistance for the psychosocial issues she is having following this trauma. I will ask her about this and make a referral if she is not."

 ## Clinical Reasoning in Occupational Therapy Practice

Edema Assessment Selection

Expanding on Mrs. A.'s case example information, you are performing her initial evaluation 10 days postoperatively and note significant edema to the right wrist, hand, and digits. She has multiple open, sutured, and healing lacerations to her hands and arms from falling during her attack. What methods would you use to evaluate and specify the extent of her edema? Would you do anything differently at her reevaluation once the lacerations have fully healed?

Summary Review Questions

1. Where does the assessment of ROM, strength, and endurance fit within the role of occupational therapy and the OTPF?
2. What does it mean if AROM is less than PROM?
3. Describe a situation where a screening of motion and strength may be more appropriate than taking formal measurements at each joint and muscle group.
4. How is a break test used to determine strength?
5. An individual has decreased function with ADL, IADL, work, and leisure tasks 8 weeks post–wrist fusion operation with limited AROM at the MCP, PIP, and DIP joints of the dominant hand and decreased hand grip strength 70 pounds less than the contralateral side. The person specifically mentions decreased ability to complete meal preparation, dressing, office administrative work, and golfing. Write appropriate short- and long-term goals.
6. Describe the standardized procedures for testing muscle strength.
7. An individual demonstrates 4−/5 MMT for the right, dominant hand, wrist, and digital extension while recovering from a radial nerve entrapment. The client states that he cannot write for more than 10 minutes or type for more than 15 minutes, which is impacting his role as a college student. Describe appropriate intervention planning for this individual.
8. An individual demonstrates decreased endurance following amputation of the left leg below the knee with an extended period of immobility from surgical complications. She is now being fit with a prosthesis, but the surgeon is concerned with safety from the decreased cardiovascular and muscular endurance. The client enjoys cooking, puzzles, and baseball. What intervention planning would you recommend?
9. What is your maximum heart rate?
10. Select a diagnosis that would impact ROM, strength, or endurance. If you were impacted by that diagnosis, what would be your short- and long-term goals? What sort of intervention planning would help you accomplish those goals?

Glossary

Active range of motion (AROM)—The amount of movement possible at a joint when it is voluntarily moved by muscle contraction.

Anatomical position—Standing straight with feet together and flat on the floor, with arms by the sides and palms of the hands facing forward. The zero position for ROM measurement.

Calibrate—To set an instrument at a known value according to a standard.

Contracture—Inability to move a body part because of soft tissue shortening.

Limits of motion—The beginning and ending positions of movement at a joint.

Maximum voluntary contraction (MVC)—The greatest amount of tension a muscle can generate and hold only for a moment, such as in muscle testing.

Mechanical advantage—The position in which the muscle is able to generate the greatest tension, that is, when it is longer than the resting length of the muscle. In this position, the passive tension generated by the viscoelastic properties of the muscle and its tendon combine with the active tension generated by the contraction of the muscle fibers to produce a maximum voluntary contraction. When the muscle is fully lengthened or shortened, the viscoelastic, or passive, tension is reduced.

Metabolic equivalent (MET) level—One MET (the unit of measure) equals basal metabolic rate. Basal metabolic rate is the amount of oxygen consumption necessary to maintain the metabolic processes of the body at rest and is quantified as 3.5 mL of oxygen per kilogram of body weight per minute (American College of Sports Medicine, 2010a). The energy cost of activities or exercise can be rated using multiples of METs.

Passive range of motion (PROM)—The amount of movement possible at a joint when an outside force moves the limb.

Reliability—Characteristic of an instrument indicating that the instrument consistently produces the same results including stability (intrarater), internal consistency, and equivalence (interrater) when properly administered under similar circumstances (Yancosek & Howell, 2009). Reliability is usually defined by a correlation coefficient (r) or an interclass correlation coefficient (ICC). An r or ICC of 1 indicates a perfect linear relationship between one variable (e.g., rater A's scores) and another variable (e.g., rater B's scores). An r of 0.85 or ICC of 0.75 is considered acceptable for measuring instruments. Reliability can be increased by controlling all variables that affect the scores other than the one being measured (e.g., change in ROM). Control is gained by keeping everything the same or by deleting some variables.

Standard deviation (SD)—A measure of dispersion indicating the variability within a set of scores. Low variability within the scores of a set of therapists indicates that the therapists are following the same protocol and the phenomenon being measured is unchanging; high variability indicates that the phenomenon being measured is unstable or that the therapists should control their test administration better. To interpret a score, the therapist often compares it with norms (averages and SDs). The SD tells you where your patient's score falls in relation to the norm because you can relate it to the normal curve. In the bell-shaped normal curve, 1 SD is equal to approximately 68% of the area under the curve (34% on each side of the mean); 2 SD is equal to approximately 95% of the area under the curve; and 3 SD is equal to approximately 99% of the area under the curve. A score of 2–3 SD below the mean normative score indicates a limitation and need for treatment.

Tenodesis—The mechanical effect caused by the length of extrinsic finger flexors and extensors. When the wrist is flexed, the fingers tend to extend because the extensors are too short to allow full finger flexion and wrist flexion at the same time. Similarly, when the wrist is extended, the fingers tend to flex.

References

American College of Sports Medicine. (2010a). *ACSM's resource manual for guidelines for exercise testing and prescription* (6th ed.). Philadelphia: Lippincott Williams & Wilkins.

American College of Sports Medicine. (2010b). *Guidelines for exercise testing and prescription* (8th ed.). Baltimore: Lippincott Williams & Wilkins.

American Occupational Therapy Association. (2008). Occupational therapy practice framework: Domain & process (2nd ed.). *American Journal of Occupational Therapy, 62,* 625–683.

Anderson, L. R., III, & Bohannon, R. W. (1991). Head and neck position does not influence maximum static elbow extension force measured in healthy individuals tested while prone. *Occupational Therapy Journal of Research, 11,* 121–126.

Awan, R., Smith, J., & Boon, A. J. (2002). Measuring shoulder internal rotation range of motion: A comparison of 3 techniques. *Archives of Physical Medicine and Rehabilitation, 83,* 1229–1234.

Bohannon, R. W. (1988). Make tests and break tests of elbow flexor muscle strength. *Physical Therapy, 68,* 193–194.

Bohannon, R. W., Warren, M., & Cogman, K. (1991). Influence of shoulder position on maximum voluntary elbow flexion force in stroke patients. *Occupational Therapy Journal of Research, 11,* 73–79.

Boone, A. J., & Smith, J. (2000). Manual scapular stabilization: Its effect on shoulder rotational range of motion. *Archives of Physical Medicine and Rehabilitation, 81,* 978–983.

Borg, G. A. V. (1985). *An introduction to Borg's RPE-Scale.* New York: Movement.

Brandsma, J. W., Schreuders, T. R., Birke, J. A., Piefer, A., & Oostendorp, P. (1995). Manual muscle strength testing: Intraobserver and interobserver reliabilities for the intrinsic muscles of the hand. *Journal of Hand Therapy, 8,* 185–190.

Chen, M. J., Fan, I., & Moe, S. T. (2002). Criterion-related validity of the Borg ratings of perceived exertion scale in healthy individuals: A meta-analysis. *Journal of Sports Sciences, 20,* 873–899.

Clarkson, H. M. (2000). *Musculoskeletal assessment: Joint range of motion and manual muscle strength* (2nd ed.). Philadelphia: Lippincott Williams & Wilkins.

Clerke, A., & Clerke, J. (2001). A literature review of the effect of handedness on isometric grip strength differences of left and right hands. *American Journal of Occupational Therapy, 55,* 206–211.

Coldham, F., Lewis, J., & Lee, H. (2006). The reliability of one vs. three grip trials in symptomatic and asymptomatic subjects. *Journal of Hand Therapy, 19,* 318–327.

Dehn, M. M., & Mullins, C. B. (1977). Physiologic effects and importance of exercise in patients with coronary artery disease. *Cardiovascular Medicine, 2,* 365–371, 377–387.

De Smet, L., & Decramer, A. (2006). Key pinch force in children. *Journal of Pediatric Orthopedics B, 15,* 426–427.

Dewey, W. S., Hedman, T. L., Chapman, T. T., Wolf, S. E., & Holcomb, J. B. (2007). The reliability and concurrent validity of the figure-of-eight method of measuring hand edema in patients with burns. *Journal of Burn Care & Research, 28,* 157–162.

Dodds, R. L., Nielsen, K. A., Shirley, A. G., Stefaniak, H., Falconio, M. J., & Moyers, P. A. (2004). Test-retest reliability of the commercial volumeter. *Work, 22,* 107–110.

Ellis, B., & Bruton, A. (2002). A study to compare the reliability of composite finger flexion with goniometry for measurement of range of motion in the hand. *Clinical Rehabilitation, 16,* 562–570.

Farrar, J. T., Berlin, J. A., & Strom, B. L. (2003). Clinically important changes in acute pain outcome measures: A validation study. *Journal of Pain and Symptom Management, 25,* 406–411.

Fess, E. E. (1987). A method of checking Jamar dynamometer calibration. *Journal of Hand Therapy, 1,* 28–32.

Fess, E. E. (1992). Grip strength. In J. S. Casanova (Ed.), *Clinical assessment recommendations* (2nd ed., pp. 41–45). Chicago: American Society of Hand Therapists.

Fike, M. L., & Rousseau, E. (1982). Measurement of adult hand strength: A comparison of two instruments. *Occupational Therapy Journal of Research, 2,* 43–49.

Finucane, L., Fiddler, H., & Lindfield, H. (2005). Assessment of the RPE as a measure of cardiovascular fitness in patients with low back pain. *International Journal of Therapy and Rehabilitation, 12,* 106–111.

Fletcher, G. F., Balady, G. J., Amsterdam, E. A., Chaitman, B., Eckel, R., Fleg, J., Froelicher, V. F., Leon, A. S., Piña I. L., Rodney, R., Simons-Morton, D. G., Williams, M. A., & Bazzarre, T. (2001). AHA Scientific Statement: Exercise standards for testing and training: A statement for healthcare professionals from the American Heart Association. *Circulation, 104,* 1694–1740.

Florence, J.M., Pandya, S., King, W.M., Robison, J.D., Baty, J., Miller, J.P., Schierbecker, J., & Signore, L.C. (1992). Intrarater reliability of manual muscle test (medical research council scale) grades in Duchenne's muscular dystrophy. *Physical Therapy Journal, 72,* 115–122.

Fong, P. W. K., & Ng, G. Y. F. (2001). Brief report: Effect of wrist positioning on the repeatability and strength of power grip. *American Journal of Occupational Therapy, 55,* 212–216.

Gerhardt, J., Cocchiarella, L., & Lea, R. (2002). The practical guide to range of motion assessment. Chicago: American Medical Association.

Greene, W. B., & Heckman, J. D. (Eds.). (1994). *The clinical measurement of joint motion.* Rosemont, IL: American Academy of Orthopaedic Surgeons.

Groth, G. N., VanDeven, K. M., Phillips, E. C., & Ehretsman, R. L. (2001). Goniometry of the proximal and distal interphalangeal joints: Part III. Placement preferences, interrater reliability and concurrent validity. *Journal of Hand Therapy, 14,* 23–29.

Gunal, I., Kose, N., Erdogan, O., Gokturk, E., & Seber, S. (1996). Normal range of motion of the joints of the upper extremity in male subjects, with special reference to side. *Journal of Bone and Joint Surgery, 78-A,* 1401–1404.

Hall, C. M., & Brody, L. T. (1999). *Therapeutic exercise: Moving toward function.* Philadelphia: Lippincott Williams & Wilkins.

Hayes, K., Walton, J. R., Szomor Z. L., & Murrell, G. A. C. (2002). Reliability of 3 methods for assessing shoulder strength. *Journal of Shoulder and Elbow Surgery, 11,* 33–39.

Herbison, G. J., Issac, Z., Cohne, M. E., & Ditunno, J. F. (1996). Strength post-spinal cord injury: Myometer versus manual muscle test. *Spinal Cord, 34,* 543–548.

Hislop, H., & Montgomery, J. (Eds.). (1995). *Daniel's and Worthingham's muscle testing* (6th ed.). Philadelphia: W. B. Saunders Co.

Hockenberry, M. J., & Wilson, D. (2009). *Wong's essentials of pediatric nursing* (8th ed.). St. Louis: Mosby.

Howell, J. W., Rothstein, J. M., Lamb, R. L., & Merritt, W. H. (1989). An experimental investigation of the validity of the manual muscle test positions for the extensor pollicis longus and flexor pollicis brevis muscles. *Journal of Hand Therapy, 3,* 20–28.

Jensen, M. P., Chen, C., & Brugger, A. M. (2003). Interpretation of visual analog scale ratings and change scores: A reanalysis of two clinical trials of postoperative pain. *The Journal of Pain, 4,* 407–414.

Johannson, C. A., Kent, B. E., & Shepard, K. F. (1983). Relationship between verbal command volume and magnitude of muscle contraction. *Physical Therapy, 63,* 1260–1265.

Karagiannopoulos, C., Sitler, M., & Michlovitz, S. (2003). Reliability of 2 functional goniometric methods for measuring forearm pronation and supination active range of motion. *Journal of Orthopaedic & Sports Physical Therapy, 33,* 523–531.

Kendall, F. P., McCreary, E. K., Provance, P. G., Rodgers, M. M., & Romani, W. A. (2005). *Muscles: Testing and function with posture and pain* (5th ed.). Baltimore: Lippincott Williams & Wilkins.

Lamb, K. L., Eston, R. G., & Corns, D. (1999). Reliability of ratings of perceived exertion during progressive treadmill exercise. *British Journal of Sports Medicine, 33,* 336–339.

LaStayo, P. C., & Wheeler, D. L. (1994). Reliability of passive wrist flexion and extension goniometric measurements: A multicenter study. *Physical Therapy, 74,* 162–176.

Leard, J. S., Breglio, L., Fraga, L., Ellrod, N., Nadler, L., Yasso, M., Fay, E., Ryan, K., & Pellecchia, G. L. (2004). Reliability and concurrent validity of the figure-of-eight method of measuring hand size in patients with hand pathology. *Journal of Orthopaedic and Sports Physical Therapy, 34,* 335–340.

Lindstrom-Hazel, D., Krat, A., & Bix, L. (2009). Interrater reliability of students using hand and pinch dynamometers. *American Journal of Occupational Therapy, 63,* 193–197.

Long, C. (1968). Intrinsic-extrinsic muscle control of the fingers. *Journal of Bone and Joint Surgery, 50A,* 973–984.

Long, C., & Brown, M. E. (1962). EMG kinesiology of the hand: Part III. Lumbricales and flexor digitorum profundus to the long finger. *Archives of Physical Medicine and Rehabilitation, 43,* 450–460.

Ma, H., & Trombly, C. A. (2002). A synthesis of the effects of occupational therapy for persons with stroke: Part II. Remediation of impairments. *American Journal of Occupational Therapy, 56,* 260–274.

MacDermid, J. C., Evenhuis, W., & Louzon, M. (2001). Inter-instrument reliability of pinch strength scores. *Journal of Hand Therapy, 14,* 36–42.

Maihafer, G. C., Llewellyn, M. A., Pillar, W. J., Scott, K. L., Marina, D. M., & Bond, R. M. (2003). A comparison of the figure-of eight method and water volumetry in measurement of hand and wrist size. *Journal of Hand Therapy, 16,* 305–310.

Massy-Westropp, N. M., Gill, T. K., Taylor, A. W., Bohannon, R. W., & Hill, C. L. (2011). Hand grip strength: Age and gender stratified normative data in a population-based study. *BMC Research Notes, 4,* 127.

Mathiowetz, V., Kashman, N., Volland, G., Weber, K., Dowe, M., & Rogers, S. (1985). Grip and pinch strength: Normative data for adults. *Archives of Physical Medicine and Rehabilitation, 66,* 69–74.

Mathiowetz, V., Vizenor, L., & Melander, D. (2000). Comparison of baseline instruments to Jamar dynamometer and the B & L Engineering pinch gauge. *Occupational Therapy Journal of Research, 20,* 147–162.

Mathiowetz, V., Weber, K., Volland, G., & Kashman, N. (1984). Reliability and validity of grip and pinch strength evaluations. *Journal of Hand Surgery, 9A,* 222–226.

Medical Research Council. (1976). *Aids to the examination of the peripheral nervous system.* London: Her Majesty's Stationary Office.

Milner-Brown, H. S., Mellenthin, M., & Miller, R. G. (1986). Quantifying human muscle strength, endurance and fatigue. *Archives of Physical Medicine and Rehabilitation, 67,* 530–535.

Ottenbacher, K. J., Branch, L. G., Ray, L., Gonzales, V. A., Peek, M. K., & Hinman, M. R. (2002). The reliability of upper- and lower-extremity strength testing in a community survey of older adults. *Archives of Physical Medicine and Rehabilitation, 83,* 1423–1427.

Pellecchia, G. L. (2004). Figure-of-eight method of measuring hand size: Reliability and concurrent validity. *Journal of Hand Therapy, 16,* 300–304.

Petersen, C. M., & Hayes, K. W. (2000). Construct validity of Cyriax's selective tension examination: Association of end-feels with pain at the knee and shoulder. *Journal of Orthopaedic & Sports Physical Therapy, 30,* 512–527.

Pollard, H., Lakay, B., Tucker, F., Wilson, B., & Bablis, P. (2005). Interexaminer reliability of the deltoid and psoas muscle test. *Journal of Manipulative and Physiological Therapy, 25,* 52–56.

Pollock, M. L., Franklin, B. A., Balady, G. J., Chaitman, B. L., Fleg, J. L., Fletcher, B., Limacher, M., Piña, I. L., Stein, R. A., Williams, M., & Bazzarre, T. (2000). Resistance exercise in individuals with and without cardiovascular disease: Benefits, rationale, safety, and prescription. *Circulation, 101,* 828–833.

Roberts, H. C., Denison, H. J., Martin, H. J., Patel, H. P., Syddall, H., Cooper, C., & Sayer, A. A. (2011). A review of the measurement of grip strength in clinical and epidemiological studies: Towards a standardised approach. *Age and Ageing, 40,* 423–429.

Russell, W. D. (1997). On the current status of rated perceived exertion. *Perceptual and Motor Skills, 84,* 799–808.

Rybski, M. (2004). *Kinesiology for occupational therapy.* Thorofare, NJ: Slack.

Sabari, J. S., Maltzev, I., Lubarsky, D., Liszkay, E., & Homel, P. (1998). Goniometric assessment of shoulder range of motion: Comparison of testing in supine and sitting positions. *Archives of Physical Medicine and Rehabilitation, 79,* 647–651.

Shechtman, O., Gestewitz, L., & Kimble, C. (2005). Reliability and validity of the DynEx dynamometer. *Journal of Hand Therapy, 18,* 339–347.

Schwartz, S., Cohen, M. E., Herbison, G. J., & Shah, A. (1992). Relationship between two measures of upper extremity strength: Manual muscle testing compared to hand held myometry. *Archives of Physical Medicine and Rehabilitation, 73,* 1063–1068.

Somers, D. L., Hanson, J. A., Kedzierski, C. M., Nestor, K. L., & Quinlivan, K. Y. (1997). The influence of experience on the reliability of goniometric and visual measurement of forefoot position. *Journal of Orthopedic Sports Physical Therapy, 25,* 192–202.

Stark, T., Walker, B., Phillips, J. K., Rejer, R., & Beck, R. (2011). Hand-held dynamometry correlation with the gold standard isokinetic dynamometry: A systematic review. *Physical Medicine & Rehabilitation, 3,* 472–479.

Tietjen-Smith, T., Smith, S. W., Martin, M., Henry, R., Weeks, S., & Bryant, A. (2006). Grip strength in relation to overall strength and functional capacity in very old and the oldest old females. *Physical & Occupational Therapy in Geriatrics, 24,* 63–78.

Ting, W., Wessel, J., Brintnell, S., Maikala, R., & Bhambhani, Y. (2001). Validity of the Baltimore therapeutic equipment work simulator in the measurement of lifting endurance in healthy men. *The American Journal of Occupational Therapy, 55,* 184–190.

Triffitt, P. D., Wildin, C., & Hajioff, D. (1999). The reproducibility of measurement of shoulder movement. *Acta Orthopaedica Scandinavica, 70,* 322–324.

Trombly, C. A., & Quintana, L. A. (1985). Differences in response to exercise by post-CVA and normal subjects. *Occupational Therapy Journal of Research, 5,* 39–58.

van de Pol, R. J., van Trijffel, E., & Lucas, C. (2010). Inter-rater reliability for measurement of passive physiological range of motion of upper extremity joints is better if instruments are used: A systematic review. *Journal of Physiotherapy, 56,* 7–17.

Williamson, A., & Hoggart, B. (2005). Pain: A review of three commonly used pain rating scales. *Journal of Clinical Nursing, 14,* 798–804.

Wilmore, J. H., & Costill, D. L. (1999). *Physiology of sport and exercise* (2nd ed.). Champaign, IL: Human Kinetics.

Yancosek, K. E., & Howell, D. (2009). A narrative review of dexterity assessments. *Journal of Hand Therapy, 22,* 258–270.

Yen, T. Y., & Radwin, R. G. (2000). Comparison between using spectral analysis of electrogoniometer data and observational analysis to quantify repetitive motion and ergonomic changes in cyclical industrial work. *Ergonomics, 43,* 106–132.

Acknowledgments

Thank you to the staff of Ireland Army Community Hospital for their contributions in collecting resources and contributing to the photography in this chapter.

8

Assessing Abilities and Capacities: Motor Planning and Performance

Khader Almhdawi, Virgil Mathiowetz, and Julie D. Bass

Learning Objectives

After studying this chapter, the reader will be able to do the following:

1. Contrast the reflex-hierarchical and systems models of motor control.
2. Describe various types of motor dysfunction seen in persons with central nervous system lesions.
3. Compare the neuromaturational and systems theories of motor development.
4. Contrast the assumptions of the neurophysiological and task-related approaches to treatment.
5. Describe the different evaluation strategies that are used by the neurophysiological and task-related approaches.
6. Describe some additional evaluation strategies that are not associated directly with either approach related to motor ability including balance, reach and manipulation, functional gait, apraxia, and motor neglect.

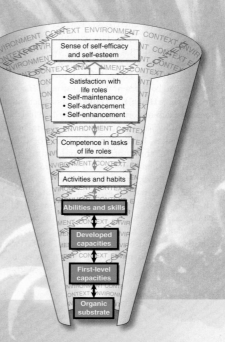

Our understanding of motor behavior and motor control, motor development, motor learning, and motor skill continues to evolve (Shumway-Cook & Woollacott, 2012). Sophisticated technology has led to an explosion of information about the control, development, and acquisition of movement (Fee & Long, 2011; Ingram & Wolpert, 2011). Human movement scientists, neurophysiologists, neuropsychologists, and others contribute to this effort. In an attempt to impose order on the many pieces of information, they deduce models and theories of motor behavior. As these models and theories change, therapeutic approaches and their evaluations also must change.

As a result of changes in the motor behavior literature, some (Rao, 2011; Shumway-Cook & Woollacott, 2012) have questioned the assumptions underlying the neurophysiological approaches, which include Rood's (1954) sensorimotor approach, Knott and Voss's (1968) proprioceptive neuromuscular facilitation, Brunnstrom's (1970) movement therapy, and Bobath's (1978, 1990) neurodevelopmental treatment. See web chapters A, B, C for further description of these approaches. Two task-related approaches, a task-oriented approach (Horak, 1991; Mathiowetz & Bass Haugen, 1994) and Carr and Shepherd's approach (1987, 2011), are proposed as alternatives to the neurophysiological approaches.

Definition 8-1 contrasts the assumptions of the neurophysiological and task-related approaches, the models and theories of motor behavior that they are based on, and the evaluation strategies associated with each approach. The evaluation strategies used by the neurophysiological approaches still continue to influence clinical practice as well. However, task-related evaluation strategies have an increasing influence on current practice.

When assessing motor behavior for clients recovering from neurological disorders, the therapist needs to consider both function and impairment. This evaluation should be applied individually, emphasizing each client's specific role performance and functional participation (Almhdawi, 2011). Following the World Health Organization definition of functioning, disability, and health (World Health Organization [WHO], 2001), the therapist can assess the body function or impairment, measuring the client's physical abilities such as range of motion and strength. Activity limitations or functional abilities are measured by examining the client's quality of movements and functional performance during real-life activities consistent with each client's specific roles and functional needs.

NEUROPHYSIOLOGICAL APPROACHES

Assumptions of the Neurophysiological Approaches

Definition 8-1 includes the assumptions of the four neurophysiological approaches as described by their original proponents. It is recognized that some of these approaches have evolved over time, adopting the assumptions of the task-related approaches (Howle, 2002). As a result, the theoretical differences between some of these approaches are much smaller today than they were 20 years ago. Unfortunately, clinical practice tends to lag behind changes in theory. To understand the neurophysiological approaches, one must understand the reflex-hierarchical model of motor control and neuromaturational theories of motor development from which these treatment approaches originated.

Reflex-Hierarchical Model of Motor Control

Figure 8-1 illustrates a reflex-hierarchical model (Trombly, 1989) that synthesizes the basic science literature of the 1970s and 1980s. This model evolved from earlier separate reflex and hierarchical models, both of which were unsuccessful in explaining the variety of movements available to human beings. This combined model assumes that the central nervous system (CNS) is hierarchically organized and that movement is controlled by central programs or elicited by sensory input.

As can be seen in Figure 8-1, the first step of purposeful movements is motivation by internal or external stimuli such as thirst (Marsden, 1982). Following this, a person utilizes his long-term memory to select a prestored generalized movement program that can enable reaching to a water bottle (Marsden, 1982). The person then adjusts the prestored motor programs to fit the context being faced (such as determining the specific muscles needed, the force of the contractions, and the overall duration of the movement) and then forwards these orders for execution (Marsden, 1982).

As the program for reaching a bottle of water is executed, the movements are monitored via cutaneous input, visual and auditory cues, and ongoing proprioceptive input (Brooks, 1986). The program being executed would be changed only if the movement was sensed to be wrong or in the case of an unexpected event. When the motor program is executed, the α- and γ-motor neurons are coactivated and excite the extrafusal and intrafusal muscle fibers according to the plan. A discrepancy in the length of these fibers would be sent to the higher centers when active movement is stopped unexpectedly. Stretch reflexes are activated in response to this discrepancy (Brooks, 1986). The outcome of the movement determines whether the motor plan needs to be adapted for future use through the use of knowledge of results feedback (Gazzaniga, Ivry, & Mangun, 2009; Wei & Körding, 2009). Finally, the successful movements whose sensory feedback matches the intended movements at the time of generating the motor program are stored in the long-term memory system for future use (Adkins et al., 2006; Gentile, 1972). The learned motor skill must be practiced to be retained at the same level of expertise (Halsband & Lange, 2006). Expertise is improved by practice with intention to improve (Cano-de-la-Cuerda et al., 2012; Latash et al., 2010).

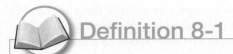

Definition 8-1

Comparison of the Neurophysiological and System-Based Task-Related Approaches

Neurophysiological Approaches	Systems-Based Task-Related Approaches

Models of Motor Control

Reflex-Hierarchical Systems

- Movements are elicited by sensory input or controlled by central programs.
- Open-loop and closed-loop controls are used.
- Feedback and feed-forward influence movements
- Central nervous system (CNS) is hierarchically organized, with higher centers controlling lower centers.
- Reciprocal innervation is essential for coordinated movement.

Systems

- The movements are organized by the functional needs/goals.
- Movement emerges from the interaction of many systems.
- Systems are dynamical, self-organizing, and heterarchical.
- The proffered movement pattern is the most efficient to achieve the functional goal.
- Changes in one or more systems can alter behavior.

Theories of Motor Development/Redevelopment

Neuromaturational Systems

- Changes are due to CNS maturation.
- Development follows a predictable sequence (e.g., cephalocaudal, proximal-distal).
- CNS damage leads to regression to lower levels and more stereotypical behaviors.

Systems

- Changes are due to interaction of multiple systems.
- Progression varies because person and environmental contexts are unique.
- CNS damage leads to attempts to use remaining resources to achieve functional goals.

Assumptions of Therapeutic Approaches

- CNS is hierarchically organized.
- Sensory stimuli inhibit spasticity and abnormal movement and facilitate normal movement and postural responses.
- Repetition of movement results in positive permanent changes in CNS.
- Recovery from CNS damage follows a predictable sequence.
- Behavioral changes after CNS damage have a neurophysiological basis.

- Personal and environmental systems, including the CNS, are heterarchically organized.
- Intensive and variable functional task practice improves the motor behavior.
- The environment interacts with the individual influencing the occupational performance.
- Individuals' functional relearning strategies are not necessarily the same.
- Recovery is variable because personal characteristics and environmental contexts are unique.
- Behavioral changes reflect attempts to compensate and to achieve task performance.

Evaluation

Primary Focus on Performance Components

- Abnormal muscle tone.
- Abnormal reflexes and stereotypical movement patterns leading to incoordination.
- Postural control.
- Sensation and perception.
- Memory and judgment.
- Stage of recovery or developmental level.

Secondary Focus: Occupational Performance

Primary Focus on Occupational Performance Using a Client-Centered Perspective

- Task analysis to determine performance components and contexts that limit function and to identify preferred movement patterns for specific tasks in varied contexts.
- Variables that cause transitions to new patterns.

Secondary Focus: Selected Performance Components and Contexts That Limit Function

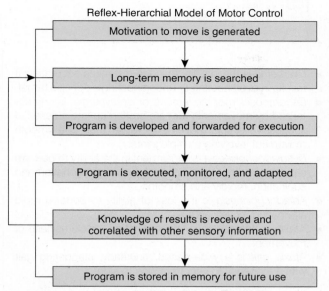

Reflex-Hierarchial Model of Motor Control

Motivation to move is generated

Long-term memory is searched

Program is developed and forwarded for execution

Program is executed, monitored, and adapted

Knowledge of results is received and correlated with other sensory information

Program is stored in memory for future use

Figure 8-1 Reflex-hierarchical model of motor control, includes both open-loop and closed-loop control. (Adapted from Trombly, C. A. [1989]. Motor control therapy. In C. Trombly [Ed.], *Occupational therapy for physical dysfunction* [3rd ed., pp. 72–95]. Baltimore: Williams & Wilkins.)

Reflex-hierarchical models of motor control have been challenged by three interrelated questions: (1) How can the CNS control the many degrees of freedom of each movement (i.e., the large number of joints, planes of motion within each joint, muscles that control each joint, and single motor units within each muscle) without specifying the details of the muscle activation pattern (Bernstein, 1967)? If the CNS does specify the details, each motor program would be extremely complex. (2) How many motor programs would be needed to perform the numerous tasks that humans perform in everyday life? It is likely that an extremely large number would be necessary, which creates a storage problem for the brain. (3) How many motor programs would be needed to perform a given task in varied contexts? Studies (Marteniuk, MacKenzie, & Jeannerod, 1987; Mathiowetz & Wade, 1995) have demonstrated that even small changes in environmental context can result in unique movement patterns during simple reaching tasks. Thus, the environment has a larger role in motor control than the reflex-hierarchical model would suggest, and it seems that an incomprehensible number of motor programs would be necessary to respond to various contexts (Newell, 2003). Does the brain have unlimited storage capacity to accommodate all of the motor programs that would be needed, even generalized motor programs? The answer is probably not, which indicates the need for an alternative explanation of motor behavior such as the task-related approaches.

Neuromaturational Theory of Motor Development

The neuromaturational theory of motor development (Gesell, 1954; McGraw, 1945) has influenced the neurophysiological approaches in various ways (Heriza, 1991).

It suggests that changes in motor development are due to maturation of the nervous system. In other words, changes in neural structures cause changes in motor function (McGraw, 1945). This implies that the environment plays a minimal role in motor development. Current research suggests the opposite—sensorimotor experiences in response to environmental opportunities or problems organize or reorganize the CNS (Kleim & Jones, 2008; Nudo, 2011).

Motor Dysfunction Caused by Central Nervous System Lesions

The view of the neurophysiological approaches is that motor dysfunctions that follow CNS damage (Definition 8-2) are understood best by knowing the site and extent of the lesions (Cheney, 1985). It is assumed that specific areas of the brain serve specific functions. Therefore, if a given area of the brain is damaged, its associated function is expected to be impaired.

View of Recovery after Central Nervous System Lesions

The view of the neurophysiological approaches is that motor recovery after CNS lesions is due to changes in the CNS. Recovery from cortical lesions is believed to follow a developmental sequence from reflex to voluntary control, from mass to discrete movements, and from proximal to distal control. After stroke, clients typically demonstrate synergistic movement patterns when attempting either an isolated single joint movement or a multijoint coordinated task. Brunnstrom (1970) referred to a stereotyped sequence of stages during motor recovery post stroke: (1) flaccidity (i.e., no voluntary movements), (2) basic components of synergies with some spasticity, (3) some voluntary control of synergies with increased spasticity, (4) movement out of synergies and decreased spasticity, (5) synergies no longer have dominance over motor acts and increased coordinated movement, and (6) movement coordination approaches normal.

A conservative definition suggests that motor recovery has been achieved when the person is able to perform functional tasks in a manner similar to before the injury. (Shumway-Cook & Woollacott, 2012). Traditionally, the neurophysiological approaches adopted this restricted view of recovery. Recovery, according to these approaches, can stop at any level along the continuum, and this is not totally predictable. The speed of early spontaneous recovery offers a clue to the ultimate level of function to be gained (Twitchell, 1951). This view of recovery is not supported by current neuroscience research (Kleim, 2011; Warraich & Kleim, 2010). The neurophysiological approaches have increasingly incorporated modern concepts of motor learning and control such as neuroplasticity and the specificity of motor learning; however, this has created some confusion in applying their treatment principles (Rao, 2011).

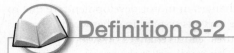

Definition 8-2

Motor Dysfunction Caused by Central Nervous System Lesions

Cortical Lesions

- *Hemiplegic posture or pattern of spasticity* includes retraction and depression of the scapula; internal rotation of the shoulder; flexion of the elbow, wrist, and fingers; pronation of the forearm; lateral flexion of the trunk toward the involved side; elevation and retraction of the pelvis; internal rotation of the hip; extension of the hip and knee; supination of the foot; and plantar flexion of the ankle and toes (Bobath, 1990).

- *Hypotonia* (decreased muscle tone or flaccidity) is less than normal resistance to passive elongation; the affected limb feels limp and heavy.

- *Hypertonia* (increased muscle tone) is more than normal resistance of a muscle to passive elongation. Both neural (spasticity) and mechanical (soft tissue stiffness) factors contribute to this.

- *Spasticity*, the neural component of hypertonus, is characterized by a velocity-dependent increase in tonic stretch reflexes and exaggerated tendon reflexes (Nagaoka & Kakuda, 2008). It is commonly accompanied by muscle clonus and the clasp knife reflex.

- *Clonus* is the oscillating contraction and relaxation of a limb segment caused by the alternating pattern of stretch reflex and inverse stretch reflex of a spastic muscle.

- *Clasp knife phenomenon or reflex* is resistance to passive stretch of a spastic muscle that suddenly gives way, like the blade of a jackknife.

- *Weakness* is the inability to generate the necessary force for effective motor action.

- *Loss of fractionation* is the inability to move a single joint without producing unnecessary movements in other joints resulting in stereotyped movement patterns instead of selective, flexible movement patterns.

- *Apraxia* is the inability to perform goal-directed motor activity in the absence of paresis, ataxia, sensory loss, or abnormal muscle tone. Apraxia is characterized by omissions, disturbed order of submovements within a sequence, clumsiness, perseveration, and inability to gesture or use common tools or utensils.

- *Lead pipe rigidity* is characterized by hypertonus in both agonist and antagonist muscles, with resistance to movement that is not velocity dependent and that is felt throughout the range of motion.

Cerebellar Lesions

- *Intention tremor* is the rhythmic oscillating movement that develops during precise intentional movements caused by involuntary alternating contractions of opposing muscles.

- *Dysmetria* is the inability to judge distances accurately; it results in overshooting or undershooting a specific target.

- *Decomposition of movement*, or *dyssynergia*, is characterized by movements that are broken up into a series of successive simple movements rather than one smooth movement involving multiple joints.

- *Dysdiadochokinesia* is impairment in the ability to perform repeated alternating movements, such as pronation and supination, rapidly and smoothly.

- *Adiadochokinesia* is the loss of ability to perform rapid alternating movements.

- *Ataxia* is unsteadiness, incoordination, or clumsiness of movement.

- *Ataxic gait* is a wide-based, unsteady, staggering gait with a tendency to veer from side to side.

Lesions of the Basal Ganglia

- *Tremors at rest* or *nonintention tremors* stop at the initiation of voluntary movement but resume during the holding phase of a motor task when attention wanes or is diverted to another task. Tremors at rest are fatiguing.

- *Cogwheel rigidity* is characterized by rhythmic interrupted resistance of the muscles being stretched when the wrist or elbow is flexed quickly.

- *Hypokinesia* is slowness or poverty of movement. It includes *akinesia*, difficulty initiating voluntary movements, and *bradykinesia*, slowness in carrying out movements. These symptoms are reflected in lack of facial expression, monotone speech, reduced eye movements, diminished arm swing during walking, and decreased balance and equilibrium responses seen in Parkinson's disease.

- *Festinating gait* is characterized by small, fast, shuffling steps that propel the body forward at an increasing rate and by difficulty stopping or changing directions.

- *Athetosis* is characterized by slow, writhing involuntary movements, particularly in the neck, face, and extremities. Muscle tone may be increased or decreased. Athetosis ceases during sleep.

- *Dystonia* is characterized by powerful, sustained contractions of muscles that cause twisting and writhing of a limb or of the whole body, often resulting in distorted postures of the trunk and proximal extremities.

- *Chorea* is characterized by sudden involuntary purposeless, rapid, jerky movements and/or grimacing, primarily in the distal extremities and face (e.g., Huntington's chorea).

- *Hemiballismus* is unilateral chorea in which there are violent, forceful, flinging movements of the extremities on one side of the body, particularly involving the proximal musculature.

From Fredericks, C. M., & Saladin, L. K. (Eds.). (1996). *Pathophysiology of the motor systems: Principles and clinical presentations*. Philadelphia: Davis.

Evaluations Used by Neurophysiological Approaches

Given the assumptions of the neurophysiological approaches (Definition 8-1), patient evaluation focuses primarily on abilities and capacities impaired by CNS damage. These include muscle tone, abnormal reflexes and movement patterns, postural control, sensation (see Chapter 9), perception (see Chapter 5), and cognition (see Chapter 6). In addition, it is important to determine the patient's stage of recovery or developmental level. Finally, occupational performance (see Chapter 4) is evaluated secondarily on the assumption that any deficits in these areas are due to impaired performance components. This bottom-up evaluation framework is not consistent with the Model of Occupational Functioning (see Chapter 1).

The evaluations used by the neurophysiological approaches still provide valuable information concerning the abilities and capacities of patients who have not recovered to the level required to engage in task-related approaches. For example, the constraint-induced movement therapy (CIMT), a task-related approach, requires voluntary, minimal range of motion abilities in the affected hand (Wolf et al., 2006). Evaluating muscle tone, strength, and sensation can help researchers assemble homogenous and specific research groups and helps clinicians to address their clients' specific motor behavior challenges to enhance treatment individualization.

Muscle Tone Assessment

Muscle Tone and Associated Factors. Muscle tone is defined as the resistance of a muscle to passive elongation or stretching (Shumway-Cook & Woollacott, 2012). Slight resistance in response to passive movement characterizes normal muscle tone. When the therapist moves the arm, it feels relatively light, and if the therapist lets go of it, it is able to maintain the position. Hypotonia is less than normal resistance to passive elongation. When the therapist moves the arm, it feels floppy and heavy. If the therapist lets go of it, it cannot maintain the position or resist the effects of gravity. Hypertonia, more than normal resistance of a muscle to passive elongation, is due to neural and mechanical factors. The neural factor (i.e., spasticity) is due to hyperactive stretch reflexes frequently seen after CNS damage. In a spastic muscle, there is a range of free movement, then a strong contraction of the muscle in response to stretch (i.e., stretch reflex), and free movement again when the muscle suddenly relaxes (i.e., clasp knife phenomenon or reflex) (Bellamy & Shen, 2007; Gillen, 2011). Thus, spasticity is not synonymous with hypertonus or muscle tone (Burridge et al., 2005). The mechanical factors of hypertonus are the elastic properties of connective tissue and the viscoelastic properties of muscle. The mechanical factors change if a muscle is immobilized in a shortened or lengthened position (i.e., there is increased or decreased resistance to passive stretching) (Stolov, 1966). The neural changes after CNS damage—spasticity—contribute to abnormal positioning of limbs, which causes secondary changes in the mechanical factors. Together, the neural and mechanical factors account for increased resistance to passive elongation—hypertonus—that is seen after CNS damage (Burridge et al., 2005).

Muscle tone is measured clinically by observing the response of a muscle to passive stretch. A problem in measuring hypertonus, especially the neural factor, is the high variation in spasticity from day to day in the same patient. Furthermore, the reliability of a test is affected by the speed of the passive test movement because the tonic stretch reflexes are velocity dependent (Nagaoka & Kakuda, 2008). Reliability is also affected by effort, emotional stress, temperature, fatigue, changes in concurrent sensory stimulation, urinary tract infections, and posture. These factors make spasticity measurements context dependent. This could explain some reported instances of low levels of interrater reliability in clinical scores such as the Ashworth and the Modified Ashworth Scales even with well-trained therapists (Bhimani et al., 2011). Rigid standardization of the test procedure must be the rule; otherwise, the findings may be misleading (Burridge et al., 2005; Platz et al., 2005). Poor evaluation techniques that allow high test–retest variability may obscure therapeutic effectiveness. Although there are many assessments of muscle tone and spasticity described in the literature (Bhimani et al., 2011; Platz et al., 2005), most are not practical for clinical use, and the Modified Ashworth Scale (MAS) is the most widely used (van Wijck et al., 2001).

Modified Ashworth Scale. Ashworth (1964) proposed a qualitative scale for assessing the degree of spasticity as part of a drug study. The resistance encountered to passive movement through the full available range was rated on a 5-point scale (from 0 to 4). Although it was developed and described as a measure of spasticity, it is a measure of muscle tone or the resistance to passive movement (Burridge et al., 2005; Pandyan et al., 2002). Bohannon and Smith (1987) modified the Ashworth Scale (Procedures for Practice 8-1) by adding an additional level (1+), by incorporating the angle at which resistance first appeared, and by controlling the speed of the passive movement with a 1-second count. The examiner performs five to eight repetitions of the movement before assigning the rating. Assessment Table 8-1 describes the psychometric properties of the MAS, which has modest evidence of concurrent validity.

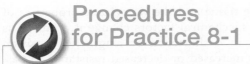

Procedures for Practice 8-1

Modified Ashworth Scale for Grading Spasticity

Grade	Description
0	No increase in muscle tone
1	Slight increase in muscle tone manifested by a catch and release or by minimal resistance at the end of the range of motion when the affected part or parts are moved in flexion or extension
1+	Slight increase in muscle tone manifested by a catch, followed by minimal resistance throughout the remainder (less than half) of the ROM
2	Marked increase in muscle tone through most of the ROM, but affected parts are easily moved
3	Considerable increase in muscle tone; passive movement difficult
4	Affected part or parts rigid in flexion or extension

Reprinted with permission from Bohannon, R. W., & Smith, M. B. (1987). Interrater reliability of a Modified Ashworth Scale of muscle spasticity. *Physical Therapy, 67,* 207. Copyright 1987 by American Physical Therapy Association.

Recently, the MAS was modified to be the Modified Modified Ashworth Scale (MMAS). This modification deleted the additional grade of 1+ between 1 and 2 from MAS and changed evaluation criteria (Ansari et al., 2006) to enhance the validity and reliability of the MAS. The MMAS has five categories scored 0–4 like the original Ashworth Scale. The scoring criteria for categories 1 and 2 reflect slight or marked increase in tone, but the MMAS includes additional stipulations about catch and resistance, which is similar to the MAS. The MMAS scoring criteria is as follows: 0 = no increase in muscle tone; 1 = slight increase in muscle tone, manifested by a catch and release or by minimal resistance at the end of the range of motion when the affected part(s) is moved in flexion or extension; 2 = marked increase in muscle tone, manifested by a catch in the middle range and resistance throughout the remainder of the range of motion, but affected part(s) easily moved; 3 = considerable increase in muscle tone, passive movement difficult; and 4 = affected part(s) rigid in flexion or extension. However, it seems that both MAS and MMAS have very good interrater reliability with no superiority for one over the other, as indicated in a study evaluating elbow flexor spasticity post stroke (Kaya et al., 2011).

SYSTEMS-BASED TASK-RELATED APPROACHES

The occupational therapy task-oriented approach (Almhdawi, 2011; Mathiowetz, 2011), the Carr and Shepherd Motor Learning Programme for Stroke (Carr & Shepherd, 2011), and CIMT (Wolf et al., 2006) are examples of the systems-based task-related approaches. The assumptions of these approaches are listed in Definition 8-1. They originate from a systems model of motor behavior, a systems view of motor development, an ecological view of action and perception, and motor learning theories related to the stages of learning, practice schedule, feedback, and learning transfer as discussed in Chapter 13. To understand the evaluation framework of the systems-based task-related approaches, it is important to understand the origins of their assumptions.

Systems Model of Motor Control

Over the past 35 years, a model of motor control has evolved from the ecological approach to perception and action (Gibson, 1979; Turvey, 1977) and from the study of complex dynamical systems in mathematics and the sciences (Gleick, 1987). The new model emphasizes the interaction between persons and environments and suggests that motor behavior emerges from persons' multiple systems interacting with unique task and environmental contexts (Newell, 1986). Thus, the systems model of motor control is more interactive or heterarchical and emphasizes the role of the environment more than the reflex-hierarchical model.

In this newer model, the nervous system is only one system among many that influence motor behavior. The nervous system itself is thought to be organized heterarchically so that higher centers interact with the lower centers but do not control them. Closed-loop and open-loop systems work cooperatively, and both feedback and feed-forward control are used to achieve task goals. The CNS interacts with multiple personal and environmental systems as a person attempts to achieve a goal.

Ecological Approach to Perception and Action. The ecological approach to perception and action emphasizes the study of interaction between the person and the environment during every day functional tasks and the close linkage between perception and action (i.e., purposeful movement). Gibson recognized the role of functional goals and the environment in the relationship between perception and action. He stated that direct perception entails the active search for *affordances* (Gibson, 1977), defined as the functional use of objects for persons and their unique characteristics (Warren, 1984). Thus, Gibson's concept of affordances explains the close relationship between perception and action in terms of what the information in the environment means to a specific person.

Assessment Table 8-1 — Psychometric Properties of Assessments of Muscle Tone or Resistance to Passive Movement.

Instrument and Reference	Description	Time to Administer	Validity	Reliability	Sensitivity	Strengths and Weaknesses
Modified Ashworth Scale (Bohannon & Smith, 1987)	Ordinal scale with score for each motion from 0 (normal muscle tone) to 4 (rigid in flexion or extension). Modification is the addition of one additional rating level (1+).	1–2 minutes per motion tested	Concurrent validity: r_s = 0.39–0.49 with quantitative spasticity measures (Allison & Abraham, 1995); r = 0.50 with motor and activity scores (Sommerfeld et al., 2004); r_s = 0.51 with resistance to passive movement (Pandyan et al., 2003); r_s = 0.40 with the H-reflex (Pizzi et al., 2005).	Interrater reliability: K_w[1] = 0.49–0.54 for shoulder, elbow, wrist, knee, and ankle joints (Mehrholz et al., 2005). Test–retest reliability: K_w = 0.77–0.94 for elbow, wrist, and knee flexors; K_w = 0.59–0.64 for ankle plantarflexors (Gregson et al., 2000) Interrater reliability: K_w = 0.868 for elbow flexor spasticity post stroke (Kaya et al., 2011) Both inter- and intrarater reliability K_w > 0.8 and ICC > 0.8) for subjects with developmental disabilities (Waninge et al., 2011).	Findings regarding sensitivity are mixed. One study found significant reduction in Modified Ashworth Scale scores after treatment with botulinum toxin (Bakheit et al., 2000, 2001) while another found nonsignificant reduction in Modified Ashworth Scale scores after treatment with botulinum toxin (Pandyan et al., 2002).	Strengths: It is a valid measure of muscle tone or resistance to passive movement (Pandyan et al., 2002); administration time is relatively brief; reliability is better for upper extremity than lower extremity joints. Moderate to good interrater reliability; moderate to very good test–retest reliability. Weakness: Only moderate concurrent validity with measures of spasticity; therefore, it is questioned as a measure of the neural component of muscle tone.

[1] Kw, weighted kappa.

Bernstein (1967) recognized the importance of the environment and personal characteristics (beyond the CNS) in motor behavior. He suggested that the role a particular muscle plays in a movement depends on the context or circumstances. Bernstein identified three possible sources of variability in muscle function. A first source is anatomical factors. For example, from kinesiology you know that the pectoralis major muscle will either flex or extend the shoulder, depending on the initial position of the arm. A second source of variability is mechanical factors. Many nonmuscular forces, such as gravity and inertia, determine the degree to which a muscle must contract. For example, a muscle must exert much more force to contract against gravity than in a gravity-eliminated plane. A third source of variability is physiological factors. When higher centers send down a command for a muscle to contract, middle and lower centers have the opportunity to modify the command. Lower and middle centers receive peripheral sensory feedback. Thus, the effect of the command on the muscle varies depending on the context and degree of influence of the middle and lower centers. As a result, the relationship between higher center or executive commands and muscle action is not one to one. The context can influence the movement patterns. Goal-directed, object-present activity has been shown to elicit different and more efficient movement patterns than non–goal-directed exercise (Lin et al., 2007; Trombly & Wu, 1999)

Thus, postures and movements are not triggered by external stimulation or central commands, as suggested by the reflex-hierarchical model, but are coordinative structures, capable of adapting to changing circumstances. Coordinative structures are groups of muscles, usually spanning several joints that are constrained to act as a single functional unit (Bockemühl, Troje, & Dürr, 2010; Magill, 2004). When learning a new task, a person tends to constrain or stiffen many joints to reduce the degrees of freedom to be controlled. This use of a coordinative structure enables the person to focus on controlling a limited number of joints. Natural tenodesis grasp and release is an example of a coordinative structure. The long flexor and extensor muscles of the forearm are constrained to work together for functional grasp and release. The coordinative structures can be modulated by sensory feedback in response to changes in the task context or demand (Safavynia & Ting, 2012; Ting et al., 2009)

Dynamical Systems Theory. The study of dynamical systems originated in mathematics, physics, biology, chemistry, psychology, and kinesiology, and it has been applied to OT, physical therapy, nursing, adapted physical education, and some areas of medicine (Burton & Davis, 1992; Lister, 1991). It has influenced the systems model of motor control as well. Dynamical systems theory proposes that behaviors emerge from the interaction of many systems. Because the behavior is not specified but emergent, it is considered to be self-organizing (Lewis, 2000). This concept of self-organization

is not compatible with the assumptions of the reflex-hierarchical model, which suggests that higher centers or motor programs prescribe movements. Evidence of self-organization is seen in the relatively stable patterns of motor behavior seen in many tasks in spite of the many degrees of freedom available to a person (Perry, 1998; Thelen & Ulrich, 1991). When we eat or write, we have many choices of ways to perform these tasks, yet we tend to use preferred patterns.

Behavior can change from stable to less stable as a result of aging or CNS damage. In fact, throughout life, behaviors shift between periods of stability and instability. It is during unstable periods, characterized by a high variability of performance, that new types of behaviors may emerge, either gradually or abruptly. These transitions in behavior, called phase shifts, are changes from one preferred pattern of coordinated behavior to another. An example of a gradual phase shift is when individuals with impaired gait post stroke change their stable inefficient gait pattern into more efficient ones in response to gait training. An example of an abrupt phase shift is when a person in a hurry walks faster and faster and suddenly changes to a running pattern.

In the dynamical systems view, control parameters are variables that shift behavior from one form to another. They do not control the change but act as agents for reorganization of the behavior to a new form (Perry, 1998). Control parameters are gradable in some way to simplify the motor tasks or to add some therapeutic challenge. This challenge should be appropriate to the client's level of motor performance, which is well known as the "just-right challenge." Therapists can influence motor behavior by manipulating the external control parameters, such as task variables (tools characteristics, success requirements, or time) or features in the environment (such as the physical space and the item setup). Internal control parameters also can be manipulated such as body alignment, muscle length, and muscle strength to influence the motor behavior. This change in motor behavior is described as a nonlinear system where the output is not proportional to the input (Harbourne & Stergiou, 2009).

Explanations of changes in motor behavior in the systems model of motor control are quite different from earlier neurophysiological models. Thelen (1989) stated that an important characteristic of a systems perspective is that the shift from one preferred movement pattern to another is marked by discrete, discontinuous transitions. These transitions in motor behavior are the result of changes in only one or a few personal or environmental systems (i.e., control parameters) (Davis & Burton, 1991). The dynamic systems theory also emphasizes the role of variability in controlling movements. Optimum movement variability is required to guarantee having flexible adaptive motor strategies that could accommodate for contextual change (Shumway-Cook & Woollacott, 2012). Thus, two important points are (1) systems themselves are subject to change, and (2) there is no inherent ordering of systems in terms of their influence on motor behavior.

Systems Model of Motor Behavior

Figure 8-2 depicts the theoretical basis of the systems-based task-oriented approach. It illustrates the interaction between the systems of the *person* (cognitive, psychosocial, and sensorimotor) and the systems of the *environment* (physical, socioeconomic, and cultural). Ability to accomplish occupational tasks and activities of daily living (ADL), work, or play/leisure emerges from the interaction between the person and the environment. Changes in any one of these systems can affect occupational performance tasks and ultimately role performance. In some cases, only one primary factor may determine occupational performance. In most cases, occupational performance emerges from the interaction of many systems. The ongoing interactions among all components of the model reflect its heterarchical nature.

In addition, any occupational performance task affects the environment in which it occurs and the person acting. For example, a client with hemiplegia who has just become independent in making his own lunch may free his spouse from coming home from work during her lunch hour. It also may mean that certain objects in the kitchen must be kept in accessible places, and the kitchen may not be as orderly as the spouse is used to. Thus, the task of making lunch affects people and objects in the environment. It also affects the person and the associated performance skills and patterns. The ability to be less dependent on his spouse may improve the client's self-esteem (i.e., psychosocial subsystem). The process of making lunch provides the client the opportunity to solve problems and to discover optimal strategies for performing tasks. This influences a client's cognitive and sensorimotor subsystems and the ability to perform other functional tasks. The various parts of the systems model of motor behavior can be related to the Occupational Therapy Practice Framework (OTPF) (American Occupational Therapy Association [AOTA], 2008) and the Occupational Functioning Model (OFM) (see Chapter 1).

View of Recovery after Central Nervous System Dysfunction

A client with a damaged CNS attempts to compensate for the lesion to achieve functional goals. Recovery from brain damage is a process of discovering what abilities and capacities remain to enable performance of activities and tasks. CNS damage affects each system differently relative to occupational performance. Therapists must consider all systems as potential variables to explain the behavior of each client at a specific time. For example, the flexor pattern commonly seen after a stroke is due to various factors in addition to spasticity, such as the inability to recruit appropriate

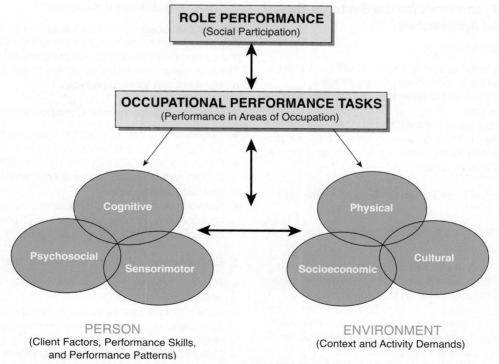

Figure 8-2 Systems model of motor behavior offer some of the theoretical bases of the task-related approaches. The occupational performance tasks and role performance emerge from an interaction of the person and environment. (Adapted with permission from Mathiowetz, V., & Bass Haugen, J. [2008]. Assessing abilities and capacities: Motor behavior. In M. V. Radomski & C. A. Trombly Latham [Eds.], *Occupational therapy for physical dysfunction* [6th ed., pp. 186–211]. Baltimore: Lippincott Williams & Wilkins.)

muscles, weakness, soft tissue tightness, and perceptual deficits (Bourbonnais & Vanden Noven, 1989; Shumway-Cook & Woollacott, 2012). This pattern may become obligatory because of abnormal positioning and decreased use in functional contexts. Because each client is a unique person and functions in a unique environment, therapists should expect recovery for each client to vary even if the CNS damage is similar (Almhdawi, 2011). In contrast with the neurophysiological approaches, the systems-based task-related approaches adopt a more flexible definition of recovery to include achieving tasks or goals using efficient and effective techniques or methods of performance not necessarily matching the ones used before the CNS injury (Shumway-Cook & Woollacott, 2012; Wittenberg, 2010).

There is increasing evidence that neural reorganization after a brain lesion reflects the functional demands on the CNS. For example, forced use of the involved limb has improved functional performance in persons more than a year post stroke (Gauthier et al., 2008; Liepert et al., 2000). These changes cannot be attributed to spontaneous recovery. Thus, providing appropriately challenging tasks and environments for those with CNS dysfunction, both in the hospital and at home, appears critical to the maximal rehabilitation of our clients (Bach-y-Rita, 1993; Nudo, 2011).

Evaluation Using the Systems-Based Task-Related Approaches

Evaluation is conducted using a top-down approach consistent with the Model of Occupational Functioning (see Chapter 1). A framework for evaluating motor behavior is described in Procedures for Practice 8-2 and illustrated in Figure 8-3.

First, evaluation focuses on role performance. A thorough understanding of the roles that a client wants, needs, or is expected to perform and of the tasks needed to fulfill those roles enables therapists to plan meaningful and motivating treatment programs. Although role definition and expectations can be assessed using a nonstandardized, semistructured interview, a standardized assessment tool such as the Role Checklist (Barris, Oakley, & Kielhofner, 1988; Hemphill-Pearson, 2007) is recommended. The Role Checklist is a written inventory designed for adolescents and adults with physical dysfunction. With clients undergoing major role

---

 Procedures for Practice 8-2

Evaluation Framework for the Systems-Based Task-Related Approaches

1. Role Performance

- Determine interest in, and definition of, self-maintenance, self-advancement, and self-enhancement roles
- Identify past roles and whether they can be maintained or must be changed.
- Determine how future roles will be balanced: worker, student, volunteer, home maintainer, hobbyist, amateur, participant in organizations, friend, family member, caregiver, religious participant, other.

2. Occupational Performance Tasks: Areas of Occupation

Determine abilities in the following areas of occupation (AOTA, 2008).

- Activities of daily living (ADL): feeding, grooming, functional mobility, dressing, oral and toilet hygiene, bowel and bladder management, and bathing/showering.
- Instrumental ADL: care of others and/or pets, communication device use, community mobility, home management, meal preparation and clean-up, safety procedures, shopping, and others unique to the patient.
- Work-related tasks: employment seeking and acquisition; job performance; volunteer exploration and participation; and retirement preparation and adjustment.
- Play-leisure: exploration and participation.

3. Task Selection and Analysis

The therapist observes a functional task important to the client to identify which performance components and/or performance contexts limit or enhance occupational performance. The task setup should be as similar to the client's natural environment and tools as possible.

4. Person: Performance Components

- Cognitive: orientation, attention span, memory, problem solving, learning, and generalization.
- Psychosocial: values, interests, self-concept, interpersonal skills, self-expression, coping skills, time management, and self-control.
- Sensorimotor: strength, endurance, range of motion, coordination, sensory awareness and processing, perceptual processing, and postural control.

5. Environment: Performance Context

- Physical: objects, tools, devices, animals, and built and natural environments.
- Socioeconomic: social supports, including family, friends, caregivers, social groups, and community and financial resources.
- Cultural: ethnicity, family, attitudes, beliefs, values, customs, and societal expectations.

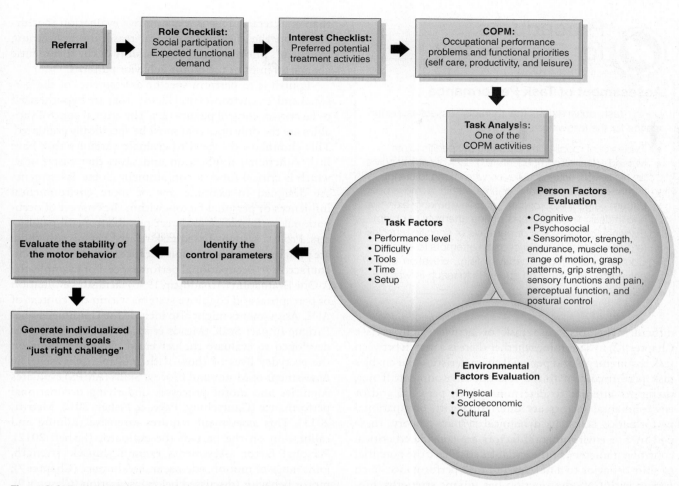

Figure 8-3 The occupational therapy task-oriented approach suggested evaluation flowchart. COPM, Canadian Occupational Performance Measure. (Adapted with permission from Almhdawi, K. A. [2011]. *Effects of occupational therapy task-oriented approach in upper extremity post-stroke rehabilitation* [Doctoral dissertation]. Retrieved from University of Minnesota Digital Conservancy.)

changes and when there is sufficient time for a comprehensive assessment, the Role Change Assessment for older adults (Rogers & Holm, 2007) or Client-Oriented Role Evaluation (CORE) (Toal-Sullivan & Henderson, 2004) are recommended.

Second, evaluation focuses on the assessment of occupational performance tasks: ADL, instrumental ADL, work, and play-leisure (Procedures for Practice 8-2). Because tasks, activities, and their contexts are unique to each role of each person, a client-centered assessment tool such as the Canadian Occupational Performance Measure (COPM) (Law et al., 1998) is recommended. It was designed to measure a client's perception of his or her occupational performance over time. A semistructured interview is used to administer the COPM. First, clients are asked to identify problem areas in self-care, productivity, and leisure. Second, the client rates the importance of each problem area. Third, clients rate their own performance and their satisfaction with the performance. The importance ratings assist therapists in setting treatment priorities. The information elicited by the COPM is unique to each client

and his or her environmental context, which is a critical facet of the systems-based task-related approaches.

While evaluating occupational performance tasks, therapists must observe both the outcome and the process (i.e., the preferred movement patterns, their stability or instability, the flexibility to use other patterns, efficiency of the patterns, and ability to learn new strategies) to understand the motor behaviors used to compensate and to achieve functional goals. It is important to determine the stability of the motor behavior, because it will help determine the feasibility of achieving behavioral change in treatment. Behaviors that are very stable require a great amount of time and effort to change. Behaviors that are unstable are in transition, the optimal time for eliciting behavioral change. Thus, a compensatory approach may be most appropriate when behaviors are stable, and a remediation approach may be more appropriate when behaviors are unstable.

Third is task selection and analysis (see Procedures for Practice 8-3). The tasks selected for observation should be ones that the client has identified as important but

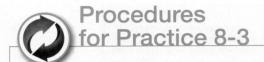

Procedures for Practice 8-3

Assessment of Task Performance

During task observation, the therapist assesses performance for the following:

- Evidence of mobility impairments at specific joints
- Missing or limited components (e.g., lack of anterior pelvic tilt, hip flexion, ankle dorsiflexion when rising to stand)
- Incorrect timing of components within a movement pattern (e.g., inappropriate interplay among extrinsic and intrinsic finger muscles during attempts at grasp)
- Evidence of weakness or paralysis of specific muscles (e.g., weakness in quadriceps on attempts to stand up)
- Compensatory motor behavior (e.g., elevation of the entire shoulder girdle on attempts to reach forward)

difficult. Therapists use task or activity analysis (see Chapter 12) to determine whether there is a match between task requirements and personal characteristics that enables task performance within a relevant environment. If not, therapists attempt to determine which personal and/or environmental factors are interfering with occupational performance tasks. In dynamical systems theory, these personal or environmental factors are considered critical control parameters, or the variables that have the potential to shift behavior to a new level of task performance. Each person with CNS dysfunction has unique strengths, limitations, and environmental context. As a result, the critical control parameters that limit or support occupational performance tasks are also unique. Case studies by Flinn (1995) and Gillen (2000, 2002) illustrate the search for critical control parameters.

In its simplest form, this search consists of observing a functional task of high priority for the client via a task analysis process. The therapist hypothesizes reasons for poor motor behavior performance. When noticing an inefficient movement pattern (i.e., one that requires unaffordable energy or time), the therapist needs to list the reasons for that pattern. Poor grasp patterns (in poststroke rehabilitation, for example) are inefficient movement patterns that might be related to spasticity, tremor, learned nonuse, weakness, impaired sensations, and/or soft tissue tightness. Once the therapist accurately identifies the reasons for poor movement patterns, the therapy process can be much more focused, effective, and individualized (Almhdawi, 2011).

After identifying the variables that support or constrain occupational performance, the therapist must assess the interactions of these systems. For example, a carpenter whose occupation requires overhead nailing would be more affected by a small shoulder flexion limitation

than a secretary. This is a qualitative evaluation that depends on the therapist's clinical reasoning concerning the client's priorities and the feasibility of the therapeutic change attempt of the motor behavior patterns.

Fourth is to perform specific assessments of the personal and/or environmental factors that are hypothesized to be critical control parameters. The critical control variables are the only ones that must be specifically evaluated. This eliminates the need to evaluate variables that have little functional implication and saves therapists' time, which is critical for cost containment. Some assessments are designed to examine one or more environmental influences or personal factors within the context of occupational performance to detect possible control parameters. From a systems-based task-related perspective, these are preferred assessment tools because they closely link client factors to occupational performance. For example, the A-One Evaluation (Arnadottir, 1990) facilitates evaluation of perceptual and cognitive systems within the context of ADL. Assessments might also include the Unidimensional Fatigue Impact Scale (Meads et al., 2009). This scale was developed to evaluate the perceived effect of fatigue on the everyday lives of those with multiple sclerosis. The Assessment of Motor and Process Skills (AMPS) evaluates cognitive and motor processes underlying occupational performance (Gantschnig, Page, & Fisher, 2012; Merritt, 2011). This assessment requires extensive training and calibration on the part of the evaluator (Fisher, 2012). Personal factor assessments examine muscle strength, joint range of motion, edema, and endurance (Chapter 7); motor behavior (discussed below); sensation (Chapter 9); coordination (Chapter 37); and/or the cognitive and visual abilities discussed in Chapters 5 and 6, independent of occupational context.

Evaluation of a client's environment may include assessment of physical, social, cultural, personal, or temporal environments, which the AOTA (2008) practice framework acknowledges as important influences on occupational performance. Chapters 3 and 10 review assessments for these variables.

Assessments of Motor Behavior and Motor Function

Motor Assessment Scale. Carr et al. (1985) developed the Motor Assessment Scale (MAS) as an easily administered and relatively brief (15–30 minutes) assessment relevant to everyday motor activities (Procedures for Practice 8-4). The original version of the MAS included a ninth subtest, muscle tone, which has been deleted because it had poor reliability and questionable validity. The psychometric properties of MAS are described in Assessment Table 8-2. Because reliability and validity data for individual subtests of the MAS are available, one or more subtests can be used independently with each client.

Procedures for Practice 8-4

Abridged Criteria for Scoring Motor Assessment Scale

The score assigned on each item is the highest criterion met on the best performance of three. A 0 score is assigned if the patient is unable to meet the criteria for a score of 1.

0 1 2 3 4 5 6

Supine to Side-Lying to Intact Side

1. Pulls self into side-lying with intact arm, moving affected leg with intact leg.
2. Moves leg across actively and lower half of body follows. Arm is left behind.
3. Lifts arm across body with other arm. Moves leg actively; body follows in a block.
4. Actively moves arm across body; rest of body follows in a block.
5. Rolls to side, moving arm and leg; overbalances. Shoulder protracts and arm flexes.
6. Rolls to side in 3 seconds. Must not use hands.

Supine to Sitting on Edge of Bed

1. After being assisted to side-lying, lifts head sideways; cannot sit up.
2. Side-lying to sitting on edge of bed with therapist assisting movement.
3. Side-lying to sitting on edge of bed with standby help assisting legs over side of bed.
4. Side-lying to sitting on edge of bed with no standby help.
5. Supine to sitting on edge of bed with no standby help.
6. Supine to sitting on edge of bed within 10 seconds with no standby help.

Balanced Sitting

1. Sits only with support after therapist assists.
2. Sits unsupported for 10 seconds.
3. Sits unsupported with weight well forward and evenly distributed.
4. Sits unsupported with hands resting on thighs; turns head and trunk to look behind.
5. Reaches forward to touch floor 4 inches in front of feet and returns to starting position.
6. Sitting on stool, reaches sideways to touch floor and returns to starting position.

Sitting to Standing

1. Gets to standing with help (any method).
2. Gets to standing with standby help.
3. Gets to standing with weight evenly distributed and with no help from hands.
4. Gets to standing; stands for 5 seconds, weight evenly distributed, hips and knees extended.
5. Stands up and sits down with no help; even weight distribution; full hip and knee extension.
6. Stands up and sits down with no help 3 times in 10 seconds; even weight distribution.

Walking

1. Stands on affected leg with hip extended; steps forward with other leg (standby help).
2. Walks with standby help from one person.
3. Walks 10 feet alone. Uses any walking aid but no standby help.
4. Walks 16 feet with no aid in 15 seconds.
5. Walks 33 feet, picks up small sandbag from floor, turns around, walks back in 25 seconds.
6. Walks up and down four steps with or without an aid three times in 35 seconds. May not hold rail.

Upper Arm Function

1. Supine, protracts shoulder girdle. Tester places arm in 90° flexion and supports elbow.
2. Supine, holds shoulder in 90° flexion for 2 seconds. (Maintains 45° external rotation and 20° elbow extension.)
3. From position in level 2, flexes and extends elbow to move palm to forehead and back.
4. Sitting, holds arm in 90° shoulder flexion with elbow extended, thumb pointing up, for 2 seconds. No excess shoulder elevation.
5. Achieves position in level 4; holds for 10 seconds; lowers arm. No pronation allowed.
6. Standing, arm abducted 90°, with palm flat against wall. Maintains hand position while turning body toward wall.

Hand Movements

1. Sitting, lifts cylindrical object off table by extending wrist. No elbow flexion allowed.
2. Sitting, forearm in midposition. Lifts hand off table by radially deviating wrist. No elbow flexion or forearm pronation allowed.
3. Sitting, elbow into side, pronates and supinates forearm through three-quarters of range.
4. Sitting, reaches forward to pick up 5-inch ball with both hands and puts ball down. Ball placement requires elbow extension. Palms stay in contact with ball.
5. Sitting, picks up plastic foam cup from table and puts it on table across other side of body.
6. Sitting, continuous opposition of thumb and each finger more than 14 times in 10 seconds.

Advanced Hand Activities

1. Reaches forward arm's length; picks up pen top; releases it on table close to body.
2. Picks up a jellybean from teacup with eight jellybeans and places it in another cup. Cups are at arm's length.
3. Draws horizontal lines to stop at a vertical line 10 times in 20 seconds.
4. Makes rapid consecutive dots with a pen on a sheet of paper. (Picks up and holds pen without assistance; at least 2 dots per second for 5 seconds; dots, not dashes).
5. Takes a dessert spoon of liquid to the mouth, without spilling. (Head cannot lower toward spoon).
6. Holds a comb and combs hair at back of head. (Shoulder is externally rotated, abducted at least 90°; head is erect.)

Used with permission from J. Carr & R. Shepherd, personal communication (1994).

Assessment Table 8-2   Psychometric Properties of Assessments of Motor Behavior and Function

Instrument and Reference	Description	Time to Administer	Validity	Reliability	Sensitivity	Strengths and Weaknesses
Motor Assessment Scale (MAS) (Carr et al., 1985)	Eight areas of motor function are rated on a 7-point hierarchical scale: 0 = easiest task and 6 = hardest task.	15–30 minutes for total MAS (Carr et al., 1985); 18–60 minutes for total MAS (Malouin et al., 1994).	Concurrent validity: $r_s = 0.88$ with the total FMA[1]; $r_s = 0.91$ for total upper extremity; $r_s = 0.28$ for balanced sitting (Poole & Whitney, 1988); $r_s = 0.96$ with the total FMA (Malouin et al., 1994). Predictive validity: arm function at 1 week ($r_s = .84$) and at 1 month ($r_s = .91$) are good predictors of arm function at discharge (Loewen & Anderson, 1990). Discriminates between different levels of motor recovery post stroke (Miller et al., 2010).	Interrater reliability: $r = 0.95$ and average of 87% agreement between raters (Carr et al. 1985); $r_s = 0.99$ between raters (Poole & Whitney, 1988); Test-retest reliability: $r = 0.96$ on clients post stroke (Miller et al., 2010).	Significant improvements for clients post stroke on all subtests as a result of clinical interventions (Ada & Westwood, 1992; Dean & Mackey, 1992).	Strengths: Items are functionally relevant; administration time is short. Evidence supports its reliability, validity, and sensitivity. Weaknesses: Sequence of the scoring hierarchy of the hand function and advanced hand activities scales is questioned (Dean & Mackey, 1992; Sabari et al., 2005)
Arm Motor Ability Test (AMAT) (Kopp et al., 1997)	Thirteen unilateral and bilateral functional tasks scored on performance time, functional ability, and quality of movement	30–45 minutes	Concurrent validity: $r_s = 0.92–0.94$ with FMA[1] (Chae, Labatia, & Yang, 2003); $r_s = 0.45–0.61$ with Motricity Index: arm score (Kopp et al., 1997). Appeared to be valid in a literature review (O'Dell et al., 2011)	Interrater reliability: $r_s = 0.97–099$; $K = 0.68–0.77$. Test-retest reliability: $r = 0.93–0.99$ Internal consistency: $K = 0.94–0.99$ (Kopp et al., 1997)	Significant improvement in scores after 1 or 2 weeks of intensive therapy (Kopp et al., 1997); significant improvement in scores after constraint-induced movement therapy (Kunkel et al., 1999)	Strengths: Use of functional tasks; excellent reliability; evidence of validity. Weaknesses: Ceiling and floor effects for performance time (Chae, Labatia, & Yang, 2003); less sensitive to change than the WMFT[2] (Morris et al., 2001)

Test	Description	Administration time	Validity	Reliability	Responsiveness	Strengths and Weaknesses
Wolf Motor Function Test (WMFT) (Wolf et al., 2001; Morris et al., 2001)	Seventeen tasks: 2 measure strength; 15 are sequenced according to joints involved and level of difficulty (Edwards et al., 2012). Six timed upper extremity movements and nine timed functional tasks (Wolf et al., 2001). Functional Ability Scale (FAS) added (Morris et al., 2001). Yields three scores: speed of performance (seconds), quality of performance (6-point ordinal scale), and strength of grip (kilogram) (Edwards et al., 2012).	30–45 minutes	Discriminates between healthy persons and those post stroke (Wolf et al., 2001). Sensorimotor and kinematic measures of reach and grasp support the construct validity (Edwards et al., 2012). Concurrent validity with the Action Research Arm Test (ARAT): time ≥ 0.64, FAS ≥ 0.75 (Edwards et al., 2012)	Interrater reliability: r = 0.95–0.99 (Wolf et al., 2001). ICC ≥ 0.93 and agreement between raters ≥ 0.88 performance time and FAS (Morris et al., 2001). Test-retest reliability: r = 0.95 for FAS and 0.90 for performance time (Morris et al., 2001). Internal consistency: Cronbach's α=0.86–0.92 for performance time and functional ability (Morris et al., 2001); Cronbach's α ≥ 0.96 for both FAS and time scores (Edwards et al., 2012).	Significant improvement in scores after CIMT (Kunkel et al., 1999; Wolf et al., 2006). The FAS score is sensitive to clinical change in the acute stage of stroke recovery (Edwards et al., 2012) and in the chronic stage (Morris et al., 2001).	Strengths: Combination of simple and complex movements; excellent interrater and test–retest reliability for performance time; excellent internal consistency; more sensitive to change than the AMAT (Morris et al., 2001). First estimate of minimal clinically important differences were grip strength (5.0 and 6.2 kg) and FAS (1.0 and 1.2) for dominant and nondominant hands, respectively (Lang et al., 2008). Weakness: Nine individual items had less than adequate interrater reliability on the FAS (Morris et al., 2001).
Motor Activity Log (MAL) (Taub et al., 1993)	Thirty common daily life tasks tested for the affected post-stroke upper extremity. Two scales: amount of use (AOU) and quality of movement (QOM). It is a self-report instrument.	20–30 minutes	High concurrent validity of the QOM scale with an objective accelerometer-based measure of arm movement: r = 0.91; good internal consistency of both scales: Cronbach's α > 0.81 (Uswatte et al., 2005)	High (test–retest) reliability of the QOM scale: r > 0.91 (Uswatte et al., 2005)	Significant improvement in scores following CIMT (Kunkel et al., 1999; Wolf et al. 2006).	Strengths: Measures the actual use of the post-stroke affected upper extremity in real life situations; strong reliability and sensitivity. Minimal therapist time to score. Weaknesses: Subjective because it is a self-report measure. AOU not found reliable (Uswatte et al., 2005).
Fugl-Meyer Motor Assessment (FMA) (Fugl-Meyer et al., 1975)	Test of motor and sensory impairment after stroke. Most items are scored on a 3-point ordinal scale (0 = cannot be performed; 1 = performed partly; and 2 = performed faultlessly).	34–110 minutes for total FMA; 30–45 minutes for the upper and lower extremity subtests; 8–12 minutes for the upper extremity subtest alone	Actual motor recovery post stroke parallels the test items (Fugl-Meyer et al., 1975). Concurrent validity: r_s = 0.88 with total Motor Assessment Scale (Poole & Whitney, 1988) and r = 0.68–0.85 with the Barthel Index (Wood-Dauphinee, Williams, & Shapiro, 1990) and Spearman's rank correlation (ρ = 0.91–0.96) among FMA, Motor Status Scale, and ARAT (Wei, Tong, & Hu, 2011).	Interrater reliability: r = 0.79–0.99 for the upper and lower extremity subtests (Duncan, Propst, & Nelson, 1983). Interrater reliability for trainees versus an expert rater: ICC 0.91–0.99 for motor scores and 0.87–0.96 for sensory scores (Sullivan et al., 2011). Intrarater (test-retest) reliability: r = .86 to .99 across three test times (Duncan, Propst, & Nelson, 1983). For an expert rater, over a 12-month time difference: ≥0.95 for motor and sensory scores (Sullivan et al., 2011).	Significantly greater improvement in experimental versus control group at 6- and 12-month follow-ups (Feys et al., 1998).	Strengths: Administration time for upper extremity is acceptable; evidence supports its reliability, validity, and sensitivity. Weaknesses: Administration time for total FMA is lengthy; items have little relevance to everyday activities; validity of balance subscale was questioned (Malouin et al., 1994) and is rarely used.

[1] FMA, Fugl-Meyer Motor Assessment
[2] WMFT, Wolf Motor Function Test

The Arm Motor Ability Test. The Arm Mobility Ability Test (AMAT) was developed as an assessment of functional ability and quality of movement as a result of CIMT (Kopp et al., 1997). Some of the 13 functional tasks are simulated (e.g., "cut meat" uses Play-Doh®) and thus are not as natural as most functional assessments. The psychometric properties are described in Assessment Table 8-2.

The Wolf Motor Function Test. The Wolf Motor Function Test (WMFT) "quantifies upper extremity movement ability through timed single- or multiple-joint motions and functional tasks" (Wolf et al., 2001, p. 1635). It was also developed to assess the effects of CIMT. Figure 8-4 shows an example of one of the WMFT 17 upper extremity tasks. The psychometric properties are described in Assessment Table 8-2.

The Motor Activity Log. The Motor Activity Log (MAL) is a structured interview that assesses the persons' post-stroke insight of how much they use the affected UE to perform 30 common functional activities (Taub et al., 1993). There are two other versions of the test, 1 with 14 tasks (Uswatte et al., 2005) and 1 with 28 (Uswatte et al., 2006). This test has two subscales: the Amount of Use Scale and the Quality of Movement Scale, where the average of 0–5 scale scores are computed for common upper extremity daily life tasks. Its psychometric properties are described in Assessment Table 8-2.

The Fugl-Meyer Motor Assessment. The Fugl-Meyer Assessment (FMA) was developed to evaluate motor function, balance, some aspects of sensation, and joint function in persons post stroke (Fugl-Meyer et al., 1975). The items were based on earlier studies on the sequential stages of motor recovery post stroke (Brunnstrom, 1970; Twitchell, 1951). The maximum points are 66 for the upper extremity, 34 for lower extremity, 14 for balance, 24 for sensation, 24 for position sense, 44 for range of motion, and 44 for joint pain (total possible score, 250). Each section can be scored separately (see Fugl-Meyer et al. [1975] for test procedures and scoring criteria). The procedures for the upper extremity subtest are described in Table 8-1. Assessment Table 8-2 describes the psychometric properties of the FMA. The FMA is the second most frequently used assessment of motor deficits of persons with CNS impairments (van Wijck et al., 2001), is widely used in outcome studies, and was a recommended assessment of motor function in the Agency for Health Care Policy and Research clinical practice guidelines for post-stroke rehabilitation (Gresham et al., 1995).

Assessments of Balance

Balance is assessed through observational analysis as the person performs self-initiated movements in sitting and standing. These include the following:

- Looking in a variety of directions (e.g., up at the ceiling, behind oneself)
- Reaching forward, sideways, and down to the floor to pick up objects
- Walking in various conditions

Forward reach in sitting entails (1) anterior movement of the pelvis, (2) flexion of the trunk at the hips, and (3) active use of the legs to aid in balancing by creating an active base of support. Reaching sideways while sitting is more challenging than reaching forward, because the base of support is smaller. Reaching while standing requires (1) establishment of an appropriate base of support with one's feet and (2) shifting body weight and center of mass toward the direction of the goal object.

The Berg Balance Scale. The Berg Balance Scale (BBS) (Berg et al., 1992) evaluates a client's performance on 14 items common in everyday life. The items include "the subject's ability to maintain positions of increasing difficulty by diminishing the base of support from sitting, to comfortable stance, to standing with feet together, and finally tandem standing (i.e., one foot in front of the other) and single leg stance, the two most difficult items. Other items assess how well the subject is able to change positions from sitting to standing, transfer from chair to chair, turn, pick up an object from the floor, and sit down" (Berg et al., 1992, p. 1074). The psychometric properties of the

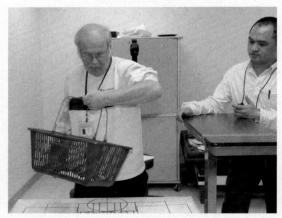

Figure 8-4 Task #17 in the Wolf Motor Function Test (WMFT): Lifting a basket loaded with a weight of 3 pounds. (Used with permission from Almhdawi, K. A. [2011]. *Effects of occupational therapy task-oriented approach in upper extremity post-stroke rehabilitation* [Doctoral dissertation]. Retrieved from University of Minnesota Digital Conservancy.

| Table 8-1 | Fugl-Meyer Assessment of Motor Function: Upper Extremity Subtest | | |

Stage	Instruction	Response	Scoring Criteria
Shoulder/Elbow/Forearm: Subtotal Score (36 points)			
I & II: Reflex activity	Tap the biceps and finger flexor tendons Tap the triceps tendon	Stretch reflex at elbow and/ or fingers Stretch reflex	0 = no reflex can be elicited 2 = reflex can be elicited
III: Voluntary movement within synergy	Flexor synergy "Turn your affected hand palm up and touch your ear." Extensor synergy "Turn your hand palm down and reach to touch your unaffected knee."	Shoulder retraction Shoulder elevation Shoulder abduction to 90° Shoulder external rotation Elbow flexion Forearm supination Shoulder adduction and internal rotation Elbow extension Forearm pronation	(For each of nine details) 0 = cannot perform 1 = can perform partly 2 = can perform faultlessly
IV: Voluntary movement mixing flexor and extensor synergies	"Show me how you would put a belt around you [or tie an apron]." "Reach forward to take [object held in front of patient]." "Put your arm to your side and bend your elbow. Turn your palm up and down."	Affected hand moves to lumbar spine area Reaches into 90° of shoulder flexion Pronates and supinates forearm with elbow at 90° and shoulder at 0°	0 = cannot perform 1 = hand must actively pass anterior-superior iliac spine 2 = faultless 0 = elbow flexes or shoulder abducts immediately 1 = if these occur later in motion 2 = faultless 0 = if cannot position arm or cannot pronate or supinate 1 = shoulder and elbow joints correctly positioned and supination seen 2 = faultless
V: Voluntary movement outside of synergies	"Turn your palm down and reach over here to touch [object held out to side]." "Reach as high as you can toward the ceiling." "Reach your arm directly forward and turn your palm up and down."	Abducts shoulder to 90° with elbow extended to 0° and forearm pronated Flexes shoulder from 90° to 180° with elbow in 0° Flexes shoulder to 30°–90°; extends elbow to 0°; and supinates and pronates	0 = initial elbow flexion or loss of pronation 1 = partial motion or elbow flexes and forearm supinates later in motion 2 = faultless 0 = elbow flexes or shoulder abducts immediately 1 = if these occur later in motion 2 = faultless 0 = if cannot position arm or cannot rotate 1 = correct position and beginning rotation 2 = faultless
VI: Normal reflex activity (tested if patient scores 6 in stage V tests)	Tap on biceps, triceps, and finger flexor tendons	Normal reflex response	0 = 2 reflexes are markedly hyperactive 1 = 1 reflex hyperactive or 2 reflexes lively 2 = no more than 1 reflex lively and none hyperactive

(continued)

| Table 8-1 | **Fugl-Meyer Assessment of Motor Function: Upper Extremity Subtest** *(continued)* | | |

Stage	Instruction	Response	Scoring Criteria
Wrist: Subtotal Score (10 points)			
Wrist stability with elbow flexed	Put the shoulder in 0° flexion and abduction, elbow in 90° flexion, and forearm pronated. "Lift your wrist and hold it there."	Patient extends wrist to 15°. Therapist can hold upper arm in position.	0 = cannot extend 1 = can extend, but not against resistance 2 = can maintain against slight resistance
Wrist stability with elbow extended	Put the elbow in 0°. "Lift your wrist and hold it there."	As above	As above
Active motion with elbow flexed and shoulder at 0°	"Move your wrist up and down a few times."	Patient moves smoothly from full flexion to full extension. Therapist can hold upper arm.	0 = no voluntary movement 1 = moves, but less than full range 2 = faultless
Active motion with elbow extended	"Move your wrist up and down a few times."	As above	As above
Circumduction	"Turn your wrist in a circle like this" [demonstrate].	Makes a full circle, combining flexion and extension with ulnar and radial deviation.	0 = cannot perform 1 = jerky or incomplete motion 2 = faultless
Hand: Subtotal Score (14 points)			
III: Mass flexion	"Make a fist."	Patient flexes fingers.	0 = no flexion 1 = less than full flexion as compared to other hand 2 = full active flexion
III: Hook grasp	"Hold this shopping bag by the handles."	Grasp involves MCP extension and PIP and DIP flexion.	0 = cannot perform 1 = active grasp, no resistance 2 = maintains grasp against great resistance
IIIB–VI: Finger extension	"Let go of the shopping bag." "Open your hand wide."	From full active or passive flexion, patient extends all fingers.	0 = no extension 1 = partial extension or able to release grasp 2 = full range of motion as compared to other hand
IV: Lateral prehension	"Take hold of this sheet of paper [or playing card]."	Patient grasps between thumb and index finger.	0 = cannot perform 1 = can hold paper but not against tug 2 = holds paper well against tug
V: Palmar prehension	"Take hold of this pencil as if you were going to write."	Therapist holds pencil upright and patient grasps it.	Scoring as above
V: Cylindrical grasp	"Take hold of this paper cup [or pill bottle]."	Therapist holds the object and patient grasps with first and second fingers together.	Scoring as above
VI: Spherical grasp	"Take hold of this tennis ball [or apple]."	Patient grasps with fingers abducted.	Scoring as above

Table 8-1	Fugl-Meyer Assessment of Motor Function: Upper Extremity Subtest *(continued)*		
Stage	**Instruction**	**Response**	**Scoring Criteria**
Coordination/Speed: Subtotal Score (6 points)			
VI: Normal movement	"Close your eyes. Now, touch your nose with your fingertip. Do that as fast as you can five times."	Patient does finger-to-nose test	
		Tremor	*Tremor:* 0 = marked
			1 = slight
			2 = none
		Dysmetria	*Dysmetria:* 0 = pronounced or unsystematic
			1 = slight and systematic
			2 = none
		Speed (compare to unaffected side)	*Speed:* 0 = >6 seconds slower
			1 = 2–5 seconds slower
			2 = <2 seconds slower
TOTAL UPPER EXTREMITY SCORE (66 points)			

Adapted from Fugl-Meyer, A. R., Jäasko, L., Leyman, I., Olsson, S., & Steglind, S. (1975). The post-stroke hemiplegic patient: A method for evaluation of physical performance. *Scandinavian Journal of Rehabilitation Medicine, 7,* 13–31.

BBS are described in Assessment Table 8-3. The BBS was a recommended assessment of balance in the Agency for Health Care Policy and Research's clinical practice guidelines for post-stroke rehabilitation (Gresham et al., 1995).

Functional Reach Test. The Functional Reach Test (Duncan et al., 1990) was developed as a quick, clinical measure of dynamic balance that uses a continuous scoring system to assess the risk of falls in the elderly. It was intended to be an alternative to sophisticated laboratory-based assessments of falls, which are not feasible for clinical use. The psychometric properties are described in Assessment Table 8-3 (for a broader review of balance assessments, see Tyson and Connell [2009]).

Assessment of Gait

Walking, a critical component of daily task engagement, is a reasonable expectation for many individuals with CNS dysfunction. Occupational therapists work with patients who wish to improve their performance in kitchen and bathroom activities and in leisure or work pursuits. In each of these contexts, the occupational therapist must help patients reach their optimal walking potential. Physical therapists determine initial walking goals based on observation and comparison of each patient's performance against the critical kinematic features of walking that have been determined through descriptive research. Although observational gait analysis cannot provide information about the kinetics of a person's gait, spatiotemporal and kinematic variables provide clues about the underlying kinetic dynamics (such as information provided by force plates that record exact loading and unloading during stepping).

For purposes of description, the gait cycle for each leg is divided into a stance phase and a swing phase. Definition 8-3 shows the subdivision of these phases of the gait cycle. Basic knowledge about the motor requirements during each phase of the gait cycle guides therapists in their interventions for patients with CNS dysfunction.

Reach and Manipulation

The arm and hand function as a single unit in reach and manipulation, with the hand beginning to open for grasp at the start of a reaching action (Karok & Newport, 2010). In many activities, the upper body, or even the entire body, is an integral component of this single coordinated unit. Clearly, reach and grasp are not exclusively upper limb activities. All reaching actions from sitting or standing are preceded and accompanied by postural adjustments. When objects are beyond the arm's reach, shifts in total body alignment contribute to functional performance (Aimola et al., 2011).

Clinical assessment of reach and manipulation is achieved through detailed observation of each patient's attempts to perform selected functional tasks. Therapists use their knowledge about the kinetics and kinematics of upper limb function to develop hypotheses as to which deficits may be serving as control parameters in

Assessment Table 8-3		Psychometric Properties of Assessments of Balance				
Instrument and Reference	**Description**	**Time to Administer**	**Validity**	**Reliability**	**Sensitivity**	**Strengths and Weaknesses**
Berg Balance Scale (Berg et al., 1992)	Fourteen items common in everyday life are "graded on a five-point scale, 0 to 4. Points are based on the time the position can be maintained, the distance the arm is able to reach forward, or the time to complete the task" (Berg et al., 1992, p. 1075)	About 15 minutes to administer and requires only a stopwatch and ruler	Concurrent validity: $r = 0.91$ with the Tinetti Balance Subscale (Tinetti, 1986); $r = -0.81$ with Timed Up-and-Go Test (TUG) (Podsiadlo & Richardson, 1991) or $r = -0.74$ with the TUG (Salavati et al., 2012). Discriminant validity: discriminates among persons using various types of walking aids (Berg et al., 1992).	Interrater reliability: ICC = 0.98 for total scale; ICC = 0.71–0.99 for individual items (Berg et al., 1992). For total scale: ICC = 0.97 (Blum & Korner-Bitensky, 2008) and 0.95 (Wirz, Müller, & Bastiaenen, 2010). Test–retest reliability: ICC = 0.99 for total scale (Berg et al., 1992). ICC for tests 1 week apart = 0.98 (Blum & Korner-Bitensky, 2008) and 0.96 (Learmonth et al., 2012). Internal consistency: Cronbach's $\alpha = 0.96$ (Berg et al., 1989) and 0.92–0.98 (Blum & Korner-Bitensky, 2008).	Significant changes in scores at 6 and 12 weeks post stroke (Wood-Dauphinee et al., 1997). Minimal detectable change value = 7 points (Learmonth et al., 2012)	Strengths: Measures many aspects of balance; consistent reports of excellent reliability; evidence of validity. Foreign versions have been studied and found psychometrically sound (Azad, Taghizadeh, & Khaneghini, 2011; Salavati et al., 2012; Scalzo et al., 2009). Weaknesses: Long administration time. Has floor and ceiling effects (Blum & Korner-Bitensky, 2008). Not predictive of falls (Blum & Korner-Bitensky, 2008; Wirz, Müller, & Bastiaenen, 2010).
Functional Reach Test (Duncan et al., 1990)	"The maximal distance one can reach forward beyond arm's length while maintaining a fixed base of support in the standing position" (Duncan et al., 1990, p. M192).	1–2 minutes to administer and requires a 48-inch leveled ruler, mounted on the wall at shoulder height (Weiner et al., 1993)	Concurrent validity: $r = 0.71$ with center of pressure excursion (Duncan et al., 1990). Discriminant validity: Significant difference between persons with high and low risk of falls. Predictive validity: score ≤ 6 inches predictive of falls in elderly (Duncan et al., 1992)	Interrater reliability: $r = 0.98$ Test–retest reliability: ICC = 0.92 (Duncan et al., 1990)	Marginal significant change ($p = 0.07$) after physical rehabilitation, responsiveness index = 0.97 (Weiner et al., 1993)	Strengths: Brief, functional test; excellent reliability, evidence of validity. Weakness: Sensitivity is borderline.

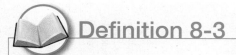

Definition 8-3

The Gait Cycle

Stance Phase

- Weight-load acceptance: from heel contact to foot flat on ground
- Midstance: from foot flat on ground to heel off of ground
- Push-off: weight moving forward onto toes and foot preparing to leave ground

Swing Phase

- Liftoff (early swing): leg swings forward with foot clearing the ground
- Reach (late swing): leg decelerates and prepares for heel contact

their hypotheses through direct assessment of muscle strength and length and through patients' responses to interventions designed to modify adaptive strategies.

Assessment of Praxis

Apraxia is the inability to implement purposeful movement that cannot be explained by deficits in sensation, movement, or coordination (Gazzaniga, Ivry, & Mangun, 2009). We will discuss limb, constructional, and dressing types of apraxia. There are two additional apraxia types: verbal and buccofacial, which are usually evaluated by a speech and language pathologist and will not be discussed in this chapter.

Limb Apraxia. Limb apraxia is usually associated with left brain damage (LBD) in right-handed patients and right brain damage (RBD) in left-handed patients, although variations have been described (Marchetti & Della Sala, 1997). As can be seen in Table 8-2, there are many types of limb apraxia including ideomotor, ideational, dissociation, conduction, and conceptual (Heilman, Rothi, & Watson, 1997; Unsworth, 2007). Limb kinetic apraxia is characterized by a loss of ability to make finely graded precise finger movements and is thought to be a motor problem rather than a true apraxia (Heilman, Watson, & Rothi, 2003).

Psychometric properties of limb apraxia tests can be found in Assessment Table 8-4. This testing requires

limiting the versatility or efficiency of motor strategies. Most motor dysfunction can be attributed to specific muscle weakness, muscle stiffness and length changes, and/or adaptive strategies developed to compensate for these impairments. Shoulder pain may also be a significant control parameter to efficient reach. Therapists test

Table 8-2 Types of Limb Apraxia

Type of Apraxia	Error Type	How Elicited	Functional Example
Ideomotor	Production errors	Most errors are made on pantomiming transitive tasks, improves with imitation and usually does best with the actual object.	Movements will be awkward but bear a resemblance to the intended movement. Able to use tools to complete tasks, but may appear clumsy or awkward.
Conceptual	Content errors: • Tool-action knowledge • Tool-association knowledge • Mechanical knowledge • Tool fabrication	Use of tools; actions associated with specific tools, association between tool and object.	Patient has obvious difficulty with tool use: may use a tube of toothpaste to brush teeth, comb hair with fork, etc.
Disassociation	Thought to be a disconnection between hemispheres; therefore, there is no recognizable movement on command.	Pantomime to command is impaired; imitation and use of object will be much better.	Unable to pantomime movements, but since able to imitate and use tools, minimal effect on functional activities.
Conduction	Difficulty decoding and understanding gestures	Impaired imitation of gestures; does better when asked to pantomime	A client with aphasia might have difficulty understanding and using gestures.
Ideational	Difficulty with a series of tasks	Tasks requiring a series of activities (e.g., clean pipe, put in tobacco, and light pipe)	Task may be completed more skillfully than with ideomotor apraxia, but client will have difficulty sequencing steps in the correct order (e.g., client might try to light the empty pipe, then put the tobacco in, and then clean it).

Adapted from Heilman, K. M., Watson, R. T., & Rothi, L. G. (2003). Disorders of skilled movements: Limb apraxia. In T. E. Fineberg & M. J. Farah (Eds.), *Behavioral neurology and neuropsychology* (2nd ed.). New York: McGraw-Hill.

Assessment Table 8-4 | Psychometric Properties of Assessments for Limb Apraxia

Instrument and Reference	Description	Time to Administer	Validity	Reliability	Sensitivity	Strengths and Weaknesses
Florida Apraxia Screening Test-Revised (FAST-R) (Rothi, Raymer, & Heilman, 1997)	Thirty items, gesture to verbal command test: 20 transitive, 10 intransitive pantomime; scored on multiple error types; normal cutoff score is 15 out of 30 correct.	Unknown; includes time to train and practice pantomime and then to complete a 30-item test	Not established	Not established Recommend that the responses are videotaped for later scoring	Not established	Strength: Can be completed with one hand only. Weakness: Psychometrics not established. Coexisting aphasia can be a problem because of verbal presentation. Relates to limb apraxia only. Scoring can be difficult and requires too much time for clinic use.
Screening for Apraxia (Almeida, Black, & Roy, 2002)	Five gestures (three transitive, two intransitive) five dimensions for each task is scored on a 3-point scale (see Roy et al., 1998 for scoring)	Authors feel that this can be used to detect apraxia and then a decision can be made to follow-up with a more comprehensive assessment battery	Not established	Not established on screen; κ coefficient for interrater reliability ranged from 0.71 to 0.78 on the full battery (Roy et al., 1998)	Not established	Strength: Short five-item screening test. Weakness: Scoring is unclear and requires knowledge and practice on the part of the examiner. Validity, test–retest reliability and sensitivity data are missing
Assessment of Apraxia (Van Heugten et al., 1999a)	Two subtests: demonstration of object use (three sets of objects presented under three different conditions) and imitation of gestures (six gestures to be imitated). Each is scored from 0 (movement not recognizable) to 3 (performance is correct and appropriate). Maximum subscore for object use is 54, for imitation of gestures is 36 with a total score of 90. Total score below 86 is considered to identify apraxia.	Unknown	Not established	Internal consistency good (Cronbach's $\alpha = 0.96$; Mokken coefficient of reliability $\rho = 0.96$). Interrater reliability $\kappa > 0.60$ on all but three items (Zwinkels, et al., 2004)	A cutoff score of 86 (mean score – one standard deviation) sensitivity was 91%	Strength: Uses common gestures and objects Weaknesses: Validity and test-retest reliability data are missing. Includes items for ideational and ideomotor apraxia only.
Assessment of Disabilities in Stroke Patients with Apraxia (van Heugten et al., 1999b)	Set of standard activities of daily living (ADL) observations for assessment of disabilities caused by apraxia: personal hygiene, dressing, preparing food, and another of the therapist's choice. Scoring: four measures (independence, initiation, execution and control) scored from 0 (no observable problems) to 3 (therapist has to take over). Then they can be added together to get a total score.	Unknown, but could easily be observed during the occupational therapist's evaluation of ADL	Not established	Coefficient of reliability $\rho = 0.94$ Interrater reliability κ value highest for independence scores (0.81–0.97)	Not established	Strength: Can be easily incorporated into the therapist's ADL evaluation; task specifically related to the client can be addressed; allows therapist to determine where the breakdown is occurring (initiation, execution, or control) to develop treatment program. Weaknesses: Validity, test-retest reliability, and sensitivity data are missing. Training is recommended to improve reliability

| Table 8-3 | Apraxia Testing Methods |

Method	Example
Gesture to command: should include both transitive movements (tool use) and intransitive movements (nonverbal communication).	Transitive: "Show me how you would open the door with a key" or "use a hammer." Intransitive: "Show me how you hitchhike, salute, wave good-bye."
Gesture to imitate	Examiner produces a gesture and asks the client to "do it the same way I do it; do not name the gesture and do not start until I'm finished"; can be familiar gestures or nonsense gestures (e.g., hand to the forehead).
Gesture in response to tool	Visual: Examiner shows the tool and says, "Show me how you use this." Tactile: Eyes closed or covered, client examines the tool by feeling and examiner says, "Show me how you use this."
Gesture in response to seeing object on which the tool acts: tool selection task	Examiner presents client with object representing an incomplete action (e.g., if the target is sawing, client is shown a partially cut piece of wood); client must choose the correct tool from a choice of three, one of which is the saw.
Actual tool use	Patient is given a tool (e.g., hammer) and asked, "Show me how you use this."
Gesture decision: discrimination between correctly and incorrectly pantomimed movements	Examiner makes a gesture and asks the client, "Is this the correct way to . . ." (e.g., use a pair of scissors).
Gesture comprehension	Examiner makes a gesture and asks the client, "Tell me what I am doing." "What tool am I using?" "Am I using a hammer or a saw?"
Serial acts	Examiner tells client, "Fold letter, put it in envelope, seal envelope, and place stamp on it."

Adapted from Rothi, L. J. G., Raymer, A. M., & Heilman, K. M. (1997). Limb praxis assessment. In L. J. G. Rothi & K. M. Heilman (Eds.), *Apraxia: The neuropsychology of action* (pp. 61–73). East Sussex, UK: Psychology Press Publishers.

gesture production where the client is asked to pantomime a task on command (e.g., "Show me how you wash your face"), to imitate the therapist, or to use an object. Transitive gestures are especially sensitive to apraxia (Enticott et al., 2010; Trojano, Labruna, & Grossi, 2007). Generally, clients with apraxia would have the least difficulty with proximal intransitive gestures away from the body (e.g., waving goodbye) and most difficulty with distal transitive gestures on the body (e.g., putting on makeup) (Helm-Estabrooks & Albert, 2004; Trojano, Labruna, & Grossi, 2007). Gesture comprehension and discrimination have been added to the list of apraxia testing methods (Table 8-3) (Heilman, Watson, & Rothi, 2003; York & Cermak, 1995).

Apraxia often occurs in conjunction with aphasia, and it is sometimes difficult to distinguish between the two (Unsal Delialioglu et al., 2008). Therefore, it is important when evaluating a client with aphasia to include (in addition to the regular commands, e.g., "show me how you would . . .") questions that can be answered by yes/no responses or by pointing at the correct answers. If the client performs poorly but can answer yes/no questions, he or she may be apraxic. Similarly, if the client is unable to respond to yes/no questions, failure to make the appropriate movement to command may be due to a language problem rather than apraxia.

There are few standardized tests available for limb apraxia (see Assessment Table 8-4). Rothi, Raymer, and Heilman (1997) have developed the Florida Apraxia Screening

Test-Revised (FAST-R) for use in the research of neurologically impaired patients. This test consists of 30 items that are presented verbally (Table 8-4). The patient uses the dominant arm if possible. Prior to testing, patients practice pantomiming such that they pretend to hold the imagined tool and act on the imagined object. This rehearsal is important to discourage use of a body part as the imagined tool itself. Normal subjects may use a body part as tool, but with instruction, they correct their performance, whereas apraxic patients continue to do so even with the instruction (Raymer et al., 1997). Scoring for the FAST-R includes multiple error types based on content of the pantomime, timing and sequencing of the response, and spatial features (Table 8-5).

| Table 8-4 | Sample Items from the Florida Apraxia Screening Test (Revised) |

Show me:
- how to salute
- how to use a saw to cut a piece of wood out in front of you
- how to hitchhike
- stop
- how to use a salt shaker to salt food on a table out in front of you
- how to use a spoon to stir coffee on a table out in front of you

From Rothi, L. J. G., Raymer, A. M., & Heilman, K. M. (1997). Limb praxis assessment. In L. J. G. Rothi & K. M. Heilman (Eds.), *Apraxia: The neuropsychology of action* (pp. 61–73). East Sussex, UK: Psychology Press Publishers.

Table 8-5 **Apraxia Error Types**

Error Type	Description
Content Errors	
Perseveration	Patient's response includes all or part of a previously produced pantomime.
Related	Pantomime is correctly produced but is only related to that requested (e.g., playing the trombone instead of playing a bugle as requested).
Nonrelated	Pantomime is accurately produced but unrelated to request (e.g., playing the trombone for shaving).
Hand	Performs the action without use of a real or imagined tool (e.g., turning a screw with the fingers rather than an imaginary screwdriver).
Temporal	
Sequencing	Addition, deletion, or transposition of the movement elements of a sequence.
Timing	Any alteration in the timing or speed of a pantomime: abnormally increased, decreased, or irregular rate of production.
Occurrence	Any multiplication of characteristically single-cycle movements (e.g., unlocking a door) or reduction of a characteristically repetitive cycle (e.g., screwing in a screw) to a single event.
Spatial	
Amplitude	Any increase, decrease, or irregularity of the characteristic movement.
Internal configuration	Any abnormality of the required finger/hand posture and its relationship to the target tool (e.g., when pretending to brush the teeth, the hand may be closed tightly into a fist with no space allowed for the imagined toothbrush handle).
Body part as tool	Patient uses finger, hand, or arm as the imagined tool even when requested to pretend they are holding the object (e.g., uses the finger to brush the teeth).
External configuration	Difficulties orienting the fingers/hand/arm to the object or in placing the object in space (e.g., brushing teeth with the hand so close to the mouth as to not allow room for the imagined toothbrush).
Movement	Any disturbance of the characteristic movement used when acting on an object (e.g., activates movement at incorrect joint; when pantomiming a screwdriver and rotation occurs at the shoulder rather than at the forearm).
Other	
Concretization	Patient performs pantomime not on an imagined object but instead on a real object not normally used in the task (e.g., instead of pretending to saw wood, they pantomime sawing on their leg).
No response	
Unrecognizable	Response shares no temporal or spatial features of the target, it is unrecognizable.

Adapted from Rothi, L. J. G., Raymer, A. M., & Heilman, K. M. (1997). Limb praxis assessment. In L. J. G. Rothi & K. M. Heilman (Eds.), *Apraxia: The neuropsychology of action* (pp. 61–73). East Sussex, UK: Psychology Press Publishers.

Some researchers suggest that there be more than one observer or even videotaping the response during testing. Butler (2002) advises not to rely on one test of apraxia, but rather to consider functional indices in ADL tasks as more clinically relevant. van Heugten et al. (1999b) developed an assessment of disability in stroke patients with apraxia that looks at an independence measure and three aspects (initiation, execution, and control) of four activities (personal hygiene, dressing, preparing food, and another activity that is chosen by the therapist). This allows the therapist to determine in what area the person is having difficulty and better focus treatment.

Constructional Apraxia. Constructional apraxia is a specific deficit in spatial-organizational performance (Chaikin,

2007) Patients with constructional apraxia have difficulty with copying, drawing, and constructing designs in two and three dimensions. Constructional apraxia was found to correlate with deficits of ADL (Neistadt, 1993; Poole, Sadek, & Haaland, 2009). It can be seen functionally as difficulty with such activities as setting a table, making a sandwich, and making a dress and with any mechanical activity in which parts are to be combined into a whole.

There are two types of constructional activities used in assessment: graphic tasks (e.g., copying line drawings and drawing to command) and assembly tasks (e.g., block and stick designs). Both types are included in an evaluation of constructional apraxia. The most common example of a graphic task is copying geometric shapes (from simple to complex)

Table 8-6	Scoring for Drawing to Command	
Shape	**Instruction**	**Scoring**
Clock	"Draw the face of a clock showing the numbers and the two hands."	0 to 3: 1 point each for approximately circular face, symmetry of number placement, and correctness of numbers
Daisy	"Draw a daisy."	0 to 2: 1 point each for general shape (center with petals around it) and symmetry of petal arrangement
Elephant	"Draw an elephant"	0 to 2: 1 point each for general shape (legs, trunk, head, body) and relative proportions correct
Cross	"You know what the Red Cross looks like? Draw an outline of it without taking your pencil off the paper."	0 to 2: 1 point each for basic configuration and ability to form all corners adequately with a continuous line
Cube	"Draw a cube-shaped block in perspective, as it would look if you could see the top and two sides."	0 to 2: 1 point each for grossly correct attempt and correctness of perspective
House	"Draw a house in perspective, so you can see the roof and two sides."	0 to 2: 1 point each for grossly correct features of house and accuracy of perspective

and drawing without a model (e.g., house, clock, or flower). It is best to use a simple task (e.g., simple geometric figures, three-dimensional block design), because a more complex task involves a greater number of skills, and interpretation becomes less specific (Cooke, McKenna, & Fleming, 2005). Goodglass and Kaplan (1983) described the test of drawing to command without a model. This test includes having the client draw a clock, daisy, elephant, cross, cube, and house; scoring criteria are given in Table 8-6. Assembly tasks include such activities as stick arrangement and three-dimensional block designs. Common errors on stick arrangement include selecting sticks of incorrect length; failing to reproduce parts of the model, especially lateral; making lines more oblique than the model indicates; tending to remove part of the model to make the copy; and crowding in (the client's copy rests on top of or touches the model) (Critchley, 1966). In general, assembly tasks are not standardized and rely on subjective judgment of the results. It is important to note the client's method of completing the task; the client's comments; any emotional display, hesitancy, indecision, and change of mind; and the type of errors made.

The Lowenstein Occupational Therapy Cognitive Assessment (LOTCA) battery was standardized on brain-injured adults and contains a section on visuomotor organization containing block design, copying, drawing, and pegboard design. The test has another updated version called the Dynamic Lowenstein Occupational Therapy Cognitive Assessment (DLOTCA) (Katz et al., 2012). See chapter 6 for more information about cognitive assessment in occupational therapy.

Dressing Apraxia. Dressing apraxia refers to an inability to dress oneself. It is usually due to RBD and secondary visuospatial disorganization. It is evaluated functionally by watching clients dress themselves. The underlying problem needs to be determined (e.g., visual deficits, unilateral neglect, apraxia, or constructional apraxia) rather than evaluating dressing apraxia per se.

Motor Neglect

Motor neglect presents as impaired initiation or execution of movement into contralateral hemispace by either limb (Bisiach et al., 1990; Tegner & Levander, 1991). Heilman, Watson, and Valenstein (2003) described several types of motor neglect (Definition 8-4). It is often difficult to differentiate between sensory and motor neglect because tests of motor neglect entail some form of sensory input. Consequently, therapists wonder whether clients fail to respond to a stimulus on the involved side because they do not see it or because they cannot initiate movement toward it. If motor neglect is suspected, one way to distinguish between the two entails contrasting a task that requires a hand response with one that has minimal motor response (e.g., naming letters on the involved side as opposed to pointing to the same letters). In other words, the stimulus (letters on the involved side) stays the same, and the motor response is varied (Arnadottir, 2011).

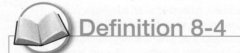 Definition 8-4

Motor Neglect

- Limb akinesia—Failure to move limb.
- Hypokinesia—Limb moves but only after a long delay and much encouragement.
- Hypometria—Movements are of decreased amplitude.
- Impersistence—Inability to maintain a movement or posture.
- Motor perseveration—Inability to disengage from a motor activity.
- Motor extinction—Delay or failure to move the contralesional limb when also required to move the ipsilateral limb.

Adapted from Heilman, K. M., Watson, R. T., & Valenstein, E. (2003). Neglect: Clinical and anatomic aspects. In T. E. Fineberg & M. J. Farah (Eds.), *Behavioral neurology and neuropsychology* (2nd ed.). new York; McGraw-Hill.

Although there are no standardized tests of motor neglect (Appelros et al., 2003), observations of clients and how they use the affected extremity can provide insight into the presence of motor neglect. One may note reluctance to move the arm or movement only after a delay (hypokinesia) or movement only with strong encouragement (akinesia), a tendency to undershoot a target when asked to move along a given line (hypometria), or inability to sustain a posture (impersistence) (Heilman, Watson, & Valenstein, 2003). Different limbs can be observed, as can the direction of the movement required (ipsilateral versus contralateral) and the hemispace in which the movement is to occur (ipsilateral versus contralateral).

SUMMARY

All therapeutic approaches evolve over time. Clinical practice and research will continue to test the assumptions and treatment principles of each approach. Evaluating motor behavior and performance will keep evolving as the therapeutic approaches evolve. The task-related approaches are more supported in current literature than the older neurophysiological approaches. The task-related approaches have

their unique evaluative procedures that emphasize the roles of the environmental, task, and individual factors on motor behavior. However, many of the neurophysiological assessments are used when using the task-related approaches, particularly when assessing the individual's factors related to motor behavior such as strength and muscle tone. Development of more evaluation tools and measures of change (with better clinical usefulness and stronger psychometric properties) is critical, particularly for individuals with poor motor abilities (Connell & Tyson, 2012). Identification of critical factors influencing occupational performance and measures of motor behavior will lead to more effective and client-centered treatment strategies. Further testing of the assumptions and treatment principles for persons having CNS dysfunction and other motor behavior problems will provide additional support for use of the systems and task-related approaches in practice. When using a clinical measure that captures a change in motor behavior, it is fundamental to make sure that this change is clinically meaningful for the clients. A clinically meaningful change is one that exceeds the minimal requirements for real life occupational performance (Lang et al., 2008).

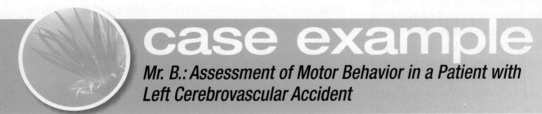

case example

Mr. B.: Assessment of Motor Behavior in a Patient with Left Cerebrovascular Accident

Occupational Therapy Assessment Process	Clinical Reasoning Process	
	Objectives	Examples of Therapist's Internal Dialogue
Patient Information Mr. B. is a 55-year-old man who worked as an administrator at a junior college until a week ago, when he had a left cerebral vascular accident with resultant right hemiparesis. His medical history includes insulin-dependent diabetes mellitus and two heart attacks in the past 5 years. He lives with his wife in a ranch-style house. She works as a middle manager at an electronics firm. They have two adult children who do not live nearby.	Understand the patient's diagnosis or condition	"Mr. B. has right hemiparesis and moderate disability 1 week post stroke. Because his right arm is not flaccid and he is able to do some self-care already, his prognosis for recovery of functional ability appears to be good."
	Know the person	"Given his age and type of job, I expect that he will be motivated to return to work, but I cannot assume that."
The acute-care occupational therapist reported that he is independent in feeding, grooming, oral hygiene, and wheelchair mobility for short distances. He needs assistance with bathing, toilet hygiene, and dressing. Other occupational performance tasks were not assessed in acute care. He has weakness throughout his dominant right arm, with grade 2 muscle tone on the Modified Ashworth Scale for scapular depression, shoulder internal rotation, and elbow, wrist, and finger flexors. Passive range of motion (PROM) is within normal limits except for a 20° limitation in shoulder external rotation and elbow extension.		"I wonder how his wife is reacting to his various health problems. Will she support his return to work or will she try to protect him? I wonder about the accessibility of his home and work environment."
	Develop provisional hypotheses	"Given his diagnosis and history, I presume that sensorimotor, psychosocial, and cognitive client factors and the physical environment at home and/or work might limit his ability to perform occupational performance tasks and to resume his usual roles. Given his early recovery, he should be able to benefit from an intensive rehabilitation program."

Assessment Process

The Role Checklist was used to identify which roles were most important to him and to identify the tasks and activities that are associated with those roles. The Canadian Occupational Performance Measure (COPM) was used to determine the occupational performance tasks he wanted or needed to do and to determine his perception of his ability. Task analysis was used with specific tasks he perceived as difficult or impossible. The therapist observed him for client factors that might be limiting function and explored environmental factors that could support or limit his performance.

Assessment Results

It was clear from the Role Checklist that Mr. B.'s work role was important to him. His concerns about returning to work included problems with writing, word processing, and removing heavy manuals from shelves above his desk. His wife, however, was pushing him to consider early retirement because of his increasing health problems. He and his wife enjoyed entertaining friends at home, for which he was the primary chef. This was an important activity for both of them. Although he was responsible for many home and yard maintenance tasks, they were not important to him. He thought friends would help them or they could hire help. On the COPM, return to work was ranked as most important, followed by cooking, toilet hygiene, dressing, and driving. He rated his performance and satisfaction for all of these tasks as very low.

His performance on several work-related, cooking, and self-care tasks were observed. He had difficulty holding a regular pen. However, a trial with an enlarged pen with a rubber grip enabled him to hold a pen for about 3 minutes and write with very poor legibility. He was unable to use his right hand for keyboarding because he could not isolate individual fingers. He became frustrated while performing a simple cooking task (i.e., making pudding) because he could not walk and had difficulty using his right hand for bilateral tasks. He was able to toilet himself with verbal cueing and standby assistance. During dressing, he had difficulty raising his right arm, reaching down to put on his socks (concerned appropriately about balance), and difficulty performing bilateral tasks (e.g., tying his shoelaces). He complained about the time and energy needed to complete functional tasks. He used his right hand in half of the bilateral tasks he attempted. Thus, it appeared that sensorimotor client factors might be the cause of the difficulty performing occupational performance tasks, so these were evaluated further.

There was no evidence of unilateral visual neglect on a line bisection test (see Chapter 5). Sensory testing indicated loss of protective sensation and diminished light touch in the right hand (Semmes-Weinstein monofilaments) and impaired proprioception in the wrist and fingers only (see Chapter 9). Selective muscle testing indicated grade 3+ in scapular elevation, elbow flexion, and extension; 3− in shoulder flexion, abduction, and external rotation; and wrist flexion and extension. Grip strength was 5 pounds in the right hand and 80 pounds in the left hand; key pinch was 3 pounds on the right and 19 pounds on the left (see Chapter 7). He was able to reach forward 9 inches on the Functional Reach Test.

Consider evaluation approach and methods

"The primary aim of the assessment in the rehabilitation unit was to determine which roles and occupational performance tasks were most important to Mr. B. and to determine his ability on those tasks. The secondary aim was to determine whether specific client or environmental factors were supporting or limiting his functional performance."

Interpret observations

"It is clear that work and cooking tasks are priorities for this client, followed by self-care tasks. It is not yet clear whether he will be able to return to work. Decreased strength and impaired sensation are limiting the function of the right hand. Decreased PROM of the shoulder external rotation is a concern because it is often associated with development of a painful shoulder. There is no evidence of cognitive or perceptual deficits. He has a mild deficit in balance. I chose the Functional Reach Test instead of the Berg Balance Scale to assess balance because it was specific to the balance problems observed and administration time is brief. Selected subscales of the MAS were considered because they are more functional than the other motor function assessments. However, the two subscales—Hand Movements and Advanced Hand Activities—that would have provided the most useful information on Mr. B. have questionable validity. Therefore, I chose not to use the MAS with this client."

Occupational Therapy Problem List

1. Decreased ability to perform work, cooking, and self-care tasks because of sensorimotor impairments
2. Decreased strength, PROM, sensibility, and dexterity in his right upper extremity; decreased endurance for activity; mild impairment of sitting balance
3. Insufficient information on home environments to prepare adequately for discharge

Synthesize results

"Although I have sufficient information to begin treatment with Mr. B., I will need additional information from him and his employer about job requirements and work environment. In addition, more details about the home environment, home management roles and responsibilities, and other leisure interests are necessary."

 ## Clinical Reasoning in Occupational Therapy Practice

The Use of Neurophysiological Assessments While Implementing the Task-Related Approaches

You are evaluating Mr. J. in an outpatient facility for subacute post-stroke rehabilitation. Mr. J. was excited about constraint-induced movement therapy and asked you whether you could apply its principle in his treatment. What types of neurophysiological assessments would help you to determine whether Mr. J. is eligible for CIMT? How would other neurophysiological assessments help you in customizing Mr. J.'s therapy in general?

 ## Clinical Reasoning in Occupational Therapy Practice

Identifying the Control Parameters

You are using the occupational therapy task-oriented approach with Mr. J. for subacute post-stroke rehabilitation. Mr. J.'s COPM score indicated that he wants to play cards with his friends (importance score = 9 out of 10, performance score = 2 out of 10, and satisfaction score = 3 out of 10). How would you analyze the card playing task to identify the activity control parameters? How would you customize the treatment to offer the "just-right challenge"?

Summary Review Questions

1. How do the reflex-hierarchical and systems models of motor control differ?
2. How do neuromaturational and systems theories of motor development differ?
3. What types of motor dysfunction are associated with cortical, cerebellar, and basal ganglia lesions of the CNS?
4. What might account for the recovery seen after CNS damage?
5. What are at least four assumptions of the neurophysiological approaches?
6. How would you evaluate abnormal muscle tone and movement patterns?
7. What are at least four assumptions of the task-oriented approach?
8. How do evaluations used by the neurophysiological and task-related approaches differ?
9. Your client has LBD with resultant right hemiparesis and nonfluent aphasia. Why and how would you evaluate for the presence of apraxia?
10. When should you include evaluation of apraxia in a client?
11. How would you differentiate between motor and sensory neglect?

Glossary

Apraxia—The inability to carry out skilled movement in the presence of intact sensation, movement, and coordination.

Closed-loop system—A control system that uses feedback to correct movement errors in order to achieve the planned movement (Schmidt & Wrisberg, 2008).

Control parameter—A variable that changes behavior from one pattern of behavior to another. It does not control the change but acts as an agent for the shift in behavior (Perry, 1998).

Coordinative structures—Groups of muscles, usually spanning several joints, that are constrained to act as a single functional unit (Magill, 2004).

Degrees of freedom—Elements of a control system that are free to vary.

Heterarchical system or model—A system in which control is distributed among many systems; control emerges from the interaction of various subsystems; there is no strict order of command; subsystems in charge vary with task requirements.

Hierarchical system or model—A system with several levels of control, each level subordinate to the one above it.

Intransitive gestures—Movements expressing an idea not associated with a particular object such as waving good-bye (Enticott et al., 2010).

Knowledge of results—Awareness of the outcome of movement in relation to the goal.

Muscle tone—Resistance of a muscle to passive elongation or stretching.

Open-loop system—A control system that uses preprogrammed instructions (i.e., anticipatory, or feed-forward, control) to an effector; does not use feedback or error-detection processes (Schmidt & Wrisberg, 2008).

Phase shift—Change, which is often nonlinear, from one preferred coordinated pattern to another (Heriza, 1991).

Self-organization—The idea that a system composed of a number of subsystems can organize itself through the dynamic interaction of the subsystems (i.e., no higher level control or motor program is required) (Perry, 1998).

Transitive gestures—Goal-directed movements expressing an idea that entail object use, such as grasping a cup (Enticott et al., 2010).

References

Ada, L., & Westwood, P. (1992). A kinematic analysis of recovery of the ability to stand up following stroke. *Australian Physiotherapy, 38,* 135–142.

Adkins, D. L., Boychuk, J., Remple, M. S., & Kleim, J. A. (2006). Motor training induces experience-specific patterns of plasticity across motor cortex and spinal cord. *Journal of Applied Physiology, 101,* 1776–1782.

Aimola, E., Santello, M., La Grua, G., & Casabona A. (2011). Anticipatory postural adjustments in reach-to-grasp: Effect of object mass predictability. *Neuroscience Letters, 502,* 84–88.

Allison, S. C., & Abraham, L. D. (1995). Correlation of quantitative measures with the *Modified Ashworth Scale* in the assessment of plantar flexor spasticity in patients with traumatic brain injury. *Journal of Neurology, 242,* 699–706.

Almhdawi, K. A. (2011). *Effects of occupational therapy task-oriented approach in upper extremity post-stroke rehabilitation* (Doctoral dissertation). Retrieved from University of Minnesota Digital Conservancy.

Almeida, Q. J., Black, S. E., & Roy, E. A. (2002). Screening for apraxia: A short assessment for stroke patients. *Brain and Cognition, 48,* 253–631.

American Occupational Therapy Association. (2008). Occupational therapy practice framework: Domain and process (2nd ed.). *American Journal of Occupational Therapy, 62,* 625–683.

Ansari, N. N., Naghdi, S., Moammeri, H., & Jalaie, S. (2006). Ashworth Scales are unreliable for the assessment of muscle spasticity. *Physiotherapy Theory and Practice, 22,* 119–125.

Appelros, P., Nydevik, I., Karlsson, G. M., Thorwalls, A., & Seiger, A. (2003). Assessing unilateral neglect: Shortcomings of standard test methods. *Disability and Rehabilitation, 25,* 473–479.

Arnadottir, G. (1990). *The brain and behavior: Assessing cortical dysfunction through activities of daily living.* St. Louis: Mosby.

Arnadottir, G. (2011). Impact of neurobehavioral deficits on activities of daily living. In G. Gillen & A. Burkhardt (Eds.), *Stroke rehabilitation: A function-based approach.* (3rd ed., pp. 456–500). St. Louis: Mosby.

Ashworth, B. (1964). Preliminary trial of carisoprodol in multiple sclerosis. *Practitioner, 192,* 540–542.

Azad, A., Taghizadeh, G., & Khaneghini, A. (2011). Assessments of the reliability of the Iranian version of the Berg Balance Scale in patients with multiple sclerosis. *Acta Neurologica Taiwanica, 20,* 22–28.

Bach-y-Rita, P. (1993). Recovery from brain damage. *Journal of Neurological Rehabilitation, 6,* 191–199.

Bakheit, A. M., Pittock, S. Moore, A. P., Wurker, M., Otto, S., Erbguth, F., & Coxon, L. (2001). A randomized, double-blind, placebo-controlled study of the efficacy and safety of botulinum toxin type A (Dysport) in upper limb spasticity in patients with stroke. *Journal of Neurology, 8,* 559–565.

Bakheit, A. M., Thilmann, A. F., Ward, A. B., Poewe, W., Wissel, J., Muller, J., Benecke, R., Collin, C., Muller, F., Ward, C. D., & Neumann, C. (2000). A randomized, double-blind, placebo-controlled, dose-ranging study to compare the efficacy and safety of three doses of botulinum toxin type A (Dysport) with placebo in upper limb spasticity after stroke. *Stroke, 31,* 2402–2406.

Barris, R., Oakley, F., & Kielhofner, G. (1988). The Role Checklist. In B. J. Hemphill (Ed.), *Mental health assessment in occupational therapy* (pp. 73–91). Thorofare, NJ: Slack.

Bellamy, S., & Shen, E. (2007). Genetic disorders: A pediatric perspective. In D. A. Umphred (Ed.), *Neurological rehabilitation* (5th ed., pp. 386–417). St. Louis: Mosby Elsevier.

Berg, K., Maki, B., Williams, J. I., Holliday, P. J., & Wood-Dauphinee, S. (1992). Clinical and laboratory measures of postural balance in an elderly population. *Archives of Physical Medicine & Rehabilitation, 73,* 1073–1080.

Berg, K., Wood-Dauphinee, S., Williams, J. I., & Gayton, D. (1989). Measuring balance in the elderly: Preliminary development of an instrument. *Physiotherapy Canada, 41,* 301–311.

Bernstein, N. (1967). *The coordination and regulation of movements.* Elmsford, NY: Pergamon.

Bhimani, R. H., Anderson, L. C., Henly, S. J., & Stoddard, S. A. (2011). Clinical measurement of limb spasticity in adults: State of the science. *Journal of Neuroscience Nursing, 43,* 104–115.

Bisiach, E., Geminiani, G., Berti, A., & Rusconi, M. L. (1990). Perceptual and premotor factors of unilateral neglect. *Neurology, 40,* 1278–1281.

Blum, L., & Korner-Bitensky, N. (2008). Usefulness of the Berg Balance Scale in stroke rehabilitation: A systematic review. *Physical Therapy, 88,* 559–566.

Bobath, B. (1978). *Adult hemiplegia: Evaluation and treatment* (2nd ed.). London: Heinemann Medical.

Bobath, B. (1990). *Adult hemiplegia: Evaluation and treatment* (3rd ed.). Oxford: Butterworth Heinemann.

Bockemühl, T., Troje, N. F., & Dürr, V. (2010). Inter-joint coupling and joint angle synergies of human catching movements. *Human Movement Science, 29,* 73–93.

Bohannon, R. W., & Smith, M. B. (1987). Interrater reliability of a modified Ashworth scale of muscle spasticity. *Physical Therapy, 67,* 206–207.

Bourbonnais, D., & Vanden Noven, S. (1989). Weakness in patients with hemiparesis. *American Journal of Occupational Therapy, 43,* 313–319.

Brooks, V. B. (1986). *The neural basis of motor control.* New York: Oxford University.

Brunnstrom, S. (1970). *Movement therapy in hemiplegia.* New York: Harper & Row.

Burridge, J. H., Wood, D. E., Hermens, H. J., Voerman, G. E., Johnson, G. R., van Wijck, F., Platz, T., Gregoric, M., Hitchcock, R., & Pandyan, A. D. (2005). Theoretical and methodological considerations in the measurement of spasticity. *Disability and Rehabilitation, 27,* 69–80.

Burton, A. W., & Davis, W. E. (1992). Optimizing the involvement and performance of children with physical impairments in movement activities. *Pediatric Exercise Science, 4,* 236–248.

Butler, J. A. (2002). How comparable are tests of apraxia? *Clinical Rehabilitation, 16,* 389–398.

Cano-de-la-Cuerda, R., Molero-Sánchez, A., Carratalá-Tejada, M., Alguacil-Diego, I. M., Molina-Rueda, F., Miangolarra-Page, J. C., & Torricelli, D. (2012). Theories and control models and motor learning: Clinical applications in neuro-rehabilitation. *Neurología.* Advance online publication.

Carr, J. H., & Shepherd, R. B. (1987). *A motor relearning programme for stroke* (2nd ed.). Rockville, MD: Aspen.

Carr, J. H., & Shepherd, R. B. (2011). *Neurological rehabilitation: Optimizing motor performance* (2nd ed.). New York: Churchill Livingstone

Carr, J. H., Shepherd, R. B., Nordholm, L., & Lynne, D. (1985). Investigation of a new Motor Assessment Scale for stroke patients. *Physical Therapy, 65,* 175–180.

Chae, J., Labatia, I., & Yang, G. (2003). Upper limb motor function in hemiparesis. *American Journal of Physical Medicine & Rehabilitation, 82,* 1–8.

Chaikin, L. R. (2007). Disorders of vision and visual perceptual dysfunction. In D. A. Umphred (Ed.), *Neurological rehabilitation* (5th ed., pp. 973–1004). St. Louis: Mosby Elsevier.

Cheney, P. D. (1985). Role of cerebral cortex in voluntary movements: A review. *Physical Therapy, 65,* 624–635.

Connell, L. A., & Tyson, S. F. (2012). Clinical reality of measuring upper-limb ability in neurologic conditions: A systematic review. *Archives of Physical Medicine and Rehabilitation, 93,* 221–228.

Cooke, D. M., McKenna, K., & Fleming, J. (2005). Development of a standardized occupational therapy screening tool for visual perception in adults. *Scandinavian Journal of Occupational Therapy, 12,* 59–71.

Critchley, M. (1966). *The parietal lobes.* New York: Hafner.

Davis, W. E., & Burton, A. W. (1991). Ecological task analysis: Translating movement behavior theory into practice. *Adapted Physical Activity Quarterly, 8,* 154–177.

Dean, D., & Mackey, F. (1992). *Motor Assessment Scale* scores as a measure of rehabilitation outcome following stroke. *Australian Journal of Physiotherapy, 38,* 31–35.

Duncan, P. W., Propst, M., & Nelson, S. G. (1983). Reliability of the Fugl-Meyer Assessment of the sensorimotor recovery following cerebrovascular accident. *Physical Therapy, 63,* 1606–1610.

Duncan, P. W., Studenski, S., Chandler, J., & Prescott, B. (1992). Functional reach: Predictive validity in a sample of elderly male veterans. *Journal of Gerontology, 47,* M93–M98.

Duncan, P. W., Weiner, D. K., Chandler, J., & Studenski, S. (1990). Functional reach: A new clinical measure of balance. *Journal of Gerontology, 45,* M192–M195.

Edwards, D. F., Lang, C. E., Wagner, J. M., Birkenmeier, R., & Dromerick, A. W. (2012). An evaluation of the Wolf Motor Function Test in motor trials early after stroke. *Archives of Physical Medicine and Rehabilitation, 93,* 660–668.

Enticott, P. G., Kennedy, H. A., Bradshaw, J. L., Rinehart, N. J., & Fitzgerald, P. B. (2010). Understanding mirror neurons: Evidence for enhanced corticospinal excitability during the observation of transitive but not intransitive hand gestures. *Neuropsychologia, 48,* 2675–2680.

Fee, M. S., & Long, M. A. (2011). New methods for localizing and manipulating neuronal dynamics in behaving animals. *Current Opinion in Neurobiology, 21,* 693–700.

Feys, H. M., De Weerdt, W. J., Selz, B. E., Steck, G., Spichiger, R., Vereeck, L. E., Putman, K. D., & van Hoydonck, G. A. (1998). Effect of a therapeutic intervention for the hemiplegic upper limb in the acute phase after stroke. *Stroke, 29,* 785–792.

Fisher, A. G. (2012). Assessment of Motor and Process Skills (AMPS), Center for Innovative OT Solutions Web Site. Retrieved May 2, 2012 from http://www.ampsintl.com/AMPS/.

Flinn, N. (1995). A task-oriented approach to the treatment of a client with hemiplegia. *American Journal of Occupational Therapy, 49,* 560–569.

Fredericks, C. M., & Saladin, L. K. (Eds.). (1996). *Pathophysiology of the motor systems: Principles and clinical presentations.* Philadelphia: Davis.

Fugl-Meyer, A. R., Jäasko, L., Leyman, I., Olsson, S., & Steglind, S. (1975). The post-stroke hemiplegic patient: A method for evaluation of physical performance. *Scandinavian Journal of Rehabilitation Medicine, 7,* 13–31.

Gantschnig, B. E., Page, J., & Fisher, A. G. (2012). Cross-regional validity of the assessment of motor and process skills for use in middle Europe. *Journal of Rehabilitation Medicine, 44,* 151–157.

Gauthier, L. V., Taub, E., Perkins, C., Ortmann, M., Mark, V. W., & Uswatte, G. (2008). Remodeling the brain: Plastic structural brain changes produced by different motor therapies after stroke. *Stroke, 39,* 1520–1525.

Gazzaniga, M., Ivry, R., & Mangun, G. (2009). *Cognitive neuroscience: The biology of the mind* (3rd ed.). New York: W. W. Norton & Company.

Gentile, A. M. (1972). A working model of skill acquisition with application to teaching. *Quest, 17,* 3–23.

Gesell, A. (1954). The ontogenesis of infant behavior. In L. Carmichael (Ed.), *Manual of child psychology* (2nd ed., pp. 335–373). New York: Wiley.

Gibson, J. J. (1977). The theory of affordances. In R. Shaw & J. Bransford (Eds.), *Perceiving, acting, and knowing* (pp. 67–82). Hillsdale, NJ: Erlbaum.

Gibson, J. J. (1979). *The ecological approach to visual perception.* Boston: Houghton Mifflin.

Gillen, G. (2000). Improving activities of daily living performance in an adult with ataxia. *American Journal of Occupational Therapy, 54,* 89–96.

Gillen, G. (2002). Improving mobility and community access in an adult with ataxia. *American Journal of Occupational Therapy, 56,* 462–466.

Gillen, G. (2011). Upper extremity function and management. In G. Gillen & A. Burkhardt (Eds.), *Stroke rehabilitation: A function-based approach* (3rd ed., pp. 218–279). St. Louis: Mosby.

Gleick, J. (1987). *Chaos: Making a new science.* New York: Penguin.

Goodglass, H., & Kaplan, E. (1983). *The assessment of aphasia and related disorders* (2nd ed.). Philadelphia: Lippincott Williams & Wilkins.

Gregson, J. M., Leathley, M. J., Moore, A. P., Smith, T. L., Sharma, A. K., & Watkins, C. L. (2000). Reliability of measurements of muscle tone and muscle power in stroke patients. *Age and Ageing, 29,* 223–228.

Gresham G. E., Duncan, P. W., Stason, W. B., Adams, H. P., Adelman, A. M., Alexander, D. N., Bishop, D. S., Diller, L., Donaldson, N. E., Granger, C. V., Holland, A. L., Kelly-Hayes, M., McDowell, F. H., Myers, L., Phipps, M. A., Roth, E. j., Siebens, H. C., Tarvin, G. A., & Trombly, C. A. (1995). *Post-stroke rehabilitation: Clinical practice guidelines no. 16* (AHCPR Publication 95-0662). Rockville, MD: U.S. Department of Health and Human Services.

Halsband, U., & Lange, R. K. (2006). Motor learning in man: A review of functional and clinical studies. *Journal of Physiology, 99,* 414–424.

Harbourne, R. T., & Stergiou, N. (2009). Movement variability and the use of nonlinear tools: Principles to guide physical therapist practice. *Physical Therapy, 89,* 267–282.

Heilman, K. M., Rothi, L. J. G., & Watson, R. T. (1997). Apraxia. In S. C. Schachter & O. Devinsky (Eds.), *Behavioral neurology and the legacy of Norman Geschwind* (pp. 171–182). Philadelphia: Lippincott-Raven.

Heilman, K. M., Watson, R. T., & Rothi, L. G. (2003). Disorders of skilled movements: Limb apraxia. In T. E. Fineberg & M. J. Farah (Eds.), *Behavioral neurology and neuropsychology* (2nd ed.). New York: McGraw-Hill.

Heilman, K. M., Watson, R. T., & Valenstein, E. (2003). Neglect: Clinical and anatomic aspects. In T. E. Fineberg & M. J. Farah (Eds.), *Behavioral neurology and neuropsychology* (2nd ed.). New York: McGraw-Hill.

Helm-Estabrooks, N., & Albert, M. L. (2004). *Manual of aphasia & aphasia therapy* (2nd ed.). Austin, TX: PRO-ED.

Hemphill-Pearson, B. J. (Ed.). (2007). *Assessments in occupational therapy mental health: An integrated approach* (2nd ed.). Thorofare, NJ: Slack.

Heriza, C. (1991). Motor development: Traditional and contemporary theories. In M. J. Lister (Ed.), *Contemporary management of motor control problems: Proceedings of the II STEP Conference* (pp. 99–126). Alexandria, VA: Foundation for Physical Therapy.

Horak, F. B. (1991). Assumptions underlying motor control for neurologic rehabilitation. In M. J. Lister (Ed.), *Contemporary management of motor control problems: Proceedings of the II STEP Conference* (pp. 11–27). Alexandria, VA: Foundation for Physical Therapy.

Howle, J. (2002). *Neurodevelopmental treatment approach: Theoretical foundations and principles of clinical practice.* Laguna Beach, CA: Neurodevelopmental Treatment Association.

Ingram, J. N., & Wolpert, D. M. (2011). Naturalistic approaches to sensorimotor control. *Progress in Brain Research, 191,* 3–29.

Karok, S., & Newport, R. (2010). The continuous updating of grasp in response to dynamic changes in object size, hand size and distractor proximity. *Neuropsychologia, 48,* 3891–3900.

Katz, N., Bar-Haim Erez, A., Livni, L., & Averbuch, S. (2012). Dynamic Lowenstein Occupational Therapy Cognitive Assessment: Evaluation of potential to change in cognitive performance. *The American Journal of Occupational Therapy, 66,* 207–214.

Kaya, T., Karatepe, A. G., Gunaydin, R., Koc, A., & Altundal Ercan, U. (2011). Inter-rater reliability of the modified ashworth scale and Modified Ashworth Scale in assessing poststroke elbow flexor spasticity. *International Journal of Rehabilitation Research, 34,* 59–64.

Kleim, J. A. (2011). Neural plasticity and neurorehabilitation: Teaching the new brain old tricks. *Journal of Communication Disorders, 44,* 521–528.

Kleim, J. A., & Jones, T. A. (2008). Principles of experience-dependent neural plasticity: Implications for rehabilitation after brain damage. *Journal of Speech, Language, and Hearing Research, 51,* S225–S239.

Knott, M., & Voss, D. E. (1968). *Proprioceptive neuromuscular facilitation* (2nd ed.). New York: Harper & Row.

Kopp, B., Kunkel, A., Flor, H., Platz, T., Rose, U., Mauritz, K.-H., Gresser, K., McCulloch, K. L., & Taub, E. (1997). The Arm Motor Ability Test: Reliability, validity, and sensitivity to change of an instrument for assessing disabilities in activities of daily living. *Archives of Physical Medicine & Rehabilitation, 78,* 615–620.

Kunkel, A., Kopp, B., Muller, G., Villringer, K., Villringer, A., Taub, E., & Flor, H. (1999). Constraint-induced movement therapy for motor recovery in chronic stroke patients. *Archives of Physical Medicine & Rehabilitation, 80,* 624–628.

Lang, C. E., Edwards, D. F., Birkenmeier, R. L., & Dromerick, A. W. (2008). Estimating minimal clinically important differences of upper-extremity measures early after stroke. *Archives of Physical Medicine and Rehabilitation, 89,* 1693–1700.

Latash, M. L., Levin, M. F., Scholz, J. P., & Schöner G. (2010). Motor control theories and their applications. *Medicina, 46,* 382–392.

Law, M., Baptiste, S., Carswell, A., McColl, M., Polatajko, H., & Pollock, N. (1998). *Canadian Occupational Performance Measure* (3rd ed.). Ottawa: Canadian Association of Occupational Therapists.

Learmonth, Y. C., Paul, L., McFadyen, A. K., Mattison, P., & Miller, L. (2012). Reliability and clinical significance of mobility and balance assessments in multiple sclerosis. *International Journal of Rehabilitation Research, 35,* 69–74.

Lewis, M. D. (2000). The promise of dynamic systems approaches for an integrated account of human development. *Child Development, 71,* 36–43.

Liepert, J., Bauder, H., Wolfgang, H., Miltner, W., Taub, E., & Weiller, C. (2000). Treatment-induced cortical reorganization after stroke in humans. *Stroke, 31,* 1210–1216

Lin, K., Wu, C., Chen, C., Chern, J. S., & Hong, W. H. (2007). Effects of object use on reaching and postural balance: A comparison of patients with unilateral stroke and healthy controls. *American Journal of Physical Medicine & Rehabilitation, 86,* 791–799.

Lister, M. J. (Ed.). (1991). *Contemporary management of motor control problems: Proceedings of the II STEP Conference.* Alexandria, VA: Foundation for Physical Therapy.

Loewen, S. C., & Anderson, B. A. (1990). Predictors of stroke outcome using objective measurement scales. *Stroke, 21,* 78–81.

Magill, R. A. (2004). *Motor learning and control: Concepts and applications* (7th ed.). Boston: McGraw-Hill.

Malouin, F., Pickard, L., Bonneau, C., Durand, A., & Corriveau, D. (1994). Evaluating motor recovery early after stroke: Comparison of the Fugl-Meyer Assessment and the Motor Assessment Scale. *Archives of Physical Medicine & Rehabilitation, 75,* 1206–1212.

Marchetti, C., & Della Sala, S. (1997). On crossed apraxia: A description of a right-handed apraxic patient with right supplementary motor area damage. *Cortex, 33,* 341–354.

Marsden, C. D. (1982). The mysterious motor function of the basal ganglia: The Robert Wartenberg lecture. *Neurology, 32,* 514–539.

Marteniuk, R. G., MacKenzie, C. L., & Jeannerod, M. (1987). Constraints on human arm trajectories. *Canadian Journal of Psychology, 41,* 365–368.

Mathiowetz, V. (2011). Task-oriented approach to stroke rehabilitation. In G. Gillen (Ed.), *Stroke rehabilitation: A function-based approach* (3rd ed., pp. 80–99). St. Louis: Elsevier Mosby.

Mathiowetz, V., & Bass Haugen, J. (1994). Motor behavior research: Implications for therapeutic approaches to CNS dysfunction. *American Journal of Occupational Therapy, 48,* 733–745.

Mathiowetz, V., & Bass Haugen, J. (2008). Assessing abilities and capacities: Motor behavior. In M. V. Radomski & C. A. Trombly Latham (Eds.), *Occupational therapy for physical dysfunction* (6th ed., pp. 186–211). Baltimore: Lippincott Williams & Wilkins.

Mathiowetz, V. G., & Wade, M. (1995). Task constraints and functional motor performance of individuals with and without multiple sclerosis. *Ecological Psychology, 7,* 99–123.

McGraw, M. B. (1945). *The neuromuscular maturation of the human infant.* New York: Hafner.

Meads, D. M., Doward, L., McKenna, S., Fisk, J., Twiss, J., & Eckert, B. (2009). The development and validation of the Unidimensional Fatigue Impact Scale (U-FIS). *Multiple Sclerosis, 15,* 1228–1238.

Mehrholz, J., Major, Y., Meissner, D., Sandi-Gahun, S., Koch, R., & Pohl, M. (2005). The influence of contractures and variation in measurement stretching velocity on the reliability of the Modified Ashworth Scale in patients with severe brain injury. *Clinical Rehabilitation, 19,* 63–72.

Merritt, B. K. (2011). Validity of using the Assessment of Motor and Process Skills to determine the need for assistance. *American Journal of Occupational Therapy, 65*, 643–650.

Miller, K. J., Slade, A. L., Pallant, J. F., & Galea, M. P. (2010). Evaluation of the psychometric properties of the upper limb subscales of the motor assessment scale using a Rasch analysis model. *Journal of Rehabilitation Medicine, 42*, 315–322.

Morris, D. M., Uswatte, G., Crago, J. E., Cook, E. W., & Taub, E. (2001). The reliability of the Wolf Motor Function Test for assessing upper extremity function after stroke. *Archives of Physical Medicine & Rehabilitation, 82*, 750–755.

Nagaoka, M., & Kakuda, N. (2008). [Neural mechanisms underlying spasticity]. [Japanese]. *Brain and Nerve, 60*, 1399–1408.

Neistadt, M. E. (1993). The relationship between constructional apraxia and meal preparation skills. *Archives of Physical Medicine & Rehabilitation, 74*, 144–148.

Newell, K. M. (1986). Constraints on the development of coordination. In M. G. Wade & H. T. A. Whiting (Eds.), *Motor development in children: Aspects of coordination and control* (pp. 341–360). Dordrecht: Martinus Nijhoff.

Newell, K. M. (2003). Schema theory (1975): Retrospectives and prospectives. *Research Quarterly of Exercise & Sport, 74*, 383–389.

Nudo, R. J. (2011). Neural bases of recovery after brain injury. *Journal of Communication Disorders, 44*, 515–520.

O'Dell, M. W., Kim, G., Finnen, L. R., & Polistena, C. (2011). Clinical implications of using the arm motor ability test in stroke rehabilitation. *Archives of Physical Medicine and Rehabilitation, 92*, 830–836.

Pandyan, A. D., Price, C. I. M., Barnes, M. P., & Johnson, G. R. (2003). A biomechanical investigation into the validity of the Modified Ashworth Scale as a measure of elbow spasticity. *Clinical Rehabilitation, 17*, 290–294.

Pandyan, A. D., Vuadens, P., van Wijck, F., Stark, S., Johnson, G. R., & Barnes, M. P. (2002). Are we underestimating the clinical efficacy of botulinum toxin (type A)? Quantifying changes in spasticity, strength and upper limb function after injections of Botox® to the elbow flexors in a unilateral stroke population. *Clinical Rehabilitation, 16*, 654–660.

Perry, S. B. (1998). Clinical implications of a dynamic systems theory. *American Physical Therapy Association Neurology Report, 22*, 4–10.

Pizzi, A., Carlucci, G., Falsini, C., Verdesca, S., & Grippo, A. (2005). Evaluation of upper-limb spasticity after stroke: A clinical and neurophysiologic study. *Archives of Physical Medicine & Rehabilitation, 86*, 410–415.

Platz, T., Eickhof, C., Nuyens, G., & Vuadens, P. (2005). Clinical scales for the assessment of spasticity, associated phenomena, and function: A systematic review of the literature. *Disability and Rehabilitation, 27*, 7–18.

Podsiadlo, D., & Richardson, S. (1991). The timed "up and go": A test of basic mobility for frail elderly persons. *Journal of the American Geriatrics Society, 39*, 142–148.

Poole, J. L., Sadek, J., & Haaland, K. Y. (2009). Ipsilateral deficits in 1-handed shoe tying after left or right hemisphere stroke. *Archives of Physical Medicine & Rehabilitation, 90*, 1800–1805.

Poole, J. L., & Whitney, S. L. (1988). Motor Assessment Scale for stroke patients: Concurrent validity and interrater reliability. *Archives of Physical Medicine & Rehabilitation, 69*, 195–197.

Rao, A. K. (2011). Approaches to motor control dysfunction: An evidence-based review. In G. Gillen & A. Burkhardt (Eds.), *Stroke rehabilitation: A function-based approach* (3rd ed., pp. 117–155). St. Louis: Mosby.

Raymer, A. M., Maher, L. M., Foundas, A. L., Heilman, K. M., & Rothi, L. J. (1997). The significance of body part as tool errors in limb apraxia. *Brain and Cognition, 34*, 287–292.

Rogers, J. C., & Holm, M. B. (2007). Role change assessment: An interview tool for older adults. In B. J. Hemphill-Pearson (Ed.), *Assessments in occupational therapy mental health: An integrated approach* (2nd ed., pp. 49–60). Thorofare, NJ: Slack.

Rood, M. S. (1954). Neurophysiological reactions as a basis for physical therapy. *Physical Therapy Review, 34*, 444–449.

Rothi, L. J. G., Raymer, A. M., & Heilman, K. M. (1997). Limb praxis assessment. In L. J. G. Rothi & K. M. Heilman (Eds.), *Apraxia: The neuropsychology of action* (pp. 61–73). East Sussex, UK: Psychology Press Publishers.

Roy, E. A., Black, S. E., Blair, N., & Dimeck, P. (1998). Analyses of deficits in gestural pantomime. *Journal of Clinical and Experimental Neuropsychology, 20*, 628–643.

Sabari, J. S., Lim, A. L., Velozo, C. A., Lehman, L., Kieran, O., & Lai, J. (2005). Assessing arm and hand function after stroke: A validity test of the hierarchical scoring system used in the Motor Assessment Scale for stroke. *Archives of Physical Medicine & Rehabilitation, 86*, 1609–1615.

Safavynia, S. A., & Ting, L. H. (2012). Task-level feedback can explain temporal recruitment of spatially fixed muscle synergies throughout postural perturbations. *Journal of Neurophysiology, 107*, 159–177.

Salavati, M., Negahban, H., Mazaheri, M., Soleimanifar, M., Hadadi, M., Sefiddashti, L., Hassan Zahraee, M., Davatgaran, K., & Feizi, A. (2012). The Persian version of the Berg Balance Scale: Inter and intra-rater reliability and construct validity in elderly adults. *Disability & Rehabilitation, 34*(20), 1695–1698.

Scalzo, P. L., Nova, I. C., Perracini, M. R., Sacramento, D. R., Cardoso, F., Ferraz, H. B., & Teixeira, A. L. (2009). Validation of the Brazilian version of the Berg Balance Scale for patients with Parkinson's disease. *Arquivos de Neuro-psiquiatria, 67*, 831–835.

Schmidt, R. A., & Wrisberg, C. A. (2008). *Motor learning and performance: A situation-based learning approach* (4th ed.). Champaign, IL: Human Kinetics.

Shumway-Cook, A., & Woollacott, M. (2012). *Motor control: Translating research into clinical practice* (4th ed.). Baltimore: Wolters Kluwer/Lippincott Williams & Wilkins.

Sommerfeld, D. K., Eek, E., Svensson, A., Holmqvist, L. W., & von Arbin, M. H. (2004). Spasticity after stroke: Its occurrence and association with motor impairments and activity limitations. *Stroke, 35*, 134–140.

Stolov, W. C. (1966). The concept of normal muscle tone, hypotonia, and hypertonia. *Archives of Physical Medicine & Rehabilitation, 47*, 156–168.

Sullivan, K. J., Tilson, J. K., Cen, S. Y., Rose, D. K., Hershberg, J., Correa, A., Gallichio, J., McLeod, M., Moore, C., Wu, S. S., & Duncan, P. W. (2011). Fugl-Meyer assessment of sensorimotor function after stroke: Standardized training procedure for clinical practice and clinical trials. *Stroke, 42*, 427–432.

Taub, E., Miller, N. E., Novack, T. A., Cook, E. W. 3rd, Fleming, W. C., Nepomuceno, C. S., Connell, J. S., & Crago, J. E. (1993). Technique to improve chronic motor deficit after stroke. *Archives of Physical Medicine & Rehabilitation, 74*, 347–354.

Tegner, R., & Levander, M. (1991). Through a looking glass: A new technique to demonstrate directional hypokinesia in unilateral neglect. *Brain, 114*, 1943–1951.

Thelen, E. (1989). Self-organization in developmental processes: Can systems approaches work? In M. R. Gunnar & E. Thelen (Eds.), *Systems and development* (pp. 77–117). Hillsdale, NJ: Erlbaum.

Thelen, E., & Ulrich, B. D. (1991). Hidden skills. *Monograph of the Society for Research in Child Development, 56* (Serial 223). Chicago: University of Chicago.

Tinetti, M. E. (1986). Performance-oriented assessment of mobility problems in elderly patients. *Journal of American Geriatrics Society, 34*, 119–126.

Ting, L. H., van Antwerp, K. W., Scrivens, J. E., McKay, J. L., Welch, T. D., Bingham, J. T., & DeWeerth, S. P. (2009). Neuromechanical tuning of nonlinear postural control dynamics. *Chaos, 19*, 026111–026111-12.

Toal-Sullivan, D., & Henderson, P. R. (2004). Client-Oriented Role Evaluation (CORE): The development of a clinical rehabilitation instrument to assess role change associated with disability. *American Journal of Occupational Therapy, 58*, 211–220.

Trojano, L., Labruna, L., & Grossi, D. (2007). An experimental investigation of the automatic/voluntary dissociation in limb apraxia. *Brain and Cognition, 65*, 169–176.

Trombly, C. A. (1989). Motor control therapy. In C. Trombly (Ed.), *Occupational therapy for physical dysfunction* (3rd ed., pp. 72–95). Baltimore: Williams & Wilkins.

Trombly, C. A., & Wu, C. (1999). Effect of rehabilitation tasks on organization of movement after stroke. *American Journal of Occupational Therapy, 53,* 333–344.

Turvey, M. T. (1977). Preliminaries to a theory of action with reference to vision. In R. Shaw & J. Bransford (Eds.), *Perceiving, acting, and knowing* (pp. 211–265). Hillsdale, NJ: Erlbaum.

Twitchell, T. E. (1951). The restoration of motor function following hemiplegia in man. *Brain, 74,* 443–480.

Tyson, S. F., & Connell, L. A. (2009). How to measure balance in clinical practice. A systematic review of the psychometrics and clinical utility of measures of balance activity for neurological conditions. *Clinical Rehabilitation, 23,* 824–840.

Unsal Delialioglu, S., Kurt, M., Kaya, K., Culha, C., & Ozel, S. (2008). Effects of ideomotor apraxia on functional outcomes in patients with right hemiplegia. *International Journal of Rehabilitation Research, 31,* 177–180.

Unsworth, C. (2007). Cognitive and perceptual dysfunction. In S. O'Sullivan & T. Schmitz (Eds.), *Physical rehabilitation* (5th ed., pp. 1149–1188). Philadelphia: F. A. Davis Company.

Uswatte, G., Taub, E., Morris, D., Light, K., & Thompson, P. A. (2006). The Motor Activity Log-28: Assessing daily use of the hemiparetic arm after stroke. *Neurology, 67,* 1189–1194.

Uswatte, G., Taub, E., Morris, D., Vignolo, M., & McCulloch, K. (2005). Reliability and validity of the upper-extremity Motor Activity Log-14 for measuring real-world arm use. *Stroke, 36,* 2493–2496.

van Heugten, C. M., Dekker, J., Deelman, B. G., Stehmann-Saris, J. C., & Kinebanian, A. (1999a). A diagnostic test for apraxia in stroke patients: Internal consistency and diagnostic value. *The Clinical Neuropsychologist, 13,* 182–192.

van Heugten, C. M., Dekker, J., Deelman, B. G., Stehmann-Saris, J. C., & Kinebanian, A. (1999b). Assessment of disabilities in stroke patients with apraxia: Internal consistency and inter-observer reliability. *Occupational Therapy Journal Research, 19,* 55–73.

van Wijck, F. M. J., Pandyan, A. D., Johnson, G. R., & Barnes, M. P. (2001). Assessing motor deficits in neurological rehabilitation: Patterns of instrument usage. *Neurorehabilitation and Neural Repair, 15,* 23–30.

Waninge, A., Rook, R. A., Dijkhuizen, A., Gielen, E., & van der Schans, C. P. (2011). Feasibility, test-retest reliability, and interrater reliability of the Modified Ashworth Scale and modified Tardieu Scale in persons with profound intellectual and multiple disabilities. *Research in Developmental Disabilities, 32,* 613–620.

Warraich, Z., & Kleim, J. A. (2010). Neural plasticity: The biological substrate for neurorehabilitation. *PM&R: The Journal of Injury, Function and Rehabilitation, 2(Suppl. 2),* S208–S219.

Warren, W. H. (1984). Perceiving affordances: Visual guidance of stair climbing. *Journal of Experimental Psychology: Human Perception and Performance, 10,* 683–703.

Wei, K., & Krding, K. (2009). Relevance of error: What drives motor adaptation? *Journal of Neurophysiology, 101,* 655–664.

Wei, X., Tong, K., & Hu, X. (2011). The responsiveness and correlation between Fugl-Meyer Assessment, Motor Status Scale, and the Action Research Arm Test in chronic stroke with upper-extremity rehabilitation robotic training. *International Journal of Rehabilitation Research, 34,* 349–356.

Weiner, D. K., Bongiorni, D. R., Studenski, S. Duncan, P. W., & Kochersberger, G. G. (1993). Does functional reach improve with rehabilitation? *Archives of Physical Medicine & Rehabilitation, 74,* 796–800.

Wirz, M., Müller, R., & Bastiaenen, C. (2010). Falls in persons with spinal cord injury: Validity and reliability of the Berg Balance Scale. *Neurorehabilitation and Neural Repair, 24,* 70–77.

Wittenberg, G. F. (2010). Experience, cortical remapping, and recovery in brain disease. *Neurobiology of Disease, 37,* 252–258.

Wolf, S. L., Catlin, P. A., Ellis, M., Archer, A.L., Morgan, B., & Piacentino, A. (2001). Assessing Wolf Motor Function Test as outcome measure for research in patients after stroke. *Stroke, 32,* 1635–1639.

Wolf, S. L., Winstein, C. J., Miller, J. P., Taub, E., Uswatte, G., Morris, D., Giuliani, C., Light, K. E., & Nichols-Larsen, D. (2006). Effect of constraint-induced movement therapy on upper extremity function 3 to 9 months after stroke: The EXCITE randomized clinical trial. *Journal of the American Medical Association, 296,* 2095–2104.

Wood-Dauphinee, S., Berg, K., Bravo, G., & Williams, I. (1997). The Balance Scale: Responsiveness to clinically meaningful changes. *Canadian Journal of Rehabilitation, 10,* 35–50.

Wood-Dauphinee, S. L., Williams, J. I., & Shapiro, S. H. (1990). Examining outcome measures in a clinical study of stroke. *Stroke, 21,* 731–739.

World Health Organization. (2001). *International Classification of Functioning, Disability and Health (ICF).* Geneva: World Health Organization.

York, C. D., & Cermak, S. A. (1995). Visual perception and praxis in adults after stroke. *American Journal of Occupational Therapy, 49,* 543–550.

Zwinkels, A., Geusgens, C., van de Sande, P., & van Heugten, C. (2004). Assessment of apraxia: Inter-rater reliability of a new apraxia test, association between apraxia and other cognitive deficits and prevalence of apraxia in a rehabilitation setting. *Clinical Rehabilitation, 18,* 819–827.

Acknowledgment

Thanks to Lee Ann Quintana, MS, OTR/L, for her work on apraxia evaluation in the previous editions of this text. Thanks to Joyce Shapero Sabari, PhD, OTR/L, FAOTA, for her work on the task-related assessments in the previous editions of this text. Thanks to Nancy Flinn, PhD, OTR/L, who uses the OT task-oriented approach in her clinical practice and has provided constructive feedback.

9

Assessing Abilities and Capacities: Sensation

Jennifer L. Theis

Learning Objectives

After studying this chapter, the reader will be able to do the following:

1. Describe the effects of sensory loss on occupational function.
2. Predict the pattern of sensory loss based on diagnosis or described lesion in the somatosensory system.
3. Demonstrate appropriate sensory testing techniques for tactile sensation when provided with appropriate tools or equipment.
4. Differentiate standardized and nonstandardized tactile tests.
5. Choose appropriate sensory testing techniques for a given patient or situation.
6. Correctly interpret the results of sensory testing for treatment planning.

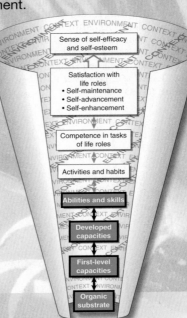

The American Occupational Therapy Association (AOTA) (2008, p. 675) defines sensory-perceptual skills as "actions or behaviors a client uses to locate, identify, and respond to sensations, interpret, organize, and remember sensory events via sensations that include visual, auditory, proprioceptive, tactile, olfactory, gustatory, and vestibular sensations." In this chapter, tactile, thermal, and proprioceptive sensations will be discussed, and methods of evaluating these senses will be described. The tactile sense throughout the body is necessary for competent occupational functioning, but tactile sensation is especially important in the hands. Moberg described hands without sensation as being like eyes without vision (Dellon, 1988).

Immediately after birth, an infant is bombarded with tactile sensations that are different from those in utero. Within a few weeks, the infant learns to interpret a multitude of tactile stimuli, such as soothing touch from a parent that brings comfort and contentment. This developed capacity supports further development of abilities and skills as the infant uses touch to grasp an object, bring two hands together at midline, and reach out to stroke a parent's face. These abilities are necessary for self-maintenance, self-enhancement, and self-advancement roles in childhood and throughout adulthood.

ROLE OF SENSATION IN OCCUPATIONAL FUNCTIONING

The role of sensation in occupational functioning is dramatically described in Cole's (1991) account of Ian Waterman, who at 19 years of age acquired a rare neurological illness that resulted in the loss of all sensation of touch in his body from the neck down. He had no awareness of the positions of his arms, legs, or body. Although his muscles were not affected, any attempt at movement was wildly uncontrolled. Ian's initial attempt at standing up resulted in him falling "in a heap . . . like a pile of wet clothes" (Cole, 1991, p. 11). He was unable to feed himself, get dressed, or do any functional activity requiring control of movement. Over several years, Waterman learned how to complete functional activities by substituting vision for his lost sensation. Every movement had to be carefully watched and consciously controlled. The high level of concentration required and the energy expended to complete daily self-care and work activities led Cole to name the account of Waterman's life, *Pride and a Daily Marathon.*

Although a loss of sensation like Waterman's without any motor loss is unusual, it exemplifies the close connection between the motor and sensory systems. With sensory loss in the hand, fine motor coordination is impaired, and manipulative ability is decreased (Carr & Shepherd, 2010). The amount of force needed to maintain grasp on an object also depends on sensory feedback. Usually, we use force that is just sufficient to overcome the pull of gravity,

taking into account the amount of friction afforded by the surface texture. Without adequate tactile sensation, the force used to grip an object is either lower or higher than the force needed, resulting in objects slipping from grasp, delicate objects (such as a plastic foam cup) being crushed by excessive grip force, or muscles developing fatigue from overactivity (Johansson, 1996).

Some activities require sensory feedback because they are totally dependent on the sense of touch, such as determining the temperature of a bowl taken from the microwave. Tactile sensations let us know whether the food is warm and whether the bowl is too hot to carry to the table. Haptic perception, active touch, helps to determine the three-dimensional characteristics of objects (Norman et al., 2011). Finding coins or other objects in a pocket and fastening a necklace or closing a back zipper are examples of activities for which vision is not used; therefore, we rely entirely on sensory feedback. It is the tactile sense that tells us when our new shoes are a bit too tight and we had better remove them or we will get a blister. Impairment in the somatosensory system not only hinders movement but also increases the risk of injury.

PURPOSES OF SENSORY EVALUATION

The purposes of sensory testing, as defined by Cooke (1991), are as follows:

- Assess the type and extent of sensory loss
- Evaluate and document sensory recovery
- Assist in diagnosis
- Determine impairment and functional limitation
- Provide direction for occupational therapy intervention
- Determine time to begin sensory re-education
- Determine need for education to prevent injury during occupational functioning
- Determine need for desensitization

Before considering sensory evaluation, therapists need a good understanding of the neural structures responsible for tactile sensation.

NEUROPHYSIOLOGICAL FOUNDATIONS OF TACTILE SENSATION

Receptors for tactile sensation are present within skin, muscles, and joints. Each tactile receptor is usually specialized for a single type of sensory stimulation such as touch, temperature, or pain (Ropper & Samuels, 2009). The types of sensation, specific kinds of receptors, and corresponding neurons that connect the sensory receptors with the spinal cord and ultimately with the cerebral cortex appear in Table 9-1. Neural impulses follow the described pathways to the brain, where the sensations are perceived and interpreted.

Table 9-1 Neural Pathways of Sensory Stimuli

Type of Sensation	Sensory Receptor	Type of Afferent Neuron	Pathway	Termination of Pathway
Constant touch or pressure Moving touch or vibration	Merkel's cell Ruffini's end organ Meissner's corpuscles Pacinian corpuscles Hair follicles	Type A-beta slowly adapting I and II myelinated neurons Type A-beta rapidly adapting I and II myelinated neurons	Ascend in dorsal column and medial lemniscus of spinal cord in posterior pyramidal tract, cross to opposite side in medulla	Thalamus and somatosensory cortex
Proprioception and kinesthesia	Same as both moving and constant touch or vibration plus touch receptors found in skin and joint structures Muscle spindles Golgi tendon organs	Same as for moving touch or vibration plus A-alpha myelinated neurons	Same as for moving touch or vibration plus spinocerebellar tract	Same as for moving touch or vibration plus cerebellum
Pain (pinprick) Pain (chronic) Temperature	Free nerve endings Free nerve endings Free nerve endings Warm receptors Cold receptors	Type A-delta myelinated neurons Type C unmyelinated fibers Type A-delta myelinated neurons and type C unmyelinated fibers	Immediately cross to opposite side and pass upward in anterior spinothalamic tracts of spinal cord	Brainstem, thalamus, and somatosensory cortex

Based on information in Dellon, A. L. (2000). *Somatosensory testing and rehabilitation*. Baltimore, MD: The Institute for Peripheral Nerve Surgery; Chapman, C. E., Tremblay, F., & Ageranioti-Bélanger, A. (1996). Role of primary somatosensory cortex in active and passive touch. In A. M. Wing, P. Haggard, & J. R. Flanagan (Eds.), *Hand and brain: The neurophysiology and psychology of hand movements* (pp. 329–347). San Diego: Academic; Fredericks, C. M. (1996a). Basic sensory mechanisms and the somatosensory system. In C. M. Fredericks & L. K. Saladin (Eds.), *Pathophysiology of the motor systems: Principles and clinical presentations* (pp. 78–106). Philadelphia: F. A. Davis; Fredericks, C. M. (1996c). Disorders of the spinal cord. In C. M. Fredericks & L. K. Saladin (Eds.), *Pathophysiology of the motor systems: Principles and clinical presentations* (pp. 394–423). Philadelphia: F. A. Davis.

Each sensory neuron and its distal and proximal terminations can be considered a sensory unit. Each sensory unit serves an area of skin that encompasses its defined receptive field. A stimulus anywhere in the field may evoke a response, but stimuli applied to the center of the receptive field produce sensations more easily. In other words, the center of a receptive field has a lower threshold than the periphery. Adjacent receptive fields overlap; therefore, a single stimulus evokes a profile of responses from overlapping sensory units.

The variation in the number of sensory units in a given area of skin is called innervation density. The face, hand, and fingers have high innervation densities. Areas with high innervation density are highly sensitive and have a proportionately large representation area within the somatosensory area of the cortex, the postcentral gyrus of the parietal lobe (Bear, Connors, & Paradiso, 2007; Ropper & Samuels, 2009). Figure 9-1 shows the organization within the cortex of sensory receptors from various regions of the body.

Table 9-1 and the description of sensory pathways simplify a complex process. For example, tactile stimuli of sufficient strength elicit responses from both constant and moving touch receptors and perhaps also from the pain receptors (Fredericks, 1996a). Extremes of hot and cold stimuli activate the pain receptors rather than the temperature receptors (Lindblom, 1994). Perception of joint motion (kinesthesia) and joint position (proprioception) appear to be a result of information from multiple kinds of receptors. Researchers disagree about the relative contributions of joint, muscle, and skin receptors to proprioception and kinesthesia (Fredericks, 1996a; Jones, 1996).

Therapists use a solid understanding of the neurophysiology of the tactile system to choose evaluation and treatment techniques for sensory deficits. They combine this understanding with knowledge of typical patterns of impairment from injury and illness prior to implementing assessment of sensation.

SOMATOSENSORY DEFICIT PATTERNS

Any interruption along the ascending sensory pathway or in the sensory areas of the cortex can lead to a decrease or loss of sensation. The extent and severity of the sensory deficit can generally be predicted in accordance with the mechanism and location of the lesion or injury. Patterns of sensory impairment are directly related to the involved neuroanatomical structures, which could be anywhere in the central or peripheral nervous system. Somatosensory and perceptual impairments contribute to poor motor control and may have an impact on participation in rehabilitation (Carr & Shepherd, 2010).

Cortical Injury

Patients with brain lesions caused by stroke or acquired brain injury demonstrate sensory losses related to loss of

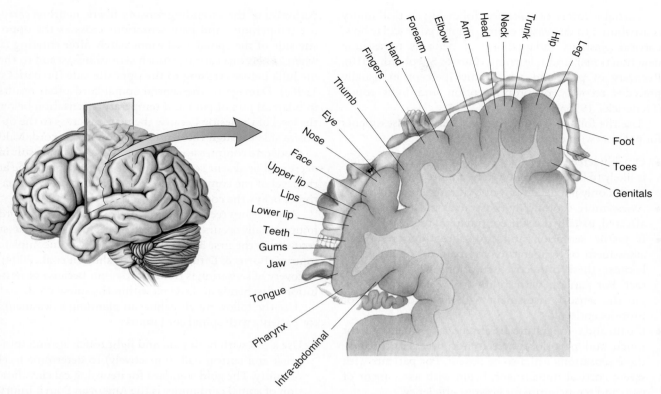

Figure 9-1 The areas responsible for sensation of body parts within the postcentral gyrus of the cerebral cortex. (Reprinted with permission from Bear, M. F., Connors, B. W., & Paradiso, M. A. [2007]. *Neuroscience: Exploring the brain* [3rd ed.]. Baltimore: Lippincott Williams & Wilkins.)

functioning of specific neurons within the central nervous system. One study found that tactile sensory loss is more common than loss of proprioception (Tyson et al., 2008), whereas another found that loss of both proprioception and stereognosis were more prevalent than loss of tactile sense (Connell, Lincoln, & Radford, 2008). The discrepancy between the two studies may be accounted for in the methods chosen to test sensory abilities, or it may simply be that one study reported ranges of sensory capacities affected, whereas the other reported the averages of those same sensory capacities. This means that the discrepancy between the two studies may actually not be a true discrepancy because Connell's ranges encompass Tyson's reported averages of type of sensory loss. In another study, approximately half of those patients presenting for rehabilitation after stroke experienced decreased discriminatory sensation (both touch discrimination and proprioception) in both the contralesional and ipsilesional hands (Carey & Matyas, 2011). For patients with either stroke or brain injury, perception of fine touch and proprioception are most affected, temperature sensation is affected less, and pain sensibility is affected least (Fredericks, 1996a). Effects of stroke on sensation depend on specific disruption of blood supply. For instance, occlusion of the middle cerebral artery (the most common site of stroke) is often associated with contralateral impairment of all sensory modalities

on the face, arm, and leg. Massive infarction in the distribution of the anterior and middle cerebral arteries may present with dense sensory deficits (Stein & Brandstater, 2010). Occlusion of the anterior cerebral artery tends to cause more loss of sensation in the contralateral leg than in the face and arm because of this artery's supply to the medial aspect of the cerebral cortex (Fig. 9-1) (Stein & Brandstater, 2010). Lesions to the posterior thalamus tend to result in loss or impaired cold sensation and central pain response (Kim et al., 2007). Patterns of sensory loss following head trauma are less predictable because of the more diffuse areas of brain damage associated with this condition (Saladin, 1996).

Sterzi et al. (1993) compared patients with left and right stroke and found that loss of proprioception and pain perception were more common following right stroke than left stroke. Patients with stroke also demonstrated decreased performance with visual deprivation (Scalha et al., 2011). Left neglect, an inability to recognize and use perceptions from the left side of the body and environment, was proposed as a factor underlying this difference. A study by Beschin et al. (1996) provides evidence to support the existence of tactile neglect; patients with right brain damage tend to ignore left space during active tactile exploration. Movement time is positively correlated with tactile sensitivity, $r = 0.604$, $p < 0.05$ (Gao et al., 2010).

Partial recovery of sensation following cortical injury is attributed to decreased edema, improved vascular flow, cortical plasticity (adaptability of neurons to assume new functions), and relearning (Carr & Shepherd, 2010). Recovery of pain and temperature perception usually precedes recovery of proprioception and light touch (Fredericks, 1996a).

Use the following guidelines in planning assessments for patients with cortical injury:

- Quickly screen those areas of the body where sensation is likely to be intact, followed by a more thorough evaluation only if a deficit is found during screening.
- Assess more thoroughly those areas most likely to be affected, usually the side contralateral to the injury.
- If tactile sensation and proprioception are intact, assessment of temperature and pain is not necessary, because these protective sensations will also be intact. For patients with mild cortical impairment, begin the sensory assessment with light touch and/or proprioception.
- If pain and temperature are absent, assessment of light touch and proprioception is not necessary because these sensations will also be absent. For patients with severe cortical impairment, begin with assessment of pain and temperature for greatest efficiency.
- During reassessment to document recovery, remember that pain and temperature sensation recover before light touch and proprioception.

Spinal Cord Injury

Patients with complete lesions of the spinal cord demonstrate a total absence of sensation in the dermatomes (Fig. 9-2) below the level of the lesion. The level of the lesion determines the extent of the sensory loss, with the greatest loss occurring in patients with lesions in the highest cervical regions of the spinal cord. Paresthesia (tingling or pins and needles sensation) may occur in the dermatome associated with the level of the lesion (Burns & Ditunno, 2001; Fredericks, 1996c).

Incomplete spinal cord lesions result in sensory losses that are related to damage within specific spinal tracts. For instance, damage to the anterior part of the spinal cord usually results in loss of pain and temperature sensation below the level of the lesion, whereas touch, vibration, and proprioception remain intact. Conversely, patients who have damaged the posterior portion of the spinal cord cannot feel light touch and vibration but can feel differences in temperature and painful stimuli. Patients with damage to one side of the spinal cord (Brown-Sequard syndrome) display loss of touch, vibration, and proprioception on the side of the lesion and loss of temperature and pain sensation on the side opposite the lesion. This occurs because of the differences in the pathways of the ascending sensory fibers; neurons carrying temperature and pain sensations cross to the opposite side of the spinal cord immediately after entering it, whereas neurons carrying touch sensations ascend to the medulla before crossing to the opposite side (Fredericks, 1996c). Damage to the central spinal cord often results in bilateral loss of pain and temperature sensation below the level of the lesion because the neurons cross to the opposite side through the central portion of the cord. Mild to moderate compression of the spinal cord may result in decreased or absent sensation in the single dermatome at the level of the compression or could also involve dermatomes below the compressed area (Fredericks, 1996c).

Any sensory recovery following traumatic spinal cord injury usually occurs within the first year, with the greatest recovery in the first 3–6 months, especially in incomplete injuries (Burns & Ditunno, 2001; Kirshblum et al., 2004). Recovery of sensation is thought to occur because of resolution of ischemia and edema within the spinal cord.

Use the following guidelines in planning assessments for patients with spinal cord injury:

- Use a test with both pain and light touch stimuli (pinprick and cotton ball, respectively) to determine level of injury. The gold standard for neurological classification of spinal cord injury is the American Spinal Injury Association's (ASIA) Impairment Scale (Consortium for Spinal Cord Medicine, 2008).
- Apply stimuli to key sensory points within each dermatome when assessing neurological level in a rostral to caudal direction (Fig. 9-3) (Consortium for Spinal Cord Medicine, 2008). The full neurological classification also involves muscle strength testing at key motor points (see Chapter 38 on Spinal Cord Injury for further details).
- Test bilaterally because results may differ from side to side.
- Do complete testing of pinprick and light touch for patients with complete lesions where sacral sparing is absent to determine the zone of partial preservation, which provides more comprehensive information to the therapist regarding the intervention and education needed regarding sensory concerns after spinal cord injury.
- Test for multiple sensory modalities, including at least one pain or temperature assessment and at least one measure of touch, vibration, or proprioception in patients with incomplete or unknown lesions. To determine spinothalamic function, select a thermal threshold test (Savic et al., 2007). To determine posterior column involvement, select a vibration threshold test (Savic et al., 2007). Finally, to test both spinothalamic and posterior column function, the electrical threshold Quantitative Sensory Test (QST) may be used (Savic et al., 2007). However, quantitative sensory testing is typically used in research settings rather than clinical

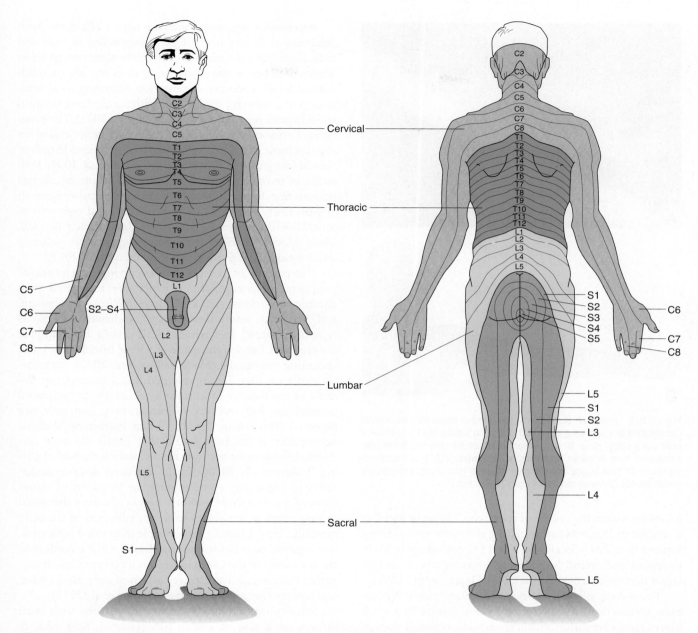

Figure 9-2 Typical dermatome distribution. (Reprinted with permission from Bear, M. F., Connors, B. W., & Paradiso, M. A. [2007]. *Neuroscience: Exploring the brain* [3rd ed.]. Baltimore: Lippincott Williams & Wilkins.)

therapy settings because of the cost of the instrument and the time required to administer the test.

Peripheral Nerve Injury

Patterns of sensory loss following peripheral nerve injury vary with the nerve or nerves involved. Damage to a single nerve root as it exits the spinal cord affects sensation on one side of the body within a single dermatome (Fig. 9-2). Damage to a peripheral nerve distal to the brachial plexus affects sensation within the appropriate peripheral nerve

distribution (Fig. 9-4) (Ropper & Samuels, 2009). For instance, in carpal tunnel syndrome, compression of the median nerve at the wrist produces sensory symptoms in the thumb, index, middle, and half of the ring finger on the affected side with the greatest changes in two-point discrimination being found in the middle finger (Comtet, 2005; Elfar, Stern, & Kiefhaber, 2010). Furthermore, compression of peripheral nerves in the upper limb can be characterized by the following: (1) pathology is observed primarily at anatomical locations where compression is more likely, (2) pathology may involve one or several specific nerves and

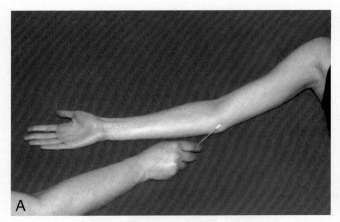

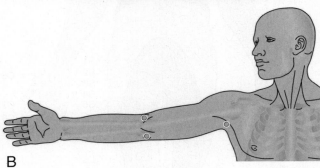

Figure 9-3 Light touch testing using key sensory points for neurological classification of spinal cord injury. **A.** Light touch testing of T1 key sensory point using cotton swab. **B.** Key sensory points of the arm. (Reprinted with permission from American Spinal Injury Association. [2011]. *International standards for neurological classification of spinal cord injury: Key sensory points.* Atlanta, GA: American Spinal Injury Association.)

locations within the course of the nerves, (3) pathology has a smaller or larger extension along the nerve versus being limited to a small focal point, and (4) pathology is likely to spread and extend over time and involve several and/or larger nerve segments (Comtet, 2005; Jepsen et al., 2009).

The severity of the sensory loss can vary widely. A complete transection of a peripheral nerve results in a total loss of tactile sensation within the region, especially loss of two-point discrimination and cutaneous pain sensibility (Karabeg, Jakirlic, & Dujso, 2009). A mild nerve compression, such as in early stages of carpal tunnel syndrome, produces a slightly elevated threshold for sensing light touch or vibration (O'Conaire, Rushton, & Wright, 2011). As the compression persists or increases in severity, further loss of sensation will occur, the threshold of light touch and vibration sensation will be further elevated (Tucker et al., 2007), and the patient will begin to report symptoms such as frequently dropping items from the hand. Eventually, if the compression is not relieved, numbness and loss of protective sensation will develop, and furthermore, prolonged loss of peripheral sensation results in cortical reorganization of the body part (Lundborg & Rosén, 2007), further disrupting sensory interpretation.

Recovery of sensation following release of a nerve from compression is very likely if the compression is brief and mild. Significant recovery following prolonged compression is common, but sensory perception does not always reach normal levels. Recovery of sensation following total transection of a nerve is possible only with surgical intervention and adequate regrowth of neurons (Smith, 2011). The prognosis of sensory recovery for the transected peripheral nerve appears most correlated with length of graft and length of time before grafting (Karabeg, Jakirlic, & Dujso, 2009). Sensation of temperature and pain generally (but not always) recovers first, followed by touch sensation, because regrowth of pain fibers averages 1.08 mm per day, and regrowth of touch fibers averages 0.78 mm per day (Waylett-Rendall, 1988). Moving touch recovers before light touch. Accurate touch localization recovers last (Callahan, 2002/2011).

The pattern of sensory loss occurring as a result of peripheral polyneuropathies, which are associated with chronic conditions such as diabetes mellitus, alcoholism, and acquired immunodeficiency syndrome (AIDS), is typically bilateral and symmetrical, usually beginning in the feet and hands (glove-and-stocking distribution) and spreading proximally (MedicineNet.com, 2012). Paresthesia and pain may accompany peripheral neuropathy. Because of the chronic conditions associated with peripheral neuropathy, full recovery of sensation is generally not expected (Fredericks, 1996b). When examining diabetic neuropathy, it has been found that tactile direction discrimination is more accurate than vibration threshold testing (Loken et al., 2010). Tactile direction discrimination refers to the ability to determine the direction of movement of touch across the skin, whereas vibratory threshold testing refers to the ability to detect vibration of the skin, typically using a tuning fork. People diagnosed with complex regional pain syndrome tested using QST according to the standards of the German Research Network on Neuropathic Pain revealed a distinct pattern of generalized bilateral sensory loss and hyperalgesia (Huge et al., 2011).

Sensory loss can also be found in persons with burn injuries at a rate of about 10% (Gabriel, Kowalske, & Holavanahalli, 2009). Furthermore, this neuropathy is characterized similarly to that found in conditions such as diabetes, systemic lupus erythematosus, and rheumatoid arthritis; however, sensory loss in burn patients may show better spontaneous recovery, as documented by a pilot study of nerve conduction testing (Gabriel, Kowalske, & Holavanahalli, 2009).

Sensory loss can also be found with amputation injuries involving the peripheral nerves. Haas et al. (2011) found that tactile sensation, as tested by Semmes-Weinstein monofilaments, was decreased in crush/avulsion injuries to the thumb compared with clean cut injuries. Finally, sensory loss in the peripheral nerves can be found in people with cancer as a result of neurotoxicity to various chemotherapy interventions (Cavaletti & Marmiroli, 2012).

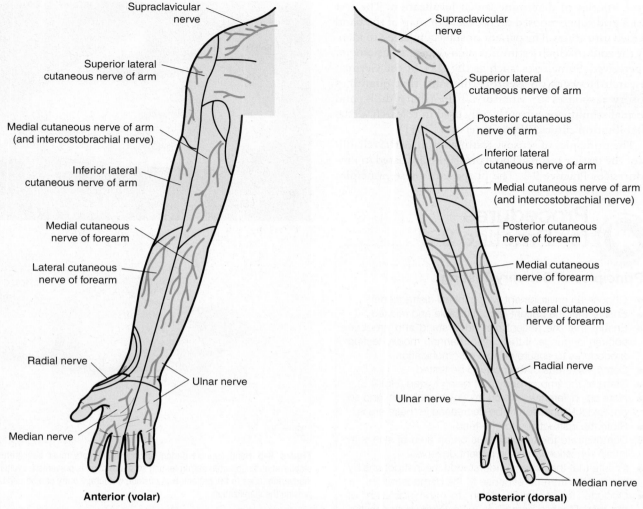

Figure 9-4 Typical sensory distribution of peripheral nerves within the upper extremity. (Reprinted with permission from Sieg, K. W., & Adams, S. P. [2009]. *Illustrated essentials of musculoskeletal anatomy* [5th ed.]. Gainesville, FL: Megabooks Inc.)

Use the following guidelines in planning assessments for patients with peripheral nerve injury:

- The purpose of evaluation in clients with peripheral polyneuropathy is to establish the impact of disease on protective sensation, so choose an assessment of protective sensation.
- The desired outcome of sensory evaluation in clients with involvement of a single peripheral nerve is an accurate map of both the body area and severity of sensory loss.
- Evaluation of nerve compression and subsequent recovery requires measures that are highly sensitive to show small changes in sensory function.
- Because functional tests of sensation requiring object or texture identification are completed with the thumb, index, and middle fingers, these assessments provide information about the functioning of the C6, C7, and C8 nerve roots and the median nerve.

- In documenting recovery of peripheral nerve function, keep in mind the recovery sequence of pain → moving touch → light touch → touch localization.

EVALUATION TECHNIQUES

There are numerous methods of testing sensation. Some are intended to evaluate a specific type of sensory receptor, such as the test for vibration awareness using a tuning fork that is believed to be specific to the Meissner's and Pacinian corpuscles (Dellon, 2000). Some are intended to evaluate the use of sensation in skills that support occupational functioning, such as the use of the hand to identify objects by touch in the test of stereognosis. Some are designed to detect very small changes in sensory perception, such as the touch threshold test using monofilaments (fine nylon strands). The locognosia test, described by Jerosch-Herold, Rosen, and Shepstone (2006) can be used after peripheral nerve injuries to determine touch localization. The test uses a grid superimposed on the hand or map of the hand divided into zones. The patient or subject is asked to identify the zone in which a stimulus such as an aesthesiometer is perceived. Some tests, such as the QST of the German Research Network on Neuropathic Pain that quantifies sensory responses to vibratory, pain (sharp/dull), and thermal stimuli are currently only used in research versus rehabilitation clinics (Blumenstiel et al., 2011).

The principles of sensory testing optimize the reliability of the testing results. These principles are listed in Procedures for Practice 9-1. The purpose of these principles

Procedures for Practice 9-1

Principles of Sensory Testing

- Choose an environment with minimal distractions.
- Ensure that the patient is comfortable and relaxed.
- Ensure that the patient can understand and produce spoken language. If the patient cannot, modify testing procedures to ensure reliable communication.
- Determine areas of the body to be tested.
- Stabilize the limb or body part being tested (Fig. 9-5).
- Note any differences in skin thickness, calluses, and so on. Expect sensation to be decreased in these areas.
- State the instructions for the test.
- Demonstrate the test stimulus on an area of skin with intact sensation while the patient observes.
- Ensure that the patient understands the instructions by eliciting the correct response to the demonstration.
- Occlude the patient's vision for administration of the test. Place a screen or a file folder between the patient's face and area being tested (Fig 9-6), blindfold the patient, or ask the patient to close his or her eyes.
- Apply stimuli at irregular intervals or insert catch trials in which no stimulus is given.
- Avoid giving inadvertent cues, such as auditory cues or facial expressions, during stimulus application.
- Carefully observe the correctness, confidence, and promptness of the responses.
- Observe the patient for any discomfort relating to the stimuli that may signal hypersensitivity (exaggerated or unpleasant sensation).
- Ensure that the therapist who does the initial testing does any reassessment.

From Brand, P. W., & Hollister, A. (1999). *Clinical mechanics of the hand* (3rd ed.). St. Louis: Mosby; Callahan, A. D. (2002/2011). Sensibility assessment for nerve lesions-in-continuity and nerve lacerations. In E. J. Mackin, A. D. Callahan, T. M. Skirven, L. H. Schneider, A. L. Osterman, & J. M. Hunter (Eds.), *Rehabilitation of the hand and upper extremity* (5th ed., pp. 214–239). St. Louis: Mosby. Archived online in T. M. Skirven, A. L. Osterman, J. M. Fedorczyk, & P. C. Amadio (Eds.). (2011). *Rehabilitation of the hand and upper extremity* (6th ed.). Philadelphia: Mosby, Inc./Elsevier; Reese, N. B. (2011). *Muscle and sensory testing* (3rd ed.). Philadelphia: Saunders/Elsevier Health Sciences Division.

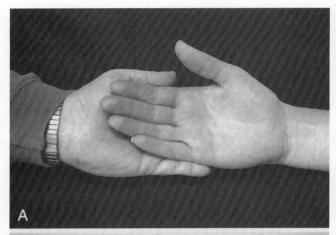

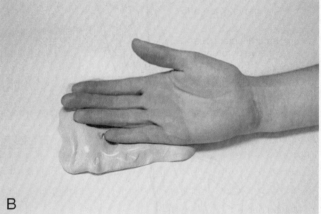

Figure 9-5 Hand support during testing. **A.** Fingers must be carefully stabilized and supported during testing so that motion is prevented, avoiding inadvertent cues to the patient. **B.** A cushion of therapy putty can be used to provide the stabilization.

is to eliminate nontactile cues and to ensure that the responses from the patient accurately reflect actual sensation. Because many of the tests require subjective reports from the patient, results can be either deliberately or unconsciously manipulated by the patient to make the deficit appear better or worse. Careful attention to test administration and patient responses can minimize the possibility of test manipulation by patients. For cases where the patient's responses are questionable and a determination of testing manipulation must be made, therapists may use a forced-choice testing methodology and statistical analysis described by Greve, Bianchini, and Ameduri (2003) in which patients are required to identify whether they are touched with one finger or two. A statistically low percentage of correct choices suggests an invalid response, because someone without sensation who merely guessed would be likely to get approximately 50% correct.

Fess (1995), in her article "Guidelines for Evaluating Assessment Instruments," describes four essential criteria for all assessment instruments. The first is reliability, which

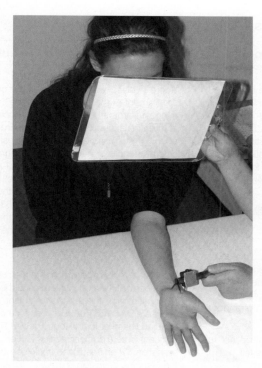

Figure 9-6 Sensory testing using an aesthesiometer for static or two-point discrimination. Vision must be occluded during testing. Using a screen, file folder, or clipboard such as this is usually more comfortable for patients than closing their eyes or being blindfolded.

includes accuracy of the instrument measurements as well as test–retest stability and interrater repeatability. Second, she describes validity as the tool's ability to measure the sensory modality for which it was designed. Third, standards for the manufacture, administration, and scoring of the assessment and interpretation of the results must be set and followed. Finally, there must be normative data and, ideally, diagnosis-specific normative data.

Specific descriptions of the administration of commonly used sensory evaluations are shown in Tables 9-2 and 9-3. The more standardized evaluations of sensation appear in Table 9-2, and the less standardized evaluations are shown in Table 9-3. Sensory testing tools have been the target of much criticism for their lack of standardization, reliability, and validity. Although the sensory tests are divided into standardized and nonstandardized tests in Tables 9-2 and 9-3, few of the tests in Table 9-2, presented as standardized, meet all of the criteria described by Fess (1995). Assessment Table 9-1 provides a summary of psychometric data regarding selected assessments. Resources 9-1 lists companies that provide assessment instruments.

Therapists must consider the various qualities of the types of sensory tests as they choose and administer them. Threshold tests determine the smallest stimuli that can be noticed by the patient. They are the most sensitive and have numeric results that can easily be compared over time. Two-point discrimination measures innervation density

in the fingers and is quite sensitive to change. Touch localization evaluates not only sensation but also whether that sensation is accurately perceived. Touch, temperature, vibration, and pain awareness are simple to administer but are not very sensitive to change. Tests of kinesthetic and proprioceptive sensations are less commonly used and are not very sensitive to change but are believed to be related to the specific type of sensory feedback required for coordinated movement. The Moberg Pick-Up Test and stereognosis test are more functional but require combined motor and sensory function in the hand. Both the DASH (Disabilities of the Arm, Shoulder, and Hand) and Quick DASH Outcome Measures are questionnaires designed to look at changes in motor and sensory function of the upper extremity (Institute for Work & Health, 2006). The HASTe (Hand Active Sensation Test) is a functional tool designed to assess the haptic perception of people who have sustained a stroke (Williams et al., 2006).

Computerized evaluations of sensation are often used for research and are becoming available in a limited number of clinics (Benton, 1994; Dellon, 2000; Riggle, 1999). The Pressure Specified Sensory Device measures pressure threshold for one- and two-point discrimination (Williams et al., 2009). The prototype Robotic Monofilament Inspector has been found to be a more sensitive screen of diabetic neuropathy than manual tests. It is only used in research and is not yet available to occupational therapists in clinic settings (Wilasrusmee et al., 2010). The QST of the German Research Network of Neuropathic Pain involves a protocol as well as instruments to test somatosensation to determine sensory loss (small and large nerve fiber functions) or gain (hyperalgesia, allodynia, and hyperpathia) as well as cutaneous and deep pain sensitivity. The QST tests vibration, pain, and mechanical thresholds at the face, hands, and feet (Rolke et al., 2006).

Although sensory tests are usually administered with the patient rested and in a comfortable, supported position, exceptions to this principle occur in the case of patients with peripheral nerve compression. For those patients, provocative testing, which determines whether increases in symptoms occur as a result of additional stress or compression on the peripheral nerve, is used. Increased sensory loss in the median nerve distribution with the wrist in flexion implicates compression of that nerve in the carpal tunnel area. Elbow flexion is the stress position for suspected cubital tunnel syndrome, which is compression of the ulnar nerve in the elbow area. Manual pressure over the nerve can be combined with the provocative position to further increase stress on the nerve (Callahan, 2002/2011; Novak & Mackinnnon, 2005; Szabo et al., 1999).

Recording Assessment Results

Documentation should include the type of test, the skin area tested, and the response. One easy way to document

Table 9-2 Standardized Sensory Testing Techniques

Sensory Test	Test Instrument	Stimulus (S) and Response (R)	Scoring and Expected Results
Touch threshold Measure of threshold of light touch sensation (Bell-Krotoski, 2011; Bell-Krotoski & Tomancik, 1987; Stoelting Company, 2001)	Semmes-Weinstein monofilaments OR Weinstein Enhanced Sensory Test (WEST)	Semmes-Weinstein S: Begin testing with filament marked 2.83; hold filament perpendicular to skin, apply to skin until filament bends (Fig. 9-7). Apply in 1.5 seconds, and remove in 1.5 seconds. Repeat three times at each testing site, using thicker filaments if the patient does not perceive thin ones (except for filaments marked >4.08, which are applied one time to each site). R: Patient says, "yes" upon feeling the stimulus. WEST S: Patient is prompted to stimulus, and then filament is applied perpendicular to skin and held for 1 second, then slowly lifted. Catch trials consisting of prompt without filament applications are randomly inserted within test sequence. R: Patient responds with "yes" or "no" to indicate whether stimulus was felt.	Semmes-Weinstein Score involves recording the number of the filament or the actual force of the thinnest filament detected at least once in three trials; results are usually recorded according to a standard color code using colored pencils or markers and a diagram of the hand/limb (Table 9-4 and Fig. 9-4; see also Fig. 9-9 in the case example). Normal touch threshold for adults is the perception of the filament marked 2.83 (force, 0.08 g) except for the sole of the foot, where the normal threshold is the filament marked 3.61 (force, 0.21 g). WEST Results are recorded according to the color of the filament. Normal touch threshold is perception of the thinnest monofilament. There are two WEST devices, one for the hand and another for the foot. The WEST is meant to be a quick screening tool of sensation. When needing to track recovery, the Semmes-Weinstein is used.
Static two-point discrimination Measures innervation density of slowly adapting fibers of the hand (Callahan, 2002/2011; Dellon, 2000)	Disk-Criminator OR aesthesiometer (Fig. 9-8)	S: Begin with a 5-mm separation of points. Lightly (just to the point of blanching) apply one or two points (randomly sequenced) in a transverse or longitudinal orientation on the hand; hold for at least 3 seconds or until patient responds. Gradually adjust distance of separation to find least distance that patient can correctly perceive two points. R: Patient responds by saying, "one," "two," or "I can't tell."	Score is smallest distance at which perception of one or two points is better than chance. When the patient's responses become hesitant or inaccurate, require two of three, four of seven, or seven of ten correct responses. Norms 3–5 mm in fingertips ages 18–70 years (Bell-Krotoski, 2011); 5–6 mm in fingertips ages 70 and above (Desrosiers et al., 1996) 5–9 mm for middle and proximal phalanges in adults age 18–60 years, 0–12 mm middle and proximal phalanges of those age 60 years and older (Shimokata & Kuzuya, 1995)
Moving two-point discrimination Measures innervation density of quickly adapting fibers of fingertips (Callahan, 2002/2011; Dellon, 1988, 2000)	Disk-Criminator OR aesthesiometer (Fig. 9-8)	S: Beginning with a 5- to 8-mm distance, move one or two points randomly from proximal to distal on the distal phalanx with points side by side and parallel to the long axis of the finger. Use just enough pressure for the patient to appreciate the stimulus. Gradually adjust distance of separation to find least distance that patient can correctly perceive. R: Patient responds by saying, "one," "two," or "I can't tell."	Score is smallest distance at which perception of one or two points is better than chance. When the patient's responses become hesitant or inaccurate, require 2 of 3, 4 of 7, or 7 of 10 correct responses. Norms 2–4 mm for ages 4–60 years (Dellon, 2000) 4–6 mm for ages 60 years and older (Dellon, 2000; Desrosiers et al., 1996)
Touch localization Measures spatial representation of touch receptors in the cortex (Nakada, 1993)	Semmes-Weinstein monofilament number 4.17, pen, or pencil eraser	S: Apply touch to patient's skin with vision occluded. R: Patient remembers location of stimulus. With vision no longer occluded, patient uses index finger or marking pen to point to spot just touched.	Score is the measured distance in millimeter between location of the stimulus and location of the response. Normal response is approximately 3–4 mm in digit tips, 7–10 mm in palm of hand, 15–18 mm in forearm (Schady, 1994; Sieg & Williams, 1986).

Table 9-2	Standardized Sensory Testing Techniques *(continued)*		
Sensory Test	**Test Instrument**	**Stimulus (S) and Response (R)**	**Scoring and Expected Results**
Touch localization or locognosia Measures ability to localize touch in hand (Jerosch-Herold, Rosen, & Shepstone, 2006)	Semmes-Weinstein monofilament number 6.65 or black filament on WEST, grid superimposed on the hand or a drawn map of the hand divided into zones	S: While vision is occluded, apply touch to patient's skin on palmar side of tips of fingers for 2 seconds followed by an interval of 3 seconds before next stimulus. Test the unaffected hand first. Each zone is stimulated twice. R: Patient identifies the location of the stimulus by calling out the corresponding number on the map.	A score of 2 points is given for each zone identified correctly. When localization is correct orientation but in an adjacent finger or correct finger but adjacent zone, a score of 1 is given. When zone cannot be identified, but correct digit is perceived, a score of 1 is also given. Anything worse or nonresponse is scored 0. Maximum score is 56 points for the area of the median nerve and 24 points for the area of the ulnar nerve.
Vibration threshold Measures threshold of rapidly adapting fibers (Callahan, 2002/2011; Dellon, 2000)	Vibrometer: biothesiometer, Vibratron II, automated tactile tester, Case IV System	Protocols vary with instrument S: Generally, vibrating head is applied to area to be tested. Stimulus intensity is gradually increased or decreased R: Patient indicates when vibration is first felt or no longer felt	Scoring varies with instrument; norms usually provided by manufacturer
Modified Pick-Up Test Dellon's modification of the Moberg Pick-Up Test measures the interpretation of sensation in the distribution of the median nerve (Dellon, 1988).	A small box and 12 standard metal objects: wing nut, screw, key, nail, large nut, nickel, dime, washer, safety pin, paper clip, small hex nut, and small square nut	Part 1 S: Tape small and ring digits to palm to prevent use. With patient using vision, have him or her pick up and place objects in a box as quickly as possible; time performance on two trials R: Patient picks up each object and deposits it in the box as quickly as possible Part 2 S: With patient's vision occluded, place one object at a time between three-point pinch in random order and measure speed of response R: Patient manipulates object and names it as rapidly as possible	Part 1 Score is total time to pick up and place all 12 objects in the box for each of two trials Normal response Trial 1, 10–19 seconds Trial 2, 9–16 seconds Part 2 Score is time to recognize each object on each of two trials (up to a maximum of 30 seconds) Normal response: 2 seconds per object
Erasmus MC Revised Nottingham Sensory Assessment Quantitative functional measure of sensation after stroke. Sensations assessed include: light touch, pinprick, pressure, two point discrimination, and proprioception (Stolk-Hornsveld et al., 2006)	A blindfold, cotton wool balls, neurotips, cocktail stick, aesthesiometer	S: Subjects are tested for light touch, pinprick, sharp-blunt discrimination, pressure, two-point discrimination, and proprioception. Areas tested are the face, trunk, shoulder, elbow, wrist, hand, hip, knee, ankle, and foot. Each stimulus is assessed three times on each area to the left and right sides in random order. For proprioception, the body part is moved by the researcher/therapist, and the subject is asked to replicate the position. R: Subjects indicate whether the stimulus is same as on unaffected side, different, or absent either by verbal response or movement of body.	All areas are scored based on 2 for normal response, 1 for impaired response, or 0 for absent response. For all categories, it is expected that the subject score "2 for normal response" for all areas

(continued)

Table 9-2	Standardized Sensory Testing Techniques *(continued)*		
Sensory Test	**Test Instrument**	**Stimulus (S) and Response (R)**	**Scoring and Expected Results**
Hand Active Sensation Test (HASTe) Quantitative functional measure of haptic perception in the hand (Williams et al., 2006)	Objects of various weights and textures	S: To complete the HASTe, subjects use one hand to manually explore objects that vary by weight and texture by using a match-to-sample forced choice recognition task without visual assistance R: Subjects indicate their choice without identifying or describing the matching object property	Eighteen trials are completed; nine test objects are matched twice, once to texture and once to weight. The total number of accurate matches (0–18) is recorded.
Quick DASH (Institute for Work & Health, 2006). Self-report tool for people with musculoskeletal disorders of the upper extremities. Measures perceived abilities to do tasks requiring sensory feedback.	None	S: Survey of 11–19 items provided to patient to complete. R: Patient fills out items on the scale and grades ability on a scale of 1–5 (no difficulty to unable, respectively).	At least 10 of the 11 items must be completed for a score to be calculated. Assigned values for completed responses are summed and then averaged, producing the score. This score is then converted to a 100 scale by subtracting 1 from the average score and multiplying by 25. A higher score indicates greater disability. The optional modules, which look at items more specific to athletes, musicians, or people whose work is physically demanding, are scored similarly to above.

touch threshold testing with monofilaments is to use a color code or a pattern code on a drawing of the body part (Fig. 9-4; see also Fig. 9-9 in the Case Example). The standard colors and patterns used to document results for the Semmes-Weinstein monofilaments and Weinstein Enhanced Sensory Test (WEST) are indicated in Table 9-4. A series of sensory maps completed over time can easily and quickly demonstrate sensory recovery.

For standardized tests, results can be compared with norms; however, age should be taken into account because studies show a decline in sensation with age (Desrosiers et al., 1996; Norman et al., 2011). Normative monofilament expectations for adults older than age 60 years are shown

in Table 9-5. For both standardized and nonstandardized tests, results from the affected area of the patient can be compared with results from the corresponding, contralateral unaffected area to determine the individual's "norms."

Sensory evaluation findings are often summarized as absent, intact, or impaired. *Absent* describes a total loss of sensation or inability to detect a specific sensory modality. *Intact* describes normal sensation. Sensation is *impaired* when the patient is able to detect some but not all of the stimuli or when the perception of the stimulus is different from that of an area of skin that has intact sensation.

(text continued on page 298)

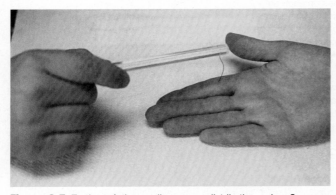

Figure 9-7 Testing of the median nerve distribution using Semmes-Weinstein monofilaments.

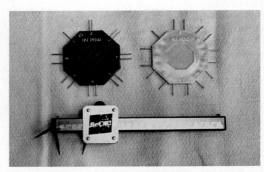

Figure 9-8 Tools used in two-point discrimination tests: Disk-Criminators (*top*) and an aesthesiometer (*bottom*).

| Table 9-3 | **Nonstandardized Sensory Testing Techniques** |

Sensory Test	Test Instrument	Stimulus (S) and Response (R)	Scoring and Expected Results
Touch awareness Measures general awareness of light touch input (Ropper & Samuels, 2009)	Cotton ball or swab, fingertip, pencil eraser	S: Light touch to a small area of the patient's skin. R: Patient says "yes" or makes agreed-upon nonverbal signal each time stimulus is felt.	Score is number of correct responses in relation to number of applied stimuli. Expected score is 100%.
Pinprick or pain awareness Measures discrimination of sharp and dull stimuli, which indicates protective sensation (Brand & Hollister, 1999; Reese, 2011)	New or sterilized safety pin	S: Randomly apply sharp and blunt ends of safety pin, perpendicular to skin, at the pressure that was necessary to elicit correct response on uninvolved side of body. R: Patient says "sharp" or "dull" after each stimulus.	Score is number of correct responses divided by number of stimuli. Expected score is 100%. Correct responses to sharp stimuli indicate intact protective sensation; incorrect responses to sharp stimuli indicate some awareness of pressure but absent protective sensation.
Temperature awareness Measures discrimination of warm and cool stimuli (Waylett-Rendall, 1988)	Hot and cold discrimination Kit or glass test tubes filled with warm and cool water	S: Apply cold (40°F) or warm (115°F–120°F) stimulus to patient's skin. R: Patient indicates hot or cold after each stimulus.	Score is number of correct responses divided by number of stimuli. Normal response is 100%.
Vibration awareness Measures awareness of input to rapidly adapting alpha-beta (α, β) fibers (Dellon, 1988)	Tuning forks: 30 cycles per second 256 cycles per second	S: Strike tuning fork with force to cause vibration; place prong tangentially to fingertip of injured and then uninjured hand; ask patient, "Does this feel the same or different?" R: Patient responds same or different and describes difference in perception.	Scoring is normal if stimuli to both hands feel the same, altered if stimuli feel different. The 30 cycles per second tuning fork is used to test the Meissner afferents, and the 256 cycles per second tuning fork is used to test the Pacinian afferents.
Stereognosis Measures the ability to identify objects, which requires interpretation of sensory input. Motor function is prerequisite. (Eggers, 1984).	A number of small objects known to the patient	S: Place a small object in the hand to be tested. R: Patient may manipulate object within the hand, patient names object.	Scoring is number of correct responses divided by total number of objects presented or time to identify each object. Normal response is correct identification of almost all objects within 2–3 seconds (Lederman & Klatzky, 1996).
Moberg Pick-Up Test Measures the function of slowly adapting alpha-beta (α, β) fibers in medial nerve injury (Callahan, 2002/2011; Dellon, 1988)	An assortment of small objects and a small box	S: Instruct patient to pick up objects as rapidly as possible and place them In the box, using right and left hands, with and without vision. R: Patient quickly picks up objects and places them in box.	Scoring is total time to pick up objects. Compare scores of left and right hands and those with and without vision. Mean times for 12 standard objects were found by Ng, Ho, and Chow (1999) to be 10–12 seconds with vision and 20–23 seconds without vision.
Proprioception Measures sense of joint position, which relies on input from an unknown combination of muscle, joint, and skin receptors (Ropper & Samuels, 2009)	None	S: Hold body segment being tested on the lateral surfaces; move the part into different positions and hold. R: Patient duplicates position with opposite extremity.	Graded as intact, impaired, or absent. Usually, reproduction of position can be accomplished within a few degrees. One study of the knee joint found on average 4° of error in normal subjects younger than age 30 years and 7° of error in normal subjects older than age 60 years (Kaplan et al., 1985).
Kinesthesia Measures sense of joint motion, which relies on input from an unknown combination of muscle, joint, and skin receptors (Ropper & Samuels, 2009)	None	S: Hold body segment being tested on the lateral surfaces; move the part through angles of varying degrees. R: Patient indicates whether part is moved up or down.	Graded as intact, impaired, or absent. Nearly 100% correct identification is expected.

Assessment Table 9-1	Summary of Assessments of Sensation				

Instrument and Reference	Description	Time to Administer	Validity	Reliability	Sensitivity	Strengths and Weaknesses
Monofilaments Available from AliMed, North Coast Medical, or Patterson Medical (see Resources 9-1)	Measures low threshold of touch perception on an ordinal scale. Results can be documented with a color-coded drawing or with numbers. 2.83 represents normal sensation, and >6.65 represents absent sensation.	5–30 minutes or more, depending on area tested	Using Semmes-Weinstein monofilaments, diminished light touch associated with longer response time for object identification (King, 1997). Weinstein Enhanced Sensory Test (WEST) monofilament testing compared with distal motor latency using electoneurometer revealed $r = 0.659$–0.886 for individual fingers (Schulz, Bohannon, & Morgan, 1998).	Repeatability of the force of application was demonstrated by Bell-Krotoski and Buford (1997). Test-retest reliability reported by Novak et al. (1993) $r = 0.78$–0.89 and interrater reliability ICC = 0.965.	Seventy-two percent sensitive in diagnosis of carpal tunnel syndrome (MacDermid & Wessel, 2004).	Strengths: Excellent reliability and validity. Widely used. Weaknesses: Relies on subjective responses from patient. Filaments are easily damaged. WEST test not helpful in tracking nerve regeneration.
Prototype Robotic Monofilament Inspector (Wilasrusmee et al., 2010).	Measures touch threshold including protective sensation. Created for detecting diabetic neuropathy.	Not reported but presumably more accurate and quicker than manual administration	Not established; however, strong agreement with Semmes-Weinstein monofilament test as well as vibration threshold perception test. Accurately identified diabetic neuropathy.	Not established	Not established	Strengths: The current model is simple to implement. Pressure application is consistent compared with manual administration, which can vary based on rater. Weaknesses: Requires training and an instrument. Psychometrics are incomplete.

Instrument	Description	Time	Reliability	Validity	Strengths/Weaknesses
Locognosia Test (Jerosch-Herold, Rosen, & Shepstone, 2006). Available from Dr. C. Jerosch-Herold; email: c.jerosch-herold@uea.ac.uk	Measures touch localization on an ordinal scale	5–10 minutes per hand, but recommended to wait 30 minutes between hands	The test-retest ICC for the median nerve zone was 0.924 (95% confidence interval 0.848–1.00), indicating a very high level of reproducibility. For the ulnar nerve zone, the ICC was 0.859 (95% confidence interval 0.693–1.00) again showing a high level of reproducibility.	Discriminant validity was measured by looking at the difference in scores between unaffected and affected hands. For the median nerve zone, the mean difference between the affected and unaffected hands was 11.1 (with a range of 1–33 and a standard deviation of 7.40). This difference was statistically significant ($p < 0.0001$; effect size $d = 1.2$). For the ulnar nerve zone, the mean difference was 4.75 (range = 1–13.5; standard deviation = 3.16), which again was a statistically significantly difference between hands ($p < 0.0001$; effect size $d = 1.3$).	Strengths: Valid and reliable tool to determine touch localization in fingers. Decreased ceiling and floor effects compared with Semmes-Weinstein and WEST. Weaknesses: If comparing scores of affected hand with those of unaffected hand, it is time consuming to wait the recommended 30 minutes in between testing of hands. Discriminant validity was determined based on the correlation between subjects' unaffected hand and the matched control hand of subjects with no nerve injuries.
Disk-Criminator and aesthesiometer Available from Lafayette Medical Instruments, North Coast Medical, or Patterson Medical	Measures two-point discrimination in millimeters, a ratio scale.	5–10 minutes	Test-retest reliability for two-point discrimination using the Disk-Criminator was reported as $r = 0.961$ for static and 0.922 for moving by Dellon, Mackinnon, and Crosby (1987) Interrater reliability ICC = 0.989 for static and 0.991 for moving (Novak et al., 1993).	The dynamic threshold values were lower than the static scores. The two-point discrimination values obtained correlated significantly with the arm grade of the overall disability sum score (static values: $r = 0.33$, $p = 0.04$; dynamic values: $r = 0.37$, $p = 0.02$) and the scores of the Weinstein Enhanced Sensory Test in patients (static values: $r = 0.58$, $p = 0.0001$; dynamic values: $r = 0.55$, $p = 0.0002$) (van Nes et al., 2008).	Study by MacDermid & Wessel (2004) reported static testing has 24% sensitivity and 62% specificity in diagnosis of carpal tunnel syndrome. The sensitivity values for the static and dynamic threshold values were 28% and 33%, respectively, for normal aging and those with polyneuropathy (Van Nes et al., 2008). Strengths: Excellent reliability. Widely used. Inexpensive, durable. Useful in documenting nerve regeneration. Most useful on fingertips. Weaknesses: Variation in force of application has been shown by Bell-Krotoski and Buford (1997), which may affect results.

(continued)

Assessment Table 9-1 | Summary of Assessments of Sensation (continued)

Instrument and Reference	Description	Time to Administer	Validity	Reliability	Sensitivity	Strengths and Weaknesses
Tuning forks (128 Hz frequency) Available from Patterson Medical	Indicates whether or not vibration is perceived, a nominal scale.	5 minutes	Concurrent validity using Pearson's product moment correlation was moderate to strong (0.515–0.634) between the tuning fork and Vibrameter, supporting concurrent validity (O'Conaire, Rushton, & Wright, 2011).	Moderate interrater reliability for median nerve was determined for the Vibrameter ICC = 0.798 and for the tuning fork Icc = 0.520 (O'Conaire, Rushton, & Wright, 2011).	Sensitivity for diagnosis of carpal tunnel syndrome is reported at 55% and specificity at 81% (MacDermid & Wessel, 2004).	Strength: Low-frequency tuning fork is useful to document regeneration of nerve Weaknesses: Relies on subjective responses from patient. Application techniques are not standardized.
Hot and cold temperature probes Available from Patterson Medical	Indicates whether or not temperature is perceived; a nominal scale.	5 minutes	Not established	Not established	Not established	Strengths: Assesses functional sensation. Is useful to identify loss of protective sensation. Weaknesses: Relies on subjective responses from patient. Tool does not test fine gradations of temperature discrimination and therefore may not be sensitive to change.
Vibrometer Biomedical Instrument Company, Sensortek, Inc., or WR Medical Electronics	Determines lowest intensity of vibration that can be perceived, an interval scale	20 minutes	Not established	Interrater reliability using Vibratron II, ICC = 0.982 (Novak et al., 1993).	In diagnosis of carpal tunnel syndrome, sensitivity is 50% and specificity is 73% (MacDermid & Wessel, 2004).	Strengths: Multiple kinds of instruments. The manufacturers provide protocols for testing. Instruments score small gradations. Weaknesses: Limited availability in occupational therapy clinics. Expense.

Assessment	Description	Time	Validity	Reliability	Sensitivity	Strengths and Weaknesses
Pressure-specified sensory device Neurotherapy DX	Measures pressure threshold and ability to feel and distinguish the distance between two points with results graphically generated by a computer and quantified on an interval scale with a range of 0.1–100 g/mm² for touch threshold	10–20 minutes	Results correlate well with timed object identification, $r = 0.691$ (Dellon, 2000).	Test-retest reliability is $r = 0.93$ for moving two-point discrimination, $r = 0.97$ for single-point static touch threshold test. Interrater reliability is $r = 0.61$. (Dellon, 2000).	In diagnosis of nerve entrapment, sensitivity is 100% (Tassler & Dellon, 1995).	Strengths: Computerized. Quantifiable. Measures both threshold and innervation density. Excellent sensitivity. Weaknesses: Limited availability in occupational therapy clinics. Expense.
Moberg Pick-Up Test (Dellon, 1988; Ng, Ho, & Chow, 1999) Available from Lafayette Instrument Company or Patterson Medical	Timed picking up of objects and timed identification of objects, resulting in an interval scale score	10 minutes	Performance of young, middle aged, and elderly subjects with carpal tunnel syndrome as denoted by nerve conduction study found to have significantly decreased performance on Moberg Pick-Up Test ($p < 0.05$). (Amirjani et al., 2011).	Interrater reliability $r = 0.67$ with patient's eyes open and $r = 0.80$ with eyes closed. (Ng, Ho, & Chow, 1999) Test-retest reliability found in people with carpal tunnel syndrome: ICC = 0.91 (95% confidence interval = 0.87–0.95), was highly significant ($p < 0.001$) (Amirjani et al., 2011).	Not established	Strengths: Simple, quick to administer. Functional. Easy to replicate. Inexpensive. Useful to assess function of median nerve. Weaknesses: Useful for limited diagnostic category. Lack of standardized protocol.
Erasmus MC modifications to Nottingham Sensory Assessment (Stolk-Hornsveld et al., 2006)	Measures light touch, pinprick, pressure, sharp-blunt discrimination, two-point discrimination, and proprioception	10–15 minutes	Not established	Interrater Weighted κ values ranged 0.66–1.00 for good to excellent agreement; except two-point discrimination was −0.10 at the fingertips. Intrarater Weighted κ values ranged 0.77–0.96 good to excellent agreement except for two-point discrimination, which was 0.11–0.63 poor to fair agreement.	Not established	Strengths: Quick and portable to administer. Provides sensory information about several areas. Weaknesses: Although validity of original Nottingham Sensory Assessment has been established, it has not been established for the Erasmus MC NSA. Reliability for two-point measures is poor to fair.

(continued)

Assessment Table 9-1	Summary of Assessments of Sensation (*continued*)

Instrument and Reference	Description	Time to Administer	Validity	Reliability	Sensitivity	Strengths and Weaknesses
Hand Active Sensation Test (HASTe) In pilot research stage available from University of Ohio through Williams et al., 2006	Measures haptic perception of the hand	Maximum of 90 minutes to complete 18 trials. For the stroke/experimental group, the average time to complete was 25 minutes (range 11–55 minutes) and for the control group, time to complete was 14 ± 3 minutes (range 10–20 minutes)	HASTe accuracy discriminated between stroke survivors and controls ($p < 0.001$) with mean accuracy scores of 14.86 ± 1.53 for controls and 8.46 ± 3.51 for stroke survivors. Both groups scored significantly higher ($p < 0.001$) on the nine texture trials (6.36 ± 2.50) than the nine weight trials (5.30 ± 2.31); however, the HASTe discriminated between stroke survivors and controls for discrimination of weight and texture ($p < 0.001$). HASTe showed moderate negative correlation with Wrist Position Sense Test (WPST) and two-point discrimination tests (because the scores of these tests decrease with improvement, whereas the score of the HASTe increases with improvement).	Test–retest reliability for the HASTe across all subjects was strong (ICC = 0.77, Pearson $r = 0.78$), indicating that the scores for the test and the retest were both correlated and in agreement despite a significant difference found for the paired t-test analysis of actual scores ($p = 0.03$). Internal consistency of the 18-item instrument was also strong (Cronbach's α coefficient = 0.82).	Not established	Strength: Uses functional objects to determine sensory recognition for people with no apparent sensory deficit, including those with stroke and the normal population. Weaknesses: Time consuming to perform. Still in pilot/research stage. Despite the quality of results, to be useful, the HASTe needs to provide unique information about hand function not currently available to the clinician.

Quick DASH				
The Quick DASH Outcome Measure is available free of charge (for noncommercial purposes) and may be downloaded from the DASH website at www.dash.iwh.on.ca. Information on scoring is also available on-line.	Survey of 11–19 items are rated on a 1–5 scale by patient with upper limb involvement.	Not stated	Internal consistency: Cronbach's α = 0.94 Test–retest reliability: ICC = 0.94	Convergent construct validity with a visual analog scale (VAS) of patient's estimation of overall problem $r = 0.70$. Convergent validity with VAS of patient's estimation of overall pain $r = 0.73$. Convergent validity with VAS of patient's estimation of ability to function $r = 0.80$. Convergent validity with VAS of patient's estimation of ability to work $r = 0.76$.	Responsiveness: Change in group of patients undergoing treatment; expected to improve SRM = 0.79. Change in those rating their problem as better SRM = 1.03. Strengths: Quick to perform and quantifies patient's perceived severity of problems. Appears to be useful in demonstrating improvements or change in overall rating of problem. Weaknesses: Scoring does not give adequate treatment planning guidance because a higher score only indicates increased problems but not specifically what problem. Responsiveness is measured by SRM, which is a weak measure of sensitivity to change (Stratford & Riddle, 2005).

ICC, intraclass correlation (Shrout & Fleiss, 1979); SRM, standardized response mean (Stratford & Riddle, 2005).

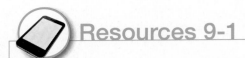

Resources 9-1

Sensory Evaluation Instrument Suppliers

AliMed

(aesthesiometers, monofilaments, Disk-Criminator, and touch test sensory evaluation kits)
297 High Street
Dedham, MA 02026
Phone: 800-225-2610
www.alimed.com

Bio-Medical Instrument Co.

(biothesiometer and vibrometer)
15764 Munn Road
Newbury, OH 44065
Phone: 440-564-5450
Fax: 440-564-5170
www.biothesiometer.com

Institute for Work & Health

(Quick DASH)
481 University Avenue, Suite 800
Toronto, Ontario, Canada
Phone: 416-927-2027, extension 2173
Fax: 416-927-4167
E-mail: dash@iwh.on.ca
Website: www.dash.iwh.on.ca

Lafayette Instrument Company

(Disk-Criminator and aesthesiometer)
P.O. Box 5729
Lafayette, IN 47903
Phone: 800-428-7545
Fax: 765-423-4111
www.lafayetteinstrument.com

North Coast Medical, Inc.

(hand screening forms, monofilaments, Disk-Criminator, aesthesiometer, sensory testing shield, touch test sensory evaluator, touch test two-point discriminator, and tuning forks)
8100 Camino Arroyo
Gilroy, CA 95020
Phone 800-821-9319
Fax: 877-213-9300
www.ncmedical.com

Patterson Medical (formerly Sammons Preston Rolyan)

(adolescent/adult sensory profile kit, monofilaments, aesthesiometer, tuning forks, pick-up test, hot and cold discrimination kit, sensory testing shield, stereognosis kit)
1000 Remington Boulevard, Suite 210
Bolingbrook, IL 60440-5117
Phone: 800-323-5547
Fax: 800-547-4333
www.sammonspreston.com

Sensortek, Inc.

(Vibratorn II)
2528 Vassar Place
Costa Mesa, CA 92626
Phone: 714-444-2276
Fax: 714-444-2278
www.sensortek.com

WR Medical Electronics Co.

(Case IV Quantitative Sensory Testing System)
1700 Gervais
Maplewood, MN 55109
Phone: 800-635-1312
Fax: 800-990-9733
www.wrmed.com

Interpretation of Evaluation Findings and Treatment Planning

In analyzing sensory evaluation findings, compare the results with those expected based on the patient's diagnosis. If the results differ from what was expected, further testing might be recommended. Individual sensory distributions sometimes vary from the illustrations of typical sensory distributions included in this and other texts. Furthermore, although there are clear lines of demarcation on the illustrations, humans generally have some overlapping areas of innervation along the borders of sensory receptive areas (Ropper & Samuels, 2009).

Consider whether the actual and expected results are different enough to suggest that there might be neural issues other than the diagnosis. If a peripheral nerve is compressed at one site, it is more sensitive to compression at other sites. Double and multiple neural compression sites can produce unexpected patterns of sensory impairment (Novak & Mackinnon, 2005).

Touch threshold testing with monofilaments can be interpreted based on categories of sensory loss as indicated in Table 9-4. With decreased light touch, patients often do not realize that they have a loss of sensation. There is no effect on the motor use of the hand, and patients can identify temperatures, textures, and objects by touch.

Table 9-4	Semmes-Weinstein and Weinstein Enhanced Sensory Test Hand Monofilaments					
Filament Number	Diameter (mm)	Mean Force (g)	Color Code	Alternate Code	Interpretation	Hand Function and Use
2.83	0.127	0.076	Green	White	Normal	Normal
3.61	0.178	0.209	Blue	Dotted	Diminished light touch	Stereognosis and perception of temperature and pain are good, close to normal use of hand
4.31	0.305	2.35	Purple	Horizontal lines	Diminished protective sensation	Decreased recognition of objects and painful stimuli, difficulty in manipulating objects
4.56	0.356	4.55	Red	Crisscrossed	Loss of protective sensation	Greatly impaired perception of pain, temperature, and object recognition; no manipulation of object without vision; marked decrease in spontaneous hand use
6.65	1.143	235.61	Red-orange	Black	Loss of all sensation except deep pressure	Unable to identify objects and temperature; hand use only with visual guidance
No response to 6.65	—	—	Red lines		Absence of all sensation	Unable to identify objects, temperature, and pain; minimal hand use

Based on information in Bell-Krotoski and Tomancik (1987), Stoelting Company (2001), and Bell-Krotoski (2011).

Diminished protective sensation results in decreased motor coordination, as evidenced by slower manipulation and dropping objects from grasp, whereas identification of temperatures and painful stimuli are intact. Loss of protective sensation causes an inability to use the hand when it is not in view. Patients will feel pinpricks and deep pressure but will be less able or unable to determine temperatures. Those patients who cannot feel the thickest monofilament may or may not be able to feel a pinprick but have no other feeling and require visual guidance for all hand function (Bell-Krotoski, 2011).

In planning treatment, diminished or lost protective sensation or absence of sensation indicates that the patient is at risk for injury of the affected body part or parts. The patient must be taught to use vision and an adapted environment to compensate for lost sensation and avoid injury. Results that indicate impaired sensation need further investigation to determine the appropriate course of intervention. If there is hypersensitivity or hyperesthesia of the body part, a program of desensitization is indicated. If there is a decrease but not total loss of sensation within an area, the patient may be a candidate for sensory retraining, as long as the diagnostic prognosis indicates that there is a potential for improvement. Chapter 22 describes each of these interventions in detail.

Table 9-5	Semmes-Weinstein Results for Subjects Older Than Age 60 Years: Median Monofilament Marking Number by Gender and Age		
Age	Women	Men
60–69	3.22	3.61
70–79	3.61	3.61
80+	3.61	3.84

Based on information from Desrosiers, J., Hébert, R., Bravo, G., & Dutil, A. A. E. (1996). Hand sensibility of healthy older people. *Journal of the American Geriatrics Society, 44*, 974–978.

CHOOSING EVALUATION METHODS

Therapists use clinical reasoning to select appropriate sensory evaluation techniques for each patient. Diagnostic and procedural reasoning suggests that certain tests are best at answering certain kinds of clinical questions. Ethical reasoning suggests that the tests should be the best available for each patient and that the practitioner has developed competence in test administration and interpretation. Pragmatic reasoning suggests that tests should be readily available and quickly administered (Schell, 2009).

Before choosing an evaluation method, decide why the test is necessary and what information is needed. Consider the diagnosis and the patient's description of the problem. For instance, for a patient with spinal cord injury, it is important to know whether sensation is intact, impaired, or absent in each sensory dermatome. A light touch awareness and pinprick test is common, with the results recorded on a schematic of the sensory dermatomes (Consortium for Spinal Cord Medicine, 2008).

If the purpose is to assist in the diagnosis of a nerve compression, such as carpal tunnel syndrome, it is necessary to use a highly sensitive test, such as a monofilament test. Sensation can be evaluated in positions that are likely to provoke more symptoms, for example with the wrist flexed (Szabo et al., 1999). A self-report of sensory loss has also been found useful in the diagnosis of carpal tunnel syndrome (Katz & Stirrat, 1990).

During observation of dressing or grooming by a patient with a diagnosis of stroke, a suspicion may arise that the observed errors are related to a loss of proprioception. An evaluation of proprioception can confirm or refute this hypothesis. For this same patient, it is important to know whether there is a risk of injury because of a loss of pain and temperature sensation (protective sensation). Either a pinprick and temperature test or monofilament test can provide this information. The monofilament test is more standardized and therefore a better choice, although it usually takes more time.

A test of stereognosis is most appropriate to predict, for example, whether a patient with a hand injury who is an auto mechanic can feel for and locate unseen automobile parts. The result of a two-point discrimination test or a monofilament test correlates with but does not totally predict the ability to identify objects with vision occluded, also known as stereognosis or haptic perception (Bell-Krotoski, 2011).

Optimal Assessment of Sensation

Ideally, patients are thoroughly assessed using standardized, reliable assessments that are easy to perform and that provide a complete understanding of sensation. A battery of tests is recommended if it is desirable to get a complete understanding of tactile sensation because no one test can assess this complex sense (Reese, 2011; Rosen, 1996). In clinical practice, however, therapists must sometimes balance the ideal with practical constraints. Schell (2009) described pragmatic constraints that affect sensory assessment in occupational therapy. These include the availability of equipment and supplies, time availability, team roles and responsibilities, reimbursement constraints, and the therapist's clinical competencies or preferences. Brand and Hollister (1999) charge that much time is wasted in sensory testing and that the results are open to question. Therapists should carefully assess their practices periodically to ensure that they are providing intervention that is as close to the ideal as possible despite pragmatic constraints. Great improvements can and should be made in tests of sensation so that they are meaningful, quantitative, and meet the criteria for good test instruments (Peripheral Neuropathy Association, 1993).

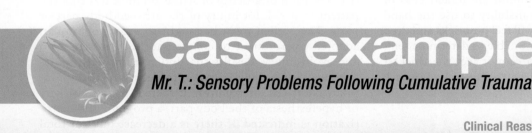

case example
Mr. T.: Sensory Problems Following Cumulative Trauma

Occupational Therapy Assessment Process	Clinical Reasoning Process	
	Objectives	Examples of Therapist's Internal Dialogue
Patient Information Mr. T. is a 45-year-old man who presented to his primary care physician with progressive weakness, pain, and sensory changes in his arms. Mr. T. works full-time as a quality assurance inspector for a machine shop. He needs to travel to various locations to inspect equipment to ensure that it is functioning correctly. He also inspects final products before they can be distributed to clients.	Understand the patient's diagnosis or condition	"I suspect that the issues Mr. T. is experiencing in his arms, especially his hands, are stemming from repetitive compression of his peripheral nerves. He describes himself as healthy and active. His job inspecting equipment requires that he keep his elbows flexed and propped up on the equipment. This positioning, as well as repetitive movement, has probably compressed his nerves (medial antebrachial cutaneous, median, and ulnar)."

When not working, Mr. T. spends time with his teenage son, for whom he functions as a single parent. They spend lots of time working around the house on various projects, especially fixing and maintaining cars. Mr. T. is the primary caregiver to two cats and one dog. He is having the most difficulty with walking his dog because he sometimes drops the leash as a result of numbness and weakness in his hands.

Mr. T. is unable to recall a specific traumatic event that coincides with the changes in function but instead reports that he has been noticing changes for more than a year. He reports pain in his forearm when it is pronated for a long time. He reports numbness and tingling in his hand especially when sleeping and when using his arms overhead. Mr. T. says that opening and manipulating small objects has become more challenging. He sometimes loses his grip on things, especially if he is not looking at his hands. At the end of a long workday, Mr. T. reports that he needs to take a long rest break as well as pain medication to stop his elbows from hurting.

Know the person	"Mr. T. appears to be hardworking. His work demands both gross and fine motor control. In work and his leisure, he needs to rely on the sensory capacity and grip of his hands. I wonder how he has been dealing with the progressive changes to his function over the past year."
Appreciate the context	"I wonder how the progressive changes to his upper extremities has affected his performance at work as well as his activities with his son?"
Develop provisional hypotheses	"Given Mr. T.'s history, I would expect that I will find changes to his peripheral nerve function, specifically that of the median and ulnar nerves. Furthermore, I would expect to find decreased proprioception, light touch, pinprick, and possibly thermal and vibratory sensory dysfunction not only because of the troubles he reports but also based on my understanding of sensory deficits after prolonged compression of peripheral nerves."

Assessment Process

The occupational therapist selected the following sensory evaluation tools:

- Touch threshold test using Semmes-Weinstein monofilaments
- Static and moving two-point discrimination
- Touch localization
- Dellon's modification of the Moberg Pick-Up Test
- Pinprick Test
- Thermal threshold test
- Vibrometer threshold test
- The Quick DASH

Consider evaluation approach and methods	"This is a good time to do a thorough sensory assessment because it will determine objectively what has happened over the past year to his peripheral nerve function. The monofilaments will give reliable information about all areas of the hand and indicate whether protective sensation is present or reduced. We need to determine whether perception of moving touch is involved, so we will also use static and moving two-point discrimination. The touch localization test will show how the brain is interpreting tactile sensations and how accurate the interpretation is. The pick-up test relates sensation to functional hand use. The pinprick test will show interpretation and accuracy of pain responses. The thermal threshold test will determine concerns about thermal discrimination. The vibrometer will help determine involvement as well as potential severity of the median nerve damage (Konchalard, Suputtitada, & Sastravaha, 2011). The Quick DASH is useful in determining Mr. T.'s subjective rating of his sensory and functional changes. These tests will provide good information for what is going on with Mr. T. and for treatment planning. The results will provide a baseline to demonstrate sensory recovery over time."

Assessment Results

The results of the Semmes-Weinstein monofilament test for bilateral forearms, palms, and fingers are shown in Figure 9-9. Mr. T. was not able to feel the Disk-Criminator anywhere on the fingertips in the moving test nor on the fingers or thumb in the static test. Touch localization in the lateral portion of bilateral forearms was 15–18 mm (normal). For the medial portion of the left forearm, touch localization measured 18–20 mm, and it measured 25–30 mm on the right forearm. The radial portion of the right palm measured 18–25 mm; that of the left palm measured 12–16 mm. Touch localization in the ulnar portion of the right palm measured 15–20 mm; that of the left palm measured 11–15 mm.

Interpret observations	"Sensation is severely compromised in the right, dominant hand as well as the medial forearm, consistent with involvement of the ulnar and medial nerves. The left side is also affected but not as severely as the right. Loss of protective sensation indicates potential for harm, especially when Mr. T. is working on cars with his son or completing his work. The incoordination found with the Moberg Pick-Up Test could be the result of motor and/or sensory deficits. Because of lack of sensation in the fingertips, object identification as well as protective responses are not possible now. I hope that we can intervene and help with return of both sensation and function. It is no wonder that Mr. T. is having difficulty with both his work and leisure pursuits."

Touch Test® Sensory Evaluators
Hand Screening Form

Patient _____Mr. T._____ Chart Number ___02134___ Date ___5/18/2012___

Evaluator Size	Target Force(g)	Representation	Thresholds	Comments
1.65 - 2.83	0.008 - 0.07	green ▢	Normal	
3.22 - 3.61	0.16 - 0.4	blue ▦	Diminished Light Touch	
3.84 - 4.31	0.6 - 2	purple ▤	Diminished Protective Sensation	
4.56 - 6.45	4 - 180	red ▦	Loss of Protective Sensation	
6.65	300	red ▪	Deep Pressure Sensation	
		red lined	Tested with No Response	

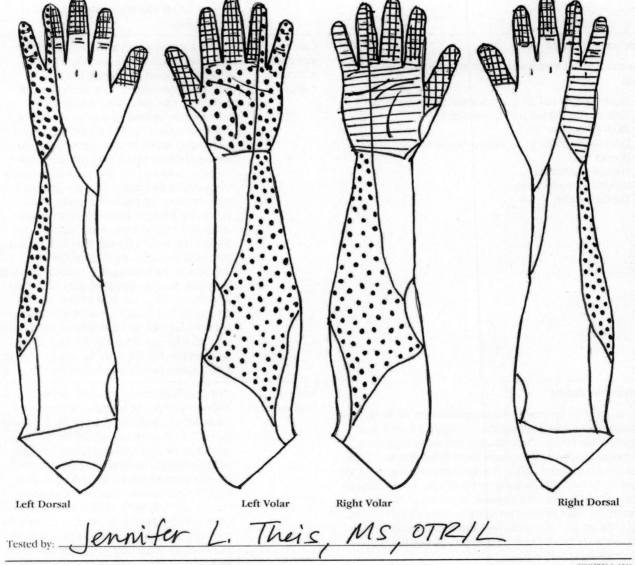

Left Dorsal   Left Volar   Right Volar   Right Dorsal

Tested by: ___Jennifer L. Theis, MS, OTR/L___

Figure 9-9 Results of initial monofilament testing for Mr. T. (see Case Example). (Reprinted with permission from North Coast Medical, Inc. [2011]. *Touch test sensory evaluator's hand screening form.* Gilroy, CA: North Coast Medical, Inc.)

Mr. T.'s scores on Dellon's modification of the Pick-Up Test were as follows:

Part 1: Left/Right
Trial 1: 30 seconds/70 seconds
Trial 2: 35 seconds/75 seconds

Part 2 No objects could be identified without vision.

Both the pinprick and thermal threshold tests showed moderate to severe impairment for the right medial forearm and hand, especially at the digits, and mild impairments for the left forearm and hand and moderate impairments at the digits. The vibrometer threshold was elevated bilaterally consistent with neuropathy. The score for the first 11 questions of the Quick DASH was 63.54, and the score was 75 for the questions pertaining to work-related problems. These results indicate moderate to severe issues with perceived function.

Occupational Therapy Problem List		
1. Absent and decreased protective sensation in the first through fifth digits and entire palm on the right hand. 2. Mislocalization of touch sensations in the entire palm, right worse than left. Mislocalization of touch on medial forearms bilaterally. 3. Decreased ability to pick up and manipulate objects; unable to pick up objects without vision. 4. Decreased use of the right hand in functional activities, which is affecting job performance.	Synthesize results	"Mr. T. is probably at some risk for injury to the fingertips, because he lacks any protective sensation in the digit tips, a likely place for thermal injuries or lacerations. The presence of some protective sensation in the palm and the mislocalization of touch stimuli suggests that retraining of sensation in this area may be effective. He might have a tendency to avoid using his right hand because of his decreased coordination. I'll need to provide functional activities to encourage bilateral functional use. Perhaps some work simulation or leisure activities will be motivating for Mr. T. I'll need to set up a plan for reducing further job-related cumulative trauma to prevent further compression of the median and ulnar nerves."

Adapted from Theis, J. L. (2011). Clinical decision making: Case studies for the occupational therapy assistant. New York: Delmar Cengage Learning. (Used with permission, www.cengage.com/permissions).

Clinical Reasoning in Occupational Therapy Practice

Interpretation and Treatment Planning for Peripheral Sensory Problem

Mr. T.'s touch threshold test is shown in Figure 9-9. After you provide intervention, how will the mapping likely change when Mr. T. is reassessed after 6 more weeks? What kind of sensation, pain or touch, will he be able to feel first in his fingertips? Compare his current functional hand use with his expected hand use when his fingertips regain touch sensation. What would you anticipate he will still have difficulties with as a quality assurance inspector, father, and pet owner? After 2 months of treatment, Mr. T. is still experiencing moderate issues with both nerves and is a candidate for surgery to both the median and ulnar nerves. What would you expect to change and, when cleared by neurosurgery, what assessments would you select and why?

Summary Review Questions

1. What pattern of sensory loss would be expected in a patient with a T10 spinal cord injury? In addition to performance and findings of the ASIA Impairment Scale, the gold standard in neurological classification after spinal cord injury, which tests light touch and pinprick/pain of key sensory points, what additional quantitative sensory tests could be performed and why?

2. What pattern of sensory loss would be expected in a patient with peripheral polyneuropathy?

3. Which patient will have a better prognosis for recovery of sensation: one with a peripheral nerve compression or one with a middle cerebral artery stroke?

4. Name and describe the purposes of at least three standardized and three nonstandardized sensory tests.

5. Describe or demonstrate the administration and scoring of a touch threshold test, a pain awareness test, and a touch localization test.

6. Which sensory test or tests would you select for a patient with peripheral polyneuropathy? Justify your response.

Glossary

Aesthesiometer—Instrument designed for sensory testing. The term usually indicates a tool consisting of a ruler type of scale and two prongs that can be moved progressively closer or farther apart that is used for assessing two-point discrimination (Figs. 9-6 and 9-8). Monofilaments are occasionally called pressure aesthesiometers in the literature.

Allodynia—A condition of pain caused by a stimulus that does not normally provoke pain (Gilron et al., 2011).

Haptic Perception—The process of recognizing objects through active touch. It involves a combination of somatosensory and proprioceptive input.

Hyperalgesia—An increased response to stimulus that is normally painful (Gilron et al., 2011).

Hyperpathia—An abnormally painful reaction to a stimulus, especially a repetitive stimulus, as well as an increased threshold (Gilron et al., 2011).

Hypersensitivity—Increased sensitivity to stimulation (Gilron et al., 2011).

Kinesthesia—The ability to identify active and passive movement of a body part (Ropper & Samuels, 2009).

Monofilament—Thin nylon strand resembling fishing line, of graded thicknesses, attached to a handle and used in testing the threshold of light touch sensation.

Paresthesia—An abnormal sensation such as a feeling of pins and needles, tingling, or tickling in the absence of tactile stimulation or in response to tactile stimuli that ordinarily do not evoke tingling or tickling.

Proprioception—Awareness of body position in space (AOTA, 2008, p. 635).

Stereognosis—The tactile identification of common objects. It involves the recognition of physical characteristics such as texture (Carr & Shepherd, 2010). Astereognosis is the term used to describe the absence of this ability.

Vibrometer—Instrument designed to test the threshold of vibration sensation. It consists of a vibrating head that is applied to the patient's skin and a control unit that allows for gradual changes in the amplitude and frequency of vibration.

Zone of partial preservation—In spinal cord injury, a region where there may be only partial damage to spinal nerves, including one to three spinal segments below the level of injury. Only calculated for people with complete spinal cord injuries (i.e., no sacral sparing or motor movement below the level of injury).

References

American Occupational Therapy Association. (2008). Occupational Therapy Practice Framework: Domain and Process (2nd ed.). *American Journal of Occupational Therapy, 62,* 625–682.

American Spinal Injury Association. (2011). *International standards for neurological classification of spinal cord injury: Key sensory points.* Atlanta, GA: American Spinal Injury Association.

Amirjani, N., Ashworth, N. L., Olson, J. L., Morhart, M., & Chan, K. M. (2011). Discriminative validity and test-retest reliability of the Dellon-modified Moberg Pick-up Test in carpal tunnel syndrome patients. *Journal of the Peripheral Nervous System, 16,* 51–58.

Bear, M. F., Connors, B. W., & Paradiso, M. A. (2006). *Neuroscience: Exploring the brain* (3rd ed.). Baltimore, MD: Lippincott Williams & Wilkins.

Bell-Krotoski, J. A. (2011). Sensibility testing: History, instrumentation, and clinical procedures. In T. M. Skirven, A. L. Osterman, J. M. Fedorczyk, & P. C. Amadio (Eds.), *Rehabilitation of the hand and upper extremity* (6th ed., pp. 132–151), St. Louis: Mosby.

Bell-Krotoski, J. A., & Buford, W. L. (1997). The force/time relationship of clinically used sensory testing instruments. *Journal of Hand Therapy, 10,* 297–309.

Bell-Krotoski, J., & Tomancik, E. (1987). Repeatability of testing with Semmes-Weinstein monofilaments. *Journal of Hand Surgery, 12A,* 155–161.

Benton, S. (1994). Computerized assessment holds promise. *Rehab Management, 7,* 37.

Beschin, N., Cazzani, M., Cubelli, R., Sala, S. D., & Spinazzola, L. (1996). Ignoring left and far: An investigation of tactile neglect. *Neuropsychologia, 34,* 41–49.

Blumenstiel, K., Gerhardt, A., Rolke, R., Bieber, C., Tesarz, J., Friederich, H.-C., Eich, W., & Treede, R.-D. (2011). Quantitative sensory testing profiles in chronic back pain are distinct from those in fibromyalgia. *Clinical Journal of Pain, 27,* 682–690.

Brand, P. W., & Hollister, A. (1999). *Clinical mechanics of the hand* (3rd ed.). St. Louis: Mosby.

Burns, A. S., & Ditunno, J. F. (2001). Establishing prognosis and maximizing functional outcomes after spinal cord injury. *Spine, 26,* 137–145.

Callahan, A. D. (2002/2011). Sensibility assessment for nerve lesions-in-continuity and nerve lacerations. In E. J. Mackin, A. D. Callahan, T. M. Skirven, L. H. Schneider, A. L. Osterman, & J. M. Hunter (Eds.), *Rehabilitation of the hand and upper extremity* (5th ed., pp. 214–239), St. Louis: Mosby. Archived online in T. M. Skirven, A. L. Osterman, J. M. Fedorczyk, & P. C. Amadio (Eds.). (2011). *Rehabilitation of the hand and upper extremity* (6th ed.). Philadelphia: Mosby, Inc./Elsevier.

Carr, J. H., & Shepherd, R. B. (2010). *Neurological rehabilitation: Optimizing motor performance* (2nd ed.). New York: Churchill Livingstone.

Carey, L. M., & Matyas, T. A. (2011). Frequency of discriminative sensory loss in the hand after stroke in a rehabilitation setting. *Journal of Rehabilitation Medicine, 43,* 257–263.

Cavaletti, G., & Marmiroli, P. (2012). Evaluation and monitoring of peripheral nerve function. *Handbook of Clinical Neurology, 104,* 163–171.

Chapman, C. E., Tremblay, F., & Ageranioti-Bélanger, A. (1996). Role of primary somatosensory cortex in active and passive touch. In A. M. Wing, P. Haggard, & J. R. Flanagan (Eds.), *Hand and brain: The neurophysiology and psychology of hand movements* (pp. 329–347). San Diego: Academic.

Cole, J. (1991). *Pride and a daily marathon.* Cambridge, MA: MIT.

Comtet, J. J. (2005). Aetiology and pathophysiology of nerve compression. In R. Tubiana & A. Gilbert (Eds.), *Surgery of disorders of the hand and upper extremity series: Tendon, nerve and other disorders* (pp. 303–312). New York: Taylor & Francis.

Connell, L. A., Lincoln, N. B., & Radford, K. A. (2008). Somatosensory impairment after stroke: Frequency of different deficits and their recovery. *Clinical Rehabilitation, 22,* 758–767.

Consortium for Spinal Cord Medicine. (2008). Early acute management in adults with spinal cord injury: A clinical practice guideline for health-care professionals. *Journal of Spinal Cord Medicine, 31,* 403–479.

Cooke, D. (1991). Sensibility evaluation battery for the peripheral nerve injured hand. *Australian Occupational Therapy Journal, 38,* 241–245.

Dellon, A. (1988). *Evaluation of sensibility and re-education of sensation in the hand.* Baltimore: Lucas.

Dellon, A. L. (2000). *Somatosensory testing and rehabilitation.* Baltimore, MD: The Institute for Peripheral Nerve Surgery.

Dellon, A. L., Mackinnon, S. E., & Crosby, P. M. (1987). Reliability of two-point discrimination measurements. *Journal of Hand Surgery, 12A,* 693–698.

Desrosiers, J., Hébert, R., Bravo, G., & Dutil, A. (1996). Hand sensibility of healthy older people. *Journal of the American Geriatrics Society, 44,* 974–978.

Eggers, O. (1984). *Occupational therapy in the treatment of adult hemiplegia.* Rockville, CO: Aspen Systems.

Elfar, J. C., Stern, P. J., & Kiefhaber, T. R. (2010). Individual finger sensibility in carpal tunnel syndrome. *Journal of Hand Surgery, 35A,* 1807–1812.

Fess, E. E. (1995). Guidelines for evaluating assessment instruments. *Journal of Hand Therapy, 8,* 144–148.

Fredericks, C. M. (1996a). Basic sensory mechanisms and the somatosensory system. In C. M. Fredericks & L. K. Saladin (Eds.), *Pathophysiology of the motor systems: Principles and clinical presentations* (pp. 78–106). Philadelphia: F. A. Davis.

Fredericks, C. M. (1996b). Disorders of the peripheral nervous system: The peripheral neuropathies. In C. M. Fredericks & L. K. Saladin (Eds.), *Pathophysiology of the motor systems: Principles and clinical presentations* (pp. 346–372). Philadelphia: F. A. Davis.

Fredericks, C. M. (1996c). Disorders of the spinal cord. In C. M. Fredericks & L. K. Saladin (Eds.), *Pathophysiology of the motor systems: Principles and clinical presentations* (pp. 394–423). Philadelphia: F. A. Davis.

Gabriel, V., Kowalske, K. J., & Holavanahalli, R. K. (2009). Assessment and recovery from burn related neuropathy by electrodiagnostic testing. *Journal of Burn Care Research, 30,* 668–674.

Gao, K. L., Ng, S. S. M., Kwok, J. W. Y., Chow, R. T. K., & Tsang, W. W. N. (2010). Eye-hand coordination and its relationship with sensorimotor impairments in stroke survivors. *Journal of Rehabilitation Medicine, 42,* 368–373.

Gilron, I., Attal, N., Bouhassira, D., & Dworkin, R. H. (2011). Assessment of neuropathic pain. In D. C. Turk & R. Melzack (Eds.), *Handbook of pain assessment* (3rd ed., pp. 326–353). New York: The Guilford Press.

Greve, K. W., Bianchini, K. J., & Ameduri, C. J. (2003). Use of a forced-choice test of tactile discrimination in the evaluation of functional sensory loss: A report of 3 cases. *Archives of Physical Medicine and Rehabilitation, 84,* 1233–1236.

Haas, F., Hubmer, M., Rappl, T., Koch, H., Parvizi, I., & Parvizi, D. (2011). Long term subjective and functional evaluation after thumb replantation with special attention to the Quick DASH questionnaire and a specially designed trauma score called modified Mayo score. *The Journal of Trauma Injury, Infection, and Critical Care, 71,* 460–466.

Huge, V., Lauchart, M., Magerl, W., Beyer, A., Moehnle, P., Kaufhold, W., Schelling, G., & Azad, S. C. (2011). Complex interaction of sensory and motor signs and symptoms in chronic CRPS. *PLoS One, 6,* 1–13.

Institute for Work & Health. (2006). The quick DASH outcome measure. Retrieved October 2, 2011 from www.dash.iwh.on.ca.

Jepsen, J. R., Laursen, L. H., Kreiner, S., & Larsen, A. I. (2009). Neurological examination of the upper limb: A study of construct validity. *The Open Neurology Journal, 3,* 54–63.

Jerosch-Herold, C., Rosen, B., & Shepstone, L. (2006). The reliability and validity of the locognosia test after injuries to peripheral nerves in the hand. *Journal of Bone and Joint Surgery, 88B,* 1048–1052.

Johansson, R. S. (1996). Sensory control of dexterous manipulation in humans. In A. M. Wing, P. Haggard, & J. R. Flanagan (Eds.), *Hand and brain: The neurophysiology and psychology of hand movements* (pp. 381–414). San Diego: Academic.

Jones, L. (1996). Proprioception and its contribution to manual dexterity. In A. M. Wing, P. Haggard, & J. R. Flanagan (Eds.), *Hand and brain: The neurophysiology and psychology of hand movements* (pp. 349–362). San Diego: Academic.

Kaplan, F. S., Nixon, J. E., Reitz, M., Rindfleish, L., & Tucker, J. (1985). Age-related changes in proprioception and sensation of joint position. *Acta Orthopaedica Scandinavia, 56*, 72–74.

Karabeg, R., Jakirlic, M., & Dujso, V. (2009). Sensory recovery after forearm median and ulnar nerve grafting. *Medicinski Arhiv, 63*, 97–99.

Katz, J. N., & Stirrat, C. R. (1990). A self-administered hand diagram for the diagnosis of carpal tunnel syndrome. *Journal of Hand Surgery, 15A*, 360–363.

Kim, J. H., Greenspan, J. D., Coghill, R. C., Ohara, S., & Lenz, F. A. (2007). Lesions limited to the human thalamic principal somatosensory nucleus (ventral caudal) are associated with loss of cold sensations and central pain. *The Journal of Neuroscience, 27*, 4995–5005.

King, P. (1997). Sensory function assessment: A pilot comparison study of touch pressure threshold with texture and tactile discrimination. *Journal of Hand Therapy, 10*, 24–28.

Kirshblum, S., Millis, S., McKinley, W., & Tulsky, D. (2004). Late neurologic recovery after traumatic spinal cord injury. *Archives of Physical Medicine and Rehabilitation, 85*, 1811–1817.

Konchalard, K., Suputtitada, A., & Sastravaha, N. (2011). Vibrometry in carpal tunnel syndrome: Correlations with electrodiagnostic parameters and disease severity. *Journal of the Medical Association of Thailand, 94*, 801–806.

Lederman, S. J., & Klatzky, R. L. (1996). Action for perception: Manual exploratory movements for haptically processing objects and their features. In A. M. Wing, P. Haggard, & J. R. Flanagan (Eds.), *Hand and brain: The neurophysiology and psychology of hand movements* (pp. 431–446). San Diego: Academic.

Lindblom, U. (1994). Analysis of abnormal touch, pain, and temperature sensation in patients. In J. Boivie, P. Hansson, & U. Lindblom (Eds.), *Touch, temperature, and pain in health and disease: Mechanisms and assessment* (pp. 63–84). Seattle: IASP.

Loken, L. S., Lundblad, L. C., Elam, M., & Olausson, H. W. (2010). Tactile direction discrimination and vibration detection in diabetic neuropathy. *Acta Neurologica Scandinavica, 121*, 302–308.

Lundborg, G., & Rosen, B. (2007). Hand function after nerve repair. *Acta Physiologica, 189*, 207–217.

MacDermid, J. C., & Wessel, J. (2004). Clinical diagnosis of carpal tunnel syndrome: A systematic review. *Journal of Hand Therapy, 17*, 309–319.

MedicineNet.com. (2012). Peripheral neuropathy. Retrieved January 28, 2012 from http://www.medicinenet.com/peripheral_neuropathy/article.htm.

Nakada, M. (1993). Localization of a constant-touch and moving-touch stimulus in the hand: A preliminary study. *Journal of Hand Therapy, 6*, 23–28.

Ng, C. L., Ho, D. D., & Chow, S. P. (1999). The Moberg Pick-Up Test: Results of testing with a standard protocol. *Journal of Hand Therapy, 12*, 309–312.

Norman, J. F., Kappers, A. M. L., Beers, A. M., Scott, A. K., Norman, H. F., & Koenderink, J. J. (2011). Aging and the haptic perception of 3D surface shape. *Attention, Perception, and Psychophysics, 73*, 908–918.

Novak, C. B., & Mackinnon, S. E. (2005). Evaluation of nerve injury and nerve compression in the upper quadrant. *Journal of Hand Therapy, 18*, 230–240.

Novak, C. B., Mackinnon, S. E., Williams, J. I., & Kelly, L. (1993). Establishment of reliability in the evaluation of hand sensibility. *Plastic and Reconstructive Surgery, 92*, 311–322.

O'Conaire, E., Rushton, A., & Wright, C. (2011). The assessment of vibration sense in the musculoskeletal examination: Moving towards a valid and reliable quantitative approach to vibration testing in clinical practice. *Manual Therapy, 16*, 296–300.

Peripheral Neuropathy Association. (1993). Quantitative sensory testing: A consensus report from the Peripheral Neuropathy Association. *Neurology, 43*, 1050–1052.

Reese, N. B. (2011). *Muscle and sensory testing* (3rd ed.). Philadelphia: Saunders/Elsevier Health Sciences Division.

Riggle, M. (1999). Review of the book *Somatosensory Testing and Rehabilitation. American Journal of Occupational Therapy, 53*, 412.

Rolke, R., Magerl, W., Campbell, K. A., Schalber, C., Caspari, S., Birklein, F., & Treede, R. D. (2006). Quantitative sensory testing: A comprehensive protocol for clinical trials. *European Journal of Pain, 10*, 77–88.

Ropper, A. H., & Samuels, M. A. (2009). Adams and Victor's *Principles of neurology* (9th ed.). New York: McGraw-Hill.

Rosen, B. (1996). Recovery of sensory and motor function after nerve repair: A rationale for evaluation. *Journal of Hand Therapy, 9*, 315–327.

Saladin, L. K. (1996). Traumatic brain injury. In C. M. Fredericks & L. K. Saladin (Eds.), *Pathophysiology of the motor systems: Principles and clinical presentations* (pp. 467–485). Philadelphia: F. A. Davis.

Savic, G., Bergstrom, E. M. K., Davey, N. J., Ellaway, P. H., Frankel, H. L., Jamous, A., & Nicotra, A. (2007). Quantitative sensory tests (perceptual thresholds) in patients with spinal cord injury. *Journal of Rehabilitation Research & Development, 44*, 77–82.

Scalha, T. B., Miyasaki, E., Lima, N. M. F. V., & Borges, G. (2011). Correlations between motor and sensory functions in upper limb chronic hemiparetics after stroke. *Arquivos de Neuropsichiatria, 69*, 624–629.

Schady, W. (1994). Locognosia: Normal precision and changes after peripheral nerve injury. In J. Boivie, P. Hansson, & U. Lindblom (Eds.), *Touch, temperature, and pain in health and disease: Mechanisms and assessment* (pp. 143–150). Seattle: IASP.

Schell, B. B. (2009). Professional reasoning in practice. In E. B. Crepeau, E. S. Cohn, & B. B. Schell (Eds.), *Willard & Spackman's occupational therapy* (11th ed., pp. 314–327). Philadelphia: Lippincott.

Schulz, L. A., Bohannon, R. W., & Morgan, W. J. (1998). Normal digit tip values for the Weinstein Enhanced Sensory Test. *Journal of Hand Therapy, 11*, 200–205.

Shimokata, H., & Kuzuya, F. (1995). Two-point discrimination test of the skin as an index of sensory aging. *Gerontology, 41*, 267–272.

Shrout, P. E., & Fleiss, J. L. (1979). Intraclass correlations: Uses in assessing rater reliability. *Psychological Bulletin, 35*, 420–428.

Sieg, K. W., & Adams, S. P. (2009). *Illustrated essentials of musculoskeletal anatomy* (5th ed.). Gainesville, FL: Megabooks Inc.

Sieg, K., & Williams, W. (1986). Preliminary report of a methodology for determining tactile location in adults. *Occupational Therapy Journal of Research, 6*, 195–206.

Smith, K. L. (2011). Nerve response to injury and repair. In T. M. Skirven, A. L. Osterman, J. M. Fedorczyk, & P. C. Amadio (Eds.), *Rehabilitation of the hand and upper extremity* (6th ed., pp. 601–610). St. Louis: Mosby.

Stein, J., & Brandstater, M. E. (2010). Stroke rehabilitation. In W. R. Frontera (Ed.), *DeLisa's rehabilitation and physical medicine: Principles and practice* (5th ed., Vol. 1, pp. 551–571). Philadelphia: Lippincott.

Sterzi, R., Bottini, G., Celani, M. G., Righetti, E., Lamassa, M., Ricci, S., & Vallar, G. (1993). Hemianopia, hemianesthesia, and hemiplegia after right and left hemisphere damage: A hemispheric difference. *Journal of Neurology, Neurosurgery, and Psychiatry, 56*, 308–310.

Stoelting Company. (2001). *Touch Test™ sensory evaluators: Semmes-Weinstein Von Frey aesthesiometers catalog number 58011*. Wood Dale, IL: Stoelting Company.

Stolk-Hornsveld, F., Crow, J. L., Hendriks, E. P., van der Baan, R., & Harmeling-van der Wel, B. C. (2006). The Erasmus MC modifications to the (revised) Nottingham Sensory Assessment: A reliable somatosensory assessment measure for patients with intracranial disorders. *Clinical Rehabilitation, 20*, 160–172.

Stratford, P. W., & Riddle, D. L. (2005). Assessing sensitivity to change: Choosing the appropriate change coefficient. *Health Quality Life Outcomes, 3*, 23.

Szabo, R. M., Slater, R. R., Farver, T. B., Stanton, D. B., & Sharman, W. K. (1999). The value of diagnostic testing in carpal tunnel syndrome. *Journal of Hand Surgery, 24A*, 704–714.

Tassler, P. L., & Dellon, A. L. (1995). Correlation of measurements of pressure perception using the pressure-specified sensory device with electrodiagnostic testing. *Journal of Occupational and Environmental Medicine, 37,* 862–866.

Theis, J. L. (2011). Clinical decision making: *Case studies for the occupational therapy assistant.* New York: Delmar Cengage Learning.

Tucker, A. T., White, P. D., Kosek, E., Pearson, R. M., Henderson, M., Coldrick, A. R., Cooke, E. D., & Kidd, B. L. (2007). Comparison of vibration perception thresholds in individuals with diffuse upper limb pain and carpal tunnel syndrome. *Pain, 127,* 263–269.

Tyson, S. F., Hanley, M., Chillala, J., Selley, A. B., & Tallis, R. C. (2008). Sensory loss in hospital-admitted people with stroke: Characteristics, associated factors, and relationship with function. *Neurorehabilitation and Neural Repair, 22,* 166–172.

van Nes, S. I., Faber, C. G., Hamers, R. M., Harschnitz, O., Bakkers, M., Hermans, M. C., Meijer, R. J., van Doorn, P. A., & Merkies, I. S. (2008). Revising two-point discrimination assessment in normal aging and in patients with polyneuropathies. *Journal of Neurology, Neurosurgery, and Psychiatry, 79,* 832–834.

Waylett-Rendall, J. (1988). Sensibility evaluation and rehabilitation. *Orthopedic Clinics of North America, 19,* 43–56.

Wilasrusmee, C., Suthakorn, J., Guerineau, C., Itsarachaiyot, Y., Sa-Ing, V., Proprom, N., Lertsithichai, P., Jirasisrithum, S., & Kittur, D. (2010). A novel robotic monofilament test for diabetic neuropathy. *Asian Journal of Surgery, 33,* 193–198.

Williams, E. H., Detmer, D. E., Guyton, G. P., & Dellon, A. L. (2009). Non-invasive neurosensory testing used to diagnose and confirm successful surgical management of lower extremity deep distal posterior compartment syndrome. *Journal of Brachial Plexus and Peripheral Nerve Injury, 4,* 4.

Williams, P. S., Basso, D. M., Case-Smith, J., & Nichols-Larsen, D. S. (2006). Development of the Hand Active Sensation Test: Reliability and validity. *Archives of Physical Medicine and Rehabilitation, 87,* 1471–1477.

Acknowledgment

I would like to thank Mary Vining Radomski for her ongoing mentorship and for encouraging me to undertake numerous opportunities for professional development. Thanks to Karen Bentzel for her original work on this chapter. It remains well written and thought provoking.

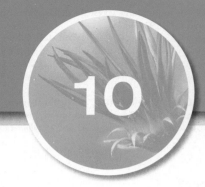

10

Assessing Environment: Home, Community, and Workplace Access and Safety

Patricia Rigby and Oana Craciunoiu

Learning Objectives

After studying this chapter, the reader will be able to do the following:

1. Describe the roles and responsibilities of the occupational therapist in the evaluation of environmental access.
2. Identify factors that act as environmental or contextual enablers or barriers/hindrances to occupational performance.
3. Identify environmental features that influence the safety of the client and the occupational therapist.
3. Apply critical appraisal when selecting assessment instruments appropriate for use in evaluating access to home, community, and workplace.
4. Explain how legislation and building standards influence the degree of environmental access that is available for people with disabilities.

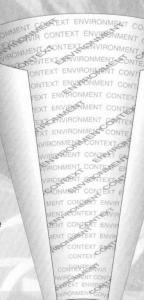

The environment influences human behavior and provides the context within which all occupational roles are performed. The environment is viewed broadly in prominent frameworks and models that guide occupational therapy practice (e.g., American Occupational Therapy Association [AOTA], 2008; Kielhofner, 2008; Law et al., 1996; Townsend & Polatajko, 2007; Trombly Latham, 2005). Most authors agree that the environment has physical, social, cultural, institutional, and temporal dimensions that can influence the performance and engagement in occupations at a personal, community, and societal level. Central to these models of practice are the notions that (1) environmental barriers or hindrances to occupational performance for people with disabilities can be modified or eliminated more easily than most other negative influences, and (2) environmental supports or enablers promote optimal engagement in occupations.

What makes occupational therapy assessment unique, compared with other disciplines, is the analysis of the person-environment-occupation (PEO) relationship and the level of congruency in this relationship or PEO fit as it affects occupational performance (Law et al., 1996). The better the PEO fit, the more optimal the occupational performance. Occupational therapists are frequently called upon to determine the degree of congruence between people with disabilities, their chosen occupations and roles, and the various environments in which they live, work, and play. Thus, assessment of the performance context is a critically important step in the occupational therapy assessment process. According to the Occupational Functioning Model, the therapist assesses whether the environment enables or hinders occupational functioning (Trombly Latham, 2005). These assessment findings can guide the therapist to develop strategies to eliminate or ameliorate barriers and to use resources and supports to improve occupational functioning. To assess the environment and the PEO relationship, the therapist should:

- identify and evaluate environmental hindrances or barriers that may challenge the competency and ability of individuals to carry out their chosen occupations and roles;
- identify and evaluate environmental resources that will support occupational performance and occupational functioning.

This chapter focuses on the assessment of the environment for occupational performance. Specifically, it will consider the environment that is external to the client when assessing occupational functioning: the physical, social, and institutional attributes of the environment. The assessment measures selected are those that the authors consider the best available and that reflect the transactive nature of the PEO relationship among people, their chosen occupations, and the occupational environment.

EVALUATION OF THE ENVIRONMENT

The environment provides the context for occupational functioning. Consequently, an assessment of its attributes should also include information about those who will use the environment and the functions they will carry out there. In the practice of occupational therapy, it is important to begin this process with the person.

Client-Centered Approach

The client is central to all occupational therapy services, and much has been written about the need to engage and involve clients in all stages of the occupational therapy process (Townsend & Polatajko, 2007). The client–therapist interaction begins with an interview and assessment so that the therapist can gain an understanding of the client's occupational profile (AOTA, 2008). This involves determining what roles and occupations the client previously had and what the client currently wants or is expected to be able to do. Collaborative goal setting is an important stage in establishing client-centered occupational therapy (AOTA, 2008; Townsend & Polatajko, 2007).

Once the occupational profile is established, the occupational therapist then completes an analysis of occupational performance to better understand the client's performance skills, patterns, and challenges, considering the contexts within which activities and roles will be carried out. This is also when environmental assessment is undertaken. For example, a therapist and client could focus on community mobility and access because it is important to the client to continue participating in a volunteer role at the local public library. The therapist would consider the client's abilities by assessing his or her mobility using a wheelchair in the hospital setting, assessing the client's ability to access community transportation systems, and assessing the library's accessibility to ensure that the client could negotiate the entrances, work areas, and public washrooms.

Roles

The roles carried out by clients address purposeful activities related to self-maintenance, self-enhancement, and self-advancement (Trombly Latham, 2005). Each individual ascribes different meaning to his or her roles.

Environmental Barriers and Enablers

The occupational therapist must be able to identify the key environmental barriers and enablers that influence the fulfillment of valued roles and occupational functioning of clients. In clinical practice, barriers and enablers are broadly defined. However, this chapter discusses barriers and enablers in the external environment; the personal, social, cultural context, and payer reimbursement are described in Chapter 3.

The International Classification of Functioning, Disability and Health (ICF) classifies environmental factors as the natural and human-made environments; assistive products and technology; supports and relationships; attitudes; and services, systems, and policies (World Health Organization, 2001). The therapist is encouraged to consider these factors during assessment. For example, physical barriers in the natural environment can prevent or impede a person with a disability from participating in daily activities, whereas human-made resources can improve accessibility. Consider the challenge that stairs or rocky paths impose on a person using a wheelchair. These barriers can be removed or reduced by adding enablers such as elevators or ramps to replace stairs and a ramped bridge across the rocks to allow access for a wheelchair.

Access that is discriminatory or inconvenient, such as forcing persons with physical disabilities to use freight elevators or ramped entrances at the back of buildings, is no longer considered a viable solution to eliminating access barriers (World Health Organization, 2011). Improved accessibility through the use of universal design (UD) and barrier-free design is preferred. These two terms are similar but not synonymous. UD refers to features of the built environment that enhance optimal function and convenience for everyone, regardless of ability. Barrier-free design refers to features of the built environment that remove physical barriers to allow full and equal accessibility for all persons with disabilities. UD can encompass barrier-free design, but the converse is not necessarily true. For this reason, it is preferable to promote the use of UD (see Resources 10-1).

Influences on Environmental Accessibility and Safety

Various societal and cultural attitudes influence the degree to which the physical environment is made accessible, inclusive, and safe for people with disabilities. Occupational therapy practice standards also reflect these global views. These influences manifest as national and state or provincial legislation, building standards, and professional practice requirements.

Legislation

Over the past two decades, great strides have been made around the world in enacting laws to protect the rights of persons with disabilities and to ensure their full and effective participation and inclusion in society. The United Nations Convention on the Rights of Persons with Disabilities was adopted in December 2006 and came into force in May 2008. The convention is a great achievement after decades of work by the United Nations to change attitudes and approaches to persons with disabilities. The convention adopts a broad categorization of persons with disabilities, and its purpose is to promote, protect, and ensure the full and equal enjoyment of all human rights and fundamental freedoms by all persons

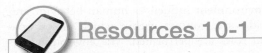

Resources 10-1

Internet Resources for Assessing Home, Community, and Workplace Access

- Adaptive Environments: Institute for Human-centered Design (http://www.adaptenv.org) provides access to resources on universal design and on accessibility and the ADA (e.g., book titled, *Achieving Physical and Communication Accessibility*).
- Americans with Disabilities Act (ADA) (http://www.ada.gov/) provides information and technical assistance on the ADA and the ADA standards for accessible design.
- Canadian Mortgage and Housing Corporation (http://www.cmhc-schl.gc.ca/en/) provides many resources about housing accessibility for persons with disabilities, including funding options; very useful resources for therapists and clients.
- Centre for Universal Design (http://www.ncsu.edu/project/design-projects/udi/) includes overviews of the principles of universal design, publications and information on Fair Housing and home modifications.
- Fair Housing Accessibility FIRST (http://www.fairhousingfirst.org) provides information and resources to support implementation of the Fair Housing Act amendments, such as the Fair Housing Act Design Manual.
- International Code Council (www.iccsafe.org/safety/Pages/accessibility-1.aspx) provides resources on accessibility, safety, etc.
- Job Accommodation Network (JAN) (http://askjan.org/).
- U.S. Department of Labor Occupational Safety and Health Administration (http://www.osha.gov/index.html).
- U.S. Department of Transportation (http://www.dot.gov).
- National Highway Traffic Safety Administration (http://www.nhtsa.gov/).

with disabilities and to promote respect for their inherent dignity (United Nations, 2001).

In the United States, the Americans with Disabilities Act (ADA) (1990), and, in Canada, the Ontarians with Disabilities Act (2001) were both designed to enable the participation and inclusion of people with disabilities in society. Key to these laws is the obligation of society to provide reasonable accommodations to ensure that public services, facilities, transportation, employment, accommodations, and telecommunications are accessible. Reasonable accommodations ensure that no person with a disability is excluded from or denied services. Titles II and III of the ADA provide detailed steps to be taken by public and private sector services, programs, and facilities to comply with and implement the requirements of the ADA. They address the accommodations required and the availability of resources; modifications to policies, practices, and procedures; the removal of barriers; and alternative forms of services, such as accessible transit services when mainline public facilities are unavailable. In addition, the ADA Amendments Act (2008) provides a revised definition of "disability" to more broadly encompass impairments that substantially limit participation in major life activity, such as work. The 2010 ADA Standards for Accessible Design outline how both public and private-sector services, programs, and facilities should comply with and implement accessibility requirements (see http://www.ada.gov/2010ADAstandards_index.htm). Titles II and III of the ADA have undergone revisions recently to provide greater clarity and guidance about requirements in the ADA amendments (see http://www.ada.gov/regs2010/ADAregs2010.htm), particularly with respect to their limited authority over private sector services. Changing the physical environment can be expensive and complicated to implement. Under the ADA, employers are expected to make "reasonable accommodations" for employees with disabilities, as long as these do not cause "undue hardship" to the employer. In Ontario, Canada, the Accessibility for Ontarians with Disabilities Act (2005) provides timelines and more specific requirements toward achieving full accessibility across the province by 2025.

These laws are expected, over time, to eliminate barriers and improve accessibility for people with disabilities. However, analysis of the impact of the ADA is mixed. Social policy analysis demonstrates changes in the attitudes and practices of Americans and shows that the ADA has improved the quality of life for persons with disabilities (Harrison, 2002). A large representative survey of small business owners shows that their businesses comply with the ADA by accommodating customers with disabilities and disabled employees who are already on the job (Moore, Moore, & Moore, 2007). They also report that the benefits have outweighed the costs. Hopefully the amendments to the ADA will continue to improve accessibility for persons with disabilities, because the view from persons with disabilities was not promising a decade ago. They reported that the ADA had not been very effective in improving accessibility (Hinton, 2003) (see Resources 10-1 for further information on the ADA).

Although the ADA and similar legislation in many jurisdictions does not mandate professional involvement in achievement of the criteria set forth, occupational therapists, skilled in occupational analysis, environmental assessment, and determining PEO fit are well suited to assist with meeting the requirements of the legislation. Because these laws are critical for improving accessibility, independence, and empowerment of persons with physical disabilities, occupational therapists must take action to become familiar with and use these laws.

Building Standards

In 2004, the U.S. Access Board released the updated ADA-ABA (Architectural Board Act) Accessibility Guidelines for new or altered buildings, which provide the accessibility requirements for public and private facilities (U.S. Access Board, 2004). The specifications in these guidelines are based on adult and child dimensions and anthropometrics and should be applied during the design and construction or alteration of buildings and facilities covered by titles II and III of the ADA. Specifications are provided for most aspects of the built environment, including space required for maneuvering wheelchairs in corridors and rooms (Figs. 10-1 and 10-2), washrooms, building entrances, and parking lots.

Other standards have been developed for specific environments such as the workplace. For example, the National Institute of Occupational Safety and Health (NIOSH; see http://www.cdc.gov/NIOSH/) publishes criteria directed at reducing the rate of workplace injuries. Occupational therapists who work in these environments must become familiar with the standards and guidelines relevant to their area of practice.

The Americans with Disabilities Act Checklist for Readily Achievable Barrier Removal (Adaptive Environments Center, 1995) was developed for owners and managers of public buildings and businesses to identify barriers in their facilities. Although this survey tool is based on the original ADA Accessibility Guidelines, it is still relevant and easy to use to identify accessibility barriers, along

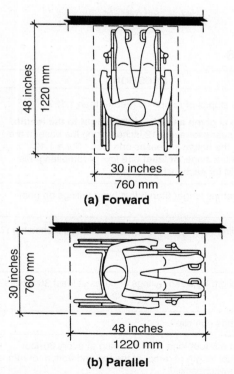

Figure 10-1 Accessibility requirements indicate that a person maneuvering a wheelchair needs a clear space of a minimum of 30 × 48 inches (760 × 1220 mm) for either forward or parallel approach in a corridor or doorway. (Adapted from the U.S. Access Board. [2004]. ADA-ABA accessibility guidelines. Retrieved August 23, 2011 from http://www.access-board.gov/ada-aba/final.cfm.)

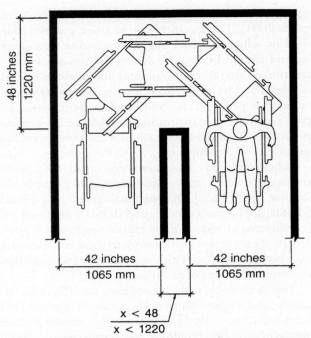

Figure 10-2 Accessibility requirements indicate that a person maneuvering a wheelchair needs a clear width of a minimum of 42 inches (1065 mm) at the approach to a turn, and 48 inches (1220 mm) at the turn. (Adapted from U.S. Access Board. [2004]. ADA-ABA accessibility guidelines. Retrieved August 23, 2011 from http://www.access-board.gov/ada-aba/final.cfm.)

with suggestions for "readily achievable" access solutions. For example, requirements for a ramped entrance to a building are shown in the checklist in Figure 10-3. The occupational therapist can assist businesses to use this tool and set priorities for achieving accessibility.

Professional Practice Requirements

The practice of occupational therapy is also guided by professional regulations. Standards of practice, core competencies, and functions expected of therapists are developed at the national and state or provincial levels and provide performance evaluation criteria. These guidelines are usually generic in nature, and apply to all therapists, regardless of the area, setting, or focus of practice (AOTA, 2009; Canadian Association of Occupational Therapists, 2007). Knowledge of, and ability to perform assessments of context or environment are considered to be core competencies and functions of practice for all occupational therapists (AOTA, 2010; Association of Canadian Occupational Therapy Regulatory Organizations, 2012).

ENVIRONMENT ASSESSMENT

Ideally, the occupational therapist should select instruments with standardization that assess PEO fit, in order to take into consideration the relationship between the

RAMPS

QUESTIONS	MEASUREMENT	YES	NO	POSSIBLE SOLUTIONS
Are the slopes of ramps no greater than 1:12? **Slope is given as ratio of the height to the length.** 1:12 means for every 12 inches along the base of the ramp, the height increases one inch. For a 1:12 maximum slope, **at least** one foot of ramp length is needed for each inch of height.	slope = _____			☐ Lengthen ramp to decrease slope. ☐ Relocate ramp. ☐ If available space is limited, reconfigure ramp to include switchbacks.
Do all ramps longer than 6 feet have railings on both sides?				☐ Add railings.
Are railings sturdy, and between 34 and 38 inches high?	height = _____			☐ Adjust height of railing if not between 34 and 38 inches. ☐ Secure handrails in fixtures.
Is the width between railings or curbs at least 36 inches?	width = _____			☐ Relocate the railings. ☐ Widen the ramp.
Are ramps non-slip?				☐ Add non-slip surface material.
Is there a 5-foot-long level standing at every 30-foot horizontal length of ramp, at the top and bottom of ramps and at switchbacks?	length = _____			☐ Remodel or relocate ramp.
Does the ramp rise no more than 30 inches between landings?	rise = _____			☐ Remodel or relocate ramp.

Figure 10-3 Requirements for an accessible approach ramp to a building. (Adapted from Adaptive Environments Center. [1995]. Americans with disabilities Act checklist for readily achievable barrier removal. Boston: Adaptive Environments Center. Retrieved August 23, 2011 from http://www.ada.gov/checkweb.htm.)

personal factors and the characteristics of the environment and the occupation. The PEO relationship is dynamic, complex, and interwoven and therefore more difficult to measure than interactions that can be understood by assessing discrete components. Because very few measures have been developed to assess this complex PEO relationship, we have included not only the measures in this chapter but also an array of useful tools that measure the person–environment relationship or specific characteristics of the environment.

In this chapter, the assessments have been categorized by setting: those suitable for assessing homes (Assessment Table 10-1), the community (Assessment Table 10-2), and the workplace (Assessment Table 10-3). Key information about each assessment, including an analysis of the tool's strengths and weaknesses, is included in the tables to assist occupational therapists to identify the most appropriate tool(s) for their purposes. The critique of each tool was guided by using the Outcomes Measures Rating Form and Guidelines (Law, 2004). Most tools included here have established measurement properties. We have, however, included some unique measures that have good content validity and clinical use but for which formal studies of measurement properties are unavailable or incomplete.

Assessment of Access to Home

A home assessment completed by an occupational therapist can be an important component of the occupational therapy process, particularly during the discharge planning process for clients going home from a hospital or rehabilitation setting. Assessment of occupational performance in the client's home is contextually relevant (Ngyard et al., 2004). In a study comparing assessment results among home, client, or proxy report and clinic-based performance assessment, Rogers et al. (2003) found that home-based performance assessment provides an accurate reflection of the clients' ability to manage in that setting, which cannot be replaced by self-report, caregiver proxy, or clinic-based performance assessments. During a home assessment, therapists can assess the degree of fit for the person, the completion of his or her daily roles, and the home environment. This individualized approach is critically important, because the factors influencing PEO fit will vary across health conditions and disabilities. For example, the nature of safety and accessibility issues in the home will be quite different for a person with Alzheimer's disease compared with a person with a spinal cord injury. Thus, therapists can identify barriers to participation and recommend modifications to the environment that ensure optimal independence and safety for each individual client.

Ensuring that clients' home environments are able to provide them with the supports they need is vitally important to enable them to continue living safely at home. Also critical is that therapists recognize that people have great attachment to their home. Both their belongings and the way their home looks are meaningful for them (Cristoforetti,

Gennai, & Rodeschini, 2011). Although the therapist may see specific features as barriers and hindrances to occupational performance and safety, the client may have a different view about the significance of those features. Thus, therapists should demonstrate sensitivity to their clients' perspectives about their homes during home assessments.

Several standardized home assessments are available for occupational therapists to use with clients and families to identify occupational performance problems in the home and environmental barriers and potential resources. Researchers have discussed the limited use of standardized home assessments by occupational therapists (Mitchell & Unsworth, 2004). In clinical practice, where service provision needs to be justified, the use of standardized home assessments can be important to ensure that a comprehensive assessment is completed both to meet the needs of the client and to justify requests for equipment and home modifications. A review of assessment tools to guide home adaptations (Rousseau et al., 2001) presented information on 16 assessments; however, only 6 of those tools included evidence for their measurement properties. Although some home assessments focus almost exclusively on the physical environment (e.g., accessibility and home hazards), a number are now available that take into consideration such factors as personal preferences for environmental resources, social supports provided by caregivers, and caregiver attitudes.

Home assessments typically involve the examination of PEO fit for a client within his or her home environment and recommendations related to home modifications and suggestions for environmental supports. The Housing Enabler (Slaug & Iwarsson, 2001) addresses environmental factors explicitly in relation to clients' needs and abilities. It includes separate components that first address the client's abilities and disabilities and then examines the home environment in relation to these factors. It is administered through an interview and observations of the physical environment. The Home Falls and Accidents Screening Tool (HOME FAST) (Mackenzie, Byles, & Higginbotham, 2000), the In-Home Occupational Performance Evaluation (I-HOPE) (Stark, Somerville, & Morris, 2010), the SAFER-HOME (Chiu & Oliver, 2006), and the Westmead Home Safety Assessment (Clemson, 1997) are also useful tools that require clinicians to integrate information about the client's abilities with observations about the environment. For example, when using the SAFER-HOME to determine the extent to which an item such as toileting is a problem, the therapist must consider the client's ability to safely transfer onto and use the toilet while simultaneously considering the availability of physical supports (such as grab bars) and social supports (family caregiver assistance), as well as how willing the client is to make use of the supports available (Fig. 10-4 is an example of the SAFER-HOME tool). The Home Safety

(text continued on page 327)

Assessment Table 10-1   Access to Home Assessments

Assessment	Description	Time to Administer	Validity[b]	Reliability[b]	Sensitivity[c]	Strengths and Weaknesses
The Housing Enabler (Slaug & Iwarsson, 2001) Ordering and pricing information available from: http://www.enabler.nu/index.html	Questionnaire to assess the congruence or fit between an individual with a functional impairment and his or her home environment. Measures functional limitations (15 items) and physical environmental barriers (188 items). Available in several languages. Scoring level: Dichotomous ratings for steps 1 and 2; step 3 ordinal scale (4-point predetermined Likert scale). Summary scores are best calculated with the use of The Housing Enabler Software. Range of scores: Dependent on the number of functional limitations, use of mobility aids, and the number of environmental barriers.	Up to 2 hours, depending on functional limitations and physical environment. In particular, step 2 can be time consuming to administer because 188 environmental items are reviewed.	Content: Item selection based on literature review and expert opinion; adjusted after pilot studies. Convergent: Swedish accessible housing standards provide the gold standard against which the environmental assessments are measured. Construct: Established theoretical agreement for person–environment relationship and for construct of housing accessibility. References: Fange & Iwarsson, 2003; Iwarsson & Isacsson, 1998; Iwarsson, Isacsson, & Lanke, 1998.	Interrater: Studies report excellent results ranging from 81% to 100% agreement; pilot 2 ($n = 440$ occupational therapists, 26 cases) overall mean $\kappa = 0.76$ for person and 0.55 for environment; pilot 3 ($n = 430$ occupational therapists, 30 cases) mean $\kappa = 0.82$ for person, 0.68 for environment (188 items), and 0.87 for accessibility problems; interclass correlation coefficient (ICC) range = 0.92–0.98. A multinational study with raters with different professional backgrounds ($n = 64$) resulted in moderate to good overall interrater reliability; sample of 422 housing adaptation cases, mean $\kappa = 0.62$ (good interrater reliability). Test-retest: Strong; ICC = 0.92–0.98. References: Fange, Risser, & Iwarsson, 2007; Iwarsson & Isacsson, 1998; Iwarsson, Nygren & Slaug, 2005.	In two separate studies, person–environment fit scores captured significant differences between baseline and follow-up by means of the Sign and McNemar's tests, respectively (Fange & Iwarsson, 2003; Iwarsson, 2005).	Strengths: Meticulous development and testing. Up-to-date website. Widely used in Europe. Step 3 provides a predictive score of accessibility problems and measure of handicap. Useful for both clinical and research purposes. Weaknesses: Rater training more difficult to arrange outside Europe. Step 2 can be time consuming to administer.

Home Falls and Accidents Screening Tool (HOME FAST) (Mackenzie, Byles, & Higginbotham, 2000). The appendix of the article includes all items of the HOME FAST along with definitions.	20–30 minutes	Health care provider completed questionnaire; designed to identify risk of falls as a result of home hazards, may be used as an outcome measure to evaluate interventions for improving function in the home environment. Scoring level: Nominal (items are scored as a hazard, not a hazard, or not applicable). Range of scores: 0–25 (indicating the number of items for which hazards are identified).	Content: Based on the literature, field testing with 83 older adults; review of content and field testing data by an expert panel reduced number of items; content further examined in a cross-national validation (Australia, Canada, and United Kingdom) where occupational therapists, physiotherapists, and nurses responded to a survey regarding the content and weighting of items. Construct: Initial evidence suggests that the *HOME FAST* may be useful in identifying relative risk for falls associated with exposure to home hazards (99% confidence intervals). Predictive: Longitudinal study (*n* = 727, community dwelling veterans) suggests HOME FAST may predict falls in older adults Responsiveness: Initial data (*n* = 727) HOME FAST items can identify change in home hazards over time. References: Mackenzie, Byles, & D'Este, 2009; Mackenzie, Byles, & Higginbotham, 2000, 2002a.	Interrater: Evaluated (*n* = 40) using κ for individual items and weighted κ for the total number of hazards; overall weighted κ was 0.56 (considered fair to good agreement); κ values for individual items indicated that 4 items had excellent reliability, 20 items had fair to good reliability, and 1 item (hazardous outside paths) had poor reliability (Mackenzie, Byles, & Higginbotham, 2002b).	Sensitivity shown by comparison of expert ratings and second ratings of home hazards; 68.6% agreement (95% confidence interval [CI] 63·4–73·6) (*n* = 844 sample ratings) (Mackenzie, Byles, & Higginbotham, 2002b). Strengths: Can be quickly administered as a screening assessment. Research has been conducted in various countries. Initial psychometric research is positive. Initial evidence suggests the HOME FAST may potentially be useful as an outcome measure. Weakness: Further examination of the predictive validity, responsiveness, and test–retest reliability would strengthen our understanding of the measure.

(continued)

| Assessment Table 10-1 | Access to Home Assessments (continued) |

Assessment	Description	Time to Administer	Validity[a]	Reliability[b]	Sensitivity[c]	Strengths and Weaknesses
Safety Assessment of Function and the Environment for Rehabilitation-Health Outcome Measurement (SAFER-HOME V3) (Chiu et al., 2006) VHA Rehab Solutions 477 Mount Pleasant Road, Suite 500, Toronto, Ontario M4S 2L9, Canada Phone: 416-489-753 E-mail: info@vha.ca Order form can be downloaded from http://www.vha.ca/SaferHome OrderForm.pdf	SAFER-HOME based on SAFER tool: Designed to measure intervention effectiveness and changes in safety intervention over time (12 domains: living situation; mobility; environmental hazards; kitchen; household; eating; personal care; bathroom and toilet; medication, addiction, and abuse; leisure; communication and scheduling; and wandering). Scoring level: SAFER-HOME – Ordinal (4-point rating scale [0 – 3]: No problem, mild problem, moderate problem, severe problem) Range of scores: SAFER-HOME: 0–228.	45–90 minutes	Content: For both the SAFER and the SAFER-HOME content validity has been established through review by experts and clinicians as well as statistical analysis of completed measures. Construct: For SAFER, total scores have been associated with cognitive status and independent living in houses, but not directly to ADL or instrumental ADL. For SAFER HOME, total scores were compared to functional status scores; Cronbach's α coefficient = 0.26 (weak correlation) confirmed that the SAFER HOME is measuring more than functional abilities. References: Chui & Oliver, 2006; Letts et al., 1998.	SAFER - Interrater: κ or percentage of agreement: Acceptable to excellent for 92 items. Test-retest: κ or percentage of agreement: Acceptable to excellent for 90 items. References: Letts et al., 1998. SAFER-HOME - Internal consistency: Cronbach's α for total scores = 0.8593; subscales ranged from 0.539 to 0.789 References: Chui & Oliver, 2006.	No formal studies have directly examined sensitivity to detect change; preliminary investigations show promising results; occupational therapists (n = 95) administered the SAFER-HOME V1 twice; 76% indicated the assessment measured changes in the client (Chui & Oliver, 2006).	Strengths: Comprehensive coverage of home safety. Both tools developed and tested rigorously. Comprehensive training manual provided. Weaknesses: Length of administration may be problematic in some clinical situations. Further research on responsiveness to change needed.

Instrument	Description	Time	Validity[a]	Reliability[b]	Sensitivity to Change[c]	Strengths/Weaknesses
Westmead Home Safety Assessment Co-ordinates Publications, a division of Co-ordinates Therapy Services Pty. Ltd., P.O. Box 59, West Brunswick, Victoria 3055, Australia Phone: 6139-380-1127 Fax: 6139-387-4829 http://www.therapybookshop.com/coordinates.html	Assessment to identify fall hazards in the home environments of older adults. Scoring level: Nominal (dichotomized relevant or not; each relevant item is rated as a hazard or not; hazards are presented by type).	One home visit	Content: Established through content analysis of the literature and a rigorous expert review process (Clemson, Fitzgerald, & Heard, 1999). Criterion: Not established (as no gold standard exists).	Interrater: Tested in a sample of 21 clients' homes; κ values of >0.75 for 34 items and between 0.4 and 0.75 for 31 items; κ could not be calculated for some items (Clemson et al., 1999).	Not established	Strengths: Comprehensive and systematic assessment of home hazards specific to falls in older adults. Manual is helpful and provides operational definitions for key hazards. Weaknesses: Does not address home hazards besides falls; further psychometric testing required.
The Safe Living Guide: A Home Hazard Checklist for Seniors (Public Health Agency of Canada, 2007; http://www.phac-aspc.gc.ca/seniors-aines/alt-formats/pdf/publications/public/injury-blessure/safelive-securite/safelive-securite-eng.pdf)	Self-completed questionnaire; designed to identify potentially hazardous areas in the home. Scoring level: Dichotomous (yes/no checklist).	20–30 minutes	Content: Items identified using literature review, consultation with seniors, seniors' agencies, and professionals. References: Clark, Shaw, & Kahn, 2002; Sorcinelli et al., 2007.	Interrater: Average κ between expert raters (n = 76) = 0.73 (substantial agreement); average κ between expert raters and seniors (n = 76) = 0.51 (moderate agreement) References: Sorcinelli et al., 2007.	Not established	Strengths: Captures the client's perspective on hazardous areas. Manual is comprehensive; provides operational definitions for key terms. Weakness: Limited evidence of measurement properties.

n, number; κ, kappa; α, alpha

[a] Validity is the ability of an instrument to measure what it is intended and presumed to measure. Criterion validity is determined by comparing its results to an agreed-on *gold standard* (accepted test). Predictive validity is its ability to predict future outcomes.

[b] Reliability is a measure of an instrument's stability. Interobserver or interrater reliability refers to the ability of two different individuals to administer the instrument to a particular person and achieve similar results. Test-retest reliability refers to the constancy of results over repeated use of the instrument in the absence of change in the patient.

[c] Sensitivity to change is the ability of an instrument to detect clinically important changes.

Assessment Table 10-2 Access to Community Assessments

Assessment	Description	Time to Administer	Validity	Reliability	Sensitivity	Strengths and Weaknesses
Craig Hospital Inventory of Environmental Factors (CHIEF and CHIEF Short Form)	Assessment of the frequency and magnitude of environmental characteristics that act to impede accomplishment of daily activities and social roles. Five categories: attitude and support, services and assistance, physical and structural, policy, and work and school.	Self-administered: 10 minutes; short form, 5 minutes. Interviewer administered: 15 minutes; short form, 10 minutes	Content: Established by literature review and consultation with experts. Four advisory panels involved.	Internal consistency: Moderate to high ratings for total score (0.93) and subscales (ranging from 0.76 to 0.81).	The authors recommend that multiple measurements using CHIEF be taken over the course of a person's lifetime to assess changes with adaptation to the disability and to gain insight into changes in environmental barriers that may occur over time.	Strengths: Based on ICF. Comprehensive inventory of environmental factors. Quick and easy to administer and score.
The Centre for Outcome Measurement in Brain Injury at Craig Hospital: http://tbims.org/combi/chief/ http://www.tbims.org/combi/chief/CHIEF.pdf	Self-administered or administered by interview. Full CHIEF: 25 items. Short form: 12 items.		Construct: Shows differences in reported frequency and magnitude of environmental barriers between groups with different impairments and activity limitations (e.g., Whiteneck, Gerhart & Cusick, 2004; Whiteneck et al., 2004). Discriminitive: Established with persons with polio (Lund & Lexell, 2009)	Authors recommend that proxies should not be used to complete CHIEF. Test-retest: Showed an overall inter-class correlation (ICC) of 0.92 for total score, and ICCs for individual items ranged from 0.33– to 0.88 (Whiteneck et al., 2004).	Sensitivity to change shown in scores for sample of persons living with AIDS (Nichols et al., 2009)	Appropriate for both population-based or individual-focused assessment and research. Weaknesses: Further evaluation of measurement properties needed. Scale for assessing magnitude of barriers has only two points (little vs. big problem).

Instrument	Description	Time	Reliability	Validity	Strengths/Weaknesses
Facilitators and Barriers Survey/ Mobility (FABS/M) (Gray et al., 2008)	A self-report survey of environmental facilitators and barriers to participation by people with mobility impairments (e.g., stroke, cerebral palsy, polio, and spinal cord injury). 133 items in six domains: personal mobility device, home built features, community built and natural features, community destinations access, community facilities access, and attitudes.	40–60 minutes	Internal Consistency: (n = 604 people with mobility impairments from five diagnostic groups; a range of mobility devices used) ranged from low to high internal consistency across the domains (moderate to high for community destinations and facilities). Test–retest: With same sample; showed moderate to high reliability across the domains (Gray et al., 2008).	Not established	Content: Established through interviews and 15 focus groups; 5 with persons with various mobility impairments (5 diagnostic groups), 5 with significant others from the first 5 groups, and 5 with health professions serving various diagnostic groups. The qualitative data formed the content for the FABS/M. Discriminative: Able to distinguish differences between different diagnostic and device user groups (Gray et al., 2008).	Strengths: Designed specifically for people with lower limb impairments and mobility impairments. Used at the individual level to develop community participation interventions. Can be used as an outcome measure of the effectiveness of those interventions. Scores can be aggregated across diagnostic groups and/or mobility device groups for broader view of environmental factors influencing participation. Weaknesses: Only applicable to targeted diagnostic groups. Further measurement studies needed.

(continued)

Assessment Table 10-2 Access to Community Assessments (continued)

Assessment	Description	Time to Administer	Validity	Reliability	Sensitivity	Strengths and Weaknesses
Measure of Quality of the Environment (MQE) Version 2 Long version: 84 items Short version: 26 items (Fougeyrollas et al., 2008; RIPPH/INDCP 525, boul. Wilfrid-Hamel Est, A-08 Québec (Québec) Canada G1M 2S8 (http://www.ripph.qc.ca/?rub2=4&rub=18&lang=en).	Measures environmental facilitators and obstacles to social participation and accomplishment of daily activities (7-point scale from major facilitator to major obstacle). Six categories: Support and attitudes of family, job and income security, government and public services, physical environment and accessibility, technology, and equal opportunity and political orientations. Interview format.	Long version, less than 30 minutes Short version, less than 10 minutes	Content: Based conceptually on the Disability Creation Process model and input from individuals with spinal cord injury and clinicians (Fougeyrollas, Noreau, & Boschen, 2002). Construct: Has been demonstrated (Noreau, Fougeyrollas & Boschen, 2002).	Internal consistency: Moderate concordance scores across items. Test-retest: Good (Boschen, Noreau & Fougeyrollas, 1998).	Not established	Strengths: Applicable for people with and without disabilities. It covers a broad scope of environmental factors. Manual with questionnaire and score sheets available. Tool is easy to administer. Used at the individual level; can be applied at population level. Some evidence of validity and reliability. Weakness: Further examination of measurement properties is recommended.
The Multidimensional Scale of Perceived Social Support (MSPSS) (Zimet et al., 1988)	Assessment of perceptions of social support from three sources: family, friends, and significant other. Inventory/list of 12 statements of relationships; each item rated on 7-point Likert scale.	2–5 minutes	Content: Established through factor analysis. Construct: Established through multiple studies with numerous health constructs, psychopathology, suicidal behavior, anxiety, and depression. Marginalized groups demonstrate lower perceived social support.	Internal consistency: Good with Cronbach's α's ranging from 0.81 to 0.91 in multiple studies. Test-retest: in study with undergraduate psychology students, good for total score (0.85) and subscales (0.72, 0.85, and 0.75) (Zimet et al., 1988). Good reliability shown in study with older adults (Stanley, Beck, & Zebb, 1998).	Not established	Strengths: Simple to use and score in a short time. Has been used primarily with mental health populations; appears to have use for populations with physical disability. Weaknesses: Need to be wary of socially desirable responses. Requires evaluation of sensitivity to change and use as an outcome measure.

Assessment Table 10-3 | Access to Workplace Assessments

Assessment	Description	Time to Administer	Validity	Reliability	Sensitivity	Strengths and Weaknesses
Checklist of Health Promotion Environments at Worksites (CHEW) (Oldenburg et al., 2002); contact Sallis, J. Department of Psychology, San Diego State University. 6363 Alvarado Court, #103 San Diego, CA 92120 USA. (http://www .drjamessallis.sdsu .edu/measures.html)	An observational measure of environments (in and around work sites); designed to assess environmental influences on health behaviors and evaluate health promotion programs. Scoring level: Separate scores computed for each content areas (physical, information, neighborhood, and surroundings); summary scores are computed for physical and information domains.	20–50 minutes; administration time can vary according to size of work site	Construct: Items selected based on multiple revisions from focus group consultation and pilot testing at 20 work sites (Oldenburg et al., 2002).	Interrater: ICC = 0.80–1.00 (n = 2, tested at 12 work sites) (Oldenburg et al., 2002).	Not established	Strengths: Can be used to assess changes over time in health-promoting environment characteristics. Manual with procedures and scoring key provided at no cost. Weaknesses: Further testing of measurement properties would strengthen our understanding of the measure.
Environmental Assessment Tool (EAT) (DeJoy et al., 2008) Department of Health Promotion & Behavior, College of Public Health, University of Georgia, Athens, GA 30602-6522 dmdejoy@uga.edu The appendix of the article (articleplus version) includes a copy of the measure.	Observation-based assessment; designed to measure work site physical, social, and institutional environment supports that may influence healthy behaviors and capture change across time. Scoring level: dichotomous (yes/no responses). Scores: Range from 0 to 100 points (divided among three subscales); scores weighted within each subscale.	Variable with work site	Content: Items selected based on literature review, contextual analysis of work environments, pilot testing, multiple revisions; weighted scoring values decided by field experts. Concurrent: Agreement with the Leading by Example questionnaire Predictive: Captured changes in workplace environments over time (n = 12). References: Baker Parker et al., 2010; DeJoy et al, 2008.	Inter-rater: Agreement ranged from 83% to 100% across 2 raters for 12 work sites (κ scores for individual items ranged from 0.56–1.00) (DeJoy et al., 2008).	Changes in EAT scores shown over time and across work sites (n = 12) for one of three subscales (Baker Parker et al., 2010)	Strengths: A more inclusive measure (incorporates the social/administrative environments). Initial evidence supports its use as a quantitative measure to track changes over time. Weakness: A more extensive manual and testing measurement properties would strengthen our understanding of the measure.

(continued)

Assessment Table 10-3 | Access to Workplace Assessments (continued)

Assessment	Description	Time to Administer	Validity	Reliability	Sensitivity	Strengths and Weaknesses
Work Environment Scale (WES) Version 4 (Moos & Insel, 2008) Mind Garden, 855 Oak Grove Avenue, Suite 215, Menlo Park, CA 94025 U.S.A. Phone: 650-322-6300 Fax: 650-322-6398 Available from: http://www.mindgarden.com/products/wes.htm#ms	Measures the social environment of all types of work settings. It comprises 10 subscales or dimensions, which are divided into three sets: the relationship dimensions, the personal growth or goal orientation dimensions, and the system maintenance and system change dimensions. For evaluation of productivity, employee satisfaction, employee expectations, and programs.	15–20 minutes per form; 5–10 minutes to score	Face: Established in manual; tools based on social climate scales. Multiple studies demonstrate construct validity. References: Moos & Insel, 2008; Staten et al., 2003	Test-retest: At 1 month, Cronbach's α coefficients = 0.69–0.83; at 12 months, test-retest coefficients = 0.51–0.63; intraclass coefficients >0.70. Internal consistency: Pearson $r > 0.60$. Reference: Moos, 1994.	Not established	Strengths: Standardized; established measurement properties; readily available, portable. Promotes discussion and identifies clients' views. Useful on an individual basis, groups, or with organizations. Weaknesses: Scores alone should not provide direction for intervention. Need further study with populations with physical disability.
Work Experience Survey (Roessler & Gottcent 1994; Roessler, 1996) Available from the National Clearinghouse of Rehabilitation Training Materials http://library.ncrtm.org/pdf/193.054A.pdf	Interview used to identify job accommodation needs (work site accessibility, performance of essential functions, job mastery and job satisfaction).	30–60 minutes	Face: Based on relevant tools and sources of information (Roessler & Gottcent, 1994) Has been used across groups of clients with a range of diagnoses (i.e., MS, blindness, diabetes, arthritis) and frequently cited as a valid tool, although specific psychometric data could not be located.	Cronbach's α values for assessing job mastery and assessing job satisfaction reported as 0.74 and 0.78, respectively, in one study (Roessler, 1996).	Not established	Strengths: Facilitates identification of barriers and reasonable accommodations. Assists in empowering clients to address work barriers with employers. Has been used with individuals with a variety of disabilities. Weaknesses: Need to look at use of WES in follow-up interviews. Additional measurement data required.

Workplace Environment Impact Scale (WEIS) V. 2.0 (Moore-Corner, Kielhofner, & Olson, 1998). Model of Human Occupation Clearinghouse, University of Illinois at Chicago www.moho.uic.edu/ Order form available from: http://www .moho.uic.edu/assess/ weis.html	Semistructured interview; addresses individuals' experiences and perceptions of their work environments. Designed for use with individuals with physical or psychosocial disabilities; for use with individuals who are employed or are planning to return to work after an interruption in employment (caused by injury/illness). Scoring level: 4-point ordinal scales (17 items).	30–45 minutes to conduct interview (depending on interviewer's abilities and the client) 15 minutes to complete scoring	Construct: Established (based on Rasch analysis in which infit MnSq = 1.6 and Zstd = 3.0). Found to measure a single construct (none of seventeen items fit criteria for misfit) Found to be valid across two distinct cultures. References: Corner, Kielhofner, & Lin, 1997; Kielhofner et al., 1998.	Rasch analysis: Item separation statistic was 2.77 (reliability of 0.88); items were consistently separated into distinct (nonoverlapping) groups. Found to lack ability to discriminate groups in another study, although population was found to be homogeneous. References: Corner, Kielhofner, & Lin, 1997; Kielhofner et al., 1998.	Kielhofner et al. (1998) report that this scale can separate and group subjects into many levels of psychosocial ability to return to work.	Strengths: Items work well to measure the construct of work environment impact. The scale is suitably matched to the clients and effectively discriminates different levels of work environment. Both Swedish and English language versions of the WEIS are equal and free of cultural bias. Manual includes suggested questions. Weaknesses: Need to be very familiar with interview and scale to ensure appropriate use.

(continued)

Assessment Table 10-3 Access to Workplace Assessments (*continued*)

Assessment	Description	Time to Administer	Validity	Reliability	Sensitivity	Strengths and Weaknesses
Worker Role Interview V. 10.0 (WRI) (Braveman et al., 2005) Order form available from: http://www.uic.edu/depts/moho/assess/wri.html Model of Human Occupation Clearinghouse, University of Illinois, Chicago, Department of Occupational Therapy Phone: 800-377-8555	Semistructured interview; designed to identify potential barriers that will interfere with return to work. Scoring level: 4-point ordinal scale (17 content areas).	40–60 minutes	Content: Item selection based on literature review, expert clinical input, extensive pilot testing from multiple studies and multiple revisions. Construct: in agreement with the Model of Human Occupation's conceptualization of behavior; Rasch analysis (n = 119) results separate participants into different levels of ability. Predictive: (n = 53; 24-month period), overall correct prediction = 81%–96% Internal: Thirteen of 17 content areas demonstrate acceptable fit in Rasch measurement model (n = 440) References: Ekbladh, Thorell, & Haglund, 2010; Forsyth et al., 2006; Velozo et al., 1999.	Interrater: ICC = 0.46–0.92 (n = 30). Test–retest: High reliability (ICC = 0.86–0.94; n = 20) Reference: Biernacki, 1993.	Scale items significantly separated the potential of clients (n = 146) of differing psychosocial ability to return to work into three distinct levels; however, a "ceiling effect" was observed (21% of measured ability) (Fenger & Kramer, 2007).	Strengths: Comprehensive manual and training videotape with case example available. Reliability and validity testing across multiple populations and cultures. Translated into multiple languages. Weakness: Further testing of measurement properties within populations with chronic disability needed.

MnSq, mean square, a measure of "item fit" in a Rasch Model; Zstd, standardized z value, another "item fit" statistic in a Rasch Model.

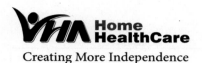

Creating More Independence

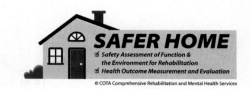

Client Name: Mrs. P.

Date of Assessment: Nov. 3, 2011

Type of housing: **x** Apartment
___ House
___ Other

No identified problem	Following observation, interview and/or task performance, no safety concern was identified at time of assessment, including not applicable items.
Mild problem	When an identified safety concern has never been a problem and is unlikely to be so in the future. (1% - 33% chance of negative consequences)
Moderate problem	A safety problem that needs to be addressed but is not likely to cause immediate danger to the client and/or the environment. (34% - 66% chance of negative consequences)
Severe problem	When a safety problem requires urgent attention or when it could put the client, others or their environment in immediate danger. (67% - 100% chance of negative consequences)

		No	Mild	Moderate	Severe	COMMENTS
LIVING SITUATION (3)						
1	Security & screen /admit visitors		x			Unable to answer door when husband away
2	Living conditions/occupants	a				Lives with husband.
3	Availability/quality of support	a				Daughter lives nearby – very supportive.
	Total	2	1			
MOBILITY (10)						
4	Walking/devices		x			Uses a quad cane & supervision with walking
5	Wheelchair/scooter/transfers				x	Sometimes forgets to put brakes on wheelchair during transfers.
6	Chair/bed transfers		x			
7	Positioning/repositioning	a				
8	Accessibility of entrances	a				Level entrance to suite
9	Indoor stairs/ramps/railings	a				
10	Outdoor stairs/ramps/railings		x			Small rise at front entrance to building
11	Venturing outdoors	a				Husband drives.
12	Public/accessible transportation				x	No disabled persons parking permit.
13	Vehicle/driving/transfers	a				License under medical suspension.

Figure 10-4 Home assessment using the SAFER tool. This example relates to the case study of Mrs. P. (Reprinted with permission from Chiu, T., Oliver, R., Ascott, P., Choo, L., Davis, T., Gaya, A., Goldsilver, P., McWhirter, M., & Letts, L. [2006]. *Safety assessment of function and the environment for rehabilitation: Health outcome measurement and evaluation (SAFER-HOME) version 3 manual.* Toronto, Canada: VHA Rehab Solutions.)

		No	Mild	Moderate	Severe	COMMENTS
	Total	5	3	2		
ENVIRONMENTAL HAZARDS (13)						
14	Clutter				x	Hallway rug – corners curled.
15	Electric blanket/heating pad	a				
16	Electrical wiring/plugs/outlets	a				
17	Fire exit	a				
18	Furnace/heater/fireplace	a				
19	Infestation/unhygienic conditions	a				
20	Lighting/night lights				x	No night light.
21	Pets	a				
22	Scatter rugs/flooring	a				
23	Smoke/carbon monoxide detectors				x	No batteries in smoke detector. No carbon monoxide detector.
24	Smoking/candles/signs of burns	a				
25	Storage of dangerous substances	a				
26	Trailing wires/cords	a				
	Total	10			3	
KITCHEN (8)						
27	Kettle - manual/electric/auto-off	a				
28	Toaster/small appliances	a				
29	Microwave	a				
30	Stove - gas/electric				x	Has forgotten to turn off stove 2 times
31	Storage - accessible/safe	a				(and has turned on wrong element 3 times).
32	Knives/scissors - storage/use	a				
33	Food supply/storage	a				Husband cooks.
34	Garbage storage/disposal	a				
	Total	7			1	
HOUSEHOLD (9)						
35	Hot drink preparation				x	Spilled hot tea & soup on self on 2 occasions.
36	Meal preparation	a				
37	Carrying drinks/meals				x	Not safe carrying drinks/meals.
38	Bed making	a				
39	Cleaning	a				Husband/daughter does cleaning.
40	Laundry/ironing	a				Husband/daughter does laundry.

Figure 10-4 (Continued)

		No	Mild	Moderate	Severe	COMMENTS
41	Indoor/outdoor maintenance	a				Daughter shops for them.
42	Shopping	a				
43	Money management	a				Husband manages money – Mrs. P. satisfied with this arrangement.
	Total	7			2	

EATING (2)

		No	Mild	Moderate	Severe	COMMENTS
44.	Feeding/swallowing	a				
45.	Nutrition	a				
	Total	2				

PERSONAL CARE (8)

		No	Mild	Moderate	Severe	COMMENTS
46	Dress/undress		x			Mr. P. provides minimal assistance for dressing – safe & comfortable with this.
47	Appropriate clothing	a				
48	Appropriate footwear		x			If uses slippers for transfers/walking
49	Hair care	a				Not currently using curling iron due to left arm paralysis.
50	Nail care	a				
51	Oral hygiene	a				
52	Shaving	a				
53	Feminine hygiene	a				
	Total	6	2			

BATHROOM & TOILET (11)

		No	Mild	Moderate	Severe	COMMENTS
54	Bath/shower method	a				Moderate assistance provided by husband for bathing – no concerns.
55	Bath/shower transfers	a				
56	Seating equipment	a				Uses bath bench
57	Bath/shower grab bars			x		Sometimes forgets to use grab bars
58	Non-slip aids				x	No non-skid aid.
59	Bladder/bowel continence	a				
60	Toileting method	a				
61	Toileting transfers			x		Difficulty getting up from toilet.
62	Raised toilet seat				x	No aid on toilet.
63	Toilet grab bar/safety frame				x	
64	Lock/unlock door				x	No emergency unlocking mechanism for door.

Figure 10-4 *(Continued)*

		No	Mild	Moderate	Severe	COMMENTS
	Total	5		2	4	

MEDICATION, ADDICTION & ABUSE (3)						
65	Prescribed/non-prescribed drugs			x		Mr. P. reminds Mrs. P. regularly to take medication.
66	Addictive behaviour	a				
67	Abuse of client/self/others	a				
	Total	2		1		

LEISURE (1)						
68	Hobby safety/tools/method	a				
	Total	1				

COMMUNICATION & SCHEDULING (3)						
69	Telephone use/emergency no.				x	Not posted.
70	Ability to tell time				x	Complains of visual problems. Not checked in 6 years. Problems reading.
71	Ability to schedule				x	Doesn't use memory aids; forgets appointments.
	Total				3	

WANDERING (3)						
72	Supervision	a				
73	Environment	a				
74	Wandering Registry/return plan				x	No personal emergency response system.
	Total	2			1	

SAFER-HOME Summary Table

Categories (Number of items)	Number of safety problems			
	No	Mild	Moderate	Severe
Living situation (3)	2	1		
Mobility (10)	5	3	2	
Environmental Hazards (13)	10			3
Kitchen (8)	7			1
Household (9)	7			2
Eating (2)	2			
Personal Care (8)	6	2		
Bathroom & Toilet (11)	5		2	4
Medication, Addiction & Abuse (3)	2		1	
Leisure (1)	1			
Communication & Scheduling (3)				3
Wandering (3)	2			1
Total	**6**	**5**	**14**	
	X 1	X 2	X 3	
Weighted Score	= 6	= 10	= 42	

SAFER-HOME score = 58

Summary

Susan Smith, OT Reg (Ont.)	Susan Smith	11/03/11
Occupational Therapist's signature & designation	Occupational Therapist's name (Please print)	Date (mm/dd/yy)

Figure 10-4 *(Continued)*

Self Assessment Tool (HSSAT) Version 3 is a promising new assessment designed to identify home hazards and reduce the occurrence of falls and is available from the authors' website (Tomita et al., 2011). Evaluation of the measurement properties of this tool is currently underway. The I-HOPE is also a promising new performance-based assessment of activities that a client finds challenging to perform at home and includes ratings of environmental barriers that influence performance (Stark, Somerville, & Morris, 2010).

Ideally, all of these assessments should be conducted in the client's home. However, in clinical settings where it is not possible to visit the home, the occupational therapist may choose to conduct an interview using the items of the SAFER-HOME with the client and/or a family member or friend selected by the client who knows the client's home well. However, the interview cannot definitively determine whether or not a client can manage safely at home or what modifications may be needed. Rather, it can be used to highlight issues that clients and/or caregivers need to consider in the home. Other very good options include self-assessment guides to home adaptation, which can be used in collaboration with a client (e.g., *Maintaining Seniors' Independence: A Guide to Home Adaptations* [Canadian Mortgage and Housing Corporation, 1989/2008a], *Maintaining Seniors' Independence through Home Adaptation: A Self-assessment Guide* [Canadian Mortgage and Housing Corporation, 2008b], and *A Consumer's Guide to Home Adaptation* [Adaptive Environments Center, 2002]). These tools provide practical suggestions for home adaptations in relation to functional problems, such as difficulty entering the shower stall/bathtub, as shown in Figure 10-5. The therapist helps the client to select solutions that best fit his or her situation (see overview of home assessments in Assessment Table 10-1). Figure 10-6 shows an example of the Functional Independence Measure (FIM™), which can help assess a client's abilities.

Home Safety and Fall Prevention

A home assessment, such as those described above, can also provide occupational therapists and their clients with specific details to enable the prevention of injuries resulting from home hazards or unsafe practices. Research on the effectiveness of home assessments to prevent falls in older adults demonstrates that home assessments reduce the risk of falls, especially in people who have a history of past falls (Pighills et al., 2011). There is considerable research evidence that shows the effectiveness of home environmental interventions for the prevention of falls in older adults, particularly those who are at high risk for falls (e.g., people who had been hospitalized for a fall and those who showed functional decline) (Clemson et al., 2008; Gillespie et al., 2009). The consequences of falls have been well established and can include long-term

disability and the need for long-term care, loss of confidence, depression, social isolation, and even premature death. Thus, the role of OT to address home safety and fall prevention is of critical importance.

Housing Options

Housing options can also be reviewed with home assessments to determine the best fit for the client. Options are numerous, and most communities have innovative, barrier-free housing with access to attendant care and other support services, meals, and recreation. Many seniors and persons with severe physical disabilities choose to live in these housing projects because they can more easily achieve independence within the supportive system. Transitional housing programs also assist clients to cultivate both independent living skills and knowledge of available resources. The occupational therapist can use assessment tools such as The Housing Enabler (Slaug & Iwarsson, 2001) to evaluate the need or probable benefit of such solutions.

The U.S. Office of Fair Housing and Equal Opportunity administers the federal laws and policies that make sure persons with physical disabilities have equal access to the housing of their choice (U.S. Department of Housing and Urban Development, 2011). Specific accessibility requirements have been established to ensure that the design and construction of new residential buildings comply with the Fair Housing Act (e.g., buildings must have an accessible entrance on an accessible route). Occupational therapists conducting an environmental assessment of an apartment should also remember to evaluate building access, parking, halls, facilities, and fire routes to ensure that these requirements have been met. Many of the home assessments presented in this chapter offer suggestions relevant for single-family as well as multi–unit dwellings.

Therapists are often unaccompanied during home visits, so therapist and client safety must be considered. Although a therapist may be very confident about her or his safety with the client, other occupants of the home, building, or even the neighborhood (including animals) may put the therapist at risk. Home and community settings can present risks because they are complex and often unfamiliar to the therapist. Therefore, it is always advisable for therapists to maintain vigilance about their personal safety when conducting home visits. The points in Safety Note 10-1 have become standard practice in many communities and are useful to ensure that the therapist and client are safe during home visits.

Assessment of Community Access

Occupational therapists are involved in changing environments to enable their clients' participation and fulfillment of community roles. As noted earlier in this chapter, community businesses, services (including public transportation)

A   **Do you perform the following activities alone and without difficulty:**

Taking a shower ☐ N.A. ⎯⎯⎯⎯⟶ go to question 28

24. Get in/out of shower stall/bathtub?

☐ No   ☐ Yes   ☐ N.A.

Functional Limitations	Home Check-List	Recommendations Housing	Other
	Check:		
☐ Poor coordination (lower limbs)	■ Height of step	☐ Eliminate/reduce step	☐ Supervision
☐ Poor balance	■ Existence of non-slip surface in and outside shower	☐ Install vertical grab bar	☐ Assistance
☐ Limited range (lower limbs)	■ Existence of grab bars or support	☐ Slip resistant flooring inside/outside shower stall (or bath) via non slippery coating, abrasive strips or rubber mats	
☐ Muscle weakness		☐ Add transfer board	
☐ Reduced mobility		☐ Improve floor drainage	
☐ Wheelchair dependent		☐ Change tub or shower stall if possible	
☐ Obesity			

B   **Do you have any difficulty stepping into or out of the bathtub?**

☐ **No** ➤ If no, go to next question

☐ **Yes**   If yes, check the adaptations below which would help you

☐ Install a vertical and an horizontal or angled grab bar by the tub

☐ Install non-slip flooring throughout the bathroom

☐ Install a non-slip surface in the bathtub

☐ Install a commercial or custom-made transfer bench so that the tub can be entered from a seated position

☐ Replace bathtub with a shower stall, if difficulty is severe

☐ Install a separate shower stall, if difficulty is severe

☐ Other (describe)

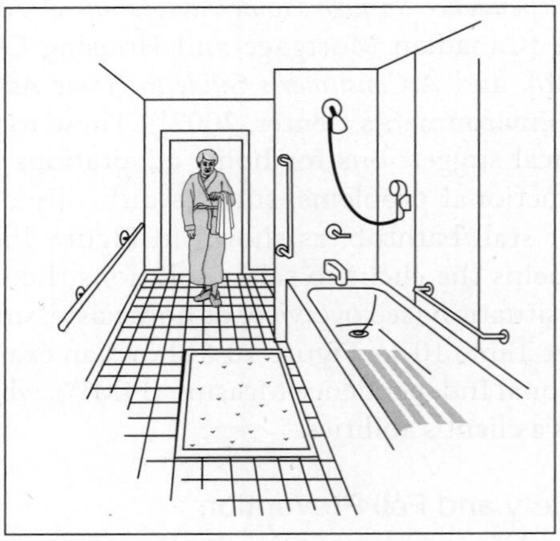

A vertical grab bar provides support when entering the tub, while an horizontal (or angled) bar helps you to complete the entrance and lower yourself onto a shower seat or to the bottom of the tub.

Figure 10-5 Using the bathroom: getting in/out of the shower stall/bathtub. (Adapted from Canadian Mortgage and Housing Corporation. [1989/2008a]. Maintaining seniors' independence: A guide to home adaptations. Retrieved October 9, 2011 from https://www.cmhc-schl.gc.ca/odpub/pdf/61042.pdf.)

FIM™ instrument

LEVELS		
7 Complete Independence (Timely, Safely) 6 Modified Independence (Device)		**NO HELPER**
Modified Dependence 5 Supervision (Subject = 100%+) 4 Minimal Assist (Subject = 75%+) 3 Moderate Assist (Subject = 50%+) **Complete Dependence** 2 Maximal Assist (Subject =25%+) 1 Total Assist (Subject = less than 25%)		**HELPER**

	ADMISSION	DISCHARGE	FOLLOW-UP
Self-Care			
A. Eating	5	6	
B. Grooming	3	4	N/A
C. Bathing	2	3	
D. Dressing - Upper Body	3	4	
E. Dressing - Lower Body	2	4	
F. Toileting	4	5	
Sphincter Control			
G. Bladder Management	5	7	
H. Bowel Management	5	7	
Transfers			
I. Bed, Chair, Wheelchair	3	5	
J. Toilet	3	5	
K. Tub, Shower	1	4	
Locomotion			
L. Walk/Wheelchair	2 W (W Walk, C Wheelchair, B Both)	6 B (W Walk, C Wheelchair, B Both)	(W Walk, C Wheelchair, B Both)
M. Stairs	2	5	
Motor Subtotal Score	40	65	
Communication			
N. Comprehension	7 B (A Auditory, V Visual, B Both)	7 B (A Auditory, V Visual, B Both)	(A Auditory, V Visual, B Both)
O. Expression	7 B (V Vocal, N Nonvocal, B Both)	7 B (V Vocal, N Nonvocal, B Both)	(V Vocal, N Nonvocal, B Both)
Social Cognition			
P. Social Interaction	7	7	
Q. Problem Solving	4	5	
R. Memory	5	6	
Cognitive Subtotal Score	30	32	
TOTAL FIM Score	70	97	

NOTE: Leave no blanks. Enter 1 if patient not testable due to risk

Figure 10-6 Case example of FIM™ assessment. (Reprinted with permission from Uniform Data Systems. [1993]. *Guide for the Uniform Data Set for medical rehabilitation.* Buffalo, NY: University of Buffalo Foundation.

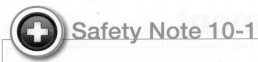

Safety Note 10-1

Therapist Safety on Home Visits

- Ensure that someone knows the location and approximate times for your home visit. If you are aware the visit will be challenging, request the presence of a case manager, second therapist, or a member of the client's family, if possible. When a visit is conducted outside of normal business hours, it is good practice to phone someone when you have completed a visit and are on your way home, to let him or her know that you are safe.
- Carry a mobile phone to use in case of emergency during the travel and home visit. Keep the battery charged.
- When you arrive at the home, assess the surroundings and inside the home to identify any potential hazards.
- Throughout the visit, be aware of exits and escape routes.
- If you feel unsafe or uncomfortable at any time, leave immediately.
- Have the client lead you to different areas of the home, including up and down stairways.
- Park as close as you safely can to the client's home.
- If traveling by car, ensure that it is in good repair and prepared for emergencies. Be cautious about leaving items in the car that may attract attention.
- If taking public transportation, follow safety recommendations related to its use.
- Adhere to any policies or procedures of your employer, including conducting joint visits, and report any unusual or unsafe situations immediately.

and programs must be made accessible for persons with disabilities in many jurisdictions. For example, it is unacceptable for wheelchair users to have to use a freight elevator at the back of a building, take safety risks to maneuver sidewalk curbs, or need someone to lift them up even just a few stairs to enter a building. In order for persons with physical disabilities to fully engage in and feel included in community life, they should experience easy, convenient, and safe access to the places, services, and programs they wish to use or participate in. Occupational therapists can assume consultation or advocacy roles with groups seeking to make educational, cultural, commercial, and religious facilities accessible. Therefore, they should become familiar with and can refer to the ADA-ABA Accessibility Guidelines (U.S. Access Board, 2004, 2007).

UD principles are now being applied across most community settings, and occupational therapists can play an important role in promoting this mainstream approach to design (Ostroff, 2001). UD is a philosophy and practice of creating products and environments that are usable by everyone, regardless of age or ability.

A variety of tools are now available to assess community environments. Three subjective measures developed

for rehabilitation practitioners are the Craig Hospital Inventory of Environmental Factors (CHIEF), the Facilitators and Barriers Survey (FABS/M), and the Measure of Quality of the Environment (refer to Assessment Table 10-2 for details). All can be used to obtain the perspective of persons with disabilities (through self-report or interview) about a breadth of environmental enablers and barriers (i.e., physical, social, institutional and attitudinal) to their participation in community life.

Two tools that facilitate discussion with a client about environmental factors influencing participation are the Multidimensional Scale of Perceived Social Support (MSPSS) (Zimet et al., 1988) and the Home and Community Environment Instrument (HACE) (Keysor, Jette, & Haley, 2005). The MSPSS targets the social environment and is useful for quickly identifying a client's perception of social supports available from family and friends to lead into a discussion of social resources enabling greater community participation. The HACE targets person–environment fit and enables a client to describe aspects of the home and community environment that hinder participation (i.e., physical characteristics and social attitudes).

Another aspect of community participation that is drawing attention is the walkability of community settings in relation to access, physical activity, and safety. Although a number of tools have been developed to evaluate walkability of neighborhoods, two are mentioned here: the Neighbourhood Walkability Scale (NEWS) (Saelens & Sallis, 2002), and the Irvine Minnesota Inventory (IMI) (Day et al., 2005). These tools measure built environmental features associated with physical activity and walking and include architectural, traffic, and aesthetic features as well as proximity of services and retailers. These features can have a positive impact on the ability of persons with disabilities to access their neighborhood community. In addition, the transportation needs of persons with disabilities should not be overlooked in communities. The Travel Chain Enabler was successfully piloted in Sweden (Iwarsson, Jensen, & Stahl, 2000); however, no recent studies have been published to support this tool.

Assessment of Access to Workplace

Occupational therapists play an important role in enabling clients to fulfill self-advancement roles by assisting them to seek or return to work. On-site assessment of workplace safety and accessibility is critical, insofar as workplace environments can differ significantly, and the needs of clients will differ depending on the nature of their condition. For example, a client with a cognitive impairment from a traumatic brain injury will have very different needs from a person returning to work following a spinal cord injury. Workplace assessment is a key step in helping the occupational therapist to learn how workplace factors impact work performance and safety (Bootes & Chapparo, 2002) (see Procedures for Practice 10-1 and 10-2 for suggestions related to conducting work site assessments).

Knowledge of the ADA and the supporting guidelines are critical for guiding workplace assessment. For practical assessment purposes, the occupational therapist may wish to use the guidelines together with the ADA Checklist for Readily Achievable Barrier Removal (Adaptive Environments Center, 1995). Other tools, such as the ADA Work-Site Assessment (Jacobs, 1999a) and the Job Analysis during Employer Site Visit (Jacobs, 1999b), may also be used to help the therapist focus on specific environmental factors in addition to work demands that may influence work performance and safety. Note, however, that these checklists have not undergone measurement studies.

Occupational therapists recognize that there is a range of environmental factors that can affect one's ability to work. Therefore, it is also important to assess the sociocultural environment, including social supports, staff interactions, and attitudes of coworkers and supervisors (Dekkers-Sánchez et al., 2010). Tools such as the Work Environment Scale, Work Experience Survey and the Workplace Environment Impact Scale (refer to Assessment Table 10-3 for details) are not limited to physical access issues because they also address such areas as social environments and resources.

Persons with disabilities may also face challenges while volunteering or attending school. Many of the tools previously discussed to address work environments or community access may be of use in these instances. Occupational therapists may also use tools such as the St. Lawrence College Accessibility Checklist (St. Lawrence College, 2005). This informal checklist briefly addresses physical, policy/programmatic, information, and attitudinal environments from a post–secondary school perspective.

Through partnering with clients and employers, occupational therapists help identify environmental factors that can affect clients' ability to work. The Job Accommodations Network website (http:/askjan.org/) can assist the team in identifying workplace modifications to address specific challenges a person with a disability might experience in the workplace. For example, workstation modifications and assistive technologies can be implemented to reduce performance barriers (see Chapter 31 for discussion of specific strategies).

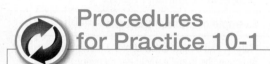

Procedures for Practice 10-1

Preparing for a Site Visit

When the occupational therapist is asked to perform a work site assessment to determine accommodations that may be necessary for a client's successful return to work, the following preparations should be made:

- Obtain a description of the job (e.g., duties, responsibilities, sequence, temporal patterns, risks, variations in complexity of tasks, and essential functions) from both employer's and employee's perspectives, if possible.
- Obtain a description of the workstation and the work site (e.g., structure, ambience, layout, environmental hazards, and location).
- Obtain written consent from employer/business/industry representatives and client (including the nature of client's wishes regarding information to be shared) both for completing the assessment and for using any digital recording devices (if applicable).
- Gain an understanding of worker's and employer's perspectives (e.g., expectations, issues, abilities, etc.).
- Make arrangements for the visit, including consent and preparatory planning, with appropriate personnel (e.g., client's supervisor) well in advance of visit.
- Ensure the presence of a contact person during the visit (e.g., client's supervisor and occupational health personnel).
- Prepare an evaluation framework including list of questions, activities, safety concerns, etc.
- Prepare and bring charts/assessment forms to record findings.
- Consider contributions from a second person (e.g., physiotherapist), depending on nature of assessment.
- Consider relevant workplace legislation (e.g., from the U.S. Department of Labor, Occupational Safety and Health Administration, and the Workplace Safety and Insurance Act in Canada).

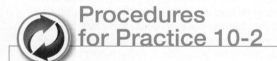

Procedures for Practice 10-2

Supplies and Materials Required for Work Site Visit

Planning with employer (including a preliminary understanding of the work site) may help to determine with greater accuracy in advance of the visit what supplies and materials may or may not be required. Recommendations include:

- tools for data recording (e.g., forms, paper, pens, laptop, or tablet computer)
- measuring tape and wheeled measuring device
- stopwatch
- force gauge dynamometer
- push-pull gauge
- personal protective equipment as appropriate (e.g., steel-toed footwear and protective glasses)
- thermometer
- digital camera (with video recording capacity); tripod, if necessary
- photo release forms (to protect confidentiality and privacy of workplace and client)

General Comments on Assessing Access to Home, Community, and Workplace

Many occupational therapists rely mainly on experience, observation, and interviews when called on to evaluate the environment. Although these strategies are necessary components of good practice, they cannot stand alone.

The use of standardized instruments that have evidence of acceptable measurement properties is also necessary. In this chapter, we have described a number of home, community, and workplace environmental assessments that will assist the occupational therapist identify suitable interventions to enable and optimize client occupational functioning.

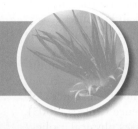

case example
Mrs. P.: Safe Environment-Person-Occupation Fit Assessment

Occupational Therapy Assessment Process	Clinical Reasoning Process	
	Objectives	Example of Internal Dialogue
Patient Information Mrs. P. is an 80-year-old woman who sustained a right-sided cerebrovascular accident (CVA) 2 months ago, resulting in left-sided hemiparesis. She was recently discharged from the rehabilitation center to an apartment that she has shared with her husband for more than 30 years. Results from the Functional Independence Measure FIM™ (Uniform Data Systems, 1993), which were conducted at time of discharge, are available from the referral. Her total FIM™ score improved from 70 (at time of admission) to 97 on discharge. Mr. P. and their daughter are presently doing the housekeeping and most of the meal preparation. Mr. P. would like to hire an attendant to work a few hours a day to assist with Mrs. P.'s personal care and to help with the housekeeping, but financial constraints do not allow for this. Both Mr. P. and their daughter have reported becoming increasingly frustrated and fatigued. They both say that they do not believe that they can leave Mrs. P. alone because of their concerns about her safety and independence. Prior to her stroke, Mrs. P. prided herself on her ability to care for her husband and her home. Mrs. P. is becoming increasingly concerned about becoming too much of a burden on her family and thinks that they are being overly protective. Mrs. P. has been referred to the community occupational therapist to address concerns about her independence and safety in her home environment.	Understand the patient's diagnosis or condition	"Mrs. P. had a right-sided stroke 2 months ago. Although she is still early in her recovery, I would expect that her hemiparesis still limits her basic personal care, homemaking and community living skills, and safety. I also need to be aware of any cognitive and perceptual changes that may be affecting her abilities. Depression is also possible after stroke, so I will need to be on the lookout for any mood changes as well."
	Know the person	"It sounds like her ability to care for herself and her family was extremely important to her. I wonder how she is coping now. Because she may have been the person who took care of everything and everyone at home, I wonder how well the daughter and husband are able to pick up the slack. Not having worked with many older people, I know that I may have some stereotyped expectations of her readiness to change; I will need to be careful, as I could very well be wrong about this. However, I am a bit concerned about how willing she will be to make modifications to her home if I suggest them."
	Appreciate the context	"I want to know more about her relationship with her husband and her daughter. Are they supportive, or have they been negatively affected by the changes? I also wonder how well she is able to get around her small apartment with the quad cane she uses at home. Although I have not worked with many older adults, I have worked with many adults who have had strokes, so I may need to consult my colleague/supervisor who has more experience with this age group. I may also want to consult the occupational therapist who worked with Mrs. P. at the rehabilitation center for more information."
	Develop provisional hypotheses	"Given her diagnosis, I am assuming that there may be cognitive and perceptual impairments in addition to the more obvious physical problems that will impact Mrs. P.'s occupational performance. I also think that the environment will play a big role in how independent and safe she is at home."

Assessment Process

The therapist decided to use the Canadian Occupational Performance Measure (COPM) (Law et al., 2005) to identify Mrs. P.'s perceptions and priorities for therapy. The SAFER-HOME was chosen to assess Mrs. P.'s ability to safely engage in occupations in her home. The SAFER-HOME allowed both Mrs. P. and her family to discuss her abilities and challenges and demonstrate a variety of occupations in her home. Use of the SAFER-HOME assisted the occupational therapist to identify areas of concern and make recommendations to enhance safety and independence.

Consider evaluation approach and methods

"I would like to get a sense of her priorities from her perspective. I want to learn more about her abilities to advocate for herself and make her ideas heard. The COPM will give me a better understanding of her awareness and priorities. The SAFER-HOME will provide me with information about her home environment and safety."

Assessment Results

Based on the COPM, Mrs. P. indicated that her priorities were to bathe, prepare meals, complete housekeeping, and do the laundry. The SAFER-HOME highlighted areas of safety concern that Mrs. P. had not raised previously, including issues associated with medication use, vision, and remembering to turn off appliances (refer to Fig. 10-4, the SAFER-HOME results for this case study).

Interpret observations

"Mrs. P. seems to have limited awareness of possible cognitive, visual, or perceptual changes since her stroke. However, she is very aware of physical changes. Further assessment may be helpful to explore cognitive, visual, and perceptual difficulties impacting occupational performance. I was surprised that Mrs. P. was having difficulties remembering to turn off the stove, because she does not seem to have memory problems in more social situations. She is occasionally missing things on the left, so I am wondering whether she has any visual attention difficulties as well."

Occupational Therapy Problem List

1. Decreased independence in self-care, particularly in bathing and toileting.
2. Decreased independence in instrumental activities of daily living including meal preparation, laundry, and housekeeping.
3. Physical barriers to independence and safety identified in home (particularly kitchen and bathroom).
4. Limited funds available for assistive devices, home modifications, and support services.
5. In addition to changes in motor function since the CVA, cognitive, visual, and perceptual difficulties may also be impacting safety and independence in daily occupations.

Synthesize results

"Overall, Mrs. P. seems to be able to benefit from occupational therapy intervention. She clearly has many areas she would like to address and is very motivated to work on these areas. The safety concerns I have identified will need to be addressed as priority areas as soon as possible. Although Mrs. P. does not seem to be as concerned about the safety issues, she is open to addressing them if only to help her husband and daughter feel a bit better. I will need to develop a plan to address the areas where I suspect that more assessment would be beneficial. I should consult with a colleague regarding options for funding. I wonder what programs Mrs. P. may qualify for in order to help supplement funding for equipment I may recommend. I am glad that I used the SAFER-HOME and the COPM because I can reuse both of these tools in the future as part of my outcome evaluation."

 # Clinical Reasoning in Occupational Therapy Practice

Assessing Mobility within the Home and Fall Prevention

In the case example of Mrs. P., the 80-year-old woman with left-sided hemiparesis, you have observed that she can walk short distances using a cane (see Case Example). Her husband would like to leave her alone for an hour or so during the day so that he can go out for groceries and other errands. Typically, Mrs. P. sits in a comfortable chair in the living room during the day, not in her wheelchair. She may need to use the toilet when her husband is out. What environmental factors might help or hinder her when she is left alone? What are the safety issues? What environmental enablers would you suggest to address this issue?

Clinical Reasoning in Occupational Therapy Practice

Assessing Community Mobility and Accessibility

In the case example of Mrs. P., she has indicated that she would like to go out shopping with her husband to get groceries at the nearby supermarket and to stop for lunch or coffee at a nearby café that they had previously frequented. Mrs. P. can walk short distances using a cane (see Case Example).

What are the environmental factors that could impact her occupational functioning and how might they help or hinder her engagement in this outing? What environment assessment tool(s) would you use to address the various occupations within this outing?

Summary Review Questions

1. Why would an occupational therapist assess the environment?
2. List seven examples of environmental barriers that a person with mobility impairment might encounter when returning to work. Now list seven examples of environmental barriers that a person with cognitive impairments following a traumatic brain injury might encounter. Compare and contrast the types of environmental barriers each might encounter and discuss any differences. How would these differences influence your choice(s) of assessments of the environment?
3. List seven examples of environmental supports that would allow an older adult with arthritis to continue to live at home.
4. Identify two home assessments that address fall prevention and safety in the home. Look around your own home and describe environmental features that would put you at risk for a fall if you had a balance or mobility impairment.
5. What assessments would you use to evaluate whether a client with a spinal cord injury can live independently in the community?
6. As a consultant to an assisted-living facility, what assistance could you offer the facility's administration regarding their plans to renovate the building?
7. If you, as an occupational therapist, were making a home visit to a client's apartment, what precautions would you take for your visit to protect your own safety?

Glossary

Accessibility—The ease with which the physical environment may be reached, entered, and used by all individuals.

Accommodations (environmental)—Removal of environment barriers and provision of environmental supports and resources to enable a person with a disability to enjoy equal opportunity.

Barrier-free design—Design features of the built environment that remove physical barriers to full and equal accessibility for all persons with disabilities.

Environmental barrier—Any component of the environment that impedes optimal occupational functioning.

Environmental support—Any component of the environment that encourages, facilitates, or provides assistance to allow a person to achieve optimal occupational functioning.

PEO fit—Person-environment-occupation fit. The level of congruency across personal factors (e.g., functional, social,

and psychological), the characteristics of the environment (e.g., barriers and enablers), and the characteristics of the chosen occupation.

Physical environment—The natural or human-made (built) features of the environment within which occupational functioning occurs.

Standardization—The process of making an assessment available in a manual with standard procedures for testing, scoring, and interpreting the results. Environmental assessments do not usually undergo a normative process because of the variability in environments, yet many are based on standards or perspectives of persons with disabilities.

Transactive—Dynamic, reciprocal relationship; integrated.

Universal design (UD)—Design features of the built environment that enhance optimal function and convenience for all individuals, regardless of their ability.

References

Accessibility for Ontarians with Disabilities Act, S.O. 2005, Chapter 11, 429/07. (2007). Retrieved May 28, 2013 from http://www.e-laws.gov.on.ca/html/statutes/english/elaws_statutes_05a11_e.htm.

ADA Amendments Act of 2008, Pub. L. No. 110-325 (2008). Retrieved August 23, 2011 from http://www.ada.gov/pubs/ada.htm.

Adaptive Environments Center. (1995). *Americans with Disabilities Act checklist for readily achievable barrier removal.* Boston: Adaptive Environments Center. Retrieved August 23, 2011 from http://www.ada.gov/checkweb.htm.

Adaptive Environments Center. (2002). *A consumer's guide to home adaptation.* Boston: Adaptive Environments Center. Retrieved October 10, 2011 from http://www.adaptenv.org/documents/aepuborder.html.

Americans with Disabilities Act of 1990, Pub. L. No. 101-336, 42 U.S.C. § 12101 (1990).

American Occupational Therapy Association. (2008). Occupational therapy practice framework: Domain and process (2nd ed.). *American Journal of Occupational Therapy, 62,* 625–683.

American Occupational Therapy Association. (2009). *The reference manual of the official documents of the American Occupational Therapy Association, Inc.* (14th ed.). Bethesda, MD: AOTA Press.

American Occupational Therapy Association. (2010). Standards of practice for occupational therapy. *American Journal of Occupational Therapy, 64 (Suppl.),* S10–S11.

Association of Canadian Occupational Therapy Regulatory Organizations. (2012). *The essential competencies of practice for occupational therapists in Canada* (3rd ed.) Retrieved May 22, 2013 from http://acotro-acore.org/sites/default/files/uploads/ACOTRO_EC_3rd_ed.pdf.

Baker Parker, K., DeJoy, D., Wilson, M., Bowen, H., & Goetzel, R. (2010). Application of the environmental assessment tool (EAT) as a process measure for a worksite weight management intervention. *Journal of Occupational and Environmental Medicine, 52,* S42–S51.

Biernacki, S. (1993). Reliability of the worker role interview. *American Journal of Occupational Therapy, 47,* 797–803.

Bootes, K., & Chapparo, C. J. (2002). Cognitive and behavioural assessment of people with traumatic brain injury in the work place: Occupational therapists' perceptions. *Work, 19,* 255–268.

Boschen, K., Noreau, L., & Fougeyrollas, P. (1998). A new instrument to measure the quality of the environment for persons with physical disabilities. *Archives of Physical Medicine and Rehabilitation, 79,* 1331.

Braveman, B., Robson, M., Velozo, C., Kielhofner, G., Fisher, G., Forsyth, K., & Kerschbaum, J. (2005). *Worker role interview (WRI)* (Version 10.0). Chicago: Model of Human Occupation Clearinghouse, University of Illinois at Chicago.

Canadian Association of Occupational Therapists. (2007). Profile of occupational therapy practice in Canada. Retrieved October 9, 2011 from http://www.caot.ca/pdfs/otprofile.pdf.

Canadian Mortgage and Housing Corporation. (1989/2008a). Maintaining seniors' independence: A guide to home adaptations. Retrieved October 9, 2011 from http://www.cmhc-schl.gc.ca/odpub/pdf/61042.pdf.

Canadian Mortgage and Housing Corporation. (2008b). Maintaining seniors' independence through home adaptations: A self-assessment guide. Retrieved October 9, 2011 from https://www03.cmhc-schl.gc.ca/catalog/search.cfm.

Chiu, T., & Oliver, R. (2006). Factor analysis and construct validity of the SAFER-HOME. *OTJR: Occupation, Participation & Health, 26,* 132–142.

Chiu, T., Oliver, R., Ascott, P., Choo, L., Davis, T., Gaya, A., Goldsilver, P., McWhirter, M., & Letts, L. (2006). *Safety assessment of function and the environment for rehabilitation: Health outcome measurement and evaluation (SAFER-HOME) Version 3 Manual.* Toronto, Canada: VHA Rehab Solutions.

Clark, J., Shaw, L., & Kahn, K. (2002). *Use of the safe living guide to identify fall hazards.* Paper presented at the Canadian Association of Occupational Therapists Conference, St. John, New Brunswick.

Clemson, L. (1997). *Home fall hazards: A guide to identifying fall hazards in the homes of elderly people and an accompaniment to the assessment tool. The Westmead Home Safety Assessment.* West Brunswick, Australia: Co-ordinates Publication.

Clemson, L., Fitzgerald, M. H., & Heard, R. (1999). Content validity of an assessment tool to identify home fall hazards: The Westmead home safety assessment. *British Journal of Occupational Therapy, 62,* 171–179.

Clemson, L., Fitzgerald, M. H., Heard, R., & Cumming, R. G. (1999). Inter-rater reliability of a home fall hazards assessment tool. *Occupational Therapy Journal of Research, 19,* 83–100.

Clemson, L., Mackenzie, L., Ballinger, C., Close, J. C. T., & Cumming, R. G. (2008). Environmental interventions to prevent falls in community-dwelling older people: A meta-analysis of randomized trials. *Journal of Aging & Health, 20,* 954–971

Corner, R., Kielhofner, G., & Lin, F. L. (1997). Construct validity of a work environment impact scale. *Work, 9,* 21–34.

Cristoforetti, A., Gennai, F., & Rodeschini, G. (2011). Home sweet home: The emotional construction of places. *Journal of Aging Studies, 25,* 225–232

Day, K., Boarnet, M., Alfonzo, M., & Forsyth, A. (2005). Irvine Minnesota Inventory. Retrieved October 9, 2011 from https://webfiles.uci.edu/kday/public/index.html.

Dejoy, E., Wilson, M., Goetzel, R., Ozminkowski, R., Wang, S., Baker, K., Bowen, H., & Tully, K. (2008). Development of the Environmental Assessment Tool (EAT) to measure organizational physical and social support for worksite obesity prevention programs. *Journal of Occupational and Environmental Medicine, 50,* 126–137.

Dekkers-Sánchez, P., Wind, H., Sluiter, J., & Frings-Dresen, M. (2010). A qualitative study of perpetuating factors for long term sick leave and promoting factors for return to work: Chronic work disabled patients in their own words. *Journal of Rehabilitation Medicine, 42,* 544–552.

Ekbladh, E., Thorell, L., & Haglund, L. (2010). Return to work: The predictive value of the worker role interview (WRI) over two years. *Work, 35,* 163–172.

Fange, A., & Iwarsson, S. (2003). Accessibility and usability in housing: Construct validity and implications for research and practice. *Disability and Rehabilitation, 25,* 1316–1325.

Fange, A., Risser, R., & Iwarsson, S. (2007). Challenges in implementation of research methodology in community-based occupational therapy: The housing enabler example. *Scandinavian Journal of Occupational Therapy, 14,* 54–62.

Fenger, K., & Kramer, J. (2007). Worker role interview. Testing the psychometric properties of the Icelandic version. *Scandinavian Journal of Occupational Therapy, 14,* 160–172.

Forsyth, K., Braveman, B., Kielhofner, G., Ekbladh, E., Haglund, L., Fenger, K., & Keller, J. (2006). Psychometric properties of the Worker Role Interview. *Work, 27,* 313–318.

Fougeyrollas, P., Noreau, L., St. Michel, G., & Boschen, K. (2008). *Measure of the Quality of the Environment* (Version 2). Quebec City, Canada: International Network on the Disability Creation Process.

Fougeyrollas, P., Noreau, L., & Boschen, K. (2002). Interaction of environment with individual characteristics and social participation: Theoretical perspectives and applications in persons with spinal cord injury. *Topics in SCI Rehabilitation, 7,* 1–16.

Gillespie, L. D., Robertson, M. C., Gillespie, W, J., Lamb, S. E., Gates, S., Cumming, R. G., & Rowe, B. H. (2009). Interventions for preventing falls in older people living in the community. *Cochrane Database of Systematic Reviews,* Issue 2, Art No. CD007146, DOI:10.1002/14651858.CD007146.pub2.

Gray, D. B., Hollingsworth, H. H., Stark, S., & Morgan, K. A. (2008). A subjective measure of environmental facilitators and barriers to participation for people with mobility limitations. *Disability and Rehabilitation, 30,* 435–457.

Harrison, T. C. (2002). Has the Americans with Disabilities Act made a difference? A policy analysis of quality of life in the post-Americans with Disabilities Act era. *Policy, Politics, & Nursing Practice, 3,* 333–347.

Hinton, C. A. (2003). The perceptions of people with disabilities as to the effectiveness of the Americans with Disabilities Act. *Journal of Disability Policy Studies, 13,* 210–220.

Iwarsson, S. (2005). A long-term perspective on person-environment fit and ADL dependence among older Swedish adults. *The Gerontologist, 45,* 327–337.

Iwarrsson, S., & Isacsson, A. (1998). Housing standards, environmental barriers in the home, subjective general apprehension of housing situation among the rural elderly. *Scandanavian Journal of Occupational Therapy, 3,* 52–61.

Iwarsson, S., Isacsson, A., & Lanke, J. (1998). ADL dependence in the elderly: The influence of functional limitations and physical environmental demand. *Occupational Therapy International, 5,* 173–193.

Iwarsson, S., Jensen, G., & Stahl, A. (2000). Travel chain enabler: Development of a pilot instrument for assessment of urban public transportation accessibility. *Technology and Disability, 12,* 3–12.

Iwarsson, S., Nygren, C., & Slaug, B. (2005). Cross-national and multiprofessional inter-rater reliability of the Housing Enabler. *Scandinavian Journal of Occupational Therapy, 12,* 29–39.

Jacobs, K. (1999a). Americans with Disabilities Act work-site assessment. In K. Jacobs (Ed.), *Ergonomics for Therapists* (2nd ed., pp. 345–354). Boston: Butterworth-Heinemann.

Jacobs, K. (1999b). Job analysis during employer site visit. In K. Jacobs (Ed.), *Ergonomics for Therapists* (2nd ed., pp. 356–364). Boston: Butterworth-Heinemann.

Keysor, J. J., Jette, A. M., & Haley, S. M. (2005). Development of the Home and Community Environment (HACE) instrument. *Journal of Rehabilitation Medicine, 37,* 37–44.

Kielhofner, G. (2008). *Model of human occupation: Theory and application.* Philadelphia: Lippincott Wilkins & Williams.

Kielhofner, G., Lai, J., Olson, L., Haglund, L., Ekbadh, E., & Hedlund, M. (1998). Psychometric properties of the work environment impact scale: A cross-cultural study. *Work: A Journal of Prevention, Assessment, and Rehabilitation, 12,* 71–77.

Law, M. (2004). *Outcome measures rating form and guidelines.* Hamilton, Canada: CanChild Retrieved August 23, 2011 from http://www .canchild.ca/en/canchildresources/resources/measguid.pdf.

Law, M., Baptiste, S., Carswell, A., McColl, M., Polatajko, H., & Pollock, N. (2005). *Canadian occupational performance measure* (4th ed.). Ottawa, Canada: CAOT Publications ACE.

Law, M., Cooper, B., Strong, S., Stewart, D., Rigby, P., & Letts, L. (1996). The Person-Environment-Occupation Model: A transactive approach to occupational performance. *Canadian Journal of Occupational Therapy, 63,* 9–23.

Letts, L., Scott, S., Burtney, J., Marshall, L., & McKean, M. (1998). The reliability and validity of the Safety Assessment of Function and the Environment for Rehabilitation (SAFER) tool. *British Journal of Occupational Therapy, 61,* 127–132.

Lund, M., & Lexell, J. (2009). Associations between perceptions of environmental barriers and participation in persons with late effects of polio. *Scandinavian Journal of Occupational Therapy, 16,* 194–204

Mackenzie, L., Byles, J., & D'Este, C. (2009). Longitudinal study of the Home Falls and Accidents Screening Tool in identifying older people at increased risk of falls. *Australasian Journal on Ageing, 28,* 64–69

Mackenzie, L., Byles, J., & Higginbotham, N. (2000). Designing the Home Falls and Accidents Screening Tool (HOME FAST): Selecting the items. *British Journal of Occupational Therapy, 63,* 260–269.

Mackenzie, L., Byles, J., & Higginbotham, N. (2002a). Professional perceptions about home safety: Cross-national validation of the Home Falls and Accidents Screening Tool (HOME FAST). *Journal of Allied Health, 31,* 22–28.

Mackenzie, L., Byles, J., & Higginbotham, N. (2002b). Reliability of the Home Falls and Accidents Screening Tool (HOME FAST) for identifying older people at increased risk of falls. *Disability and Rehabilitation, 24,* 266–274.

Mitchell, R., & Unsworth, C. A. (2004). Role perceptions and clinical reasoning of community health occupational therapists undertaking home visits. *Australian Occupational Therapy Journal, 51,* 13–24.

Moore, D. P., Moore, J. W., & Moore, J. L. (2007). After fifteen years: The response of small businesses to the Americans with Disabilities Act. *Work, 29,* 113–126.

Moore-Corner, R., Kielhofner, G., & Olson, L. (1998). *A user's guide to work environment impact scale (WEIS)* (Version 2.0). Chicago: The Model of Human Occupation Clearinghouse, University of Illinois at Chicago.

Moos, R. H. (1994). *Work Environment Scale manual* (3rd ed.). Palo Alto, CA: Consulting Psychologists Press.

Moos, R. H., & Insel, P. M. (2008). *Work Environment Scale manual* (4th ed.). Menlo Park, CA: Mind Garden, Inc.

Nichols, L., Tchounwou, P. B., Mena, L., & Sarpong, D. (2009). The effects of environmental factors on persons living with HIV/AIDS. *International Journal of Research and Public Health, 6,* 2041–2054.

Noreau, L, Fougeyrollas, P., & Boschen, K. (2002). Perceived influence of the environment on social participation among individuals with spinal cord injury. *Topics in SCI Rehabilitation, 7,* 56–72.

Ngyard, L., Grahn, U., Rudenhammar, A., & Hydling, S. (2004). Reflecting on practice: Are home visits prior to discharge worthwhile in geriatric inpatient care? *Scandinavian Journal of Caring Science, 18,* 193–203.

Oldenburg, B., Sallis, J., Harris, D., & Owen, N. (2002). Checklist of health promotion environments at worksites (CHEW): Development and measurement characteristics. *American Journal of Health Promotion, 16,* 288–299.

Ontarians with Disabilities Act, S.O. 2001, Chapter 32 (2001). Retrieved October 2, 2011 from http://www.e-laws.gov.on.ca/html/statutes /english/elaws_statutes_01o32_e.htm.

Ostroff, E. (2001). Universal design: The new paradigm. In W. F. E. Preiser & E. Ostroff (Eds.), *Universal design handbook.* New York: McGraw Hill.

Pighills, A., Torgerson, D., Sheldon, T., Drummond, A., & Bland, M. (2011). Environmental assessment and modification to prevent falls in older people. *Journal of the American Geriatrics Society, 59,* 26–33.

Public Health Agency of Canada. (2007). The safe living guide. Retrieved September 1, 2011 from http://www.phac-aspc.gc.ca/seniors-aines/ publications/public/injury-blessure/safelive-securite/index-eng.php.

Roessler, R. T. (1996). The role of assessment in enhancing vocational success of people with multiple sclerosis. *Work, 6,* 191–201.

Roessler, R. T., & Gottcent, J. (1994). The Work Experience Survey: A reasonable accommodation/career development strategy. *Journal of Applied Rehabilitation Counseling, 25,* 16–21.

Rogers, J. C., Holm, M. B., Beach, S., Schulz, R., Cipriani, J., Fox, A., & Starz, T. W. (2003). Concordance of four methods of disability assessment using performance in the home as the criterion method. *Arthritis & Rheumatism (Arthritis Care & Research), 49,* 640–647.

Rousseau, J., Potvin, L., Dutil, E., & Falta, P. (2001). A critical review of assessment tools related to home adaptation issues. *Occupational Therapy in Health Care, 14,* 93–104.

Saelens, B. E., & Sallis, J. F. (2002). Neighborhood Environment Walkability Scale (NEWS). Retrieved May 22, 2013 from http://www.activelivingresearch.org/node/10649.

Slaug, B., & Iwarsson, S. (2001). *Housing Enabler 1.0: A tool for housing accessibility analysis. Software for PC.* Staffenstorp & Navlinge: Slaug Data.

Sorcinelli, A., Shaw, L., Freeman, A., & Cooper, K. (2007). Evaluating the safe living guide: A home hazard checklist for seniors. *Canadian Journal on Aging, 26,* 127–138.

Stanley, M. A., Beck, J. G., & Zebb, B. J. (1998). Psychometric properties of the MSPSS in older adults. *Aging & Mental Health, 2,* 186–193.

Stark, S., Somerville, S., & Morris, J. (2010). In-home occupational performance evaluation (I-HOPE). *American Journal of Occupational Therapy, 64,* 580–589.

Staten, D. R., Mangalindan, M. A., Saylor, C., & Stuenkel, D. L. (2003). Staff nurse perceptions of the work environment: A comparison among ethnic backgrounds. *Journal of Nursing Care Quality, 18,* 202–208.

St. Lawrence College. (2005). St. Lawrence College Accessibility Checklist. Retrieved October 30, 2011 from http://www.stlawrencecollege.ca/_files/accessibilityplan.pdf.

Tomita, M., Nochajski, S., Schweitzer, J., Lenker, J., Russ, L., Rajendran, S., & Sumandeep, S. (2011). *Home Safety Self Assessment Tool (HS-SAT)* (Version 3). Retrieved May 22, 2013 from www.agingresearch.buffalo.edu.

Townsend, E. A., & Polatajko H. J. (Eds.). (2007). *Enabling Occupation II: Advancing an occupational therapy vision for health, well-being and justice through occupation.* Ottawa, Canada: CAOT Publications ACE.

Trombly Latham, C. A. (2005). Conceptual foundations for practice. In M. A. Radomski & C. A. Trombly Latham (Eds.) *Occupational therapy for physical dysfunction* (6th ed.). Philadelphia: Lippincott Williams & Wilkins.

Uniform Data Systems. (1993). *Guide for the Uniform Data Set for medical rehabilitation.* Buffalo, NY: University of Buffalo Foundation.

United Nations. (2011). United Nations Convention on the Rights of Persons with Disabilities and Optional Protocol. Retrieved May 22, 2013 from http://www.un.org/disabilities/documents/convention/convoptprot-e.pdf.

U.S. Access Board (2004). ADA-ABA accessibility guidelines. Retrieved August 23, 2011 from http://www.access-board.gov/ada-aba/final.cfm.

U.S. Access Board. (2007). Proposed ABA Accessibility Guidelines for Outdoor Developed Areas. Retrieved August 23, 2011 from http://www.access-board.gov/outdoor/nprm/.

U.S. Department of Housing and Urban Development. (2011). Fair housing and equal opportunity: People with disabilities. Retrieved August 23, 2011 from http://www.hud.gov/offices/fheo/disabilities/sect504.cfm.

Velozo, C., Kielhofner, G., Gern, A., Lin, F., Azhar, F., Lai, J., & Fisher, G. (1999). Worker role interview. Toward validation of a psychosocial work-related measure. *Journal of Occupational Rehabilitation, 9,* 153–168.

Whiteneck, G. G., Gerhart, K. A., & Cusick, C. P. (2004) Identifying environmental factors that influence the outcomes of people with traumatic brain injury. *Journal of Head Trauma Rehabilitation, 19,* 191–204.

Whiteneck, G. G., Harrison-Felix, C. L., Mellick, D. S., Brooks, C. A., Charlifue, S. B., & Gerhart, K. A. (2004). Quantifying environmental factors: A measure of physical, attitudinal, service, productivity and policy barriers. *Archives of Physical Medicine & Rehabilitation, 85,* 1324–1335.

World Health Organization. (2001). International classification of functioning, disability and health. Retrieved August 21, 2011 from http://www.who.int/classification/icf/.

World Health Organization. (2011). World Report on Disability. Retrieved August 21, 2011 from http://www.who.int/disabilities/world_report/2011/report/en/.

Zimet, G. D., Dahlem, N. W., Zimet, S. G., & Farley, G. K. (1988). The Multidimensional Scale of Perceived Social Support. *Journal of Personality Assessment, 52,* 30–41.

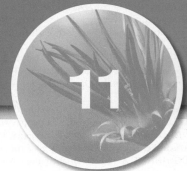

11

Occupation: Philosophy and Concepts

Catherine A. Trombly Latham

Learning Objectives

After studying this chapter, the reader will be able to do the following:

1. Define occupation.
2. Discuss the importance of occupation in people's lives.
3. Discuss the concept of occupational balance.
4. Discuss occupation as a therapeutic medium.
5. Characterize occupation-as-end and occupation-as-means.
6. Discuss the therapeutic qualities of occupation: purposefulness and meaningfulness.
7. Cite evidence that supports the use of occupation as therapy.
8. Describe how therapeutic occupation is implemented in practice.

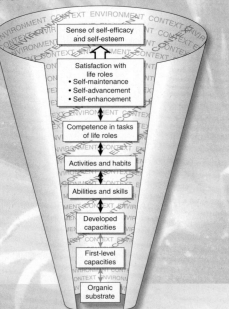

OCCUPATION DEFINED

Occupation is both the center of human experience and the core of our profession (Harris, 2008). Occupation is defined by the general public as an activity in which one engages, especially the principal business of one's life (vocation) (Merriam-Webster Online, 2012). Occupational therapists define occupation in various ways, but all definitions include the idea of activities of everyday life that are meaningful to individuals (American Occupational Therapy Association [AOTA], 2008). "Occupation is everything people do to occupy themselves, including looking after themselves, enjoying life and contributing to the social and economic fabric of their communities" (Law et al., 1997, p. 32). Personal identity emerges from a harmonious balance of the many meaningful occupations in which a person engages over time (Christiansen, 1999/2011; Häggblom-Kronlöf et al., 2007; Unruh, 2004). People engaged in occupation not only define their identity but also achieve a sense of competence and report a sense of satisfaction and fulfillment (AOTA, 2008).

Although the terms occupation and purposeful activity are used interchangeably by most therapists, the Occupational Therapy Practice Framework (OTPF) (AOTA, 2008) distinguishes between occupation and purposeful activity on the basis of meaningfulness. The key difference is that occupations are central to a person's identity, and they influence how one spends time and makes decisions (AOTA, 2008), whereas purposeful activity is a class of human actions that are goal directed and allow a person to develop skills that enhance occupational engagement but do not assume a place of central importance or meaning to the life of the person (AOTA, 2008; Rogers, 2007). Each occupation is composed of several purposeful activities. Purposeful activity is circumscribed; it demands particular responses within particular contexts and is used therapeutically to facilitate change in impairments and functional limitations. In this text, occupation-as-end is equated to occupation, and occupation-as-means is equated to purposeful activity.

IMPORTANCE OF OCCUPATION IN PEOPLE'S LIVES

Occupational engagement contributes to the experience of a life worth living (Hammell, 2004). Engagement in positive occupations (e.g., care of self, others, and property and creative or productive endeavors) that the person has the capability to accomplish and chooses to accomplish regulates the rhythm of personal and community life. Such occupations absorb attention and evoke creativity, promote feelings of satisfaction with achievement, and contribute to a sense of self-esteem and self-efficacy (Fig. 11-1). These occupations are potentially therapeutic.

Time-use studies indicate that people who are mentally able to envision goals fill their time with activities and tasks (Grady, 1992; McKinnon, 1992; Pentland et al., 1999; Yerxa & Baum, 1986; Yerxa & Locker, 1990). Beyond the organization and positive feelings generated by engagement in occupation, there is evidence that social and productive occupations are independently associated with survival (Glass et al., 1999). Failure to engage in meaningful occupation by older Swedish adults was found to be associated with a reduced sense of hope (Borell et al., 2001). In the absence of social and productive occupation (as occurs, for example, early in retirement, in the acute stage of motor disability, or immediately after a profound loss [Hoppes, 2005]), a person may experience a sense of disorganization, depression, and loss of a sense of self-worth.

Not all occupation or purposeful activity is beneficial. Attempts to engage in occupations beyond one's capabilities can lead to frustration, anxiety, and depression (Rebeiro & Polgar, 1998). Engagement in negative occupation (e.g., crime and destruction) disrupts personal and community life. Doing the same activity repetitively beyond the requirements of the task, as seen in obsessive-compulsive disorder (OCD), reinforces pathology. Imposition of unsuitable, negatively meaningful activities (e.g., children's games as therapy for elderly patients) fails to build a sense of self-esteem and satisfaction. These types of occupation are not therapeutic. Therapeutic occupation, a special type of occupation, is defined as the use of positive, relevant, meaningful, and purposive activities to improve a person's ability to participate in his life (Strzelecki, 2009), or to improve abilities and capacities to enable improved occupational functioning.

Occupational Balance

Occupational therapy subscribes to the belief that the balance of engagement in life occupations, including rest, is basic to health and wellness (Meyer, 1922/1977; Rogers, 1984; Strzelecki, 2009). The ideal configuration of this balance changes as the person matures from infancy to old age (Rogers, 1984) and is individually defined, consisting of occupations that are meaningful to the particular person and that promote wellness (Hammell, 2009; Stamm et al., 2009; Wilcock, 1997). What is considered "balance" by one person may not be seen that way by another. As part of the occupational history interview, the therapist can ascertain whether the patient feels that he or she is in occupational balance or not and on what basis the person defines that balance.

Balance may be defined on the basis of a mixture of challenging versus relaxing occupations, a mixture of activities meaningful to the individual versus those meaningful to society, or a mixture of activities intended to care for oneself versus those intended to care for others (Stamm et al., 2009). Other gradients on which to establish balance

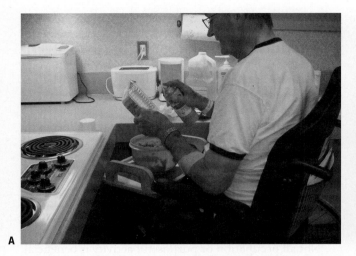

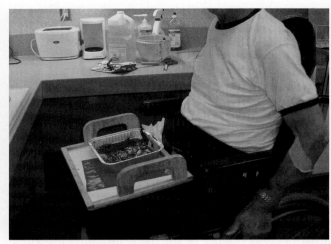

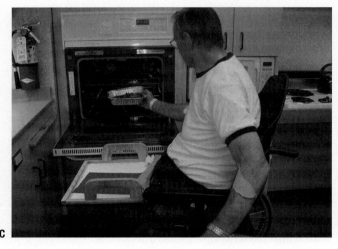

Figure 11-1 Occupation-as-end. Baking brownies again under new circumstances (after spinal cord injury). **A.** Preparing the pan. **B.** Transporting to the oven. **C.** Putting the brownies into the oven.

include allotment of time among physical, mental, social, and rest occupations or mixing physically taxing occupations with light, relaxing occupations (also called pacing, which is commonly used in the treatment of persons with arthritis, cumulative trauma, or cardiopulmonary disorders), or balancing occupations of doing with occupations of being (Wilcock, 1997).

If the balance is skewed toward one end of the continuum or the other, then the person suffers occupational dysfunction. For example, if too much time is spent in self-enhancement activities (e.g., video gaming) to the detriment of other roles or rest, then the person's work, social life, and/or self-care suffers, and he is occupationally "out of balance." If the person engages in mentally challenging occupations without balance with rest or lesser challenging occupations, then the person becomes stressed ("burned out"), unhealthy, and ineffective in other areas of his life (Wilcock, 1997). If the person engages in physically stressful occupations or movements without rest, damage occurs to the body structures involved (cumulative trauma) (Barcenilla et al., 2012; Walker-Bone et al., 2012).

OCCUPATION AS THERAPY

Occupational therapists work with people who have experienced, or are in danger of experiencing, significant occupational dysfunction secondary to changes in their physical, cognitive, emotional, or social well-being or their environments. It is the role of the occupational therapist to help the person to grieve his or her loss and to reconstruct an acceptable occupational identity (Unruh, 2004).

Occupation is used to create or promote health, to remediate impairments or restore an ability or skill, to modify or adapt performance, to maintain performance capabilities, or to prevent disability (AOTA, 2008). To be therapeutic, occupation must involve the patient in active participation, must evoke in the patient a willingness to participate and must hold meaning for the person to engage in it. The appropriate occupation results in a sense of mastery by the participant (Laws, 2012). Occupational intervention becomes therapeutic when it is guided by theory (Dooley, 2009). In this text, the theoretical guideline is the Occupational Functioning Model, but therapists may choose to use other guidelines or frames of reference.

Occupation is the unique therapeutic medium of occupational therapy (National Society for the Promotion of Occupational Therapy, 1917; Reilly, 1962/2011; Slagle, 1914). Occupation is both intervention and outcome (Amini, 2010; Trombly, 1995/2011).

What about occupation maintains or restores health? That question is still debated, but one suggestion is that occupation is therapeutic when it appeals to the patient (has meaning for the patient); when it advances therapeutic goals (makes demands on the system needing improvement); and when it is carried out in the space, time, and sociocultural conditions that it would be in real life (fulfills a purpose in the person's life) (Dooley, 2009; Pierce, 1998). The notion that purpose is necessary for the therapeutic effect has persisted throughout the history of therapeutic occupation, whereas the ideal of meaningfulness of occupation got lost temporarily after World War II, during the biomechanical era of occupational therapy, which, for efficiency's sake, promoted exercising using the motions of an activity—thereby "preserving" meaningfulness—without true meaning (e.g., "weaving" on a floor loom for exercise without thread on the loom) (Laws, 2012). Another aspect of therapeutic occupation is the "just right" challenge, the optimal fit between demands of the occupation and the skills of the person (Lowenstein, 2009; Rebeiro & Polgar, 1998). An occupation is therapeutic when it requires effort for the patient to accomplish but is possible for the patient to accomplish. By accomplishing it, the patient improves the impaired ability or capacity being challenged. By succeeding

in the challenge, the patient is motivated to continue or repeat the experience (Rebeiro & Polgar, 1998). A successful therapeutic occupation results in feelings of self-efficacy, self-esteem, and self-satisfaction, as well as improved occupational functioning.

Today, as in the past, occupational therapists help people achieve satisfying occupational competence in several ways. One way is to adapt the environment or tools and teach the person how to use these contextual adaptations or other adapted methods to accomplish activities and tasks of daily life (Clark et al., 1997; Jackson et al., 1998; Moyers & Dale, 2007). In this case, occupation is both the treatment and the end goal (occupation-as-end). Occupation-as-end may remediate impairments, but this benefit is serendipitous, and the occupation is not chosen for that purpose. The second way is to remediate impaired capacities and abilities that prevent successful performance of activities and tasks required of a patient's roles (Moyers & Dale, 2007). In this case, occupation is the means to remediate impairment (occupation-as-means) (Fig. 11-2). The occupation used may actually be the same, for instance, chopping apples to make a pie. If the goal is to relearn how to make an apple pie, then we consider it occupation-as-end. If the goal is to improve strength of grasp to enable multiple other life occupations, then we consider chopping apples occupation-as-means.

The key skill of the occupational therapist is the ability to analyze activities in terms of the required skills, abilities and capacities; what influence the social and physical environments have on the likelihood of successful

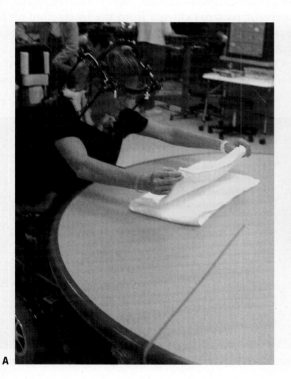

A

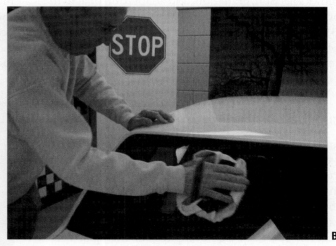

B

Figure 11-2 Occupation-as-means. **A.** Folding towels as a means to improve sitting balance for a person with spinal cord injury. **B.** Polishing the car to gain movement control of a weak arm after a stroke.

Procedures for Practice 11-1

What is occupation? What is occupational therapy?

Many people will ask you, over your working lifetime, what do you mean by "occupation"? Those who are not occupational therapists equate occupation *only* with a job or work (Thomas, 2012). They often ask whether it is your job as an occupational therapist to find work for people with disabilities. You need to develop your own brief answer that clarifies those concepts for people who have no inkling of the profession and are usually only casually interested, such as people you would meet on a bus or at a cocktail party. However, you may also want to embellish your answer if your grandfather asks about your chosen profession. Points to consider include:

- Historical aspect, i.e., why we use the term occupation. You can seek your answer at the Wilma L. West Library of the American Occupational Therapy Foundation (http://www.aotf.org).
- Current usage. You can seek your answer in published position papers and guidelines of the American Occupational Therapy Association (www.aota.org) or other occupational therapy associations.
- Research evidence of the effectiveness of engagement in occupation on wellness, the recovery of health, and the

reorganization of the brain. You can refer to studies cited in this chapter and textbook or other publications that provide evidence that occupation organizes one's brain, one's life, and/or one's behavior or that occupation motivates engagement in life. Conversely, you can cite studies that indicate that the lack of occupation is disorienting, results in failure to develop, and depression.

Then you can add for your grandfather: We study the science of engaging in activity and the effects that has on the body, brain, and psychological and emotional well-being of people from birth to old age. If he asks you, "What science?" you will be prepared to answer because you have studied the research. If he asks you, "Who thought that up?" you will have the answer because you have studied the history of occupational therapy.

I am a retired "phys dys" occupational therapist, so my "elevator speech" goes like this: Occupational therapy helps people who have had an accident or an illness, like a stroke, to recover their ability to take care of themselves, their homes, and any other life activities that they need to, or want to, or are expected to do. We use various activities, which we call occupations, to help people recover lost skills, or we teach them to do activities in new ways or change their surroundings so that they can succeed even if they have some disability.

---

occupational performance; and what abilities and capacities the person brings to the therapeutic encounter. Analysis allows selection, gradation, and adaptation of activities to promote a therapeutic outcome (Watson & Wilson, 2003). Chapter 12 describes the analysis, gradation and adaptation processes. Procedures for Practice 11-1 discusses how one might explain the skills and responsibilities of an occupational therapist.

Occupation-as-End

Occupation-as-end is the complex of activities and tasks that comprise roles (Figs. 11-3 and 11-4). It is a person's functional goal that he or she tries to accomplish in a given environment using what abilities and capacities he or she has and any adaptations that may be necessary. Relearning the occupation within the customary environment is the goal. The occupational therapist uses a person-environment-occupation focused analysis (see Chapter 12), sometimes referred to as PEO fit (Thomas, 2012). Successful intervention involves a match among the client's goals and abilities, the task itself, the client's perception of the challenge of the task, the client's sense of self-efficacy regarding the task (Lowenstein, 2009; Lowenstein & Tickle-Degnen, 2008), and the environment in

which the task is to be carried out. This view is consonant with dynamical motor control theory, which suggests that movement patterns emerge from the interaction among the person's abilities, the environment, and the goal of the occupation (Mastos et al., 2007).

Occupation-as-end is more or less equivalent to *areas of occupation* of the OTPF (AOTA, 2008) and *activities*

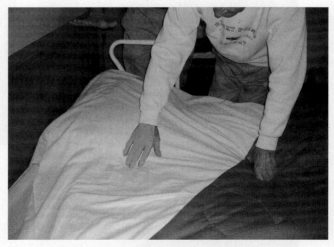

Figure 11-3 Occupation-as-end. Relearning to make the bed after stroke.

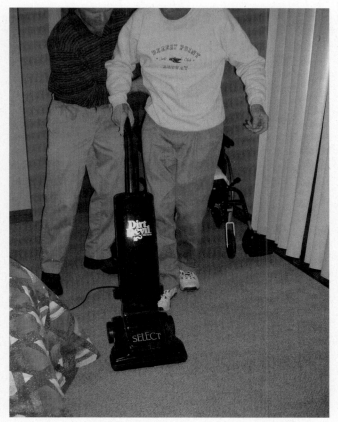

Figure 11-4 Occupation-as-end. Relearning to vacuum after stroke.

Purposeful occupation-as-end organizes a person's behavior, day, and life (Meyer, 1922/1977; Slagle, 1914; Yerxa & Baum, 1986; Yerxa & Locker, 1990). Occupation-as-end is purposeful by virtue of its focus on accomplishing activities and tasks, on accomplishing goals. Client-centered goal setting focuses the patient's attention and enthusiasm on occupations that matter. The patient will need the therapist's help to develop his or her more general goals into SMART goals, that is, ones that are **s**pecific, **m**easureable, **a**ttainable, **r**ealistic, and **t**ime specified (Mastos et al., 2007). From such goals, both patient and therapist can estimate progress.

Occupation-as-end is not only purposeful but also meaningful because it is the performance of activities or tasks that a person sees as important. Only meaningful occupation remains in a person's life repertoire. Meaningfulness of occupation-as-end is based on a person's values and context. Context includes the physical, social, cultural, temporal, personal, and sometimes virtual milieu in which occupation occurs (AOTA, 2008; Coppola et al., 2006). Meaningfulness also springs from a person's desire to preserve his or her personal integrity, defined as a satisfying sense of wholeness (Leidy & Haase, 1999); from a sense of the importance of participating in certain occupations or performing in a particular manner; from the person's estimate of his or her reward in terms of success or pleasure; or possibly from a threat of bad consequences if the occupation is not engaged in. Meaning is individual (Bruner, 1990; Harmer & Orrell, 2008), and although the occupational therapist can guess what may be meaningful to the patient based on the person's life history, the therapist must verify with each patient that the particular occupation *is* meaningful to that person *now* and verify that the person sees value in relearning it. What a person finds meaningful may not only have to do with occupational history but may be a function of where he or she is on the recovery/adaptation trajectory. That is, even if someone has an occupational history of loving to cook, she may not be ready emotionally to take on cooking tasks

and participation of the World Health Organization's International Classification of Functioning (ICF) (World Health Organization, 2001) (see Chapter 1).

Occupation-as-end achieves its therapeutic effect from the qualities of purposefulness and meaningfulness (Definition 11-1). Purposefulness is hypothesized to organize behavior, and meaningfulness is hypothesized to motivate performance (Trombly, 1995/2011).

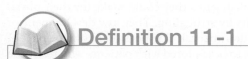 Definition 11-1

Therapeutic Characteristics and Effects of Occupation-as-Means and Occupation-as-End

	Occupation-as-Means	Occupation-as-End
Purposefulness	**Organizes** abilities and capacities, e.g., movement, cognition, and perception	**Organizes** capacities and abilities into activities, tasks, and roles
Meaningfulness	**Motivates** engagement in therapeutic occupation	**Motivates** engagement in activities, tasks, and life roles
Effect	Occupation, through task demand, remediates capacities and abilities	Occupation, through adaptation or education, restores activities and tasks of life roles

after a devastating injury or illness because that occupation would force her to confront her loss and therefore would not be positively meaningful to her. Occupational therapists practice a client-centered approach that involves the patient choosing the occupational goals of most importance at this time. The therapist cannot substitute his or her own values or judgments based solely on occupational history in selecting appropriate occupational goals for the patient. A new assessment, the Meaningful Activity Participation Assessment (MAPA) appears to be a valid and reliable measure of meaningful activity (Eakman, 2007; Eakman, Carlson, & Clark, 2010a, 2010b). The MAPA measures the time spent doing 28 types of activity (respondent can add to the list), how much each matters or is personally fulfilling, how much each contributes to physical or mental health, and the reason why the person does the activity (needs to, seeks new experience, connects with people, or gives sense of accomplishment).

Meaningfulness is not only a psychological term but also a mechanism of change. It affects neurological functioning, as was seen in a positron emission tomography (PET) study by Decety et al. (1997), who discovered that brain activation differed with the meaning of an action regardless of subjects' strategies. Newman-Norlund et al. (2010) discovered, using functional magnetic resonance imaging, that certain neurons in the brain, the human mirror neuron system, distinguishes between meaningful and meaningless actions.

Habits and Routines as Components of Occupation-as-End

Most self-maintenance and many self-advancement and self-enhancement roles depend on habits and routines, which are long practiced and automatic. Injury, disease, environmental change, and significant life changes (e.g., moving, marriage, birth of a child, death of a spouse, retirement, or first job) disrupt useful routines and habits which may cause occupational dysfunction.

Clark and colleagues (2007) synthesized literature pertaining to habits. They described nine types of habits, ranging from tics (spasmodic recurrent actions of a body part) to habitus (a person's disposition or usual manner of acting in society). Occupational therapists who treat persons with physical dysfunction are interested in habit as an everyday activity, such as brushing the teeth, and routine, defined as a well-defined pattern of behavior, a string or sequence of activities that enable complex action to be completed efficiently and with little attention, such as driving or bathing and dressing in preparation for going to work. Routines are performance patterns that give life order (AOTA, 2008; Clark et al., 2007; Segal, 2004). Both habit and routine are automatic, controlled without conscious thought, until either they are disturbed by change in the environment or person's capabilities or they fail to

accomplish the goal, at which time the person must pay attention and modify actions. Both habit and routine free the mind to pay attention to more complex occupations (Clark et al., 2007).

Habits are learned through repetition of an action under particular cue conditions, and the action results in a reward that can be as simple as successfully shaving one's face cleanly in the morning. In the beginning, the person must focus on the action, but with repetition and consistency of context, little to no attention is necessary.

Habits and routines may be preserved after injury or illness if the patient is placed in the customary context or environment that provides the cues to enactment of the habitual action. Such preservation would enable the person to engage in formerly important, albeit automatic, occupations when he may not be able to learn new methods easily because of brain damage. Therapists would be interested in determining whether such habits were preserved in patients with brain injury by setting the context in such a way that it might trigger the habitual response.

When habits or routines are disturbed, for example moving to a nursing home or after a sudden trauma, life suddenly becomes chaotic and confusing, unlike the orderliness of morning preparation, commuting, working routines, etc., that contributed to an efficient and goal-directed life prior to the change (AOTA, 2008; Segal, 2004). The therapist will acknowledge this loss with the patient and prepare to develop new habits and routines, given the new circumstances. To develop new routines or habits, therapists can manipulate the environment as well as teach the person in a consistent manner new strings of actions tied to a cue that will evoke the sequenced action.

In a study of Swedish adults aged 42–82 years old who had suffered a stroke, patients were frustrated in their daily occupations because they were not able to carry out their former habits because of their impairments (Wallenbert & Jonsson, 2005). However, they resisted making adaptations or developing new habits because they feared doing so would diminish gains they could make for their physical impairments by struggling. They saw development of new habits as detrimental. The possibility of this type of thinking needs to be explored with patients who resist the benefits of learning new habits.

Some habits or routines are not health promoting and need to be changed, for example, sitting for long periods without changing positions to relieve pressure on insensitive skin. The context may trigger habitual action even when the person intends to act differently (Clark et al., 2007), such as engaging in attention-absorbing activities, such as playing video games. In that case, therapists would attempt to interrupt the habitual aspect of the action (prolonged sitting in this case) by (1) changing the cues (environment/context) and/or (2) changing the reward, that is, ensuring that the habitual action does not accomplish the goal the person expected. For example, the therapist could install a pressure-sensitive switch that has a timer under the wheelchair cushion that would turn off the computer if pressure is not relieved after so many minutes.

Occupation-as-Means

Occupation-as-means is the use of occupation as a treatment to improve a person's impaired capacities and abilities to enable eventual occupational functioning. Occupation-as-means refers to occupation acting as the therapeutic change agent. An occupational therapist uses the client-focused activity analysis (see Chapter 12) in prescribing therapeutic occupation. It is important to remember that whereas the linkage between occupation-as-means and the remedial goal is crystal clear to the therapist, it is likely not to the patient. Therefore, when using occupation-as-means, the therapist must *repeatedly* and clearly explain why a given activity is being recommended or used in therapy. Various arts, crafts,

games, sports, exercise routines (Figs. 11-5 and 11-6), and daily activities that are systematically selected and tailored to each individual are used as occupation-as-means (Cynkin & Robinson, 1990).

Occupation-as-means is therapeutic when the activity has a purpose or goal that makes a challenging demand to the capacities and abilities that need to be improved yet has a prospect for success and that engages the person repeatedly in the action. Because the central nervous system (CNS) is organized to accomplish goals (Granit, 1977), the goal or purpose seems to organize the most efficient response, given the constraints of person and context (Wisneski & Johnson, 2007; Wu et al., 2000). Furthermore, if an activity has meaning and relevance to the individual who is to change, it motivates the will to learn and improve (Cynkin & Robinson, 1990).

Meaningfulness in the sense of occupation-as-means has an immediate aspect. Choice to participate in an activity at the moment is based on immediate motivation that is guided by currently perceived needs, feelings, and desires that may or may not be related to life goals.

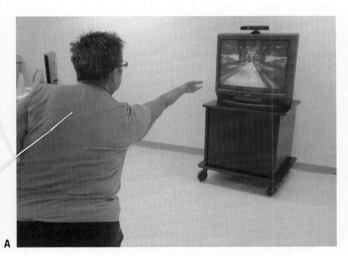

A

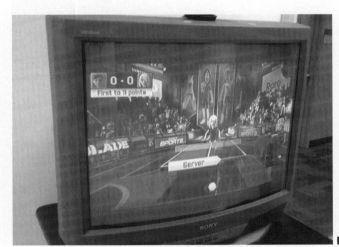

B

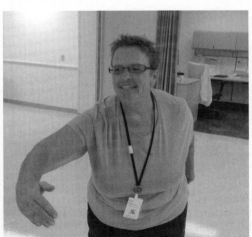

C

Figure 11-5 Occupation-as-means. Lady playing virtual reality games on X-Box 360 Kinect to improve dynamic balance and use of affected upper extremity. **A.** Bowling. **B.** Table tennis game on TV showing the "opponent." **C.** Patient laughing about a good return.

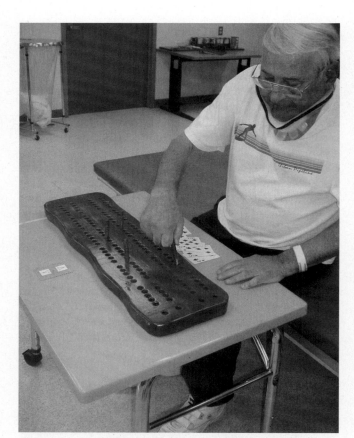

Figure 11-6 Occupation-as-means. Playing cribbage using an adapted board to improve coordination.

The meaningful aspect of occupation-as-means may be the emotional value that an interesting and creative experience offers the patient (Ayres, 1958). Meaningfulness may also stem from familiarity with the occupation, its power to arouse positive associations, the likelihood

that completion of it will elicit approval from others who are respected and admired, its value in learning a prized skill, or its potential to contribute to recovery (Cynkin & Robinson, 1990; Grady, 1992). Thus, the therapeutic aspects of occupation used as a means to change impairments are purposefulness and meaningfulness (Definition 11-1).

Evidence That Occupation-as-Means Organizes Responses

Evidence of changes in organization of emotions, cognition, and perception secondary to engagement in occupation or activity having the therapeutic quality of purposefulness is not easily obtained. However, evidence concerning the organization of movement can be easily gained using instruments designed to track the spatial–temporal aspects of movement. Movement organization can be detected from the shape of the velocity profile (Georgopoulos, 1986; Wisneski & Johnson, 2007). Different velocity profiles, which indicate differences in movement organization and CNS control, emerge for particular goals or purposes (Jeannerod, 1988; Nelson, 1983) (Fig. 11-7). Some of that evidence will be reported here.

In 1987, Marteniuk et al. demonstrated for the first time the effect of goal on the organization of movement as detected from velocity profiles. They found that five university students organized movement differently when they reached for the same object for different purposes. One goal was to pick up a 4-cm disk and *place it* into a slot. The other goal was to pick up the disk and *throw it* into a basket. They measured the reach *to* the disk, not the placing or throwing motion. The distance and biomechanical demands were exactly the same under both conditions. Only the intent after reach was different.

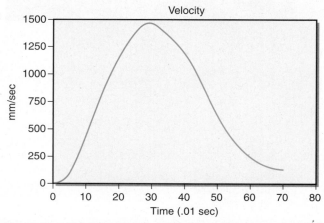

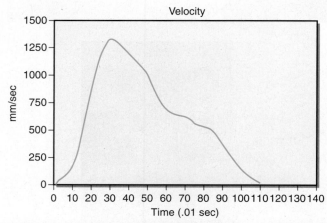

Figure 11-7 Velocity profiles of reaches to two different targets. The profile on the left is symmetrical and bell-shaped, which is commonly seen in planned reach to a stationary, large target or to a familiar object. The peak of the velocity profile (end of the acceleration phase) occurs between 33% and 50% of the reach. The profile on the right is left-shifted, which is commonly seen in guided reach to a small target or to an imaginary place on the table (rote exercise). The peak velocity occurs early in the reach, and the deceleration phase is extended as the person guides the hand to the target.

The two goals produced different velocity profiles for reaching for the disk, indicating different movement organizations.

Goal or purpose is generated from the patient's own intention, from the therapist's directions (Fasoli et al., 2002; Fisk & Goodale, 1989; Massie & Malcolm, 2012), or from the context, including what objects are available, the relevance of the objects, and what the objects afford the person in terms of action. We are familiar with generation of goals by the person and by the therapist, but contextual indication of goal may be unfamiliar, so a few studies concerning this will be reviewed.

Wu et al., (2000) used a counterbalanced repeated-measures design to examine the effects of context on reaching performance in neurologically impaired and intact populations. Context was varied by the presence or absence of objects used to complete a task. Each participant was tested under two conditions: presence of the object, in which the participant reached forward with the impaired, or corresponding, arm to scoop coins off the table into the other hand; and absence of the object, in which the participant reached forward to a place where the coins would be placed if the object were present. The kinematics of reaching to the coins or point on the table were significantly better ($p < 0.0055$) when the object was present as compared with when the object was absent. Better performance was defined as faster (shorter movement time), more direct (less total displacement), more planned and less guided (greater percentage of reach where peak velocity occurs), and smoother (fewer movement units).

Evidence that full context or presence of real functional objects affect the trajectory of reach, as opposed to imagined or absent objects, has been verified in other studies (Cattaneo et al., 2009; Ma, Trombly, & Robinson-Podolski, 1999; Mathiowetz & Wade, 1995; Trombly & Wu, 1999; Wisneski & Johnson, 2007; Wu et al., 1998, 2000), implying that the goal, as defined by the object, organizes movement.

Filippi and colleagues (2010) mapped gray matter volume changes associated with motor learning of goal-directed motor sequences and nonpurposeful motor actions in 31 healthy subjects. The goal-directed action group showed gray matter volume increase of the hippocampi as compared with those who learned nonpurposeful action, whereas the grey matter of the ones who learned nonpurposeful action increased in the inferior parietal lobule as compared with the goal-directed group. The researchers concluded that motor learning results in structural changes of the brain, the specific areas depending on whether learning involves a goal.

The speed or complexity parameters of the task also changes the organization of movement, as found through kinematic analysis of checker playing, in a sample of healthy elders (Ma & Trombly, 2004) and kinematic analysis of target pointing by 11 poststroke survivors (Massie & Malcolm, 2012).

In terms of motor responses, then, purposiveness, as transmitted by context, does appear to organize behavior and may affect brain structure and function. Of course, much more study is required to verify these ideas and confirm them to be true for other performance skills.

Evidence That Occupation-as-Means Motivates Participation

Although the meaningfulness of occupation to a person must be determined by interview and discussion with that person, *meaningfulness* has been operationalized in occupational therapy research in four ways: (1) provide enjoyment, (2) offer a choice, (3) offer the end product to keep, and (4) enhance the context or make the context more applicable to the person's life. The response, *motivation*, is operationally defined as the number of repetitions or length of time engaged in the occupation or the effort expended.

Fun or Enjoyment. Fun is immediately motivating. Several studies confirm that fun or enjoyment derived from play motivates attempts to perform an action or prolongs engagement in an action (Hoppes, 1997; King, 1993; Melchert-McKearnan et al., 2000; Omar, Hegazy, & Mokashi, 2012).

Choice. Provision of a choice presumably creates emotional value because the person is likely to choose an activity that is interesting and creative and/or arouses positive associations from the past. LaMore and Nelson (1993) found a significant increase in repetitions when 22 adult subjects with mental disabilities were given a limited choice of which ceramic object to paint (26 repetitions) as compared with being told to paint a particular one (17 repetitions). Zimmerer-Branum and Nelson (1995) gave 52 elderly nursing home residents a choice between a simulated basketball game chosen to encourage shoulder flexion and rote shoulder flexion exercises. After trying both, 69% chose the game for the actual treatment session. Choice or perceived control was also found to result in more effective and efficient performance in both younger and older adults whether the task was familiar or novel (Dickerson & Fisher, 1997). Pride of performance may be part of the motivating force when choice is offered.

Keeping an End Product. Presumably, letting a patient make a product that he or she can keep may motivate by arousing positive emotions or through the potential of gaining approval from others (Davis, 2010; Murphy et al., 1999).

Enriched Context. Enriched or natural contexts motivate through the positive emotions associated with familiarity and arousal of positive associations with one's home, culture, or previous life. Lang, Nelson, and Bush (1992) tested the responses of 15 elderly nursing home residents under three conditions: kicking a red balloon as one might do as a child, kicking a described imagined balloon, and exercise in which they kicked as demonstrated. A significantly greater number of repetitions was associated with really kicking the balloon (54) versus in the imagery or exercise conditions (26 and 18, respectively). This study was later replicated by DeKuiper, Nelson, and White (1993) with similar results. A number of other researchers demonstrated significantly greater numbers of repetitions or duration of performance under enhanced context conditions (Bloch, Smith, & Nelson, 1989; Kircher, 1984; Miller & Nelson, 1987; Steinbeck, 1986; Thomas, Vander Wyk, & Boyer, 1999; Yoder, Nelson, & Smith, 1989). Meaningfulness, as operationalized by fun and enjoyment, enriched or natural context, and possibly choice, appears to motivate continued performance, but much more research is needed.

EFFECTIVENESS OF THERAPEUTIC OCCUPATION

Long before there was scientific evidence, occupational therapists believed, based on personal experience and observation, that occupation maintained or restored health and gave meaning and quality to one's life through its organizational and attention demanding aspects (Laws, 2012; Rebeiro, 1998; Reilly, 1962/2011). Later, on the basis of deductive reasoning and anecdotal accounts, that belief was extended to include restoration of physical function through the biomechanical aspects of engagement in occupation. Occupational therapy started as a philosophically based profession and is now in the process of becoming a scientific, evidence-based profession (AOTA, 2007; Holm, 2000/2011; Laws, 2012). Although existing knowledge is primarily theoretical and little empirical support can be found in occupational therapy literature to substantiate the effectiveness of particular interventions (Orellano, Colón, & Arbesman, 2012; Stav et al., 2012), as occupational therapy approaches its 100th year, the research efforts of occupational and other scientists have begun to establish a solid experimental basis for the health-regaining action of occupation. For example, advances in technology have enabled neuroscientists, over the past 20 years, to examine brain function of humans engaged in functional occupations. This has resulted in remarkable advances in knowledge that the cortex is functionally and structurally plastic throughout life and that engaging—or not engaging—in behavioral experiences [occupation] modifies the brain's topography

and physiology (Nudo, 2007). To change the brain in a positive direction, that is, to enhance brain reorganization toward enabling better performance, the occupation must be meaningful and require effort or be challenging to the outer limits of one's capabilities but still within possibility (Nudo, 2007).

There is, however, an urgent need to experimentally verify the effects of occupation to cause particular changes and to promote a sense of well-being (Hammell, 2009; Orellano, Colón, & Arbesman, 2012). This is especially true concerning *how* occupational interventions cause the therapeutic change (Stav et al., 2012).

Evidence That Occupation Restores a Sense of Self-Efficacy or Self-Esteem

The qualitative study by Rebeiro and Cook (1999) provides the best evidence we have at this time that engagement in occupation restores a sense of self-efficacy and self-esteem. The participants were eight long-time members of an outpatient women's group at a mental health facility who engaged in a cooperative occupational project—making a quilt. On interview after 25 weeks of participation, the participants reported that engagement in the occupation gave them a sense of self-confidence and competency because of their accomplishment, which they did not have before the introduction of occupation to the group. The qualitative study of 12 persons with chronic obstructive pulmonary disease (COPD) by Leidy and Haase (1999) also found that purpose and meaning through activity resulted in a satisfying sense of wholeness and preservation of personal integrity.

Evidence That Occupation-as-End Restores Self-Maintenance, Self-Enhancement, and Self-Advancement Roles

Research Note 11-1 describes a review of studies on the effectiveness of occupational therapy to restore the role of independent person poststroke. In addition, Orellano, Colón, and Arbesman (2012) reviewed 38 studies, of which 82% offered level I evidence, to determine the effectiveness of occupation- and activity-based interventions on performance of instrumental activities of daily living (IADL) basic to role engagement by community-dwelling elders. They concluded that the evidence was moderate to strong in support of these interventions. Another systematic analysis of studies (Trombly & Ma, 2002) determined from 15 studies involving 895 elderly persons poststroke that there was a 16% increase in success rate for improved IADL and a 30% increase in success rate for improved basic activities of daily living or self-care as a result of home-based, task-specific, occupation-based training as compared with control conditions. Trombly, Radomski, and Davis (1998) and Trombly et al. (2002) studied the

Research Note 11-1

Legg, L., Drummond, A., Leonardi-Bee, J., Gladman, J. R. F., Corr, S., Donkervoort, M., Edmans, J., Gilbertson, L., Jongbloed, L., Logan, P., Sackley, C., Walker, M., & Langhorne, P. (2007). Occupational therapy for patients with problems in personal activities of daily living after stroke: Systematic review of randomised trials. *British Medical Journal, 335,* 922–929.

Abstract

Objective: To determine whether occupational therapy focused specifically on personal activities of daily living [occupation-as-end] improves recovery for patients after stroke.

Design: Systematic review and meta-analysis.

Data sources: The Cochrane stroke group trials register, the Cochrane central register of controlled trials, Medline, Embase, CINAHL, PsychLIT, AMED, Wilson Social Sciences Abstracts, Science Citation Index, Social Science Citation Index, Arts and Humanities Citation Index, Dissertations Abstracts register, Occupational Therapy Research Index, reference lists, personal communication with authors, and manual reference searching.

Review methods: Trials were included if performance in personal activities of daily living was the target of occupational therapy intervention, delivered or supervised by a qualified occupational therapist, to a stroke population. Original data were obtained from authors of eight studies and reanalyzed to standardize outcomes.

Results: Out of a possible 14,593 studies, 9 randomized trials, which included 1,258 participants, met the inclusion criteria. Participants who received occupational therapy after stroke were significantly more independent in personal activities of daily living than those who received no intervention or "usual care." Performance scores increased (standardized mean difference = 0.18, 95% confidence interval = 0.04–0.32, p = 0.01) as a result of treatment (equivalent to approximately 1 point on the Barthel Index). The odds of a poor outcome were significantly lower in those who received occupational therapy as opposed to 42% of control participants who experienced poor outcome, defined as death, deterioration of ability to perform personal care, or requiring institutional care.

Conclusions: Occupational therapy that focuses on improving personal activities of daily living after stroke can improve performance and reduce risk of deterioration in these abilities.

Application to practice:

- Intervention using occupation-as-end to improve self-care in persons who have suffered stroke is effective.
- Persons who have suffered a stroke and do not receive targeted occupation-as-end intervention may become or remain dependent in self-care.
- Client-centered goal setting and task-specific practice are successful interventions. The studies reviewed included these interventions: teaching and practice of new skills for dressing, bathing mobility, etc.; provision and teaching the use of adapted equipment and/or clothing; practice of energy conservation methods; and homework to increase the intensity of practice.
- Some patients benefit more than others, so key predictive variables need to be determined.

achievement of valued IADL goals in persons with mild to moderate brain injury and found that goal-directed, occupation-based therapy resulted in achievement of 81% of all goals named by the participants. Levine and Gitlin (1993) reported that 17 randomly selected chronically disabled community-living elders engaged in a greater range of tasks such as wine making, visiting relatives, attending church, and cleaning after receiving home-based occupational therapy as compared to before the intervention. As a result of that program, they became more engaged in life, as shown by their volunteerism and increased social activities.

Evidence That Occupation-as-Means Remediates Impairments

Studies of the effects of occupation-as-means on persons with physical impairments are few and scattered. Some are presented as case reports. While offering the lowest level of evidence, case reports do serve as models for clinical reasoning (Earley, Herlache, & Skelton, 2010; Earley & Shannon, 2006).

One systematic review (Ma & Trombly, 2002) of 29 studies with 892 participants on the effects of occupational therapy on psychosocial, cognitive-perceptual, and sensorimotor impairments poststroke concluded that homemaking tasks resulted in greater improvement in cognitive ability than paper-and-pencil drills and that practice of movement to achieve a specific action goal had small to moderate positive effects (r = 0.27) compared with control conditions. Two studies of particular interventions that found positive outcomes are described in Evidence Table 11-1. Other studies of constraint-induced movement therapy, also successful for selected patients poststroke, are described in other chapters of this textbook. However, two studies in Evidence Table 11-1 failed to

Evidence Table 11-1   Best Evidence Regarding Occupation

Intervention	Description of Intervention Tested	Participants	Dosage	Type of Best Evidence and Level of Evidence	Benefit	Statistical Probability and Effect Size of Outcome	Reference
Occupation-as-end: Goal-specific training to achieve valued occupational goals	Experimental: Long-term activities of daily living (ADL) goals valued by the participants and carers and considered amenable by the staff were worked toward via a series of written contracts that specified interim and short-term goals. Carried out in homes, day centers, and work place by two occupational therapists, one physical therapist (PT), one speech-language pathologist, one psychologist, and one social worker. Control: Booklet that listed resources with those particular to the participant highlighted.	One hundred ten (75.5% male) community-dwelling persons with moderate to severe traumatic brain injury (TBI) aged 16–65 years, in acute to chronic stages of recovery. Randomized to group. Ninety-four (85%) available at 2-year follow-up, but only 75 (68%) available for analysis of BICRO-39.[a]	Two to 6 hours per week for a mean of 27 weeks for experimental group and one visit for control group. The independent variable was compromised because some of the patients in the control group received up to 1 month of experimental treatment before randomization.	Randomized controlled trial. Level IA3a	Yes. Practice of valued goal activities in a community setting yielded benefits to persons with severe TBI that outlived the active treatment period by at least 18 months.	Thirty-five percent of the experimental participants versus 20% of the control group improved from baseline to follow-up on the Barthel Index (Mann-Whitney $U = 831$, $p < 0.05$). The experimental participants scored significantly better at posttest than the control on the total BICRO-39 score (Mann-Whitney $U = 517$, $p < 0.05$) and self-organization (Mann-Whitney $U = 474$, $p < 0.05$) and psychological well-being (Mann-Whitney $U = 469$, $p < 0.05$) subscales. No improvements and no significant differences between groups on subscales of socializing or productive employment. Effect sizes could not be calculated from data provided.	Powell, Heslin, & Greenwood (2002)
Occupation-as-end: Group-based and individual task-specific dressing retraining	Group-based for outer garment dressing retraining supervised by two occupational therapists + individual occupational therapy (OT) treatments for training with underclothing and particular dressing problems. Multiple repetitions were encouraged.	Consecutive cohort of 119 patients; ~2 weeks poststroke, medically stable	Group: 1 hour twice weekly during admission. Mean = 4.0, 1-hour group sessions. No record of number of individual treatments.	Pretest-posttest design; retrospective analysis of data. Level IIIA3a	Yes. Task-specific practice of dressing tasks made a clinically important difference to dressing performance.	Three subgroups: upper body dressing, lower body dressing, and both upper and lower body dressing. All groups improved significantly ($p = 0.0001$) on the questions relating to dressing on the Functional Independence Measure (FIM). The effect size is estimated to be small to medium ($r = 0.34$).	Christie, Bedford, & McCluskey (2011)

Intervention	Description	Participants	Dosage	Design/Level	Occupation-supported?	Statistical results	Author
Occupation-as-end: Occupation- and activity-based health management and health maintenance interventions	Interventions were within the scope of occupational therapy practice and included an activity- or occupation-based component	Twenty-eight articles met inclusion criteria of targeting health routines; 24 were level I randomized controlled trials.	NA	Systematic review. Level I	Yes. There is moderate to strong evidence that occupational therapy improves occupational performance related to health management.	NA; not a meta-analysis.	Arbesman & Mosley (2012)
Occupation-as-means: Game to increase arm reach	Condition #1: Participant reached to a point 3 inches above the center of the table placed to require full forward reach. Condition #2: Participant reached the same distance to play the Simon® computer-controlled game of flashing lights and sounds.	Twenty (17 men; 3 women) brain-injured adults with mild to moderate spasticity of the upper extremity	Ten trials of each condition in a laboratory setting	Nonrandomized, counterbalanced design. Level IIIC2c	Yes. The use of the game elicited significantly more range of motion of the affected upper extremity than the rote exercise. The results support the use of an occupationally embedded intervention.	$t_{(19)} = 5.77, p < 0.001, r = 0.80$.	Sietsema et al. (1993)
Occupation-as-means: Game to decrease pronator spasticity and to increase supination (external rotation) range of motion	Experimental: Bilaterally assisted supination exercise in the context of a dice game that required the subjects to supinate to dump out the dice for a score. Control: Bilaterally assisted supination exercise using the same apparatus without the game.	Twenty-six women in acute stage after stroke (11 LCVA[b]; 15 RCVA[c]; mean age = 68.4 years. Participants were randomly assigned in a stratified balanced way to either the experimental or the control condition.	Two sets of 10 trials for each condition; different days	Randomized controlled trial. Level IC2c	Yes. Those who participated in the game demonstrated significantly greater handle rotation (supination) (95.3°) than the controls (81.9°).	Mean gain of 13.4° in handle rotation by the experimental group was significant ($p = 0.016, r = 0.42$).	Nelson et al. (1996)
Occupation-as-means: Hand Dance Pro™ gaming system to reduce upper extremity (UE) impairment and improve function	High repetitions (mean = 1,118 per session) of unilateral and bilateral reaching to targets coordinated to music and visual prompts with immediate performance feedback. Subjects seated at table; the up/down target buttons aligned with affected shoulder and placed to encourage maximum elbow extension. Trunk restrained to prevent substitution.	Nine persons post-stroke (chronic), categorized by Fugl-Meyer Upper Extremity Motor Assessment to mild (>50/66; n = 3), moderate (26–50/66; n = 5), or severe (<26/66). All able to actively raise the involved arm from side (0°) to 45° in any plane.	Fifteen 2-minute songs per session with at least 1-minute rest between songs; 18 sessions over 6 weeks.	Single group cohort pretest–posttest design. Level IIIC2b	Partially. The gaming intervention improved UE movement kinematics, but not clinical measures in this group. The subjects enjoyed playing the game and were motivated to improve scores. Carryover of kinematic improvements to functional tasks may require concurrent practice of those tasks.	Statistically significant ($p < 0.05$) improvements and medium to large effect sizes in kinematic measures of movement duration ($d = 0.67$,[d] velocity ($d = 0.97$), and elbow excursion ($d = 0.45$). Some subjects improved in performance time, grip strength, and hand function, but no significant differences for Wolf Motor Function Test ($d = 0.04$–0.17) or Stroke Impact Scale ($d = 0.08$–0.34).	Combs et al. (2012)

(continued)

Evidence Table 11-1   Best Evidence Regarding Occupation (continued)

Intervention	Description of Intervention Tested	Participants	Dosage	Type of Best Evidence and Level of Evidence	Benefit	Statistical Probability and Effect Size of Outcome	Reference
Occupation-as-means: Purposeful activities to improve gross and fine manual dexterity	Experimental: Task-oriented intervention to enhance arm function supervised by an occupational therapist. Patients identified activities they wanted to improve. If patients had voluntary movement, they actively practiced the tasks; if not, the therapist guided the limb through the tasks and modalities to facilitate muscle tone. Control: Walking program of 10 functional tasks supervised by a physical therapist All subjects had a home program to be done 15 minutes/day.	Ninety-one persons post-stroke (chronic) discharged from nine hospitals and two rehab centers; 44 were randomized to the control condition, and 47 were assigned to the arm training program. No requirement for voluntary movement in the arm for inclusion.[e]	Ninety-minute sessions, 3 times/week for 6 weeks. One on one.	Randomized controlled trial. Level IB3a	No. Those assigned to arm training did not improve their arm function to a greater extent than people assigned to walking training.	There was no significant difference in improvement between groups on Box & Block Test ($\chi^2 = 0.09$,[f] $df = 3$); the arm intervention group improved in measures of arm impairment, but not significantly more than controls and not a clinically significant amount.	Higgins et al. (2006)

[a] BICRO-39 is the Brain Injury Community Rehabilitation Outcome-39, a self-report that measures level of activity, participation, and psychological aspects of functioning in the community.
[b] Left cerebrovascular accident (LCVA) usually results in weakness to the right side of the body.
[c] Right cerebrovascular accident (RCVA) usually results in weakness to the left side of the body.
[d] d, Cohen's d effect size; small, 0.20, medium, 0.50, and large, 0.80.
[e] This is considered a prerequisite for regaining voluntary control through therapy.
[f] There was an error in the report, corrected here, using the data supplied.
df, degrees of freedom

find improvement in clinical measures of motor function. The study by Higgins et al. (2006) had many limitations, the most serious being that patients without any voluntary control of arm movement were included in the sample; some voluntary movement control is a basic prerequisite to regaining motor function. This study needs to be repeated under more controlled conditions. The study by Combs et al. (2012) found improvement in the organization of movement but not in clinical measures. The authors suggested that task-specific training may need to be combined with reaching training. It also may be that the intervention period was too brief (18 treatments) for the improvements in movement organization to translate into the more gross and observable improvements that the clinical measures assess. Clearly, much more research is needed.

IMPLEMENTATION OF THERAPEUTIC OCCUPATION IN PRACTICE

Occupation-as-end is implemented by teaching the activity or task directly, using whatever abilities the patient has or by providing whatever adaptations are necessary to enable performance. Because occupation occurs within a person-task-environment interaction, change in any one of these variables may result in successful performance. Implementation of occupation-as-end focuses on changing the task demands and/or the environment, whereas occupation-as-means focuses on changing the person. Therapeutic principles for application of occupation-as-end derive from cognitive information processing and learning theories. It was once called the rehabilitative approach (Trombly & Scott, 1977). In this approach, occupations are analyzed to ensure that they are within the capabilities of the patient, but they are not used to bring about change in these capabilities per se. The patient learns, with the help of the therapist as teacher and adaptor of the task demands and context. In the therapeutic encounter, the therapist:

- analyzes the task and environment to determine whether the task is within the person's capabilities in that environment
- organizes or modifies the environment or task demands to facilitate success
- organizes the subtasks to be learned so the person will succeed
- provides clear instructions
- provides feedback to promote successful outcome

- structures the practice to ensure improved performance and learning

To implement occupation-as-means, occupations of interest are analyzed to determine that they demand particular responses from the person and that the responses demanded are slightly more challenging than what the person can easily produce (see Chapter 12). The therapist provides the opportunity to engage in the potentially therapeutic occupation (Meyer, 1922/1977; Yerxa, 1966/2011), and as the person makes the effort and succeeds, the particular impairment the occupation-as-means was chosen to remediate is reduced. In the therapeutic encounter, the therapist:

- ascertains the patient's interests
- selects occupations that reflect those interests
- analyzes the occupations to determine which would be appropriate to achieve the patient's goal
- lets the patient choose from among several offered occupations
- instructs the patient in the correct procedure for doing the activity to derive the most therapeutic benefit
- grades the occupation to increase the challenge as the patient improves

Lyons, Phipps, and Berro (2004) described ways they organized one clinic to efficiently use occupation therapeutically. The treatment areas in the clinic were rearranged to resemble a homelike environment (e.g., bedroom, living room, and nursery). The therapists prepared "occupation kits," which were large plastic boxes containing all the props necessary to engage in an occupation. Occupation kits were made for gardening, letter writing, pet care, fishing, scrapbooking, and car care, which were the most commonly named activities by their clients. Furthermore, therapists in this clinic were encouraged to work with the patients in the various areas of the hospital campus and surrounding environment, the larger community, and the client's own community (e.g., barbershop, market, or place of worship) to provide meaningful occupation-based interventions in the clients' natural contexts. Davis (2010) also described her method of choosing meaningful and purposeful client-centered activities that successfully addressed the specific impairments of her patients.

The processes involved in using occupation therapeutically are activity analysis, selection and gradation, and adaptation. Guidelines for these processes are presented in Chapter 12.

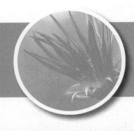

case example
Ms. C.: Using Occupation Therapeutically

Occupational Therapy Intervention Process	Clinical Reasoning Process	
	Objectives	**Examples of Therapist's Internal Dialogue**

Patient Information

Ms. C. is a 55-year-old, right-handed woman who began inpatient rehabilitation after a left cerebral vascular accident (LCVA). She was originally from the Philippines, where she worked as a school teacher. For the past few years, she has been living in the United States with one of her daughters.

Evaluation:

1. *Occupational history interview.* Ms. C. described her life through a series of stories, allowing her self-story to become evident. Several themes of meaning and important occupations emerged: (1) the theme of being a teacher, which was evident in her communication style, her previous role as teacher, and the educational play she described with her grandchildren; (2) the theme of cleanliness and efficiency, which was evident through her report that she had to finish all the housework before playing with her grandchildren; and (3) the theme of spirituality when she discussed the importance of daily church attendance.

2. *Description of a typical day* in chronological sequence revealed that her routine consisted of cooking breakfast for her granddaughters, doing housework, playing with her grandchildren, going to church in the evening, and sending text messages to her friends in the Philippines.

3. *Evaluation of impairments* revealed (1) decreased motor control but developing volitional movement throughout her right arm; (2) decreased sensation; (3) poor muscle tone of the right side of her body, although she was able to stand for short periods of time; (4) impaired but improving expressive language; and (5) poor executive cognitive functioning.

Appreciate the context

"Ms. C. is a relatively young woman who has experienced a stroke affecting her dominant side. She is depressed because she fears the loss of important roles and occupations. I chose to use a narrative approach to begin the evaluation so that I can understand Ms. C. as an occupational being and so that she can gain hope that someone is going to help her resume her life activities. Three themes of meaning emerged as she talked—teaching, home management, and spirituality. These will become important components of the treatment planning process."

Develop intervention hypotheses

"Occupation-based treatment will initiate the development of Ms. C.'s new view of herself as someone who could now continue to participate in her roles and occupations. This new vision of herself will lighten her depression and assist her in setting goals for her future. I notice that by providing Ms. C. with the opportunity to make decisions regarding her goals and preferences for treatment, she is becoming empowered and demonstrates increased motivation to participate in therapy."

Select an intervention approach

"I will use a client-centered, occupation-based approach."

Reflect on competence

"I have treated many patients of Ms. C.'s age with similar disability. My client-centered, occupation-based approach has been universally successful with them; therefore, I am competent to treat Ms. C."

Recommendations

Ms. C. will attend inpatient occupational therapy for 60- to 90-minute treatment sessions, six times a week for 3 weeks.

The long-term goal is to return home and resume valued roles of grandmother, homemaker, and church attendee.

Consider the patient's appraisal of performance

"I have helped Ms. C. notice that she is able to incorporate her returning motor, cognitive, and language skills directly into occupation-based treatment so that her impairments will improve as she relearns the activities and tasks of her valued roles. This pleases her."

Consider what will occur in therapy, how often, and for how long

"Intensive therapy during her brief inpatient hospitalization is warranted. Ms. C. agrees with this plan."

Ascertain the patient's endorsement of plan

Summary of Short-Term Goals and Progress

Goal setting was accomplished using the COPM (Canadian Occupational Performance Measure). Ms. C.'s goals included the following most valued occupations:

1. performing household chores
2. cooking
3. storytelling with her grandchildren
4. sending text messages to the Philippines
5. going to church

The initial occupation-based session with Ms. C. involved engaging in household management occupations. To prepare for engaging in these roles at home, she began cleaning, vacuuming, and doing laundry in a homelike setting within the clinic.

A subsequent intervention session was held in a simulated living room environment. Her daughter brought her two children, along with some of their storybooks. During the session, Ms. C. had difficulty maintaining the attention of the children and physically calming them down. She then used her teaching skills to explain to her grandchildren her new participation level in her role as grandmother and taught them to help hold her right hand as they played together.

One of Ms. C.'s final intervention sessions involved going on a market outing to prepare for a cooking activity. This session provided Ms. C. with opportunities to relearn how to push a grocery cart, reach for and manipulate items in the store, attend to tasks despite increased ambient noise, and practice mobility within the store.

Next Steps

Again, using the COPM, these short-term goals were identified for outpatient rehabilitation:

1. clean the bottom of her bathtub
2. clean the bathroom sink
3. carry a heavy laundry basket
4. carry heavy grocery bags long distances
5. cut vegetables with her right dominant hand
6. write letters to friends in the Philippines
7. find transportation to attend church daily
8. kneel to pray and read the Bible in church

Know the person	"We are using occupation-as-means, so by performing valued activities, Ms. C. is improving motor control by incorporating her right arm into activity completion. She is also learning how to structure her day to complete the activities she wants to include in her day. She is using the household management occupation kit to practice opening containers of laundry products, which promotes fine motor skills as well as prepares her for an important activity. Vacuuming is challenging her dynamic balance. Ms. C. told me that she saw her new role as an assistant in home management so, through the use of occupation-as-end, Ms. C. is beginning to form a new self-identity and vision for her future."
Appreciate the context	"In the play session with her grandchildren, Ms. C. gained insight into the process of role resumption for this activity at home. In addition, her family was able to see her potential for participating in the children's play." "The shopping session allowed Ms. C. to carry over some of the skills that she had learned in the clinic into the real world. The experience supported her continual formation of herself as an occupational being, and it provided her with hope for participation in this role."
Anticipate present and future patient concerns Analyze patient's comprehension Decide whether he or she should continue or discontinue therapy and/ or return in the future	"At discharge from inpatient rehabilitation, Ms. C. believed she would be able to return to her chosen occupations, such as self-care, light household management, playing with her grandchildren, and preparing light meals. She was able to initiate and integrate the use of her right side, so she expected she could participate in her typical day when she returned home. Armed with strategies and ideas regarding how to more fully participate in her life roles and occupations, she felt that she had a good foundation to return home. However, Ms. C. found that the transition from the structure of the inpatient rehabilitation setting to home and community settings presented greater challenges to her participation than she had anticipated. She was tearful about diminished participation in occupations that held considerable meaning for her life. Outpatient occupational therapy was required, and I recommended that she be seen for 60- to 120-minute sessions, once a week for 4 weeks to facilitate the transition."

Adapted with permission from Lyons, A., Phipps, S. C., & Berro, M. (2004). Using occupation in the clinic. *OT Practice, 9,* 11–15. American Occupational Therapy Association.

Clinical Reasoning in Occupational Therapy Practice

Implementing Therapeutic Occupation in Practice

One way to efficiently incorporate occupation into practice is to use "occupation kits" (Lyons, Phipps, & Berro, 2004; Rogers, 2007). Occupation kits are used to implement occupation-as-means or purposeful activity. Kits are made up of objects pertaining to a certain occupation, all contained in a box. They enable an occupational therapist to engage a person in valued activity without having to spend time in assembling the paraphernalia needed for that activity. For example, an occupation kit for the activity of wrapping gifts may include wrapping paper, tissue, ribbon, scissors, tape,

and boxes. Using the kit, the patient would practice wrapping and tying gift packages (Rogers, 2007). Describe the contents of occupation kits and the activity(ies) to be practiced for these interests:

- home repair
- baking
- grooming (male or female)

Design a kit for one of your favorite activities and share with the class.

Summary Review Questions

1. Define occupation and purposeful activity.
2. State some reasons why occupation is important in a person's life.
3. Are you in occupational balance? Which basis would you use to evaluate your own occupational balance—time, level of challenge, sociability, self/others, etc.?
4. Define occupation-as-end.
5. Define occupation-as-means.
6. Therapeutic occupation is both purposeful and meaningful. What effects do these qualities produce?
7. List two examples of evidence that occupation is therapeutic.

Glossary

Activity analysis—A process by which properties of a given activity, task, or occupation are identified for their ability to elicit targeted responses or enable a person to accomplish successfully.

Constraints—Limitations imposed on purposeful movement or the completion of occupational performance. Extrinsic constraints include the physical and sociocultural contexts and environments and task demands. Intrinsic constraints include personal factors such as biomechanical and neuromuscular aspects of a person's body (Newell, 1986), vision, sensation, cognition-perception, cardiorespiratory capacity, and so on (AOTA, 2008).

Habit—A habit is a performance pattern that is automatic (AOTA, 2008). It is a behavior pattern acquired by frequent repetition or physiologic exposure that shows itself in regularity or increased facility of performance (Merriam-Webster Online, 2012).

Occupation—The profession of occupational therapy uses the word, occupation, to capture the breadth and meaning of everyday activity (AOTA, 2008, p. 628). The term *occupation* encompasses activity (p. 629). Occupations have specific meaning and relevance to the client (Greening, 2009).

Purposeful activity—Purposeful activity is a general class of human actions that are goal directed. Purposeful activity involves specific components of occupations that help the client develop skills to enhance occupational engagement (Greening, 2009). They are activities that are goal directed and characterized by purpose and meaning as determined by the person participating in the activity (Omar, Hegazy, & Mokashi, 2012).

Task demands (activity demands)—The specific features of an activity that influence the type and amount of effort to perform the activity or that evoke certain maneuvers required to accomplish the goal of the task (AOTA, 2008). The features or context of an activity include the shape, size, texture, number of objects; the visual, auditory, physical or emotional impact of surroundings; the meaning of ritual associated with the activity; the size, shape, weight, configuration of tools; and the colors, textures, weight, familiarity, etc., of materials.

Velocity profile—A graph of time (e.g., seconds) versus speed of movement (e.g., mm/second), the latter being derived from position data recorded by kinematic instrumentation.

References

American Occupational Therapy Association. (2007). AOTA centennial vision and executive summary. *American Journal of Occupational Therapy, 61,* 613–614.

American Occupational Therapy Association. (2008). Occupational therapy practice framework: Domain and process (2nd ed.). *American Journal of Occupational Therapy, 62,* 625–688

Amini, D. (2010). Defining the term *occupation. OT Practice, 15,* 6.

Arbesman, M., & Mosley, L. J. (2012). Systematic review of occupation- and activity-based health management and maintenance interventions for community-dwelling older adults. *American Journal of Occupational Therapy, 66,* 277–283.

Ayres, A. J. (1958). Basic concepts of clinical practice in physical disabilities. *American Journal of Occupational Therapy, 12,* 300–302, 311.

Barcenilla, A., March, L. M., Chen, J. S., & Sambrook, P. N. (2012). Carpal tunnel syndrome and its relationship to occupation: A meta-analysis. *Rheumatology (Oxford), 51,* 250–261.

Bloch, M. W., Smith, D. A., & Nelson, D. L. (1989). Heart rate, activity, duration, and affect in added-purpose versus single-purpose jumping activities. *American Journal of Occupational Therapy, 43,* 25–30.

Borell, L., Lilja, M., Sviden, G. A., & Sadlo, G. (2001). Occupations and signs of reduced hope: An explorative study of older adults with functional impairments. *American Journal of Occupational Therapy, 55,* 311–316.

Bruner, J. (1990). *Acts of meaning.* Cambridge, MA: Harvard University.

Cattaneo, L., Caruana, F., Jezzini, A., & Rizzolatti, G. (2009). Representation of goal and movements without overt motor behavior in the human motor cortex: A transcranial magnetic stimulation study. *Journal of Neuroscience, 29,* 11134–11138.

Christiansen, C. H. (1999/2011). Defining lives: Occupation as identity: An essay on competence, coherence, and the creation of meaning. *American Journal of Occupational Therapy, 53,* 547–558. Reprinted in Padilla, R., & Griffiths, Y. (2011). *A professional legacy: The Eleanor Clarke Slagle lectures in occupational therapy, 1955–2010* (3rd ed.). Bethesda, MD: AOTA Press.

Christie, L., Bedford, R., & McCluskey, A. (2011). Task-specific practice of dressing tasks in a hospital setting improved dressing performance post-stroke: A feasibility study. *Australian Occupational Therapy Journal, 58,* 364–369.

Clark, F., Azen, S. P., Zemke, R., Jackson, J., Carlson, M., Mandel, D., Hay, J., Josephson, K., Cherry, B., Hessel, C., Palmer, J., & Lipson, L. (1997). Occupational therapy for independent-living older adults: A randomized controlled trial. *Journal of the American Medical Association, 278,* 1321–1326.

Clark, F., Sanders, K., Carlson, M., Blanche, E., & Jackson, J. (2007). Synthesis of habit theory. *OTJR: Occupation, Participation and Health, 27* (Suppl.), 7S–23S.

Combs, S. A., Finley, M. A., Henss, M., Himmler, S., Lapota, K., & Stillwell, D. (2012). Effects of a repetitive gaming intervention on upper extremity impairments and function in persons with chronic stroke: A preliminary study. *Disability and Rehabilitation, 34,* 1291–1298.

Coppola, S., Berger, S. E., Elliott, S, J., Horowitz, B. P., & Knotts, V. J. (2006). Occupational therapy for older adults: A reflection on advanced practice. *OT Practice, 11,* 14–18.

Cynkin, S., & Robinson, A. M. (1990). *Occupational therapy and activities health: Toward health through activities.* Boston: Little, Brown.

Davis, J. (2010). Our time is now. *OT Practice, 15,* 14–17.

Decety, J., Grezes, J., Costes, N., Perani, D., Jeannerod, M., Procyk, E., Grassi, F., & Fazio, F. (1997). Brain activity during observation of actions: Influence of action content and subject's strategy. *Brain, 120,* 1763–1777.

DeKuiper, W. P., Nelson, D. L., & White, B. E. (1993). Materials-based occupation versus imagery-based occupation versus rote exercise: A replication and extension. *Occupational Therapy Journal of Research, 13,* 183–197.

Dickerson, A. E., & Fisher, A. G. (1997). Effects of familiarity of task and choice on the functional performance of younger and older adults. *Psychology and Aging, 12,* 247–254.

Dooley, N. R. (2009). Application of activities in practice. In J. Hinojosa & M.-L. Blount (Eds.), *The texture of life: Purposeful activities in the context of occupation* (3rd ed., pp. 229–252). Bethesda, MD: AOTA Press.

Eakman, A. M. (2007). *A reliability and validity study of the meaningful activity participation assessment.* Doctoral dissertation. Graduate School of the University of Southern California, Los Angeles, CA.

Eakman, A. M., Carlson, M. E., & Clark, F. A. (2010a). Factor structure, reliability and convergent validity of the engagement in meaningful activities survey for older adults. *OTJR: Occupation, Participation and Health, 30,* 111–121.

Eakman, A. M., Carlson, M. E., & Clark, F. A. (2010b). The Meaningful Activity Participation Assessment: A measure of engagement in personally valued activities. *International Journal of Aging and Human Development, 70,* 299–317.

Earley, D., Herlache, E., & Skelton, D. R. (2010). Use of occupations and activities in a modified constraint-induced movement therapy program: A musician's triumphs over chronic hemiparesis from stroke. *American Journal of Occupational Therapy, 64,* 735–744.

Earley, D., & Shannon, M. (2006). The use of occupation-based treatment with a person who has shoulder adhesive capsulitis: A case report. *American Journal of Occupational Therapy, 60,* 397–403.

Fasoli, S. E., Trombly, C. A., Tickle-Degnen, L., & Verfaellie, M. H. (2002). Effect of instructions on functional reach in persons with and without cerebrovascular accident. *American Journal of Occupational Therapy, 56,* 380–390.

Filippi, M., Ceccarelli, A., Pagani, E., Gatti, R., Rossi, A., Stefanelli, L., Falini, A., Comi, G., & Rocca, M. A. (2010). Motor learning in healthy humans is associated to gray matter changes: A tensor-based morphometry study. *PLoS One, 5,* e10198.

Fisk, J. D., & Goodale, M. A. (1989). The effects of instructions to subjects on the programming of visually directed reaching movements. *Journal of Motor Behavior, 21,* 5–19.

Georgopoulos, A. P. (1986). On reaching. *Annual Review of Neurosciences, 9,* 147–170.

Glass, T. A., Mendes de Leon, C., Marottoli, R. A., & Berkman, L. F. (1999). Population based study of social and productive activities as predictors of survival among elderly Americans. *British Journal of Medicine, 319,* 478–483.

Grady, A. P. (1992). Nationally speaking: Occupation as vision. *American Journal of Occupational Therapy, 46,* 1062–1065.

Granit, R. (1977). *The purposive brain.* Cambridge, MA: MIT.

Greening, E. (2009). Occupations and activities. *OT Practice, 14,* 8.

Habit. (2012). In *Merriam-Webster Online.* Retrieved August 15, 2013 from http://www.merriam-webster.com/dictionary/habit

Häggblom-Kronlöf, G., Hultberg, J., Eriksson, B. G., & Sonn, U. (2007). Experiences of daily occupations at 99 years of age. *Scandinavian Journal of Occupational Therapy, 14,* 192–200.

Hammell, K. W. (2004). Dimensions of meaning in the occupations of daily life. *Canadian Journal of Occupational Therapy, 71,* 296–305.

Hammell, K. W. (2009). Self-care, productivity, and leisure, or dimensions of occupational experience? Rethinking occupational categories. *Canadian Journal of Occupational Therapy, 76,* 107–114

Harmer, B. J., & Orrell, M. (2008). What is meaningful activity for people with dementia living in care homes? A comparison of the views of older people with dementia, staff and familiy carers. *Aging and Mental Health, 12,* 548–558.

Harris, E. (2008). The meanings of craft to an occupational therapist. *Australian Occupational Therapy Journal, 55,* 133–142.

Higgins, J., Salbach, N. M., Wood-Dauphinee, S., Richards, C. L., Côté, R., & Mayo, N. E. (2006). The effect of task-oriented intervention on arm function in people with stroke: A randomized controlled trial. *Clinical Rehabilitation, 20,* 296–310.

Holm, M. B. (2000/2011). Our mandate for the new millennium: Evidence-based practice. *American Journal of Occupational Therapy, 54,*

575–585. Reprinted in Padilla, R., & Griffiths, Y. (2011). *A professional legacy: The Eleanor Clarke Slagle lectures in occupational therapy, 1955–2010* (3rd ed.). Bethesda, MD: AOTA Press.

Hoppes, S. (1997). Can play increase standing tolerance? A pilot study. *Physical and Occupational Therapy in Geriatrics, 15,* 65–73.

Hoppes, S. (2005). When a child dies the world should stop spinning: An autoethnography exploring the impact of family loss on occupation. *American Journal of Occupational Therapy, 59,* 78–87.

Jackson, J., Carlson, M., Mandel, D., Zemke, R., & Clark, F. (1998). Occupation in lifestyle redesign: The well elderly study occupational therapy program. *American Journal of Occupational Therapy, 52,* 326–336.

Jeannerod, M. (1988). *The neural and behavioral organization of goal-directed movements.* Oxford, UK: Clarendon.

King, T. I. (1993). Hand strengthening with a computer for purposeful activity. *American Journal of Occupational Therapy, 47,* 635–637.

Kircher, M. A. (1984). Motivation as a factor of perceived exertion in purposeful versus nonpurposeful activity. *American Journal of Occupational Therapy, 38,* 165–170.

LaMore, K. L., & Nelson, D. L. (1993). The effects of options on performance of an art project in adults with mental disabilities. *American Journal of Occupational Therapy, 47,* 397–401.

Lang, E. M., Nelson, D. L., & Bush, M. A. (1992). Comparison of performance in materials-based occupation, imagery-based occupation, and rote exercise in nursing home residents. *American Journal of Occupational Therapy, 46,* 607–611.

Law, M., Polatajko, H., Baptiste, W., & Townsend, E. (1997). Core concepts of occupational therapy. In E. Townsend (Ed.), *Enabling occupation: An occupational therapy perspective* (pp. 29–56). Ottawa, Canada: Canadian Association of Occupational Therapists.

Laws, J. (2012). Crackpots and basket-cases: A history of therapeutic work and occupation. *History of the Human Sciences, 24,* 65–81.

Legg, L., Drummond, A., Leonardi-Bee, J., Gladman, J. R. F., Corr, S., Donkervoort, M., Edmans, J., Gilbertson, L., Jongbloed, L., Logan, P., Sackley, C., Walker, M., & Langhorne, P. (2007). Occupational therapy for patients with problems in personal activities of daily living after stroke: Systematic review of randomised trials. *British Medical Journal, 335,* 922–929.

Leidy, N. K., & Haase, J. E. (1999). Functional status from the patient's perspective: The challenge of preserving personal integrity. *Research in Nursing & Health, 22,* 67–77.

Levine, R. E., & Gitlin, L. N. (1993). A model to promote activity competence in elders. *American Journal of Occupational Therapy, 47,* 147–153.

Lowenstein, N. (2009). A self-management approach to Parkinson's disease. *OT Practice, 14,* 14–17.

Lowenstein, N., & Tickle-Degnen, L. (2008). Developing an occupational therapy home program for patients with Parkinson's disease. In M. Trail, E. J. Protas, & E. C. Lai (Eds.), *Neurorehabilitation in Parkinson's disease: An evidence-based treatment model* (pp. 231–243). Thorofare, NJ: Slack.

Lyons, A., Phipps, S. C., & Berro, M. (2004). Using occupation in the clinic. *OT Practice, 9,* 11–15.

Ma, H.-I, & Trombly, C. A. (2002). A synthesis of the effects of occupational therapy for persons with stroke: Part I. Remediation of impairments. *American Journal of Occupational Therapy, 56,* 260–274.

Ma., H.-I., & Trombly, C. A. (2004). Effects of task complexity on reaction time and movement kinematics in elderly people. *American Journal of Occupational Therapy, 58,* 150–158.

Ma, H., Trombly, C. A., & Robinson-Podolski, C. (1999). The effect of context on skill acquisition and transfer. *American Journal of Occupational Therapy, 53,* 138–144.

Marteniuk, R. G., MacKenzie, C. L., Jeannerod, M., Athenes, S., & Dugas, C. (1987). Constraints on human arm movement trajectories. *Canadian Journal of Psychology, 41,* 365–378.

Massie, C. L., & Malcolm, M. P. (2012). Instructions emphasizing speed improves hemiparetic arm kinematics during reaching in stroke. *NeuroRehabilitation, 30,* 341–350.

Mastos, M., Miller, K., Eliasson, A. C., & Imms, C. (2007). Goal-directed training: Linking theories of treatment to clinical practice for improved functional activities in daily life. *Clinical Rehabilitation, 21,* 47–55.

Mathiowetz, V., & Wade, M. G. (1995). Task constraints and functional motor performance of individuals with and without multiple sclerosis. *Ecological Psychology, 7,* 99–123.

McKinnon, A. L. (1992). Time use for self care, productivity, and leisure among elderly Canadians. *Canadian Journal of Occupational Therapy, 59,* 102–110.

Melchert-McKearnan, K., Dietz, J., Engel, M., & White, O. (2000). Children with burn injuries: Purposeful activity versus rote exercise. *American Journal of Occupational Therapy, 54,* 381–390.

Meyer, A. (1922/1977). The philosophy of occupational therapy. *Archives of Occupational Therapy, 1,* 1–10; Reprinted in *American Journal of Occupational Therapy, 31,* 639–642.

Miller, L., & Nelson, D. L. (1987). Dual-purpose activity versus single-purpose activity in terms of duration of task, exertion level, and affect. *Occupational Therapy in Mental Health, 1,* 55–67.

Moyers, P. A., & Dale, L. M. (2007). *The guide to occupational therapy practice* (2nd ed.). Bethesda, MD: AOTA Press.

Murphy, S., Trombly, C. A., Tickle-Degnen, L., & Jacobs, K. (1999). The effect of keeping as end-product on intrinsic motivation. *American Journal of Occupational Therapy, 53,* 153–158.

National Society for the Promotion of Occupational Therapy. (1917). *Constitution of the National Society for the Promotion of Occupational Therapy.* Baltimore: Sheppard Hospital.

Nelson, D. L., Konosky, K., Fleharty, K., Webb, R., Newer, K., Hazboun, V. P., Fontane, C., & Licht, B. C. (1996). The effects of an occupationally embedded exercise on bilaterally assisted supination in persons with hemiplegia. *American Journal of Occupational Therapy, 50,* 639–646.

Nelson, W. L. (1983). Physical principles for economies of skilled movements. *Biological Cybernetics, 46,* 135–147.

Newell, K. M. (1986). Constraints on the development of coordination. In M. G. Wade & H. T. A. Whiting (Eds.), *Motor development in children: Aspects of coordination and control* (pp. 341–360). Boston: Martinus Nijhoff.

Newman-Norlund, R., van Schie, H. T., van hoek, M. E., Cuijpers, R. H., & Bekkering, H. (2010). The role of inferior frontal and parietal areas in differentiating meaningful and meaningless object-directed actions. *Brain Research, 1315,* 63–74.

Nudo, R. J. (2007). The role of skill versus use in the recovery of motor funtion after stroke. *OTJR: Occupation, Participation and Health, 27* (Suppl.), 24S–32S.

Occupation. (2012). In Merriam-Webster Online. Retrieved August 4, 2012 from http://www.merriam-webster.com/dictionary/occupation

Omar, M. T. A., Hegazy, F. A., & Mokashi, S. P. (2012). Influences of purposeful activity versus rote exercise on improving pain and hand function in pediatric burn. *Burns, 38,* 261–268.

Orellano, E., Colón, W. I., & Arbesman, M. (2012). Effect of occupation- and activity-based interventions on instrumental activities of daily living performance among community-dwelling older adults: A systematic review. *American Journal of Occupational Therapy, 66,* 292–300.

Pentland, W., Harvey, A. S., Smith, T., & Walker, J. (1999). The impact of spinal cord injury on men's time use. *Spinal Cord, 37,* 786–792.

Pierce, D. (1998). The Issue Is: What is the source of occupation's treatment power? *American Journal of Occupational Therapy, 52,* 490–491.

Powell, J., Heslin, J., & Greenwood, R. (2002). Community based rehabilitation after severe traumatic brain injury: A randomized controlled trial. *Journal of Neurology, Neurosurgery, and Psychiatry, 72,* 193–202.

Rebeiro, K. L. (1998). Occupation-as-means to mental health: A review of the literature, and a call for research. *Canadian Journal of Occupational Therapy, 65,* 12–19.

Rebeiro, K. L., & Cook, J. V. (1999). Opportunity, not prescription: An exploratory study of the experience of occupational engagement. *Canadian Journal of Occupational Therapy, 66,* 176–187.

Rebeiro, K. L., & Polgar, J. M. (1998). Enabling occupational performance: Optimal experiences in therapy. *Canadian Journal of Occupational Therapy, 65,* 14–22.

Reilly, M. (1962/2011). Occupation can be one of the great ideas of 20th century medicine. *American Journal of Occupational Therapy, 16,* 1–9. Reprinted in Padilla, R., & Griffiths, Y. (2011). *A professional legacy: The Eleanor Clarke Slagle lectures in occupational therapy, 1955–2010* (3rd ed.). Bethesda, MD: AOTA Press.

Rogers, J. C. (1984). Why study human occupation? *American Journal of Occupational Therapy. 38,* 47–49.

Rogers, S. (2007). Occupation-based intervention in medical-based settings. *OT Practice, 12,* 10–16.

Segal, R. (2004). Family routines and rituals: A context for occupational therapy interventions. *American Journal of Occupational Therapy, 58,* 499–508.

Sietsema, J. M., Nelson, D. L., Mulder, R. M., Mervau-Scheidel, D., & White, B. E. (1993). The use of a game to promote arm reach in persons with traumatic brain injury. *American Journal of Occupational Therapy, 47,* 19–24.

Slagle, E. C. (1914). History of the development of occupation for the insane. *Maryland Psychiatric Quarterly, 4,* 14–20.

Stamm, T., Lovelock, L., Stew, G., Nell, V., Smolen, J., Machold, K., Jonsson, H., & Sadlo, G. (2009). I have a disease but I am not ill: A narrative study of occupational balance in people with rheumatoid arthritis. *OTJR: Occupation, Participation and Health, 29,* 32–39.

Stav, W. B., Hallenen, T., Lane, J., & Arbesman, M. (2012). Systematic review of occupational engagement and health outcomes among community-dwelling older adults. *American Journal of Occupational Therapy, 66,* 301–310.

Steinbeck, T. M. (1986). Purposeful activity and performance. *American Journal of Occupational Therapy, 40,* 529–534.

Strzelecki, M. V. (2009). An uphill climb. *OT Practice, 14,* 7–8.

Thomas, H. (2012). *Occupation-based activity analysis.* Thorofare, NJ: Slack.

Thomas, J. J., Vander Wyk, S., & Boyer, J. (1999). Contrasting occupational forms: Effects on performance and affect in patients undergoing phase II cardiac rehabilitation. *The Occupational Therapy Journal of Research, 19,* 187–202.

Trombly, C. A. (1995/2011). Occupation: Purposefulness and meaningfulness as therapeutic mechanisms. *American Journal of Occupational Therapy, 49,* 960–972. Reprinted in Padilla, R., & Griffiths, Y. (2011). *A professional legacy: The Eleanor Clarke Slagle lectures in occupational therapy, 1955–2010* (3rd ed.). Bethesda, MD: AOTA Press.

Trombly, C. A., & Ma, H.-I. (2002). A synthesis of the effects of occupational tehrapy for persons with stroke: Part I. Restoration of roles, tasks and activities. *American Journal of Occupational Therapy, 56,* 250–259.

Trombly, C. A., Radomski, M. V., & Davis, E. S. (1998). Achievement of self-identified goals by adults with traumatic brain injury: Phase I. *American Journal of Occupational Therapy, 52,* 810–818.

Trombly, C. A., Radomski, M. V., Trexel, C., & Burnett-Smith, S. E. (2002). Occupational therapy and achievement of self-identified goals by adults with acquired brain injury: Phase II. *American Journal of Occupational Therapy, 56,* 489–498.

Trombly, C. A., & Scott, A. D. (1977). *Occupational therapy for physical dysfunction.* Baltimore: Williams & Wilkins.

Trombly, C. A., & Wu, C. (1999). Effect of rehabilitation tasks on organization of movement after stroke. *American Journal of Occupational Therapy, 53,* 333–344.

Unruh, A. M. (2004). Reflections on: "So . . . what do you do?" Occupation and the construct of identity. *Canadian Journal of Occupational Therapy, 71,* 290–295.

Walker-Bone, K., Palmer, K. T., Reading, I., Coggon, D., & Cooper, C. (2012). Occupation and epicondylitis: A population-based study. *Rheumatology (Oxford), 51,* 305–310.

Wallenbert, I., & Jonsson, H. (2005). Waiting to get better: A dilemma regarding habits in daily occupations after stroke. *American Journal of Occupational Therapy, 59,* 218–224.

Watson, D. E., & Wilson, S. A. (2003). Task analysis: An individual and population approach (2nd ed.). Bethesda, MD: AOTA Press.

Wilcock, A. A. (1997). The relationship between occupational balance and health: A pilot study. *Occupational Therapy International, 4,* 17–30.

Wisneski, K. J., & Johnson, M. J. (2007). Quantifying kinematics of purposeful movements to real, imagined, or absent functional objects: Implications for modelling trajectories for robot-assisted ADL tasks. *Journal of Neuroengineering and Rehabilitation, 4,* 7–22.

World Health Organization. (2001). *International Classification of Functioning, Disability and Health (ICF).* Geneva, Switzerland: World Health Organization.

Wu, C., Trombly, C. A., Lin, K., & Tickle-Degnen, L. (1998). Effects of object affordances on reaching performance in persons with and without cerebrovascular accident. *American Journal of Occupational Therapy, 52,* 447–456.

Wu, C., Trombly, C. A., Lin, K., & Tickle-Degnen, L. (2000). A kinematic study of contextual effects on reaching performance in persons with and without stroke: Influences of object availability. *Archives of Physical Medicine and Rehabilitation, 81,* 95–101.

Yerxa, E. J. (1966/2011). Authentic occupational therapy. *American Journal of Occupational Therapy, 21,* 1–9. Reprinted in Padilla, R., & Griffiths, Y. (2011). *A professional legacy: The Eleanor Clarke Slagle lectures in occupational therapy, 1955–2010* (3rd ed.). Bethesda, MD: AOTA Press.

Yerxa, E. J., & Baum, S. (1986). Engagement in daily occupations and life satisfaction among people with spinal cord injuries. *Occupational Therapy Journal of Research, 6,* 271–283.

Yerxa, E. J., & Locker, S. (1990). Quality of time use by adults with spinal cord injuries. *American Journal of Occupational Therapy, 44,* 318–326.

Yoder, R. M., Nelson, D. L., & Smith, D. A. (1989). Added-purpose versus rote exercise in female nursing home residents. *American Journal of Occupational Therapy, 43,* 581–586.

Zimmerer-Branum, S., & Nelson, D. L. (1995). Occupationally embedded exercise versus rote exercise: A choice between occupational forms by elderly nursing home residents. *American Journal of Occupational Therapy, 49,* 397–402.

Acknowledgments

I thank former students and colleagues for our conversations about occupation and for their ongoing research to support the efficacy of therapeutic occupation. I am also especially indebted to the occupational therapists and patients of the Sister Kenny Institute in Minneapolis, Minnesota, for allowing me to photograph them or for facilitating the photography. Specifically, I thank Cindy Bemis, Arlan Berg, Michelle Brown, MEd, OTR/L, Larry Chaney, Anthony Drong, Larry Larkin, Robb Miller, OTR/L, Mary Radomski, PhD, OTR/L, Cheryl Smith, Jennifer Theis, MS, OTR/L, Sharon E. Gowdy Wagener, OTR/L, and Matthew White, OTR/L.

12

Occupation as Therapy: Selection, Gradation, Analysis, and Adaptation

Catherine Verrier Piersol

Learning Objectives

After studying this chapter, the reader will be able to do the following:

1. Select occupation-as-means to achieve particular client-centered therapeutic outcomes.
2. Grade occupations/activities/tasks to challenge the person's abilities to improve performance.
3. Analyze occupations/activities/tasks to determine their therapeutic value for remediation of decreased abilities.
4. Analyze occupations/activities/tasks to determine whether they are within the capabilities of a particular person.
5. Adapt occupations/activities/tasks to increase their therapeutic value or to bring them within the capability of a person.
6. Apply the evidence that supports activity analysis and occupation as therapy.

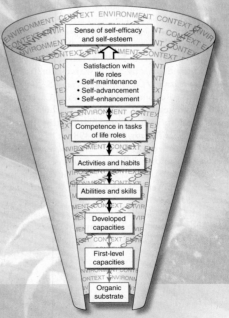

Occupations are central to an individual's identity and competence and offer meaning and value (American Occupational Therapy Association [AOTA], 2008). As described in the previous chapter, occupation is the therapeutic medium of occupational therapy with the outcome of facilitating the patient's health and participation in life (AOTA, 2008). The therapist must select the appropriate occupation for the patient that will remediate a skill or ability (occupation-as-means) or enable performance of valued occupations (occupation-as-end) (AOTA, 2008; Trombly, 1995/2011). To be able to select an appropriate occupation, the therapist must be able to analyze activities. To improve decreased abilities, the occupation must appropriately challenge those abilities and continually be adjusted as the patient's performance changes. The therapist controls the challenge by grading the activity along particular therapeutic continua and/or by adapting the method. When the patient's impairments and limitations prevent usual engagement in the occupation, therapists adapt the activity demands and/or the contexts and environments in order to enable performance in a desired occupation (occupation-as-end). This chapter instructs how to select, analyze, grade, and adapt occupation.

SELECTION AND GRADATION

The therapist skilled in activity analysis can match the patient's abilities with activities and tasks the patient needs or wants to do (occupation-as-end) and select the most appropriate activity for remediation from those that are available and are of interest to the patient (occupation-as-means).

Selection of Occupation-as-End

Occupation-as-end activities and tasks are those that comprise the patient's perceived life roles. The patient and therapist identify key tasks and activities that would enable the patient to engage in his or her desired roles within a particular context and environment. Through activity analysis, the therapist matches the particular patient's capabilities and skills to the demand level of each activity and task. The comparison between activity demands within the usual context and environment and the patient's skills determines whether the patient will be able to perform the activity independently, with adaptation, or not at all. A person feels best when engaging in activity if his or her skills match the situational challenges posed by the activity and the challenge of the activity matches the person's skills—called "flow" by Csikszentmihalyi (1990; Engeser & Rheinberg, 2008; Moneta & Csikszentmihalyi, 1996).

Selection and Gradation of Occupation-as-Means

An activity that is to be used to restore one or more skills must be within the patient's capacity and challenge the patient's level of ability so that, through effort and/or practice, the patient's performance improves (see Definition 12-1). Some specific characteristics of the goals commonly addressed by occupational therapists who treat persons with physical disabilities are listed here and are summarized in Procedures for Practice 12-1. The dimensions along which the activity is to be graded are also listed. When more than one dimension is listed, the therapist should be careful to grade the changes one dimension at a time so that change in each dimension can be monitored and the patient has more of a chance at success. The best activity for remediation is one that intrinsically demands the exact response that has been determined to need improvement and that allows incremental gradations starting where the patient can be successful. Contrived methods of doing an ordinary activity to make it therapeutic may diminish the value of the activity in the eyes of the patient. Contrived methods also require the patient constantly to focus directly on the process rather than the goal of the activity, undermining the therapeutic value.

To Retrain Sensory Awareness and/or Discrimination

The activity must provide components that offer a variety of textures, shapes, and sizes, graded from large, distinct, common shapes to small, less common shapes with less distinct differences between them. The texture of the various objects should be graded from diverse to similar and coarse to smooth materials. The therapist must also involve the patient in a teaching–relearning interactive experience in which the characteristics of the objects are discussed and correct identification by touch is rewarded.

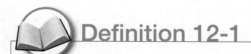

Definition 12-1

Characteristics of Therapeutic Occupation

Generally, activities should:
- have the necessary inherent characteristics to evoke the desired response
- allow gradation of response to progress the patient to the next level of performance
- be within the patient's capabilities
- be meaningful to the person
- be as repetitive as required to evoke the therapeutic benefit

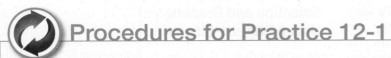

Procedures for Practice 12-1

Selecting and Grading Therapeutic Occupation-as-Means

Remediation Goal	Key Factors of the Activity
To retrain sensory awareness and/or discrimination	Offer various textures, sizes, shapes. Grade from diverse to similar, coarse to smooth, large to small.
To decrease hypersensitivity	Offer various textures and degrees of hardness or softness. Grade from acceptable to barely tolerable.
To relearn skilled voluntary movement	Require sought-after, purposeful movement; allow feedback. Grade from simple to complex movements.
To increase coordination and dexterity	Require skilled motor actions the patient can control. Grade from slow, gross movement involving limited number of joints to fast, precise movement involving a greater number of joints.
To increase active range of motion (ROM)	Require repeated movement to the limit of range, graded to demand greater amounts of movement.
To increase passive ROM or elongate soft tissue contracture	Provide controlled stretch or traction. Grade from lesser to greater ROM.
To increase strength	Require movement or holding against resistance. Grade from lesser to greater resistance or from slow to fast movement.
To increase cardiopulmonary endurance	Use activities rated at the patient's current metabolic equivalent (MET) level. Grade by increasing duration, frequency, then intensity (METs).
To increase muscular endurance	Require repetitive movement or holding against 50% or less of maximal strength. Grade by increasing repetitions or duration.
To decrease edema	Allow use of the extremity in an elevated position and require isotonic contraction.
To improve perceptual impairments	Perform activities that require perceptual processing at the outside edge of current skill. Grade by complexity of stimuli.
To increase attention	Practice activities that are graded from less distracting to more distracting and from less time demand to more time demand.
To increase memory	Practice activities that are graded from simple to complex in terms of demand on the patient's ability to remember.
To improve problem solving	Practice activities that are graded from simple (one step) to complex (multiple steps), concrete to abstract, and familiar to un-familiar. Higher level activity should include unexpected challenge.

To Decrease Hypersensitivity

The activity should involve objects or media whose textures can be graded from those that the patient perceives to be least noxious to textures perceived to be tolerably noxious. Another plan grades textures and objects from soft to hard to rough and grades the contact with the objects from touching them to rubbing them to tapping them.

To Relearn Skilled Voluntary Movement

Organization of voluntary movement depends both on the unique problem or purpose to be addressed and the constraints operating at a given time (Jordan & Newell, 2004; Newell, 1986). The activity must have a clear goal or purpose, demand the sought-after movement or movements, and offer the opportunity to self-monitor success (feedback). The contextual and task constraints should support natural responses. Grading should provide increasingly more difficult motor challenges (e.g., moving the body in various directions, moving the limbs in various directions, isolated movement of particular joints, faster movement, more accurate movement in more challenging contexts, or greater number of submovements [Ma & Trombly, 2004]). Constraint-induced movement therapy (CIMT) is an approach used to progressively increase the function of a hemiplegic extremity in which the unaffected limb is purposefully restrained, thus forcing the use of the affected limb (Bolduc & Lawrence, 2011). Evidence supports a reduced level of disability, improved ability to use the paretic upper extremity, and enhanced spontaneity of movement in patients who receive a modified CIMT protocol (Shi et al., 2011). However, some kinematic data indicate that improved performance may be due to learned compensation rather than improved motor control (Kitago et al., 2012).

Sensorimotor learning requires practice, so opportunities for vast amounts of varied practice should be provided in treatment sessions and in a home program. The activity may provide an opportunity for practice simply through the accomplishment of the intended purpose. For example, weaving requires multiple passes of the shuttle to produce the desired product and offers repetitive practice of bilateral horizontal abduction and adduction. For other activities, the specific movement may be achieved quickly, so practice is sought through repetition of the whole action, as with ironing, polishing silverware, throwing a ball, putting cans on a shelf, and other activities of daily living. Variable practice promotes learning. Unvaried (blocked) practice improves performance within a session but does not generalize to long-term learning. Blocked practice is used, however, to begin to develop a new movement or skill (see Chapter 13).

To Increase Coordination and Dexterity

The activity should allow as much active range of motion (ROM) or skilled motor actions as the patient can control and allow grading from slow, gross motions to precise, fast movements involving greater skilled movement at more joints. At first, if the therapist is grading along the continuum of increasing speed, expect accuracy to suffer. A speed-accuracy trade-off is basic to the organization of the central nervous system (CNS) (Fitts, 1954).

To Increase Active Range of Motion

The activity must require that the part of the body being treated repeatedly move to its limit and is graded, naturally or through adaptations, to demand greater amounts of movement as the patient's limit changes.

To Increase Passive Range of Motion or Elongate Soft Tissue Contracture

The activity must provide controlled stretch or traction to the part being treated and be held at the end of range

for several seconds. *Safety Message: Stretch should be slow and gentle to avoid tearing the tissue, causing inflammation, or increasing abnormal muscle tone*. Grade from lesser to greater range of motion (ROM).

To Increase Strength

Stress to muscle tissue increases strength. Stress can be graded by activities that increase the velocity and/or resistance needed to complete the activity or, for very weak muscles, by increasing the number of repetitions of an isotonic contraction or the amount of time an isometric contraction is held while performing the activity.

To Increase Cardiopulmonary Endurance

The metabolic demand of the activity (metabolic equivalent [MET] level) should match the patient's health status. The demand can be graded by increasing the duration of an activity, by increasing the frequency of doing the activity, by changing the muscles used in the activity (smaller muscles increase metabolic demand), or by increasing the intensity (METs). The metabolic intensities (METs) of 605 physical activities, including activities of daily living and sexual activity, occupation (work), transportation, volunteering, religious activities, and sports and recreational activities, have been measured and reported (Ainsworth et al., 1993, 2011).

To Increase Muscular Endurance

The activity must be repetitious over a controlled number of repetitions or duration. To increase muscle endurance, the resistance provided should be held to 50% or less of maximal strength.

To Decrease Edema

The activity should entail repetitive isotonic contractions of the muscles in the edematous portion of the body structure. An activity that requires repeated movement of the extremity into an elevated position helps to drain the fluid out of the extremity.

To Improve Perceptual Impairments

The activity should involve varied practice of information processing or perceptual processing at the outside edge of the person's capability. For example, if the person has impaired figure-ground discrimination skill, practice may start with detecting one object from a plain background (white sock on a black table) and progress through finding multiple objects on a plain background (various clothing items on a dark surface) or finding one object in more complex backgrounds (white sock in a drawer filled with clothes) until the person has developed the skill he or she requires (e.g., able to find the scissors in a kitchen "junk" drawer). Gradation is along a continuum of increasing complexity (more stimuli).

To Increase Attention

Attention involves multiple capacities including noticing an environmental cue, sustaining attention over time, attending to relevant stimuli, alternating attention between different tasks, and keeping track of two or more items during an ongoing activity (Toglia, Golisz, & Goverover, 2009). An activity can be graded by increasing the demand in one or more of these capacity domains. For example performing an activity in a quiet room without distraction and increasing the demand by introducing extraneous noises. The amount of time the patient is able to sustain attention can be measured.

To Increase Memory

Memory is described as a multistep process including the encoding, storing, and retrieving of information (Levy, 2005). There are four types of memory that individuals use: working memory (e.g., temporary storage of information during an event or task), declarative memory (e.g., conscious memory of events and facts), procedural memory (e.g., unconscious memory of how to perform an activity), and prospective memory (e.g., remembering information for the future) (Toglia, Golisz, & Goverover, 2009). An activity should increasingly challenge the patient to encode, store, and retrieve information based on the type of memory needing remediation. Gradation occurs on a continuum from simple to complex. For example, remembering increasingly more activity steps or number of items/events.

To Improve Problem-Solving Strategies

Practice may start with simple activities that present concrete problems involving objects that the patient can see and touch, such as asking the patient to get soup out of a can, with soup can, manual can opener, and electrical can opener in clear view. The patient must determine that the can must be opened to get the soup, select a can opener, and figure out through exploration how to use the can opener. Gradation involves proceeding to more complex activities that require a higher level of abstraction, such as asking the person to make soup in an unfamiliar kitchen without obvious supplies. Further gradation can involve unexpected challenges for which the patient must solve a problem. For example, while preparing soup, something spills on the floor. Another example of an activity is to have a patient figure out how many pills he or she needs for the week if he or she should take one (or two or more) pill(s) every day. The pill bottle, calendar, and weekly pill minder container are present. The patient may solve the problem in one of several ways: using arithmetic (unlikely, because the patient may have other cognitive deficits); using a calendar; taking out the pill or pills for each day and lining them up on the calendar and counting them; or putting a pill in each compartment of the pill minder and then counting them. Gradation is along a continuum of concrete to abstract and few objects or ideas to multiple objects or ideas (see Chapter 24 for suggestions for particular impairments).

ANALYSIS

Activity analysis, or task analysis, is a fundamental skill of occupational therapists. Occupational therapists analyze an activity because they want to know (1) whether the patient, given certain abilities, can be expected to do the activity and (2) whether the activity can challenge latent abilities or capacities and thereby improve them. Through activity analysis, one gains an appreciation of the activity's components and characteristics (Greene, 1990).

Activity analysis developed from industrial time-and-motion study methods. Military occupational therapists applied these methods to rehabilitation of injured soldiers during World War I (Creighton, 1992) at the suggestion of Gilbreth and Gilbreth (1920), industrial engineers who observed injured soldiers in military hospitals. Gilbreth (1911) listed these steps for analyzing a task: "(1) Reduce practice to writing; (2) enumerate motions used; (3) enumerate variables which affect each motion" (p. 5). Variables considered were characteristics of the worker, the surroundings, and the motion. This method has been used by occupational therapists for many years when focusing the analysis on the activity. Other methods of occupational analyses that focus on the performance of the patient are performance analysis (Fisher & Bray Jones, 2010), ecological task analysis (Burton & Davis, 1996; Davis & Burton, 1991), and dynamic performance analysis (Polatajko, Mandich, & Martini, 2000), described below. Both activity and performance analyses entail unnesting the component tasks and activities that constitute the occupation and determining what abilities and skills are needed to do the specified activity or that may improve through the person's performance of the activity (Mayer, Keating, & Rapp, 1986; Trombly, 1995/2011).

The therapist begins the activity analysis by stating the purpose and by identifying the task demands, that is, the constraints that will control or impinge on performance. Some constraints to be considered are the size and type of tools, placement of the selected tools and equipment in relation to the patient, the speed at which the activity is to be accomplished, the complexity of the task, and the physical and/or social environment in which it will be carried out. Changes in any of these variables change the task demands and require a different analysis. The prerequisite abilities and capacities for accomplishing the whole activity are identified. If these prerequisite abilities are lacking and the goal is to accomplish the activity (occupation-as-end), then the way the goal is to be accomplished would have to be modified (e.g., if the patient is blind). Alternatively, if the goal is to improve one or more of the required abilities (occupation-as-means), then the activity would be adapted to reduce the demands to just challenge the patient's level of performance.

In order to capture different types of activity analysis, three perspectives are helpful: (1) activity-focused analysis, (2) client-focused activity analysis, and (3) environment-client focused activity analysis. *Activity-focused analysis* focuses on the activity itself without considering the characteristics of the client or his or her environment and is used to develop a repertoire of therapeutic activity interventions (see Procedures for Practice 12-2 and 12-3). *Client-focused*

activity analysis focuses on the therapeutic utilization of the activity for a particular client toward a specific therapeutic goal, an occupation-as-means intervention (see Procedures for Practice 12-4 and 12-5). Alternately, the *environment-client focused activity analysis* is an occupation-as-end approach that focuses on the fit between the person and the environment with regard to the activity in order to determine and/or optimize the potential for successful performance (see Procedures for Practice 12-6 and 12-7).

Analyzing the activity in order to determine the abilities and capacities required to carry out the activity presupposes that activities have reliably identifiable inherent therapeutic qualities. This belief is stated in a position paper of the AOTA (1995): "Whether physical or mental in nature, the behaviors necessary for completion of tasks in daily occupations can be analyzed according

Procedures for Practice 12-2

Activity-Focused Analysis

1. Describe the activity
2. Describe the task demands
   - Objects used: What are the properties of the utensils, tools, and materials and their locations relative to the person?
   - Environmental demands: What are the characteristics of the environment in which the activity is usually performed, including possible environmental barriers and enablers?
   - Social demands: What is the nature of and extent to which the activity involves others and/or holds particular meaning associated with social roles?
   - Contextual demands
   - Sequencing and timing
   - Required actions: What are the steps of the activity?
   - Prerequisite capabilities, abilities, and skills (sensorimotor, visual-perceptual, cognitive, or emotional/relational)
   - Safety precautions
3. Identify the primary therapeutic aspects of the activity/adapt activity demands to align with therapy goals
   - Sensorimotor (ROM, strength, motor control, postural control, endurance, or coordination/dexterity). If analysis of specific muscular requirements is required, complete a biomechanical activity-focused analysis, which describes the biomechanical internal constraints for the most therapeutic or repetitive step, using the table below. Include what must be stabilized to enable doing this activity and how that stabilization will be provided. If appropriate, estimate the MET level of the activity.

Motions	ROM	Primary Muscles	Gravity Assists, Resists, No Effect	Minimal Strength Required	Type of Contraction

   - Visual-perceptual (visual scanning, perception of objects in space, and awareness of extrapersonal space)
   - Cognitive (attention, memory, executive functioning, problem solving, and awareness)
   - Emotional/relational (mood, engagement, and interactions with others)
4. Modify the activity demands to calibrate difficulty level
   - Objects used
   - Space demands
   - Social demands
   - Contextual demands
   - Sequencing and timing

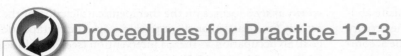

Procedures for Practice 12-3

Activity-Focused Analysis: Vacuuming the Hallway Carpet

Task Analysis Process			Example
Describe the task demands	Objects used	Properties of the utensils, tools, and materials and their locations relative to the person	*Lightweight upright vacuum cleaner with 25-foot cord* *Stored in closet next to the area to be cleaned*
	Environmental demands	Characteristics of the environment in which the activity usually is carried out, including possible environmental barriers and enablers	*The hallway is 30 feet long and 3 feet wide* *The electrical outlet is halfway between the two ends of the hallway, 5 inches from the floor* *No furniture is in the way* *The carpet is a low pile type*
	Social demands	Nature of and extent to which the activity involves others and/or holds particular meaning associated with social roles	*Does not require the participation of others* *Vacuuming may fulfill a valued role*
	Contextual demands	Nature of and extent to which the activity or the way it is carried out holds particular meaning to certain cultures or age groups	*The person takes pride in a clean, well-vacuumed home* *The person is not willing to switch to a lighter, nonmotorized carpet sweeper because of the belief that it does not do a thorough job*
	Sequencing and timing	Monological task (requiring a singular sequence in order to be performed correctly) or a multilogical task in which a variety of sequences will work Extent to which the task involves temporal requirements or timing requirements	*Monological—there are not many alternative approaches or sequences that will satisfy the task requirements* *Can be completed in one therapy session* *There is no limiting time factor involved in the activity under normal circumstances*
	Required actions	Steps that comprise the activity	*1. Retrieve the vacuum cleaner from the closet* *2. Unwind the electric cord* *3. Plug cord into wall outlet* *4. Adjust height of vacuum cleaner for carpet use* *5. Turn on vacuum cleaner* *6. Push vacuum cleaner back and forth* *7. Move vacuum on carpet to complete entire carpet* *8. Unplug cord from outlet* *9. Wind cord on vacuum cleaner* *10. Place vacuum cleaner in closet*

Procedures for Practice 12-3 *(continued)*

Activity-Focused Analysis: Vacuuming the Hallway Carpet

Task Analysis Process			Example
	Prerequisite capacities, abilities, and skills necessary to successful task performance	Sensorimotor: range of motion, strength, motor control, postural control, endurance, and coordination/dexterity	*Volitional function of at least one upper extremity to move against gravity with moderate resistance; shoulder flexion/extension, elbow flexion/extension, scapular protraction/retraction, cylindrical grasp, and wrist stabilization* *Trunk flexion/extension* *Standing balance* *Ambulation forward/backward* *Estimated required 2–3 MET level*
		Vision-perception: visual acuity, visual scanning, visual perception, and awareness of extrapersonal space	*Visual proficiency in acuity, scanning, and perception (figure-ground, spatial relations)*
		Cognitive: attention, memory, executive functioning, problem solving, and self-awareness	*Procedural memory of how to use a vacuum cleaner* *Ability to sustain attention for 10–15 minutes* *Ability to complete multistep activity* *Ability to problem solve*
		Emotional, relational	*The person takes pride in a clean, well-vacuumed home* *Performed without social interaction*
	Safety precautions	Nature of safety considerations if performed in a therapy context	*Patients may need guarding/supervision and rest periods related to balance and/or endurance* *Patients may need cueing related to cognition* *Patient my need adaptations because of low back pain*
Identify the primary therapeutic aspect of the task; adapt task demands to align with therapy goals	Sensorimotor Refer to The biomechanical activity-focused analysis mentioned later in this table for specific muscular requirements	Range of motion	*Upper extremity is moved to its limit while vacuuming*
		Strength, motor control	*Use a heavier vacuum cleaner* *Vacuum a thicker pile carpet* *Lift objects out of the way to vacuum*
		Postural control, endurance	*Bend to reach outlet and behind furniture* *Increase the time spent vacuuming*
		Coordination, dexterity	*Place furniture in the area so patient has to change directions of the vacuum to go around obstacles* *Larger or smaller handled vacuum cleaner* *Type of on/off switch*

(continued)

Procedures for Practice 12-3 (continued)

Task Analysis Process			Example
	Vision-perception	Visual scanning	*Find vacuum cleaner in cluttered closet*
			Items that need to be picked up before vacuuming are placed on the carpet
		Visual perception, extrapersonal space	*Spread "dirt" that is in contrast or similar to the color of the carpet*
			Place objects that cannot be moved on the carpet so the patient must move around them
	Cognition	Attention, memory	*Add distractions during the vacuuming activity, e.g., additional noise in the room*
			Interrupt the patient during the activity, e.g., someone asks the patient a question
		Executive functioning, problem solving, awareness	*Use an unfamiliar vacuum cleaner so patient must figure out how to use it*
			Have the patient predict performance before task performance and analyze the performance after completion of task
	Emotional-relational	Mood, engagement, interactions with others	*Patient expresses pride in accomplishment*
Modify task demands to calibrate difficulty level	Objects used		*Weight and size of vacuum cleaner*
			Type of vacuum cleaner handle and control switches
			Low or high pile carpet
	Space demands		*Size of space to be vacuumed, e.g., hallway and living room*
	Social demands		*NA*
	Contextual demands		*Set personal goal to complete vacuuming activity by a certain time*
	Sequencing and timing		*Set specific time parameters to vacuum a certain amount of carpet in a designated amount of time*

Biomechanical Activity-Focused Analysis

Motions	ROM (degrees), Distances	Primary Muscles	Gravity Assists, Resists, No Effect	Minimal Strength Required	Type of Contraction
Shoulder flexion	0–75	Anterior deltoid, coracobrachialis, pectoralis major	Resists	4− to 4	Concentric
Elbow extension	90–0	Triceps	Assists	4− to 4	Concentric
Scapular protraction	1.5 inches	Serratus anterior	No effect	4− to 4	Concentric

Procedures for Practice 12-3 *(continued)*

Biomechanical Activity-Focused Analysis

Motions	ROM (degrees), Distances	Primary Muscles	Gravity Assists, Resists, No Effect	Minimal Strength Required	Type of Contraction
Shoulder extension	0–45	Posterior deltoid Latissimus dorsi Teres major	Assists No effect Resists	4– to 4	Concentric
Elbow flexion	90–120	Biceps, brachialis	Resists	4– to 4	Concentric
Scapular retraction	1.5 inches	Middle trapezius	No effect	4– to 4	Concentric
Cylindrical grasp		Finger flexors, finger extensors, interossei	No effect	4– to 4	Isometric
Wrist stabilize		All wrist muscles	No effect	4– to 4	Isometric
Trunk flexion	0–30	Back extensors	Assists	3+ to 4–	Eccentric
Trunk extension	30–0	Back extensors	Resists	4– to 4	Concentric

Procedures for Practice 12-4

Client-Focused Activity Analysis

1. Specify the primary goal that this task is intended to advance through client performance
2. Specify which primary ability and/or capacity the task is intended to challenge:
   - ROM
   - strength
   - motor behavior
   - praxis
   - sensation
   - vision-visual perception
   - cognition
3. Evaluate the therapeutic value of activity based on these characteristics:
   - inherently evoke desired response
   - be gradable to progress the patient to higher function
   - be within patient's capabilities
   - be meaningful
   - be repetitive
4. Specify task parameters to calibrate difficulty level of the task:
   - method of instruction
   - nature and level of cueing
   - objects and their properties (materials and equipment)
   - environmental demands
   - social demands
   - sequence and timing
   - required actions and performance skills
   - required body functions
   - required body structures
   - context or environment

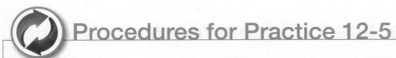

Procedures for Practice 12-5

Client-Focused Activity Analysis: Meal-Preparation Task to Improve Ability to Compensate for Memory Problems

Patient Information

D.B. (a 26-year-old man, 3 months post-traumatic brain injury) participated in an outpatient occupational therapy (OT) assessment, and these problems were identified: (1) decreased initiation of activities of daily living (ADL) and instrumental ADL (IADL), (2) decreased productivity because of poor stamina and limited appropriate avocational outlets, (3) memory impairment and inadequate repertoire of memory compensation strategies, and (4) decreased awareness of cognitive deficits interfering with compensatory strategy use. The therapist decided to incorporate task performance into the intervention plan to help advance D.B.'s progress toward the following goal: *D.B. will independently initiate note-taking when presented with occupational therapy homework (at least 60% of the time) and thereby improve his follow-through on intended tasks.*

Task Analysis Process	Intervention Planning	Clinical Transactions: Preparation for and Interactions at the OT Session	Clinical Reasoning: Example of Therapist's Internal Dialogue
S E L E C T I O N Specify the primary goal that performing this task is intended to advance	Improve ability to follow novel instructions after a time delay	The therapist selected a meal preparation task as a venue for building note-taking skills. The therapist decided to focus on the instruction giving/taking aspect of the meal preparation task.	"The therapeutic aim of this task is to develop the skills of note-taking. I am not specifically training D.B. to cook but am using a meal preparation task as occupation-as-means as one way to help him learn when and how to take effective notes. That said, he has told me in the past that he would like to learn more about cooking, and so I thought that this task would be of some interest to him." "I want to create a situation in which D.B. needs to take effective notes in order to successfully complete a task that he is interested in. I believe that this experience will help him learn to compensate for his memory problems and heighten his appreciation of the need to take notes with adequate detail."
Specify the primary abilities and capacities that the task is intended to challenge: • ROM • Strength • Motor behavior • Praxis • Sensation • Vision-visual perception • Cognition	Cognition	The therapist built memory demands into the task in order to build D.B.'s skills with cognitive compensatory strategies.	"I am not at all concerned about the physical challenges of this task, but I am setting it up so that it challenges self-awareness and D.B.'s note-taking and organizational skills."

Procedures for Practice 12-5 *(continued)*

Task Analysis Process		Intervention Planning	Clinical Transactions: Preparation for and Interactions at the OT Session	Clinical Reasoning: Example of Therapist's Internal Dialogue
A N A L Y S I S	Evaluate the therapeutic value of activity based on these characteristics: • Inherently evoke desired response • Be gradable to progress the patient to higher function • Be within patient's capabilities • Be meaningful • Be repetitive	Use of multi-step, multi-ingredient task that relates to D.B.'s personal goal and involves structured, personal choice	Prior to the session, the therapist preselected five main dish recipes that D.B. could likely prepare in 30 minutes or less. Each involved less than six ingredients and involved some details that will be new to D.B. At the OT session, the therapist asked D.B. which of the five main dishes he wanted to prepare at a subsequent session. He selected a stovetop pasta dish involving sautéed shrimp and vegetables.	"I thought it was important that I set up the parameters of this task so that D.B. could be challenged and yet successful. I have learned from past experience that with too much choice, some patients select food to prepare that is way beyond their skill level or the time available for the treatment session." "I used unfamiliar recipes because I hope that he will remember that when faced with an unfamiliar task, he should take detailed notes to guide future performance."
G R A D A T I O N & A D A P T A T I O N	Specify task parameters to calibrate difficulty level of the task: • Method of instruction • Nature and level of cueing • Objects and their properties (materials and equipment) • Space demands • Social demands • Sequence and timing • Required actions and performance skills • Required body functions • Required body structures • Context or environment	Oral instructions evoke the desired response of awareness of the need to take notes as will building in a delay between instruction and performance.	After discussing that D.B. would prepare the dish at his next outpatient OT session, the therapist orally presented the task (recipe) instructions. Grocery items that D.B. was to purchase and bring to the session were also orally presented. In order to make the task simpler, the therapist ensured that the treatment sessions were carried out in a quiet place where interruptions were minimal. If D.B. had too much difficulty with note-taking, the therapist planned to grade the task to make it easier by giving him written recipes that included some but not all of the details. If the task of taking and relying on notes was easily accomplished by D.B., the therapist was prepared to grade the task difficulty by adding nonobvious substeps to the cooking task that D.B. would likely perform only if he had taken notes with adequate detail and thought to refer to them.	"I am using oral instructions (rather than providing a written copy of the recipe) so that the task will challenge D.B.'s awareness that he needs to take notes that are usable in the future. I am also building in a delay by providing the instructions at one session and asking him to actually perform the task at a session next week. This will increase the likelihood that he will realize that he needs to rely on his notes rather than his memory and that the notes need to be of a quality that will enable performance." "It can be very difficult or stressful for some people to take written notes on a lot of unfamiliar information. If this is the case with D.B., he can use a written copy of some bare-bones notes that I have prepared and add any additional information that he needs. This will also give me a sense of how aware he is of his need for note-taking." "If this task proves to be too easy for D.B., I will add some prospective memory demands by asking him to step away from the task after sautéing the vegetables and call my voice mail to leave me a message about how it is going and then return to the task. I am trying to create a situation in which D.B. must rely on his notes rather than proceeding on his own instincts."

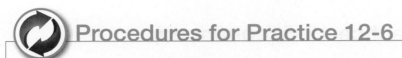

Procedures for Practice 12-6

Environment-Client-Focused Activity Analysis

1. Specify the task that the person wants or needs to perform in a given environment
2. Specify the performance environments (e.g., environment in which the client will perform the desired activity or environment in which the therapy session with occur)
3. Evaluate the barriers or enablers to performance of this activity in this environment:
   - task
   - environment
   - person
4. Determine solutions that will enable performance:
   - person
   - environment
   - task

5. Specify task and environmental parameters to calibrate difficulty level:
   - method of instruction
   - nature and level of cueing
   - objects and their properties (materials, equipment)
   - space demands
   - social demands
   - sequence and timing
   - required actions and performance skills
   - required body functions
   - familiar or novel task or environment
   - known adaptations or specifics to design & build the needed adaptation

Procedures for Practice 12-7

Environment-Client Focused Activity Analysis: Advancing Homemaker Role

Patient Information

Mrs. B. is a 45-year-old woman who sustained a right-sided cerebrovascular accident 2 months ago. After inpatient rehabilitation, she was discharged home. She lives with her husband, who works full-time, and daughter who is a senior in high school. Mr. B. would like to hire a housekeeper to help with the housekeeping, but finances are tight. Both he and their daughter are managing to do the household tasks now, but Mrs. B. realizes that they are fatigued by this extra burden. Prior to her stroke, Mrs. B. prided herself on her ability to care for her family and home. She has been referred to home care and is working with an occupational therapist to address her desire to recover her role as homemaker.

Task Analysis Process		Intervention Planning	Therapeutic Transactions: Preparation for and Interactions at the OT Session	Clinical Reasoning: Example of Therapist's Internal Dialogue
S E L E C T I O N	Specify the task that the person needs or wants to perform in a given environment	Mrs. B. wants to assist daughter in meal preparation activities (occupation-as-end) in her own home and to eventually regain her homemaker role, of which meal preparation is a key task. Mrs. B. likes to cook and has been feeling bad that her daughter has been doing the meal preparation.	In consultation with Mrs. B., the therapist selected preparation of bagged lunches for Mrs. B.'s daughter and husband and making lunch for herself.	"Mrs. B. is aware of the burden that her family feels because they have to do so many of the tasks she ordinarily did before her stroke. It is important to her to lessen that burden as well as to recover her homemaker role."
	Specify the performance environments (environment in which the patient will perform the desired activity; environment in which the therapy session will occur)	The therapy session will occur in the kitchen of Mrs. B.'s home, which is where she will ultimately perform the task.		"Being able to work with Mrs. B. in her home will eliminate any potential performance problems associated with an unfamiliar environment."

Procedures for Practice 12-7 *(continued)*

Task Analysis Process	Intervention Planning	Therapeutic Transactions: Preparation for and Interactions at the OT Session	Clinical Reasoning: Example of Therapist's Internal Dialogue
A N A L Y S I S Evaluate the barriers or enablers to performance of this activity in this environment: • Task • Environment • Person Determine solutions that will enable performance: • Person • Environment • Task	Barriers: • Mrs. B.'s left hand is weak for grasping objects and her standing tolerance is limited to 10 minutes. • Mrs. B. has a throw rug in front of her sink, which may be a hazard. • Mr. B. is very interested in supporting his wife, but his presence in the kitchen appears to distract the client. Enablers: • Mrs. B. has intact visual perception and cognition. • Her kitchen has ample counter space with utility drawers located under the counter where Mrs. B. could work. A refrigerator is located to the left of the counter space. • Selected task is time limited, and adaptations can be used to minimize effects of poor standing tolerance and weak left hand Solutions: • Sit to work to relieve fatigue and increase safety • Use a cutting board with corner guards to compensate for weak left hand • Use a mounted jar opener to compensate for weak left hand • Ensure that the countertop is uncluttered to ease performance (remove clutter if necessary)	Materials required: • High stool • Cutting board with corner guards • Bread • Condiments • Luncheon meat • Fruit • Napkins • Knife • Dishes • Paper bags • Mounted jar opener Safety precautions: • Guard Mrs. B. when she gets onto stool and when she walks to refrigerator • Cover the spikes on the cutting board with corks to prevent cuts	"Before we get started, I want to optimize some aspects of the work environment. I have asked Mrs. B. if we can remove the throw rug and asked that Mr. B. join us in the kitchen at the end of our session. I need to instruct Mrs. B. in the use of the cutting board with guards to 'trap' the bread while she spreads the condiments on each slice and how to use the mounted jar opener, which will compensate for the weakness in her left hand. As she is right-hand dominant, I will encourage her to use her left arm and hand as an assist during the activity. I need to teach Mrs. B. how to use her body to hold the refrigerator door open as she gets the items out. I will watch Mrs. B. carefully as she moves about the kitchen and gets onto the stool. I will not 'hover,' but allow Mrs. B. to solve some of the problems she will encounter if she can. In that way, she will gain confidence, and the learning will generalize to other activities."

(continued)

Procedures for Practice 12-7 *(continued)*

Task Analysis Process	Intervention Planning	Therapeutic Transactions: Preparation for and Interactions at the OT Session	Clinical Reasoning: Example of Therapist's Internal Dialogue
G R A D A T I O N Specify task and environmental parameters to calibrate difficulty level: • Method of instruction • Nature and level of cueing • Objects and their properties (materials and equipment) • Space demands • Social demands • Sequence and timing • Required actions and performance skills • Required body functions • Familiar or novel task or environment • Known adaptations or specifics to design and build the needed adaptation	To advance Mrs. B. toward greater involvement in her valued role as homemaker, food preparation activities can be graded by changing the number of objects and their properties (size, weight, shape, and texture), by changing required actions and performance skills (stand for longer periods of time), and later by changing the novelty of the recipe.	Challenge Mrs. B. to include sliced tomato and lettuce in the sandwiches, using the cutting board to hold the tomato and a proper knife. Materials needed: • Cutting board • Tomato • Several knives from which to choose the correct one • Sandwich materials as above • Stool Challenge Mrs. B. to prepare a salad that requires handling and preparing different sizes and shapes of vegetables or fruits and a large bowl. Materials needed: • Large bowl • Variety of vegetables or fruits • Cutting board • Knives • Stool	"I want to see if Mrs. B. will remember to use the cutting board. If she does not, I will coach her. I will coach her to use the safest knife for cutting the tomato." "When preparing the salad, I will want to see her solve how to position each differently shaped fruit or vegetable to cut it. I will coach her to move the large bowl by sliding rather than lifting."

to specific components related to moving, perceiving, thinking, and feeling" (p. 1015). Although tasks and activities require particular performance skills, abilities, and capacities, identification of these (activity analysis) is a high-level skill that requires practice under supervision.

Activity-Focused Analysis

Using an analytical approach, the therapist examines an activity to determine its components and the level of ability and skill demanded. The outcome can be used to select activities for remediation or to match a particular person's skills with the demands of the activity.

All analyses should occur within some conceptual framework to give them direction, coherence, and meaning (Mosey, 1981). For example, planting a tulip bulb in a plant pot can be analyzed from various frames of reference. The biomechanical approach prompts the therapist to examine the physical requirements, such as grasp, coordination, and ROM, whereas the cognitive-perceptual approach examines the activity according to its cognitive or perceptual demands, such as attention, problem-solving, and spatial requirements.

Whereas biomechanical analysis observes joint ROM and estimates muscle contraction used to carry out the activity based on knowledge of anatomy and kinesiology, electromyographic (EMG) and kinematic research indicates that this type of analysis may not be wholly valid because of individual differences in muscle action and differences in movement strategies secondary to learning, maturation, injury, and perception of goal (Illyes & Kiss, 2005; Jordan & Newell, 2004; Kelly et al., 2005; Trombly & Quintana, 1983) that are not detectable by an observer without instrumentation. Each person's CNS plans movement to accomplish the goal with the resources the person has. Reaching for a glass of milk on the table may or may not activate the anterior deltoid. If that muscle is weak, the patient may accomplish the goal by substituting other muscles or strategies, such as turning sidewise to the table to make use of the stronger middle deltoid to reach the glass. The substitutions listed in the muscle testing section are common ways people accomplish the movement goal when the prime mover is weak. The idea that doing a certain activity will always exercise a certain weak muscle may be naive. If it is essential that a particular muscle of a particular patient be contracting to a certain level of activity, as may be the case in tendon transfer rehabilitation, it is best to monitor the muscle directly using EMG biofeedback as the patient does the activity (Trombly & Cole, 1979; Trombly & Quintana, 1983) (see Chapter 19).

On average, certain motions and muscle actions are more probable than others, and therefore, an analysis can be based on observation if the therapist realizes that actual performance of a particular patient must be verified and not assumed. As instrumentation to measure human movement is too complex to be used clinically at this time; by default, the traditional biomechanical activity-focused analysis continues to be the method used by practicing therapists and is described in Procedures for Practice 12-2 and 12-3.

The first step of an activity analysis is to identify the exact activity. Next, a detailed description of the task demands is completed, followed by the primary therapeutic aspects of the task, and finally the gradations to task demands that can calibrate the level of difficulty or challenge. If analysis of specific motor requirements is required (e.g., ROM and strength), a specialized biomechanical analysis should be completed, as done in Procedures for Practice 12-3, in which the potential repetitions of each motion are noted. Only the sixth step of the activity, pushing the vacuum cleaner back and forth, would be analyzed biomechanically if vacuuming were going to be used as occupation-as-means because it is the repetitive, therapeutic aspect of this activity. The other steps occur too infrequently to be therapeutic. Each repetitive step is subdivided into motions. For

example, pushing the vacuum back and forth involves shoulder flexion with elbow extension, shoulder extension with elbow flexion, and trunk flexion and extension, although trunk movement may be eliminated, depending on how the person moves in relation to the machine. Wrist stabilization (cocontraction) in extension and cylindrical grasp are also "motions" associated with vacuuming.

The range of each motion is estimated by observing another person or by doing the activity oneself. Each motion is further analyzed to determine which muscle or muscles are likely responsible, based on anatomical, kinesiological, and electromyographical knowledge. Examining the effect of gravity allows estimation of the minimal strength necessary to do the motion. The kind of contraction demanded for each muscle group in each motion is established by definition.

Activities selected to restore motor function must also take into account the person's cognitive and perceptual skills, emotional status, cultural background, and interests. An analysis of the cognitive functions required for the activity should include the number and complexity of the steps involved in doing the activity, the requirements for organizing and sequencing of the steps or stimuli, and the amount of concentration and memory required. Some perceptual factors to be considered are whether the activity requires the patient to distinguish figure from ground, determine position in space, construct a two- or three-dimensional object, or follow verbal or spatial directions. Other cognitive-perceptual considerations are found in Chapters 23 and 24. Some psychosocial aspects of an activity that may be important to patients include whether the activity must be done alone or in a group, the length of time required to complete the activity, whether fine detailed work or large expansive movements are involved, how easily errors can be corrected, the value of the activity from the person's particular cultural and social background, and the likelihood of producing a satisfying outcome.

Other methods of analysis of activities have been published. Gentile (2000) has provided a detailed taxonomy of task analysis to be used for evaluation and selection of functionally relevant activities. The taxonomy is related to the learning of motor tasks. Her taxonomy is briefly described here, although the reader should see the original material for a complete description and rationale. The taxonomy consists of 16 categories composed of movement types and environmental regulatory constraints. The dimensions of environmental regulation and movement type are presented separately in Definition 12-2 for the sake of clarity, but they are meant to be combined. The easiest tasks are repetitive ones done in a stationary environment with the body in a stable position, such as sitting and brushing one's hair. Tasks are

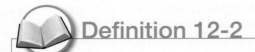

Definition 12-2

Examples of Tasks Described According to the Taxonomy of Gentile

Environmental Regulatory Dimension		
Environmental Regulatory Conditions during Performance	*No Differences in Performance between Trials*	*Differences in Performance between Trials*
Stationary: objects, people, and/or apparatus do not move	Closed tasks Climbing stairs at home Brushing teeth Unlocking the front door Turning on the bedroom light	Tasks in which objects are different but stationary during performance: Walking on different surfaces Drinking from mugs, glasses, cups Putting on shirt, sweater
Motion: objects, people, and/or apparatus move	Tasks in which objects move consistently over repeated encounters: Stepping onto an escalator Lifting luggage from the conveyer belt at the airport Moving through a revolving door	Open Tasks Propelling a wheelchair down a crowded hall Catching a ball Carrying a wiggling child

Movement Type Dimension		
Body Orientation	*No Manipulation*	*Manipulation*
Stability: body is positioned in one place	Body stability: Sit Stand Lean on table	Body stability plus manipulation: Hold object while standing Reach for hairbrush while sitting Using a keyboard while sitting at a computer
Transport: body is moving through space	Body transport: Walk Run Drive an automobile Propel wheelchair	Body transport plus manipulation: Run to catch a ball Dial phone while walking

Adapted with permission from Gentile, A. M., Higgins, J. R., Miller, E. A., & Rosen, B. (1975). Structure of motor tasks. In *Mouvement actes du 7e symposium Canadien en appentissage psycho-motor et psychologie du sport* (pp. 11–28). Quebec, Canada (out of print). Also in Gentile, A. (2000). Skill acquisition: Action, movement and neuromotor processes. In J. H. Carr, R. B. Shepherd, J. Gordon, A. M. Gentile, & J. M. Held (Eds.), *Movement science: Foundations for physical therapy in rehabilitation* (2nd ed., pp. 111–187). Rockville, MD: Aspen Systems.

graded by changing the various parameters one at a time (e.g., environmental regulatory conditions, differences in performance between trials, body orientation, and manipulation demands). The most demanding tasks are those done in an environment that changes with the performance, with requirements that change between trials, and with the body in motion while manipulating an object, such as playing basketball.

Some therapists keep files of activity-focused analyses, which they can adapt to client-focused, based on particular patients, whereas others prefer to use an environment-client activity analysis, focusing on a particular patient in a particular context. Over the years, activity-focused analyses have been published for general use by therapists: Hi-Q game (Neistadt et al., 1993); macramé (Chandani & Hill, 1990); planting a small garden (Nelson, 1988); using a computer for skill development, education, and prevocational training (Okoye, 1993); hand activities (Trombly & Cole, 1979); donning a sock (Greene, 1990); and bilateral inclined sanding (Spaulding & Robinson, 1984). Watson and Wilson (2003) published a task-analysis form based on the American Occupational Therapy Association's Occupational Therapy Practice Framework.

Performance-Focused Analysis (Client-Focused and Environment-Client Focused Activity Analyses)

Using an analytic approach, the therapist observes the patient's performance of role-related occupations. Figure 12-1 and Procedures for Practice 12-8 depict analysis of role performance within the environment using the Occupational Functioning Model as the basis (Trombly, 1993). The first step is to determine whether the person is accomplishing the role as he or she wants, needs, or expects to do. If not, the patient identifies the tasks and activities within the role that are not being accomplished to criterion. Observing the person's attempt to do an activity gives the therapist clues about which abilities and capacities may need further evaluation and treatment. This is the assessment described in Chapter 1. It is similar to the Dynamic Performance Analysis (DPA) proposed by Polatajko, Mandich, and Martini (2000). The DPA is described as a performance-based dynamic iterative process of analysis that is carried out as the client performs an occupation. The steps are: (1) establish whole-task performer prerequisites (motivation and knowledge of the task), (2) analyze observed performance to identify where the patient demonstrates performance difficulties, and (3) establish the source of the difficulties within the relationship between client abilities and the environmental or occupational supports or demands. Analysis according to the Occupational Functioning Model is also similar to

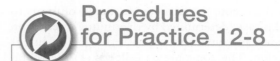

Procedures for Practice 12-8

Performance-Focused Analysis According to the Occupational Functioning Model

1. Name the role
2. List the tasks the person identifies as important to this role
3. List the activities the person identifies as part of a key task
4. Describe the environment and context in which the person will be performing the activity
5. Observe the person performing one of the activities within the environment
6. If the person is able to perform the activity, observe another of the activities. When the person is unable to do an activity, one of three directions can be taken:
   - Teach the person adapted methods to accomplish the activity
   - Modify/simplify the environment to allow the person to perform the activity
   - Remediate impaired abilities and capacities to enable performance
7. If remediation is chosen, analyze what ability limitations are interfering with performance
8. After identifying particular ability limitations, measure those abilities to confirm the limitation
9. If the ability is significantly limited, analyze what deficit capacities are causing that limitation
10. Measure those capacities and treat when verified

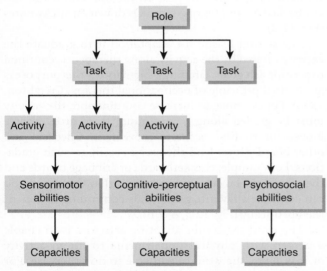

Figure 12-1 Performance-focused analysis according to the Occupational Functioning Model. One role is composed of several tasks. Each task consists of several activities. Each activity depends on varying degrees of sensorimotor, cognitive-perceptual, and psychosocial abilities. Those abilities depend on supporting capacities. The performance-focused analysis examines these components of the model from the top down by observing the patient. When the patient has difficulty performing, the therapist examines the next lower levels and/or the environment as possible constraints to the performance.

the analysis based on the Occupational Therapy Practice Framework, 2nd ed. (Watson & Wilson, 2003) but is less complicated.

The performance analysis proposed by Fisher and Bray Jones (2010) involves observational evaluation of the "transaction between the client and the environment as the client performs a task that is familiar, meaningful, purposeful and relevant" (p. 517). To do this, Fisher uses a standardized performance analysis, the Assessment of Motor and Process Skills (AMPS) (Fisher & Bray Jones, 2010; Merritt & Fisher, 2003), although it can also be done by informal observation. The quality of performance, not the patient's underlying capacities, is graded, although the capacities are considered when interpreting the outcome and planning treatment.

The Ecological Task Analysis (ETA) is based on ideas of the dynamical systems theory of movement and Gibson's (1977) theory of affordances (Burton & Davis, 1996; Davis & Burton, 1991). This environment-client activity analysis examines the interacting constraints (limitations and enablers) of performer, environment, and task as the occupation is undertaken. The ETA is based on the premise that there are many solutions to a particular task, determined by the unique interaction of performer and environment with the goal or intent of the action. The steps are as follows: (1) the therapist selects and establishes the task goal, structures the physical and social environments, and provides verbal and other cues to allow for an understanding of the task goal by the patient; (2) the patient practices the task, with the therapist allowing the patient to choose movement solutions; (3) the therapist manipulates the performer, environment, or task variables to find the optimal performance; (4) the therapist identifies specific contexts in which the person can always (sometimes, never) accomplish the task and discovers by perturbation (e.g, increase speed, force, or other potentially controlling variable) the importance of performer or environmental variables on the performance of the task or movement; and (5) the therapist provides direct instructions of other possibilities of movement solutions (see Chapter 21 for application of this analysis and teaching process).

ADAPTATION

Activity adaptation is the process of modifying an activity of daily living, craft, game, sport, or other occupation to enable performance, prevent cumulative trauma injury, or accomplish a therapeutic goal (Definition 12-3). Although we may like to think that occupational therapists devised this process, actually Gilbreth devised it in the early 1900s (Creighton, 1992, 1993). He proposed adapting activity to suit the anatomy of workers to make work more efficient (Gilbreth, 1911).

There are four reasons to adapt an activity in the treatment of patients with physical disabilities. One is to modify the activity to make it therapeutic when ordinarily it would not be so. Many examples of this can be seen in

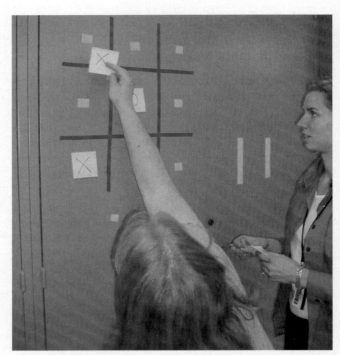

Figure 12-2 Therapist and patient playing tic-tac-toe in an adapted way that requires reaching up.

occupational therapy clinics. For example, in wall checkers, the board is mounted on the wall and has pegs at each square to hold the checkers. Tic-tac-toe can be adapted similarly by drawing the grid on the wall and using Velcro-backed Xs and Os or Xs and Os drawn on sticky notes (Fig. 12-2).

The second reason for adaptation is to graduate the exercise offered by the activity along therapeutic continua to accomplish goals. Grading of activity for this purpose is an original principle of occupational therapy (Creighton, 1993). For example, to increase coordination, the activity must be graded along a continuum from gross, coarse movement to fine, accurate movement. Checkers and other board games lend themselves easily to such gradations. For example, checkerboards or cribbage boards and the pieces can be changed in size so that the aficionado can continue a favorite game while continuing to benefit therapeutically (Fig. 12-3, A & B).

The third reason for adapting activities is to enable a person with physical impairments to do an activity or task he or she would be unable to do otherwise. For example, after having a stroke that causes paresis of one upper limb, a patient can learn a new method of putting on a shirt that requires only one hand. Or the environment in which a favorite activity was accomplished can be modified to allow engagement. For example, a gardener who undergoes bilateral lower extremity amputation because of diabetes can continue to garden from a wheel-

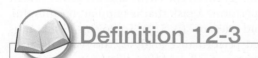

Definition 12-3

Characteristics of a Good Adaptation

A good adaptation:

- accomplishes the specific goal
- does not encourage or require odd movements or postures
- is not dangerous to the patient
- intrinsically demands a certain response on which the patient does not have to concentrate
- does not demean the patient (some contrived adaptations may seem ridiculous to the patient and thus are embarrassing and nontherapeutic)

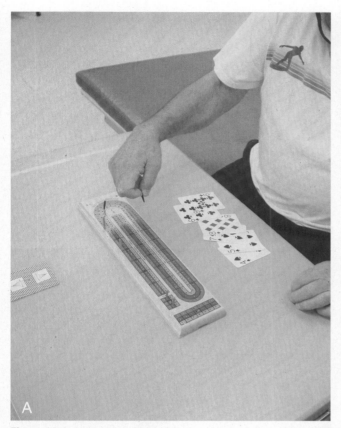

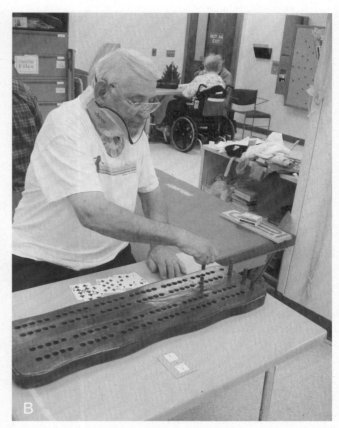

Figure 12-3 **A.** Standard-sized cribbage board demands fine coordination. **B.** Enlarged cribbage board and pegs allow a person with deficient fine coordination to play (occupation-as-end) or demand greater range of motion of reaching (occupation-as-means).

chair if the beds are raised (Harnish, 2001). Figures 12-4 and 12-5 (A & B) show other examples of contextual adaptation to enable performance. Chapters 25–28 outline ways to compensate for particular disabilities to enable role performance.

The fourth reason for adapting activities, especially work activities that are engaged in for long periods of time, is to prevent cumulative trauma injury. Examples of such adaptation are changing the table height to reduce strain on the back or upper extremities or doing the work task while seated to reduce stress on the lower back.

As with all therapeutic techniques, for patients that are cognitively intact, it is vital for the patient to understand the reason why an activity is adapted (Peloquin, 1988). For patients who have cognitive impairment, it is important to determine their cognitive capacity to process complex and/or abstract information and explain the reason for an activity at the level they will understand (McCraith, Austin, & Earhart, 2011).

Using the activity demands described in the Occupational Therapy Practice Framework (AOTA, 2008), specific methods to modify activities for therapeutic purpose are described here and listed in Procedures for Practice 12-9.

Parameters Used to Adapt or Modify Activities

Activity Demand: Required Body Functions

This group of adaptations focus on specific body functions that support the actions used to perform activities (e.g., muscle strength and standing balance).

Position the Activity Relative to the Person. The position of the person relative to the work to be done dictates the movement demanded by the activity and therefore which muscle groups are likely to be used (McGrain & Hague, 1987). Poor positioning of work equipment relative to the size of the person may result in musculoskeletal discomfort or repeated stress injuries (Sung et al., 2003). Adaptation by positioning refers to changes in incline of work surface, height of work surface, location of work equipment, or placement of pieces to be added to the project in order to require a specific body function that is the target of the therapeutic activity.

Activities that are usually done on a flat surface, such as finger painting, board games, and sanding wood, can be made more or less resistive by changing

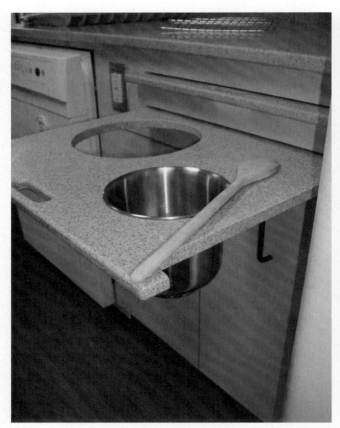

Figure 12-4 A pull-out shelf with cut-outs that accommodate bowls or pots enables a person to cook efficiently from a sitting postion, e.g., when in a wheelchair.

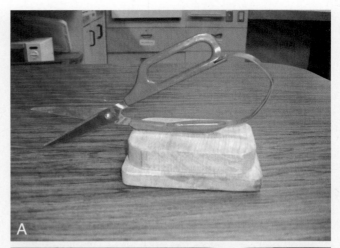

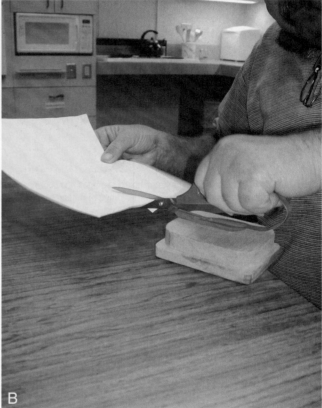

Figure 12-5 A, B. Scissors have been stabilized in a wooden block to enable cutting by a person who lacks finger dexterity.

the incline of the surface. For example, if the surface is inclined down and away from the patient, resistance is given to shoulder extension and elbow flexion. If the incline is up and toward the patient, resistance is given to shoulder flexion and elbow extension. Similarly, the standard horizontal work surface itself can be raised or lowered to make demands on certain muscle groups or to alter the effect of gravity. For example, a table raised to axilla height allows flexion and extension of the elbow on a gravity-eliminated plane and may enable a person with grade 3+ muscles to eat independently. The purpose of these changes in position would be to increase joint strength and ROM or enable performance.

Placing items, such as nails, mosaic tiles, pieces of yarn, beads, darts, bean bags, and paint brushes, in various locations changes the motion required to reach them when performing the activity in an otherwise standard manner. Placement may be high enough to encourage shoulder flexion or abduction; lateral to encourage shoulder rotation, trunk rotation, or horizontal motion; or low to encourage trunk

flexion or lateral trunk flexion. All of the placements would encourage improvement in dynamic balance (Fig. 12-6).

Arrange Objects Relative to Each Other. To grade an activity for improving perceptual skills (e.g., figure-ground discrimination or unilateral neglect), the arrangement of objects to be used, the printing on a

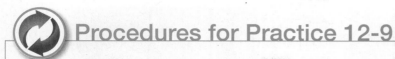

Procedures for Practice 12-9

Adaptations for Therapeutic Purpose

Activity Demand	Adaptation	Therapeutic Purpose
Body function	Position the task relative to the person	Increase ROM Target specific muscles, motions Enable performance
Body function	Arrange objects relative to each other	Improve perceptual skills Require specific movements Decrease energy expenditure Enable performance
Body function	Change lever arms	Increase strength Reduce required strength Prevent injuries
Required actions	Change method of doing the activity	Enable performance Increase strength Increase ROM Increase coordination and dexterity Increase cognitive-perceptual skills
Required actions	Change level of difficulty	Increase cognition Increase perception Increase motor planning Enable performance
Required actions	Change materials or texture of materials	Increase strength Increase coordination Challenge sensory system
Object properties	Change handles of tools and utensils	Reduce stress on painful joints Enable performance

Activity Demand	Adaptation	Therapeutic Purpose
Object properties	Change the size or shape of objects	Improve dexterity Enable performance Increase strength Increase ROM
Object properties	Change color contrast between objects	Improve figure-ground discrimination Enable performance
Object properties	Modify or use supplemental tools and utensils	Enable performance Prevent deformity Prevent cumulative trauma disorders
Object Properties	Add weights	Increase strength Reduce incoordinated movements Provide passive range of motion (PROM)
Object properties	Add springs or rubber bands	Increase strength Reduce incoordinated movements Provide PROM Assist weak muscles
Sequence and timing	Modify steps	Enable performance Increase attention and concentration Increase memory
Sequence and timing	Modify time	Enable performance Increase attention and concentration Increase muscular endurance

page, and so on can be graded from sparse to dense (i.e., fewer objects or words with space between versus many objects or words with no space between). Putting game pieces on the right side of the game board encourages use of the right hand, while placement on the left encourages use of the left hand. Placement of ingredients on a kitchen counter across the room from the mixing bowl encourages walking in the kitchen that would not occur if all were together. On the other hand, placing all objects needed for a task together reduces the energy required to do the task.

Change Length of the Lever Arm The amount of work a muscle or muscle group is doing depends on

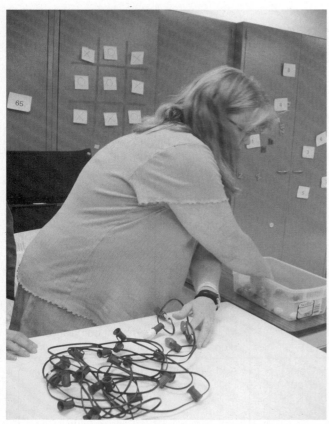

Figure 12-6 Christmas tree lights are placed to the left of a right-handed person to encourage reaching and development of dynamic standing balance.

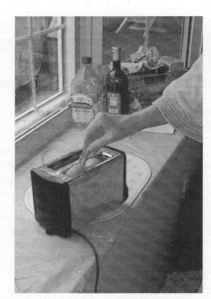

Figure 12-7 Retrieving toast with a spring clothespin.

with decreased strength to use them (Fig. 12-8). Furthermore, this idea guides workers in methods of lifting and handling on their jobs to avoid musculoskeletal injuries (see illustrations of lever arms in Chapter 20).

the resistance. Resistance is determined by the pull of gravity on the limb and the implements the patient is using, which together act as the resistance lever arm. The effect of a given amount of resistance can be altered by lengthening or shortening the resistance arm. The longer the resistance arm, the greater the force required to counterbalance it. The resistance arm can be altered by shortening or lengthening the limb; for example, flexing the knee, which shortens the limb, offers less resistance to hip extension than if the knee were extended. Another example is carrying an object close to the body, which requires less involvement of back muscles than if the object is carried at arm's length.

On the other hand, increasing the length of the force lever arm decreases the muscle activity needed to accomplish a task. For example, in Figure 12-7, if the clothespin were adapted to have longer handles, less pinch would be required to open it to the same width.

Attention to lengths of lever arms is important not only in adapting the required body functions of an activity to make it more therapeutic but also in adapting objects used in daily activities to enable patients

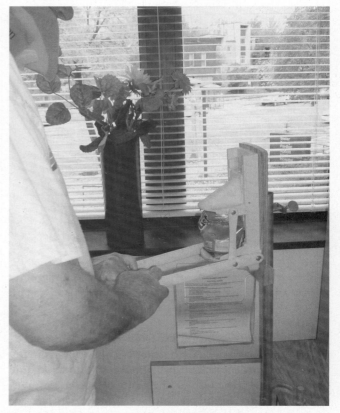

Figure 12-8 A patient who has weak upper extremities is able to crush cans for recycling because the handle (force arm) of the crusher has been elongated.

Activity Demand: Required Actions and Performance Skills

This group of adaptations focuses on methods used for adapting the actions and skills that are required to carry out the activity.

Change Method of Doing the Activity; Change Physical Context. Change of method is used both for occupation-as-means (Fig. 12-2) and for occupation-as-end (Figures 12-3B; 12-4; 12-9, A & B; 12-10, A & B; and 12-11). Such compensatory adaptation allows performance of an activity that would otherwise be impossible because of the person's disability. Bowling, basketball, and many other sports can be done seated instead of standing. A change of rules adapts some sports, such as track and field events, to certain requirements of the physically impaired. Sewing and needlework, normally bilateral activities, can be made unilateral by adaptations that hold the material steady for the working hand (Fig. 12-12). Books, notebook computers, or other tools can be transported via a rolling backpack or rolling table instead of carrying them.

By altering the physical context, individuals are able to move at the edge of their competence (Nilsen, Kaminiski, & Gordon, 2003). For example, if a person cannot flex his shoulder against gravity, by placing him in a side-lying position, the effects of gravity are minimized, allowing the movement. Movement organization in a gravity-eliminated plane, however, differs from movement in an against-gravity context.

Movement organization is also different in simulated contexts using simulated objects compared with natural contexts with actual objects (Dunn, Brown, & McGuigan, 1994; Flinn, 1999; Ma, Trombly, & Robinson-Poldolski, 1999; Mathiowetz & Wade, 1995; Trombly & Wu, 1999; Wu et al., 1998, 2000). Because movement organization is sensitive to contextual changes (Nilsen, Kaminiski, & Gordon, 2003), some rehabilitation centers now have manufactured "real" environments or have renovated their clinic spaces to allow patients to practice in realistic contexts to enable best performance and to facilitate carry over to actual contexts (Fig. 12-13).

Change Level of Difficulty Patterns for craft activities, game rules, extent of task (e.g., prepare instant coffee versus espresso), and level of creativity can be downgraded to enable the patient to succeed or upgraded to demand performance at higher levels. Changing the difficulty entails changing the number of pieces or the ideas that must be

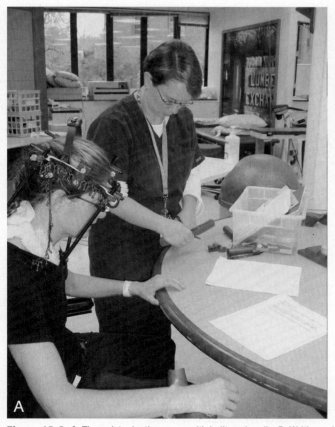
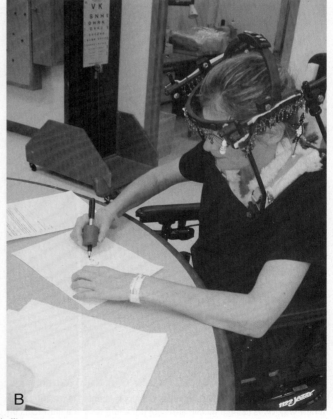

Figure 12-9 **A.** Therapist adapting a pen with built-up handle. **B.** Writing using built-up pen.

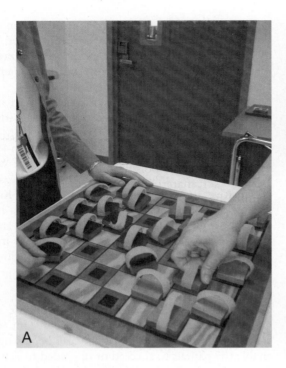

A

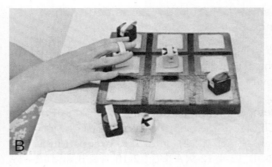

B

Figure 12-10 **A, B.** Checkers and tic-tac-toe pieces adapted with looped handles. This enables a person to play who otherwise could not (occupation-as-end) or challenges abilities not used when playing standard games (occupation-as-means).

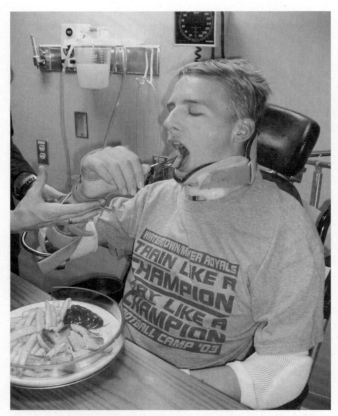

Figure 12-11 A patient with spinal cord injury is learning to feed himself in a new way. He is using a mobile arm support, a fork held in a universal cuff, and a plate guard to prevent food from being pushed off the plate.

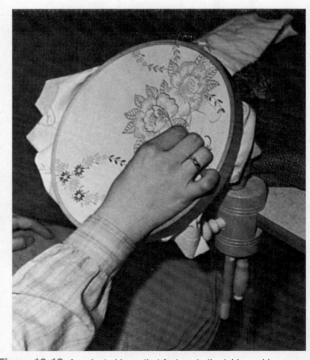

Figure 12-12 An adapted hoop that fastens to the table enables a person with the use of only one hand to embroider.

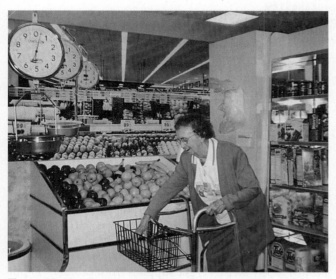

Figure 12-13 "Shopping" at Independence Square Market, a manufactured "real" environment to promote best performance in preparation to return to the community. (Photo by Mary Vining Radomski.)

manipulated, changing the problem-solving level from concrete reasoning to abstract reasoning, changing the directions from specific to general, and so on. For example, a patient with traumatic brain injury may be unable to pay the bills if the top of the desk is littered with bills and papers but may be able to manage if one bill is taken out at a time. A patient with low cardiopulmonary endurance may not be able to stand for long periods of time to prepare a simple meal in the kitchen; however, would be able to complete a kitchen activity while sitting on a stool. As endurance increases, the level of difficulty can be increased to include standing positions during portions of the activity.

Activity Demand: Objects and Their Properties

This next group of adaptations moves the focus of adaptation to the tools, materials, and equipment that are used to perform the activity.

Change Materials or Texture of Materials. Gradation along the strengthening continuum may be accomplished by selection of material by type and also by variations of texture or density to change resistance. Resistance can be changed, for example, by starting a cutting project with tissue paper and then progressing to heavier materials. Metal tooling can be graded for resistance by choosing materials in grades from thin aluminum to thick copper. Sandpaper is graded from extra fine to coarse, and resistance increases as the grade coarsens. Mixing can be graded from making gelatin dessert to scrambled eggs to biscuit batter and so on. If materials are graded in the opposite direction, that is, from heavy to light, the activity demands increased coordination from the patient. Weaving may begin using thicker material

like rug roving and be graded toward fine linen threads as the patient progresses in coordination.

Cutaneous stimulation changes with the amount of texture of objects or surfaces. By making balls from yarn or terry toweling, carpeting the surfaces the person works on, padding handles with textured material, and so on, the therapist adapts the activity to increase sensory stimulation.

Change Handles of Tools or Utensils. Padding the handles of utensils or tools with high-density foam or other firm but soft material (Fig. 12–9, A & B) reduces stress on painful finger joints and/or enables persons with poor grip to use the utensil or tool.

Change Size or Shape of Objects. Playing pieces of board games can vary in size and shape and can therefore offer a therapeutic benefit that the standard objects would not. For example, checkers, which are usually flat pieces approximately 2.5 cm in diameter, can be cylinders, squares, cubes, or spheres; can range in size from tiny to as large as a person's grasp permits; or can have handles attached (Fig. 12-10, A & B).

Reducing the size or changing the shape of the pieces being worked on facilitates the goals of increased dexterity and fine coordination. Therapists creatively change sizes of craft materials (e.g., weaving thread, tiles, paint-by-number guidelines, and ceramic pieces) and recreational materials (e.g., puzzle pieces, chess pieces, and target games) to increase coordination. Tools and utensils can be adapted by changing the length, diameter, or shape of their handles or by adding handles to tools that do not normally have them.

The actual size of the tool can be chosen to offer more or less resistance. For example, saws range in size from small coping saws and hacksaws to large cross-cut and rip saws. The resistance of saws can also be graded by the number of teeth per inch on the blade; the fewer the teeth, the greater the resistance. Woodworking planes vary in size, and the amount of exposed blade can be adjusted to provide resistance. Size of scissors, screwdrivers, stirring spoons, and other tools and utensils can also be varied.

Change Color Contrast between Objects. Neistadt et al. (1993) suggested grading challenge to figure-ground discrimination ability by changing game objects from contrasting colors to increasingly similar colors.

Modify or Use Supplemental Tools and Utensils Using tools when normally none are used or modifying tools or utensils enables a person to accomplish activities and tasks that he or she would not be able to do otherwise. For example, toast can be retrieved from a toaster by use of a wooden spring clothespin when sensory precautions are in effect (Fig. 12-7). Angling the handles on carving knives allows a person with rheumatoid arthritis to cut meat or vegetables without putting deforming forces on the wrist and fingers. Changing keyboard or mouse designs can prevent carpal tunnel syndrome. Including the tool in a specially designed splint can reduce symptoms caused by prolonged holding (Bockman, 2004). Although manufacturers are offering tools and household utensils designed to enable persons with weak grasp or arthritic pain to use them comfortably, therapists must not assume that tools labeled "ergonomic" produce better positioning or less discomfort than nonadapted tools. Patients' perceptions of comfort and ease of use need to guide the selection (Tebben & Thomas, 2004).

Add Weights. The addition of weights adapts an activity to meet such goals as increase of strength, promotion of cocontraction, and increase of passive ROM by stretch. Some nonresistive activities can be made resistive by adding weights to the apparatus directly or by use of pulleys; others may be made resistive by adding weights to the person, as with weighted cuffs (Fig. 12-14). Tools also are weights, and they can be selected or adjusted to offer graded resistance; for instance, hammers range from lightweight tack hammers to heavy claw hammers.

Add Springs or Rubber Bands. Springs and rubber bands are means of adapting activity to increase strength through resistance, to assist a weak muscle, or to stretch muscle and other soft tissue to increase passive ROM. When offering resistance, the spring or rubber band is positioned so that its pull is opposite to the pull of motion of the target muscle group, whereas if used for assistance, the spring or rubber band is set to pull in the same direction as the contracting muscle group. Springs and rubber bands applied for the purpose of stretching are placed so the pull is against the tissue to be stretched.

Springs of graduated tensions may be applied directly to larger pieces of equipment. Rubber bands can be added to smaller pieces of equipment and can be graded from thin with light tension to thick with heavy tension. For example, a rubber band can be wrapped around the pincer end of a spring-type clothespin to add resistance when it is used in games involving picking up small pieces.

Activity Demand: Sequence and Timing

This final group of adaptations involves changing demands related to the steps involved in an activity including the sequence of the steps and the time required to complete the steps

Modify Steps. An activity can be modified by increasing the number of steps to complete the activity. Grading the number of steps from one or two steps to multiple steps can be used to increase attention and concentration skills and memory. For example, the activity of "brushing teeth" can be graded from two steps: (1) brush teeth and (2) rinse mouth to five steps: (1) get supplies from cabinet, (2) put toothpaste on brush, (3) brush teeth, (4) rinse mouth, and (5) return supplies to cabinet.

To enable occupation-as-end, the activity can be adapted to include a sequential checklist of the steps to perform the activity. Depending on the person's cognitive ability, the checklist can be written or pictorial. Using the same example above, a written checklist for the steps involved in brushing teeth could be posted on the mirror in the bathroom (Fig. 12-15, A & B).

Conversely, the patient may receive a singular instruction to a multi-step task (such as prepare and clean up a light lunch within 30 minutes) to engage decision-making and problem-solving skills.

Modify Time. Changing and monitoring the length of time to complete the individual steps of an activity or the entire activity can be used to increase attention and concentration skills. For example, making a peanut butter and jelly sandwich can be graded by increasing the required time to make additional sandwiches. Devices can be used to promote a therapeutic goal or enable performance such as the use of a kitchen timer or alarm clock.

EVIDENCE PERTAINING TO OCCUPATIONAL ANALYSIS, GRADATION, AND ADAPTATION

Additional helpful information is listed in Resources 12-1. However, evidence concerning the effectiveness of gradation and adaptation of activity to accomplish therapeutic goals is sparse. The three practice skills of activity analysis, gradation, and adaptation discussed here are basic to the practice of occupational therapy and as such have been practiced with success clinically and universally accepted with little objective study. Some studies, other than the classic ones mentioned in this chapter, are described in Evidence Table 12-1. Continued research is needed in this area in order to support the efficacy of occupational therapy practice.

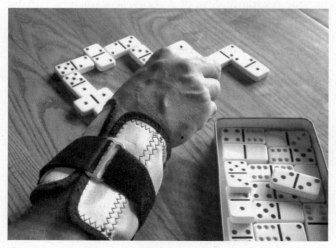

Figure 12-14 Weight cuff used to add resistance to an action that is not normally resistive.

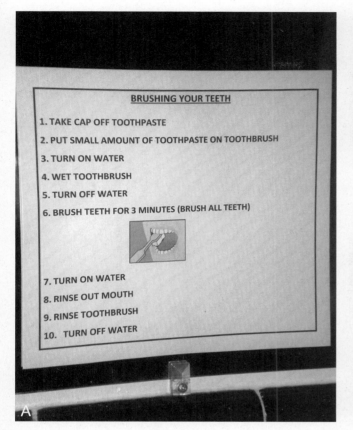

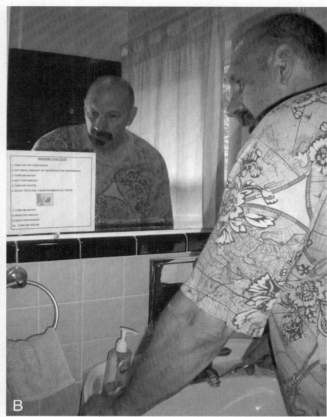

Figure 12-15   **A.** A written checklist for brushing teeth posted on the mirror in the bathroom. **B.** Brushing teeth using the checklist

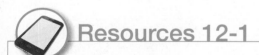 Resources 12-1

Additional Sources of Information Concerning Activity Analysis

Capasso, N., Gorman, A., & Blick, C. (2010). Breakfast group in an acute rehabilitation setting. *OT Practice, 15,* 14–18.
A restorative program for incorporating clients' hemiparetic upper extremities for function.

Davis, J. (2009). Treatment ideas and strategies in stroke rehabilitation. *OT Practice, 14,* 13–18.
A step-by-step approach for selecting and using activities based on patient impairments and goals.

Fecko, A., Errico, P., & Jacobs, K. (2004). Everyday ergonomics for therapists. *OT Practice, 9,* 16–18.
A detailed list of ergonomic considerations for everyday life.

Harnish, S. (2001). Gardening for life: Adaptive techniques and tools. *OT Practice, 6,* 12–15.
A compilation of adapted techniques and tools to enable gardening.

Latella, D., & Langford, S. (2008). Hippotherapy: An effective approach to occupational therapy intervention. *OT Practice, 13,* 16–20.
Description of hippotherapy as an intervention to address motor, process, and interaction skills to enhance occupational performance.

Lyons, A., Phipps, S. C., & Berro, M. (2004). Using occupation in the clinic. *OT Practice, 9,* 11–15.
Description of one facility's readoption of a focus on occupation. Excellent case example.

Thomas, H. (2012). *Occupation-based activity analysis.* Thorofare, NJ: Slack Incorporated.
A detailed look at activity analysis.

Walters, L. (2001). One-hand typing: Adapt the technology or the client? *OT Practice, 6,* 20–21.
Suggested adaptations to enable one-handed typing or keyboarding.

| Evidence Table 12-1 | Best Evidence for Occupational Therapy Practice Regarding Selection, Gradation, and Adaptation of Occupation |

Intervention	Description of Intervention Tested	Participants	Dosage	Type of Best Evidence and Level of Evidence	Benefit	Statistical Probability and Effect Size of Outcome	Reference
Task constraints: #1: Different sized handles #2: Different weight cups	#1: Three ceramic cups 12 cm high, weighing 309.0 g, having handles of 2, 4, and 8 cm #2: Two cups, 12 cm high with 2-cm handles, weighing 309.0 g and 705.9 g when filled with water	Thirty healthy women aged 20–45 years	Three trials for each cup; carried out in a laboratory	One group, repeated-measures design, randomized of condition; Level: 1B1b	Mixed #1: Yes. The size of the handle significantly affected the number of fingers being placed through the handle; the larger the handle, the more fingers. #2: No. Weight did not significantly affect the number of fingers used to support the cup.	#1: $x^2_{(2)} = 49.8$, $p < 0.001$; effect size could not be calculated #2: Not significant	Fuller & Trombly (1997)
Exercise apparatus adapted into a game	Experimental: Exercise using a game apparatus that required supination to dump dice out to score Control: Exercise using the same apparatus without the game	Thirty patients with acute stroke, mean age = 68.4 years	Two sets of 10 trials for each condition; different days	Randomized controlled trial; Level: IC2c	Yes. The game significantly increased the degrees of handle rotation (supination) achieved. Mean of 13.4° more in experimental group compared with control group.	$p = 0.016$, $r = 0.42$, indicating a 42% improvement caused by meaningfulness of game as compared with rote exercise	Nelson et al. (1996)
Functional activity (goal object present) versus rote exercise (goal object absent)	Present: Reach to scoop coins off the table in the laboratory Absent: Reach forward without functional goal	Fourteen patients with chronic stroke, mean age = 61.8 years; 24 healthy persons, mean age = 63.2 years	Ten trials within 1 day; in a laboratory	Randomized controlled trial; Level: IC1c	Yes. Both groups demonstrated significantly better movement organization with goal object present. The results are reported for the stroke patients only.	Overall effect size = 0.63. Speed, $p = 0.003$, $r = 0.70$; straightness of path, $p = 0.002$, $r = 0.72$; smoothness, $p = 0.005$, $r = 0.66$; automaticity of movement, $p = 0.001$, $r = 0.75$. Force of movement, $p = 0.28$, $r = 0.17$	Wu et al. (2000)

Grade speed of action; grade work surface	Condition: #1: Rest #2: Unilateral horizontal sanding at 15 cycles/min #3: Same as #2 at 30 cycles/min #4: Unilateral sanding with board inclined to 15° at 15 cycles/min #5: Same as #4 at 30 cycles/min	Eight patients with stroke of unknown chronicity, mean age = 67.6 years	Three minutes each of five conditions with rests between; all conditions within 1 day	One group, repeated-measures design without randomization of condition; Level: IIC2c	Mixed. When tested together, speed and angle significantly increased cardiopulmonary measures above resting. When separated, only different velocities affected the outcome.	$p < 0.01$; effect size could not be calculated; no statistical information available concerning the tests of angle and speed separately	Muraki et al. (1990)
Weighted cuff	Weighted cuff applied to forearm to decrease tremors and increase functional feeding in adults. Each person ate half the meal with the weighted cuff and half without the cuff. Weight determined individually by trial and error.	Five adults aged 30–81 years; all had tremor secondary to various diagnoses	Eight or 16 meals	AB single-case design; conditions alternated randomly; Level: IVC3b	Partial benefit for some participants. Time to acquire food on utensil decreased significantly for four of five participants. The number of spills decreased significantly for two of five participants. The amount of food consumed did not change significantly.	Time to acquire food on utensil: $p < 0.013$; effect size, $r = 0.97$. Number of spills: $p < 0.012$; effect size, $r = 0.96$.	McGruder et al. (2003)

Clinical Reasoning in Occupational Therapy Practice

Adaptation and Gradation

The occupational therapy department in a busy rehabilitation hospital received a donation of 25 new jigsaw puzzles from a grateful patient. The donation included a variety of puzzles, ranging from 100- to 500-piece puzzles, small- to large-sized puzzle pieces, and various types of themes from landscapes to sports teams. For her patient, the therapist chose a 100-piece puzzle of medium-sized pieces that pictured, in a simple way, a Golden Labrador dog. For what impaired ability and skill competence might this activity have been chosen? What are three types of adaptations the therapist can use to adapt this activity to address different therapeutic goals? State the type of adaptation, the therapeutic purpose (goal) of the adaptation, and how the therapist could grade the activity to accomplish the goal.

Clinical Reasoning in Occupational Therapy Practice

Adaptation

Joan has hemiplegia in her right upper extremity because of a recent cerebrovascular accident (CVA) and cannot use her right arm or hand, which are flaccid and supported in an arm trough positioned on her wheelchair. She is right-handed. Joan's sitting balance is impaired; she can sit unsupported only for short periods of time. Her cognitive abilities are intact. She has fair cardiopulmonary endurance. Joan is currently receiving occupational therapy in a skilled nursing facility. During the occupational therapy evaluation, Joan told her therapist that she loves to do needlepoint and is currently working on a very special project for her "soon-to-arrive" granddaughter. She is very upset that she will not be able to finish the project.

How can the activity of needlepoint be adapted so Joan could resume this meaningful occupation?

How can needlepoint activity be used therapeutically in Joan's occupational therapy treatment?

Summary Review Questions

1. What is the difference between occupation-as-end and occupation-as means? Give an example of each type of therapeutic use of occupation.
2. What would a therapist need to know in order to select an appropriate occupation-as-end for a particular patient?
3. What would a therapist need to know about the patient and activity to select occupation-as-means?
4. List the general required characteristics of an activity used as occupation-as-means for the following impairments.
   - Voluntary movement
   - Active ROM
   - Cardiopulmonary endurance
   - Memory
   - Problem solving
5. Describe how the process of activity analysis relates to selection of an occupation or activity for a particular patient.
6. What therapeutic purpose and goal(s) might be accomplished by engaging a patient in occupation-as-means that requires moving at different speeds?
7. What are two reasons for adapting an occupation used as means? An occupation used as end?
8. What are the five characteristics of good adaptations?
9. What therapeutic goals can be accomplished by the following?
   - Changing the position of the task relative to the person
   - Adding weights to tools or game pieces
   - Adding springs or rubber bands to craft equipment or tools
   - Changing the length of lever arms of tools, equipment, or the limb itself
   - Changing the material to be used in a project
   - Modifying the steps of the activity

Glossary

Activity analysis—A systematic process through which activities, tasks, and occupations are analyzed in order to understand "their component parts, their possible meaning to clients, and their therapeutic potential" (Crepeau & Schell, 2009, p. 360). This chapter describes three approaches to activity analysis: (1) activity-focused analysis, which focuses on the activity itself without considering the characteristics of the client or his or her environment to build a repertoire of activity knowledge; (2) client-focused activity analysis, which focuses on the therapeutic utilization of the activity for a particular client toward a specific therapeutic goal, an occupation-as-means approach; and (3) environment-client focused activity analysis, which is an occupation-as-end approach that focuses on the fit between the person and the environment with regard to the activity in order to determine and/or optimize the potential for successful performance.

Activity demands—See *Task demands*.

Closed task—A closed task involves the least interaction with the environment (Gentile, 2000). A closed task is one in which the task demands remain constant and for which habits can develop so that little conscious control is required once learned.

Constraints—Limitations imposed on purposeful movement or the completion of occupational performance. Extrinsic constraints include the physical and sociocultural environment and task demands. Intrinsic constraints include biomechanical and neuromuscular aspects of a person's body, as well as other personal contextual factors (Newell, 1986).

Electromyographic—Pertaining to recording the electrical activity produced by a contracting muscle. When a muscle is at rest, no electrical activity is recorded. As the muscle contracts, the electrical activity increases proportionately.

Kinematic—The branch of mechanics that studies the motion of a body or a system of bodies without consideration given to its mass or the forces acting on it (*American Heritage Dictionary of the English Language*, 2009). Kinematics describe motion in terms of displacement (position), velocity (a derivative of position), and acceleration (a derivative of velocity). For example, by recording the displacement of the wrist in space, the velocity or acceleration of reach can be derived. Kinematic analysis allows detection of strategies for the organization of movement (Georgopoulos, 1986; Jeannerod, 1988).

MET (metabolic equivalent)—The amount of energy expended when a person is engaged in activity. At rest in a semireclined position and with the extremities supported (basal state), that amount is 3.5 mL of oxygen per minute per kilogram of body weight (1 MET). Energy expenditure of activities is rated in terms of multiples of METs.

Occupation-as-end—Activities and tasks that constitute the roles of a given individual (Trombly, 1995/2011).

Occupation-as-means—Activities and tasks chosen to remediate deficient abilities or capacities (Trombly, 1995/2011).

Open task—Task with most interaction between the performer and environment (Gentile, 2000). An open task is one for which the environment and/or objects may vary during performance and between trials. Open tasks require attention and vigilance.

Task analysis—Similar to activity analysis; term used primarily in relation to work assessment (ergonomics). Analysis of the dynamic relationship among a person, a selected task or occupation, and a specific context or environment (Watson & Wilson, 2003).

Task demands—The context (e.g., objects, surroundings, and ritual) that evokes certain maneuvers required to accomplish the goal of the activity or task.

References

Ainsworth, B. E., Haskell, W. L., Hermann, S. D., Meckes, N., Bassett, D. R., Jr., Tudor-Locke, C., Greer, J. L., Vezina, J., Whitt-Glover, M. C., & Leon, A. S. (2011). Compendium of physical activities: A second update of activity codes and MET values. *Medicine and Science in Sports and Exercise, 43,* 1575–1581.

Ainsworth, B. E., Haskell, W. L., Leon, A. S., Jacobs, D. R., Montoye, H. J., Sallis, J. F., & Paffenbarger, R. S. (1993). Compendium of physical activities: Classification of energy costs of human physical activities. *Medicine and Science in Sports and Exercise, 25,* 71–80.

American Heritage Dictionary of the English Language (4th ed.). (2009). Boston: Houghton Mifflin Company. Retrieved April 26, 2012 from www.thefreedictionary.com/kinematics.

American Occupational Therapy Association. (1995). Position paper: Occupation. *American Journal of Occupational Therapy, 49,* 1015–1018.

American Occupational Therapy Association. (2008). Occupational therapy practice framework: Domain and process (2nd ed.). *American Journal of Occupational Therapy, 62,* 625–683.

Bockman, T. (2004). Splinting the tool to the worker. *OT Practice, 9,* 22.

Bolduc, J. J., & Lawrence, S. (2011). Constraint Induced Movement Therapy: Treating hemiplegia and apraxia following an acute stroke. *OT Practice, 16,* 12–16.

Burton, A. W., & Davis, W. E. (1996). Ecological task analysis: Utilizing intrinsic measures in research and practice. *Human Movement Science, 15,* 285–314.

Chandani, A., & Hill, C. (1990). What really is therapeutic activity? *British Journal of Occupational Therapy, 53,* 15–18.

Creighton, C. (1992). The origin and evolution of activity analysis. *American Journal of Occupational Therapy, 46,* 45–48.

Creighton, C. (1993). Looking back: Graded activity: Legacy of the sanatorium. *American Journal of Occupational Therapy, 47,* 745–748.

Crepeau, E. B., & Schell, B. A. B. (2009). Analyzing occupations and activity. In E. B. Crepeau, E. S. Cohn, & B. A. B. Schell (Eds.), *Willard and Spackman's occupational therapy* (11th ed., pp. 359–374). Philadelphia: Lippincott Williams & Wilkins.

Csikszentmihalyi, M. (1990). *Flow: The psychology of optimal experience.* New York: Harper & Row.

Davis, W. E., & Burton, A. W. (1991). Ecological task analysis: Translating movement behavior theory into practice. *Adapted Physical Activity Quarterly, 8,* 154–177.

Dunn, W., Brown, C., & McGuigan, A. (1994). The ecology of human performance: A framework for considering the effect of context. *American Journal of Occupational Therapy, 48,* 595–607.

Engeser, S., & Rheinberg, F. (2008). Flow, performance and moderators of challenge-skill balance. *Motivation and Emotion, 32,* 158–172.

Fisher, A. G., & Bray Jones, K. (2010). *Assessment of Motor and Process Skills. Vol. 1: Development, standardization, and administration manual* (7th ed.). Fort Collins, CO: Three Star Press.

Fitts, P. M. (1954). The information capacity of the human motor system in controlling the amplitude of movement. *Journal of Experimental Psychology, 47,* 381–391.

Flinn, N. A. (1999). Clinical interpretation of "Effect of rehabilitation tasks on organization of movement after stroke." *American Journal of Occupational Therapy, 53,* 345–347.

Fuller, Y., & Trombly, C. A. (1997). Effect of object characteristics on female grasp patterns. *American Journal of Occupational Therapy, 51,* 481–487.

Gentile, A. (2000). Skill acquisition: Action, movement and neuromotor processes. In J. H. Carr, R. B. Shepherd, J. Gordon, A. M. Gentile, & J. M. Held (Eds.), *Movement science: Foundations for physical therapy in rehabilitation* (2nd ed., pp. 111–187). Rockville, MD: Aspen.

Gentile, A. M., Higgins, J. R., Miller, E. A., & Rosen, B. (1975). Structure of motor tasks. In *Actes du 7e symposium Canadien d'apprentissage psycho-moteur et psychologie du sport* (pp. 11–28). Montreal, Quebec, Canada: Association des professionales de l'activité physiologic du Québec. C. Bard, M. Fleury, & J. Salmela (Eds.).

Georgopoulos, A. P. (1986). On reaching. *Annual Review of Neurosciences, 9,* 147–170.

Gibson, J. J. (1977). The theory of affordances. In R. E. Shaw & J. Bransford (Eds.), *Perceiving, acting, and knowing: Toward an ecological psychology* (pp. 67–82). Hillsdale, NJ: Lawrence Erlbaum.

Gilbreth, F. B. (1911). *Motion study.* New York: Van Nostrand.

Gilbreth, F. B., & Gilbreth, L. M. (1920). *Motion study for the handicapped.* London: Routledge.

Greene, D. (1990). A clinically relevant approach to biomechanical analysis of function. *Occupational Therapy Practice, 1,* 44–52.

Harnish, S. (2001). Gardening for life: Adaptive techniques and tools. *OT Practice, 6,* 12–15.

Illyes, A., & Kiss, R. M. (2005). Shoulder muscle activity during pushing, pulling, elevation and overhead throw. *Journal of Electromyography and Kinesiology, 15,* 282–289.

Jeannerod, M. (1988). *The neural and behavioral organization of goal-directed movements.* Oxford, UK: Clarendon.

Jordan, K., & Newell, K. M. (2004). Task goal and grip force dynamics. *Experimental Brain Research, 156,* 451–457.

Kelly, B. T., Williams, R. J., Cordasco, F. A., Backus, S. I., Otis, J. C., Weiland, D. E., Altchek, D. W., Craig, E. V., Wickiewicz, T. L., & Warren, R. F. (2005). Differential patterns of muscle activation in patients with symptomatic and asymptomatic rotator cuff tears. *Journal of Shoulder and Elbow Surgery, 14,* 165–171.

Kitago, T., Liang, J., Huang, V. S., Hates, S., Simon, P., Tenteromano, L., Lazar, R. M., Marshall, R. S., Mazzoni, P., Lennihan, L., & Krakauer, J. W. (2012). Improvement after constraint-induced movement therapy: Recovery of normal motor control or task-specific compensation? *Neurorehabilitation and Neural Repair, 27,* 99–109. DOI: 10.1177/1545968312452631.

Levy, L. L. (2005). Cogntive information processing. In Katz, N. (Ed.), *Cognition, occupation, and participation across the life span: Neuroscience, neurorehabilitation, and models of intervention in occupational therapy* (3rd ed., pp. 93–115). Bethesda, MD: American Occupational Therapy Association.

Ma, H., & Trombly, C. A. (2004). Effects of task complexity on reaction time and movement kinematics in elderly people. *American Journal of Occupational Therapy, 58,* 150–158.

Ma, H., Trombly, C. A., & Robinson-Podolski, C. (1999). The effect of context on skill acquisition and transfer. *American Journal of Occupational Therapy, 53,* 138–144.

Mathiowetz, V., & Wade, M. G. (1995). Task constraints and functional motor performance of individuals with and without multiple sclerosis. *Ecological Psychology, 7,* 99–123.

Mayer, N. H., Keating, D. J., & Rapp, D. (1986). Skills, routines, and activity patterns of daily living: A functional nested approach. In B. Uzzell & Y. Gross (Eds.), *Clinical neuropsychology of intervention* (pp. 205–222). Boston: Martinus Nijhoff.

McCraith, D. B., Austin, S. L., & Earhart, C. A. (2011). The Cognitive Disabilities Model in 2011. In Katz, N. (Ed.), *Cognition, occupation, and participation across the life span: Neuroscience, neurorehabilitation, and models of intervention in occupational therapy* (3rd ed., pp. 374–406). Bethesda, MD: American Occupational Therapy Association.

McGrain, P., & Hague, M. A. (1987). An electromyographic study of the middle deltoid and middle trapezius muscles during warping. *Occupational Therapy Journal of Research, 7,* 225–233.

McGruder, J., Cors, D., Tiernan, A. M., & Tomlin, G. (2003). Weighted wrist cuffs for tremor reduction during eating in adults with static brain lesions. *American Journal of Occupational Therapy, 57,* 507–516.

Merritt, B. K., & Fisher, A. G. (2003). Gender differences in the performance of activities of daily living. *Archives of Physical Medicine and Rehabilitation, 84,* 1872–1877.

Moneta, G. B., & Csikszentmihalyi, M. (1996). The effect of perceived challenges and skills on the quality of subjective experience. *Journal of Personality, 64,* 275–310.

Mosey, A. C. (1981). *Occupational therapy: Configuration of a profession.* New York: Raven.

Muraki, T., Kujime, K., Su., M., Kaneko, T., & Ueba, Y. (1990). Effect of one hand sanding on cardiometabolic and ventilatory functions in the hemiplegic elderly: A preliminary investigation. *Physical and Occupational Therapy in Geriatrics, 9,* 37–48.

Neistadt, M. E., McAuley, D., Zecha, D., & Shannon, R. (1993). An analysis of a board game as a treatment activity. *American Journal of Occupational Therapy, 47,* 154–160.

Nelson, D. L. (1988). Occupation: Form and performance. *American Journal of Occupational Therapy, 42,* 633–641.

Nelson, D. L., Konosky, K., Fleharty, K., Webb, R., Newer, K., Hazboun, V. P., Fontane, C., & Licht, B. C. (1996). The effects of an occupationally embedded exercise on bilaterally assisted supination in persons with hemiplegia. *American Journal of Occupational Therapy, 50,* 639–646.

Newell, K. M. (1986). Constraints on the development of coordination. In M. G. Wade & H. T. A. Whiting (Eds.), *Motor development in children: Aspects of coordination and control* (pp. 341–360). Boston: Martinus Nijhoff.

Nilsen, D. M., Kaminiski, T. R., & Gordon, A. M. (2003). The effect of body orientation on a point-to-point movement in healthy elderly persons. *American Journal of Occupational Therapy, 57,* 99–107.

Okoye, R. L. (1993). Computer applications in occupational therapy. In H. L. Hopkins & H. D. Smith (Eds.), *Willard and Spackman's occupational therapy* (8th ed., pp. 341–353). Philadelphia: Lippincott.

Peloquin, S. M. (1988). Linking purpose to procedure during interactions with patients. *American Journal of Occupational Therapy, 42,* 775–781.

Polatajko, H. J., Mandich, A., & Martini, R. (2000). Dynamic performance analysis: A framework for understanding occupational performance. *American Journal of Occupational Therapy, 54,* 65–72.

Shi, Y. X., Tian, J. H., Yang, K. H., & Zhao, Y. (2011). Modified constraint-induced movement therapy versus traditional rehabilitation in patients with upper extremity dysfunction after stroke: A systematic review and meta-analysis. *Archives of Physical Medicine and Rehabilitation, 92,* 972–982.

Spaulding, S. J., & Robinson, K. L. (1984). Electromyographic study of the upper extremity during bilateral sanding: Unresisted and resisted conditions. *American Journal of Occupational Therapy, 38,* 258–262.

Sung, C. Y. Y., Ho, K. K. F., Lam, R. M. W., Lee, A. H. Y., & Chan, C. C. H. (2003). Physical and psychosocial factors in display screen equipment assessment. *Hong Kong Journal of Occupational Therapy, 13,* 2–10.

Tebben, A. B., & Thomas, J. J. (2004). Trowels labeled ergonomic versus standard design: Preferences and effects on wrist range of motion during a gardening occupation. *American Journal of Occupational Therapy, 58,* 317–323.

Toglia, J. P., Golisz, K. M., & Goverover, Y. (2009). Evaluation and intervention for cognitive perceptual impairments. In E. B. Crepeau, E. S. Cohn, & B. A. B. Schell (Eds.), *Willard and Spackman's occupational therapy* (11th ed., pp. 739–776). Philadelphia: Lippincott Williams & Wilkins.

Trombly, C. A. (1993). The issue is: Anticipating the future: Assessment of occupational function. *American Journal of Occupational Therapy, 47,* 253–257.

Trombly, C. A. (1995/2011). Occupation: Purposefulness and meaningfulness as therapeutic mechanisms. *American Journal of Occupational Therapy, 49,* 960–972. Reprinted in Padilla, R., & Griffiths, Y. (2011). *A professional legacy: The Eleanor Clarke Slagle Lectures in Occupational Therapy, 1955–2010* (3rd ed., pp. 399–414). Bethesda, MD: AOTA Press.

Trombly, C. A., & Cole, J. M. (1979). Electromyographic study of four hand muscles during selected activities. *American Journal of Occupational Therapy, 33,* 440–449.

Trombly, C. A., & Quintana, L. A. (1983). Activity analysis: Electromyographic and electrogoniometric verification. *Occupational Therapy Journal of Research, 37,* 104–120.

Trombly, C. A., & Wu, C. (1999). Effect of rehabilitation tasks on organization of movement after stroke. *American Journal of Occupational Therapy, 53,* 333–344.

Watson, D. E., & Wilson, S. A. (2003). *Task analysis: An individual and population approach* (2nd ed.). Bethesda, MD: American Occupational Therapy Association.

Wu, C., Trombly, C. A., Lin, K., & Tickle-Degnen, L. (1998). Effects of object affordances on reaching performance in persons with and without cerebrovascular accident. *American Journal of Occupational Therapy, 52,* 447–456.

Wu, C., Trombly, C. A., Lin, K., & Tickle-Degnen, L. (2000). A kinematic study of contextual effects on reaching performance in persons with and without stroke: Influences of object availability. *Archives of Physical Medicine and Rehabilitation, 81,* 95–101.

Acknowledgements

I wish to acknowledge the contribution of Catherine Trombly Latham, ScD, OTR to previous versions of this chapter. We are especially indebted to the occupational therapists and patients at Sister Kenny Institute (Minneapolis, Minnesota), for their assistance with photography for this chapter. Specifically, we thank Jake Beckstrom, Cindy Bemis, Arlan Berg, Tricia Bonavoglia, OTR/L, Michelle Brown, MEd, OTR/L, Krista Elfink, MS, OTR/L, Larry Larkin, Mary Vining Radomski, PhD, OTR/L, Jennifer Theis, MS, OTR/L, and Valerie Wheeler.

13

Learning

Nancy Ann Flinn

Learning Objectives

After studying this chapter, the reader will be able to do the following:

1. Differentiate between patient performance and patient learning.
2. Outline clinical considerations necessary for planning patient-specific teaching.
3. Explain the roles of context, feedback, and practice in the acquisition of both task-specific skills and general strategies.
4. Identify strategies for facilitating caregiver education and training.
5. Identify the guiding principles of motivational interviewing.

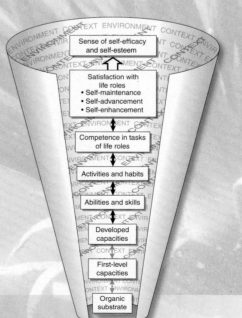

Learning is a primary therapeutic mechanism underlying many, if not all, occupational therapy interventions. Occupational therapists teach patients to perform activities of daily living (ADL), teach family members home programs, teach other therapists new techniques, and teach the public in community education courses. Each teaching opportunity requires preparation: the physical environment needs to be prepared; any needed materials, props, or equipment needs to be gathered; and most importantly, the learner must be prepared for the session. Teaching strategies need to be consciously designed to maximize learning, using methods designed to support different learning styles (e.g., visual, aural, read/write, or kinesthetic learners) (Lofland, 2009). Any handouts should address health literacy concerns and are developed with an understanding of the cultural, social, and cognitive issues that might affect the teaching session (DeWalt et al., 2010). All of these concerns need to be addressed in order for effective teaching to take place.

Finally as teachers, therapists must determine whether learning has taken place. For example, after a 30-minute dressing session, a patient who has had total knee replacement surgery is able to don his pants, socks, and shoes. From a traditional learning perspective, the patient's performance at the end of the session reflects the extent to which he has learned the desired skill or strategy. However, what if a nurse later reports that the patient is unable to carry out the activities he demonstrated proficiency with the day before? One can easily see that although within-session performance was buoyed by cues and practice, true learning did not occur.

Schmidt and Lee's (2011) contemporary definition of motor learning allows us to differentiate learning from within-session performance: ". . . motor learning is a set of processes associated with practice or experience leading to relatively permanent changes in the capability for responding" (p. 327). Based on this definition of learning, we would expect the patient with knee replacement to demonstrate similar levels of proficiency after the occupational therapy session as during. The term *performance* is used to describe what is seen during training, that is, short-term capabilities resulting from instruction, cues, or assistance. For occupational therapy to help patients resume occupational roles, therapists must understand the process of transforming performance into learning and use teaching methods that help the patient learn new skills.

This chapter discusses the role of information processing in learning and then summarizes the array of variables that affect the patient-specific teaching plan. Key influences on learning are detailed, and the chapter concludes with specific applications to occupational therapy practice. Regarding issues of learning, there has been a traditional division in the research between motor and cognitive tasks. In clinical practice, however, it is unusual to find motor tasks that do not have a cognitive component

or the reverse. Because this distinction does not translate into practice and because principles in the two areas are similar, the principles are combined in this chapter.

HUMAN INFORMATION PROCESSING MODEL OF LEARNING

Learning is inextricably linked to memory, specifically the encoding and retrieval of information. As explained in Chapter 6, people hold environmental stimuli very briefly in a series of short-term sensory stores before transferring it to limited-capacity working memory (Atkinson & Shiffrin, 1971). In working memory, sometimes called short-term memory, people may use control processes to encode information for storage in long-term memory (Schneider & Shiffrin, 1977). These control processes include techniques such as rehearsal, coding, and imaging (Atkinson & Shiffrin, 1971). Rehearsal is rote repetition of information, whereas coding entails linking the new information to something meaningful. Imaging transforms verbal information to visual images that are stored in memory. Craik and Tulving (1975) found that the durability of the memory trace is a function of depth of processing. That is, deep processing, as in the time-consuming process of linking new information to personally relevant old knowledge, results in better retention than shallow processing, such as rote rehearsal. If the learner does not use some form of conscious control, the memory trace quickly fades from working memory and cannot be recovered (Atkinson & Shiffrin, 1971). From the standpoint of human information processing, learning is the transfer of information from short-term or working memory to long-term memory (Shiffrin & Schneider, 1977).

Controlled versus Automatic Information Processing

Consider the attentional resources required of you the first time you drove a car compared with the attention required for the same task now. After years of experience, the car seems to drive itself, freeing the driver to concentrate on plans for the day or talk to a passenger. This example typifies the difference between controlled and automatic processing.

Controlled Processing

Controlled processing is technically a temporary activation of a series or sequence of elements in long-term memory under the attention and control of the thinker (Schneider & Shiffrin, 1977). For example, the new driver must actively recall specific rules and instructions and direct his attention to each motor sequence of the task. Controlled processing is limited by the capacity of working memory and is therefore effortful but flexible in handling novel situations. When learning a new task or skill that requires effortful concentration, people employ controlled processing. Thus, patients learning new skills or behaviors can process only a limited number of inputs (instructions, cues, and environmental distractions) at a time.

Automatic Processing

With enough controlled processing, a task requires less and less concentration to carry out (Shiffrin & Schneider, 1977). That is, the task becomes increasingly automatic, as in the example of the proficient driver. Automatic processing occurs when specific contextual stimuli internal or external to the person trigger the activation of a specific learned sequence in long-term memory (Schneider & Shiffrin, 1977). Given enough repetition, the individual performs the skill or task in a consistent manner with little or no attention. Sternberg (1986) suggested that development of a full level of automatization requires at least 200 trials of a task but that automatization begins in as few as 10 trials, so long as those trials are consistent. With fully automatic skills, people cannot stop themselves from performing the overlearned sequence unless control processes are employed to override it. Definition 13-1 discusses implications related to helping patients with memory impairment to reacquire skills. According to Giles (2005), overlearning is practice of a skill or strategy well beyond demonstration of learning or proficiency; it increases the likelihood that the skill or strategy will become automatic. These automatic skills and strategies become the easiest behaviors to initiate from an array of possible behaviors (Giles, 2005), minimizing demands on attention and decision making. Habits and routines are examples of automatic motor sequences that, according to Kielhofner, Barris, and Watts (1982), organize a person's tasks, space,

and time. Characteristic of automatic skills and strategies, habits and routines are responsive to the environmental conditions under which they are learned and develop with repetition (Kielhofner, Barris, & Watts, 1982; Wood, Quinn, & Kashy, 2002). Habit learning is a form of implicit learning, which is described in Definition 13-2. Occupational therapists often help patients resume or relearn self-maintenance tasks so that they are once again automatic.

Implications of the Information Processing Memory Model

Attention and memory play important roles in many aspects of learning, and so occupational therapists assess these domains before they try to teach patients skills or

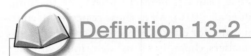

Definition 13-2

Implicit and Explicit Learning

People learn through two key processes that are supported by separate brain structures and have very different characteristics.

Explicit learning (sometimes called declarative learning) refers to the conscious encoding and recollection of specific events, task rules, and facts (Deckersbach et al., 2002; Eldridge, Masterman, & Knowlton, 2002). It relies on the integrity of the medial temporal lobe and diencephalic structures, particularly the hippocampus (Eldridge, Masterman, & Knowlton, 2002). It can be facilitated by a therapist through direct instruction about key environmental features, task-relevant feedback, and cues (Reber & Squire, 1994). Explicit learning is more flexible than implicit learning and has been shown to generalize more easily, probably because it is not as context dependent (Squire, 1994).

Implicit learning (also called procedural learning) refers to an unconscious change in behavior resulting from repetition within a stable context. There appear to be several forms of implicit learning including skill and habit learning, some forms of conditioning, and the phenomenon of priming (Squire, Knowlton, & Musen, 1993). Much of the learning of a motor task is thought to be implicit, including the dynamics of force production in the task, which is the interaction of active and passive components of the multiple joints involved in the task. The therapist facilitates implicit learning by structuring the environment to create consistent cues and frequent opportunities for appropriate task practice (Gentile, 1998). Implicit learning is more robust than explicit learning and retains its strength even when the explicit knowledge about a task has decayed (Lee & Vakoch, 1996). The basal ganglia support implicit learning rather than the medial temporal lobe (Packard & Knowlton, 2002). This suggests that even people with impaired explicit memory systems (e.g., Alzheimer's disease) are capable of implicit learning (Eldridge, Masterman, & Knowlton, 2002).

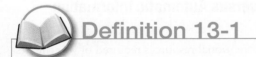

Definition 13-1

Errorless Learning

Errorless learning is a technique that involves encoding new information without error (Tailby & Haslam, 2003). Learners are helped to do it right each time the new skill is performed by introducing and then fading preemptive cues and/or assistance. Wilson and Evans (1996) propose errorless learning methods for persons with severe memory impairments. They suggest that these individuals have difficulty remembering what they learned if they made errors during the training process. Guessing and trial-and-error are avoided, and because training generally occurs in the context in which the new skills will be used, expectations of transfer are minimized. In a clinical trial, individuals with cognitive impairment and transtibial amputations benefited from an errorless learning protocol for donning their prosthesis, both in remembering more steps and making fewer errors (Donaghey, McMillan, & O'Neill, 2010).

strategies. Therapist awareness of distractions, such as pain, fatigue, and noise, allows therapists to plan sessions so that patients can use limited-capacity cognitive resources to hold and store stimuli related to the new skills or strategies. Therapists do this by helping patients use effective control processes, such as linking the new information to something they already know. Finally, therapists recognize that, for many skills, the learning end point is not proficiency but automaticity. Therapists ultimately enable their patients to carry out these tasks with accuracy and ease if they encourage consistency in performance (consistent environment and consistent sequence of steps).

CLINICAL CONSIDERATIONS IN TEACHING CLIENTS

In advance of every teaching intervention, occupational therapists make deliberate decisions regarding appropriate teaching methods. These decisions are based on the characteristics of the learner, anticipated length of intervention, desired learning outcome (specific task versus general strategy), and expectations for transfer and generalization. Evidence Table 13-1 lists some of the best evidence of the positive effects of learning- and teaching-related intervention.

Learner Characteristics

A client's learning potential is determined by many factors. Variables affecting cognitive status (reviewed in Chapter 6) are critical contributors to learning potential. Remember, these considerations apply to family caregivers as well as patients (see Procedures for Practice 13-1). Literacy is one important dimension of the experiential sociocultural influence on learning, with many implications regarding teaching methods (see Chapter 3). Neistadt (1995) suggested that occupational therapists attempt to answer four questions regarding patients' learning capacities during the course of their traditional evaluation. These questions include the following:

1. What modes of input (e.g., visual, auditory, and tactile) can this patient process most easily?
2. What approaches to tasks (outputs or behaviors) are still available to this patient?
3. What tasks remain meaningful or are most likely to facilitate learning for this patient?
4. How well is this patient able to transfer learning, that is, apply specific skills to a variety of tasks under a variety of circumstances?

Anticipated Length of Treatment

Occupational therapists also consider how many teaching sessions are likely to be available, as dictated by expected length of stay at the hospital, rehabilitation center,

or nursing facility; insurance coverage of rehabilitation services; acuteness of medical condition; and learning potential of the patient. The clinician selects learning goals based on this awareness of the constraints on teaching. Discharge planning then incorporates recommendations for continuing and extending the learning that began in treatment.

Stages of Learning

In 1967, Fitts and Posner described three sequential stages of learning, or acquisition, of motor skills: cognitive, associative, and autonomous. Each of the stages requires different kinds of attention resources (Eversheim & Bock, 2001). During the cognitive stage, the patient tries to understand the requirements of the task. The patient uses conscious control to acquire the new skill or strategy: thinking through or verbalizing the steps, attending to visual and verbal feedback from the therapist, and determining what cues to heed. In the associative stage, the patient is able to generally perform the task but now begins to make refinements in performance. The learner relies less on vision and verbal feedback and begins to use internal feedback mechanisms. During this stage, practice takes on primary importance; this important dimension of learning is discussed in more detail later in this chapter.

During the autonomous stage, the new skill or strategy becomes increasingly automatic or habitual. The patient can accurately perform most of the skill or strategy without thinking about it and is less subject to interference from other activities or environmental distractions.

Desired Learning Outcomes: Task-Specific Skills versus General Strategy Related to Expectations for Transfer and Generalization

Occupational therapy clients have a variety of learning needs. Therapists deliberately determine the patient-specific learning end point because it dictates teaching methods, length of treatment, and expectations for transfer and generalization.

Task-Specific Skills and Transfer of Training

After a stroke, many patients receive occupational therapy services to learn task-specific skills such as how to dress themselves using only one hand. For example, a client who receives home-based treatment may learn techniques specific to donning her housecoat and slippers (her usual attire) at the side of her bed, which rests on shag carpeting. Teaching in this situation (within the environment and context that the skill will be used) is task-specific. The learning process is embedded in the performance environment, with surroundings and objects becoming cues. The therapist does not expect the client to apply skills learned

Evidence Table 13-1 | Best Evidence for Learning–Teaching-Related Intervention

Intervention	Description of Intervention Tested	Participants	Dosage	Type of Best Evidence and Level of Evidence	Benefit	Statistical Probability and Effect Size of Outcome	Reference
Training in reaching tasks using either task-related or movement-related instructions	Participants practiced three reaching tasks with two types of instructions. One set of instructions focused on the task, and the second set of instructions focused on their arm movement.	Sixteen stroke survivors and 17 age-matched adults without neurological impairments were taught three reaching tasks with different instructions.	Forty-eight training trials on 1 day; eight trials for each task condition on each of three tasks	Counterbalanced repeated measure design, with random assignment to AB or BA sequence of task performance; Level: 1B1a	Participants directed to focus on the task had shorter movement times and greater peak velocity than participants directed to focus on the movement itself.	Can task: CVA group movement time $p = 0.002$, $r = 71$; peak velocity $p = 0.002$, $r = 61$. Control group movement time $p = 0.009$, $r = 0.61$; peak velocity $p = 0.0001$, $r = 0.79$. Mug task: CVA group movement time $p = 0.027$, $r = 0.68$; peak velocity $p = 0.013$, $r = 0.61$; control group movement time $p = .003$, $r = .68$; peak velocity $p = 0.003$, $r = 0.68$	Fasoli et al. (2002)
Training in a task in a natural or simulated context	Participants practiced an eating task using chopsticks in a natural or simulated context.	Forty right-handed college students without disabilities and without previous experience with using chopsticks. Mean age = 23.75 years.	Sixty training trials on 1 day; 24-hour retention measured on a transfer task	Randomized controlled study; Level: IB1c	Participants in natural context performed better than those in a simulated context on the transfer task.	Natural context: $p = 0.03$, $r = 0.30$ for success rate at retention trial in the transfer task.	Ma, Trombly, & Robinson-Podolski (1999)
Effect of goal-directed action	Experiment 1: Subjects reached in a goal-directed action or to a spatial location. Experiment 2: Subjects reached for phone, disconnected receiver, and a stick.	Fourteen stroke survivors (nine LCVA, four RCVA, and one bilateral CVA). Mean age = 65 years; average time since onset of stroke = 39 months	Each participant tested under several conditions	Randomized controlled repeated measures counterbalanced design; Level: IC1b	Participants reaching for an object were faster, smoother, and took less time to reach peak speed than when they reached for a point in space.	Experiment 1: number of movement units, $p = 0.05$, $r = 0.55$; movement time $p = 0.02$, $r = 0.62$; percentage of reach to peak velocity, $p = 0.04$, $r = 0.57$; peak velocity, $p = 0.01$, $r = 0.66$; Experiment 2: no effect	Trombly & Wu (1999)
Presence or absence of objects used in movements	Participants were evaluated for movements with object or without object.	Fourteen stroke survivors (nine LCVA, five RCVA, and one bilateral CVA) and twenty-five neurologically intact adults	Each participant was tested under two conditions: reaching to scoop up coins and reaching to where the coins would have been	Randomized controlled repeated measures counterbalanced design; Level: IC1b	Using real objects elicited better performance of reaching, as measured by decreased movement time, decreased displacement, higher velocity, and fewer movement units.	Stroke survivor data: movement time, $p = 0.0028$, $r = 0.70$; total displacement, $p = 0.0019$, $r = 0.72$; percentage of reach where peak velocity occurs, $p = 0.0011$, $r = 0.75$; movement units, $p = 0.0055$, $r = 0.66$	Wu et al. (2000)

RCVA, right cerebral vascular accident; LCVA, left cerebral vascular accident; CVA, cerebral vascular accident.

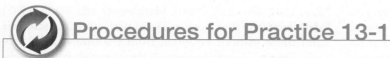

Procedures for Practice 13-1

Caregiver Education and Training

Ever-decreasing hospital lengths of stay continue to increase the demands and responsibilities of family caregivers (Clark et al., 2004). Occupational therapists and other rehabilitation professionals can contribute to clients' quality of life by providing multidimensional education and training to their caregivers (Chee et al., 2007; Kalra et al., 2004; Pasacreta et al., 2000). Here are some important considerations and strategies:

- Acknowledge and validate the pivotal role that family caregivers play in the recovery and quality of life of your client. Make sure that your occupational therapy intervention plan incorporates specific goals, strategies, and timelines for caregiver training.
- Appreciate the complex demands placed on people when they assume caregiver roles. Remember that family caregivers typically have to juggle the needs of other family members and their own jobs and activities in addition to their caregiving responsibilities (Carter & Nutt, 1998; Pasacreta et al., 2000). Adjust your teaching methods in consideration of these demands and distractions on caregivers and expect that you will need to repeat information and instructions more than once.
- Empathize with the emotional burden often carried by family caregivers. Appreciate that they carry an array of worries about their loved one's condition, the quality of care their loved one is receiving, and what the future holds in terms of their caregiving responsibilities (Hong, 2005). Make a point of structuring your education and training efforts to address these worries.

- Incorporate caregiver education and training into your intervention from day 1 by showing family members how to participate in providing care. Ask family members to attend therapy sessions and include them as active participants. Show them how they can extend the benefits of occupational therapy intervention by, for example, prompting and assisting with ADL or reinforcing the use of adaptive equipment.
- Often, therapists are well acquainted with the client's medical and social history, but the caregiver's situation may be less well known. Caregiver factors that are important to investigate include the caregiver's health and their understanding of the client and the client's condition (Chee et al., 2007). When caregiver health is a concern, the caregiver may need to be encouraged to address their personal health concerns.
- Collaborate with other health care professionals to ensure that caregiver education and training is multifaceted and ongoing. Appreciate that current and premorbid family functioning is an important predictor of caregiver stress and adjustment (Clark et al., 2004). Refer caregivers and their family members to counselors, psychologists, and social workers when necessary (Nabors, Seacat, & Rosenthal, 2002).
- Take responsibility for helping family caregivers to transfer what they have learned in the hospital or clinic setting to their home and family contexts. Consider making a home visit before discontinuing your services to review information and techniques within the client's home environment.

---

in this sequence to new tasks, and therefore training time is minimized. The therapist plans that with consistent repetition, the routine will be carried out automatically.

However, occupational therapy intervention, such as ADL training, often begins while the patient is hospitalized. Patients learn one-handed dressing techniques from hospital beds in rooms that are very different from those of their homes. For the intervention to improve the patient's level of independence after discharge, the therapist must train to transfer. That is, therapists employ teaching techniques that optimize patients' chances of being able to apply the task-specific dressing skills learned at the hospital when they get home.

Transfer of learning refers to a person's ability to carry out the same task in a different environment. According to Toglia (1998), transfer is not an all-or-nothing phenomenon. She described three levels of transfer—near, intermediate, and far—based on the number of differences in the surface characteristics between the learning and real-life environments. In general, near transfer requires the person to apply the same skill in very similar circumstances,

whereas far transfer implies greater differences in application environment (Perkins, 1995). Transfer is associated with perceptual similarities of tasks, not similarities in underlying principles (Perkins, 1995). Therefore, transfer places minimal demands on metaprocessing abilities and requires less training time than generalization of newly learned strategies (Saloman & Perkins, 1989).

Strategies and Generalization of Learning

Whereas acquisition of task-specific skills involves learning targeted behavioral sequences, the acquisition of strategies entails learning rules or principles that can be broadly applied. For example, many therapists expect persons with stroke to learn this general strategy: dress the weak side first. This rule or principle enables patients to don sweatshirts, dress shirts, slacks, and outerwear, but it presumes generalization of learning.

Generalization occurs when the person is able to apply the newly learned strategy to a new task in a new environment. For example, the patient who demonstrates the ability to get dressed one-handed in the hospital can use the same strategies to put on a raincoat at home. Generalization, as it is here defined, depends on the learner's mindful abstraction of a principle and is based on conceptual similarities between the learning task and environment and the real-world application (Perkins, 1995). Generalization of learning places greater demands on patients' metaprocessing abilities (Saloman & Perkins, 1989).

FUNDAMENTALS OF THE TEACHING–LEARNING PROCESS

Clearly, the value of occupational therapy intervention will largely be judged by the extent to which new skills and strategies are carried out in patients' real-life environments. Therapists interested in helping patients achieve transfer and generalization objectives incorporate research findings about critical constructs in teaching–learning theory. These constructs relate to the therapeutic use of context, feedback, and practice.

Therapeutic Use of Context

The term "context" broadly refers to the setting in which an event or activity occurs. Many conceptions of context as a facilitator or barrier to function can be found in the occupational therapy and rehabilitation literature (American Occupational Therapy Association [AOTA], 2008; Fisher, 1998; World Health Organization, 1997) (see Chapters 3 and 10). The Occupational Therapy Practice Framework (AOTA, 2008) suggests that context has many dimensions: cultural, physical, social, personal, temporal, and virtual. It also defined activity demands in terms of objects and their properties, space demands, social demands, sequencing and timing, and required actions as influencing the performance of skills and patterns. A brief discussion of the influence of environmental context and activity demands on learning follows.

Role of Context in Learning

Research strongly supports that objects used in activities, the characteristics of those objects, and the goals of the activities performed have a strong influence on motor performance and must be carefully manipulated in treatment. Wu et al. (2000) demonstrated that stroke survivors and nonimpaired individuals elicited smoother, faster, and more coordinated arm movements when using real objects in movement tasks. Participants were asked to scoop money from a table or reach to a point on the table in the scooping position. The use of real objects has been found to elicit different movements and learning than imagery-based tasks or rote exercise in persons with disabilities such as cerebral palsy, stroke, and multiple sclerosis (Mathiowetz & Wade, 1995; Trombly & Wu, 1999; van der Weel, van der Meer, &

Lee, 1991; Wu et al., 2000). Mathiowetz and Wade (1995) demonstrated that both subjects with multiple sclerosis and those without benefited from the information provided by real objects. Subjects in the materials-based condition were asked to eat applesauce with a spoon, bowl, and applesauce available; in the partial-support condition, they pretended to eat applesauce with a spoon and bowl available; and in the imagery-based condition, they pretended to eat applesauce without a spoon or bowl. Again, the movement patterns in the three conditions were significantly different. These findings support occupational therapy approaches that emphasize the significance of real-life objects and tasks in optimizing function (Mathiowetz & Haugen, 1994) (see Chapters 8 and 21 for more about this approach.) These and previous findings are likely explained by two important principles: encoding specificity and contextual interference.

Encoding Specificity

The principle of encoding specificity suggests that events are stored in memory along with their contexts (Smith & Vela, 2001). That is, people encode features of the learning task and environment along with the newly acquired skill or strategy. Encoding specificity limits transfer and generalization because new tasks and environments do not have the same cueing properties as those present during original learning, making retrieval from long-term memory more difficult. For example, imagine that a patient practices the same grasp and release task every day; even the work space is consistent. Although the patient improves performance on the task, the information about control of grasp and release is stored along with the context of the practice task and environment, and he or she may not be able to demonstrate the skills during functional activities or away from the practice space.

Contextual Interference

One way to mitigate the influence of encoding specificity on learning is to employ high contextual interference training (Battig, 1978). Low contextual interference occurs when the context and training task are invariant, allowing the learner to perform the same task repetitively in a consistent environment, as in the previous example. On the other hand, high contextual interference occurs when the task and environment keep changing throughout the learning process. This principle asserts that task and environmental variation force people to use multiple and varied information processing strategies, which makes retrieval easier. Contextual interference forces elaborate processing strategies, and transfer is facilitated. As a result, the patient will be more likely to use the newly learned skills to solve problems within the inevitable variety of the real world. Therefore, to facilitate transfer of task-specific skills and generalization of newly learned strategies, therapists deliberately vary the learning tasks and environments.

Therapeutic Use of Feedback

Feedback also can enhance or interfere with learning. Occupational therapists understand the functions of feedback and deliberately select the types and schedules of feedback in designing a patient's learning experience.

Functions of Feedback

Feedback regarding performance has several functions (Salmoni, Schmidt, & Walter, 1984). It has a temporary motivating or energizing effect and a guidance effect that informs the learner how to correct an error on the next trial. However, feedback can permanently impair motor learning if provided beyond the point that the person has a rough idea of the desired motion, because it becomes a part of the environment and is then needed for performance.

Types of Feedback

To help patients learn and sustain skills and strategies, therapists initially provide extrinsic feedback on performance but ultimately must facilitate the development of intrinsic feedback.

Extrinsic Feedback: Knowledge of Results and Knowledge of Performance. Therapists typically provide feedback about performance in verbal form. Extrinsic information presented after task completion falls into two categories, knowledge of results and knowledge of performance. This feedback allows subjects to alter or adapt their responses or behaviors on subsequent trials. *Knowledge of results* provides information about outcome, such as "You've got your shirt on" or "You took the cap off the jar." A second type of feedback, *knowledge of performance*, is related to qualitative descriptions of a performance, such as "You shifted your weight too far to the left" or "You bent your elbow." This information directs patients' attention not to outcome but to components of movement that they need to change or attend to. This type of feedback duplicates information patients already have but may serve to focus their attention to specific parts of the movement. Other external information provided to patients during practice falls into the category of encouragement. It is important that therapists not confuse encouragement ("Keep going") with feedback ("You're doing great"), especially if the latter is not true, because incorrect feedback is highly detrimental to learning (Buekers, Magill, & Hall, 1992).

Intrinsic Feedback. Intrinsic feedback, or internal feedback, is information that patients receive through their own senses, such as seeing an egg break as it hits the floor after dropping it or feeling the pain of hitting the ground

after an unsuccessful transfer. Although this information is available to patients, they may need cueing to focus on the most important components of a skill or strategy, such as using vision when moving a limb with impaired sensation. Intervention that incorporates self-monitoring and self-estimation (task difficulty, completion time, accuracy score, amount of cueing, or assistance needed) enables patients to create mechanisms for self-generated feedback (Cicerone & Giacino, 1992; Toglia, 1998), lessening dependence on therapists for successful performance.

Feedback Schedules

The frequency and content of feedback are critical to the learning process and must be considered when a teaching situation is planned.

Immediate and Summary Feedback. The frequency and timing of feedback can profoundly influence the acquisition and learning of task-specific skills and strategies. Studies in this area evaluate learning during a "retention trial," which is done some time after teaching is completed. For example, Lavery (1962) wanted to know which schedule of feedback best facilitated learning: immediate feedback provided after each trial was completed, also referred to as constant feedback; summary feedback provided after a number of trials were completed; or both. Lavery found that subjects who received immediate or combined feedback improved their performance of the task more quickly during the training than the group receiving only summary feedback. However, when tested for retention of the task 4, 37, and 93 days after training, the subjects who received only summary feedback did significantly better than those who received either immediate feedback or both types.

Lavery (1962) hypothesized that people who received immediate feedback came to rely on it when performing the task and those that received only summary feedback were forced to analyze their own movements. The subjects who received both immediate and summary feedback did just as poorly as those who received only immediate feedback, suggesting that the immediate feedback interfered with the processing of the summary feedback. Beyond its implications about the schedule of feedback, these findings support the idea that performance during the training phase does not reflect actual learning of the skill and that learning can only be assessed after the training session.

Faded Feedback. Therapists are often concerned that providing only summary feedback after a series of trials will not help their patients understand tasks that are complex or new. Winstein and Schmidt (1990) evaluated the effectiveness of feedback given on 50% and 100% of trials on the learning of a task by college students. The 50% feedback was faded, with the feedback given on every trial initially and then decreased to no feedback at the end of training, with feedback being given on an overall average of 50% of all the trials. They found a slight advantage for the 100% feedback group during acquisition of the skill, but the group that received faded feedback performed significantly better than the immediate feedback group on the retention trials. These findings point out an important irony in teaching: factors that degrade performance during acquisition often improve learning.

Bandwidth Feedback. With bandwidth feedback, an acceptable range of performance is defined, and the subject receives feedback only when performance is outside of that range. As the subject's performance improves, feedback is provided less frequently.

Therapeutic Use of Practice

In addition to planning feedback, the design of a treatment session factors in the nature of instructions and a plan for practicing the material.

Internally or Externally Focused Instructions

Research supports instruction that is focused on the task rather than on the patient's performance. For example, Fasoli et al. (2002) found that patients with strokes reached faster and more smoothly when cued to focus on the object and what they were going to do with it rather than focusing on their arm as they did the task. This means that the instructions given to patients should focus their attention on the objects and the task, rather than on the movements that they will be using to achieve the goal.

Blocked versus Random Practice

As discussed earlier, traditional models of learning did not distinguish between learning and performance. These models also promoted blocked forms of practice, such as drill, as the most efficient schedule for learning a task. Using a blocked format, the same skill or strategy is practiced over a number of repetitions, after which the next skill or strategy is rehearsed. As such, blocked practice is a form of practice with low contextual interference.

Shea and Morgan (1979) studied whether increasing the contextual interference by random practice during skill acquisition leads to improved retention and transfer of motor skills. Their experiments entailed knocking over wooden barriers with a tennis ball held in the hand. In brief, they found that blocked practice provided low contextual interference, whereas random practice provided high contextual interference, requiring subjects to formulate a new movement plan for each trial. Subjects who practiced with high contextual interference demonstrated better retention and transfer than those who used blocked practice. This study demonstrated two important findings: (1) performance during acquisition of a skill does not necessarily relate to later learning and

(2) conditions that may improve performance during acquisition do not necessarily create better learning. In fact, structuring training to improve performance during practice by using blocked practice schedules can actually decrease task retention and transfer (Brady, 2004).

The advantage of random practice over blocked practice was also demonstrated for patients with hemiplegia (Hanlon, 1996). Patients practiced a multistep functional activity that consisted of reaching for a cupboard door, opening it, picking up a coffee cup by the handle, transferring it to a counter, and releasing the handle. The subjects practiced these steps in either a blocked or a random pattern. The random pattern group performed significantly better than either the blocked or control group on both the 2- and 7-day retention trials.

Part-Whole Practice

Therapists also decide whether patients practice the whole task or components of a task (referred to as part-whole training). Ma and Trombly (2004) evaluated the characteristics of movement under part and whole task conditions. The task involved reaching for a pen, bringing the pen to paper, and signing their name. The three segments of movement were performed separately and then as a single task for each individual. The performance of the whole task elicited greater efficiency of movement, greater force during the task, and smoother movements. Winstein et al. (1989) examined the effect of part-task practice with gait training. One group of patients with hemiplegia received traditional physical therapy gait training. The second group received traditional physical therapy and specific training in standing balance symmetry (proposed as a reasonable critical component of symmetrical gait). After several weeks of training, the group that had practiced symmetry in standing showed improvement in that component of the activity, but there was no carryover to the whole task of gait. There was no significant difference in gait symmetry between the two groups.

These findings demonstrate that in some situations whole practice is more effective than part practice. It will require much more research to identify the components that will transfer to the whole task before part-task training can be the preferred method. Winstein et al. (1989) suggested that tasks that are continuous and cannot be easily separated into component parts may not be appropriate for part training. Examples of this type of movement include walking or driving a car—tasks that require many adjustments with components that occur simultaneously and cannot be easily separated.

Intensity of Practice

Much focus in motor rehabilitation over the last several years has been on techniques such as constraint-induced movement treatment for people with upper extremity dysfunction. This intervention has been found to drive neuroplasticity and improve functional use of the arm after stroke (Wolf et al., 2006). Intensive practice has now been identified as an active component in a variety of other interventions, including partial weight supported gait training for people with stroke (Duncan, Sullivan, & Behrman, et al., 2011), and Lee Silverman Voice Treatment® Big and Loud Therapy (BIG) for people with Parkinson's Disease (Farley & Koshland, 2005). BIG is an intensive intervention specifically designed to remediate movement disorders in clients with Parkinson's Disease. Intensity of practice includes a number of features of practice, including practice of difficult tasks that are directly related to the performance objective, high rates of repetition, a focus on transfer of the skill to the performance environment, and choosing tasks with meaning to the client (Kleim & Jones, 2008). Incorporating these principles into occupational therapy treatment will increase the effectiveness of treatment, but the number of these principles that can be implemented will depend on the client's diagnosis, endurance, and the treatment environment (see Research Note 13-1).

MAKING PERSONAL CHANGE

Employing a newly learned skill or strategy is fundamentally a personal change depending not only on recall, transfer, or generalization but also on learners' beliefs about their competence and their stage in the change process.

Bandura (1977) posited that people's beliefs about their ability to handle a new situation largely determine whether they attempt the new task and their ultimate performance. Self-percepts of efficacy (self-perceptions of competence) predict success with a wide range of acquired health behaviors, including smoking cessation (Stewart, Borland, & McMurray, 1994), exercise maintenance (McAuley, 1993), medication compliance (DeGeest et al., 1994), and use of energy-conservation techniques to manage fatigue (Mathiowetz, Matuska, & Murphy, 2001). Bandura (1977) demonstrated that people make judgments about their competence (self-efficacy) by thinking about past accomplishments, vicarious experience (observing others who are similar), verbal persuasion, and emotional arousal, such as anxiety. Because self-percepts of competence seem to explain the discrepancy between what people can do and what they actually do (Bandura, 1982), occupational therapists actively create opportunities for patients to demonstrate to themselves that they are indeed competent with the new skill or strategy.

Many patients served by occupational therapists have had recent changes in physical functioning. Persons who are insulated from ramifications of these changes (perhaps those who have been hospitalized continuously since onset) may not fully appreciate the need for the skills and strategies therapists are attempting to teach them. The Stages of

Research Note 13-1

Lo, A. C., Guarino, P.D., Richards, L.G., Haselkorn, J. K., Wittenberg, G. F., Federman, D. G., Ringer, R. J., Wagner, T. H., Krebs, H. I., Volpe, B. T., Bever, C. T. Jr., Bravata, D. M., Duncan, P. W., Corn, B. H., Maffucci, A. D., Nadeau, S. E., Conroy, S. S., Powell, J. M., Huang, G. D., Peduzzi, P. (2010). Robot-assisted therapy for long-term upper-limb impairment after stroke. *New England Journal of Medicine, 362,* 1772–1783.

Abstract

Lo and colleagues investigated the effects of robot-assisted therapy in subjects with upper limb impairment who were at least 6 months post stroke. One hundred twenty-seven participants with moderate to severe arm impairment were randomized to three intervention groups. Group 1, who enrolled an average of 3.6 years after their stroke, received 36 1-hour sessions of intensive robot-assisted therapy focused on four modules. They included a shoulder–elbow movement focusing on horizontal movements, an antigravity unit for vertical movements, a wrist unit for wrist movements, and a grasp-hand unit focused on hand opening and closing. Group 2, who enrolled an average of 4.8 years after their stroke, received 36 1-hour sessions over 12 weeks of intensive comparison therapy, including a structured high repetition protocol of assisted shoulder stretching,

arm exercises, shoulder-stabilization activities, and functional reaching tasks. Group 3, who enrolled an average of 6.2 years after their stroke, received usual and standard care that was available to all clients and was not dictated by the research project. The robot-assisted therapy and intensive comparison therapy were matched for repetitions per session, at about 1,000 repetitions per 1-hour session. At the end of the 12-week intervention period, robot-assisted therapy did not produce significantly better motor outcomes than usual care or intensive comparison therapy. However, over the 36-week study period, robot-assisted therapy was significantly better than usual care but not significantly better than the intensive comparison therapy. This study provides evidence that intensive models of rehabilitation may benefit patients even years post stroke.

Implications for Practice

- The intensity of practice, as determined by the number of repetitions, is a critical feature of a therapy intervention and needs to be included in the plan for therapy.
- Provision of therapy, even years post stroke, can provide clinically significant improvements in arm function, and potential long-term benefits from rehabilitation. This finding challenges the clinical belief that long-term stroke survivors cannot make significant improvements in upper extremity function.

Change Model (Prochaska & DiClemente, 1982) helps therapists target their teaching–learning interventions to address the learning predispositions of the client and family.

This model identifies five stages of change: precontemplation, contemplation, determination, action, and maintenance. During the precontemplation stage, clients are not even aware of the problem. In the contemplation stage, they become aware of the problem or concern, and in the determination stage, they resolve to do something about it. During the action stage, clients work to address the problem or issue. During the maintenance stage, clients must still put forth some degree of effort to sustain the desired skill or behavior. Prochaska and DiClemente (1982) suggested that verbal intervention strategies are most appropriate during the first three stages (pointing out the problem and discussing possible approaches), whereas action-oriented behavioral interventions are most helpful during the last two stages. For example, before a client routinely employs strategies for scanning the left visual field, he must believe that he is missing those parts of the environment or that personal safety is in jeopardy. Attempting to verbally convince a patient that they have a particular problem is estimated to be effective in generating behavior change in only about 15% of the time (Kottke et al., 1988). Once the patient is convinced that he has a problem and is motivated to change, he can be taught specifically how to manage the problem.

Motivational Interviewing

Motivational interviewing (MI) is a method designed to help clients make behavior changes. MI was developed in the field of chemical dependency and has been very effective in helping clients implement behavior change across a broad range of health conditions including musculoskeletal diagnoses, asthma, diabetes, hypertension, cardiovascular disease, and increasing the effectiveness of family education (Byers, Lamanna, & Rosenberg, 2010; Rollnick, Miller, & Butler, 2008; Shannon & Hillsdon, 2007). The central feature of MI is development of a client–clinician relationship that is collaborative, evocative, and honors the client's autonomy. MI's effectiveness is based on activation of the clients' own motivation for change while acknowledging their ambivalence about those changes. In the management of many chronic conditions, the problem is not necessarily an issue of knowledge about the condition: clients often know that they should take their medication, exercise, or quit smoking but are not motivated to make those changes today. MI helps clients develop the motivation to make those changes by helping them articulate the arguments for the change.

There are four guiding principles for therapists using MI: **R**esist the righting reflex, **U**nderstand the client's own motivations, **L**isten with empathy, and **E**mpower the patient through encouraging hope and optimism (Rollnick & Heather, 1992). The righting reflex (or the reflex to resist change) is a normal psychological response to being told what to do: resisting the change. This creates a conversation that includes statements like "Yes, . . . but," in which clients articulate the reasons *not* to change. As they restate the reasons they cannot change, clients become further convinced by their own arguments. Thus, this conversation actually decreases the likelihood that clients will implement the change. The goal of MI is to switch the conversation so that clients make the arguments for change. In order to do that, the occupational therapist must resist the tendency to tell clients what to do, and instead, collaborate with them to develop their own arguments for change (Rollnick & Heather, 1992). This is done primarily through the use of a communication style that is "guiding" (Rollnick, Miller, & Butler, 2008).

MI requires that occupational therapists be aware of their communication styles and have the skills to move between them as they work with clients (Rollnick, Miller, & Butler, 2008). The three communication styles used in MI are the following:

- Guiding—characterized by recognition by the occupational therapist that the client has the answers about how to change his or her own behavior and that the client is in charge of making those changes.
- Following—seeks to understand the client's story, focuses on listening, encouraging the client to talk, and asking questions only to clarify. When using a "following" style, there is no agenda other than to understand the client's perspective and experience. A following style is often appropriate when initially trying to understand clients' lives.
- Directive—used when there is a clear difference in knowledge, expertise, or power between the occupational therapist and the client. This is appropriate when we are instructing clients in techniques, strategies, or providing specific information. However, when the focus is on creating motivation for behavior change, a directive approach may trigger the righting reflex. The appearance of "Yes, . . . but" statements are a cue for the occupational therapist that she is using a directive style (Rollnick, Miller, & Butler, 2008).

The second guiding principle is to focus on the client's understanding, values, and motivations (Rollnick, Miller, & Butler, 2008). The client's situation is unique, and it is only through focusing on the client's perspective that his or her motivation can be awakened. This client-centered focus aligns well with the principles of occupational therapy.

The third guiding principle involves using open-ended questions, reflective statements, and summaries, with particular attention to statements that indicate a **D**esire for change, **A**bility to change, **R**easons for change, and **N**eed for change (DARN) (Rollnick, Miller, & Butler, 2008). DARN statements are forms of "change talk," in which clients talk about their understanding of the pro-behavior-change side of their ambivalence. DARN statements indicate that they are in a precommitment state and reveal their values. The occupational therapist reflects these statements back to the client, which helps the client clarify desires, abilities, reasons, needs, and values. Therapists also pay particular attention to statements about committing to change and statements about taking behavioral steps (Rollnick, Miller, & Butler, 2008). As clients engage in self-talk, they strengthen their own motivation to make change.

The final guiding principle of MI is to empower clients to make changes in their behavior. The therapist may know that a client needs to do home exercises or be more active, but the client is the one who knows how to make those changes within the context of his or her daily life. By helping clients think out loud about how they might implement change within their lives, the small steps that they might take, we can help clients improve their health (Rollnick, Miller, & Butler, 2008).

While MI focuses on clients' control of their behavior, the therapist structures the interaction so that clients begin to identify the need for change through the agenda-setting process (Rollnick, Miller, & Butler, 2008). At this point, clients are presented with a variety of possible behavior change topics, always leaving the opportunity for clients to pick other areas if their target is not present. For example, you might present a number of behaviors such as exercise or losing weight, depending on the client's situation. Then the client is asked which, if any, he or she would like to work on. When the client picks his or her target behavior, the therapist continues to ask open-ended questions, reflect back the client's statements, and work toward commitment to change. If the client is not able to pick a target behavior, the therapist continues to elicit change talk. In this way, the power of behavior change is held by the client, and the therapist is there to help him or her implement those changes (Rollnick, Miller, & Butler, 2008).

OCCUPATIONAL THERAPIST AS TEACHER

The extent to which occupational therapy contributes to a client's resumption of roles depends to a large extent on the effectiveness of the therapist as a teacher. The principles of teaching parallel therapy are the following: assessment, goal setting, intervention, and evaluation (Redman, 1997). Although this process rarely follows a predictable, orderly sequence, these steps serve as a checklist to ensure that therapists consider variables affecting the outcome of their teaching efforts (Redman, 1997).

Assess Learning Needs and Readiness

Based on the therapist assessment of the client and identification of barriers to learning, the therapist determines who will be the subject or subjects of the teaching—the patient, family member, or both (Vanetzian, 1997).

Set Client-Specific Learning Goals

Therapists use the results of their assessments and estimates of the treatment time available to set learning and cognitive objectives for each patient. Therapists plan treatment around transfer and generalization goals by identifying reinforcements in the natural environment and incorporating into the treatment stimuli common to both training and real-world environments (Sohlberg & Raskin, 1996). If the intervention ultimately is to change an existing routine, skill, or strategy, the therapist attempts to identify the client's stage of change. For example, a patient with no awareness of a memory problem will see little value in learning to use compensatory memory techniques. Therefore, the therapist sets goals that move the patient toward the contemplative stage of change by allowing him or her to take the consequences of forgetting. Finally, therapists merely recommend learning goals. Goals that direct teaching–learning efforts are set in collaboration with patients and their families.

Create Learning Opportunities Throughout Intervention

Therapists deliberately use context, feedback, and practice to help patients meet learning goals (Procedures for Practice 13-2). They enhance motivation and recall by linking new skills or strategies with patients' specific interests, knowledge, and abilities. Effective teachers also make an effort to overcome barriers to learning. Clinicians recognize that literacy affects comprehension and use written materials that minimize the demand for reading (DeWalt et al., 2010). Citing the results of the 2003 National Adult Literacy Survey, Schneider (2005) reported that 13% of all Americans had "below basic" English literacy for prose material. This means that 30 million Americans cannot do much more than sign a form or review a document to see what they are allowed to drink before a medical procedure (Schneider, 2005). Another 22% had only "basic" literacy, meaning, at best, they can find information in a pamphlet about how jurors were selected for a jury pool (National Center for Education Statistics, 2005). Therefore, clinicians create and use written materials that are well organized and limit the demands on reading (Procedures for Practice 13-3).

Develop Plan to Promote Patient Adherence

As a part of teaching, therapists need to explicitly address issues of patient adherence, defined as the degree to which patients act in accord with advice of a health

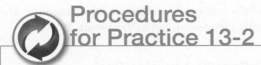

Procedures for Practice 13-2

Therapeutic Use of Context, Feedback, and Practice to Promote Transfer and Generalization

- Vary the training environmental context to achieve transfer; vary training tasks and environments to achieve generalization of new strategies.
- Provide extrinsic feedback just until the learner understands the desired movement, skill, or strategy. Use cueing and the patient's own performance prediction and analysis to help the learner increasingly rely on intrinsic feedback.
- Provide summary feedback when possible. Tolerate a slower or longer acquisition phase of learning, appreciating the later benefits in terms of retention, transfer, and generalization.
- Fade therapist feedback and cues so that these elements of training do not get encoded with the new skill or strategy.
- Attempt to teach movement, skills, and strategies within whole tasks. Address components or subskills only when they are critical to whole-task performance.

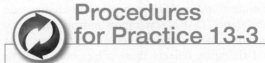

Procedures for Practice 13-3

Addressing Low Literacy in Patient Teaching

Problems with literacy pervade all socioeconomic and ethnic groups (Thomas, 1999). People with low literacy tend to be ashamed of their difficulties with reading and are reluctant to admit the problem, even to family members (Parikh et al., 1996). Thomas (1999) and DeWalt et al. (2010) offer the following suggestions for addressing this issue in occupational therapy:

- Incorporate a brief evaluation of literacy into the occupational therapy assessment process (see Chapter 3).
- Limit the quantity of information to the most important messages. Collaborate with the patient, family, and other team members to establish priorities.
- Reduce the reading level of printed materials by using one- or two-syllable words, shortening sentences to 10–15 words, and targeting materials to the fifth- or sixth-grade reading level.
- Make sure text and graphics are well organized. DeWalt et al. (2010) recommend chunking information, using paragraph headings, and having white space between sections.
- Use materials that are racially and culturally sensitive. As recommended by Thomas (1999), "make sure that patients can 'see themselves' in materials provided. (p. 3)."

professional (Moseley, 2006). Critically, when therapists acknowledge the normal problems with adherence that the average client has, they give clients license to admit whether adherence is a problem at the time of future sessions (Radomski, 2011). Acknowledging that compliance is difficult also helps client and therapist set up an adherence plan at the time of the recommendations, by linking the home program to a specific point in the daily routine and purposely simplifying the recommendations. In developing this adherence plan, clients and therapists identify any social, technological, or environmental supports available to shore up adherence, such as family members who can cue the client, either in person or through text messaging, alarms that could be set, or checklists that could be followed. Finally, clients are more likely to comply with adherence plans when there is a clear benefit (Radomski, 2011). By addressing the

issue of adherence as recommendations are made, the likelihood of the recommendations being carried out is increased.

Evaluate Achievement of Learning Goals

Effective teachers routinely assess clients' progress toward learning goals, typically by changing the training task or environment and evaluating carryover. Family members perform return demonstrations of new techniques, such as transfers. Based on performance or other changes in learning status, therapists adjust learning goals throughout the intervention.

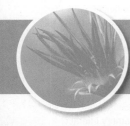

case example

Learning as Part of Clinic-Based Intervention for a Client with Mild Stroke

Occupational Therapy Intervention Process	Clinical Reasoning Process	
	Objectives	**Examples of Therapist's Internal Dialogue**

Client Information

Mrs. B. is a 45-year-old woman who had a mild stroke 3 weeks ago. She is married with three grown children. She had an episode of expressive aphasia and right-sided weakness while at work. She was admitted to the hospital and given anticoagulants, and most symptoms resolved over the next 48 hours. She was hospitalized for 2 days, and hyperlipidemia and high blood pressure were identified as the causes of her stroke. She was discharged to the care of her family physician and has been off work since her discharge. She works as an executive assistant in a large insurance company.
ADL: She is able to do her self-cares but rates her fatigue, as 10/10 in severity. Currently, she tries not to rest during the day: "No pain, no gain," but becomes so exhausted by 2:00 that she falls asleep wherever she is. When asked about taking more rest breaks when she was tired, she said, "I'd be sleeping all the time—I'm tired at 9:00 in the morning!"
Upper extremity function: Mrs. B. had noticed some right upper extremity weakness on the day of her stroke but has had no difficulty since then. Mrs. B.'s arm function has normal strength and range of motion, and she uses it well in activities. Walking and mobility: Mrs. B. reports no problems with gait or balance. IADL: She is struggling with managing her low-fat diet and feels like she needs to "learn a whole new way to cook." She has been told she cannot drive for 3 months and is relying on family and friends for transportation. Cognitive function: Mrs. B. complains that sometimes her thinking is "not right," whereas at other times, she has no problems. She says she forgets things and is struggling to learn her new diet and take her new medications. She scores within normal limits on a cognitive screen. Work: She is anxious to return to work as soon as possible, but her physician has said she cannot go back for at least another month. She is afraid that her boss will not hold her job for her while she is on medical leave.
Patient's safety: Mrs. B.'s judgment and memory are intact, she is a good historian. However, the severe fatigue could lead to problems with safety, particularly while cooking or walking.

Appreciate the context

"This is a young woman who had no real health concerns prior to this stroke, so it must have been quite a shock to her. She also has other new diagnoses with major consequences, so there are lots of changes in her life right now. I think if I can help her understand her fatigue and its implications, she will be able to get back to her usual tasks. She seems very anxious to return to her life and motivated to make changes, but these are big changes and will be difficult to implement."

Develop intervention hypotheses

"I think that instruction in energy conservation principles might be helpful, but they will need to be integrated into her life. Given her level of fatigue, it is going to be difficult to balance her therapy schedule with her capacity to attend therapy. Return-to-work issues will need to be discussed, and the willingness of her employer to make adaptations for her could be a problem."

Consider the evidence

"I have read that fatigue after stroke occurs in about 50%–70% of stroke survivors (Lerdal et al., 2009) and can have a profoundly limiting effect on stroke survivors' function (Flinn & Stube, 2009). Energy conservation techniques have been shown to be promising in a pilot study (Clarke, Barker-Collo, & Feignin, 2012)."

Select an intervention approach

"I will use these intervention approaches: teach compensatory skills for fatigue, change the physical environment/context as needed to decrease fatigue, and further evaluate her work situation."

Reflect on competence

"These new diagnoses are going to be a challenge for Mrs. B. to manage and have changed how she needs to do previously automatic tasks, such as cooking. The need to change so many things at once is going to be difficult for Mrs. B. She needs to understand the role of fatigue in memory function. I know some information about reducing cholesterol through diet, but I should have Mrs. B. bring in the materials she has been given so that I am sure that what I say is consistent with what she has learned elsewhere."

Recommendations

Clinic-based occupational therapy two times a week for 2 weeks and then once a week for 4 weeks. This therapy schedule will allow Mrs. B. to practice energy conservation techniques and accommodate her overwhelming fatigue. Short-term goals for therapy include (1) client will report fatigue of 7/10 at the end of the day in her daily diary; (2) client will explain her fatigue to her husband and gain his help in making accommodations; (3) in the next 2 weeks, the client will cook three new meals that accommodate her high cholesterol diet; and (4) Mrs. B. will find out how long they will hold her job and how to go about making accommodations.

| Consider the client's appraisal of performance | "Mrs B.'s fatigue is overwhelming to her, and she does not really understand how her cognitive symptoms relate to fatigue. She is so overwhelmed by all the changes in her life that she has not made changes in her diet. She will need help dealing with that additional change." |

| Consider what will occur in therapy, how often, and for how long | "We will meet for eight 1-hour sessions over 6 weeks, first addressing how fatigue and memory interact to allay some of Mrs. B.'s concerns. I am going to have her keep a diary so that she can record what she is doing, her fatigue levels, and how well she is implementing rest periods. In preparation for return to work, where she may need to ask for accommodations, I want her to start practicing how to explain her fatigue to her husband as way to build those skills." |

| Ascertain the client's endorsement of the plan | "I think that Mrs. B. is uncertain that she can learn to manage her fatigue but will be convinced if she starts to be successful." |

Summary of Short-Term Goals and Progress after 3 Weeks

Once Mrs. B. understood how her fatigue affected her memory, she began to compensate for it by adding two rest breaks a day. Mrs. B. has established a routine for being home during the week that includes taking her medications and planning low cholesterol meals. She reports taking her medication regularly and has incorporated some dietary changes into her cooking. She has said that she talked to her husband about her fatigue and that she feels he understands, but she does not always tell him she is tired when they go out. She then gets overtired, and it takes her a day or two to recover. She continues to be anxious to return to work, but did talk to her employer, and got assurances that her job would be held until she is released to return to work by her physician.

| Assess the client's comprehension | "It was really helpful to describe the components of memory and how fatigue and anxiety can sabotage memory function." |

| Understand what she is doing | "She has started to implement some principles of energy conservation, adding rest breaks at midmorning and midafternoon. She reports that her fatigue is usually about 5/10 at the end of the day, which is a big improvement. She has been inconsistent in implementing energy-saving strategies like using a tub bench or asking to rest when she and her husband go out to run errands." |

| Compare actual to expected performance | "Mrs. B. is not consistently implementing energy conservation strategies, and she will need to do that when she returns to work." |

| Know the person Appreciate the context | "I'm not sure how much Mr. B. really understands about her fatigue. Mrs. B. continues to need to ask him to make adjustments in their activities. I need to explore this further." |

Next Steps

In the next three weekly sessions, continue to reinforce other energy conservation techniques by focusing on activities that she finds particularly fatiguing. Identify strategies that she could use at work to conserve energy. Encourage further changes in diet. Explore her reticence to ask her husband to accommodate her fatigue, perhaps using motivational interviewing.

    Continue with revised goals.

    After the first 3 weeks of treatment, new goals for therapy were set. They included the following: (1) Mrs. B. will report fatigue rating of 3/10 at the end of the day, (2) client will gain her husband's assistance in accommodating her fatigue, and (3) client will consistently modify her cooking to reduce cholesterol.

| Anticipate present and future client concerns | "Mrs. B. is doing well, making changes and seeing benefit. She is reassured about her cognition and understands the impact of post-stroke fatigue. I think that post-stroke fatigue is going to be a major challenge to her return to work. I believe that she will be a safe driver but am recommending a driving evaluation when her physician allows her to drive again." |

| Analyze client's comprehension Decide if he or she should continue or discontinue therapy and/or return in the future | "Mrs. B. will be off work for another month or two. Mrs. B. and I have discussed the return-to-work services that are available through the state, and she has reluctantly applied for them. I am not suggesting continued therapy but have suggested that she return to therapy just prior to returning to work to review energy conservation strategies for work." |

Clinical Reasoning in Occupational Therapy Practice

Designing Strategies to Increase Task Transfer and Generalization

Mrs. B.'s assessment suggested a number of learning needs related to energy conservation. List Mrs. B.'s learning needs. For two needs, give examples of how you can teach these skills to encourage transfer and generalization to other situations. Explain the difference in Mrs. B.'s learning processes for task-specific skills and general strategies in terms of speed and ease of acquisition and teaching methods.

Teaching to Increase Transfer and Generalization

For the examples listed above, explain the difference in Mrs. B.'s learning processes for task-specific skills and general strategies in terms of speed and ease of acquisition and teaching methods.

Summary Review Questions

1. List the types of practice patterns and discuss the advantages and disadvantages of each.
2. Design two ADL training sessions, one for learning a specific task and the second for learning a general strategy.
3. Discuss the different feedback schedules and compare their advantages and disadvantages.
4. Identify Fitts and Posner's (1967) three stages of learning. Describe the characteristics of performance that you might see as patients learn to use a piece of adaptive equipment.
5. List characteristics of practice most likely to facilitate transfer and generalization of practice.
6. Describe the influences on the learning readiness of a family caregiver. What will you do to optimize the learning process in response to these influences?

Glossary

Automaticity—The phase of learning resulting from numerous consistent repetitions in which a person accurately carries out a skill or task with little or no cognitive effort (Sternberg, 1986).

Contextual interference—Changes across trials in intrinsic and extrinsic factors that force learners to use multiple and variable processing strategies (Shea & Morgan, 1979).

Encoding specificity—A phenomenon of information processing wherein we store a given memory along with information about the context in which the memory occurred, and as a result, elements of the context may trigger recall and recognition of that memory in the future.

Feedback—Intrinsic or extrinsic information that patients receive while learning to perform a new skill or strategy.

Generalization—The ability to apply a skill or strategy to an altogether new task in an environment that is different from the one in which the original training occurred.

Health literacy—The cognitive and communication skills that allow individuals to access, understand, and use information in ways that promote and maintain good health (DeWalt et al., 2010).

Learning—The result of processes associated with practice or experience that leads to relatively permanent changes in a person's knowledge, skills, and behavior (Schmidt & Lee, 2011).

Performance—Temporary changes in response during practice.

Practice—The repetition of a to-be-learned task, a key ingredient in the learning of skills and strategies.

Retrieval—The search for and location of information stored in long-term memory that occurs when people remember (recall or recognize) something that they have learned (Eysenck & Keane, 1990).

Transfer—The ability to perform a new skill in an environment that is different from the training environment.

References

American Occupational Therapy Association. (2008). Occupational therapy practice framework: Domain and process (2nd ed.). *American Journal of Occupational Therapy, 62,* 625–683.

Atkinson, R. C., & Shiffrin, R. M. (1971). The control of short-term memory. *Scientific American, 225,* 82–90.

Bandura, A. (1977). Self-efficacy: Toward a unifying theory of behavior change. *Psychological Review, 84,* 191–215.

Bandura, A. (1982). Self-efficacy mechanism in human agency. *American Psychologist, 37,* 122–147.

Battig, W. F. (1978). The flexibility of the human memory. In L. S. Cermak & F. I. M. Craik (Eds.), *Levels of processing and human memory* (pp. 23–44). Hillsdale, NJ: Erlbaum.

Brady, F. (2004) Contextual interference: A meta-analytic study. *Perceptual and Motor Skills, 99,* 116–126.

Buekers, M. J. A., Magill, R. A., & Hall, K. G. (1992). The effect of erroneous knowledge of results on skill acquisition when augmented information is redundant. *Quarterly Journal of Experimental Psychology, 44,* 105–117.

Byers, A. M., Lamanna, L., & Rosenberg, A. (2010). The effect of motivational interviewing after ischemic stroke on patient knowledge and patient satisfaction with care: A pilot study. *Journal of Neuroscience Nursing, 42,* 312–322.

Carter, J. H., & Nutt, J. G. (1998). Family caregiving: A neglected and hidden part of health care delivery. *American Academy of Neurology, 51,* 1245–1246.

Chee, Y. K., Gitlin, L. N., Dennis, M. P., & Hauck, W. W. (2007). Predictors of adherence to a skill-building intervention in dementia caregivers. *The Journals of Gerontology, 62A,* 673–678.

Cicerone, K. D., & Giacino, J. T. (1992). Remediation of executive function deficits after traumatic brain injury. *NeuroRehabilitation, 2,* 12–22.

Clark, P. C., Dunbar, S. B., Shields, C. G., Viswanathan, B., Aycock, D. M., & Wolf, S. (2004). Influence of stroke survivor characteristics and family conflict surrounding recovery on caregivers' mental and physical health. *Nursing Research, 53,* 406–413.

Clarke, A., Barker-Collo, S. I., & Feignin, V. L. (2012). Poststroke fatigue: Does group education make a difference? A randomized pilot trial. *Topics in Stroke Rehabilitation, 19,* 32–39.

Craik, F. I. M., & Tulving, E. (1975). Depth of processing and retention of words in episodic memory. *Journal of Experimental Psychology: General, 104,* 268–294.

Deckersbach, T., Savage, C. R., Curran, T., Bohne, A., Wilhelm, S., Baer, L., Jenike, M. A., & Rauch, S. L. (2002). A study of parallel implicit and explicit information processing in patients with obsessive-compulsive disorder. *American Journal of Psychiatry, 159,* 1780–1782.

DeGeest, S., Abraham, I., Gemoets, H., & Evers, G. (1994). Development of the long-term medication behavior self-efficacy scale: Qualitative study for item development. *Journal of Advanced Nursing, 19,* 233–238.

DeWalt, D. A., Callahan, L. F., Hawk, V. H., Broucksou, K. A., Hink, A., Rudd, R., & Brach, C. (2010). *Health literacy universal precautions toolkit* (AHRQ Publication No. 10-0046-EF). Rockville, MD: Agency for Healthcare Research and Quality.

Donaghey, C. L., McMillan, T. M., & O'Neill, B. (2010). Errorless learning is superior to trial and error when learning a practical skill in rehabilitation: A randomized controlled trial. *Clinical Rehabilitation, 24,* 195–201.

Duncan, P. W., Sullivan, K. J., Behrman, A. L., Azen, S. P., Wu, S. S., Nadeau, S. E., Dobkin, B. H., Rose, D. K., Tilson, J. K., Cen, S., & Hayden, S. K. (2011) "Body-weight–supported treadmill rehabilitation after stroke". *The New England Journal of Medicine, 364,* 2026–2036.

Eldridge, L. L., Masterman, D., & Knowlton, B. J. (2002). Intact implicit habit learning in Alzheimer's disease. *Behavioral Neuroscience, 116,* 722–726.

Eversheim, U., & Bock, O. (2001). Evidence for processing stages in skills acquisition: A dual-task study. *Learning and Memory, 8,* 183–189.

Eysenck, M. W., & Keane, M. R. (1990). *Cognitive psychology: A student's handbook.* East Sussex, UK: Lawrence Erlbaum.

Farley, B. G., & Koshland, G. F. (2005). Training BIG to move faster: The application of the speed-amplitude relation as a rehabilitation strategy for people with Parkinson's disease. *Experimental Brain Research, 167,* 462–467.

Fasoli, S. E., Trombly, C. A., Tickle-Degnen, L., & Verfaellie, M. H. (2002). Effect of instructions on functional reach in persons with and without cerebrovascular accident. *American Journal of Occupational Therapy, 56,* 380–390.

Fisher, A. G. (1998). Uniting practice and theory in an occupational framework. *American Journal of Occupational Therapy, 52,* 509–521.

Fitts, P. M., & Posner, M. I. (1967). *Human performance.* Belmont, CA: Brooks/Cole.

Flinn, N. A. & Stube, J. E. (2009). Post-stroke fatigue: Qualitative study of three focus groups. *Occupational Therapy International, 17(2),* 81-91.

Gentile, A. M. (1998). Implicit and explicit processes during acquisition of functional skills. *Scandinavian Journal of Occupational Therapy, 5,* 7–16.

Giles, G. M. (2005). A neurofunctional approach to rehabilitation following severe brain injury. In N. Katz (Ed.), *Cognition and occupation across the life span* (pp. 139–165). Bethesda, MD: American Occupational Therapy Association.

Hanlon, R. E. (1996). Motor learning following unilateral stroke. *Archives of Physical Medicine and Rehabilitation, 77,* 811–815.

Hong, L. (2005). Hospitalized elders and family caregivers: A typology of family worry. *Journal of Clinical Nursing, 14,* 3–8.

Kalra, L., Evans, A., Perez, I., Melbourn, A., Patel, A., Knapp, A., & Donaldson, N. (2004). Training carers of stroke patients: Randomised controlled trial. *British Journal of Medicine, 328,* 1099.

Kielhofner, G., Barris, R., & Watts, J. H. (1982). Habits and habit dysfunction: A clinical perspective for psychosocial occupational therapy. *Occupational Therapy in Mental Health, 2,* 1–21.

Kleim, J. A., & Jones, T. A. (2008). Principles of experience-dependent neural plasticity: Implications for rehabilitation after brain damage. *Journal of Speech, Language and Hearing Research, 51,* S225–S239.

Kottke, T., Battista, R. N., Degriese, G., & Brekke, M. (1988). Attributes of successful smoking cessation interventions in medical practice: A meta-analysis of 30 controlled trials. *Journal of the American Medical Association, 259,* 2882–2889.

Lavery, J. J. (1962). Retention of simple motor skills as a function of type of knowledge of results. *Canadian Journal of Psychology, 16,* 300–311.

Lee, Y., & Vakoch, D. A. (1996). Transfer and retention of implicit and explicit learning. *British Journal of Psychology, 87,* 637–651.

Lerdal, A., Bakken, L. N., Kouwenhoven, S. E., Pedersen, G., Kirkevold, M., Finset, A., & Kim, H. S. (2009). Poststroke fatigue: A review. *Journal of Pain and Symptom Management, 38,* 928–949.

Lo, A. C., Guarino, P. D., Richards, L. G., Haselkorn, J. K., Sittenberg, G. F., et al[1]. (2010). Robot-assisted therapy for long-term upper-limb impairment after stroke. *New England Journal of Medicine, 362,* 1772–1783.

Lofland, S. (2009). Determining learning styles to increase client participation. *OT Practice, 14,* 13–17.

Ma, H., Trombly, C. A., & Robinson-Podolski, C. (1999). The effect of context on skill acquisition and transfer. *American Journal of Occupational Therapy, 53,* 138–144.

Ma, H. I., & Trombly, C. A. (2004). Effects of task complexity on reaction time and movement kinematics in elderly people. *American Journal of Occupational Therapy, 58,* 150–158.

Mathiowetz, V., & Haugen, J. B. (1994). Motor behavior research: Implications for therapeutic approaches to central nervous system dysfunction. *American Journal of Occupational Therapy, 48,* 733–745.

Mathiowetz, V., Matuska, K., & Murphy, M. E. (2001). Efficacy of an energy conservation course for persons with multiple sclerosis. *Archives of Physical Medicine and Rehabilitation, 82,* 449–456.

Mathiowetz, V., & Wade, M. G. (1995). Task constraints and functional motor performance of individuals with and without multiple sclerosis. *Ecological Psychology, 7,* 99–123.

McAuley, E. (1993). Self-efficacy and the maintenance of exercise participation in older adults. *Journal of Behavioral Medicine, 16,* 103–113.

Moseley, G. L. (2006). Do training diaries affect and reflect adherence to home programs? *Arthritis and Rheumatism, 55,* 662–664.

Nabors, N., Seacat, J., & Rosenthal, M. (2002). Predictors of caregiver burden following traumatic brain injury. *Brain Injury, 16,* 1039–1050.

National Center for Education Statistics. (2005). *National Assessment of Adult Literacy (NAAL): A first look at the literacy of America's adults in the 21st century* (Department of Education, Institute of Education Sciences Publication No. NCES 2006-470). Pittsburgh, PA: U.S. Government Printing Office.

Neistadt, M. E. (1995). Assessing learning capabilities during cognitive and perceptual evaluations for adults with traumatic brain injury. *Occupational Therapy in Health Care, 9,* 3–16.

Packard, M. G., & Knowlton, B. J. (2002). Learning and memory functions of the basal ganglia. *Annual Review of Neuroscience, 25,* 563–593.

Parikh, N. S., Parker, R. M., Nurss, J. R., Baker, D. W., & Williams, M. V. (1996). Shame and health literacy: The unspoken connection. *Patient Education and Counseling, 27,* 33–39.

Pasacreta, J. V., Barg, F., Nuamah, I., & McCorkle, R. (2000). Participant characteristics before and 4 months after attendance at a family caregiver cancer education program. *Cancer Nursing, 23,* 295–303.

Perkins, D. (1995). *Outsmarting IQ: The emerging science of learnable intelligence.* New York: Free Press.

Prochaska, J. O., & DiClemente, C. C. (1982). Transtheoretical therapy: Toward a more integrative model of change. *Psychotherapy: Theory, Research and Practice, 19,* 276–288.

Radomski, M. V. (2011). More than good intentions: Advancing adherence to therapy recommendations. *American Journal of Occupational Therapy, 65,* 471–477.

Reber, P. J., & Squire, L. R. (1994). Parallel brain systems for learning with and without awareness. *Learning and Memory, 1,* 217–229.

Redman, B. K. (1997). *The practice of patient education.* St. Louis: Mosby.

Rollnick, S., & Heather, N. (1992). Negotiating behavior change in medical settings: The development of brief motivational interviewing. *Journal of Mental Health, 1,* 25–37.

Rollnick, S., Miller, W. R., & Butler, C. C. (2008). *Motivational interviewing in health care: Helping patients change behavior.* New York: The Guilford Press.

Salmoni, A. W., Schmidt, R. A., & Walter, C. B. (1984). Knowledge of results and motor learning: A review and critical reappraisal. *Psychological Bulletin, 95,* 355–386.

Saloman, G., & Perkins, D. N. (1989). Rocky roads to transfer: Rethinking mechanisms of a neglected phenomenon. *Educational Psychologist, 24,* 113–142.

Schmidt, R. A., & Lee, T. D. (2011). *Motor control and learning: A behavioral emphasis* (5th ed.) Champaign, IL: Human Kinetics.

Schneider, M. (2005). 2003 National Assessment of Adult Literacy (NAAL) results. Retrieved June 2, 2006 from http://nces.ed.gov/whatsnew/commissioner/remarks2005/12_15_2005.asp.

Schneider, W., & Shiffrin, R. M. (1977). Controlled and automatic human information processing: I. Detection, search, and attention. *Psychological Review, 84,* 1–66.

Shannon, R., & Hillsdon, M. (2007) Motivational interviewing in musculoskeletal care. *Musculoskeletal Care, 5,* 206–215.

Shea, J. B., & Morgan, R. L. (1979). Contextual interference effects on the acquisition, retention and transfer of a motor skill. *Journal of Experimental Psychology: Human Learning and Memory, 5,* 179–187.

Shiffrin, R. M., & Schneider, W. (1977). Controlled and automatic human information processing: II. Perceptual learning, automatic attending, and a general theory. *Psychological Review, 84,* 127–190.

Smith, S. M., & Vela, E. (2001). Environmental context-dependent memory: A review and meta-analysis. *Psychonomic Bulletin and Review, 8,* 203–220.

Sohlberg, M. M., & Raskin, S. A. (1996). Principles of generalization applied to attention and memory interventions. *Journal of Head Trauma Rehabilitation, 11,* 65–78.

Squire, L. R. (1994). Declarative and nondeclarative memory: Multiple brain systems support learning and memory. In D. Schacter & E. Tulving (Eds.), *Memory systems 1994* (pp. 203–231). Cambridge, MA: MIT.

Squire, L. R., Knowlton, B. J., & Musen, G. (1993). The structure and organization of memory. *Annual Review of Psychology, 44,* 453–495.

Sternberg, R. J. (1986). *Intelligence applied: Understanding and increasing your intellectual skills.* New York: Harcourt Brace Jovanovich.

Stewart, K., Borland, R., & McMurray, N. (1994). Self-efficacy, health locus of control, and smoking cessation. *Addictive Behaviors, 19,* 1–12.

Tailby, R., & Haslam, C. (2003). An investigation of errorless learning in memory-impaired patients: Improving the technique and clarifying theory. *Neuropsychologia, 41,* 1230–1240.

Thomas, J. J. (1999). Enhancing patient education: Addressing the issue of literacy. *Physical Disabilities Special Interest Section Quarterly, 22,* 3–4.

Toglia, J. P. (1998). A dynamic interactional model to cognitive rehabilitation. In N. Katz (Ed.), *Cognition and occupation in rehabilitation.* Bethesda, MD: American Occupational Therapy Association.

Trombly, C. A., & Wu, C. (1999). Effect of rehabilitation tasks on organization of movement after stroke. *American Journal of Occupational Therapy, 53,* 333–344.

van der Weel, F. R., van der Meer, A. L. H., & Lee, D. N. (1991). Effect of task on movement control in cerebral palsy: Implications for assessment and therapy. *Developmental Medicine and Child Neurology, 33,* 419–426.

Vanetzian, E. (1997). Learning readiness for patient teaching in stroke rehabilitation. *Journal of Advanced Nursing, 26,* 589–594.

Wilson, B. A., & Evans, J. J. (1996). Error-free learning in the rehabilitation of people with memory impairments. *Journal of Head Trauma Rehabilitation, 11,* 54–64.

Winstein, C. J., Gardner, E. R., McNeal, D. R., Barto, P. S., & Nicholson, D. E. (1989). Standing balance training: Effect on balance and locomotion in hemiparetic patients. *Archives of Physical Medicine and Rehabilitation, 70,* 755–762.

Winstein, C. J., & Schmidt, R. A. (1990). Reduced frequency of knowledge of results enhances motor skill learning. *Journal of Experimental Psychology: Learning, Memory, and Cognition, 16,* 677–691.

Wolf, S. L., Winstein, C. J., Miller, J. P., Taub, E., Uswatte, G., Morris, D., Giuliani, C., Light, K. E., & Nichols-Larson, D. (2006). Effect of constraint-induced movement therapy on upper extremity function 3 to 9 months after stroke: The EXCITE randomized clinical trial. *Journal of the American Medical Association, 296,* 2095–2104.

Wood, W., Quinn, J. M., & Kashy, D. A. (2002). Habits in everyday life: Thought, emotion, and action. *Journal of Personality and Social Psychology, 83,* 1281–1297.

World Health Organization. (1997). *ICIHD-2: International Classification of Impairments, Activities, and Participation (Beta-1 draft for field trials).* Geneva, Switzerland: World Health Organization.

Wu, C., Trombly, C. A., Lin, K., & Tickle-Degnen, L. (2000). A kinematic study of contextual effects on reaching performance in persons with and without stroke: Influences of object availability. *Archives of Physical Medicine and Rehabilitation, 81,* 95–101.

14

Therapeutic Rapport

Linda Tickle-Degnen

Learning Objectives

After studying this chapter, the reader will be able to do the following:

1. Define high therapeutic rapport.
2. Describe how rapport influences intervention and the client's occupational functioning.
3. Describe how collaboration between therapist and client contributes to achieving high therapeutic rapport.
4. Select methods to enhance rapport with a client.
5. Identify therapists' and clients' attributes that can influence the development of rapport.
6. Apply knowledge of ethics of practice to the therapeutic relationship.

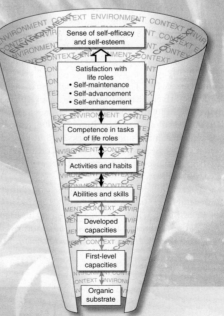

The term *rapport* reflects an emphasis on communication, connection, mutual understanding, and harmony between individuals (*Oxford English Dictionary Online*, 2011). Although rapport can occur in any social situation, the type of rapport developed in therapy has its own special characteristics. Rapport is one *mechanism*, or means, by which a client achieves positive therapeutic outcomes, or in the case of occupational therapy, confident and competent occupational functioning. High therapeutic rapport involves interpersonal influences between client and therapist that support the client's desire to try occupational therapy, to maintain continued involvement in therapy despite the need for considerable effort and courage, and to participate with the therapist in constructing a new vision of life possibilities that projects into the client's occupational future (Mattingly, 1998; Peloquin, 2005; Price & Miner, 2007). The therapist and client work as a unit performing the *cooccupation* (Pierce, 2009) of therapy by immediately, spontaneously, and warmly responding to one another. This mutual responsiveness supports their occupations-as-means toward achieving therapeutic goals.

This chapter defines behaviors and feelings associated with therapeutic rapport, describes conditions affecting its development, and discusses the ethics of a therapeutic relationship. Although this chapter focuses on therapeutic rapport with a single client, its content can be applied to developing rapport with caregivers, family members, and others important in the client's social network (American Occupational Therapy Association [AOTA], 2008; Klein & Liu, 2010; Sherer et al., 2007).

DEFINITION OF HIGH THERAPEUTIC RAPPORT

High therapeutic rapport (Definition 14-1) is a function of the mutual experience and behavior of the client and therapist as they interact with each other plus the outcome of the interaction for the client (Tickle-Degnen, 2006):

1. It is an optimal interpersonal *experience* for both the client and the therapist that involves concentration, masterful communication, and enjoyment.

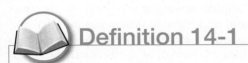

Definition 14-1

High Therapeutic Rapport

Qualities of Experience	
Concentration	Client and therapist experience deep and effortless concentration on the interaction. Distractions, worries, and self-concern disappear.
Masterful communication	They are challenged by the interaction yet feel skillful in meeting the challenge. The goals of the interaction and the effectiveness of the progress toward them are experienced as clear and shared by both.
Enjoyment	They experience the interaction with deep satisfaction.
Qualities of Verbal and Nonverbal Behavior	
Attentiveness	Client and therapist demonstrate verbally and nonverbally that their attention is focused on the other.
Interpersonal coordination	They demonstrate responsiveness to each other—behavior and emotional expression are highly coordinated between them.
Positivity	They demonstrate verbally and nonverbally that their feelings are positive toward one another and the interaction.
Beneficial Effects for the Patient	
Enhanced client performance	Qualities of the client–therapist interaction are beneficial if they improve client performance during evaluation and intervention.
Client follow-through with therapeutic activities	Qualities of the client–therapist interaction are beneficial if they support the clients' continued involvement in activities that enable them to make progress toward their goals.

2. It occurs with *behavior* that reflects high levels of mutual attentiveness, interpersonal coordination, and mutual positivity.
3. It has a *beneficial effect* on client performance and follow-through with intervention plans.

MUTUALITY AND THERAPEUTIC RAPPORT

Mutuality in the relationship between client and therapist is relatively new in the espoused philosophy of occupational therapy. In early- to mid-20th century, the American Occupational Therapy Association (AOTA, 1948) promoted friendliness and cheerfulness but not intimacy between therapists and clients. The two were not to affect each other through the force of their personal attributes. Over a decade later, *therapeutic use of self* (Frank, 1958) became a prevailing philosophical orientation. Therapists recognized that besides modalities their own selves and role modeling, with some level of professional detachment, could be agents of change in clients. In the late 1960s, occupational therapy's view of the therapeutic relationship underwent a major transformation, marked by the view that the relationship involves an exchange between equals. Yerxa (2011) stated, "The therapist allows himself to feel real emotion as he enters into mutual relation with the client. . . . The authentic occupational therapist is involved in the process of caring and to care means to be affected just as surely as it means to affect" (p. 8). In the current philosophy of the therapeutic relationship, the occupational therapist is an engaged, committed partner with the client. As coparticipants, *together* they engage in satisfying and productive interaction as they create daily life (Burke, 2010; Peloquin, 2005). The relationship between client and therapist embodies mutual respect and caring similar to that of friends or coworkers, yet it has unique qualities:

- It is client centered with focus on the client's health, perception of meaningful occupation, and social, cultural, and physical contexts of daily living (AOTA, 2008; Egan et al., 1998; Shaw et al., 2007).
- It is part of a therapeutic skill set put into service to improve client occupational performance (Burke, 2010; Taylor et al., 2009).
- The client is not expected to contribute equally to the development of rapport, especially if suffering or impairment makes the contribution difficult (Rosa & Hasselkus, 2005).
- The therapist usually is paid for services and is accountable to institutional and professional systems that are charged with monitoring therapy and tracking client outcomes.

Despite a therapeutic focus on the client, clients and therapists mutually influence one another. Evidence suggests that, if either the client or the therapist is not attentive, responsive, or positive or is perceived as such by the other, high therapeutic rapport is difficult to achieve (Crepeau & Garren, 2011; Hall et al., 2009; Shaw et al., 2007; Tickle-Degnen, 2006). Evidence Table 14-1 explains more about the benefits and practice of therapeutic rapport.

THE EXPERIENCE AND COMMUNICATION OF THERAPEUTIC RAPPORT

There are innumerable means by which one can attend, coordinate, or express positive affiliation with another person. Therapists draw on clinical reasoning and social skills to determine ways to interact with a particular client in a given context. However, evidence supports that there are fundamental and universal principles of communication that span culture, race, gender, and other qualities of human diversity, whereas simultaneously there are specific forms of communication that vary by diversity in norms and practices (Tickle-Degnen, Zebrowitz, & Ma, 2011) (Research Note 14-1). Adherence to a practice that is client centered, self-reflective, and congruent with current models of clinical reasoning may help the therapist to be sensitive and responsive to differences in verbal and nonverbal behavioral meanings during therapy and to evaluate and adjust accordingly as the interaction emerges (Bonder, Martin, & Miracle, 2004; Katz & Alegría, 2009). Nonetheless, it can be challenging to develop rapport because of (1) differences in the cultural and social identities, norms, and statuses of the therapist and client; (2) structural differences in the world views of the societies and institutions in which therapy takes place; and (3) difficulty in perceiving and evaluating implicit and automatic operation of human differences (Iwama, 2003; Kantartzis & Molineux, 2010; Pooremamali, Persson, & Eklund, 2011; Tickle-Degnen, Zebrowitz, & Ma, 2011). This chapter does not attempt to address variation among cultural and social groups, but rather to advocate for an experiential and behavioral stance to therapy that will help the therapist negotiate individual variation in all its forms. Health care research findings and client autobiographical accounts, primarily from the literature of Western culture, are used in the following sections to illustrate therapist and client rapport qualities and how these qualities affect therapy processes and outcomes.

Therapist Concentration and Attentiveness

Verbal and nonverbal attentiveness and engagement have been found to be positively associated with client disclosure about the experience of illness (Duggan & Parrott, 2000), participation in therapy (Crepeau & Garren, 2011; Mattingly, 1998; Price & Miner, 2007), client satisfaction (Feinberg, 1992; Hall et al., 2009), and occupational

Evidence Table 14-1 | Best Evidence for Occupational Therapy Practice Regarding Therapeutic Rapport

Intervention	Description of Intervention Tested	Participants	Dosage	Type of Best Evidence and Level of Evidence	Benefit	Statistical Probability and Effect Size of Outcome	Reference
Therapeutic alliance	Therapeutic relationship characterized by an affective bond, shared therapy tasks, and goals	4,771 clients, 66% female, with psychiatric, neurological conditions	Average of 22.18 sessions (standard deviation = 18.76)	Meta-analysis of 79 studies	Yes. Stronger therapeutic alliance yields better client outcomes.	Mean weighted effect size was $r = 0.22$, equivalent to a 22% success rate over control treatment	Martin, Garske, & Davis (2000)
Therapeutic nonverbal behavior	Physical therapist (PT) distancing behavior (not smiling, looking away, and remaining seated)	Twenty-eight women and 20 men inpatients, ≥75 years old, mobility disorders, 11 PTs	Average of 9.3 single sessions of inpatient therapy	correlational design Level: IIB3a	Yes. Less distancing PT behavior yields better ADL, cognition, and depression outcomes.	ADL: $p < 0.001$, $r = -0.34$ Confusion: $p < 0.05$, $r = 0.29$; Depression: $p < 0.05$, $r = -0.27$ Mobility: $p > 0.05$, $r = 0.02$	Ambady et al. (2002)
Interview context	Woman or man interviewer asked open-ended questions about (1) frustrating event in past week and (2) enjoyable event in the past week.	Thirty-two women, 74 men in the community, average age 67 years, moderate Parkinson's disease severity, one woman, one man interviewer	Thirty-minute interview session	compared two types of interview questions, gender composition of the interview dyad Level: IIA3a	Yes. Enjoyable question elicited more expressiveness and positivity than frustrating question. Women participants more talkative than men.	Positive words: $p < 0.01$, $r = 0.85$ Smiling: $p < 0.01$, $r = 0.38$ Expressivity: $p < 0.01$, $r = 0.28$ Gender, talkativeness: $p < 0.05$, $r = 0.23$	Takahashi et al. (2010)

Research Note 14-1

Tickle-Degnen, L., Zebrowitz, L. A., & Ma, H. (2011). Culture, gender and health care stigma: Practitioners' response to facial masking experienced by people with Parkinson's disease. *Social Science & Medicine, 73,* 95–102.

Abstract

The purpose of this study was to evaluate the effect of masking, culture, and gender on practitioners' impressions of patient psychological attributes. Practitioners ($n = 284$) in the United States and Taiwan judged 12 Caucasian American and 12 Asian Taiwanese women and men patients in video clips from interviews. Half of each patient group had a moderate degree of facial masking, and the other half had near-normal expressivity. The results indicated that practitioners in both countries judged patients with higher masking to be more depressed and less sociable, less socially supportive, and less cognitively competent than patients with lower masking. Practitioners were more biased by masking when judging the sociability of the American patients and the cognitive competence and social supportiveness of the Taiwanese patients. In response to masking, American practitioners' perceptions of patient sociability were more negatively biased than were those of Taiwanese practitioners, and the Taiwanese practitioners' judgments of patient cognitive competence were more negatively biased than were those of American practitioners. The negative response to higher masking was stronger in practitioner judgments of women than men patients, particularly American patients. The findings suggest local cultural values as well as ethnic and gender stereotypes operate on practitioners' use of facial expressivity in clinical impression formation.

Implications for Practice

- Practitioners must learn how their clinical impressions can influence therapeutic rapport with their client by understanding their own cultural values, implicit biases and stereotypes, and their expectations for what constitutes appropriate demeanor and behavior.
- Practitioners should strive to translate immediate impression into hypotheses rather than conclusions and to test these hypotheses by triangulating information from the patient, family members, and research literature.
- Practitioners can draw upon patients' storytelling and self-advocacy capacities by letting go of their sole reliance on facial cues when a person has a motor-based facial expressiveness disorder and asking about and attending to what matters most for people living with the disability.
- Practitioners should receive training that addresses the processes underlying accurate and faulty impression formation.

performance outcomes (Ambady et al., 2002). Therapists can show that they are paying attention to clients by taking the time to sit down and talk with them (Figs. 14-1 and 14-2). Attentive behavior, such as orienting the body and eyes toward the client, enables the therapist to watch the client and to pick up emotion and thought cues from the client's face and body. A serious demeanor, often with a slightly furrowed brow, may signal engaged interest and concern to the client (Sharpley, Jeffrey, & McMah, 2006). Crepeau and Garren (2011) report how Dan experienced his hand therapist, Leah, as deeply caring, with one example described by Dan

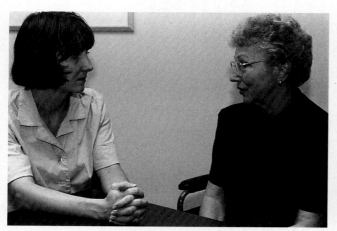

Figure 14-1 Mutual attentiveness by therapist and client forms the basis for effective communication and the development of a successful working relationship.

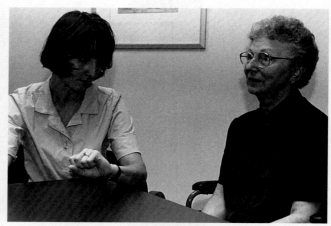

Figure 14-2 The therapist who is distracted by time pressure or other concerns loses the interpersonal connection with the client.

as Leah's unwavering focus on him during multiclient sessions:

> . . . there were exercises that I didn't do properly and bang, she was there saying, "Hey, you're not doing this the way I showed you." . . . Her attention's never ending, even though there were other patients there. . . . So that you knew she was watching what you were doing. (p. 879)

Paying attention to a client goes beyond physical attention. It requires listening carefully to what the client has to say about his or her life, the illness, and the experience of intervention (Crepeau & Garren, 2011; Fisher et al., 2007; Verbeek et al., 2004) and remaining open to changing one's own therapeutic ideas in response to what is heard (Jack & Estes, 2010; Shaw et al., 2007). If the therapist applies an intervention incongruent with the client's values and perceptions, the client may fail to engage in therapy. Despite strong collaborative ethics in occupational therapy, research finds that therapists often fall short of collaborative decision making, and divergence rather than convergence of therapist and patient perspective is common (Maitra & Erway, 2006; Peoples, Satink, & Steultjens, 2011; Rosa & Hasselkus, 2005; Shaw et al., 2007). One study found that clients have strong preference for shared decision making, particularly related to occupational performance compared to basic medical home care or preventative physical intervention such as exercise (van den Brink-Muinen, Spreeuwenberg, & Rijken, 2011). However, the client participants experienced the least involvement in shared decision making in the area of occupational performance intervention. An example of possible mismatched perspectives occurred in the stroke rehabilitation of McCrum (1998), who unhappily felt like a child when the therapist gave him plastic letters used to teach children the alphabet:

> . . . with my Day-Glo letter-blocks I could not escape reflecting on the irony of the situation. If only Milan Kundera, Kazuo Ishiguro, or Mario Vargas Llosa, whose texts I had pored over with their authors, could have seen their editor at that moment! (p. 139)

The plastic letters themselves do not create the potential problem here. Therapeutic rapport involves the therapist learning the client's meanings surrounding occupational processes and outcomes in order to build a therapeutic alliance. If the client views elements of therapy to be negative or unimportant, the therapist and client may decide to change the processes or outcomes, or the therapist can guide the client toward a reframing of the meanings involved. Mattingly's (1998, pp. 48–71) description of a session between a therapist and two young men in spinal cord rehabilitation demonstrates how a seemingly inconsequential and childish checker game can be transformed into an occupation that points toward more consequential adulthood occupations. As the young men increase their skilled use of mouthsticks and splints while playing the game, the three partners in therapy engage in banter that solidifies the young men's adult status, and interspersed throughout the conversation is strategic planning about performing near-future occupations (a school prom, a visit home). The game is an engaging choreographed therapeutic event that takes the young men one step closer to their desired occupational lives.

Client Concentration and Attentiveness

Therapists need attention from their clients as well. A client who does not attend to the therapist cannot give or get important information from him or her and may appear to have low commitment to therapy. Pathological conditions, such as traumatic brain damage or anxiety, can affect the ability to engage attentively with the therapist. Rehabilitation therapists rate cognitive issues as a frequent barrier to clients' ability to engage in therapy (Lequerica, Donnell, & Tate, 2009). Evidence suggests that there is a positive relationship between the attention capacity of clients with brain injury and the development of a good therapeutic alliance (Schönberger, Humle, & Teasdale, 2007). The more that these clients actively engage in early therapy sessions, the more likely they are to complete their therapeutic programs (Sherer et al., 2007) and to have more effective occupational performance outcomes (Prigatano et al., 1994).

Therapist Communication and Interpersonal Coordination

Because of their uniqueness as individuals, it is impossible for even the most attentive therapists and clients to fully apprehend one another's experiences or role obligations. However, they can maximize the exchange of their perspectives through optimal verbal and nonverbal communication (Burke, 2010; Crepeau & Garren, 2011). After the therapist focuses attention on the client, the next step is to *interpret* accurately the client's verbal and nonverbal behavior. Accurate interpretation of behavior has been found to relate to therapeutic rapport (Hall et al., 2009) and to predict occupational therapy students' clinical performance during fieldwork experiences (Tickle-Degnen, 1998). The interpretation process occurs very rapidly and involves first the observation of the behavior and then its translation into an impression, accurate or not, about the other's thoughts and emotions (Fig. 14-3) (Blanch-Hartigan, 2011; Tickle-Degnen, Zebrowitz, & Ma, 2011). Accuracy can be enhanced if the therapist encourages the client to be active in giving feedback about the accuracy of the therapist's impressions (Street & Haidet, 2011). If the client cannot give verbal feedback because of impairment, the therapist may be able to learn what the client is feeling simply by reflecting on what the therapist's own emotions are. What the therapist and client feel may be similar because of their subtle mimicry of one another's facial and bodily movements (Chartrand & van

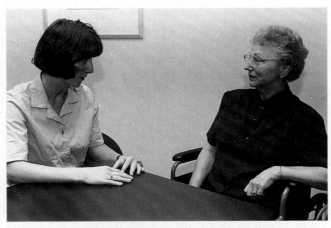

Figure 14-3 The client's backward lean may indicate that she is withdrawing from the therapist or from the information the therapist is giving her. The therapist must determine whether or not the client's behavior is a sign of withdrawal and then whether to adjust her own behavior to maintain rapport. This therapist may decide to become less confrontational, relaxing her posture and making less intense eye contact.

Baaren, 2009) and the effect of this mimicry on their own feelings (Hatfield, Rapson, & Le, 2009). For example, while working with a client with stooped posture, a therapist may develop a stooped posture through mimicry and begin to feel dejection in response to the client's own bodily pattern of dejection. If therapists are aware of the possibility of this form of emotional influence, they may more accurately detect the unspoken emotions of clients.

After accurate interpretation of a client's message, the next step in effective communication is for the therapist clearly to *express* emotions and thoughts in a manner that is beneficial for the client (Tickle-Degnen & Gavett, 2003). Clients may respond favorably to genuine expressions of feelings conducive to rapport (Fig. 14-4)

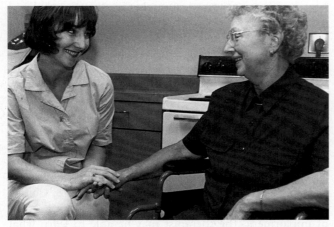

Figure 14-4 The therapist and client show mutual positivity through their facial expressions and physical contact. Social physical contact, like holding a client's hand, is appropriate if it is an expression of professional warmth and the client gains comfort from it. Not all clients like being touched in this manner.

(Ambady et al., 2002; Di Blasi et al., 2001). Such was the case for Watt (1996), a man in severe pain:

> I believed [the nurse] would make things better. It was never anything she said. It was something in her face. (p. 13)

Facial expressiveness is one of the most impactful and rapid mediums of communication related to social and therapeutic rapport (Collins et al., 2011; Sharpley et al., 2006).

The combination of verbal and nonverbal behavior that the therapist uses to express feelings and attitudes toward the client can be profoundly moving for the client and strengthen their bond as they move through set-backs and difficulties. Brack (Brack & Collins, 1981), a woman with multiple sclerosis, could not suppress her tears of despair and shame at not being able to regain her ability to walk. Her therapist quickly wheeled her wheelchair down to the therapy office, where together they wept:

> Our eyes met. "Do you want to quit?" [the therapist] said. "I know it's tough and you know you may never get any better. But shall we try a little longer?" Right away I knew I had to. I smiled damply and dried my eyes. What a friend! (pp. 71–72)

Because the therapist had worked with Brack for a long time, she could express her genuine feelings by weeping with the client. Subsequently, they worked hard in therapy until Brack regained her mobility. The act of continuing therapy, even when it seems that hope is lost, is a message itself. In the case of Brack, the message was that hope is *not* lost.

Likewise, messages are conveyed through the objects of therapy. When an occupational therapist gives the client a buttonhook, the message can be that the client is capable of using adaptive tools, that dressing independently is a valued goal of the client, and so on. Hanlan (1979), a man with amyotrophic lateral sclerosis, wanted to maintain his daily functioning:

> Of increasing importance to me is the help of occupational therapists. . . . My first OT, a man with a direct and kind manner, provided me with a buttonhook, so I could button and unbutton my clothing. I had an almost childlike, happy response to discovering this little tool. (p. 40)

In effective therapy, the client experiences a bond with the therapist, is in agreement with the intervention methods, and is working toward goals that are important to both the client and the therapist (Martin, Garske, & Davis, 2000; Schönberger, Humle, & Teasdale, 2006b).

Client Communication and Interpersonal Coordination

Some clients, especially those with neurological conditions, have difficulty accurately interpreting a therapist's emotions or social behavior (e.g., Gray & Tickle-Degnen, 2010). Those clients with a receptive form of aphasia may be unable to understand the therapist's speech.

The therapist should make frequent attempts and multimedia adaptations to communicate with these clients (Redman, 2007). Moreover, problems of motor expression, such as that found in right brain damage and Parkinson's disease, interfere with an individual's ability to show interpretable emotions (Brozgold et al., 1998; Tickle-Degnen, Zebrowitz, & Ma, 2011). However, these individuals may be able to verbally express their emotions and preferences quite well when talking about meaningful activities (DeGroat, Lyons, & Tickle-Degnen, 2006). The case of Sofia illustrates this effect (Sunvisson et al., 2009). Sunvisson, a nursing researcher, noted that Sofia's decline in mobility and expressive capacity after moving into a nursing home was augmented by nursing staff who did not think that Sofia could either understand or express messages. Therefore, they did not try communicating with her. During one of her visits, Sunvisson activated the seemingly unresponsive Sofia by asking her if she recalled a sermon that Sofia had earlier reported as a major influence on her life:

> Then I see her erecting her body, her face opens up and she says with a quite loud voice. "Yes I do. It was a wonderful sermon." Surprised, I see her return to her former self, and we laugh and exchange thoughts. . . . (pp. 247–248)

On the other hand, if clients have low capacity to verbally communicate yet are able to nonverbally communicate, therapists can guide them to convey their thoughts and needs via various means. The medium of communication could be facial and bodily expression, use of meaningful objects or audio-video media, and family and friends as proxy self-reporters.

Therapist Enjoyment and Positivity

The expression of positive feelings, warmth, and respect is elemental to therapeutic rapport (Palmadottir, 2006; Roter et al., 2011; Sharpley et al., 2006; Shaw et al., 2007) and clinical effectiveness (Tickle-Degnen & Puccinelli, 1999). Leaning forward and spontaneous smiles of enjoyment are simple behaviors that express warmth and liking (Fig. 14-4), and a furrowed brow can express caring (Ambady et al., 2002; Sharpley et al., 2006). Most important is that the therapist's expression of positivity toward clients is derived from genuine feelings of respect and caring (Peloquin, 2005; Shaw et al., 2007). In addition, moderate degrees and changing levels of enjoyment versus serious behavior appear to be more indicative of beneficial therapy than unchanging high degrees and levels (Sharpley et al., 2001; Tickle-Degnen, 2006).

Occupational therapists strongly endorse humor, such as bantering, joke books, and shaving cream fights, as having positive therapeutic effects as long as it is embedded in a respectful relationship (Leber & Vanoli, 2001). Humor is a deeply complex medium of human relationship, as exemplified in Mattingly's (1998) description of the style of interchange between two young men with quadriplegia, Matt and John. The style was one of "muted desire, of anger turned into an informal omnipresent derision, of extreme truth-telling in the jocular mode" (Mattingly, 1998, p. 55). When the men's therapist suggested a checker game, Matt asked "How are we going to jump one another?" in a manner that clearly infused the word *jump* with sexual innuendo (Mattingly, 1998, p. 65) and the irony that the two young men were unable to jump in any of several senses of the physical meaning of the word—sexually, by feet or by hand. The therapist, Lin, retorted "wise guy" as she laughed, thus accepting multiple meanings of the word, the cleverness of the self-put-down, and the status of these young men as adults learning to live with severe disability. Lin expertly framed the men's bantering humor with serious occupation-as-means to attaining their goals. Bantering humor was a therapeutic medium also depicted by Crepeau and Garren (2011) in their study of how a therapist, Leah, established rapport with her client, Dan. In their first encounter, Dan was negative about his previous experiences with therapy and was expecting more of the same. Leah surprised him by agreeing with his assessment, and they both laughed. Their therapy progressed in a mutually caring and respectful relationship that included teasing and laughter. As Leah stated, ". . . nothing hurts as bad when you're laughing" (Crepeau & Garren, 2011, p. 876).

Research studies are rare on the incidence or nature of harmful or disrespectful behavior by occupational therapists. As a result, we know very little about this end of the therapeutic rapport spectrum. Palmadottir (2006) interviewed 20 clients who mostly characterized their current occupational therapy experiences as satisfying. Satisfying dimensions included the therapist concern, direction, fellowship, guidance, or coalition. Some, however, had experienced neutral detachment or overt rejection, lack of interest, or humiliation. One client said that his therapist

> often spoke to me as I was a little kid . . . sometimes when I was shaving myself I forgot to turn off the water and then she would say with disdain; well, did we forget something? (p. 398)

More evidence is needed to determine the magnitude of this type of behavior, under what conditions it occurs, and what can be done to remedy harmful occupational therapy relationships.

Client Enjoyment and Positivity

Occupational therapists report feeling good about compliments from clients and enjoying their memory of them (Taylor et al., 2009), suggesting that client satisfaction and enjoyment are not rare. Therapists enjoy clients who are enthusiastic (Rosa & Hasellkus, 2005). As therapist Leah told Crepeau and Garren (2011) about her client Dan, "he just made me feel good inside" (p. 879) and had a significant impact on her life. However, because of the effects of their health condition, some clients may have lowered capacity to experience enjoyment or satisfaction. Clients who are very anxious or depressed may demonstrate little warmth nonverbally, perhaps by infrequent smiles or eye contact, and health-related misery or pain may cause outbursts of anger.

Therapy itself may be frustrating or overly challenging to some clients, especially if they perceive the tasks as simple ones (Darragh, Sample, & Krieger, 2001). For example, Puller (1991), a Vietnam veteran with bilateral upper extremity amputations, reported that he "felt like screaming" (p. 181) when trying to learn how to button clothes or thread a needle in therapy. Such frustration should not be ignored. The therapist should reevaluate the balance of emotional costs to physical benefits of some activities as related to client goals.

Ethics and professionalism prescribe practitioners to rise above petty responses to unpleasant client behavior and to not take unpleasant behavior personally or to respond with resentment and harmful behavior (Rosa & Hasselkus, 2005). Furthermore, practitioners must be careful not to view all negative expressions as confirmation of pathology. These expressions may be indeed signs of a pathological process that requires diagnosis, or they may be normal responses to the experience of illness and intervention. Finally, seemingly pathological behavior of a client may be exacerbated through implicit features of the context. For example, the content of questions posed to clients as well as the gender of the interviewer have been found to elicit more or less expressive movement in clients with Parkinson's disease (Takahashi et al., 2010). Asking clients about enjoyable events in their lives elicited more expressiveness, particularly of a positive emotional nature, than asking them about frustrations.

BENEFICIAL EFFECT AND HIGH THERAPEUTIC RAPPORT

Possible reasons that attentive, coordinated, and positive client–therapist interactions may have a beneficial effect on client occupational outcomes and health include the following:

1. The interaction scaffolds skill development by directing attention to important features of a task problem, communicating information necessary to solve the problem, generating trust in the therapist and therapy process, giving motivational support for pursuing problem solution, and facilitating adherence to treatment recommendations (Radomski, 2011; Street et al., 2009; Tham & Kielhofner, 2003; Tickle-Degnen, 2006).
2. The interaction improves physiological and emotional health, thus enabling individuals to focus energy and effort on occupation (Di Blasi et al., 2001; Street et al., 2009). The health effects of positive therapeutic relationships, including direct effects on immune and physiological functioning and indirect effects on adherence to health interventions, are similar to the health effects of social support provided by positive familial relationships (DiMatteo, 2004).
3. The interaction creates a self-fulfilling prophecy of improved performance (Ambady et al., 2002). The therapist communicates his or her expectations for the progress of a client, with the effect that the client's actual performance conforms to those expectations. Informative, warm, and respectful behavior may affirm to clients that they are capable and valued human beings, which mobilizes clients' psychological and physical resources toward fulfillment of those qualities. Affirmation of values has been found to help change the performance of individuals who feel insecure or have low self-efficacy and reverse negative self-fulfilling prophecies (Stinson et al., 2011).

DEVELOPMENT OF A HIGH THERAPEUTIC RAPPORT RELATIONSHIP

Evidence suggests that the critical development of rapport and a working alliance begins within minutes of the first session and is achieved within the first three to five sessions of therapy (Horvath & Luborsky, 1993; Roter et al., 2011; Schönberger, Humle, & Teasdale, 2006a). First meetings tend to be somewhat superficial and rigidly constrained by role expectations around the assessment process. Through close adherence to cultural scripts of polite behavior, therapist and client offer their identities to one another as valuable and likable. In the first meeting, the client may convey private information to the therapist, but the depth of intimacy, working alliance, and mutuality continues to grow over subsequent interactions (Schönberger, Humle, & Teasdale, 2006a). The development of the relationship is not necessarily linear. A dialectical tension between the desires for intimacy and autonomy appears to manifest itself in a cyclical pattern of intimate and more distant behavior (Tickle-Degnen, 2006). The client and therapist may try out different patterns of relating to one another. There are also patterns of shifting between therapeutic work and socializing with chit-chat that may provide off-task opportunity for rest and reaffirmation of the bond between therapist and client (Crepeau & Garren, 2011; Hall, Roter, & Milburn, 1999).

Therapists' and clients' characteristics and conditions in the therapy setting can facilitate or inhibit the development of rapport. Different interpersonal styles and skills appear to be beneficial for therapeutic effectiveness in physical versus mental health settings or children versus adult populations, suggesting that therapists should adapt their styles to the specific therapeutic context (Tickle-Degnen, 1998). Through self-reflection, feedback from supervisors, colleagues, and clients, and reflective clinical experience and training, the therapist should be able to learn how to make these adaptations (Cohn, Schell, & Crepeau, 2010). Based on the evidence presented here, Procedures for Practice 14-1 gives guidelines

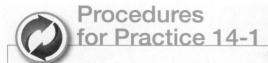

Procedures for Practice 14-1

Therapist Guidelines for Facilitating the Development of High Therapeutic Rapport

Create Conditions That Maximize Concentration and Attention

1. Reduce distractions and potential for embarrassment or anxiety in the therapy setting.
2. Position bodies of therapist and client for seeing and hearing each other clearly.
3. Give time for meaningful engagement, and attend to issues that are important to the client.

Create Conditions That Maximize Masterful Communication and Interpersonal Coordination

1. Provide assistance as needed for the client to express emotions and thoughts.
2. Remain open and sensitive to verbal and nonverbal messages from the client.
3. Clearly express emotions and thoughts that are consistent with the needs and goals of the client.
4. Check to make sure that each is interpreting the other accurately.
5. Create a challenging, interesting, and effective interaction for the client.
6. Involve the client collaboratively in the development of goals and the planning of intervention.

Create Conditions That Maximize Enjoyment and Positivity

1. Find a satisfying, fulfilling aspect to every interaction with a client.
2. Express genuine concern and caring for the client through verbal and nonverbal behavior.
3. Resolve personal problems and worries outside of the client–therapist interaction.
4. Provide opportunities for the client to engage in activities that he or she finds enjoyable.
5. Provide opportunities for rest and off-task recovery during potentially frustrating activities.
6. Determine the source of client negativity and respond appropriately.
7. Manage negativity and disagreements to generate a constructive and collaborative relationship.

for enhancing the development of rapport. It is not the client's responsibility to change to enhance the rapport; it is the therapist's. Therefore, the guidelines are directed at therapist actions.

Clients and therapists can experience events in their therapy sessions that create negative emotions and

threaten to "rupture" their rapport and their working alliance (Safran, Muran, & Eubanks-Carter, 2011). Safran, Muran, and Eubanks-Carter (2011) found in psychotherapy that the more patients and therapists experienced "repairs" to ruptures, the more successful their outcomes. The following rupture repair strategies are adapted to occupational therapy for physical dysfunction from the suggestions of Safran, Muran, and Eubanks-Carter:

- Be attentive to possible problems as they arise.
- Be open for disagreement or negative emotions from clients.
- Remain nondefensive and talk directly about disagreements and problems in the therapy process.
- Validate the client bringing up differences of opinion or negative feelings.
- Use clinical reasoning and client collaboration to determine whether it is more therapeutic to change the tasks or goals of the intervention without exploring the rupture in depth or to deal in depth with the cause of the rupture and getting help as needed in doing so.

Typically, therapeutic relationships work toward a planned end to the relationship as goals are achieved or services are no longer needed. As discharge approaches, the therapist should work actively with the client to transform their relationship appropriately, so that the client does not feel abandoned (e.g., Klein, 1995). The form this transformation takes depends on the setting. For example, the therapist may help the client to develop other fulfilling relationships in the community or may keep in contact with the client through the phone or occasional clinic visits.

ETHICS AND THE THERAPEUTIC RELATIONSHIP

The four principles of the Occupational Therapy Code of Ethics (AOTA, 2010) that are most relevant to the therapeutic relationship are the following ones:

Principle 1 (Beneficence): Occupational Therapy Personnel Shall Demonstrate a Concern for the Well-being and Safety of the Recipients of Their Services

Beneficence refers to kindness, humaneness, and actions that benefit others. Although there is no ethical imperative to feel rapport with clients, the imperative to demonstrate a concern for the well-being of the recipient of services is consistent with developing high therapeutic rapport with the client as defined in this chapter. To maximize benefit, the therapist should use current knowledge and research in practice, evaluate the effect of services periodically, and terminate services in collaboration with the client when the needs and goals of the client have been met or when services no longer produce changes as intended. As a therapist works to create rapport, it is important that the therapist realize that his or her own beliefs about what is important for well-being and occupation are not necessarily equivalent to the beliefs held by the client, particularly those with cultures and backgrounds different from the therapist's (Iwama, 2003; Kantartzis & Molineux, 2010; Tickle-Degnen, Zebrowitz, & Ma, 2011).

Principle 2 (Nonmaleficence): Occupational Therapy Personnel Shall Intentionally Refrain from Actions That Cause Harm

Negative therapist feelings may result in negative client outcomes. Therapists should consider changing jobs or clinical specialization if they are unable to overcome negative feelings with clients typically seen in a setting or specialization area. After an honest but unsuccessful attempt to support high therapeutic rapport, therapists may consider referring the client to a different therapist, perhaps one that is a specialist in such cases (Rosa & Hasselkus, 2005). One element of this principle is to not exploit the client sexually, physically, emotionally, financially, socially, or in any other manner. Therapists must understand how to set professional boundaries in their therapeutic relationships in order to create a friendly and engaged relationship that does not involve the same reciprocity, casualness, and interdependency of many close personal friendships. For example, therapists are selective about sharing their own personal information, and do not complain about their coworkers or supervisors. They should be careful about accepting or exchanging gifts and be aware of institutional policies that may prohibit staff members from accepting gifts of any kind. Therapists who become dependent on a client for meeting a personal need are exploitive because of their higher power relative to the clients' position of vulnerability. Furthermore, although the therapist is ethically responsible for helping the client, the client is not expected to help the therapist in any manner.

Principle 3 (Autonomy and Confidentiality): Occupational Therapy Personnel Shall Respect the Right of the Individual to Self-determination

Respect for the client's autonomy requires therapeutic relationships in which clients, including families, significant others, and caregivers, collaborate to the best of their ability in the determination of goals and priorities during intervention. Collaboration requires that the therapist must inform clients about the nature, risks, and potential outcomes of the intervention and that clients have the opportunity to suggest, reject, or refuse services or elements of services. Therapists facilitate communication and comprehension as needed in order to aid collaboration.

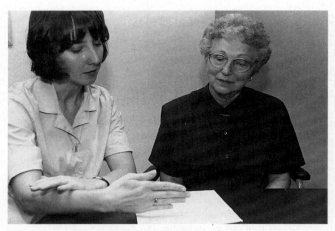

Figure 14-5 In a collaborative relationship, the therapist and client discuss the benefits and risks of participating in various occupational therapy interventions so that the client can make informed decisions about participating in these interventions.

Collaborative decisions are carried out not because of external pressures but because the client has an active feeling of personal control and responsibility (Fig. 14-5).

Other elements of this principle are privacy and confidentiality. During a relationship of high therapeutic rapport, the client may tell the therapist about matters that are private and confidential. The therapist must protect the confidentiality of information by not discussing it in an inappropriate context, for example, in a public elevator conversation, or inappropriate manner, for example, laughing at the client's capabilities with a colleague or any other person.

Principle 4 (Social Justice): Occupational Therapy Personnel Shall Provide Services in a Fair and Equitable Manner

Therapists are called upon to uphold the altruistic responsibilities of the profession to help ensure the common good, to advocate for just and fair treatment for all clients, and to provide services in an equitable manner to all individuals. A therapist may have fears or negative attitudes about a particular client population. Despite these feelings, therapists should provide services in an impartial manner and based on the development of an effective and health-promoting therapeutic relationship. Therapists are responsible for understanding how services can be affected by factors such as economic status, age, ethnicity, race, geography, disability, marital status, sexual orientation, gender, gender identity, religion, culture, and political affiliation.

SUMMARY

High therapeutic rapport develops as the therapist and client are mutually attentive, coordinated to one another, and mutually positive. It is one mechanism by which the client achieves confident and competent occupational functioning. It supports the client's desire to try occupational therapy, to maintain continued involvement in therapy, and to participate with the therapist in constructing a new vision of life possibilities. Although rapport is based on a perspective of mutuality and collaboration between client and therapist, it is the therapist's responsibility to manage oneself, guide the client, and modify the environment to support attentiveness, coordination, and positivity. Through self-reflection, feedback from others, reflection about clinical practice, and careful adherence to ethical standards, the therapist can learn to facilitate therapeutic rapport with a variety of clients in a variety of practice settings.

In this chapter, the focus has been directed on individual therapist responsibility for developing therapeutic relationships. However, it is important to recognize that the therapist works in a larger health care system and that the development of therapeutic rapport is not only a function of therapist behavior but also the societal and structural constraints operational in the health care system. It is not easy to achieve a high level of attention, concern, and caring in today's health care system, which emphasizes cost containment and adherence to protocol and provides little recognition for caring involvement (Cohn, Schell, & Crepeau, 2010). A supportive system composed not only of the therapist's personal commitment to caring but also of an institutional and societal commitment to caring are needed to sustain a therapeutic level of caring. As part of their ongoing commitment to offer services that are maximally beneficial for clients, therapists should consider advocating to their institutions and health policy bodies for resources and infrastructure that support beneficial therapeutic relationships.

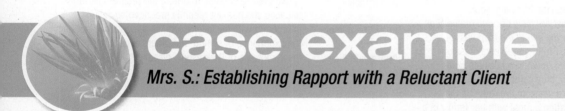

case example
Mrs. S.: Establishing Rapport with a Reluctant Client

	Clinical Reasoning Process	
Occupational Therapy Intervention Process	**Objectives**	**Examples of Therapist's Internal Dialogue**
Client Information Mrs. Smith, a 75-year-old woman (widowed) with Parkinson's disease, was referred to the adult day program by her physician and her children because of concern about her social isolation and reluctance to do basic self-care despite adequate physical and cognitive capacity. The diagnosis of depression was ruled out. Assessment identified the following: (1) rigidity, bradykinesia, and moderate facial masking (hypomimia) caused by the motor disorder; (2) self-reported stigmatization and difficulty with family and friend interactions although these were her favorite activities; and (3) no learned compensatory strategies for handling the community and social aspects of parkinsonian symptoms.	Appreciate the context	"Because Mrs. Smith did not have cognitive or emotional impairment, I expected that she would be able to reflect upon and discuss her occupational functioning. In order to understand her limited functioning, it was important to hear and understand her perspective. A quality of life assessment procedure was appropriate for eliciting her reflection and generating a client-centered discussion."
	Develop intervention hypotheses	"Mrs. Smith's problems may be due to stigmatizing aspects of reduced motor expressiveness in her face and body. She looks apathetic and unfriendly, and interacting with her is difficult because of slowed responses. She becomes more active and quick when talking about enjoyable activities. Pleasurable activities may reduce symptoms and activate social participation."
	Select an intervention approach	"I can engage Mrs. Smith's interest through my eye contact, body positioning, and listening to her perspective. I will develop a strong therapeutic alliance to gain her commitment to working on her occupational functioning."
	Reflect on competence	"I have not worked with many clients with Parkinson's disease. Mrs. Smith can teach me what it is like to live with the disease."

Recommendations

Because of a high risk of Mrs. Smith refusing intervention, the occupational therapist suggested to her that they meet once per week for 3 weeks in order to get to know one another better before starting the day program. The immediate goal was to establish rapport and a strong working alliance, after which they could address directly her occupational functioning needs.

Consider the patient's appraisal of performance

Consider what will occur in therapy, how often, and for how long

Ascertain the patient's endorsement of plan

"Mrs. Smith is willing to meet with me for no more than three weekly 1-hour sessions before deciding about whether or not to participate in the day program. I plan to meet with her in an area where she can see what other participants in the program, who have similar interests to hers, are doing. I believe that if she became familiar with the day program in a nonpressured manner, she might start to see how it might be helpful for her."

Summary of Short-Term Goals and Progress

(1) *Mrs. Smith and the therapist will complete a task that is interesting to both.*

The therapist and Mrs. Smith each completed an interest checklist and then discussed their responses with one another. They noted five mutual interests, one being an interest in poetry. They each brought a favorite poem to the following session to read to the other. At the end of the task, both agreed that they found the task interesting and then selected another task to do with one another in the following week.

(2) *Mrs. Smith and the therapist will have decided mutually on one goal of intervention by the end of the third session.*

The therapist and Mrs. Smith ended each session with discussing and writing down two possible goals of intervention. Tentatively, they selected one potential goal by the end of the third session: the reduction of stigma associated with eating a meal with her family in a restaurant. Mrs. Smith did not see this goal as the one that she wanted to make a commitment to achieving as of yet.

(3) *Mrs. Smith and the therapist will have at least one positive experience during each session.*

The therapist and Mrs. Smith agreed to try to do something that made them feel good or happy at least once during each session. They would assess their achievement of this goal during each session. At each session, they identified several times in which they experienced positive feelings.

Therapeutic rapport was developing in a satisfactory manner by the third session. Mrs. Smith continued to be reluctant to make a commitment to attend the day program but agreed to try it out for an additional 4-week period at two half-day sessions per week.

Assess the patient's comprehension

Understand what she is doing

Compare actual to expected performance

Know the person

Appreciate the context

"Mrs. Smith has come to every scheduled session. It has gotten easier to work with her as I have learned what cues indicate that she is happy, sad, angry, or frightened. Her positive attributes are easiest to see whenever we discuss or do things related to her favorite activities and interests. Mrs. Smith appears to understand my role and the tasks involved in intervention. She responds positively to clear explanations and my undivided attention."

"I think her reluctance to attend the program is partly because she has not recently practiced socially interacting with her peers, and, as a result, has not had the experience of seeing that others accept her despite the symptoms of Parkinson's disease."

Next Steps

Revised short-term goals:

(1) *Mrs. Smith will express interest in participating in a group activity on identifying goals for daily living.*
(2) *Mrs. Smith will communicate about her ideas with the group members.*
(3) *Mrs. Smith will have a pleasant social interaction with at least one of the other group members.*

Anticipate present and future patient concerns

Analyze patient's comprehension

Decide whether he or she should continue or discontinue therapy and/or return in the future

"I feel that Mrs. Smith and I have developed a good rapport with one another and that now she understands she may be able to participate in friendly interactions with other people. She is ready to try a group activity in the day program. I must prepare for the possibility that Mrs. Smith will decide not to continue the program after 1 month. I will discuss her concerns about the day program with her family and physician to determine how best to support her involvement in goal setting, and to determine what alternatives are available for helping Mrs. Smith to participate fully in her life activities."

Clinical Reasoning in Occupational Therapy Practice

When to Refer to Another Therapist

The therapist suspects that one reason that Mrs. Smith does not want to be involved in the day program is because the therapist is of a different ethnicity than that of Mrs. Smith, who seems to have a negative attitude toward the therapist's ethnic group. How should the therapist attempt to deal with this possibility? What can be done to promote rapport? At what point and under what conditions should the therapist attempt to refer the client to another therapist or program?

 ## Clinical Reasoning in Occupational Therapy Practice

Managing Challenging Family Involvement

Mrs. Smith's son and his wife would like to increase Mrs. Smith's commitment to and involvement in the day program. On the first visit, they accompany Mrs. Smith. When the occupational therapist asks Mrs. Smith what her favorite activities are, the son and wife answer the question. They also answer the next question that the therapist asks of Mrs. Smith. Mrs. Smith listens passively. How can the therapist manage family communication in order to obtain a direct answer from Mrs. Smith?

 ## Clinical Reasoning in Occupational Therapy Practice

An Ethical Dilemma

Mrs. Smith refuses involvement in the day program despite the therapist's, the family members', and the physician's encouragement for her to participate. What should the therapist do? What is the therapist's ethical responsibility? How will the therapist's decision affect the therapeutic relationship with Mrs. Smith?

Summary Review Questions

1. What are the elements of high therapeutic rapport?
2. How has the view of the client–therapist relationship changed over time?
3. How are the therapist's experience and behavior related to rapport?
4. How are the client's experience and behavior related to rapport?
5. What are three reasons high rapport may be beneficial for clients?
6. How can the therapist facilitate the development of high therapeutic rapport?
7. What are two ethical responsibilities that a therapist holds in a relationship with a client?

Glossary

Mutuality—Interaction between the client and therapist in which they influence one another.

Nonverbal communication—Interpreting another's nonverbal behavior and expressing one's own thoughts and emotions through nonverbal behavior. Nonverbal behavior includes positions and movements of the face and body, as well as vocal tone, intensity, and speed.

Therapeutic rapport—The qualities of experience and behavior between client and therapist that affect the client's performance and involvement in therapy.

Verbal communication—Interpreting another's words and expressing one's own thoughts and emotions through words.

Working or therapeutic alliance—Working together to achieve agreed upon goals through agreed upon methods of intervention. A positive affective bond promotes the alliance.

References

Ambady, N., Koo, J., Rosenthal, R., & Winograd, C. H. (2002). Physical therapists' nonverbal communication predicts geriatric patients' health outcomes. *Psychology and Aging, 17,* 443–452.

American Occupational Therapy Association. (1948). Professional attitudes. *American Journal of Occupational Therapy, 2,* 97–98.

American Occupational Therapy Association. (2008). Occupational therapy practice framework: Domain and process (2nd ed.). *American Journal of Occupational Therapy, 62,* 625–683.

American Occupational Therapy Association. (2010). Occupational therapy code of ethics. *American Journal of Occupational Therapy, 60,* 652–658.

Blanch-Hartigan, D. (2011). Measuring providers' verbal and nonverbal emotion recognition ability: Reliability and validity of the Patient Emotion Cue Test (PECT). *Patient Education and Counseling, 82,* 370–376.

Bonder, B. R., Martin, L., & Miracle, A. W. (2004). Culture emergent in occupation. *American Journal of Occupational Therapy, 58,* 159–168.

Brack, J., & Collins, R. (1981). *One thing for tomorrow: A woman's personal struggle with MS.* Saskatoon, Canada: Western Producer Prairie.

Brozgold, A. Z., Borod, J. C., Martin, C. C., Pick, L. H., Alpert, M., & Welkowitz, J. (1998). Social functioning and facial emotional expression in neurological and psychiatric disorders. *Applied Neuropsychology, 5,* 15–23.

Burke, J. P. (2010). What's going on here? Deconstructing the interactive encounter. *American Journal of Occupational Therapy, 64,* 855–868.

Chartrand, T. L., & van Baaren, R. B. (2009). Human mimicry. In M. P. Zanna (Ed.), *Advances in experimental social psychology* (Vol. 41, pp. 219–274). San Diego: Academic Press.

Cohn, E. S., Schell, B. A. B., & Crepeau, E. B. (2010). Occupational therapy as a reflective practice. In N. Lyons (ed.), *Handbook of reflection and reflective inquiry: Mapping a way of knowing for professional reflective inquiry* (pp. 131–157). New York: Springer.

Collins, L. G., Schrimmer, A., Diamond, J., & Burke, J. (2011). Evaluating verbal and non-verbal communication skills, in an ethnogeriatric OSCE. *Patient Education and Counseling, 83,* 158–162.

Crepeau, E. B., & Garren, K. R. (2011). I looked to her as a guide: The therapeutic relationship in hand therapy. *Disability and Rehabilitation, 33,* 872–881.

Darragh, A. R., Sample, P. L., & Krieger, S. R. (2001). "Tears in my eyes 'cause somebody finally understood": Client perceptions of practitioners following brain injury. *American Journal of Occupational Therapy, 55,* 191–199.

DeGroat, E., Lyons, K. D., & Tickle-Degnen, L. (2006). Verbal content during favorite activity interview as a window into the identity of people with Parkinson's disease. *Occupational Therapy Journal of Research: Occupation, Participation, and Health, 26,* 56–68.

Di Blasi, Z., Harkness, E., Ernst, E., Georgious, A., & Kleijnen, J. (2001). Influence of context effects on health outcomes: A systematic review. *Lancet, 357,* 757–762.

DiMatteo, M. R. (2004). Social support and patient adherence to medical treatment: A meta-analysis. *Health Psychology, 23,* 207–218.

Duggan, A. P., & Parrott, R. L. (2000). Research note: Physician's nonverbal rapport building and patients' talk about the subjective component of illness. *Human Communication Research, 27,* 299–311.

Egan, M., Dubouloz, C.-J., von Zweck, C., & Vallerand, J. (1998). The client-centered evidence-based practice of occupational therapy. *Canadian Journal of Occupational Therapy, 55,* 191–199.

Feinberg, J. (1992). Effect of the arthritis health professional on compliance with use of resting hand splints by patients with rheumatoid arthritis. *Arthritis Care and Research, 5,* 17–23.

Fisher, G. S., Emerson, L., Firpo, C., Ptak, J., Wonn, J., & Bartolacci, G. (2007). Chronic pain and occupation: An exploration of lived experience. *American Journal of Occupational Therapy, 61,* 290–302.

Frank, J. D. (1958). The therapeutic use of self. *American Journal of Occupational Therapy, 12,* 215–225.

Gray, H., & Tickle-Degnen, L. (2010). A meta-analysis of performance on emotion recognition tasks in Parkinson's disease. *Neuropsychology, 24,* 176–191.

Hall, J. A., Roter, D. L., Blanch, D. C., & Frankel, R. M. (2009). Observer-rated rapport in interactions between medical students and standardized patients. *Patient Education and Counseling, 76,* 323–327.

Hall, J. A., Roter, D. L., & Milburn, M. A. (1999). Illness and satisfaction with medical care. *Current Directions in Psychological Science, 3,* 96–99.

Hanlan, A. J. (1979). *Autobiography of dying.* New York: Doubleday.

Hatfield, E., Rapson, R. L., & Le, Y.-C. (2009). Emotional contagion and empathy. In J. Decety and W. Ickes (Eds.), *The social neuroscience of empathy* (pp. 19–30). Cambridge, MA: MIT.

Horvath, A. O., & Luborsky, L. (1993). The role of the therapeutic alliance in psychotherapy. *Journal of Counseling and Clinical Psychology, 61,* 561–573.

Iwama, M. (2003). Toward culturally relevant epistemologies in occupational therapy. *American Journal of Occupational Therapy, 57,* 582–588.

Jack, J., & Estes, R. I. (2010). Documenting progress: Hand therapy treatment shift from biomechanical to occupational adaptation. *American Journal of Occupational Therapy, 64,* 82–87.

Kantartzis, S., & Molineux, M. (2010). The influence of Western society's construction of a healthy daily life on the conceptualization of occupation. *The Journal of Occupational Science.* Advance online publication. Retrieved August 29, 2011 from http://www.jos.edu.

Katz, A. M., & Alegría, M. (2009). The clinical encounter as local moral world: Shifts of assumptions and transformation in relational context. *Social Science & Medicine, 68,* 1238–1246.

Klein, B. S. (1995). Reflections on . . . An ally as well as a partner in practice. *Canadian Journal of Occupational Therapy, 62,* 283–285.

Klein, J., & Liu, L. (2010). Family-therapist relationships in caring for older adults. *Physical & Occupational Therapy in Geriatrics, 28,* 259–270.

Leber, D. A., & Vanoli, E. G. (2001). Therapeutic use of humor: Occupational therapy clinicians' perceptions and practices. *American Journal of Occupational Therapy, 55,* 221–226.

Lequerica, A. H., Donnell, C. S., & Tate, D. G. (2009). Patient engagement in rehabilitation therapy: Physical and occupational therapy impressions. *Disability and Rehabilitation, 31,* 753–760.

Maitra, K. K., & Erway, F. (2006). Perception of client-centered practice in occupational therapists and their clients. *American Journal of Occupational Therapy, 60,* 298–310.

Martin, D. J., Garske, J. P., & Davis, M. K. (2000). Relation of the therapeutic alliance with outcome and other variables: A meta-analytic review. *Journal of Consulting and Clinical Psychology, 68,* 438–450.

Mattingly, C. (1998). *Healing dramas and clinical plots: The narrative structure of experience.* Cambridge, UK: Cambridge University Press.

McCrum, R. (1998). *My year off.* New York: Norton.

Oxford English Dictionary Online. (2011). Oxford University Press. Retrieved August 30, 2011 from http://www.oed.com.

Palmadottir, G. (2006). Client-therapist relationships: Experiences of occupational therapy clients in rehabilitation. *British Journal of Occupational Therapy, 69,* 394–401.

Peloquin, S. M. (2005). The 2005 Eleanor Clarke Slagle Lecture: Embracing our ethos, reclaiming our heart. *American Journal of Occupational Therapy, 59,* 611–625.

Peoples, H., Satink, T., & Steultjens, E. (2011). Stroke survivors' experiences of rehabilitation: A systematic review of qualitative studies. *Scandinavian Journal of Occupational Therapy, 18,* 163–171.

Pierce, D. (2009). Co-occupation: The challenges of defining concepts original to occupational science. *Journal of Occupational Science, 16,* 203–207.

Price, P., & Miner, S. (2007). Occupation emerges in the process of therapy. *American Journal of Occupational Therapy, 61,* 441–450.

Prigatano, G. P., Klonoff, P. S., O'Brien, K. P., Altman, I. M., Amin, K., Chiapello, D., Shepherd, J., Cunningham, M., & Mora, M. (1994). Productivity after neuropsychologically oriented milieu rehabilitation. *Journal of Head Trauma Rehabilitation, 9,* 91–102.

Pooremamali, P., Persson, D., & Eklund, M. (2011). Occupational therapists' experience of working with immigrant clients in mental health care. *Scandinavian Journal of Occupational Therapy, 18,* 109–121.

Puller, L. B. (1991). *Fortunate son.* New York: Grove Weidenfeld.

Radomski, M. V. (2011). The issue is . . . More than good intentions: Advancing adherence to therapy recommendations. *American Journal of Occupational Therapy, 65,* 471–477.

Redman, B. K. (2007). *The practice of patient education: A case study approach* (10th ed.). St. Louis: Mosby.

Rosa, S. A., & Hasselkus, B. R. (2005). Finding common ground with patients: The centrality of compatibility. *American Journal of Occupational Therapy, 59,* 198–208.

Roter, D. L., Hall, J. A., Blanch-Hartigan, D., Larson, S., & Frankel, R. M. (2011). Slicing it thin: New methods for brief sampling analysis using RIAS-coded medical dialogue. *Patient Education and Counseling, 82,* 410–419.

Safran, J. D., Muran, J. C., & Eubanks-Carter, C. (2011). Repairing alliance ruptures. *Psychotherapy, 48,* 80–87.

Schönberger, M., Humle, F., & Teasdale, T. W. (2006a). The development of the therapeutic working alliance, patients' awareness and their compliance during the process of brain injury rehabilitation. *Brain Injury, 20,* 445–454.

Schönberger, M., Humle, F., & Teasdale, T. W. (2006b). Subjective outcome of brain injury rehabilitation in relation to the therapeutic working alliance, client compliance and awareness. *Brain Injury, 20,* 1271–1282.

Schönberger, M., Humle, F., & Teasdale, T. W. (2007). The relationship between clients' cognitive functioning and the therapeutic working alliance in post-acute brain injury rehabilitation. *Brain Injury, 21,* 825–836.

Sharpley, C. F., Halat, J., Rabinowicz, T., Weiland, B., & Stafford, J. (2001). Standard posture, postural mirroring and client-perceived rapport. *Counselling Psychology Quarterly, 14,* 267–280.

Sharpley, C. F., Jeffrey, A. M., & McMah, T. (2006). Counsellor facial expression and client-perceived rapport. *Counselling Psychology Quarterly, 19,* 343–356.

Shaw, L., McWilliam, C., Sumsion, T., & MacKinnon, J. (2007). Optimizing environments for consumer participation and self-direction in finding employment. *OTJR: Occupation, Participation & Health, 27,* 59–70.

Sherer, M., Evans, C. C., Leverenz, J., Stouter, J., Irby, J. W., Lee, J. E., & Yablon, S. A. (2007). Therapeutic alliance in post-acute brain injury rehabilitation: Predictors of strength of alliance and impact of alliance on outcome. *Brain Injury, 21,* 663–672.

Stinson, D. A., Logel, C., Shepherd, S., & Zanna, M. P. (2011). Rewriting the self-fulfilling prophecy of social rejection: Self-affirmation improves relational security and social behavior up to 2 months later. *Psychological Science.* Advance online publication, 22(9), 1145-1149. doi:10.1177/0956797611417725.

Street, R. L., & Haidet, P. (2011). How well do doctors know their patients? Factors affecting physician understanding of patients' health beliefs. *Journal of General Internal Medicine, 26,* 21–27.

Street, R. L., Jr., Makoul, G., Arora, N. K., & Epstein, R. M. (2009). How does communication heal? Pathways linking clinician-patient communication to health outcomes. *Patient Education and Counseling, 74,* 295–301.

Sunvisson, H., Habermann, B., Weiss, S., & Benner, P. (2009). Augmenting the Cartesian medical discourse with an understanding of the person's lifeworld, lived body, life story and social identity. *Nursing Philosophy: An International Journal for Healthcare Professionals, 10,* 241–252.

Takahashi, K., Tickle-Degnen, L. Coster, W., & Latham, N. (2010). Expressive behavior in Parkinson's disease as a function of interview context. *American Journal of Occupational Therapy, 64,* 484–495.

Taylor, R. R., Lee, S. W., Kielhofner, G., & Ketkar, M. (2009). Therapeutic use of self: A nationwide survey of practitioners' attitudes and experiences *American Journal of Occupational Therapy, 63,* 198–207.

Tham, K., & Kielhofner, G. (2003). Impact of the social environment on occupational experience and performance among persons with unilateral neglect. *American Journal of Occupational Therapy, 57,* 403–412.

Tickle-Degnen, L. (1998). Working well with others: The prediction of students' clinical performance. *American Journal of Occupational Therapy, 52,* 133–142.

Tickle-Degnen, L. (2006). Nonverbal behavior and its functions in the ecosystem of rapport. In M. L. Patterson & V. Manusov (Eds.), *Handbook of nonverbal communications* (pp. 381–399). Thousans Oaks, CA: Sage.

Tickle-Degnen, L., & Gavett, E. (2003). Changes in nonverbal behavior during the development of therapeutic relationships. In P. Philippot, R. S. Feldman, & E. J. Coats (Eds.). *Nonverbal behavior in clinical settings* (pp. 75-110). Oxford: Oxford University Press.

Tickle-Degnen, L., & Puccinelli, N. (1999). The nonverbal expression of negative emotions: Peer and supervisor responses to occupational therapy students' emotional attributes. *Occupational Therapy Journal of Research, 19,* 18–39.

Tickle-Degnen, L., Zebrowitz, L. A., & Ma, H. (2011). Culture, gender and health care stigma: Practitioners' response to facial masking experienced by people with Parkinson's disease. *Social Science & Medicine, 73,* 95–102.

van den Brink-Muinen, A., Spreeuwenberg, P., & Rijken, M. (2011). Preferences and experiences of chronically ill and disabled patients regarding shared decision-making: Does the type of care to be decided upon matter? *Patient Education and Counseling, 84,* 111–117.

Verbeek, J., Sengers, M., Riemens, L., & Haafkens, J. (2004). Patient expectations of treatment for back pain: A systematic review of qualitative and quantitative studies. *Spine, 29,* 2309–2318.

Watt, B. (1996). *Patient.* New York: Grove.

Yerxa, E. J. (2011). The 1966 Eleanor Clarke Slagle Lecture: Authentic occupational therapy. In R. Padilla & Y. Griffiths (Eds.), *A professional legacy: The Eleanor Clarke Slagle lectures in occupational therapy, 1955–2010* (3rd ed.). Bethesda, MD: AOTA Press.

Acknowledgments

Thank you to Irene Zombek, Melissa Muns, and Shantelle Carmichael who helped to compile and develop elements of this chapter. The photographer for this chapter was Robert Littlefield.

15

Upper Extremity Orthoses

Lisa D. Deshaies

Learning Objectives

After studying this chapter, the reader will be able to do the following:

1. Define and discuss key concepts and terms related to orthoses.
2. Identify major purposes for using orthoses.
3. Explain general precautions relative to the use of orthoses.
4. Identify key factors to consider when selecting the most appropriate orthosis.
5. Given a photograph or illustration, identify the orthosis and a clinical problem for which it may be used.
6. Select an appropriate orthosis for a given diagnosis based on a specific clinical need.

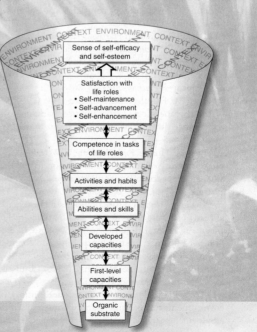

O rthoses are often an integral component of occupational therapy for clients with physical dysfunction. Orthotics entails prescription, selection, design, fabrication, testing, and training in the use of these special devices.

Successful use of orthoses is made possible only through an integrated team approach including the client, his or her significant others, and health care providers. Several rehabilitation professionals may bring their expertise to different aspects of the orthotic process. The physician typically prescribes the device. The certified orthotist is an expert in the design and fabrication of permanent orthoses, especially complicated spinal, lower extremity, and upper extremity orthoses used to restore function. The rehabilitation engineer is an expert in technical problem solving involving mechanical and/or electrical solutions to unique needs of clients.

The occupational therapist, as an expert in the adaptive use of the upper extremities in occupational performance tasks, has the major responsibility for the recommendation of appropriate orthoses, the testing and training in the use of orthoses for the upper extremities, and the selection, design, and fabrication of thermoplastic splints. Occupational therapists often collaborate with orthotists and rehabilitation engineers to solve problems encountered by clients in performing their occupations and activities of daily life. The therapist presents the parameters of the problem to these professionals in terms of the client's abilities and limitations and the functional and psychological goals that the prescribed device should meet or allow. The orthotist or engineer then proposes technical solutions, and together they apply them to the client and evaluate the outcome.

Finally, and possibly most importantly, the client and caregivers bring key physical, psychological, social, and functional characteristics to the orthotic process and should be considered the primary members of the team. For the orthosis to be successful, all team members must work in close collaboration.

KINDS OF ORTHOSES

The numerous kinds of upper extremity orthoses vary according to the body parts they include, their mechanical properties, and whether they are custom-made or prefabricated.

Classification Systems

An orthosis is an externally applied device used to modify the structural and functional characteristics of the neuromuscular and skeletal systems (Condie, 2008). Orthoses may also be called splints; the American Society of Hand Therapists (ASHT) (1992) validated that the two terms may be used interchangeably. Brace and support are other commonly used terms for orthoses. One challenge when discussing orthoses is the lack of uniform terminology in the medical literature, which makes it difficult to compare and contrast features and outcomes when a single orthosis may be known by many names.

Before the 1970s, there was no standard system for classifying orthoses, and orthoses were identified by proper names or eponyms based on the place of origin or the developer. A classification system was later developed to describe orthoses using acronyms based on the major joints or body parts they include. For example, a thumb carpometacarpal (CMC) support is a hand orthosis (HO); a wrist cock-up splint is a wrist–hand orthosis (WHO); an elbow brace is an elbow orthosis (EO); and a complete support for an arm is a shoulder–elbow–wrist–hand orthosis (SEWHO) (Condie, 2008). Each classification may contain several types of splints. A wrist cock-up splint and a flexor hinge hand splint are both WHOs, although they serve different purposes.

To simplify, organize, and describe a standardized professional nomenclature, the ASHT developed the ASHT Splint Classification System in 1992. It classifies splints in terms of their function and the number of joints they secondarily affect. According to this system, a wrist cock-up splint is a wrist extension immobilization, type 0, because no other joints are affected. Although the intent was to serve as a universal language for referral, reimbursement, communication, and research, the system has not been widely used outside of the hand therapy community.

This chapter uses the traditional or most commonly used names for the splints it describes.

Basic Types of Orthoses

Mechanical splint properties fall into three categories: static, static progressive, and dynamic (Colditz, 2002/2011). The static splint, which has no moving parts, is used primarily to provide support, stabilization, protection, or immobilization. Serial static splinting can be used to lengthen tissues and regain range of motion by placing tissues in an elongated position for prolonged periods (Bell-Krotoski, 2011; Colditz, 2011). With this process, splints are remolded as range of motion increases. Because immobilization causes such unwanted effects as atrophy and stiffness, a static splint should never be used longer than physiologically required and should never unnecessarily include joints other than those being treated.

Static progressive splints use nondynamic components, such as Velcro®, hinges, screws, or turnbuckles, to create a mobilizing force to regain motion. This type of splinting, termed inelastic mobilization, offers benefits not available with serial static or dynamic splinting because the same splint can be used without remolding, and adjustments can be made more easily as motion improves (Fess et al., 2005).

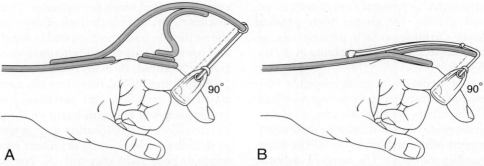

Figure 15-1 Outriggers directing proper 90° line of pull. **A.** High profile. **B.** Low profile. (Adapted with permission from Hunter, J. M., Mackin, E. J., & Callahan, A. D. [Eds.]. [1995]. *Rehabilitation of the hand: Surgery and therapy* [4th ed.]. St. Louis: Mosby.)

Dynamic splints use moving parts to permit, control, or restore movement. They are primarily used to apply an intermittent, gentle force with the goal of lengthening tissues to restore motion. Forces may be generated by springs, spring wires, rubber bands, or elastic cords. This type of splinting is termed elastic mobilization (Fess et al., 2005).

With dynamic splinting to increase range of motion, two concepts are critical. The first is that the force must be gentle and applied over a long time (Bell-Krotoski & Breger-Stanton, 2011; Fess et al., 2005). Safe force must be determined based on tissue tolerances. Excessive force results in tissue trauma, inflammation, and necrosis (Fess & McCollum, 1998).

The second concept is that, to be effective and prevent skin problems, the line of pull must be at a 90° angle to the segment being mobilized (Fess, 2011). To ensure this, forces are directed by an outrigger, a structure extending outward from the splint.

Outriggers may be high profile or low profile (Fig. 15-1). Each design has distinct advantages and disadvantages. Selection of outrigger design must be based on the specific client's needs and abilities. High-profile outriggers are inherently more stable and mechanically efficient, require fewer adjustments to maintain a 90° angle of pull, and require less effort for the client to move against the dynamic force. Low-profile outriggers are less bulky but require more frequent adjustments and greater strength to move against the dynamic force (Fess, 2011; Fess et al., 2005).

By allowing motion in the opposite direction, dynamic splints reduce the risk of joint stiffness from immobility, as seen with static splinting. If successful, an increase in passive joint mobility can be expected within 2 weeks (Fess & McCollum, 1998).

In addition to gaining motion, dynamic splints can be used to assist weak or paralyzed muscles. These dynamic splints may be intrinsically powered by another body part or by electrical stimulation of the client's muscles.

Orthotic Selection

Splinting is one of the most useful modalities available to therapists when used correctly and appropriately. Remember, the end result of splinting should always relate to the client's function (Figs. 15-2–15-5). McKee and Rivard (2004) caution that orthotic intervention may have become an end unto itself in the minds of therapists and clients rather than the means to enable occupational performance. The outcome of successful splinting is that the splint serves its purpose and that the client accepts and wears it. To meet these ends, the therapist must think critically and often creatively. Orthotic intervention should always be individualized with careful consideration of each client's unique physical and psychosocial needs, as well as personal factors and contexts (Amini & Rider, 2008; McKee & Rivard, 2011).

The therapist's multifaceted role is to evaluate the need for a splint clinically and functionally; to select the most appropriate splint; to provide or fabricate the splint; to assess the fit of the splint; to teach the client and caregivers the purpose, care, and use of the splint;

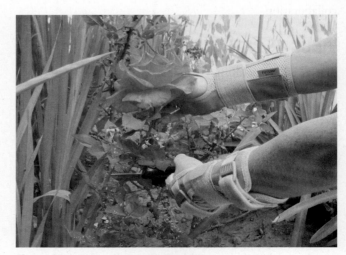

Figure 15-2 Wrist splints enabling gardening.

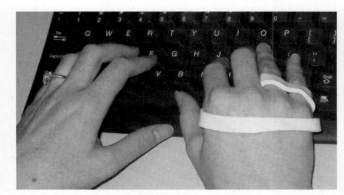

Figure 15-3 Hand splint enabling keyboarding.

and to provide related training as needed. The therapist must take a leadership role to ensure that the treatment team, including the client and caregivers, work collaboratively in every phase of the orthotic process. A client-centered, occupation-based approach empowers the client and caregivers to participate actively. This also positions them as the experts in the client's occupations, lifestyle, values, image, and activity contexts, which complements the expertise that the health care professionals bring. The therapist should clearly explain rationales, make clinically sound recommendations, and offer choices to the client whenever possible. This helps establish each team member's accountability and increases the likelihood that the client will actually use the splint.

A problem-solving approach to splinting directs the therapist to answer several key questions before splinting proceeds:

- What is the primary clinical or functional problem?
- What are the indications for and goals of splint use?
- How will the orthosis affect the problem and the client's overall function?
- What benefits will the splint provide?

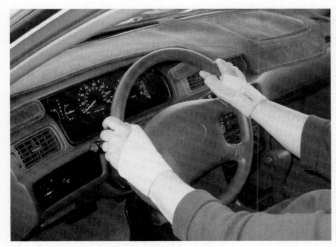

Figure 15-4 Thumb splints enabling driving.

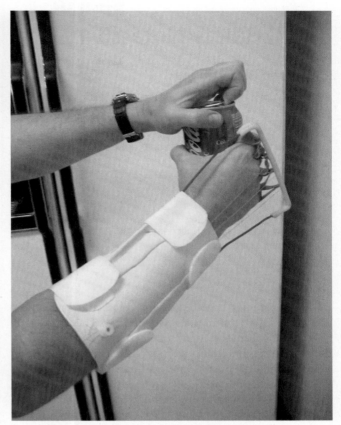

Figure 15-5 Wrist–hand splint enabling function in the kitchen.

- What limitations will the splint impose?
- What evidence is available related to the splint?

Based on these considerations, the therapist must select or design the most appropriate orthosis. In some cases, the best choice is no orthosis at all.

The growing array of commercial products has led to a greater number of choices. The first choice to be made is whether the orthosis should be custom fabricated or prefabricated. Materials must also be considered. The therapist must be familiar with properties, benefits, and drawbacks of each. Options abound, with rigid, semi-rigid, and soft materials available (see Chapter 16).

When making a splint selection, several key factors must be carefully weighed:

- Among the splint-related factors are type, design, purpose, fit, comfort, cosmetic appearance, cost to purchase or fabricate, weight, ease of care, durability, ease of donning and doffing, effect on unsplinted joints, and effect on function.
- Client-related factors include clinical and functional status, attitude, lifestyle, preference, occupational roles, living and working environments, social support, issues related to safety and precautions, ability to understand and follow through, and financial or insurance status.

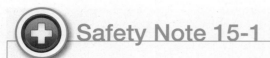

Safety Note 15-1

Orthotic Precautions

The therapist must consider, carefully monitor, and teach the client and caregiver to report any of these problems related to orthotic use:

- Impaired skin integrity (pressure areas, blisters, maceration, dermatological reactions)
- Pain
- Swelling
- Stiffness
- Sensory disturbances
- Increased stress on unsplinted joints
- Functional limitations

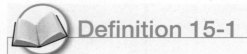

Definition 15-1

Purposes of Orthoses

Orthoses may be used to:

- support a painful joint
- immobilize for healing
- protect tissues
- provide stability
- restrict unwanted motion
- restore mobility
- substitute for weak or absent muscles
- prevent contractures
- modify tone

Several studies have been done on clients' preferences and factors that contribute to splint wear. They show that the following factors may encourage splint wear: flexibility of the splinting regimen and vigorous teaching to enable clients to understand the purpose and wearing schedule (Pagnotta, Baron, & Korner-Bitensky, 1998), individualized prescriptions focusing on the client's comfort and preference (Callinan & Mathiowetz, 1996; Stern et al., 1996), strong family support (Oakes et al., 1970), positive attitudes and behaviors exhibited by health care providers (Feinberg, 1992), and benefits that are immediately obvious to the client (Groth & Wulf, 1995). Rapport, trust, sensitivity to individual client's learning styles, trial evaluations, and giving clients the opportunity to voice their concerns and frustrations can also greatly enhance the collaborative process and outcome (Collins, 1999). A systematic review of adherence to splint wear in adults with acute upper limb injuries found little published scientific evidence and concluded that existing studies were of varied quality (O'Brien, 2010). With the relatively small base of literature on orthotics, therapists must continue to put their clinical judgments and experience to the test and strive to develop evidence-based practice related to observed outcomes and factors that influence successful orthotic intervention.

Should problems with splint wear arise (Safety Note 15-1), the therapist should examine both the splint and the wearing schedule. The splint itself may not fit properly or comfortably. The client's functional demands may outweigh the benefits of splint wearing, or the wearing schedule may be too complex. Actively engaging the client in the problem-solving process is likely to improve the outcome. Although it is important to strive for the ideal, therapists must remain realistic in the scope of the client's daily life.

PURPOSES OF ORTHOSES

In this chapter, orthoses are categorized according to several purposes (Definition 15-1). Although a specific orthosis is discussed under the category for which it is most commonly used, that purpose may not be its only one. Also, a single orthosis may fulfill several functions simultaneously. The orthoses presented here are by no means an exhaustive list but a representative sampling of commonly used or historically significant orthoses. Inclusion of specific orthoses should not be interpreted as an endorsement of one type over another. Whenever possible, published evidence-based data have been included. Because the intent of this chapter is to provide an overview of orthotics, the reader is encouraged to explore the references and resources for more detailed information.

Support a Painful Joint

Pain in a joint or soft tissues can result from a wide variety of causes, including acute trauma (such as sprains and strains), nerve irritation (such as carpal tunnel syndrome and ulnar nerve neuritis at the elbow), inflammatory conditions (such as tendonitis and rheumatoid arthritis [RA]), and joint instability (such as degenerative arthritis, ligamentous laxity, and shoulder subluxation). When resting a joint is indicated to relieve pain, protect joint integrity, and/or decrease inflammation, supportive orthoses can be used. These orthoses are often worn all day, all night, or both to provide the maximum benefit, or they may be worn only during selected activities. Unless contraindicated, the orthosis should be removed at least once a day for skin hygiene and gentle range-of-motion exercises to prevent loss of joint mobility. The following are common examples of orthoses used for pain relief.

Support a Painful Shoulder or Elbow

Arm slings have been developed to prevent or correct shoulder subluxation or reduce pain in clients who have subluxation caused by brachial plexus injuries, hemiplegia, or central cord syndrome injuries. Sling designs are numerous, with some commercially available and others fabricated by the therapist (see Resources 15-1).

Certain slings support and immobilize the whole arm. These slings, such as the standard pouch and the

Resources 15-1

Vendors of Splints and Splint Supplies

AliMed, Inc.

297 High Street
Dedham, MA 02026
Phone: 800-225-2610
www.alimed.com

Bioness, Inc.

25103 Rye Canyon Loop
Valencia, CA 91355
Phone: 800-211-9136
www.bioness.com

DeRoyal

200 DeBusk Lane
Powell, TN 37849
Phone: 800-251-9864
www.deroyal.com

Empi, Inc.

599 Cardigan Road
St. Paul, MN 55126
Phone: 800-328-2536
www.empi.com

JAECO Orthopedic Specialties, Inc.

214 Drexel
Hot Springs, AR 71901
Phone: 501-623-5944
www.jaeco-orthopedic.com

Joint Active Systems, Inc.

2600 South Raney
Effingham, IL 62401
Phone: 800-879-0117
www.jointactivesystems.com

North Coast Medical, Inc.

8100 Camino Arroyo
Gilroy, CA 95020
Phone: 800-821-9319
www.ncmedical.com

Otto Bock Medical

14630 28th Avenue North
Minneapolis, MN 53447
Phone: 800-328-4058
www.ottobockus.com

Patterson Medical

1000 Remington Boulevard
Suite 210
Bolingbrook, IL 60440
Phone: 800-323-5547
www.pattersonmedical.com

Restorative Care of America, Inc.

12221 33rd Street North
St. Petersburg, FL 33716
Phone: 800-627-1595
www.rcai.com

Saebo, Inc.

2725 Water Ridge Parkway
Suite 320
Charlotte, NC 28217
Phone: 888-284-5433
www.saebo.com

Silver Ring Splint Company

1140 East Market Street
Charlottesville, VA 22902
Phone: 800-311-7028
www.silverringsplint.com

3-Point Products, Inc.

118 Log Canoe Circle
Stevensville, MD 21666
Phone: 888-378-7763
www.3pointproducts.com

UE Tech

P.O. Box 2145
Edwards, CO 81632
Phone: 800-736-1894

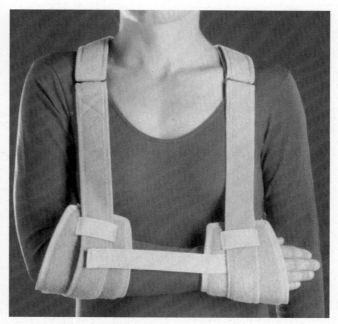

Figure 15-6 Rolyan® Figure-of-8 sling.

double arm cuff sling (Fig. 15-6), restrict motion by keeping the humerus in adduction and internal rotation and the elbow in flexion. Although these slings may take some of the weight off the affected shoulder, downsides are that they place the extremity in a nonfunctional position, reinforce synergy patterns, and fail to provide the client with the opportunity for motor and sensory feedback (Bobath, 1990). Other sling designs support the shoulder but leave the rest of the arm free for function, such as a humeral cuff sling (Fig. 15-7).

Arm troughs, lapboards, and half-lapboards are also used to support the painful shoulder when the client is seated in a wheelchair. These may be more acceptable to

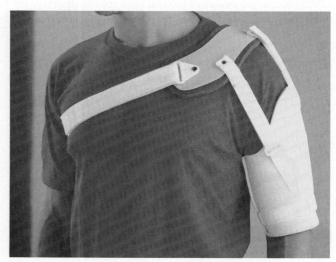

Figure 15-7 Hemi Shoulder Sling, a type of humeral cuff sling.

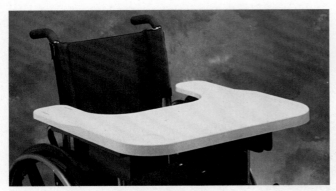

Figure 15-8 Rolyan® slide-on adjustable lap tray.

clients than slings, and they allow the arm to be ideally positioned with the scapula pulled forward and the hand supported (Bobath, 1990). It is important to remember that these supports lack the constant relationship between the client and the support as exists with slings. Any change in postural alignment will alter forces and the support effectiveness (Spaulding, 1999). Lapboards (Fig. 15-8) are generally indicated for clients with poor trunk control or visual field deficits and for those who require greater variability of upper extremity positioning or a work surface. Arm troughs (Fig. 15-9) are used for clients who need a device that does not interfere with wheelchair propulsion or transfer activities. The half-lapboard (Fig. 15-10) combines the positive features of both the arm trough and the full lapboard (Walsh, 1987). Full and half-lapboards can be purchased commercially or custom fabricated from acrylic or wood. Some designs allow the half-lapboard to be rotated up and out of the way instead of having to be removed from the wheelchair when the client needs to transfer. Arm troughs are also commercially available or can be custom-made.

The use of supports in reducing shoulder subluxation remains controversial and lacks empirical evidence. A systematic review by Ada, Foongchomcheay, and Canning (2005) found no evidence to conclude that supportive devices are effective in preventing or reducing subluxation

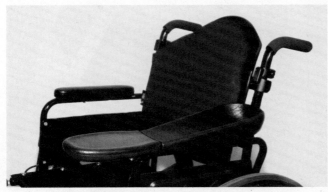

Figure 15-9 Otto Bock™ Arm Trough.

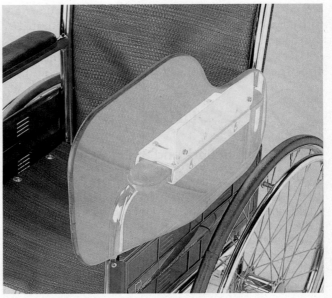

Figure 15-10 Clear flip-away armrest in upright position.

or in decreasing pain after stroke. In addition, whether subluxation has a causal relationship to shoulder pain is in question (Zorowitz et al., 1996). There is no consensus as to which type of support is the best in the treatment of shoulder subluxation or whether a support should be used at all. The effects of various sling and support designs have proved variable in multiple studies over the years as summarized by Zorowitz et al. (1995) and Turner-Stokes and Jackson (2002).

Ultimately, it is agreed upon that if a support is to be used, several types should be evaluated on the client to optimize the reduction of shoulder pain, the function of the affected extremity, and the ease of donning and doffing (Zorowitz et al., 1995). Therapists need to consider the different mechanical forces each support produces on the shoulder complex (Spaulding, 1999). The client's acceptance of the sling also must be considered. Relative ease of donning and doffing the sling is imperative so the limb is not damaged further from improper wearing. More definitive research on the effectiveness of slings and orthoses in the management of the flaccid or subluxed shoulder is needed, and therapists should carefully consider all options before prescribing slings.

A gunslinger orthosis is another means of supporting a painful shoulder, such as from a brachial plexus injury. This type of orthosis is commercially available or can be custom fabricated for the client. A commercial gunslinger (Fig. 15-11) can be easily adjusted to position the shoulder and elbow for maximal pain relief. A custom-fabricated gunslinger (Fig. 15-12) has the benefit of a much more streamlined design, allowing the client to wear it under clothing as desired with minor garment adaptations (Lunsford & DiBello, 2008). Also, this orthosis is much

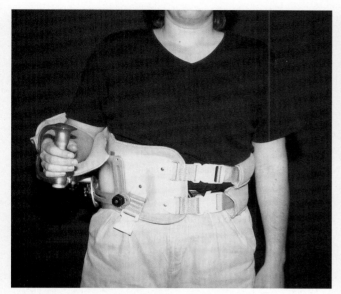

Figure 15-11 Commercial gunslinger orthosis.

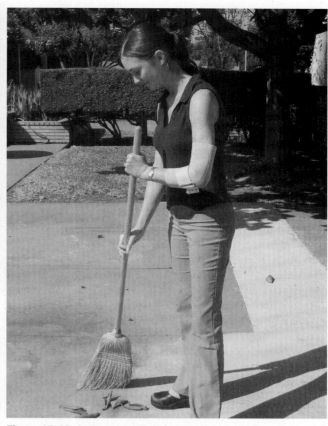

Figure 15-13 Commercial soft elbow support.

easier to don and doff. It is often the best solution for clients who require long-term or permanent use of a shoulder orthosis.

Commercial neoprene sleeves that provide neutral warmth, gentle compression, and soft dynamic support to the shoulder or elbow (Fig. 15-13) are often used to relieve pain from arthritis, tendinitis, sprains, and strains. *Safety Message: As occupational therapists are expanding their use of supports fabricated from neoprene, it is important to be aware of the potential for dermatological reactions to the material and to teach clients to discontinue use of the support should symptoms develop (Stern et al., 1998).*

The treatment of lateral and medial epicondylitis often entails the use of orthoses to relieve pain and prevent further stress to affected tissues. In both conditions, pain reduces grip strength and function. Counterforce braces (Fig. 15-14), of which there are several commercial models,

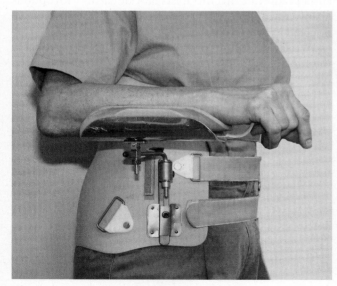

Figure 15-12 Custom-fabricated gunslinger orthosis.

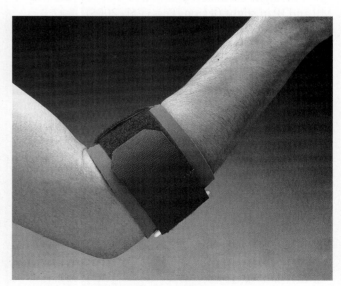

Figure 15-14 VariPad tennis elbow support.

are wide, nonelastic bands designed to limit full expansion of the forearm extensor or flexor muscle masses during contraction (Fedorczyk, 2011). These braces can also be custom fabricated from thermoplastic or strapping materials. The literature reports wide variation in the success of braces (Borkholder, Hill, & Fess, 2004; Wuori et al., 1998). *Safety Message: Instruct the client that complications can result from the brace being applied too tightly, including nerve compression syndromes. The client must be carefully taught accordingly.*

A wrist splint placing the wrist in 35°–40° of extension and worn alone or in conjunction with a counterforce brace is often prescribed to rest the forearm musculature (Fedorcczyk, 2011). A study by Jafarian, Demneh, and Tyson (2009) found that use of a counterforce brace resulted in immediate increase in pain-free grip strength, whereas a wrist splint did not. Conversely, Garg et al. (2010) found that pain relief was significantly better with a wrist splint than with a counterforce brace. The prescription of orthoses must be based on the client's symptoms. It is vital that the cause of the problem and the biomechanics of loading forearm musculature are also addressed in relation to all activity demands.

Support a Painful Wrist or Hand

Resting hand splints are used to support the wrist, fingers, and thumb. The normal resting position of the hand is determined anatomically by the bony architecture, capsular length, and resting tone of the wrist and hand muscles. This is typically 0°–20° of wrist extension, 20°–30° of metacarpophalangeal (MCP) joint flexion, 10°–30° of proximal interphalangeal (PIP) joint flexion, and slight distal interphalangeal (DIP) joint flexion, the thumb CMC in slight extension and abduction, and the thumb MP and IP in slight flexion (Fess et al., 2005).

A resting hand splint is commonly prescribed for clients with RA (see Chapter 39). Resting splints can reduce stress on joint capsules, synovial lining, and periarticular structures, thereby decreasing pain (Melvin, 1989). A randomized controlled trial also found that in addition to pain relief, nighttime use of resting hand splints improved hand strength and functional status (Silva et al., 2008). With RA, splinting should be in a position of comfort regardless of whether this is the ideal anatomical position (Fess et al., 2005). During an acute exacerbation of the disease, splints are generally worn at night and during most of the day and removed at least once for hygiene and gentle range-of-motion exercises. It is recommended that splint use continue for at least several weeks after the pain and swelling have subsided (Fess et al., 2005; Melvin, 1989).

Resting hand splints can be volar or dorsal, depending on needs and preferences. Commercial splints, such as those fabricated from wire-foam (Fig. 15-15) or a malleable

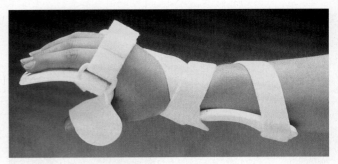

Figure 15-15 LMB economical resting splint.

metal frame covered by dense foam padding (Fig. 15-16), may be used if the limited adjustments they allow for can provide the client with a proper fit. This becomes more difficult if the client has established joint deformities. Custom-fabricated splints (Fig. 15-17) allow for a precise, individualized fit.

If the thumb or IP joints of the fingers are not painful, a modified resting hand splint (Fig. 15-18) will keep these joints free. This often results in less stiffness related to splint wear, some degree of hand function while the splint is worn, and improved splint wear and comfort.

Although health care professionals generally agree on the benefits of using splints to rest inflamed and painful joints, studies have shown approximately 45% compliance in wearing resting hand splints as prescribed which is less than optimal (Feinberg, 1992). Callinan and Mathiowetz (1996) compared soft versus hard resting hand splints on pain and hand function. Their results showed that pain was significantly decreased with splint wear and that 57% of clients preferred the soft splint, 33% preferred the hard splint, and 10% preferred no splint. The rate of compliance was greater for the soft splint (82%) than for the hard splint (67%). The authors advocate that therapists provide clients with options relative to comfort and preference to ensure client satisfaction and improved outcome.

Wrist extension, or cock-up, splints are probably the most commonly prescribed type of orthosis for the upper extremity. Indications for use include sprains,

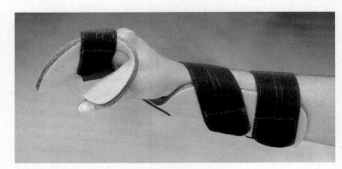

Figure 15-16 Progress™ functional resting splint.

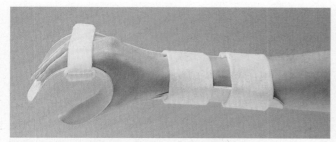

Figure 15-17 Custom thermoplastic resting hand splint.

strains, tendonitis, arthritis, carpal tunnel syndrome, following cast removal of wrist fractures, and other conditions that cause pain. A wrist splint typically positions the wrist in 10°–30° of extension, which is thought to be the best position for hand function (Fess et al., 2005). A well-fitting splint is one that clears the distal palmar and thenar creases to allow for unrestricted mobility of the fingers and thumb and that conforms to the palm to support the arches of the hand. Wrist splints may be volar (Fig. 15-19), dorsal (Fig. 15-20), or circumferential (Figs. 15-2 and 15-21) and can be custom fabricated or prefabricated. Because these splints are intended to provide wrist support while allowing functional use of the hand, fit and comfort are crucial.

A growing variety of commercial splints are available, with designs and materials offering a range of soft to rigid support. Elasticized wrist orthoses with an adjustable metal stay that slides into a volar pocket (Fig. 15-22) are commonly used because they are cost-effective and readily available. The drawbacks of these splints are that they do not fully support the palmar arches, they do not completely clear the palmar and thenar creases, and the metal stay is often prepositioned at a 35°–45° angle of extension. Therefore, it is critical to fit and adjust the stay to the desired angle before issuing the splint. Other commercial products are made of wire-foam, neoprene, leather, canvas, and other fabric blends, all of which offer features having distinct advantages and disadvantages.

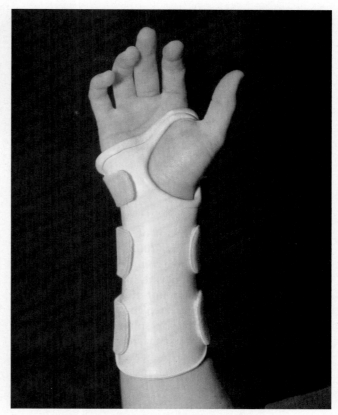

Figure 15-19 Custom thermoplastic volar wrist extension splint.

Several studies have been conducted on the effects on hand function of different styles of wrist extension splints. Stern (1991) studied hand function speed in normal subjects who wore three styles of custom-fabricated wrist splints and a commercial elastic wrist splint. She found that although all of the splints significantly slowed hand speed, the commercial elastic splint allowed for faster speeds and dexterity than the others. A later study on grip strength and dexterity across five styles of commercial wrist splints concluded that each style impeded power grip and dexterity but to different extents (Stern, 1996).

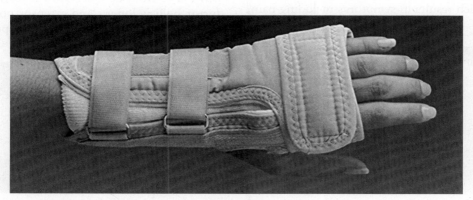

Figure 15-18 Rolyan® D-Ring™ wrist brace with MCP support.

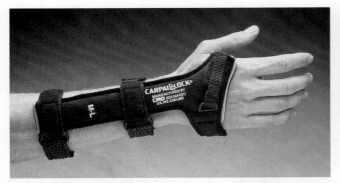

Figure 15-20   Carpal Lock® splint.

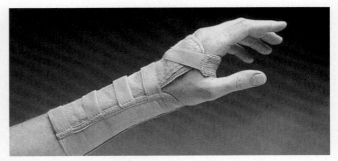

Figure 15-22   Norco™ wrist brace.

Splints vary in the amount of motion they allow or restrict. Collier and Thomas (2002) compared range of motion at the wrist with three commercial supports and a custom-made volar thermoplastic splint. The commercial splints allowed the same amount of motion (wrist flexion to about neutral and wrist extension to about 26°–31°). In contrast, the thermoplastic splint allowed less wrist flexion (not past 14° of wrist extension) and more wrist extension (about 40°). This suggests a custom thermoplastic splint may be more appropriate for conditions where limited wrist flexion is desired.

Elastic wrist orthoses have been widely used in the treatment of arthritis to stabilize wrists, decrease pain, and improve function. Again, studies have shown conflicting results across different styles of orthoses in grip strength, dexterity, hand function, pain reduction, comfort, security during task performance, and adverse effects of stiffness or muscle atrophy caused by orthotic wear (Pagnotta, Baron, & Korner-Bitensky, 1998; Stern et al., 1996). In a related study, most of 42 subjects knew their preferred orthosis within a few minutes of wear when given three styles to try (Stern et al., 1997). These studies reinforce the importance of task analysis, having a wide variety of splints to try with each client, and a careful weighing of the benefits and limitations of splinting.

Another common indication for wrist splinting is carpal tunnel syndrome, a condition caused by median nerve compression, which results in symptoms including pain, sensory disturbances, muscle weakness, swelling, stiffness, and frequent dropping of items. Symptoms often are worse at night or with repetitive activity involving wrist flexion (see Chapter 37). For pain and related symptoms caused by carpal tunnel syndrome, conservative or postoperative treatment often uses wrist splints to prevent the elevation of carpal tunnel pressure by restricting wrist motion (Evans, 2011b).

The ideal position of the wrist to minimize pressure in the carpal tunnel varies, according to sources, from 10°–15° of extension (Melvin, 1989) to neutral (Weiss et al., 1995) to slight flexion (Gelberman et al., 1988). There is a consensus that commercial wrist splints, which often place the wrist in excessive extension, may not be of any benefit unless they are modified to a less extended position. Dorsal wrist splints (Fig. 15-20) are often recommended because they do not create external pressure over the volar wrist. A systematic review of splinting for carpal tunnel syndrome showed benefits from splinting across splint types and wrist angles, with evidence suggesting custom splints and full-time splint wear promote better results (Piazzini et al., 2007). Splinting is most effective when initiated early after symptom onset. Control of wrist position alone may be insufficient, and blocking the MPs in slight flexion may also be needed to decrease intratunnel pressure (Evans, 2011b).

A long opponens splint (Fig. 15-23), also known as a long thumb spica, can relieve pain from wrist and thumb arthritis or from de Quervain's tenosynovitis of the abductor pollicis longus and extensor pollicis brevis. This splint is typically based on the radial aspect of the forearm

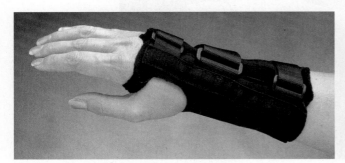

Figure 15-21   Comfort Cool™ D-ring wrist splint.

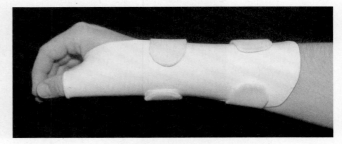

Figure 15-23   Custom thermoplastic long thumb spica splint.

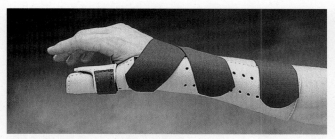

Figure 15-24 Liberty™ wrist and thumb splint.

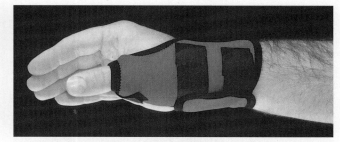

Figure 15-26 AliMed® custom-molded thumb splint.

and extends distally to immobilize the thumb CMC and MP joints. The wrist is generally splinted in slight extension, with the thumb in slight flexion and palmar abduction to enable opposition to the index and middle fingers (Lohman, 2008b). If the thumb IP joint or the extensor pollicis longus tendon is involved, the IP joint can be included in the splint as well (Fig. 15-24). Prefabricated splints often provide a softer support, whereas custom-made thermoplastic splints give more rigid immobilization.

A thumb CMC stabilization splint, or a short thumb spica, is a static splint that encompasses the first metacarpal to provide stability, reduce pain, and increase hand function. It restricts motion of the CMC and MP joints but leaves the wrist relatively mobile and the thumb IP free. A static thumb MP splint allows for CMC and IP motion and can be used when the disorder is localized to the MP joint alone.

Indications for short thumb splints include RA or osteoarthritis (OA) of the thumb CMC or MP joints or trauma to soft tissues, such as the ulnar collateral ligament of the MP. The thumb is generally positioned to enable opposition to the fingers for function while in the splint, and the splint is most often worn during functional activities that cause or aggravate pain (Melvin, 1995). Commercially prefabricated rigid CMC and MP stabilization splints are often ineffectual because they fit poorly (Melvin, 1995). For a precise fit and rigid support, splints can be custom fabricated from thermoplastic materials (Fig. 15-25).

Newer commercial products made of soft, breathable elastic material have moldable thermoplastic stays to enable a custom fit, combining comfort and ease of fabrication with the required individualized rigid support (Fig. 15-26). Rigid support may not always be needed. In comparing a custom-made thermoplastic splint and a soft neoprene support for OA of the thumb CMC joint, Weiss et al. (2004) found that the prefabricated neoprene splint (Fig. 15-27) provided greater pain relief and function and was preferred over the thermoplastic splint by 72% of the subjects. Sillem et al. (2011) similarly found that clients preferred a soft prefabricated splint even though a more rigid custom splint decreased pain slightly more. Systematic reviews found evidence for the effectiveness of splinting to relieve pain and improve function in CMC OA, found evidence of varying client splint preferences, but found no evidence of splint design superiority (Egan & Brousseau, 2007; Kjeken et al., 2011).

If the thumb or finger IP joints are painful from trauma or arthritis, lateral, dorsal, or volar gutter splints (Fig. 15-28) may be used for pain relief. Silicone-lined sleeves or pads (Fig. 15-29) can protect painful joint nodules from external trauma.

Pain, volar subluxation, and ulnar deviation of the MCPs are common sequelae of RA. MCP ulnar deviation supports may be used to provide stability, realign joints, reduce joint

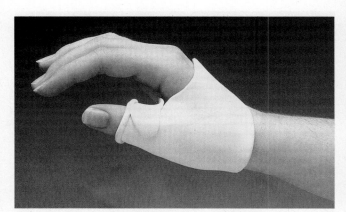

Figure 15-25 Custom thermoplastic short thumb splint.

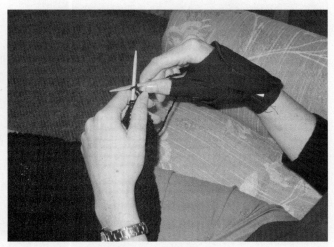

Figure 15-27 Commercial soft thumb splint.

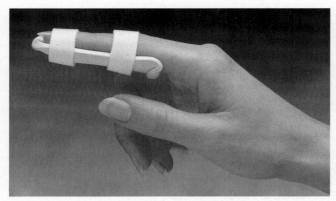

Figure 15-28 Custom thermoplastic volar gutter splint.

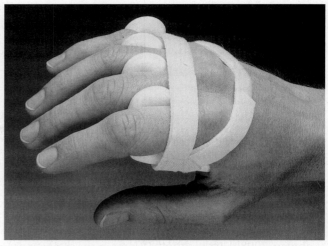

Figure 15-30 LMB Soft-Core™ Wire-Foam™ ulnar deviation splint.

stress, and relieve pain. They may delay the progression of deformity but do not correct or prevent it (Beasley, 2011b; Melvin, 1995). These supports may be worn alone or incorporated into a resting hand splint.

Prefabricated and custom-designed orthoses with dividers or straps to align the digits include dynamic and static and soft and rigid. Rigid static splints (Fig. 15-30) used to achieve passive correction of deformity can create focal pressure points on the digits. It is therefore important not to try to achieve ideal alignment at the risk of creating pressure problems (Melvin, 1989).

Despite the variety of splint materials and designs, MCP ulnar deviation supports are reported to be infrequently prescribed or used by clients for a variety of reasons (Rennie, 1996). For some clients, immobilization of the MCPs impairs functional use of the hand and may increase stress and pain on the adjacent PIP joints (Melvin, 1995). Additionally, bulky or volar-based splints interfere with palmar sensation and impede the ability to grasp objects.

Some clients, however, benefit from the improved digital alignment and pain reduction that supports offer. High client satisfaction rates have been reported for a custom dorsal-based design (Rennie, 1996). Soft ulnar deviation splints are commercially available (Fig. 15-31) or can be custom fabricated (Gilbert-Lenef, 1994). The prime indicator for use and selection of an MCP ulnar deviation support should be the client's preference (Harrell, 2006; Melvin, 1995).

Immobilize for Healing or to Protect Tissues

Many of the orthoses previously discussed for pain relief can also be used to immobilize for healing or protection following injury or surgery. For example, a gunslinger orthosis used to relieve traction pain associated with a brachial plexus injury can also protect the nerve structures from overstretching during the healing phase. A thumb MP splint that relieves pain from arthritis may also be used while an acutely injured collateral ligament heals. These orthoses are not discussed in detail again; different ones are reviewed.

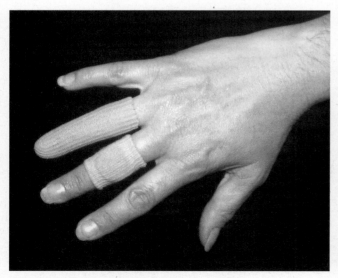

Figure 15-29 Silicone-lined digital sleeve and pad.

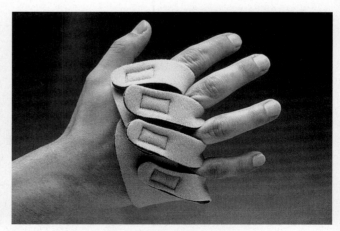

Figure 15-31 Norco™ soft MP ulnar deviation support.

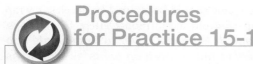

Procedures for Practice 15-1

How to Adjust a Sling

- Place the client upright.
- Ensure that the elbow is flexed to 90° and is seated properly in the sling, with the hand and wrist also supported as the design allows.
- Adjust the strap or straps so that the arm is comfortably supported.
- Check for comfort.
- Teach the client and caregiver about proper donning and doffing of the sling.
- Monitor the axilla and areas where sling straps cross the body for signs of skin breakdown.
- Monitor for signs of edema and joint stiffness.

Immobilize or Protect the Shoulder, Upper Arm, or Elbow

The sling is the simplest and most commonly used device for the upper extremity when there is a need to limit motion of the shoulder yet allow for some motion of the arm on the thorax. The basic arm sling consists of a forearm pouch or cuffs, a strap, and a mechanism for adjusting and securing the strap. Guidelines for sling adjustment are in Procedures for Practice 15-1.

To further limit mobility, shoulder immobilizers (Fig. 15-32) can be used. These devices, which relatively immobilize the shoulder and elbow, are typically used following shoulder surgical reconstructions, arthroplasty, and rotator cuff repair. Immobilizers are more complex than slings, involving strapping that wraps the body to stabilize the arm against the trunk. Several commercial designs are available.

Foam abduction pillows or wedges may be used to maintain the arm at a certain elevation from the body. Abduction braces, sometimes called airplane splints, are commercially

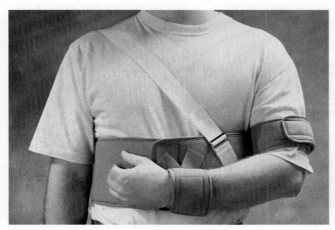

Figure 15-32 Rolyan® universal shoulder immobilizer.

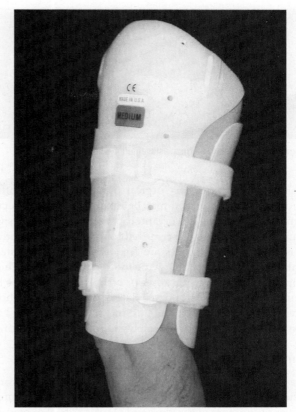

Figure 15-33 Commercial humeral fracture brace.

available or custom fabricated from thermoplastics. These devices are based on the trunk and can position the shoulder in varying degrees of abduction or rotation and the elbow in varying degrees of flexion or extension. Commercial braces offer ease of adjustability with the use of wrenches but may need extra padding to prevent skin breakdown. Indications for use include postoperative shoulder repairs, burns, and skin grafts to the axillary region.

The treatment of humeral shaft fractures often involves functional fracture bracing (see Chapter 36). A humeral fracture brace (Fig. 15-33) provides external stabilization and alignment of the fracture by compressing surrounding soft tissues while allowing for early mobilization of the shoulder and elbow. These braces may be prefabricated or custom fabricated by the therapist from low-temperature thermoplastics. They are circumferential in design, with D-ring straps to allow for a secure closure and size adjustments as edema subsides. They should be lightweight and made of a perforated material for ventilation. *Safety Message: Whether the brace is prefabricated or custom, the therapist should ensure that its distal end does not block elbow flexion motion and that its proximal end does not unnecessarily limit shoulder motion.* Excellent results with the use of functional fracture bracing of the humerus have been reported (Ekholm et al., 2006).

Casts, splints, and hinged braces can be used to immobilize and protect the elbow following fractures, burns,

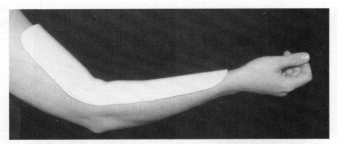

Figure 15-34 Custom thermoplastic anterior elbow extension splint.

ligamentous injuries, or surgical procedures. Casts offer rigid immobilization and may be made according to a circumferential, posterior, or anteroposterior bivalve design that allows the cast to be removed for wound care or range of motion. Hinged braces are frequently used to protect healing ligaments while allowing motion of the elbow. Thermoplastic splints may be anterior or posterior and may be secured by Velcro® straps or an elastic wrap. Anterior elbow extension splints (Fig. 15-34) are most commonly used to immobilize and position the elbow following skin grafting.

Immobilize or Protect the Wrist or Hand

The maintenance of normal hand function requires strong tissue repair with free gliding between neighboring structures. Proper positioning of the wrist and hand is critical to prevent complications caused by injury, edema, and tissue healing. Splinting in the early stages of healing can counteract the typical joint contractures of the injured hand that produce common deformities of wrist flexion, MCP extension, IP flexion, and thumb adduction. It is essential to position joints correctly and keep uninvolved joints moving so that they will not stiffen (Pettengill, 2011). *Safety Message: Incorrect application of a splint or improper positioning while in a splint may lead to both joint limitations and tissue damage.*

Unless specifically contraindicated, the antideformity, or safe, position of immobilization for most hand conditions is with the wrist in 10°–30° of extension, the MCPs in 70°–90° of flexion, the IPs in 0°–15° of flexion, and the thumb in palmar abduction (Fess et al., 2005; Pettengill, 2011). This is most often accomplished through a volar custom-fabricated low-temperature thermoplastic splint (Fig. 15-35). If edema

is present, the splint should be secured by an elastic wrap or gauze wrap to avoid a tourniquet effect from straps. *Safety Message: It is crucial never to force joints into the ideal position but to position joints as closely as possible to the ideal and serially revise the splint until the optimal position is realized.*

Antideformity splints are integral to the treatment of acute dorsal hand burns (see Chapter 40). An investigation of the literature found an overall lack of consensus on the design of these splints (Richard et al., 1994). The most commonly recommended positions for joints is with the wrist in 15°–30° of extension, the MCPs in 50°–70° of flexion, the IPs in full extension, and the thumb in palmar abduction or midway between palmar and radial abduction with the MP and IP in slight flexion to full extension to prevent common burn-related contractures (Richard & Staley, 1994; Tufaro & Bondoc, 2011). Preformed splints are commercially available and may be used if adequate fit can be obtained given the size of the hand and any edema. Custom-fabricated splints, preferably of a perforated material, ensure the best fit. Splints may have to be adjusted daily for optimal fit and maintenance of proper joint positioning. For the grafting and rehabilitation phases of burn treatment, splint design varies with the positions necessary to counteract the contractile forces of the scars.

Wrist splints, as discussed in the previous section, may be used for protection or immobilization of wrists following cast removal or to treat soft tissue injuries. Athletic injuries to the wrist and hand, such as contusions, sprains, strains, fractures, and joint dislocations, often require the use of protective splints to enable the client to continue participation in sports. As with other splints, selection of material and design should be carefully tailored to the client's needs. Materials may be thermoplastic, silicone rubber, plaster, fiberglass, cloth tape, or neoprene. Selection should be based on the degree of immobilization required, material durability and breathability, the player's sport position, governing rules of the sport, and the safety of other players.

Treatment of tendon injuries and repairs may involve static positioning to immobilize the tendon for healing or dynamic splinting to protect the tendon while allowing controlled motion to increase tendon repair strength and gliding. Flexor tendon repair protocols vary, but a

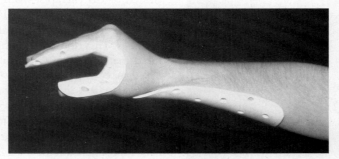

Figure 15-35 Custom thermoplastic "safe position" wrist–hand splint.

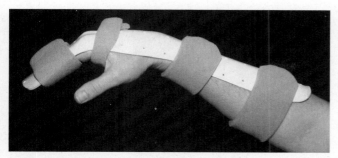

Figure 15-36 Custom thermoplastic dorsal blocking splint.

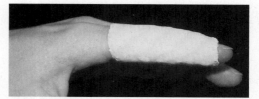

Figure 15-37 Plaster digit cast.

protective dorsal blocking splint (Fig. 15-36) positioning the wrist and MCPs in flexion and blocking the IP joints at 0° of extension is typically used. Rubber band traction may be added to hold the digits in a flexed position or to enable resistive extension and passive flexion exercises. The splint is usually custom fabricated from low-temperature thermoplastic and is often worn for as long as 6 weeks (Pettengill & van Strien, 2011).

Extensor tendon injuries involve treatment and splinting based on the level of injury. For injuries at the DIP level that may result in a mallet finger deformity, the DIP is immobilized for 6–8 weeks in a slightly hyperextended position (Evans, 2011a). The PIP joint is left free. The splints used may be volar or dorsal and may be prefabricated or custom fabricated from padded aluminum strips or thermoplastics. Excellent results for the treatment of mallet finger have been reported with various splints (Pike et al., 2010). For injuries

at the PIP level, treatment includes digital cast (Fig. 15-37) or splint immobilization with the PIP in absolute 0° of extension for 6–8 weeks to prevent boutonniere deformity. For more proximal tendon injuries, splinting may involve static positioning, dynamic assists, or both (Evans, 2011a).

Splinting is an integral part of postoperative MCP arthroplasty treatment. Early positioning and motion following arthroplasty often uses a dynamic MCP extension assist (Fig. 15-38) to support the wrist, control MCP position and alignment, allow guided motion, and assist with extensor power. This controlled stress allows for joint capsule remodeling over time (Lubahn, Wolfe, & Feldsher, 2011). Dynamic MCP extension assists may use high-profile or low-profile outrigger designs. They have slings to support the MCPs in neutral extension and deviation and to provide rotatory alignment. Outrigger kits are commercially available, or the outrigger may be hand fabricated. The dynamic extension splint may be supplemented by a static positioning splint at night (Fess et al., 2005; Lubahn, Wolfe, & Feldscher, 2011).

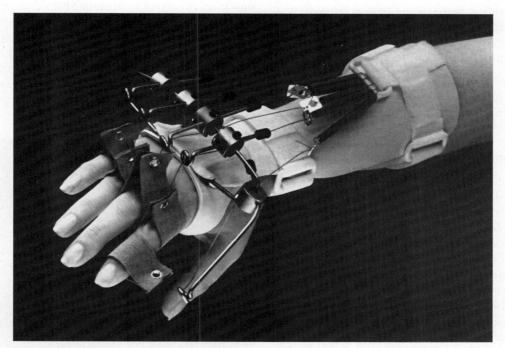

Figure 15-38 Custom thermoplastic low-profile dynamic MCP extension splint using Rolyan® adjustable Outrigger kit.

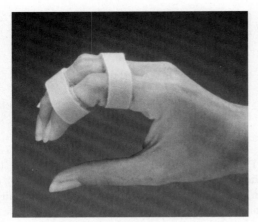

Figure 15-39 Rolyan® buddy straps.

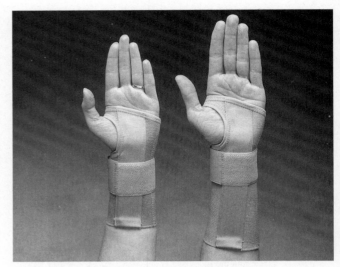

Figure 15-40 Liberty™ short and long elastic wrist braces.

To protect digits but allow for stabilization or controlled motion of the MCP, PIP, or DIP joints following injury or surgery, buddy straps (Fig. 15-39) (Jensen & Rayan, 1996), buddy sleeves (Bassini & Patel, 1994), or buddy splints (Lamay, 1994), which connect an injured finger to an adjacent finger, can be used. Common indications for these include stable fractures, PIP joint dislocations, collateral ligament injuries, and staged flexor tendon reconstructions (Beasley, 2011a; Fess et al., 2005)

Provide Stability or Restrict Unwanted Motion

Orthoses can be helpful in stabilizing joints when their integrity has been compromised by an acute injury or a chronic disease such as arthritis. Stabilization or restriction of motion can often greatly facilitate functional use of a limb.

Stabilize or Restrict Motion of the Shoulder or Elbow

In addition to the purposes previously described, slings, gunslingers, and hinged elbow orthoses can also be used to provide proximal stability that may enable improved distal function.

Stabilize or Restrict Motion of the Wrist or Hand

It is essential to determine the position in which a joint is to be supported relative to hand dominance and task requirements because specific functional demands vary greatly among individual clients. The wrist is considered by many to be the key to ultimate hand function, and wrist splints are commonly prescribed to provide stability. Dorsal wrist splints allow for the greatest palmar sensation but are least supportive, volar wrist splints are most commonly prescribed and provide a moderate amount of stability, and circumferential wrist splints provide the greatest amount of stability (Lohman, 2008a).

For optimum mechanical advantage to support the weight of the hand, the forearm portion of the splint

should be two-thirds the length of the forearm (Fess et al., 2005; Lohman, 2008a). Although greater length is believed to add to stability, studies have shown that a longer splint can decrease grip strength, slow finger dexterity, and decrease hand function speeds compared with a shorter wrist splint (Stern, 1996). For smaller or lighter hands and for clients who do not use their hands for high-demand activities, a shorter wrist support (Fig. 15-40) can increase comfort while being less obtrusive than a long splint (Melvin, 1995).

A lumbrical bar is a hand-based orthosis that extends over the dorsal aspect of the proximal phalanges to restrict unwanted hyperextension of the MCPs that can result from an ulnar nerve or combined median and ulnar nerve injury. By blocking this motion, IP flexion contractures can be prevented and functional hand opening can be improved as the power of the long finger extensors is transferred to the IPs for extension. Lumbrical bar orthoses using spring wire are commercially available (Fig. 15-41), but they tend

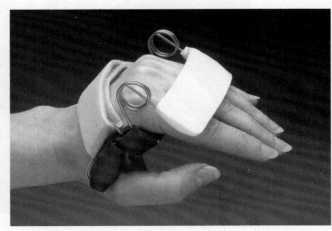

Figure 15-41 LMB MP flexion spring.

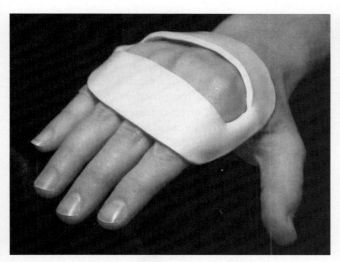

Figure 15-42 Custom thermoplastic lumbrical bar splint.

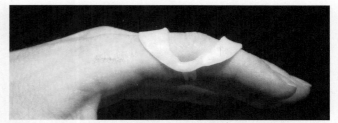

Figure 15-43 Custom thermoplastic PIP hyperextension block.

to be bulky and limit the ability to grasp objects. Custom-fabricated thermoplastic splints (Figs. 15-3 and 15-42) provide for a more intimate and streamlined fit (Duff & Estilow, 2011).

This same principle of restricting undesired motion is used in a PIP hyperextension block, also known as a swan-neck splint. Swan-neck deformities are common sequelae of RA and a possible complication following an extensor tendon injury or repair. These deformities often cause difficulty with hand closure, as PIP tendons and ligaments can catch during motion, and the finger flexors have less of a mechanical advantage to initiate flexion when the PIP is hyperextended. By blocking the PIP in a slightly flexed position, the client can flex the PIP more quickly and easily (Beasley, 2011b; Harrell, 2006).

For short-term use or for trial purposes, custom-fabricated thermoplastic swan-neck splints (Fig. 15-43) may suffice. For long-term use or for use on adjacent digits, commercial swan-neck splints are often recommended because they are more durable, less bulky, more easily cleaned, and more cosmetically appealing. Custom-ordered ring splints made of silver or gold (Fig. 15-44) are attractive, durable, streamlined, and adjustable for variations in joint swelling, but they are more costly. Silver splints have also been shown to improve dexterity (Zijlstra, Heijnsdijk-Rouwenhorst, & Rasker, 2004). Prefabricated splints made of polypropylene (Fig. 15-45), also available commercially, offer some of the benefits of silver splints with less cost. In a study comparing commercial silver and polypropylene splints, both were equally effective and acceptable to clients (van der Giesen et al., 2009). Heavy-duty metal splints, such as Murphy ring splints, may benefit clients who use their hands in highly demanding tasks. Swan-neck splints can also be used to provide lateral stability to unstable IP joints of the fingers or thumb.

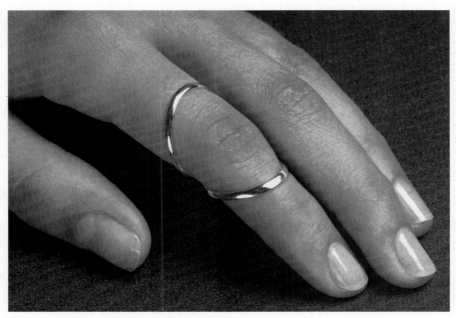

Figure 15-44 Siris™ Silver Swan neck splint.

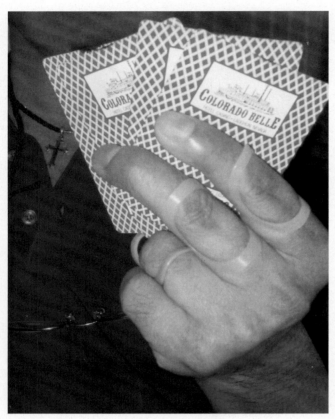

Figure 15-45 Oval-8™ commercial ring splints.

Flexible boutonniere deformities may benefit from boutonniere splinting to block the PIP in a more extended position to allow for greater functional hand opening. These may also be custom-made by the therapist or custom ordered from the companies that fabricate swan-neck splints (Fig. 15-46). Because there is direct pressure over the PIP, the dorsal skin must be carefully monitored for signs of breakdown.

Thumb stability is a requirement of almost all prehensile activities, so splinting of unstable thumb joints may have a particular value for function (Fess et al., 2005). Instability of the CMC often requires a long thumb splint that crosses the wrist because shorter splints may not adequately support the CMC. Short thumb spica splints (Fig. 15-25), also known as thumb posts or opponens splints, can provide MP stability and a stable post for pinching. Although a circumferential design is commonly used, problems with marked MP deformity can make donning and doffing of the splint difficult, and direct pressure over the MP may lead to breakdown of fragile skin.

Restore Mobility

Orthoses play an integral role in the restoration of mobility by correcting soft tissue or joint contractures that can occur as a result of poor positioning, trauma, scarring, or increased muscle tone, and there is evidence to support their use (Michlovitz, Harris, & Watkins, 2004). Devices providing low-load, prolonged stretch have proven to be effective in the contracture management of clients having a neurological or orthopedic disorder (Hill, 1994; Nuismer, Ekes, & Holm, 1997). As described earlier in this chapter, different types of splinting may be used: serial static plaster or thermoplastic, dynamic, and static progressive.

A therapist implementing a splinting program to regain motion must understand how splints work to affect positive change. Range of motion is gained not by tissue stretching but by actual tissue elongation from new cell

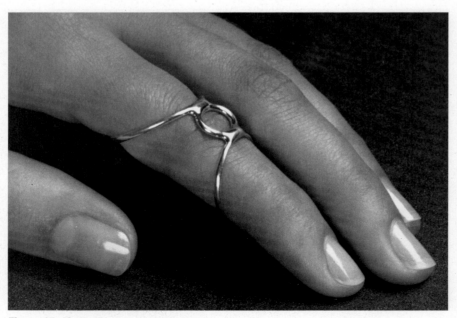

Figure 15-46 Siris™ silver boutonniere splint.

growth (Bell-Krotoski & Figarola, 1995; Fess et al., 2005). *Safety Message: The forces used must be gentle and carefully applied, and the tissue must be closely monitored for signs of excessive stress, such as redness and inflammation, which are indicators to change or stop treatment.* Inelastic mobilization applies constant forces needed to remodel tissues and is the most effective means for gaining motion in chronically stiff joints. Elastic mobilization is most indicated for acute joint stiffness or more supple joints because forces can be more easily controlled and fine adjustments made (Fess et al., 2005).

Fixed contractures and chronically stiff joints often respond best to inelastic mobilization from serial casting. Plaster is an ideal material because it conforms intimately and is more rigid than thermoplastics. Casts are changed as motion gains are achieved. In a systematic review of upper extremity casting in central nervous system disorders, there was insufficient high quality evidence on the long-term benefits from casting, and there was high variability in casting protocols (Lannin, Novak, & Cusick, 2007); therefore, it is not possible to make recommendations for practice.

Dynamic splinting is more effective when used for early contractures (Bell-Krotoski & Figarola, 1995; Glasgow et al., 2011). It allows for motion in the opposite direction, which helps prevent unwanted stiffness. Splints can also be removed for hygiene and function. Often, dynamic splints are worn at night so as not to interfere with use of the limb. This decrease in wearing time, however, means that tissues are not kept under constant tension, and less rapid gains may result. The amount and direction of force must be carefully monitored and adjusted as joint angles change.

Static progressive splinting is often indicated for fixed contractures. It has the advantage of being worn for shorter periods throughout the day, allowing for motion and functional use of the limb.

Restore Mobility of the Shoulder, Elbow, or Forearm

A serial static abduction splint can be used to apply pressure to and elongate burn scars in the axilla. The benefits of wearing this type of splint must be carefully weighed against the complete lack of function that it imposes. For flexion contractures of the elbow, thermoplastic anterior elbow extension splints (Fig. 15-34), serial casts or dropout casts, and dynamic elbow extension or static progressive elbow extension splints can be used.

Serial casting, which typically entails changing the cast weekly, can safely reposition joints without providing undue stress to tissues (Bell-Krotoski, 2011; Colditz, 2011). When the contracture is a result of increased tone, such as in the client with a brain injury, casting is often used in conjunction with nerve blocks or surgical procedures. *Safety Message: Great care must be taken with casting in the presence of severe tone, because pressure areas may develop.*

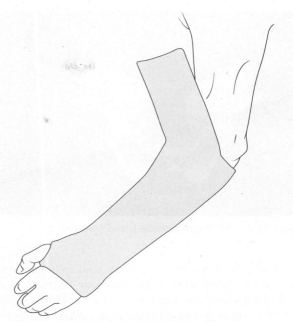

Figure 15-47 Plaster elbow dropout cast.

Dropout casts (Fig. 15-47) use the force of gravity to assist in reducing an elbow flexion contracture. The posterior portion of the cast above the elbow is removed, allowing the forearm to drop into extension. This type of casting is effective only if the client is upright most of the day.

A bivalved cast, also known as an anteroposterior splint (Fig. 15-48), is often used to maintain range of motion once it is achieved through casting or other means. This splint is well padded, with several straps holding the two halves together. The caregiver must be thoroughly trained so that it is applied properly and in the correct alignment to prevent pressure problems and skin breakdown.

Dynamic or static progressive splints (Fig. 15-49) have been reported to be successful in the treatment of elbow burn flexion contractures when static splinting was not effective. An average of 5°–10° can be gained per day (Richard, Shanesy, & Miller, 1995). They have also proven to be effective in the treatment of orthopedic and neurological flexion contractures (Marinelli et al., 2010; Nuismer, Ekes, & Holm, 1997). Elbow extension contractures, which are less commonly seen, can be treated with serial casting into flexion, dynamic flexion splinting, or static progressive splinting.

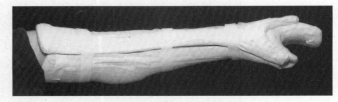

Figure 15-48 Fiberglass anteroposterior elbow splint with wrist and digits included.

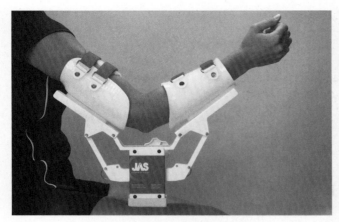

Figure 15-49 JAS Static Progressive Elbow™ orthosis.

Loss of forearm rotation, often seen following spinal cord injury, peripheral nerve injury, or fracture, can be treated with dynamic forearm rotation splinting. Splints can be custom fabricated (Fess et al., 2005) or obtained commercially as a preformed product or kit (Fig. 15-50). Altering the direction of force when using these splints can produce supination or pronation. A static progressive supination splint described by Murphy (1990) achieved favorable results.

Restore Mobility of the Wrist or Hand

Serial short arm casts, with or without the fingers or thumb included, can be used in the treatment of flexion or extension contractures related to increased muscle tone. Serial plaster slab splinting (Bell-Krotoski, 2011) can be especially effective in the presence of muscle–tendon unit shortening that can result in the inability to compositely flex or extend the wrist and fingers. Long flexor tightness can develop as a result of the wrist being in a prolonged position of flexion, such as with wrist drop from radial

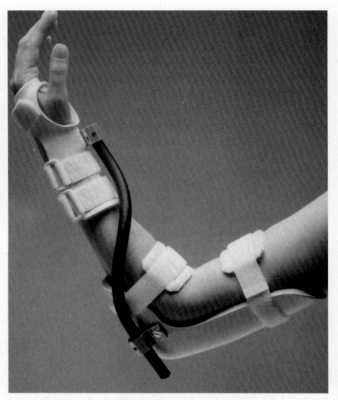

Figure 15-50 Rolyan® preformed dynamic pronation/supination splint.

nerve palsy, wrist fracture immobilization, and protective positioning following flexor tendon repair. A plaster slab splint or a volar thermoplastic splint that positions the wrist and fingers in maximum composite extension can help to correct tightness of the long finger flexors.

Serial static thermoplastic wrist splints, dynamic wrist splints (Fig. 15-51), and static progressive wrist splints can be used for limitations in wrist flexion or extension. These may be custom fabricated or preformed. Dynamic or

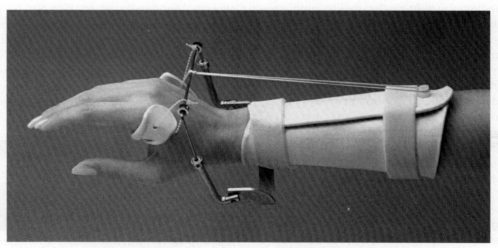

Figure 15-51 Custom thermoplastic dynamic wrist extension splint using Phoenix wrist hinge.

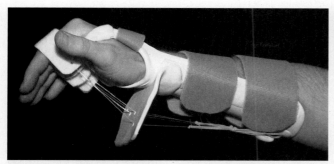

Figure 15-52 Custom thermoplastic dynamic MCP flexion splint.

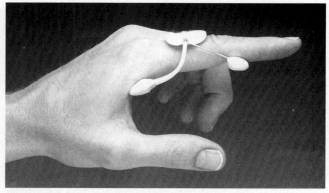

Figure 15-54 LMB spring finger extension assist.

static progressive component kits can also be purchased commercially. This allows the therapist to custom mold the splint bases while more easily assembling force units.

Lack of MCP flexion can devastate hand function. Many dynamic splint designs to regain MCP motion are available. Custom-fabricated thermoplastic splints use individual finger loops over the proximal phalanx (Fig. 15-52). Attached to these loops are rubber bands or springs that provide the needed force for sustained tension. An outrigger is used to direct the line of pull at 90°. It is important to clear the distal palmar crease so as not to block full flexion range of motion. These splints may be forearm based or hand based, depending on the mechanical advantage needed, any adhesions, and the client's wrist strength and stability (Fess et al., 2005).

Commercial hand-based dynamic splints use springs, coiled spring wire (Fig. 15-41), or rubber bands to provide flexion force to the MCPs as a unit. These splints are effective only if all MCPs are uniformly stiff. Some force adjustments can be made, but individual finger force amount or angle adjustments are not possible, as they are with custom-made thermoplastic splints having separate finger loops. Finger flexion gloves (Fig. 15-53), which incorporate

rubber band traction, can be used to gain composite flexion of all joints, but they have the most effect on the MCPs.

Limited PIP flexion makes grasp difficult, and limited PIP extension interferes with the ability to open the hand in preparation for grasp or to release objects. PIP flexion contractures are a frequent complication of trauma or poor positioning, and extension contractures can be seen following dorsal hand burns or prolonged immobilization for fracture management.

To address these contractures, forearm- or hand-based dynamic thermoplastic splints similar to those designed for MCP flexion and extension can be used by extending the distal part of the splint across the MCP to just proximal to the PIP joint. Immobilizing the MCP applies force to the PIP.

Prefabricated spring wire and spring coil splints are also available to gain flexion or extension range of motion. In a study of prefabricated spring wire (Fig. 15-54) and spring coil (Fig. 15-55) extension splints by Fess (1988), exerted forces were found to vary in the same splint design and to vary also according to the degree of joint contracture. Some forces were alarmingly high, well above recommended limits. Callahan and McEntee (1986) found similar

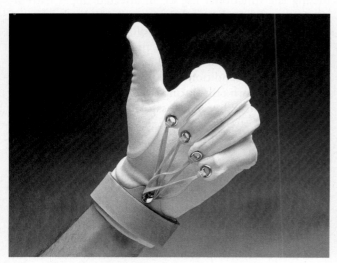

Figure 15-53 Finger flexion glove.

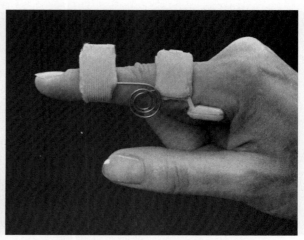

Figure 15-55 Rolyan® Sof-Stretch coil extension splint.

results and expressed concern about whether these splints fit accurately and about forces being distributed over small surface areas as compared with custom-fabricated splints. Designs have since been improved so that tension can be somewhat modified. If used, these splints must be carefully monitored to avoid further joint or tissue damage.

Spring coil extension splints, sometimes called Capener splints, may be custom fabricated and are described in the literature (Callahan & McEntee, 1986; Colditz, 2011). A study of dynamic splinting in the management of PIP flexion contractures using Capener and low-profile hand-based outrigger splints found the two to be equally effective, suggesting that the client may prefer the less bulky Capener splint if offered a choice (Prosser, 1996). Additional findings concluded that the longer the flexion contracture was present, the less it resolved and that splint wearing time was a significant factor affecting outcome. Glasgow et al. (2012) also found the duration of dynamic orthotic use to be a key factor in PIP joint contracture resolution, with flexion motion obtained more quickly than extension.

A commercial neoprene dynamic finger extension tube (Fig. 15-56) provides circumferential pressure and a dynamic force into extension via an angled seam on its volar surface. It may also offer other therapeutic values, such as heat, mild joint distraction, and longer tolerable wearing times (Clark, 1997). PIP extension can also be gained though serial plaster casting or splinting.

Thermoplastic gutter (Fig. 15-28) or circumferential splinting and dynamic traction splinting are useful in the treatment of mild contractures, whereas serial plaster digital casting (Fig. 15-37) has been advocated for moderate to severe contractures (Bell-Krotoski, 2011). Plaster casting offers the advantages of intimate conformity, rigidity, breathability, and uniform distribution of pressure. Casting does require the client's cooperation in keeping the cast dry, and casts have the disadvantage of not being removable for function or motion. For most effective results,

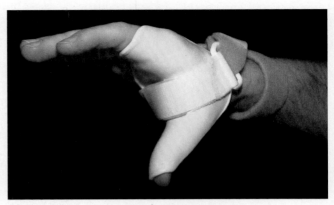

Figure 15-57 Custom thermoplastic thumb abduction splint.

casts should be changed every 2–7 days (Bell-Krotoski & Figarola, 1995) or sooner if they become loose or wet. The DIP joint may be left free if its motion is not limited. It is at times beneficial to involve the DIP in the cast if increased mechanical advantage is desired for PIP extension. Variations of many of these splints can be used for the treatment of DIP contractures or contractures of the thumb MP or IP.

Adduction contractures of the thumb, which are commonly seen in burns and nerve injuries, are most often treated with serial static thumb abduction splints, which conform to the first web space (Fig. 15-57). It is important to ensure that abduction forces are directed to the CMC joint by involving as much of the distal aspect of the first metacarpal as possible (Fess et al., 2005). Strapping must be designed to apply pressure in the proper direction and to prevent distal migration of the splint. This often requires a strap that crosses the wrist.

Substitute for Weak or Absent Muscles

Orthoses are commonly used to assist clients in maximizing the functional use of an affected upper extremity. Orthoses may be used temporarily, as in the case of recovering nerve injuries or neurological diseases such as Guillain-Barré, or they may be prescribed for long-term use, such as in complete spinal cord injury or progressive neuromuscular conditions like postpolio syndrome. They are generally worn only during the day or for specific functional tasks. An orthosis successful in improving the ability to function is often much more accepted and appreciated by the client than orthoses prescribed for other purposes.

Substitute for Weak or Absent Shoulder or Elbow Muscles

Proximal arm devices can support the shoulder and forearm to encourage motion of weak proximal musculature, allow for distal function, and enable occupational performance as well as prevent loss of motion and provide pain relief.

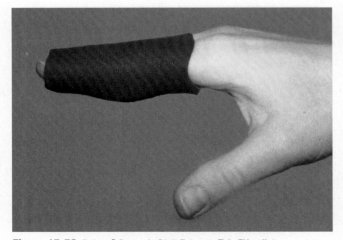

Figure 15-56 Rolyan® Dynamic Digit Extensor Tube™ splint.

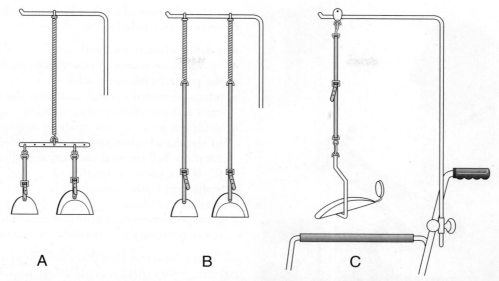

Figure 15-58 Suspension arm devices. **A.** Suspension sling with horizontal bar. **B.** Suspension sling without horizontal bar. **C.** Suspension arm support. (Adapted with permission from Redford, J. B. [Ed.]. [1986]. *Orthotics etcetera* [3rd ed.]. Baltimore: Williams & Wilkins.)

Suspension arm devices (Fig. 15-58) suspend from above the head, generally on an overhead rod that is mounted to a wheelchair. The arm swings as in a pendulum from straps attached to the overhead rod. *Safety Message: Contraindications to use include glenohumeral joint instability, and care must be used to ensure that the humeral head does not sublux or impinge on the supraspinatus when the arm is in the device.*

The suspension sling with a single strap suspended from the overhead rod has a horizontal balance bar with multiple holes for adjustment of the fulcrum and supports separate wrist and elbow cuffs. The suspension sling without horizontal bar has two straps that originate directly from the overhead rod with cuffs to support the elbow and wrist. The suspension arm support has a forearm trough suspended from a single point on the overhead rod. These can be easily attached to the wheelchair upright or to an overhead frame on the client's bed. Springs of various tensions may be added to the straps that support the limb, allowing a client with only slight active motion to produce accelerated shoulder movement by bouncing the arm up and down. Suspension devices can be adjusted to allow for certain motions (Procedures for Practice 15-2) but lack the fine adjustment that extremely weak clients may need.

A mobile arm support (MAS) (Fig. 15-59) is a mechanical device that supports the weight of the arm and provides assistance to shoulder and elbow motions through a linkage of ball-bearing joints (Mulcahey, 2008; Yasuda, Bowman, & Hsu, 1986). The MAS is

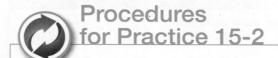

Procedures for Practice 15-2

How to Adjust Suspension Arm Devices

Suspension Arm Sling

- For horizontal abduction, rotate the overhead rod laterally.
- For horizontal adduction, rotate the overhead rod medially.
- For external rotation, move the arm cuffs back on the balance bar to shift weight toward the elbow.
- For internal rotation, move the arm cuffs forward on the balance bar to shift weight toward the hand.
- For elbow flexion, move the point of suspension backward on the overhead rod to put the hand toward the client's face.
- For elbow extension, move the point of suspension forward on the overhead rod to put the hand away from the client's face.
- For height adjustments, vary the length of the strap or straps that connect to the overhead rod, or raise or lower the bracket on the wheelchair upright.

Suspension Arm Support

- For horizontal motion and height adjustments, see list under Suspension Arm Sling.
- For elbow flexion, move the rocker arm farther from the trough elbow dial.
- For elbow extension, move the rocker arm closer to the trough elbow dial.

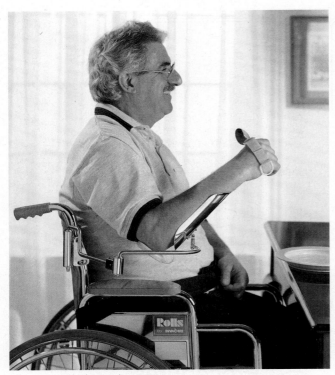

Figure 15-59 Mobile arm support.

typically mounted to a client's wheelchair, but it can also be attached to a tabletop or even a floor stand for trial use (Fig. 15-60). The mechanical principles are three-fold: (1) use of gravity to assist weak muscles, (2) support of the arm to reduce the load on weak muscles,

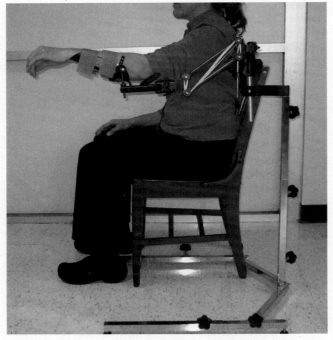

Figure 15-60 JAECO/Rancho MultiLink MAS with elevation assist on floor stand.

and (3) reduction of friction by using ball-bearing joints. Criteria for use include:

- a defined functional need
- an adequate source of power from neck, trunk, shoulder girdle, or elbow muscles
- adequate motor control such that the client can contract and relax functioning muscles
- sufficient passive joint range of motion, with 0°–90° of shoulder flexion and abduction, 0°–30° of external rotation, full internal rotation and elbow flexion, and 0°–80° of pronation preferred
- stable trunk positioning
- a motivated client
- a supportive environment that provides the client with the opportunity and assistance to use the device

Clients who may benefit include those with cervical spinal cord injury (Atkins et al., 2008), muscular dystrophy, Guillain-Barré syndrome, amyotrophic lateral sclerosis, poliomyelitis, and polymyositis.

Selection of MAS components, assembly of parts, and balance and adjustment of the MAS generally requires postgraduate hands-on training. Balance and adjustment principles are presented in Procedures for Practice 15-3 to give the reader a basic overview and appreciation for what is possible. This does not negate the need for additional training or consultation with experienced therapists to ensure that the best possible adjustments are made to give the client maximal mechanical advantage.

The standard MAS assembly described in this chapter consists of an adjustable arm positioner bracket (also known as a semireclining bracket), standard proximal and distal arms, a standard rocker arm assembly, and a basic forearm trough (Fig. 15-61). The many commonly used special MAS component parts include the outside rocker arm assembly and the elevating proximal arm (Fig. 15-62). The outside rocker arm (or offset swivel) has a ball-bearing joint that allows for greater freedom in vertical motion, thus facilitating hand-to-mouth or hand-to-table movements. The elevating proximal arm is useful for a client with poor to fair deltoid strength. As the client initiates the elevating motion, the rubber band assists, allowing the client to flex and abduct the humerus to a higher level.

A newer MAS system that is less complicated and more user friendly is available in standard (Fig. 15-63) and elevating models (Fig. 15-60). Advantages are their more contemporary appearance, streamlined design, and ease of adjustments (JAECO, 2008).

For a client who can walk, a gunslinger orthosis can provide both proximal stability and mobility. This type of shoulder–elbow orthosis consists of a metal forearm trough that is mechanically coupled to a plastic hemigirdle anchored on the client's pelvis. This device is most useful for clients having good distal function but proximal weakness from brachial plexus injuries, spinal cord injuries, or postpolio syndrome. Prefabricated gunslingers

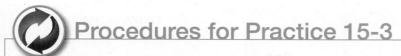

Procedures for Practice 15-3

Mobile Arm Support Assembly and Training Principles

How to Assemble and Balance the Standard Mobile Arm Support Assembly

- Assemble tools (Phillips and flathead screwdrivers and Allen wrenches) and mobile arm support (MAS) parts (bracket, proximal arm, distal arm, rocker arm, and trough).
- Inspect ball-bearing components for smooth operation.
- Ensure that the client is seated properly in the wheelchair, with pelvis well back in chair and trunk in good vertical alignment.
- Fit the trough to the client's arm by bending the elbow dial toward the radial side of the trough.
- Attach the rocker arm to the trough by placing the screws in the third and fifth holes from the dial.
- Attach the bracket to the wheelchair at approximately the midhumerus level so that it is neutrally rolled[1] and pitched.[2]
- Attach the proximal arm to the bracket.
- Attach the distal arm to the proximal arm.
- Attach the trough to the distal arm.
- Balance the arm support to neutral by adjusting the pitch of the bracket and the distal end of the proximal arm so that the bearing tubes are perpendicular to the floor.
- Place the client's arm in the trough.
- Observe for abnormal shoulder elevation, and adjust the height of the bracket as needed to correct it.

Mobile Arm Support Hand-to-Mouth Movement Pattern

Instructions to Client
- Push down on the trough dial while adducting your humerus.
- Externally rotate your shoulder.
- Shift your body weight toward the MAS.
- Straighten up or lean back in your chair.
- Rotate your trunk toward the MAS.
- Turn your head toward the MAS.

Equipment Adjustments to Aid This Motion
- Move the rocker arm farther from the trough elbow dial.
- Pitch the MAS at the bracket assembly toward the wheelchair back.
- Raise the bracket assembly on the wheelchair upright.

[1] Roll is the rotation of the bracket assembly on the wheelchair upright governing the side-to-side (horizontal) slope. The name comes from the side-to-side swaying of a ship.
[2] Pitch is the tilt of the ball-bearing tube on the bracket assembly governing the upward-downward (vertical) slope. The name comes from the backward-forward pitch of a ship as it goes over waves.

Mobile Arm Support Hand-to-Table Movement Pattern

Instructions to Client
- Lift and internally rotate your shoulder to lower your hand.
- Shift your body weight away from the MAS.
- Roll your shoulder forward.
- Rotate your trunk away from the MAS.
- Tilt or turn your head away from the MAS.

Equipment Adjustments to Aid This Motion
- Move the rocker arm closer to the trough elbow dial.
- Pitch the MAS at the bracket assembly toward the client's feet.
- Lower the bracket assembly on the wheelchair upright.

Mobile Arm Support Horizontal Abduction and Adduction Movement Patterns

Instructions to Client
- Shift your body weight in the direction you want to move.
- Rotate your trunk toward the direction you want to move.
- Turn your head briskly in the direction you want to move.

Equipment Adjustments to Aid This Motion

- Roll the bracket assembly on the wheelchair upright toward the client for adduction.
- Roll the bracket assembly on the wheelchair upright away from the client for abduction.

Mobile Arm Support Controls Training and Use Training

Controls Training
- Teach the client the effects of head, trunk, and proximal movements on the movement of the MAS.
- If bilateral MASs are used, begin with one side first.
- Begin with horizontal motions by having the client practice moving the MAS as far as possible from side to side and front to back.
- Proceed with vertical motions by having the client practice moving the hand to the table and up to the mouth at various points within the horizontal range.

Use Training
- Teach the client to use the MAS for specific desired functional activities, such as eating, grooming, writing, keyboarding, texting, page turning, and power wheelchair driving.
- Encourage practice and independent problem-solving skills.

(Fig. 15-11) are commercially available, but for long-term use, a custom-designed orthosis (Fig. 15-12) is indicated.

Depending on the client's proximal muscle status and specific functional needs, the coupling between the trough and hemigirdle base can be customized to permit a variety of motions, such as glenohumeral internal–external rotation and flexion–extension. It can also be made to hold a very weak shoulder in a static position for function, which may be with the hand in midline. If the wrist also has weakness, the trough can be extended to support the hand. Usefulness must be determined for each individual case, considering factors

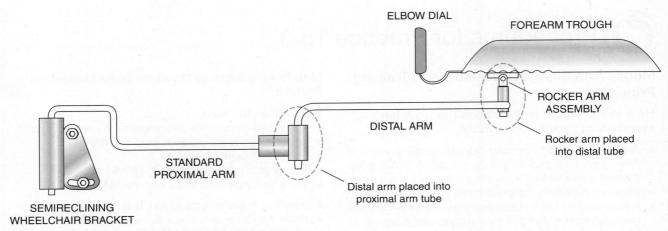

Figure 15-61 Standard components of a mobile arm support.

such as acceptance by the client, ease of donning, cost, and especially, functional benefit.

Substitute for Weak or Absent Wrist or Hand Muscles

The combination of sensory loss and motor imbalance caused by a peripheral nerve injury greatly impairs normal hand function. As Colditz (2002/2011) points out, it is impossible to build an external device that can substitute for the intricately balanced muscles that a splint attempts to replace. In splinting nerve palsies, the key concept is to understand the client's condition and neuromuscular status so as to prescribe or design an appropriate splint to increase function. Splints should keep areas of intact

sensibility free if possible, should be as simple as possible, and should not immobilize joints unnecessarily. The splinting program must be closely monitored and altered in response to nerve recovery as the client's muscle status changes (see the Case Example). In a study to assess factors that influenced splint wear in peripheral nerve lesions, the only significant variable was a positive effect as perceived by the client; 52% of clients reported terminating wear because splints hindered their daily life and 23% reported terminating wear because splints had not been of any use. Interestingly, the highest effectiveness score was for day splints for the dominant hand aimed at replacing function (Paternostro-Sluga et al., 2003).

Radial nerve palsy, commonly associated with humeral fractures, can result in the complete loss or partial weakness

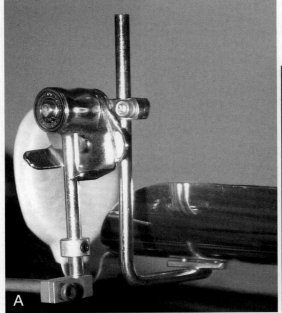

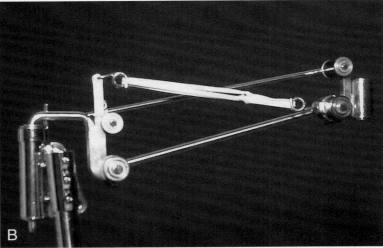

Figure 15-62 Special mobile arm support components: **A.** Outside rocker arm. **B.** Elevating proximal arm.

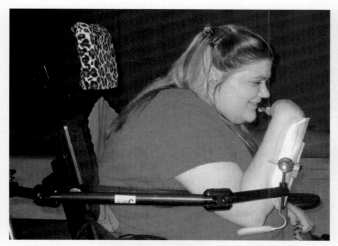

Figure 15-63 JAECO/Rancho MultiLink MAS.

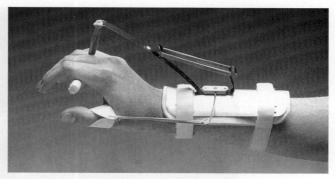

Figure 15-64 Bunnell™ Thomas suspension splint.

of wrist, finger, and thumb extensors and weakness of forearm supination and thumb abduction. The loss of wrist extensor strength devastates hand grasp. Not only is the client unable to position the hand properly, but the inability to stabilize the wrist in extension impairs normal function of the long finger flexors. Loss of extrinsic finger extension is much less of a functional problem, because the unaffected intrinsic muscles can actively extend the IPs. Supporting the wrist in extension is the primary goal of radial nerve splinting, and the use of a simple static wrist splint may suffice in improving hand function (Fess et al., 2005).

Prefabricated radial nerve splints, such as a Thomas suspension splint (Fig. 15-64) or a wire-foam splint, are designed to dynamically extend the wrist, MCPs, and thumb. It is usually preferable not to include the thumb because of the limitation in intrinsic motion it imposes and

the danger of stressing the MP collateral ligament through poorly directed forces. Adding individual finger loops to the palmar bar, thus removing bulk in the palm and allowing individual finger motion, can enhance the Thomas suspension splint. The palmar bulk of the wire-foam splint often impedes the ability to grasp large objects. *Safety Message: Caution should be used when prescribing a dynamic orthosis because strong unopposed flexors may easily overcome the dynamic forces trying to hold the wrist and hand in extension, negating functional benefits.*

A custom-fabricated radial nerve splint, also known as a Colditz splint, has been designed to allow for partial wrist and full finger motion and a facsimile of a normal tenodesis effect (Fig. 15-65). This splint consists of a low-profile outrigger attached to a dorsal forearm base (Figs. 15-5 and 15-66). Nonelastic cords connect the splint base to finger loops. The cord length is adjusted so that, when the MCPs actively flex, the wrist is brought into extension. Conversely, when the wrist flexes, the cord

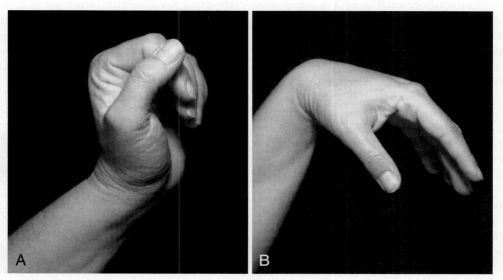

Figure 15-65 Normal tenodesis effect. **A.** When the wrist is extended, the fingers flex. **B.** When the wrist is flexed, the fingers extend.

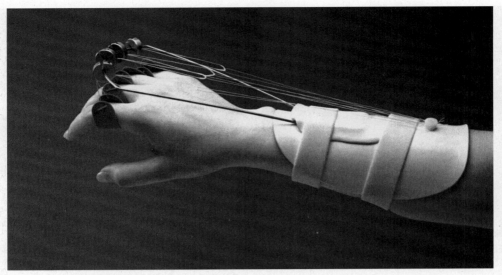

Figure 15-66 Custom thermoplastic radial nerve splint using low-profile Phoenix extended outrigger.

tension causes the MCPs to extend. Little training is required for the client to be able to use the splint functionally, and grasp and release of objects is greatly enhanced. Further advantages of this splint are the maintenance of normal hand arches, the absence of splinting material covering the palm, the low-profile design, and the facilitation of wrist extensor strength as return of nerve function occurs (Colditz, 2002/2011). Preformed splints and outrigger kits are commercially available.

Splinting in median nerve palsy is geared toward substituting for weak or absent thenar muscles that render the thumb unable to pull away from the palm and oppose to the fingers. This is most often accomplished through a custom-fabricated thermoplastic opponens splint, which stabilizes the thumb in a position of abduction and opposition to enable pulp-to-pulp pinch (Fig. 15-25). Although such a splint often greatly improves fine motor prehension, this must be individually assessed, because substitution patterns from unaffected thumb muscles may provide sufficient thumb function (Colditz, 2002/2011; Fess et al., 2005). Clients may choose to wear an opposition splint for selected activities only.

In the presence of ulnar nerve palsy, the hand assumes a claw position, or intrinsic-minus position, with ring and small finger hyperextension of the MCPs and flexion of the IPs. This is a result of weakness or loss of lumbrical and interossei muscles, which are responsible for MCP flexion and IP extension. The prime splinting objective is to assist in grasp and release of objects by preventing the claw position. This is accomplished by a lumbrical bar splint, which blocks the MCPs in slight flexion, allowing the force of the unaffected long finger extensors to extend the IPs.

Dynamic splints, such as prefabricated spring wire splints (Fig. 15-41), do not work well because the spring tension is usually not sufficient to hold the MCPs in flexion when the

client actively opens the hand. Thus, the MCPs hyperextend against the force, which actually strengthens the long extensors and encourages deformity (Colditz, 2002/2011).

A static custom-molded thermoplastic splint is advocated as the best solution. It should be nonbulky, carefully molded to distribute pressure evenly over the dorsum of the proximal phalanges, and designed so as not to obstruct full flexion of all joints (Colditz, 2002/2011; Fess et al., 2005). The splint may include just the affected ring and small fingers (Figs. 15-3 and 15-67) or may include all fingers to distribute pressure more effectively and comfortably (Fig. 15-42). The latter splint is used in the treatment of combined median and ulnar nerve injuries, which result in the clawing of all four fingers.

For a client who has only radial nerve function, a custom-fabricated Rehabilitation Institute of Chicago (RIC) tenodesis splint (Fig. 15-68) may be used. This splint can provide minimal hand grasp by harnessing the power of the wrist extensors to bring the thumb, index finger, and long finger into a functional pinch. It has three molded thermoplastic pieces: one to position the thumb, one to position the index and long fingers, and a wrist cuff to

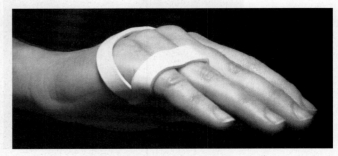

Figure 15-67 Custom thermoplastic lumbrical bar splint for ring and small fingers.

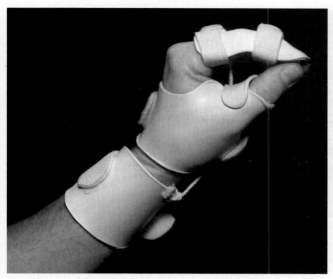

Figure 15-68 Custom thermoplastic RIC tenodesis splint.

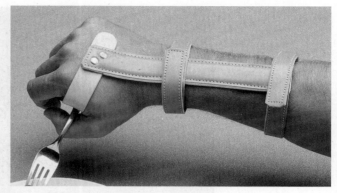

Figure 15-69 Wrist support with universal cuff.

serve as the base for connecting a static line from the wrist to the fingers (Colditz, 2002/2011).

Static orthoses, which allow passive holding of functional implements such as utensils or pens, may also be used in the presence of wrist or hand weakness. Examples include a hand-based universal cuff, a wrist support with universal cuff (Fig. 15-69), and a short or long design Wanchik writing splint (Fig. 15-70).

For clients with long-term or permanent loss of muscle function, as is the case of complete spinal cord injury or progressive neuromuscular disease, permanent functional orthoses may be used. These orthoses are fabricated by experienced orthotists from metal and are recommended by occupational therapists for individual clients based on neuromuscular status and specific functional needs. Often, these distal orthoses are used in conjunction with

proximal ones (such as a MAS) if proximal weakness is also present. Although they are now less frequently used than in years past, they remain an option for select circumstances.

A ratchet WHO (Fig. 15-71) may be used for clients with weak (below grade 3) wrist extension and finger strength, such as that seen with C5 tetraplegia (see Chapter 38). A thumb post positions the thumb in abduction and in alignment with the index and long fingers, and a finger piece assembly maintains the index and long fingers in a position for pinch. A ratchet system is used to close the hand in discrete increments. Closing is accomplished by manually pushing the finger piece to flex the fingers against the thumb using the contralateral hand, the chin, or the side of a table or chair. Release is accomplished by a spring that is activated by the press of a release button (Lunsford & DiBello, 2008).

For clients with the potential for neurological return at the C6 level, a wrist-action WHO (Fig. 15-72) can be used as a transition system (Lunsford & DiBello, 2008). This orthosis allows for free wrist motion, with stops that can be adjusted to limit motion to a prescribed range. When no wrist extensors are present, the wrist is locked into a set position.

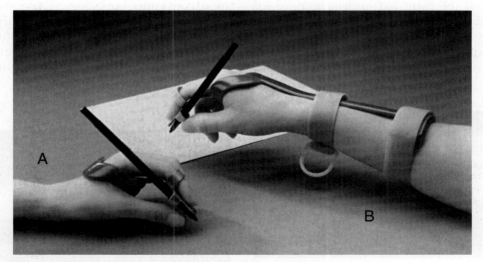

Figure 15-70 Wanchik writing splints. **A.** Short design. **B.** Long design.

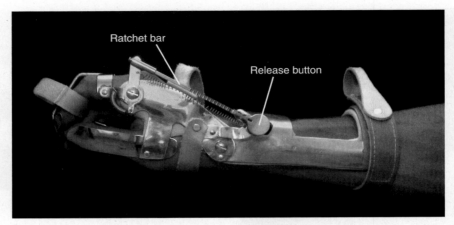

Figure 15-71 Custom metal ratchet wrist–hand orthosis.

As recovery occurs and strength increases, progressive range of motion is allowed. Rubber bands are often attached to provide an extensor assist to weak muscles.

A wrist-driven wrist–hand orthosis (WDWHO) (Fig. 15-73) may be indicated for clients having 3+ or greater wrist extensor strength, such as a client with C6 tetraplegia. Using the principle of tenodesis (Fig. 15-65), this type of flexor hinge orthosis transfers wrist extensor power to the fingers for grasping. Active wrist extension operates a mechanical linkage transferring power to flex the index and long fingers against the thumb. A properly adjusted orthosis allows for 1 pound of pinch for every 2 pounds of wrist extensor force. Gravity-assisted wrist flexion opens the hand for release. An activating lever at the wrist controls the size of the opening and the resultant position of prehension to allow for grasp of various size objects and different pinch forces.

Fitting the client with bilateral WDWHOs is rare and requires a highly motivated client (Lunsford & DiBello, 2008). Bilateral orthoses are difficult to use, requiring a great deal of balance, coordination, and practice to become successful. If the client has inadequate proximal strength, it may be difficult to bring the arms into midline. If sensation has been lost, the client must rely on visual compensation, which also makes bilateral orthotic use difficult. A client generally uses one WDWHO, with the contralateral hand serving as a gross assist. Training principles are listed in Procedures for Practice 15-4.

Given the cost and complexity of fabrication and training, follow-up studies have been done to assess whether clients use WDWHOs over the long term after discharge from therapy. Knox, Engel, and Seibens (1971) reported a 51% continued use rate; Shepherd and Ruzicka (1991) reported a 50% rate; and Allen (1971) reported a 43% rate. Factors that were reported to contribute to continued use were education, commitment, and involving the client in the orthotic decision-making process (Knox, Engel, & Seibens, 1971); the ability to don the orthosis easily (Allen, 1971); and adequate training, acceptance, internal motivation, and strong functional or vocational goals (Shepherd & Ruzicka, 1991). In these same studies, reasons for orthotic discontinuation were stated by subjects to be improvement in muscle strength, use of alternative methods or equipment to perform tasks previously done with the WDWHO, poor fit, bulk, and the orthosis taking too long to put on. Orthotic intervention remains a mainstay in spinal cord injury, but lack of evidence and inadequate clinician education in how to train clients in permanent functional orthoses have limited their use (Mulcahey, 2008).

Newer orthoses are now available aimed at facilitating distal motion and motor reeducation in neurologically

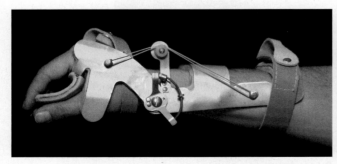

Figure 15-72 Custom metal wrist-action wrist–hand orthosis with rubber band assist.

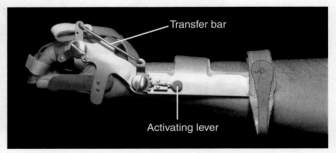

Figure 15-73 Custom metal wrist-driven wrist–hand orthosis.

Procedures for Practice 15-4

Wrist-Driven Wrist–Hand Orthosis Controls Training and Use Training

Controls Training

- The client needs to become proficient in basic orthotic skills, such as picking up, placing, and releasing objects of various sizes, textures, densities, and weights.
- Soft medium-sized objects or 1-inch firm, semirough objects are often best to start with; progress to more difficult objects as skill level increases.
- Encourage skills practice from a variety of heights because the client may have to learn to abduct and internally rotate the shoulder to approach and handle objects appropriately.

Use Training

- Teach the client to use the wrist-driven wrist–hand orthosis to perform specific functional tasks, such as writing, eating, and oral hygiene.
- Have the client practice activities under various conditions to encourage independent problem solving and spontaneous use of the orthosis.

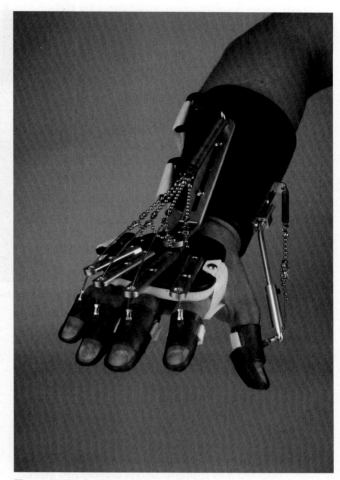

Figure 15-74 SaeboFlex dynamic orthosis.

imparied upper extremities. The SaeboFlex (Fig. 15-74) dynamic orthosis uses a fixed wrist support and a finger/thumb spring system that assists with opening the hand during grasp and release activities. The Ness H200 Hand Rehabilitation System (Fig.15-75) supports the wrist in a functional position and uses low-level electrical stimulation to assist finger and thumb motion. Specialty training in fitting and use of these devices is required, and evidence of their efficacy is limited pending more independent studies (Alon, Levitt, & McCarthy, 2007; Farrell et al., 2007).

Prevent Contractures or Modify Tone

Careful attention to positioning in the presence of wound healing, muscle imbalance, abnormal muscle tone caused by stroke or brain injury, or motor disorders such as cerebral palsy is critical in the prevention of loss of range of motion, which can lead to functional or skin hygiene problems. Many of the static splints, casts, and orthoses previously mentioned for immobilization, stabilization, or substitution can be used for this purpose. Examples of these orthoses include acute burn immobilization splints to prevent wrist and digital contractures, wrist extension splints to prevent contractures caused by wrist drop, thumb abduction splints to prevent thumb adduction contractures, and lumbrical bar splints to prevent MCP hyperextension and IP flexion contractures.

Ideally, these splints should not limit function, exert excessive stress on soft tissues, or interfere with movement of uninvolved joints. If splints are not required for functional use, often it is possible for clients to wear static positioning splints at night only. In addition to the prevention of contractures, splints may be used to prevent shortening of the muscle–tendon unit. For example, a volar thermoplastic or

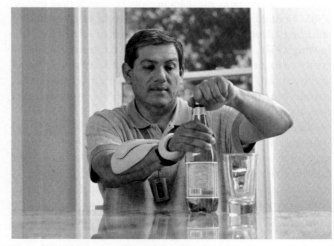

Figure 15-75 Ness H200® hand rehabilitation system.

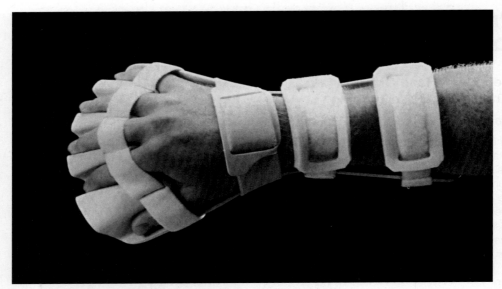

Figure 15-76 Rolyan® antispasticity ball splint with slot and loop strapping.

plaster splint worn at night to position the wrist and fingers in maximum composite extension can help to prevent tightness of the long finger flexors (Bell-Krotoski, 2011).

Lapboards, arm troughs, and suspension arm slings can help to position the upper extremities properly. Bivalved plaster casts or anteroposterior splints (Fig. 15-48) can be used to maintain range of motion, especially in the presence of increased tone. *Safety Message: Care must be taken to avoid pressure problems by ensuring that casts are properly padded and that the skin is closely monitored.*

The use of splinting in the modification of tone in the wrist and hand continues to be controversial in the literature and in practice. A survey of occupational therapists clearly demonstrated the conflicting practices in splinting (Neuhaus et al., 1981). Opponents of splinting argue that splinting may lead to increased muscle tone, joint stiffness, and muscle atrophy and may interfere with treatment aimed at facilitation and functional use. Proponents of splinting contend that splinting can reduce tone (McPherson, Becker, & Franszczak, 1985; Neuhaus et al., 1981). In a systematic review of hand splinting to prevent contracture and reduce spasticity following stroke, Lannin and Herbert (2003) found insufficient evidence to either support or refute its effectiveness. Tyson and Kent (2011) concluded from their systemtic review that current evidence suggests splinting does not improve function, motion, or pain following stroke.

Literature regarding optimal thermoplastic splint designs and wearing times shows no consensus. Static designs may be volar or dorsal, and comparative studies have been done in attempts to determine quantitatively which design is more effective in tone reduction. A study by McPherson et al. (1982) demonstrated no significant difference between the two basic splint designs and encouraged therapists to reexamine the amount of wearing time prescribed so that tonal reduction occurs without unwarranted secondary stiffness.

A design clinically studied by McPherson (1981) used a dorsal forearm base, volar finger and thumb pans, and finger abductors to position the wrist in 30° of extension, the MCPs in 45° of flexion, the IPs in full extension, the fingers fully abducted, and the thumb in extension and abduction. McPherson reported that splint wearing resulted in a reduction of tone related to the length of time that subjects wore the splint and that the effects of splint wearing were not necessarily permanent.

Garros, Gagliardi, and Guzzo (2010) also studied a volar dorsal orthosis worn by clients with wrist and hand spasticity post stroke. The results showed an increase in client-rated occupational performance at 3 months, but no longer term follow-up was done.

Common static splint designs include resting pan splints, finger spreaders or abduction splints, and cone splints (Coppard & Lohman, 2008). Several preformed splints are commercially available (Figs. 15-76 and 15-77), but no clinical studies have been done to establish their fit and effectiveness.

Dynamic splint designs have also been developed to reduce tone in the wrist and hand. In a study of eight

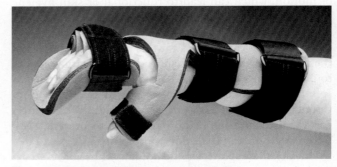

Figure 15-77 Progress™ dorsal antispasticity splint.

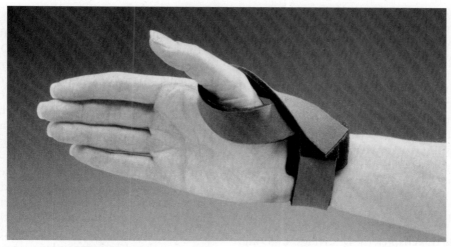

Figure 15-78   Rolyan® thumb loop.

subjects, the finding was a greater reduction in hypertonus using a dynamic splint as compared with static splints and passive range of motion (McPherson, Becker, & Franszczak, 1985). Scherling and Johnson (1989) studied the effects of their dynamic splint design on 18 subjects, with all subjects achieving varying degrees of tone reduction with a minimum of 4 hours of splint use per day.

Soft splints made of neoprene can be custom fabricated (Casey & Kratz, 1988) or purchased commercially. A hand-based thumb loop can be used to decrease tone and position the thumb out of the palm for function (Fig. 15-78). To position the forearm, a long neoprene strap can be added to the hand splint.

A thermoplastic hand-based inhibitive weight-bearing splint described in the treatment of children with increased flexor tone (Coppard & Lohman, 2008; Kinghorn & Roberts, 1996) can also be used with adult clients having hypertonicity. This volar splint is custom fabricated to hold the fingers in extension and thumb in radial abduction to enable the hand to be in an optimum position for upper extremity weight-bearing activities (Fig. 15-79).

Splinting may be an effective means of providing a low-cost, noninvasive method for decreasing tone in some clients but may not be effective in others (Langlois, Pederson, & Mackinnon, 1991). Continued research on the long-term effectiveness of splinting for tone reduction and the key client variables that contribute to that effectiveness is needed. Meanwhile, therapists must carefully decide on splint use and monitor outcomes client by client.

SPECIALIZED PERMANENT FUNCTIONAL ORTHOSES

Permanent functional orthoses represent a great investment of time, cost, expertise, and commitment to fabrication, fit, training, and use by the client-therapist-orthotist team. Proper fit, training, and successful functional use are accomplished only through close collaboration and communication among all who participate in the process. As with all orthoses, this process should begin with careful consideration of functional needs, achievable goals, and education of the client and significant others in orthotic purpose and selection. Providing the client with opportunities to interact with experienced users of similar equipment can be quite helpful to the client, both before the prescription and during training.

A permanent orthosis that is useful to the client must be valued, accepted, and incorporated into the client's body image. A prime prerequisite to acceptance is that the orthosis allows the client to do something meaningful that cannot otherwise be done without it (Yasuda, Bowman, & Hsu, 1986). Because the orthosis will be used over the long term, the client and caregivers must also be

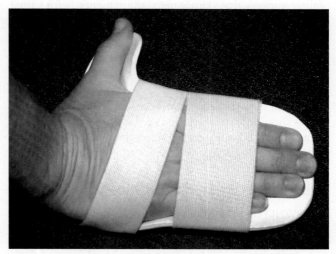

Figure 15-79   Custom thermoplastic hand-based weight-bearing splint.

educated about whom to contact should problems arise after the therapy program has ended.

The principles of orthotic training are similar to those of prosthetics. They include testing of fit and mechanics, teaching the client the names and functions of component parts, care of the orthosis, donning and doffing of the orthosis, controls training, and functional use training. Intensive practice under various conditions to encourage independent problem solving by the client and skilled spontaneous use is a key element of training. Following is a closer look at two commonly used permanent functional orthoses.

Mobile Arm Supports

As described earlier in this chapter, the MAS (Figs. 15-59 and 15-61) is a mechanical device prescribed to support the weight of an arm and assist weak proximal muscles for function.

Client and Caregiver Education

If the client has been actively involved in the decision making, a brief review of the MAS's purpose and capabilities should be sufficient. The client and caregiver should be oriented to key component names and how they operate. Finally, they should know how to care for and maintain the orthosis.

Assembling and Balancing

Procedures for Practice 15-3 has instructions on how to assemble and balance the standard MAS assembly.

Training and Adjusting

Adaptive equipment or a WHO is commonly used in conjunction with the MAS and should be integrated during all phases of MAS training and adjusting. Once the client is proficient with basic movement patterns, MAS training with all of the occupations that the client is interested in performing should be done. Any of these activities may require various fine component adjustments before final MAS adjustments are completed. Periodic follow-up may be required. Procedures for Practice 15-3 has information related to MAS training and adjusting.

Orthotic Checkout

Once final adjustments have been completed, bolts and screws should be checked for a secure fit. A MAS appraisal form (Fig. 15-80) can be used to ensure that all important details are assessed.

Wrist-Driven Wrist–Hand Orthosis

A WDWHO (Fig. 15-73), as previously described, is used to enhance hand function in the presence of distal muscle weakness by using wrist extensor power to enable prehension.

Orthotic Checkout

The therapist must begin with a careful inspection of the orthosis both on and off the client. Optimal fit is crucial for maximum function. Ensuring smooth operation of mechanical parts, proper positioning of the digits for pad to pad prehension, and proper location of splint joint axes at the wrist and second MCP is essential. The strength of pinch should be assessed, and the length of the transfer bar should be changed by the orthotist to increase pinch strength as needed.

Straps should facilitate independent application and removal of the orthosis. Loops added to the ends of the straps enable the client to use the thumb of the other hand to fasten and unfasten them with increased ease.

The client's ability to don and doff the orthosis is strongly related to independence in activities and to the client's ultimate acceptance of the device. This is true especially if the client must remove the orthosis to perform other activities such as propulsion of a wheelchair. Removal of the WDWHO is typically easier than application of it. Initially, the orthosis should be placed on the client for no more than 30 minutes. Upon removal, the skin should be carefully checked for any areas of redness. These red areas should be reassessed in half an hour, and if they are still present, the orthosis requires adjustment before the client can use it. Once pressure problems have been resolved, wearing time can be gradually increased.

Client and Caregiver Education

A brief review of the WDWHO's purpose and capabilities should be provided. The client and caregivers should be instructed in the importance of skin inspection to prevent excessive pressure and skin breakdown. Accordingly, they should also be taught wearing tolerance and the schedule. They should be oriented to key component names and how the components operate prior to orthotic controls training. Finally, they should know how to care for and maintain the orthosis. Education in these areas should be reinforced throughout the orthotic training process.

Controls Training and Functional Use Training

Procedures for Practice 15-4 shows WDWHO controls training and use training.

EFFICACY AND OUTCOMES

Although the use of upper extremity orthoses is an accepted practice with much clinical and intuitive support, the state of best evidence about upper extremity orthoses is limited (Evidence Table 15-1). Most published materials are anecdotal, based on clinical experience, are of varying study quality, and/or outdated. Good, valid studies of current practice are needed to enhance our knowledge of splinting efficacy and variables that lead to optimum outcomes.

Rancho Los Amigos National Rehabilitation Center   Occupational Therapy Department

MOBILE ARM SUPPORT APPRAISAL

Patient's Name_____   Type of MAS (L)_____

Date Fitted_____   Type of MAS (R)_____

I. PATIENT'S POSITION IN WHEELCHAIR

YES	NO	N/A	Are hips well back in wheelchair?
YES	NO	N/A	Is spine in good vertical alignment?
YES	NO	N/A	Does patient have lateral trunk stability?
YES	NO	N/A	Is wheelchair set-up providing adequate comfort and stability?
YES	NO	N/A	Is patient sitting in maximum upright position possible?
YES	NO	N/A	Does patient have needed hand splints on?
YES	NO	N/A	Does patient meet requirements for passive range of motion?

II. MECHANICAL CHECKOUT

YES	NO	N/A	Are all screws tight?
YES	NO	N/A	Is bracket tightly secured on wheelchair?
YES	NO	N/A	Are all MAS arms and joints freely movable?
YES	NO	N/A	Is proximal arm inserted completely in bracket bearing tube?
YES	NO	N/A	Is distal arm inserted completely in proximal arm bearing tube?
YES	NO	N/A	Is bracket at proper height so shoulder is not forced into elevation?
YES	NO	N/A	Does elbow dial clear lapboard when trough is in "up" position?
YES	NO	N/A	Is patient's hand (in "up" position) as close to mouth as possible?
YES	NO	N/A	Can patient obtain maximum active reach?
YES	NO	N/A	Is patient's arm secured in trough?
YES	NO	N/A	Is trough long enough to give maximum support to forearm?
YES	NO	N/A	Is trough short enough to allow wrist flexion if desired?
YES	NO	N/A	Are trough edges rolled so that they do not contact forearm?
YES	NO	N/A	Is elbow secure and comfortable in elbow dial?
YES	NO	N/A	Is trough balanced correctly?
YES	NO	N/A	During vertical motion, is elbow dial free of distal arm?
YES	NO	N/A	Are vertical stops correctly placed for both up and down motions?
YES	NO	N/A	Are rubber band hooks secured?
YES	NO	N/A	Are rubber bands securely attached?

Figure 15-80 Mobile arm support appraisal form.

III. CONTROL CHECKOUT

YES	NO	N/A	Can patient control motion of proximal arm from either extreme?
YES	NO	N/A	Can patient control motion of distal arm from either extreme?
YES	NO	N/A	Can patient control vertical motion from either extreme?
YES	NO	N/A	Have stops been applied to limit motion, if necessary?
YES	NO	N/A	Does patient accomplish maximum horizontal reach in front of body?
YES	NO	N/A	Can patient easily reach mouth?
YES	NO	N/A	Can patient easily reach tabletop?
YES	NO	N/A	Can patient horizontally adduct arm sufficiently to clear doorways?
YES	NO	N/A	Is performance consistent from day to day?

IV. USE CHECKOUT

YES	NO	N/A	Are fine adjustments necessary to enable patient to perform different activities?
YES	NO	N/A	Are there some tasks that patient can perform better without MAS?
YES	NO	N/A	Is patient able to instruct caregivers in how to assemble MAS components?
YES	NO	N/A	Have patient and caregivers been instructed in care of MAS?

Figure 15-80 *(continued).*

Evidence Table 15-1 | Best Evidence for Occupational Therapy Practice Regarding Upper Extremity Orthoses

Intervention	Description of Intervention Tested	Participants	Dosage	Type of Best Evidence and Level of Evidence	Benefit	Statistical Probability and Effect Size of Outcome	Reference
Hand splinting to prevent contracture and reduce spasticity following stroke	Different types of splints and splint designs	Two hundred thirty patients	Splint wear for unknown time up to 11 weeks, various wearing patterns	Meta-analysis of 21 studies	Insufficient evidence to either support or refute the effectiveness of hand splinting for adults following stroke	Heterogeneity of study design, methods, splint design and regimen, and outcomes prevented the pooling of data to determine effect size	Lannin & Herbert (2003)
Splinting for lateral epicondylitis	Six splint designs	Three hundred sixty-two participants (277 patients and 85 healthy subjects)	Splint wear for test session up to 4 weeks	Systematic review of 11 studies	Yes. Early positive, but not conclusive, effectiveness of splinting	Not reported	Borkholder, Hill, & Fess (2004)
Splinting for carpal tunnel syndrome	Different types of splints and various angles of immobilization	Four hundred four patients (452 hands)	Splint wear for night only or full-time for 2–8 weeks	Systematic review of six studies	Yes. Significant benefits from splinting across different splint types and wrist angles, especially if used full-time	Not reported	Piazzini et al. (2007)
Splinting for osteoarthritis of thumb carpometacarpal (CMC)	Different types of splints and splint designs	Three hundred forty-eight patients with physician-diagnosed osteoarthritis of the first CMC	Splint wear for 2 weeks up to 7 years, various wearing schedules	Systematic review of 12 studies	Yes. Significant decrease in pain short term (≤45 days) and long term (≥3 months)	Heterogeneity of study design, methods, splint design and regimen, and outcomes prevented the pooling of data to determine effect size	Kjeken et al. (2011)
Adherence to splint wear	Different types of splints and splint designs	Four hundred ninety patients with acute hand, wrist, or forearm injuries	Follow-up from unknown duration to 12 months	Systematic review of six studies	Higher overall adherence rates found in acute injuries (≥75%) than comparable literature for chronic conditions (25%–65%); some evidence that immediacy of benefit, comfort, and minimizing of interference with daily tasks improve adherence	Because of heterogeneity of studies, synthesis was narrative rather than quantitative	O'Brien (2010)

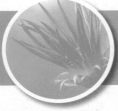

case example
Ms. N.: Orthotic Intervention in a Client with Peripheral Nerve Injury

Occupational Therapy Intervention Process	Clinical Reasoning Process	
	Objectives	Examples of Therapist's Internal Dialogue

Patient information

Ms. N., a 22-year-old woman 8 weeks post motor vehicle collision, was referred to outpatient occupational therapy for evaluation and splinting of her left arm. She had a brachial plexus traction injury and a humeral fracture, treated with a closed reduction and fracture brace (purpose: to immobilize for healing). Prior to her injury, she was right-hand dominant and employed full time as a secretary.

On initial assessment, the following problems were identified as related to her left upper extremity: (1) poor positioning of the entire arm, with Ms. N. using her right arm to help to support the left arm; (2) absent motor function and impaired sensation throughout; (3) limited passive range of motion of the shoulder in all planes, forearm supination, MCP flexion, and thumb abduction; (4) traction pain in the shoulder; and (5) lack of functional use for any activities.

Objectives	Examples of Therapist's Internal Dialogue
Appreciate the context	"Ms. N. is dealing with a significant injury with an enormous impact on her life. I am concerned not only about the status of her left arm but also about the disruption of her routines and roles. She is obviously frustrated about not being able to work and having to ask her mother to help with most tasks. I need to help her feel empowered and instill hope for her future."
Develop intervention hypotheses	"I think that poor left arm positioning is the factor contributing most to her lack of occupational functioning. If I can free up her right arm for function, I believe this will go a long way in helping her cope with her injury."
Select an intervention approach	"Orthoses will be an integral part of Ms. N.'s treatment and will need to be carefully selected based on her clinical and functional status. From reviewing the literature, I know that collaborating with the client closely throughout the splinting process is crucial to a successful outcome. I also understand that recovery may occur at a slow rate, and orthoses will need to be durable."
Reflect on competence	"I have treated clients having similar peripheral nerve injuries in the past and have seen good functional recovery occur in many cases. These past experiences have also taught me that I have to do what I can to help Ms. N. be patient because recovery time with these types of injury can be frustratingly slow."

Summary of Short-Term Goals and Progress

Ms. N. was fitted with a standard pouch sling that was easy to don and doff and supported the weight of her arm with the goals of pain relief and freeing her right arm for functional use (purposes: to support a painful joint and to protect tissues); she was also fitted with a custom-fabricated static wrist extension–thumb abduction splint to prevent the loss of wrist extension and to regain MCP flexion and thumb abduction range of motion (purposes: to prevent contractures and to restore mobility).

Objectives	Examples of Therapist's Internal Dialogue
Assess the client's comprehension	"I think it is important to begin with an intensive program that will quickly address Ms. N.'s clinical and functional needs. Even though they have to travel a good distance from home, Ms. N. and her mother understand the importance of early therapy intervention to improve the prognosis for recovery. I acknowledge the hardship this causes for them, so I promise to minimize the therapy visits as much as possible."
Understand what he or she is doing	
Ascertain the client's endorsement of plan	
Compare actual to expected performance	
Know the person	
Appreciate the context	

Next Steps

As Ms. N.'s neuromuscular recovery progressed, the following orthoses were used in response to new problems and functional potential identified:

Week 11: The sling was discontinued, because shoulder and elbow strength had improved to 3 to 3+ and traction pain had resolved. Ms. N. continued to use the wrist extension–thumb abduction splint during the day. At night, Ms. N. wore a custom-fabricated composite wrist and finger extension static splint to prevent long flexor tightness from unopposed finger flexors that had regained 3+ strength (purpose: to prevent contractures).

Week 17: At night, Ms. N. wore a custom-fabricated serial static elbow extension splint to regain elbow extension range of motion lost to initial positioning from the sling, an ineffective home range-of-motion program, and return of unopposed 3+ elbow flexor strength (purpose: to restore mobility).

Week 21: A Colditz radial nerve splint was fabricated to substitute for weak muscles supplied by the radial nerve and to enhance hand function as long finger flexors and wrist flexors recovered to sufficient strength of 3+. Ms. N. wore this splint during the day to allow functional use of the hand during light tasks (purpose: to substitute for weak or absent muscles).

Week 26: The Colditz radial nerve splint was discontinued, because wrist and long finger extensors had regained 3+ strength. A custom-fabricated thermoplastic lumbrical bar splint for the ring and small fingers was issued to address residual weakness of intrinsic muscles innervated by the ulnar nerve, leading to clawing. Ms. N. wore this splint during the day to assist with hand opening and prevent IP flexion contractures (purposes: to restrict unwanted motion and to prevent contractures).

Week 28: A dynamic forearm rotation splint was fabricated from a commercial kit; Ms. N. wore it at night to regain full supination range of motion initially lost from positioning and an imbalance of forearm rotator muscle strength (purpose: to restore mobility).

Week 36: No further splinting was required, as Ms. N. had full neuromuscular recovery. Ms. N. was able to return to her previous employment with full functional use of her left arm.

Anticipate present and future client concerns	"I need to be ready to respond to Ms. N.'s unique needs. I need to closely monitor for changes in range of motion, motor function, and sensory function and be on the lookout for development of deformity that may occur from muscle imbalance. I want to optimize her ability to use her left arm as soon as her clinical status allows. To enable an optimum functional and clinical outcome, I need to discontinue orthoses as soon as they become unnecessary and implement new orthoses as different needs arise."
Analyze the client's comprehension	"It is important to continuously educate Ms. N. on her status so she can see her recovery progressing and understand how important the various orthoses are to optimize her functional outcome."
Decide if she should continue or discontinue therapy and/or return in the future	"I also need to give Ms. N. the opportunity to voice her questions, concerns, and preferences so that we can work together to select the most appropriate orthoses and design optimal wearing schedules."

 Clinical Reasoning in Occupational Therapy Practice

Addressing Issues with Splint Wear

During the course of Ms. N.'s outpatient therapy program, the therapist suspects that Ms. N. is not wearing some splints as often as recommended.

How might this problem be evident to the therapist? What can the therapist do to address this issue?

Summary Review Questions

1. What is the role of the occupational therapist in orthotic rehabilitation?
2. Define orthosis.
3. Name the purposes for which splinting may be used.
4. What are key factors for selecting an orthosis for a particular client?
5. Discuss factors that may enhance splint wearing and those that may interfere with it.
6. Discuss why a static splint may be chosen and the precautions related to such splints.
7. Describe two dynamic splints and the purposes for which they are used.
8. Select an orthosis to decrease an elbow flexion contracture, discuss the reasons for your choice, and state the principle or principles that it implements.
9. Discuss two types of finger or hand orthoses that assist in restoring function while stabilizing a joint.
10. For which type of client would you choose a WDWHO?
11. Name the basic components of a standard MAS and two diagnostic categories of candidates who may benefit from its use.
12. Describe a treatment session to improve a client's hand-to-mouth and hand-to-table control of a MAS and basic adjustments that can be made to the MAS to facilitate these motions.
13. What are the pros and cons of various orthoses designed to modify tone?

Glossary

Arm sling—An orthosis that supports the proximal upper extremity to restrict motion, reduce pain, or prevent or reduce shoulder subluxation.

Arm trough—An upper extremity positioning device attached to a wheelchair armrest.

Dynamic splint—Orthosis that has moving parts; primarily used to regain joint mobility or facilitate function.

Lapboard—A portable tabletop that is applied to a wheelchair to provide a working surface or support an upper extremity; also known as a lap tray.

Mobile arm support—A mechanical device that uses ball-bearing joints, gravity, and sometimes rubber bands to support the arm and assist in movement when proximal muscles are weak; may be mounted onto a wheelchair or table; also known as a balanced forearm orthosis, ball-bearing arm support, or ball-bearing feeder.

Orthosis—Any externally applied device added to a person's body to support, align, position, immobilize, prevent or correct deformities, assist weak muscles, or improve function; also known as a splint, brace, or support.

Serial casting—Applying casts at routine intervals as range of motion improves, with the goal of restoring joint mobility.

Serial static splinting—Remolding or fabricating new static splints as range of motion improves, with the goal of restoring joint mobility.

Static splint—Orthosis that has no moving parts; primarily used to support, stabilize, protect, or immobilize.

Static progressive splint—Orthosis that uses nondynamic forces; primarily used to regain joint motion.

Wrist-driven wrist–hand orthosis—Flexor hinge orthosis that uses tenodesis to accomplish palmar pinch.

References

Ada, L., Foongchomcheay, A., & Canning, C. G. (2005). Supportive devices for preventing and treating subluxation of the shoulder after stroke. *Cochrane Database of Systematic Reviews,* Issue 1, Art No. CD003863.

Allen, V. (1971). Follow-up study of wrist-driven flexor-hinge-splint use. *American Journal of Occupational Therapy, 25,* 420–422.

Alon, G., Levitt, A. F., & McCarthy, P. A. (2007). Functional electrical stimulation enhancement of upper extremity functional recovery during stroke rehabilitation: A pilot study. *Neurorehabilitation and Neural Repair, 21,* 207–215.

American Society of Hand Therapists. (1992). *Splint classification system.* Chicago: American Society of Hand Therapists.

Amini, D., & Rider, D. A. (2008). Occupation-based splinting. In B. M. Coppard & H. Lohman (Eds.), *Introduction to splinting: A clinical reasoning and problem-solving approach* (3rd ed., pp. 15–28). St. Louis: Mosby.

Atkins, M. S., Baumgarten, J. M., Yasuda, Y. L., Adkins, R., Waters, R. L., Leung, P., & Requejo, P. (2008). Mobile arm supports: Evidence-based benefits and criteria for use. *Journal of Spinal Cord Medicine, 31,* 388–393.

Bassini, L. B., & Patel, M. R. (1994). Buddy sleeves. *Journal of Hand Therapy, 7,* 257–258.

Beasley, J. (2011a). Soft orthoses: Indication and techniques. In T. M. Skirven, A. L. Osterman, J. M. Fedorczyk, & P. C. Amadio (Eds.), *Rehabilitation of the hand and upper extremity* (6th ed., pp. 1610–1619). Philadelphia: Mosby.

Beasley, J. (2011b). Therapist's examination and conservative management of arthritis of the upper extremity. In T. M. Skirven, A. L. Osterman, J. M. Fedorczyk, & P. C. Amadio (Eds.), *Rehabilitation of the hand and upper extremity* (6th ed., pp. 1330–1343). Philadelphia: Mosby.

Bell-Krotoski, J. A. (2011). Tissue remodeling and contracture correction using serial plaster casting and orthotic positioning. In T. M. Skirven, A. L. Osterman, J. M. Fedorczyk, & P. C. Amadio (Eds.), *Rehabilitation of the hand and upper extremity* (6th ed., pp. 1599–1609). Philadelphia: Mosby.

Bell-Krotoski, J. A., & Breger-Stanton, D. (2011). The forces of dynamic orthotic positioning: Ten questions to ask before applying a dynamic orthosis to the hand. In T. M. Skirven, A. L. Osterman, J. M. Fedorczyk, & P. C. Amadio (Eds.), *Rehabilitation of the hand and upper extremity* (6th ed., pp. 1581–1587). Philadelphia: Mosby.

Bell-Krotoski, J. A., & Figarola, J. H. (1995). Biomechanics of soft tissue growth and remodeling with plaster casting. *Journal of Hand Therapy, 8,* 131–137.

Bobath, B. (1990). *Adult hemiplegia: Evaluation and treatment* (3rd ed.). London: William Heinemann Medical.

Borkholder, C. D., Hill, V. A., & Fess, E. E. (2004). The efficacy of splinting for lateral epicondylitis: A systematic review. *Journal of Hand Therapy, 17,* 181–199.

Callahan, A. D., & McEntee, P. (1986). Splinting proximal interphalangeal joint flexion contractures: A new design. *American Journal of Occupational Therapy, 40,* 408–413.

Callinan, N. J., & Mathiowetz, V. (1996). Soft versus hard resting splints in rheumatoid arthritis: Pain relief, preference, and compliance. *American Journal of Occupational Therapy, 50,* 347–353.

Casey, C. A., & Kratz, E. J. (1988). Soft splinting with neoprene: The thumb abduction supinator splint. *American Journal of Occupational Therapy, 42,* 395–398.

Clark, E. N. (1997). A preliminary investigation of the neoprene tube finger extension splint. *Journal of Hand Therapy, 10,* 213–221.

Colditz, J. C. (2002/2011). Splinting the hand with a peripheral nerve injury. In E. J. Mackin, A. D. Callahan, T. M. Skirven, L. H. Schneider, & A. L. Osterman (Eds.), *Rehabilitation of the hand and upper extremity* (5th ed., pp. 622–634). St. Louis: Mosby. Archived online in T. M. Skirven, A. L. Osterman, J. M. Fedorczyk, & P. C. Amadio (Eds.). (2011). *Rehabilitation of the hand and upper extremity* (6th ed.). Philadelphia: Mosby.

Colditz, J. C. (2011). Therapist's management of the stiff hand. In T. M. Skirven, A. L. Osterman, J. M. Fedorczyk, & P. C. Amadio (Eds.), *Rehabilitation of the hand and upper extremity* (6th ed., pp. 894–921). Philadelphia: Mosby.

Collier, S. E., & Thomas, J. J. (2002). Range of motion at the wrist: A comparison study of four wrist extension orthoses and the free hand. *American Journal of Occupational Therapy, 56,* 180–184.

Collins, L. (1999). Helping patients help themselves: Improving orthotic use. *OT Practice, 4,* 30–34.

Condie, D. N. (2008). International organization for standardization (ISO) terminology. In J. D. Hsu, J. W. Michael, & J. R. Fisk (Eds.), *AAOS atlas of orthoses and assistive devices* (4th ed., pp. 3–7). Philadelphia: Mosby.

Coppard, B. M., & Lohman, H. (2008). *Introduction to splinting: A clinical reasoning and problem-solving approach* (3rd ed.). St. Louis: Mosby.

Duff, S. V., & Estilow, T. (2011). Therapist's management of peripheral nerve injury. In T. M. Skirven, A. L. Osterman, J. M. Fedorczyk, & P. C. Amadio (Eds.), *Rehabilitation of the hand and upper extremity* (6th ed., pp. 619–633). Philadelphia: Mosby.

Egan, M. Y., & Brousseau, L. (2007). Splinting for osteoarthritis of the carpometacarpal joint: A review of the evidence. *American Journal of Occupational Therapy, 61,* 70–78.

Ekholm, M. D., Tidermark, J., Törnkvist, H., Adamil, J., & Ponzer, S. (2006). Outcome after closed functional treatment of humeral shaft fractures. *Journal of Orthopaedic Trauma, 20,* 591–596.

Evans, R. B. (2011a). Clinical management of extensor tendon injuries: The therapist's perspective. In T. M. Skirven, A. L. Osterman, J. M. Fedorczyk, & P. C. Amadio (Eds.), *Rehabilitation of the hand and upper extremity* (6th ed., pp. 521–554). Philadelphia: Mosby.

Evans, R. B. (2011b). Therapist's management of carpal tunnel syndrome: A practical approach. In T. M. Skirven, A. L. Osterman, J. M. Fedorczyk, & P. C. Amadio (Eds.), *Rehabilitation of the hand and upper extremity* (6th ed., pp. 666–677). Philadelphia: Mosby.

Farrell, J. F., Hoffman, H. B., Snyder, J. L., Giuliani, C. A., & Bohannon, R. W. (2007). Orthotic aided training of the paretic upper limb in chronic stroke. *NeuroRehabilitation, 22,* 99–103.

Fedorczyk, J. M. (2011). Elbow tendinopathies: Clinical presentation and therapist's management of tennis elbow. In T. M. Skirven, A. L. Osterman, J. M. Fedorczyk, & P. C. Amadio (Eds.), *Rehabilitation of the hand and upper extremity* (6th ed., pp. 1098–1108). Philadelphia: Mosby.

Feinberg, J. (1992). Effect of the arthritis health professional on compliance with use of resting hand splints by patients with rheumatoid arthritis. *Arthritis Care and Research, 5,* 17–23.

Fess, E. E. (1988). Force magnitude of commercial spring-coil and spring-wire splints designed to extend the proximal interphalangeal joint. *Journal of Hand Therapy, 1,* 86–90.

Fess, E. E. (2011). Orthoses for mobilization of joints: Principles and methods. In T. M. Skirven, A. L. Osterman, J. M. Fedorczyk, & P. C. Amadio (Eds.), *Rehabilitation of the hand and upper extremity* (6th ed., pp. 1588–1598). Philadelphia: Mosby.

Fess, E. E., Gettle, K. S., Philips, C. A., & Janson, J. R. (Eds.). (2005). *Hand and upper extremity splinting: Principles and methods* (3rd ed.). St. Louis: Mosby.

Fess, E. E., & McCollum, M. (1998). The influence of splinting on healing tissues. *Journal of Hand Therapy, 11,* 157–161.

Garg, R., Adamson, G. J., Dawson, P. A., Shankwiler, J. A., & Pink, M. M. (2010). A prospective randomized study comparing a forearm strap brace versus a wrist splint for the treatment of lateral epicondylitis. *Journal of Shoulder and Elbow Surgery, 19,* 508–512.

Garros, D. S., Gagliardi, R. J., & Guzzo, R. A. (2010). Evaluation of performance and personal satisfaction of the patient with spastic hand after using a volar dorsal orthosis. *Arquivos de Neuro-Psiquiatria, 68,* 385–389.

Gelberman, R. H., Rydevik, B. L., Pess, G. M., Szabo, R. M., & Lundborg, G. (1988). Carpal tunnel syndrome: A scientific basis for clinical care. *Orthopedic Clinics of North America, 19,* 115–124.

Gilbert-Lenef, L. (1994). Soft ulnar deviation splint. *Journal of Hand Therapy, 7,* 29–30.

Glasgow, C., Fleming, J., Tooth, L. R., & Hockey, R. L. (2012). The long-term relationship between duration of treatment and contracture resolution using dynamic orthotic devices for the stiff proximal interphalangeal joint: A prospective cohort study. *Journal of Hand Therapy, 25,* 38–47.

Glasgow, C., Tooth, L. R., Fleming, J., & Peters, S. (2011). Dynamic splinting for the stiff hand after trauma: Predictors of contracture resolution. *Journal of Hand Therapy, 24,* 195–206.

Groth, G. N., & Wulf, M. B. (1995). Compliance with hand rehabilitation: Health beliefs and strategies. *Journal of Hand Therapy, 8,* 18–22.

Harrell, P. B. (2006). Splinting of the hand. In S. J. Bartlett (Ed.), *Clinical care in the rheumatic diseases* (3rd ed., pp. 261–266). Atlanta: Association of Rheumatology Health Professionals.

Hill, J. (1994). The effects of casting on upper extremity motor disorders after brain injury. *American Journal of Occupational Therapy, 48,* 219–224.

Hunter, J. M., Mackin, E. J., & Callahan, A. D. (Eds.). (1995). *Rehabilitation of the hand: Surgery and therapy* (4th ed.). St. Louis: Mosby.

JAECO Orthopedic, Inc. (2008). *Set-up instructions for multilink mobile arm support.* Hot Springs, AR: JAECO.

Jafarian, F. S., Demneh, E. S., & Tyson, S. F. (2009). The immediate effect of orthotic management on grip strength of patients with lateral epicondylitis. *Journal of Orthopaedic and Sports Physical Therapy, 39,* 484–489.

Jensen, C., & Rayan, G. (1996). Buddy strapping of mismatched fingers: The offset buddy strap. *Journal of Hand Surgery, 21,* 317–318.

Kinghorn, J., & Roberts, G. (1996). The effect of an inhibitive weight-bearing splint on tone and function: A single-case study. *American Journal of Occupational Therapy, 50,* 807–815.

Kjeken, I., Smedslund, G., Moe, R. H., Slatkowsky-Christensen, B., Uhlig, T., & Hagen, K. B. (2011). Systematic review of design and effects of splints and exercise programs in hand osteoarthritis. *Arthritis Care and Research, 63,* 834–848.

Knox, C., Engel, W., & Seibens, A. (1971). Results of a survey on the use of a wrist-driven splint for prehension. *American Journal of Occupational Therapy, 15,* 109–111.

Lamay, G. (1994). Buddy splint. *Journal of Hand Therapy, 7,* 30–31.

Langlois, S., Pederson, L., & Mackinnon, J. (1991). The effects of splinting on the spastic hemiplegic hand: Report of a feasibility study. *Canadian Journal of Occupational Therapy, 58,* 17–25.

Lannin, N., & Herbert, R. (2003). Is hand splinting effective for adults following stroke? A systematic review and methodological critique of published research. *Clinical Rehabilitation, 17,* 807–816.

Lannin, N. A., Novak, I., & Cusick, A. (2007). A systematic review of upper extremity casting for children and adults with central nervous system disorders. *Clinical Rehabilitation, 21,* 963–976.

Lohman, H. (2008a). Splints acting on the wrist. In B. M. Coppard & H. Lohman (Eds.), *Introduction to splinting: A clinical reasoning and problem-solving approach* (3rd ed., pp. 119–155). St. Louis: Mosby.

Lohman, H. (2008b). Thumb immobilization splints. In B. M. Coppard & H. Lohman (Eds.), *Introduction to splinting: A clinical reasoning and problem-solving approach* (3rd ed., pp. 156–187). St. Louis: Mosby.

Lubahn, J., Wolfe, T. L., & Feldscher, S. B. (2011). Joint replacement in the hand and wrist: Surgery and therapy. In T. M. Skirven, A. L. Osterman, J. M. Fedorczyk, & P. C. Amadio (Eds.), *Rehabilitation of the hand and upper extremity* (6th ed., pp. 1376–1407). Philadelphia: Mosby.

Lunsford, T. R., & DiBello, T. V. (2008). Principles and components of upper limb orthoses. In J. D. Hsu, J. W. Michael, & J. R. Fisk (Eds.), *AAOS atlas of orthoses and assistive devices* (4th ed., pp. 179–190). Philadelphia: Mosby.

Marinelli, A., Bettelli, G., Guerra, E., Nigrisoli, M., & Rotini, R. (2010). Mobilization brace in post-traumatic elbow stiffness. *Musculoskeletal Surgery, 94,* S37–S45.

McKee, P., & Rivard, A. (2004). Orthoses as enablers of occupation: Client-centered splinting for better outcomes. *Canadian Journal of Occupational Therapy, 71,* 306–314.

McKee, P. R., & Rivard, A. (2011). Biopsychosocial approach to orthotic intervention. *Journal of Hand Therapy, 24,* 155–162.

McPherson, J. J. (1981). Objective evaluation of a splint designed to reduce hypertonicity. *American Journal of Occupational Therapy, 35,* 189–194.

McPherson, J. J., Becker, A. H., & Franszczak, N. (1985). Dynamic splint to reduce the passive component of hypertonicity. *Archives of Physical Medicine and Rehabilitation, 66,* 249–252.

McPherson, J. J., Kreimeyer, D., Aalderks, M., & Gallagher, T. (1982). A comparison of dorsal and volar resting hand splints in the reduction of hypertonus. *American Journal of Occupational Therapy, 36,* 664–670.

Melvin, J. L. (1989). *Rheumatic disease in the adult and child: Occupational therapy and rehabilitation* (3rd ed.). Philadelphia: Davis.

Melvin, J. L. (1995). Orthotic treatment of the hand: What's new? *Bulletin on the Rheumatic Diseases, 44,* 5–8.

Michlovitz, S. L., Harris, B. A., & Watkins, M. P. (2004). Therapy interventions for improving joint range of motion: A systematic review. *Journal of Hand Therapy, 17,* 118–131.

Mulcahey, M. J. (2008). Upper limb orthoses for the person with spinal cord injury. In J. D. Hsu, J. W. Michael, & J. R. Fisk (Eds.), *AAOS atlas of orthoses and assistive devices* (4th ed., pp. 203–217). Philadelphia: Mosby.

Murphy, M. S. (1990). An adjustable splint for forearm supination. *American Journal of Occupational Therapy, 44,* 936–939.

Neuhaus, B. E., Ascher, E. R., Coullon, B. A., Donohoe, M. V., Einbond, A., Glover, J. M., Goldberg, S. R., & Takai, V. L. (1981). A survey of rationales for and against hand splinting in hemiplegia. *American Journal of Occupational Therapy, 35,* 83–90.

Nuismer, B. A., Ekes, A. M., & Holm, M. B. (1997). The use of low-load prolonged stretch devices in rehabilitation programs in the Pacific Northwest. *American Journal of Occupational Therapy, 51,* 538–543.

Oakes, T. W., Ward, J. F., Gray, R. M., Klauber, M. R., & Moody, P. M. (1970). Family expectations and arthritis patients' compliance to a resting hand splint regimen. *Journal of Chronic Diseases, 22,* 757–764.

O'Brien, L. (2010). Adherence to therapeutic splint wear in adults with acute upper limb injuries: A systematic review. *Hand Therapy, 15,* 3–12.

Pagnotta, A., Baron, M., & Korner-Bitensky, N. (1998). The effect of a static wrist orthosis on hand function in individuals with rheumatoid arthritis. *Journal of Rheumatology, 25,* 879–885.

Paternostro-Sluga, T., Keilani, M., Posch, M., & Fialka-Moser, V. (2003). Factors that influence the duration of splint wear in peripheral nerve lesions. *American Journal of Physical Medicine and Rehabilitation, 82,* 86–95.

Pettengill, K. M. (2011). Therapist's management of the complex injury. In T. M. Skirven, A. L. Osterman, J. M. Fedorczyk, & P. C. Amadio (Eds.), *Rehabilitation of the hand and upper extremity* (6th ed., pp. 1238–1251). Philadelphia: Mosby.

Pettengill, K. M., & van Strien, G. (2011). Postoperative management of flexor tendon injuries. In T. M. Skirven, A. L. Osterman, J. M. Fedorczyk, & P. C. Amadio (Eds.), *Rehabilitation of the hand and upper extremity* (6th ed., pp. 457–478). Philadelphia: Mosby.

Piazzini, D., Aprile, I., Ferrara, P., Bertolini, C., Tonali, P., Maggi, L., Rabini, A., Piantelli, S., & Padua, L. (2007). A systematic review of conservative treatment of carpal tunnel syndrome. *Clinical Rehabilitation, 21,* 299–314.

Pike, J., Mulpuri, K., Metzger, M., Ng, G., Wells, N., & Goetz, T. (2010). Blinded, prospective randomized clinical trial comparing volar, dorsal, and custom thermoplastic splinting in treatment of acute mallet finger. *Journal of Hand Surgery, 35,* 580–588.

Prosser, R. (1996). Splinting in the management of proximal interphalangeal joint flexion contracture. *Journal of Hand Therapy, 9,* 378–386.

Redford, J. B. (Ed.). (1986). *Orthotics etcetera* (3rd ed.). Baltimore: Williams & Wilkins.

Rennie, H. J. (1996). Evaluation of the effectiveness of a metacarpophalangeal ulnar deviation orthosis. *Journal of Hand Therapy, 9,* 371–377.

Richard, R., Shanesy, C. P., & Miller, S. F. (1995). Dynamic versus static splints: A prospective case for sustained stress. *Journal of Burn Care and Rehabilitation, 16,* 284–287.

Richard, R., & Staley, M. (1994). *Burn care and rehabilitation: Principles and practice.* Philadelphia: Davis.

Richard, R., Staley, M., Daugherty, M. B., Miller, S. F., & Warden, G. D. (1994). The wide variety of designs for dorsal hand burn splints. *Journal of Burn Care and Rehabilitation, 15,* 275–280.

Scherling, E., & Johnson, H. (1989). A tone-reducing wrist-hand orthosis. *American Journal of Occupational Therapy, 43,* 609–611.

Shepherd, C. C., & Ruzicka, S. H. (1991). Tenodesis brace use by persons with spinal cord injuries. *American Journal of Occupational Therapy, 45,* 81–83.

Sillem, H., Backman, C. L., Miller, W. C., & Li, L. C. (2011). Comparison of two carpometacarpal stabilizing splints for individuals with thumb osteoarthritis. *Journal of Hand Therapy, 24,* 216–226.

Silva, A. C., Jones, A., Silva, P. G., & Natour, J. (2008). Effectiveness of a night-time hand positioning splint in rheumatoid arthritis: A randomized controlled trial. *Journal of Rehabilitation Medicine, 40,* 749–754.

Spaulding, S. J. (1999). Biomechanical analysis of four supports for the subluxed hemiparetic shoulder. *Canadian Journal of Occupational Therapy, 66,* 169–175.

Stern, E. B. (1991). Wrist extensor orthoses: Dexterity and grip strength across four styles. *American Journal of Occupational Therapy, 45,* 42–49.

Stern, E. B. (1996). Grip strength and finger dexterity across five styles of commercial wrist orthoses. *American Journal of Occupational Therapy, 50,* 32–38.

Stern, E. B., Callinan, N., Hank, M., Lewis, E. J., Schousboe, J. T., & Ytterberg, S. R. (1998). Neoprene splinting: Dermatological issues. *American Journal of Occupational Therapy, 52,* 573–578.

Stern, E. B., Ytterberg, S. R., Krug, H. E., & Mahowald, M. L. (1996). Finger dexterity and hand function: Effect of three commercial wrist extensor orthoses on patients with rheumatoid arthritis. *Arthritis Care and Research, 9,* 197–205.

Stern, E. B., Ytterberg, S. R., Larson, L. M., Portoghese, C. P., Kratz, W. N. R., & Mahowald, M. L. (1997). Commercial wrist extensor orthoses: A descriptive study of use and preference in patients with rheumatoid arthritis. *Arthritis Care and Research, 10,* 27–35.

Tufaro, P. A., & Bondoc, S. L. (2011). Therapist's management of the burned hand. In T. M. Skirven, A. L. Osterman, J. M. Fedorczyk, & P. C. Amadio (Eds.), *Rehabilitation of the hand and upper extremity* (6th ed., pp. 317–341). Philadelphia: Mosby.

Turner-Stokes, L., & Jackson, D. (2002). Shoulder pain after stroke: A review of the evidence base to inform the development of an integrated care pathway. *Clinical Rehabilitation, 16,* 276–298.

Tyson, S. F., & Kent, R. M. (2011). The effect of upper limb orthotics after stroke: A systematic review. *NeuroRehabilitation, 28,* 29–36.

van der Giesen, F. J., van Lankveld, W. J., Kremers-Selten, C., Peters, A. J., Stern, E. B., Le Cessie, S., Nelissen, R. G., & Vliet Vlieland, T. P. (2009). Effectiveness of two finger splints for swan neck deformity in patients with rheumatoid arthritis: A randomized, crossover trial. *Arthritis Care and Research, 61,* 1025–1031.

Walsh, M. (1987). Half-lapboard for hemiplegic patients. *American Journal of Occupational Therapy, 41,* 533–535.

Weiss, N. D., Gordon, L., Bloom, T., So, Y., & Rempel, D. M. (1995). Position of the wrist associated with the lowest carpal tunnel pressure: Implications for splint design. *Journal of Bone and Joint Surgery, 77-A,* 1695–1699.

Weiss, S., La Stayo, P., Mills, A., & Bramlet, D. (2004). Splinting the degenerative basal joint: Custom-made or prefabricated neoprene? *Journal of Hand Therapy, 17,* 401–406.

Wuori, J. L., Overend, T. J., Kramer, J. F., & MacDermid, J. (1998). Strength and pain measures associated with lateral epicondylitis bracing. *Archives of Physical Medicine and Rehabilitation, 79,* 832–837.

Yasuda, Y. L., Bowman, K., & Hsu, J. D. (1986). Mobile arm supports: Criteria for successful use in muscle disease patients. *Archives of Physical Medicine and Rehabilitation, 67,* 253–256.

Zijlstra, T. R., Heijnsdijk-Rouwenhorst, L., & Rasker, J. J. (2004). Silver ring splints improve dexterity in patients with rheumatoid arthritis. *Arthritis and Rheumatism, 51,* 947–951.

Zorowitz, R. D., Hughes, M. B., Idank, D., Ikai, T., & Johnston, M. V. (1996). Shoulder pain and subluxation after stroke: Correlation or coincidence? *American Journal of Occupational Therapy, 50,* 194–201.

Zorowitz, R. D., Idank, D., Ikai, T., Hughes, M. B., & Johnston, M. V. (1995). Shoulder subluxation after stroke: A comparison of four supports. *Archives of Physical Medicine and Rehabilitation, 76,* 763–771.

Acknowledgments

I acknowledge the following contributions:

- Figures 15-2–15-5, 15-9, 15-11–15-13, 15-19, 15-23, 15-24, 15-27, 15-29, 15-33–15-37, 15-42, 15-43, 15-45, 15-48, 15-52, 15-56, 15-57, 15-60, 15-62, 15-63, 15-65, 15-67, 15-68, 15-71–15-73, 15-79, and 15-80 courtesy of Rancho Los Amigos National Rehabilitation Center, Downey, CA
- Figures 15-6–15-8, 15-10, 15-17, 15-18, 15-32, 15-38, 15-39, 15-50, 15-51, 15-55, 15-59, 15-66, 15-70, 15-76, and 15-78 courtesy of Patterson Medical, Bolingbrook, IL
- Figure 15-14–15-16, 15-20–15-22, 15-25, 15-28, 15-30, 15-31, 15-40, 15-41, 15-53, 15-54, 15-64, 15-69, and 15-77 courtesy of North Coast Medical, Inc., Gilroy, CA
- Figure 15-26 courtesy of AliMed, Inc., Dedham, MA
- Figures 15-44 and 15-46 courtesy of Silver Ring Splint Company, Charlottesville, VA
- Figure 15-49 courtesy of Joint Active Systems, Inc., Effingham, IL
- Figure 15-74 courtesy of Saebo, Inc., Charlotte, NC
- Figure 15-75 courtesy of Bioness, Inc., Valencia, CA

16

Construction of Hand Splints

Charles D. Quick and Priscillia D. Bejarano

Learning Objectives

After studying this chapter, the reader will be able to do the following:

1. Describe the anatomical, biomechanical, and mechanical principles applied to splint construction.
2. List the six primary reasons to use splinting as a therapeutic intervention.
3. Recognize factors affecting splint wear compliance.
4. Explain design, pattern making, and construction for three splints.
5. Describe the components of a splint checkout.

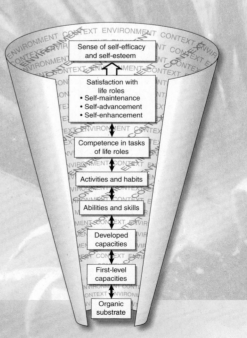

In order to effectively construct hand splints, one must appreciate the significance, biomechanics, and anatomy of the human hand. Mary Reilly (1962) described the significance of hand function in her 1961 Eleanor Clarke Slagle lecture when she suggested, "That man, through the use of his hands as they are energized by mind and will, can influence the state of his own health" (p. 88). Others have suggested that hands are among the features that distinguish human beings from other living creatures; hands are most certainly important to occupational performance. Many medical conditions result in hand impairments involving weakness, swelling, and/or decreased range of motion. Occupational therapists often address these issues by incorporating a splint into the intervention plan.

In this chapter, we first introduce the biomechanical and anatomical structures of the hand that occupational therapists consider in making splints. We then provide basic information about splint construction, appreciating that practice and further training is required to develop expertise in this area.

ANATOMICAL AND BIOMECHANICAL CONSIDERATIONS FOR SPLINT MAKING

A functional understanding of the human body requires the appreciation of three major areas of study; musculoskeletal anatomy, neuromuscular physiology, and biomechanics (Hamilton, Weimer, & Luttgens, 2011). Recovery of hand function following disease or injury can be optimized when the above sciences are combined with understanding of function in occupation and splinting.

Anatomy

The anatomy of the hand informs the concept, design, and construction of hand splints. Such consideration requires a basic review of the macrostructure of tissues and component structures that contribute to functional interaction with the environment. Anatomical principles that are foundational to splinting are described in Definition 16-1.

Bone

The specific functions of bone considered for splinting include structural support, levers for body movement, and protection of underlying structures. Bones are categorized according to shape and size. Long bones have a shaft that acts as a rigid tube; each end of the shaft is expanded, creating a basic component of a joint. Short bones are cube shaped, as long as they are wide. Flat bones are broad and thin with flat or curved surfaces, and sesamoid bones are round (Muscolino, 2011). The three primary arches of the hand are assured by the structural anatomy of the bones. A splint must conform to these arches to support a functional position of the hand (see Fig. 16-1).

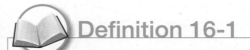

Definition 16-1

Anatomic Principles Applied to Splint Construction

- Bones create structural support and arches of the hand. Splints conform to structure and arches to create dual obliquity and support functional position.
- Joints create levers for movement. The more stable a joint, the less motion; the more actual degrees or planes of motion, the less stable.
- Muscles create movement of joints. Splint design is intervention specific, encouraging motion, stability or immobilization of tissue and joints.
- Neuromuscular physiology is the organ system that drives function. Splint design must allow neuron to muscle fiber communication to be a beneficial intervention.
- Integumentary system encapsulates the body. Understanding the relationship of skin creases to joints is important for splint design and construction.

The metacarpals of the fingers vary in length and height. Metacarpals of the radial fingers are longer than those of the ulnar fingers of the hand. The metacarpal heads on the radial side are higher than those on the ulnar side of the hand, an effect more pronounced when the hand is closed. The therapist must apply this concept of dual obliquity to the construction of a splint. That is, the splint must be longer and higher on the radial side of the hand (Fess et al., 2004) (Fig. 16-2).

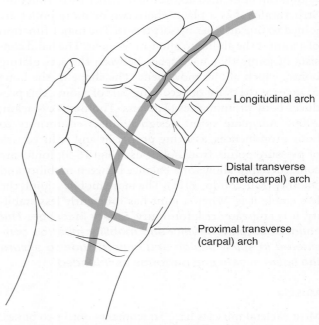

Figure 16-1 Arches of the hand must be supported in splinting.

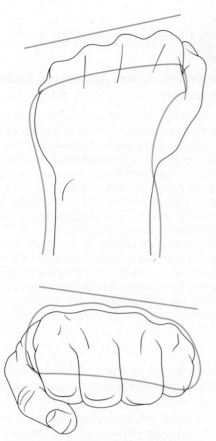

Figure 16-2 Concept of dual obliquity applied to splinting.

Joints

A joint can be defined according to structure or function. Structurally, it is a place where two or more bones are joined to one another by soft tissue. The major function of a joint is the ability to allow movement. The hand consists of joints that have space between the articulating bones, which allows movement. The shape of the bone changes at the point of becoming part of a joint; this produces bony prominences (Tubiana, Thomine & Mackin, 2006). Adequate splint design requires conformity to bony prominences, assuring proper fit and reduced risk of pressure points from splint use (Fig. 16-3). Joints are constructed to allow for a balance between mobility and stability (Muscolino, 2011). The more mobile a joint, the less stable it is. When a joint has inherently less stability, it is at greater risk for injury. *Safety Message: The concept of joint stability and mobility must be considered in splint design and construction to assure the splint is safe and performs as intended.*

Muscle

Most skeletal muscles have attachments onto two bones, the origin, where it begins, and the insertion, where it ends. Musculotendinous structure crosses a joint or joints that are located between the origin and insertion. When a muscle contracts, it shortens toward its center; when the contraction force is sufficient, one or both of the bones to which the muscle is attached will be pulled toward the center of the muscle (Muscolino, 2011). The joint or joints between the muscle's origin and insertion function to allow movement. Understanding the action of a joint caused by the forces applied by muscle and other generated forces is critical to splint design.

Integumentary System

As the largest organ system of the human body, skin encapsulates the body uninterrupted and permits unrestricted mobility (Hedman et al., 2009). Dorsal hand skin is relatively thin with creases directly over articulations. Volar skin is fibrous and thick with more defined creases. As in the dorsal digital creases, the volar digital creases directly correlate to joint location. The palmar creases do not relate directly to the associated joints (Williams et al., 1995). The relationship of skin creases to the joints of the hand and digits is important to splint design because the creases of the hand can provide landmarks for splint fabrication (Coppard & Lohman, 1996) (Fig. 16-4).

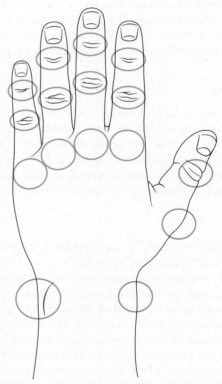

Figure 16-3 Bony prominences can lead to pressure points, especially over the back of the hand. Careful contouring of the splinting material can minimize this problem.

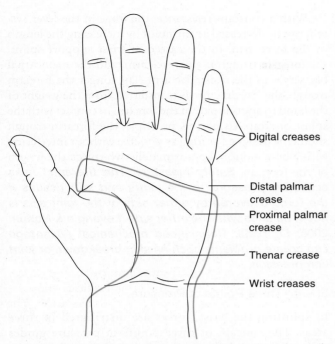

Figure 16-4 Creases of the hand provide landmarks for the distal ends of the splint. For a wrist support splint, the distal end of the splint should not block the thenar eminence or distal palmar crease.

Digital creases

Distal palmar crease

Proximal palmar crease

Thenar crease

Wrist creases

Biomechanical Principles Applied to Splint Construction

Biomechanics is the study of mechanics focused on the human body and is divided into two areas of study: statics and dynamics (Hamilton, Weimer, & Luttgens, 2011; Levangie & Norkin, 2005). Statics or kinematics study forces as though they are in balance and the body in equilibrium. There are five

variables considered in the process of applied biomechanics. The therapist considers each variable to determine how a splint will affect hand function in the transmission of forces from the unsplinted to the splinted hand (see Table 16-1).

The dynamic component of biomechanics, kinetics, introduces the application of forces on a given body (Hamilton, Weimer, & Luttgens, 2011). The force can be gravity, weight, or a choice of a dynamic or static splint that contacts the hand, wrist, or forearm to create a desired position with a desired motion during use. The therapist's understanding of biomechanical principles will allow the desired mechanics to be applied to the design of a splint.

Mechanical Principles Applied to Splint Construction

Mechanics is a branch of physics that examines cause and effect such as the force on an object and the motion or response that results (Hamilton, Weimer, & Luttgens, 2011). As exemplified in the following list, therapists use biomechanical principles to assess function of the hand and apply mechanical principles to the splint design.

- The therapist must be aware of the natural postures of the hand that affect function. For instance, when the hand is held in supination, the wrist is in neutral to slight radial deviation. When the hand is held in pronation, the wrist is more ulnarly deviated. If a splint is fitted in supination for a patient who will be using the hand primarily in pronation, the splint may not be comfortable.
- During flexion in normal biomechanics, the fingers converge toward the scaphoid bone; splint mechanics must incorporate this property for best splint function (Fig. 16-5).

Table 16-1	**Biomechanical Considerations for Splint Design**
Biomechanical Variables	**Implications for Splint Design**
Type of motion: linear, rotary, or a combination, known as general motion	Splints can create or restrict motion to enhance function. When joint motion is to be enhanced through splinting, the motion or combination of motion must be identified. Rotary motion considers movement of a joint around an axis, and linear motion considers the distraction (or separation of joint articulations) of a joint. The therapist considers the forces required to retain balance between the two motions to obtain maximum benefit without creating joint irritation or damage.
Axis of motion considering anatomical position	When there is a therapeutic need to generate motion through static progressive or dynamic splinting, the axis of motion indicates the direction of introduced forces. Applied forces can be calculated to overcome the antagonistic forces required through the axis of motion.
Direction of displacement: flexion, extension, abduction, adduction, etc.	Consider the normal ranges of movement and desired directional motion of the joints affected by the splint.
Magnitude of displacement: range of motion	The initial and overall desired degree of motion of the affected joints from the splint applications.
Rate of displacement: speed	This pertains to the rate of motion over time desired from application of the splint. The rate can vary according to the type of splint (static, dynamic, or static progressive) and the patient's needs or goals.

(Adapted from Hamilton, N., Weimer, W., & Luttgens, K. [2011]. *Kinesiology: Scientific basis of human motion* [12th ed., Rev.]. Boston: McGraw Hill, Inc.)

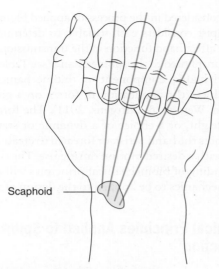

Scaphoid

Figure 16-5 Fingers flex toward the scaphoid.

- In dynamic splints or static progressive splints, the line of pull (force) must be at a 90° angle to the joint at which motion is intended (Fig. 16-32).

The therapist designing and constructing a splint considers the following principles of force distribution for best possible outcomes.

Increase the Mechanical Advantage to Reduce Pressure and Increase Comfort

Upper extremity anatomy consists of several basic lever systems. The first class lever system is the basis of mechanical principles for splinting the hand (Fig. 16-6). In a first class lever system, the combined forces in one direction must be opposed by an equal opposite force at the axis (Li, 1999). The musculoskeletal system of the hand allows forces to be transferred to and through the splinted area. Therefore, the design and construction of the splint requires the use of a favorable force delivery system (Li, 1999). One key principle is that mechanical advantage is equal to the force arm divided by the resistance arm.

With a constant resistance, the force in the lever system can be decreased at any point by increasing the length of the force arm. In the case of a wrist support splint, the forearm trough is the force arm, and the metacarpal bar serves as the resistance arm. The longer the forearm trough, the less pressure is transferred from the weight of the hand to any one part of the forearm in contact with the splint or strap. Using this principle, the forearm trough should be designed as long as possible without interfering with elbow motion, approximately two-thirds the length of the forearm. *Safety Message: The therapist risks excessive pressure to the joints and soft tissues if the force delivered by either side of the joint axis is not in balance with the other side (Levangie & Norkin, 2005; Li, 1999). Unbalanced mechanical advantage can create problems such as skin breakdown or joint compression.*

Ensure Three Points of Pressure

In splinting the wrist, forces are distributed in three areas. The concept of three points of pressure guides splint design and directs placement of straps for proper force application (Fig. 16-6). The splint acts as a counterforce proximally and distally to the forces of the forearm and hand, respectively. A strap securing the splint at the axis position provides a reciprocal parallel force (Li, 1999).

Increase the Area of Force Application to Disperse Pressure and Increase Comfort

Splints apply external forces to all areas of contact. The concept of pressure dispersion suggests that the larger the contact area, the less overall pressure for any area, given a constant resistance (Li, 1999). This means that a wide, long splint applies less pressure in any one area than a narrow, short splint. A contoured splint requires more material and surface area contact than an uneven or point-pressured design over a prominence. *Safety Message: Padding may actually increase pressure to the hand if the splint is not well molded.*

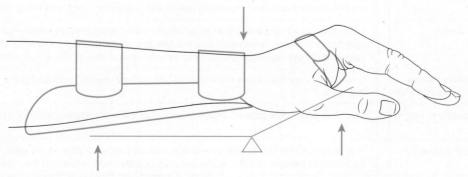

Figure 16-6 The splint as a class 1 lever system.

Add Strength through Contouring Tensile Characteristics

The response that a material has to stress and the degree of strain produced in an elastic body is described in Hooke's law of elasticity. This law suggests that if the same material is curved, the level of energy stored is greater, and the material can more effectively withstand force (*American Heritage Science Dictionary*, 2005). This means that contour mechanically increases a material's strength. Therefore, splints should be constructed with contour and extend midway around the part being splinted to create increased strength and maximum comfort (Fess et al., 2004). Curved and contoured edges are preferred over square edges.

CONSIDERATIONS REGARDING SPLINT MATERIALS

You may become biased toward certain materials that are relatively easy to work with, but with experience, you will learn to appreciate a variety of materials, each with its own benefits and limitations. The properties of various splint materials determine their suitability for use in specific and varied splint applications (Canelon, 1995). These properties have significant bearing on any splint construction: material strength or its ability to bear stress, density or thickness, conformability or drape, self-adherence or surface texture, durability or the ability to repeatedly tolerate stress, ease of fabrication, cost, and availability (Canelon, 1995).

A material's strength describes its ability to bear stress, and rigidity identifies the amount of bend or compression that occurs in response to the stress (Canelon, 1995). When heavy activity is anticipated, the ability to repeatedly tolerate stress is an important consideration, particularly if the splint is to be used for long periods of time with stress and nonstress cycles throughout the wear period (Canelon, 1995). Splint materials are also available in a variety of thicknesses. The most commonly used thicknesses are 1/8 and 1/16 inch. Thick material is preferred for rigid splints, whereas thin material is suited for finger-based or circumferential splint designs.

Available materials have varying levels of elasticity, and the demand placed on the splint is vital in selecting a material. Low-temperature thermoplastics have plasticlike, rubber, or rubberlike bases that give the splinting material its individual characteristics (Breger-Lee et al., 1993; Breger-Lee & Buford, 1992). In choosing thermoplastics, consideration must be given to these characteristics, because they are the basis for the specific physical and mechanical variations of the materials (Canelon, 1995). Materials with a plastic (polycaprolactone) base, such as Polyform™ (Patterson Medical) and NCM Clinic (North Coast Medical), may have fillers that affect their drape and durability. Materials with a rubber (polyisoprene) base, such as Orthoplast (North Coast Medical), have less drape and require firmer handling. Some

of these materials, such as Aquaplast (Patterson Medical), have memory that allows them to stretch and return to their original shape with reheating (see Resources 16-1 for information about suppliers).

The degree of conformability of the splint material determines the handling techniques required (McKee & Morgan, 1998). A material with a high degree of conformability, or drape, molds easily to the contours of the hand. Conformability is suitable when an intimate contour is desired; a material with decreased drape is preferred for firm handling techniques.

A material's self-adherence or bonding strength is considered when splint design requires attaching two or more pieces of material together. Polyform (Patterson Medical) is an example of a material that has a coating, or laminate, on the surface that resists self-adherence until it is modified. This coating must be removed before attaching straps or other permanent attachments; common techniques include using a solvent or scraping the surface. If a bonding solvent is not available to remove the laminate, a cotton towel pressed into the contact sites of the heated material works well to remove the laminate from various materials.

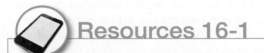

Resources 16-1

Resources for Locations of Suppliers

Each of the resources listed has online and mail order catalogs to assist in acquiring specific materials and accessories for splinting. It is recommended to have these resources readily available to equip your splint workshop.

AliMed Inc.

297 High Street
Dedham, MA 02026-9135
Phone: 800-225-2610
Fax: 800-437-2966
www.alimed.com

DeRoyal Industries

200 DeBusk Lane
Powell, TN 37849
Phone: 800-251-9864
Fax: 800-543-2182
www.deroyal.com

North Coast Medical, Inc.

18305 Sutter Boulevard
Morgan Hill, CA 95037-2845
Phone: 800-821-9319
Fax: 877-213-9300
www.ncmedical.com

Patterson Medical Holdings, Inc (formerly Sammons Preston Rolyan)

1000 Remington Blvd.,
Suite 210
Bolingbrook, Illinois
60440-5117
Phone: 800-323-5547
Fax: 800-547-4333
www.pattersonmedical.com

UE Tech

P.O. Box 2145
Edwards, CO 81632
Phone: 800-736-1894 or
970-926-8867
Fax: 970-926-8870

Once the laminate is removed, the adhesive qualities are vastly improved.

Some materials are susceptible to fingerprints. A controlled technique of smooth, gentle, stroking during molding can prevent fingerprinting. Surface textures vary as well.

Ease of fabrication is multifactorial. It includes the time, equipment, and skills or techniques used to build the splint from design to creation (Canelon, 1995). Material cost and availability should be considered based on effectiveness for a particular splint design.

Soft lightweight splint materials, such as neoprene or thickened closed cell foam are also available. These materials provide light restriction, which may be desirable for patients who do not tolerate hard thermoplastic splints. The disadvantages of these splints may be their bulk, lack of rigidity, and relatively short durability (Breger-Lee & Buford, 1991). *Safety Message: Sensitivity to various materials, such as an allergic contact dermatitis to neoprene has been reported in the literature (Stern et al., 1998).* The therapist should consider the patient's tolerance to any material being used in splinting.

Technological advances have allowed engineers to incorporate an antimicrobial agent into several splinting materials. Splints are often worn continuously against the skin; a moist environment can lead to bacteria and an unpleasant smell over time. Antimicrobial protection may make it easier to clean and maintain splints that are worn continuously. High-temperature thermoplastics are also available for rigid splinting. They require use of a band saw for cutting and an oven for heating (Fess et al., 2004). These high-temperature thermoplastics have high-impact strength but do not contour well, making them unsuitable for hand splinting.

PATIENT CONSIDERATIONS IN SPLINTING

As with any intervention, the therapist considers many patient factors in determining the appropriateness of splinting (see Procedures for Practice 16-1). The therapist should evaluate the patient's neurovascular status (sensation and blood supply), mobility, motor function, edema, tone, and cognition prior to splint design and construction. Sensory deficit in the hand creates a concern: the patient may not be able to feel pressure points or areas of irritation from the splint, which can lead to skin breakdown or injury. In the case of hypersensitivity, the use of a splint can protect the fingertip or hand from unpleasant stimuli. Edema may also indicate the need for close monitoring of splint fit and comfort. As edema diminishes, the splint requires modification or remolding to maintain proper fit. Deficits in mobility may change during the course of splinting, so the splint may have to be modified. Weakness may indicate the need for a dynamic assist splint to prevent muscle imbalance or deformity. As muscle strength improves, the force of the dynamic assist should

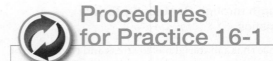

Procedures for Practice 16-1

Considerations for Designing a Splint

- What is the patient's provisional diagnosis?
- Is there a good reason to splint? If so, what should the splint accomplish?
- Does the benefit of splinting outweigh the benefits of not using a splint?
- Does the clinical evaluation support the provisional diagnosis and intervention of splinting?
- What are the implications of splinting for various anatomical factors (e.g., affected structures, number of joints, etc.)?
- Biomechanically should the splint be static, static progressive, or dynamic?
- What are the mechanical considerations? Forearm or hand based? Volar or dorsal design?
- Can the goals be achieved with a commercial splint?
- Does the patient understand the purpose and benefits of the splint?
- Can the patient don and doff the splint as required?
- What can be done to support patient adherence?

be adjusted to the patient's needs. Increased or decreased tone may indicate the need for splinting to maintain balance and prevent contracture. As tone changes, the therapist should modify the splint as necessary to meet the goals of treatment. Ongoing assessment helps the therapist identify any need for changes in the splint.

In designing a splint that includes functional positioning of the thumb, the therapist notes the position of the thumb for prehension to the index and middle finger (Fig. 16-20). Typically, the thumb is held in palmar abduction and opposition to these fingers for effective prehension. While forming the splint, the therapist may have the patient hold a pen or other object in the hand to test the ability of the thumb to achieve functional prehension. When designing a splint for the patient with carpal tunnel syndrome, the therapist should be aware of the position of the wrist that produces the lowest pressure in the carpal canal. The ideal position for the wrist is close to neutral, with $2 \pm 9°$ of dorsiflexion and $2 \pm 6°$ of ulnar deviation (Weiss et al., 1995).

Primary Reasons to Use Splinting as a Therapeutic Intervention

There are many reasons to introduce splinting into a patient's therapeutic program (see Definition 16-2). By understanding the body's response to trauma and the healing process, the therapist can better identify the patient's splinting needs. Trauma to the body creates

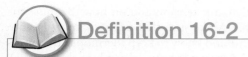

Definition 16-2

Reasons to Splint (Fess, 2002)

Reasons to splint include:

- to improve function
- avoid deformity
- to correct deformity
- to protect healing structures
- to limit motion
- to allow tissue proliferation and remodeling

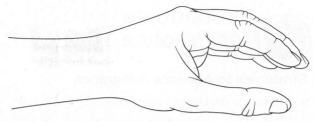

Figure 16-8 Functional position of the hand.

an inflammatory response, creating increased capillary permeability that results in tissue edema (Hedman et al., 2009). To determine the most appropriate management technique, the therapist must understand the integrity of the tissue involved. If the integrity of the tissue involved is stable, motion can be used for edema reduction and functional recovery; the stress of active motion to unstable structures can cause edema production and delay the recovery process.

Tissue Healing

The therapist should be aware of the phases of wound healing when selecting the splint design for the patient with an injured hand. Splinting applies gentle stress to healing tissues to influence change (Fess & McCollum, 1998). During the inflammatory phase, the therapist may use a splint to immobilize and protect the healing tissues (Fig. 16-7). A splint in the position of safe immobilization, also known as the intrinsic-plus position, is considered during this phase to reduce risks of collateral ligament shortening at the metacarpal phalangeal (MCP) joints and tissue contracture throughout the area of insult. The MCP joints are placed in flexion, and the interphalangeal (IP) joints are in extension, whereas the wrist is placed in extension to the degree of function (Coppard & Lohman, 1996).

During the fibroblastic phase of healing, splints may be used to mobilize healing tissues while protecting them. As the strength of the healing tissue increases, the scar tissue matures in the maturation phase. Low-load force may be applied with splinting as in the use of a static progressive splint, which is designed to lengthen contracted tissues through the application of incrementally adjusted static force. As maturation progresses, the tissues can tolerate an increased amount of stress (Schultz-Johnson, 2002).

A therapist must recognize these changes in healing tissues with appropriate changes in the splinting program. A splint incorporating the functional position may be considered in the later two phases of tissue healing (Fig. 16-8). This places the wrist in extension as in the intrinsic-plus splint, decreases the MCP joint flexion to approximately 20° and flexes the IP joints to approximately 10° each, while placing the thumb in palmar abduction with the MCP joint and the IP joint of the thumb in extension (Coppard & Lohman, 1996). Exercise programs for tissue preparation and functional activity must begin simultaneously with splinting to maximize therapeutic benefit.

Influence of Splinting on Scar Remodeling

When immobilization is required to heal damaged tissue, collagen fibers develop increased intermolecular bonds, which result in dense tissue with relatively little mobility (Bell-Krotoski & Figarola, 1995). This response causes tissues to shorten, resulting in contracture. Such a limitation in mobility may be treated with splinting. Current research suggests that ideal tissue remodeling occurs with gentle elongation of tissues (Boccolari & Tocco, 2009). Tissues lengthen and grow if gentle stress is applied (Boccolari & Tocco, 2009). This process is not stretching but rather tissue proliferation to accommodate the stress placed on them (Bell-Krotoski & Figarola, 1995; Brand, 2002).

Patient Adherence to Splint Wearing

Patient adherence has a profound influence on the effectiveness of any intervention. Even the most expertly

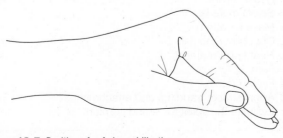

Figure 16-7 Position of safe immobilization.

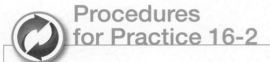

Procedures
for Practice 16-2

Strategies to Advance Adherence

- Incorporate the patient's preferences (as able) in splint design.
- When possible, educate family members of the importance of splint use.
- Educate the patient in benefits of splint use and the possible outcomes if splint is not used.
- Instruct in proper splint wear and care to include splint hygiene.
- Make sure the splint fits properly and feels comfortable.
- Incorporate aesthetics into the splint design for improved cosmesis.
- Offer splint options to the patient if possible.
- Provide for easy application and removal of the splint.
- If feasible, collaborate with the patient on a wearing schedule.

designed and constructed splint will not benefit the patient if it is not worn. Adherence to a therapeutic program is influenced by intrinsic and extrinsic factors. Intrinsic factors are derived from the patient's perception of hand function, the seriousness of the injury, and the perceived efficacy of the treatment or rehabilitation (Sandford, Barlow, & Lewis, 2008). The therapist must understand that a patient's perception of the effectiveness of the splint in achieving the goals of rehabilitation can influence his or her willingness to wear a splint (McKee & Rivard, 2011; O'Brien, 2010). An informed patient takes ownership and adheres to splint use.

Extrinsic factors likely to influence adherence include time restriction, discomfort or pain, forgetting to perform the program or splint application, interference with family or social activities, and a lack of positive feedback (Sandford, Barlow, & Lewis, 2008). It is helpful to collaborate with the patient to identify effective options that are also acceptable to the patient (see Procedures for Practice 16-2 for strategies to advance adherence).

Education

Patients must be taught the goal and purpose of splinting. It may also be helpful to inform the patient of the consequences of failing to comply with splint wear. Provide written instructions on wear and care, which may include a diagram of proper application. If the patient has a cognitive deficit, instruct a caregiver in the proper application of the splint. Patients or caregivers also receive instructions to watch for pressure points, edema,

and excessive dynamic tension and on how to adjust the splint, if feasible. Make sure that patients know how to clean their splints and know to keep thermoplastic splints away from heat (so that splints do not lose their shape). Schedule a follow-up visit if you anticipate needing to modify the splint.

SPLINT CONSTRUCTION

Methods to construct splints from thermoplastic materials are described here. An overview of this process is provided in Procedures for Practice 16-3, as well as in the figures on the pages that follow. Figures 16-9 through 16-18 depict the process of making a resting splint, Figures 16-19 through 16-21 depict the process of making a thumb splint, and Figures 16-22 through 16-32 depict the process of making a dynamic extension splint.

Splint Design

As discussed above, the primary determination of a splint design is identified by the provisional diagnosis. Total design is multifactorial, requiring an appropriate assessment of the patient and clinical condition. Design decisions are also informed by relevant biomechanical and physiological factors and the therapeutic goals of the patient, therapist, and physician (Fess, 1995). The clinician weighs options by also considering costs related to custom splint construction. If there is a commercial splint that achieves the same purpose, it may be more cost effective to provide the commercial splint.

Material Selection

As discussed earlier, occupational therapists become familiar with the properties of various thermoplastics in order to select the material that best meets the patient's needs

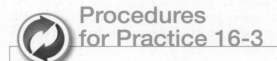

Procedures
for Practice 16-3

Steps in Splint Construction

1. Design splint.
2. Select material.
3. Make a pattern.
4. Cut splint material.
5. Heat splint material.
6. Form splint.
7. Finish edges.
8. Apply straps, padding, and attachments.
9. Evaluate the splint for fit and comfort.

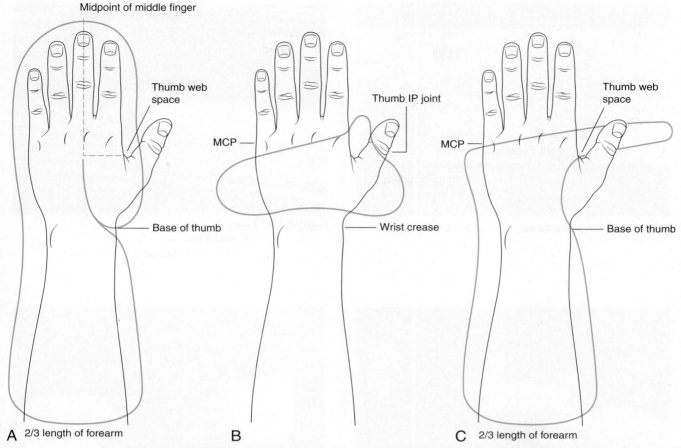

Figure 16-9   Patterns. **A.** Resting splint. **B.** Hand-based thumb splint. **C.** Dorsal wrist splint. IP, interphalangeal; MCP, metacarpophalangeal.

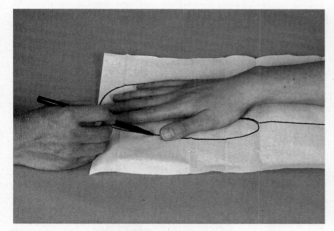

Figure 16-10   Making the pattern for a resting splint on a patient.

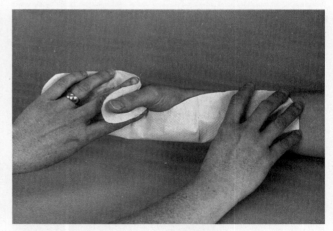

Figure 16-11   Fitting the pattern on the patient.

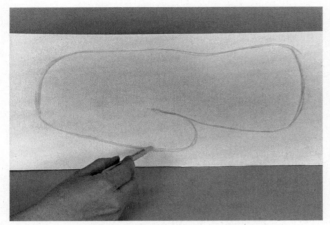

Figure 16-12 Transferring the pattern to the thermoplastic.

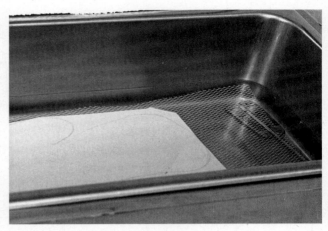

Figure 16-13 Heating the thermoplastic.

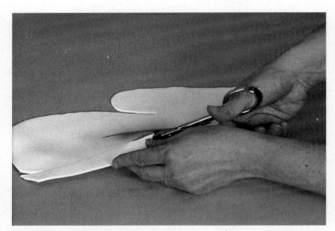

Figure 16-14 Cutting the thermoplastic.

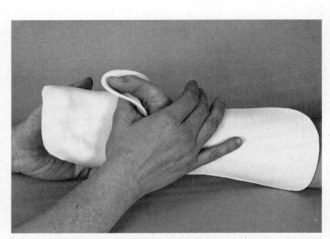

Figure 16-15 Forming the splint on the patient.

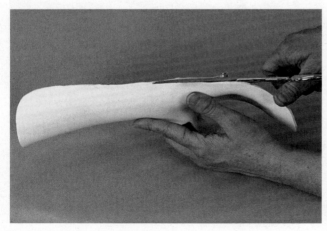

Figure 16-16 Trimming the splint.

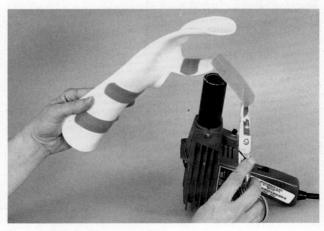

Figure 16-17 Applying straps.

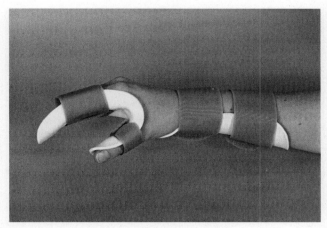

Figure 16-18 Finished resting splint on the patient.

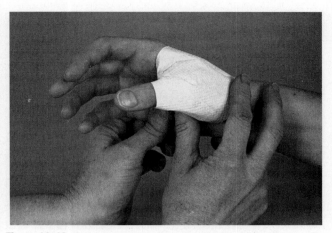

Figure 16-19 Fitting the pattern on the patient for a hand-based thumb splint.

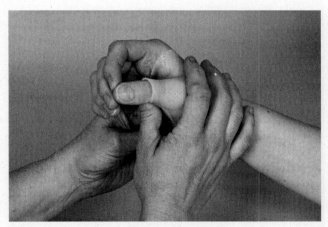

Figure 16-20 Forming the splint on the patient.

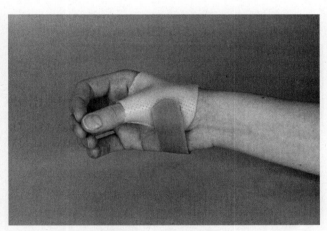

Figure 16-21 Finished splint on the patient.

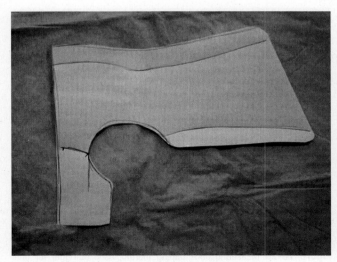

Figure 16-22 Pattern for a dynamic finger extension splint.

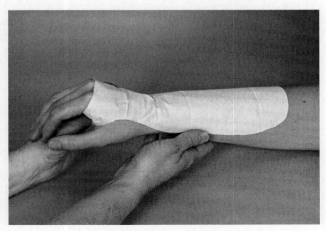

Figure 16-23 Fitting the pattern for the wrist splint base on the patient.

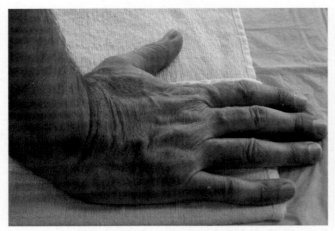

Figure 16-24 Pressing into heated plastic with a cotton towel removes the material laminent, which prepares it for self-bonding.

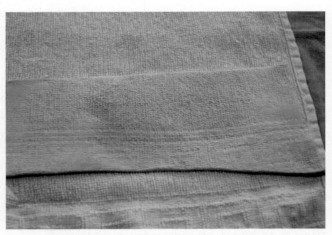

Figure 16-25 Towel impressions indicate that enough pressure was applied to remove the laminent from the splinting material.

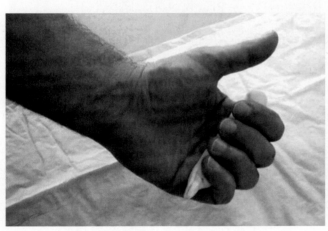

Figure 16-26 Shaping the thermoplastic into a tube.

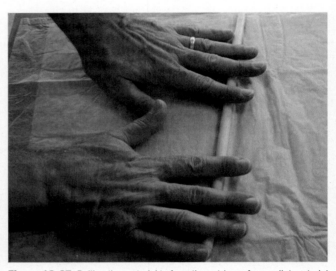

Figure 16-27 Rolling the material to form the outrigger from splint material scraps.

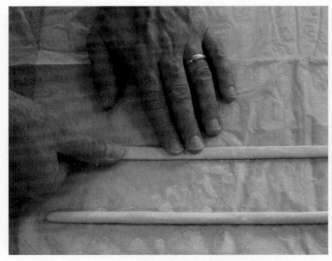

Figure 16-28 Pressing thermoplastic into flattened outrigger.

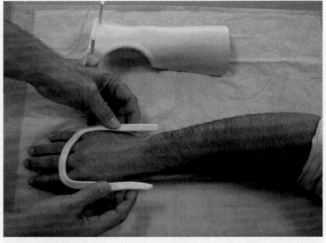

Figure 16-29 Measuring and shaping thermoplastic outrigger for final construction.

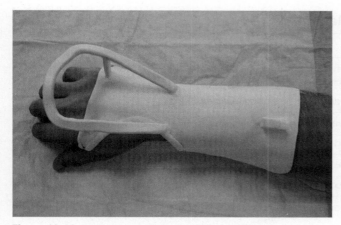

Figure 16-30 Placing thermoplastic outrigger on splint base.

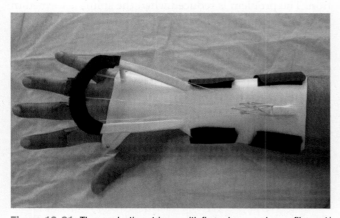

Figure 16-31 Thermoplastic outrigger with finger loops and monofilament/rubber band dynamics placed on splint base.

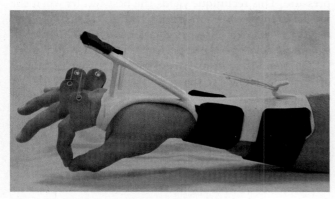

Figure 16-32 Proper dynamic angle of the outrigger.

and aligns with the purpose of the splint (see Table 16-2 for pros and cons of some commonly used materials).

Pattern Making

Once the splint design and material are determined, the splint should be well visualized, and you can create a pattern. A well-designed splint pattern leads to a functional, well-fitted splint. The pattern provides a two-dimensional guide for the three-dimensional splint that helps minimize waste of time and splint material. Three common splint patterns are illustrated in Figure 16-9. Paper towels provide an excellent moldable pattern, but any type of paper can be used for the pattern. Place the patient's hand directly on the paper and mark the anatomical landmarks according to the design being used (Fig. 16-10).

The pattern must extend beyond the lateral borders of the hand and forearm to allow the splint to form a trough, which will extend halfway around the surface being splinted for adequate support. When creating a forearm-based splint—dorsal, volar, or lateral—extend the forearm trough two-thirds the length of the forearm. Once drawn, cut out the pattern and place it on the patient in the design of the splint to assure it does not block joints unnecessarily (see Figs. 16-11, 16-19, and 16-23).

Modifications can be achieved by reducing the pattern, adding paper for extra length or width as needed. If the patient is unable to lay the hand flat for pattern drawing because of deformity or spasticity, use the uninvolved hand for pattern making and flip the pattern over for the contralateral side. A pattern can be adjusted for edema or other variations before transferring. When the pattern fits as designed, trace it onto the splinting material (Fig. 16-12).

A pen or pencil can be used to draw the pattern on the thermoplastic material. Cut away the marks as you cut out the splint. An awl can also be used to scratch the pattern onto the plastic.

Cutting

Cut the splinting material to a size that will fit the pattern; this provides a manageable sheet of plastic. Cut the full sheet with a utility knife by scoring it and bending it; turn the material over and score it again from the other side. Heat the thermoplastic once the pattern is marked (see Fig. 16-13). When the material is soft, cut the splint pattern out with sharp straight-edged scissors (see Fig. 16-14).

Cutting the material after heating eliminates rough edges, saving time in the finishing step. Minimize fingerprinting by maintaining the material on the work surface, handling it by sliding your flattened hand under the material, lifting as little as possible, and retaining the material horizontally while cutting to avoid stretching.

Table 16-2	**Pros and Cons of Various Splint Materials**
Splint Material	**Pros and Cons**
Rolyan® Polyform™ Patterson Medical	Pros: Stretches easily, conforms well for intimate fit, minimal handling, rigid, excellent self-bonding, used for hand-based splints, creating dynamic outriggers Cons: When overheated, it is difficult to control; no memory
Rolyan® Aquaplast® Patterson Medical	Pros: Stretches easily, excellent memory, excellent for serial splints or fracture bracing Cons: Additional work required to smooth edges
Orthoplast® North Coast Medical	Pros: Excellent for reuse in serial splints, good for forearm-based splints, edges smooth easily Cons: Limited long-term self-bonding
LMB Blend DeRoyal	Pros: Controlled stretch, good drape ability, excellent for reuse in serial splints, static positioning splints Cons: No self-bonding, additional effort to apply attachments

Heating Splinting Material

Electric fry pans, splint pans, and hydrocollators can be used to heat thermoplastic materials. If using a fry pan, the recommended depth of water is at least 1 inch. If using a hydrocollator, prevent material from stretching or dropping to the bottom; heat pan liners are helpful. Water temperature is usually kept at 150°F–160°F for most materials, but the recommended temperature varies among materials. Consult the manufacturer's recommendations for specific materials. Use a thermometer in the water to ensure consistent temperature. Heating time for most materials is about 1 minute. The therapist should check the material to make sure it is heated uniformly before forming the splint on the patient. The working time for splinting materials varies from 1 to 6 minutes depending on thickness or filler. Thin materials cool more rapidly than thick. Because heat guns do not uniformly soften splinting material, they are recommended only for spot heating when attachments are required, minor adjustment, and edge finishing.

Forming the Material into a Splint

Once the entire piece of material is heated, remove it from the water with a spatula or tongs, being careful not to stretch the pattern. The entire piece should feel soft and easily moldable. Lay the material on a towel to dry briefly. If you are rolling the edges to finish them, do so before forming the splint on the patient. If the material is too hot, let it cool slightly before placing it on the patient to assure tolerance and comfort. When using a material with draping qualities, it is best to let gravity assist the positioning.

Proper Positioning

Proper upper extremity positioning during splint construction can make the difference between use of the splint and noncompliance. If the splint is formed with the patient's forearm in supination, the trough of the splint may impose undue pressure on the forearm when it is moved toward the more common functional position of pronation. The problem is reduced when the splint is formed in neutral, creating enhanced comfort during splint use. The therapist must find a position that is comfortable for the patient to maintain. This may require some creativity, such as using a plinth so the patient can lay supine if he or she exhibits restricted shoulder or elbow motion.

After placing the patient's hand and forearm in the desired position, place the heated splint material on the patient. Avoid gripping or squeezing the thermoplastic (Figs. 16-15 and 16-20).

Finishing the Edges

Smooth edges are important to prevent pressure points. Cutting the material at the required temperature allows the edges to seal smoothly without requiring additional work (Fig. 16-16).

With some perforated materials or rough-cut thermoplastics, it may be necessary to smooth the edges by dipping the edge of the splint into the hot water and cutting it to produce a smooth edge or smooth it lightly with fingertip pressure. This technique yields the best results when the fingers are wet while smoothing. *Safety Message: The heat gun produces a very hot stream of dry heat. It should never be directed toward the patient's skin.*

Set the heat gun on a cool setting before turning it off to avoid damage to the motor. If edges remain slightly rough, apply a thin piece of moleskin along the edge to seal it for comfort.

Applying the Straps

Straps attach the splint to the patient. Their location must be planned to achieve optimal surface contact for pressure dispersion and positional stability. Apply adhesive-hook

Velcro® to the splint and use loop or foam strapping material to hold the splint securely on the patient. Hook Velcro® adheres well to the splint if the surface is prepared for the bond. Remove the nonstick finish on the thermoplastic by using a heat gun to spot heat the part of the splint to receive the Velcro® hook and press a cotton towel into the material. Then spot heat the sticky side of the Velcro® with a heat gun before applying it to the thermoplastic (Fig. 16-17).

Other techniques are to apply a solvent or scrape the plastic with the sharp edge of scissors. There are variations to the application of Velcro® hook. A full piece of sticky-back Velcro® can be used on the splint running the width of the trough or two pieces on the splint's edges for each strap. There are advantages and disadvantages to each technique. If the material has been properly prepared to accept the Velcro®, either technique will be adequate. Strapping materials include Velcro®, durable foam, neoprene, and elastic strapping in a variety of widths. It is best to round the corners of the strapping material to avoid bending and "dog ears."

Splint Attachments

Outriggers and pulleys can be attached to splints when the splint base is complete. An outrigger is best considered an extension to the splint base, providing the desired angle to direct a static progressive or dynamic force. An outrigger can be made by rolling or pressing thermoplastic into shape, by using prefabricated tubes, or by bending wire to the desired position (Coppard & Lohman, 1996) (see Procedures

for Practice 16-4). Commercial outriggers are also available. The therapist should consider the requirements of the outrigger, be it high or low profile (Austin et al., 2004), single or multiple finger, static progressive, or dynamic. If the requirements of the outrigger are of a very specific or complex application, it is best to custom construct it from thermoplastic. Begin with a splint base to support the outrigger.

Attach the outrigger or pulley by preparing the surface of the splint first for optimal bond. Use a heat gun to spot heat the material to receive the outrigger or pulley and press a cotton towel into the material, removing the laminate. Spot heat the post or area of the outrigger that will contact the base and attach it to the base while both pieces are heated (Fig. 16-30).

Bonding solvent or scraping the surface of the base can also remove the laminate. The outrigger or pulley attachment points should be treated similarly. Use a heat gun as described above and press them together. To increase the material bond, gently pull and push the base and outrigger enough to stress the material, gradually forcing them tighter together but not enough to separate or shift the position of attachment. As the material cools, hold the pieces together for adequate bonding. They can be cooled with cool water or a cold spray before starting the next attachment.

The described technique will omit the need for additional reinforcement. If an alternate technique is used, heat another piece of thermoplastic and apply it over the outrigger base attachment. Always prepare surfaces with dry heat for effective bonding. Dynamic splints may be prone to slide distally because of the traction on the splint. You can control this migration with appropriate strap placement and a friction-enhanced material that is in contact with the skin. Silicone gel or Microfoam tape (available through Patterson Medical) provides light friction to keep the splint in place. Rubber bands, coil springs, or elastic thread provide the tension to a dynamic splint. They can be attached to the splint with a thermoplastic hook, Velcro® tabs, or thumbscrews placed proximal to the outrigger on the splint base. Pulleys or line guides such as Velcro® hook and loop can redirect the line of pull as needed for dynamic or static progressive flexion splinting. Monofilament (fishing line) attached to the rubber band creates a smooth excursion for the rubber band tension as it pulls over the outrigger or under the pulley (Fig. 16-32).

The monofilament attaches to a finger sling, fingernail hook, or tab to provide the appropriate tension and angle of pull. Dynamic splints may incorporate hinges, which provide a movable axis at a joint. Hinges are available commercially or can be made from rivets (Byron, 1994), crimped thermoplastic tubing, or brass fasteners (Dennys, Hurst, & Cox, 1992). Static progressive splints use locking hinges and various types of inelastic components such as Velcro® strips, monofilament line, MERiT components,

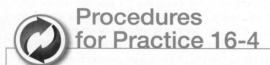

Procedures for Practice 16-4

Process for Creating a Custom Outrigger

A technique to create a custom outrigger with thermoplastic material such as Polyform™ is described here. It is best to use the same material used for the splint base.

1. Heat a piece of material and place it on a cotton towel.
2. Cover the material on all surfaces with the towel and press the towel into the material (Fig. 16-24).
3. The impression of the towel indicates the removal of laminate from the material (Fig. 16-25).
4. Remove the material from the towel and press the warm material into the shape of a solid tube (Fig. 16-26).
5. The material can be reheated in the splint pan as needed and rolled into a tube and then flattened (Figs. 16-27 and 16-28).
6. Reheat the material to allow flexibility to conform it to the hand for precise construction (Fig. 16-29).

and Click Strips (Vazquez, 2002). Hinges and turn screws may also be used for static progressive splinting to provide adjustable positioning of stiff joints in the optimal position tolerated by the patient. These components allow for adjustments as the patient achieves increased mobility (Schultz-Johnson, 2002).

The Use of Padding

When padding a splint (static or dynamic), allow extra space in the design and molding phases to contour over a bony prominence, avoiding additional pressure in this area. Some padding can be applied before forming the splint. When applying the padding after splint construction, ensure that the material padding is measured to fit only the splint formed to accept padding (Fig. 16-33). Cut the padding before removing the pad backing, reducing damage to the scissors. Place padding over the splint area to be padded, assuring proper placement, then remove the backing, and apply padding to the splint (Fig. 16-34).

If the padding is applied to the thermoplastic before heating, the excess water should be squeezed out before applying the material to the patient. You can use stockinette liners instead of padding for light protection, or sticky-back moleskin is also available for a thin, soft padding material. Padding should never substitute for a well-fitting splint.

Evaluating Splint Fit and Comfort

Once the splint is completed, the therapist performs a checkout to verify its fit and comfort and to assure that the patient understands its use and care (see Figs. 16-18, 16-21, and 16-31 and Procedures for Practice 16-5).

In summary, orthotic intervention (such as splint construction) requires a client-centered approach by a skilled therapist. Splinting is an important component in

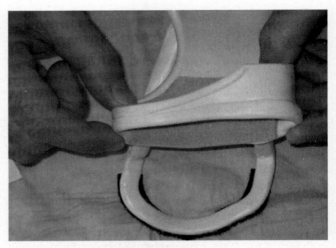

Figure 16-34 Placing padding on the splint.

the rehabilitation process to meet the occupational performance goals of the patient, not just the application of a device. By combining applicable knowledge, principles of splinting, skill, and creativity with the patient's needs, the therapist can meet the challenges imposed to meet the goals of rehabilitation.

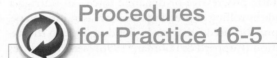

Procedures for Practice 16-5

Splint Checkout

Ask the patient to wear the splint for about 20 minutes, and then remove it. If redness or blanching is identified and does not readily resolve, it may be an indication that the pressure of the splint is too much (Brand, 2002). Modify the splint if signs of excessive pressure are present then reevaluate fit and comfort.

Prior to sending the splint home with the patient, consider the following questions:

- Does the splint achieve the purpose?
- Does the splint maintain proper position at rest and perform as required with stress?
- Does the splint contour to and fit the hand considering arches and bony prominences?
- Does the splint extend beyond necessary structures causing undue restrictions?
- Is the splint long enough to support splinted structures?
- Is the splinting finished with smooth edges and resolved pressure points?
- Can the patient apply and remove the splint?
- Does the patient understand wear and care instructions?
- Does the splint design have maximum patient acceptability for compliance?

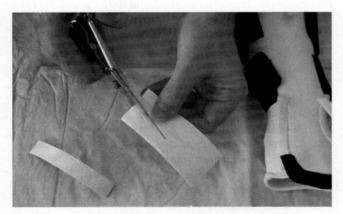

Figure 16-33 Cutting padding prior to removing backing.

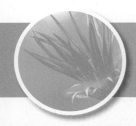

case example

Mr. J.: Construction of a Resting Splint for a Patient with Hemiparesis

Occupational Therapy Assessment Process	Clinical Reasoning Process	
	Objectives	Examples of Therapist's Internal Dialogue
Patient Information Mr. J. is a 67-year-old man who sustained a left cerebral vascular accident (CVA) 4 weeks ago resulting in right hemiparesis. He is medically stable. Hypertonicity of finger flexors limits grasp and release of his right hand. There is limited passive range of motion (PROM) in wrist and finger extension caused by mild hypertonicity. Mr. J. was referred for outpatient occupational therapy to address residual impairments impeding his occupational performance.	Obtain information about the patient	"Hemiparesis will limit the patient's strength, active range of motion, and endurance. Hypertonicity will affect grip strength, active and passive range of motion, gross motor coordination, and dexterity. Flexor inhibition will help weak extensors overcome flexion."
Interview Mr. J. is right-hand dominant, married and lives with his wife in a two-story home. He is retired but has remained socially active through hobbies, including golf and bridge. He misses the many close and supportive friends he has developed through his leisure activities. Currently, his wife assists him with basic activities of daily living (ADL) and community mobility.	Evaluate to identify the problem(s)	"The patient is highly motivated to retain his current hobbies, which require functional grasp and release."
Assessment The therapist tested upper extremity muscle tone, functional range of motion, and sensation during the initial assessment. Using the Modified Ashworth Scale, Mr. J. scored 3: considerable increase in muscle tone with full passive movement difficult to achieve (Bohannon & Smith, 1987). Mr. J. demonstrated right upper extremity active and passive range of motion (A/PROM) within functional limits with the exception of the right wrist and digits. He presented in Brunnstrom stage III: able to perform mass grasp, hook grasp, lateral prehension, but no release or voluntary extension of digits (Trombly, 2008). His right upper extremity sensation is normal.		"The patient values his roles as an independent person, husband, friend, and sportsman. Increased ability to participate in leisure activities will improve his occupational performance, quality of life, and self-esteem."
Mr. J. and his wife were provided instruction on splint purpose, precautions, wear and care, plus consequences of noncompliance. He stated the splint was comfortable and was able to don and doff it independently. Mr. J. received a home exercise program of tactile simulation, weight-bearing, A/PROM, strengthening, and functional activity.	Implement the intervention	"He will need a resting hand splint to help normalize muscle tone, maintain soft tissue length, and prevent painful contractures (Milazzo & Gillen, 2011). I will arrange follow-up appointments to monitor tone and make splint modifications as necessary."
Mr. J. exhibited decreased hypertonicity of the finger flexors and scored 1 on the Modified Ashworth Scale. Testing revealed improved right grip strength and full PROM of fingers. Patient had progressed to Brunnstrom stage V and demonstrated ability to voluntarily grasp and release objects (Trombly, 2008). Mr. J. was able to perform all ADLs to include leisure activities. He discontinued splint use at 6 months post CVA.	Evaluate the result	"I believe that the splint helped inhibit flexor spasticity and prevent contractures following his CVA. It likely helped that Mr. J. adhered to his splint wear schedule and home program."

 Clinical Reasoning in Occupational Therapy Practice

Hemiparesis and Flexor Hypertonicity-Resting Hand Splint

What important factors must be considered in the construction of Mr. J.'s resting splint? What properties should the splinting material selected include? How should the therapist position the wrist and in the splint and why?

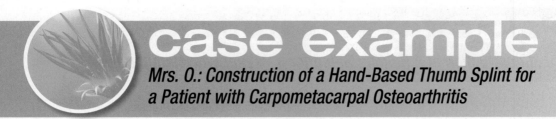

case example

Mrs. O.: Construction of a Hand-Based Thumb Splint for a Patient with Carpometacarpal Osteoarthritis

Occupational Therapy Intervention Process	Clinical Reasoning Process	
	Objectives	Examples of Therapist's Internal Dialogue

Patient Information

Mrs. O. is a 55-year-old right-hand–dominant female with carpometacarpal (CMC) osteoarthritis of the trapeziometacarpal joint of the right hand. Mrs. O. was referred to outpatient occupational therapy for conservative management to reduce hand pain and increase function.

Objectives: Obtain information about the patient

Examples of Therapist's Internal Dialogue: "She can reduce pain by using thermal modalities, applying joint protection principles, wearing a hand-based thumb splint, modifying her activities, and using adaptive equipment when necessary."

Interview

Mrs. O. lives alone in her one-story home. She is employed as a part-time librarian. Her leisure activities include reading and gardening. She is independent in all ADL. She describes pain with tasks like turning a key, grasping books, writing, and using gardening tools. She experiences swelling and redness at the base of her right thumb after prolonged use. Mrs. O. greatly values her self-advancement and self-enhancement roles of independent person, worker, and gardener. Her supervisor has revised her schedule to help lessen pain during work. She will spend more time at the checkout counter and less time shelving books. On her days off, Mrs. O. loves working on her favorite horticulture projects.

Objectives: Evaluate to identify the problem(s)

Examples of Therapist's Internal Dialogue: "Mrs. O. values all her roles. She is highly motivated to make changes that will allow her to continue in these roles."

"Mrs. O. gets so involved in her gardening that she works until her thumb pain is quite severe. She can find ways to manage her time and adapt her gardening."

"Mrs. O. needs to work with her employer to find ways to manage her demands at work by rotating tasks and taking minibreaks."

Assessment

Mrs. O. reported her pain was a 2/10 at rest and 7/10 with activity on the visual analog scale. Ligament stress testing revealed slight joint instability and tenderness with palpation at her right thumb CMC joint. Her sensation was intact, and there was no redness or inflammation present. Right-hand AROM was within functional limits (Biese, 2007).

Mrs. O. is fitted with a custom-fabricated hand-based thumb splint made from a 1/16-inch thermoplastic. She received instruction on her program of splint wear, superficial heat or cold, pain-free thenar eminence strengthening, and AROM exercises. Joint protection, energy conservation, and the benefits of adaptive equipment use are introduced (Kurtz, 2006). She states her splint feels comfortable and is able to don and doff it without difficulty. A follow-up appointment is scheduled for a splint check and review of all instructions.

Objectives: Implement the intervention

Examples of Therapist's Internal Dialogue: "She will benefit from use of a splint during her work day and as needed in the garden. She will modify her work day by taking minibreaks for exercises and alternating tasks that may be stressful to her thumbs. Setting a timer while in the garden to remind her to take breaks will help her pain awareness. Adaptive tools and joint protection techniques may be helpful in daily tasks as well as in the garden."

Mrs. O. tolerates the splint well and wears it as needed during the day. She is able to work and garden with the splint on. She is compliant with her home exercise program and has integrated joint protection strategies and adaptive equipment into her daily routine. Mrs. O. reports home paraffin baths help alleviate her joint pain.

Objectives: Evaluate the results

Examples of Therapist's Internal Dialogue: "She may need splint adjustments over time as changes occur in her hand. She may require different splints for different activities: one for work and one for gardening."

Clinical Reasoning in Occupational Therapy Practice

Carpometacarpal Osteoarthritis and Hand-Based Thumb Splint Wear Compliance

During the assessment, Mrs. O. reveals that she does not understand how wearing a splint will decrease her thumb pain. In fact, she fears that it will be uncomfortable and interfere with her ability to use her hand. How can the therapist address Mrs. O.'s concerns and persuade her as to the effectiveness of the splint in helping her achieve her rehabilitation goals?

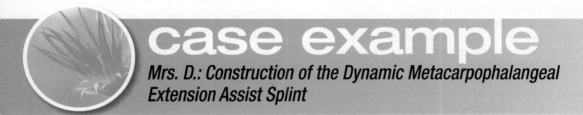

case example

Mrs. D.: Construction of the Dynamic Metacarpophalangeal Extension Assist Splint

Occupational Therapy Intervention Process	Clinical Reasoning Process	
	Objectives	**Examples of Therapist's Internal Dialogue**
Patient Information Mrs. D. is a 41-year-old, right-hand–dominant woman with a 12-year history of rheumatoid arthritis. Her surgeon performed left-hand metacarpophalangeal (MCP) arthroplasties with the surgical goals of restoring normal joint alignment and extensor tendon balance for improved hand function (Theisen, 2006). Mrs. D. was referred to occupational therapy 5 days postoperative for splinting, therapy, and activities of daily living (ADL) adaptations.	Obtain information about the patient	"Initially, Mrs. D. will have limited left-hand use; she will need assistance with ADL and must learn to perform many tasks one-handed. Her family will help with household tasks. She has taken a medical leave from work to devote the next month to therapy. The surgeon was pleased with the surgical result and wants her to follow his standard protocol. Mrs. D. is healthy and should do well."
Interview Mrs. D. lives in a two-story home with her husband and three teenage daughters. She is employed as a part-time receptionist and remarks that her hand deformity has made keyboarding extremely hard. Cooking is her favorite social and creative outlet, but her hand makes this hobby difficult. She cannot lay her hand flat, wash her face, or put her hand in her pocket. She has trouble turning keys, opening doors, and cutting with a knife. Mrs. D. values her self-advancement and self-enhancement roles of worker and cook. She will return to work but is happy her leave of absence will permit her to focus on her rehabilitation. Her daughters will assist with household chores.	Evaluate to identify the problem(s)	"Ms. D. values her roles as an independent person, wife, mother, friend, and worker. She wants to retain those roles." "During the recovery process, her activity requirements will be reviewed. Joint protection techniques and kitchen adaptations may be suggested."

Assessment

The patient's left-hand sensation is normal. Mrs. D. exhibits no signs of infection. There is mild edema localized to the dorsum of her left hand. Active range of motion (AROM) measurements are MCP extension of 0° and flexion 25°.

The therapist applies a light dressing and fabricates a dynamic extension splint for daytime wear and a resting splint for night use. Mrs. D. can actively flex her MCPs in the dynamic splint, and then the rubber bands passively return her MCPs to a neutral position. She and her husband are given verbal and written instructions to perform active MCP flexion exercises in the dynamic splint 10 times each waking hour, allowing the rubber bands to return her MCPs to full extension. Additional instructions describe splint wear and care, edema control techniques, wound care, and scar management. The surgeon told Mrs. D. that light ADL can be resumed while wearing the dynamic extension splint at postoperative week 3. She wears the dynamic splint for 4 weeks. She receives joint protection, energy conservation, work simplification, and adaptive device education to facilitate improved occupational performance.

Mrs. D. returns to work 4 weeks after surgery to answer phones with the use of a wireless headset and is learning to use a voice-activated keyboarding system. She gradually increases work demands and resumes full duties at 6 weeks after surgery. She continues to use the night resting splint for 3 months. Mrs. D. is very happy with her outcome. Her occupational performance is greatly improved because of her improved hand function and willingness to apply joint protection, work simplification, and energy conservation principles.

"She must wear a dynamic splint during the day and a resting splint at night per postoperative protocol."

Implement the intervention	"Mrs. D. will follow a standard protocol for postoperative MCP arthroplasty. She needs review of joint protection, work simplification, and energy conservation principles. Information on adaptive devices that will enable her to perform daily tasks more efficiently will be provided; she should be open to any suggestions."
Evaluate the results	"Mrs. D. has had uneventful recovery and outstanding functional outcome."

Clinical Reasoning in Occupational Therapy Practice

Patient with Rheumatoid Arthritis: Ensuring a Positive Postoperative Outcome

Mrs. D. has had rheumatoid arthritis for 12 years. How does her diagnosis affect the therapist's splinting intervention?

Summary Review Questions

1. Name the steps of splint making in order.
2. Name the creases of the hand and describe their importance in splint construction.
3. What is the difference between the functional position of the hand and the position of safe immobilization in splinting? Give an example of when you would use each.
4. Describe the concept of dual obliquity as applied to splinting.
5. What does mechanical advantage mean in splinting?
6. What are some strategies to enhance compliance with splint wear?
7. What does a splint checkout include?
8. What are the top six cited reasons to introduce splinting as a therapeutic intervention?

Glossary

Dual obliquity—The difference, or variance between the length and the height of the metacarpals, with the radial side longer and higher than the ulnar side. This difference must be considered when designing splints for the hand.

Dynamic splint—A splint that applies a mobile force, applied with rubber bands or springs, in one direction while allowing active motion in the opposite direction.

Fibroblastic phase—Stage of wound healing that follows the inflammatory phase, during which fibroblasts proliferate and initiate collagen production in the healing of tissues.

Inflammatory phase—Phase of wound healing immediately following injury or surgery, characterized by edema and infiltration of leukocytes and macrophages to begin healing tissue.

Maturation phase—Stage of wound healing that follows the fibroblastic phase; characterized by wound contraction, remodeling, and maturation of the healed tissues.

Splint—A device applied to the body to provide protection, positioning, immobilization, restriction, correction, or prevention of deformity for the splinted part; an orthosis.

Static progressive splint—A splint designed to stretch contractures through the application of incrementally adjusted static force to promote lengthening of contracted tissues.

References

American Heritage Science Dictionary. (2005). Boston: Houghton Mifflin.

American Occupational Therapy Association. (2008). Occupational therapy practice framework: Domain and process (2nd ed.). *American Journal of Occupational Therapy, 62,* 625–683.

Austin, G. P., Slamet, M., Cameron, D., & Austin, N. M. (2004). A comparison of high-profile and low-profile dynamic mobilization splint designs. *Journal of Hand Therapy, 17,* 335–343.

Bell-Krotoski, J. A., & Figarola, J. H. (1995). Biomechanics of soft-tissue growth and remodeling with plaster casting. *Journal of Hand Therapy, 8,* 131–137.

Biese, J. (2007). Arthritis. In C. Cooper (Ed.), *Fundamentals of hand therapy: Clinical reasoning and treatment guidelines for common diagnoses of the upper extremity* (pp. 348–375). St. Louis: Mosby Elsevier.

Boccolari, P., & Tocco, S. (2009). Alternative splinting approach for proximal interphalangeal joint flexion contractures: No profile static progressive splinting & cylinder splint combo. *Journal of Hand Therapy, 22(3),* 288–293

Bohannon, R., & Smith, M. (1987). Interrater reliability of a modified Ashworth scale of muscle spasticity. *Physical Therapy, 67,* 206.

Brand, P. (2002). The forces of dynamic splinting: Ten questions before applying a dynamic splint to the hand. In J. Hunter, E. Macking, & A. Callahan (Eds.), *Rehabilitation of the hand* (5th ed., pp. 1811–1817). St. Louis: Mosby.

Breger-Lee, D. E., & Buford, W. L., Jr. (1991). Update in splinting materials and methods. *Hand Clinics, 7,* 569–585.

Breger-Lee, D. E., & Buford, W. L., Jr. (1992). Properties of thermoplastic splinting materials. *Journal of Hand Therapy, 5,* 202–211.

Breger-Lee, D. E., Voelker, E. T., Giurintano, D., Novick, A., & Browder, L. (1993). Reliability of torque range of motion: A preliminary study. *Journal of Hand Therapy, 6,* 29–34.

Byron, P. (1994). Splinting the arthritic hand. *Journal of Hand Therapy, 7,* 29–32.

Canelon, M. (1995). Material properties: A factor in the selection and application of splinting materials for athletic wrist and hand injuries. *Journal of Orthopedic & Sports Physical Therapy, 23,* 164–172.

Coppard, B. M., & Lohman, H. (1996). *Introduction to splinting: A critical-thinking and problem solving approach.* St. Louis: Mosby, Incorporated.

Dennys, L. J., Hurst, L. N., & Cox, J. (1992). Management of proximal interphalangeal joint fractures using a new dynamic traction splint and early active motion. *Journal of Hand Therapy, 5,* 16–24.

Fess, E. E. (1995). Splints: Mechanics versus convention. *Journal of Hand Therapy, 8,* 124–130.

Fess, E. E. (2002). A history of splinting: To understand the present, view the past. *Journal of Hand Therapy, 15,* 97–132.

Fess, E. E., Gettle, K., Philips, C., & Janson, R. (2004). *Hand and upper extremity splinting: Principles and methods* (3rd ed.). St. Louis: Mosby.

Fess, E.E., McCollum, M., The influence of splinting on healing tissues. *Journal of Hand Therapy,* 1998 Jul; 11(3):163–236.

Hamilton, N., Weimer, W., & Luttgens, K. (2011). *Kinesiology: Scientific basis of human motion* (12th ed., Rev.). Boston: McGraw Hill, Inc.

Hedman, T.L., Quick, C.D., Richard, R.L., Renz, E.M., Fisher, S.V., Rivers, E. A., Casey, J.C., Chung, K.K., Desocio, P.A., Dewey, W.S., Drook, J.L., Lehnerz, N.J., Maani, C.V., Montalvo, A.E., Shields, B.A., Smith, M.Z. Thompson, C.K., White, A.F., Williams, J.F., And Young, A.W., (2009). Rehabilitation of burn casualties. In *Textbooks of Military Medicine: Care of the Combat Amputee* (pp. 277–379). Office of the Surgeon General Department of the Army, United States of America and U. S. Army Medical Department Center and School, Fort Sam Houston Texas.

Kurtz, P. (2006). Conservative management of arthritis. In S. Burke, J. Higgins, M. McClinton, R. Saunders, & L. Valdata (Eds.), *Hand and upper extremity rehabilitation: A practical guide* (3rd ed., pp. 649–658). St. Louis: Elsevier Churchill Livingstone.

Levangie, P., & Norkin, C. (2005). *Joint structure & function: A comprehensive analysis* (4th ed.). Philadelphia: F. A. Davis Company.

Li, C. (1999). Force analysis of the belly gutter and capener splints. *Journal of Hand Therapy, 12,* 337–343.

McKee, P., & Morgan, L. (1998). *Orthotics in rehabilitation.* Philadelphia: Davis.

McKee, P., & Rivard, A. (2011). Biopsychosocial approach to orthotic intervention. *Journal of Hand Therapy, 24,* 155–163.

Milazzo, S., & Gillen, G. (2011). Splinting applications. In A. Burkhard & G. Gillen (Eds.), *Stroke rehabilitation a function-based approach* (3rd ed., pp. 326–349). St. Louis: Mosby.

Muscolino, J. E. (2011). *Kinesiology: The skeletal system and muscle function* (2nd ed.). St. Louis: Mosby.

O'Brien, L. (2010). Adherence to therapeutic splint wear in adults with acute upper limb injuries: A systematic review. *Hand Therapy, 15,* 3–12.

Reilly, M. (1962). Occupational therapy can be one of the greatest ideas of 20th century medicine. *American Journal of Occupational Therapy, 16,* 87–105.

Sandford, F., Barlow, N., Lewis, J., A Study to Examine Patient Adherence to Wearing 24-Hour Forearm Thermoplastic Splints after Tendon Repairs. *Journal of Hand Therapy,* 2008 Jan; 21(1):44-53.

Sandford, F., Barlow, N., & Lewis, J. (2008). A study to examine patient adherence to wearing 24-hour forearm thermoplastic splints after tendon repairs, *Journal of Hand Therapy, 21*, 44–51.

Schultz-Johnson, K. (2002). Static progressive splinting. *Journal of Hand Therapy, 15,* 163–178.

Stern, E. B., Callinan, N., Hank, M., Lewis, E. J., Schousboe, J. T., & Ytterberg, S. R. (1998). Neoprene splinting: Dermatological issues. *American Journal of Occupational Therapy, 52,* 573–578.

Theisen, L. (2006). Metacarpophalangeal joint arthroplasty. In S. Burke, J. Higgins, M. McClinton, R. Saunders, & L. Valdata (Eds.), *Hand upper extremity rehabilitation: A practical guide* (3rd ed., pp. 625–631). St. Louis: Elsevier Churchill Livingstone.

Trombly, C. (2008). Optimizing motor behavior using the Brunnstrom movement therapy approach. In M. Radomski & C. Trombly (Eds.), *Occupational therapy for physical dysfunction* (6th ed., pp. 668–689). Baltimore: Lippincott.

Tubiana, R., Thomine, J. M., & Mackin, E. (1996). *Examination of the hand and wrist.* St. Louis: Mosby-Year Book.

Vasquez, N. (2002). Introduction to a new method for inelastic mobilization. *Journal of Hand Therapy, 15,* 205–209.

Weiss, N.D., Gordon, L., Bloom, T., So, Y., Rempel, D.M., Position of the wrist associated with the lowest carpal-tunnel pressure: implications for splint design. *Journal of Bone and Joint Surgery of America,* 1995 Nov; 77(11):1695-9.

Williams, P. L., Bannister, L. L., Collins, P., Dyson, M., & Ferguson, M. W. J. (1995). *Gray's Anatomy* (38th ed.). New York: Churchill Livingstone.

Acknowledgements

Collectively, we would like to thank Nancy Callinan for establishing a wonderfully educational chapter in the sixth edition. Her use of timeless resources made our job much easier. —C. D. Q. and P. D. B.

I would like to thank my amazing wife, Ginger, who shouldered additional responsibilities and supported and inspired the development of this chapter. I also must recognize my teacher, mentor, and friend, Steve Luster, for his amazing vision and application of the extraordinary. —C. D. Q.

I wish to thank my wonderful, loving husband, Robert, for his tireless encouragement throughout this project. —P. D. B.

Wheelchair Selection

Brian J. Dudgeon, Jean C. Deitz, and Margaret Dimpfel

Learning Objectives

After studying this chapter, the reader will be able to do the following:

1. Describe the factors that should be considered in wheelchair selection and explain how they interrelate.
2. Describe the three basic types of wheelchairs and reasons for each to be chosen.
3. Specify measurements typically taken to determine wheelchair and related seating system configurations for a particular individual.
4. Demonstrate knowledge of the components common to many wheelchairs, and describe why each merits consideration in wheelchair selection.
5. Discuss the roles and responsibilities of the occupational therapist in wheelchair selection.
6. Suggest how the occupational therapist can acknowledge user preferences and facilitate the user's participation in wheelchair selection.

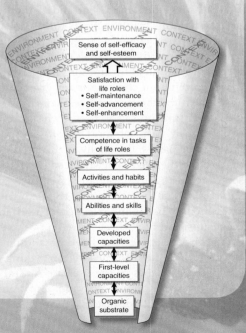

> Mobility is a fundamental part of living. Being able to move about, to explore, under one's volitional control is a keystone of independence. (Warren, 1990, p. 74)

Mobility is a major part of daily living, facilitating participation in home, work, and community settings. Mobility difficulties are one of the most commonly reported functional difficulties, a problem that is commonly addressed by use of special devices or equipment (Dudgeon et al., 2008). Walking aids and wheelchair selection and use are also frequent needs arising for either short- or long-term adaptation to disability. As such, wheelchair selection and training necessitate consideration of the user's preferences and current as well as anticipated performance needs, capacities, and environments. The process of evaluating and choosing a wheelchair system involves the user, an interdisciplinary team, and equipment suppliers or vendors. Also, family members, primary care providers, and others from the user's work and leisure environments may contribute important information useful in choosing an appropriate wheelchair system to meet needs for mobility within and between environments. Such information could affect choices regarding seating and positioning, controls used, and supports for engagement in activities at home as well as mobility and transport in community settings.

Wheelchair selection has a functional orientation and involves multiple factors including the user's (1) needs and goals; (2) home, work, recreational, and other community environments; (3) physical and cognitive status and anticipated course of impairments; (4) financial and community resources; (5) views about appearance, maintenance, and social acceptability; and (6) needs for interface of the wheelchair system with other assistive technology and care provider or assistant requirements. A selection process includes issues, such as current and changing needs of the user and family, training needs for use and maintenance, and anticipated changes in technology. A wide range of wheelchair options are available, yet funding and community-based resources for training and servicing of mobility devices often limit choices for any given individual.

Some individuals use wheelchairs only occasionally to meet brief transportation needs, whereas others use them continuously to meet most day-to-day positioning and mobility demands. Especially in the latter case, the events that lead to the need for a wheelchair may be dramatic. For some, acquiring a wheelchair system may create stress or confusion, and this can hinder their contributions to the assessment of needs and selection of a system. Others view the acquisition of a wheelchair as a positive move toward greater independence and freedom and make substantial efforts to become informed about making choices. In either case, the needs of the user are central to the overall process of selection, prescription, and training, with the wheelchair viewed not just as a means for mobility but as

a highly personal device to be chosen with care and precision (Steins, 1998).

In contributing to the selection process, the occupational therapist must have a thorough understanding of the user's medical needs and personal factors, including environment, daily routines, goals related to activities and participation, and assistance or care provided by others. In addition, the therapist should understand the seating and positioning needs of the individual and wheelchair types, control mechanisms, features, and accessories. Knowledge of product resources and local area vendors is also important in creating device choice options. Although this information is presented as separate components, all of these factors interrelate in comprehensive planning for functional mobility through a clinical reasoning process.

EVALUATION OF THE INDIVIDUAL

During evaluation, primary attention is given to user and family goals for use of the wheelchair as part of a functional mobility system. Further, the therapist evaluates the skills of the user, the user's ability to develop new skills, and changes expected from the diagnosis (e.g., declining sensorimotor skills). How the user plans to transport the system is also an important consideration. Priorities of users should be considered and are likely to include concerns about both comfort as well as functioning with user satisfaction typically being most related to comfort and ease of use (Ward et al., 2010). Evaluation of needs should include interview, observation, and examination. Trials with seating simulators, trial seating systems, self-propulsion methods, and/or other control systems are often needed to confirm appropriate prescription of these systems. Figure 17-1 outlines evaluation needs; patient-specific information relates to Lisa (Case Example 17-1).

The evaluation typically involves both sitting posture and mobility needs. The therapist can best assist in seating and wheelchair selection by understanding the client's personal capacity and needs and medical conditions.

Personal Capacity and Needs

The evaluation of the client includes attention to factors such as age and stature, developmental status, living environment, educational or work routines and plans, recreational pursuits, other assistive technology needs or uses, and future anticipated needs. Special attention is given to seating and operation of the chair in both private and public environments. Specifically, the therapist should consider factors such as floor surfaces, outdoor terrain, climate, doorways, hall spaces, restroom dimensions, workspace design, transportability, and parking. If a client has already used an adaptive mobility device before, it is important for the therapist to determine

Sample Wheelchair Evaluation: Needs of the Individual

Client information: Lisa, 17-year-old high school senior with recent C7 level tetraplegia from traumatic SCI in MVC. Attends evaluation with mother during inpatient stay in acute rehabilitation unit.

Functional Needs and Goals

Environments of use (home, school, work, community at large): Full-time at home, at school, and in other community locations. Has interest in athletics, high school programs.

Seating needs (time, pressure relief, transfers): Postural support needs for trunk and thighs, cushioning for neurogenic skin, and armrests for upper limb support.

Able to perform push-up pressure relief and can do independent transfers to/from wheelchair to same level bed or other surface.

Control or propulsion methods (attendant, manual needs, power controls): With postural support and seat belt, self-propels using friction push rims and wheel brakes. May benefit from grade aids for propelling up inclines.

Methods of wheelchair transport (car, van, truck; ground travel, air travel): Family owns full-sized truck and minivan. Lisa has driver's license, but has not yet explored or been oriented to adaptive driving.

Physical Examination

Head control: Now using a Minerva brace for cervical spine immobilization that will be discontinued in several weeks with healing. Otherwise, no limitations in head movements when trunk is stabilized.

Sitting balance and spinal deformity: Propped wheelchair seating, enables good head control when neck immobilization is discontinued.

Pelvic rotation or obliquity: Symmetrical at this time, mobile pelvis, lumbar support through wheelchair seating back contour and lateral trunk supports.

Lower limb mobility: Full PROM, flaccid at rest with periodic spasms into hip adduction, knee extension and ankle plantarflexion. Neurogenic skin below C8 level.

Upper limb mobility: Full PROM, good to normal strength in shoulder, elbow flexion 5/5, extension 4/5, forearm rotation 4/5, wrist extension 4/5, flexion 3/5, finger extension 3/5. Neurogenic skin lateral hand, 4th and 5th fingers.

Sitting and Balance Needs

Postural support: Now using brace for stability, lateral trunk supports for midline positioning. Seat belt and chest harness necessary for support and safety. Explore back cushion contouring when brace is discontinued.

Cushioning: Solid base of support needed with cushion contour. Tried low-profile Roho and Jay Cushion. Lisa preferred latter for balance, good cushioning effects.

Wheelchair Training Needs

Control or propulsion: Manual propulsion with seating components in place. Enlarged and rubberized friction rim tried and preferred over plain rim or knobs. Wheel camber may assist in hand placement. Needs training for propulsion on level surfaces, maneuvering corners and doorways, all outdoor settings.

Transfers to and from wheelchair and chair, bed, toilet, bathing tub or shower, floor, car: Is beginning transfer training wheelchair to bed using sliding board. Removable armrests and swing-away footrests will enable independence. Will need car transfer training, tub transfer, and floor to wheelchair instruction later.

Wheelchair Maintenance Resources
Lisa expresses interest in learning maintenance routine; father willing to assist as reported by Lisa and her mother. Wheelchair vendor is within 15 miles from this family's home.

Figure 17-1 Evaluation overview. Clinicians address these issues by interview, observation, and physical examination. MVC, motor vehicle collision; PROM, passive range of motion; SCI, spinal cord injury.

the user's assessment of pros and cons regarding that mobility method or system. A blending of walking aids and wheelchair use may be planned. Therapists should recognize that uses of adapted mobility systems often conflict with personal spaces and public accessibility. Public accessibility is based in part on human factors design, in which the typical wheelchair user sits at a 19-inch height and propels a manual wheelchair through a 32-inch wide opening and turns around in a 5-foot open floor space. Many people are served well by environments that accommodate this type of user, but others continue to be constrained by the environment and need individual guidance about making appropriate selection and accommodations. For example, some power mobility devices have a larger turning radius or excessive weight that puts limits on the user's access to some buildings, assistance that can be provided by others, and/or load limits of transportation systems.

Medical Conditions

Evaluation of a user's medical conditions includes a review of medical history and physical assessment. The therapist should be aware of the user's diagnosis and prognosis; that is, whether the medical condition is temporary, stable, or progressive (i.e., declining capacity). Such factors influence choices related to complexity of options and need for adjustment as well as preferences for rental, lease, or purchase. For example, if a condition is temporary, a chair may be selected with greater concern for cost factors. In contrast, if a client's condition is chronic, stable, and necessitates full-time use of a wheelchair, durability and individualization to meet needs are priorities. If a condition is progressive, a chair that permits a range of adjustments for both seating and wheelchair control may be indicated in order to meet a client's changing needs and maximize function and independence for as long as possible. The physical assessment should focus on neuromuscular status (e.g., muscle tone, postural control, reflexes, and coordination), musculoskeletal status (e.g., range of motion, deformity, strength, and endurance), sensory status (e.g., anesthetic skin and skin integrity), and physiological status (e.g., temperature regulation, respiration, and cardiopulmonary). Cognitive skills are also considered relative to capacity and safety in using and operating a wheelchair mobility system.

Wheelchair products are currently evaluated using standards put forth by the American National Standards Institute (ANSI) and the Rehabilitation Engineering and Assistive Technology Society of North America (RESNA), an interdisciplinary association for the advancement of rehabilitation and assistive technologies. Such standards enable direct product comparisons regarding features such as stability, safety, durability, and cost (Cooper et al., 1997). These standards are changing and call for uses of new terminologies as well as design elements that impact choices regarding seating and positioning options, wheelchair frame styles, and various control and equipment attachment options.

SEATING AND POSITIONING

Critical to selection of a wheelchair system is the attention given to the seating and posture needs of the user. Seating systems have a significant effect on the ability of the user to perform functional activities and on basic decisions about choice of mobility base types and components. Effective seating has several broad goals, including (1) enhancing posture, comfort, respiration, and skin protection; (2) preventing injury; (3) accommodating existing and preventing future deformity; (4) enabling vision readiness and limb use; (5) attending to cosmetic appearance and social acceptance; and (6) assisting with or enabling functional access and performance in specific settings or environments. Evaluation and intervention related to positioning often entails participation by team members, such as physical therapists to address postural supports, speech therapists to address augmentative communication, and family members and others to address daily routines and schedules. Occupational therapists may coordinate these concerns by incorporating the needs and goals of the user and family with medical care concerns in making recommendations and by analysis of functional issues so that recommendations optimize the individual's access to activities and participation. The roles of team members may vary somewhat in different locations and in different organizations.

Seating Principles: Solid Base of Support

Seating strategies and particular techniques can be specific to age groups and diagnoses, although some principles can be applied to meet a variety of needs. One such principle is the need to provide the individual with a solid base of support that begins with appropriate pelvic positioning. The sling seat, common to folding and unlocked wheelchair cross-brace frames, is a seating element that tends to promote pelvic instability and malalignment of the thighs. A solid seating base is accomplished by stabilizing the pelvis on a firm surface with pressure distributed throughout the buttocks and nearly the full length of each thigh. Seating pressure mapping can be used to assess distribution of pressure and peak pressure problems that may exist (Stinson, Crawford, & Porter-Armstrong, 2008). Although these systems give feedback to both clinicians and users, who can then visualize pressure difficulties and how effective pressure relief techniques may be, specific uses of such technology remain somewhat uncertain (see Fig. 17-2).

Postural Supports

Postural control is influenced by the seat and back contact surfaces and by orientation adjustments to the seat-back angle and the angle in space (Fig. 17-3). There are three commonly used seating positions. First is a sitting position with 90° hip, knee, and ankle positions. Second is a slight anterior (forward) tilt of the upper pelvis to distribute weight through the buttocks and thighs and, for some individuals, to inhibit abnormal reflexive responses (Fig. 17-4). Third is a 95° seat-back angle with a 3°–5° angle-in-space recline. Adjustable hardware that

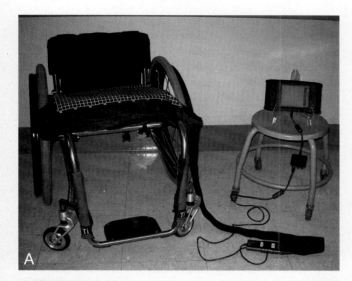

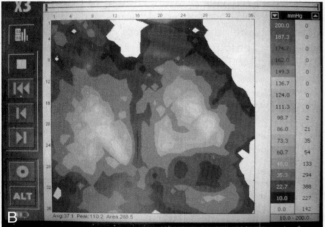

Figure 17-2 A. Flexible pressure maps are placed over cushions to measure body contact pressures. High and low readings are displayed continuously and can be saved for record keeping. **B.** Pressures are shown in color, in grayscale, or graphed. Dynamic readings can be shown or summed over variable lengths of time.

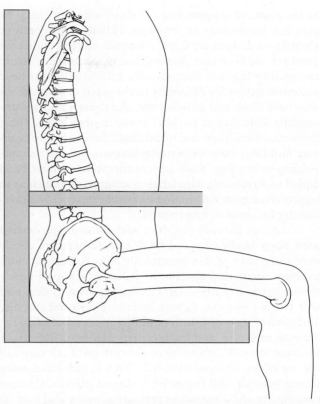

Figure 17-4 Pelvic positioning with slight anterior tilt helps to distribute tissue pressure throughout the buttock and thigh.

secures the seat and the back components to the frame are often used to adjust these positions.

Seat Surfaces and Cushioning

The seat and back contact surfaces can be planar, precontoured, or custom contoured. Single-plane or flat surfaces are typically appropriate only for those who need little

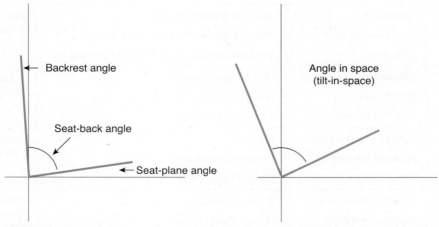

Figure 17-3 Adjustment of seat-back angle and angle in space helps to support posture and provide appropriate pressure distribution.

or no postural support and for those who can easily re-position themselves to maintain balance and comfort. Contoured designs are used to provide added contact for postural support and distribution of pressure. Custom contouring is often necessary for individuals who need accommodation for deformity of the pelvis or spine, those who have abnormal muscle tone, and those who have discomfort from lack of support at the lumbar spine. These customized cushions are individually fabricated by bead-seat molding, foam-in-place techniques, or other shape-sensing technology. Such devices are often fabricated and added to an existing wheelchair seating system, such as to improve seatback cushioning or enable better pelvic positioning for comfort and control.

Cushions are used to reduce peak pressures associated with bony landmarks and to distribute pressure evenly over a large area of skin contact. Shearing forces that compromise circulation also can be reduced by appropriately shaped cushions. Although cushioning relieves skin and soft tissue pressures, factors including postural stability and control, ease of transfers, ability to accommodate deformity, moisture, and maintenance may be as important for some users. Cushioning of the seat and back may call for use of one or more materials, such as variable-density foams, gels, air, and honeycomb-shaped plastics. Custom contouring and alternating pressure systems also may be considered. Table 17-1 lists advantages, disadvantages, and examples of each. Selection of cushion coverings, for both contact with the user and contact with wheelchair seating surface, also should take into account factors such as heat and moisture, friction, durability, and cosmetic appearance. The actual pressure characteristics of cushions are being evaluated and compared with a focus on both compression and sheering forces that are encountered with use (Akins, Karg, & Brienza, 2011). Regardless of cushion types, the techniques of pressure relief described next are vital to consider as part of pressure management.

Skin should be monitored closely for tolerance when use of any new positioning or cushion system is started. Progressive sitting time schedules along with ongoing skin inspection routines are essential, because no cushion provides sufficient pressure relief during regular use. Properties of materials vary, yet no cushion is considered sufficient in relieving pressure enough to preserve capillary blood flow to compressed tissues while a person is seated. Pressure on sitting surfaces can be greatest during manual propulsion, and users should be informed about dynamic factors that may put at risk the health of skin tissues. Although cushions help to reduce skin pressures, other means of pressure relief are necessary. Assisted or user-performed wheelchair push-ups, side leans, or forward leans for pressure relief are typically

Table 17-1 Cushion Types and Examples

Classification	Advantages	Disadvantages	Example
Foam	Lightweight Easily sized, shaped Low cost	Uneven pressure relief Poor durability Hard to clean	T-Foam by Alimed®
Gel-filled	Self-contouring Posture control Sitting balance	Heavy to move Temperature sensitive Leaking, maintenance	Jay® Cushion by Jay Medical
Air-filled	Lightweight Even pressure relief Little shear	Reduced control/balance Requires attention to air-pressure tending Potentially requires repair of puncture/air leaking	High or Low Profile by Roho®
Honeycomb	Lightweight Easy to clean Low maintenance	Uneven pressure relief Difficult to shape Excessive thickness	Supracor Stimulite® Contoured
Custom-contoured foam	Surface area coverage Reduced shearing Better postural control	Expense Longevity with change Reduced weight shift	Contour U® Pindot by Invacare
Alternating pressure systems	Scheduled relief cycle Reduces user effort Self-contouring	Cost and availability Uneven pressure relief Unsteady sitting balance	Bellows Air Support Equipment™ by Talley Medical

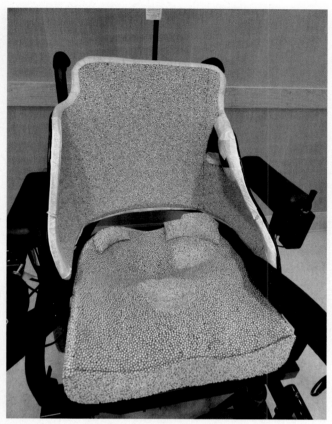

Figure 17-5 Custom contouring. Specialty manufacturers make custom cushions and backrests from a direct cast molding of the individual, through an electronic sensing system or by foam-in-place methods. These systems are typically used with individuals whose unique postural needs cannot be well supported by premade cushions or backrests.

needed or recommended every 15–30 minutes. Alternatively, technologies for pressure relief include tilt-in-space mechanisms, use of alternating pressure cushions that continuously cycle varying pressure segments of a cushion, and custom contouring of cushions (Fig. 17-5). Options of powered tilt and recline systems are growing and available for lesser cost and impact on the weight of wheelchair systems (Dicianno et al., 2009).

Adding Seating System Components

A seat belt is often recommended because it serves an important role in stabilizing the pelvis as part of therapeutic positioning in the seating system. This anterior support is typically mounted on the wheelchair frame so that it pulls on the pelvis at a 45° angle to the base of the seat back, fitting just under the anterior superior iliac spines. Additional seating supports should be used as needed to improve posture, restrict abnormal movements, and promote head control and voluntary use of

the limbs. For example, if sitting balance and abnormal postures are problematic, lateral trunk and thigh supports may be suggested. Use of anterior supports, in addition to the seat belt, may be necessary across the upper trunk, knee, or ankle for balance and stabilization. Neck and head supports are used to promote head and neck alignment and are sometimes recommended for safety. Upper extremity positioning also may be a concern, in which case specialized armrests or lap trays can be recommended.

Justification of Seating Systems

Because sitting is a dynamic rather than a static state, seating devices should allow some element of pressure relief and freedom of movement. The principle of *less is more* is recommended when applying specialized seating systems because as more seating apparatuses are used, freedom of movement tends to diminish. Therefore, only components that maximize individuals' abilities to function, correct their positions, and maintain comfort should be applied. When considering additions to wheelchair systems, trade-offs between support and function need to be carefully considered.

Expense justification with a health insurance third-party payer must relate to medical necessity. Inappropriate seating and mobility base selection can exacerbate complications and result in decline for the user. Functional accessibility and protection of the user from secondary complications that come with immobility or physiological risks with seating may be cited as part of insurance justifications.

To justify specialized seating with users and families, the experienced therapist can employ clinical observation and literature evidence. Improved motor skills, comfort and participation, physiological supports, and functional independence are widely hoped for as part of specialized seating and wheelchair selection. Some goals should be viewed cautiously, however, because wheelchair and seating configurations can be considered specific to certain diagnostic groups and mostly provide a prosthetic effect, meaning that these benefits are largely limited to the time that the person spends in the seating system. Although more wheelchair seating research is now being conducted, methodological challenges and studies with small samples have led to calls for a more focused research effort. Geyer et al. (2003) assembled a variety of stakeholders who reviewed existing work addressing wheelchair seating and called for future research efforts aimed to address wheelchair transportation, postural control, comfort, and tissue integrity. Inclusion of the user in research regarding wheelchair uses and consequences of use should be considered (Sprigle, Cohen, & Davis, 2007) (see Evidence Table 17-1, which is related to selection and uses of powered postural controls.)

Evidence Table 17-1 Best Evidence for Powered Seating Posture Features

Intervention	Description of Intervention Tested	Participants	Dosage	Type of Best Evidence and Level of Evidence	Benefit	Statistical Probability	Reference
Monitoring of power seating activations	Tilt, recline, and/or height adjustments recorded and appraised for patterns of use	Eleven adult power wheelchair users, ages 18–70 years	Seating Function Data Logger used to monitor self-actuated seating functions over approximately 12 hours of use for a 2-week period of typical daily use	Description of seating activations and likely purposes of such self-actuated changes in sitting posture; Level: N	Users made frequent use of power seating adjustments, with >50 times in at least partial tilt or recline positions. This increased reported comfort but did not achieve pressure relief guidelines.	Descriptive statistics on each user's frequency and duration of seating posture change activations	Ding et al. (2008)
Tilt-in-space seating use and outcomes for nonambulatory users	Systematic literature review (19 studies) appraising use ot tilt by those children and adults with neurological impairment	Nineteen selected studies addressing neurological impairments (e.g., CP [n = 8] and SCI [n = 8])	NA	Systematic review with meta-analysis; citing level I and level II research studies. Level: I	Statistically significant reduction in pressure under ischial tuberosities when tilted backward (20°–45°); evidence lacking regarding effects of tilt on function and seating use	Varied per article reviewed	Michael, Porter, & Pountney (2007)
Participation and activity measurement approach used with wheeled mobility users	Nonintervention study; semistructured, prompted recall interview about wheeled mobility at home and in community; objective use measures and, satisfaction report as well	Five adult power tilt-in-space wheelchair users with various neurological disorders	NA; system use recall reported; 2 weeks of objective use measures	Descriptive study and systematic interview; Level N	Comfort was a common reason for tilt activation. Varied uses and places of use of tilt feature were part of participation in varied activities.	Descriptive summaries and satisfaction change reported.	Harris et al. (2010)
Relieving contact pressure & obtaining tissue perfusion with wheelchair push-ups or dynamic seating system	Contact pressure measurement changes and improve ischial tissue health with wheelchair push-ups or use of a dynamic seating system device	Twenty individuals with paraplegic SCI, 20 with tetraplegic SCI, and 20 nondisabled participants	Laboratory setting appraising hour-long sitting protocols and pressure as well as tissue health changes with use of push-ups or dynamic seating systems	Repeated measures design; Level IIIB	Contact pressure relief achieved with wheelchair push-up or dynamic device, but tissue recovery poor with push-up method; good with dynamic system device	Descriptive statistics on contact pressure reduction and tissue reoxygenization Skin contact pressure reduction $p \leq 0.05$; tissue perfusion varied with poorer success for those with SCI who did not significantly improve $p \geq 0.05$	Makhsous et al. (2007)

Aim	Intervention	Sample	Method	Design	Results	Author
Evaluate biomechanical responses in seated pressure and blood flow with body tilt	Interface pressure reduction at ischial tuberosity and oxygenated blood flow with tilt sequences from upright to 45° tilt recline	Eleven participants with SCI who used tilt-in-space wheelchairs and had no current pressure ulcers	Laboratory-based appraisal in different tilt sequences, single-session testing	One-group, repeated measures design. Level: IIIC	Highly variable responses to tilt, with increased blood flow observed only with maximum (45° tilt). Maximal (45°) tilt in wheelchairs can best assure peak and mean pressure relief and tissue health, although less than maximal tilt may have some benefit.	Varied success with 30° recline and better success with maximal 45° tilt recline ($p \leq 0.05$) — Sonenblum & Sprigle (2011)
Study of wheelchair users with SCI perception of wheeled mobility behaviors and development of pressure ulcer	Multiple participant observations with structured and unstructured interviews regarding wheelchair use over approximately 1.5 years of use	Twenty community-dwelling adults with SCI who used manual wheelchairs	NA	Qualitative, descriptive study. Level IVB.	Pressure ulcer risk episodes are described relative to wheelchair and cushion use routines. Lifestyle choices, equipment selection and adjustments, and lifestyle contexts influence risks. Variable risks are acknowledged and based on minute-to-minute decision making regarding wheelchair use; pressure ulcers viewed as a failure in one or more components.	NA — Fogelberg et al. (2009)

CP, Cerebral palsy; NA, not applicable; SCI, spinal cord injury.

WHEELCHAIR TYPES: MOBILITY BASES

Once the therapist has a full understanding of the user's personal capacities and medical issues, seating needs, and environments of expected use (Karmarkar et al., 2011), it is important to understand the types and uses of wheelchair systems. Wheelchairs used in everyday activity can be divided into three general categories: (1) attendant-propelled chairs, (2) manual chairs, and (3) power mobility devices. Special-use chairs and attachments to standard mobility bases for participation in recreation and sports also can be considered.

Attendant-Propelled Chairs

Attendant-propelled chairs are designed to be pushed by another individual because of the user's inability to propel or operate a manual or power wheelchair in a functional or safe manner. This may be necessary for some users on a temporary or circumstantial basis, for example, as a means to be mobile during community outings. Attendant assistance also may be a full-time need for individuals who have diminished cognitive capacities, severe judgment difficulties, or severely restricted physical capacities. These chairs may be full size (e.g., those used in skilled nursing facilities) or may be smaller and created for use in limited spaces (e.g., folding stroller types). Attendant-propelled chairs also are used as a substitute for power mobility when the individual's typical mobility system is being repaired or when space constraints preclude power mobility use. When assisting a user in selecting an attendant-propelled chair, it is necessary to consider not only the fit and comfort of the chair for the person who will be seated but also the sizing needs of the person most likely to be pushing it. As with all wheelchairs, attention to transportation of the user and the wheelchair device between environments needs attention and planning. In addition to chairs specifically designed to be attendant propelled, many manual wheelchairs (described next) can be propelled by an attendant. In both situations, the capacities of care providers, who may be family members, become important considerations. For example, it is important to consider needs of a partner assisting a patient in going to doctors' appointments, shopping malls, family events, and various other settings. If a chair must be lifted into the trunk of a car, consider the ability of the primary care provider to do this. Consider not only the weight of the chair but also the ergonomics involved in picking it up and positioning it in a specific vehicle.

Manual Chairs

Manual wheelchairs are for those who can propel and brake using the upper limbs (Fig. 17-6). These chairs have a variety of frame types, weights, and transport features. In general, manual wheelchairs have rigid box frames or

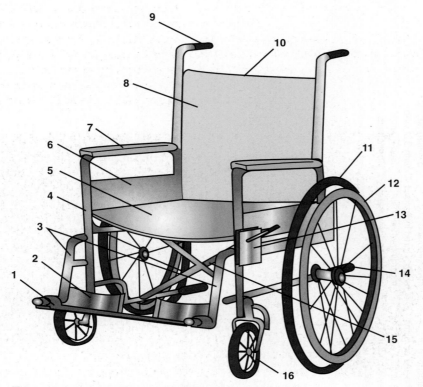

1. Footrest
2. Legrest
3. Front Rigging
4. Frame
5. Seat
6. Metal Skirt
7. Armrests
8. Backrest
9. Push Handles
10. Push Axle
11. Rear Wheels
12. Handrims
13. Brakes
14. Tipping Lever
15. Crossbars
16. Caster Wheels

Figure 17-6 Conventional manual wheelchair with component parts.

folding frames; folding frames are either free or locking lever–secured. Quick-release wheels can also be selected. Folding, locking-secured frames with quick-release wheels and detachable front rigging may offer the greatest flexibility for transporting the wheelchair. Rigid-frame chairs may provide greater energy efficiency with propulsion, and, with quick-release wheels, users can find this style to be either easier or more difficult to transport, depending on the type of vehicle used. Manual wheelchairs may be primarily user operated for most activities and many environments, but consideration of how others may help propel the wheelchair should be considered as well.

The conventional manual wheelchair frame has large rear wheels, which are used to propel the chair, with smaller caster wheels in the front. Wheelchairs of this design are highly maneuverable and easy to propel, and they allow freedom for tilting and wheeling pop-ups that can be learned for ascending or descending curbs (see Chapter 26). Standard designs, sometimes called depot or institutional wheelchairs (Cooper, 1998), weigh at least 50 pounds without specialized seating systems. A distinction can be made between multiuser chairs, often found in health care settings or places of public transportation (e.g., depot wheelchairs), and single-user or rehabilitation chairs, usually designated as lightweight and ultralight chairs. In recent years, sturdy lightweight metals and designs have been adapted from sport wheelchairs, resulting in lightweight and ultralightweight wheelchairs ranging from less than 25 to 40 pounds. Lightweight chairs are often used on a full-time basis. Many enable adjustable wheel positions and seat heights, which can help optimize biomechanical efficiency for the user. Along with reduced weight, these changes serve to enhance propulsion and ease transport and also may reduce strain on user's upper limbs.

Other types of manual wheelchair designs include the amputee frame for the person with loss of or severely reduced weight of the lower limbs. In this design, the rear axle is offset farther behind the seat back than is standard. This concentrates a person's weight farther in front of the rear axle, reducing the risk of the chair tipping backward. Another type of manual wheelchair, although not commonly recommended, is the indoor frame. It has large front wheels, which are used for propulsion, with smaller casters in back. This design rolls easily over door sills and rug edges, but larger barriers such as curbs are difficult to traverse; transfers may be awkward because of the forward placement of the large wheels; and access to tables and the use of lap trays can be more awkward.

In the conventional manual wheelchair, manual propulsion is typically accomplished through hand rims attached to the outside of each large wheel. The user is seated so that, with shoulders slightly extended and elbows partially flexed, each hand rests approximately at the 12 o'clock position of each hand rim. Contact with rims generally occurs between the 11 and 2 o'clock positions on each side. Circular steel tube hand rims are common. For users who have difficulty with grip, hand rims can be covered with vinyl coating, knobs or other projections can be added as part of the rims so that grip is not required, and/or gloves or mitts can be worn for traction and to protect the hands. Hand rims vary in size. Small hand rims, often used on racing chairs, result in a slower and more difficult start but may provide for a high top speed that is sustainable with relatively little effort. For most users, the push wheel axle is in line with the fingertip of the middle finger with the arm at one's side.

Foot propulsion can also be considered as an option, particularly indoors, making seat height considerations important for foot placement on ground surfaces. This may also be a common consideration for steering and propelling with hemiparesis. Manual propulsion by a person with hemiplegia or unilateral upper limb use necessitates additional adaptations. Commonly, the person with hemiplegia uses the more capable side for the hand rim and the leg and foot to steer and provide additional propulsion and braking. This requires removal of the unused footrest and lowering the seat height or using small-diameter wheels to optimize foot contact with the floor. For the user who plans to propel the wheelchair using only one arm, a chair can be ordered with both hand rims on one side so that each wheel can be controlled independently or together. Learning to maneuver dual hand rims on the same side can be perceptually and mechanically difficult. Another option for unilateral control is the single-lever drive. This less commonly used device option uses a forward-and-backward motion to propel the chair and rotation of the lever to turn the chair.

Parking brakes are used on each large wheel and are engaged through a variable length single- or dual-action lever, depending on reach and force capabilities of the user. Such levers press on the tire to resist rolling and require that tires be fully inflated with periodic tightening after tire wear. Brakes restrict wheel turning when the chair is parked but are not typically recommended for slowing or stopping. In addition, antirotation locks also can be used on casters.

Augmentation of manual propulsion and braking systems is available. As an aid to propelling on inclines, hill climbers or grade aid devices restrict the rearward movement of wheels through a friction stop engaged by a lever on each tire. Speed control and braking to a stop simply depend on slowing wheel rotation by use of the arms or legs. New devices that augment propulsion through electrical or mechanical means can also be considered. Such devices provide supplemental power from an electric motor that amplify the user's effort (e.g., Superwheel™ and e-motion®) or give mechanical advantage through a gear system and wheel changes (e.g., HandMaster™ and Magic Wheels™). Another option for manual wheelchairs is to provide power through add-on devices (e.g., viamobil® and e-fix®). Such systems can be engaged and disengaged to switch between manual and power mobility. Because a significant amount of weight is added to the chair and units are not easily taken on and off the frame, this option is most commonly suggested as a trial for a transition to a regular power wheelchair.

Power Mobility Devices: Motorized Wheelchairs

Power mobility devices are used by individuals (1) who cannot propel a chair using either the hands or the feet; (2) for whom the energy expenditure required to walk or propel a manual chair is contraindicated; (3) who have musculoskeletal complications, such as arthritis in upper limb joints; (4) who are prone to repetitive stress injury; and/or (5) who have neuromuscular dysfunction that may cause associated reactions in the lower extremities when the upper extremities are used for manual wheelchair propulsion. There are a number of types of power mobility devices. Selection of power mobility can be a complex task because of the variety of user needs and the many options for wheels, controls, and environmental designs.

Power Wheelchairs

Most power wheelchairs have a power-base design so that the wheels are, in effect, independent of the seating components. Such bases may have front-, middle-, or rear-wheel drive, with a variety of wheel diameters. For each type of design, the wheels may be coupled to motors through exposed or concealed chains or gear systems. Middle-wheel–drive chairs generally have a smaller turning radius, which improves maneuverability. Power-base wheelchair designs are noted for being sturdy and appropriate for the full-time user both indoors and outdoors. These designs generally allow for ease in changing seating dimensions, such as for a growing child or for an individual with changing seating system needs. Typically, the rear wheels are powered, but some designs have front wheel drive (e.g., Permobil) or, as noted, middle-wheel power (e.g., Invacare).

Several power-base chairs have options that enable the user to change seat height or elevate toward a standing position independently. Similarly, some manual wheelchairs have manual lever systems that allow the user to rise to a near standing position. These allow the person greater vertical flexibility in environmental accessibility, enabling face-to-face communication and easing performance in reaching books in a library, accessing a high counter, or reaching and operating controls. All environments of functioning should be considered as wheelchairs best for use outdoors may not work as well for indoor mobility (e.g., front wheel drive). Tilt, recline, and elevating leg-rest equipment are powered by wheelchair batteries and can be controlled by separate or integrated controls. Power seating controls enable users to sit more dynamically and can improve comfort and function (Dicianno et al., 2009).

The primary disadvantages of power wheelchairs are that (1) they can be large and heavy and may be difficult to maneuver in small spaces and transport from one place to another and (2) a 5 × 5–foot turning space, as part of standard barrier-free design, may not be sufficient for some power wheelchairs. Typically, van or bus transport of the individual sitting in a power mobility device requires special lifts or ramp devices, and the sizes of some chairs necessitate a raised roof in these vehicles. Alternatively, the user can transfer into the vehicle, and an attendant can load the chair separately by use of a lift or by breakdown into components. Some lightweight power wheelchairs are designed to be taken apart for automobile transport (e.g., the At'm Take-Along- Power Chair™). Some of these chairs are built on folding frames and/or have low-powered motors, making hill climbing and use on uneven surfaces more challenging. Assistance with taking apart and reassembling the chair often is required.

Scooter

Another popular power mobility device is the scooter. Scooters typically have three wheels, although four-wheeled designs are available, and may have either rear- or front-wheel drive. Most of these designs are characterized by tiller control, wherein the user steers the scooter by rotating the front wheel while using a lever-style switch for forward or reverse power. This type of chair is appropriate for the marginal walker and is often used to compensate for a person's inability to travel comfortably within the community. Scooters are sometimes modular and can be disassembled and loaded in and out of the trunk of a car or the back of a station wagon or van more easily. Steering and control of scooters can be difficult, so individuals with marginal control may be better served by use of a power wheelchair with a variety of control options. Scooters may also not be appropriate for individuals with significant posture control needs because special seating and other components are difficult to attach. In addition, scooters require a larger turning radius and may limit maneuverability indoors or not fit vehicle lifts and van and bus tie-down systems.

Power Mobility Considerations

Specific factors unique to power mobility require consideration. The therapist should determine whether the device will be used primarily indoors or both indoors and outdoors. A device that is to be used in both settings must have more stability, power, distance capability, and durability than an indoor-only model. User's planned operating distances, slopes, and outdoor conditions such as rain, temperature, and sunlight should be considered as part of selection and training. In addition, the therapist should consider the use and maintenance of the batteries that provide power. Various sizes of deep-cycle lead-acid batteries and sealed cell gel types have different expense, longevity, and needs for recharging. Other power wheelchair characteristics to consider include noise, braking systems, ride quality, and portability, including ease of assembly and disassembly. If the device can be disassembled, the weight and size of each part should be carefully evaluated for transportability. Nonleaking sealed cell or gel batteries are preferred for added safety in airline transportation, with wet-cell lead-acid wheelchair batteries becoming somewhat obsolete. Such batteries require special handling as part of airline travel.

Selection of appropriate controls for driving is critical, and a graded approach to controls training is often needed. Wheelchair seating posture is key to determining the most reliable and effective motor actions for control. Programmable controls are most common and enable careful selection of torque and speed control based on wheeling surface resistance and safety. Power devices are driven using one of two types of options: proportional or discrete control. Most commonly, a proportional joystick is used, in which directions and speeds are linked to angle and magnitude of stick displacement. Proportional control also may be achieved through proximity-sensing devices that, for example, sense the position of the head. The user moves his or her head as a joystick, and the wheelchair's speed and directional control are proportional to the head displacement. Another alternative is discrete microswitch control activated with a joystick, a multiple-switch array, or a single-switch scan. Each switch activation engages a preset or programmed speed and direction. Microswitch systems require less skilled movement to achieve control, although control of the wheelchair is often less precise than that provided by proportional control. Also, learning to use microswitch control is not simple. Each direction may be controlled by activating a microswitch using a body part (i.e., hand, arm, chin, foot, head, mouth, lips, or tongue), and control may be organized through a combination of special techniques such as sip and puff, scanning, or switches imbedded in headrests (Fig. 17-7). For instance, breath may be used for forward and reverse control, and proximity-sensing switches may be used to activate turning control. When selecting controls, the therapist should consider adjustment options provided by various systems in relation to the needs of the individual. For example, clients with poor motor control may benefit from adjustment of programmable electronics that enable wheelchair speeds to be automatically restricted when turning or that enable several levels of control to be programmed for new learning and controls training in various environments.

Power wheelchairs and scooters electronically brake, meaning that drive wheels do not rotate except under power and with activation. Gears are then released by levers that allow the chair to roll freely.

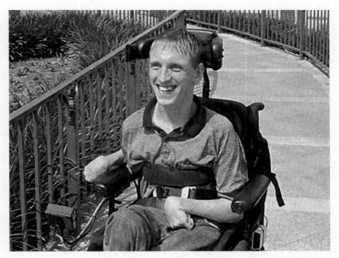

Figure 17-7 College student uses a power wheelchair controlled with proximity switches in a head array. The display in front of right armrest provides feedback regarding drive selection, electronic aids to daily living (EADL) functions, and battery level. A switch on the right side of the head array permits selection of drive and EADL functions. (Courtesy of Adaptive Switch Laboratories, Inc., Spicewood, TX.)

Activity- or Environment-Specific Wheelchairs

For everyday use, attendant-propelled, manual, or power wheelchairs are selected. Many users may also need mobility to overcome unique barriers or for use in recreation and leisure activities that require activity- or location-specific technology. Special power-wheel configurations have been designed for ascending or descending stairs, although market availability for such models has been inconsistent. Other special designs for wheelchairs, including those for use at the beach and on other soft and uneven surfaces, are available commercially or may be custom made. For recreation, cycling configurations may be requested. Row cycles are large, low to the ground three-wheeled cycles propelled by a rowing action that activates chain-driven rear wheels. Cycling action also can be added to manual wheelchairs (Fig. 17-8) or be

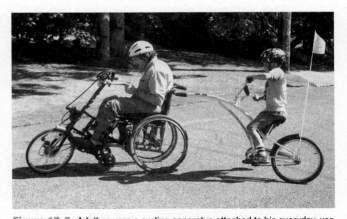

Figure 17-8 A father uses a cycling apparatus attached to his everyday-use manual wheelchair for outdoor activity with his children.

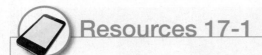

Resources 17-1

Wheelchairs and Accessories

AbleData

8630 Fenton Street
Suite 930
Silver Spring, MD 20910
www.abledata.com

Ability Magazine

1001 West 17th Street
Costa Mesa, CA 92627
www.abilitymagazine.com

Assistive Technology, RESNA

1700 North Moore Street
Suite 1540
Rosslyn, VA 22209
www.resna.org
The Boulevard

jjMarketing, Inc.

1205 Savoy Street, Suite 101
San Diego, CA 92107
www.blvd.com/Wheelchairs
_and_Accessories/

Disabled World: towards tomorrow; Assistive Technology

173 D'Youville
Chateauguay, Quebec J6J
5R1, Canada
www.disabled-world.com
/assistivedevices/mobility
/wheelchairs

disABILITY Information and Resources

http://www.makoa.org
/mobility.htm

Mainstream Magazine-Online

www.mainstream-mag.
com

New Mobility

23815 Stuart Ranch Road
P.O. Box 8987
Malibu, CA 90265
www.newmobility.com

Paraplegia News & Sports 'N Spokes

http://pvamag.com/sns/

Paralyzed Veterans of America

801 18th Street, NW
Washington, DC,
20006-3517
http://www.pva.org

USA Tech Guide

United Spinal Association
75-20 Astoria Boulevard
East Elmhurst, NY 11370
http://www.usatechguide
.org/reviews.php

configured as a separate chair for outdoor sport. Sport wheelchairs for racing, basketball, and other competitions are commercially available, but often they require customized sizing and expert instruction. For a thorough review of options for using activity-specific or sport and recreation chairs, see Cooper (1998) and *Paraplegia Sports 'N Spokes* (Resources 17-1). As described later, health insurance funding for wheelchairs is most often restricted to one device purchased for up to 5 years or more of use, and so most second wheelchairs, for any purpose, are funded privately.

WHEELCHAIR SIZING AND ERGONOMIC CONSIDERATIONS

Modern wheelchairs are engineered as modular systems and are assembled to match the specific physical dimensions of the user. Measurements of the individual form the basis for determining wheelchair frame size, adjustable component parts, and other customization to meet special needs.

Sizing

Appropriate size determinations of the wheelchair frame, seat, back, leg rests, and armrests are based on measurements typically taken with the user in an optimally seated position. Alternatively, the therapist can evaluate the individual on a mat in a supine or side-lying position and take careful measurements of distances between key landmarks. These measurements are confirmed for accuracy with the user seated. The user's typical or specialized clothing needs should be considered during measurement. If thoracolumbar bracing or lower limb orthotics and prosthetics are likely to be used in the wheelchair, they should be worn during sizing measurements. Manufacturers of wheelchairs and seating systems have differing standards for measurement and sizing. Typically included are measures of pelvic or hip width; upper and lower leg lengths; midback, midscapula, and top of shoulder heights; chest and shoulder widths; elbow height; and overall sitting height (Fig. 17-9).

- Seat width: The therapist determines the widest point across the hips and thighs and may add a total of 5 cm (2 inches) for adequate clearance on the sides for clothing and positioning comfort. However, the seat width is kept as narrow as possible because overall wheelchair width is dictated by the seat-width measure. Wheelchairs should be as narrow as possible while allowing for comfort, easy repositioning, clothing needs, and transfers. For manual users, narrower wheelchairs are likely to improve ease of hand-rim propulsion and maneuverability.

- Seat depth: The therapist, for both the left and right sides, measures the distance from the most posterior part of the buttocks under the thigh to the popliteal fossa crease of each knee. About 5 cm (2 inches) is subtracted from the measure. This allows as much weight bearing through the thigh as possible without the front edge of the seat pressing into the back of the knee. Right and left leg length discrepancies can be caused by hip dislocation, pelvic rotation, or other anatomical factors. The shorter side may be used to determine seat depth, or if a greater than 1-inch discrepancy is found, the front seat edge may be offset to accommodate the length of each side. Individuals who use their feet to propel or steer will need greater front-edge seat clearance.

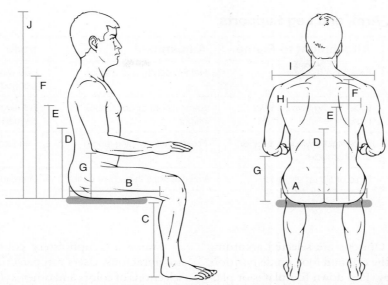

Figure 17-9 Seating measurements. For **B** to **G**, all measurements are taken on both right and left sides. **A.** Hip and thigh width. **B.** Thigh length. **C.** Leg length. **D.** Back height to below scapula. **E.** Back height to midscapula. **F.** Back height to top of shoulder. **G.** Elbow and forearm height. **H.** Chest width. **I.** Shoulder width. **J.** Sitting height.

Selected seat cushion height should be taken into account with further measurement of trunk, arm, and leg positioning components.

- Back height and width: The therapist generally takes three measures from the seat surface upward: (1) to the midback just under the scapula, (2) to the midscapula or axilla, and (3) to the top of the shoulder. Back height is affected by seat cushions, which should be considered in sizing decisions. Height of the chair back is based on the need for postural stability and freedom of arm movements for propulsion or other functions. For those who exclusively self-propel, a chair back height of 2–5 cm (1–2 inches) under the tip of the scapula may be preferred. For sporting activities, the optimal back height may be even lower. By contrast, for power wheelchair users, back heights to midscapula or the top of the shoulder may be necessary to allow use of postural supports for the upper trunk and the head. Chest and shoulder width should be measured in cases of deformity or to determine the space requirements for lateral trunk supports or other trunk-positioning devices. Alterations of the standard sling back may be necessary for improving trunk posture by using an adjustable or flexible sling back, curved backs, or additions of lateral trunk supports or custom-contoured backs.
- Seat height and leg rests: Seat height is based on positioning of the individual such that footrests have at least a 5-cm (2-inch) clearance from the floor. Use of seat cushions affects this measurement by raising overall seat height. Seat height is determined with the individual's knees and ankles positioned at about 90°.

Measurements are taken from under the distal thigh to the heel of the individual's commonly used footwear or shoe. Several inches of adjustment are typically available in leg rest lengths. Unusual leg lengths or hip or knee deformity may necessitate special ordering. Overall seat height may be determined and measured from the ground with considerations of needs for interactions with those who are standing, versus lower height to aid propelling, and considerations for transfer height surfaces.

- Armrest height: The therapist measures from under each elbow to the cushioned seating surface with the shoulder in neutral, the arms hanging at the sides, and the elbows flexed to 90°. Armrests must provide forearm support with neutral shoulder position but should not obstruct reach to hand rims for propulsion or to brake levers.

Common and Special Components

In addition to overall sizing and seat and back surface, the team and user should consider selection of head and neck rests, armrests, leg rests, and other options. Table 17-2 lists options for head, neck, arm, leg, and foot support. Users should consider armrest stability for performing wheelchair push-ups for pressure release. Detachable or swing-away styles may allow greater ease in sliding board and other sideways transfers and improve access to tables and desks. Guards can be used on armrests to keep clothes from coming in contact with wheels. Attachment of lap trays may require use of full-length armrests or other specialized hardware. The front rigging consists of

Table 17-2	Head, Arm, and Leg Supports		
Component	**Attachment to Frame**	**Adjustment**	**Style**
Head and neck supports	Fixed or removable	Height, depth, and rotation	Flat, winged, lateral, occipital, or wedged
Armrests	Fixed, swing away, and/or removable	Same height or adjustable height	Full length or desk length, rigid or padded
Leg rests	Fixed rigid, swing away, and/or detachable	Fixed or telescoping length	Fixed angle or elevating
Calf pad and footplate	Rigid or flip up, flip away	Variable sizes in pads or straps	Plate, tubular, rigid, or padded

leg rests and footplates. Options are selected according to needs for elevation of the calf and foot, ankle position, and stabilization of the leg. Flip-down footplates or platforms are common and popular because they can reduce the overall length of the chair. Swing-away or detachable front rigging enables easy transfers, approach to tables and desks, and ease of transportability of the wheelchair in and out of vehicles.

Tires can be either pneumatic (air filled), semipneumatic (airless foam inserts), or solid-core rubber and are mounted on spoke or molded wheels. Air-filled tires are lightweight with low rolling resistance, providing a well-cushioned ride and shock-absorber function that tends to improve comfort and prolong the life of the chair, but they do require regular maintenance. Semipneumatics provide good cushioning and less maintenance, but tire wear may be more of a problem. Solid-core tires are noted for minimal maintenance and approach the weight and low rolling resistance of high-pressure pneumatic tires but without concerns for getting a flat and becoming stranded.

Casters, as either front or rear wheels, vary in diameter, and small ones better enable maneuverability. Pneumatic and semipneumatic caster tires provide some shock absorption for use outdoors and on rough surfaces. Solid-core caster tires are best for use indoors and on smooth surfaces. Special designs (e.g., Frog Legs™) for manual wheelchairs and power wheelchairs are promoted for shock absorption and enhanced maneuverability.

Seat belts, safety vests, and harnesses vary in design and are used for both safety and positioning. These devices should be considered for individuals who have severe neuromuscular impairments and need control for posture and safety. Restraints may be considered with individuals who have poor judgment but should be avoided whenever possible and be regarded separately from seating postural needs. Restraint reduction efforts in long-term care facilities may be enhanced by use of appropriate and comfortable seating, and because there are risks associated with wheelchair seating restraints, planning for client's control of releasing belts and straps should be considered (Chaves et al., 2007).

Frame and upholstery color and material options are numerous. Users can personalize their chair through selections of colors and other styling. Durability, cleaning, ease of repair, and compatibility of materials with temperature regulation, friction, moisture, and skin protection requires careful planning. Trial use of the wheelchair seat and back may be suggested with special consideration for surface stability and handling of moisture and heat.

Other special considerations are specific to different wheelchair mobility bases. On most manual wheelchairs, placement of the rear axles can be fixed or adjustable, especially with newer manual lightweight and ultralight styles. Backward placement of the axle tends to increase stability; by contrast, forward placement of the axle decreases stability but increases maneuverability and shortens turning radius. Sometimes rear wheels have a camber adjustment. This orients the hand rim for easier propulsion and slightly widens the wheel base for better stability. Although users often prefer a 6° camber, such configurations do not appear to impact ease of propulsion or handling (Perdios, Sawatzky, & Sheel, 2007). Antitipping extensions can be used on a wheelchair to prevent the chair from tipping backward or forward. Typically used on the back, these fixed or adjustable extensions can improve safety, particularly during mobility training.

Recline and tilt-in-space options, considered with attendant-propelled and power mobility, enable postural changes for rest and pressure relief. In attendant-propelled wheelchairs, semireclining up to 30° from upright or full reclining up to 90° from upright can be considered. In tilt-in-space systems, the seat and back assembly pivot together. This feature makes the use of postural seating components more stable because the angle between the seat and the back remains unchanged, reducing or eliminating the problem of shear. Power recline systems can be used with conventional or power-base designs. Such systems may involve tilt-in-space and/or low-shear back recline, both of which can be used to provide pressure relief and rest positioning. Tilt-in-space chairs that go back 45°–60° can achieve effective pressure relief under the buttock and thigh and may have other benefits such as improved breathing These systems, however, add to costs and increase wheelchair size and weight.

Other considerations are accessories that optimize use and performance. Lap trays can be used for postural support of the upper limbs and serve a variety of purposes related to function. Other accessories include mounting bags or baskets for storage and carrying, cup or bottle holders for taking fluids, and storage attachments for a reacher or walking aids to enhance access and mobility. Communication devices or electronic aids to daily living may be mounted on the wheelchair and operated independently of wheelchair controls or can be integrated with power wheelchair controllers. Other medical equipment such as ventilators, oxygen tanks, or other devices need to mount within the wheelchair mobility system.

MOBILITY TRAINING

Mobility training with the wheelchair system can be essential and often involves interdisciplinary team members, such as the physical therapist. Most users benefit from instruction and practice beyond the training provided by vendors. Once the chair has been provided, a check should be conducted, and appropriate training of the user and attendants should commence. This includes review of the user's goals for mobility along with a check of the device for fit and adjustment. Instruction also should be provided regarding (1) use of the chair indoors and outdoors and on a variety of surfaces (e.g., level, carpeted, incline, and uneven), (2) transfers (e.g., bed, toilet, and car), (3) transport of the wheelchair (e.g., cars, trucks, vans, and buses), and (4) maintenance of the wheelchair (e.g., cleaning the chair, lubricating moving parts, monitoring tire pressure and wear, adjusting brakes, and caring for batteries). Troubleshooting with the wheelchair system ultimately becomes the responsibility of the user and equipment supplier or vendor, but the therapist may advise about problem-solving strategies and organization of maintenance routines and schedules. Throughout training, the therapist emphasizes safety issues because accidents during day-to-day wheelchair use do occur and are preventable (Chen et al., 2011).

For more than a decade, functional skill evaluation with wheelchair use has received increasing attention (Kikens et al., 2003). Manual wheelchair skills assessment (Fliess-Douer et al., 2010; Mortenson, Miller, & Auger, 2008) has received the greatest attention, and overall, increasing emphasis is also being placed on participation (Kikens et al., 2005).

Manual wheelchair users can benefit from instruction about propelling, braking, and transport. Hand placement and trunk lean for effective and efficient wheeling can be explored. General consumer use guidelines are available for the user and trainer (Axelson et al., 1998). Power wheelchair users also need guidance about power functions, such as controllers, batteries, and accessory devices. With all wheelchair users, the therapist should provide initial checks; periodic follow-up to address safety issues, fit, and adjustment; and updated information about new options to meet the changing needs of the user.

Transportability of the wheelchair system between environments can be especially challenging. Loading and unloading should be trialed with the vehicle most likely to be used. As noted, car transfers of the user and loading and unloading of the wheelchair need careful planning. Breakdown of the wheelchair for portability or the addition of special lift accessories to vehicles should be considered during selection. The weight of the wheelchair and its component parts may be limiting to users as well as care providers who assist with vehicle transfers. Lifts are often used with vans or buses. In these vehicles, wheelchair tie-downs are necessary as safety mechanisms to keep chairs stabilized when traveling. The style needed is determined by wheelchair design. Such devices secure the wheelchair to the base of the vehicle; the individual is independently secured in the wheelchair seat or in another seating device within the vehicle.

WHEELED MOBILITY AND PARTICIPATION

As part of the wheelchair selection process, the impact of devices on the users' roles and participation needs to be considered relative to home, work, and community contexts. User roles and social interactions have implications for positioning, speed of mobility, and ease of access within and between settings. For example, wheeling may necessitate using different routes of travel to gain access, and this may detract from user's or other's feelings of inclusion. Slow mobility speed may hinder shopping trips within and between stores or with movements at work. Armrest or other features of the wheelchair may preclude positioning with peers at dinner or meeting room tables. Professional rating tools that address needs (Miller et al., 2004) and consumer rating tools that address satisfaction with wheeled mobility devices are being proposed and address issues and interactions among the person, the technology, and the environment (Mills et al., 2002).

Greater success in matching devices with environments of participation is needed. Although wheelchair mobility can lead to successful independence, challenges continue regarding integration of wheelchair users in various settings. For example, data on disability and workplace accommodation (http://www.infouse.com/disabilitydata /workdisability/2_1.php) reveal that less than 25% of wheelchair users are employed. Studies involving wheelchair users often indicate that obstacles created by use of wheeled mobility devices are seen as a major reason for lack of community participation and as a source of frustration (Chaves et al., 2004; Hoenig et al., 2003). Nevertheless, use of wheelchairs, and powered mobility devices in particular, is often credited with enhancing occupational performance and participation (Buning, Angelo, & Schmeler, 2001; Davies, DeSouza, & Frank, 2003). Although the built environment is a major reason for obstacles, attention also should be given to associated factors, such as wheelchair user fitness and health, use of assistants and other assistive technologies, social interactions in the community, and the natural environment's weather conditions.

FINAL DETERMINATION

In making a final determination regarding seating components, style, size, and control systems, the user and team take a comprehensive and functional view, simultaneously considering the current and future needs, desires, and resources of the user; environments of participation; and anticipated changes in technology. This can certainly be a challenge in matching a client's current needs with a wheelchair mobility system, as well as forecasting future needs in the weeks and months and years ahead in terms of independence, participation, and well-being.

Decision Making and Justification

Costs and related funding issues are critical components of the decision-making process. Expensive technology and options should not be ordered unless justifiable for increased function, health, user satisfaction, or safety. When expensive choices are being considered, it is important to rule out the feasibility of using less costly alternatives. For example, before selecting power mobility, it is important to rule out the feasibility of using a manual chair because the cost of providing and maintaining a powered system may be much more costly than getting and using a manual system. In such cases, appropriate justification must be clearly delineated for users and third-party payers. Some users decide to purchase devices or features on their own or seek funding through other sources when the feature is denied by the third-party payer.

A comprehensive functional mobility system for an individual often includes more than one means of mobility and selective use in different environments (Hoenig et al., 2002). For example, an individual may use limited walking skills within some settings (e.g., walking from the kitchen table to the refrigerator), benefit from a manual chair for traveling longer distances within indoor environments (e.g., moving from room to room within the home), and use a power chair for traveling longer distances in the community and at school or work. Funding sources will typically pay for only one of these options, but with mobility being unique to different activities, negotiation of options may be explored with health insurance providers as well as educational and vocational support programs. In many cases, the expected term of use for a wheelchair by medical insurance funding policies is 5 years, although expected uses and benefits for that period of time may be difficult to predict. Private pay for assistive technology, including wheelchairs, is common (Carlson & Ehrlich, 2006).

The Clinician's Responsibilities

Therapists have a responsibility to keep abreast of new technology, new products, and new product evaluation research. They must be able to provide users with appropriate and updated information on the advantages and disadvantages of wheelchair options and components. In addition, they must have current knowledge of issues related to availability, serviceability, and performance of various wheelchairs and options. Professional and consumer sources of information about wheelchairs, related options, and manufacturers of mobility systems, controls, and seating systems are useful for product information (see Resources 17-1). Therapists also are encouraged to explore wheelchair standards developed by the ANSI, the RESNA, and the International Standards Organization (http://www.wheelchairstandards.pitt.edu/). These voluntary standards for wheelchair developers and manufacturers provide guidelines for product specifications based on uniform measurements and testing. Use of these standards facilitates product comparisons. In addition to being aware of wheelchair standards, the therapist also is responsible, along with the interdisciplinary team, for developing relationships with appropriate vendors of seating and wheelchair systems in order to make trial equipment available.

Wheelchairs, selected through a user-led team, can facilitate participation in multiple environments. Selection of an appropriate wheelchair system results from a clinical reasoning process that considers multiple variables, particularly best fit, function, and the user's preferences. Consumers' satisfaction with seating and mobility systems can be incorporated in critical program evaluations that address outcomes. Ragnarsson (1990) stated, "Ultimately, the most important factor in the success of a wheelchair prescription is the user's total level of acceptance and satisfaction with [the] chair as it combines looks, comfort, and function" (p. 8).

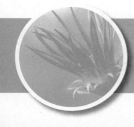

case example

Ms. Lisa: Wheelchair Selection for a Student Who Has Tetraplegia

Occupational Therapy Intervention Process	Clinical Reasoning Process	
	Objectives	Examples of Therapist's Internal Dialogue

Patient Information

Lisa is a 17-year-old high school senior with C7-level tetraplegia from a traumatic spinal cord injury (SCI) that she experienced in an automobile crash. She is expected to be a long-term wheelchair user. In the hospital, she demonstrates the ability to propel a manual ultralight wheelchair using coated push rims. Lisa previously was active in soccer and other sports and would like to match her school colors with her wheelchair frame. She was intrigued to learn about competitive wheelchair sports but is inexperienced with independent mobility.

Appreciate the context — See Chapter 38 for a review of SCI rehabilitation.

Develop intervention hypotheses — "Lisa may not endorse her need for long-term use of a wheelchair but may agree to the interim reality and specific wheelchair choices related to return to home and school."

Consider the evidence — "My recommendations to Lisa are based on prior experiences with this level of SCI and supported by literature regarding manual versus power mobility uses with SCI (Hastings et al., 2011) and skills obtained with manual wheelchair uses (Lemay et al., 2012)."

"Ultralight wheelchair styles have good longevity and can be customized in various ways for her size and needs. A vendor and options for wheelchair choices from such a vendor should be introduced to Lisa and her family."

Select an intervention approach — "A rehabilitative approach matches her adaptive capacities and skills with training for use of appropriate assistive technology, environmental accommodations, and care providers."

Reflect on competence — "My own knowledge of wheelchair needs is strong, but my awareness of currently available products will be augmented through the vendor and product representatives. Accessibility needs at home, in school, and in the community will need to be explored specifically for Lisa and her support network."

Recommendations

The care team is preparing a wheelchair prescription and considering these features:

Wheelchair
- Manual ultralight cross-brace folding frame
- Purple frame with black upholstery
- Adjustable axle position with camber control
- Lift-off desk-length tubular armrests
- Swing-away fixed-angle foot rests with heel loops on flip-up footplates
- Vinyl-coated push rims with pneumatic tires and nonpneumatic front casters
- Grade aids and standard rubber-coated brake levers

Seating
- Cloth-covered Jay seat cushion with flexible sling back, midscapular height
- Seat belt and chest strap

Consider the patient's appraisal of performance — "Lisa may regard the wheelchair as a short-term versus a long-term strategy but seems interested in resuming independent mobility, as seen in her use of a loaner wheelchair. Helping her learn about customization of size, cushioning, colors, and other features may encourage her use of the wheelchair."

Consider what will occur in therapy, how often, and for how long — "Her new wheelchair may not be available until after inpatient hospital discharge."

Ascertain the patient's endorsement of plan — "Options to review with her for selection of chair include frame type, cushioning, arm and leg rest features, frame and upholstery color, and a variety of hand rim and brake features."

"Gel cushion is encouraged for sitting balance and pressure relief. Air cushions demonstrated good pressure relief but can impair sitting balance and necessitates tending to air pressure. Foam or silicone cushions have less even pressure distribution but are lighter weight and do not need regular maintenance. Gel has the precaution of cooling/freezing with low outdoor temperature and could puncture and leak."

Summary of Short-Term Goals and Progress

A loaner rehabilitation wheelchair has been provided to Lisa, and she makes use of this self-propelled device to go to and from therapy and other appointments. When she is with visitors, she is often pushed to other locations on the hospital campus.

Sitting tolerance times have been increasing daily with skin inspection performed by Lisa with nursing or therapy supervision and guidance. Sitting tolerance and travel distances are being staggered and staged to increase time and range of mobility. By discharge, up to 6 hours of wheelchair time is expected before bed rest relief. Indoor mobility independence is expected, including use of doorways and elevators. Outdoor mobility is supervised initially to assure safety with ramps, curb cuts, and cross-slopes.

Wheelchair-to-bed transfer training is proceeding with use of a lightweight sliding board and standby supervision for safety. Toilet and tub transfer skills are being introduced, and she currently receives moderate assistance. Independence in wheelchair transfers is expected with standby supervision anticipated.

Assess the patient's and family's comprehension	"Trial use of a loaner wheelchair has Lisa experiencing transfers, self-propulsion, and environmental access on hospital grounds. She is taking responsibility to go to and from therapy sessions but is seen being pushed by family and friends at other times."
Compare actual to expected performance	"Staging of wheelchair sitting time is scheduled, and Lisa seems willing to observe this precaution and is accepting of reminders to attempt pressure relief routines. She does not appear to attend to time of day on a regular basis, so she will likely need an external cue of some sort."
Know the person	"Lisa monitors her progress carefully in both occupational and physical therapy with high hopes of regaining strength. Nevertheless, she also is aware of her functional mobility and capacity to self-propel and transfer."
Appreciate the context	"Self-initiated goals for functional mobility in and around the hospital campus are being suggested by her. These are being encouraged with use of appropriate standby supervision."

Next Steps

Lisa will be using the wheelchair full-time at home, at school, and in other community locations. Her own wheelchair is being ordered and will be available at discharge or soon after her return home. Accessibility at home and school need to be assessed with Lisa and her family.

Loading her wheelchair into a personal vehicle as well as public transportation need to be considered. Driver retraining with adaptive hand controls also is being explored.

Anticipate present and future patient concerns	"Lisa has become aware and has concerns about accessibility at home and school, where stairs are an issue to enter and move between levels."
Analyze patient's comprehension	"An accessibility audit of home and school through interview will be conducted, and a home visit with Lisa and family members is anticipated before inpatient discharge. School access may be appraised in conjunction with the school therapist."
	"Lisa continues to hope that she will again be able to walk, but as weeks progress, she has focused increasingly on her wheelchair skills."
Determine what referrals may be needed to appropriate community-based services for advice regarding community mobility and driving	"Referral to and follow-along in community-based therapy or outpatient visits to the SCI program are anticipated. Goals will be safe mobility; community transportation; and full participation in school, work, and community settings. Consideration for airline travel and sports participation might be anticipated in coming years."

 Clinical Reasoning in Occupational Therapy Practice

Wheelchair Selection with a Student Who Has Tetraplegia

What else should be considered related to wheelchair selection and mobility training with Lisa? Consider uses of wheelchair accessories, capacity to carry items, performance in transfers, transportation with the wheelchair, and maintenance of the wheelchair. Under what circumstances might power mobility be considered?

case example

Mr. R.: Dependent Mobility with Amyotrophic Lateral Sclerosis

Occupational Therapy Intervention Process	Clinical Reasoning Process	
	Objectives	Examples of Therapist's Internal Dialogue

Patient Information

Mr. R. is a 48-year-old husband and father with amyotrophic lateral sclerosis (ALS). He is near the end of his ability to walk safely and has quit driving a car. He teaches in a public school and expects to retire at the end of the month. He coaches his children's youth baseball teams. He lacks sufficient strength in his arms to self-propel a wheelchair. To address his needs now for mobility at home, at work, and in the community, a prescription for a wheelchair is being written. Family financial resources are limited.

	Objectives	Examples of Therapist's Internal Dialogue
	Appreciate the context	See related assessment and intervention in Chapter 35 regarding adults with neurodegenerative disorders.
	Consider the evidence	"Power wheelchair prescriptions for those with ALS appear to address needs (Ward et al., 2010), yet a full spectrum of equipment and devices is likely needed in the latter half of this disease process (Bromberg et al., 2010)."
		"Mr. R.'s walking difficulty combined with upper limb weakness will necessitate power wheelchair mobility and/or dependent wheelchair use. Use of power mobility in homes is problematic for maneuverability and will likely necessitate a dependent wheelchair for function and care."
		"Medicare funding would address wheeled mobility for at-home use and perhaps transportation to and from medical appointments. Other community mobility needs should be addressed separately."
	Select an intervention approach	"A rehabilitative approach will attempt to match devices and environments with abilities to address Mr. R.'s family goals. Wheelchair use will take place along with uses of other assistive devices and environmental accommodations planned for home."
	Reflect on competence	"As a therapist, I am familiar with dependent mobility devices and need to carefully match size and adjustment options for the client's home environment. Loaner equipment or used devices are sometimes preferred for cost savings. The ALS Association or other assistive technology recycling programs could be explored."

Recommendations

To address needs within the home, an attendant-propelled wheelchair is needed. A tilt-in-space manual chair that permits full upright position to 45° recline is selected, along with a foam seat cushion and flexible sling back with a winged headrest. A lap tray is added to enable positioning of the arms and for attachment of communication devices. This chair is requested through health insurance, and once Mr. R. is unable to walk safely, it will be used at home and for attending medical appointments. Community mobility may be served by this device, but other options will need to be explored as well.

	Objectives	Examples of Therapist's Internal Dialogue
	Consider the patient's appraisal of performance	"Mr. R. is knowledgeable about his condition but is reluctant to give up walking. Presenting the wheelchair as an option rather than an exclusive device for mobility might be best."
	Consider what will occur in therapy, how often, and for how long	"Selecting, fitting, and brief training are specifically needed with the wheelchair device. Operation of brakes, recline mechanism, and other features should be reviewed with Mr. R. and his care providers."
	Ascertain the patient's endorsement of plan	"Mr. R. is in agreement but views the wheelchair as being a further indicator of his decline."

Summary of Short-Term Goals and Progress

Mr. R. needs consumer education about wheelchair products and options that he could use. Funding mechanisms need careful review in terms of requirements, dollar allowances, and costs of options.

Client and family training in use of the wheelchair is a service goal, with Mr. R. having informed options about wheelchair use and the family being educated about community mobility with wheeled mobility devices.

Assess the patient's comprehension	"Mr. R. recognizes his mobility needs and is aware of and concerned about costs and access within his home, such as installation of ramps and widening of doorways."
Understand what the patient is doing	"Adjustable cushioning for comfort and function should be devised. Foam cushions are likely the most cost-effective and flexible option, both for seating and transport. He will likely adjust his position easily on his own at first. With more static seating later on, air cushioning could be considered. This will then necessitate adjustment and tending of the cushion relative to air pressure. Gel cushions could be considered, but they are heavy and may make Mr. R.'s own adjustment of his position more challenging."
Appreciate the context	"Resting and functional settings at home are likely to include his bed, wheelchair, and another chair or couch location. Transfer training with family care providers should take place soon."

Next Steps

Mr. R. obtains and uses the mobility devices, which appear to meet his present needs. Occupational therapy is put on hold, with plans for reassessment in 6 weeks.

Anticipate present and future patient concerns	"Monitoring of wheelchair operation and use, along with other assistive devices, should occur as part of outpatient follow-up, perhaps every 6 weeks depending on the speed of Mr. R.'s decline. Coordination with home-health or hospice care also may be considered."
Decide if patient should continue or discontinue therapy and/ or return in the future	

 Clinical Reasoning in Occupational Therapy Practice

Selection of Other Mobility Options

Mr. R. and his family also recognize his need for functional mobility outside the home. His extended family are discussing pooling resources to purchase another mobility device he can use outdoors for coaching baseball, shopping, and other activities. Given the progressive decline expected with ALS, what might you suggest in terms of powered mobility? What kind of comprehensive mobility system would you recommend, and why, if financial resources were not an issue?

Summary Review Questions

1. Who should participate in the wheelchair selection process?
2. What are the three basic types of wheelchairs, and why would each be selected?
3. What factors should be taken into consideration in wheelchair selection and use by adults and older adults?
4. Describe a situation in which the optimal decision for an individual might involve the selection of more than one mobility device.
5. What are the six broad goals of wheelchair seating and positioning?
6. In determining wheelchair and related seating system sizes for a particular individual, what measurements typically are taken?

7. Contrast the benefits and limitations of various manual and power mobility frame types.
8. Name and describe two types of controls for power mobility devices. Which would be preferable for a person with cerebral palsy and extremely poor upper extremity control? Why?
9. How can an occupational therapist keep abreast of new product development and research related to these products?
10. How can the occupational therapist facilitate the client's participation in wheelchair selection?

Glossary

Angle in space—Angle of the seat back in relation to the true vertical when the seat and back are rotated counter-clockwise as a unit. Sometimes called tilt-in-space or orientation, this position may be altered for postural control.

Camber—The amount of angle on the wheels, creating flare-out at the bottom. A 6° camber is recommended for push-rim convenience and wheelchair width.

Locking lever–secured—A locking mechanism on the frame that holds folding frame parts in place for smoother ride with less frame migration and reduced wheel and caster flutter.

Pelvic rotation—Asymmetrical position of the pelvis with forward position of one side, typically because of low back rotation, muscle asymmetry, or spinal deformity.

Proximity-sensing devices—Devices or systems that remotely sense the position of a body part (e.g., head) and use that position to control the wheelchair without physical contact between the part of the body used for control and the switch.

Scanning—Control option that presents choices one at a time, grouped or singly, until the desired choice is offered for the user to select by switch activation.

Seat-back angle—The angle of the seat surface relative to the back surface. This angle is typically 90°–100°. Backrest angles and seat-plane angles may be designated separately.

Sip and puff—A system typically involving a dual-action switch, in which one action is controlled by the user sipping on a tube held in the mouth and the second action is controlled by puffing on the same tube. (In wheelchair operation, the chair functions can be controlled by patterns of switch closures.)

Third-party payer—Individual or organization (i.e., insurance company) other than the person receiving services that pays for services or equipment.

References

Akins, J., Karg, P. E., & Brienza, D. M. (2011). Interface shear and pressure characteristics of wheelchair seat cushions. *Journal of Rehabilitation Research and Development, 48,* 225–234.

Axelson, P. W., Chesney, D. Y., Minkel, J., & Perr, A. (1998). *The manual wheelchair training guide.* Santa Cruz, CA: PAX Press.

Bromberg, M. B., Brownell, A. A., Forshew, D. A., & Swenson, M. (2010). A timeline for predicting durable medical equipment needs and interventions for amyotrophic lateral sclerosis patients. *Amyotrophic Lateral Sclerosis, 11,* 110–115.

Buning, M. E., Angelo, J. A., & Schmeler, M. R. (2001). Occupational performance and the transition to powered mobility: A pilot study. *American Journal of Occupational Therapy, 55,* 339–344.

Carlson, D., & Ehrlich, N. (2006). Sources of payment for assistive technology: Findings from a national survey of persons with disabilities. *Assistive Technology, 28,* 77–86.

Chaves, E. S., Boninger, M. L., Cooper, R., Fitzgerald, S. G., Gray, D. B., & Cooper, R. A. (2004). Assessing the influence of wheelchair technology on perception of participation in spinal cord injury. *Archives of Physical Medicine and Rehabilitation, 85,* 1854–1858.

Chaves, E. S., Cooper, R. A., Collings, D. M., Karmarkar, A., & Cooper, R. (2007). Review of the use of physical restraints and lap belts with wheelchair users. *Assistive Technology, 19,* 94–107.

Chen, W. Y., Jang, Y., Wang, J. D., Huang, W. N., Change, C. C., Mao, H. F., & Wang, Y. H. (2011). Wheelchair-related accidents: Relationship with wheelchair-using behavior in active community wheelchair users. *Archives of Physical Medicine and Rehabilitation, 92,* 892–898.

Cooper, R. A. (1998). *Wheelchair selection and configuration.* New York: Demos.

Cooper, R. A., Gonzalez, J., Lawrence, G., Renschler, A., Boninger, M. L., & VanSickle, D. P. (1997). Performance of selected lightweight wheelchairs on ANSI/RESNA tests. *Archives of Physical Medicine and Rehabilitation, 80,* 1138–1144.

Davies, A., DeSouza, L. H., & Frank, A. O. (2003). Changes in the quality of life in severely disabled people following provision of powered indoor/outdoor chairs. *Disability and Rehabilitation, 25,* 186–290.

Dicianno, B. E., Margaria, E., Arva, J., Lieberman, J. M., Schmeler, M. R., Souza, A., Kevin Phillips, K., Lange, M., Cooper, R., Davis, K., Kendra L., & Betz, K. L. (2009). RESNA position on the application of tilt, recline, and elevating legrests for wheelchairs. *Assistive Technology, 21,* 13–22.

Ding, D., Leister, E., Cooper, R. A., Cooper, R., Kelleher, A., Fitzgerald, S. G., & Boninger, M. (2008). Usage of tilt-in-space, recline, and elevation seating functions in natural environment of wheelchair users. *Journal of Rehabilitation Research and Development, 45,* 973–984.

Dudgeon, B. J., Hoffman, J. M., Ciol, M. A., Shumway-Cook, A., Yorkston, K. M., & Chan, L. (2008). Managing activity difficulties at home: A survey of Medicare beneficiaries. *Archives of Physical Medicine Rehabilitation, 89,* 1256–1261.

Fliess-Douer, O., Vanlandewijck, Y. C., Manor, G. L., & Van Der Woude, L. H. (2010). A systematic review of wheelchair skills tests for manual wheelchair users with a spinal cord injury: Towards a standardized outcome measure. *Clinical Rehabilitation, 24,* 867–886.

Fogelberg, D., Atkings, M., Blanche, E. I., Carlson, M., & Clark, F. (2009). Decisions and dilemmas in everyday life: Daily use of wheelchairs by individuals with spinal cord injury and the impact on pressure ulcer risk. *Topics in Spinal Cord Injury Rehabilitation, 15,* 16–32.

Geyer, M. J., Brienza, D. M., Bertocci, G. E., Crane, B., Hobson, D., Karg, P., Schmeler, M., & Trefler, E. (2003). Wheelchair seating: A state of the science report. *Assistive Technology, 15,* 120–128.

Harris, F., Sprigle, S., Sonenblum, S. E., & Maurer, C. L. (2010). The Participation and Activity Measurement System: An example application among people who use wheeled mobility devices. *Disability & Rehabilitation: Assistive Technology, 5,* 48–57.

Hastings, J., Robins, H., Griffiths, Y., & Hamilton, C. (2011). The differences in self-esteem, function, and participation between adults with low cervical motor tetraplegia who use power or manual wheelchairs. *Archives of Physical Medicine and Rehabilitation, 92,* 1785–1788.

Hoenig, H., Landerman, L. R., Shipp, K. M., & George, L. (2003). Activity restriction among wheelchair users. *Journal of the American Geriatrics Society, 51,* 1244–1251.

Hoenig, H., Pieper, C., Zolkewitz, M., Schenkman, M., & Branch, L. G. (2002). Wheelchair users are not necessarily wheelchair bound. *Journal of the American Geriatrics Society, 50,* 645–654.

Karmarkar, A. M., Dicianno, B. E., Cooper, R., Collins, D. M., Matthews, J. T., Koontz, A., Teodorski, E. E., & Cooper, R. A. (2011). Demographic profile of older adults using wheeled mobility devices. *Journal of Aging Research,* Article ID 560358.

Kikens, O. J., Post, M. W., Dallmeijer, A. J., Seelen, H., & van der Woude, L. H. (2003). Wheechair skills tests: A systematic review. *Clinical Rehabilitation, 17,* 418–430.

Kikens, O. J., Post, M. W., Dallmeijer, A. J., van Asbeck, F. W., & van der Woude, L. H. (2005). Relationship between manual wheelchair skill performance and participation of person with spinal cord injuries 1 year after discharge from inpatient rehabilitation. *Journal of Rehabilitation Research and Development, 42(Suppl. 1),* 65–73.

Lemay, V., Routhier, F., Noreau, L., Phang, S. H., & Martin-Ginis, K. A. (2012). Relationship between wheelchair skills, wheelchair mobility and level of injury in individuals with spinal cord injury. *Spinal Cord, 50,* 37–41.

Makhsous, M., Priebe, M., Bankard, J., Rowles, D., Seigler, M., Chen, D., & Lin, F. (2007). Measuring tissue perfusion during pressure relief maneuvers: Insights into preventing pressure ulcers. *Journal of Spinal Cord Medicine, 30,* 497–507.

Michael, S. M., Porter, D., & Pountney, T. E. (2007). Tilted seat position for non-ambulant individuals with neurological and neuromuscular impairment: A systematic review. *Clinical Rehabilitation, 21,* 1063–1074.

Miller, W. C., Miller, F., Trenholm, K., Grant, D., & Goodman, K. (2004). Development and preliminary assessment of the measurement properties of the Seating Identification Tool (SIT). *Clinical Rehabilitation, 18,* 317–325.

Mills, T., Holm, M. B., Trefler, E., Schmeler, M., Fitzgerald, S., & Boninger, M. (2002). Development and consumer validation of the Functional Evaluation of a Wheelchair (FEW) instrument. *Disability and Rehabilitation, 24,* 38–46.

Mortenson, W. B., Miller, W. C., & Auger, C. (2008). Issues for the selection of wheelchair-specific activity and participation outcome measures: A review. *Archives of Physical Medicine and Rehabilitation, 89,* 1177–1186.

Perdios A., Sawatzky, B. J., & Sheel, A. W. (2007). Effects of camber on wheeling efficiency in the experienced and inexperienced wheelchair user. *Journal of Rehabilitation Research and Development, 44,* 458–466.

Ragnarsson, K. T. (1990). Prescription considerations and a comparison of conventional and lightweight wheelchairs. *Journal of Rehabilitation Research and Development: Clinical Supplement, 2,* 8–16.

Sonenblum, S. E., & Sprigle, S. H. (2011). The impact of tilting on blood flow and localized tissue loading. *Journal of Tissue Viability, 20,* 3–13.

Sprigle, S., Cohen, L., & Davis, K. (2007). Establishing seating and wheeled mobility research priorities. *Disability Rehabilitation Assistive Technology, 2,* 169–172.

Steins, S. A. (1998). Personhood, disablement, and mobility technology. In D. B. Gray, L. A. Quatrano, & M. L. Lieberman (Eds.), *Designing and using assistive technology: The human perspective* (pp. 29–49). Baltimore: Paul H. Brooks.

Stinson, M. D., Crawford, S. A., & Porter-Armstrong, A. P. (2008). Interface pressure measurements: Visual interpretations of pressure maps with MS clients. *Disability and Rehabilitation, 30,* 618–624.

Ward, A. L., Sanjak, M., Duffy, K., Bravver, E., Williams, N., Nichols, M., & Brooks, B. R. (2010). Power wheelchair prescription, utilization, satisfaction, and costs for patients with amyotrophic lateral sclerosis: Preliminary data for evidence-based guidelines. *Archives of Physical Medicine and Rehabilitation, 91,* 268–272.

Warren, C. G. (1990). Powered mobility and its implications. *Journal of Rehabilitation Research and Development: Clinical Supplement, 2,* 74–85.

Suggested Readings

Batavia, M. (2010). *The wheelchair evaluation: A clinician's guide* (2nd ed.). Sudbery, MA: Jones and Bartlett Publishers.

Cooper, R. A. (1998). *Wheelchair selection and configuration.* New York: Demos.

Croteau, C. (1998). *Wheelchair mobility: A handbook.* Worcester, MA: Park Press.

Karp, G. (1998). *Choosing a wheelchair: A guide to optimal independence.* Sebastopol, CA: O'Reilly & Associates.

Acknowledgements

We thank and acknowledge clinicians from the University of Washington Medicine Systems for contributing their knowledge and expertise.

18

Technology for Remediation and Compensation of Disability

Mary Ellen Buning

Learning Objectives

After studying this chapter, the reader will be able to do the following:

1. Apply occupational therapy concepts and skills for evaluation, planning, and treatment to the process of incorporating digital technologies for treatment-as-means for remediation and treatment-as-end as compensation for impaired or missing body structures and functions.
2. Understand the interdisciplinary nature of assistive technology (AT) assessment and treatment, the roles of other professionals, and the unique contribution of occupational therapy to the process.
3. Use knowledge of unimpaired abilities and features of digital technologies to determine the required features of a user interface and to optimize settings and use of digital devices to accomplish therapeutic goals.
4. Recognize clients who should be referred to AT experts.
5. Define primary categories of AT and give examples of AT use to support occupational functioning.

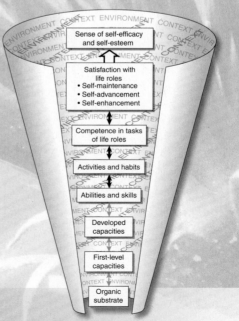

Occupational therapists use assistive technology (AT) to remediate and/or compensate for disability. Descriptions of assistive devices and various adaptations are given throughout this text. This chapter focuses on digital technology. Computerized technology is a central reality in society today because it underlies most of the tasks of modern life and increasingly influences human communication and transactions. Computer technologies are rapidly changing societal patterns around the world. In the developed world, it is difficult to find a school setting or a job that does not incorporate computer-based technology. Microprocessor technology underlies so many aspects of life today that it is almost impossible to think of a way that it does not affect human occupations. It is found in home appliances, shopping, banking, learning and acquiring information, transportation, and all types of business and commerce. People now carry Wi-Fi–enabled smartphones that have features far beyond those found in expensive computers 5 years ago (Mack, 2011).

In many ways, technology has significant advantages for an individual with a disability. In addition to managing many of the tasks of daily life, technology has the additional capacity to support compensation. AT brings an array of options for alternate access in addition to new technologies that increase capacity and enable occupations in new ways. The rapidly increasing availability and creativity of consumer technology is expanding the application of AT by occupational therapists beyond adaptation for disability. Occupational therapists use this technology to remediate impairment, prevent disability, and maintain health.

THE ORIGINS OF TECHNOLOGY IN OCCUPATIONAL THERAPY

OT as a profession has been using technology as a treatment modality since its earliest days. Wikipedia (2011) describes technology as making, using, and knowing about tools, machines, techniques, crafts, systems or methods of organization in order to solve a problem or perform a specific function. Further, humans have always used technology to control and adapt to their natural environments. Early therapists used technology to adapt looms, build bicycle jigsaws, and teach leather crafts to develop eye–hand coordination. Using technology, they facilitated emotional expression and improved problem solving and sequential task behavior. These outcomes can occur with digital technologies.

Today's technologies include microprocessors and sensors that increasingly influence employment, education, human interactions, and all types of instrumental activities of daily living (IADL). These technologies enable human capacity in ways that range from instant access to information and communication to real-time feedback on movement trajectory, speed, and accuracy. This capacity can support group interaction in virtual or simulated environments and motivate users to stay engaged as they repeat and refine their movements. This ability to generate multisensory environments can be used to customize therapeutic amounts of visual, auditory, kinesthetic, and proprioceptive input while challenging a patient to learn new skills in an emotionally stimulating activity. These digital interventions demand that occupational therapists use and be comfortable with microprocessor-based or digital technologies. Such occupational therapists will then learn to apply activity analysis and treatment planning skills combined with critical thinking and creativity to successfully incorporate digital technologies into therapy. When knowledge of technology and media tools are combined with knowledge of a patient's pretreatment occupations and interests, therapists will easily bring digital technologies into occupational therapy practice.

OVERVIEW OF THIS CHAPTER

Several challenges arose in attempting to organize the content of this chapter. Some occupational therapists have been intrigued by the potential of technology and quickly embraced it as a modality for treatment and remediation. This is a key characteristic of the diffusion of innovations (Rogers, 2003). Innovators incorporated digital technologies into their practice because they recognized its potential for motivating patients with fun, "just right" challenges and the ability to provide knowledge of results. Now that evidence of positive outcomes is appearing in the literature (see Evidence Table 18-1 for examples), other early adopters who are comfortable with technology will adopt it and lead more therapists to acknowledge its usefulness.

For this reason, it seems important to create some common language and categories and provide some organizing concepts that will help to guide increased interest and usage of technology for remediation. Because this topic will be emerging as you read this chapter and begin to practice, it is also important to offer suggestions for staying current with developments.

TECHNOLOGY AS A TOOL FOR REMEDIATION: OCCUPATION-AS-MEANS

The core occupational therapy treatment skills (evaluation, goal-setting, selecting activities based on task analysis to help a patient achieve a treatment goal, and evaluating the outcome) will also guide therapists as they incorporate digital devices into occupational therapy treatment. Therapists have quickly recognized the potential of home entertainment devices such as Nintendo's Wii®, Sony's PlayStation®, and Microsoft's Xbox 360 with Kinect® as treatment activities. Using activity analysis to recognize

Evidence Table 18-1 | Best Evidence for Occupational Therapy Practice Using Technology for Remediation and Compensation

Intervention	Description of Intervention Tested	Participants	Dosage	Type of Best Evidence and Level of Evidence	Benefit	Statistical Probability and Effect Size of Outcome	Reference
Remediation: Robot-assisted (RA) upper limb therapy following CVA in acute rehabilitation settings	Mirror Image Movement Enabler (MIME) robot combines bimanual movements with unilateral passive, active-assisted, and resisted movements of hemiparetic upper limb. Both RA groups could see their limbs, used physical objects, and did goal-directed tasks. Control received conventional therapy to improve the paretic upper limb plus 5 minutes of exposure to the robot without forces applied. FMA (for randomization) plus FIM™, WMFT, Motor Power, and Ashworth at intake, completion, and at 6-month follow-up	Fifty-four subjects at three VA Medical Center sites randomized to three groups: low dose, high dose, and control. Acute ischemic CVA with some upper extremity sensory or motor recovery. Exclusion: joint pain on movement, no proprioception, scored <22 Mini Mental Status Exam, and other comorbidities that preclude exercise. First, stratified by FMA score into high, medium, and low impairment and then randomized to high- or low-dose RA or conventional therapy.	All three groups got 5 minutes of preparatory and terminal (undescribed) therapy. Low-dose group = 8.6 hours; high-dose group = 15.8 hours of RA therapy. Control group = 9.4 hours of conventional therapy.	Randomized, controlled, multisite study; Level: IC2b	Yes. RA training is equal to or better than conventional therapy. RA can increase intensity and dose at lower cost.	Randomization created equivalent groups. Analysis of covariance (ANCOVA) used to control for scores, age, and chronicity. Robot high-dose group improved significantly more than control ($p = 0.04$) on FIM™. No group differences in any other outcome measure. Dose of RA therapy positively correlated with gains in FMA ($r = 0.34$, $p = 0.04$), possibly because of intensity (intensity and FMA: $r = 0.45$, $p = 0.005$).	Burgar et al. (2011)
Compensation: Use of automatic speech recognition (ASR) as a means of computer access	Collected performance data via interview and task measures from experienced ASR users on (1) computer use, (2) type of ASR, (3) reasons for ASR use, and (4) measures of performance on six ASR tasks (e.g., file management, transcription rate, etc.). For 18 users who had a choice: comparison between ASR and alternative method.	Twenty-four users of ASR with >6 months experience; 5 participants could use ASR only, and 19 used ASR plus keyboard.	Exploration of the ASR experience for variety of experienced users. Results varied widely because of (1) limitations of the technology and (2) limitations in user's ability to maximize effective use of ASR.	One group, descriptive statistics; Level: VC3a	Of participants with choice, 48% used ASR for ≤25% of computer tasks, and 37% used ASR for >50% of computer tasks; 63% reported overall satisfaction with ASR. Text entry rate ranged from 3 to 32 words per minute with accuracy of 72%–94%. Best users had best correction strategies. Typists with speed >15 words per minute got less benefit from ASR.	Those with higher recognition accuracy had higher satisfaction scores, $p = 0.027$. For non-text-entry tasks, ASR plus keyboard was 61% slower, $p < 0.05$. For study participants, more agreed with (1) I can enter text more quickly with ASR than with any other method, (2) ASR is easy to use, and (3) I can enter text more accurately ($p < 0.05$).	Koester (2004)

Conventional therapy included soft tissue mobilization, joint mobilization, use of reeducation strategies, isolated progressive resistive exercises, and progression to functional activities of daily living (ADL).
CVA, cerebrovascular accident; FMA, Fugl-Meyer Assessment; FIM™, Functional Independence Measure; MMSE, Mini-Mental State Exam; WMFT, Wolf Motor Function Test.

task characteristics, they use these technologies to motivate patients for purposeful movement within interesting and satisfying goal-directed activities that allow self-challenge and tracking of progress. Clients are drawn to the novelty of these forms of digital play and are motivated to interact with technology to restore function and maintain health.

All indicators point toward even greater use of technology within the realm of occupation-as-means (i.e., use of Wii® bowling to develop tolerance for standing and simple balance and progressing to adding dynamic balance paired with the need for eye–hand coordination). Additionally, quantitative data gathering is within the capability of a digital device to measure frequency, accuracy, and duration. Robotic arm devices such as the Rice Robot (Fig. 18-1) sense increasing strength and accuracy and escalate the task demands for range or complexity to further challenge developing strength and coordination. Even digital media such as video cameras in cell phones and the face-to-face communication enabled on tablets and laptops make it easier to document progress, substantiate the need for a device, or provide a remote home accessibility consultation.

Digital devices even find a role in wellness or prevention. With GameWheel®, a computerized arm ergometer attached to a video game, hand-cycling motion on a pivoting base translates into racecar control. Faster cycling speeds one's car, and pivoting the crank arm in the frontal plane translates into right and left steering motions. Soon, the user is absorbed in cycling to avoid other cars or barricades on the track as he engages in bilaterally integrated activity and gets a moderate aerobic workout (O'Connor et al., 2000).

With this new domain for applying task and activity analysis skills, occupational therapists can help with the selection of entertainment platforms based on the types of user controls offered by particular platforms. These

same skills may even enable occupational therapists to collaborate on the design of games and activities or on improved or customizable user interfaces. The next generation of activities and games could help improve carryover of skills performed with digital devices into the actual performance of activities of daily living (ADL) in the real world. Occupational therapists who are comfortable with technology will be ready to use it in their practice both as a means and as an end—both to treat and support recovery and as a compensation to enable return to performance of the activities that comprise valued roles. The next section of this chapter focuses on use of computerized technology for remediation (technology as means).

Early Visions of Technology for Remediation

Older therapists can visualize their first exposure to virtual reality (VR) innovations. Humans, strangely outfitted with goggles or helmets and special gloves, worked in special settings or immersive environments in which they felt like they were actually opening doors or trekking on a challenging pathway. This technology of the mid-1990s motivated some rehabilitation researchers to actually conduct trials to determine whether VR environments could be used to create situations that were dynamic and interactive and provided opportunities for challenge to motor and sensory systems (Sveistrup et al., 2003). In their study, using a new commercially available rehabilitation product with 14 individuals with traumatic brain injury (TBI), Sveistrup and colleagues (2003) demonstrated that those who used VR had greater improvement in functional balance and mobility than the conventional exercise or control groups. These researchers even wondered whether someday VR might provide a tool for rehabilitation at a distant location or a motivating tool for maintaining the gains of rehabilitation (Sveistrup et al., 2003). This research article actually discusses many of the positives that therapists using technology for treatment today consider as advantages for this approach, which are discussed next.

Ability to Control the Level of Stimulus

VR can offer characteristics of good therapeutic intervention: repeated opportunities for tasks using multiple sensory modalities (vision, touch, and manipulation or haptics, proprioception, and audition) with a focus on function (Sveistrup, 2004). Because parameters can be set ahead of time, therapy can be provided within a context that provides just the right challenge and stimulus to support recovery of performance skills. Therapeutic activities need to be engaging and rewarding at the same time that they require patients to repeatedly move weak limbs or increase ranges of motion or strength. Novel, multisensory environments are adept at this. Therapists and users benefit from the ability to grade challenge and document the outcome of intervention in various scenarios.

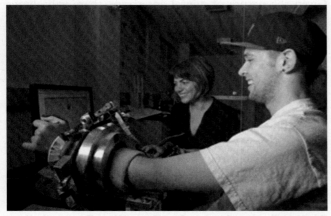

Figure 18-1 The Rice Robot, a fully articulated exoskeleton for spinal cord injury (SCI) rehabilitation, mimics upper extremity joints from shoulder to hand. (Courtesy of the Mechatronics and Haptic Interfaces Lab, Department of Mechanical Engineering & Materials Science, Rice University, Houston, TX.)

Control of the Environment

Digital or virtual environments can simulate a functional or realistic context while presenting a purposeful task or goal. For example, walking on a treadmill can increase endurance—a reasonable goal in therapy—but the activity could be more realistic and motivating if it were set to simulate walking a sidewalk to the corner store to get eggs and milk for breakfast. Meanwhile, the client is not actually dealing with weather, outdoor temperature, or risk of falls on uneven sidewalks. Activities in VR can be repeated and additional components or interactions added to increase the level of challenge or complexity as endurance and problem-solving skills develop.

Environments and activities that exist in VR allow a therapy team to preplan and modify treatment activities in interesting ways to maintain motivation. Solo activities can become group activities. The visual interface can range from a desktop monitor to a head-mounted display that creates a 180° sense of actually being in the middle of an environment. Gloves and controllers can provide a haptic interface that allows users to interact with virtual objects in real time. Opportunities for object manipulation and movable platforms challenge body movement in variable degrees that are perceived as real-world situations.

Fine Motor and Eye–Hand Coordination

A key feature of all VR applications is purposeful interaction within the surroundings. Virtual environments not only use spaces and surfaces to challenge a user's balance responses and coordination but also to interact with virtual objects within that space. This can occur when the user sees a representation of her hand that is linked to her own movement pattern as she reaches for and touches objects or even as she watches her movements as if she were a third person observing her body in action.

Repetition with a Level of Novelty

Technology-based interventions do not fatigue! They can vary tasks within parameters or at the direction of the therapist. Reaching into a cabinet to put away dishes is a common activity that changes in important ways when the dish is a cup versus a plate or whether the dish goes on a high or low shelf. In the natural environment, opportunity to practice this movement is limited by cabinet space, but in a virtual environment, the cabinet can always accept more dishes. Playing Wii® tennis offers opportunities for repetition of variable responses because the path and speed of the oncoming ball are different with each play, similar to the variation that is an important characteristic of similar activities in natural environments.

Data Collection

Digital technologies because of their very nature require precise settings, require specific amounts of time, and are set to count or measure the behavior or response for which they are designed. This makes it easy to see progress and display results in formats that motivate patients with evidence of progress—such as increases in strength, speed, or time. This, of course, frees the therapist to coach on quality of movement or optimal use of a body segment.

Transferability

Some worried that skills learned in VR would not transfer to the real world. To test this concept, Zhang et al. (2003) developed an immersive virtual kitchen in which patients with TBI could cook. Her researchers asked subjects to prepare a multistep meal both in a VR kitchen and in an actual kitchen twice over a 3-week period. Performance in the VR environment was actually a good predictor for performance in the actual kitchen assessment ($r = 0.63$, $p < 0.01$). The VR system showed adequate reliability and validity as a method of assessment in persons with brain injury (Zhang et al., 2003). This study shows the role that occupational therapists can play in contributing to the design of tasks for emerging VR tools. Activity simulations relating to common therapeutic goals and containing task elements that can be graded to increase challenge and complexity will be even more useful to occupational therapists.

Home-Based Activities

Because so many of these technology-based interventions are based on mass-marketed home entertainment systems, it becomes easier to encourage activity carryover as part of a home program or postdischarge activities. Older adults are often pleased to learn that being savvy about video games elevates their status with children and younger family members. Wii® golf, for example, recreates the experience of golf games shared with others but occurs within the safety and environmental predictability of the family room.

Range of Therapeutic Virtual Reality Activities

Given the nature of digital enterprise, there will always be new and improved products and interfaces for games and activities. A laptop computer purchased 5 years ago may have cost $1,500, but spending the same amount today buys one with faster processors, better graphics, more storage, etc. Observing the explosion of "apps" to entertain and support tasks on various smartphones and tablets suggests that there will be no shortage of software developers interested in working with therapists to develop therapeutic games and activities. The demand for apps appropriate for rehabilitation outcomes will only increase, so developing for this market will create opportunities for both entrepreneurial therapists and developers.

Digital Technologies for Cognitive Remediation

Compensation has always been an emphasis in treatment for cognitive impairment. We already know that compensatory strategies and devices are very helpful for functioning in the presence of memory and executive function impairments (Gentry, 2011). We know that individuals with TBI often cannot remember to use calendars or notes nor attend to a task through to its completion. Digital devices have some key advantages over low-technology strategies. They have interactive multisensory user interfaces that are well designed and so intuitive that task sequences are easy to learn. Most devices allow easy customization for user needs so that once set up, retrieving data or responding to reminders can be made consistent and predictable.

Knowledge gained from perceptual or neuropsychological testing can be very helpful in setting up these devices for a specific client. Interfaces on smartphones and tablets offer features such as text-to-speech, distinctive icons/sounds, and immediate knowledge of results in a nonjudging interaction. Thus, mainstream, "cool looking" products can offer reminders for medications or appointments with one or more alert sounds, offer a map and directions, a photo of a landmark, the list of four steps in a task, or a phone number linked to help. Remediation is supported by repetition of steps for setup or response to device prompts. This new learning stimulates the development of neural pathways and opens the door to even more opportunities for learning and restoration (Dowds et al., 2011).

As personal mobile technology becomes more and more part of daily life and a tool used for all kinds of IADL, the tasks that support device management will be even more imbedded in common procedural memory. However, professionals specializing in cognitive rehabilitation seem clear that considering context is essential when retraining cognitive processes, skills, or functional abilities (Sohlberg & Mateer, 2001). Individuals who used devices in one way prior to TBI will need individualized instruction to reestablish patterns of use, develop new strategies for seeking help, and get consistent reinforcement for appropriate response to cues.

With high interest in neuroplasticity and recovery, there is new interest in determining whether digital technologies support remediation. Evidence from well-designed studies must show whether using today's digital technologies can stimulate dendritic regrowth and actually support repair and improved motor function following acquired or TBIs.

Motor Recovery with Electrical Stimulation

Forty years of research with functional electrical stimulation (FES) has led to the development of a number of interventions and devices for treatment, although most are in the realm of neuroprostheses (Peckham & Knutson, 2005). Efficacy in the remediation of neuromuscular deficits is still preliminary. Electrical stimulation is being used in combination with goal-oriented repetitive movement therapy to augment motor learning in hemiplegia, and it has been helpful for treatment of shoulder subluxation and pain in hemiplegia (Sheffler & Chae, 2007). Neuromuscular electrical stimulation is effective in strengthening muscles, preventing muscle atrophy (see chapters 15, 19 and 21), preventing deep vein thrombosis, improving tissue oxygenation and hemodynamics, and facilitating cardiopulmonary conditioning (Sheffler & Chae, 2007). Current outcomes research on using FES in activity-based therapy for treatment of spinal cord injury (SCI) suggests that even when FES was withdrawn, there was evidence of sustained improvement when FES was used along with other interventions to elicit adaptability within a damaged nervous system (Behrman & Harkema, 2007).

Therapeutic Robots

Robots have been part of future fantasy for years but were only considered useful for rehabilitation starting in the early 1990s (Dijkers et al., 1991). Initially, developers thought robots could serve as intelligent assistants for those with high levels of impairment. High cost, regulation policy, and reluctance were effective barriers (Seelman, Kelleher, & Grindle, 2010).

Rehabilitation of stroke has been the area of first focus for robotics researchers. Stroke is prevalent, and helping individuals to achieve maximal recovery is very labor intensive, generally involving one-on-one interaction with an occupational therapist for a prolonged episode of care. Because rehabilitation for stroke recovery had always used this model of care, it is interesting to note that patients, once introduced to the idea of a robot helper, were enthusiastic about its use in treatment (Dijkers et al., 1991). Robots are novel and clearly report progress, which can increase patient motivation (Fig. 18-2). In the past 10 years, there have been many studies to demonstrate efficacy. An early, randomized clinical trial (RCT) showed significant differences in motor outcome when comparing conventional therapy with a robotic intervention. However, investigators could not report whether greater strength and motor control led to improved functional ability (Volpe et al., 2000). Since then, many studies have demonstrated that robotic stimulation leads to improvements in movement patterns that can be trained so that motor patterns are regained and the improvement is sustained over time (Hogan & Krebs, 2011; Krebs et al., 2008; Volpe et al., 2008).

Not all studies to date have had rosy reports. The most comprehensive clinical trial to date regarding the effectiveness of robot-assisted therapy reported mixed evidence for the use of robot-assisted therapy for upper arm rehabilitation after stroke (Lo et al., 2010). The main conclusions indicated that following 36 1-hour high-intensity robotic therapy sessions (with horizontal, vertical, wrist, and hand modules), stroke survivors 6 months post with moderate to severe upper limb impairment and with lesions caused by single and multiple strokes did not improve significantly more than nonrobot control groups of usual care or intensive therapy. They did have modest improvements over 36 weeks.

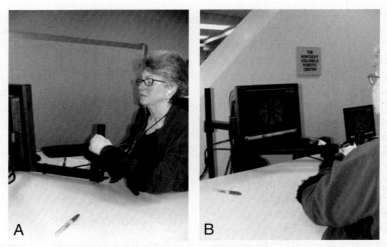

Figure 18-2 **A, B.** Patients recovering from cerebrovascular accident (CVA) like accuracy-challenge games presented by a computer and robotic arm.

A review of RCTs on the use of robotics suggests that motor improvements are greater when used earlier in post-stroke treatment and that research should focus on whether upper limb robots should be used in place of, or in addition to, standard of care interventions (Masiero, Armani, & Rosati, 2011).

Looking for ways to increase the improvement attributed to robotic devices has led to adding other modalities to robotic interventions, such as FES. The goal of therapeutic FES is to improve voluntary function by inducing physiological changes that remain after the stimulation is discontinued (Kowalczewski & Prochazka, 2011; Peckham & Knutson, 2005; Sheffler & Chae, 2007). Newer studies of robotic treatment are introducing pharmaceuticals as well. As we learn more about the biochemistry of neurological dysfunction, researchers look to pharmacology to modify blocked receptors and speed recovery following neurological trauma (Aravamudhan & Bellamkonda, 2011).

Researchers are looking, too, at the importance of attention, emotion, novelty, or reward in the recovery process. Often, incoming stimuli are reduced as a consequence of neurological loss and resulting inactivity. This makes increasing stimuli in the ascending brainstem pathways even more important so that learning is enhanced. It appears that combining robotics and highly stimulating interventions is essential to creating neuroplastic changes. These stimuli can range from engagement in highly valued tasks, to VR or FES, or the addition of neuromodulating drugs; their specific combination is the focus of current research (Volpe et al., 2009). Initial RCTs have yielded promising results (Knecht, Hesse, & Oster, 2011).

Occupational therapists have always associated recovery of function with the use of meaningful, repetitive, and task-specific activities that provide strong sensory input to the nervous system. It is affirming that research studies in

SCI, with both animals and humans, show that this kind of intervention is very effective in the treatment of SCI. Using the intrinsic physiological properties of the nervous system in combination with frequent, intensive sensory input to spinal networks is facilitating the recovery of function below the level of injury (Barbeau, Nadeau, & Garneau, 2006; Behrman & Harkema, 2007). The neurological system responds with plasticity as the spinal cord integrates supraspinal and afferent information arising from repetitive practice to improve motor output within the central pattern generators of the spinal cord. Training interventions based on the innate processing capacity of the spinal cord are leading to recovery of ambulation and improved respiratory function (McKay et al., 2011). The SCI recovery model has increased expectations for recovery of upper extremity (UE) functions for those with cervical injuries as therapeutic robots designed for SCI work to maintain normal range of motion (ROM), augment weak muscles, and gradually add resistance to increase strength to start, stop, and touch targets. In tandem with UE robotics and FES orthotic devices, outpatient occupational therapists use intensive, focused repetitive grasp and release tasks. Publications on development of robotic devices and case studies on outcomes for SCI are just beginning to emerge (Kadivar et al., 2011; Pehlivan, Celik, & O'Malley, 2011). YouTube videos of robot demonstrations are found with a search for "rehabilitation robot."

There are several reasons why research and development are so intensely focused on digital strategies to support functional motor recovery. Health care reform is seeking better treatment outcomes at lower costs. Robotic technologies have already helped to identify fundamental properties of brain function. This success is attributed to the fact that robots are able to control the position of, or forces applied to, limbs while having the ability to easily, objectively, and reliably quantify sensorimotor behavior (Loureiro et al., 2011; Scott & Dukelow, 2011). Robots do not fatigue or give up and through variability in tasks and modifiable resistance and movement parameters help maintain focus and interest.

Researchers recognized that robots had potential to reduce cost of stroke rehabilitation (Dijkers et al., 1991). Since then, forces for change—the coming flood of aging baby boomers, the rising cost of health care, and the remarkable advances in neuroscience and computer technology—have increased the interest in robotics for improved economic and health outcomes. The success with stroke recovery has also increased the interest in robotics for treatment of other significant conditions too—multiple sclerosis (MS), cerebral palsy (CP), peripheral nerve injuries, burns, etc.

Telerehabilitation and the Portability of Therapeutic Activities

The development of these digital tools and interventions that support recovery or remediation are also creating greater interest in consultation with experts or therapy that can be provided remotely with central oversight through telerehabilitation. It is an extension of the use of wireless audio and video communication technology (with secure signal transmission to protect health care information) that allows rehabilitation services to be delivered in client's homes. A document on telerehabilitation from the American Occupational Therapy Association (AOTA) cites many studies in which this technology is used for evaluation and intervention (AOTA, 2010a). Because digital technologies enable data collection and assessment with computer-based tools, therapists can measure progress even at a distance. They are using VR techniques with computer-based simulations and telemonitoring with real-time video and using apps on smartphones to take advantage of digital motion sensors imbedded in them. The quality of data collected via telerehabilitation has been shown to have excellent correlation with in-person assessment (Kim et al., 2008). Therapists save the time and expense of travel, and clients receive remotely supervised, individualized care in the comfort of their home or local environment. After all, performing ADL safely and effectively within the daily context is precisely the goal of occupational therapy care.

Being engaged in the therapeutic process does not necessarily require use of telerehabilitation. Many people with disabilities live in small communities far from the accessible health club facilities or resources of larger towns. They can also use digital technologies to maintain health and wellness. The sedentary lifestyle of many with SCI makes cardiovascular disease a major health concern, whereas a suitable exercise program could improve their cardiovascular fitness level.

One such concept is a hand-crank ergometer linked to a computer and its display. The individual controls a computer game with the direction and intensity of arm rotations. In the research that led to its development, physiological data were collected, and the subjects' oxygen consumption and heart rate were analyzed. Analysis showed that the system enabled nine subjects to reach their training zone, defined as 50%–60% of their maximum O_2 consumption and heart rate, respectively (O'Connor et al., 2001). Using this digital exerciser, now sold as GameCycle™, which is fun yet enables an effective training response, individuals can take a greater role in health self-maintenance.

The Big Question: Evidence of Effectiveness

These new digital technologies for treatment will challenge tomorrow's OT practitioners to develop the critical thinking skills and decision algorithms needed to select, modify, and use them appropriately with their clients. The current complexity of setup and adjustment of rehabilitation technologies will be refined and improved just as the human technology interface has for all digital technologies. Evidence of effectiveness will be easier to measure, yet occupational therapists will need to be clear in their treatments goals, choose appropriate tools, and ensure that measurable gains demonstrated on devices translate to real improvements in everyday tasks that are part of life in natural and desired environments. The chapter focus will now transition to another role of technology in OT.

ASSISTIVE TECHNOLOGY FOR COMPENSATION: OCCUPATION-AS-END

Occupational therapists have been interested in "high tech" AT, since the early 1980s when the Adaptive Firmware Card and Unicorn Board showed up to modify input for the Apple IIe computer (Bates et al., 1993). Early adopters recognized the ability of a modified computer to compensate for absent or impaired abilities and enable occupational performance. A consumer with significant physical or sensory limitation could suddenly create a document, a spreadsheet, or "speak" text using a home computer. In addition, therapists quickly recognized the value of computer technology to speed documentation and establish peer networks for their own sharing of information and resources.

Now that computers are more powerful, AT supports even more sophisticated activities. Today, a consumer with tetraplegia can use a hands-free interface to make video phone calls, design and distribute documents, or control the environment. AT enables consumers with limitations to participate in activities and make choices based on their goals and desired roles that motivate them. AT clearly fits within the model of occupation-as-end (i.e., an alternate way to complete an activity).

As stated in Chapter 1, competent role performance leads to life satisfaction; this is a prime goal of AT. Occupational therapists interact with the clients to identify current and future life roles and the tasks and activities those roles require. They analyze the individual's skills and abilities to build on strengths. They use their knowledge of intact body structures and functions to identify categories of AT with features that offer user interfaces and have functions that can replace missing capacities. They recognize that training as well as human and environmental supports are necessary to learn to use AT and integrate it into the tasks and activities of life roles. AT devices that match consumers' goals and abilities help them assume or return to meaningful roles and lives even in the presence of physical, sensory, or cognitive disabilities. Let us look at some specific examples of ways that ATs help individuals perform the activities and tasks of occupations and roles to support self-maintenance, self-advancement, and self-enhancement roles.

Self-Maintenance Roles

Enabling ADL performance is a familiar reason for OT referral. Simple technologies such as electric toothbrushes and shavers can increase efficacy and safety in personal care ADL tasks. However, IADL clearly benefit from AT solutions. Video relay services that use smartphones and video devices to enable remote American Sign Language (ASL) interpreters to speak to the recipients of phone calls are quickly replacing the text telephones and relay operator previously used by those who are deaf. Bluetooth headsets enable voice dialing on cell phones for those with paralysis who need to schedule a paratransit ride, shop for groceries, or request technical assistance over the telephone. Closed-circuit televisions (CCTVs) that enlarge objects help those with low vision pay bills and balance checkbooks. Even more IADL, such as banking, shopping, and e-mail, are supported with adaptations to computers and tablets.

Individuals with significant impairment can independently control lights, fans, or the TV volume within their living space with electronic aids to daily living (EADL) or even with smartphones equipped with apps and add-on transmitters that enable smartphones to function like universal remotes. The signaling technologies used in EADL are the same as those used in typical remotes: radio frequency (RF) and infrared (IR) light. Figure 18-3 illustrates the concept for categorizing simple and complex EADL.

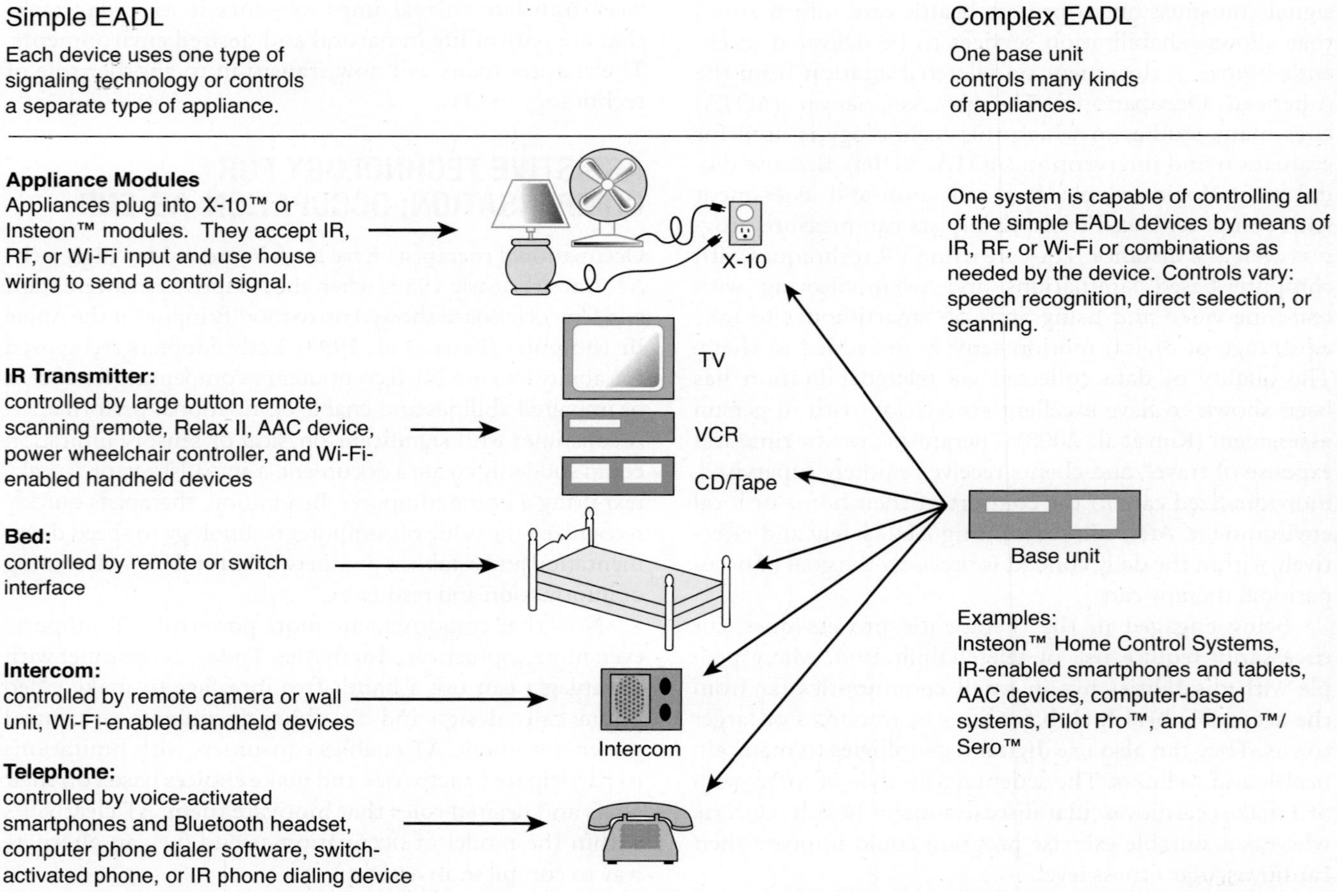

Simple EADL

Each device uses one type of signaling technology or controls a separate type of appliance.

Complex EADL

One base unit controls many kinds of appliances.

Appliance Modules
Appliances plug into X-10™ or Insteon™ modules. They accept IR, RF, or Wi-Fi input and use house wiring to send a control signal.

One system is capable of controlling all of the simple EADL devices by means of IR, RF, or Wi-Fi or combinations as needed by the device. Controls vary: speech recognition, direct selection, or scanning.

IR Transmitter:
controlled by large button remote, scanning remote, Relax II, AAC device, power wheelchair controller, and Wi-Fi-enabled handheld devices

Bed:
controlled by remote or switch interface

Intercom:
controlled by remote camera or wall unit, Wi-Fi-enabled handheld devices

Telephone:
controlled by voice-activated smartphones and Bluetooth headset, computer phone dialer software, switch-activated phone, or IR phone dialing device

Examples:
Insteon™ Home Control Systems, IR-enabled smartphones and tablets, AAC devices, computer-based systems, Pilot Pro™, and Primo™/ Sero™

Figure 18-3 EADL devices are classified as simple or complex and use a variety of signal transmission methods that now include Wi-Fi and the internet. AAC, augmentative and alternative communication; EADL, electronic aids to daily living; IR, infrared; RF, radio frequency.

Powered mobility, for those who cannot propel a manual wheelchair, contributes greatly to self-maintenance tasks. Independent mobility not only communicates curiosity, interest in participating, or the wish to be alone, it also supports independence with basic ADL such as eating, toileting, and bathing, and instrumental activities such as shopping for groceries. Powered mobility can increase the capacity of individuals to engage in the activities of role performance, although the availability of accessible environments is a key requirement (Buning, Angelo, & Schmeler, 2001). Home modification is usually necessary for using a wheelchair to cook a meal in a kitchen or approach a toilet in the bathroom. Universal design, which offers seven principles to guide inclusive design, considers the needs of a broad range of individuals by creating people-friendly spaces that are safer and more easily modified for those with severe impairment (Center for Universal Design, 2012). (See further discussion of powered mobility in Chapters 17 and 26 and more information regarding universal design in Chapter 31).

Augmentative and alternative communication (AAC) devices can incorporate synthesized or digitized speech devices for those who are unable to speak or whose speech is difficult to understand. Some AAC devices support the capacity to engage in full conversations; others store only a few messages. AAC devices allow consumers who have been taught to use them to socialize, call for assistance, direct caregivers, inform health care providers about health issues, initiate plans for activities, make food or clothing choices, and even gain employment.

Self-Advancement Roles: Work, School, or Community Volunteer

AT enables self-advancement roles for those with disability that range from volunteering by retirees to working full-time in paid employment or to students acquiring education. Wheelchairs and scooters allow travel on neighborhood sidewalks, commuting on accessible public transportation, and access to schools, stores, and workplaces with accessible entrances. Four-wheel drive wheelchairs give mobility on farms, on ranches, and in the backwoods.

Wireless internet communication technologies make information exchange easier and faster for everyone. When clients with sensory, motor, and language impairments can use these technologies, they reap huge benefits. Desktop and tablet computers commonly enable listening to text, writing, searching the Internet, managing finances and data, working remotely, and making video phone calls for work or leisure. Real-time closed captioning of a speaker's words at a conference and captioned multimedia and distance learning software create access for those with sensory impairment.

AAC devices are an essential part of communication and participation in school or workplace. Making choices, demonstrating knowledge, asking questions, forming peer relationships, and getting the job done all occur when alternative or augmentative communication devices are used.

Self-Enhancement Roles: Recreation and Leisure

Recreational choices often have symbolic meaning and clearly reveal our interests and our tolerance for challenge (Kielhofner, 1997). Recreational choices, made for their intrinsic and symbolic qualities, allow individuals to take on valued images of self as adventurer, connoisseur, or creator (see Chapter 29). AT enables activities ranging from alternate controls for video games to adapted reels for one-handed fishing. Recreational AT includes wheelchairs designed for beaches, tennis courts, or mountain trails. Water sit-skis and adaptive snow skis like mono- or bi-skis allow full participation and agility in mainstream recreations.

Many enjoy using home computers for leisure. Adapted computer access allows browsing sites on the Internet, pursuing interests like genealogy or collecting, and engaging in creative art activities and puzzles. The Internet allows researching destinations, finding accessible accommodations, and renting accessible vans. With this increased accessibility, even traveling is now a form of recreation and play.

THE ASSISTIVE TECHNOLOGY ASSESSMENT PROCESS

The potential contribution of AT devices is remarkable. However, the real contribution of AT only occurs as a result of a skilled, thoughtful, and thorough assessment that centers on the client's goals. A discussion of the elements of this process follows. Figure 18-4 is an overview of the AT assessment and intervention sequence.

Assessments are driven by the consumer's goals and needs (Bain & Leger, 1997). Family members or caregivers, speaking on behalf of a consumer with communication impairment, may also identify goals and needs. Occupational therapists, because of their knowledge of functional impairment and adaptations, are often an entry point for exploring the possibilities created by ATs (Hammel & Smith, 1993). As a member of an AT team, the occupational therapist attempts to understand the reason for the client referral, seeks to recognize the role that AT might play in compensating for impairment, and assists individuals in forming realistic expectations.

Consumers, family members, and caregivers come to an OT assessment with various needs and motivations. For example, a young adult transitioning to college may need computer technology and training in order to more efficiently complete assignments and participate in online class discussions or project development. A working adult

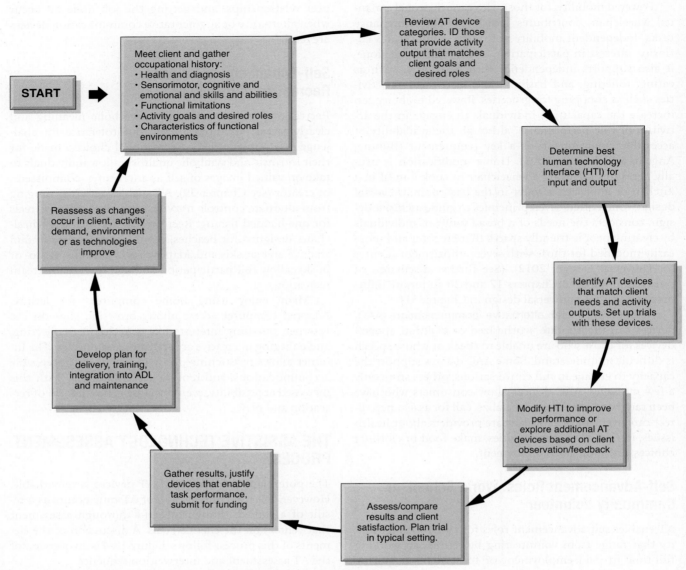

Figure 18-4 The AT assessment process. ADL, activities of daily living; AT, assistive technology; ID.

with a newly acquired motor impairment may need to learn about technologies, such as a trackball or speech recognition in order to return to work.

In addition to their goals and priorities, the assessment focuses on consumer and family attitudes toward AT. Some people easily adopt technology and incorporate it into tasks and routines; others resist and even fear it. Some feel that the latest high-technology equipment is not necessary and prefer simpler, more familiar devices. Consumers' religious and cultural background and personal tastes may also influence their choice of devices. Devices that fit within the personal, social, and cultural context of the consumer are more likely to be used than those outside the consumer's comfort zone.

Multiple factors need to be considered because consumer dissatisfaction leads to AT abandonment (Batavia & Hammer, 1990). Putting aside personal values, the therapist concentrates on addressing the consumer's goals and preferences.

As new occupational therapists who have grown up with technology and are already comfortable with a variety of digital devices and the internet begin to practice, digital solutions will become more common in OT practice. Some therapists will discover that they enjoy a more specialized focus on technology and will seek opportunities to work with an AT team in order to meet the needs of clients who would benefit from more specialized types of AT devices.

Team Members

Because of the wide variety of AT devices available, AT services are often delivered with the help of a multidisciplinary team that consists of a variety of professionals and stakeholders. The consumer, family, and caregivers have key roles because they will use the equipment on a daily basis. Professionals on the team vary according to the consumer's needs.

- A seating expert, an occupational or physical therapist, understands maximizing fine motor function when sitting. With the consumer's activities in mind, this expert assesses posture and ROM and specifies seat, back and foot support angles, and cushion type (e.g., support or pressure relief or accommodation to abnormal posture). If the consumer uses a wheelchair, assessment includes a trial with his or her wheelchair. The decision to use a manual or powered wheelchair can affect selection and use of other AT devices (see Chapter 17 for information on wheelchairs and assessment).
- An access specialist, typically an occupational therapist, focuses on finding the best method for controlling an AT device. The access specialist works with the rehabilitation technology supplier (RTS) and/or the rehabilitation engineer in selecting and developing control for specific devices, such as computers, AAC devices, and EADL.
- A teacher or special educator, if the consumer is a student, describes schoolwork tasks and helps ensure that AT solutions support educational tasks and school participation.
- A vocational rehabilitation counselor, if the consumer works or is preparing for work, will approve AT solutions and help with funding.
- A speech–language pathologist (SLP) with expertise in AAC leads the team when communication is the focus. The SLP evaluates a consumer's potential for verbal and written communication, determines the symbol set to be used (alphabet, pictures, etc.), and collaborates with the access specialist.
- A rehabilitation engineer may be on the team if the consumer has complex needs and off-the-shelf solutions are not likely to be effective. The engineer may integrate several types of AT when consumers have few options for control. For example, a consumer with reliable control of only a finger would need an integrated control system that allows this small movement to drive a wheelchair, operate a computer, and control an AAC device.
- A social worker may help locate funding sources or provide counseling as consumers and significant others come to terms with disability.
- RTSs (often called vendors) are equipment experts. Because they sell devices, an RTS may be able to provide demonstration equipment for evaluations.

The RTS knows product features and can help with selecting components, customizing products, and handling warranty issues following delivery. Suppliers with specialty certification have advanced training, skill with assessment, and commitment to ethical practices.

The Assistive Technology Assessment

Prior to an AT assessment, the team needs to understand the consumer's goals related to roles and the performance of activities to support roles. This client-centered approach, a key feature of OT assessment, can be accomplished either through a structured interview or an intake questionnaire (AOTA, 2008). For some clients, goals are actually expressed by family members or caregivers. Once goals are established, the door is open for focusing on a particular area of AT and categories of solutions and for assessing current skills and abilities to determine potential access methods. During this part of the assessment, it is important to gather a realistic picture of the consumer's motor control, social skills, and cognitive and sensory abilities, as well as the environments where the consumer will use the devices. Areas commonly addressed in AT assessments follow.

Seating

Optimal seating is mandatory to achieve the best results during the rest of the assessment. If the client uses a seating system that does not provide adequate support, the performance observed during subsequent AT evaluation activities will not accurately show the consumer's ability.

Sometimes it is not possible to address seating issues before the rest of the assessment. When this happens, a seating simulator with an adjustable back, sides, armrests, and lateral trunk and foot supports can be used to meet a broad range of postural support needs. The optimal solution is to assess consumers in their own appropriately fitting seating system.

Another important factor to determine early in the assessment is where and in what positions the consumer spends the most time. Asking these questions at the beginning of the assessment avoids recommending access methods that the consumer can use with accuracy in their wheelchair only to find out that, at home, the consumer spends the most time in bed or a lounge chair. Once seating issues have been resolved, motor control for access is addressed.

Motor Control

Ideally, an access method (e.g., touch-typing on a keyboard) is effortless. Effortlessness comes after practicing and refining a skill and allows attention to be directed to thoughts rather than to keystrokes. To reach effortlessness, access methods that the consumer is able to activate consistently, reliably, and with endurance are needed.

To plan for physical control of an AT device, the therapist needs to identify optimal body segments usable for reaching, touching, turning, tapping, etc. This leads to a functional evaluation of ROM, coordination, and endurance. Often, consumers and their family members and caregivers know a consumer's best controlled body segments and can provide this information. Usually, the hands and fingers are assessed first because humans prefer them for interacting with objects (Cook & Polgar, 2007). If not hands or fingers, assess head movement next. Consumers with limited control over their UEs sometimes have excellent control of head movements. If the head is only partly successful, consider use of eye movements. Some find best or preferred control through the feet or knees. The best two or three sites should become the focus at this point in the assessment (Cook & Polgar, 2007).

Evaluating accuracy, ROM, and endurance helps to determine the active range a consumer has for accessing a keyboard, a switch, or other input devices. It is helpful to quantify this function. Using a vertical or horizontal checkerboard or a spare computer keyboard can be very useful when assessing this capacity. It may be necessary to do a series of trials with various body parts in order to determine which one moves reliably with the least effort. This serves to narrow options for access devices that can be explored further. For example, overshooting or dragging a finger on a typical computer keyboard indicates a need for bigger targets or the use of keys with less sensitivity. Conversely, if the consumer has good accuracy but can only reach targets close to the midline, consider small keyboards or a joystick to reach all keys or to control a cursor. Coordination can also be assessed in this simple manner by asking the consumer to point to specific squares on a board. If precise pointing is not possible, the occupational therapist may add a control enhancer (to be discussed) or a more specialized control interface to ensure accuracy.

Once pointing and reaching trials are completed with several body segments, compare the results to determine which body segment offered the best control. It is important to ask the consumer whether he or she agrees. If the consumer feels more comfortable using another body part despite less accuracy, the therapist and consumer should discuss this and come to agreement about the primary access site. Skill can develop in time.

Having said all of this, it seems important to note that speech recognition and eye gaze technology have improved greatly in the last few years. These technologies create the possibility that a consumer may need no physical contact with an input device in order to control it. Depending on a consumer's cognitive abilities and goals, it may be possible to use speech recognition, eye gaze, or scanning to move past the need for good motor control.

Direct versus Indirect Selection Methods. With motor skill assessed, the occupational therapist is ready to determine whether direct or indirect selection will be used (Definition 18-1). If a consumer can point, touch, or move accurately, direct selection is appropriate. Target size and device placement will still be factors. Use indirect selections only when some form of accurate pointing to select from a set of options (e.g., keyboard or number pad) is not possible or is too inefficient. Indirect selection is very demanding. The consumer must be able to plan a sequence as well as anticipate the choice and activate the switch at exactly the right time.

Switch Assessment. Selecting and mounting the optimal switch is critical for success with indirect selection, Morse code, or other controls (Table 18-1 for options and sources). Consistent, comfortable, and reliable switch pressing increases accuracy. The body segment that is most reliable guides switch choice. A consumer with muscular dystrophy who has finger weakness should be offered a small, sensitive switch. In contrast, someone with CP may need a rugged foot switch mounted on a wheelchair footrest. For an anatomical site that is bony, such as the back of the hand, a padded or pillow switch is appropriate.

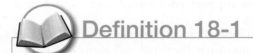

Definition 18-1

Direct and Indirect Selection

Selection set refers to the universe of options from which an individual can choose. In *direct selection*, all of the items in the selection set are available all the time. Examples of direct selection are computer keyboards, telephone keypads, and calculators. Direct selection is very intuitive; if K is pressed on a keyboard, K will appear on the display. The disadvantage is that direct selection demands hand–eye coordination, range of motion, and endurance.

If the consumer is unable to reliably press the desired keys even with a performance enhancer, the option often becomes *indirect selection* or scanning. In this mode, only a subset of all possible choices are available at a given time, for example, setting the time on a digital clock and waiting for the correct number to appear. The advantage of indirect selection is that a consumer needs only one reliable movement (i.e., an eyebrow, elbow, or toe) to activate a switch indicating choice. However, this process is demanding because a user must wait for an item to be presented, accurately time switch activation, have the cognition to focus on an objective, and sequence the steps to achieve it. Additionally, error correction is frustrating and very time consuming.

Table 18-1   Common Switches and Activation Methods

Category and Switch Name	Image	How and Where It Works
No Physical Contact (requires battery or external power source (e.g., power wheelchair battery)		
Self-Calibrating Auditory Tone Infrared (SCATIR) switch from AbleNet		Activates with small movement (i.e., eyelid, facial muscle, or finger) that interrupts an IR beam. Provides auditory feedback.
Proximity switch from Adaptive Switch Laboratory		Activates when body part moves into a preset but adjustable range. Does not provide sensory feedback.
Physical Contact, No Pressure		
Pneumatic (or sip and puff) from AbleNet and others		Activates as a dual switch with minimal force; internal membrane detects in or out air pressure delivered through closed lips. Gives no feedback.
Physical Contact with Pressure		
Micro Light switch from AbleNet		Activates with minimal force; for use with small or weak body part. Gives auditory and tactile feedback.
Ribbon switch from AbleNet		Activates with minimal force; moisture proof for use at chin, hand, or other body part. Gives no feedback when the flexible ribbon is bent >10°.
Plate switch from AbleNet		Activates with minimal force; thin and moisture proof for use by hand, arm, knee, or foot. Gives no feedback when touched.
Pillow switch from AbleNet		Activates with moderate force; soft foam padding makes it best for bony areas. Gives auditory and tactile feedback.

| Table 18-1 | Common Switches and Activation Methods *(continued)* |

Category and Switch Name	Image	How and Where It Works
Big Red (5 inches), Jelly Bean (2.5 inches), and Spec (1.4 inches) switches from AbleNet		Activate with moderate to maximum force; match size to finger, hand, arm, knee, or foot. Gives auditory and tactile feedback.
Big Beamer or Jelly Beamer switches from AbleNet		Activates with moderate to maximum force; sends wireless signal 30 feet to the receiver plugged into target device; can be pressed by hand, arm, or foot. Gives auditory and tactile feedback.
Rocker switch from AbleNet		Activates as a dual switch with moderate force; use with small body part for row/column scanning or Morse code. Gives auditory and tactile feedback.

Switches need to be mounted so they remain in place and in line with the angle of activation. Wheelchair and desk mounts with solid, one-way connections are far more likely to be used correctly than those that are adjustable. A switch mount must also be easily removable so it does not interfere with transfers or eating.

Regardless of the type of switch selected, it should give the consumer feedback about successful movement. Usually, this feedback is auditory or tactile, but it can also occur through the instant response of the device being controlled. Switches activated with head movements need less auditory feedback, because a noisy switch mounted near the ear can be annoying. Six occupational therapists with expertise in AT participated in a focus group to develop a list of the 10 most important considerations for switch access (Angelo, 2000). In the control category, the therapists indicated that the most important considerations were reliability of response, ability to perform timed responses, ability to activate and deactivate the switch within

a given time frame, and endurance (the ability to sustain a force and to apply that force repeatedly over time). In the ease of movement category, therapists said that tasks should be performed volitionally, easily, and efficiently and that past performances with positive outcomes should be considered. Because context was considered important, assessments should occur in the environment where tasks are routinely performed. Finally, switch safety should be considered. Switches should have rounded corners, and all wires should be secured or avoided so that they do not become entangled with fingers, pointing devices, or other equipment (Procedures for Practice 18-1).

Cognition

Cognition is usually evaluated informally during AT assessment (Cook & Polgar, 2007). During the assessment activities and interaction, it is possible to estimate the consumer's attention span, reading level, short- and long-term

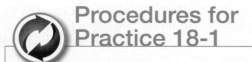

Procedures for Practice 18-1

Switch Assessment

1. Identify the anatomical sites over which the consumer has most control for switch activation. No timing is involved in this step. Cause-and-effect software games can make this a fun activity.
2. Evaluate the consumer's ability to wait a specific length of time before activating the switch. This skill is critical for effectively using indirect selection. Errors in selection occur when the switch is released too soon or too late. Cause-and-effect games that introduce timing (e.g., Frog and Fly) are useful for determining this ability.
3. Evaluate the consumer's ability to maintain contact with the switch and to release the switch on command. This information will help to identify the best scanning mode, for example, automatic, inverse, or step scanning.
4. When one or more anatomical sites have been identified for accurate switch activation, the AT team determines which body part and type of switch is most appropriate and how and where to mount the switch. This concept is further described by Cook and Polgar (2007).

memory, and ability to follow instructions and sequence tasks. A neuropsychological evaluation can also be very helpful. Knowing more about cognitive functioning helps the AT team determine which devices have the features and performance characteristics that will match the consumer's cognitive ability (see Chapter 6). A consumer with a learning disability or an intellectual disability associated with cerebrovascular accident (CVA) or TBI should be assessed for visual perception. Knowledge about figure-ground problems or form constancy helps the team ensure that a visual display is usable. Icons, words, or symbols may need to be placed farther apart or the background may need to be simplified to reduce visual stimulation.

Visual Acuity and Visual Perception

The AT evaluation team should always consider vision because many impairments affect acuity, occulomotor skills, or visual perception. Visual acuity will affect the size of symbols used for communication boards and the sizes of letters and icons on a computer display. Decreasing the distance from the eye to the display (typically one arm's length) can help. It is also possible to use options in the computer control panel to alter brightness or screen resolution or add magnification or change contrast.

Eye ROM, conjugate eye movements, visual field cuts, and tracking should be noted (see Chapter 5). Knowing the extent of eye movement and whether the eyes work together is especially important when consumers are using indirect selection methods. This method requires the eye to track or follow a cursor and scan options to find a specific item. If imbalance is noted, then eye preference should be established, and this information should be used during the assessment and later during equipment setup. Information about a visual field loss helps to determine the location of visual displays and may influence choice of font, font size, or contrast to help compensate. If visual tracking is impaired, remedial work with single switch and cause-and-effect software may help to develop this skill for users who have limited experience with controlling their environment.

Finalizing the Match between User and Technology

By this time in the assessment, an AT team has a clear idea of the consumer's motor, cognitive, visual, and visual perception abilities. The AT team should have begun to narrow the range of options down to a few devices with activity outputs, user controls, mounts, and control enhancers that match the consumer's needs and abilities.

Once options are narrowed to two or three, it is time to conduct a more extensive trial with each. Trials of two to three devices with the control interface and control enhancers allow the consumer to become familiar with the equipment and determine level of comfort when using it. As previously mentioned, this trial, if not the entire assessment, should occur in the environment where the consumer will use the equipment. Using the system in the actual or intended environment—home, workplace, or school—uncovers problems that may not emerge during center-based trials (Angelo, 2000). Noise, desks that are too small for devices, tables that are too low for rolling under with a wheelchair, and lights that are too dim or that glare on the display can be addressed and resolved. Trials should occur before making recommendations and submitting a final equipment list because this increases the likelihood that the devices will actually be used and not abandoned. With the reauthorization of the Tech Act of 1988, each state is required to develop an AT device-lending library. AT teams should make use of this resource (Bailey, Weber, & Meidenbauer, 2012).

THE ASSISTIVE TECHNOLOGY INTERVENTION PROCESS

An AT device recommendation is guided first by a consumer's activity goals with the AT device features based on the consumer's abilities, capacities, and preferences. The broad categories of AT solutions include control enhancers, computer modifications, AAC devices, and EADL, and each of these will be briefly discussed in turn.

It may be helpful to think of an AT solution as a complex assistive device. Because of its complexity, four critical components must be considered: (1) a user interface (how the client will interact with it), (2) a processor that converts the user input into the desired action, (3) the product or activity output, and (4) an environmental interface that influences its adoption and effectiveness. The environmental interface includes the physical, social, and cultural environments in which a device will be used.

Occupational therapists, by their education and interest in human function, are already familiar with this kind of consideration, because they have already learned a process for recommending assistive devices to their clients. However, interdisciplinary AT team members are usually acquainted with a service delivery model called the HAAT (Human Activity and Assistive Technology) model (Cook & Polgar, 2007). The HAAT model is based on systems theory, in which a change at any point in the process requires readjustment in other components of the system to rebalance and ensure continuity (von Bertalanfy, 1968). This model (Fig. 18-5) will look familiar to occupational therapists. Because AT practice demands greater knowledge of devices with processors, more customizable user interfaces and activity outputs, occupational therapists with an interest in AT must typically invest additional time and effort in continuing education or self-directed learning with a mentor to develop competence with specific elements of the HAAT model.

Hierarchy of Access

When consumers with impairments cannot use digital devices in standard ways, a principle called hierarchy of access is used (Schmitt, 1992). This principle reminds us that simple solutions should be considered before those that are complex. Less complex solutions are less costly and easier to implement. The goal is to optimize control without burdening consumers with more technology than they need.

Control

One of the key approaches to reducing complexity is to consider how typical or mainstream user interfaces can be enhanced using low-tech aids or assistive devices that consider the consumer's limitations and address barriers to use. This concept has been referred to as control enhancers. This term refers to aids that enhance or extend a consumer's physical control (Cook & Polgar, 2007). Control enhancers include head pointers, handheld pointing devices (pencils, pointers with built-up handles, and typing sticks), mouth sticks, wrist rests, and arm supports (Fig. 18-6). Control enhancers also include devices that modify placement of user interfaces such as easels, flexible switch mounts, and flat-panel monitor arms. For example, a lever-adjustable keyboard tray can increase keyboarding comfort or an easel can position a regular keyboard for a consumer using a mouth stick and eliminate the need for a special keyboard. Control enhancers also support using devices efficiently with less fatigue. Comparing outcomes with several control enhancers helps determine the best fit between the consumer and his or her AT device.

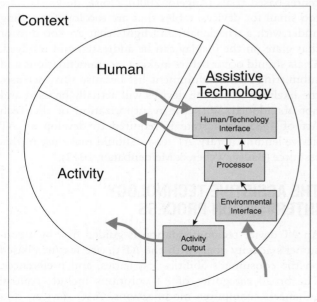

Figure 18-5 The HAAT (Human Activity and Assistive Technology) Model helps to conceptualize factors in an assistive technology (AT) device system.

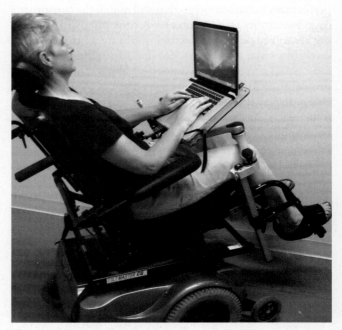

Figure 18-6 Often performance or control can be enhanced by repositioning an assistive technology device or the orientation of the person using the device (Photo courtesy of Blue Sky Designs, Inc., Minneapolis, MN).

Adaptive Computer Access

In general, adaptations for computer use fall into two categories—changing how information is put into a computer (input) or changing how a computer's information is delivered (output). Depending on impairment, consumers who want to use computers may have difficulty with one or the other or even both input and output. Typically, input is accomplished with keyboard, mouse, or trackpad, and output is accomplished through computer display, sound, or a printer. However, technology continues to offer new modes of input and output such as automatic speech recognition and soon, brain-computer interface (BCI).

Adapting access to a computer should always start with the accessibility options (Fig. 18-7) in the control panel of the computer operating system (OS). Because these options are included in all computers at no additional cost, they are the first step in the "hierarchy of access." Accessibility or universal access options allow any user to modify input and outputs such as setting the size and speed of the mouse cursor, latching modifier keys on the keyboard to aid one-handed typing, reducing keyboard sensitivity to reduce errors caused by tremor, increasing the contrast or size of fonts on the menus and icons, and controlling basic computer functions with speech. Both Microsoft and Apple websites offer extensive tutorials and step-by-step guides for these features.

Modifications to Computer or Device Input

There are a variety of ways that specialized and even mainstream software and hardware can modify computer input. Because the goal of this chapter is to acquaint occupational therapy practitioners with the range of possibilities

for adapting computers, the descriptions that follow will serve as encouragement to search and learn more about specific products.

Keyboarding. A standard keyboard should be the first device tried. Using accessibility options or a keyguard to reduce unintended key hits may be all that is needed. If not, then consider alternative keyboards. Most alternative keyboards provide transparent computer access; that is, the computer thinks the input is coming from a standard computer keyboard. Additionally, most of these keyboards are equipped with Universal Serial Bus (USB) connectors so they can be exchanged without rebooting and will work on either Windows or Macintosh platforms.

Several commercial products are included in this category. Some are adaptable and can be used in a variety of ways; others have narrow applications. One keyboard, shown in Figure 18-8, crosses computer platforms. It comes with a set of standard overlays that are instantly detected by the keyboard via bar code readers. The layouts of these overlays range from simple enough for those with low cognitive ability to those for advanced computer users. Key press acceptance rates are easily adjusted, and keyguards can facilitate key pressing accuracy. The keyboard also allows arrow keys to control mouse movements. The keyboard is 11 × 17 inches, so good ROM is needed to reach all of the keys. These features make this a good device to use in an OT setting where therapists are providing basic adaptive access for a variety of diagnoses.

Another option that is available on all computers is an on-screen keyboard. In this adaptation, a physical keyboard is not used. Rather, a keyboard is represented on the computer display and the consumer uses a device that can move an arrow cursor to point to keys on the virtual keyboard (Fig. 18-9). This method is the equivalent

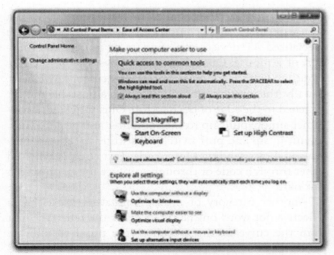

Figure 18-7 First, consider accessibility options within a computer operating system.

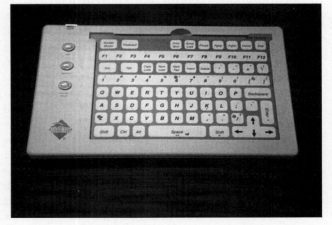

Figure 18-8 Intellikeys keyboard allows easy modification when the user needs large keys or decreased sensitivity.

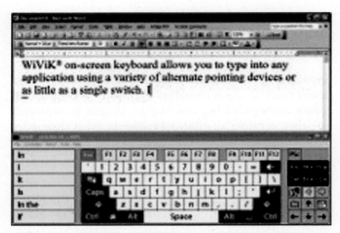

Figure 18-9 A resizable, on-screen keyboard with word prediction allows text entry by mouse, trackball, or any device that moves the cursor on a computer display.

of one-finger typing, but it makes typing possible for someone without the endurance to hold fingers over a keyboard. On-screen keyboards are usually packaged with word prediction and abbreviation expansion software. Word prediction software uses rules of recency, frequency, and grammar to anticipate the next word. Optimally configured, word prediction saves keystrokes, but it works especially well with the on-screen keyboard because the consumer's eyes are looking at the screen where the predicted words are displayed. A second click or dwell chooses a whole word and enters it into the text document. Abbreviation expansion lets the consumer establish shortcuts to represent frequently used phrases or personal information, such as BTW for "by the way." As you will see shortly, there are many mouse pointing options.

There are also variations in keyboard layout that can help a one-handed typist be more efficient. Balance the usefulness of this approach with the time needed to relearn a keyboard layout. The ability to electronically select an alternate keyboard layout is much easier now because of the sophistication of control panels or system preferences that are part of today's computer OS. Keyboard keys can be relabeled with stickers or popped off and rearranged on a spare keyboard. In this approach, the hand stays in a home position and uses reaches from the home row to type all letters and numbers.

The process for determining a best option for a keyboard modification is to determine existing skill and familiarity with keyboarding and the places where keyboarding will need to occur. Then expose the consumer to use of some adaptive options that consider his or her activity and task needs, determine a keyboard rate for comparison, and then discuss the usability of each approach across settings. Remember unlearning a familiar skill is not easy, and success in use of all new methods will be slow in the beginning.

Mousing. A mouse is still the most common pointing device, and pointing is still an essential means of directing a computer's action. The actions of pointing and clicking can be completed with a range of devices. One mainstream product with features that make it useful for consumers with limitations is a trackball. A trackball offers both the advantage of remaining stationary in a base as well as separating the actions of pointing and clicking. This allows more accurate cursor control and reduces the frustrating movement that can occur when initiating a mouse click. The ability to rest the wrist on the base of the trackball increases proximal stability for the fingers. Many consumers with poor coordination who cannot control a mouse can control a trackball. Furthermore, a trackball is sturdy enough for control via elbow, wrist, or foot movements. Trackball software allows adjusting the ratios between ball movement and cursor speed and clicks and double clicks can be linked to buttons on the right or left side of the trackball base.

Trackpads are common on computers. They can be customized to change the number of fingertips or the direction of their movement required to scroll or flip through pages in a photo collection. This mainstream customization can function to simplify computer input for some.

A touch screen is also a mouse substitute. Selecting or interacting with a touch screen is as simple as touching an icon to select it or dragging a finger to draw in a paint program. This reality is basis for the revolution created by touch screen devices. Some touch screen devices work by creating contact between two membranes with the pressure of touch. Other touch screens work because the screen is coated with a material that detects the small electrical charge in human skin. The device processor translates the xy coordinates of the consumer's touch or the mouse location on the screen for conversion to action outputs.

Mouse Emulation. When hands or feet cannot control a mouse or cursor, more complex AT devices are used. These specialized AT devices can emulate or imitate the function of a mouse. One category is a joystick operated by mouth to provide for quick and precise cursor movement. Usually, the joystick is mounted on an adjustable mount attached to the edge of the desktop. Once adjusted, a consumer simply pulls up to the computer and gets to work. A built-in sip and puff switch substitutes for mouse buttons or allows sending Morse code. Text entry is achieved either through code or through software for an on-screen keyboard.

Another category of mouse emulators use either a reflective dot worn on the forehead or the reflected light from the curve of the eyeball at the pupil to indicate pointing. Solid-state photo sensors in a camera attached to a computer or AAC device detect small movements and convert them into *xy* coordinates. Selecting or mouse clicking and dragging are produced with an external switch or with associated software. Another means of selecting occurs through the use of dwell. This feature allows choice making by floating the cursor over an icon or key for a predetermined amount of time. Mouse emulation enables typing with an on-screen keyboard or using computer-aided design (CAD) or illustration software. This technology allows pixel-to-pixel accuracy and smooth cursor movement.

Of course, using a mouse or any other pointing technology is very challenging if not impossible for a consumer without vision. With a touch screen device, they will, at a minimum, need auditory feedback through a speech synthesizer to know what they are touching on the screen and the associated function of that position. For most other devices that commonly use a mouse for pointing, an entirely different user interface will be needed.

Automatic Speech Recognition. Automatic Speech Recognition (ASR) technology, a mainstream technology developed to enable data entry in settings where hands were busy, was quickly recognized as valuable for those with motor impairment (Koester, 2001). Consumers with significant motor limitations but with speech were able to write independently using a computer. Although early versions required each word to be spoken separately, the technology now works with continuous speech. The leading product, Dragon Naturally Speaking™ (Simpson & Koester, 1999) uses sophisticated algorithms to compare speech sounds with likely or logical phrases, a process that requires a computer with sufficient RAM and processor speed. Most ASR applications require good literacy skills, because the user must compare the displayed text to the text he or she intended to write. Auditory playback, however, make this much more feasible for most users. SpeakQ™, another speech recognition application, removes this obstacle for individuals with learning disabilities or low literacy skills. Its user interface is easy to customize and tends to work well with users whose voices have unique characteristics.

With ASR technology, it is important to consider both the user and the environment. This technology requires learning and using a very different approach to writing. The user must mentally compose a sentence and then speak it without "ums" or incidental comments. Users who cannot use their hands or a mouse must recall specific command phrases, although on-screen help has reduced this cognitive load. The user needs to be able to work in an environment that is tolerant of someone speaking at conversational volume; that is to say not in a classroom or a typical office cube environment. Also, loud environmental sounds can interfere with ASR. Individuals should use a high-quality, noise-cancelling microphone connected to the USB port rather than the sound card.

Good instruction in proper correction strategies is essential for continuously improving recognition accuracy and the efficiency of ASR (Koester, 2006).

At present, speech recognition offers good access to well-designed Internet websites, launching applications, and performing general computer tasks. Computer OS and handheld devices are rapidly moving in the direction of allowing individuals to have voice control over complex processing tasks.

Optical Character Recognition. Optical character recognition (OCR), a mainstream technology that converts pages of print into computer documents, can also serve as an adaptive input method. OCR uses a page scanner to capture text and software to analyze the image and recognize it as text. This creates a significant compensation for those with visual impairment or learning disability because this text can be read with a speech synthesizer as text-to-speech, converted to large print, or sent to a Braille printer. OCR is used in stand-alone products such as the SARA™ (scanning and reading appliance) or with software on a personal computer. Naturally, recognition accuracy is critical for success, but excellent accuracy is achieved with high-quality printed materials.

Use of Single Switches for Input: Morse and Scanning. Single switches can be used for direct selection. The consumer needs control and endurance at one motor site (e.g., a finger or eyebrow) and the cognitive ability to learn and recall codes, which can be sent via one or two switches. Those with the motor ability to send both long and short signals use one switch. Those unable to vary switch closure must use two switches, one for dit and one for dah. Once the code is sent, computer software converts signals into alphanumeric characters, keyboard shortcuts, or OS macros. Morse code supports writing, using spreadsheets, and Internet browsing. Using a body part that can be moved quickly, it is possible to text at 30 words per minute. No other input method for a person with severe motor limitation allows writing at this rate of speed (Anson, 1997). Higher word-per-minute rates are claimed for ASR, but Koester (2006) found that those with motor impairment rarely achieve these rates.

Scanning is the input method of last resort and has already been described. When a consumer lacks the ability to accurately choose one item from a set of all options (e.g., a key on a keyboard or touch screen), an array with subsets of options is offered. The individual chooses by activating a switch, but the time spent waiting makes it very inefficient. This delay increases further when the consumer cannot see. In this case, auditory scanning is used, and the consumer listens for an announcement of each choice just before it is available for selection. Scanning arrays can be used to control computers, EADL, and AAC

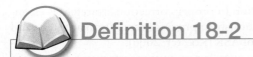

Definition 18-2

Basic Scanning Modes

Automatic—The consumer presses the switch to initiate scanning and bring up an array of choices. The cursor highlights items in the selection set one at a time. The consumer presses the switch to choose when the desired item is highlighted.

Inverse—The consumer presses the switch to initiate scanning. The consumer must maintain pressure or switch activation to enable the cursor to move through the selection set or array of choices. When the desired item is highlighted, the consumer releases the switch to choose it.

Step—The consumer presses the switch to bring up the array and to move the cursor to the next item in the selection set or array. The highlighted area moves to the next item each time the switch is pressed. A selection is made when the cursor dwells on an item for a preset amount of time and the consumer refrains from pressing the switch.

devices. Information on scanning modes is provided in Definition 18-2.

New Input Technologies. Work continues on development of a BCI. This topic is related to neural prosthetics in which an artificial device replaces the function of an impaired nervous system or sensory organ, for example, a cochlear or retinal implant. Currently, BCI occurs primarily through noninvasive techniques that capture brain signals through electroencephalogram (EEG) or with sensors located with the help of functional magnetic resonance imaging (MRI) or magnetic encephalography. Products suited for consumers have begun to appear but rely on extensive training for any level of reliable performance. Successful BCI would aid those locked in as a result of brainstem stroke or the late stages of motor neuron diseases such as amyotrophic lateral sclerosis (ALS) or MS.

Modifications to Computer Output

Once a computer receives input, the central processing unit (CPU) and the OS software perform the requested task. The CPU delivers output as words, images, or video on the display, as a printed page, or as a sound. Output can be a dialogue box, a finished product, or an alert sound. Individuals with sensory impairment are most affected by computer output, and this leads to the other broad category: adaptations to computer output for sensory or learning disabilities.

Screen. For most, output via the computer display is interpreted quickly via the visual system; those with impairment will need adaptation. Visual impairments range from field deficits and color blindness to low vision and the inability to perceive light; likewise, there is a range of adaptations. Some are as simple as reducing the amount of light coming from the display. Use the accessibility options in the control panel or preferences to reverse screen contrast so that letters are light on a dark background. Likewise, increase the size of objects on a display by reducing monitor resolution. To illustrate, if the resolution on a 17-inch display is set to 1280 × 1024, then changing it to 640 × 480 will make text and icons appear twice the size.

Those with more significant vision issues will need screen enlargement software that can magnify the screen 2 to 16 times. One product, ZoomText™, shown in Figure 18-10, creates a virtual magnifying glass for a section of the screen. The user shifts between the normal display and a magnified area to see parts of the screen that are of interest, for example, a radio button. Screen enlargement software offers the option of highlighting words as a speech synthesizer reads them. Listening while seeing larger text allows hearing to support weak vision. Software also allows users to set up default colors for text and background, which supports usable vision.

When consumers have no usable vision, they need software to completely substitute for seeing, not just in application software but also in the OS. Specialized software, generically called a screen reader (e.g., JAWS™, WindowEyes™), allows a consumer to send the cursor around the display as they listen to a speech synthesizer

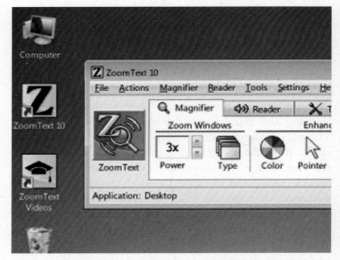

Figure 18-10 ZoomText™ (here with 3× magnification) offers customizable enlargement of part of the screen, with or without text-to-speech option. (Courtesy of Ai Squared, Manchester Center, VT.)

read menu choices, dialogue boxes, and paragraphs in word-processed documents. All cursor and reading functions are controlled via the keyboard's number pad or by a separate keypad. Consumers can set up preferences for speech rate, pronunciation of proper nouns, etc. Similar adaptations are used when consumers have learning disabilities. Solutions include text-to-speech tools that highlight text as it is spoken and extensive resources for writing organization, spelling, and grammar.

Refreshable Braille Display. Braille is an important tool for literacy, although audio recordings and speech synthesis are increasingly common. Today, few learn Braille, although it is highly correlated with literacy and academic achievement. Refreshable Braille on a computer lets a user "see" information on a display and read and correct errors (Cook & Polgar, 2007). The Braille display sits beneath a computer keyboard, extending beyond its front edge. Movable pins rise and fall, making tactile dots that change as the cursor moves. Proficient users easily move between keyboard and Braille display. As adaptive output, a Braille display gives access to text in web pages, numbers in a column, text in a table, and notation in a math formula. A Braille embosser prints documents by pressing dots into heavy paper, which makes it easy to make Braille resources, restaurant menus, etc.

Large Print. Consumers with low vision often use large print. Computers make it easy to change font size. Some fonts are considered easier to read. Serif fonts (with a small cap or foot) are considered better than sans serif fonts. However, OCR devices more accurately recognize sans serif fonts. Luckily, it is easy to select text in a document and change a font or size before printing.

Auditory Signals. Hearing impairment requires modification to computer output such as flashing menu bar instead of alert sounds. Otherwise, users with hearing loss usually do not require other adaptations. It is important that multimedia videos, ads, and distance learning software offer captioning and text descriptions of sound features—especially when they convey meaning.

Augmentative and Alternative Communication Devices

AAC intervention is the process of facilitating functional communication across all types of activities and environments. AAC intervention should be considered when *motor* impairments such as CP, ALS, and apraxia or when *language* impairment such as aphasia, autism, and TBI affect speech production or communication. Using an AAC device is very different from speech because it requires learning a language representation system and mastering a complex user interface.

Augmentative and Alternative Communication Intervention

SLPs with specialized training are responsible for this form of AT. Successful use requires device selection, a user interface designed to maximize speed and efficiency, extensive teaching, and practice in retrieving and using language in ADL (Beukelman & Mirenda, 2006; U.S. Society for Augmentative and Alternative Communication [USSAAC], 2012).

Occupational therapists will also encounter consumers who use *unaided* communication systems, such as sign languages, gestures, facial expressions, and looking up for yes and down for no, as well as *aided* communication systems. Aided systems use physical objects such as picture and letter boards and voice output devices such as dedicated AAC devices or apps on tablets or smartphones to convey thoughts, needs, and wants. Both types are useful depending on setting and communication partner familiarity. There are situations when paper and pencil and alphabet, symbol or picture boards and books are very appropriate. However, speech output devices allow a user to get the attention of others and communicate easily with voice output—especially to unfamiliar partners.

Most complex, dedicated AAC devices offer speech output along with a microprocessor-based storage and retrieval system. This allows messages to be prepared ahead of time, stored, retrieved, and then delivered as either synthesized or digitized speech as needed. Dedicated AAC devices have highly adaptive user interfaces and many options for customizing vocabulary for various users. They allow Internet access, use of computer applications, and control of IR devices in the environment.

Reimbursement for AAC devices has greatly improved. The Centers for Medicare and Medicaid Services (CMS) pays for them as speech-generating devices, a type of durable medical equipment (Kander, 2012).

The Occupational Therapy Practitioner's Role in Augmentative and Alternative Communication

Occupational therapists are key partners with SLPs because they often recognize individuals who could benefit from AAC evaluation and work with SLPs to identify the best access method. In addition to pointing with a finger, access methods include use of a performance enhancer, head or eye pointing, joystick, or scanning. Occupational therapists can advise on best motor patterns and on device layout. The most frequently used items should be located where the consumer has the best accuracy because this facilitates success with the device and speeds communication. Occupational therapists can advise on single-switch selection, placement, mounting, and design of scanning arrays. Arrays should be designed so that the most commonly used items are offered as the first or second choice. Finally, occupational therapists often help with placement or mounting of an AAC device and the configuration of environments and interactions to encourage AAC device use. Occupational therapists are often the lead advocates for setting up AAC devices so patients can control IR devices in home as EADL.

Future Trends with Augmentative and Alternative Communication

There has been tremendous interest in the use of Wi-Fi–enabled touch screen tablets and handheld devices for AAC. They are attractive and not associated with disability. Additionally, they are much less expensive and available without professional assistance. Care in selection is needed because of the highly variable quality of the software for language representation, storage, and retrieval. Do-it-yourself enthusiasm can overlook the expertise of an SLP for teaching device use, developing language and literacy skills, and the pragmatic skills needed for social communication.

Electronic Aids to Daily Living

EADLs create independent control of electrically powered devices in a home environment. The name changed from environmental control unit (ECU) to EADL because it is a more accurate description of adaptive function (Lange, 2002). Instead of emphasizing the item controlled (i.e., television, telephone), the focus is the outcome (i.e., increased independence, safety, communication, leisure). EADL create access to lights, telephones, home entertainment, beds, intercoms, thermostats, door locks, and window curtains.

EADL have clearly benefitted from the surge of interest in home automation and mass-marketed technologies designed to save effort or money by remotely regulating lights, security, thermostats, and sprinklers. These same products with or without an adaptive user interface increase the capacity for independent living and safety for those with disability. Good examples are products that turn on lights in response to a clap or a house robot that vacuums and washes floors while conserving energy for those with chronic illness or pain (Drew, 2012).

New home automation products let Wi-Fi–enabled devices and tablets function as control centers when loaded with free apps and hardware that can send IR signals (Fig. 18-11). Operating an iOS or Android device with a finger or with a special stylus or mouth

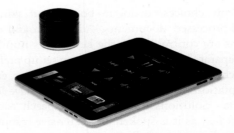

Figure 18-11 The Gear 4 Unity Remote is an example of a wireless link between tablet and IR emitter that enables customized control of entertainment appliances and other X-10™ or Insteon™ devices. (Courtesy of Disruptive USA, Inc., Seattle, WA.)

stick gives control of most household systems. There may always be a need for specialized EADL systems that allow advanced customization of the human technology interface for those with complex needs, but it is clear that EADL technology is more within reach than ever before.

Characteristics of Electronic Aids to Daily Living Control Technology

Occupational therapists often see consumers who are unable to reach or manipulate knobs, dials, and buttons or who are limited by pain or fatigue. Like other forms of AT, EADL can be controlled either through direct (speaking a command or pressing a button) or indirect (scanning) methods. Most direct-selection devices are developed for the mass market and therefore are inexpensive and found in electronics stores. If direct selection is not possible, even with control enhancers, a specialized AT product may be needed. The same criteria previously discussed for computers or AAC devices apply to choosing an access method for EADL.

Appliances vary in complexity of the control signals they require. For example, turning on a light requires only an on/off signal, but reshuffling the songs on the CDs in a five-disc player requires a complex control signal. Control signals can be transmitted by several methods: through the electrical wiring in a house, by IR or RF, or by a combination of these. Transmission technologies are often associated with control of specific types of devices.

Using a building's electrical wiring for control of electrical appliances is excellent for controlling appliances, such as lights or fans, which require only simple on/off or dimming signals. Technology called X-10™ has long been used for this function. X-10™ transmits a signal through the pathway of the house wiring. A newer technology, Insteon™, uses the same approach but is faster and more reliable while still compatible with X-10™. Both types offer command centers that plug into the house wiring and receiver modules that are controlled by IR or RF signals.

Both types send a coded signal that is intended for a module with a specific address, for example, a light at the far end of the house. Insteon™ modules offer an important additional feature because they respond to Wi-Fi or internet communication. This allows control of modules in its home automation system via Wi-Fi–enabled smartphones and tablets or even from a remote location outside the home.

IR signals are invisible to the human eye and are used to control things within line of sight. Television remote controls use this technology because the user is typically sitting directly in front of the television. The IR signal is interpreted by an IR receiver, which translates the signal into an output or function. Various patterns of IR light are coded for various devices and functions. IR tends to be used in applications that require multiple adjustments, such as television sets, DVRs, and CD players. Insteon™ and X-10™ have receivers that can convert IR signals into house wiring signals for control by AAC devices, power wheelchair controllers, etc.

RF signals, another transmission technology, do not require line of sight and are not affected by obstacles such as walls. Devices using RF offer consumers a choice of bands in order to bypass heavily used channels. That is, the consumer can change the frequency band so as not to turn on devices in the neighbor's house. RF signals are typically used to open garage doors and unlatch front doors. They are also used in Insteon™ or X-10™ systems equipped with an RF receiver that converts the signal for transmission through house wiring.

Simple or Complex Electronic Aids to Daily Living

A simple EADL gives alternate control over one electrical device. It can take the form of a large-button remote control or a household appliance plugged into an AbleNet PowerLink®4 (Fig. 18-12). This type of EADL

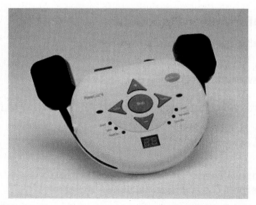

Figure 18-12 The redesigned PowerLink®4 gives customizable, single-switch control of any plug-in device such as a blender, fan, etc. (Courtesy of AbleNet, Inc., Roseville, MN.)

is useful for teaching cause and effect, increasing personal control, or developing responsibility. Simple EADL can be set up to work in momentary mode (i.e., work only as long as the switch is activated) or latched mode (i.e., stay on until the switch is pressed again to turn off the device). A device like the PowerLink®4 appliance interface can be easily incorporated into a group participation activity. Similarly, an AAC device that sends an IR signals to an Insteon™ module can turn on a bedroom light and give control over personal space. Picture phones with large buttons and speed dial or phones that scan phone numbers give modified phone access with simple interfaces. AbleNet offers an EADL selection guide that provides an overview of options (Resources 18-1).

Consumers with a desire for control over more devices within their environment will need a system that offers complex EADL functions (see Fig. 18-3). These systems exist as dedicated EADL devices, as a feature of an AAC device, and through computer-, Internet-, or Wi-Fi–enabled systems. Dedicated devices perform complex adjustments to multiple systems within a consumer's environment. Some use voice commands; others use scanning input to take commands. They respond to user input and use a combination of transmission technologies based on what is best for the appliance being controlled.

The rapid development of home automation devices has created the potential for the same AT device that enables speech or powered mobility or use of a Wi-Fi–enabled tablet to monitor security cameras, change the thermostat, and turn on the home theater. Of course, those relying on home automation must plan for power loss with an uninterruptible power supply for safety.

Sensory Accommodations

Many therapists find opportunities to suggest technology for vision loss because of the older adults they treat for hemiplegia, movement disorders, and orthopedic impairments. Often, these adults are unfamiliar with digital technologies and so are not necessarily ready to adopt the microprocessor-based aids that are available. Simpler forms of AT devices are needed.

Closed-Circuit Television

Consumers with low vision and limited interest in computer-based adaptations may benefit from CCTV systems. CCTVs use a camera mounted downward facing so it focuses on a surface where the individual places the item of interest—greeting card, recipe, invoice, or magazine article. The camera sends the image to a flat-panel display positioned at eye level for which the user sets magnification, color, and contrast. This same

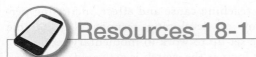

Resources 18-1

Vendors

AbleNet, Inc.

Phone: 800-322-0956
http://www.ablenetinc.com/
Assistive technology products

Adaptive Switch Laboratories, Inc.

Phone: 800-626-8698
http://www.asl-inc.com/

Don Johnston Incorporated

Phone: 800-999-4660
http://www.donjohnston.com/

School-Based AT Hardware and Software

EnableMart

Phone: 888-640-1999
http://www.enablemart.com/
Resells most AT products

Freedom Scientific

Phone: 800-444-4443
http://www.freedomscientific.com/
Products for blindness and low vision

GoQ

Phone: 877-674-7687
http://www.goqsoftware.com/
WordQ and SpeakQ™

Humanware

Phone: 800-722-3393
http://www.humanware.com/
Products for blindness, low vision, and learning disabilty

IntelliTools

Phone: 800-547-6747
http://www.intellitools.com/
School-based AT hardware and software

Kensington Technology Group

Phone: 800-535-4242
http://www.kensington.com/
Universally designed computer accessories

Madentec, Inc.

Phone: 877-623-3682
http://www.madentec.com/
Head pointers, on-screen keyboards, and scanning

Nuance Communications, Inc.

Phone: 781-565-5000
http://www.nuance.com/
Dragon Naturally Speaking™ and Omnipage

RJ Cooper and Associates

Phone: 800-752-6673
http://www.rjcooper.com/
Unique cause-and-effect, switches, and adaptations

SmartHome

Phone: 800-762-7846
http://www.smarthome.com/LearningCenter.html

Research and Development Centers

Center for Applied Special Technology (CAST) and the National Center on Accessible Instructional Materials

Phone: 781-245-2212
http://www.cast.org/
http://aim.cast.org/

Center for Assistive Technology and Environmental Access

Phone: 404-894-4960
http://www.catea.org/

National Center for Technology Innovation

Phone: 202-403-5323
http://www.nationaltechcenter.org/

Trace Research and Development Center

Phone: 608-262-6966
http://www.trace.wisc.edu/

AT Information Resources

Alliance for Technology Access

Phone: 707-778-3011
http://www.ataccess.org/

Assistive Technology Industry Association (ATIA)

Phone: 877-687-2842
http://www.atia.org/

California State University Northridge Center on Disabilities (CSUN)

Phone: 818-677-2578
http://www.csun.edu/cod/

(continued)

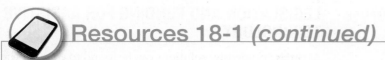

Resources 18-1 *(continued)*

Closing the Gap

Phone: 507-248-3294
http://www.closingthegap.com/

DO-IT: Disabilities, Opportunities, Internetworking and Technology

Phone: 888-972-3648
http://www.washington.edu/doit/

EASI: Equal Access to Software and Information

Phone: 949-916-2837
http://people.rit.edu/easi/

Job Accommodation Network

Phone: 800-526-7234
http://askjan.org/

LD Online

Phone: 703-998-2600
http://www.ldonline.org/

National Assistive Technology Technical Assistance Partnership (NATTAP)

Phone: 703-524-6686
http://www.resnaprojects.org/nattap/

National Center for Accessible Media

Phone: 617-300-3400
http://ncam.wgbh.org/

Rehabilitation Engineering and Assistive Technology Society of North America (RESNA)

Phone: 703-524-6686
http://resna.org/

RERC on Telerehabilitation

http://www.rerctr.pitt.edu/

Technology Special Interest Section within AOTA

Phone: 301-652-2682
http://www.aota.org/ (within the member login area)

U.S. Society for Augmentative and Alternative Communication (USSAAC)

http://www.ussaac.org/

World Wide Web Consortium–Web Accessibility Initiative

http://www.w3.org/WAI/

---

technology exists as small, portable handheld units that are easy to use for reading a menu or a price tag when shopping.

Reading Appliances

OCR technology (previously described as computer input) is offered for those who are not interested in or ready for computer use. These "reading machines" provide an extremely simple user interface with bright, textured buttons that control the process. A camera photographs the image of a page of print placed on top of the device. Using amazingly intelligent OCR, the internal processor recognizes the text on the printed page and immediately begins to read it. A speech synthesizer reads at a user-selected speed and volume in the language of the text.

For consumers with visual impairment, portable microprocessor-based note takers function like personal digital assistants (PDAs). Consumers can choose between models with a six-key Braille keyboard or a full QWERTY keyboard. Some models offer speech feedback via earphone; others allow review via a refreshable Braille display. Consumers can record notes from class or a meeting and later upload them to a computer or print them directly to a paper or Braille printer. These devices function as smartphones with calendars, contacts, and reminders, with the ability to access the Internet.

Closed Captioning

Real-time closed captioning is an important technology for those with hearing impairment who do not understand ASL. Early systems required a stenographer who could capture spoken language and a computer to process and display the text. A speaker's words then appeared as they were spoken. Speech recognition technology has advanced to the point that a stenographer is not always needed. This makes it more useful when groups need to accommodate those with hearing impairment.

ENVIRONMENTAL ACCESS AND UNIVERSAL DESIGN

AT devices enable participation and control only when the human and nonhuman environments create access for consumers and their devices. Independent power mobility is only an advantage in places with ramps and doorways that are wide enough to allow entry. Consumers using AAC devices can only communicate if people will take the time to interact with them. Within AOTA, this philosophy is evident in the skills and practice document produced for technology and environmental interventions (AOTA, 2010b). If architects and product designers truly consider human variability, many barriers can be eliminated. This concept, universal design, means that products and environments are designed to be usable by all people, to the greatest extent possible, without the need for adaptation or specialized design (Center for Universal Design, 2012).

LEGISLATION AND FUNDING FOR ASSISTIVE TECHNOLOGY

At times, inexpensive solutions can be found to enhance the consumer's occupational performance, but sometimes AT equipment is costly. Although cost should be considered, the consumer's abilities, needs, and specific occupational goals should drive the assessment, and the compelling need for an AT device or service should drive the search for funding (Table 18-2). If the best solution facilitates the consumer's occupation but is expensive, the AT team needs to document its contribution and present a strong case to the funding agency or to a community nonprofit or advocacy group.

Justification Letter

This documentation is an important component of getting AT devices and services funded. Occupational therapists use the knowledge gained from the consumer-centered assessment, trial use of a device, interviews with significant others, and, possibly, a home visit to justify the need for AT devices. In medical settings, a physician's prescription is needed for all requests and generally accompanies the

---

Table 18-2 Sources of Assistive Technology Funding for Adults

Funding Source	Available to	Notes
Private health insurance	Employees and dependents	Vary by policy benefits
Medicaid	Those with low income or with a waiver, for example, for brain injury	Limited devices, may pay for services
Medicare	Those who qualify for disability or older than 65 years of age	Limited devices, may pay for services
PASS Plan (Plan to Achieve Self Sufficiency)	Individuals receiving Social Security Disability	Social Security benefits can be sheltered and saved for AT
Public/private agencies	Vary by community but are often diagnosis related	For example, ALS Society, Muscular Dystrophy Association
Grants/trust funds/legal settlements	Applicants, beneficiaries, and plaintiffs	Must meet funding or inclusion criteria
Friends, relatives	Families with resources who can organize an appeal	AT devices and home modifications are tax deductible
Clubs, churches, service organizations	Members or individuals who match fund-raising focus	For example, Lions Club's interest in visual impairment
Vocational rehabilitation	AT devices and training needed to prepare for or return to work	Vocational rehabilitation services are available in all 50 states
Worker's compensation	Employers insurance that covers those injured at work	Restore independent living and possible return to work
Veterans' Administration	Covers in service-related injuries for military	Generous benefits, also covers recreational AT
Low-interest consumer loans and device lending libraries	Available through Tech Act Projects located in all 50 states and U.S. territories	(Bailey, Weber, & Meidenbauer, 2012; U.S. Congress, 1988/1998, 2004)

therapist's letter of justification. For work-related funding sources, another form of "prescription" may be needed.

To develop a report, the occupational therapist uses knowledge gained in clinical assessment, knowledge of product features, and the expected outcomes for the consumer. Clear writing, case data, and sometimes photographs or videotape footage of the consumer using the device are used to show that the cost of AT devices will be offset by an increase in function, employability, and/or greater independence. The report needs to be tailored to the funding source; for example, Medicaid requests must use medical necessity to justify AT devices and services.

A denial letter does not always mean "no" as a system of appeals is used to weed out groundless requests. Always get a denial in writing, and then prepare an appeal letter while honoring deadlines. The mandate to pay for AT is clear, but payers still raise objections to avoid obligations. A clear, logical letter of appeal can win payment for AT devices and services.

ROLES OF OCCUPATIONAL THERAPISTS IN ASSISTIVE TECHNOLOGY INTERVENTION

AOTA (2010b) has published a specialized knowledge and skills document for the practice of AT and environmental interventions that provides the foundation for this section. The document presents guidelines for entry- and advanced-level skills that define minimum levels of knowledge and skills for practice in the area of technology. Of course, therapists have an ethical responsibility to do no harm and be aware of their level of competence. Novice therapists should seek supervision, mentoring, and continuing education opportunities to build their level of skill and competence.

Most occupational therapists should be able to assist with AT for common needs or topics covered in this chapter such as modifications to accessibility settings in the computer OS, trials with performance enhancers, and knowledge of general categories of AT intervention. They should also be able to discuss and describe the benefits of AT with their clients and give them hope for regaining occupations by means of AT solutions available through specialized AT evaluation and service delivery. Consumers with complex needs and goals should be referred to an occupational therapist with advanced practice skills or to an interdisciplinary AT center such as one supported by a university, Easter Seals, or a Tech Act project. Referrals can also occur via telerehabilitation. Telerehabilitation research has demonstrated equivalence between remote and in-person services (AOTA, 2010a; Schein et al., 2011). Referring to experts creates an opportunity for OT practitioners to increase their knowledge about AT. Additionally, they can contribute to the process with in-depth knowledge of consumer skills, abilities, and needs and position themselves to collaborate in follow-up as the consumer

begins to integrate an AT solution into everyday tasks and routines. We discussed roles for the professionals within the AT assessment team, and now we present possible roles for occupational therapists.

Assistive Technology Specialist

Occupational therapists with AT service delivery expertise usually strive for the assistive technology professional (ATP) credential. This certification, offered through the Rehabilitation Engineering and Assistive Technology Society of North America (RESNA), sets a standard for entry-level expertise for AT knowledge and experience. RESNA is an interdisciplinary professional association of those with a desire to improve the potential of people with disabilities to achieve their goals through the use of technology. Professionals with the ATP credential adhere to a code of ethics, practice within their scope of knowledge, practice in a consumer-centered manner, and stay current in their area of AT specialty. RESNA now offers a specialty credential for seating and mobility and anticipates offering specialty credentials for other types of AT (RESNA, 2011).

Product Development Team and Product Testing

Occupational therapists contribute significantly to engineering and research teams because of their broad clinical knowledge of impairment and their comfort with functional tasks and environments. They can help engineers conceptualize consumer needs as well as the device's output features and user interfaces. Occupational therapists are also excellent partners for testing prototypes and measuring the efficacy of devices for treatment and compensation.

Continuing Education for Keeping Current

AT for remediation and compensation will be constantly changing, so occupational therapists practicing with technology must commit to continuing education. Device manufacturers and professional organizations continuously offer education (see Resources 18-1). University courses, sessions at annual conferences, weekend workshops, online courses, journal articles (Research Note 18-1), and thoughtful consideration of the application of consumer and entertainment electronics allow practitioners to gain the knowledge and skills needed to incorporate technology into a range of practice settings. Listservs, like those offered by AOTA, RESNA, and university programs, allow novice practitioners to use the expertise and help of experienced AT practitioners to solve practical problems or develop effective plans for referral.

Research Note 18-1

Masiero, S., Armani, M., & Rosati, G. (2011). Upper-limb robot-assisted therapy in rehabilitation of acute stroke patients: Focused review and results of new randomized controlled trial. *Journal of Rehabilitation Research and Development, 48,* 355–366.

Abstract

The successful motor rehabilitation of stroke patients requires early intensive and task-specific therapy. A recent Cochrane review, although based on a limited number of randomized controlled trials (RCTs), showed that early robotic training of the upper limb (i.e., during acute or subacute phase) can enhance motor learning and improve functional abilities.

Purpose

To determine whether training with the Neuro-Rehabilitation-roBot (NeReBot) resulted in comparable reductions in motor impairment and enhancements of upper limb function as compared to conventional upper limb exercise (control).

Method

Twenty-one patients, aged 18–85 years, within 20 days of a first, single ischemic or hemorrhagic cerebrovascular accident with paralysis or paresis and with sufficient cognitive and language capacities to understand directions were randomized to the experimental or control group. For the experimental group ($n = 11$), NeReBot was used as an alternative to standard treatment 35% of the total treatment time. NeReBot assists movement of the upper limb in three-dimensional space, simulating hand-over-hand therapy. The patient is told to anticipate the trajectory to add the necessary active contribution to the movement of the limb. The NeReBot provides visual and auditory feedback. Each session lasted 20 minutes; number of sessions per day or week are not reported; total treatment lasted 5 weeks. Therapy for the control group ($n = 10$) was not described.

Results

An evaluator, blind to group assignment, evaluated each patient at the end of the 5-week treatment period and at 3-month follow-up. Before-after training improvements in motor and functional scales within each group were all statistically significant at the 5-week mark, indicating that both groups improved. However, because of ethical considerations, a no-treatment group to control for spontaneous recovery was not possible, so it cannot be said for certain that therapy, with or without robotic enhancement, was responsible for the improvement. The between-group comparisons revealed no significant differences between groups either at the end of therapy or at follow-up. All patients in the experimental group voiced favor of including NeReBot training in the post-stroke rehabilitation program.

Implications for Practice

- Therapy appears to enhance recovery that is occurring spontaneously post stroke.
- Patients enjoy engaging in therapy that involves novelty (robot assistance).
- Repetitive, active movement therapy for 20 minutes per day for 5 weeks results in improvement of motor impairments and function as measured by the FIM™ and the Box & Block Test.

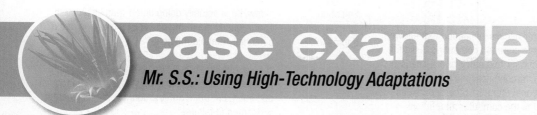

case example

Mr. S.S.: Using High-Technology Adaptations

Occupational Therapy Assessment Process	Clinical Reasoning Process	
	Objectives	Examples of Internal Dialogue

Patient Information

Mr. S.S. is a 29-year-old male who is 4 months post-traumatic brain injury (TBI) sustained in a bicycle crash with injury to his right motor cortex. He is left-hand dominant and has worked hard in rehab to regain strength, range of motion (ROM), and fine motor skills. He has a positive attitude and is eager to return to his work as a civil engineer and reduce his dependence on his wife. Although very eager to return to work, Mr. S.S. is concerned that continued limitations in his left hand prevent writing and keyboarding and that he has occasional gaps in task sequencing and recall of recent events. Mr. S.S. is being referred for an assistive technology (AT) assessment to identify compensations for these remaining deficits and to support his return to work. Mr. S.S. and his wife both like technology and use computers intensively at work and to manage their household.

Objectives	Examples of Internal Dialogue
Understand the patient's diagnosis or condition	"I can see that Mr. S.S. is eager to change his focus from rehab to getting back to work. It is great to have a client who had an active healthy lifestyle and is so well supported by his wife, his vocational rehabilitation counselor, and his employer. His desire to return to work definitely links him to vocational rehabilitation funding."
Know the person	"Both Mr. S.S. and his wife use and like computers, so 'talking computers for work' is a nice change from rehabilitation topics."
Appreciate the context	"AT devices and environmental modifications can help him **compensate** for motor and cognitive impairment. I expect there will be **remediation** of cognitive deficits through graded return to familiar work tasks. Computers are predictable and sequential, and reengaging in work-related tasks could support recovery."
Develop provisional hypotheses	

AT/OT Intervention Process

Based on this information, it is clear that AT should focus on finding an adaptive computer-access strategy so that a keyboard and software could help support compensation for and remediation of memory and sequencing skills. Although his task sequencing for self-care skills has progressed, a computer-access assessment will show his ability to retain and use new learning. Mr. S.S. and his wife were pleased that the occupational therapist will make a workplace visit to identify barriers or needed modifications to increase the possibility of success. With Mr. S.S. and his wife, these AT goals were agreed on:

1. Return to productive computer use with an adaptive computer-access method
2. Use Outlook® calendar, tasks, and contacts synched with his smartphone as a cognitive support for work events and tasks
3. Determine need for workplace modifications to optimize safety, independence, and social supports

Mr. S.S. and his wife like this plan, which begins to move their life back toward "normal."

Objectives	Examples of Internal Dialogue
	"It seems like Mr. S.S. and his wife are grateful for his recovery to this point. Although they expect more, they are willing to compensate now."
	"I'm not sure that Mr. S.S. and his wife know what is ahead, but at this point both are relieved to be moving beyond treatment to achieve medical stability and into activities that focus on return to function."
Consider intervention approach and methods	"I think an intensive approach is needed so a return to work can happen as soon as possible. I would like to increase the amount of time at work and the complexity of tasks, but we will go ahead and get started."
Consider what will occur in therapy, how often, and for how long	"I have tried to devise a plan that will allow one skill to build on another. I want to avoid overwhelming him. The emphasis will be on developing one skill at a time and taking one day at a time."
	"Occupational therapy (OT) sessions will need to happen about three times a week to ensure continuity and sufficient opportunities for teaching, learning, and practicing."

Computer-Access Assessment

They returned for a 2-hour computer-access evaluation that allowed the occupational therapist to observe common computing tasks for reach, finger isolation, pointing accuracy, text entry, and success with three-step instructions and to introduce several hardware and software adaptations. The occupational therapist recorded results of task trials and Mr. S.S.'s opinion of the computer adaptations presented. The results pointed to three strong tactics: learning to use a trackball with his left hand to include his impaired side yet increase pointing accuracy, learning to use the HalfQWERTY™ keyboard for simple text writing, and learning Dragon Naturally Speaking™ (DNS™) speech recognition for writing reports and longer e-mails. The plan will involve 3 weeks of AT sessions for learning and skill development, followed by another 3 weeks of transition into the workplace as direct services fade to direct services only as needed.

Because Mr. S.S. reported during the assessment that his work desk is in a cube environment, the occupational therapist needs to consult with Mr. S.S.'s supervisor before finalizing use of DNS™ or proceeding with training. A noisy environment can affect recognition accuracy. Training will begin with a trackball and HalfQWERTY™. With this decided, Mr. S.S will have occupational therapy training in these adaptations three times per week for 3 weeks with follow-up activities for practice and learning at home. AT devices will be loaned for home use to support continuity and practice. This will assure confidence when asking purchase approval from vocational rehabilitation. His wife will attend as many sessions as possible so that she can help bridge between occupational therapy and home practice.

Select an intervention approach	"Wow, he is actually doing better than I expected. That reminds me of the power of motivation and a personally meaningful goal." "I must remind Mr. S.S.: Be sure you have the right tool before you proceed. DNS™ is a powerful tool for text entry, but there are just some contexts where it is doomed to failure!" "I am so glad his wife is a willing partner in this process. That will help Mr. S.S. be successful. His vocational rehabilitation counselor is really pleased with his enthusiasm and focus, too."
Interpret observations	"I think the fact that Mr. S.S. is an engineer makes him a good AT client and problem solver. He likes using technology to solve problems. This is a familiar concept to him and one that he uses to solve his client's problems, too."

Computer Access Results

In his first training session, Mr. S.S. really liked the four-button trackball. He realized immediately that a trackball separates the actions of pointing and clicking. His earlier efforts at mouse use were frustrating because trying to click the mouse button with his left index finger caused an involuntary arm movement that moved the mouse cursor off its intended target.

The occupational therapist introduced him to the trackball with computer solitaire, where he used new movement patterns to point, click, and drag cards to appropriate locations. The occupational therapist observed the intense effort he made to isolate his little finger for left button clicks. The occupational therapist moved the function of the left-sided button to the lower thumb side button, which reduced his distraction and increased his efficiency.

Once confident with this new skill, he appeared to transfer it directly to more accuracy with desktop and file management activities.

The occupational therapist sent Mr. S.S. home with a loaner trackball to practice the new motor skill with a simple graphics application on his home computer. She knew that concentrating on a game would help increase his attention span and make demands on his procedural memory.

Select an intervention approach	"I hope that he and his wife have fun with this trackball approach. I whispered to his wife the suggestion that she help him find a practical goal for using the drawing app. Could he draw up plans for a ramp for their garage door?" "Can you believe he was able to draw up the plans for a simple 1:2 sloped ramp for the 4-inch step up in their garage?" "Motor learning theory in action! I am so glad that I took the time to explain the concept underlying HalfQWERTY™. I think that I really liked the idea that he had this basic motor pattern in his brain and that he just needed to modify it." "It is so important to remind clients about the complexity of what they are trying to accomplish. A bright perfectionist like Mr. S.S. needs encouragement to be focused on process and not solely on results." "I am really starting to feel confident that I am on the right path with Mr. S.S. Each person with a TBI is so unique. He has an amazing ability to self-assess, and this is a skill so often missing in the presence of TBI. This bodes well for his future."

In the second training session, the results of home practice were reviewed prior to starting work with HalfQWERTY™. The occupational therapist recorded how well he used the trackball in a 5-minute demonstration with solitaire. She knew he had practiced, retained skill, and regained confidence with his new abilities.

The recommendation for using HalfQWERTY™ was based on the fact that Mr. S.S. was a strong touch-typist. During the AT assessment, he had shown that he understood the concept of using his right hand to type assigned keys and using his right hand as it held down the space bar to type keys on the left side of the keyboard. During this session, Mr. S.S. began formal instruction in using the software. The occupational therapist used the tutorial that comes with HalfQWERTY™ to introduce the new motor patterns needed for letters previously typed with the left hand. Repetition of motor patterns, gradual introduction of new letter combinations, and avoiding any concern for speed allowed Mr. S.S. to end the occupational therapy session typing at a rate of 8–10 words per minute—as fast as writing long hand.

The occupational therapist gave his wife instructions so she could download the demo software to enable home practice before his next visit. The goal was to return with two approximately 100-word paragraphs typed by his right hand alone.

At the next visit, Mr. S.S. met the goal but reported that it had gone very slowly. The occupational therapist praised and reassured him that he was doing extremely well. The occupational therapist reminded Mr. S.S. to pursue accuracy over speed, assuring him that new motor patterns would develop and speed would return.

The next two sessions were spent with more focus on a "drill and practice" approach intended to develop proficiency and speed. Each session ended with a home assignment to start writing a personal journal about his recovery.

On the fifth session, Mr. S.S. was able to type 17 words per minute and was pleased to have more than met his goal of 15 words per minute. He reported he was expending less cognitive effort and had started pressing the correct keys without conscious thought.

Just prior to his sixth session, Mr. S.S.'s supervisor responded to my questions about the noise level in the cube. The company will not only move his desk to an enclosed office space but reported that the IT manager will integrate any needed software into his computer system.

This allowed training to begin in use of DNS™. His success with the trackball and strong progress with HalfQWERTY™ gave him tools that he would be able to use instead of having to learn voice commands. Many editing actions can be done by keyboard or mouse.

Select an intervention approach

"Great, I am very relieved that I can proceed with teaching DNS™. His interest in learning and adopting other adaptive computer-access methods gives me assurance about his potential for success with this application. The cube environment was my major worry."

"I am so pleased that Mr. S.S. is grasping the big picture and is able to see how these adaptive strategies work together for a comprehensive approach."

"I'm really starting to see progress. Each time Mr. S.S. comes in with a finished assignment, I see his confidence grow too. He has used my incremental approach, and that makes me feel good too."

"Who knew that engineering firms commonly encourage team problem solving? Mr. S.S. even seemed to appreciate Joe's presence and exceeded my expectations."

"Many people have ended up rejecting automatic speech recognition because of this issue. I hope he can adopt this trackball strategy."

The occupational therapist used the next four sessions to introduce DNS™ and develop his confidence with using his voice to write. First, they created a voice file and then, using a quick-start menu, started writing text using speech and voice commands. The occupational therapist showed that the keyboard and trackball can substitute for a voice command. The trackball gives access to menus and HalfQWERTY™ allows typing (rather than speaking) to correct recognition errors. The occupational therapist focused intervention on training recognition accuracy and building vocabulary. These skills actively build voice files and refine recognition accuracy. The next session was focused on developing a pattern that is important when using DNS™—"preparing to write" or silently developing an idea before speaking it.

During prior conversations, the occupational therapist had learned that a coworker and friend, Joe, also used DNS™. Mr. S.S. really liked the idea that Joe could be a DNS™ resource at work. He agreed to have Joe come to one of their DNS™ training sessions so that he could understand how Mr. S.S. used DNS™. By the end of the session with Joe, Mr. S.S. had written 200 words and corrected six recognition errors as Joe watched. Mr. S.S. had learned to pause and think before speaking and had adopted a speech pattern that is clear and deliberate when using his voice for writing.

"Hmmm, what about his pal, Joe? Would Mr. S.S. allow a colleague at work to give him some assist?"

The occupational therapist had given Mr. S.S. the home practice task of using DNS™ to dictate 100 words per day in his daily journal documenting his recovery.

"He is so proud that his journal is growing in pages and that his sentences are longer . . . like they used to be."

Synch Outlook® with Smartphone

The occupational therapist knew that when DNS™ got installed on Mr. S.S.'s workstation that it would integrate well with Microsoft Office® and Outlook®. The DNS™ version selected for Mr. S.S. includes commands for immediate use with Microsoft Office®. As a first action, the occupational therapist directed DNS™ to import the vocabulary and the names stored in Word and Outlook® documents. This instantly customizes DNS™ and makes it more powerful for writing and managing daily tasks and calendars. Mr. S.S. will be able to add new information either with DNS™ or with HalfQWERTY™ based on which is more suited to the task.

Select an intervention approach

"Now the process gets a little more complicated as I start to transition him back to the work site from our weeks of AT sessions. I am going to need people at the firm to help me with the systems issues there. I should better make a list."

Mr. S.S. had been using a smartphone for several years but had not put any effort into synching with his work computer. His situation was suddenly different, now that he was dealing with the consequences of a TBI. He needed to have calendars, contacts, and tasks synched to his smartphone. The occupational therapist will record the steps for the synching process and create a step-by-step guide in the notes section of Outlook®.

Appreciate the context

"I need the IT manager to confirm that Mr. S.S.'s phone is compatible with the network, and I need help with passwords and access to directories. I need the DNS™ and HalfQWERTY™ software loaded onto his workstation. His smartphone needs to have proper security for synching with the network and using the office Wi-Fi connection."

The occupational therapist will recruit his wife to create medication reminders and set up other personal reminders like birthdays or holidays and scheduled appointments for the household.

"Mr. S.S. does not need the challenges of learning or resolving these issues right now, he just needs it all to be ready to go! He will learn more as he is ready and as recovery becomes more solidified."

"It is great that technology that helps so much at work will help in his personal life, too."

The occupational therapist looked for Joe while at the engineering firm and told him that Mr. S.S. would soon be starting a daily schedule but for only 4 hours per day. The occupational therapist gave Joe AT center contact information and asked him to call if he saw that Mr. S.S. was having unexpected problems with new computer skills.

"Oops! I need to remind his wife to create a personal calendar for home events so they do not get imported to his work calendar."

"Glad to know that Joe already synchs his smartphone with the firm's Outlook® calendar, contacts, and task lists. Another resource for Mr. S.S."

Assess the Workplace for Accessibility

The occupational therapist was pleased with the results of the workplace visit. The engineering company is located in a fairly new building, which brought several benefits:

- Handicapped parking and accessible bathrooms are available.
- The new enclosed office space made available to Mr. S.S. is close to Joe's cube. This office is one that was previously used by visiting staff so Mr. S.S. will have to share this office space occasionally. This will allow him to measure the interference created by others' conversations and perhaps lead to returning to a cube as microphones and recognition continue to improve.

Vocational rehabilitation has agreed to pay for future occupational therapy visits to address changes in his access method or office software. The vocational rehabilitation counselor will also be checking on Mr. S.S. and will alert the occupational therapist if more intensive support is needed. Mr. S.S. and his wife will return to the AT center for a follow-up visit in 6 weeks to assess progress and any new issues.

Understand the patient's diagnosis or condition	"Mr. S.S. has regained so much of his mobility that his mobility issues are now actually pretty minimal. He will be adequately served by standard Americans with Disabilities Act (ADA) accessibility accommodations for bathroom and parking."
Appreciate the context	"Mr. S.S. must really be a valuable employee because his company really went out of the way to meet his needs and reintegrate him into the office."
	"With three vocational rehabilitation-approved AT visits remaining, I know I have approval for follow-up to help him succeed."
	"It is hard to see my collaboration with Mr. S.S and his wife come to an end. We have all worked hard, and it feels great to see his progress."

 ## Clinical Reasoning in Occupational Therapy Practice

Assistive Technology Related to Self-Maintenance Roles

Claire, a 65-year-old widow, is increasingly frustrated by the effects of macular degeneration on her activities of daily living (ADL) routines. She has become dependent on her daughter, Jean, to stop by her apartment daily to assist her with visual tasks. Claire is upset because Jean's husband has taken a new job in another state, and they will be moving soon. Jean has heard that there are low-vision aids that might help restore her mother's confidence and self-sufficiency and wants to help her mother find resources. Claire's goals include restoring her independence with food preparation, bill paying, and reading correspondence; feeling safer at home; and feeling better about herself.

1. What kind of assistive technology (AT) solution might allow Claire to regain some of her self-sufficiency and ease her daughter's mind about moving away?
2. What pieces of equipment would assist Claire in her apartment?
3. What would help ensure a better "fit" between Claire and this equipment?

 ## Clinical Reasoning in Occupational Therapy Practice

Assistive Technology Related to Self-Advancement Roles: Return to Employment

Charles is a 55-year-old psychologist discharged 2 weeks ago from an acute inpatient rehabilitation stay. He has made a significant recovery from his second Guillain-Barré syndrome (G-B) episode, an acute polyneuropathy that affects the peripheral nervous system. In his work as a counselor, he always makes session notes at the end of each patient visit and for efficiency uses a laptop computer. Actually, he explored Dragon Naturally Speaking™ (DNS™) following his first episode of G-B but did not have the confidence to adopt it as a tool without support. This episode, his hands have been more affected, and he has not yet recovered quick, independent finger movements like those used in keyboarding. His outpatient occupational therapist, Jeanne, has experience with DNS™ because she used it when writing long documents back in college. She immediately recognized the value of automatic speech recognition as an adaptive strategy for Charles. Not only would it allow him to return to work more quickly and help to restore his professional identity, but it would also enable him to log his recovery from this second G-B episode and restore his ability to communicate with friends and colleagues by e-mail.

1. What environmental characteristics of Charles's office space make automatic speech recognition a good AT solution?
2. How should Jeanne set up her outpatient occupational therapy (OT) treatment sessions so that she can charge for instruction in the use of an AT solution?
3. How long should treatment persist, and how will Jeanne know when she has met a treatment goal for this activity that affects both Charles's professional and personal lives?

Summary Review Questions

1. What social, reimbursement, and scientific factors have driven interest in using technology for remediation?
2. What is a key challenge for occupational therapists using VR and robotic interventions in rehabilitation for neurological diagnoses?
3. What is a minimal level of AT competence needed by a therapist providing services to adults with physical dysfunction?
4. How do occupational therapy activity analysis skills guide a therapist in exploring AT solutions for a particular consumer?
5. For adaptive computer use, list two input and two output devices (other than a keyboard or standard mouse or display), and describe consumers who might need these modifications.
6. What are the differences between RF and IR control interfaces that make them more suitable for one EADL versus another?
7. Where and how can occupational therapists learn more about recommending AT devices and services?

Glossary

Abbreviation expansion—Software designed to decrease keystrokes, increase efficiency, and decrease errors. For example, OT is the abbreviation for occupational therapy. The abbreviation is entered instead of the words, and software expands the abbreviation into the words or phrases it represents.

Array—When indirect selection is used, the array is the set of options that are presented in sequence. The user selects from an array by waiting until the desired item is offered and then activates a switch. Some items in an array may branch to a secondary array, for example, when a punctuation array is opened from an alphabet array.

Augmentative and alternative communication (AAC)—A communication system that requires using something external to the body. Examples include pen and paper, letter or picture communication boards, and communication devices. Gestures and vocalizations are often used to enhance communication when using an AAC device. Devices may be manual or electronic. AAC devices use a language representation system, for example, letters grouped into words or picture symbols.

Automatic Speech Recognition (ASR)—Software that enables recognition of spoken words through a sophisticated process of sound pattern recognition, predicting the likeliest phrase or pair of words, and analysis of user writing style and vocabulary; sometimes called speech-to-text.

Bluetooth—The short-range wireless interconnection of cellular phones, computers, and other electronic devices.

Brain-computer interface (BCI)—Technology that creates a pathway between neurological signals and an external device to enable direct control of impaired sensorimotor functions such as vision, hearing, and movement; also referred to as neuroprosthetics.

Computer-aided design (CAD)—Software used to design, draft, or lay out technical projects ranging from home design and architecture to manufacturing. CAD makes modifications and estimating construction costs much easier.

Digital—Continuous data or signals represented by digits. Digital devices rely on microprocessors, which express data in binary code as a series of 0s and 1s and offer output in ways that are useful for analysis, storage in databases, and entry into electronic medical records.

Digitized speech—Speech that is converted from sound wave to digital form for playback at a later time.

Dwell—This input method interprets hovering over a key or an object for a user-adjusted amount of time. It is equivalent of a mouse click and allows selection without needing an external switch.

Electronic aids to daily living (EADL)—Devices that give consumers control of appliances in their environment. This term is favored over the alternative, environmental control unit (ECU), because it focuses on the task (i.e., safety, communication, and independence) rather than the device (i.e., television, telephone, and lights). The term EADL accurately describes the technology and has helped acquire funding, both here and in Europe.

Home automation—Using digital devices to enable remote control and/or monitoring of entertainment appliances, lights, heating, sprinkler systems, security cameras, etc.

Infrared (IR) light—Light wave outside of (longer than) the spectrum normally detected by the human eye. Sequences of IR signal are interpreted as unique instructions by an IR receiver, which executes the associated instruction, for example, power on, volume up.

Microprocessor—Integrated circuit board that processes digital signals to complete a set operation and are common in all of today's technologies including AT devices.

Pixel—The smallest unit of visual display on a computer screen; a dot. These dots combine to form words and images. Pixels-per-square-inch is a measure of resolution or pixel density, for example, 640 × 480. Higher numbers indicate more pixels thus more information shown on a display.

Pneumatic—Refers to control activation by changing the amount or direction of air pressure. Sip n' Puff switches commonly are pneumatic switches.

QWERTY—Common layout for computer keyboards in which the letters in the top left row are QWERTY. This layout originated with mechanical typewriters when it was important to slow down typists so that the strike arms that printed each letter had time to avoid each other.

Radio frequency (RF)—A signaling technology that uses private radio bands to control appliances, open doors, or communicate with other AT devices.

Rehabilitation engineer—This term includes those with various engineering degrees who develop, test, customize, and support use of sophisticated digital devices by rehabilitation teams for remediation or compensation of impairment.

Scanning—A selection method in which the consumer watches an array and waits for a choice to be offered rather than actively choosing. Activating a single switch indicates choice.

Universal design—A concept used to make built space or consumer products accessible or highly usable for most people. For example, a universally designed airport considers not only persons using wheelchairs but also those who have auditory or visual impairments or who do not speak English.

Universal Serial Bus (USB)—A standard interface commonly used for connections between two or more devices (e.g., mouse, printer, or keyboard) connected to a computer. USB II supports high-speed data transfer and works on Windows and Apple computers.

Wi-Fi—An abbreviation for wireless fidelity, which is a group of technical standards enabling the transmission of data over wireless networks.

Word prediction—Software that uses rules of recency and frequency to anticipate the word the consumer is beginning to spell. It is designed to decrease keystrokes and errors but does not increase typing speed.

References

American Occupational Therapy Association. (2008). Occupational therapy practice framework: Domain and process (2nd ed.). *American Journal of Occupational Therapy, 62,* 625–683.

American Occupational Therapy Association. (2010a). Telerehabilitation. [Official Document]. *American Journal of Occupational Therapy, 64,* S106–S111.

American Occupational Therapy Association. (2010b). Specialized knowledge and skills in technology and environmental interventions for occupational therapy practice. [Official Document]. *American Journal of Occupational Therapy, 64,* 544–556.

Angelo, J. (2000). Factors affecting single switch efficiency in assistive technology. *Journal of Rehabilitation Research and Development, 37,* 591–598.

Anson, D. (1997). *Alternative computer access: A guide to selection.* Philadelphia: F. A. Davis, Inc.

Aravamudhan, S., & Bellamkonda, R. V. (2011). Toward a convergence of regenerative medicine, rehabilitation, and neuroprosthetics. *Journal of Neurotrauma, 28,* 2329–2347.

Bailey, N., Weber, A., & Meidenbauer, N. (2012). National assistive technology technical assistance partnership (NATTAPP Comprehensive website). Retrieved January 18, 2012 from http://www.resnaprojects.org/nattap/at/stateprograms.html.

Bain, B., & Leger, D. (1997). *Assistive technology: An interdisciplinary approach.* Philadelphia: Churchill Livingston.

Barbeau, H., Nadeau, S., & Garneau, C. (2006). Physical determinants, emerging concepts, and training approaches in gait of individuals with spinal cord injury. *Journal of Neurotrauma, 23,* 571–585.

Batavia, A. J., & Hammer, G. S. (1990). Toward the development of consumer-based criteria for the evaluation of assistive devices. *Journal of Rehabilitation Research and Development, 27,* 425–436.

Bates, P. S., Spencer, J. C., Young, M. E., & Rintala, D. H. (1993). Assistive technology and the newly disabled adult: Adaptation to wheelchair use. *American Journal of Occupational Therapy, 47,* 1014–1021.

Behrman, A. L., & Harkema, S. J. (2007). Physical rehabilitation as an agent for recovery after spinal cord injury. *Physical Medicine and Rehabilitation Clinics of North America, 18,* 183–202.

Beukelman, D. R., & Mirenda, P. (2006). *Augmentative & alternative communication: Supporting children & adults with complex communication needs* (3rd ed.). Baltimore: Paul H. Brookes.

Buning, M. E., Angelo, J. A., & Schmeler, M. R. (2001). Occupational performance and the transition to powered mobility: A pilot study. *American Journal of Occupational Therapy, 55,* 339–344.

Burgar, C. G., Lum, P. S., Scremin, A. M., Garber, S. L., Van der Loos, H. F., Kenney, D., & Shor, P. (2011). Robot-assisted upper-limb therapy in acute rehabilitation setting following stroke: Department of

Veterans Affairs multisite clinical trial. *Journal of Rehabilitation Research and Development, 48,* 445–458.

Center for Universal Design. (2011). The principles of universal design. Retrieved March 14, 2012 from http://www.ncsu.edu/project/design-projects/udi/center-for-universal-design/the-principles-of-universal-design/.

Cook, A. M., & Polgar, J. M. (2007). *Cook and Hussey's assistive technologies: Principles and practices* (3rd ed.). St. Louis: Mosby.

Dijkers, M. P., deBear, P. C., Erlandson, R. F., Kristy, K., Geer, D. M., & Nichols, A. (1991). Patient and staff acceptance of robot technology in occupational therapy: A pilot study. *Journal of Rehabilitation Research and Development, 28,* 33–44.

Dowds, M. M., Lee, P. H., Sheer, J. B., O'Neil-Pirozzi, T. M., Xenopoulos-Oddsson, A., Goldstein, R., Zainea, K. L., & Glenn, M. B. (2011). Electronic reminding technology following traumatic brain injury: Effects on timely task completion. *The Journal of Head Trauma Rehabilitation, 26,* 339–347.

Drew, C. (2012). For iRobot, the future is getting closer. Technology Review. *New York Times.* Retrieved from http://www.nytimes.com/2012/03/03/technology/for-irobot-the-future-is-getting-closer.html?scp=1&sq=for iRobot the future is getting closer&st=cse.

Gentry, T. (2011). Assistive technology for people with neurological disability. *NeuroRehabilitation, 28,* 181–182.

Hammel, J. M., & Smith, R. O. (1993). The development of technology competencies and training guidelines for occupational therapists. *American Journal of Occupational Therapy, 47,* 970–979.

Hogan, N., & Krebs, H. I. (2011). Physically interactive robotic technology for neuromotor rehabilitation. *Progress in Brain Research, 192,* 59–68.

Kadivar, Z., Sullivan, J. L., Eng, D. P., Pehlivan, A. U., O'Malley, M. K., Yozbatiran, N., & Francisco, G. E. (2011, Jun). *Robotic training and kinematic analysis of arm and hand after incomplete spinal cord injury: A case study.* Paper presented at the IEEE International Conference on Rehabilitation Robotics (ICORR), Zurich.

Kander, M. (2012). Coverage policy on speech-generating devices. *Medicare coverage of speech-language pathologists and audiologists.* Retrieved Jan 11, 2012 from http://www.asha.org/practice/reimbursement/medicare/sgd_policy.htm.

Kielhofner, G. (1997). *Conceptual foundations of occupational therapy* (2nd ed.). Philadelphia: F. A. Davis.

Kim, J. B., Brienza, D. M., Lynch, R. D., Cooper, R. A., & Boninger, M. L. (2008). Effectiveness evaluation of a remote accessibility assessment system for wheelchair users using virtualized reality. *Archives of Physical Medicine and Rehabilitation, 89,* 470–479.

Knecht, S., Hesse, S., & Oster, P. (2011). Rehabilitation after stroke. *Deutsches Arzteblatt International, 108,* 600–606.

Koester, H. H. (2001). User performance with speech recognition: A literature review. *Assistive Technology, 13,* 116–130.

Koester, H. H. (2004). Usage, performance and satisfaction outcomes for experienced users of automatic speech recognition. *Journal of Rehabilitation Research and Development, 41,* 739–754.

Koester, H. H. (2006). Factors that influence the performance of experienced speech recognition users. *Assistive Technology, 18,* 56–76.

Kowalczewski, J., & Prochazka, A. (2011). Technology improves upper extremity rehabilitation. *Progress in Brain Research, 192,* 147–159.

Krebs, H. I., Mernoff, S., Fasoli, S. E., Hughes, R., Stein, J., & Hogan, N. (2008). A comparison of functional and impairment-based robotic training in severe to moderate chronic stroke: A pilot study. *NeuroRehabilitation, 23,* 81–87.

Lange, M. L. (2002). The future of electronic aids to daily living. *American Journal of Occupational Therapy, 56,* 107–109.

Lo, A. C., Guarino, P. D., Richards, L. G., Haselkorn, J. K., Wittenberg, G. F., Federman, D. G., . . . Peduzzi, P. (2010). Robot-assisted therapy for long-term upper-limb impairment after stroke. *New England Journal of Medicine, 362,* 1772–1783.

Loureiro, R. C., Harwin, W. S., Nagai, K., & Johnson, M. (2011). Advances in upper limb stroke rehabilitation: A technology push. *Medical & Biological Engineering & Computing, 49,* 1103–1118.

Mack, C. A. (2011). Fifty years of Moore's Law. *IEEE Transactions on Semiconductor Manufacturing, 24*(2), 202–207 doi: 10.1109/TSM.2010.2096437.

Masiero, S., Armani, M., & Rosati, G. (2011). Upper-limb robot-assisted therapy in rehabilitation of acute stroke patients: Focused review and results of new randomized controlled trial. *Journal of Rehabilitation Research and Development, 48,* 355–366.

McKay, W. B., Ovechkin, A. V., Vitaz, T. W., Terson de Paleville, D. G., & Harkema, S. J. (2011). Long-lasting involuntary motor activity after spinal cord injury. *Spinal Cord, 49,* 87–93.

O'Connor, T. J., Cooper, R. A., Fitzgerald, S. G., Dvorznak, M. J., Boninger, M. L., VanSickle, D. P., & Glass, L. (2000). Evaluation of a manual wheelchair interface to computer games. *Neurorehabilitation and Neural Repair, 14,* 21–31.

O'Connor, T. J., Fitzgerald, S. G., Cooper, R. A., Thorman, T. A., & Boninger, M. L. (2001). Does computer game play aid in motivation of exercise and increase metabolic activity during wheelchair ergometry? *Medical Engineering & Physics, 23,* 267–273.

Peckham, P. H., & Knutson, J. S. (2005). Functional electrical stimulation for neuromuscular applications. *Annual Review of Biomedical Engineering, 7,* 327–360.

Pehlivan, A. U., Celik, O., & O'Malley, M. K. (2011, Jun). *Mechanical design of a distal arm exoskeleton for stroke and spinal cord injury rehabilitation.* Paper presented at the IEEE International Conference on Rehabilitation Robotics (ICORR) Zurich.

Rehabilitation Engineering and Assistive Technology Society of North America. (2011). SMS Certification. Retrieved April 1, 2011 from http://resna.org/certifications/

Rogers, E. M. (2003). *Diffusion of innovations* (5th ed.). New York: Free Press.

Schein, R. M., Schmeler, M. R., Holm, M. B., Pramuka, M., Saptono, A., & Brienza, D. M. (2011). Telerehabilitation assessment using the Functioning Everyday with a Wheelchair-Capacity instrument. *Journal of Rehabilitation Research and Development, 48,* 115–124.

Schmitt, D. (1992). *Hierarchy of access.* Paper presented at the Closing the Gap Conference, Bloomington, MN. Sponsored by Closing the Gap, Inc., Henderson, MN.

Scott, S. H., & Dukelow, S. P. (2011). Potential of robots as next-generation technology for clinical assessment of neurological disorders and upper-limb therapy. *Journal of Rehabilitation Research and Development, 48,* 335–353.

Seelman, K. D., Kelleher, A. R., & Grindle, G. G. (2010, June). *Social enablers and barriers to adoption of assistive robots: Case studies of the iBOT and PerMMA.* Paper presented at the Second International Symposium on Quality of Life Technology associated with the 2010 Rehabilitation Engineering and Assistive Technology Society of North America Annual Conference, Las Vegas, NV.

Sheffler, L. R., & Chae, J. (2007). Neuromuscular electrical stimulation in neurorehabilitation. *Muscle and Nerve, 35,* 562–590.

Simpson, R., & Koester, H. H. (1999). Adaptive one-switch row-column scanning. *IEEE Transactions on Rehabilitation Engineering, 7,* 464–473.

Sohlberg, M. M., & Mateer, C. A. (2001). *Cognitive rehabilitation: An integrative neuropsychological approach.* New York: The Guilford Press.

Sveistrup, H. (2004). Motor rehabilitation using virtual reality. *Journal of NeuroEngineering and Rehabilitation, 1,* 10–18.

Sveistrup, H., McComas, J., Thornton, M., Marshall, S., Finestone, H., McCormick, A., . . . Mayhew, A. (2003). Experimental studies of virtual reality-delivered compared to conventional exercise programs for rehabilitation. *Cyberpsychology & Behavior, 6,* 245–249.

U.S. Congress. (1988/1998). Technology-related Assistance for Individuals with Disabilities Act ("Tech Act"). Public Law 100-407 (1988) & 105-394 (1998).

U.S. Congress. (2004). The Assistive Technology Act of 2004. Public Law 108-364.

U.S. Society for Augmentative and Alternative Communication. (2012). AAC devices. Retrieved January 15, 2012 from http://www.ussaac.org/.

Volpe, B. T., Huerta, P. T., Zipse, J. L., Rykman, A., Edwards, D., & Dipietro, L. (2009). Robotic devices as therapeutic and diagnostic tools for stroke recovery. *Archives of Neurology, 66,* 1086–1090.

Volpe, B. T., Krebs, H. I., Hogan, N., Edelstein, L., Diels, C., & Aisen, M. (2000). A novel approach to stroke rehabilitation: Robot-aided sensorimotor stimulation. *Neurology, 54,* 1938–1944.

Volpe, B. T., Lynch, D., Rykman-Berland, A., Ferraro, M., Galgano, M., Hogan, N., & Krebs, H. I. (2008). Intensive sensorimotor arm training mediated by therapist or robot improves hemiparesis in patients with chronic stroke. *Neurorehabilitation and Neural Repair, 22,* 305–310.

von Bertalanfy, K. L. (1968). *General system theory: Foundations, development, applications.* New York: George Braziller.

Wikipedia. (2011). Technology. Retrieved January 29, 2012 from http://en.wikipedia.org/w/index.php?title=Technology&oldid=473844228.

Zhang, L., Abreu, B., Seale, G. S., Masel, B., Christiansen, C., & Ottenbacher, K. (2003). A virtual reality environment for evaluation of a daily living skill in brain injury rehabilitation: Reliability and validity. *Archives of Physical Medicine and Rehabilitation, 84,* 1118–1124.

Acknowledgements

Thank you, Frazier Rehab Institute team members! You have taught me so much.

19

Physical Agent Modalities and Biofeedback

Christine M. Wietlisbach and F. D. Blade Branham

Learning Objectives

After studying this chapter, the reader will be able to do the following:

1. Describe the phases of tissue healing.
2. Identify the professional and regulatory issues related to physical agents.
3. Describe the appropriate indications for use of superficial thermal agents, deep thermal agents, and electrotherapeutic agents.
4. List the precautions and contraindications in the use of select physical agents.
5. Discuss the current evidence and its implications for using physical agents as part of a comprehensive occupational therapy treatment plan.
6. Describe how surface electromyography (EMG) biofeed-back can be used as an adjunct to occupational therapy to restore motor control.

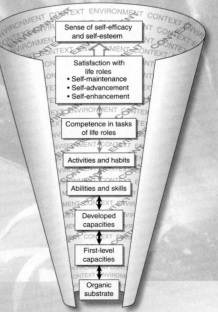

Physical agent modalities are interventions or procedures that produce a response in soft tissue through the use of light, water, temperature, sound, electricity, or mechanical devices. They are applied to modify specific client factors and prepare clients for engagement in occupations when neurological, musculoskeletal, or skin conditions limit occupational performance. Physical agent modalities are used in preparation for or concurrently with purposeful and occupation-based activities (American Occupational Therapy Association [AOTA], 2012). There are four primary classifications of physical agents: superficial thermal agents, deep thermal agents, electrotherapeutic agents, and mechanical devices. Superficial thermal agents include hydrotherapy/whirlpool; cryotherapy; Fluidotherapy®; hot packs; and paraffin, water, and infrared heating. Deep thermal agents include therapeutic ultrasound, phonophoresis, and short-wave diathermy. Electrotherapeutic agents include biofeedback, neuromuscular electrical stimulation (NMES), functional electrical stimulation (FES), transcutaneous electrical nerve stimulation (TENS), high-voltage galvanic stimulation (HVGS), high-voltage pulsed current, direct current, and iontophoresis. Mechanical devices may include vasopneumatic devices and continuous passive motion devices (AOTA, 2012).

The overall purpose of occupational therapy is to support health and participation through engagement in occupation (AOTA, 2008). Physical agent modalities are used as part of a comprehensive occupational therapy treatment plan as preparatory interventions to facilitate outcomes in our clients as quickly and as cost effectively as possible. The focus is always on helping our clients engage in their occupations. Physical agents can help increase soft tissue extensibility, reduce pain and inflammation, and improve muscle performance to help clients more successfully engage in occupational activity. Although other health professions may also use physical agents as part of their treatment, the occupational therapy profession's distinct approach always focuses on occupational performance.

This chapter provides a broad overview of the physical agents most commonly used by occupational therapists. This chapter reviews superficial thermal agents, such as hydrotherapy, hot packs, paraffin, and cryotherapy; and deep thermal agents, such as ultrasound, along with their biophysiological effects. A discussion of the principles and clinical application of electrotherapy and surface electromyographic biofeedback is included. This chapter also discusses tissue healing. This information, often overlooked by therapists, is vital to determine which type of agent would be most efficacious and at which point in treatment and healing it should be applied.

It is beyond the scope of this chapter to present all of the information needed to use physical agents safely and effectively. The intent of this chapter is to provide a basic description of the most commonly used physical agents and their potential for incorporation into clinical practice to facilitate engagement in occupation.

COMPETENCY AND REGULATORY ISSUES

The profession of occupational therapy has a long and colorful history, adapting and changing in response to internal and external issues and challenges. The use of physical agent modalities in clinical practice has not always been embraced within the occupational therapy professional community. However, when the new accreditation standards for occupational therapy education programs went into effect in 2008, all entry-level occupational therapy and occupational therapy assistant students were, for the first time, required to demonstrate some knowledge of physical agents upon graduation (AOTA, 2007a, 2007b, 2007c). The implementation of this educational requirement symbolized the widespread acceptance of using physical agents in occupational therapy practice. Physical agents are now an accepted tool for preparing clients for occupational performance.

Although physical agents are now accepted in occupational therapy, the use of this intervention is associated with some risk in terms of both client safety and professional liability. Occupational therapy practitioners must carefully consider three issues when deciding whether or not to use a particular physical agent modality in clinical practice: (1) the American Occupational Therapy Association's (AOTA) position on the use of physical agent modalities; (2) personal competency in the specific physical agent; and (3) federal, state, and institutional rules and guidelines surrounding use of physical agents in occupational therapy practice.

AOTA asserts that physical agents are preparatory and are to be used by occupational therapy practitioners before or during therapeutic activities that ultimately enhance engagement in occupation (AOTA, 2008, 2012). AOTA clarifies this point by stating, "The exclusive use of (physical agents) as a therapeutic intervention without application to occupational performance is not considered occupational therapy" (AOTA, 2012). Therefore, an occupational therapist who uses a physical agent modality must always do so relative to an occupational outcome. Occupational therapists who use physical agents without any application to occupational performance could be viewed by regulatory agencies as practicing outside the scope of occupational therapy (Definition 19-1).

Personal competency in using specific physical agents is another consideration for clinicians who want to use this type of intervention. AOTA states that physical agents may only be applied by occupational therapy practitioners who have documented evidence of possessing the theoretical background and technical skills for safe and competent integration of the modality into an occupational therapy intervention plan (AOTA, 2012). This sentiment is echoed

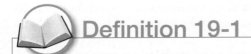

Definition 19-1

Is It Occupational Therapy?

Consider the following scenarios: Because there is evidence that electrical stimulation helps reduce post-stroke spasticity in the upper extremity (Hardy et al., 2010; Sahin, Ugurlu, & Albayrak, 2012), a therapist decides to use electrical stimulation when treating a client with stroke-related hand spasticity.

Scenario A: The therapist applies electrical stimulation to reduce spasticity and then works with the client on using the hand for grooming. The client is pleased because she is more successful using the hand for grooming if spasticity is first reduced through electrical stimulation.

Scenario B: The therapist applies electrical stimulation at the end of a treatment session to reduce hand spasticity. The client is pleased because the electrical stimulation helps reduce spasticity, and she leaves the clinic with less hand pain.

Question: Which scenario is considered an appropriate occupational therapy intervention using a physical agent modality?

Answer: Scenario A meets the criteria established by the American Occupational Therapy Association (AOTA) to be considered an occupational therapy intervention. Physical agents should always be used in preparation for, or concurrently with, purposeful and occupation-based activities. Scenario B would not be considered occupational therapy because although the client did receive some benefit (pain relief) from using electrical stimulation to reduce spasticity, the physical agent was applied without any application to occupational performance.

in the Occupational Therapy Code of Ethics and Ethics Standards, which states, "Occupational therapy personnel shall provide occupational therapy services that are within each practitioner's level of competence and scope of practice (e.g., qualifications, experience, the law)" (AOTA, 2010). Although occupational therapy programs educate students about physical agents, each institution has discretion about the depth and breadth of instruction in this area. Entry-level therapists are advised to seek additional education and training, as needed to supplement their knowledge basis, in each modality they plan to use in clinical practice. Education and training in these interventions can be accomplished through in-service training or professional education, such as continuing education or accredited higher education programs and courses.

Occupational therapists that use physical agents as part of their clinical practice also need to know federal, state, and institutional rules and guidelines, which may restrict or limit the use of physical agents. Many states have statutes and regulations related to the use of physical agents by occupational therapy practitioners. It is illegal to apply physical agent modalities without meeting the regulatory requirements outlined in a particular state's laws. Some state guidelines may also regulate or limit specific applications by occupational therapy assistants. It is the responsibility of all occupational therapy practitioners to stay up to date concerning any regulatory issues related to practice in one's state. All occupational therapy practitioners who anticipate using physical agents should contact their respective state regulatory board to obtain the most current information and should be able to document and defend their education and training in meeting regulatory requirements.

EVIDENCE-BASED PRACTICE, PHYSICAL AGENT MODALITIES AND CLINICAL DECISION MAKING

In its Centennial Vision (AOTA, 2007d), the American Occupational Therapy Association has identified evidence-based practice as a key component in linking education, research, and practice. It is imperative that we occupational therapists substantiate the efficacy of our interventions to preserve the long-term viability of our profession. Our professional literature has seen a rise in the number of research reports, including randomized controlled trials and systematic reviews, over the past 10 years, but there is still much work to be done. Many interventions used in clinical practice still need to be studied and validated. The use of physical agent modalities is one such area that requires more research. For the most part, the evidence in peer-reviewed literature is contradictory when it comes to the efficacy of most physical agents. In the absence of definitive external evidence, however, we must remember that the founders of the evidence-based medicine movement never intended for high-level research to be the *only* evidence upon which we base clinical decision making.

David L. Sackett, a pioneer in the evidence-based medicine movement, and his colleagues clarified the widespread misconception that evidence-based medicine is some sort of "cookbook" approach to patient care. In fact, evidence-based medicine is the integration of *three* distinct components: (1) current best evidence, (2) clinical expertise, and (3) patient choice (Sackett et al., 1996). It is important to note that the founders of evidence-based medicine embraced clinician expertise and patient choice as valid components of sound clinical decision making. Effective clinicians combine knowledge of the best published evidence with their own clinical skills and judgment, as well as patient preference, to develop the most appropriate plan of care for each individual patient. Therefore, it is perfectly acceptable, in the face of contradictory literature, for a clinician to use a physical agent to prepare a client to more successfully participate in an occupation-based activity if, in the therapist's experience or anecdotal knowledge, the agent has been successful with another similar client. The therapist must carefully observe the client's reaction. Improved performance is evidence of treatment efficacy.

This chapter contains both external evidence from peer-reviewed journals and expert clinical opinion. The chapter presents evidence supporting the use of physical agents when that evidence exists and could be located by the authors (see Evidence Table 19-1). Critical consumers of this information would do well to remember that contradictory evidence abounds. We make a plea to our colleagues to conduct more high level research in this area.

TISSUE HEALING

High-level evidence supporting the use of physical agents for tissue healing is mixed. Definitive guidance will require considerably more research. However, many occupational therapists do use physical agents for this purpose, and there is widespread opinion by experienced therapists that physical agents are effective for tissue healing. Occupational therapists that choose to use these modalities need a basic understanding of normal tissue healing and an appreciation for the sequence of events that follows an injury to determine the appropriate physical agent to facilitate healing at each stage of the healing process.

Tissue healing is a complex series of events affected by both physical and psychological components. In the healthy individual, the body's attempt to heal itself in response to an injury is well ordered and sequenced. Factors such as advanced age, the presence of foreign objects, infection, poor nutrition, and medications may slow the healing process (Mulder, Brazinsky, & Seeley, 2010). Traditionally, tissue healing is thought of in terms of healing damaged epithelial tissue in the form of an open wound on the surface of the body. However, understanding tissue healing is also important in the case of internal soft tissue traumas that occur with musculoskeletal overuse injuries causing tissue inflammation and degeneration, or after surgical repair of internal soft tissue structures. In both internal and external tissue healing, the healing sequence is similar (with some minor differences depending on the internal structure and tissue involved). A basic understanding of the phases of tissue healing and how physical agents may influence each phase is helpful when addressing tissue injuries, both internal and external. The stages of healing and repair may overlap, but they consist of three primary phases: inflammation, proliferation, and maturation/remodeling.

Phase I: Inflammatory Phase

Inflammation is the initial response to tissue injury; it is both vascular and cellular. At this point, the body is working to control blood loss and to clean the wounded area.

The inflammatory response may be associated with changes in skin color (red, blue, or purple), temperature (heat), edema (swelling), sensation (pain), and loss of function. The inflammatory phase begins from the moment the injury is sustained and continues until the injured area is free from debris such as bacteria, foreign matter, and dead tissue. It is a normal and necessary phase of tissue healing. The acute inflammatory phase lasts a couple of days to a couple of weeks. Physical agents that help manage pain and control excessive edema are cryotherapy and pulsed wave ultrasound. It is important to remember that elimination of all inflammation and edema in the acute phase of tissue injury is not only unrealistic but unwarranted. Some amount of inflammation and swelling are needed to prepare the wound for the proliferative phase of healing. Inflammation becomes an issue only when it is unrelenting. Chronic inflammation indicates an abnormality in the body's healing response, and the cause of this abnormality must then be identified by a physician. Edema becomes a problem when it is excessive because it is painful and can reduce blood flow, which is critical for bringing nutrients to healing cells. *Safety Message: The use of heat during the acute inflammatory phase of healing is contraindicated because it causes physiological responses that increase edema.*

Phase II: Proliferative Phase

Once the injured area is clean, the body starts working on repairing the damaged tissue site. This repair stage is known as the proliferative phase of tissue healing. Proliferation consists of granulation, angiogenesis, wound contraction, and epithelialization. Granulation occurs when the body forms a matrix of connective tissue, including collagen, in the wound bed. This tissue is known as granulation tissue and builds on itself to fill the tissue defect, or "hole" of the wound.

Angiogenesis is the growth of new blood vessels. Very small capillary networks are formed in the matrix of connective tissue in the wound bed and give healthy wounds their distinctive reddish color. Wound contraction occurs when specialized cells in the wound bed act to pull the edges of the wound together. Finally, the wound is covered with epithelial cells that migrate across the top of the wound bed. This is known as epithelialization. The proliferation phase may take up to a few weeks to complete. Physical agents that help speed new tissue formation (proliferation) are therapeutic ultrasound and electrical stimulation.

Phase III: Remodeling/Maturation Phase

Newly healed tissue is still quite fragile and must go through the remodeling (also called the maturation) phase of tissue healing. During this final phase, collagen fibers in the wounded tissue are produced, broken down, changed,

| Evidence Table 19-1 | | Best Evidence for Use of Physical Agent Modalities | | | | |

Intervention	Description of Intervention Tested	Participants	Dosage	Type of Best Evidence and Level of Evidence	Benefit	Statistical Probability	Reference
Functional electrical stimulation (FES)	Use of FES to supraspinatus and posterior deltoid muscles in addition to conventional therapy versus conventional therapy only. Active electrode placed over the posterior deltoid (see the article for specifics of FES parameters).	Fifty hemiplegic patients with shoulder subluxation and shoulder pain. Mean age 60.7 years in study group, 62.0 years in control group; no statistically significant difference for age, gender, etiology, hemiplegic duration, or side affected; randomized to group	FES to affected extremity five times per day, 1 hour daily for 4 weeks for a total of 20 sessions	Randomized controlled trial (RCT) Level: 1B2a (greater intensity of therapy to control group)	Yes. FES treatment to the supraspinatus and posterior deltoid muscles, in addition to conventional treatment (not described), reduced subluxation in hemiplegic patients more than conventional treatment alone. No significant change in pain in the study group after treatment as compared to before, but the control group experienced significantly less pain after treatment ($p < 0.016$).	Statistically significant difference between the pre- and postrehabilitation shoulder subluxation values of the study group (10-mm subluxation reduced to 5 mm; $p = < 0.001$) but nonsignificant in the control group (10 mm both pre- and postrehabilitation; $p = 0.077$). Between-group comparison of change from pre- to postrehabilitation indicated a significant difference ($p = 0.025$) in favor of the study group.	Koyuncu et al. (2010)
Iontophoresis	Iontophoresis with dexamethasone sodium phosphate compared to a saline solution (placebo) for the treatment of epicondylitis	One hundred ninety-nine patients from 11 centers with diagnosis of acute elbow epicondylitis; mean age = 49.9 years (17–70 years) in study group and 50.9 years (21–70 years) in the placebo group; symptom duration ranged from 3 to 150 days. All patients had prior treatment and medications; randomized to group	40 mA-minute dosage at a maximum current of 3–4 mA of either active medication or placebo for six treatments, 1–3 days apart within 15 days	Randomized, double-blinded, placebo-controlled study (RCT) Level: 1A2a	Yes. Iontophoresis treatment was effective in reducing symptoms of epicondylitis at short-term follow-up. Dexamethasone produced a significant 23-mm improvement on the 100-mm patient visual analog pain scale (VAS) ratings compared with 14 mm for the placebo at 2 days and 24.5 mm compared with 19.5 mm at 1 month	Statistically significant ($p = 0.012$; effect size $r = 0.16$) difference between the groups in pain reduction at 2 days but not at 1 month ($p = 0.249$). Patients completing six treatments in 10 days or less had better results than those treated over a longer period. Mild adverse effects were reported for both the study ($n = 12$) and the placebo ($n = 11$) groups.	Nirschl et al. (2003)

	Purpose	Subjects	Design/Level	Procedure	Best evidence	Results	Citation
Ultrasound and Phonophoresis	Comparison of effect of ultrasound, phonophoresis, and placebo ultrasound therapies in the treatment of myofascial pain syndrome	Sixty subjects (48 females, 12 males; 20–73 years) who had a diagnosis of myofascial pain syndrome with at least one active trigger point in the upper trapezius and symptom duration for 1 month; randomized to three groups	Randomized, double-blind, placebo controlled study Level: 1B1a	Groups received either (1) phonophoresis (diclofenac gel), (2) ultrasound, or (3) placebo ultrasound over trigger points. Dosage = 1 MHz, 1.5 watt/cm² for 10 minutes per day, five times per week for 15 treatments in 3 weeks. All groups received a home-based neck exercise program.	Yes. Both the ultrasound and phonophoresis were effective in treatment of patients with myofascial pain syndrome.	Both groups showed statistically significant improvements in the VAS for pain ($p = 0.000$; $r = 0.80$, a large effect); number of trigger points ($p = 0.000$, $r = 0.80$); pain pressure threshold ($p = 0.007$; $r = 0.55$, a large effect); cervical ROM ($p < 0.05$); neck pain disability index NPDI ($p = 0.000$, $r = 0.80$). There was no difference between the ultrasound and phonophoresis groups. Significant improvement in the placebo group was limited to increased cervical rotation and lateral flexion ($p \leq 0.0456$) and improved pain pressure threshold ($p = 0.000$). No adverse effects observed.	Ay et al. (2011)
EMG biofeedback to learn relaxation	Comparison of the effect of EMG biofeedback and sham biofeedback on pain reduction and number of tender points in patients with fibromyalgia	Thirty subjects (21 females, 9 males) with diagnosis of fibromyalgia; average age 39 years; randomized to group	RCT Level: 1C1b	Both groups received six 45-minute sessions of treatment to forearm extensors, upper trapezius and frontalis. One group received EMG biofeedback. The other group received a sham treatment that provided visual feedback to the participant irrespective of muscle activity. Both groups were taught relaxation techniques.	Yes. EMG biofeedback as a treatment modality reduces pain in patients with fibromyalgia.	There was a significant decrease in pain ($p = 0.09$; $r = 0.24$, small effect) and number of tender points ($p = 0.002$, $r = 0.53$, large effect) for the EMG group as compared to the sham group. EMG group mean change for VAS was −4.3 (CI: −5.3, −3.3); for the sham group, −2.6 (CI: −4.4, −1). Group mean change for number of tender points for the EMG group was −8.6 (CI: −10.9, −6.3) and for the sham group was −4.4 (CI: −5.9, −2.9).	Babu et al. (2007)

CI, confidence interval; VAS, visual analog scale, often used to measure pain. EMG, electromyography, recording of the electrical signal generated by muscle when it contracts.

and reoriented to become what we know as scar tissue. Gradually, the wound cover—a combination of scar tissue and epithelial tissue—gets stronger. The maturation phase can take up to 2 years to complete. Even when it is fully remodeled, this new wound covering is only about 80% as strong as the original tissue's strength. Additionally, this new tissue is relatively inelastic and "tight" compared to the original tissue. Physical agents that help improve connective tissue extensibility in preparation for tissue stretch and ultimately improved function are superficial heating agents and the use of continuous wave ultrasound that provides deep heat.

INCORPORATING PHYSICAL AGENTS INTO A TYPICAL OCCUPATIONAL THERAPY TREATMENT

Physical agents are used as a precursor to, or during, functional activity to facilitate occupational performance. The therapist determines which physical agents will help achieve the patient's goals. Physical agents address pain and other biophysiological client factors that interfere with engagement in occupation. For example, a patient with osteoarthritis of the hand may have joint pain. Any physical agent that relieves the pain of hand osteoarthritis may help improve function (Barthel et al., 2010). Therapeutic ultrasound, for example, has been shown to have beneficial effects on pain and functional outcomes in patients with osteoarthritis (Srbely, 2008). An occupational therapist might use ultrasound to alleviate the patient's hand pain prior to training with adaptive equipment for self-care activities.

Patients with lateral epicondylitis report pain at the elbow that interferes with grip strength and function. The cause of this condition is degeneration of the common extensor tendon fibers where they originate on the lateral epicondyle, and it is closely associated with overuse and inflammation. A number of studies support using a specialized type of electrical stimulation—called iontophoresis—to reduce pain and thus improve grip strength and function in patients with lateral epicondylitis (Nirschl et al., 2003; Stefanou et al., 2012). Iontophoresis uses electrical charges to drive medication through the skin and into the body. Occupational therapists might use iontophoresis to deliver anti-inflammatory medication to chronically inflamed tissues in the elbow to reduce pain and promote healing in preparation for return to work activity.

Patients who have experienced a stroke may struggle with increased spasticity that interferes with functional use of the arm and hand. There is evidence to support the use of electrical stimulation to reduce spasticity in the hemiplegic upper extremity (Hara et al., 2008; Sahin, Ugurlu, & Albayrak, 2012). An occupational therapist could use electrical stimulation to reduce spasticity in the patient's arm in preparation for having that patient perform a dressing activity. Before administering any

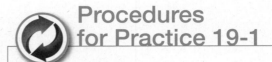

Procedures for Practice 19-1

Documenting Physical Agent Interventions

Documentation of physical agent interventions should include the following:

- Physical agent applied and treatment parameters
- Site of application or placement
- Treatment duration
- Physiological responses elicited from treatment
- Subjective responses from the patient, such as tolerance, reaction, and clinical effectiveness
- Reason for using the physical agent with respect to the ultimate functional goal

modality, the therapist should question the patient about any negative response to physical agents applied in previous treatment and review whether the patient has any contraindications for the selected agent. Prior to administering the physical agent, the therapist should inform the patient as to the procedure, expected outcome, and subjective sensation that the patient may feel during the treatment. Skin integrity should always be evaluated prior to administration of physical agents and immediately following the intervention. Documentation should be clear and concise (Procedures for Practice 19-1). Therapists should also assess the effectiveness of the modality on a session-by-session basis. If the modality fails to provide the desired outcome or if the patient has discomfort or negative results, the modality should be discontinued.

THERMOTHERAPY

Thermotherapy is the term used to describe the therapeutic application of heat. A thermotherapy agent is any modality applied to the body that increases tissue temperature. These agents are further classified as either superficial-heating agents or deep-heating agents. Superficial agents heat tissues at depths of up to 1 cm (Kaul, 1994). Commonly used superficial-heating agents include warm whirlpool baths, Fluidotherapy®, hot packs, and paraffin. Deep-heating agents heat tissues at depths up to 5 cm. Therapeutic ultrasound is commonly used to deliver deep heat.

The four primary biophysiological effects of thermotherapy are analgesic, vascular, metabolic, and connective tissue responses.

- The analgesic effect reduces pain symptoms. Heat acts selectively on free nerve endings, tissues, and peripheral nerve fibers, which directly or indirectly reduces pain, elevates pain tolerance, and promotes relaxation.

- Vascular effects aid in pain relief and in decreasing muscle spasm and spasticity. As the temperature of tissue elevates, substances such as histamines are released into the bloodstream, resulting in vasodilation. This increased blood flow reduces ischemia, muscle spindle activity, tonic muscle contractions, spasticity, and pain.
- Metabolic effects influence tissue repair and aid pain relief. In addition to the vascular effect of increased circulation, thermal agents affect inflammation and healing because of chemical reactions. Increases in blood flow and oxygen within the tissues bring a greater number of antibodies, leukocytes, nutrients, and enzymes to injured tissues. Pain is reduced by the removal of by-products of the inflammatory process. Nutrition is enhanced at the cellular level, and repair occurs.
- The connective tissue response to heat refers to the fact that biological tissues are more easily stretched after heating. Collagen is the primary component protein of skin, tendon, bone cartilage, and connective tissue. Those tissues containing collagen can become shortened because of immobilization or limited range of motion (ROM) as a result of weakness, injury, or pain. Improvement in the properties of collagen and extensibility of tissues occurs when heat is combined with passive or active mobilization and/or engagement in occupation. This ultimately results in reduced joint stiffness and increased ROM.

Selection of Superficial Thermal Agents

Thermotherapy is used when an increase in tissue temperature is the intended effect. General dosage guidelines provide a starting point for selection of an agent and for application parameters. Dosage refers to the amount of heat applied to the tissue that then elevates the tissue temperature. A positive therapeutic effect occurs when the temperature of soft tissue is increased to the range of 102°F–113°F (38°C–45°C). If the soft tissue is heated to a temperature less than 102°F (38°C), cell metabolism may not be stimulated adequately enough to elicit a therapeutic response. If tissue is heated to a temperature greater than 113°F (45°C), tissue damage may occur.

Application of a mild dose of heat elevates tissue temperature 4°F–5°F (2.2°C–2.78°C). For example, if the average skin surface temperature is 91°F (32.8°C), a change of 4°F would elevate the skin temperature to 95°F (35°C). The primary benefit of a mild application of heat is relaxation and pain relief. Many conservative home remedies (for example, a dry heating pad) provide this mild dosage. A moderate dose of heat causes an increase in tissue temperature of approximately 6°F (3.3°C) and a moderate increase in blood flow. A vigorous dose elevates the tissue up to 14°F (9.78°C) and results in a marked increase in blood flow. Moderate to vigorous doses of heat are needed to cause vascular, metabolic, and connective tissue responses. The therapist should

be especially vigilant with moderate and vigorous doses of heat by monitoring skin color and the patient's reported perception of comfort during the heating process. Patients can be burned during the application of therapeutic heat. This usually occurs when tissue temperatures have been elevated beyond 113°F (45°C). However, individual sensitivity to heat varies from patient to patient. *Safety Message: It is important that heat be applied only to patients who can feel the sensation of heat and only to patients who can understand and communicate to the therapist if the heating process becomes uncomfortable.* Therapeutic heating should always be discontinued if a patient reports pain or burning during application. Safety Note 19-1 lists precautions and contraindications of thermotherapy.

Regardless of the type of heating modality applied to the tissue (paraffin, hot pack, etc.), the biophysiological effects will be the same. However, the choice of heating modality determines *how* the heat will be transferred. There are three primary mechanisms of heat transfer within the body: conduction, convection, and radiation. Conduction occurs when heat transfers from a stationary heat source that has direct contact with body tissue, such as hot packs and paraffin baths. Convection occurs when heated particles or molecules continuously move across body tissue causing a

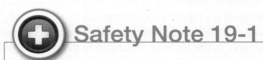

Safety Note 19-1

Superficial Thermal Agents

Precautions

- Edema
- Diminished sensation
- Compromised circulation
- Use of anticoagulant medications

Contraindications

- Impaired sensation caused by skin graft or scar
- Tumors or cancer
- Advanced cardiac disease (body inadequately dissipates heat)
- Acute inflammation or acute edema
- Deep vein thrombophlebitis
- Pregnancy (systemic effects of circulating blood on fetus are unclear)
- Bleeding tendencies
- Infection
- Primary repair of tendon or ligament
- Semicoma or impaired cognitive status
- Rheumatoid arthritis: vigorous dosages of heat can exacerbate joint inflammation

Adapted from Schmidt, K. L., Ott, V. R., Rocher, G., & Schaller, H. (1979). Heat, cold, and inflammation. *Zeitschrift fur Rheumatologie, 38*, 391–404.

heat transfer, such as with the use of whirlpool baths and Fluidotherapy®. Radiation occurs when there is a transfer of radiant energy through the air from a warmer source to a cooler source, such as with the use of infrared lamps.

The therapist must remember that the temperature of the heating agent is not necessarily the temperature to which the body tissue will rise. For example, setting the Fluidotherapy® to 118°F (47.7°C) will not increase tissue temperature to 118°F (47.7°C). The ultimate rise in tissue temperature depends on the mechanism of heat transfer (conduction versus convection versus radiation), the dosage of heat applied, and the time period tissue is exposed to the heating agent. More research is needed to identify the optimal combination of dosage, mechanism, and timing guidelines for reaching specific tissue temperatures. However, the guiding principle for heating tissue is that deeper tissues require longer periods of heat application to reach therapeutic temperatures. When heat must be applied for longer periods, it cannot be so intense as to overheat the skin layer before tissues at greater depths (i.e., muscle, tendon) are adequately heated. Also, we know that adipose tissue is an excellent insulator, so heating tissue located below body fat requires a longer application of heat. Likewise, heating more superficial body structures that are generally devoid of adipose tissue (such as the hand) will require shorter time periods of heat application for tissue to reach therapeutic temperatures.

The choice of a superficial heating agent depends on the treatment objective, the location of the involved structure, and the desired ultimate tissue temperature. Other considerations include whether moist or dry heat is desired, the positioning of the extremity in a nondependent or intermittently dependent position, and whether active or passive participation by the patient is desired (Earley, 1999). The acuity or chronicity of the patient's condition is also an important factor. It is important to understand that while heat can be beneficial to tissue healing in the case of a prolonged inflammatory phase (for example, as the body tries to reabsorb a large hematoma), heat tends to worsen acute inflammation and edema. Injuries in the early inflammatory phase should be treated with cryotherapy, not heat, to avoid increased edema. Tissues in the remodeling stage of recovery would be treated with heat to facilitate the remodeling process of collagen alignment and differentiation.

Common Superficial Heating Modalities in the Occupational Therapy Clinic

Whirlpool Baths

Whirlpool treatment is performed in a tank equipped with a water circulating mechanism that draws water out and pushes it into the tank at varying speeds (whirlpool bath). Water temperature is usually set between 99°F and 104°F (37.2°C–40°C) and should never exceed 110°F (43.3°C).

Treatment time is approximately 20 minutes. Advantages of whirlpool use are that the client can actively exercise the extremity as the tissue heats up, the therapist has easy access to the extremity for providing active-assistive and passive mobilization, and the degree of agitation of the water can be controlled to act as a soft tissue massage or resistance for exercise. *Safety Message: However, the use of whirlpool is contraindicated when significant edema is present. The heat as well as the unavoidable and prolonged dependent position of the extremity in the whirlpool bath almost always increases edema. Additionally, whirlpool is contra-indicated when open wounds are present. Cross-contamination and risk for infection is significant because it is difficult to adequately disinfect all parts of the whirlpool bath between patients.*

Fluidotherapy®

Fluidotherapy® uses fine particles of organic cellulose blown around in a hot air stream inside a containing unit to heat an extremity. The force of the air and particles circulating within the machine can be graded via the blower speed. It is like a dry whirlpool bath. Temperature is controlled by a thermostat and is generally set between 105°F and 118°F (40.5°C–47.7°C). Treatment time is approximately 20 minutes. The advantage of Fluidotherapy® is the ease of implementation, the client can actively exercise the extremity as the tissue heats up, the therapist has easy access to the extremity for providing active-assistive and passive mobilization, and the dry cellulose particles can provide desensitization therapy during the heating process. *Safety Message: Extremities with open wounds should not be placed in the Fluidotherapy® machine and all clients should wash the area to be treated with soap and water prior to using this modality.*

Hot Packs

Hot packs are canvas cases of material stored in a thermostatically controlled container of hot water called a hydrocollator. Water temperature is kept at approximately 165°F (73.8°C). When the pack is removed from the water, its temperature is typically between 104°F and 113°F (40°C–45°C). The pack is then wrapped in dry padding with appropriate towel use and applied to the body to provide moist heat. Treatment time is approximately 20 minutes. The advantages to hot packs are that they are simple to use, are widely available, and can heat large surface areas. Disadvantages include the heaviness of hot packs—which can be uncomfortable for the patient—as well as their difficulty in conforming to small multisurface body parts such as the hand. Another disadvantage to hot packs is that the area being treated must be nonmobile and covered. This limits active and active-assistive mobilization during the heating process, although a joint can be placed on passive stretch while being heated with a hot pack. *Safety Message: It is important to ensure that six to eight layers of dry padding is used between the hot pack and the skin to avoid burns. Toweling is commonly used to cover hot packs. Commercially available terry cloth "hot pack covers" are also available and are the equivalent of three to four layers of toweling. If toweling and hot pack covers become damp from repeated use throughout the day, more heat is transferred from the hot pack to the body. Therefore, padding should be rotated and allowed to dry, or more layers of moist padding will be needed to avoid tissue burns.* The therapist should also remember to rotate the hot packs inside the hydrocollator because packs cool during use. It takes approximately 30 minutes to adequately reheat a hot pack to a therapeutic temperature between uses.

Paraffin

Therapeutic paraffin baths consist of a thermostatically controlled heating unit filled with a commercial mixture of paraffin wax and mineral oil. Mineral oil is used to lower the melting point of the paraffin. Paraffin baths are kept at temperatures between 120°F and 130°F (48.8°C–54.4°C). Paraffin is often the heating agent of choice for occupational therapists working with hand dysfunction. This is because paraffin easily conforms to the contours of the hand and therefore provides even distribution of heat to all surfaces. The patient immerses the hand in the bath for 1–2 seconds and withdraws it to allow the paraffin to harden. This gloving process is repeated 8–10 times, and then the hand is wrapped in a plastic bag followed by a towel to retain the heat. The paraffin, bag, and towel are left on for 20 minutes (Fig. 19-1). At the end of treatment, the paraffin is removed and discarded. A disadvantage to this

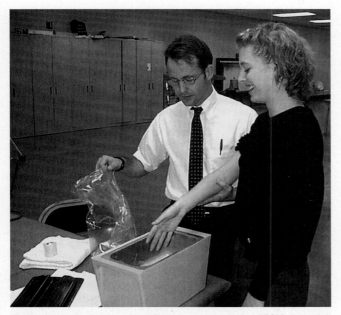

Figure 19-1 Application of paraffin to increase pain-free AROM of the digit interphalangeal joints. The extremity will be wrapped in a plastic bag and then a towel.

form of paraffin treatment is that the hand needs to remain still during the heating process, and this limits active and active-assistive mobilization. *Safety Message: The therapist should always check the temperature of the paraffin before each use to ensure a safe temperature and avoid burns. Paraffin is not appropriate to use when open wounds are present at the treatment site, and the client should wash the entire extremity with soap and water before using the paraffin bath.*

CRYOTHERAPY

Cryotherapy–also called "cold therapy"—is the therapeutic application of physical agents to lower tissue temperatures. Cryotherapy is classified as a superficial thermal agent because it moves heat out of the body. Cold therapy agents can affect tissue temperatures to a depth of 2 cm (Bracciano, 2008). Commonly used cooling agents include commercial and homemade ice packs and ice massage. The primary biophysiological effects of cryotherapy are analgesic, vascular, metabolic, and neuromuscular.

- The analgesic effect influences pain symptoms. Cold elevates the pain threshold through counterirritation and by reducing nerve conduction velocity in the more superficial sensory nerves (Algafly & George, 2007; Herrera et al., 2010).
- Vascular effects include both vasoconstriction (when cold is applied for less than 15 minutes) and vasodilation (when cold is applied for longer than 15 minutes) (Bracciano, 2008). Short-term application of cold therapy can help reduce edema.
- Metabolic effects influence inflammation and tissue repair. Application of cold therapy slows down the metabolic processes of tissue repair and should therefore be used thoughtfully. We do not want to interfere with the normal healing process, but cold therapy can be useful to control excessive inflammation and edema in the very early stages of healing.
- Neuromuscular effects influence muscle tone. Cold therapy can temporarily reduce spasticity in patients with upper motor neuron lesions (dos Santos & de Oliveira, 2004).

Selection of Cryotherapy Agents

Cryotherapy involves the application of a cooling agent to cause heat to move *out* of the body. As with superficial heating agents, where the goal of therapy is to transfer heat *into* the body, heat energy can be transferred out of the body for the purposes of cooling through conduction and convection. Application of a cold pack is an example of conduction cryotherapy. Immersing an extremity in a cold water bath is an example of convection cryotherapy. In addition to these methods of application, heat can also be transmitted out of the body through evaporation.

Therapeutic cold sprays applied to the body in the form of liquid absorb heat from the skin and then evaporate.

The temperature of the cooling agent is certainly not the temperature to which the body tissues will fall. Tissue temperature change and biophysical effects of cooling are related to the specific cooling agent used, the time of exposure, and the conductivity of the tissue. It is important to ensure that target tissues are completely covered by the cooling agent in order to achieve the desired results. The location and size of target tissues will help guide the selection of an appropriate cooling agent. A large area of target tissue is more effectively cooled with a large cold pack or cold water immersion, whereas a smaller area of target tissue might be best cooled with an ice massage.

Another guiding principle for cooling tissue is that deeper tissues, and tissues located under body fat, require longer periods of cold application to reach therapeutic temperatures. When deeper tissues need to be cooled, the method of applying cold therapy must be adjusted to reduce the intensity of cold against the skin so that longer treatment times can be tolerated. In the case of a conductive cold agent like a crushed-ice cold pack, this can be achieved by covering the cold pack with dry material. Ice packs covered with wetted material will cool superficial tissues at a faster rate and may not be tolerated well by patients who need deeper tissues cooled (Dykstra et al., 2009). *Safety Message: Care must be used when applying cold agents because changes in skin temperature occur quickly, and tissue may be damaged before the desired biophysical effects are achieved. As with superficial heating agents, monitoring of the skin for tissue damage is essential, and caution is advised for patients with decreased sensation or mentation. Cold therapy normally turns the skin a pink or light red color. It should be immediately discontinued if the skin turns bright red, white, pale, or grayish yellow or develops welts.* Safety Note 19-2 lists contraindications to cryotherapy.

Common Cooling Modalities in the Occupational Therapy Clinic

Cold Packs

Cold packs come in a variety of shapes and sizes. They are commercially available as cold therapy machines and gel packs, or they can be homemade. Cold therapy machines circulate cold water through an insulated cooler and special sleeve that covers the body part (Fig. 19-2). Commercial gel packs are generally made from gel covered with a type of plastic. They can be kept in a standard household or industrial freezer between uses. Cold packs can also be made from crushed ice wrapped in toweling or placed in a plastic bag. An unopened bag of frozen peas can serve as a cold pack and works well to conform to small rounded areas like the hand. Cold packs can also be made by combining three parts water to one part isopropyl alcohol in a plastic zip-seal bag and freezing. The alcohol will keep the mixture from fully freezing, resulting in a slushy soft cold pack similar in consistency to some commercial gel packs. Cold packs should always be covered with a material such as toweling or a pillow case. A dry covering will make the initial contact with the patient more comfortable and slow the cooling process. Wetted cold pack covers cause more rapid cooling of tissues. Treatment time can be up to 20 minutes, but the patient should be monitored for signs of cold intolerance or tissue damage.

The advantages of cold packs are that they are inexpensive, are easy to find or make, and can cover large areas. A disadvantage of some cold packs is that they can be difficult to conform to smaller, multisurface areas such as the hand.

Ice Massage

Ice massage requires holding ice directly against the skin and moving it in slow circles over the target tissue. This technique is normally used for cooling small areas such as

---

✚ Safety Note 19-2

Cryotherapy

Avoid cryotherapy with patients who exhibit the following:

- Peripheral vascular disease or any circulatory compromised area
- Cold sensitivity or Raynaud's phenomenon
- Multiple myeloma, leukemia, or systemic lupus (cryoglobinemia is a disorder of abnormal protein formation that can lead to ischemia in these individuals)
- Cold urticaria/intolerance; can occur with rheumatic diseases, or following crush injuries or amputations

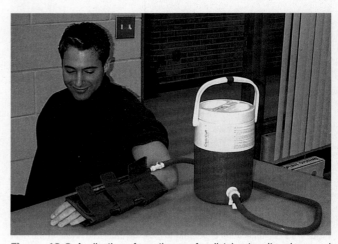

Figure 19-2 Application of cryotherapy for distal extremity edema and inflammation.

tendon insertion sites and hyper-irritable muscle spots to produce an analgesic effect. Because tissues are cooled so rapidly during ice massage, this treatment generally takes no longer than 10 minutes, and treatment time should be guided by how the patient feels. The patient can expect to experience the sensation of cold, then burning, then aching, and finally numbness. Once the patient experiences numbness, the ice massage should be discontinued.

It can become uncomfortable for the therapist to hold a piece of ice in his or her bare hands for the duration of the treatment, so ice cubes can be held with a folded wash cloth. Alternatively, small Styrofoam or paper cups can be filled with water and frozen. Prior to starting an ice massage, the top rim of the cup is peeled off to expose the ice tip. The therapist then holds the cup part while performing the massage. This protects the therapist's hands from the ice. As the ice melts during the massage, more cup can be peeled away to expose more ice.

Advantages to ice massage include ease of use, little expense, and quick inducement of analgesia in appropriate tissues. A disadvantage to ice massage is that it is not tolerated well by people who do not want to endure the sensations of burning and aching prior to reaching the stage of numbness. Additionally, ice massage can be messy as the ice melts, so protect your patients' clothing with dry toweling during this procedure.

THERAPEUTIC ULTRASOUND

Ultrasound is acoustic energy (sound waves) used in medicine for diagnosis and in rehabilitation to help restore and heal soft tissues. Therapeutic ultrasound is classified as a deep-heat modality. Ultrasound is inaudible high frequency acoustic vibration that produces thermal and/or nonthermal (mechanical) physiologic effects on tissue. Thermal effects refer to those biophysiological changes produced by cellular heating, whereas nonthermal, or mechanical effects, refer to biophysiological changes produced by the cellular effects of cavitation, microstreaming, or acoustic streaming. Both thermal and nonthermal ultrasound can be used to facilitate healing and ultimately improve occupational function.

Physical Principles

Standard ultrasound units consist of a power supply, generator, coaxial cable, transducer, and crystal. The generator produces a high frequency alternating current at 1–3 million cycles per second (MHz). The alternating current travels through the coaxial cable into the transducer. The transducer houses the vibrating crystal and converts electrical energy into ultrasonic or acoustic energy (Fig. 19-3). The vibration of the crystal generates the sound waves, which are transmitted to a small volume of tissue, causing molecules within the tissue to move. Ultrasound travels poorly

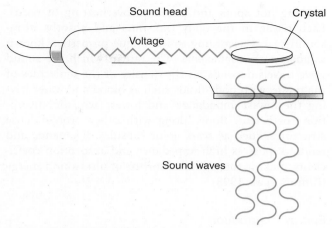

Figure 19-3 Production of ultrasound.

through air, so a lubricant is used to maintain contact between the transducer and the tissue, ensuring that the energy is dispersed into the tissue (Draper, 2010) (Fig. 19-4).

When the sound waves are generated rapidly and dispersed into the tissue, the molecules in the waves' path are pushed back and forth by the alternating phases of successive waves until the wave runs out of energy. This type of wave, moving in one direction and compressing and decompressing the molecules in its way, is termed a *longitudinal wave*. When the wave encounters bone, the sound energy is transferred along the periosteum and is then deflected up at a right angle causing a *shear wave*. Shear waves occur when the sound energy strikes a solid substance. This may cause heating of the outer covering of the bone but is negligible in terms of tissue temperature elevation (Bracciano, 2008; Cameron, 2012). A *standing wave* occurs when the sound head is not moved adequately enough, and the incoming sound waves encounter the reflected sound waves moving back up toward the surface,

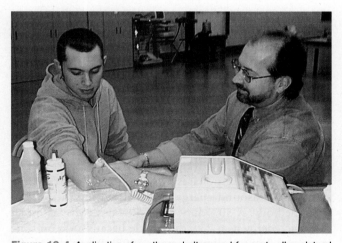

Figure 19-4 Application of nonthermal ultrasound for acute elbow lateral epicondylitis.

creating hot spots and potential overheating of tissue. Each tissue in the body transmits and absorbs ultrasound energy according to its unique properties, known as absorption coefficients. The rate at which the sound wave travels depends on the density of the molecules of the tissue, with body fluids such as blood and water having the lowest impedance and lowest acoustic absorption coefficient. Bone, along with other protein-dense structures, such as scars, joint capsules, ligaments, and tendons, possess high impedance and absorption coefficients, making them good absorbers of ultrasound energy (Kimura et al., 1998)

Energy Distribution

The spread of ultrasound waves into tissue is affected by the frequency (produced by the generator) and size of the crystal (mounted inside the transducer head). The frequency of the ultrasound (the number of times per second that the crystal changes shape) determines the depth of penetration and rate of heating. At 1 MHz, the depth of penetration is 2.5–5 cm, and at 3 MHz, the depth is surface to 2.5 cm. Three MHz will also heat three times faster than 1 MHz (Draper, 2010).

The intensity of the beam of energy varies within the sound wave; this phenomenon is called the beam nonuniformity ratio (BNR). The BNR is a measure of the homogeneity of the therapeutic ultrasound wave (Venes, 2009). The BNR of a transducer refers to the ratio (ideal is 1:1) between its spatial peak and the average intensities in the output wave. Higher areas of intensity are in part responsible for hot spots, which can be prevented by moving the sound head during treatment. Smaller ratios refer to a more uniform ultrasound beam (Johns, Straub, & Howard, 2007). The intensity of the beam of energy is a significant factor in determining tissue response. In general, there is greater tissue temperature elevation with higher intensities. Intensity is documented as watts per square centimeter (W/cm²). Ultrasound energy will decrease as it passes through different layers of tissue. This is related to the absorption of energy by tissue and the scattering of the beam.

To simplify, ultrasound is absorbed into tissue, causing tissue molecules to rotate and bounce, resulting in heat or nonthermal effects depending on parameter settings (frequency, intensity, continuous or pulsed, and time), treatment goals (thermal/nonthermal), and the area being treated. The duty cycle determines the overall amount of acoustic energy a patient receives and plays a role in determining tissue response (Fig. 19-5). The duty cycle (refers to pulsed or continuous) is a percentage or ratio of time that the ultrasound energy is actually being introduced into the body. A 50% duty cycle provides twice as much acoustic energy as a 25% duty cycle because the on-time is twice as long (Kollmann et al., 2005). When the sound wave is on 100%, the sound wave and energy are constant.

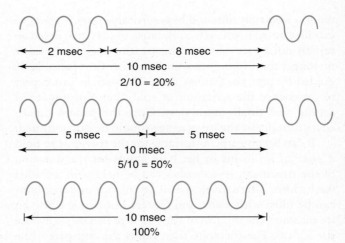

Figure 19-5 Duty cycles determine the on time of the ultrasound.

When the sound energy is turned on and off rapidly, the sound wave is pulsed and is described in terms of a ratio of the cycle. Whether to use continuous or pulsed ultrasound depends on the pathology, stage of wound healing, and the area being treated (Bracciano, 2008).

Effects on Tissue: Thermal Versus Nonthermal Ultrasound

In the thermal mode, ultrasound is a deep-heating agent capable of elevating tissue temperatures to a depth of 5 cm. Thermal effects are typically achieved with continuous sound waves (as in a 100% duty cycle). Nonthermal ultrasound exerts mechanical effects at the cellular level such as increased cellular permeability and diffusion but does not elevate tissue temperature. It typically involves delivering the ultrasound at a 20% duty cycle (on 20%, off 80% of each cycle) (Fig. 19-5). Clinicians may use ultrasound to achieve thermal or nonthermal effects and must select the effect considering a patient's given problem and the therapeutic effect that is desired. Table 19-1 summarizes the thermal and nonthermal effects of therapeutic ultrasound (Draper, 2010).

Table 19-1	Thermal and Nonthermal Effects of Therapeutic Ultrasound
Thermal Effects	**Nonthermal Effects**
• Increases extensibility of collagen fibers • Decreases muscle stiffness • Reduces muscle spasm • Alters nerve conduction velocity/diminishes pain perception • Increases metabolism and blood flow • Provides all of the effects of nonthermal ultrasound	• Increases phagocytic activity of macrophages/attracts immune cells to tissue • Increases protein synthesis • Increases capillary density • Regenerates tissue • Heals wounds

Nonthermal effects of pulsed ultrasound occur at the cell membrane because of stable cavitation, acoustic streaming, and micromassage (Apfel, 1982; Hauptmann et al., 2012). Acoustic streaming occurs with the unidirectional movement of the body fluids that cause currents that exert force and structural changes in the cell membrane along with increased permeability. Second-order effects of nonthermal ultrasound are due to the destabilization of the cellular membrane. With destabilization, more molecules are able to enter the cell and facilitate increased intercellular calcium and protein synthesis and the release of histamine. All this contributes to the enhancement of the inflammatory response to accelerate tissue healing.

Clinical Use of Ultrasound

A thorough evaluation of the patient is necessary to determine the location, stage of healing, depth, and anatomical location of the injury and the area and type of tissue to be treated. Superficial conditions, for example epicondylitis, are best treated using a frequency of 3 MHz. Deeper conditions, such as adhesive capsulitis, are better treated with a 1-MHz frequency. This will allow the ultrasound to be more effectively and efficiently absorbed into the desired tissue.

The thermal dose of the ultrasound should be set according to treatment goals. When treating subacute inflammation, the thermal effect should be mild, that is an increase in tissue temperature of approximately 1°C (1.8°F). A moderate thermal effect is used for pain modulation/altered nerve conduction velocity, muscle relaxation/stiffness, muscle spasm, and chronic inflammation. A vigorous increase in tissue temperature (approximately 4°C [7.2°F]) is used when the goal is to heat in order to stretch collagen (positional stretch, splinting, manual therapy) and increase blood flow. It is important to respect the stretching window following high intensity applications as the tissue temperature will cool approximately 2°C (3.6°F) within 5–10 minutes (Draper, 2010).

Patients should feel gentle warmth with thermal treatments. Remember that 3 MHz heats faster than 1 MHz, so treatment times will be longer (at the same intensity level) with 1 MHz in order to obtain the same desired increase in tissue temperature. Because application of the ultrasound requires a medium or lubricant between the sound head and the skin to avoid interference of the transmission from air, water immersion is appropriate for small areas when the sound head cannot lie flat (bony prominences). With water immersion, the sound head should be held approximately 0.5 cm away from and perpendicular to the area being treated. The water temperature should be warm and close to body temperature.

With application of ultrasound in general, the size of the treatment area should be limited to twice the size of the sound head. Transducer movement should cover approximately 4 cm per second using back and forth or circular strokes. The goal is to keep the face of the sound head flat. The treatment duration (time per application) and number of treatments depends on the treatment goals, size of the area treated, and the intensity, frequency, and efficacy of the modality. Preset intensities should be avoided because they will likely not be as effective in generating desired treatment outcomes and benefits of therapeutic ultrasound (Draper, 2010).

Phonophoresis

Phonophoresis is the use of ultrasound to facilitate the delivery of topically applied drugs or medication to selected tissue. Although it is used by some practitioners, there are questions as to its effectiveness because of variability in outcomes associated with inconsistent treatment parameters, such as intensity of sound waves and transmission characteristics of the conducting medium (typically hydrocortisone cream or a dexamethasone sodium phosphate sonic gel mixture). Therapists should review current literature prior to selecting phonophoresis as the treatment modality of choice (for example, see Evidence Table 19-1).

Precautions for Use of Ultrasound

Patients should be monitored during ultrasound, and any pain or discomfort may indicate that the intensity is too high or that there is an inadequate amount of gel. When using ultrasound as a thermal agent, one must follow general contraindications and precautions for any thermal modality. Safety Note 19-3 lists precautions and contraindications specific to ultrasound.

ELECTROTHERAPY

The growth of the use of electrical stimulation in recent years is due to advances in technology. Electrical stimulation is used in the clinical setting to increase muscle strength, decrease muscle spasm, decrease swelling, improve tissue healing, decrease pain, and provide an option for longer lasting analgesia. Frequently used applications include NMES, TENS, electrical stimulation for tissue repair (ESTR), FES, electrical muscle stimulation (EMS), interferential current therapy (IFC), and iontophoresis. Surface electromyography biofeedback monitors the level of electrical activity in muscles (helps determine how well somebody is able to recruit muscle activity on their own) and is often paired with NMES. The various applications will be described now, and certain clinical applications will be discussed later.

- NMES uses pulsating, alternating current to activate muscles through stimulation of intact peripheral nerves to cause a motor response. Stimulation of the nerve is used to decrease muscle spasm, to strengthen muscle,

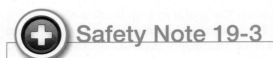

Safety Note 19-3

Ultrasound

Precautions

- Unhealed fracture sites
- Early stages of tendon or ligament repair
- Marked demineralization/osteoporosis
- Plastic and metal implants
- When using phonophoresis, be aware of drug allergies

Contraindications

- Suspected deep vein thrombophlebitis
- Bleeding and edema; areas with tendency to hemorrhage
- Where sensation is reduced or if a person cannot report heat sensations accurately
- In the very old and very young, because of compromised body temperature regulation
- Skin or lymphatic cancers; tumors or malignancies
- Over a cardiac pacemaker or surrounding adjacent tissue
- Pregnancy
- Infected areas
- Epiphyses of growing bone (high intensity, needs to be less than 1.0 W/cm²)
- In conjunction with radium or radioactive isotopes treatment for cancer within 6 months
- Over the heart, eyes, or testes
- Over carotid sinus and cervical ganglion
- Over the spinal column or where there is inadequate protection over the spinal cord, such as after laminectomy

Adapted from Draper, D. (2010). *Syllabus for enhancing treatment outcomes with therapeutic modalities: Electrotherapy and ultrasound.* Brentwood, TN: Cross country Education; Sicard-Rosenbaum, L., Lord, D., & Danoff, J. (1995). Effects of continuous therapeutic ultrasound growth and metastasis of subcutaneous murine tumors. *Physical Therapy, 75*, 3–13.

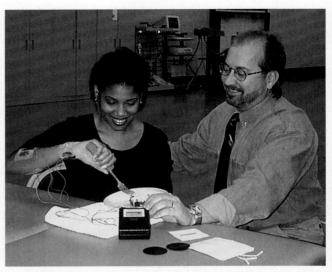

Figure 19-6 FES for the extrinsic finger flexor and extensor muscle groups to facilitate grasp for self-feeding.

and fibrosis of the fibers. EMS facilitates nerve regeneration and muscle reinnervation.

- IFC utilizes two channels (four electrodes placed in a vector pattern) simultaneously with different frequencies. This allows for a more comfortable surface and deeper tissue penetration to help with pain reduction and edema management.
- Iontophoresis is the use of low-voltage direct current to ionize topically applied medication into the tissue. Iontophoresis is often used in the treatment of inflammatory conditions or for scar formation and management.
- ESTR, also known as high-voltage galvanic stimulation, has been used for tissue healing. Because of its complexity, use requires highly advanced training, and therefore it is not reviewed in this chapter.

Principles of Electricity

To use electrotherapy in occupational therapy practice, clinicians need working knowledge of the principles of current, duration, frequency, duty cycle, and current modulation and ramp time.

Current

Electric current is the movement of ions or electrons, which are charged particles, from one point to another to equalize the charge. Current, measured in amperes, occurs when there is an imbalance in the number of electrons in two distinct locations. Voltage is the potential or electromotive force that drives the current and is measured in volts. Current flows from an area of high electron concentration (cathode, or negative pole) to an area of less concentration (anode, or positive pole). Opposition or resistance to current flow is measured in ohms. Ohm's law states that

and to cause muscle pumping that can reduce edema. NMES stimulation applied directly to innervated muscle is used for muscle reeducation and to prevent atrophy.

- FES is electrical stimulation used to activate targeted muscle groups for orthotic substitution or to facilitate performance of functional activities or movements (Fig. 19-6). FES is often used with individuals who have shoulder subluxation or foot drop after a stroke (see Evidence Table 19-1).
- TENS operates on the gate theory (to be discussed later in this chapter) and describes the wide variety of stimulators used for pain control. TENS uses surface electrodes placed strategically over regions of pain to stimulate specific afferent nerve fibers with the goal of sensory analgesia rather than a motor response.
- EMS is electrical stimulation of denervated muscle to facilitate viability and to prevent atrophy, degeneration,

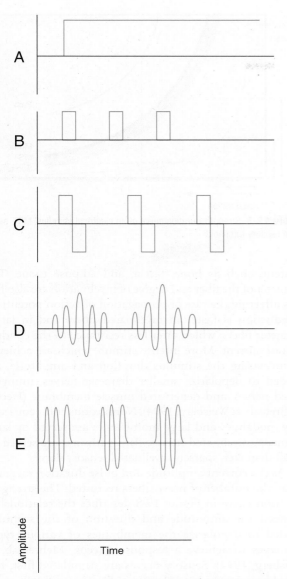

Figure 19-7 Commonly used electrotherapeutic current wave forms. **A.** Direct current. **B.** Monophasic pulsed. **C.** Biphasic pulsed. **D.** Interferential beats. **E.** Russian bursts.

voltage (*V*) is proportional to both current (*I*) and resistance (*R*), such that $V = I \times R$. Three specific forms of current: direct current (DC), alternating current (AC), and pulsatile current, are used in clinical applications (Fig. 19-7).

Direct Current. Direct current (DC) is unidirectional, with the electrons moving continuously in one direction, and the electrodes maintaining their polarity. DC flow, characterized by the square wave, can cause chemical reactions in the body and facilitate the ionization of medication through the skin (iontophoresis).

Alternating Current. Alternating current (AC) is characterized by periodic changes in the polarity of the current flow

(sinusoidal wave form). The current is uninterrupted and bidirectional, without any true positive or negative pole. Household electricity uses AC.

Pulsed Current. Pulsed current is the term used when the electron flow is periodically interrupted for very short periods of milliseconds or microseconds. These interrupted currents can flow in one phase (monophasic), two phases (biphasic), or in many phases (polyphasic). Most current modulation output is pulsed DC or continuous repetitive series of AC pulses.

- Monophasic waveforms have a single phase to each pulse, with the current flow being unidirectional and either negative or positive.
- Biphasic currents have two opposing phases in a single pulse, and the current flows in both directions.
- Polyphasic waveforms consist of a burst of three or more phases, a series of pulses delivered as a single charge. IFC and Russian NMES currents are examples of polyphasic waveforms. There have been many claims as to the uniqueness of this type of current, although there are no confirmed physiological advantages to this type of waveform.

Duration

For monophasic current, phase and pulse duration are synonymous and refer to the length of time between the beginning and end of one phase of the pulse. For biphasic currents, the pulse duration is equal to the total of the two phase durations, including the intrapulse interval. As pulse width increases, more muscle fibers are stimulated because the current is available for longer periods of time. Short pulses are less than 150 microseconds, and longer durations are greater than 200 microseconds. A narrow pulse width is typically better for pain control (Draper, 2010).

Stimulus Frequency

The number of pulses or wave forms repeated at regular intervals is the pulse or stimulus frequency. The pulse frequency consists of the number of cycles or pulses per second (pps) delivered to the body. Low frequency is less than 1,000 pps, and high frequency is greater than 10,000 pps. Low frequency is typically used for pain management, but skin resistance may require higher intensities. Frequency controls the strength of the muscle contraction (number of motor units being stimulated in the muscle) and relative recovery time before the muscle can be stimulated again. The higher the intensity and frequency of pulses, the stronger the muscle contraction will be.

Duty Cycle

Duty cycle is the proportion of time between the stimulation period and the rest period. That is, it is the ratio of the time the current is on to the time the current is off. For example, a treatment protocol in which electrical stimuli are delivered for 10 seconds followed by a 50-second off period is expressed as a 1:5 duty cycle. Duty cycle is important in determining muscle fatigue because muscles need recovery time. As the patient's condition improves, the duty cycle can be gradually increased so that the stimulus delivery is a greater proportion of the duty cycle.

Current Modulation and Ramp Time

Changes to the current or to the pulse characteristics are referred to as modulation. Current can be modulated by modifying the frequency, amplitude (intensity), or duration. Ramping is a change of the pulse intensity or duration of the current. Ramp time is the time required for successive current stimuli to reach the desired amplitude and plateau. Ramp-down, the gradual decrease of the intensity, describes the movement of the peak amplitude back to zero. Ramp time is important for muscle comfort during recruitment of fibers, contraction time, and recovery time. A gradual ramp is usually more comfortable and effective with general strengthening applications, but a steep ramp may be necessary when the desired plateau needs to be accomplished more quickly with functional activities.

Physiology of Nerve and Muscle Excitation

In addition to a working knowledge of electrical principles, clinicians using electrotherapy must understand the physiology of nerve and muscle excitation. The application of electrical current causes physiological changes at both a local and a cellular level; these changes can occur segmentally or systemically. The application of electrical current modifies the body's physiological response and has physiochemical effects (Hess, Howard, & Attignger, 2000).

Human tissue is either excitable or nonexcitable. Excitable tissues, such as nerves and muscles, can initiate and propagate an action potential if the stimulation parameters are sufficient. Stimuli must be sufficiently intense and last long enough to cause the ions to shift across the resting cell membrane to depolarize the cell. Depolarization of a neural or muscle cell occurs quickly, and the sudden alteration in the cell membrane's electrical potential is known as an action potential. Action potentials are an all-or-none occurrence and, once started, are carried along the cell membrane to depolarize it. Following depolarization, a period of hyperpolarization occurs, making the cell briefly unable to be stimulated.

Following stimulation and generation of an action potential in a nerve cell membrane, the membrane needs a short period to recover its excitability. This recovery time is known as the absolute refractory period.

Propagation

Tissues with high water content, such as muscle and nerve, transmit electricity better than those with lower water

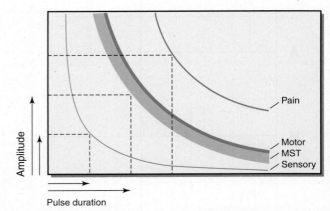

Figure 19-8 Strength-duration curve of an electrical stimulus. MST, maximum sensory threshold.

content, such as bone, fascia, and adipose tissue. The diameter of the fiber and degree of myelination are also factors affecting the rate of propagation of action potentials. Conduction is faster in myelinated fibers and in large-diameter fibers, which offer less resistance to the conduction of current. More intense stimuli, which are achieved by increasing the stimulus duration and amplitude, are needed to depolarize smaller diameter nerves, unmyelinated nerves, and denervated muscle membrane (Hecox, Mehreteab, & Weisberg, 1994). Nonnoxious cutaneous sensory modalities and large motor units are served by large diameter, myelinated nerves. Pain pathways are served by small-diameter, sparsely myelinated sensory nerves.

As the current amplitude and pulse duration increase, so do the number of nerve fibers recruited. The strength-duration curve in Figure 19-8 describes the relationship between the amplitude and duration of the stimulus needed to depolarize the membranes of various types of nerves to achieve a response (Hecox, Mehreteab, & Weisberg, 1994). Sensory nerves are stimulated first, followed by motor nerves, then pain fibers, and finally muscle fibers. Although pain fibers are superficial in relation to motor nerves, they also have a smaller diameter and a greater resistance to electrical current flow.

When the cell membrane or tissue receives an unchanging stimulus over time, the cell membrane begins to adapt to the stimulus and requires higher levels of stimulation to trigger an action potential; this is termed accommodation.

Electrically Stimulated Movement

The diameter of the nerve, depth of the nerve, and duration of the pulse affect a nerve's response to electrical stimulation (Baker, Bowman, & McNeal, 1988; Bennie et al., 2002). If there is sufficient intensity of electrical stimulation to cause the motor nerve to reach threshold, contraction of all muscle fibers attached to that nerve (motor unit) occurs. If the stimulus frequency is sufficient, the muscle twitch contractions become fused in synchronous rapid succession, and the contraction becomes tetanic, leading to a complete contraction of the muscle and movement at the specified joint. In a voluntary contraction, smaller motor units are recruited first, followed by the larger motor units as contraction strength increases. This gradual, asynchronous sequence allows for fine motor control, with larger fibers recruited as increased strength or speed is needed. This type of recruitment allows smooth, controlled movement. In electrically stimulated movement patterns, however, the reverse occurs, with larger motor units recruited first in a synchronous pattern. This causes electrically stimulated muscle to fatigue more rapidly and limits the finely controlled quality of functional movement.

Treatment Planning Specific to Electrotherapy

Before incorporating electrotherapy into treatment, clinicians make decisions about the type of electrical stimulator to use and placement and size of electrodes.

Parameters of Electrical Stimulation Devices

Because research has been equivocal, the clinician must critically evaluate the claims made for various outcomes of electrotherapeutic interventions. Prior to use, the therapist should be familiar with the specific capabilities of the available stimulators and their stimulation parameters (types of current offered, frequencies, intensities, treatment guidelines, etc.).

Electrodes

Electrodes are the contact point providing the current flow from the stimulation device to the body. The electrode interfaces with the skin surface at the point where the electron–ion conversion occurs. Electrodes should offer little resistance to the current flow. A variety of electrodes are commercially available (see Resources 19-1). Commonly used electrodes include carbon-rubber electrodes, which are silicon rubber impregnated with small

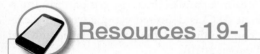 Resources 19-1

Physical Agent Modalities and Biofeedback Equipment Vendors

Allegro Medical

www.allegromedical.com
Phone: 800-861-3211
Electrotherapy, ultrasound, and biofeedback machines and supplies; cold and hot packs; paraffin units

Amrex Electrotherapy Equipment

www.amrexusa.com
Phone: 800-221-9069
Electrotherapy and ultrasound machines and supplies

Chattanooga Medical Supply, Inc.

www.chattmed.com
Phone: 423-870-9030
Electrotherapy, ultrasound, biofeedback, and Fluidotherapy® machines and supplies; cold and hot packs; paraffin units

Comfort Technologies, Inc.

www.comforttechnologies.com
Phone: 800-321-STIM (7846)
TENS units

Dynatronics

www.dynatronics.com
Phone: 800-874-6251
Electrotherapy/iontophoresis, ultrasound, biofeedback and fluidotherapy machines and supplies; cold and hot packs; paraffin units

Empi, Inc.

www.empi.com
Phone: 800-328-2536
Electrotherapy machines and supplies

Mettler Electronics Corp.

www.mettlerelectronics.com
Phone: 800-854-9305
Electrotherapy and ultrasound machines and supplies; cold and hot packs

North Coast Medical

www.ncmedical.com
Phone: 800-821-9319
Electrotherapy/iontophoresis, ultrasound, and fluidotherapy machines and supplies; cold and hot packs; paraffin units

Patterson Medical

www.pattersonmedical.com
Phone: 800-343-9742
Electrotherapy/iontophoresis, ultrasound, biofeedback and fluidotherapy machines and supplies; cold and hot packs; paraffin units

carbon particles; metal- or foil-backed electrodes; sponges over metal plates; and self-adherent polymer electrodes (Draper, 2010). The self-adhering electrodes may be reusable and do not require strapping or taping, making them convenient to use. Full contact with the skin is crucial, which is facilitated by use of electrode gel.

Electrodes should be examined before each use and changed when necessary. Electrodes degrade with use and become unable to conduct the current efficiently. Therapists should look for cracking and worn spots in the carbon-rubber electrodes or excessive dryness in self-adhering electrodes and replace them as needed. With frequent use, carbon-rubber electrodes may develop non-conductive areas because of the absorption of dirt, skin oil, or electrode gel and depletion of the carbon rubber. This may cause "hot spots," areas of high current density that may be uncomfortable for the patient and cause skin burns. When uneven conductivity causes a biting or stinging sensation during electrical stimulation, the electrodes should be replaced.

Regardless of the type of electrode used, it is necessary to prevent skin irritation or breakdown. This factor becomes critically important for patients who are using the stimulators on a home program or when there is prolonged placement and use of the electrodes.

Electrode Size. Current density is inversely related to the electrode size. As the electrode size decreases or the contact area of the electrode decreases, the current density increases, which can cause hot spots, as mentioned earlier. As the current density increases, there is a greater perception of the stimulation beneath the electrode along with a greater physiological response because of the charge transfer. The inverse relationship between electrode size and current density means that smaller electrodes require less current to stimulate tissue. Electrode size is therefore determined by the size of the targeted tissue.

Electrode Placement. The distance between the electrodes also influences the depth of the current flow. When the electrodes are close together, the current passes superficially, and when the electrodes are farther apart, the current penetrates deeper. Care should be taken when applying and selecting location of the electrodes because closely spaced electrodes may increase discomfort. Size of electrodes must also be considered when stimulating muscles. Small electrodes can be used to obtain an isolated contraction from smaller muscles, such as those of the hand. Larger electrodes are less specific in stimulating isolated muscles.

There are three primary methods of electrode placement for electrical stimulation: monopolar, bipolar, and quadripolar. Simply put, the terms identify whether one electrode (monopolar) is placed over the targeted tissue or if all electrodes (bipolar and quadripolar) are placed over the area. The monopolar technique uses one stimulating (active) electrode, which is placed over the targeted area. The other (dispersive) electrode completes the electrical circuit and can be placed away from the target area in the same region. The dispersive electrode is often larger, minimizing the current density and perception of sensory stimulation. Monopolar placement is used for iontophoresis, acupuncture, and trigger point stimulation.

The bipolar technique consists of both electrodes placed over the targeted area. Because both electrodes or sides of the circuit are in contact with the targeted area, the current flow is more local, and the stimulation is perceived under both electrodes. Most often, the electrodes are the same size, and this technique can be used to stimulate muscle contraction. Bipolar techniques are often used to activate muscles atrophied because of disuse, for muscle reeducation, or to obtain stronger contraction (neuromuscular facilitation) to increase limited movement.

Quadripolar placement refers to two sets of electrodes, each from its own channel. Electrodes generally surround the targeted area in a parallel or criss-cross pattern. Interferential current (IFC) is delivered via quadripolar placement and is commonly used for pain management and circulation (Draper, 2010).

Clinical Use of Electrotherapy

The unique applications and indications for each type of electrotherapy are discussed in turn. Safety Note 19-4 lists precautions and contraindications for electrotherapy.

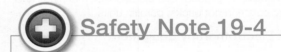

Safety Note 19-4

Electrotherapy

Precautions

- Monitor patients with epilepsy
- When used in or around healing tissue, avoid muscle contraction
- When using iontophoresis, be aware of drug allergies
- Where sensation is reduced
- Pregnancy
- Early stages of tendon repair or tenolysis

Contraindications

- Cardiac pacemaker
- Active cancer/tumor
- Transcerebral, transcranial, or transthoracic stimulation
- Danger of hemorrhage immediately following injury
- Overdamaged or denuded skin

Adapted from Draper, D. (2010). *Syllabus for enhancing treatment outcomes with therapeutic modalities: Electrotherapy and ultrasound.* Brentwood, TN: Cross Country Education.

Electrical Stimulation. Electricity has been advocated in the treatment of a variety of body systems and for a plethora of conditions, including joint swelling and inflammation, joint dysfunction, tissue healing, muscle reeducation, circulatory disorders, postural disorders, fracture healing, and pain management. There are a number of claims for electrical stimulation along with a variety of protocols and applications; some are objective, but many are unsubstantiated or anecdotal. The clinician should take a systematic and objective approach to the use of electrical stimulation.

Neuromuscular Electrical Stimulation. NMES has a variety of clinical uses as an adjunct to occupational therapy treatment. NMES is the electrical stimulation of an intact or partially intact peripheral nerve to evoke a muscle contraction (Bracciano, 2008). NMES is often erroneously referred to as "functional" electrical stimulation. Functional electrical stimulation, or FES, is a subcategory of NMES and refers to the use of NMES as a substitute for an orthosis to assist with a functional activity, such as standing or holding an object, or as a substitute for a sling.

NMES can be used for strengthening and endurance, ROM, facilitation of muscle function, management of muscle spasms and spasticity, edema reduction, and orthotic substitution (Cahe, Yu, & Walker, 2004). Clinical use of NMES requires a partially intact or intact peripheral nerve, and its use with primary muscle disease or muscular dystrophy is unwarranted.

Maintain Muscle Mass. NMES can be a successful adjunct to conventional treatment in individuals with limited traumatic or orthopedic injuries. There is a relationship between intensity and strength gains; improving muscle strength is based in part on the overload principle. The overload principle refers to the fact that the body must be subjected to greater levels of stress than it is accustomed to for strength gains to occur. To accomplish this, the therapist must increase the load, frequency, or duration of the exercise or activity. Patients who are deconditioned or have areas of weakness may benefit from NMES to improve endurance of the targeted muscle. Isometric strengthening using NMES produces better results than conventional isometric exercises alone but is most effective when paired with functional goals and movements (Baker et al., 2000).

Maintain or Gain Range of Motion. Neurologically impaired patients often develop spasticity as a consequence of their injury. Hemiplegic patients with chronic moderate spasticity in the wrist or finger flexors may be appropriate candidates for this intervention (Rosewilliam et al., 2012). For these individuals, the stimulus applied to the antagonist muscle should ramp up slowly and be sufficiently intense to allow for a slow stretch without increasing spasticity caused by a quick stretch or jerk (Baker et al., 2000). Ramp-up times should be extended to 6–8 seconds or

longer. Proper positioning or blocking of other muscles should be considered. Serial casting or splinting of the extremity can be an effective adjunct to NMES. The use of NMES is effective as part of a home program because it allows the caregiver to carry out passive ROM several times daily.

For the orthopedic patient, ROM may be limited by contractures secondary to immobilization or pain. NMES may be used to improve joint ROM if the limitation is due to intrinsic soft tissue shortening as opposed to a bony block or biomechanical limitation. The technique should maintain a low-intensity stretch for a few seconds.

Management of Spasticity. The effectiveness of NMES for the treatment of spasticity depends in part on the underlying disease causing the spasticity. The response of NMES in a patient with a spastic spinal cord injury may be different from the response in a patient with a brain injury or multiple sclerosis. The variability of abnormal tone may only result in a temporary interruption of the motor neuron excitability, with short-term treatment effects. Stimulation of a spastic muscle in the neurologically impaired client using high frequency pulses causes a tetanic response that fatigues the muscle (Vodovnik, Bowman, & Hufford, 1984).

NMES also affects spasticity by stimulating the muscle antagonistic to the spastic muscle, which inhibits the spastic muscle, allowing ROM exercise (Sabut et al., 2011; Wang, Tsai, & Chan, 1998). Heat or ice and serial casting or splinting paired with functional movements and activities may enhance the therapeutic response.

Orthopedic patients may have pain–spasm cycles caused by local spasm of a particular muscle or group. Decreasing the pain–spasm cycle through the application of NMES to the area improves and enhances ROM and occupational performance.

Facilitate Voluntary Control. NMES has been used frequently for muscle reeducation and facilitation, particularly with neurological injuries and orthopedic injuries after surgery. Facilitation and retraining can be effective for patients suffering from disuse atrophy, muscle weakness, and pain (Lewek, Stevens, & Snyder-Maackler, 2001). In neurologically involved patients, the sensory feedback loop becomes distorted or impaired.

The goal of NMES for facilitation and reeducation is to incorporate the stimulation with voluntary contraction, functional movement and activity, and sensory feedback (Bracciano, 2008). The intent of NMES for facilitation and reeducation is to flood the central nervous system with sensory and kinesthetic information linked to an anticipated motor response. A variety of functional activities incorporating the desired motor response should be used to ensure adequate carryover of the response. For example, a patient who has had a stroke who is working on grasp and release should practice a meaningful activity that requires picking up and placing a variety of objects of various shapes, sizes, and weights to various heights and locations.

Functional Electrical Stimulation. FES, the use of NMES as a replacement for orthoses, has been an effective adjunct in facilitating occupational function, most notably positional stability and mobility. Stimulation of innervated paretic or paralyzed muscles can decrease dependence on slings, splints, or other orthoses through the development of increased strength and endurance of the paretic musculature.

FES has been effectively used with hemiparetic patients who display shoulder subluxation during the flaccid phase of recovery and also to facilitate grasp-and-release activities (Thrasher et al., 2008). In the hemiplegic patient, gravity stresses the shoulder capsule, stretching it. When muscle tone and voluntary control develop at the shoulder, normal glenohumeral alignment may not recur when the arm is at rest because of this ligamentous laxity (Yu et al., 2001). Slings may be helpful to establish glenohumeral alignment, but stimulation of the posterior deltoid and supraspinatus muscles may be more effective in improving normal shoulder integrity (Koyuncu et al., 2010; Lin, Granat, & Lees, 1999; Wang, Chan, & Tsai, 2000). Use of FES for maintaining shoulder integrity can be an effective adjunct to splinting and facilitate occupational function. Clearly outlining and teaching the client and caregivers in a home program is vital to ensure continuity and carryover.

Transcutaneous Electrical Nerve Stimulation. Pain is one of the most common complaints that cause patients to seek medical care. Adequate pain management facilitates occupational function (Fig. 19-9). TENS can be used to manage pain in musculoskeletal disorders. The two primary theories on which the modulation of pain with TENS is based are the gate control theory (Melzack & Wall, 1965; Robertson et al., 2006) and the endorphin theory (Bonica, 1990). Basically described, the gate theory is the stimulation of afferent nerves to block pain by closing the gate in the spinal column to pain signals coming from slower conducting nerves. The endorphin theory specifies that natural beta endorphins are released with the application of intense beat frequency of TENS that inhibits pain signal transmission and decreases chemical irritants in the central nervous system (Draper, 2010).

Treatment applications using electrical stimulation for pain control employ pulsed or alternating current in a variety of stimulation patterns. The type of stimulation is based on the neurological response to the stimulation with the goal being pain relief and comfort. The four levels of stimulation used include subsensory level, sensory level, motor level, and noxious level. Stimulation sites

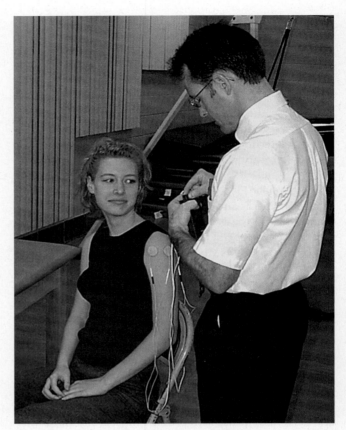

Figure 19-9 Application of transcutaneous electrical nerve stimulation (TENS) to the shoulder for acute pain.

for electrode placement are based on the problem areas. Optimal electrode placements should correlate with the structures and sources of pain and include motor points, trigger points, and acupuncture points. TENS units are often used at home, and the therapist should explain the purpose of the equipment and instruct the patient in its operations and precautions, with written and pictorial instructions. Through application of TENS for sensory analgesia, the patient may better perform functional activities and movements that foster independence and function because they are in less pain.

Iontophoresis. Iontophoresis is a method of topically delivering a medication or ionized drug to an area of tissue by using direct electrical current. Occupational therapists frequently use iontophoresis in the treatment of inflammatory conditions such as epicondylitis, carpal tunnel syndrome, glenohumeral bursitis, ulnar nerve inflammation, and wrist tendinitis and tenosynovitis (see Evidence Table 19-1). Therapists using iontophoresis should thoroughly understand the pathophysiology of the condition, the tissue healing process, the medications being used, and any potential drug interactions. *Safety Message: Caution must be used whenever using iontophoresis because medications may cause an allergic or* *anaphylactic reaction, which is a life-threatening condition and medical emergency. Patients should always be asked for a list of current medications and whether they have any known allergies, sensitivities, or reactions to foods or medications.* Documented orders should always be obtained from the patient's physician prior to using iontophoresis (Bracciano, 2008).

SURFACE ELECTROMYOGRAPHIC BIOFEEDBACK

Feedback is an important element in motor learning (Molier et al., 2011). Occupational therapists often use verbal feedback to provide encouragement and direction to patients who are performing a task. For example, the therapist may comment on the speed or accuracy of a feeding task and offer suggestions to improve functional outcomes, such as, "Good, you got the spoon to your lips without dropping anything. Now open your mouth wider." This type of therapeutic feedback is beneficial in rehabilitation, but it is limited by the therapist's ability to comment only on a result that has already occurred ("Good, you got the spoon to your lips without dropping anything.") or a result that the therapist hopes will occur next ("Now open your mouth wider.").

Biofeedback—which means biological feedback—refers to the process of using instrumentation to feed back to the patient immediate information about what the body is doing. Feedback is provided to the patient before the patient is even consciously aware of the body's action. This allows the patient to make small alterations in body functions *during* performance in order to improve the actual functional outcome. When occupational therapists use biofeedback technology, they most commonly use surface electromyographic biofeedback. This type of biofeedback helps make the patient more aware of muscle activation and is used for muscle reeducation and training. When the term "biofeedback" is used in this chapter, the authors are referring to surface electromyographic biofeedback. Biofeedback has been used to treat urinary incontinence (Herderschee et al., 2011), motor dysfunction and spasticity following stroke (Dogan-Aslan et al., 2012; Woodford & Price, 2007), chronic pain (Babu et al., 2007) (see Evidence Table 19-1), muscle dysfunction and myoclonus following spinal cord injury (De Biase et al., 2011; Sugimoto et al., 2007), focal hand dystonia (Byl, Archer, & McKenzie, 2009), and motor dysfunction in children with cerebral palsy (Bolek, 2006).

In biofeedback, small electrodes are attached to the patient's skin to detect the tiny electrical signals that are generated when skeletal muscle contracts. When the onset of a muscle contraction is detected, the biofeedback unit will alert the patient with, typically, an auditory or visual stimulus. As the muscle contraction progresses and strengthens, the auditory tone will become louder, and the visual display will become larger. Because electrical signals from skeletal muscle are detected as soon as motor units are recruited in the target muscle—before movement even occurs—biofeedback provides the patient with immediate information about desired or unwanted muscle activity.

In patients with motor dysfunction who need to relearn voluntary control over impaired muscles, biofeedback provides an early signal to the patient that his current muscle activity is either leading to the desired movement or not. The patient can then try to improve the effectiveness of muscular effort *during* activity. If a patient's arm is paralyzed, biofeedback is the only way to inform the patient who is trying to move that appropriate muscle motor units are being recruited, even if no movement in the arm can be seen yet. When chronic pain is a result of unconscious forceful or prolonged muscle contraction, biofeedback can signal the patient to relax those muscles.

Biofeedback Equipment

Biofeedback units have three major components to detect, measure, and report activity in the body: the transducer, the processing unit, and the output mechanism. The transducer is what detects the target activity in the body. In surface electromyographic biofeedback, the transducers are electrodes attached to the patient's skin to detect muscle contraction. The electrodes are placed over the muscle belly and aligned parallel to the muscle's line of pull. The electrodes are spaced according to the goal of treatment but must always stay within the margins of the target muscle. Widely spaced electrodes pick up signals from a wider area of the muscle and should be used initially to reeducate a weak muscle. If the goal is to reduce spasticity, placing the electrodes more closely together will reduce the pickup area and make it easier for the patient to relax the muscle enough to influence the biofeedback system (see Procedures for Practice 19-2 and 19-3) .

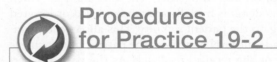

Procedures for Practice 19-2

Electromyography Biofeedback Session for Muscle Reeducation

- Begin with large, widely spaced electrodes over the muscle belly.
- Initially set the threshold at an attainable level.
- During a 10- to 15-minute treatment session, the patient voluntarily contracts the muscle to reach the threshold level.
- When possible, incorporate purposeful activities to facilitate the muscle activity desired.
- Gradually raise the threshold during the treatment session to challenge the patient to contract the muscle more strongly.

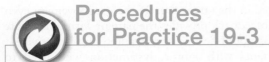

Procedures for Practice 19-3

Electromyography Biofeedback Session to Decrease Spasticity

- Begin with small, closely spaced electrodes over the muscle belly.
- Initially set the threshold at an attainable level.
- Place the limb in midrange, and keep the environment free of distractions.
- During a 10- to 15-minute treatment session, the patient attempts to maintain relaxation of the muscle below the threshold level.
- Gradually decrease the threshold as the patient learns to relax the muscle.
- In subsequent sessions, challenge the patient to maintain relaxation of the spastic muscle while contracting the antagonistic group and then while performing a functional task.

The processing unit contains electrical circuits that amplify, integrate, and otherwise prepare the messages from the electrodes for an output signal. Biofeedback units in occupational therapy departments generally have output mechanisms that give off visual, auditory, or both types of feedback. The processing unit will send a signal for visual or auditory output once a certain amount of electrode messages are received. As more motor units fire and more messages are received, more electricity flows through the circuits. When more electricity flows through the circuit, the processing unit will send a signal to increase the visual or auditory output. If the number of electrode messages is reduced, the signal for output will reduce or stop altogether. The threshold at which the output signal is initially set can be raised or lowered depending on the patient's ability. This allows the therapist to grade the level of activity the patient must achieve before he or she receives feedback. As the patient's performance improves, the threshold is set higher so that an output response is not obtained until more input signals are received. If the goal is muscle inhibition, the threshold is set so that the device will deliver the feedback response when the level of motor activity decreases below the specific setting.

Biofeedback units come in the form of small handheld devices, as well as larger units attached to video display screens. In small units, the visual output may be as simple as a red dot that turns on when an electrode signal is first detected—signaling muscle firing in the targeted muscle. The red dot might then turn into a red line that grows longer if the electrode detects more muscle firing. Audio output on handheld devices will likely be a soft "beep" that grows louder or faster as muscle firing is increased. Larger biofeedback units often come with interesting graphic visual displays and auditory tones that respond to muscle activity. On larger units, multiple electrodes can be used to simultaneously gather information about muscle activity in different areas. These multichannel units can provide a variety of visual and auditory stimuli that can be programmed in the form of a video game with sound. Some biofeedback instruments can be connected to radios, DVD players, electronic toys, etc., which provide the feedback reward for achieved muscle activity or relaxation. For example, if the patient achieves muscle inhibition to a certain preset level, his audiobook player will turn on and stay on as long as the inhibition is maintained.

Some biofeedback equipment can be synchronized with NMES to increase motor unit recruitment and movement. Biofeedback paired with NMES can be used for patients who are, for example, unable to fully complete a movement through full desired ROM. The therapist can set the threshold so that the patient receives auditory and visual feedback with activation of a selected muscle, which, when achieved, activates the NMES to complete the movement, thereby reinforcing and strengthening the response (Pullman et al., 2000; Seo et al., 2005).

Incorporating Biofeedback into the Occupational Therapy Treatment Plan

When choosing a therapy intervention for a patient, it is important to choose wisely for a successful outcome. Successful biofeedback treatment requires that the patient be able to understand the relationship between his effort and the feedback. Additionally, patients with some visible movement tend to do better with biofeedback than patients who are completely flaccid, and patients who have less spasticity tend to do better than those who are severely spastic. However, biofeedback success is not dependent on the age or sex of the patient, the side affected by injury, or the duration of injury. Biofeedback can be successful when used with both peripheral and central nervous system injuries (Bloom, Przekop, & Sanger, 2010; Vedsted et al., 2011). Because biofeedback is essentially a learning process, if the patient fails to benefit after just one session, another session is justified.

Biofeedback treatments should be conducted in a quiet environment so that the patient can concentrate on his muscle activity and the biofeedback unit's response without distraction. The first session should start with an orientation and a trial run with the biofeedback unit. The trial, using an intact limb, allows the patient to understand how muscular contractions influence the equipment's audio or visual feedback. Then the electrodes are placed over target muscle(s) in the dysfunctional extremity or area. The feedback unit is set so that no signal is produced with the baseline level of muscle activity present in the target muscles. The threshold level is then set by the therapist so that the patient must achieve that preset level of muscle contraction or relaxation to receive the feedback signal. The patient then attempts to relax or contract the target muscle (depending on the goal). Biofeedback treatment sessions are generally about 15 minutes (see Procedures for Practice 19-2 and 19-3).

Biofeedback is motivating for patients because they are provided instantaneous feedback in the form of visual and auditory modes. As the patient gains some control over target muscles, occupational therapy sessions should incorporate simple functional tasks and activities to reinforce the muscular contractions (or relaxation) relearned with biofeedback. As muscle function continues to improve, more complex movement patterns can be added to the therapy program. As with all physical modalities used in occupational therapy, biofeedback is to be performed in preparation for or concurrently with purposeful and occupation-based activities. The goal is always eventual engagement in occupation.

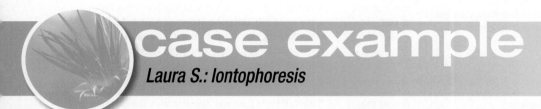

case example
Laura S.: Iontophoresis

Occupational Therapy Intervention Process	Clinical Reasoning Process	
	Objectives	Examples of Therapist's Internal Dialogue
Patient Information Laura S. is an active, and athletic, 47-year-old female who was referred to occupational therapy by her family physician. She relates that she was "painting her kitchen and family room" in the "new house" they recently purchased. After three days of painting, she developed pain in her right elbow (dominant hand), increasing inability to hold onto objects such as a gallon of milk, and further difficulty with cooking and self-care activities requiring her to use her right hand in static hold positions. She reports the pain being "constant 5 out of 10" and increasing to "8 out of 10" with use. The patient displayed pain on the lateral epicondyle with resisted wrist extension. Patient also displays point tenderness over the right lateral epicondyle. Grip strength is significantly decreased in the right hand (20 pounds) compared to her left hand (80 pounds). The patient also displays an extension lag at the elbow of 25° and lacks full elbow flexion by 20° (pain in both end ranges).	Appreciate the context	"It seems that Laura's signs and symptoms are consistent with a diagnosis of lateral epicondylitis. Her symptoms developed quickly after 3 days of repetitive use of the right upper extremity to paint her house."
	Develop intervention hypotheses	"Because of the rapidity with which her symptoms developed, the quick referral by her physician, and the lack of previous difficulties in her right upper extremity, Laura's condition is considered an acute episode. I know that the root cause of lateral epicondylitis is tendinosis—a degeneration of the tendon fibers. However, right now, Laura's elbow is inflamed and painful—a true epicondylitis. I believe that she will require a multifaceted approach to treat her condition. We will first need to reduce her inflammation and pain, and then we need to strengthen her muscles and tendons to reduce the likelihood of a recurrence in the future."
	Select an intervention approach	"Laura's problems and clinical presentation are consistent with a diagnosis of acute lateral epicondylitis. I expect that her physician will recommend some form of nonsteroidal anti-inflammatory drugs (NSAIDs) or other anti-inflammatory medications. I will be recommending static splinting of the right wrist in 30° of extension, physical agent modalities to reduce her inflammation and pain, gentle range of motion (ROM)/stretching, and modification of her daily activities until her pain and inflammation subside. Then I will introduce gradual strengthening of the upper extremity starting with isometrics and then progressing to concentric and eccentric strengthening exercises."
	Reflect on competence	"I am familiar with a number of therapeutic approaches that can be used with lateral epicondylitis. I have advanced training in iontophoresis and am permitted to use it by my state's practice act. I will need to consistently monitor Laura's response to the interventions used and modify the treatment as needed. I will also want to monitor her compliance with the splint wearing schedule and modifications to her daily routine to prevent further exacerbation of her condition."

Recommendations

The occupational therapist recommended three treatment sessions per week for 4 weeks. The following initial goals were established:

In 1 week, Laura will report:

1. Understanding of and use of activities of daily living (ADL) modification techniques to reduce stress on her elbow
2. Compliance with her splinting program

In 2 weeks, Laura will report:

1. Decreased pain at the right elbow during rest from a score of 5 out of 10 to a score of 1 out of 10
2. Decreased pain at the right elbow during daily activities from a score of 8 out of 10 to one of 3 out of 10

In 2 weeks, Laura will demonstrate

1. 25° improved elbow extension
2. 20° improve elbow flexion

Consider the patient's appraisal of performance	"From the beginning, it was apparent that Laura would follow through on all recommendations. She is highly motivated and has been very active and participated in a number of athletic activities prior to her injury. Because her children are older, I am confident that she could ask her family members to help her with those activities that require heavy lifting or static hold and release patterns. She is anxious to return to her premorbid activities, and there is a slight concern that she might 'overdo it' as she progresses in treatment and her pain begins to subside. I will ask her to come for therapy three times weekly to closely monitor and upgrade her program."
Consider what will occur in therapy, how often, and for how long	
Ascertain the patient's endorsement of plan	"Laura agreed with the goals and is eager to begin treatment to decrease the pain and loss of function in her right upper extremity. Once she understood the importance of strengthening after the pain and inflammation subsided, she was agreeable to not 'overdoing' her activities until she was stronger."

Summary of Interventions and Progress

The treatment approach and intervention will include:

1. Static extension splinting of the right wrist
2. Iontophoresis with dexamethasone to decrease the inflammatory process and pain
3. Gentle A/PROM to the right elbow
4. Education in modification of ADL and specific movements to prevent exacerbating her condition
5. Progressive upper extremity strengthening

Laura was instructed in different methods of modifying activities that required her to lift or manipulate objects as part of her daily activities. She was also provided with a static extension positioning splint for her right wrist that she was to wear at night and also initially during the day. She was aware of skin and splint care and her wearing schedule.

Laura's condition responded to the iontophoresis, and she reported a decrease in pain after the fourth treatment. As she responded to treatment, her iontophoresis dosage was increased from 40 mA/min to 60 mA/min and finally to 80 mA/min.

Assess the patient's comprehension	"I noticed that Laura was apprehensive about asking for assistance at home, but after we talked about the importance of initially resting the wrist and elbow, she allowed her family to take an active role in assisting her with her activities and responsibilities. As her pain subsided and her elbow ROM increased, I recommended that she begin wearing her wrist splint only at night, but to resume wearing the splint during the day if she noticed any return of her symptoms or pain. I know how important it is for me to monitor Laura's condition closely and to note any changes in pain or symptoms during each treatment visit, modifying the treatment and interventions as needed. If she reports a reversal back to earlier levels of pain and symptoms, I will have to figure out whether the interventions are effective or whether she is impacting the injury somehow in the performance of her daily occupations and activities."
Understand what the patient is doing	
Know the person	
Appreciate the context	

Next Steps

Revised goals (at week 2)
By week 4, Laura will report

1. Decreased pain in the right elbow during rest from 1 out of 10 to 0 out of 10
2. Decreased pain in the right elbow during activity from 5 out of 10 to 2 out of 10
3. Complete weaning from wearing the wrist splint
4. Proper understanding of resistance progression in her home strengthening program

By week 4, Laura will demonstrate

1. Proper technique for her home strengthening exercises
2. An increase in right grip strength from 20 to 50 pounds

Anticipate present and future patient concerns	"I am pleased with Laura's response to the initial 2 weeks of treatment. She was compliant with her splint wearing and modified her routine and activities to avoid overusing the right upper extremity. She noticed a marked decrease in pain (from 5 out of 10 to 1 out of 10 at rest and from 8 out of 10 to 5 out of 10 with activity) and an increase in elbow ROM to 'normal' by the end of 2 weeks. Because she responded so well to the treatment, I recommend that we continue with the iontophoresis and also begin gentle isometric strengthening exercises. If she tolerates isometrics without an increase in pain, we can wean from the iontophoresis treatments and wrist splinting and progressively strengthen with concentric and eccentric exercises. If I can strengthen Laura gradually and avoid any 'flare-ups,' Laura will be much more likely to withstand her normal activities without a recurrence of pain and inflammation in the future. I plan to transition Laura to a home strengthening program once I am sure she understands her exercises and how to upgrade the resistance cautiously. I will have her demonstrate her home exercises in the clinic so I can ensure that she understands."
Analyze patient's comprehension	
Decide whether he or she should continue or discontinue therapy and/or return in the future	

Clinical Reasoning in Occupational Therapy Practice

Determining Progress in Physical Agent Modalities

Laura's injury occurred following her engagement in a rather "normal" activity, painting her house. The signs and symptoms that she exhibited were pain in her elbow, difficulty holding onto objects, and difficulty performing activities of daily living (ADL). These symptoms are clues that an occupational therapist would use to select an appropriate treatment plan and physical agent modality. Establishing a realistic "starting point" based on the evaluation provides a mechanism for determining progress and efficacy of the therapeutic interventions, which guides modifications to the treatment.

Based on Laura's objective and subjective presentation, what physical agent modality—other than iontophoresis—could be provided in the clinic to achieve the same results of decreased pain and inflammation? If ultrasound was the modality that the therapist selected, should the therapist use a frequency of 1 or 3 MHz? Why? If Laura starts to feel better after a couple of treatments and asks to return to painting her house, what should the therapist's response be?

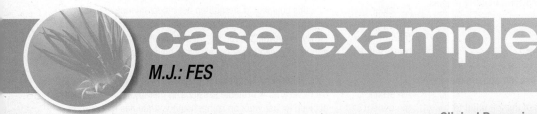

case example
M.J.: FES

Occupational Therapy Intervention Process	Objectives	Examples of Therapist's Internal Dialogue
	Clinical Reasoning Process	
Patient Information M.J. is a 36-year-old female who suffered a stroke affecting her left, nondominant, side. The stroke occurred while she was camping with her two sons (ages 12 and 9 years) and her husband. When her condition stabilized, she was referred to an inpatient rehabilitation program, where she stayed for 4 weeks. She was discharged home with the recommendation for outpatient occupational and physical therapy. Prior to the cerebrovascular accident (CVA), she was employed as a surgical nurse. She was independent in all her activities of daily living (ADL). She was accompanied by her husband for the initial evaluation. She was alert and oriented, but somewhat apprehensive and subdued. The following problems were identified during the occupational therapy assessment:	Appreciate the context	"M.J. seems to be a young, vibrant woman. All of her occupational roles have been affected by her CVA. She has gone from total independence to one of greater dependence on her family and husband. She seems apprehensive and concerned over whether she will regain function in her upper extremity. She is also in a lot of pain when she moves her arm, so is not very motivated to try to use the arm for functional activities." "M.J. seems worried about whether she will be able to return to work and was also concerned about the financial impact her disability would have on the family. Her husband and family seem extremely supportive of her, and I am pleased that they are very engaged in her rehabilitation and in facilitating her independence."
1. Decreased initiation of instrumental activities of daily living (IADL) 2. Decreased functional use of the left upper extremity (active shoulder flexion/abduction limited to 95°) 3. Subluxed left shoulder (two finger widths) 4. Painful (8 out of 10) shoulder range of motion (ROM) and use	Develop intervention hypotheses	"Despite M.J.'s encouraging family, pain is a powerful deterrent to movement and use of her left arm. I know that trying to use her left arm is extremely important in M.J.'s recovery. If I can help reduce her shoulder pain, M.J. is much more likely to participate in therapeutic activities geared toward improving function in the left arm. Shoulder subluxation is associated with shoulder pain in patients who have suffered a stroke. If I can reduce the subluxation in her left shoulder, then the pain is likely to decrease."
5. Increased tone in the left upper extremity with active grasp and weak release 6. Dependent for transportation and community mobility	Select an intervention approach	"I am proposing an intervention plan that emphasizes compensatory techniques, pain reduction strategies, remediation, and neuro-reeducation techniques to facilitate the return of function in the upper extremity. M.J. is in a lot of pain right now and not very motivated to move her left arm. However, she says she wants to 'try everything and anything to get better.'"

"I have to admit that M.J. is a challenging case because she is about my age and was extremely active prior to her CVA. She wants to try to return to work, but cannot imagine regaining use of her left arm because she is in so much pain. I know that we can use functional electrical stimulation (FES) to help reduce the amount of shoulder subluxation, and this will likely reduce M.J.'s pain. If we can reduce her left shoulder pain, M.J. will be less reluctant to move her left arm, and this will allow her to more fully participate in other treatment approaches aimed at improving left arm use."

Reflect on competence	"I have experience treating patients who present as M.J. does. Additionally, my state's occupational therapy practice act allows me to use electrical modalities. However, even though I learned about FES in school, this will be my first application of this knowledge to a patient, so I will ask my supervisor for guidance at first."

Recommendations

The occupational therapist initially recommended three outpatient treatment sessions per week for 4 weeks. In collaboration with M.J. and her family, the occupational therapist established the following long-term treatment goals:

In 6 months, M.J. will demonstrate

1. No subluxation of left shoulder joint
2. No pain in left shoulder
3. Active range of motion (AROM) in the left upper extremity within normal limits
4. Active grasp and release patterns of the left hand to manipulate large objects
5. Independence in IADL
6. A return to work
7. The ability to drive independently

Consider the patient's appraisal of performance	"M.J. seems highly motivated to attempt to return to work, and her family is supportive of this goal. In addition, because of the school and church activities that her sons are involved in and the fact that public transportation is negligible in the county that she lives in, M.J. really wants to return to driving independently. I know that this goal would strengthen her independence and ability to engage in those IADL that are so vital to an active and involved family. However, to keep her focused on these goals, even M.J. admits we need to get her shoulder pain under control."
Consider what will occur in therapy, how often, and for how long	
Ascertain the patient's endorsement of plan	"M.J.'s husband is agreeable to driving M.J. to therapy three times each week for 45-minute sessions. In therapy, M.J. and I have decided to first work on compensatory strategies for self-care and pain reduction. We will use FES in the clinic, and I will also teach M.J. how to use the FES unit at home. She agrees to follow through with using the FES at home five times each day for an hour because she is very motivated to reduce her shoulder pain."

Summary of Short-Term Goals and Progress

In 4 weeks, M.J. will demonstrate

1. Decreased subluxation of the left shoulder joint to one finger width
2. Decreased pain in the left shoulder from 8 out of 10 to 3 out of 10
3. Increased AROM of the left shoulder to 110° of flexion and abduction
4. The ability to actively grasp a plastic cup with her left hand

The therapist began treatment using FES to the supraspinatus and posterior deltoid muscles in order to decrease shoulder subluxation. FES was used both in the clinic and as part of M.J.'s home program. The therapist ordered M.J. a home FES unit and instructed M.J. in the use of the modality five times per day for 1 hour daily. When the FES unit was stimulating the muscles, M.J. was instructed to work with the stimulation in reaching for objects. She engaged in a variety of reaching activities that initially required active shoulder movement slightly below the point that would cause her pain. The amount of shoulder subluxation was monitored weekly by the therapist for 4 weeks. Gradually, the subluxation was reduced to about one finger width. As the subluxation reduced, M.J. experienced less pain. As her pain decreased, she was able to reach further and higher for objects.

Assess the patient's comprehension	"In the initial evaluations and subsequent visits in the first week of therapy, I showed M.J. how to use the FES machine. She understood how to apply the electrodes and turn on the machine, but she needed her husband's help in placing the electrodes appropriately, so her husband was instructed in helping M.J. with her FES setup. I had M.J. and her husband demonstrate to me the proper FES setup a few times over the first week of therapy."
Understand what she is doing	
Compare actual to expected performance	"M.J. is a perfect candidate for this kind of intervention. She quickly learned how to use the FES unit, and so did her husband. He will be a good support for M.J. and a source of motivation for her to follow through with her daily FES sessions."
Know the person	"I am monitoring the subluxation in M.J.'s shoulder, as well as her pain levels and shoulder AROM each week. After the first week, there was not much change, despite M.J.'s compliance with her program. I encouraged her to continue. By the end of the second week, M.J. said she was able to raise her left arm further without as much pain, and I noticed a little decrease in the shoulder subluxation. By the end of 4 weeks, M.J.'s shoulder subluxation was down to about one finger width. Her shoulder pain level was tolerable at 3 out of 10. Additionally, her active shoulder flexion was greatly improved to 110°. M.J. is getting better at grasping objects, but she still has a lot of difficulty releasing her grasp on these objects. However, she is starting to use her left arm more during self-care strategies, and I can now add some other treatment techniques to the therapy plan that will focus on further left arm improvement."
Appreciate the context	

"I am pleased to see M.J. translate her gains in upper extremity function into expansion of her IADL. She recently began testing to determine whether she could resume driving independently and ultimately succeeded. This will further her independence and resumption of IADL and eventually enable her to attempt to return to her work."

Next Steps

Continue outpatient occupational therapy for 1 month but with declining contact. Intervention will focus on weaning M.J. away from the FES and ensuring that she continues to use the extremity for functional movements. Focus will be on function and imparting the importance of a home program of exercise and movement as crucial to ensure continued progress toward the established long-term goals. The patient will also be assisted in resuming many of her social and religious activities and reintegrating into meaningful community organizations and activities. Thought will be given to potential for return to work.

Anticipate present and future patient concerns

Analyze patient's comprehension

Decide whether he or she should continue or discontinue therapy and/ or return in the future

"Because of the patient's background as a nurse, M.J. seems well aware of challenges and potential limitations based on her initial prognosis. She has always been highly motivated to 'try almost anything' if it would 'work.' I am impressed at her insight into the possible risks and difficulties she would face returning to her career as a surgical nurse, and she is starting to prepare herself for other options that might require less fine motor dexterity and endurance as her condition improves. I expect that she will work closely with her employer and physicians to adapt her work site and work requirements."

"In-clinic therapy will transition to a home-based program when M.J. has received maximum benefit from the skilled services of a therapist. Once I have taught M.J. and her family all they need to know, and they are able to follow through independently, M.J. will be discharged and continue to work toward her long-term goals."

Clinical Reasoning in Occupational Therapy Practice

Identifying Appropriate Therapeutic Goals and Interventions

M.J. was a young, active, healthy individual prior to her devastating stroke. Overnight, her life and roles changed, impacting her immediate family and employer. She was highly motivated to return to some semblance of her premorbid activities and life. The difficulty she faced, and that the therapist had to assist her prioritize, was in determining short-term, realistic goals and objectives and expanding those into long-term functional goals. As pain decreased and functional return and movement occurred in her upper extremity, refining and strengthening the motor patterns and movements available to the patient became a motivating factor for her. There are a variety of neuromuscular facilitation techniques that can be used as part of neuromuscular reeducation.

Other than FES, what other physical agent modalities could the therapist use to address M.J.'s shoulder pain? Why is FES the *best* modality choice to help manage shoulder pain associated with subluxation? What are some key points to remember when training M.J. to use the FES unit at home?

Summary Review Questions

1. Identify and discuss the three phases of tissue healing. Why is the phase of tissue healing a significant factor in selection of a specific physical agent modality as an adjunct to treatment?

2. What are the superficial and deep thermal agents discussed in this chapter?

3. List the different types and the most frequent uses of electrotherapy.

4. Discuss AOTA's position on physical agent modalities and how each modality can be used as a precursor to functional performance tasks.

5. Define and discuss therapeutic ultrasound, both its thermal and nonthermal effects.

6. List precautions and contraindications for superficial heat and cryotherapy.

7. List precautions and contraindications for use of ultrasound and electrical stimulation.

8. Why would an occupational therapist use surface electromyographic biofeedback?

9. How do licensing/regulatory issues affect an occupational therapist's use of physical agent modalities?

10. Discuss how the push for evidence-based practice may or may not influence the use of physical agents in clinical practice.

Glossary

Absorption coefficients—The ability of biological tissue to absorb and transmit energy relative to the tissue's unique properties.

Acoustic streaming—The physical forces of sound waves capable of displacing ions and small molecules.

Angiogenesis—The biological process of developing new blood vessels.

Biofeedback—Procedures or techniques that are used to provide an individual with an auditory or visual cue or "feedback" to learn and gain volitional control over a physiological response.

Cavitation—The physical forces of sound waves causing gas bubble formation, expansion, and contraction within fluid or tissue.

Conduction—Exchange of energy (for example heat or cold) when two surfaces are in direct contact with each other.

Convection—Conveyance of heat by the movement of heated particles, such as air or water molecules, across the body part being treated, creating temperature variations.

Cryotherapy—Application of a superficial cold agent to part of the body. Often used for pain relief, reducing edema, and decreasing inflammation following trauma.

Deep thermal agent—Therapeutic application of any modality to the skin and underlying soft tissue structures to cause a temperature elevation in tissue up to a depth of 5 cm.

Duty cycle—During the delivery of electrical stimulation or ultrasound, the duty cycle refers to the time that the electrical current or sound energy is on versus the time the electrical current or sound energy is off.

Electrotherapeutic agents—Therapeutic application of an electrical current to selected tissue or monitoring of endogenous electrical activity in tissue. Includes biofeedback, neuromuscular electrical stimulation, functional electrical stimulation, transcutaneous electrical nerve stimulation, electrical stimulation for tissue repair, high-voltage galvanic stimulation, and iontophoresis.

Epithelialization—The biological process of tissue healing in which a wound is covered by the proliferation of epithelial cells over the wounded area.

Impedance—Resistance of tissue to the passage of electrical current or ultrasound waves or the resistance of the electrodes used in biofeedback to detection of electrical signal generated by muscle activity.

Inflammation—Cellular and vascular response in affected tissue that follows injury or abnormal stimulation; the initial phase of the healing process; the body's attempt to rid itself of bacteria, foreign matter, and dead tissue and to decrease blood loss.

Iontophoresis—The use of electrical current to actively deliver drug ions through the skin.

Microstreaming—The microscopic fluid movement caused by cavitation.

Overload principle—In terms of gaining muscle strength, this principle refers to the fact that the body must be subjected to greater levels of stress than it is accustomed to for strength gains to occur.

Phonophoresis—The use of ultrasound to deliver topically applied medications to selected tissue.

Physical agent modality—An occupational therapy intervention, considered preparatory, that uses heat, light, sound, cold, electricity, or mechanical devices to modify specific client factors when neurological, musculoskeletal, or skin conditions may be limiting occupational performance.

Proliferation—Formation of new collagen tissue and epithelium in the intermediate stage of wound healing.

Remodeling—Third phase of tissue healing; dynamic process with maturation of new collagen tissue within the wound.

Superficial thermal agents—Therapeutic application of any modality that raises or lowers the temperature of skin and superficial subcutaneous tissue to a depth of 1–2 cm.

Thermotherapy—The therapeutic application of heat to increase tissue temperature.

Ultrasound—Deep-heat modality; application of sound waves to soft tissue, causing thermal and nonthermal effects; sound having a frequency greater than 20,000 Hz.

Wound contraction—The biological process of tissue healing where wound edges are drawn toward each other as the body attempts to heal and close the wound.

References

Algafly, A. A., & George, K. P. (2007). The effect of cryotherapy on nerve conduction velocity, pain threshold, and pain tolerance. *British Journal of Sports Medicine, 41,* 365–369.

American Occupational Therapy Association. (2007a). Accreditation standards for a doctoral-degree-level educational program for the occupational therapist. *American Journal of Occupational Therapy, 61,* 641–651.

American Occupational Therapy Association. (2007b). Accreditation standards for a master's-degree-level educational program for the occupational therapist. *American Journal of Occupational Therapy, 61,* 652–661.

American Occupational Therapy Association. (2007c). Accreditation standards for an educational program for the occupational therapy assistant. *American Journal of Occupational Therapy, 61,* 662–671.

American Occupational Therapy Association. (2007d). AOTA's Centennial Vision and executive summary. *American Journal of Occupational Therapy, 61,* 613–614.

American Occupational Therapy Association. (2008). Occupational therapy practice framework: Domain and process (2nd ed.). *American Journal of Occupational Therapy, 62,* 625–683.

American Occupational Therapy Association. (2010). Occupational therapy code of ethics and ethics standard. *American Journal of Occupational Therapy, 64,* 151–160.

American Occupational Therapy Association. (2012). *Physical agent modalities.* Retrieved September 30, 2012 from http://www.aota.org/Practitioners/Official/Position/41259.aspx?FT=.pdf.

Apfel, R. (1982). Acoustic cavitation: A possible consequence of biomedical uses of ultrasound. *British Journal of Cancer, 45,* 140–146.

Ay, S., Dogan, S. K., Evcik, D., & Baser, O. C. (2011). Comparison the efficacy of phonophoresis and ultrasound therapy in myofascial pain syndrome. *Rheumatology International, 31* (9), 1203–1208.

Babu, A. S., Mathew, E., Danda, D., & Prakash, H. (2007). Management of patients with fibromyalgia using biofeedback: A randomized control trial. *Indian Journal of Medical Sciences, 61,* 455–461.

Baker, L. L., Bowman, B. R., & McNeal, D. R. (1988). Effects of wave form on comfort during neuromuscular electrical stimulation. *Clinical Orthopedics, 223,* 75–85.

Baker, L. L., Wederich, C. L., McNeal, D. R., & Waters, R. I. (2000). *Neuromuscular electrical stimulation: A practical clinical guide* (4th ed.). Downey, CA: Rancho Los Amigos Research and Education Institute.

Barthel, H. R., Peniston, J. H., Clark, M. B., Gold, M. S., & Altman, R. D. (2010). Correlation of pain relief with physical function in hand osteoarthritis: Randomized controlled trial post hoc analysis. *Arthritis Research & Therapy, 12,* R7.

Bennie, S. D., Petrofsky, J. S., Nisperos, J., Tsurudome, M., & Laymon, M. (2002). Toward the optimal waveform for electrical stimulation of human muscle. *European Journal of Applied Physiology, 88,* 13–19.

Bloom, R., Przekop, A., & Sanger, T. D. (2010). Prolonged electromyogram biofeedback improves upper extremity function in children with cerebral palsy. *Journal of Child Neurology, 25,* 1480–1484.

Bolek, J. E. (2006). Use of multiple performance-contingent SEMG reward programming in pediatric rehabilitation: A retrospective review. *Applied Psychophysiology and Biofeedback, 31,* 263–272.

Bonica, J. J. (1990). *The management of pain* (Vols. 1 and 2, 2nd ed.). Malvern, PA: Lea & Febiger.

Bracciano, A. (2008). *Physical agent modalities: Theory and application for the occupational therapist* (2nd ed.). Thorofare, NJ: Slack.

Byl, N. N., Archer, E. S., & McKenzie, A. (2009). Focal hand dystonia: Effectiveness of a home program of fitness and learning-based sensorimotor and memory training. *Journal of Hand Therapy, 22,* 183–198.

Cahe, J., Yu, D., & Walker, M. (2004). Percutaneous, intramuscular neuromuscular electrical stimulation for the treatment of shoulder subluxation and pain in chronic hemiplegia: A case report. *American Journal of Physical Medicine and Rehabilitation, 80,* 296–301.

Cameron, M. (2012). *Physical agents in rehabilitation: From research to practice* (4th ed.). Philadelphia: Elsevier/W.B. Saunders.

De Biase, M. E., Politti, F., Palomari, E. T., Barros-Filho, T. E., & De Camargo, O. P. (2011). Increased EMG response following electromyographic biofeedback treatment of rectus femoris muscle after spinal cord injury. *Physiotherapy, 97,* 175–179.

Dogan-Aslan, M., Nakipoglu-Yuzer, G. F., Dogan, A., Karabay, I., & Ozgirgin, N. (2012). The effect of electromyographic biofeedback treatment in improving upper extremity functioning of patients with hemiplegic stroke. *Journal of Stroke and Cerebrovascular Diseases, 21,* 187–192.

dos Santos, M. T., & de Oliveira, L. M. (2004). Use of cryotherapy to enhance mouth opening in patients with cerebral palsy. *Special Care in Dentistry, 24,* 232–234.

Draper, D. (2010). *Syllabus for enhancing treatment outcomes with therapeutic modalities: Electrotherapy and ultrasound.* Brentwood, TN: Cross Country Education.

Dykstra, J. H., Hill, H. M., Miller, M. G., Cheatham, C. C., Michael, T. J., & Baker, R. J. (2009). Comparisons of cubed ice, crushed ice, and wetted ice on intramuscular and surface temperature changes. *Journal of Athletic Training, 44,* 136–141.

Earley, D. (1999). Superficial heat agents: A hot topic. *OT Practice, 4,* 26–30.

Hara, Y., Ogawa, S., Tsujiuchi, K., & Muraoka, Y. (2008). A home-based rehabilitation program for the hemiplegic upper extremity by power-assisted functional electrical stimulation. *Disability and Rehabilitation, 30,* 296–304.

Hardy, K., Suever, K., Sprague, A., Hermann, V., Levine, P., & Page, S. J. (2010). Combined bracing, electrical stimulation, and functional practice for chronic, upper-extremity spasticity. *American Journal of Occupational Therapy, 64,* 720–726.

Hauptmann, M., Struyf, H., Mertens, P., Heyns, M., De Gendt, S., Glorieux, C., & Brems, S. (2013). Towards an understanding and control of cavitation activity in 1MHz ultrasound fields. *Ultrasonics Sonochemistry, 20,* 77–88.

Hecox, B., Mehreteab, T., & Weisberg, J. (Eds.). (1994). *Physical agents: A comprehensive text for physical therapists.* Norwalk, CT: Appleton & Lange.

Herderschee, R., Hay-Smith, E. J. C., Herbison, G. P., Roovers, J. P., & Heineman, M. J. (2011). Feedback or biofeedback to augment pelvic floor muscle training for urinary incontinence in women. *Cochrane Database of Systematic Reviews, (7),* CD009252.

Herrera, E., Sandoval, M. C., Camargo, D. M., & Salvini, T. F. (2010). Motor and sensory conduction are affected differently by ice pack, ice massage, and cold water. *Physical Therapy, 90,* 581–591.

Hess, C. L., Howard, M., & Attignger, C. (2000). A review of mechanical adjuncts in wound healing: Hydrotherapy, ultrasound, negative pressure therapy, hyperbaric oxygen, and electrostimulation. *Annals of Plastic Surgery, 51,* 210–218.

Johns, L. D., Straub, S. J., & Howard, S. M. (2007). Analysis of effective radiating area, power, intensity, and field characteristics of ultrasound transducers. *Archives of Physical Medicine and Rehabilitation, 88,* 124–129.

Kaul, M. P. (1994). Superficial heat and cold. *The Physician and Sports Medicine, 22,* 65–74.

Kimura, I., Gulick, D., Shelly, J., & Ziskin, M. (1998). Effects of two ultrasound devices and angles of application on the temperature of tissue phantom. *Journal of Orthopedic and Sports Physical Therapy, 27,* 27–31.

Kollmann, C., Vacariu, G., Schuhfried, O., Fialka-Moser, V., & Bergmann, H. (2005). Variations in the output power and surface heating effects of transducers in therapeutic ultrasound. *Archives of Physical Medicine and Rehabilitation, 86,* 1318–1324.

Koyuncu, E., Nakipoglu-Yuzer, G. F., Dogan, A., & Ozgirgin, N. (2010). The effectiveness of functional electrical stimulation for the treatment of shoulder subluxation and shoulder pain in hemiplegic patients: A randomized controlled trial. *Disability and Rehabilitation, 32,* 560–566.

Lewek, M., Stevens, J., & Snyder-Mackler, L. (2001). The use of electrical stimulation to increase quadriceps femoris muscle force following total knee arthroplasty. *Physical Therapy, 81,* 1565–1571.

Lin, S. L., Granat, M. H., & Lees, K. R. (1999). Prevention of shoulder subluxation after stroke with electrical stimulation. *Stroke, 30,* 963–968.

Melzack, R., & Wall, P. D. (1965). Pain mechanisms: A new theory. *Science, 150,* 971–999.

Molier, B. I., Prange, G. B., Krabben, T., Stienen, A. H., van der Kooih, H., Buurke, J. H., Jannink, M. J., & Hermens, H. J. (2011). Effect of position feedback during task-oriented upper-limb training after stroke: Five-case pilot study. *Journal of Rehabilitation Research & Development, 48,* 1109–1118.

Mulder, G., Brazinsky, B. A., & Seeley, J. (2010). Factors complicating wound repair. In J. M. McColloch & L. C. Kloth (Eds.), *Wound healing: Evidence-based management* (4th ed.). Philadelphia: F.A. Davis.

Nirschl, R. P., Rodin, D. M., Ochiai, D. H., & Maartmann-Moe, C. (2003). Iontophoretic administration of dexamethasone sodium phosphate for acute epicondylitis. A randomized, double-blinded, placebo-controlled study. *American Journal of Sports Medicine, 31,* 189–195.

Pullman, S., Goodink, D., Marquinez, A., & Tabbal, S. (2000). Clinical utility of surface EMG: Report of the Therapeutics and Technology Assessment Subcommittee of the American Academy of Neurology. *Neurology, 55,* 171–177.

Robertson, V., Ward, A., Low, J., & Reed, A. (2006). *Electrotherapy explained: Principles and practice* (4th ed.). Philadelphia: Elsevier

Rosewilliam, S., Malhotra, S., Roffe, C., Jones, P., & Pandyan, A. D. (2012). Can surface neuromuscular electrical stimulation of the wrist and hand combined with routine therapy facilitate recovery of arm function in patients with stroke? *Archives of Physical Medicine and Rehabilitation, 93,* 1715–1721.

Sabut, S. K., Sikdar, C., Kumar, R., & Mahadevappa, M. (2011). Functional electrical stimulation of dorsiflexor muscle: Effects on dorsiflexor strength, plantarflexor spasticity, and motor recovery in stroke patients. *NeuroRehabilitation, 29,* 393–400.

Sackett, D. L., Rosenberg, W. M. C., Gray, J. A. M., Haynes, R. B., & Richardson, W. S. (1996). Evidence-based medicine: What it is and what it isn't. *British Medical Journal, 312,* 71–72.

Sahin, N., Ugurlu, H., & Albayrak, I. (2012). The efficacy of electrical stimulation in reducing the [sic] post-stroke spasticity: A randomized controlled study. *Disability and Rehabilitation, 34,* 151–156.

Schmidt, K. L., Ott, V. R., Rocher, G., & Schaller, H. (1979). Heat, cold, and inflammation. *Zeitschrift fur Rheumatologie, 38,* 391–404.

Seo, J. T., Choe, J. H., Lee, W. S., & Kim, K. H. (2005). Efficacy of functional electrical stimulation-biofeedback with sexual cognitive-behavioral therapy as treatment of vaginismus. *Urology, 66,* 77–81.

Sicard-Rosenbaum, L., Lord, D., & Danoff, J. (1995). Effects of continuous therapeutic ultrasound on growth and metastasis of subcutaneous murine tumors. *Physical Therapy, 75,* 3–13.

Srbely, J. Z. (2008). Ultrasound in the management of osteoarthritis: Part I. A review of the current literature. *The Journal of the Canadian Chiropractic Association, 52,* 30–37.

Stefanou, A., Marshall, N., Holdan, W., & Siddiqui, A. (2012). A randomized study comparing corticosteroid injection to corticosteroid iontophoresis for lateral epicondylitis. *Journal of Hand Surgery, 37,* 104–109.

Sugimoto, K., Theoharides, T. C., Kempuraj, D., & Conti, P. (2007). Response of spinal myoclonus to a combination therapy of autogenic training and biofeedback. *BioPsychoSocial Medicine, 1,* 18.

Thrasher, T. A., Zivanovic, V., McIlroy, W., & Popovic, M. R. (2008). Rehabilitation of reaching and grasping function in severe hemiplegic patients using functional electrical stimulation therapy. *Neurorehabilitation and Neural Repair, 22,* 706–714.

Vedsted, P., Søgaard, K., Blangsted, A. K., Madeleine, P., & Sjøgaard, G. (2011). Biofeedback effectiveness to reduce upper limb muscle activity during computer work is muscle specific and time pressure dependent. *Journal of Electromyography and Kinesiology, 21,* 49–58.

Venes, D. (Ed.). (2009). *Taber's Cyclopedic Medical Dictionary* (21st ed.). Philadelphia: F.A. Davis Co.

Vodovnik, L., Bowman, B. R., & Hufford, P. (1984). Effects of electrical stimulation on spinal spasticity. *Scandinavian Journal of Rehabilitation Medicine, 16,* 29–34.

Wang, R. Y., Chan, R. C., & Tsai, M. W. (2000). Functional electrical stimulation on chronic and acute hemiplegic shoulder subluxation. *American Journal of Physical Medicine and Rehabilitation, 79,* 385–394.

Wang, R. Y., Tsai, M. W., & Chan, R. C. (1998). Effects of spinal cord stimulation on spasticity and quantitative assessment of muscle tone in hemiplegic patients. *American Journal of Physical Medicine and Rehabilitation, 77,* 282–287.

Woodford, H. J, & Price, C. I. M. (2007). EMG biofeedback for the recovery of motor function after stroke. *Cochrane Database of Systematic Reviews, (2),* CD004585.

Yu, D. T., Cahe, J., Walker, M. E., & Fan, Z. P. (2001). Percutaneous intramuscular neuromuscular electric stimulation for the treatment of shoulder subluxation and pain in patients with chronic hemiplegia: A pilot study. *Archives of Physical Medicine and Rehabilitation, 82,* 20–25.

Acknowledgment

The authors acknowledge with appreciation the contributions to referencing by Dr. Catherine Trombly Latham.

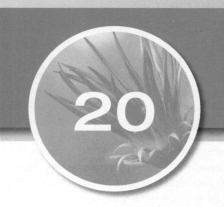

20

Optimizing Abilities and Capacities: Range of Motion, Strength, and Endurance

Andrew Fabrizio and Jose Rafols

Learning Objectives

After studying this chapter, the reader will be able to do the following:

1. State the biomechanical and physiological mechanisms that underlie therapeutic exercise and occupation.
2. Apply the methods for decreasing edema, minimizing contracture, and mobilization to prevent limitation of range of motion.
3. Apply biomechanical and physiologcial priinciples of the biomechanical approach to the selection of occupations as a means for treating range of motion, strength, and/or endurance problems as needed for occupational performance.
4. Design treatment goals and therapy for clients who have problems with range of motion, strength, and/or endurance to enhance occupational performance.

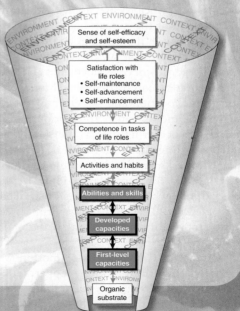

An assumption of the occupational functioning model is that the ability to carry out one's roles and activities depends on an individual's basic capacities (see Chapter 1). Three capacities necessary for performing physical activity are range of motion (ROM), strength, and endurance. Occupational therapists help clients improve these basic capacities as a preparatory means for developing higher level skills needed for the performance of everyday activities or occupations (American Occupational Therapy Association, 2008). The underlying biomechanical and physiological principles that pertain to motion, strength, and endurance are the building blocks upon which treatment for physical dysfunction is built. The principles are applied to the remediation of impairments from acute injuries; the prevention of illnesses and conditions caused by repetitive motion, cumulative trauma, or poor biomechanics; and as compensation for or adaptation to chronic disability.

MUSCULOSKELETAL SYSTEM

The following is a simple overview of the biomechanical and physiological elements of the musculoskeletal system that underlie ROM, strength, and endurance. This basic understanding enables occupational therapists to analyze and prescribe therapeutic occupations and exercise to promote occupational function. Table 20-1 illustrates the linkage between various biomechanical capacities needed for a common military activity (see Activity-Focused Case Example later in the chapter).

Biomechanical Aspects

Although mechanics is a branch of physics that deals with the study of motion produced by force, biomechanics involves taking those principles and applying them to the structure and function of the human body. Biomechanics is broken down into static (nonmoving) and dynamic (moving) systems, and the dynamic systems can be further broken down into concepts described as kinematics and kinetics.

Kinematic analysis describes human motion in relation to the location and direction of the movement, the magnitude and velocity of the motion, and the type of motion that is occurring such as translatory motion or rotary motion (Levangie & Norkin, 2011). Researchers use these quantitative kinematic descriptors to describe the act of grasping with reachers (Maitra, Philips, & Rice, 2010), the effect of elbow angles in manual wheelchair propulsion (Goins et al., 2011), and the way the three joints of the thumb move during different activities of daily living (Lin et al., 2011).

Kinetics is a description of motion with regards to the forces that cause motion (Lippert, 2006). The forces that provide movement or stability are both internal and external to the body. Internal forces consist of muscle contractions that enable us to engage in our daily occupations or the elasticity of structural and connective tissue that prevent unwanted movement. The wind that pushes against the body, the friction of a sock on the floor, or the weight of a hammer held by a construction worker are all examples of external forces on human movement. Gravity is another example of external force. Gravity is constant and unnoticeable to most of us, but it affects all human movement. It is the gravitational pull on the body and body segments that gives them weight and can be a challenge to patients who have lost the strength to overcome this weight. Researchers are studying kinetics when they measure the influence of gravity during reach and retrieval activity for subjects with spinal cord injuries (Kloosterman et al., 2010), when they study the maximum load, stress, and elongation of different tendons used for tendon grafting (Mazurek et al., 2011), or when they look at the force on the wrist and thumb during jar opening activities (Chang, Ho, & Su, 2008).

Nearly all purposeful activity can be broken down into a series of coordinated movements. Understanding the different types of movement and forces behind the motion helps therapists design the most efficient exercise programs and structure therapeutic occupation. The following is an example of force, stability, and motion in occupation. While dining, a person grasps a glass filled with a beverage and lifts it to take a sip. This task requires both stability and motion. Initially, muscles in the trunk and shoulder girdle (internal forces) co-contract to provide proximal stability, allowing for controlled distal mobility. To raise the glass, the forearm flexors contract causing rotary motion, or flexion of the elbow joint. When rotary motion occurs, each point on the bone segment (ulna and radius) moves through an arc at the same time at a constant distance from the axis (elbow joint). To cause rotation, the forearm flexors must have enough strength to overcome the external forces created by gravity and the weight of the glass.

Torque

When analyzing the movement in this scenario, one must also consider torque. Torque is the tendency of a force to produce rotation about an axis (Lippert, 2006). In rotary movements, torque depends on (1) the amount of force applied and (2) the distance of the force from the axis of movement, also known as the moment arm. Thus, in mathematical terms, torque is equal to the magnitude of a force times the perpendicular distance between the line of force and the axis of rotation [$T = (F)(D)$] (Levangie & Norkin, 2011). In relation to the example of taking and raising a glass, the torque produced by the biceps at the elbow (effort force) is equal to the force the muscles can produce times the distance between the bicep's insertion on the radius and the axis of motion or elbow joint (Fig. 20-1A).

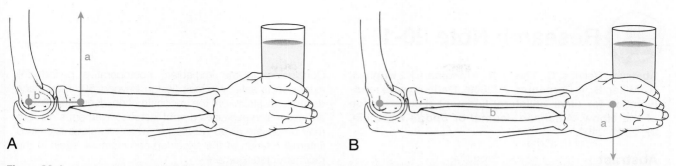

Figure 20-1 **A.** Torque of effort force. *a,* Line of pull of effort force (elbow flexors). *b,* Perpendicular distance between the insertion of the elbow flexors and the axis of rotation. **B.** Torque of resistance force. *a,* Line of pull of resistance force (weight of glass and forearm). *b,* Perpendicular distance between the resistance force and the axis of rotation.

The torque of resistance force (the glass, forearm, and hand) is equal to the resistance force (weight of the glass, forearm, and hand) times the distance between the glass and the axis of movement or elbow joint (Fig. 20-1B). For a person to flex the elbow and take a sip, the torque of the biceps has to be greater than the torque of the glass, forearm, and hand.

The concept of torque also explains why the placement of an object either closer to or farther from the axis of rotation changes the effort needed to make the movement, even though the object's weight remains constant. Therapists use this concept in a number of situations. Teaching clients to lift objects closer to the body's center of gravity, thereby reducing the moment arm and the amount of stress on the back and shoulders, is one example. Likewise, when assisting a patient to perform a stand-and-pivot transfer from the wheelchair to the bed, a therapist stands close to the patient as they both pivot, and the therapist lowers the patient to a sitting position. The patient provides less resistance torque (the weight of the patient times the perpendicular distance between the patient and the therapist's back) when he or she is close to the therapist. This in turn requires less effort force by the therapist's back muscles for raising, maintaining the position during the pivot, and lowering the patient to the bedside. Similarly, therapists use this concept to help clients increase productivity while minimizing effort. For example, by using longer tools, which increase the moment arm and thereby increase the amount of torque that is placed on the nut or bolt, manual laborers decrease the muscle force needed to turn the tool (see Research Note 20-1 for further information regarding torque and safe rehabilitation).

Lever Systems

Another way to evaluate torque in angular movement is through the description of levers. A lever system consists of a rigid bar (such as a bone), an axis of rotation (such as a joint), and two forces: effort and resistance. Effort is

the force that causes movement, and resistance is the force that tends to keep an object from moving. There are three classes of lever systems.

A first-class lever is a system where the axis of rotation lies between the effort and resistance forces (Levangie & Norkin, 2011). A common example of a first-class lever is the seesaw (Fig. 20-2A). As one can see, a seesaw would remain in balance, with no movement, if two children of the same weight sat the same distance from the axis. This balance, or equilibrium, is maintained because the torque (weight of child 1 times the perpendicular distance from child 1 to the axis of rotation) on one side of the seesaw equals the torque (weight of child 2 times the perpendicular distance from child 2 to the axis of rotation) on the opposite side of the seesaw. In essence, they balance, and there is no movement. If one of the children is heavier, he or she must move closer to the axis to maintain that balance (Fig. 20-2B).

In second- and third-class levers, the effort and resistance force lie on the same side of the axis (Lippert, 2006). A second-class lever system, such as a bottle opener or a wheelbarrow used to carry compost in a garden, is a system in which the resistance force lies closer to the axis of rotation than does the effort force (Fig. 20-3). With a bottle opener, the resistance force is the force of the cap that is tightly connected to the bottle. The effort force is a person's hand lifting the end of the opener to release the cap. This lever system allows a relatively small amount of force to overcome strong resistance. Second-class lever systems explain the type of tools used frequently in occupations when mechanical advantage is required, such as an extended handle on a faucet.

In third-class lever systems, the effort force lies closer to the axis than does the resistance force (Levangie & Norkin, 2011) (Fig. 20-4, top). The example of bringing a glass to one's mouth represents a third-class lever. The elbow joint is the axis; the biceps is the effort force; and the combined weight of the forearm and glass is the resistance force (Fig. 20-4, bottom). In contrast to the stability of first-class levers and the mechanical advantage of second-class levers, third-class levers produce greater velocity and ROM. Most body segments that are moved

Research Note 20-1

Abstract: Bernas, G., Thiele, R., Kinnaman, K., Hughes, R., Miller, B., & Carpenter, J. (2009). Defining safe rehabilitation for ulnar collateral ligament reconstruction of the elbow. *American Journal of Sports Medicine, 37*, 2392–2400.

Abstract

Background: Forces on the ulnar collateral ligament of the elbow after reconstruction are measured during a rehabilitation protocol that includes passive range of motion, isometric muscle contraction, and varus and valgus torques to help develop guidelines for safe and productive rehabilitation.

Methods: Eight cadaveric elbows underwent ulnar collateral ligament reconstruction using a gracilis tendon graft. Strain on the anterior and posterior bands of the ligament were measured with differential variable reluctance transducers during passive range of motion, isometric flexion and extension contractions, and varus and valgus torques with the arm at 90° of flexion.

Results: Range of motion from maximum extension to 50° of flexion produced 3% or less strain in both bands of the reconstructed ligament. Forearm rotation did not significantly affect strain in the ligament. Strain at 90° approached 7% in the posterior band. Isometric muscle contractions had no measurable effect on strain. Varus torques decreased and valgus torques increased strain significantly.

Conclusion: In the immediate postoperative period, full extension is safe, whereas flexion beyond 50° may place deleterious strain on the reconstruction. Isometric flexion and extension exercises do not increase ligament strain but may be unsafe at 90° of flexion, whereas valgus exercises (internal rotation at the shoulder) can increase strain in the reconstructed ligament.

Implications for Practice:

A unique expertise of occupational therapy is the design and prescription of purposeful and meaningful activity (occupation) to enhance and promote health. Along these lines, occupational therapists frequently use therapeutic occupation to improve an individual's ROM, strength, and endurance. In this example, the ulnar collateral ligament is often repaired to enable athletes who use overhead motions to return to competition. However, this study highlights the need to use biomechanical principles to design therapeutic programs that are safe and effective for patients.

Whether therapists are designing exercise programs to increase motion or strength or prescribing purposeful and meaningful activities that do the same, it is important to analyze the forces that are put on the body, as to not injure or debilitate a person who is recovering. Through activity analysis, an educational background steeped in kinetics and kinematics, and knowledge of human anatomy, occupational therapists are able to design the most appropriate methods for rehabilitation.

---

by muscular effort are third-class lever systems where the muscles provide the effort force and the joints are the axis (Hamilton, Weimar, & Luttgens, 2012). However, the potential work capacity of the various muscles of the body also depends on the amount of force they can generate and the distance over which the muscles can shorten. In other words, the ability to fully function, move, and engage in occupation depends not only on the biomechanics of the musculoskeletal system but also the physiologic principles of the muscles themselves.

Physiological Aspects

Skeletal muscle provides the power to produce movement of a bony lever around its joint axis. A muscle's strength and endurance to perform this activity depend on multiple factors including the size and type of muscle fibers, the number and frequency of motor units firing, and the length-tension relationship of the muscle. Before this discussion, it is important to understand the basic contractile elements within muscle.

The sarcomere, made up of actin and myosin, is the main contractile portion of skeletal muscle and is located within the myofibrils of the muscle. A nerve impulse sent to a motor unit, which consist of a motor neuron, an axon, and the muscle fibers supplied by the neuron, initiates a chemical reaction and the release of calcium throughout the muscle fibers. The calcium ions release the inhibition that prevents actin and myosin filaments from combining. When these thin and thick filaments are allowed to combine, cross-bridges are created. According to the sliding filament theory, muscle contraction occurs when these cross-bridges are broken, actin is pulled over the myosin, and new cross-bridges are formed (Cooke, 2004; Levangie & Norkin, 2011) (see Fig. 20-5). As this sequence continues, tension is generated, and the muscle shortens (concentric contraction). In a lengthening contraction (eccentric contraction), cross-bridges are broken and reformed as the actin is pulled away from the myosin filaments (see Definition 20-1).

The strength of a contraction depends on the number and type of muscle fibers found in a motor unit (MacIntosh, Gardiner, & McComas, 2006). Muscles that produce large contractions typically are composed of motor units that have large axons, large cell bodies, and many muscle fibers. These fibers are also typically type II fibers, which are fast twitch fibers capable of producing more power and

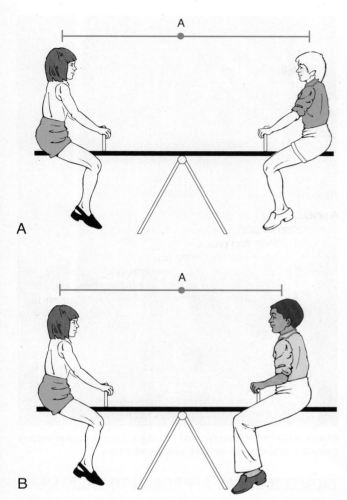

Figure 20-2 A. First-class lever system. Balanced equilibrium depicted by children on a seesaw. Both children weigh 60 pounds, and they are equidistant from the axis. **B.** First-class lever system. The heavier child must be closer to the axis of the seesaw to maintain the equilibrium.

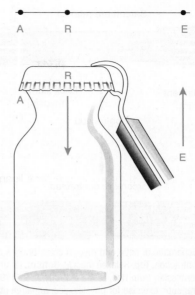

Figure 20-3 Top, Schematic drawing of a second-class lever. **Bottom,** Second-class lever depicted by using a bottle opener to remove the cap from a bottle. *A,* axis; *R,* resistance force (tightly secured cap); *E,* effort force (force from bottle opener to open cap).

are usually recruited first, but if they cannot complete the task, larger motor units are recruited to complete the action. The frequency of a motor unit's firing also affects the force modulation. For small distal muscles, there is more of a reliance on an increased frequency of motor unit firing than for larger proximal muscles that may rely more heavily on recruiting more motor units (Levangie & Norkin, 2011).

Finally, a muscle's ability to produce force depends on the length of the muscle. This is tied directly to the length and number of sarcomeres in a muscle fiber. When a muscle

a higher rate of contraction (Levangie & Norkin, 2011). Muscles that contain a majority of these types of motor units, like the bicep or hamstring, are often responsible for activities that call for large movements. On the other hand, muscles that contain motor units with small axons, smaller cell bodies, and fewer muscle fibers are more adept at smaller movements, stabilizing actions and fine motor activity. Smaller motor units typically have more type I slow twitch fibers, which are capable of prolonged activity because they do not fatigue as rapidly (see Fig. 20-7).

Other contributing factors for regulating the force of a muscle contraction are the number of motor units that are recruited and the modulation of firing rates of active motor units (Contessa, Adam, & De Luca, 2009). As the need for force increases because of the load or if motor units fatigue because of duration of contraction, other motor units are recruited (Hall & Brody, 2005). Small motor units that produce less tension and thus require less energy

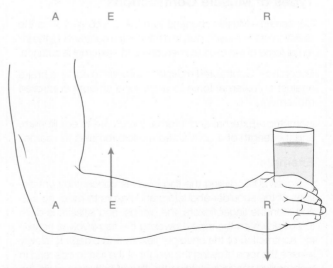

Figure 20-4 *Top,* Schematic drawing of a third-class lever. *Bottom,* Third-class lever depicted by lifting a filled glass. *A,* axis; *E,* effort force (elbow flexors); *R,* resistance force (weight of glass and forearm).

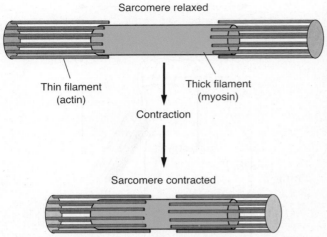

Sarcomere relaxed

Thin filament (actin)

Thick filament (myosin)

Contraction

Sarcomere contracted

Figure 20-5 Schematic of actin and myosin cross-bridges during muscle relaxation and contraction. **Top.** Relaxed muscle. **Bottom.** Contracted muscle. (Adapted with permission from Hall, C. M., & Brody, L. T. [1999]. Functional approach to therapeutic exercise for physiological impairments. In C. Hall & L. Brody [Eds.], *Therapeutic exercise: Moving toward function* (pp. 45–46). Philadelphia: Lippincott Williams & Wilkins.)

is at its optimal length, the actin and myosin filaments are positioned in such a way that the maximum number of cross-bridges are formed (Levangie & Norkin, 2011). If muscle fibers are lengthened, there is less overlap of the actin and myosin filaments, resulting in fewer cross-bridges and less tension, and when muscle fibers are shortened, the filaments do not slide as far, resulting in decreased force.

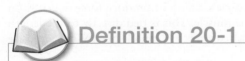

Definition 20-1

Types of Muscle Contractions

Concentric—Muscle shortens to move a limb section in the direction of the muscle pull. In a concentric contraction, the internal force of the muscle overcomes the external resistance.

Eccentric—Contracted muscle lengthens to act as a brake against an external force to allow for a smooth controlled movement.

Isometric—External and internal forces are in equilibrium, and the length of a contracted muscle remains the same.

Example

In Figure 20-6, raising the flag involves concentric contractions of the shoulder abductors and flexors to raise the arm and then the finger flexors, the biceps, and latissimus dorsi to pull down on the rope. Lowering the flag involves eccentric contraction of the shoulder flexors and biceps to slowly release the rope allowing the weight of the flag to descend in a controlled manner. Holding the flag at half mast while the rope is being tied off is an example of isometric contraction of the biceps and triceps and shoulder flexors and extensors.

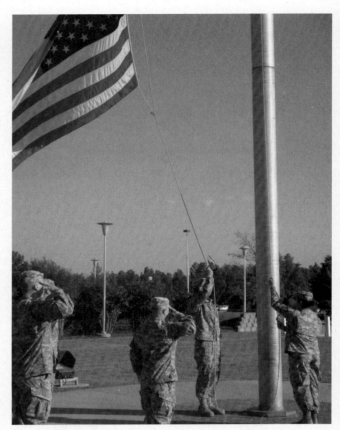

Figure 20-6 Raising, lowering, and securing a flag on a flagpole requires concentric, eccentric, and isometric muscle contractions.

BIOMECHANICAL APPROACH TO TREATMENT

Having an understanding of the biomechanical and physiologic principles of ROM, strength, and endurance helps occupational therapists design the most effective treatment programs aimed at enabling performance.

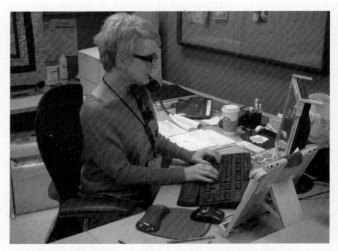

Figure 20-7 Typing or computer work is a fine motor task that uses muscles with smaller motor units that contain more type I slow twitch fibers for prolonged activity.

Remediation or prevention of limitations in these three capacities prepares an individual to fully engage in purposeful and occupation-based activities that support health and participation in life.

Maintaining or Preventing Limitation in Range of Motion

ROM is the maximal distance that bones move about a connecting joint. It involves the length and excursion of muscles as well as the extensibility of connective tissues that cross the joint. There are assessments that provide guidelines for the typical ROM available at various joints in the human body, but an individual's actual ROM at any joint is directly affected by the structures surrounding the segments that are moving. Occupational therapists are concerned with the total range allowed by these structures, but more importantly, they are concerned with functional ROM, which is the range necessary to perform daily activities. To this end, it is the therapist's responsibility to provide treatment that helps clients maintain functional motion or to help patients gain motion when there are limitations that interfere with occupation.

Factors That Limit Range of Motion

There are numerous reasons for limited ROM such as systemic, neurological, or muscular diseases that impair muscle performance (Kisner & Colby, 2007). Joint diseases such as arthritis that create pain and inflammation decrease motion, and surgical or traumatic insults that produce edema and scarring may also limit motion. Finally, simple inactivity or immobilization affects ROM.

Forces that act across a joint during motion determine the quantity, alignment, length, and structural organization of the collagen fibers that make up the majority of connective tissue around a joint (Glasgow, Tooth, & Fleming, 2010). When a joint is not put through its full ROM because of either internal factors such as pain and inflammation or external factors such as casting, splinting, or bed rest, physiological changes in the connective tissues occur. For muscle, this includes changes in the length and numbers of sarcomeres, thickening of the tissue, a loss of fibers, and potential atrophy, resulting in a muscle's inability to exert force on the bony lever. For ligaments, joint capsules, and tendons, a lack of motion results in a decrease in collagen fibers, which results in weakness, and when new collagen is formed, it is done in a shortened, disorganized fashion that results in stiffness (Levangie & Norkin, 2011). In the joints themselves, a loss of motion results in the breakdown of articular cartilage because synovial fluid is no longer moving to carry the necessary nutrients to the joint surfaces (Kisner & Colby, 2007). This in turn creates further loss of motion because of pain, inflammation, and edema.

Edema, defined as the accumulation of excessive fluid in intercellular spaces, is a natural result of trauma or injury (Guyton & Hall, 2011). The fluid (made up mostly of water and dissolved electrolytes) usually dissipates as the healing process progresses (Priganc & Ito, 2008). However, if the edema persists over time, the content of the fluid changes to a highly viscous, protein-laden material, which if not managed can increase circumference of a joint, cause fibrosis and thickening of tissues, and result in adhesions and contractures that restrict motion and limit a person's ability to engage in purposeful activity (Glasgow, Tooth, & Fleming, 2010; Hall & Brody, 2005; Kisner & Colby, 2007).

Intervention Methods

Many ROM limitations can and should be prevented. Limited motion creates a pathological cycle where the loss of motion results in pain, edema, and shortened structures that result in further loss of motion. It is important for occupational therapists to help patients break the cycle in order to remain as functional as possible. This is done by providing therapy that is aimed at decreasing edema, helping patients prevent contractures through proper positioning and/or splinting, and facilitating joint movement through as much range as possible if motion is not contraindicated.

Decreasing Edema. In order to prevent ROM limitations secondary to edema, occupational therapists commonly use techniques of elevation, cryotherapy, compression, massage, and at times electrical current (see further information on physical agent modalities in Chapter 19). The use of these techniques is dependent on the stage of the injury, the vascular status of the patient, and the desired clinical effect. During acute injuries or right after surgery, patients who do not have any arterial compromise are instructed to slightly elevate injured extremities above the heart in order to use gravity to improve venous and lymphatic flow and decrease swelling (Villeco, 2011). Cryotherapy or the use of cold application is helpful in managing edema by producing vasoconstriction, which reduces blood flow, slows down metabolic activity, and decreases the inflammatory response that causes edema (Capps, 2009). Compression limits edema by restricting the accumulation of subcutaneous fluid in tissues through external pressure. The pressure is provided by form fitting compressive garments like gloves or hosiery, tubular sleeves such as Tubigrip™ (Mark One Health Care Products, Philadelphia, PA), or elastic wraps such as Coban™ (3M, St. Paul, MN) (see Procedures for Practice 20-1 for the proper use of elastic wrap compression). There are various techniques of massage to reduce edema, including retrograde massage, which involves a constant stroking massage from the distal portion of the extremity back proximally toward the heart, and a newer technique called manual edema mobilization (discussed further in Chapter 37). Finally, although the effectiveness of high-voltage pulsed current at reducing edema has not

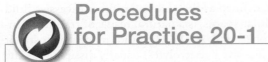

Procedures for Practice 20-1

Applying Self-Adhesive Elastic Bandages for Compression

- Choose the appropriate width of bandage, understanding that the narrower the bandage, the greater the pressure.
- Start at the distal end of the limb or digit and wrap proximally, keeping the tension constant at about 50% of the stretch of the material.
- Wrap in a spiral motion overlapping 50% so that the fluid can flow evenly back toward the body and not be trapped in pockets of unwrapped tissue.
- If wrapping a digit, leave the tip open to observe skin color and preservation of circulation.
- Instruct patient on amount of wear (nighttime, hourly, or multiple hours).
- Instruct patient to remove bandage periodically to inspect skin for color and maceration.

been established, some therapists use this technique in the belief that it helps decrease edema that may be limiting ROM. Note that use of many of these intervention techniques require specialized training and/or licensure.

Minimizing Contractures. Contractures are defined as static shortening of muscle and connective tissue that result in reduced joint mobility and an increase in resistance to passive joint movement (Fergusson, Hutton, & Drodge, 2007). People suffering from hypertonicity caused by a stroke or traumatic brain injury may develop contractures in the upper extremity when elbow or wrist flexors continually fire, resulting in a shortening of the flexors and lengthening of the extensors. Even without hypertonicity, patients with paralysis often rest with their affected arm in the lap, which predisposes the shoulder muscles and tissues to shorten. Patients with burns or deep wounds as a result of trauma may develop contractures when normal skin is replaced by scar tissue (Dewey, Richard, & Parry, 2011). As stated before, patients who are immobilized for a long period of time may also develop contractures when their soft tissues begin to shorten because of lack of movement. To counteract tissue shortening and prevent contractures and subsequent loss of motion and function, occupational therapists may use therapeutic positioning and splinting. Therapeutic positioning is designed to help with edema resolution when limbs are elevated, to help preserve function by holding limbs at a proper muscle length, and to help patients avoid positions that result in tissue shortening or contracture. For example, patients often develop tightness in the shoulder extensors, adductors, and internal rotators after stroke. Therefore, positioning the patient with the arm in shoulder flexion, abduction, and external rotation helps prevent that tightness from developing (Ada et al., 2005).

Splinting, which is an extension of positioning, is indicated when there is a need to prevent unwanted motion or when a patient does not have the capability to assume postures and positions that prevent tissue shortening (see Chapter 16). Splints can be used to hold joints in a position with optimum tissue length, and in the case of burns, they are used to prevent or limit scar contracture (Selvaggi et al., 2005). In spite of prevention, sometimes contractures and consequent ankylosis are unavoidable because of the disease process. In these instances, positioning and splinting patients in a safe, functional position that allow the patient to manage self-care and other functional tasks, is necessary. The functional position of the hand and wrist is slight (20°–30°) extension of the wrist, opposition and abduction of the thumb, metacarpal-phalangeal joints in 40°–60° of flexion and semiflexion of the finger joints (Haines & Cooper, 2007). Then, if a patient's hand contracts in that position, the person can still hold objects. If, however, the hand or digits were to contract in a fully flexed or fully extended posture, function is lost. When positioning and splinting a patient, the occupational therapist must be vigilant in anticipating eventual outcomes of prolonged immobilization that may compromise occupational performance.

Movement through Full Range of Motion. Immobilization is often necessary to protect structures such as bone and skin while they heal, but prolonged immobilization can lead to decreased strength, shortened tissues, contractures, and loss of motion (Glasgow, Tooth, & Fleming, 2010). Controlled motion applied early in the rehabilitation process helps minimize the negative effects of immobilization (Levangie & Norkin, 2011). The method used for movement through full ROM, referred to as ranging, involves teaching the patient to move the joints that are injured, immobilized, or edematous or passively moving the joints if the patient is unable to actively move the joint themselves. In active range of motion (AROM), the patient actively moves the joint through full range with their own muscle power, and in passive range of motion (PROM), the patient's limb is moved through the desired motion by an external source. If a patient has some strength but is unable to fully move a joint through its desired ROM because of weakness, a therapist may use active-assistive ROM (AAROM) to provide just enough assistance to help the patient achieve the desired motion. AROM or AAROM is preferred to PROM because the contraction of the muscles helps pump the fluid out of the extremity helping with edema and stiffness. However, if AROM is not possible, PROM and in particular the use of a continuous passive motion (CPM) machine, which electronically moves a joint through a set ROM, also reduce stiffness and edema (O'Driscoll & Giori, 2000). The extent of effectiveness of CPM versus PROM has been studied and debated (see LaStayo and Cass [2002], O'Driscoll and Giori [2000], and Schwartz and Chafetz (2008) for additional information on the use of CPM with the upper extremities).

Whatever kind of motion is being applied, therapists must pay attention to the plane of motion a joint is moving through, the structures involved with the movement of the joint, and joint biomechanics. For example, the therapist pays special attention to the scapulohumeral rhythm when ranging the shoulder girdle. By moving the scapula with one hand and the humerus with the other, the therapist ensures that they are moving in synchrony (Fig. 20-8). Attention to this alignment during movement of the scapula and humerus eliminates injury to the glenohumeral joint, bursae, capsule, and ligaments.

To maintain ROM, joints must periodically be moved through their available ranges (Kisner & Colby, 2007). As for the frequency of AROM or PROM when trying to maintain motion, there is no set protocol. Therapists constantly monitor a patient's response to any intervention and adjust treatment accordingly. The amount of motion is dependent on the patient's status (inpatient versus outpatient), time constraints during treatment, and the patient's own abilities, both physical and cognitive. If a patient has the physical and cognitive abilities, occupational therapists use activity to promote the AROM and PROM needed to prevent loss of motion. For example, using a Wii™ golf or tennis program during therapy encourages a patient who has either of those interests to move at the shoulder, elbow, and wrist. Another example is having a patient use his or her hemiplegic upper extremity in weight-bearing activities for balance and postural stability while passively stretching the wrist and fingers in extension.

Increasing Range of Motion

If limitation in ROM impairs a patient's ability to function independently or is likely to lead to joint deformity, skilled intervention to facilitate and improve ROM is warranted. Whereas some significant limitations of ROM can be improved or corrected through the use of occupation and exercise, others cannot. Problems that can be changed include contractures of soft tissues, such as skin, muscles, tendons, and ligaments. Occupational therapists may treat ROM limitations using several time-tested interventions such as moist heat, PROM with prolonged passive stretch at the patient's end range, CPM, and various splinting techniques. However, therapists universally recognize the importance of stretch in helping patients develop the capabilities needed to perform occupations. Some problems cannot be changed through these means including ankylosis or arthrodesis, long-standing contractures in which there are extensive fibrotic changes in soft tissue and severe joint destruction. If ROM limitations cannot be overcome, occupational therapy facilitates functional mobility by providing compensatory techniques through the use of equipment to enable participation in life occupations.

Stretching

Stretch is a process by which the target tissue is lengthened by an external force, usually through manual therapy or through the use of splinting, casting, or external equipment. Stretch is used to eliminate tightness that has the potential to cause contracture, even in periods of brief inactivity. Stretch produces change in the extensibility of soft tissue that dissipates when the stress is removed, so to make lasting gains, the stretch needs to be repeated or sustained over time (Katalinic, Harvey, & Herbert, 2011). Factors that determine the effectiveness of stretching are the duration, the intensity, the speed, and the frequency of the stretch being applied (Hall & Brody, 2005; Kisner & Colby, 2007).

The duration of a stretch refers to the amount of time tissues are held under an external force. According to the total end range time principle outlined by Flowers and LaStayo (1994), the longer a joint is held at the end range under adequate tension, the greater the gains will be in ROM. However, there are different types of stretching such as ballistic stretching or joint mobilization techniques that incorporate shorter stretches. It is clinically recognized that maintained stretching is more effective; however, gains are also noted using the briefly held stretches (Kisner & Colby, 2007; Michlovitz, Harris, & Watkins, 2004).

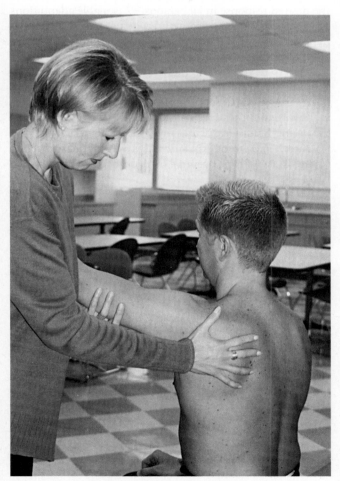

Figure 20-8 Facilitation of glenohumeral rhythm during passive ROM.

The intensity of a stretch is determined by the amount of force put on the tissues that are being stretched. Gentle, controlled stretching that achieves small increments of gain over time is thought to be more effective than vigorous stretching aimed at large, rapid gains. *Safety Message: Residual pain after stretching indicates that the stretch was too forceful and caused tearing of soft tissues or blood vessels.* The method of moving gently to the point of maximal stretch and holding that position allows connective tissue to gradually adapt to its new elongated state over time. This is the principle behind static progressive stretching. In static progressive stretching, shortened tissues are held comfortably in a lengthened position until a degree of relaxation is felt by the patient or the therapist. Once this is achieved, the newly lengthened tissues are lengthened again, and over time the accommodated tissues lengthen to a functional position.

As for the velocity of a stretch, it is generally thought that the speed should be slow to allow the tissues to adjust gradually to the forces being applied. As a protective mechanism, connective tissue resists quick vigorous stretching by evoking a stretch reflex that increases the tension in the contractile structures of muscle, thereby opposing the purpose of the stretch (Kisner & Colby, 2007).

The frequency of stretching refers to the number of sessions during a day or week that the tissues are stretched either at home, by a therapist, or during occupation. There is little evidence to define the optimal frequency of stretching, but it is known that there needs to be adequate time between stretching to allow for tissue healing and to prevent inflammation. In the case of low-load, prolonged stretching to lengthen contracture found in static progressive splinting, frequency is not an issue as much as the duration of splint wear.

Intervention Methods

There are two types of stretching: active and passive. In active stretching, contraction of muscles opposite to the direction of limitation is the source of the force, and in passive stretching, an external force is applied.

Active Stretching. An occupational therapist's clinical expertise lies in using occupation as a treatment medium and in this case, as a means for reaching the goal of increasing ROM in a given joint or mobility within a given extremity. The use of occupation for stretching is empirically based on the idea that a person involved in an interesting and purposeful activity will gain greater range because he or she is relaxed, is not anticipating pain, is motivated to complete the task, and therefore is likely to move as the activity demands (Colaianni & Provident, 2010; Earley & Shannon, 2006.)

The therapist and patient choose a life occupation that has significance to the patient. Occupations can be performed using a number of muscle patterns. Therefore, through the use of activity analysis, the therapist must determine how the patient completed the activity prior to injury. If the activity, as naturally performed by the patient, requires stretching of the soft tissues that are shortened, it can be used as a form of active stretching. Occupations used as a means to increase ROM must provide a gentle active stretch by use of slow, repetitive isotonic contractions of the muscle opposite the contracture or by use of prolonged passive stretched position of the contracted tissue. In both types of stretch, the requirement is that the range be increased slightly beyond the limitations. Grading of the task or subtasks can also be seamlessly integrated into the activity and is of great therapeutic benefit. Techniques, such as, slowing down the sequence of the task or event, increasing or decreasing the placement distance from the patient's center of gravity, and increasing the weight of the object being transferred to and from the various levels all address active stretching with ROM. These techniques not only facilitate active stretching, but also promote gross motor control, trunk balance, and weight shifting, which are all used in performing occupational tasks (Holmes et al., 2008). People move in individually characteristic ways and frequently compensate by using available ROM in adjacent joints, so the therapist must carefully monitor the patient's motions. The therapist cannot assume that the activity itself will evoke the desired response in all persons. Reasonable adaptations of the occupation may sometimes be used to elicit desired motions. Examples of adaptations include adjusting the size of a handle to stretch finger flexors or by placing an object that has to be reached up higher to increase the amount of shoulder ROM during the activity (Fig. 20-9). The Activity-Focused Analysis Case Example incorporates active stretching involved in the aforementioned task. Table 20-1 details the biomechanical capacities involved in this activity.

Another technique that increases the range of shortened tissue is the proprioceptive neuromuscular facilitation

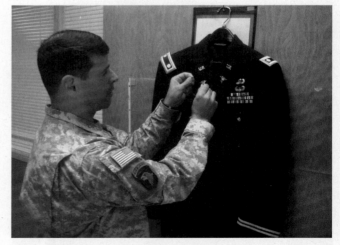

Figure 20-9 Putting together an army uniform with all decorations with the jacket hanging from a hanger will achieve more shoulder ROM than if the jacket was laying on a table.

Activity-Focused Analysis
Assembling an Army Uniform

Task Analysis Process			Example
Describe the task demands	Objects used	Properties of the utensils, tools, and materials and their locations relative to the person	U.S. Army Service Uniform jacket 8 Army ribbons and 21 decoration clasps 1 name plate, unit crest, combat service badge 2 U.S. Army insignia, branch insignia, skill badges 2 rank epaulettes Ruler Decorations placed on a table, the uniform jacket on a hanger, and the person doing the activity between the table and the uniform
	Environmental demands	Characteristics of the environment in which the activity is usually carried out, including possible environmental barriers and enablers	Indoors Decorations positioned on the table top surface within reach No obstacles between the table and uniform
	Social demands	Nature of and extent to which the activity involves others and/or holds particular meaning associated with social roles	Does not require participation of others; may hold personal meaning to those in the military or for those who wear a uniform to work such as police officers or firemen
	Contextual demands	Nature of and extent to which the activity or the way it is carried out holds particular meaning to certain cultures or age groups	Appropriate for individuals who are of work age and any cultural background
	Sequencing and timing	Monological task (requiring a singular sequence in order to be performed correctly) or a multilogical task in which a variety of sequences will work Extent to which the task involves temporal requirements or timing requirements	Assembling the decorations on the uniform jacket can be multilogical where the order of placement of the decorations on the jacket can be alternated. If working on memory or following directions, the order of placement can be written out to create a monological task. The activity can be completed within one therapy session (no specific temporal requirements).
	Required actions	Steps that comprise the activity	1. Hang the uniform jacket on a hanger at eye level. 2. Set out decorations including rank and name plates on the table. 3. Place name plate on flap of the right pocket between top of button and top of pocket. 4. Place unit awards 1/8 inch above right pocket and regimental crest 1/4 inch above awards. 5. Place combat service identification badge in the center of the right pocket. 6. Assemble ribbons on a ribbon rack according to military order of importance. 7. Place ribbons 1/8 inch above the top of the left pocket. 8. Place skill badges 1/4 inch above the ribbons and centered between sides of ribbons.

(continued)

			9. Place U.S. insignia 5/8 inch above the notch on both collars with centerline of insignia parallel to the edge of the lapel and branch insignia 1 and 1/4 inch below the U.S. insignia. 10. Place epaulettes of rank on shoulder clasps.
	Prerequisite capacities, abilities, skills necessary to successful task performance	Sensorimotor: range of motion, strength, motor control, postural control, endurance, coordination/dexterity	See Table 20-1 for biomechanical analysis of Steps 3 to 10.
		Vision-perceptual: visual acuity, visual scanning, visual perception, awareness of extrapersonal space	Visual proficiency with small objects that are within arm's reach. Ability to differentiate color, figure-ground perception, position in space Adequate spatial relations to move between table and uniform
		Cognitive: attention, memory, executive functioning, problem solving, self-awareness	Ability to sustain attention for ~20 minutes Ability to follow directions for sequence of placement of decorations and ribbons or ability to memorize steps Able to problem solve to achieve correct spacing between decorations
		Emotional, relational	Varies based on patient background with activity; can be performed with or without social interaction
	Safety precautions	Nature of safety considerations if performed in a therapy context	Patients who perform the task standing may need supervision related to balance and/or endurance. Patients with limited sensation in digits need to be aware of the sharpness of pins as they go through fabric into the clasps.
Identify the primary therapeutic aspect of the task; adapt task demands to align with therapy goals	Sensorimotor	Range of motion	Uniform decorations are positioned so that the patient has to reach for them repeatedly
		Strength, motor control	Patient may wear weight cuffs during task performance. The uniform can be hung at eye level or higher to work against gravity.
		Postural control, endurance	If postural control is problematic, activity can be done in a seated position with uniform on the table. To work on endurance, uniform can be placed further away from the patient.
		Coordination, dexterity	The activity involves multiple small items that can be increased or decreased to change the size of items or the number of repetitions.
	Vision-perceptual	Visual scanning	Rather than separating all decorations, items can be placed in one pile requiring patient to locate specific decorations working on figure-ground skills. Require exact placement of decorations according to regulations to work on position in space skills. Decorations can be scattered across table to work on visual scanning skills.
		Visual perception, extrapersonal space	
	Cognition	Attention, memory	Patient is challenged to work in an increasingly noisy, distracting environment. Therapist creates interruptions to determine whether patient is able to return to task efficiently. Decorations are placed on the uniform in a specific sequence to work on memory.

		Executive functioning, problem solving, awareness	Patient is given general instructions (assemble uniform according to regulations). Ribbons to be placed on a ribbon rack according to order of importance.
	Emotional-relational	Mood, engagement, interactions with others	Patient performs task in parallel with others or in cooperation with others.
Modify task demands to calibrate difficulty level	Objects used		Number of decorations to place on uniform Location of uniform decorations (within reach, within visual field, within clinic space) Patient can use clasps to increase physical demands or assemble without clasps.
	Space demands		Stimulus arousal properties of the environment Options to sit versus stand while working
	Social demands		Working alone versus working with others
	Contextual demands		Incorporate meaning by having the uniform inspected by another member of the military
	Sequencing and timing		Establish specific time parameters by which patient must assemble the uniform. Allow patient to assemble decorations without regard to sequence to make task easier or provide instructions on specific sequence of assembly to increase cognitive demands.

Table 20-1 **Prerequisite Biomechanical Capacities, Abilities, Skills Necessary for Placing Decoration on the Uniform**

Motions	ROM (°), Distances	Primary Muscles	Gravity Assists, Resists, No Effect	Minimal Strength Required	Type of Contraction
Shoulder flexion	0–90	Anterior deltoid, coracobrachialis, pectoralis major	Resists	4– to 4	Concentric
Elbow extension	90–0	Triceps	Assists	3+ to 4–	Eccentric
Shoulder extension	90–0	Anterior deltoid, coracobrachialis, pectoralis major	Assists	3+ to 4–	Eccentric
Elbow flexion	0–90	Biceps, brachialis	Resists	4– to 4	Concentric
Cylindrical grasp		Finger flexors, finger extensors, interossei	No effect	4– to 4	Isometric
Wrist extension	0–45	Extensor carpi radialis brevis and longus	Resists	4– to 4	Concentric
Wrist Flexion	45–0	Flexor carpi ulnaris and radialis	Assists	4– to 4	Concentric
Wrist stabilize		All wrist muscles	No effect	4– to 4	Isometric
3 Jaw Chuck Pinch		Flexor digitorum superficialis and Flexor digitorum profundus of index and middle finger; interossei; opponens; Flexor pollicus brevis and Flexor pollicus longus, abductor pollicis brevis and adductor pollicis	No effect	4– to 4	Isometric
Trunk flexion	0–30	Back extensors	Assists	3+ to 4–	Eccentric
Trunk extension	30–0	Back extensors	Resists	4– to 4	Concentric

technique called contract relax (CR) and agonist contraction (O'Hora et al., 2011; Sharman, Cresswell, & Riek, 2006) (see Web Chapter C). CR involves a maximal isometric contraction of the tight muscle, usually performed at the point of limitation. The muscle is contracted maximally for 3–10 seconds against resistance provided by the therapist and then relaxed. During the relaxation phase, the therapist moves the part in the direction opposite to the contraction and holds it. For example, if there is a contracture of the elbow flexors, the elbow is extended to its limit. The patient is instructed to contract the flexors isometrically and maximally and then relax, at which point the therapist smoothly extends the elbow into a greater range. The CR technique is repeated until as many increments of gain as possible are achieved.

Therapists have typically used a variety of stretching techniques, including those described here. Based on a review of studies spanning 20 years, Hall and Brody (2005) concluded that no one technique has been demonstrated to have greater benefit over any other.

Passive Stretching. Passive stretching is often done by an occupational therapist as a preparatory method for increasing ROM so patients are able to engage in purposeful activity. Techniques for passive stretching may include manual stretch and the use of orthotic devices, such as splints or casts, to provide controlled passive stretching (see Chapter 16). The procedures for manual stretching by the therapist are outlined in Procedures for Practice 20-2. Safety Note 20-1 lists precautions.

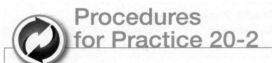

Procedures for Practice 20-2

Manual Stretching Methods

- Provide a relaxing environment for the patient.
- Describe manual stretching, noting that it involves tolerable pain.
- Use motions identical to motions used in ROM evaluation (see Chapter 7).
- Stabilize the bone proximal and distal to the joint that is to be moved to avoid any compensatory movement.
- Move the bone smoothly, slowly, and gently to the point of maximal stretch (mild discomfort indicated verbally or facially by the patient).
- Make sure the movement is in the line of pull of the muscle.
- Encourage the patient to assist in moving the limb if possible.
- Hold the limb at the point of maximal stretch for 15–60 seconds (Thompson, Gordon, & Pescatello, 2010).
- Relief of discomfort should immediately follow the release of stretch.
- If the patient complains of residual pain, future stretches should be performed more slowly and with less force.

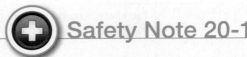

Safety Note 20-1

Safety Precautions Related to Passive Stretching

- Inflammation weakens the structure of collagen tissues. Therefore, inflamed tissues must be stretched cautiously with slow, gentle motions (Kisner & Colby, 2007).
- Sensory loss prevents the patient from monitoring pain; thus, the therapist must pay particular attention to the tension of the tissues being stretched.
- Overstretching must be avoided because it may increase pain and inflammation and cause internal bleeding and subsequent scar formation. It may also lead to heterotopic ossification.
- Resistance can be provided by weights either held in the patient's hand or strapped around the moving part. Resistance can also be provided by tools and materials of the activity. The greater the resistance that is provided, the more aggressive the stretch will be, so the therapist must take care that the stretch is slow and gentle.

There are many ways patients can perform stretching of soft tissue contractures themselves. Patients can be given a home program on specific joint stretches, or they can participate in activities such as Pilates, yoga, or the ROM dance, which includes some passive stretching and can be integrated into their daily occupations. Occupational therapists can help a patient modify these activities to provide the necessary active and passive stretches to meet the ROM needs. Therapists must remember that with any method to increase rather than maintain ROM, the patient's limb must move to the point of maximal stretch.

Strengthening

Muscle strengthening is the process of working against resistance to increase the maximum force-producing capacity of muscle or muscle groups. Strengthening is warranted if a limitation in a patient's strength prevents participation in occupation or may lead to a deformity. Weakness can be deforming if the muscles on one side of a joint are significantly weaker than their antagonists, resulting in a muscle imbalance. If the weakness prohibits a person from maintaining a functional position or moving through a regular AROM, this may lead to a contracture deformity (Tafti, Cramer, & Gupta, 2010).

It is important to realize that strengthening is a very specific and individualized process affected by age, a person's medical condition, activity level, and training or therapeutic goals (Chodzko-Zajko et al., 2009; Hall & Brody, 2005). If a patient needs to return to a specific activity or type of work, the strengthening program needs to be designed in a way that will replicate the functional demands of the activity in relation to the type and speed of contraction, the muscles involved, and the intensity of the task. If the patient just needs general strengthening, then variation is the key because the body adapts quickly to resistive training, so there needs to be some change in the process for continual progress to occur (Ratamess et al., 2009; Thompson, Gordon, & Pescatello, 2010).

Intervention Methods: Occupations and Exercise

Strengthening interventions are defined as any intervention that involves an attempt at repetitive, effortful, muscle contraction and may include biofeedback, electrical stimulation, muscle reeducation, and progressive resistance exercise (Ada, Dorsch, & Canning, 2006). Occupations or functional activity may also be used to increase strength. Therapists find that various occupations provide sufficient opportunities for muscle strengthening and are more effective at maintaining the patient's interest and motivation than exercise alone. At other times, therapists may develop an exercise program specifically targeted to strengthen certain muscles needed for occupation using other modalities. The specific targeting of groups of muscles for the sole purpose of reintegrating an injured worker to the work site is known as "work hardening." Through the measured use of work hardening and work reintegration, the injured worker, client, or patient can be allowed to slowly build up sufficient strength, gross motor coordination, and balance in a simulated setting to allow safe transition into the work site (Marois & Durand, 2009). Strengthening may be used as a warm-up to occupation, or occupation may be introduced to enhance carryover of the strength gained by exercise. Carefully prescribed therapeutic occupations can strengthen muscles in situations closely approximating their intended uses.

For some individuals, an exercise program may be a valued occupation in and of itself. In these cases, exercise can be used as a therapeutic occupation designed to address the individual nature of the performance, the meaning of exercise for that person, and the context in which that person typically exercises. In this instance, the occupational therapist may use the therapeutic occupation of exercise to remediate any performance component. For example, in the military the push-up is a common everyday activity with purpose and meaning to the soldier. Using the push-up not only increases strength but also touches on the role of a soldier in relation to discipline, physical fitness, and esprit de corp (see Fig. 20-10).

Grading Muscle Strength Parameters. Similar to stretching, there are many factors that influence the effectiveness of strengthening interventions. For strength to increase and muscle hypertrophy to occur, there must be a gradual increase of stress placed on the muscles (Ratamess et al., 2009). Parameters that may be manipulated to increase stress to muscle include exercise intensity, volume, the amount of rest between exercises, the type and velocity of contraction, and the frequency of exercise.

In order to increase the intensity of strengthening exercises, the amount of resistance imposed on the contracting muscle or muscle groups during each repetition is increased. For example, a patient recovering from a hand injury will progress from the use of soft Theraputty™, to medium, and then to firm as a way to increase intensity and improve grip. The starting point for resistance is based on a therapist's judgment or on the data ascertained through manual muscle testing or testing with standardized equipment. Another method to calculate the appropriate starting load for strength training is to determine a repetition maximum (RM). DeLorme (1945) and DeLorme and Watkins (1948) developed a progressive resistive exercise program based on the use of an RM defined as the greatest amount of weight a muscle can move through available ROM just one time. Once the RM is established, then the intensity of training can be set up based on a percentage of this maximum. Patients at the beginning of training or rehabilitation should use a lower percentage (40%–60% of 1 RM) versus those who have progressed or are well trained, where 80% of 1 RM is recommended (Ratamess et al., 2009).

Training volume refers to the number of repetitions and sets performed during a training session multiplied by the resistance (Kisner & Colby, 2007). An occupational therapist alters the training volume by changing the number of repetitions of an activity, changing the number of sets required of that one activity, or changing the number of activities done during a treatment session. The volume of strength training is also linked to the goal for treatment. If the goal is muscle strengthening, then it is recommended that fewer repetitions are done with increased resistance; if the goal is muscle endurance, then more repetitions are required with less resistance (McNair & Rice, 2010).

A rest period between exercises affects the muscle's response to strength training and is related to the intensity and volume of activity. If a patient is being asked to perform activity that requires a high degree of intensity such as lifting heavy

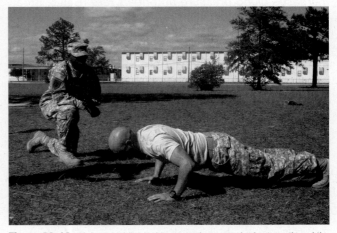

Figure 20-10   An Army soldier is demonstrating upper body strength and the strength of his triceps by performing the push-up during a physical fitness test.

boxes or if the activity demands that a box be lifted multiple times to complete a task, then the amount of rest between lifts or between tasks needs to be lengthened. If the activity involves low intensity or fewer repetitions to complete, then the rest period can be shortened. The recommendation is that for activities that call for high loads or repetitions or if the patient is very young, elderly, or easily prone to fatigue, the rest period between activity should be 3–4 minutes, and for low intensity or low repetition activity, it should be 1–2 minutes (Kisner & Colby, 2007; Ratamess et al., 2009).

The type and velocity of muscle contraction during a strengthening program is established by the demands of the task and the physical abilities of the patient. Most strengthening programs involve dynamic muscle contraction with concentric or eccentric muscle action, but isometric exercise is also a vital part of rehabilitation (review Definition 20-1). During dynamic concentric muscle contraction, the velocity of the muscle action can be manipulated to simulate the demands of functional activity that call for fast movement (sports) or slow movement (painting). The velocity of muscle contraction in training should eventually match the velocity of muscle contraction that is required in the patient's occupational routine (Ratamess et al., 2009). With dynamic eccentric muscle contraction, it is easier to control a load, meaning that it takes less effort to lower a weight than to lift a weight. This is why, when dealing with a patient who is very weak, it is better to start with active eccentric exercise (i.e., having the patient lower the weakened limb while resisting gravity) rather than lifting the limb (Kisner & Colby, 2007). Isometric strengthening is used when joint movement is not available or contraindicated, but strengthening is still warranted, such as after repair of soft tissue or to minimize atrophy during immobilization (see Fig. 20-11). Even though there is no joint movement, an isometric contraction can still produce a forceful contraction. *Safety Message: For this reason, when the patient has hypertension or cardiovascular problems, isometric contraction should be avoided because contraction of either large or small muscles increases blood pressure and heart rate* (Hall & Brody, 2005; Kisner & Colby, 2007) (see Chapter 42). Procedures for Practice 20-3 has guidelines for setting up a therapeutic exercise or occupation program. Although these guidelines are for exercise programs, the principles can be used in designing a routine of occupations to be used for strengthening.

The recommended frequency of strengthening exercises or the number of exercise sessions in a week depends on a number of variables including the patient, the patient's goals, the level of patient adherence to the home program, and the ability of the patient to come to therapy for supervised rehabilitation. The frequency of strengthening is also tied into the amount of rest that is needed for muscle or muscle groups to recover. It is recommended that people who are starting a strengthening program should exercise 2–3 days a week, which can then increase to 3–5 days a week as the strength progresses (Ratamess et al., 2009).

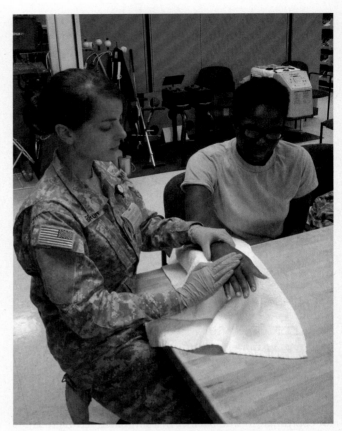

Figure 20-11 As the patient contracts her wrist extensors in an effort to raise her wrist, the therapist is resisting the movement, resulting in an isometric contraction.

For an example of grading the variables for strength during a comprehensive strengthening program, see the patient Case Example. In this example, Ms. C., who has poor musculature but needs upper extremity strengthening to accomplish her daily tasks, can begin by washing her face side-lying in bed (reduce the effect of gravity) until she can complete the task upright. Ms. C.'s occupational therapist can set up the task to be accomplished in bed while assisting Ms. C. in bringing her hand to her face so that she washes with her muscles in a gravity-eliminated plane. Ms. C. may next attempt to wash her face sitting upright in a chair in the bathroom. The therapist may bring Ms. C.'s hand to her face and then ask the patient to resist against gravity in an eccentric contraction. The next step in the progression involves having Ms. C. move the extremity against the resistance of gravity with a concentric contraction. The therapist can further increase the intensity by adding various weighted tools, such as a light puff, a washcloth, or a bar of soap. As Ms. C. gradually progresses in strength, the therapist can continue to increase the intensity and volume of strengthening by adding more resistive occupations, such as dressing, making a bed, washing a car, gardening, or playing basketball. With any of these activities, resistance can be graded by adding a load to the extremity

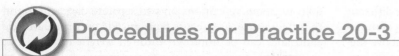

Procedures for Practice 20-3

Guidelines for a Strengthening Program

Type of Exercise	Definition	Muscle Grades	Procedures
Isometric	Exercise in which a weak muscle is isometrically contracted to its maximal force 10 times with rest periods between each contraction	Trace (0) The force of contraction is not sufficient to move the part.	Provide a stimulating environment. Explain procedures. Instruct the patient to contract the weak muscle ("hold"). External resistance applied by the therapist may help the patient isolate the contraction to the weak muscle or muscle group. Patient holds contraction at maximum effort as long as possible while breathing normally. Repeat 10 times with a rest between each contraction. Increase duration of maximal contraction as patient improves. *Safety Message: Maximal isometric contraction is contraindicated for patients with cardiac disease.*
Dynamic assistive (active assistive ROM)	Exercise in which a weak muscle is concentrically or eccentrically contracted through as much ROM as patient can achieve; therapist and/or external device provides assistance to complete motion	Poor minus (2−) Fair minus (3−) The muscle can move only through partial available range in either a gravity-eliminated or against-gravity plane.	Provide a stimulating environment. Explain procedures. For a 2− muscle, position limb to move in a gravity-eliminated plane. For a 3− muscle, position the limb to move against gravity. Patient moves weak muscle through as much range as possible. Therapist provides external force to complete motion. Although this seems similar to PROM, it differs because the patient actively contracts the weak muscle.
Dynamic active (active ROM)	Patient contracts muscle to move part through full ROM.	Poor (2) Fair (3) Muscle can move through full available range in either gravity-eliminated or against-gravity plane.	Provide a stimulating environment. Explain procedures. For a 2 muscle, position the limb to move in a gravity-eliminated plane. For a 3 muscle, position the limb to move against gravity. Patient moves weak muscle through full available ROM. Patient repeats motion for three sets of 10 repetitions with rest break between sets.
Dynamic active resistive (active resistive ROM)	Patient contracts muscle to move part through full available ROM against resistance.	Poor plus (2+) Fair (3) Fair plus (3+) Good (4) Good plus (4+)	Provide a stimulating environment. Explain procedures. For a 2+ or 3 muscle, position limb to move in a gravity-eliminated plane. For a 3+ or above muscle, position limb to move against gravity. Therapist determines appropriate amount of resistance depending on the strengthening protocol chosen. If a 1RM has been established, then a percentage of that maximum can be used starting at 40%–60% and progressing to 80% as strength increases. Patient moves weak muscle through full available ROM against resistance.[a] The patient will do three or four sets of 10 with varying resistance and rest breaks between sets.

[a]Resistance can be provided by weights either held in the patient's hand or strapped around the moving part. Resistance can also be provided by tools and materials of activity.

(i.e., tools such as washcloth, gardening utensils, or different size and weight of the ball) or by changing the plane of movement (i.e., gravity eliminated to against gravity, to above-the-shoulder work). The frequency of the sessions started at three times a day for 4–6 weeks, but Ms. C., who is starting off very weak, may not be able to finish washing her face in bed during a session. The therapist can manipulate the rest breaks during the activity or divide up the task into subtasks, allowing Ms. C. to pace herself throughout the entire task. This technique can also be used to help a deconditioned client perform household chores or any of the other activities without tiring excessively. As Ms. C. develops enough strength to complete activities, she then works to improve endurance to participate in the activities for a longer period of time.

Increasing Endurance

Exercise programs designed to increase muscle endurance rather than muscle strength require different techniques. The following describes the underlying principles and guidelines for those modifications.

Factors That Influence Muscle Endurance

Muscle endurance refers to the ability of a muscle to maintain performance over a sustained period of time (McNair & Rice, 2010). During light resistive activities, motor units within the muscles are recruited and activated asynchronously, meaning that while some motor units are working and then fatiguing, other motor units are being recruited to make up for the recovering units (Contessa, Adam, & De Luca, 2009). This allows for prolonged activity or muscle contraction. With activities that call for maximum muscle contraction, such as lifting heavy loads, more motor units must contract simultaneously without the opportunity to recover, resulting in quicker fatigue. Other factors that influence muscle endurance include the predominant type of fiber that is contracting during the activity (type I slow twitch fibers fatigue slower than type II fast twitch fibers), the energy and oxygen storage within the muscle and external factors such as room temperature, altitude, and amount of allowed recovery time during an activity (Kisner & Colby, 2007).

Intervention Methods

Grading Occupations to Increase Endurance. The key elements of endurance training are low-intensity muscle contractions, a large number of repetitions, and a prolonged time period of training to the point of muscle overload (Kisner & Colby, 2007). The American College of Sports Medicine advocates for light to moderate loads (40%–60% of 1 RM) for high repetitions (>15) using short rest periods (<90 seconds) for endurance training (Ratamess et al., 2009). Roy et al. (2011) developed a protocol for evaluating shoulder endurance where subjects performed two isotonic exercises of internal and external rotation at 50% of peak torque for

60 continuous repetitions on two separate days and found that the muscle fatigue was reproducible over time. Muscle endurance can be improved through weight training, but occupational therapists prefer to use purposeful activity to provide the same benefits. Occupational therapists provide the patients with interest-sustaining occupations that can be graded along the dimension of time or repetition. For example, for patients who are interested in computer games or sports that can be replicated on a Wii™, the therapist may increase the number of games they play or the length of time they play to get to muscle fatigue. Occupational therapists can also work with patients to schedule their everyday routines so that they gradually increase the amount of time they engage in occupations throughout the day and/or gradually increase the duration of engagement in one particular occupation. For example, increasing the time working in the garden or the amount of muscular effort put forth through repetition (picking tomatoes versus pulling weeds) is an effective way to increase muscular endurance (Fig. 20-12).

Evidence Table 20-1 shows the best evidence regarding strengthening, stretching, and endurance training. Programming for cardiovascular endurance specifically with patients who have cardiopulmonary problems is discussed in Chapter 42.

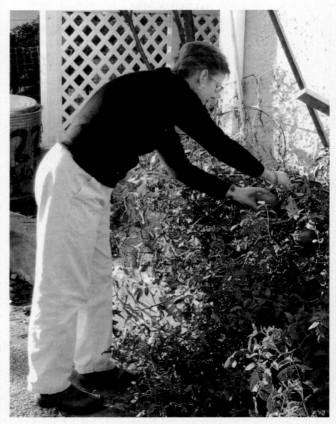

Figure 20-12 Muscular endurance can be increased by adding to the time spent on a task or adding to the resistance of the activity. In gardening, picking tomatoes could advance to weeding the garden.

Evidence Table 20-1	Best Evidence for Occupational Therapy Practice Regarding Strengthening, Stretching, and Endurance Training					
Intervention	Description of Intervention Tested	Participants	Dosage	Type of Best Evidence and Level of Evidence	Benefit	Statistical Probability and Effect Size of Outcome	Reference
Stretching to increase joint range of motion (ROM)	Experimental groups received a 6-week stretching program compared to a control group that did not.	Forty-three participants (controls and those with osteoarthritis [OA]) were randomly assigned to groups (experimental group with OA, $n = 14$; control group with OA, $n = 10$; experimental group without OA, $n = 8$; control group without OA, $n = 11$).	Experimental groups performed three 60-second stretches to all muscle groups of the leg, 5 days a week for 6 weeks with two of the days being supervised. The control group did not stretch.	Randomized controlled study Level: 1C1b	Yes. All stretching groups (OA and without OA) improved range	Statistically significant differences in posttest knee extension ROM between experimental and control groups: $p < 0.05$; effect size: $r = 0.30$ (medium effect)	Reid & McNair (2011)
Effectiveness of exercise on reducing impairment and increasing activity in people with upper limb fractures	Studies included compared various dimensions of upper extremity therapy exercise programs.	Thirteen trials involving 781 participants with an upper limb fracture were identified.	Exercise therapy programs differed in timing, intensity, frequency, duration, and exercises performed.	Systematic review with a single meta-analysis	Preliminary but inconclusive evidence to support the role of exercise regimens in reducing impairments and improving upper limb function following upper limb fractures (likely because of cointerventions used in most studies)	One meta-analysis (involving two studies) did not demonstrate effects of exercise on grip strength after distal radius fracture.	Bruder et al. (2011)
Effectiveness and safety of dynamic exercise for patients with rheumatoid arthritis (RA)	Short- and long-term, land-based exercise programs to increase muscle strength	Three hundred seventy-nine participants with RA; mean age = 52 years and disease duration between 5 and 14 years	Land-based aerobic capacity training and strength training: at least twice per week for >20 minutes, lasting at least 12 weeks for short-term programs and 24 weeks for long-term programs (muscle strengthening starting at 30%–50% of repetition maximum [RM] performed under supervision)	Systematic review and meta-analysis of four studies	Yes. There is a positive effect of combined aerobic and strength training on muscle strength after 12 weeks; nonsignificant but trending toward positive effect on muscle strength at 24 weeks.	Data pooled from two studies resulted in a significant, medium positive effect on muscle strength (standard mean difference of 0.47) immediately after the 12 weeks compared to the control groups.	Hurkmans et al. (2009)

(continued)

| Evidence Table 20-1 | Best Evidence for Occupational Therapy Practice Regarding Strengthening, Stretching, and Endurance Training (*continued*) |

Intervention	Description of Intervention Tested	Participants	Dosage	Type of Best Evidence and Level of Evidence	Benefit	Statistical Probability and Effect Size of Outcome	Reference
Effect of progressive resistance exercise program	Experimental group received progressive resistive exercise training (PRET), and a control group received a standardized therapeutic exercise protocol (TP).	Fifty-two head and neck cancer survivors were randomly assigned to two groups (experimental PRET group *n* = 27; control TP group *n* = 25)	Twelve weeks of supervised sessions meeting two times a week consisting of two sets of 10–15 repetitions of five to eight exercises progressing from 25% to 75% of 1RM strength	Randomized controlled study Level: 1C1a	Progressive resistance training provided superior upper extremity strengthening, endurance and pain reduction than traditional strengthening program consisting of ROM, stretching, postural, and general strengthening exercises.	Shoulder pain and disability $p = 0.001$ (when adjusted for baseline value, age, sex, cancer stage, pain medication use), affected shoulder strength (unadjusted) $p = 0.003$ ($r = 0.45$); upper extremity endurance (unadjusted) $p = 0.017$ ($r = 0.33$).	McNeely et al. (2008)
Effectiveness of strength training after stroke	Strengthening interventions that involved repetitive, effortful muscle contractions (including biofeedback, electrical stimulation, muscle reeducation, progressive resistance exercise, and mental practice)	Twenty-one studies met inclusion criteria with a total of 768 participants categorized as acute (<6 months) or chronic stroke and into weak and very weak categories.	Ranged from 2- to 12-week programs, 3–6 days per week and 30–90 minutes a day	Systematic review with meta-analysis of 15 studies	Yes. Strengthening interventions provided a small positive effect of strength across all stroke participants.	Posttest improvements in strength (0.33 standardized mean difference; 95% confidence interval 0.13 to 0.54, $p = 0.001$). Strengthening interventions had very little effect on spasticity ($p = 0.69$).	Ada, Dorsch, & Canning (2006)

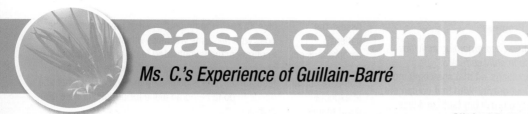

case example
Ms. C.'s Experience of Guillain-Barré

	Clinical Reasoning Process	
Occupational Therapy Assessment Process	**Objectives**	**Examples of Therapist's Internal Dialogue**

Patient Information

Ms. C. is a 40-year-old woman who was the executive administrator of a large computer company. She lives at home with her partner and her high school–aged son from a previous marriage. Her partner is a lawyer in a small law firm that requires at least 10–12-hour work days. Ms. C. is a high-powered, motivated woman who not only enjoyed but was energized by the various people with whom she interacted with at her job and the diverse assignments she supervised. When Ms. C. returned home from work, she often used household occupations as a means of changing from her high-energy level to a more relaxed state. Ms. C. shared household tasks equally with her partner and also her son. Relationships are essential in her life.

Ms. C. began to complain of tingling in her legs about 3 weeks ago. This progressed to her trunk and then to weakness in her legs and arms about 2 weeks ago. She was admitted to the hospital at that point and was then diagnosed with Guillain-Barré syndrome. She was in intensive care for about 10 days and has now been admitted to the rehab unit. At this point, she is extremely weak and has poor endurance. She is unable to lift her arms against gravity and has been up in a reclining wheelchair for about 30 minutes before she needs to go back to bed. Following an occupational therapy evaluation that included this history, the following problems were identified by Ms. C. and the therapist: (1) loss of independence in all occupations including all self-care activities and use of the phone and computer; (2) weakness throughout her arms, trunk, and legs, with manual muscle testing scores of 2–3, but very limited endurance, so that she is able to do only three or four repetitions of a motion before she is fatigued; (3) depression and anxiety because of an unpredictable future; and (4) inability to communicate with her employees, employer, and her son, which is causing considerable anxiety.

Appreciate the context

Develop intervention hypotheses

Select an intervention approach

"I think if Ms. C. reestablished some of her more important activities, such as being able to communicate with work, she would feel that she was making progress. In addition, with her endurance and strength both so low, repetition of any movements would help to increase them both."

"Ms. C. would benefit from remediation to increase strength and endurance in her extremities, which would allow her to regain independence in her occupations. However, I also think she would benefit from compensation through the use of adapted equipment to help her resume some important activities."

"Ms. C. is really having difficulty being separated from work. I think that if she could communicate with her workplace, she would feel that she was back in some control. In addition, it is difficult for her to see her son because he can only come after school, and at that point, she is usually exhausted. If she could have some other means to communicate with both work and her son, she might begin to see that she is making progress. I will need to see if she is willing to use adaptive equipment as a bridge to independence; some patients do not tolerate 'gadgets,' so I will have to check that out."

Recommendations

The occupational therapist recommended three brief treatment sessions each day for 4–6 weeks. Ms. C. and the therapist together established the following long-term treatment goals: (1) Ms. C. will carry out her hygiene, self-care, dressing, and showering independently, which would prepare her for being at home during the day; (2) Ms. C. will prepare a light meal for lunch, which will also ready her for discharge; (3) Ms. C. will learn skills and develop strategies to be able to work from home when she is discharged, for at least a few hours a day; (4) Ms. C. will be independent in a home exercise program for strengthening and endurance; and (5) Ms. C. will resume an active role as the mother of her son.

Consider what will occur in therapy, how often, and for how long

"I think that Ms. C. is so overwhelmed with what has happened that it is difficult for her to fully participate in goal-setting. It is such a change from her previous life of being in charge of everything. I think that we will need to start with things that are very important to her and that she can succeed at. Because work and her son are so important, I think that, if we used an overhead sling, she might be able to operate both a speakerphone and e-mail, and that would allow her to be involved. My one concern is that she might overdo it, so we will have to talk about that."

"I will need to maintain her passive range of motion (PROM), particularly in those antigravity positions that she cannot move into. Daily PROM exercises will be necessary until she gains enough strength to move herself. In addition, care will need to be taken to ensure that she is not developing imbalances of muscle strength around joints that would lead to contractures.

Once she has had some success, we can begin to do other activities such as strengthening activities and self-care."

Summary of Short-Term Goals and Progress

1. *Ms. C. will start assisting with hygiene and grooming activities and then advance to independence in daily self-care.*

   Ms. C. was fitted with overhead slings, so that she could move her arms without lifting them against gravity. With that equipment, Ms. C. was able to wash her face and brush her teeth and was able to drive a power wheelchair, which greatly improved her independence.

2. *Ms. C. will access a speakerphone and e-mail to make working from home possible.*

   With the overhead slings, she was able to operate both a speakerphone and her laptop computer in her room. She was able to work for about 25 minutes before she fatigued.

3. *Ms. C. will feed herself and get food in and out of the refrigerator.*

   Ms. C. was able to feed herself with a set up using the overhead slings and progressed to feeding herself without equipment. Using the power wheelchair, she was able to get items out of the refrigerator.

4. *Ms. C. will develop ways to communicate with her son more frequently.*

   She was able to access her e-mail account and sent an e-mail to her son. She also was able to call him on his cell phone over the noon hour, and he was really excited to talk to her when she was alert and awake.

5. *Ms. C. will begin an upper extremity strengthening and endurance program.*

As she gained endurance, she was able to begin doing resistive exercises to some muscles, as well as assume some responsibility for stretching. She will have to be independent in some parts of the program when she goes home.

The therapist and Ms. C. discussed that it was important that she not overdo it, and she seemed to understand that. Her endurance for activity increased considerably over the first week, as she had the opportunity to do things that were important to her on her own schedule.

Next Steps

We are also going to need to assess the accessibility of her home, because she will probably be using her wheelchair most of the time at home, particularly when she is alone.

At some point in the next several weeks, we will remove the overhead slings, progress her to a manual wheelchair, and then begin doing more activities in standing, as she can tolerate. This may be frustrating for her because occupations she is currently doing will become more difficult, so I will have to be careful of that.

We will need to plan out a typical day and make sure that Ms. C. can do all the things she will need to do at home.

Assess the patient's comprehension

Compare actual to expected performance

Know the person

Appreciate the context

"Ms. C. seems to understand that any activities she does with her arms will help with strengthening and endurance and is motivated to do more. Now that she can access her e-mail and use the phone and feed herself, she is beginning to think about what she needs to do to be home alone for periods of time after discharge."

"Ms. C. is accepting of the use of adaptive equipment as a bridge to independence, so that opens up a lot of opportunities. She is doing better than I expected, and she is tolerating all the activity well."

"We will continue to advance her to more complex activities, such as meal preparation, and more work-related tasks, such as handling files, organizing a work station, etc."

"I need to check with her partner and her son to see how things are going at home. If the partner is working 10–12 hours a day, and her son is home alone, we may need to come up with a new plan."

Anticipate present and future patient concerns

Decide whether the patient should continue or discontinue therapy and/ or return in the future

---

"Ms. C. is making very good progress and will be able to leave the hospital in several more weeks. Because her partner works and they do not have any family nearby, Ms. C. will need to be home alone for periods of time after discharge. I'm not sure Ms. C. is anticipating how isolating that can be. Although she will probably be walking short distances at that time, she will likely spend most of her time in her wheelchair. I will need to be sure that she has an emergency plan, can operate a cell phone that she has with her, and has anticipated as much as possible what things she needs to be able to do. Home care may be a very feasible option for Ms. C. for a while, and then she can consider outpatient therapy when she is no longer homebound. Transportation to and from rehab will be a challenge. She will also need to check with her doctor about when he might allow her to drive."

Clinical Reasoning in Occupational Therapy Practice

Effects of Endurance and Strength on Performing Occupations

Range of motion (ROM), strength, and endurance are needed to perform activities of daily living. How does the decline in ROM, strength, and endurance impact the patient's ability to perform house-cleaning chores? How can energy conservation be used to allow Ms. C. to engage in regular household chores? How can activity modification techniques be used to allow Ms. C. to more efficiently complete her household chores?

Clinical Reasoning in Occupational Therapy Practice

Deconstructing Activity in Order to Use Occupation-as-Means

Assembling a uniform is a common military task. What fine motor manipulation skills and bimanual dexterity are needed to accomplish this task? How does this activity directly address upper extremity positioning, active range of motion, endurance, and eye–hand coordination? How is the assembly and preparation of the army uniform considered a core occupation-based function?

Summary Review Questions

1. What are the physiological aspects of muscle contraction?
2. Give an example of a third-class lever system in the body. What is the force arm (effort force)? What is the resistance arm (resistance force)?
3. Explain turning a wrench in terms of torque.
4. Analyze the forces, stability, and motions required to put a can of soup on the shelf at nose height.
5. How should passive stretching treatment be modified if the patient acknowledges residual pain after treatment?
6. What parameters can be manipulated to alter stress on the muscle to increase strength?
7. What are the necessary characteristics of exercise or occupation required to increase muscle endurance?
8. Plan a therapeutic occupation program to strengthen a patient who has generalized poor (grade = 2) upper extremity musculature. Revise the program to accommodate changes in the patient's musculature from poor (grade = 2) to fair (grade = 3).
9. Differentiate between a therapeutic occupation program designed to strengthen muscles and one designed to increase muscle endurance.
10. Following replacement of the proximal interphalangeal (PIP) joint of the ring finger, the patient's finger and hand are edematous. What treatment choices does the occupational therapist have?

Glossary

Ankylosis—Pathological stiffening of a joint caused by fibrotic changes in the bones and/or tissues surrounding the joints.

Connective tissues—Tissues made up mostly of collagen that make up a joint structure such as bones, bursae, capsules, cartilage, discs, fat pads, labra, ligaments, and tendons.

Cross-bridge—The bonding of actin and myosin myofilaments within a myofibril that creates muscle contraction.

Guillain-Barré syndrome—An inflammatory disorder in which the body's immune system attacks the peripheral nervous system, resulting in weakness and numbness in the arms, legs, trunk, and face. Most patients make substantial improvements, but about one-third of patients still have some residual weakness 3 years after onset.

Heterotopic ossification—The process in which bone tissue forms outside the skeleton in an abnormal site, such as muscle or soft tissue.

Hypertonicity—Increased rigidity, tension, and spasticity of muscles commonly associated with high muscle tone, exaggerated reflexes, lack of selective control, and fatigability.

Kinematics—Study of the displacement or motion of a segment without regard to the forces that cause the movement.

Kinetics—Study of forces, including static forces that balance or stabilize and dynamic forces that mobilize.

Moment arm—The perpendicular distance between a muscle's point of pull and the center of the joint (axis of rotation).

Muscle hypertrophy—An increase in the size of muscle cells through mechanical, metabolic, and hormonal processes.

Rotary motion—Movement of a segment around a fixed axis also known as angular displacement.

Torque—Product of force $\times$ perpendicular distance between the force and the axis of rotation.

Translatory motion—Movement of a segment in a straight line also known as linear displacement.

References

Ada, L., Dorsch, S., & Canning, C. G. (2006). Strengthening interventions increase strength and improve activity after stroke: A systematic review. *Australian Journal of Physiotherapy, 52,* 241–248.

Ada, L., Goddard, E., McCully, J., & Stavrinos, T. (2005). Thirty minutes of positioning reduces the development of shoulder external rotation contracture after stroke: A randomized controlled trial. *Archives of Physical Medicine and Rehabilitation, 86,* 230–234.

American Occupational Therapy Association. (2008). Occupational therapy practice framework: Domain and process (2nd ed.). *American Journal of Occupational Therapy, 62,* 625–683.

Bernas, G., Thiele, R., Kinnaman, K., Hughes, R., Miller, B., & Carpenter, J. (2009). Defining safe rehabilitation for ulnar collateral ligament reconstruction of the elbow. *American Journal of Sports Medicine, 37,* 2392–2400.

Bruder, A., Taylor, N. F., Dodd, K. J., & Shields, N. (2011). Exercise reduces impairment and improves activity in people after some upper limb fractures: A systematic review. *Journal of Physiotherapy, 57,* 71–82.

Capps, S. G. (2009). Cryotherapy and intermittent pneumatic compression for soft tissue trauma. *International Journal of Athletic Therapy & Training, 14,* 2–4.

Chang, J.H., Ho, K.Y., & Su, F.C. (2008). Kinetic analysis of the thumb in jar-opening activity among female adults. *Ergonomics, 51,* 843-857.

Chodzko-Zajko, W. J., Proctor, D. N., Fiatarone-Singh, M. A., Minson, C. T., Nigg, C. R., Salem, G. J., & Skinner, J. S. (2009). Exercise and physical activity for older adults: Position stand. *Medicine and Science in Sports and Exercise, 41,* 1510–1530.

Colaianni, D., & Provident, I. (2010). The benefits of and challenges to the use of occupation in hand therapy. *Occupational Therapy in Health Care, 24,* 130–146.

Contessa, P., Adam, A., & De Luca, C. J. (2009). Motor unit control and force fluctuation during fatigue. *Journal of Applied Physiology, 107,* 235–243.

Cooke, R. (2004). The sliding filament model: 1972-2004. *Journal of General Physiology, 123,* 643–656.

Dewey, W. S., Richard, R. L., & Parry, I. S. (2011). Positioning, splinting, and contracture management. *Physical Medicine and Rehabilitation Clinics of North America, 22,* 229–247.

DeLorme, T. (1945). Restoration of muscle power by heavy resistance exercises. *Journal of Bone and Joint Surgery, 27,* 645–667.

DeLorme, T., & Watkins, A. L. (1948). Techniques of progressive resistance exercise. *Archives of Physical Medicine and Rehabilitation, 29,* 263–273.

Earley, D., & Shannon, M. (2006). The use of occupation-based treatment with a person who has shoulder adhesive capsulitis: A case report. *American Journal of Occupational Therapy, 60,* 397–403.

Fergusson, D., Hutton, B., & Drodge, A. (2007). The epidemiology of major joint contractures: A systemic review of the literature. *Clinical Orthopaedics and Related Research, 456,* 22–29.

Flowers, K. R., & LaStayo, P. (1994). Effect of total end range time on improving passive range of motion. *Journal of Hand Therapy, 7,* 150–157.

Glasgow, C., Tooth, L. R., & Fleming, J. (2010). Mobilizing the stiff hand: Combining theory and evidence to improve clinical outcomes. *Journal of Hand Therapy, 23,* 392–399.

Goins, A. M., Morgan, K., Stephens, C. L., & Engsberg, J. R. (2011). Elbow kinematics during overground manual wheelchair propulsion in individuals with tetraplegia. *Disability & Rehabilitation: Assistive Technology, 6,* 312–319.

Guyton, A., & Hall, J. (2011). *Textbook of medical physiology* (12th ed.). Philadelphia: W. B. Saunders.

Haines, B., & Cooper, C. (2007). Preventing and treating stiffness. In C. Cooper (Ed.), *Fundamentals of hand therapy: Clinical reasoning and treatment guidelines for common diagnoses of the upper extremity* (pp. 440–451). Philadelphia: Mosby.

Hall, C. M., & Brody, L. T. (2005). *Therapeutic exercise: Moving toward function* (2nd ed.). Philadelphia: Lippincott Williams & Wilkins.

Hamilton, N., Weimar, W., & Luttgens, K. (2012). *Kinesiology: Scientific basis of human motion* (12th ed.). New York: McGraw-Hill.

Holmes, W., Lam, P. Y., Elkind, P., & Pitts, K. (2008). The effect of body mechanics education on the work performance of fruit warehouse workers. *Work, 31,* 461–471.

Hurkmans, E., van der Giesen, F. J., Vliet Vlieland, T. P. M., Schoones, J., & Van den Ende, E. C. H. M. (2009). Dynamic exercise programs (aerobic capacity and/or muscle strength training) in patients with rheumatoid arthritis. *Cochrane Database of Systematic Reviews, (4),* 1–58.

Katalinic, O. W., Harvey, L. A., & Herbert, R. D. (2011). Effectiveness of stretch for the treatment and prevention of contractures in people with neurological conditions: A systematic review. *Physical Therapy, 91,* 11–24.

Kisner, C., & Colby, L. A. (2007). *Therapeutic exercise: Foundations and techniques* (5th ed.). Philadelphia: Davis.

Kloosterman, M. G., Snoek, G. J., Kouwenhoven, M., Nene, A. V., & Jannink, M. J. (2010). Influence of gravity compensation on kinematics and muscle activation patterns during reach and retrieval in subjects with cervical spinal cord injury: An exploration study. *Journal of Rehabilitation Research and Development, 47,* 617–628.

LaStayo, P. C., & Cass, R. (2002). Continuous passive motion or the upper extremity: Why, when and how. In E. J. Mackin, A. D. Callahan, T. M. Skirven, L. H. Schneider, & A. L. Osterman (Eds.), *Rehabilitation of the hand and upper extremity* (5th ed., pp. 183–193). St. Louis: Mosby.

Levangie, P. K., & Norkin, C. C. (2011). *Joint structure and function: A comprehensive analysis* (5th ed.). Philadelphia: F.A. Davis.

Lin, H. T., Kuo, L. C., Liu, H. Y., Wu, W. L., & Su, F. C. (2011). The three-dimensional analysis of three thumb joints coordination in activities of daily living. *Clinical Biomechanics, 26,* 371–376.

Lippert, L. S. (2006). *Clinical kinesiology and anatomy* (4th ed.). Philadelphia: F.A. Davis.

MacIntosh, B. R., Gardiner, P., & McComas, A. J. (2006). *Skeletal muscle: Form and function* (2nd ed.). Champaign, IL: Human Kinetics.

Maitra, K. K., Philips, K., & Rice, M. S. (2010). Grasping naturally versus grasping with a reacher in people without disability: Motor control and muscle activation differences. *American Journal of Occupational Therapy, 64,* 95–104.

Marois, E., & Durand, M. J. (2009). Does participation in interdisciplinary work rehabilitation programme influence return to work obstacles and predictive factors? *Disability and Rehabilitation, 31,* 994–1007.

Mazurek, T., Strankowski, M., Ceynowa, M., & Roclawski, M. (2011). Tensile strength of a weave tendon suture using tendons of different sizes. *Clinical Biomechanics, 26,* 415–418.

McNair, P. J., & Rice, D. (2010). Muscle endurance: A review and update. *New Zealand Journal of Physiotherapy, 38,* 2.

McNeely, M. L., Parliament, M. B., Seikaly, H., Jha, N., Magee, D. J., Haykowsky, M. J., & Courneya, K. S. (2008). Effect of exercise on upper extremity pain and dysfunction in head and neck cancer survivors. *Cancer, 113,* 214–222.

Michlovitz, S. L., Harris, B., & Watkins, M. P. (2004). Therapy interventions for improving joint range of motion: A systematic review. *Journal of Hand Therapy, 17,* 118–130.

O'Driscoll, S. W., & Giori, N. J. (2000). Continuous passive motion (CPM): Theory and principles of clinical application. *Journal of Rehabilitation Research and Development, 37,* 179–188.

O'Hara, J., Cartwright, A., Wade, C. D., Hough, A. D., & Shum, G. L. K. (2011). Efficacy of static stretching and proprioceptive neuromuscular facilitation stretch on hamstrings length after a single session. *Journal of Strength and Conditioning Research, 25,* 1586–1591.

Priganc, V. W., & Ito, M. A. (2008). Changes in edema, pain, or range of motion following manual edema mobilization: A single-case design study. *Journal of Hand Therapy, 21,* 326–334.

Ratamess, N. A., Alvar, B. A., Evetoch, T. K., Housh, T. J. Kibler, W. B., Kraemer, W. J., & Triplett, N. T. (2009). Progression models in resistance training for healthy adults: Position stand. *Medicine and Science in Sports and Exercise, 41,* 687–708.

Reid, D. A., & McNair, P. (2011). Effects of a six week lower limb stretching programme on range of motion, peak passive torque and stiffness in people with and without osteoarthritis of the knee. *New Zealand Journal of Physiotherapy, 39,* 5–12.

Roy, J. S., Ma, B., MacDermaid, J. C., & Woodhouse, L. J. (2011). Shoulder muscle endurance: The development of a standardized and reliable protocol. *Sports Medicine, Arthroscopy, Rehabilitation, Therapy & Technology, 3,* 1.

Schwartz, D. A., & Chafetz, R. C. (2008). Continuous passive motion after tenoylysis in hand therapy patients: A retrospective study. *Journal of Hand Therapy, 21,* 261–266.

Selvaggi, G., Monstrey, S., Landuyt, K. V., Hamdi, M., & Blondeel, P. (2005). Rehabilitation of burn injured patients following lightning and electrical trauma. *NeuroRehabilitation, 20,* 35–42.

Sharman, M., Cresswell, A., & Riek, S. (2006). Proprioceptive neuromuscular facilitation stretching: Mechanism and clinical implications. *Sports Medicine, 36,* 929–939.

Tafti, M. A., Cramer, S. C., & Gupta, R. (2008). Orthopaedic management of the upper extremity of stroke patients. *Journal of the American Academy of Orthopaedic Surgeons, 16,* 462–70

Thompson, W. R., Gordon, N. F., & Pescatello, L. S. (Eds). (2010). *American College of Sports Medicine's guidelines for exercise testing and prescription* (8th ed.). Philadelphia: Lippincott Williams & Wilkins.

Villeco, J. P. (2011). Edema: Therapist's management. In T. M. Skirven, A. L. Osterman, J. M. Fedorczyk, & P. C. Amadio (Eds.), *Rehabilitation of the hand and upper extremity* (6th ed., pp. 845–857). Philadelphia: Mosby.

Acknowledgements

Andy Fabrizio thanks the members of the military for volunteering to be photographed for this chapter.

21

Optimizing Motor Planning and Performance in Clients with Neurological Disorders

Joyce Shapero Sabari, Nettie Capasso, and Rachel Feld-Glazman

Learning Objectives

After studying this chapter, the reader will be able to do the following:

1. Identify how major theoretical paradigms influence task-based interventions to improve motor performance and motor planning in survivors of stroke and traumatic brain injury.[1]
2. Identify the multiple factors that contribute to optimal motor performance, and describe how occupational therapy interventions are designed to help patients improve each of these.
3. Describe how occupational therapists help patients with neuromotor impairments improve balance, functional mobility, functional arm and hand use, and motor planning.
4. Determine appropriate interventions and task challenges for patients at each of the Functional Upper Extremity Levels (FUEL).

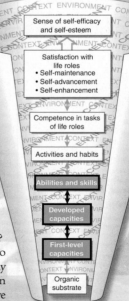

[1]NOTE. Because there are so many research studies that support both the rationale for and the effectiveness of the interventions described in this chapter, the citations to that research are interwoven within the chapter instead of being put into an evidence table as in other chapters. The reader who is contemplating using one of the interventions is advised to access the original research and consider the following: (1) Are the participants in the research study similar to the person I want to use this intervention with? (2) How was the intervention administered and at what intensity and for how long? (3) Do the results indicate statistical significance, which indicates that the outcome was unlikely caused by chance? Does the size of the effect make it worth using? Was the improvement in outcome measure clinically significant? (4) Was this study conducted validly so that I have confidence that the change in the dependent variable (outcome measure) was caused by the independent variable (treatment), or does it seem that some other factor that was not controlled by the researchers could have produced the change in the outcome measure?

ifficulty with motor performance is a critical concern for many survivors of acquired brain damage (stroke and traumatic brain injury). Occupational therapists provide intervention to assist these people in (1) optimizing their motor function and (2) integrating their improved motor skills into enhanced performance of functional activities for greater independence and engagement in their daily lives.

This chapter will

- introduce the constellation of motor impairments that are typically associated with acquired brain injury
- review the major theoretical paradigms that historically have guided neurorehabilitation interventions that are designed to improve motor performance for survivors of brain injury and stroke
- describe the multiple factors that contribute to optimal motor performance
- provide a framework for occupational therapy (OT) interventions that are geared toward improving motor performance related to
    - sitting and standing balance
    - functional mobility
    - functional arm and hand use
    - motor planning (praxis)

MOTOR CHARACTERISTICS OF CENTRAL NERVOUS SYSTEM DYSFUNCTION

Human movement is dependent on complex interactions among multiple systems, with key contributions from integrated motor centers within the brain. Damage to neural cells impacts motor, sensory, and cognitive function, and there is typically a direct relationship between anatomical pathology and functional loss. The constellation of movement problems associated with brain injury is often referred to as upper motor neuron dysfunction. This term is differentiated from lower motor neuron dysfunction, which describes the weakness and flaccidity that is associated with peripheral nerve damage.

Primary motor impairments are those deficits that are directly attributable to the brain lesion. Primary motor impairments can be further classified as positive or negative. Negative impairments include paralysis (hemiplegia or hemiparesis), sensory loss, fatigue, decreased movement speed, and difficulty organizing available movement into functional motor sequences. Spasticity (hypertonicity) and the presence of abnormal reflex activity are the hallmarks of positive impairments associated with stroke. Ataxia and intention tremor are positive impairments that are associated with cerebellar pathology. Resting tremor is a positive impairment associated with basal ganglia dysfunction such as Parkinson's disease.

Secondary motor impairments are preventable deficits that develop over time in response to immobility, inactivity,

or asymmetries in postural alignment. Limitations in joint range of motion (ROM), diminished flexibility between body segments, pain, and edema are common secondary impairments in stroke survivors.

Rehabilitation specialists may also consider another category of features associated with upper motor neuron dysfunction. Adaptive features (Carr & Shepherd, 2003) are disorders of movement that develop in response to a person's attempts to move within the constraints of limited mobility, specific weakness, or hypertonicity in specific muscles. It has long been observed that many people with hemiparesis move their limbs in characteristic patterns that typically are awkward and inefficient. Throughout the history of neurorehabilitation, these abnormal patterns, often called synergies, have been interpreted in different ways. In this chapter, we will refer to these abnormal movement constellations as maladaptive strategies.

An additional dichotomy for conceptualizing movement dysfunction in brain injury survivors is to differentiate between deficits in motor *execution*, associated with specific impairments and deficits in motor *control*, which are associated with deficits in higher order processes, such as motor planning and motor learning (Raghavan, 2007). No one would argue that motor execution is an essential prerequisite to functional movement. However, it has become increasingly clear that the ability to activate specific muscle contractions, alone, is not sufficient for functional balance, mobility, or purposeful use of the arm and hand.

Finally, the amount of use in daily activities is a critical variable for describing limb motor performance in those stroke survivors who have moderate levels of function in both motor execution and motor control. Later in this chapter, we will explore the phenomenon of learned nonuse and present compelling research findings for the efficacy of maximizing continuous, long-term recovery of motor function by helping stroke survivors to incorporate use of the paretic limb when performing routine, daily tasks.

HISTORY OF THEORETICAL PARADIGMS ASSOCIATED WITH REHABILITATION INTERVENTIONS TO IMPROVE MOTOR PERFORMANCE IN CLIENTS WITH CENTRAL NERVOUS SYSTEM DYSFUNCTION

Interventions to improve motor performance in clients with central nervous system (CNS) dysfunction are heavily influenced by underlying conceptual frameworks about movement, learning, motor control, and brain plasticity. A series of paradigm shifts in the past hundred years has led to significant fluctuations in approaches to evaluating and treating patients.

Stroke and post-stroke disability have been documented medical conditions since the time of Hippocrates. However, it was not until the 20th century that society recognized the possibility that rehabilitation interventions could improve functional capacity in stroke survivors (Pound, Bury, & Ebrahim, 1997). The earliest rehabilitation efforts recognized limb motor impairments only and took a two-pronged approach. Primarily, rehabilitation focused on ways to compensate for hemiplegia through training patients to walk with a cane and to perform activities of daily living (ADL) using the unaffected arm and hand. In addition, passive stretch was implemented in an attempt to reverse limitations in passive ROM.

Brunnstrom's Movement Therapy

In 1951, Dr. Thomas Twitchell, a neurologist, published a seminal paper in which he described the longitudinal progression of motor recovery in 121 patients. Twitchell observed that, early in recovery, these people tended to demonstrate stereotypical movement patterns. In addition, he observed that they tended to progress in their motor recovery through a consistent series of stages. Twitchell did not hypothesize why some patients recovered further than others and did not present any recommendations for therapeutic interventions that might influence motor recovery.

Signe Brunnstrom, a physical therapist, combined Twitchell's findings with her own clinical observations to develop a treatment approach that was designed to facilitate the progression through the stages of recovery that Twitchell had reported. Brunnstrom's major contributions were

- her detailed description of reflexes and associated reactions exhibited by patients with post-stroke hemiplegia
- the concept of flexor and extensor synergy patterns in the paretic arm and leg
- a postulated sequence of treatment, designed to move patients through seven stages of recovery for the arm and hand

Please see online Chapter B about Brunnstrom's Movement Therapy approach for more information about these concepts and techniques.

Many of Brunnstrom's contributions remain influential today. The associated reactions and reflexes she described are still recognized as characteristic features of motor behavior in stroke survivors with limited recovery. A major difference is that Brunnstrom advised therapists to use techniques to elicit these pathological responses in an effort to stimulate movement. Today, however, rehabilitation professionals seek to *prevent* eliciting these responses. The current understanding is that reflexive movements are *not* precursors to active, functional motor performance.

Many members of the rehabilitation community continue to consider the upper limb synergies as hallmarks of motor performance in stroke survivors. In fact, the

Fugl-Meyer Motor Assessment (FMA) (Fugl-Meyer et al., 1975), sometimes called the Brunnstrom-Fugl-Meyer Motor Function Assessment, is a widely used adaptation of Brunnstrom's Hemiplegia Classification and Progress Record. This assessment, often considered to be the "gold standard" for evaluating movement ability, is used by researchers as well as clinicians, even when Brunnstrom's approach to therapy is not used. For details about the FMA, see Chapter 8. Even though there is no research support for the premise that stroke survivors pass through the predictable stages of motor recovery that Brunnstrom described, these seven stages are still used today to facilitate communication between rehabilitation professionals. Therefore, it is valuable for occupational therapists to be familiar with these stages and comfortable in grossly categorizing a patient's general arm function as "stage I," "stage II," etc. (see Definition 21-1).

Currently, rehabilitation professionals disagree on whether to consider the limb synergies as primary sequelae of the neurological damage (as Brunnstrom and Twitchell postulated) or examples of maladaptive strategies that patients develop when they attempt to move, in spite of underlying mechanical obstacles, such as immobility at the pelvis or scapula. This may be an important distinction. Those who view the flexor and extensor synergies of the upper limb as maladaptive strategies organize therapeutic

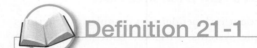 Definition 21-1

Brunnstrom Stages of Recovery for the Affected Arm

Stage I	Flaccidity: no voluntary movement, muscle tone, or reflexive responses
Stage II	Synergies can be elicited reflexively; spasticity is developing
Stage III	Beginning voluntary movement but only in synergy; spasticity may be significant
Stage IV	Spasticity begins to decrease; ability to voluntarily perform movements that deviate slightly from synergy patterns
Stage V	Increased control of isolated voluntary movements, independent of synergy patterns
Stage VI	Isolated motor control; spasticity is minimal
Stage VII	Normal speed and coordination of motor function

interventions to prevent or remove specified "obstacles to movement" that may lead the person to develop inefficient motor strategies. Those who view the synergies as unavoidable motor deficits that precede full recovery of motor function are not concerned when patients move in these stereotypical patterns of movement. There is *no* controversy, however, about the efficacy of following a therapeutic sequence in which the therapist guides the patient in moving through the six postulated stages of recovery. This paradigm for structuring motor therapy is *not* supported by current understanding of neural plasticity and recovery of motor function after stroke.

Rood and Proprioceptive Neuromuscular Facilitation Approaches

The Rood and proprioceptive neuromuscular facilitation (PNF) approaches, advanced during the mid-20th century, shared Brunnstrom's reliance on the predominant paradigms for understanding motor performance at the time. Reflecting the view that motor development and motor recovery from stroke followed a hierarchical sequence, these approaches advocated that patients "recapitulate" the movement sequence exhibited by typically developing infants during the first year of life. Hence, therapy techniques included exercises that required the person to first learn how to maintain stability and then to move, in the prone position on elbows, quadruped positions, and kneeling positions. Subsequent understanding of motor recovery in adults with acquired brain injuries has negated the value of using a developmental model. In fact, today, the emphasis is on providing movement practice to patients in natural contexts. Therefore, motor activities are performed in supine, sitting, or standing postures. Decisions about which posture is most effective at a given session with a particular patient are based on mechanical factors (such as the influence of gravity) and the patient's functional goals (such as the desire to kneel during housecleaning or gardening activities) rather than on developmental considerations.

Another hierarchical concept, also influenced by knowledge of infant development, was that stroke survivors recovered motor function in a proximal to distal sequence. Hence, therapeutic interventions always began at the pelvic and shoulder girdles. When working to improve upper limb motor function, proximal control over scapular and glenohumeral motions was considered to be a prerequisite for implementing treatment that focused on forearm and hand function. Today, it is understood that survivors of stroke or TBI may demonstrate distal voluntary movements (e.g., some capacity to flex the thumb joints) before they have achieved a particular level of proximal control of scapular and glenohumeral motions (Beebe & Lang, 2008, 2009). In addition, research about reach and grasp has revealed that, during functional performance, the neural plan begins with attention to the object that is going to be lifted or moved. Neural signals to proximal muscle groups are based on orienting the shoulder, elbow, and forearm so that the hand is in the optimal position for interacting with the goal object (Paulignan et al., 1997). Therefore, current motor intervention for patients recovering from stroke or brain injury does *not* follow a proximal to distal sequence. Instead, each patient's constellation of motor abilities guides the therapist in setting treatment goals. At the same time, however, therapists must be mindful of the kinesiological interactions between proximal and distal limb segments. Proximal alignment and stability at the scapula, trunk, and pelvis affect functional use of the arm and hand. For the purpose of minimizing mechanical constraints to pain-free movement, several interventions (described later in this chapter) focus on improving proximal function.

Like Brunnstrom's model, both the Rood and PNF approaches advocated the use of specific sensory stimuli for facilitation or inhibition of motor "firing" within selected muscles. Stimuli that facilitate the spinal level myotatic reflex, like quick stretch, or vibration over a muscle belly, were used to stimulate the stretch reflex and thus elicit a momentary increase of muscle fiber contraction. The physiological principle of reciprocal inhibition (that stimulation to a muscle will simultaneously elicit inhibitory neural signals to its antagonist) was used to relax spastic muscles. For example, a quick stretch to the triceps would elicit a momentary increase of neural signals to elicit contraction of muscle fibers in the elbow extensor muscle and also elicit a momentary decrease of neural "firing" to the muscle fibers of the biceps. The observed result was a temporary decrease in hypertonicity in the biceps and greater ease in passively or actively moving the elbow into extension. Generalized inhibitory stimuli included slow, rhythmic vestibular input (as in slow rolling) and various types of relaxing somatosensory stimuli.

Although these techniques are no longer used in neurorehabilitation as initially prescribed by the Rood and PNF approaches, there are certainly modern correlates to these ideas. Functional electrical stimulation (FES) has replaced the facilitation techniques. Medical interventions such as botulinum toxin injections and GABAergic medications (Denham, 2008; Ivanhoe et al., 2006) and generalized relaxation strategies, as applied through yoga poses, controlled breathing, guided imagery, and meditation, have replaced the reflex-based inhibitory techniques advanced by the Rood and PNF approaches. A major contribution by the PNF approach is the use of diagonal patterns of limb movement (see figures C-5 through C-8 in online Chapter C), which are consistent with well-supported kinematic and kinetic linkages (Surburg, 1997). Before PNF, rehabilitation professionals tended to view movement as occurring only through the three cardinal planes (sagittal, coronal, and transverse). Passive movement through diagonal patterns ensures safe and efficient stretch to all muscles, at all joints of the upper limb. Active and resisted movements through diagonal patterns provide exercise to groups of muscles in the limbs and trunk that are recruited synergistically by the CNS. PNF diagonals and ancillary techniques continue to be used effectively in orthopedic rehabilitation and athletic training. Their effectiveness as an intervention to improve motor function after brain injury has never been supported by research. Most likely, this is related to the fact that PNF interventions are directed toward improving motor execution, without providing task-related practice to improve motor control. Even so, occupational therapists apply a core concept of PNF, which is that functional movements comprise integrated interaction between multiple joints and muscles through an infinite number of diagonal planes. Please see online Chapter C about the Rood and PNF approaches for more information about these concepts and techniques.

Neurodevelopmental Therapy (The Bobath Approach)

Berta Bobath, a physical therapist, and her husband, Karel Bobath, a psychiatrist and neurophysiologist, began advancing a different set of ideas for enhancing motor recovery in children and adults as early as the 1940s. Their first major publication about stroke rehabilitation (Bobath, 1970) was, in several ways, a direct challenge to primary tenets espoused

by Brunnstrom. Where Brunnstrom's approach capitalized on spasticity and hyperactive reflexes as *opportunities* to elicit early movement, the Bobaths viewed hypertonicity as an *obstacle* to a person's ability to move freely. In addition, they recognized that once a person begins to move his paretic limbs in abnormal patterns, it is extremely difficult to break away from these obligatory patterns for flexible movement sequences that meet the contextual demands of activity performance.

Finally, the Bobath approach conceptualized the underlying cause of limb synergies quite differently than Twitchell and Brunnstrom. Instead of viewing the synergies as primary impairments that are directly associated with cerebral damage, they conceptualized these abnormal movement patterns as secondary maladaptive strategies. Carr and Shepherd (2003) later coined the term "adaptive features" to describe disorders of movement that develop in response to a person's attempt to move within the constraints of limited mobility, specific weakness, or hypertonicity in specific muscles. For example, Figures 21-1A and 21-1B illustrate the marked difference in scapular mobility in two people. Notice the extent to which the scapula protracts and upwardly rotates when the young man on the left flexes his shoulder. As demonstrated by the photo on the right, many stroke survivors experience limited scapula mobility (also described as impaired dissociation between the scapula and the thorax). This is a secondary impairment,

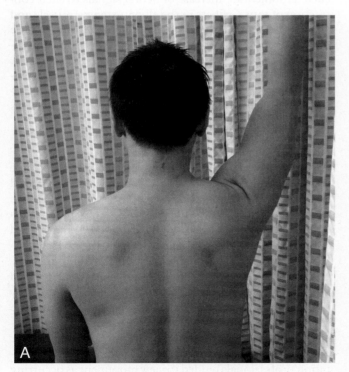
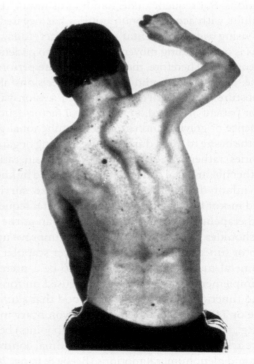

Figure 21-1 Influence of scapulohumeral kinematics on arm and trunk movement. **A.** Notice the degree of scapular protraction and upward rotation as this healthy young man reaches forward. **B.** A man with right hemiparesis is attempting to reach forward, but his scapula remains fixed in retraction and fails to upwardly rotate. Note that he attempts to compensate for his difficulty raising the arm by laterally flexing his trunk to the opposite side. (Used with permission from Davies, P. M. [2000]. *Steps to follow: The comprehensive treatment of patients with hemiplegia* [2nd ed., p. 68]. Berlin: Springer-Verlag.)

usually caused by loss of muscle length in the middle trapezius muscle. As the man in the photo tries to raise his arm into flexion, his lack of scapulohumeral rhythm interferes with efficient kinematics. To achieve the movement, he uses what motor capacities are available to him. He laterally flexes his trunk, elevates his scapula, abducts his arm away from the body, and ultimately, to achieve greater active range of motion (AROM), externally rotates at the glenohumeral joint. Compare this photo to Figure A-1 in online Chapter A, which illustrates a flexor synergy pattern.

Neurodevelopmental therapy (NDT) introduced the concept that therapy could "prevent" the development of abnormal limb synergy patterns by removing mechanical obstacles to movement. NDT training, which continues today, prepares therapists to have keen observational skills and to employ kinesiological concepts when determining motor interventions. In particular, NDT provides specific guidelines for observing a patient's postural alignment, predicting how misalignment might impact the kinematics of limb movement, and improving the patient's postural symmetry and balance.

The Bobaths were the first to articulate that motor performance problems in stroke survivors are due to factors beyond the activation of individual muscles. They stressed that many stroke survivors have "lost the feeling of normal movement" (Bobath, 1970). In today's lexicon, this concept of "normal movement" is described as motor programs or flexible attractor states (to be discussed later in this chapter). In addition, they recognized that postural alignment and postural control provide a critical foundation for functional movement.

Thanks to the foresight of Berta and Karel Bobath, the NDT approach has continued to evolve over time, in response to newer ideas about motor control and relearning. Numerous textbooks by the Bobaths and others who have studied with them provide helpful guidelines for structuring motor interventions with stroke survivors (Davies, 2000; Howle, 2002; Ryerson & Levit, 1997). However, outcome studies have not supported the efficacy of the total package of NDT intervention, as compared with other approaches to improving motor control in stroke survivors (Kollen et al., 2009). In addition, some have suggested that NDT therapists put too much emphasis on monitoring the kinematics of movement and using hands-on techniques in an attempt to prevent the person from developing "abnormal movement patterns." Because of this, NDT interventions may fail to provide patients with sufficient opportunities to actually practice using their emerging motor skills (French et al., 2010).

Influences from Neuroscience Evidence about Brain Plasticity

There has been an explosion of evidence in the past 30 years that confirms the human brain's capacity to reorganize after injury has occurred. The American Occupational Therapy Association (AOTA) Practice Guidelines for Adults with Stroke present an extensive review of research findings that support the importance of activity-based environmental challenges and repetitive practice opportunities in facilitating this neural reorganization (Sabari, 2008). Combined with advances in medical treatment of acute cerebrovascular accident (Wardlaw et al., 2003) and stroke rehabilitation (Stroke Unit Trialists' Collaboration, 2007), emerging concepts related to neuroplasticity have contributed to a heightened sense of optimism that stroke survivors have the potential to recover motor function (Gauthier et al., 2008).

Depending on the extent of neuropathology, all stroke survivors have varying potential for spontaneous recovery and reorganization of neural mechanisms. Studies of humans and other mammals have provided significant evidence that recovery of function after brain lesions is associated with recruitment of brain regions not typically activated for a specific function (Butefish, 2004; Murphy & Corbett, 2009). These studies consistently find that brain plasticity is a dynamic process that is influenced by the individual's active efforts to meet environmental and task demands (Hoffman et al., 2008). This finding has contributed significantly to changing views about neurorehabilitation. The philosophy, long held within the OT profession, that engagement in specially designed therapeutic activities can improve motor function is now supported by the scientific community. In addition, neurorehabilitation goals have been reframed from a focus on motor execution to an emphasis on helping patients improve motor control and, with regard to paretic limbs, amount of use. Several streams of research, in a variety of disciplines, have added support to incorporate these ideas into rehabilitation interventions to improve motor performance in survivors of stroke and brain injury.

Evolution from Impairment-Focused Interventions to Interventions Designed to Help Patients Develop Effective Movement Strategies

Although kinesiology has long been a core subject of study in OT and physical therapy curricula, it was not until the 1970s and 1980s that rehabilitation professionals began to seriously consider how principles from the academic disciplines of movement science and motor learning could be applicable to therapeutic interventions. Many of these principles related to stages of learning, types of feedback, and therapeutic use of practice are described in Chapter 13, "Learning." We recommend that you review this chapter, with particular emphasis on Definition 13-2 (implicit learning and explicit learning) and Procedures for Practice 13-2 (Therapeutic Use of Context, Feedback, and Practice to Promote Transfer and Generalization).

At the same time, a major paradigm shift was occurring in neuroscience. Previously, neural control of movement was explained by tracking the descent of neural signals through corticospinal pathways, delineating the direct influences from brainstem nuclei on motor neurons in the spinal cord, and describing communication between alpha motoneurons and muscle fibers (the "final common pathway"). In essence, motor performance was viewed as the collection of neural stimuli to individual muscles. Furthermore, regions of the CNS were viewed as relatively static structures, with assigned functions that did not change in response to experience or injury.

A proliferation of neuroscience research provides significant evidence that neural control of movement can best be conceptualized as a fluid, dynamic system. Through repetitive but varied practice, people develop motor programs that govern the production of generalized categories of movement. These motor programs are then adapted to suit particular features of task performance. Therefore, a unique pattern of activity with core foundational characteristics emerges whenever the motor program is executed. For example, a tennis player develops an underlying motor program that structures her posture and sequence of muscle recruitment for producing a forehand swing. This set of kinesiological relationships forms a core foundation, but the athlete alters the force characteristics, timing, and spatial details each time she returns the ball. The tennis player chooses these alterations (or variant characteristics of the motor program) based on the speed, force, and direction of the tennis ball, as well as the player's intentions regarding how to return the ball to her opponent.

The confluence between empirical findings in movement science and neuroscience research has led to increasing overlap between these two fields of study. These findings have had significant influence on rehabilitation interventions to improve motor performance in survivors of stroke and TBI. Schmidt and Lee (2011) provide useful background information about core concepts and research evidence related to human motor control and motor learning. Shumway-Cook and Woollacott (2012) provide more specific applications to OT and physical therapy practice. Winstein and Knecht (1990), Carr and Shepherd (1998, 2003), and Mathiowetz and Bass-Haugen (1994) developed practical guidelines for therapeutic intervention based on dynamic systems, ecological systems, and motor program theories.

Influences from Dynamical Systems, Ecological Systems, and Motor Program Theory

Dynamical systems theory, also known as nonlinear dynamics, provides a mathematical paradigm for conceptualizing phenomena that are subject to unpredictable changes over time (Hirsch, Smale, & Devaney, 2004). True dynamical systems theorists are mathematicians and philosophers, but in the 1980s scholars in the movement and neural sciences began to apply these ideas to explanations of motor learning, skill development, and recovery of motor function after brain injury (Schmidt & Lee, 2011).

Ecological systems theory began as an exploration of how multiple factors interact to influence child development (Bronfenbrenner, 1979). Several OT scholars have synthesized these concepts into broad-based models for OT intervention (Dunn, Brown, & McGuigan, 1994; Law et al., 1996).

Dynamical systems and ecological systems theories have significantly impacted our current understanding of how people develop motor skill and recover motor function after brain injury. The following principles guide the way rehabilitation professionals conceptualize our role in helping patients reach their maximum functional potential.

- **Dynamic systems are self-organizing.** When a system is in a state of equilibrium, all influences are in perfect balance, and the system perpetuates itself without any need for change. As occupational therapists, we are most interested in understanding systems in states of *disequilibrium*. The human CNS can be conceptualized as a dynamic system. The hypothetical "system" that plans and organizes movement can also be conceptualized as a dynamic system. Dynamic systems continuously seek to "solve problems" that are presented by internal or external challenges. Furthermore, dynamic systems have the capacity to self-organize for the purpose of meeting these challenges. For illustration purposes, when learning to water ski, a person develops a strategy that will enable him or her to rise from a crouched position to standing, and then maintain his or her balance—all while wearing skis, on the surface of a lake, and being pulled by a motor boat that will vary its speed and direction. Similarly, when recovering from brain injury, a person relearns motor strategies for skills as basic as maintaining sitting balance, rising to a standing position, and coordinating arm and hand movements to reach and grasp objects. In dynamic systems theory (DST), external challenges are described as "perturbations." Without perturbations, a system will have no reason to use its self-organizing capabilities. Just as a person learns to water ski by "solving the problems" that are presented when participating in this sport, a person recovering from brain injury needs task-based challenges to begin the active process of "figuring out" how to move, using his or her current motor capabilities.

- **Influences on dynamic systems are heterarchical rather than hierarchical.** By that we mean that responsibilities for motor control are distributed among a number of structures within and external to the CNS. Spinal level structures are not completely dependent on higher centers for direct movement commands. Instead, the role of hemispheric structures is to tune and prepare the motor system to respond most efficiently to changing environmental and task demands. Within the person, but external to the nervous system, factors such as muscle strength, ROM, and peripheral pain also contribute significantly to the choices that are made when selecting the best solution to a motor challenge. Finally, features in the environment and specific factors related to the task provide additional heterarchical influences that determine how the "motor system" will decide to adapt in order to meet a particular goal. (Refer to Chapter 12 for specific examples of how occupational therapists adapt tasks for the purpose of changing motor demands.)

- **The most efficient solutions in a dynamic system are those which present the fewest** degrees of freedom.
- **Dynamic systems inherently seek the most efficient solutions in their attempts to self-organize.** Bernstein's (1967) "degrees of freedom problem" has been supported in the literature that guides current neuromotor interventions. As you may recall from studying statistics or kinesiology, degrees of freedom in any system refer to the number of components (variables) that are free to vary. If we consider the number of degrees of freedom involved in controlling the muscles of the arm when picking up and drinking from a cup of coffee, it becomes clear that the system could not possibly be controlled via separate commands to individual muscles. Bernstein proposed that people reduce the degrees of freedom by creating linkages among muscular activities at various joints. Various terms have been used to describe these linkages: coordinative structures, function generators, and, most recently, motor programs and attractor states (Schmidt & Lee, 2011; Shumway-Cook & Woollacott, 2012).

Motor Programs and Attractor States. Two distinct concepts, advanced by different sets of theorists, provide conceptually similar descriptions of the mechanisms that are used to limit degrees of freedom during motor performance. A motor program is a memory-based schema that controls coordinated movement. Generalized motor programs (GMPs) are "prestructured sets of central commands" that govern a particular class of actions (Schmidt & Lee, 2011). They consist of both invariant and variant components. The invariant components comprise the core elements of the GMP. The variant components are flexible; they change dynamically in response to continuous changes in environmental and task parameters. For example, when a person develops a GMP for water skiing, the invariant dimensions are the muscle interactions required to maintain an appropriate posture. Variant dimensions include flexible shifts in alignment and muscle activation to meet the dynamic demands of the speed, direction, and wake created by the motorboat.

An attractor, as conceptualized in dynamic patterns theory, is a preferred pattern within a motor control system that leads to a consistent pattern of performance (Shumway-Cook & Woollacott, 2012). A preferred movement pattern

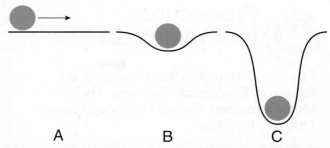

Figure 21-2 Various attractor states. **A.** No attractor state. **B.** Shallow well; stable and flexible attractor state. **C.** Deep well; stable and inflexible attractor state.

can be illustrated by how a marble moves on different surfaces (see Fig. 21-2) (Thelen, 1989). When people first attempt to learn a new motor skill, they have not yet developed an attractor state and thus do not exhibit any underlying pattern (see Fig. 21-2A). Every time they attempt to perform a task, they do it in a different way. Performance is irregular and unpredictable, and the person is not effective or efficient in achieving the goal. Think of the novice water skier who tries a different strategy every time, but at the end of the session has never succeeded in reaching a standing position. Early after stroke or head injury, people find themselves unsure of how to coordinate movement within the new constraints of their motor impairments. They are in a situation of having no attractor states for achieving functional motor performance. When people are inflexible in the way they perform a motor skill, they are demonstrating stable wells (see Fig. 21-2C). Consider a person who has learned to water ski but has been afraid to try to cross the wake or to allow the driver to vary the speed or acceleration of the boat. This person will develop a stable well, allowing her to show competence only when the task variables are unchanged. When motor learning occurs without opportunities to vary the task parameters, the person is at risk for developing stable wells. Stable wells are like "bad habits." They seem to serve a short-term purpose, but over time it becomes apparent that they are not useful in the real world where environmental and task affordances are continuously changing. The upper limb synergy patterns described by Twitchell and Brunnstrom can be conceptualized as attractor states with stable wells.

The goal in neuromotor rehabilitation is to assist patients to develop shallow wells, or flexible motor programs, for performing motor sequences that serve as the foundation for many types of functional movement. Variability in practice is a key component to helping people develop flexible attractor states. Using the terminology of dynamical systems theory, the therapist manipulates control parameters in therapeutic tasks to provide task-based challenges that will "drive" the individual to develop the most effective and versatile attractor states (see Procedures for Practice 21-1).

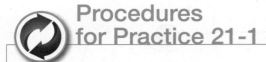

Procedures for Practice 21-1

Applying Principles from Dynamical Systems, Ecological Systems, and Motor Program Theory to Occupational Therapy Practice

- Reduce kinesiological constraints to movement performance such as limited range of motion, excessive effects of gravity, etc.
- Present task-based challenges designed to provide graded practice in using available capacities to achieve functional goals.
- Manipulate affordances/regulatory conditions within therapeutic tasks (and the environmental context) to provide varied and graded opportunities to practice incorporating effective motor programs into performance of functional tasks.
- Provide opportunities for practice and active experimentation with varied strategies in a variety of contexts to develop flexibility and skill in motor performance.

Constraints and Affordances

Motor performance is the result of a series of choices (often at the unconscious level). These choices are influenced by internal and external factors that shape the way we move. Constraints are factors that limit the choices that are available. Limitations caused by secondary impairments after stroke and brain injury impose constraints on movement choices. Although these are certainly negative constraints that therapists seek to prevent or reduce, there may also be external constraints to movement that are integral to a task. In the case of learning to water ski, having one's feet in the skis and one's hands on the tow rope imposes constraints that influence the ultimate strategy a person will use to rise to and maintain an upright posture. Affordances are factors that invite particular choices (Wu et al., 1998). An object's shape, size, perceived weight, location, and purpose all influence the constellation of movements that will be most efficient for using the object. For example, when a person sees a coffee mug, he or she immediately perceives its affordance as something to be picked up by the handle and brought to the mouth for drinking a hot beverage. The term, regulatory condition is used to describe task-related features that influence movement (Gentile, 2000). The term "control parameter" is used to describe any variable that, when changed, can cause a change in motor behavior. External control parameters, such as regulatory conditions or object affordances, influence a person's plan of action for executing a particular task. Internal control parameters, such as body alignment, muscle length, and muscle strength, also influence one's

motor tactics. Maladaptive movement strategies can be conceptualized as inefficient deep well attractor states that develop as a person attempts to move within the context of internal negative control parameters (see Fig. 21-2).

Learned Nonuse and Constraint-Induced Movement Therapy

Although the constraint-induced movement therapy (CIMT) approach is applicable to only a small population of stroke survivors who demonstrate high levels of motor ability, its underlying tenets and its methods of evaluation and intervention mark a significant paradigm shift in neurorehabilitation to improve movement performance. Edward Taub, a psychologist with little interest in the kinesiological details of human movement, developed the foundations for CIMT after making critical observations during animal lesion research.

Background and Research Findings

In studying the effects of deafferentation to the forelimbs of experimental monkeys through dorsal rhizotomy, Taub (1976) observed that the monkeys behaved as if these limbs were paralyzed, even though the animals were capable of performing voluntary movements with the affected extremities. He coined the term "learned nonuse" to describe the phenomenon in which the monkeys developed a learned behavior of relying exclusively on a single forelimb when they were faced with initial difficulty moving the contralateral limb. Taub postulated that learned nonuse developed in response to the coupling of negative reinforcers when the monkeys unsuccessfully tried to use the affected forelimb and positive reinforcers when they successfully used compensatory behavior patterns to perform tasks unilaterally with the unimpaired forelimb. Even when the animals experienced neurological recovery, they continued this behavior of relying exclusively on the unimpaired forearm for functional performance. To provide experimental evidence for his theory of learned nonuse, Taub restrained the unimpaired forelimbs of monkeys who had undergone lesion surgery. As predicted, when the restraining devices were removed after several weeks, the animals were able to use the deafferented limb and demonstrated smooth, functional motor performance.

Taub (1976) hypothesized that, in some stroke survivors, the failure to recover motor function in the affected arm and hand was due to learned nonuse rather than to specific difficulties in generating movement. To test this hypothesis, Taub and colleagues established minimal criteria for participation in constraint-based research. Although these criteria have changed slightly over time, they have always required participants to demonstrate the capacity to generate significant movements of the hand (see Definition 21-2).

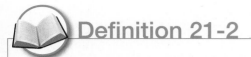
Definition 21-2

Inclusion Criteria for Participating in Constraint-Induced Movement Therapy Clinical Trials

- Paretic hand
  - ≥10° active wrist extension
  - ≥10° active thumb abduction or extension
  - ≥10° extension in at least two additional digits
  - ability to repeat these movements three times in 1 minute
- Adequate balance while wearing a restraint and transferring to and from the toilet independently
- Able to stand from a sitting position without relying on assistance from the unaffected hand
- Ability to stand for at least 2 minutes with or without upper extremity (UE) support
- Score of ≥24 on Mini-Mental State Examination
- Stamina and motivation required to participate in a 2-week program, including
  - constraint of the less impaired UE for 90% of waking hours (7 days per week)
  - 6 hours of intensive therapy per day (5 days per week)
  - at-home practice

From Wolf, S., Winstein, C. J., Miller, J. P., Taub, E., Uswatte, G., Morris, D., Giuliani, C., Light, K. E., Nichols-Larsen, D., & EXCITE Investigators. (2006). Effect of constraint-induced movement therapy on upper extremity function 3 to 9 months after stroke: The EXCITE randomized clinical trial. *Journal of the American Medical Association, 296*, 2095–2104.

In the past 30 years, Taub has collaborated with colleagues from a variety of disciplines to develop interventions that are designed to improve functional use of the arm and hand in this population. The first clinical application was the program of "forced use." In this protocol, which closely mirrors Taub's earlier work with laboratory monkeys, participants constrained their unaffected upper limb for 90% of waking hours over a 2-week period. This constraint alone, without supervised practice, resulted in clinically significant changes among individuals who had survived stroke or head injury more than 1 year prior to participation in the forced use protocol (Wolf, 1989). In the following decade, Taub and colleagues added the component of supervised practice sessions, using the technique of shaping to gradually refine task demands and coined the term constraint-induced movement therapy to describe the combined intervention of intensive practice and constraint of the unaffected upper limb. Over time, the method of constraint has shifted from restraining the entire unaffected upper limb in a sling to less restrictive hand mitts that serve as constant reminders not to use the unaffected limb. Furthermore, although it is beyond the scope of this

chapter, CIMT has been applied to other populations, most notably children with hemiparesis caused by cerebral palsy and other developmental disabilities (Hoare et al., 2007).

In the current CIMT intervention protocol, participants wear a hand mitt for 90% of their waking hours over a 2-week period, including two weekends, for a total of 14 days. On each weekday, these individuals participate in shaping and standard task training of the paretic limb for up to 6 hours per day (Wolf et al., 2006). Results from multiple studies have provided consistent evidence that, with the intended population, CIMT is effective in improving function related to motor execution, motor control, and amount of use (Shi et al., 2011; Sirtori et al., 2009). In addition, several studies have used neuroimaging techniques to provide evidence of changes in neural organization following CIMT (Liepert, 2006; Lin et al., 2010b; Murayama et al., 2011).

Of all the considerable evidence in support of CIMT, the Extremity Constraint-Induced Therapy Evaluation (EXCITE) trial is particularly noteworthy. This prospective, single-blind, randomized, cross-over, multisite clinical trial is the largest systematic outcomes study in the history of stroke rehabilitation (see Research Notes 21-1, 21-2, and 21-3). In addition to the three seminal articles reporting results from the EXCITE trial, the researchers have contributed multiple publications that delineate the study design (Morris et al., 2009; Winstein et al., 2003) and reflect on implications of findings to future research and clinical practice (Park et al., 2008; Wolf, 2007; Wolf et al., 2007). A long-term case report of one EXCITE trial participant with assessments 4 and 5 years following CIMT intervention (Rowe, Blanton, & Wolf, 2009) revealed that this individual continued to maintain the gains reported in the aggregate studies described in the Research Notes.

Modified Constraint-Induced Movement Therapy Protocols

In spite of the overwhelming research support for CIMT, two concerns limit its application: (1) issues related to clinical feasibility and (2) the small percentage of stroke survivors who can participate in the standard CIMT protocol. Therefore, several adaptations to CIMT have been proposed and evaluated. The goal is to find a level of modification that will decrease costs and improve accessibility to more stroke survivors while maintaining highly beneficial outcomes.

The high intensity of practice sessions and the significant demand of wearing a restrictive mitt for 90% of waking hours are the two critical concerns related to CIMT's clinical feasibility. Beyond staffing considerations, patient fatigue and overall preference indicate the need for shorter periods of practice, spaced over a longer time period than 2 weeks (Page et al., 2001). Regarding the constraint component of CIMT, several researchers have found that patients have difficulty complying with an intense mitt-wearing

Research Note 21-1

Wolf, S. L., Winstein, C. J., Miller, J. P., Taub, E., Uswatte, G., Morris, D., Giuliani, C., Light, K. E., & Nichols-Larsen, D. (2006). Effect of constraint-induced movement therapy on upper extremity function 3 to 9 months after stroke: The EXCITE randomized clinical trial. *Journal of the American Medical Association, 296,* 2095–2104.

Abstract

The participants were 222 individuals who had sustained a first stroke (predominantly ischemic strokes) within the previous 3–9 months. They were assigned to receive either a 2-week constraint-induced movement therapy (CIMT) program (*n* = 106; wearing a restraining mitt on the less affected hand while engaging in repetitive task practice and behavioral shaping with the hemiplegic hand) or usual and customary care (*n* = 116; ranging from no treatment after concluding formal rehabilitation to pharmacological or physiotherapeutic interventions). For group assignment, patients were stratified by gender, prestroke dominant side, side of stroke, and level of paretic function. For participants in the CIMT group, several behavioral techniques were used to enhance mitt use outside of the training sessions. These methods included behavioral contracts for participants and their caregivers, a sensor-based mitt compliance device, and formal, daily schedules. The Wolf Motor Function Test (WMFT) and Motor Activity Log (MAL) were the main outcome measures. Of all the participants, 98 completed treatment and testing in the experimental group, and 105 completed treatment and testing in the control group. Data were collected on five occasions: baseline, posttreatment, and at 4-, 8-, and 12-month follow-up. Data analysis of results revealed that "the CIMT group showed significantly larger improvements immediately after treatment than the control group in quality and speed of paretic arm movement (WMFT Functional Ability and Performance Time) and in the quality and amount of paretic arm use in daily life (MAL). . . . The advantages for the CIMT group on all primary outcomes persisted at the 12-month follow-up" (p. 2102).

Implications for Practice

Direct implications: For stroke survivors who meet inclusion criteria, a 2-week program of intensive task-related training, combined with restraint to the unaffected arm during 90% of waking hours, has immediate and lasting effects (up to 12 months after participation) on motor performance and spontaneous, functional use of the paretic arm.

Indirect implications:

- Intensive practice using the paretic arm and hand in functional tasks has the potential to improve motor performance and spontaneous use.
- Behavioral methods that ensure accountability in complying with practice schedules within and outside of treatment may have the potential to improve patients' compliance and thus contribute to improvements in motor performance and spontaneous use of the paretic upper limb.

Research Note 21-2

Wolf, S. L., Winstein, C. J., Miller, J. P., Thompson, P. A., Taub, E., Uswatte, G., Morris D., Blanton, S., Nichols-Larsen, D., & Clark, P. C. (2008). Retention of upper limb function in stroke survivors who have received constraint-induced movement therapy: The EXCITE randomized trial. *Lancet Neurology, 7,* 33–40.

Abstract

Of the 98 participants who completed treatment in the experimental group of the EXCITE Trial (described in Research Note 21-1), 70 completed additional follow-up testing at 16 months and 24 months after intervention. Follow-up tests included Wolf Motor Function Test (WMFT), Motor Activity Log (MAL), and several subtests on the Stroke Impact Scale (SIS). The findings "extend previous results by showing that the improvements in function at 12 months after a 2-week Constraint-Induced Movement Therapy (CIMT) intervention are retained or improve further" (p. 38). Statistically significant improvements at 24 months (when compared to scores at the 12-month follow-up) were on strength-related scores on WMFT, and several domains of the SIS (a self-report measure used extensively in stroke research). The SIS domains showing significant, continued improvement were strength, activities of daily living (ADL) and instrumental activities of daily living (IADL), social participation, and overall assessment of physical ability.

Implications for Practice

Direct implications: Participation in a 2-week CIMT program has long-lasting impact on motor, ADL, and social function. This finding is critical because other longitudinal follow-up studies of stroke survivors after participation in rehabilitation programs have failed to show that short-term improvements are retained over time.

Indirect implications: The findings suggest that a change in the pattern with which stroke survivors use their paretic limb may be instrumental in fostering ongoing practice in using this limb during daily activities. This ongoing practice can lead to ongoing improvements in performance, an overall sense of optimism about potential for future gains in motor function, and continuous improvements in satisfaction related to physical, ADL, IADL, and social participation.

Research Note 21-3

Wolf, S. L., Thompson, P. A., Winstein, C. J., Miller, J. P., Blanton, S. R., Nichols-Larsen, D. S., Morros, D. M., Uswatte, G., Taub, E., Light, K. E., & Sawaki, L. (2010). The EXCITE Stroke Trial: Comparing early and delayed constraint-induced movement therapy. *Stroke, 41,* 2309–2315.

Abstract

The EXCITE Trial followed a cross-over design. One year after the study, the participants who were randomized to the control group were given the opportunity to receive contraint-induced movement therapy (CIMT) intervention. The same procedures reported in Research Notes 21-1 and 21-2 for intervention and data collection were followed. Of the initial 116 members of the control group, 86 participated in this delayed CIMT intervention, 78 completed the intervention and were tested immediately posttreatment, and 61 were retested after 24 months. The results were similar to results previously reported for the original experimental group (called the "early CIMT" group in this report). Even when CIMT was initiated an additional year after the original period of 3–9 months after stroke, delayed CIMT participants showed statistically significant improvements on Wolf Motor Function Test (WMFT) and Motor Activity Log (MAL) scores. However, they did not exhibit the statistically significant improvements on Stroke Impact Scale (SIS) scores that are reported in Research Note 21-2. When comparing data from both the early and delayed participants, researchers found that, although both groups showed significant improvements, the earlier CIMT group showed greater improvement than the delayed CIMT group in WMFT performance time and the MAL, as well as in the SIS hand and activity domains.

Implications for Practice

- "CIMT can be delivered to eligible patients 3 to 9 months or 15 to 21 months after stroke. Both patient groups achieved approximately the same level of significant arm motor function 24 months after enrollment" (p. 2309).
- It may be more effective to provide CIMT earlier, rather than later, after a person has sustained a stroke. It is not clear whether this is due to factors related to neural plasticity or to the possibility that members of the delayed CIMT group may have already solidified their expectations related to motor, activities of daily living (ADL), and social function.

schedule, particularly if they are living alone (Flinn et al., 2005). Levine and Page (2004) proposed the first alternative to CIMT that meets the practical realities of reimbursement and professional staffing, as well as patient fatigue and desire to participate in work and leisure activities. Today, there are several variations of modified (or distributed) constraint-induced movement therapy (mCIMT). Typically, constraint is limited to 5 hours per day, 5 days per week for a duration of 10 weeks. Practice sessions range from 30 minutes to 3 hours, 3 days per week. Group sessions are cost-effective, and the camaraderie they promote is beneficial to the rehabilitation process (Brogårdh & Sjölund, 2006; Flinn et al., 2005). Sessions can also be modified with regard to therapist supervision. A case report (Ploughman et al., 2008) and a cohort study (Hosomi et al., 2011) have reported that dividing practice sessions into a smaller percentage of time with direct supervision and a larger percentage of time devoted to self-training yields similar outcomes to the standard CIMT protocol. Results from a number of randomized controlled trials have confirmed that outcomes of mCIMT interventions are similar to those of standard CIMT (Lin et al., 2010b; Page et al., 2008; Shi et al., 2011).

Kinematic Analyses of Constraint-Induced Movement Therapy Outcomes

The definitive EXCITE trial studies of CIMT focused on outcomes related to task performance, as measured by the Wolf Motor Function Test (WMFT) and changes in self-perceived amount and quality of movement, as measured by the Motor Activity Log (MAL). Other researchers have used motion analysis to investigate the effect of CIMT and mCIMT protocols on the kinematic aspects of movement. These studies seek to determine whether CIMT improves the *way* people use their paretic upper limb in addition to improving success in task completion. Several studies have found that, in addition to improved scores on standardized evaluations, CIMT participants also improve the following kinematic aspects of movement in the paretic upper limb:

- Ability to initiate movement more quickly and perform tasks with straighter and smoother reaching trajectories (Wu et al., 2007a)
- Improved movement speed and coordination between shoulder and elbow motions (Caimmi et al., 2008)
- Temporal and spatial improvements in the efficiency of movements and better evidence of preplanned motor control (Wu et al., 2007b)
- Improved movement time, average velocity, and stability of the reach trajectory, as well as increased shoulder flexion during reach (Massie et al., 2009).

However, it has also become apparent that, even with other improvements, CIMT participants may continue to rely on common compensatory movement patterns, such as

- excessive anterior trunk displacement with reach
- poor dissociation between the thorax, shoulder, and elbow
- maladaptive shoulder abduction during attempts at forward reach (Massie et al., 2009).

Previous researchers, investigating potential limitations to other forms of task-related training, have identified compensatory trunk movements as a contributing factor to inefficient arm and hand control in stroke survivors. Excessive trunk rotation and anterior displacement seem to be most problematic in stroke survivors with more severe upper limb impairments (Cirstea, Ptito, & Levin, 2003), who may not qualify to participate in standard CIMT protocols. Reminiscent of NDT procedures that were designed to prevent stroke survivors from using maladaptive compensatory strategies, there is a trend to provide passive trunk restraint to patients while they engage in task-based practice sessions. Trunk restraint is typically provided by using a shoulder belt attached to a chair back, similar to the seat belt in a car (but without the "give").

A few studies have investigated the short-term effects of trunk restraint combined with either task-related training (see Definition 21-3) or mCIMT (Michaelsen, Dannenbaum, & Levin, 2006; Woodbury et al., 2009; Wu et al., 2012). These studies have found some promising outcomes. In particular, the trunk restraint groups showed greater gains in shoulder flexion and elbow extension during forward reach, as well as less compensatory trunk movement and improved grasp control, when tested immediately after participation in a 2-week protocol. It is important to note that no studies have yet assessed retention of these improvements over time. Additionally, there has not been any assessment of whether trunk restraint may have negative effects on the integration between pelvic, trunk, and upper limb kinematics during functional reach that naturally requires movement at each of these body segments.

Effect of Constraint-Induced Movement Therapy Research on Paradigms for Conceptualizing Stroke Rehabilitation

Clearly, not all stroke survivors are candidates for CIMT interventions. However, several concepts and findings related to CIMT can be applied to OT intervention for *all* individuals with hemiparesis caused by stroke or brain injury.

Empirical Support for Applying Dynamic Systems Theory to Neuromotor Rehabilitation. One way to view the concepts and findings of CIMT is in relation to DST. A central tenet to DST is that all systems are capable of reorganization, but this reorganization occurs only in response to some external perturbation (or challenge). Rehabilitation therapists provide external challenge through structuring constraints and affordances during task-related practice. The constraint of not being able to rely on one's unaffected arm and hand, combined with specific affordances of activities presented during shaping sessions, provides a double dose of perturbations that challenge the motor system to reorganize itself. Furthermore, practice sessions are structured to provide the person with opportunities to "figure out" how to meet task-based challenges. This is a major paradigm shift from previous therapies that relied on exercise-based repetitions of specific movements.

Empirical Support for Motor Learning Theories Related to Practice. The success of CIMT can be attributed primarily to the wide opportunities this intervention provides for varied, intense, practice—in which the motivation to move begins with attention to objects in the environment that a person wishes to move, grasp, or manipulate. The constraint is a vehicle for ensuring that the person will participate in practicing with the paretic upper limb. Shaping sessions are similar to traditional activity-based OT: the therapist grades activity demands and creatively designs tasks and competitive games in which the patient is motivated to use her arm and hand again and again, faster and faster, further and further, and using increasingly complex patterns of proximal and distal control. A two-group, randomized study found similar improvements in stroke survivors who participated in a CIMT program and others who participated in a bilateral task-based program of equal intensity (Hayner, Gibson, & Giles, 2010). This finding, coupled with a failure to find significant differences in WMFT scores between the two groups, suggests that the nature and intensity of the practice are the key variables to CIMT's success. The challenge to occupational therapists is to find creative ways to provide this type of motor practice to patients with stroke and brain injury who are not candidates for CIMT.

A New Outcome Variable: Amount of Use. Taub introduced the notion that recovery is integrally tied to amount of use. Although there is no empirical support, to date, to confirm this relationship between amount of use and changes in motor skill, this is an intriguing hypothesis. Consistent with motor learning and dynamical systems theory, Taub highlighted that stroke survivors improve their functional movement skills when they are faced with tasks and environmental challenges to harness their available capacities. When people change their activity patterns to incorporate the paretic arm and hand, they are providing their own opportunities for practice—not only during therapy sessions but also during functional tasks performed throughout the day. Before CIMT, few interventions led to generalization of motor capacities, and they were rarely sustained over time. Changes in pattern of use lead to infinite opportunities to practice. The outstanding long-term results of the EXCITE trial studies indicate (but do not prove) that a positive cycle takes effect (see Fig. 21-3). Improved performance leads to enhanced confidence in functional success. When the person experiences pride in using the limb throughout the day, he uses it even more, and, with this further increase in practice, improves even further—developing enhanced strength and dexterity over time.

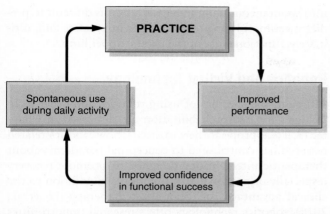

Figure 21-3 Paradigm to promote long-term, continuous improvement in motor control.

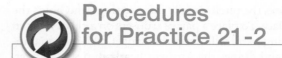

Key Principles from Constraint-Induced Movement Therapy That Can Be Applied to Occupational Therapy for All Stroke Survivors

- Prevent learned nonuse by teaching patients how to capitalize on emerging abilities to execute specific movements.
- Design/adapt activities that the person can perform with existing capabilities.
- Teach the person how to design/adapt activities for functional use of available abilities within natural contexts.

Support for the Concepts of Patient Accountability and Motivation. It is hard, frustrating work to practice using a paretic upper limb. Coupled with the fact that humans can quickly learn to perform many daily tasks with one hand only, it is not surprising that stroke survivors experience the phenomenon of "learned nonuse." The literature in motor learning consistently finds that, when learning a new skill, it is most difficult to practice during early stages, when performance is difficult and clumsy. Think about how you may have hated to practice a musical instrument when taking lessons as a child. Once a person attains a critical level of skill, further practice becomes enjoyable, and it no longer seems arduous to perfect one's skill even further (Schmidt & Lee, 2011). At the early stages of learning, internal motivation may not be forceful enough to compel the person to stick with a practice routine. Therefore, accountability to others may be critical. Several factors in the CIMT protocol enhance accountability. Patients and caregivers sign behavioral contracts before participating in the program. Patients are supervised for 6 hours per day during task-related training. To ensure compliance in wearing the mitt outside of training sessions, a sensor is embedded in each constraint mitt. The person knows that, if she fails to wear the mitt appropriately, she may be asked to terminate the CIMT program. Although these approaches may not be appropriate in clinical OT practice, we can use other behavioral strategies that increase patient accountability to practice using their emerging abilities. One tactic is to provide patients with structured homework logs and check sheets that they share with the therapist at the beginning of each session. Another strategy is to challenge patients to determine their own task goals and to share their achievements with the therapist. Most people have a competitive spirit. It is easier to practice a repetitive task when the goal is to complete a designated set of repetitions in an arbitrary amount of time. It is fun to see if you can "break your previous record."

Tasks, which might otherwise seem meaningless, become motivating if the person knows he will be recording his performance time or racing against the clock (see Procedures for Practice 21-2).

Unanswered Questions. The success of CIMT, albeit with a small subset of stroke survivors, raises two additional questions that remain unanswered for clinicians who are providing neuromotor rehabilitation.

How Important Are Kinematics during Early Learning? Perhaps because Taub is a psychologist rather than a movement scientist or rehabilitation professional, he has never articulated any interest in the kinematics of movement. Abnormal movement synergies and maladaptive movement patterns are simply not considered in Taub's theories about learned nonuse and CIMT. Intervention focuses on preventing learned nonuse and providing extensive opportunities to practice using the hemiparetic limb. Although shaping (or activity grading) is used during therapy sessions, there is no mention of kinematic analysis or any physical manipulation or guidance. Research is needed to determine the best balance between encouraging patients to move and restraining them from moving inefficiently.

Does It Matter if Task Practice Is Unilateral or Bilateral? Because the unaffected upper limb is constrained, task practice in CIMT is inherently unilateral. In reality, however, most functional task performance is bilateral—typically, with one upper limb playing a dominant role in manipulating an object while the other arm assists in stabilizing the same object or another related item. For example, a person may use his or her left hand to stabilize a piece of paper while writing on the paper with his or her right hand. When opening a water bottle, one hand may grasp the cylindrical shaft of the bottle while the other hand turns the cap. To pour water into a glass, one hand manipulates the pitcher while the assisting hand holds the glass in place. To place a pair of trousers on a closet hanger, the assisting hand will grasp the hanger while the manipulating hand drapes the garment neatly onto the hanger. Finally, while using the right hand to load dishes from a kitchen sink into the dishwasher, a person may rest her left hand on the counter—to provide overall stability while she shifts her body weight. Hayner, Gibson, and Giles (2010) compared bilateral training with CIMT, while controlling for amount of practice, and found similar results from both protocols. One potential value is that patients who do not meet the motor criteria to participate in a CIMT protocol may be candidates for a bilateral training program.

Bilateral arm training (BAT) is a therapeutic technique in which patients perform repetitive identical movements with both arms simultaneously. Some examples are

- using bilateral robotics devices, such as BATRAC (Hesse et al., 2005; Whitall et al., 2011)
- pushing/pulling with both arms (as in opening and closing a drawer with two handles or two identical drawers
- wiping a table, using both arms symmetrically
- moving two identical grocery objects from countertop to shelf with both hands (Stoykov, Lewis, & Corcos, 2009)

A comparison of unilateral versus bilateral training groups, matched for amount of practice, revealed that although both groups showed statistically significant improvements on the Motor Status Scale and measures of muscle strength, the bilateral group improved significantly more on a measure of proximal arm function (Stoykov, Lewis, & Corcos, 2009). A randomized controlled study comparing BAT to standard rehabilitation found moderate and statistically significant effects on reaching kinematics and FMA scores, but no differences between groups on ADL function, as measured by the FIM™ (Functional Independence Measure), or amount of use, as measured by the MAL (Lin et al., 2010a). Two randomized controlled studies comparing BAT to mCIMT and a control group (Lin et al., 2009; Wu et al., 2011) found that participants in the BAT group showed significantly better performance than the other groups on factors related to proximal upper limb function. However, the mCIMT group performed significantly better on the MAL and several domains of the Stroke Impact Scale. In summary, when comparing BAT to CIMT, the advantages are the following:

- More stroke survivors can participate in this type of therapy.
- It has therapeutic influence on improving proximal arm control.
- It can be used as a cost-effective enhancement to standard therapy.

A major drawback is that BAT does not impact the extent to which participants incorporate the paretic limb into spontaneous daily activity. Thus, it is difficult to predict meaningful long-term changes in practice and, ultimately, functional use of the paretic upper limb.

Robotics and Virtual Technology

Although the specifics of using robotics and other technologies for neurorehabilitation are discussed in Chapter 18, it is appropriate here to discuss how robotics-related research has contributed to conceptual paradigms about therapeutic interventions designed to promote recovery (especially of proximal arm function). In addition to the clinical advantages of robot-assisted therapy (Lo et al., 2010), robotics technology offers research opportunities to carefully control and study several variables that are difficult to operationalize when therapy is provided by human therapists. Findings from robotics research have lent support to several principles related to the nature of motor relearning and effective therapeutic practice (Hogan et al., 2006; Krebs, Volpe, & Hogan, 2009):

- Intensity of practice is a key factor to recovery of function, but it may not be more important than other factors.
- For improvements to occur, patients must be actively engaged and attempting to move for a functional purpose. Repetitive, passive movement does not improve motor control. Robotics are most effective when they are designed to provide dynamic assistance and challenges based on the robot's continuous monitoring of current performance.
- It is more effective to focus therapy on kinematic challenges rather than on muscle strengthening.
- Neural plasticity is activity dependent.
- The most relevant improvements in motor skill result from implicit rather than explicit learning.
- Treatment that continuously challenges and assists the patient to perform task-driven movements is more effective than exercise to individual muscles.

In addition, robotics researchers have explored the long-standing controversy about limb synergies and recovery. One study (Dipietro et al., 2007) found that, in patients whose arm motor function improved after robotics training, videographic movement analysis revealed that they had modified their existing maladaptive synergy patterns, rather than learning a completely new adaptive strategy. This finding may provide support for interventions that encourage patients to move, regardless of the initial kinematics of the movement.

MULTIPLE FACTORS CONTRIBUTE TO OPTIMAL MOTOR PERFORMANCE

Figure 21-4 illustrates that several sets of factors are required for a person to move in a functional way. The interaction among these variables determines the degree

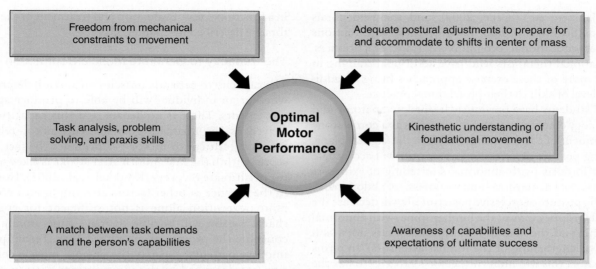

Figure 21-4 Multiple factors contribute to optimal motor performance.

to which an individual can be successful in performing daily tasks. Occupational therapists need to evaluate and intervene in all of these areas to help our patients meet their full potential.

Mechanical Requirements for Movement Execution

The most elemental requirements for motor performance are freedom from mechanical constraints. Thus, joint mobility, fluid dissociation between body segments, optimal postural alignment, the absence of limiting factors such as edema and pain, and the capacity to generate specific movements are essential to a person's capacity to develop functional motor control.

Joint Mobility

Joint mobility, the capacity for limbs to be moved passively around a joint fulcrum, is necessary for active movement and functional performance. Deficits in passive ROM are preventable, secondary, impairments associated with immobility. Histologically, soft tissues do not maintain their underlying distensibility (capacity to be stretched to maximum length) unless they are routinely lengthened by antagonist muscles or an external force. Figure 21-5

illustrates the importance of interventions that are designed to prevent pathological "shortening" of muscles, tendons, and ultimately joint capsule tissue. In survivors of stroke or TBI, spasticity may be a factor that contributes to loss of joint mobility.

Dissociation

Dissociation between body segments refers to the underlying potential for adjacent body segments to move independently of one another. When applicable to the task or movement desired, every segment within our bodies must have the capacity to move freely, without undue restraint from loss of length of multijoint or single-joint muscles. For example, in a healthy musculoskeletal system, the scapula moves freely within the thorax for a variety of passive and active motions within all planes of movement. The thorax is free to move independently of the lumbar spine and pelvis. The pelvis moves freely in all planes, with relation to the lumbar spine. Therapeutic interventions to prevent and improve impairments in dissociation between body segments are presented in the interventions section of this chapter.

Optimal Postural Alignment

Optimal postural adjustment allows a person to efficiently maintain balance against the force of gravity, to freely dissociate adjacent body segments, and to move the arms and legs on a stable foundation at the body core. In our popular culture, there are many exercise programs whose essential goals are to improve postural alignment for efficient, pain-free movement and core muscle strength. Dancers, athletes, and other individuals who wish to reduce biomechanical stress can choose from well-established interventions like Pilates (Kloubec, 2010), the Alexander technique

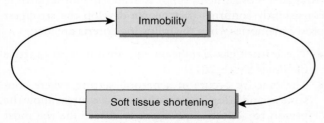

Figure 21-5 Cycle of immobility and soft tissue shortening.

(Jain, Janssen, & DeCelle, 2004), and the Feldenkrais method (Schlinger, 2006). Each of these interventions provides educational programs to train practitioners. Occupational therapists who have additional training in one or more of these exercise approaches bring an additional level of skill to their professional practice.

OT students have previously learned, in anatomy and kinesiology courses, that the pelvis serves as a cornerstone to alignment of the trunk and limbs. In the sagittal plane, a resting posture of excessive anterior tilt will accentuate lumbar lordosis (with abnormal shortening of extensors and abnormal distension—and weakness—of abdominals). A resting posture of excessive posterior tilt will decrease the normal lordotic curve of the lumbar spine (with abnormal shortening of the abdominals and latissimus dorsi and excessive lengthening of the lumbar extensors). In terms of function, this will limit the person's capacity to flex the hips, which is crucial when moving from stand to sit and when reaching forward while sitting. This posture will also accentuate the kyphotic curve of the thoracic spine, which can impact respiratory capacity and mechanics at the scapula and humerus. In the frontal plane, a resting posture of lateral tilt will accentuate lateral trunk flexion away from the weight-bearing side and lead to asymmetries in posture throughout the scapulae and upper limbs, as well as throughout the lower limbs.

When assessed in sitting, stroke survivors with impairments in postural alignment often exhibit excessive posterior pelvic tilt and excessive lateral pelvic tilt—either toward or away from the paretic side. Based on influences from the NDT approach, many clinicians refer to abnormalities in lateral pelvic tilt as problems in weight bearing. A person with excessive left lateral pelvic tilt demonstrates an abnormal pattern of weight bearing, with most of the body weight supported on the left ischium.

When assessed in standing, stroke survivors with impairments in postural alignment may vary in pelvic posture from the sagittal view but almost always exhibit asymmetries with a greater degree of weight bearing (and pelvic lateral tilt) toward the unaffected side. Typical abnormalities in scapular alignment will be discussed later in this chapter. Because postural alignment impacts all other mechanical factors that influence movement, occupational therapists and physical therapists typically assess postural alignment before administering other motor-related evaluations.

Freedom from Other Secondary Impairments

Problems with postural alignment, dissociation between body segments, and joint mobility are all preventable secondary impairments in stroke survivors. Distal edema, localized pain, and complex pain syndromes are examples of other secondary impairments that will also impede a person's capacity to use his or her available motor ability

in a functional way. Evaluation and treatment of these factors are described in Chapter 33.

The Capacity to Generate Muscle Contraction

The capacity to generate muscle contraction determines whether an individual will be able to produce specific movements. There is no debate that this capacity, long viewed as the ultimate goal in neuromotor rehabilitation, is critical to motor performance. In fact, FMA scores within the first month after stroke is a key predictor of ultimate recovery (Kwakkel et al., 2003). However, in the absence of other factors affecting motor control, motor execution alone is not sufficient for ensuring that a person will be able to move functionally or to continue the process of motor recovery. Techniques to improve patients' capacity to generate muscle contraction are described in the interventions section of this chapter.

Kinesthetic Understanding of Foundational Movement Strategies

When the neuromuscular system is functioning optimally, a person can rely on automatic kinematic and kinetic linkages to serve as a foundation for functional movements. Often, patients who are recovering from brain injury have lost the automatic kinesiological linkages associated with efficient movement (Shumway-Cook & Woollacott, 2012). This may be a result of limited mobility of body segments, weakness of specific muscular components, or loss of the motor program that links muscles or joints during a given movement sequence.

Normally, when a seated person wants to reach forward to grasp an object, the CNS calls forth a movement pattern that includes anterior pelvic tilt, hip flexion, scapular abduction, and upward rotation, as well as glenohumeral flexion and external rotation. Additionally, wrist extensors contract to establish optimal mechanical efficiency for the finger flexors. Many persons with hemiplegia cannot rely on automatic generation of these complex muscle linkages, and each attempt at movement presents the challenge of coordinating an unmanageable number of degrees of freedom.

Motor skill learning is dependent on the consolidation of motor memory that guides muscle recruitment (Krakauer & Shadmehr, 2006). Research in motor learning consistently confirms that people develop the strongest motor memories when the following criteria are met:

- The learner has significant opportunities to practice (Schmidt & Lee, 2011).
- The practice occurs in a natural setting, where constraints and affordances within a task context allow the person to actively experiment to determine the most effective strategy (Ma & Trombly, 2004).

- The learner participates in variable rather than repetitive or blocked practice schedules (Davids et al., 2003; Kantak et al., 2010).
- The learner develops an intrinsic feedback system (i.e., he or she "feels" when he or she is performing most efficiently), which lessens his or her reliance on external feedback.

Occupational therapists draw on sound knowledge of kinesiology to determine when a patient is demonstrating inefficient movement strategies. After intervening to reduce mechanical obstacles, the therapist structures therapeutic tasks so that the patient gains practice in implementing a selected motor strategy in a variety of contexts. For example, the therapeutic goal may be to develop the linkage between anterior pelvic tilt, hip flexion, and symmetrical trunk extension as a foundational motor program for forward reach in sitting, as well as standing up from a seated position. The session may begin with the therapist moving the patient's pelvis so that the person understands the kinematic model of action. The therapist may then ask the patient to sit on a therapy ball, which is rocked forward and backward using anterior and posterior pelvic movement. After this, the seemingly unrelated task of reaching for objects from the seated position will emphasize that the patient anteriorly tilt the pelvis by directing attention to "keep your back straight" and "bring your nose over your toes." Following this, the patient will practice standing up and sitting down on a variety of surfaces with an emphasis on the same lumbopelvic interactions previously practiced in different contexts. Finally, the patient may practice this same sequence but while holding a variety of objects. The size and shape of the object may require either unilateral or bilateral grasp, as well as varying configurations of the arms in relation to the body. Research findings from studies with healthy participants (Giuffrida, Shea & Fairbrother, 2002) and men with traumatic brain injury (Giuffrida et al., 2009) provide support for using this approach for learning the invariant structure of a GMP.

Lots and lots of practice is a key variable in determining whether any person will be successful in developing a new foundational movement strategy. Unfortunately, researchers have found that stroke and TBI patients in typical rehabilitation settings tend to get far fewer practice opportunities than laboratory animals in studies of neural plasticity (Kimberley et al., 2010). When opportunities for practice repetitions were increased to recommended levels, patients demonstrated statistically and clinically significant improvements in motor control, with few complaints of pain or fatigue (Birkenmeier, Prager, & Lang, 2010).

Postural Adjustments

Every time a person moves, his or her body's center of mass (COM) changes its relationship to the base of support (BOS). Postural control mechanisms enable us to maintain balance by ensuring that our body's COM remains within the BOS. Effective balance requires adequate function in sensory and motor systems. Sensory processing of visual, vestibular, tactile, and proprioceptive information allows a person to maintain continuous and dynamic awareness about the body's COM and alignment between body segments. Muscle contractions

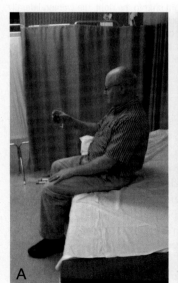
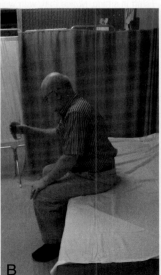
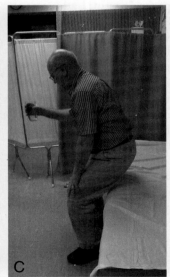
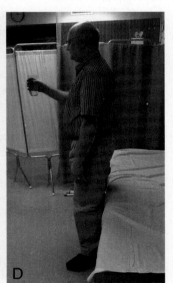

Figure 21-6 Patient practicing sit to stand with the added challenge of a glass of water in his hand. **A.** Patient is in posterior pelvic tilt. **B.** Patient shifts to anterior pelvic tilt and hip flexion in preparation to stand. **C.** Patient bears weight through both legs as he rises from the seating surface. **D.** Patient completes the sequence of moving from sit to stand.

of appropriate amplitude and timing allow for predictive and ongoing force production to match the changing influence of gravity during motor performance. Sufficient joint mobility and muscle length allow the necessary movements to be generated through their full ROM (Hall et al., 2010).

During daily activities, a person's COM can be displaced in three ways: (1) by an external force applied to the body, as occurs during contact sports; (2) by external movement of the support surface, as occurs when we sit or stand in a moving vehicle; and (3) during performance of activities requiring self-initiated movement of the head, limbs, or trunk (Carr & Shepherd, 2003). Typically, balance challenges arising from self-initiated movement are more important to daily function than are balance challenges arising from external perturbations. Postural adjustments are both task and context specific. Studies have shown that muscle activation patterns for balance control vary according to (1) the position of the person, (2) the task being performed, (3) the context in which the activity occurs, and (4) the person's perception of which body part is in contact with the more stable BOS (Dean, Shepherd, & Adams, 1999a, 1999b). Furthermore, during self-initiated movement, postural adjustments are *anticipatory* (Hall et al., 2010). Simultaneous with the motor plan to reach or even turn one's head in a particular direction, tectospinal and vestibulospinal signals are transmitted to produce tonal changes in muscles that will be necessary to counteract excessive displacement in the body's COM (Bear, Connors, & Paradiso, 2007).

Figure 21-7 shows a healthy woman using effective postural adjustments when she shifts her body weight to the right side. Notice that her trunk laterally flexes to the left. If this automatic anticipatory postural adjustment did not occur, the woman's COM would fall to the right of her BOS (her pelvis), and she would be in danger of losing her balance. Of course, trunk lateral flexion to the left cannot occur without lateral elongation of the trunk on the opposite side. As her body weight shifts further and further, she implements additional postural adjustments to keep her COM over her BOS. These adjustments include abduction of her left arm and leg. This is one illustration of significant integration between muscles of the limbs and trunk.

Postural set is a constellation of postural adjustments that precede the performance of a specified motor activity (Layne & Spooner, 1992). If you were to stand up right now, you would "posturally set" yourself by positioning both feet on the floor in an appropriate BOS. You would establish ≤90° angles at your hips and knees, and you would free your lumbar spine by anteriorly tilting your pelvis. When standing, people automatically change the configuration of their BOS in anticipation of the direction toward which they expect to shift their body weight.

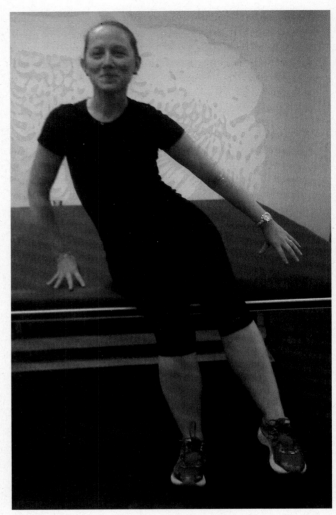

Figure 21-7 Efficient postural adjustments during self-initiated weight shift in sitting. Notice that, with weight shift to the right, the woman laterally flexes her trunk to the left and abducts her left arm and leg. These postural adjustments ensure that, even as her center of mass (COM) shifts significantly, her COM will remain safely over her base of support (BOS). Notice also that her head remains erect and her trunk is elongated on the right.

For example, if they plan to move forward, as in bowling or throwing, they will establish an anterior-posterior BOS. If they plan to shift to the left or right, as in a tennis swing, they will establish a medial-lateral BOS. In addition, when they plan to move a limb, they intuitively shift their body weight to provide the most efficient postural set. In the case of the lower limb, during gait, you shift your body weight in the opposite direction to "unweight" that side. Clearly, you cannot swing your right leg forward unless you have shifted your body weight onto the left leg.

Individuals with impairments in postural adjustments will be fearful of falling when sitting or standing without support, and, even more so, when attempting to move their limbs. They are likely to develop adaptive strategies that may seem effective in the short run but that have long-term maladaptive influence on balance and other motor function (Carr & Shepherd, 2003). When people feel unable to maintain their balance in posturally threatening situations, one such strategy is to constrain movement at selected body parts and thus decrease the number of motor elements, or degrees of freedom, the CNS must control. Individuals with postural adjustment deficits as a result of CNS dysfunction may feel insecure about their ability to maintain balance, even in routine sitting or standing positions. The strategy of fixating one's pelvis on the lumbar spine or the scapula on the thorax has short-term benefits for enhancing the person's sense of postural security. A negative consequence is that these patterns lead to soft tissue shortening and difficulty dissociating the scapula and pelvis from adjacent proximal structures. This lack of sufficient mobility at the limb girdles subsequently limits the normal kinematics of upper and lower extremity movement. Figure 21-5 illustrates how immobility and muscle shortening interact in a self-perpetuating cycle.

The strategies of shifting weight away from a paretic leg, unnecessarily widening the BOS, or using one's hands excessively for support present further obstacles to using and improving available muscle strength and sensory processing skills. In addition, these strategies contribute to additional problems in gait and in using the upper limbs to their maximum potential. Conversely, with improvements in balance, a person has greater potential to dissociate adjacent body segments and to use his or her available motor capacity for moving the upper limb.

Match between Task Demands and the Person's Capabilities

In studies of motor control using kinematic analysis, skilled performers consistently exhibit more efficient strategies than novice performers (Schmidt & Lee, 2011). Even among individuals with healthy neuromuscular systems, when the task demands exceed one's capabilities, people demonstrate a variety of maladaptive motor behaviors. Some examples are using a postural set that is ineffective in supporting the movement sequences associated with the task, assuming a stiff posture in an ineffective attempt to reduce degrees of freedom, and recruiting muscles that are not required for performance.

People with CNS dysfunction face additional problems that make their motor success even more dependent on a good match between their current capabilities and a task's demands. Muscle spasticity is highly influenced by physical, cognitive, and emotional stress. In the face of an overly strenuous or otherwise challenging task, a patient is likely to experience an increase in hypertonicity and, possibly, pathological influences of primitive reflexes. Frustration and anxiety impede anyone's performance during motor tasks. These factors are even more critical for people whose bodies are responding in unpredictable ways.

Chapter 12 provides critical information about the process occupational therapists use to select, grade, analyze, and adapt activities. We recommend that you review material in this chapter about the use of occupation-as-means. Pay particular attention to Procedures for Practice 12-5. Occupational therapists combine skills in activity adaptation and knowledge of kinesiology with their evaluation findings to develop individualized therapeutic tasks that are within the person's capability while providing just the right amount of challenge for meaningful practice that will lead to improvements in motor skill.

Awareness of Capabilities and Expectations of Ultimate Success

Early after a stroke or closed head injury, many survivors exhibit motor deficits that reflect widespread physiological impairment in the affected cerebral hemisphere. In addition to cell death in those neurons directly affected by the brain injury, indirect damage includes changes in cerebral blood flow, cerebral metabolism, edema, and cascading degeneration along neural pathways. This transient inhibition of neurons in a wide penumbra surrounding the site of infarct or hemorrhage is often referred to as diaschisis (Seitz et al., 1999). As diaschisis resolves over time, neural activities return to the temporarily suppressed regions, and the stroke survivor experiences return of function. Diaschisis is a probable explanation for the shift to spontaneous innervation of some flaccid muscles so often seen in the early weeks after a stroke.

One likely explanation for learned nonuse is that, when this recovery begins, the individual does not know how to detect the reemergence of movement capacity because he or she has already learned how to perform most activities unilaterally with the unaffected upper limb. Another explanation is that the person notices some isolated abilities to perform specific movements, but it is extremely difficult to use these movements for integrated functional performance. As a result, the person continues to rely exclusively on the unaffected upper limb and loses the opportunity to practice using his or her newly emerging capacities in the affected arm and hand.

Learned nonuse begins a negative spiral of events. Without active use, the paretic limbs are more vulnerable to developing secondary impairments associated with immobility, such as limited ROM and edema. Furthermore, practice opportunities with the affected limbs, which are essential to neural reorganization following brain injury, are lost if the person does not attempt to use the paretic arm or leg during functional activities. The theory of learned nonuse may explain why upper limb recovery often lags behind recovery of function in the paretic lower limb. Whereas each attempt to stand or walk requires bilateral activity in the legs, many upper limb activities may be accomplished by using the unaffected side exclusively.

Task Analysis, Problem Solving, and Praxis Skills

In any situation that requires motor action, we automatically "size up" the task and environmental parameters before creating the motor plan that will guide the action. In addition to preplanning postural adjustments (previously discussed in this chapter), we rely on complex interactions between the visual (striate), parietal, premotor, and primary motor cortices to match our arm and hand motions to the task requirements. Praxis, or motor planning, is the ability to

- quickly analyze the motor requirements of a task
- determine the best solution to the motor "problems" that are inherent to the task

These abilities seem to be dependent on two networks, described below, with primary functions in the dominant, left hemisphere.

Neural Networks

As described by leading theorists (Jeannerod et al., 1995), the process begins in the visual cortex and continues through two parallel networks: the ventral stream and the dorsal stream. Connections within the ventral stream, between the striate cortex and specific premotor areas, enable us to accurately determine the purpose of an object. Connections within the dorsal stream, between the striate cortex and various regions within the parietal lobe, enable us to accurately determine which physical properties of the object goal are essential to formulating the specifics of a motor plan. These parameters include information about the object's size, shape, weight, texture, and location. To use a term introduced earlier in this chapter, the essential first step in motor planning is to accurately interpret the affordances of task objects for the purpose of determining the most efficient movement strategy.

Feedforward Control

It is essential to remember that this intricate analysis of task requirements occurs *before* a person makes contact with the task objects. Control of reach and grasp is anticipatory, just as is control of postural adjustments during task performance (Frey et al., 2011). Feedforward control is much like the strategic planning process used to manage organizations. Based on previous experience and accurate interpretation of current trends, the business manager

sets forth a plan of action. Corrections, based on feedback, are necessary only when errors occur. In the case of reach and grasp, visual and somatosensory information, combined with previous experience and learning, contribute to preprogramming a general plan for the motor action. In addition to postural adjustments, this general plan includes all the variables for

- determining and presetting the hand position—for pointing, swiping, pushing, or grasping the object
- positioning the shoulder, elbow, forearm, and wrist so that the hand will be oriented in precisely the right direction at precisely the right time so that, when the hand makes contact with the target object, it is in the best position to interact with the object.

Treatment for patients with apraxia, the inability to effectively use the process described above, will be presented in the interventions section of this chapter. However, *any* individual who has experienced significant loss in motor function will need opportunities to "figure out" strategies for using the affected arm and hand in a variety of task-based situations.

FRAMEWORK FOR OCCUPATIONAL THERAPY INTERVENTIONS GEARED TOWARD IMPROVING MOTOR PERFORMANCE

The framework for OT interventions to improve motor performance in clients who are recovering from brain injury is informed by a series of general principles and a core understanding of the factors (illustrated in Fig. 21-4) that contribute to optimal motor performance.

General Principles for Occupational Therapy Interventions to Improve Motor Performance

Take a moment to review the Glossary and "Fundamentals of the Teaching–Learning Process" sections in Chapter 13. We will be applying many of these concepts in our presentation of general principles related to task-based interventions, viewing the therapist as a coach, and well-established tenets of effective practice for motor learning.

Task-Based Interventions

It is a core, historical assumption of OT practice that engagement in specially designed therapeutic activities can improve motor function. As illustrated in this chapter and throughout this entire textbook, recent literature in neuroscience, movement science, and rehabilitation provides consistent support for the efficacy of task-oriented practice in promoting motor skill development and neural plasticity in humans with movement impairments caused by CNS dysfunction. Some of the many different terms used to describe the use of activities as a therapeutic intervention to improve motor control are repetitive task training/practice (French et al., 2010), task-related training (Carr & Shepherd, 1982, 1998, 2003, 2010), activity-based therapy (Dromerick, Lum, & Hidler, 2006), task-specific training (Hubbard et al., 2009), and goal-directed training (Mastos et al., 2007).

Consistent with dynamical systems theory and ecological theory, task-based intervention capitalizes on the interrelationship between the task, environment, and the person in shaping human movement and promoting the development of new motor skills.

Definition 21-3 describes the core elements of tasks as therapeutic interventions to improve motor performance. In addition, when designing task-based intervention, the therapist appreciates the natural interdependence between balance, gross mobility, and functional limb movement. Therefore, even though we have divided our discussion of intervention into these three categories, the treatment program will strive to integrate all three types of motor demands into therapeutic tasks.

Unlike compensatory training, generalization of learning is the goal of task-based neuromotor intervention. Even though the patient practices specific tasks, the therapeutic purpose is *not* focused on fostering independence in those particular tasks. Rather, the therapeutic goal is that the patient will develop an underlying strategy (or motor program) for performing an infinite variety of tasks that require foundational skills in balance, gross mobility, and/or functional movement of a paretic limb.

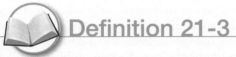

Definition 21-3

Task-Based/Task-Related/Activity-Based, Goal-Directed Training

Definition of Task-Based, Goal-Directed Training and Criteria for a Therapeutic Task

"Client-selected goals are used to provide opportunities for problem solving and to indirectly drive the movements required to meet the task demands" (Mastos et al., 2007, p. 47).

Criteria for a therapeutic task:

- The task uses natural objects whose affordances are clear to the client.
- The task inherently allows for repetitive actions that vary with natural changes in the task demands.
- The task is well matched to the client's current motor abilities and therapeutic goals.
- The client fully understands parameters related to his or her own position and the placement of task-related objects.

Therapist as Coach

The patient–therapist relationship in task-related training is an active, collaborative mentorship with regard to motor performance. Just as an athletic coach is well versed in the motor strategies that are critical to success in a particular sport, therapists bring an expertise about functional movement for performance of daily tasks. Therapists must have extensive knowledge about the kinetic and kinematic features of movement, both as performed by individuals with intact neuromuscular systems and as frequently observed in people demonstrating specific motor dysfunction, such as hemiparesis or ataxia. Therapists apply this knowledge when assessing performance, setting goals, structuring practice sessions, and providing feedback and instruction. The therapist's critical goals as coach are (1) to encourage performance of the most important mechanical features within a given category of motor tasks and (2) to discourage behavioral adaptations that have limited effectiveness (Carr & Shepherd, 2003).

As coaches, therapists structure practice sessions in order to

- direct the patient's attention to features of the task that are most salient for learning
- provide appropriate instructions
- develop each patient's ability to actively analyze his or her own performance (Carr & Shepherd, 2003).

Focusing Attention. An early step in the process of learning a motor skill is to identify the key components of the action. In other words, early learning of a motor skill requires explicit instruction to establish key parameters that will be critical for successful performance. At this stage, demonstration and instructions, which focus on one or two salient points, are important in directing the patient's efforts. Learning proceeds most smoothly when the patient has a clear idea of the motor goal and which strategies are appropriate or inappropriate for reaching that goal. Carr and Shepherd (2003) recommend that therapists routinely ask patients to describe or demonstrate, with another body segment if necessary, the specific movements required to achieve a task. This allows therapists to understand what patients think they are being asked to do. Instructions can then be modified to ensure that both patient and therapist are actually working toward the same goal.

Once an individual has internalized this "model" of an action, the next goal is to develop skill and efficiency in coordinating actions to perform the action in a smooth, efficient manner. This implicit learning is dependent on continued task practice, with increasing demands on speed, strength, and coordination. At this stage, it may be detrimental to focus a patient's attention on the details of performance (Fasoli et al., 2002). Instead, the therapist structures control parameters within the task objects to shape the intended kinematics of a movement sequence.

Instructions and Feedback. Instruction is important when the therapist's goal is to promote explicit learning. With oral instruction, words should be kept to a minimum. The therapist identifies the most important aspect of the movement and presents directions in terms of an object goal. Visual demonstration can be provided through the therapist's own performance of the task, with a focus on one or two components that are most essential to the motor strategy. Pictures and photographs are particularly helpful in clarifying procedures for "homework practice" to be completed outside of therapy sessions. Physical "handling" can also be valuable at times to convey information about postural alignment or a desired movement trajectory. This manual interaction by the therapist can help to clarify the model of action by passively guiding the patient through the path of movement or by physically constraining inappropriate components. For example, during attempts at task-related forward reach, the therapist may provide passive movement to the scapula, with simultaneous cues over the acromium for the patient to limit elevation of the entire shoulder girdle. When a patient attempts to sit down, the therapist's manual guidance behind the shoulders reinforces the concept that the individual must move the upper body forward to achieve the necessary hip and knee flexion for smooth controlled descent.

Feedback, or information about a response, can be intrinsic or extrinsic, concurrent or terminal, and can provide knowledge of performance (KP) or knowledge of results (KR). Intrinsic feedback is a result of an individual's own proprioceptive, tactile, vestibular, visual, and auditory sensory systems. Often after a stroke, somatosensory function is impaired, which limits the effectiveness of intrinsic feedback about motor performance. Extrinsic feedback from a therapist or feedback technology can provide useful supplementary information to facilitate early awareness and learning. However, the goal is for patients to return to providing their own intrinsic feedback so they can continually perfect their motor performance. Therefore, in therapy sessions, extrinsic feedback is gradually decreased, and patients are encouraged to use their own internal sensations to guide their movement.

Concurrent feedback is provided during task performance. It includes intrinsic somatosensory feedback and ongoing verbal or manual guidance by a therapist. Terminal, or summary, feedback is given after task completion. There are no published studies that compare the effectiveness of concurrent and terminal feedback, but research has established that excessive external concurrent feedback is distracting to the learner and may prevent the patient from learning to rely on his or her own internal, concurrent feedback (Schmidt & Lee, 2011).

KP feedback is information about the processes used during task performance, such as the way a person moves the pelvis or scapula. Individuals with intact proprioceptive systems receive concurrent, intrinsic KP feedback as they move. Survivors of stroke or brain injury, however, may no longer have access to this continuous supply of information. Therapists provide extrinsic KP feedback when they call a patient's attention to specific aspects of his or her postural alignment or key features of a movement trajectory. Research findings about the value of extrinsic KP feedback in stroke rehabilitation are mixed. The results of some studies indicate that a focus on internal performance factors may be counterproductive to learning (Fasoli et al., 2002). On the other hand, a randomized controlled trial of 28 chronic stroke survivors found that KP feedback was more effective than KR feedback in improving the kinematics of arm movement (Cirstea & Levin, 2007).

KR feedback is feedback about the outcome of an action. Results of laboratory research with healthy subjects indicates that frequent, accurate, immediate KR tends to promote improved performance during early learning but results in poorer retention and generalization of the learning (Schmidt & Lee, 2011). Therefore, when using technologies that provide consistent and immediate KR feedback, such as robotics, or electromyograph-triggered neuromuscular stimulation (EMG-TMS), therapists are advised to gradually "wean" patients from depending on this extrinsic feedback and help patients develop their own intrinsic feedback mechanisms.

Helping Patients Develop Skills in Analyzing Their Own Performance. Because the goal is to help patients learn to monitor their movement through intrinsic feedback, from the beginning, they must be active participants in analyzing their own performance. This practice allows therapists to see how well each person understands the salient features of the current therapeutic task. Furthermore, this process of self-analysis encourages individuals to develop insight about their own motor abilities, develop problem-solving skills, and understand the goals of the treatment program.

The Nature of Practice

Practice is a critical component to motor skill learning. Chapter 13 presents findings from several studies about practice conditions that are relevant to OT intervention. The following principles about practice are particularly important when designing therapy to improve motor skill in persons recovering from stroke or brain injury:

- Random (or variable) practice schedules lead to better generalization of learning than blocked practice schedules. Therefore, therapists structure practice tasks that require mild variations in movement patterns during successive repetitions.
- People learn what they practice. Therefore, patients must clearly understand instructions about the key kinematic components of general movement strategies they will be practicing during and outside of therapy sessions.

- Greater amounts of practice are important to skill learning and generalization. Because therapy sessions do not provide sufficient opportunities for patients to practice developing new motor skills, therapists help patients develop routines for practicing new skills on their own or with family members. It is human nature to practice more when we know that someone will hold us accountable. Therefore, patients should be responsible for keeping "homework logs" and reporting their progress to the therapist at the beginning of each session.
- Practice of specific movements leads only to improvements in motor execution but not in functional performance. Therefore, the goal of therapeutic practice is that patients learn general strategies for solving motor problems.

Self-care and leisure activities provide logical opportunities for task-based practice. Too often, occupational therapists prescribe universal methods for ADL that contradict our goals for optimum motor performance. Unless balance and limb function are routinely challenged during daily activity performance, there are no environmental challenges to stimulate brain plasticity. Unless patients have opportunities for routine practice of motor skills required for balance, mobility, and functional use of their affected limbs, time spent during therapy sessions will have little effect. *Therefore, the occupational therapist must design safe, individualized methods for each patient that continually include that person's emerging capacities into daily self-care and leisure performance.*

Interventions are Informed by the Multiple Factors that Contribute to Optimal Motor Performance

Earlier in this chapter, we presented multiple factors that contribute to optimal motor performance. These are summarized in Figure 21-4. Occupational therapists consider the effect of each of these factors on a person's ability to maintain balance during task performance, to perform gross functional movements, and to use the arm and hand. Overall, the sequence of intervention is as follows:

- Analyze a person's motor performance to determine key limiting factors that are amenable to change through therapeutic intervention.
- Prevent or reduce these key limiting factors through direct intervention and client education.
- Design activities for use as therapeutic challenges that promote development of effective movement strategies.
- Adapt the physical environment to promote maximal function.
- Assist clients in developing strategies for approaching and mastering the motor challenges of new activities they may wish to perform in the future.

Intervention to Improve Postural Alignment and Balance

Neuromotor intervention typically begins with assessment and treatment to improve alignment and balance in sitting and standing. There are two major reasons for this:

1. Some patients will never develop functional arm and hand use on the paretic side, but they can still be independent if they can develop adequate balance and gross mobility.
2. A person's abilities in gross functional mobility and use of a paretic arm and hand are highly influenced by his or her foundational balance. In other words, sitting and standing balance serve as a critical foundation for the development of other functional motor skills.

Intervention to Improve Sitting Balance

To assist patients in improving sitting balance, the occupational therapist ensures that each person achieves optimal alignment for seated task performance, develops a kinesthetic understanding of alignment and postural adjustments, and has ample opportunity for implicit learning through task-based challenges that require the person to actively shift his or her COM.

Optimal Alignment for Seated Task Performance. Earlier in this chapter, we described positions of optimal alignment in sitting, as well as common problems exhibited by patients with neuromotor impairments. One critical step in a balance intervention is to help the person develop kinesthetic awareness of efficient alignment between body segments. First, however, the therapist determines which mechanical constraints are influencing a person's posture. This assessment takes place on a surface where the trunk is unsupported, such as sitting over the side of the patient's bed or on a therapy mat (short sitting). If the person demonstrates soft tissue stiffness, leading to difficulty dissociating the thorax and the lumbar spine, the scapula and the thorax, or the lumbar spine and pelvis, then the therapist provides passive stretch before asking for active engagement in balance activities.

If, however, the "cause" for limited dissociation between body segments can be attributed to the person's postural insecurity, then the intervention will focus on providing additional external support—usually through physical "handling" by the therapist.

Gillen (2011) provides an excellent description of the "seated position of readiness for function." The pelvis is in neutral to anterior tilt, with equal weight bearing on both ischial tuberosities. The trunk is extended and in a midline orientation. Shoulders are symmetrical and positioned anterior to the hips. Hips and knees are flexed and neutrally rotated. Both feet are flat on the floor, and each foot is ready to accept body weight as the trunk moves forward.

Developing Kinesthetic Awareness. To help patients develop kinesthetic awareness of the model for optimal sitting alignment, we precede each therapeutic task with a request to the person to assume this "position of function." If the patient assumes a position in which specific elements are less than optimal, the therapist, as coach, points out these errors in alignment and challenges the person to actively correct his or her posture. Patients must also develop kinesthetic awareness of postural adjustments that accompany active shifts in their COM during activity performance. To achieve this, they must have opportunities to participate in graded, task-based challenges.

Introducing Task-Based Challenges that Involve Active Shifts in Center of Mass. Balance is the process of maintaining one's COM over the BOS. Postural adjustments involve strategic changes in alignment that will minimize changes in COM when we shift body weight in a variety of planes and directions. During functional performance, task demands may require us to move

- forward and backward (sagittal plane)
- to the left and to the right (coronal plane)
- by rotating our trunk to the left or right (transverse plane)
- in any combination of the three cardinal planes listed above (e.g., forward motion to the left) and in any combination of the cardinal planes plus the upward or downward direction

Each direction of weight shift is accompanied by its own associated postural adjustments. For example, when shifting weight forward while sitting, the hips flex, the pelvis anteriorly tilts, and the trunk extends at the lumbar, thoracic, and cervical spine. (see Fig. 21-6). Conversely, when shifting weight backward, the pelvis posteriorly tilts and the trunk flexes. When shifting weight to the right side (as illustrated in Fig. 21-7), the pelvis tilts to the right, and the left side of the pelvis lifts off of the sitting surface. The right hip externally rotates and the left hip internally rotates. The trunk laterally flexes to the right and, concomitantly, extends on the left. This lateral flexion (or concavity) may be described as "trunk shortening on the left" and the accompanying lateral extension (convexity) as "trunk lengthening on the right" (Bobath, 1990; Davies, 2000).

Research evidence shows that stroke survivors develop sitting balance in the context of task performance (Dean, Channon, & Hall, 2007; Dean & Shepherd, 1997; Shumway-Cook & Woollacott, 2012). The therapist structures activities that require the patient to shift weight in a variety of directions. These include the following:

- Looking in a variety of directions (e.g., up at the ceiling, behind oneself).
- Reaching for and moving objects that are strategically positioned (e.g., in front, to the left, and lower than the arm position in a typical seated posture to a variety of other predetermined locations). The upper limb diagonal patterns described in the PNF approach provide therapists with a helpful model for structuring activities that provide postural challenges through an infinite combination of planes and directions of movement.
- Simulated and natural performance of self-care activities, such as dressing, bathing, and grooming, with graded changes in placement of goal objects and degree of postural support.

Early in the process, the therapist may provide tactile/proprioceptive cues that provide the "model of the action" of the motor program for each associated postural adjustment. Figure 21-8 illustrates a therapist providing somatosensory cues for a patient to "shorten" his trunk on the contralateral side and "elongate" his trunk on the ipsilateral side during lateral weight shift (Davies, 2000).

Strengthening of postural muscles occurs within the context of self-initiated shifts in body COM. For example, tasks involving posterior weight shift provide strengthening "exercise" to the rectus abdominis. Tasks involving trunk movement through multiple planes provide strengthening exercise to virtually every abdominal and extensor muscle of the thoracic and lumbar spine (Gillen, 2011).

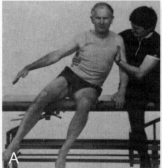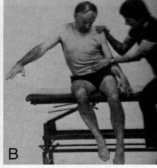

Figure 21-8 Therapist providing cues about appropriate postural adjustments during weight shift in sitting. **A.** The patient is shifting weight to his left (paretic) side as the therapist promotes trunk elongation/lateral extension on the left and lateral flexion on the right. Note that the patient appropriately abducts his unaffected right arm and leg as an automatic postural adjustment to maintain his center of mass (COM) over his base of support. Note also that the therapist is positioning his left arm to allow for some weight bearing onto his left hand as the patient shifts his weight to the left. **B.** The patient is shifting weight to his right side as the therapist promotes trunk lateral flexion on his left (paretic). (Used with permission from Davies, P. M. [2000]. *Steps to follow: The comprehensive treatment of patients with hemiplegia* [2nd ed., p. 168]. Berlin: Springer-Verlag.)

Standing Balance

There are key similarities and differences between standing balance and sitting balance.

The Goal Is to Maintain the Body's Center of Mass over Its Base of Support as We Shift Body Weight in a Variety of Directions. A key difference between standing and sitting is that, when standing, one's feet are the BOS. Although, this creates an inherently smaller foundation than the pelvis and thighs (in sitting), we have the capacity to rearrange our foot position to suit the balance demands of a particular activity. As discussed earlier in this chapter, we make quick, anticipatory judgments about how the COM will shift during task performance. If we plan to move our body weight forward or backward, we increase the anterior-posterior BOS by positioning one foot in front of the other. If we plan to move our body weight to either side, we increase the medial-lateral BOS by positioning our feet side by side. If we plan to move our body weight in a diagonal direction, we have an infinite number of options for arranging the BOS.

Another significant difference is that, in standing, the COM is further displaced superiorly from the BOS. In addition to increasing the complexity of balance adjustments in standing, this factor contributes to postural sway, the continuous displacement and correction of the COM within the BOS. In actuality, there is no such thing as static standing balance, because when standing, a person constantly "sways" over the BOS. When the postural set is anterior-posterior, we sway in a lateral-medial direction. When the postural set is medial-lateral, we sway in an anterior-posterior direction. Of course, the smaller the BOS, the greater the ongoing postural sway will be.

Optimal Alignment Contributes Significantly to Efficient Balance. Functional standing balance requires the ability to shift weight from one leg onto the other. In patients with hemiparesis caused by stroke or brain injury, an early goal is to establish bilateral weight bearing on both the left and right legs. Patients need to learn how to recognize when they are, in fact, supporting weight over their paretic leg. Key factors in postural alignment during bilateral weight bearing will be symmetrical posture at the pelvis, hips, trunk, shoulders, and head.

The next goal is for the patient to be able to shift weight onto the paretic leg—so the other leg will be free to move. However, it is not sufficient to merely be able to support body weight through the affected leg. In addition, the person must be able to quickly "unweight" that leg in order to swing it forward for functional gait. One common maladaptive strategy after stroke or brain injury is to assume a weight-bearing posture that makes the leg into a "rigid pillar" (Davies, 2000). The hallmark of this posture is hyperextension (locking) at the knee often accompanied by pelvic retraction and ankle plantar flexion.

Optimal alignment of a weight-bearing leg is characterized by

- at least 90° of ankle dorsiflexion—so the foot is flat on an even surface
- relaxed, active extension at the knee (with no locking)
- active hip extension
- neutral position of the pelvis

In addition, if weight is shifted onto the left leg

- the pelvis will be laterally tilted to the left
- the trunk should be laterally flexed to the right and elongated on the left

Sensory Awareness Is Critical to Effective Balance Adjustments. In addition to the kinesthetic awareness of postural alignment discussed earlier with regard to sitting balance, considerable research has established that a triad of sensory systems is necessary for adequate standing balance. Complex and dynamic interrelationships between somatosensory, vestibular, and visual processing ensure that we will be able to maintain standing balance in a variety of sensory conditions. For example, when walking in a dark environment, people rely more on kinesthetic cues from muscles and joints, tactile cues from the floor surface on our feet, and vestibular cues (Shumway-Cook & Woollacott, 2012). In stroke survivors, somatosensory cues from the paretic leg and arm may be disrupted. Therapeutic goals are to (1) enhance somatosensory awareness by introducing many opportunities to experience weight bearing on the affected leg (Davies, 2000) and/or (2) to promote enhanced vestibular functioning by providing task-based challenges in which vision and somatosensory cues are reduced (Bayouk, Boucher, & Leroux, 2006).

Postural Adjustments and Strength in Key Postural Muscles Are Developed through Task-Based Challenges. Extensive research supports the use of task-related training to develop muscle strength and postural adjustments needed for standing balance and gait (see, for example, Grabiner et al., 2012 and Sullivan et al., 2007). Lower limb muscles are exercised as the patient supports and shifts body weight during task performance (Carr & Shepherd, 2003). Initially, the focus may be similar to the therapeutic strategy described earlier to improve sitting balance. The therapist designs tasks that require reach, grasp, and placement of objects while the patient is standing. Later, when the goal is to provide opportunities to use the paretic limb exclusively for body weight support, the therapist selects tasks that inherently require active movement of the other leg, such as stepping forward, stepping onto a bathroom scale, or knocking down objects (such as toy bowling pins) with the unaffected foot. Choreographed dance routines that involve kicking or swinging one leg at a time also provide varied, repetitive, activity-based practice in bearing weight and then taking weight off of the paretic lower limb. As the patient gains balance control, task objects are strategically positioned so that the patient is required to actively move from place to place to complete the task. Dynamic tasks, such as ball or balloon toss games or virtual reality games, present additional challenges to standing balance (see Fig. 11-5). Familiar homemaking tasks, such as loading/unloading a dishwasher, picking up clothes from the floor, and placing them in a laundry basket are natural therapeutic activities to improve standing balance. Dolechek and Schkade (1999) found that this type of intervention was more effective in improving dynamic standing endurance than an exercise-based program that did not include meaningful tasks. In a motion analysis study, Lin et al. (2007) found that the presence of a task object in a standing reaching task contributed to factors that decrease postural sway in standing.

Functional Mobility

Functional mobility training includes task-specific interventions that enable patients to move efficiently in bed, to rise from supine to a sitting position, to move about within the sitting position through "scooting," to stand up and sit down, and to perform daily activities while standing and walking. Other authors have presented detailed analyses of the kinematics and kinetics of functional mobility tasks, as well as instructive photographs to guide therapists in assisting patients in their initial learning (Davies, 2000; Kane & Buckley, 2011). Like balance, efficient functional mobility inherently requires optimal postural alignment and dissociation between body segments. Like balance interventions, task training in functional mobility tasks provides the opportunity to strengthen core muscles and improve postural adjustments. During the rehabilitation process, therapeutic interventions to improve functional mobility and balance are rarely separated.

Moving in Bed

In the acute phase of recovery after a stroke or brain injury, patients find themselves in a body with unfamiliar sensations and an inability to control many movements. Early goals for the patient include learning to access the nurse call buzzer and learning to assist caregivers in adjusting the position in bed.

In crook lying, a person is supine with both legs flexed at the hips and knees and both feet flat on the supporting surface. From this starting position, bridging is the act of pushing weight through one's feet and lifting the buttocks off of the bed or mat. Bridging is an important component to moving vertically in bed. In addition, the task of bridging gives patients the opportunity to discover what it means to move the pelvis in isolation of the lumbar spine and to experiment with alternating between anterior and posterior pelvic tilt. This learning serves as a precursor to developing a model for optimal alignment in sitting and standing.

Rolling in bed, toward either the affected or unaffected side, requires dissociations between adjacent body segments: the scapula and thorax, the thorax and the lumbar spine, and the lumbar spine and pelvis. When rolling toward the unaffected side, the patient learns to capitalize on any available motor control in the paretic arm. He or she can also use the unaffected arm to assist, as needed.

Multiple studies have examined the kinematics of sitting up from supine, and the ultimate finding is that people choose from a variety of effective strategies (Carr & Shepherd, 2003). All the strategies involve some level of weight bearing and "push off" over one arm. When patients show potential to use the paretic arm for this function, therapists structure the activity to incorporate this challenge into the task training. To promote the best retention and generalization, training should be varied. Opportunities to practice short sitting can be alternated with opportunities to practice rising from supine to long sitting (knees extended, with feet remaining on the supporting surface). The task is easier when the ultimate short sitting position provides support to the feet (i.e., feet on the floor when sitting on a chair or chair-height therapy mat) but should also be practiced on higher surfaces when the feet will be unsupported. Finally, practice is also required to move from sitting to supine. Task demands shift to requiring concentric and eccentric contractions from different groups of muscles when the goal is to slowly lower oneself onto the bed.

Moving in the Seated Position

In our earlier discussion of interventions to improve balance, we presented concepts and strategies for helping patients improve their ability to perform activities in the seated position. One key concept is that the trunk elongates on the side toward which weight is shifted and shortens on the other side. This is an equilibrium adjustment that keeps the body's COM over the BOS. Often, we shift our weight so far laterally that the opposite ischium completely rises off of the supporting surface. This is necessary when we wish to smooth our clothing or, more importantly, when we readjust our seated BOS.

In "scooting," a seated person repositions his or her buttocks—forward, backward, or to the side. He or she achieves this by shifting all of his or her body weight over the left ischium in order to freely move the right ischium in the desired direction. This is followed by a reverse shift of body weight to the right ischium in order to move the left ischium in the desired direction. This process is repeated until the person has repositioned his or her BOS—either at the front edge of the seating surface in preparation for standing or back into the chair as the final step in sitting down. Scooting is a valuable motor skill. In addition to its importance in safely standing up and sitting down, practice in scooting provides patients with opportunities to experiment with producing pelvic movements that are independent of movement at the lumbar spine. At the same time, patients develop a motor program for the postural adjustments that accompany extreme shifts in COM. Finally, through scooting, patients implicitly learn that active movement can only be achieved when a body segment is "unweighted." This is an important precursor to functional balance in sitting and standing. Scooting practice can be incorporated creatively into games and activities on a therapy mat. The therapist places a goal object in various places on the mat, and the patient is challenged to scoot so that his or her buttocks make contact with the object. This intervention provides infinite opportunities to vary the direction of each weight shift and simultaneously affords varied challenges to balance in both the short and long sitting positions.

Standing Up and Sitting Down

Rising to a standing position, and its counterpart, sitting down safely and efficiently, are critical to performance of daily tasks. Although each must be trained separately, the components of "sit to stand" and "stand to sit" are similar enough that the abbreviation "STS" is often used to refer to both. Successful performance of STS requires the integration of

- adequate mobility at the pelvis and hips
- kinesthetic awareness of postural alignment
- automatic postural adjustments during weight shift
- sufficient strength in muscles of the lower limbs and trunk
- a motor program that guides the action.

Direct training in STS is an important component of any stroke rehabilitation program. Research shows that this intervention is effective in improving actual performance (Canning et al., 2003; Janssen et al., 2010). In addition, a systematic STS training program contributes significantly to improvements in dynamic balance, postural alignment in standing, and strength in extensor muscles of the paretic limb (Tung et al., 2010).

It is important to note that STS training is *different* from stand-pivot transfer training. The stand-pivot transfer is a compensatory approach for assisting a person into and out of a wheelchair. For individuals who have the motor potential to stand and walk, learning how to stand up and sit down has greater functional implications

and is more natural to learn than stand-pivot transfer techniques.

Successful performance of sit to stand relies on effective postural set. The body must be symmetrically aligned, with a BOS that is ready to accept weight through both legs, and the body's COM must lie directly within the BOS. Sit-to-stand training, then, is inherently related to activities (described previously) that require the person to maintain balanced sitting while shifting weight forward and in a variety of other directions. Practice moving one's buttocks in the seated position will enable a person to perform the first step of sit to stand, which is to scoot to the edge of the support surface.

A key goal for patients with hemiparesis is to perform STS with symmetrical posture through the neck, trunk, and lower limbs. This is critical because future progress related to standing balance and walking is dependent on appropriate alignment, ability to shift body weight onto and off of the paretic leg, and efficient balance adjustments. Research comparing individuals with hemiparesis after a stroke to healthy individuals has confirmed that, in addition to presenting greater asymmetry in weight bearing, stroke survivors fail to perceive that they are asymmetrically aligned (Briere et al., 2010). Therefore, it is important to provide patients with opportunities to analyze their own performance. Before standing, the therapist asks, "Are you sitting straight? Is your weight evenly distributed over both hips?" Some individuals respond well to viewing their own performance on videotape and critiquing elements that the therapist delineates for them. After this self-analysis, the person tries again, with greater awareness about specific components that will improve the efficiency and safety of future performance.

A number of biomechanical studies (reviewed in Shumway-Cook and Woollacott [2012] and in Kane and Buckley [2011]) have described the kinematics and kinetics of STS. See Procedures for Practice 21-3 for the general sequence of sit to stand and stand to sit. Many healthy older people use a strategy of pushing down with their arms to assist in standing up and sitting down. Although this strategy may be useful as a compensatory technique to reduce force requirements at the hip, knee, and ankle, there are two major drawbacks for patients recovering from stroke or brain injury:

- Extending the arm at the elbow and shoulder girdle provides a "model of action" that contradicts the essential motor strategy of moving the entire upper body in an anterior direction. In the early phase of rising to stand, reaching backward with one's arm makes it more difficult to anteriorly tilt the pelvis and flex the hips and knees. These same movements are necessary during the later stage of controlling one's descent into the chair when sitting down. Therefore, reaching backward with one's arm may contribute to an inefficient

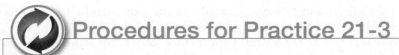

Procedures for Practice 21-3

Procedures for Improving Performance of Sit to Stand and Stand to Sit (STS)

Sit to Stand: The Sequence

1. Scoot forward on the seated surface and establish a position of "readiness to stand" (hip, knee, and ankle <90°, pelvis neutral in all planes, trunk extended and symmetrical).
2. Bring center of mass (COM) over base of support (BOS) by anteriorly tilting pelvis and flexing hips, while keeping the trunk and neck extended and symmetrical. This also establishes momentum that will assist with step 3. Mnemonic for patients: "Nose over toes."
3. Transfer momentum from the upper body and raise buttocks off the seated surface onto both legs.
4. Rise to the upright position by extending (but not locking) the hips and knees.
5. Adjust standing posture to meet environmental/task demands.

Stand to Sit: The Sequence

1. Position body directly in front of the seating surface ("feel" the seat behind both legs).

2. "Fold" body onto the chair (anterior pelvic tilt, hip and knee flexion, ankle dorsiflexion, while keeping trunk and neck extended and symmetrical). Eccentrically contract leg extensors to control the downward pull of gravity.
3. After upper thighs are resting on the seating surface, "scoot" to assume a position of "readiness for function" in seated activities.

Possible Environmental Modifications

- Raise seat to decrease lower limb force requirements (while still providing a stable surface for the feet).
- Grade seat to lower heights as strength in leg extensors improves.
- Use chair without arms if patient shows too much reliance on using hands for push-off.
- Select chair that allows for placing the feet back (knee and ankle <90°).

---

tendency to extend at the hips and "plop" onto the sitting surface.

- A patient with upper limb paresis will use only the unaffected arm as a support. This will, inherently, create an asymmetrical posture. As we have discussed previously, an asymmetrical posture during STS will change the mechanics of the movement sequence and prevent the opportunity to regain any kinesthetic awareness and motor performance in the paretic leg.

Although sitting down from standing has several similarities to standing up, it is a different activity that must be practiced as well. No momentum to reduce force requirements is present, so additional muscle strength (particularly in knee extensors) is needed just before the body mass is lowered onto the seat. Carr and Shepherd (2003) recommend that, when learning STS, patients should be instructed to stop the movement midway and reverse their directions for a few degrees. This will help them develop control over changing from concentric to eccentric muscle activity.

Functional Ambulation

Walking, a critical component of daily task engagement, is a reasonable expectation for many individuals with CNS dysfunction. Occupational therapists work with patients who wish to improve their performance in kitchen and bathroom activities, and in leisure or work pursuits.

In each of these contexts, the occupational therapist must help patients reach their optimal walking potential.

The Gait Cycle. Research on individuals with no neuromuscular or musculoskeletal impairments has revealed remarkable consistency among people in the kinematic aspects of gait. Patterns of muscle use, however, vary widely. The kinetics of gait vary between subjects and within a single subject, depending on walking speed and fatigue. Furthermore, a natural redundancy in the motor system for walking allows for compensation by stronger muscles when specific muscles are weak.

Walking forward in a uniform direction is achieved through repetitive performance of sequential gait cycles. Each cycle begins when the heel of one foot makes contact with the ground. As that leg supports the body weight, it rocks forward until its only ground contact is at the toes. Simultaneously, the other leg swings forward until its heel makes contact with the ground. Double support is the brief period when both feet are on the ground. Immediately after double support, the first leg swings forward while the second leg supports the body weight. One gait cycle is completed when the heel of the first foot touches the ground once again. For purposes of description, the gait cycle for each leg is divided into a stance phase, which comprises approximately 60% of the gait cycle, and a swing phase. Definition 21-4 shows the subdivision of these phases of the gait cycle, and Figure 21-9 provides an illustration.

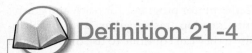

Definition 21-4

Phases of the Gait Cycle, Using the Right Leg as a Reference

Stance phase—The right foot is on the ground, supporting body weight (60% of one gait cycle).

- Heel contact
- Foot flat
- Midstance
- Heel off
- Toe off

Swing phase—The right foot is in the air and is advancing forward toward its next contact with the ground.

- Early swing
- Midswing
- Late swing

From Neumann, D. A. (2010). *Kinesiology of the musculoskeletal system: Foundations for rehabilitation* (2nd ed.). St. Louis: Mosby, Elsevier.

muscles. Neuroprosthetic devices (e.g., Ness L-300®, marketed by Bioness, Inc.) provide electrical stimulation to the tibialis anterior during gait to ensure appropriate heel strike and foot clearance during the swing phase. Research has found that the use of neuroprosthetic devices during gait has significant short-term and long-term influence on gait performance (Ring et al., 2009) as well as social participation (Laufer, Hausdorff, & Ring, 2009). Gains continue to be enhanced over time, and improvements in balance and gait velocity are apparent even when participants are no longer using the device (Laufer et al., 2009).

Occupational Therapy Contributions to Preventing and Reducing Gait Deviations. In collaboration with our physical therapy colleagues, occupational therapists contribute to the process of maximizing efficient gait patterns. Using activity-based interventions described in previous sections of this chapter about postural alignment and balance, we

- promote active ankle dorsiflexion in a closed kinematic chain through activities in sitting and standing that require the tibia to move forward over a weight-bearing foot
- promote stability mechanisms in pelvic muscles through activities in sitting and standing that require weight shift in a variety of directions
- promote appropriate postural adjustments during weight shift in standing

Physical therapists provide evaluation and intervention to prevent and reduce gait deviations that are commonly seen in patients with hemiparesis. A variety of ankle–foot orthoses (AFOs) may be prescribed to compensate for weakness in ankle dorsiflexors and foot evertor

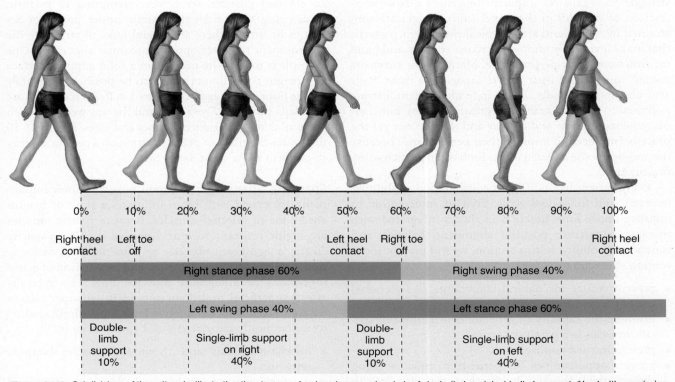

Figure 21-9 Subdivisions of the gait cycle, illustrating the stance and swing phases and periods of single-limb and double-limb support. (Used with permission from Neumann, D. A. [2010]. *Kinesiology of the musculoskeletal system: Foundations for rehabilitation*. St. Louis: Mosby, Elsevier.)

- promote a balance between stability and mobility at the pelvis, hip, knee, and ankle through standing activities that require the person to reciprocally shift body weight onto and off of the paretic leg.

Functional Ambulation. Occupational therapists contribute to maximizing walking skill during interventions that require the simultaneous performance of walking with tasks involving use of the upper limbs. This integration is inherent in naturalistic activities within home, work, and leisure environments. Think of all the things we do while walking! We *push* shopping carts and strollers. We *carry* objects, with one or both hands, positioned close to or far away from the body. We *reach* for objects at a variety of heights, while cleaning our homes or shopping. For those individuals who rely on the use of a cane, the challenge includes being able to negotiate the intermittent need to stand without any external support while using one or both upper limbs. Therapists determine interventions for functional ambulation based on our clients' identification of their daily tasks, as well as creative integration of our knowledge of activity requirements with each client's current level of motor function.

Functional Use of the Arm and Hand

Recovery of arm and hand function after stroke or brain injury is a complex and varied process. Many patients struggle to regain the capacity to generate basic contraction of muscles in the upper limb. Others are constrained by inefficient, stereotypical movement patterns that make it virtually impossible to use the arm and hand for functional task performance. Many stroke survivors remain unaware of their actual capacity to move their arm and hand. Finally, some individuals demonstrate potential to perform reach and grasp activities, but their movements are slow and clumsy and they do not get the practice they need to improve their performance because they rarely use the affected upper limb when participating in daily tasks.

Every patient has a different constellation of abilities, interests, and functional goals. Even so, intervention to improve upper limb function is always integrated with therapy to enhance postural alignment, balance, and functional mobility. In this section, we will present intervention strategies to

- prevent/reduce mechanical constraints to functional use of the arm and hand
- promote the capacity to generate contractions of specific muscles in a paralyzed arm
- prevent learned nonuse
- provide opportunities for patients to practice using their available function by matching task demands to the person's current capabilities

- develop effective motor programs for reach and grasp
- help patients develop task-analysis and problem-solving skills so they can continue to use their arm and hand in a variety of new situations, after they have completed their participation in OT rehabilitation.

Interventions to Prevent/Reduce Mechanical Constraints to Upper Limb Function

Four factors may impose mechanical constraints to upper limb function: problems with pelvic and trunk alignment and mobility, spasticity, problems with scapular alignment, and scapular immobility.

Pelvic/Trunk Alignment and Mobility. A study of 59 healthy adults showed that performance on the Jebsen Taylor Hand Function Test is significantly affected by trunk posture (Gillen et al., 2007). Specifically, speed for completing selected tasks was significantly slower when participants assumed positions of thoracic flexion (kyphotic posture) and lumbar lateral flexion (accompanied by asymmetrical pelvic alignment). This is because changes in pelvic, lumbar, and thoracic alignment have a direct effect on the resting posture of the scapulae. In turn, the relative position of the scapula within the thorax affects its stability, mobility, and the orientation of scapulohumeral muscles (Davies, 1990). Therefore, it is important for stroke and brain injury survivors to develop a core understanding of optimal postural alignment and to assume an efficient postural set before attempting to perform challenging tasks with the paretic upper limb. For activities in sitting, there are several ways to structure the environment to foster optimal proximal alignment. One example is to seat the patient on a solid support surface at a height that allows the feet to be positioned securely on the floor. Other examples (listed in Resources 21-1) are the Nada chair, the Dyna disc, and therapy wedges, which are available in a variety of shapes and sizes. Figure 21-10 illustrates the effect of pelvic position on a person's ability to perform active shoulder flexion.

Spasticity. Spasticity, a common primary motor impairment associated with brain injury, is a state of heightened tone in selected muscles. Because spastic muscles are highly resistant to quick, passive stretch, spasticity creates a significant obstacle to joint mobility, dissociation between adjacent segments, and production of active movement by antagonist muscles. Spasticity typically affects superficial, multijoint muscles in a distinct pattern for the paretic upper and lower limb. Upper limb spasticity is commonly associated with hypertonicity in

- middle trapezius and rhomboid muscles (scapula retractors)
- pectoralis major (glenohumeral adductor and internal rotator)

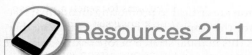

Resources 21-1

Resources for Purchasing Materials Mentioned in the Text, Figures, Boxes, and Case Examples

Nada Chair

http://www.nadachair.com/

Saeboglide

http://www.saebo.com/store/products/saeboglide.cfm

Mirror Box

http://www.mirrorboxtherapy.com/

Wedge

http://www.pattersonmedical.com/app.aspx?cmd=get_product&id=72965

Dyna Disc

http://www.pattersonmedical.com/app.aspx?cmd=get_product&id=334666

Furniture Slider

http://www.ezmoves.com/

Bar Stool

http://www.barstools-inc.com/mall/WW430-1-wooden-stool.htm

PVC Pipes

http://www.homedepot.com/h_d1/N-5yc1v/R-202300503/h_d2/ProductDisplay?langId=-1&storeId=10051&catalogId=10053

Neuro Move

http://www.neuromove.com/

Biomove

http://biomove.com/index.html

Kinesio Tape

http://www.kinesiotaping.com/kinesio/products.html

Bioness

http://www.bioness.com

Beazy Board

http://www.pattersonmedical.com/app.aspx?cmd=get_product&id=98859

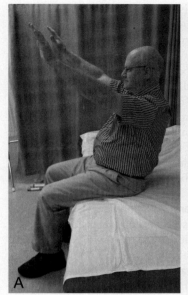
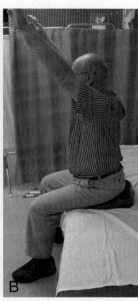

Figure 21-10 Impact of pelvic position on shoulder range of motion. **A.** The patient's pelvis is in a position of posterior tilt, which limits range of motion in shoulder flexion. **B.** With assistance from Dyna disc (see Resources 21-1), the patient aligns his pelvis into a position of anterior tilt, which enables him to increase range of motion in shoulder flexion.

- biceps brachii (elbow flexor)
- pronator teres (forearm pronator)
- flexor digitorum superficialis and profundus (wrist and finger flexors).

A number of pharmacological interventions are available to reduce spasticity. Occupational therapists must be familiar with side effects of all medications each patient is currently taking and alert the physician if a patient is exhibiting unusual levels of drowsiness or fatigue.

Because the myotatic stretch reflex is velocity dependent, spastic muscles are only hyperresponsive to quick, rather than slow, sustained stretch (Bear, Connors, & Paradiso, 2007). Therefore, intervention to prevent muscle "overshortening" and subsequent joint contractures can be provided in the form of slow, prolonged stretch to spastic muscles. Therapists use slow prolonged stretch to

- temporarily reduce tension in spastic muscles to make it easier for the person to move
- reduce muscle stiffness to prevent long-term limitations in ROM.

A recent systematic review reports that slow, prolonged stretch has a small immediate effect but no short-term or long-term effects on joint mobility (Katalinic, Harvey, & Herbert, 2011). However, two reports of preventive positioning protocols for the shoulder have generated more positive findings. Ada et al. (2005) found that positioning the shoulder in maximum external rotation reduced limitations in ROM for external rotation in acute stroke survivors. deJong, Nieuwboer, and Aufdemkampe (2006) found that limitations in shoulder abduction were minimized through the use of a similar positioning protocol.

Slow, prolonged stretch can be provided by the therapist or caregiver, by the patient, or through static positioning. When applying slow stretch, the patient must assume a posture in which the pelvis, trunk, and scapula are optimally aligned. Our experience is that slow prolonged stretch is most effective when provided simultaneously over multiple joints: protraction at the scapula, external rotation (and, if possible, abduction) at the glenohumeral joint, extension at the elbow and wrist, and supination at the forearm. Patients can learn to hold this posture immediately before beginning therapeutic activities and when resting or watching television. Engagement in yoga may also be effective in reducing abnormal muscle tension and maintaining pain-free joint mobility (Garrett, Immink, & Hillier, 2011).

Many patients with spasticity report that they experience an increase in muscle tension when they engage in activities that elicit high degrees of physical, emotional, or cognitive stress. They can learn to control this excessive tone by implementing their own slow, prolonged stretch to the spastic muscles at these times. Generalized relaxation strategies, such as deep breathing, mental imagery, and meditation may also be effective.

Scapular and Glenohumeral Alignment. In persons with healthy musculoskeletal systems, the scapula sits in the thorax in a resting position of 5° upward rotation and 30° anterior to the frontal plane (Neumann, 2010). This resting position, which allows for optimal kinematics between the scapula, the thorax, and the humerus, is often disrupted in patients with hemiplegia. The most common problems of scapula alignment, with their associated misalignments in trunk and pelvic posture, are

- depression and downward rotation (associated with asymmetrical weight bearing on the unaffected side, and trunk lateral flexion toward the affected side)
- elevation (associated with asymmetrical weight bearing on the unaffected side, accompanied by trunk lateral flexion toward the unaffected side)
- excessive protraction (associated with thoracic kyphosis)
- excessive retraction (associated with pelvic retraction and excessive shortening of muscle fibers in the middle trapezius).

Because each person may demonstrate differences in postural alignment, the therapist uses careful observational assessment to determine problems and goals.

Changes in resting alignment of the scapula are directly related to abnormal resting alignment of the humeral head at the glenohumeral joint and an alteration in the line of pull for rotator cuff muscles (Neumann, 2010). Several orthopedic impairments are associated with misalignment of the scapula and glenohumeral joint but are beyond the scope of this chapter. These include shoulder subluxation, complex regional pain syndrome (CRPS; previously called shoulder–hand syndrome), rotator cuff injury, and adhesive capsulitis (see Chapter 36).

When problems with scapular alignment are related to inefficient alignment of the pelvis and trunk, the therapist uses techniques, presented earlier in this chapter, to promote the patient's kinesthetic understanding of optimal postural set. Often, problems persist even when the patient is sitting or standing with good alignment at more proximal body segments. This indicates losses in length (distensibility) or spasticity in selected muscles. Slow, passive stretch in the directions of scapula protraction and upward rotation are critical to promoting an optimal resting position for the scapula and humeral head. The therapist provides this manual stretch before asking a patient to assume an erect aligned posture for task engagement. Therapists also teach patients how to provide appropriate stretch to themselves, in the context of enhancing scapular mobility.

Scapular Mobility. Efficient, pain-free shoulder motions are dependent on integrated movement between the clavicle, scapula, and humerus. In particular, during upward motions of the shoulder (abduction, flexion, and scaption), the scapula must upwardly rotate (Bourne et al., 2007). During forward reach, the scapula must also protract (abduct away from the vertebral column). Figure 21-1A shows how much the scapula moves in a healthy adult. Figure 21-1B shows the extent to which scapular mobility may be impaired in stroke survivors and illustrates compensatory movements this individual uses to try to achieve some arm motion, in spite of an immobile scapula. A recent motion analysis study compared scapular and humeral movement patterns between people with stroke and a group of matched healthy controls (Hardwick & Lang, 2011). The researchers found significant decreases in scapular upward rotation and glenohumeral lateral rotation in the stroke group. These findings confirm long-held assumptions, based on clinical observation, about the kinematics of shoulder movement in persons with hemiparesis.

To prevent the development of secondary orthopedic disorders and to promote a foundation for future upper limb function, therapy begins by helping patients understand how the scapula must move during passive and active shoulder motions. One early lesson takes place with the patient seated (in appropriate postural set) and his or her unaffected arm flexed forward to 90°. The person experiments to see how far he or she is able to protract his or her unaffected shoulder girdle to "make his or her arm long," and the therapist helps him or her appreciate that this change in arm length is due to movement at the scapula. Following this explicit instruction, the person learns to passively protract his or her paretic arm by holding the forearm with his or her other hand (with as much rotation as is comfortably possible at the glenohumeral joint). This can be done while lying supine (both shoulders flexed to 90° and reaching "toward the ceiling," rolling from supine to side lying (toward the unaffected side, reaching "across the mat") or sitting (reaching down and forward, or forward on a table that is slightly lower than seated height). The therapist may passively assist to ensure appropriate alignment.

In the absence of full scapular mobility, serious injury can occur as a result of active or passive shoulder motion beyond 90° (Kumar et al., 1990). It is important to adhere to all points listed in Safety Note 21-1 when implementing therapeutic programs for individuals with hemiparesis.

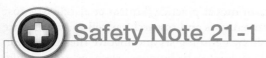

Safety Note 21-1

To Prevent Injury and Secondary Orthopedic Impairments at the Shoulder in Patients with Limited Scapular Mobility:

- Avoid passive humeral flexion or abduction without appropriate concomitant scapular motion.
- When providing passive range of motion (ROM), *always* provide manual mobilization to ensure appropriate scapular movement.
- Avoid any passive movement of the arm by individuals who are unfamiliar with scapula-humeral interactions.
- When teaching patients to perform self-ROM, focus on scapular rather than glenohumeral motion and limit glenohumeral motion to 90°.
- Do *not* use overhead pulleys as exercise.

Promoting Early Movement in the Arm and Hand

Functional use of the upper limb is dependent on an underlying ability to execute movement. For patients who are unable to generate any muscle contraction in the arm or hand, there are several options to facilitate this level of motor recovery. We will introduce several of these techniques and present information about research findings that support their efficacy: electrical stimulation, EMG-TMS, mental imagery, priming, mirror therapy, BAT, and Kinesio tape.

Functional Electrical Stimulation (FES) to Selected Muscles. We have previously discussed neuroprosthetic devices using electrical stimulation to activate contraction of ankle dorsiflexors at appropriate times during the gait cycle. The NESS H200® hand rehabilitation system from Bioness is a medical device that uses low-level electrical stimulation to activate various muscle groups in the hand and forearm, allowing patients to open and close their hand while wearing the device. Using this type of system provides patients with the opportunity to practice a variety of reach and grasp tasks that would otherwise be impossible for them to achieve. In the process, patients are able to actively use their available function at other joints in a meaningful way. In addition, it is postulated that the challenge to open and close the hand, with assistance from electrical stimulation, contributes to a process of neuroplasticity, in which intact cortical regions take on responsibility for controlling hand function (Popović, Sinkaer, & Popović, 2009). A pilot study comparing stroke survivors who used a FES device with other stroke survivors who participated in task-specific upper extremity (UE) rehabilitation found statistically significant better speed of performance on the task-based Box and Block Test and higher scores on a modified FMA.

Electromyograph-Triggered Neuromuscular Stimulation. EMG-TMS combines electrical stimulation with elements of biofeedback, in which a monitoring device provides information about an automatic bodily function. Systems such as Neuromove and Biomove monitor electromyograph (EMG) signals from target muscles and provide electrical stimulation that enables the person to produce a visible movement.

Neuromuscular stimulation is provided only when EMG signals are above a designated threshold, which is set by the therapist. Thus, the system "rewards" a person's muscular efforts with the momentary capacity to produce functional movement. In addition, the person is provided an opportunity to practice performing functional tasks that would not be possible without the presence of electrical stimulation to target muscles. There is significant evidence for the efficacy of these devices (Ivanhoe et al., 2006), and the active component to triggering the stimulation may account for better effectiveness, as compared to FES (de Kroon et al., 2005). The understanding is that these modalities must be used in conjunction with, or as immediate predecessors to, task-based interventions if the goal is to improve motor skill (Page & Levine, 2006; Page et al., 2009).

Mental Practice. "All other things being equal, more learning will occur if there are more practice trials" (Schmidt & Lee, 2011, p. 347). Mental practice is a strategy, often used by healthy individuals, to increase practice time, even when it is unfeasible to physically engage in the actual task. Thus, teachers rehearse delivering a lecture without actually talking. Athletes envision how they will perform a basketball jump shot or putt a golf ball. Neuroscience studies have recorded similar brain activity in healthy people when comparing their actual performance of a task and their mental rehearsal of the same task (Michelon, Vettel, & Zacks, 2006). A systematic review (Nilsen, Gillen, & Gordon, 2010) of multiple studies concluded that mental practice in moving one's paretic limb can be a helpful adjunct to other therapeutic interventions.

Therapists provide patients with structured directions for mental practice outside of therapy sessions. Audiotapes can consist of relaxation imagery and instructions to imagine performing particular tasks or movements with the affected arm and hand. Other protocols may involve the use of pictures, photographs, or written instructions. Patients adhere to a predetermined amount of time each day (usually 20–30 minutes) for independent mental practice, designed by the occupational therapist to capitalize on the person's level of function.

Mirror Therapy. Mirror therapy may be viewed as one example of mental practice. It is designed to help stroke

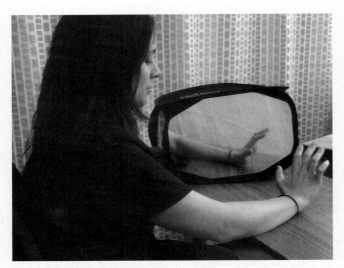

Figure 21-11 Mirror therapy.

survivors improve their ability to generate specific muscle contractions in their affected upper or lower limbs. In the case of training for motor execution in the forearm and hand, the person is seated at a table, with a mirror facing the unaffected side (see Fig. 21-11). The person places her paretic hand on the other side of the mirror, so that it is nearby, yet obstructed from view. The person's goal is to perform simultaneous, identical, bilateral movements, using both hands. Because of the mirror placement, she sees the reflection of her unaffected hand as if it were her paretic hand.

Case studies (Stevens & Stoykov, 2004) and two randomized controlled trials (Dohle et al., 2009; Yavuzer et al., 2008) provide support for mirror therapy as an adjunct to other rehabilitation interventions. The mechanisms are still hypothetical with regard to how mirror therapy helps stroke survivors relearn to generate specific movements. Aside from viewing this as a form of mental practice, another explanation is that this approach provides the person with effective visual feedback that compensates for potentially erroneous or absent proprioceptive feedback from the paretic hand. Another explanation lies in the emerging science related to "mirror neurons" (Ramachandran & Altschuler, 2009).

Mirror boxes can be constructed at a therapy site or purchased from commercial distributors. Because people can engage in mirror therapy independently, this is a cost-effective adjunct to direct therapeutic interventions. The therapist typically instructs a patient to practice using the mirror box for 20-minute sessions above and beyond OT sessions.

Priming. In the context of neurorehabilitation, priming is the use of an intervention for the specific purpose of pre-exciting the brain so that it will be easier for the person to generate a subsequent motor response and to enhance the benefits of motor practice (Stinear et al., 2008). Most clinical interventions and research related to priming are administered by neurologists and involve the application of neurophysiological techniques, such as transcranial magnetic stimulation or continuous theta burst stimulation to selected regions in the affected motor cortex (Kim et al., 2006). Simultaneous bilateral training is one priming technique that can be administered by occupational therapists.

Simultaneous Bilateral Training/Bilateral Arm Training
Neurophysiologically, optimal motor function is dependent on a balance of excitability between the left and right primary motor areas (M1) in both cortical hemipheres. Through intercallosal pathways, neural networks from each hemisphere exert inhibitory influences on the contralateral hemisphere to maintain this balance. Neuroscientists have established that, after stroke, there is an imbalance between M1 in the two hemispheres, with excessive inhibition to neurons in the affected motor cortex. Therefore, one goal is to increase excitability of neural networks within the affected motor cortex, whose purpose is to generate inhibitory signals to the contralateral hemisphere. There is evidence that, through the use of exercise technology that provides active-passive bilateral therapy, changes are seen in the balance between M1 excitability, as well as behavioral improvements in motor function in the paretic arm (Stinear et al., 2008).

Earlier in this chapter, we presented the methods and results of two clinical studies that used BAT in a task-oriented context (Lin et al., 2010a; Stoykov, Lewis, & Corcos, 2009). In addition to the potential neurophysiological benefits of BAT, performance of simultaneous bilateral movements may be of value from a motor learning perspective. When coupling the two arms as one single unit, it is possible that a single GMP can be effective in organizing performance in both arms simultaneously (Schmidt & Lee, 2011).

Kinesio Tape. Our final example of an intervention that is designed to prepare patients for therapeutic practice is not supported by research evidence. However, many therapists report that skilled use of Kinesio tape seems to make a difference in how patients respond to other interventions.

Kinesio tape is an elastic therapeutic tape. Its degree of elasticity is variable and dependent on the skilled procedure with which a practitioner applies the tape. In neurorehabilitation, Kinesio tape is most typically applied to either relax a muscle or to facilitate muscle contraction (Jaraczewska & Long, 2006). When the tape is applied with the stretch in a distal to proximal direction ("insertion to origin application"), the tape exerts an effect that seems similar to slow, sustained muscle stretch in relaxing a tight muscle. When applied with the stretch in a proximal to distal direction ("origin to insertion application"), the tape exerts an effect that seems to assist muscle contraction. Once applied, Kinesio tape can stay in place for 3–4 days and is not affected by swimming or bathing. In the case study of Mrs. M., the occupational therapist applied Kinesio tape to the woman's wrist and finger extensor muscles to help facilitate extension when she released her grasp on objects. Although this woman progressed significantly during her course of therapy, we cannot make any inferences about the influence of Kinesio tape on the improvements she exhibited.

Preventing Learned Nonuse

Although there is no direct research evidence to support interventions that prevent learned nonuse, the concept is compatible with findings from studies of CIMT, as well as the literature that supports the value of task-based practice in promoting functional recovery after stroke. During the acute and rehabilitation stages after stroke, prevention of learned nonuse is a primary goal in OT intervention (Sabari, 2008). Therapists use every opportunity to teach stroke survivors to be aware of, and to use, their paretic limbs to the limits of current, available motor function. Using the paretic leg and arm to support body weight, called "weight bearing" in some literature (Howle, 2002), is usually the first tangible way a stroke survivor can learn to rely on his hemiparetic limbs and to reincorporate them into his overall body schema. Activities requiring the person to shift body weight in a variety of directions may also play a role in preventing learned nonuse by challenging the stroke survivor to be aware of, and use, muscles on the paretic side. To prevent learned nonuse in the paretic arm, therapists continually assess motor potential in specific muscles, using external support or special positioning to detect emerging changes. In addition, occupational

therapists teach clients to understand movement linkages and to check actively for changes in their ability to recruit specific muscles. Therapy sessions become opportunities for stroke survivors to share their discoveries with their therapists. In turn, occupational therapists structure activities that enable clients to practice emerging movement capacities.

Two programs at the Rusk Institute of Rehabilitation Medicine at NYU Langone Medical Center in New York City illustrate how occupational therapists help patients maximize their awareness of capabilities and provide them with structured opportunities to successfully incorporate their paretic upper limb into performance of daily tasks. In the Use My Arm Program, therapists adapt common daily tasks according to each patient's current functional level and use homework assignment logs and behavioral contracts to ensure that patients will follow through on recommendations for practice outside of therapy sessions (Procedures for Practice 21-4). The Breakfast Group, a task-based program for four to six patients, is held Monday through Friday at 8 am in the occupational therapy clinic (Capasso, Gorman, & Blick, 2010). One therapist supervises two to three patients as they eat breakfast, using the paretic UE to the extent possible, based on the Functional Upper Extremity Levels (FUEL) described later in this chapter.

Developing Effective Motor Programs for Reach and Grasp

Humans use our upper limbs in a variety of ways. Sometimes, we use an arm and hand in a closed kinematic chain, in which proximal limb segments move over the distal components, which are stable on a supporting surface (Neumann, 2010). Two examples are (1) when rising

 ## Procedures for Practice 21-4

Welcome to the *Use My Arm Program*

- Research shows that practice using your weaker arm as much as possible after a stroke may:
  - lead to beneficial changes in the brain
  - help your recovery
  - enable you to use your arm during daily activities
- There are many ways to practice even if you are unable to move your arm and hand or have very little movement.
- Your occupational therapist will help you to practice using your arm and hand *in the best way you can right now*.
- We are giving you a photograph showing you how you can practice using your arm and hand when you are eating. We are also giving you photographs of some practice exercises we would like you do each evening for 30 minutes.

- We are giving you a check-off log, and asking you to complete the log every evening that you practice.
- It is important that you do the practice. Remember, this is a homework program, and this is your arm and hand. Like athletes that train for competition, you are now TRAINING your arm to work again. So please *do your exercises daily!*
- Part of your homework, every night, is to figure out one new way you can use your arm. Do your best to implement your idea, and report your success to your occupational therapist at your next therapy session.

Note: This is the cover sheet to materials provided to participants in *Use My Arm Program* at Rusk Institute of Rehabilitation Medicine at NYU Langone Medical Center. The packet of materials is individualized to match the capability level of each patient. As patients progress, the occupational therapist provides new photographs with directions for practicing the recommended activities.

from supine to sitting, we bear weight, first on the forearm (with the elbow flexed) and then on the hand, with the wrist extended, and (2) when supporting some body weight over a hand placed on the kitchen counter when emptying a dishwasher.

More often, the hand moves freely in space, or on a support surface, in an open kinematic chain (Neumann, 2010). We point to a target (as on a touch-screen at a bank ATM). We depress a button with a single finger (as on a telephone). We employ independent movements of our digits to depress a series of keys (as on a keyboard). We grasp objects of varying sizes, shapes, weights, and textures. We carry these objects and release them at an appropriate time and place. We maintain a grasp while using an object as a tool. We manipulate objects in our hands.

Foundational Elements to All Reach and Grasp. Although there are many variations inherent in the multiple ways of using our arms and hands, the following foundational elements are important to all reach and grasp (Duff, Shumway-Cook, & Woollacott, 2012; Neumann, 2010; Shumway-Cook & Woollacott, 2012) and influence OT interventions:

- Reaching movements are coordinated with movements of the eye and head.
- Shoulder, elbow, and forearm motions orient the hand in space to match the task demand. For example, if you reach to grasp a telephone with your right hand, with the purpose of bringing the phone to your mouth and ear, you laterally rotate the humerus and supinate the forearm so that your hand will grasp the phone from the right side.
- Active scapular movement is necessary for efficient reach. This includes protraction during forward reach and upward rotation during abduction and flexion at the glenohumeral joint.
- When reaching against the force of gravity, complex interactions between muscles of the thorax, scapula, and humerus are necessary to provide shoulder girdle stability.
- Active wrist extension is necessary to achieve an efficient length-tension ratio for the multijoint, extrinsic finger flexors.
- Early in the transport phase, a person assumes the grasp (or pointing) pattern, in anticipation of producing grasp that is best suited to the affordances of the target object.
- A variety of specific power grips and precision grasps have been identified in children and adults (and are described in the cited references). Specific kinematic and kinetic features of these grasp patterns contribute to the efficiency of task performance.

OT intervention to assist patients in relearning the elements of reach and grasp with the paretic arm and hand is highly individualized and is based on each patient's current capabilities. We use a combination of explicit learning (one example related to scapula motion during forward reach was described earlier), designing tasks to elicit specific components of functional reach and grasp, matching challenges to each person's current level of function, and providing opportunities for implicit learning through practice with a variety of tasks.

Matching Task Demands to the Person's Capabilities

One of the greatest challenges for occupational therapists is to design tasks that are well suited to a patient's motor and cognitive capabilities. This is especially important in the early weeks after the person has sustained a stroke or brain injury, when motor recovery has been limited. The FUEL categorizes motor capability from the perspective of how an individual is able to use his or her paretic arm in functional performance. These levels inherently guide the therapist in structuring therapeutic tasks for the patient to practice during and outside of therapy sessions. See Definition 21-5, Procedures for Practice 21-5, Figure 21-12, and Clinical Reasoning Box 21-1 for specific information about applying these levels of function to OT intervention to improve arm and hand use in individuals who are recovering motor skill in a paretic upper limb after stroke or brain injury.

When implementing these task-based treatment suggestions, the occupational therapist must consider several additional factors:

- People work harder and move more efficiently when there is a task goal.
- After progressing to a higher functional level, patients should continue to practice activities that are currently easier for them. People are more likely to practice when they feel capable of achieving task demands. Opportunities to practice previously learned skills make it possible for the patient to introduce his or her own challenges, related to speed, duration, or number of repetitions.
- Whatever the task, the person should be in an optimal position of postural alignment.
- When providing tasks for the person to practice outside of therapy sessions, always consider the person's safety. Structure the task to prevent falls, and follow the points in Safety Note 21-1 to prevent injury to the paretic shoulder.
- Ensure that the setup of activity objects and targets is appropriate for the person's current ability to stabilize the shoulder girdle when moving against gravity. Note that when the demands of gravity exceed a person's current muscular potential, the person will use stereotypical movement patterns. We suggest two major ways to control the effects of gravity:
  - Structure early activities with support from a surface. The person can either slide the arm along the surface (as in dusting a table, or in moving a

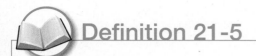

Definition 21-5

Functional Upper Extremity Levels

Level	Definition
Nonfunctional	• Involved upper extremity (UE) is not incorporated into daily activities. • Decreased awareness of involved UE. • No active range of motion (AROM) present.
Dependent Stabilizer	• Involved UE is incorporated into activities as a stabilizer but is placed by the less involved UE or by a caregiver. • Some AROM may be present (scapular, gravity eliminated); however, patient is unable to initiate placement. • Increasing awareness of involved UE during functional tasks.
Independent Stabilizer	• Some AROM is present in involved UE and able to position independently (without use of other UE) in activities. • Used primarily as a weight to stabilize. • No active hand use.
Gross Assist	• Involved arm and hand are used actively to assist in accomplishing simple functional activities. • Involved UE may still be influenced by synergistic movements or have extreme weakness. • Gross grasp may have developed but no functional release. • Fine motor coordination is not functional.
Semifunctional Assist	• Involved arm and hand are used in activities that require active motor control for pushing, pulling, stabilizing. • Gross grasp and release have developed, and some individual finger movements may be developing; however, measurements for grasp, pinch, and coordination are below norms. • Hand is able to assist with fastenings.
Functional Assist	• Involved arm and hand have full AROM. • Able to use involved UE for all activities and fine motor tasks, but it remains the assistive UE with mild awkwardness and weakness.
Fully Functional	• Involved UE has returned to complete function. • Able to use as dominant UE if premorbidly dominant. • Strength, grasp, pinch, and coordination measurements are all within normal limits.

Note: This framework is used at NYU Langone Medical Center–Rusk Institute of Rehabilitation Medicine to categorize levels of function for use of the involved arm and hand following a neurological injury. After identifying the functional UE level, the occupational therapist also notes whether the person uses the involved UE spontaneously during tasks. If the person requires verbal, visual, or tactile cues to incorporate the UE, the occupational therapist notes if the patient needs minimal, moderate, or maximal cueing.

furniture slider, Beazy Board, or Saebo-glide) or use the arm to push an object, while using the object as a support against the effect of gravity (as in tipping a bar stool or pushing a bolster or a stool on wheels) (see Fig. 21-13).

■ When necessary for optimal performance, place items below shoulder height so that the person will be reaching into gravity.

• Consider how the interplay between task variables will affect overall task difficulty. Task variables include factors affecting

■ reach (height, direction, distance of the target objects for grasp and release)

■ specificity of the target (large versus small)

■ grasp (size, shape, and texture of target objects, type of grasp pattern required)

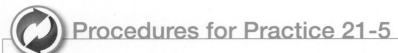

Procedures for Practice 21-5

Examples of Task-Based Practice Matched to Each of the Functional Upper Extremity Levels

Nonfunctional/Dependent Stabilizer

- Putting lotion on affected upper extremity (UE)
- Stabilize meal menu with affected UE to fill it out
- Stabilize a plate with affected UE while eating

Independent Stabilizer

- *Any activities from previous functional level*
- Washing table (with therapist's assistance)
- Stabilize bowl with the affected UE while stirring
- Push objects (such as bean bags) off a low surface (bench, wedge)

Gross Assist

- *Any activities from previous functional levels*
- Open screw-top containers (hold with affected UE and open with unaffected UE)

- Open milk container
- Squeeze toothpaste out of tube with affected UE

Semifunctional Assist

- *Any activities from previous functional levels*
- Wring out a washcloth
- Crumble paper
- Use built-up utensils to eat and cut food

Functional Assist

- *Any activities from previous functional levels*
- Typing
- Place coins into slot
- Hand writing

Note: Because patients differ in their specific movement capabilities within each of the functional levels, the therapist individualizes the program for each person.

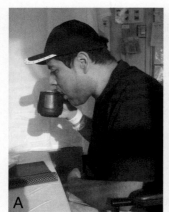
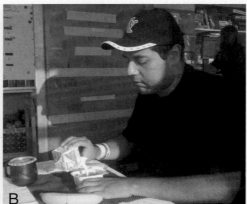
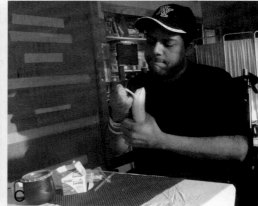
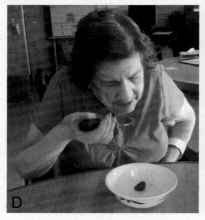
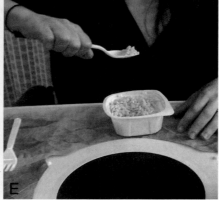

Figure 21-12 Examples of each of the levels of upper extremity (UE) function described in Functional Upper Extremity Levels (FUEL). **A.** Left nonfunctional. **B.** Left stabilizer (dependent or independent is based on whether the person can actively put the limb in the stabilizing position). **C.** Left gross assist. **D.** Right semifunctional assist. **E.** Right functional assist.

Clinical Reasoning in Occupational Therapy Practice

Adapting an Activity to Meet Different Levels of Functional Upper Extremity Use

In Figure 21-12, we have provided examples of how a person would use his or her paretic upper extremity (UE) during mealtime activities at each of the Functional Upper Extremity Levels (FUEL). The FUEL levels are described in Definitions Box 21-5. Provide your own examples for the activity of brushing teeth and for the activity of playing cards.

- release (into a small versus large container),
- speed requirements
- postural demands (sitting versus standing, changes in the BOS)
- cognitive demands.
- Never increase the difficulty level of multiple variables at once. When adding challenge to one element of upper limb performance, consider decreasing the complexity of other variables. The goal is for patients to experience success and to become aware of their progress, so they will be motivated to practice even more and to use the affected arm and hand during daily activities.

Developing Task Analysis and Problem-Solving Skills

An ultimate goal in neurorehabilitation is for individuals to learn the strategy of analyzing activities in reference to their own functional strengths and impairments. During the OT process, therapists share their strategies for activity analysis and challenge patients to develop their own skills in this area. Midway through the treatment process, therapists present new tasks and require individuals to analyze each task's inherent performance requirements. In addition, occupational therapists encourage individuals to develop their own alternative strategies for task performance. The therapist's major role at this stage is to provide feedback about the safety and efficacy of the person's ideas. Before treatment is terminated, stroke survivors should develop skill in activity analysis so that they have the confidence and capability to attempt an infinite variety of new tasks and roles.

Intervention to Improve Motor Planning in Patients with Limb Apraxia

Limb apraxia, associated primarily with left hemispheric pathology, refers to difficulties in planning and executing limb movement sequences that cannot be explained

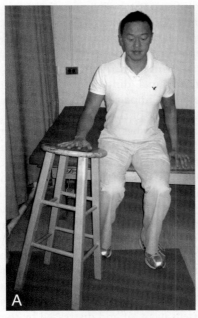
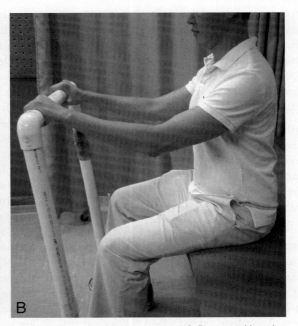

Figure 21-13 Treatment activities for patients with minimal upper extremity movement. **A.** Person pushing a bar stool tipped on two legs forward and backward. This activity reduces the impact of gravity and helps to promote initiation of shoulder and elbow flexion/extension. **B.** The same concept is used with a PVC pipe frame. This can be performed unilaterally or bilaterally.

by weakness, lack of coordination, sensory loss, comprehension deficits, memory, or motivation. Individuals with apraxia demonstrate difficulty using both the paretic and nonparetic arms. They may also have difficulty organizing gross movements during bed mobility or STS activities. If the affected (usually right) limbs are completely paralyzed, people with apraxia have difficulty using the left arm and leg during daily activities and find it exceptionally difficult to learn how to perform compensatory one-handed strategies for self-care tasks. The two types of limb apraxia are best understood by referring back to this chapter's previous discussion of the neurological processes that underlie task analysis, problem solving, and praxis skills. The capacity to plan a motor action is dependent on several neural networks, primarily in the left, dominant hemisphere, which oversee

- processing of visual information in the striate cortex
- effective communication between the striate and premotor cortex via the ventral stream to accurately determine the purposes of goal objects in order to formulate the overall plan for using these objects to achieve a functional goal
- effective communication between the striate cortex and several parietal regions via the dorsal stream to accurately determine how movements can be organized most efficiently to meet the physical/spatial properties of the object goal.

Two Types of Limb Apraxia: Ideational and Ideomotor Apraxia. Ideational apraxia (IA) is an impairment in which the individual has difficulty relating everyday objects and tools to their common usage and/or makes significant errors in sequencing multistep tasks that are performed on a daily basis. IA, in isolation of severe global aphasia and/or dementia, is rare in stroke survivors. However, Gillen (2009) and Arnadottir (2011) provide several examples of behaviors that are seen in some brain injury survivors. These behaviors may include

- using a toothbrush to comb one's hair or smearing toothpaste over the face
- using a spoon to try to "spear" a piece of food, as one would typically use a fork
- stirring coffee with one's finger
- putting trousers on before underwear and then attempting to put the underwear over the trousers

Ideomotor apraxia (IMA), which has been definitively linked to impairment in the dorsal stream (Murtha, Sainburg, & Haaland, 2010), is an inability to match the motor action to specific factors within a task such as distance of objects from the body or weight and configuration of objects. An individual with IMA has a clear understanding of the purpose of objects, but his movements are clumsy and awkward. For example, when reaching to pick up a sandwich (with an upper limb that otherwise exhibits normal movement execution), the person will approach the sandwich with an awkward orientation or an inappropriate grasp pattern. Not surprisingly, people with IMA improve their motor performance when they are performing familiar tasks and interacting with objects that have very clear affordances. Perhaps, in these situations, they are relying on information from the ventral stream to assist them in planning their motor strategy. Standardized assessments of IMA require the person to perform movements without the cues provided by task-related objects. For example, the person may be asked to "pretend" to comb his hair, without using an actual comb. In addition, the person may be asked to perform an abstract gesture, such as waving goodbye or making the "peace sign." During rehabilitation therapy sessions, commands to "raise your arm" or "turn your body" in an exercise context, without the benefit of contextual task cues, are particularly difficult for people with IMA.

Common Additional Problems Are Frequently Associated with Ideational Apraxia and Ideomotor Apraxia

Limb apraxia is rarely exhibited as an isolated deficit after stroke or brain injury (van Heugten et al., 2000). Rather, most patients present with several other impairments that present significant challenges during rehabilitation. Most commonly, patients exhibit various forms of aphasia. Ironically, the accurate use of physical gestures would be helpful as a compensatory strategy for individuals who are unable to speak. A deficit in gesture production is particularly frustrating. Therefore improving gesture use is a valuable functional goal for patients who exhibit both limb apraxia and impairments in expressive language.

Depending on the pathology, patients with IA and IMA can exhibit all the other problems associated with brain injury, including paresis, sensory loss, spasticity, visual field loss, impaired alignment, balance problems, and learned nonuse of the paretic upper limb. One important factor distinguishes people with limb apraxia from other stroke survivors who exhibit learned nonuse. Individuals with learned nonuse but intact praxis skills can still use their unaffected upper limb to perform one-handed activities. Individuals with IMA and learned nonuse are left with very few choices for functional performance of daily tasks.

Some patients with IMA have additional challenges of memory impairment and other neuropsychological deficits. Depression and poor frustration tolerance present further obstacles to function. Although there are reports in the literature of patients with apraxia who are unaware of the motor planning deficit, most individuals with IMA are acutely aware of and distressed by their difficulty performing motor tasks. Finally, some individuals demonstrate behaviors that are associated with both IMA and IA.

Evidence-Based Occupational Therapy Intervention for Patients with Ideational and Ideomotor Apraxia

To date, there are no interventions that claim to change underlying apraxia. However, three compensatory interventions have generated strong research evidence for their effectiveness in helping people resume productive task performance.

Gesture Training. Smania et al. (2000) developed a standardized protocol that teaches patients to produce transitive and intransitive gestures. Transitive gestures require an ability to understand the relationship between motor actions and task objects. Therefore, training begins by presenting the patient with a series of actual common objects and asking the person to demonstrate how he or she would use each object. When a person makes an error, the therapist corrects him or her and the person tries again. After correctly showing how he or she would use 20 common objects, the person moves on to the next phase of transitive gesture training. In phase B, the therapist presents a series of pictures, each illustrating a different, common transitive gesture (such as a person using a spoon to eat). After viewing each picture, the patient is asked to produce a pantomime of that action. In phase C, the person views a series of pictures showing an object alone and then pantomimes how he or she would use that object. When the individual is able to correctly respond to 17 out of 20 items in each phase of transitive gesture training, he or she moves on to the next level: intransitive symbolic gesture training. Resources 21-2 lists sources for picture cards.

Intransitive gesture training prepares people to perform actions without the cues associated with task objects. In the sequential steps of the intransitive symbolic gesture training program, the patient is challenged to perform pantomime actions in response to a series of pictures that show information about the action, with decreasing levels of contextual cues. These gestures are considered to be symbolic because they are related to actual actions. For example, the person might view a man pretending to eat a sandwich and attempt to pantomime the action.

During intransitive nonsymbolic gesture training, the patient imitates meaningless, intransitive gestures performed by the examiner. If the person cannot perform a particular gesture, the examiner assists him or her through verbal cueing, passive positioning, or passively moving the person through the complete action of producing the gesture.

Results of two randomized controlled trials established that the standardized protocol for gesture training led to generalization of learning. Participants in the treatment group showed statistically significant improvements on standardized apraxia tests that included gestures that were not included in the training protocol (Smania et al., 2000). Control group participants did not show any significant change in performance. Most importantly for occupational therapists, participants in the treatment group also showed

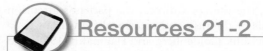

Resources 21-2

Resources for Picture Cards Used as Part of Apraxia Training

Item	Source
The Activity Card Sort	http://myaota.aota.org/shop_aota/prodview.aspx?TYPE=D&PID=763&SKU=1247 (for AOTA members only)
The Life Interests and Values Cards	www.livcards.org
Activities of daily living (ADL) and instrumental activities of daily living (IADL) picture sequence cards	Examples: http://www.speechremedy.com/products6 http://www.dysphagiaplus.com/everyday-activities-sequence-functional-photo-cards-p-221.html
Customized photos of a person performing steps within a specific task sequence	Therapists can produce these on-site (to match specific tasks)

statistically significant improvements on a questionnaire that asked caregivers to report the burden of care during performance of ADL (Smania et al., 2006).

Task-Specific Training with Errorless Support. In repeated practice of a desired ADL task, occupational therapists provide patients with the opportunity for "errorless support/learning" through cueing and assistance throughout task performance. Errorless support enables a person to complete a task when otherwise the individual's motor planning problems would prevent such achievement. Errorless learning is important in patients with apraxia, because high levels of frustration are emotionally upsetting and hinder the person's motivation to engage in continued practice. Goldenberg and Hagmann (1998) proposed that the highest level of therapist assistance is through passive "hand over hand" cueing, where the occupational therapist physically guides the person through the motor sequence. In the next degree of support, the therapist performs the action simultaneously with the patient while sitting next to him or her. As the patient progresses in learning the action steps to the task, the therapist demonstrates the action, and the patient copies the action immediately afterward. In this model, training continues until the patient achieves independent performance of the specific task.

In addition, the therapist directs the patient's attention to the details of the task and to critical features of task-associated actions. Goldenberg and Hagmann (1998) and Goldenberg, Daumuller, and Hagmann (2001) found this method to be successful in training patients with limb apraxia to perform both self-care and instrumental activities of daily living (IADL). Consistent with theories of motor learning, "direct training," in which the patient actively performed the entire activity, was effective in improving performance. However, "exploration training," which focuses on teaching about the roles of objects in a task, had no effect on performance when it was not combined with active opportunities for patients to actually perform the task. The researchers found that patients did not generalize their learning to activities they had not practiced in this manner. Evidence of retention, on long-term follow-up (6–30 months after therapy ended) was mixed. Those patients who continued to practice an activity at home, within their daily routine, preserved their ability to complete the task independently, without planning errors. Those who had stopped practicing lost their ability to perform.

Compensatory Strategy Training. A series of studies has established compensatory strategy training as the gold standard intervention for patients with limb apraxia (Donkervoort et al., 2001; Geusgens et al., 2007; van Heugten et al., 1998). This approach (summarized in Procedures for Practice 21-6 and Research Note 21-4) shares many similarities with task-specific errorless learning. However, in addition to repetitive practice, patients develop strategies that they can later generalize to compensate for limb apraxia during a variety of current and future tasks. In this approach, the occupational therapist determines how the client's deficit is impeding one of three stages required in motor planning of selected functional tasks: initiation, execution, or ongoing control. Following this, the occupational therapist teaches the client a compensatory strategy, such as verbalizing the sequence during activity performance or viewing pictures that illustrate the steps required for task execution. The therapeutic goal is to improve functioning in spite of impairment in motor planning (van Heugten et al., 1998). Evidence from both a single group pre-post design (van Heugten et al., 1998) and a randomized controlled trial (Donkervoort et al., 2001) indicates that this intervention produces statistically significant improvements in ADL function as measured by the Barthel Index. A subsequent pretest–posttest study with 29 patients provided support for the long-term and generalized effects of this compensatory strategy intervention. For stroke survivors with apraxia who were tested in their own homes after 8 weeks of training and again 7 weeks after training ended, the statistically significant improvements in ADL function made during training were maintained on retesting. In addition, patients were able to generalize their learned strategies to other tasks at home that they had never practiced during the intervention (Geusgens et al., 2007). Although apraxia is associated with other cognitive impairments, such as language comprehension, cognitive orientation, and short-term memory, this intervention to develop compensatory strategies is not influenced by cognitive comorbidities (van Heugten et al., 2000).

General Guidelines for Occupational Therapy Interventions to Improve Performance in Patients with Limb Apraxia. A few key factors differentiate OT treatment for patients with IA and IMA from other neuromotor interventions described in this chapter:

- Blocked practice is used to a greater extent than variable practice. Efficient ADL performance is the primary goal. To that end, OT sessions focus on helping the individual achieve mastery of one task at a time. Patients must have an active role in selecting therapeutic tasks. In essence, proficiency in these tasks is an end goal of intervention.
- Whenever possible, practice sessions are best held in the actual environment for task performance. Although the hope is that patients will generalize their achievements in ADL performance from a rehabilitation setting to their own home after discharge, it is important to match the context so that task performance "makes sense" to the person. For example, bathing and dressing tasks should be practiced during the routine of getting out of bed and ready for the day. Leisure tasks should be practiced with tools and materials provided by the family from the person's own home. Of course, home-based interventions would be important as well.
- Errorless learning is stressed. The therapist provides enough assistance for the person to complete the task every time. With each successive trial, the therapist fades the type of cueing and assistance provided until the individual can perform the task independently. Because many patients with limb apraxia have concomitant problems understanding language, the therapist may need to limit verbal or written directions.

In summary, however, evidence-based occupational therapy intervention for patients with limb apraxia is consistent with OT to improve other aspects of motor performance in people who are survivors of stroke or brain injury. After careful consideration of task parameters, underlying impairments and each person's activity goals, the occupational therapist structures therapy sessions to provide patients with practice, guidance, and support. As in all intervention to improve motor function in people with CNS pathology, the patient is an active participant who develops his or her own strategies through the process of engaging in challenging yet attainable therapeutic tasks.

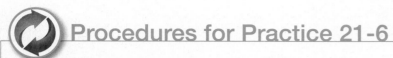 Procedures for Practice 21-6

Phases of the Motor Planning Process during Task Performance and Intervention Strategies at Each Phase

Compensatory Strategy Approach for Improving Activities of Daily Living Performance in Patients with Limb Apraxia

- The therapist observes the patient perform a selected task.
- The therapist determines the phase of task performance at which motor planning errors occur.
- The therapist implements training or assistance, targeted at the phase where errors occur.

- The therapist provides "errorless learning" (a term used to convey that the therapist's intervention enables the patient to successfully complete the task on all trials).
- The therapist selects methods (summarized on the table below) that are appropriate to the person's needs and abilities.
- The patient practices the same task many times, as the therapist gradually reduces assistance and cues.
- Training on a particular task is completed when the patient demonstrates that he can perform the task without any assistance or cueing from the therapist.

Phase	Functions	Therapist Training and Assistance
Initiation and orientation	<ul><li>Determine a general plan of action</li><li>Select appropriate objects to use in the task</li><li>Determine the sequence of steps for performing the task</li></ul>	<ul><li>Practice selecting the correct tool (from an array of three or four choices)</li><li>Provide explicit verbal, written, or pictorial directions that describe the goal, the purpose of task objects, and steps of the task</li><li>Alert the patient to the relevant objects—by placement, pointing to appropriate objects, gestures</li><li>Simplify the activity if it is too complex (select an appropriate number of task objects and performance steps)</li></ul>
Execution	<ul><li>Perform the task in an efficient manner</li></ul>	<ul><li>Provide explicit directions (e.g., "try reaching this way") through gesture, demonstration, or physical assistance</li><li>Show pictures of each step in the activity sequence</li><li>Sit next to, rather than across from the person, when providing demonstration</li><li>Physical assistance may entail prepositioning the limbs, guiding the limbs, and performing steps the patient cannot yet achieve</li></ul>
Control and correction	<ul><li>Assess how effective performance has been</li><li>Make necessary corrections</li></ul>	<ul><li>Provide extrinsic feedback (KR, KP)</li><li>Cue the person to consciously use his senses to evaluate the result (Can you taste the toothpaste on your teeth? Can you feel the comb on your scalp? Do you see a fork, knife, spoon, and plate at each table setting?)</li><li>Ask the patient to assess his or her own performance</li></ul>

KP, knowledge of performance; KR, knowledge of results.

Research Note 21-4

Geusgens, C. A. V., van Heugten, C. M., Cooijmans, P. J., Jolles, J., & van den Heuvel, W. J. A. (2007). Transfer effects of a cognitive strategy training for stroke patients with apraxia. *Journal of Clinical and Experimental Neuropsychology, 29,* 831–841.

Abstract

This study evaluated transfer effects of cognitive strategy training for stroke patients with apraxia. During 8 weeks, 29 patients with apraxia received cognitive strategy training to teach them how to perform activities of daily living (ADL). ADL functioning was assessed at the rehabilitation centre at baseline and after 8 weeks of training. Assessment also took place at the patients' homes at 8 weeks and 5 months after the start of the training. Assessment included observation of both trained and nontrained tasks. Patients were equally independent in trained tasks and nontrained tasks at the rehabilitation centre as well as at home, indicating transfer of training of effects which were stable over time.

This is a follow-up study to previous reports of a strategy training approach to teach patients with limb apraxia to compensate for their deficit in automatically developing motor plans for performing daily activities (Donkervoort et al., 2001; van Heugten et al., 1998, 2000). Using the Assessment of Motor and Praxis Skills (AMPS), each of 29 apraxic patients selected six ADL tasks from a list containing 14 tasks of similar difficulty. This selection process ensured that the individuals had a choice in determining which activities would constitute the practice sessions and which activities would be tested at a later date to determine whether improvements in motor planning generalized (transferred) to tasks that had not been practiced during therapy sessions. Over the 8-week intervention, patients practiced applying a compensatory strategy approach to performing four of the selected tasks. During therapy sessions, the therapist assisted the patient with three phases of performing each task: (1) initiation and orientation, (2) execution, and (3) control and correction. Patients were all survivors of left hemisphere stroke, and many of them exhibited other cognitive and motor deficits in addition to the limb apraxia. Standard assessments of ADL, apraxia, and motor function were administered on three occasions: before training, immediately after the 8-week training while patients still resided at the rehabilitation facility, and at home 20 weeks after the start of training. In addition to the standardized Barthel Index, assessment was of the four tasks that each patient practiced during training and the two additional tasks that the patient never practiced during training but selected as meaningful tasks prior to beginning the training. Participants showed statistically significant improvements on scores for both trained and untrained tasks at both 8-week testing and 20-week testing at home. Participants also showed statistically significant improvements on the apraxia test and the Barthel Index of ADL function after 8 weeks of training. No significant changes were found on the functional motor test.

Several findings indicate that participants developed, retained, and generalized a compensatory strategy that enabled them to perform a variety of old and new tasks—both in the rehabilitation center and in their own homes, 3 months after discharge. No significant differences were found between trained tasks and nontrained tasks, either at home or at the rehabilitation center. No significant differences were found between function at the rehabilitation center and at home. No significant differences were found between performance immediately after training and at 20-week follow-up.

Implications for Practice

- Practice performing familiar tasks, with structured and graded cueing by an occupational therapist can help people develop strategies for planning their performance of daily activities, in spite of limb apraxia associated with left hemisphere dysfunction.
- Therapists can assist patients in developing motor planning strategies by focusing on the planning requirements during three phases of action performance: initiation and orientation, execution, and control and correction.
- Patients are able to generalize the use of this compensatory strategy to tasks they have not practiced directly and in new environments, including the home setting.
- This approach is effective with patients who demonstrate significant motor and cognitive deficits in addition to limb apraxia.

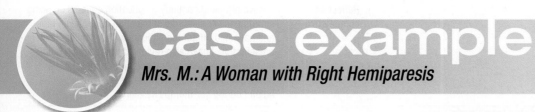

case example

Mrs. M.: A Woman with Right Hemiparesis

Occupational Therapy Intervention Process	Clinical Reasoning Process	
	Objectives	**Examples of Therapist's Internal Dialogue**

Patient Information

Mrs. M. is an 85-year-old woman who had a left middle cerebral artery stroke following a carotid endarterectomy. She was admitted to an acute inpatient rehabilitation hospital 5 days post stroke. Prior to admission, she lived alone in a building with an elevator. She was independent with all activities of daily living (ADL)/instrumental activities of daily living (IADL), functional mobility, and transfers. Mrs. M. was very active prior to admission and performed community ambulation without an assistive device. Mrs. M. is a widow and has three grown children (the closest child lives 45 minutes away from Mrs. M.'s home). One daughter offered to have Mrs. M. live in her home after discharge from the rehabilitation hospital. There are five steps to enter her daughter's home, and a first floor setup for bedroom and bathroom is possible.

During her occupational therapy assessment, the following problems were identified:

1. Hemiparesis of her right (dominant) arm. Mrs. M.'s upper extremity Fugl-Meyer Motor Assessment score was 15/66. She had active shoulder flexion to approximately half range but used compensatory shoulder and trunk movements. She had three-quarters of full range of motion (ROM) of elbow flexion and extension, but the movement was uncoordinated and effortful. Mrs. M. was able to flex her fingers into a weak gross grasp but was unable to extend her fingers (Functional Upper Extremity Levels [FUEL]–gross assist; see Definition 21-5). Her postural alignment was good but with minor thoracic kyphosis noted. Mrs. M. did not have glenohumeral subluxation, edema, or limitations in passive ROM. Testing revealed a subtle impairment in light touch sensation compared with left side (she required increased time to detect the stimuli).
2. She needed assistance to perform ADL (FIM™ scores: feeding and grooming with setup assistance; upper body dressing and toilet transfers with moderate assist; and toileting, bathing, and lower body dressing with maximal assist).
3. She exhibited mild non-fluent aphasia.
4. She had decreased standing tolerance and standing balance. Mrs. M. was able to perform bed mobility with minimal assist from sit to supine and minimal assist for transfers. She was able to maintain sitting balance with extensive weight shifts. She was able to stand without assistance but could not maintain unsupported standing balance when shifting weight. With upper extremity support, she was able to maintain standing balance with supervision. She was able to walk with no device for 50 feet with minimal to moderate assistance depending on her fatigue level. She used a wheelchair for mobility in the rehabilitation hospital because of decreased balance and endurance.

Mrs. M. demonstrated good insight into her deficits and her need to ask for assistance from nursing staff for ADL.

Appreciate the context

"At this time, it is too early to predict what functional improvements Mrs. M. will exhibit in gross mobility, arm function, and ability to stand and walk. Regarding arm function, it is promising that, 5 days after she sustained her stroke, she is able to actively execute some movements in the shoulder, forearm, and hand."

"Mrs. M. would like to return to her prior level of independence including cooking, laundry, shopping, knitting, and handwriting. She expresses frustration that the stroke impacted her right dominant hand and her speech."

Develop intervention hypotheses

"Mrs. M. expressed that her greatest frustration is related to the paresis of her right arm and hand. She seems very motivated to work on her arm movement because she already has gained back some functional movement. She sees this as one of her major obstacles to gaining back her independence with ADL and IADL. Integrating the hemiparetic arm into functional activities has been shown to be effective. Using repetition and clinical modalities should help to prevent learned nonuse and maximize the movement that she has available."

Consider the evidence

"Task-related training is an effective strategy for improving arm and hand function in stroke survivors."

"Bioness® is an orthotic device that provides neuromuscular electrical stimulation to the finger flexors and extensors. A randomized controlled trial supports the effectiveness of an interactive training program using Bioness® during patients' practice of grasping, moving, placing, and releasing objects, which resulted in better functional recovery of the upper extremity in ischemic stroke survivors than task-related exercise training alone (Alon, Levitt, & McCarthy, 2007)."

"There is no research support for the effectiveness of Kinesio tape in stroke recovery, but clinical experience at this site has been positive. Bilateral arm training with auditory cueing has been shown to improve hemiparetic arm function (Stoykov, Lewis, & Corcos, 2009)."

Select an intervention approach

"I will use a combined approach of restoration and compensation to increase Mrs. M.'s level of independence and functional use of her right arm and hand. To help her arm get better, I want her to attempt and to practice functional activities using the available movement and modalities (neuromuscular electrical stimulation and Kinesio tape). I do not want her to just rely on her left arm because this could lead to learned nonuse."

| | Reflect on competence | "I have attended continuing education courses on using neuromuscular electrical stimulation and Kinesio tape and have had numerous patients with a similar clinical presentation. I have also reviewed the research studies that have been done with these approaches. I have developed a good rapport with Mrs. M., which will be helpful during our therapy sessions." |

Recommendations

Mrs. M. will receive occupational therapy 6 days per week. She would benefit from an hour of individual occupational therapy and can also participate in a 30–60-minute group session focused on practicing using her right arm during meals and other functional activities. Mrs. M. would benefit from staying in the acute rehabilitation setting for 3 weeks with the goal of a discharge to her daughter's house.

Mrs. M. and therapist collaborated to develop the following long-term goals:

1. Mrs. M. will perform toilet transfers with supervision using a raised toilet seat.
2. Mrs. M. will perform feeding with setup assistance using built-up utensils with her right hand.
3. Mrs. M. will perform toileting with minimal assist for clothing management.
4. Mrs. M. will increase standing tolerance to 15 minutes in preparation for grooming at the sink while standing.

Consider the patient's appraisal of performance	"Mrs. M. is extremely motivated to use her right arm and hand. She reports being fiercely independent prior to the stroke and is willing to attempt any activity that is presented to her during therapy. She does not want to be a burden to her children."
Consider what will occur in therapy, how often, and for how long	"I will have to constantly ask Mrs. M. how she is feeling during therapy and determine whether she needs rest breaks. With the combination of her motivation and her difficulty speaking because of the aphasia, it is easy to forget to give her rest breaks."
Ascertain the patient's endorsement of plan	"Mrs. M. was actively involved in selecting goals that were meaningful to her."

Summary of Short-Term Goals and Progress

1. Mrs. M. will incorporate her right hand/arm into grooming and feeding activities 70% of the time.

   Functional activities: Mrs. M. was encouraged to incorporate her right arm into every activity, even if she had limited movement. She could use the weight of her arm and the limited grasp that she had to stabilize items such as her toothbrush while squeezing the toothpaste with her left hand. She was able to place her arm independently on table top surfaces because she had sufficient proximal movement.

   Modalities: Electrical stimulation with the Bioness® unit was used to help strengthen movement in her hand and assist with motor planning. The purposeful activities of reaching for grooming items with the Bioness® assisting with her grasp also strengthened the proximal movement in her arm (Fig. 21-14A). The occupational therapist applied Kinesio tape to her wrist and finger extensors to help facilitate extension during her release of objects (see Fig. 21-14B).

   Repetition: Grasp and release of items were practiced with a variety of items and in various environments including sitting and standing. Mrs. M. practiced moving colored balls from one bin to the other using her right hand while standing (see Fig. 21-14C). She had more difficulty with release than grasp. Mrs. M. required verbal cues to avoid compensatory movements and to ensure that she was focused on the quality of the movement. Mrs. M. responded well to verbal cues. A cognitive and linguistic component was added to the activity by having Mrs. M. move balls in a specific color sequence. On occasion, she dropped the balls and appeared frustrated. She benefited from a seated rest break at these times.

Assess the patient's comprehension	"Mrs. M. has aphasia. She seems to have more difficulty getting her words out than understanding what has been said. I need to consult with the speech therapist to ensure she really understands what I am saying when I give her directions. She may have more difficulty understanding or remembering what I have said than I initially expected."
Compare actual to expected performance	
	"Mrs. M. gained back motor recovery in her arm faster than I expected or that I have seen consistently in the past. I think this is due to her persistence and practice. She also demonstrated good carryover of the movements practiced both within and between therapy sessions."

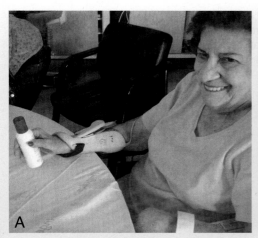
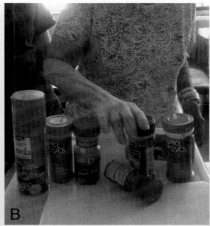
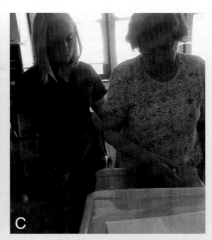

Figure 21-14 Interventions with Mrs. M. **A.** Mrs. M. using the Bioness® for grasp and release of containers. **B.** Mrs. M. reaching for spices while standing (right hand has Kinesio tape to facilitate finger and wrist extension). **C.** Mrs. M. reaching for balls to practice grasp and release while standing.

Mrs. M. participated in bilateral arm training with an auditory cue. Mrs. M. had to touch the edge of the table with both her hands at the same time as the metronome made a sound. The speed of the metronome was adjusted to match Mrs. M.'s speed of reaching the table with her right hand. She was encouraged to perform 30 repetitions and then take a rest break. This activity was completed during the group session because she only required assistance setting up the metronome and practicing the task a few times before she was able to perform the task without the therapist's continuous assistance.

2. Mrs. M. will perform upper body dressing activities with minimal assist for fasteners.

    Preparatory activities: Mrs. M. had tightness/shortening in her pectoralis minor and latissimus dorsi, which resulted in poor dissociation between the scapula and thorax. She benefited from scapular mobilization stretches in side lying as a preparatory activity. To help strengthen her arm, she performed closed chain strengthening activities in sitting and standing as well as open chain reaching activities.

    Dressing: Mrs. M. performed the task while short sitting. She learned to dress the right arm first because the shirt could be moved to accommodate the movement she had in the right arm. Mrs. M. was encouraged to use the movement in her right shoulder and elbow to push her arm through the sleeve. She was unable to fasten the buttons on her shirt, so she was encouraged to either ask for assistance or wear shirts that did not have fasteners and were looser so they were easier to don/doff.

3. Mrs. M. will perform toilet transfer with minimal assist using a raised toilet seat.

    Mrs. M. required moderate assistance to stand from a standard toilet seat due to impaired standing balance and fear of falling. Mrs. M. practiced sitting and standing from a variety of surfaces. Initially, she was resistant to the idea of having to use a raised toilet seat due to impaired standing balance and fear of falling. Mrs. M. practiced getting up from a regular height toilet and realized that she needed more assistance than when she used a raised toilet seat. Mrs. M. felt more confident performing the transfer with a grab bar on her left side so that she could hold on as well as using the raised toilet seat.

Next Steps

Mrs. M. achieved her short-term and long-term goals on discharge from inpatient rehabilitation after 3 weeks. She was able to use her right dominant hand as a FUEL semifunctional assist when grasping and releasing objects, i.e., item retrieval, pulling up pants, and feeding. Mrs. M.'s Fugl Meyer Motor Assessment score improved to 39/66. She was able to negotiate to the bathroom without a device and transfer on and off a raised toilet seat with supervision. Mrs. M.'s balance had improved, but her endurance was still limited, and she required additional assistance when she became fatigued.

Mrs. M. was provided with a home exercise programs that included pictures and descriptions of the activities she had practiced during therapy. She was encouraged to follow a daily schedule to ensure the home exercises were performed consistently upon discharge.

Mrs. M.'s daughter came in for caregiver training focused on ADL performance, safe transfers, and the home exercise program. A grab bar and raised toilet seat were ordered for her daughter's home.

The occupational therapist provided Mrs. M. with her contact information in case she had any questions once she left the hospital.

Mrs. M. is scheduled to receive home care services at her daughter's house for a few weeks. Following this, she is planning to participate in occupational therapy as an outpatient. Goals are to further improve standing balance/endurance, functional use of her right arm, and independence in daily activities.

Objectives	Examples of Therapist's Internal Dialogue
Anticipate present and future patient concerns	"Mrs. M. made great progress in her 3 weeks of acute rehabilitation. I think that Mrs. M. will continue to make an impressive recovery based on her motor return and her strong determination to get better."
Decide whether he or she should continue or discontinue therapy and/ or return in the future	"She would benefit from occupational therapy at her daughter's home to address the barriers she encounters there. Once she has adjusted to managing life outside of the hospital environment, she would benefit from outpatient occupational therapy. Mrs. M.'s goal of returning to living independently in her own apartment is still an appropriate continued long-term rehabilitation goal."

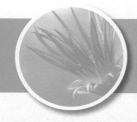

case example
Mr. S.: A Man with Left Hemiplegia

Clinical Reasoning Process

Occupational Therapy Intervention Process	Objectives	Examples of Therapist's Internal Dialogue

Patient Information

Mr. S. is a 61-year-old right-handed male admitted to an acute inpatient rehabilitation facility approximately 3 weeks after experiencing a right middle cerebral artery infarct. He has resulting dense left hemiplegia. Mr. S. is a semiretired Broadway actor who lives with his supportive wife in a New York City elevator apartment with three steps to enter. She is a retired teacher. Mr. S. was independent in activities of daily living (ADL) and instrumental activities of daily living (IADL) prior to the stroke. His short-term primary goal at this time is to return home at the most independent level as possible. Mr. S. would eventually like to return to the stage as an actor.

Objectives	Examples of Therapist's Internal Dialogue
Appreciate the context	"I believe Mr. S.'s left hemiparesis is a significant factor that is impacting his ability to function independently at home and at work. I am assessing the environmental context to which he will be returning and the social supports he will have there. Mr. S.'s primary goal at this time is to return home as independently as possible. He would like to return to his job as an actor in the more distant future."
	"It is still too early to predict the extent of Mr. S.'s motor recovery. I will do all that I can to prevent the development of secondary impairments that could limit his ability to function to his full potential."

Mr. S.'s Initial Clinical Assessment

In sitting, Mr. S. presented with a posterior pelvic tilt, right pelvic obliquity (right anterior superior iliac spine lower than the left), and left lateral trunk flexion. His left scapula was depressed, adducted, and downwardly rotated. There was a one-finger-breadth inferior subluxation of the humerus and evident supraspinatus and infraspinatus muscle atrophy. Passive range of motion was full. The more involved left upper extremity (UE) was generally hypotonic throughout except for minimal hypertonicity noted in the humeral internal rotators and adductors and elbow flexors. Right UE movement and sensation were within functional limits. Mr. S. did not report any pain.

Mr. S. did not exhibit any spontaneous UE movement against gravity; however, he was able to initiate scapular elevation in the gravity-eliminated plane. While seated with the weight of his arm displaced by the therapist, Mr. S. was also able to initiate shoulder flexion and elbow extension.

Functional use the left UE: Upon admission, Mr. S. was able to incorporate his left UE as a Functional Upper Extremity Levels (FUEL)-dependent stabilizer (see Definition 21-5) (i.e., he had enough awareness of his left UE and was able to use his less involved right UE to place his left UE on the table during functional activities such as meals) with minimal cueing from the therapist. Mr. S. was also able to use his right UE to place the left UE into the hole of the shirt sleeve and had enough movement to put the left UE down into the sleeve into the direction of gravity (i.e., sleeve placed in the direction of the floor) with moderate cueing from the therapist. He lacked the available movement at this time to move the UE against gravity during functional tasks without the support and guidance of his right UE.

Functional mobility: Mr. S. could sit unsupported, but lost his balance when attempting to turn his head or trunk. He required moderate assistance to move from supine to sitting on the edge of the bed. However, he compensated mostly with the right side of his body and made few attempts to incorporate the left side of his body (even though Mr. S. had minimal volitional movement of his left lower extremity [LE]). Mr. S. required maximal assistance to transition from sit to stand and needed maximal facilitation of his pelvis and left LE to maintain a standing position for about 30 seconds.

Sensory testing revealed impaired light touch and proprioception throughout the left UE.

Cognition/perception: Mr. S. was alert and oriented to time and place (A & 0 × 2) (he required cueing for the date). He also demonstrated moderate impulsivity and judgment (i.e., attempting to get out of bed without assistance) and had impaired insight into his deficits (i.e., stating that he does not need assistance to move from the bed to the wheelchair). Mr. S. also demonstrated moderate impairments in overall attention (able to attend to tasks for 3–5 minutes in a quiet environment) and a left spatial neglect.

Functional status: Mr. S. required minimal assistance for eating and grooming, maximal assistance for upper body dressing, and total assistance for lower body dressing, toileting, and bathing. He required maximal to total assistance for functional transfers from the bed to the wheelchair.

Develop intervention hypotheses	"I hypothesize that a combination of UE remediation interventions and compensatory strategies where necessary will facilitate Mr. S.'s return home and possible eventual return to work."
	"I also hypothesize that, to prevent future secondary impairments, it will be important for Mr. S. to improve his postural alignment in sitting. In particular, he will need to relearn how to move his pelvis into the positions of neutral and anterior tilt, and he will need to develop the ability to maintain a symmetrical trunk posture."
	"I hypothesize that improvements in sitting posture, sitting balance, and the ability to move from sit to stand and stand to sit will be important to Mr. S.'s ability to meet his ADL and functional mobility goals."
Consider the evidence	"I know that individuals with right-sided brain lesions may be impulsive and show a lack of awareness of their deficits. I also know that 'learned nonuse' is a common occurrence after stroke (Taub et al., 2006)."
	"I know that functional electrical stimulation (FES) to the supraspinatus in particular is effective in reducing shoulder subluxation."
	"I know that functional sitting balance is dependent on underlying mobility in the trunk, pelvis, and scapula."
	"I know that functional movement of the upper limb is dependent on full mobility of the scapula (for scapula-humeral rhythm), full mobility of the pelvic girdle, and the capacity to maintain sitting balance when he shifts his body weight during functional transfers."
	"Additionally, I know that I need to be particularly proactive and retrain and maintain the length of certain muscle groups, that is, humeral external rotators, which I know are currently underactive and likely to be overshadowed by the stronger and more numerous internal rotators (i.e., latissimus dorsi, pectoralis major), which are already showing some signs of hypertonicity."
	"In considering possible interventions for facilitating UE movement, I know that mental practice, mirror therapy, and FES have been shown to improve motor recovery." (Teasell et al., 2012)
Reflect on competence	"I have several ideas for how to potentially restore some UE movement. I need more information about Mr. S.'s home environment and whether his wife will need assistance in caring for Mr. S. at home."

Mr. S. participated daily in the breakfast group in the occupational therapy clinic. This group focused on ways for Mr. S. to consistently incorporate his left UE into eating at a dependent stabilizer level. During eating, Mr. S. was encouraged to place his UE on the table at all times while eating and to use it to stabilize containers as he used his right UE to open lids. He also needed to use his right UE for utensil management and bringing food to his mouth because he did not have enough movement in his left UE to do this presently. Mr. S. required moderate cueing to incorporate his left UE in this way.

Mr. S. and his wife were also given written educational materials and photos for how he could carry over these techniques in his room. Fortunately, Mr. S.'s wife was present with him for lunch and dinner, so she was able to ensure the table was set to the correct height and that Mr. S. was using his left UE as a dependent stabilizer consistently.

Still, Mr. S. had a difficult time with this concept and seemed to view the use of his left UE as an "all or nothing phenomenon," that is, if he couldn't use it the way he did before the stroke then it was "no use trying." The occupational therapist explained that there are different ways the UEs can be used and that there can be improvement with practice.

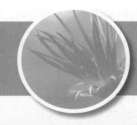

case example

Mr. J.: A Man with Right Hemiparesis and Ideomotor Apraxia

Occupational Therapy Intervention Process	Clinical Reasoning Process	
	Objectives	Examples of Therapist's Internal Dialogue

Patient Information

- Mr. J. is a 76-year-old right-handed male who sustained a left cerebrovascular accident approximately 2 weeks ago. He is now admitted to acute rehabilitation for a 3-week length of stay.
- Mr. J.'s primary deficits are aphasia (patient is nonverbal) and ideomotor apraxia (IMA).
- Mr. J. is a retired college professor who resides in a private home with two steps to enter. He was independent in activities of daily living (ADL) and instrumental activities of daily living (IADL) prior to admission and was very active in his community, travel, and sports. His wife and three children are very supportive.
- Postural alignment is WNL (within normal limits).
- Upper limb use: Mr. J. shows capacity to perform significant movement with his right upper extremity (RUE). However, he has great difficulty initiating and executing movements and tends to rely on his left upper extremity (LUE). However, movements with the LUE are far more awkward than would be expected, even for a nondominant arm. For instance, when Mr. J. was squeezing toothpaste onto a toothbrush with his left hand, he held the tube in an awkward fashion and had a hard time getting the paste onto the toothbrush.
- Gross mobility: Bed mobility and sit to stand (STS) are extremely inefficient, awkward, and unsafe. To an observer, it appears that Mr. J. is "using the wrong parts of his body at the wrong times."

Appreciate the context

"Although it is difficult to tell from Mr. J., I believe his primary goal is to return home and to function as independently as possible. His wife and children agree with this plan. However, they are open to the possibility that Mr. J. may need to go to a subacute rehabilitation facility after discharge from this facility."

"It is still too early to predict the extent of Mr. J.'s recovery. I will do all I can to promote his recovery and train and educate his family about IMA and how to help Mr. J. perform to his potential."

"I know that Mr. J.'s aphasia and IMA are very frustrating for him and for his family."

"I will need to provide all treatment in a highly functional context and use a minimum of language-based commands during therapy sessions."

- Communication/cognition: Mr. J.'s yes/no responses are unreliable either by head nod/shake or by pointing to letters or the words yes/no on a page. Gesturing is extremely difficult. He can accurately follow one-step commands about half the time during functional contextual tasks.

Develop intervention hypotheses	"A compensatory strategy training approach using errorless support techniques will help Mr. J. compensate for his IMA during performance of daily tasks. Mr. J. and his family are highly motivated to help him meet his maximum potential."
Consider the evidence	"Level I evidence exists for the efficacy of a compensatory strategy training approach to improve ADL function in people with IMA. Constraint-induced movement therapy (CIMT) research supports the value of preventing learned nonuse of a paretic upper limb, whenever possible."
Select an intervention approach	"I have decided to use a compensatory strategy training approach using errorless support techniques. We will also work toward prevention of learned nonuse of RUE."
Reflect on competence	"I have worked with other patients with IMA. I will be attuned to Mr. J.'s responses to my cueing strategies so that I can find the best approach to facilitate his performance."

Recommendations

Mr. J. will participate in 1-hour occupational therapy sessions daily for 6 days per week. In addition, he will participate in a 1-hour breakfast/UE retraining program five mornings per week. The occupational therapist will focus on teaching Mr. J. strategies for planning gross movements (STS for stand transfers, bed mobility), using his paretic RUE, and performing tasks requiring both arms/hands while sitting and standing. In addition, the occupational therapist will implement compensatory strategy training to assist him in compensating for his IMA during functional tasks.

Consider the patient's appraisal of performance	"I think Mr. J. is motivated to improve his function and movement. He tries really hard to do what I ask of him. However, I also think he is appropriately frustrated. It is difficult to explain to him the reasons why we are doing certain things because of his aphasia."
Consider what will occur in therapy, how often, and for how long	"Mr. J.'s length of stay at this acute rehabilitation facility will be about 3 weeks."

Summary of Short Term Goals and Progress

1. Mr. J. will be able to perform functional mobility tasks (i.e., supine to sit, sit to supine, and STS) with minimal prompting.
   - Task-specific training focused on STS, and later, sit to supine and supine to sit—using errorless support (teaching him to posturally set himself, using manual assistance to pelvic and trunk movements, and decreasing to tactile cues).
   - Physical therapy and nursing staff collaborated, using similar strategies during physical therapy sessions and activities on the nursing unit.
   - After 2 weeks, Mr. J. was able to perform STS, supine to sit, and sit to supine with minimal cueing.

2. Mr. J. will perform purposeful, bilateral activities—using his RUEs and LUEs.
   - Treatment initially focused on simple bilateral UE activities.
   - At times, the occupational therapist used a metronome to incorporate a timing aspect to the movements.
   - Once he was able to perform a simple, single-plane bilateral activity, treatment progressed to circular and diagonal movements. Initial interventions aimed at Mr. J. moving both UE in the same direction but progressed to him moving them in opposite directions during the first few weeks of therapy.
   - Treatment to develop foundational motor control of the right scapula enabled Mr. J. to begin to use his RUE for functional assist to his LUE during daily activities.

Assess the patient's comprehension	"At the beginning of treatment, Mr. J. was awkward and unsafe in performing gross mobility activities."

"At the beginning of treatment, Mr. J. failed to incorporate his RUE into tasks despite the presence of a considerable amount of available movement. Further, when he did try to use it, the movements were awkward, clumsy, and inefficient, and Mr. J. spilled food frequently onto his lap."

"A large part of the occupational therapy treatment was educating Mr. J.'s wife and family so that they could cue him appropriately when he was not in therapy and improve his function."

"Simple, uniplanar, bilateral UE activities were designed to give Mr. J. a chance to see that he was capable of moving both UEs in a coordinated way." |

3. Mr. J. will use his RUE to stabilize containers 75% of the time during meals (while bringing food to his mouth with his LUE) by 1 week.
   - In the breakfast group, the occupational therapist initially demonstrated how Mr. J. could stabilize a milk container with his RUE while opening it with his left. The occupational therapist used demonstration and hand-over-hand guidance to approximate the appropriate "shape" and pressure with his RUE to get the container open with his left hand. As Mr. J. improved, she decreased this cueing.
   - The occupational therapist gave Mr. J. adapted devices to assist him in eating successfully. These included a nonskid mat to prevent the plate and containers from sliding on the table while Mr. J. was attempting to open containers or eat. The occupational therapist also provided Mr. J. with a mug with a lid so he could drink without spilling.
   - The occupational therapist educated Mr. J.'s wife and the nursing staff on how Mr. J. could carry over these techniques during times outside of therapy (i.e., when he was served lunch and dinner in his room). Mr. J.'s wife was able to follow this hierarchy of cueing, that is, the use of demonstration if Mr. J. got stuck and hand-over-hand guidance when absolutely necessary.
   - After 1.5 weeks, Mr. J. was incorporating his RUE to stabilize containers about 50% of the time.
   - Mr. J. progressed to bringing food to his mouth with his RUE when there were "easier" to eat or finger foods on his tray (i.e., bananas, toast). The occupational therapist progressed to this as soon as possible because Mr. J. was right handed, and it was more natural to eat with his RUE if he could.

4. Mr. J. will use his RUE to help with clothing management during toileting with minimal cuing.
   - The occupational therapist used hand-over-hand and cueing strategies to help Mr. J. use his right arm when managing his clothing during toileting (i.e., pushing pants down and pulling them up). Mr. J. had a lot of difficulty pushing/pulling and grasping/releasing at the appropriate times. The cues were gradually decreased as Mr. J. improved. Mr. J. met this goal in about 2 weeks.

5. Mr. J. will stand symmetrically during toileting.
   - Occupational therapy improved Mr. J.'s ability to shift his weight onto his right LE during occupational therapy clinic activities.
   - Once Mr. J. was incorporating his RUE more and once he was more secure in shifting his weight during similar dynamic tasks, the occupational therapist began to encourage Mr. J. shift his weight to his right LE during the toileting activity.

At this time, Mr. J. requires setup for eating and grooming and minimal assistance for upper body dressing and toilet transfers. He requires moderate assistance for lower body dressing and toileting. These are improvements, but Mr. J. and his family would like him to be more independent.

Understand what he is doing

"Mr. J. took pride and pleasure in seeing that he could drink from a cup without spilling."

Appreciate the context

"Mr. J.'s independence in toileting was a significant goal for the patient and his family."

"Despite the fact that Mr. J. was incorporating his RUE more during functional activities such as eating and bed mobility, there was little carryover to other activities."

"Mr. J.'s recovery was about the pace that I expected considering the extent and nature of his deficits."

"I anticipate that Mr. J.'s recovery will extend into outpatient therapy and beyond. I am encouraged by Mr. J.'s motivation and the dedication of his wife and family."

Next Steps

- The goals for the next week at this facility are to continue to work on increasing Mr. J.'s independence in ADL, continue training and educating Mr. J.'s family, and ordering durable medical equipment for Mr. J.'s bathroom activities.
- Mr. J. will receive about 2–3 hours per day Monday through Friday of home health assistance through Medicare. Mr. J.'s family plans to hire help for an additional 4 hours a day (7 days a week) to assist and offer some respite to Mr. J.'s wife. She will be with him at nighttime where the plan will be for him to use a bedside commode with the assistance of his wife if needed.
- Outpatient occupational therapy services will be arranged, closer to his home, to provide ongoing opportunity to improve function in motor planning and motor control, as well as return to social and community activities.

Anticipate present and future patient concerns	"Mr. J. has another week remaining at this inpatient rehabilitation facility. After discharge, his family would like to take him home."
Decide whether he or she should continue or discontinue therapy and/ or return in the future	"I believe that home-based occupational therapy services will be essential in helping Mr. J. and his family make the transition to living at home and in training him to perform activities within his home environment."

Summary Review Questions

1. How do motor deficits associated with upper motor neuron dysfunction differ from those associated with lower motor neuron dysfunction?
2. What contributions from the Brunnstrom, Rood, NDT, and PNF approaches are still relevant in neurorehabilitation today?
3. Occupational therapists use task-based intervention to improve motor performance in people who are recovering from stroke and brain injury. In what ways is this intervention consistent with neuroscience evidence and current theories about motor learning and motor control?
4. Why is variable practice more effective than repetitive practice for developing flexible motor strategies?
5. How and why do occupational therapists use object affordances when designing treatment for persons who are recovering motor function after stroke or brain injury?
6. Identify interventions described in this chapter that have been influenced by findings in CIMT research.
7. Some researchers and clinicians believe that it is best practice to prevent patients from developing abnormal synergy patterns in their paretic upper limb. Others believe that this is merely a phase of recovery. Present arguments in support of each of these views.
8. Explain this statement: Postural alignment and motor execution are *necessary but not sufficient* for functional movement.
9. Why is it important to help patients develop balance skills in preparation for improving upper limb function?
10. In what ways are OT interventions to improve motor planning and performance in patients with IMA similar to and different from interventions with other neuromotor goals?

Glossary

Affordances—Specific characteristics of objects or environments that influence the way an individual will perform an action.

Attractor state—Preferred pattern of organization within a system.

Control parameter—Variable that, when changed, will influence changes in a system's pattern of organization.

Degrees of freedom—Number of elements that are free to vary within a system and hence must be controlled.

Explicit learning—Acquisition of information through verbal, written, pictorial, visual, or tactile/proprioceptive instructions.

Functional upper extremity levels (FUEL)—A hierarchical classification of arm and hand function that guides the choice of therapeutic tasks and challenges for patients with neuromotor disorders.

Ideational apraxia (IA)—Inability to plan movement caused by difficulty in judging the overall purpose and/or sequence of task performance.

Ideomotor apraxia (IMA)—Inability to plan movement caused by difficulty matching motor actions to physical qualities of the task objects.

Implicit learning—Skill development through active practice.

Kinematics—Description of movement in terms of direction, speed, and position of body segments.

Kinetics—Description of movement in terms of forces required.

Postural adjustments—Automatic, anticipatory, and ongoing muscle activation that enables individuals to maintain balance against gravity; optimal alignment between body parts; and optimal orientation of the head, trunk, and limbs in relation to the environment.

Practice—Opportunity to develop skill through engagement in tasks that require problem solving and implementation of effective motor strategies.

Regulatory condition—Control parameters within the task or environment.

Scaption—Movement at the glenohumeral joint within a plane that lies between the sagittal and coronal planes.

Shaping—Psychological term used to describe training that provides incremental challenges to the learner.

Skill—Goal-directed patterns of movement that efficiently address the spatiotemporal demands of a task.

References

Ada, L., Goddard, E., McCully, J., Stavrinos, T., & Bampton, J. (2005). Thirty minutes of positioning reduces the development of shoulder external rotation contracture after stroke: A randomized controlled trial. *Archives of Physical Medicine and Rehabilitation, 86,* 230–234.

Alon, G., Levitt, A. F., & McCarthy, P. A. (2007). Functional electrical stimulation enhancement of upper extremity functional recovery during stroke rehabilitation: A pilot study. *Neurorehabilitation and Neural Repair, 21,* 207–215.

Arnadottir, G. (2011). Impact of neurobehavioral deficits on activities of daily living. In G. Gillen (Ed.), *Stroke rehabilitation: A function-based approach* (pp. 456–500). St. Louis: Elsevier/Mosby.

Bayouk, J. F., Boucher, J. P., & Leroux, A. (2006). Balance training following stroke: Effects of task-oriented exercises with and without altered sensory input. *International Journal of Rehabilitation Research, 20,* 51–59.

Bear, M. F., Connors, B. W., & Paradiso, M. A. (2007). *Exploring the brain* (3rd ed.). Philadelphia: Lippincott Williams & Wilkins.

Beebe, J. A., & Lang, C. E. (2008). Absence of a proximal to distal gradient of motor deficits in the upper extremity early after stroke. *Clinical Neurophysiology, 119,* 2074–2085.

Beebe, J. A., & Lang, C. E. (2009). Active range of motion predicts upper extremity function 3 months after stroke. *Stroke, 40,* 1772–1790.

Bernstein, N. (1967). *The co-ordination and regulation of movements.* Oxford, UK: Pergamon Press.

Birkenmeier, R. L., Prager, E. M., & Lang, C. E. (2010). Translating animal doses of task-specific training to people with chronic stroke in 1-hour therapy sessions: A proof-of-concept study. *Neurorehabilitation and Neural Repair, 24,* 620–635.

Bobath, B. (1970). *Adult hemiplegia: Evaluation and treatment.* London: W. Heinemann Medical Books.

Bobath, B. (1990). *Adult hemiplegia: Evaluation and treatment* (3rd ed.). London: W. Heinemann Medical Books.

Bourne, D. A., Choo, A. M., Regan, W. D., MacIntyre, D. L., & Oxland, T. R. (2007). Three-dimensional rotation of the scapula during functional movements: An in-vivo study in healthy volunteers. *Journal of Shoulder and Elbow Surgery, 16,* 150–162.

Briere, A., Lauziere, S., Gravel, D., & Nadeau, S. (2010). Perception of weight bearing distribution during sit-to-stand tasks in hemiparetic and healthy individuals. *Stroke, 41,* 1704–1708.

Brogårdh, C., & Sjölund, B. H. (2006). Constraint-induced movement therapy in patients with stroke: A pilot study on effects of small group training and of extended mitt use. *Clinical Rehabilitation, 20,* 218–227.

Bronfenbrenner, U. (1979). *The ecology of human development: Experiments by nature and design.* Cambridge, MA: Harvard University Press

Butefish, C. M. (2004). Plasticity in the human cerebral cortex: Lessons from the normal brain and from stroke. *Neuroscientist, 10,* 163–173.

Caimmi, M., Carda, S., Giovanzana, C., Maini, E. S., Sabatini, A. M., Smania, N., & Molteni, F. (2008). Using kinematic analysis to evaluate constraint-induced movement therapy in chronic stroke patients. *Neurorehabilitation and Neural Repair, 22,* 31–39.

Canning, C. G., Shepherd, R. B., Carr, J. H., Alison, J. A., Wade, L., & White, A. (2003). Randomized controlled trial of the effects of intensive sit-to-stand training after recent traumatic brain injury on sit-to-stand performance. *Clinical Rehabilitation, 17,* 355–362.

Capasso, N., Gorman, A., & Blick, C. (2010). Breakfast group in an acute rehabilitation setting: A restorative program for incorporating clients' hemiparetic upper extremities for function. *OT Practice, 15,* 14–18.

Carr, J. H., & Shepherd, R. B. (1982). *A motor relearning programme for stroke.* Rockville, MD: Aspen.

Carr, J. H., & Shepherd, R. B. (1998). *Neurological rehabilitation: Optimizing motor performance.* Oxford, UK: Butterworth-Heinemann.

Carr, J. H., & Shepherd, R. B. (2003). *Stroke rehabilitation: Guidelines for exercise and training to optimize motor skill.* London: Butterworth-Heinemann.

Carr, J. H., & Shepherd, R. B. (2010). *Neurological rehabilitation: Optimizing motor performance* (2nd ed.). Oxford, UK: Butterworth-Heinemann.

Cirstea, M. C., & Levin, M. F. (2007). Improvement of arm movement patterns and endpoint control depends on type of feedback during practice in stroke survivors. *Neurorehabilitation and Neural Repair, 21,* 398–411.

Cirstea, M. C., Ptito, A., & Levin, M. F. (2003). Arm reaching improvements with short-term practice depend on the severity of the motor deficit in stroke. *Experimental Brain Research, 152,* 476–488.

Davids, K., Paul, G., Araujo, D., & Bartlett, R. (2003). Movement systems as dynamical systems: The functional role of variability and its implications for sports medicine. *Sports Medicine, 33,* 245–260.

Davies, P. M. (1990). *Right in the middle. Selective trunk activity in the treatment of adult hemiplegia.* Berlin: Springer-Verlag.

Davies, P. M. (2000). *Steps to follow: The comprehensive treatment of patients with hemiplegia* (2nd ed.). Berlin: Springer-Verlag.

Dean, C. M., Channon, E. F., & Hall, J. M. (2007). Sitting training early after stroke improves sitting ability and quality and carries over to standing up but not to walking: A randomised trial. *Australian Journal of Physiotherapy, 53,* 97–102.

Dean, C. M., & Shepherd, R. B. (1997). Task-related training improves performance of seated reaching tasks after stroke: A randomized controlled trial. *Stroke, 28,* 722–728.

Dean, C., Shepherd, R., & Adams, R. (1999a). Sitting balance I: Trunk-arm and the contribution of the lower limbs during self-paced reaching in sitting. *Gait and Posture, 10,* 135–144.

Dean, C., Shepherd, R., & Adams, R. (1999b). Sitting balance II: Reach direction and thigh support affect the contribution of the lower limbs when reaching beyond arms' length in sitting. *Gait and Posture, 10,* 147–153.

deJong, L. D., Nieuwboer, A., & Aufdemkampe, G. (2006). Contracture preventive positioning of the hemiplegic arm in subacute stroke patients: A pilot randomized controlled trial. *Clinical Rehabilitation, 20,* 656–657.

de Kroon, J. R., Ijzerman, M. J., Chae, J., Lankhorst, G. J., & Zilvold, G. (2005). Relation between stimulation characteristics and clinical outcome in studies using electrical stimulation to improve motor control of the upper extremity in stroke. *Journal of Rehabilitation Medicine, 37,* 65–74.

Denham, S. P. (2008). Augmenting occupational therapy treatment of upper-extremity spasticity with botulinum toxin A: A case report of progress at discharge and 2 years later. *American Journal of Occupational Therapy, 62,* 473–479.

Dipietro, L., Krebs, H. I., Fasoli, S. E., Volpe, B. T., Stein, J., Bever, C., & Hogan, N. (2007). Changing motor synergies in chronic stroke. *Journal of Neurophysiology, 98,* 757–768.

Dohle, C., Püllen, J., Nakaten, A., Küst, J., Rietz, C., & Karbe, H. (2009). Mirror therapy promotes recovery from severe hemiparesis: A randomized controlled trial. *Neurorehabilitation and Neural Repair, 23,* 209–217.

Dolechek, J. R., & Schkade, J. K. (1999). The extent dynamic standing endurance is affected when CVA subjects perform personally meaningful activities rather than nonmeaningful tasks. *Occupational Therapy Journal of Research, 19,* 40–54.

Donkervoort, M., Dekker, J., Stehmann-Saris, F. C., & Deelman, B. G. (2001). Efficacy of strategy training in left hemisphere stroke patients with apraxia: A randomized clinical trial. *Neuropsychological Rehabilitation, 11,* 549–566.

Dromerick, A. W., Lum, P. S., & Hidler, J. (2006). Activity based therapies. *Neurotherapeutics, 3,* 428–438.

Duff, S. V., Shumway-Cook, A., & Woollacott, M. (2012). Clinical management of the patient with reach, grasp, and manipulation disorders. In A. Shumway-Cook & M. Woollacott (Eds.), *Motor control: Translating research into clinical practice* (4th ed., pp. 552–594). Philadelphia: Lippincott Williams & Wilkins.

Dunn, W., Brown, C., & McGuigan, A. (1994). The ecology of human performance: A framework for considering the impact of context. *American Journal of Occupational Therapy, 48,* 595–607.

Fasoli, S. E., Trombly, C. A., Tickle-Degnen, L., & Verfaellie, M. H. (2002). Effect of instructions on functional reach in persons with and without cerebrovascular accident. *American Journal of Occupational Therapy, 56,* 380–389.

Flinn, N. A., Schamburg, S., Fetrow, J. M., & Flanigan, J. (2005). The effect of constraint-induced movement treatment on occupational performance and satisfaction in stroke survivors. *OTJR: Occupation, Participation and Health, 25,* 119–127.

French, B., Thomas, L., Leathley, M., Sutton, C., McAdam, J., Forster, A., Langhorne, P., Price, C., Walker, A., & Watkins, C. (2010). Does repetitive task training improve functional activity after stroke? A Cochrane systematic review and meta-analysis. *Journal of Rehabilitation Medicine, 42,* 9–15.

Frey, S. H., Fogassi, L., Grafton, S., Picard, N., Rothwell, J. C., Schweighofer, N., Corbetta, M., & Fitzpatrick, S. M. (2011). Neurological principles and rehabilitation of action disorders: Computation, anatomy and physiology (CAP) model. *Neurorehabilitation and Neural Repair, 25(Suppl.),* 6S–20S.

Fugl-Meyer, A. R., Jaasko, L., Leyman, I., Olsson, S., & Steglind, S. (1975). The post-stroke hemiplegic patient: I. A method for evaluation of physical performance. *Scandinavian Journal of Rehabilitation Medicine, 31,* 174–177.

Garrett, R., Immink, M. A., & Hillier, S. (2011). Becoming connected: The lived experience of yoga participation after stroke. *Disability and Rehabilitation, 33,* 2404–2415.

Gauthier, L. V., Taub, E., Perkins, C., Ortmann, M., Mark, V. W., & Uswatte, G. (2008). Remodeling the brain: Plastic structural brain changes produced by different motor therapies after stroke. *Stroke, 39,* 1520–1525.

Gentile, A. M. (2000). Skill acquisition: Action, movement and neuromotor processes. In J. H. Carr & R. B. Shepherd (Eds.), *Movement science: Foundations for physical therapy in rehabilitation* (2nd ed., pp. 111–187). Rockville, MD: Aspen.

Geusgens, C. A. V., van Heugten, C. M., Cooijmans, P. J., Jolles, J., & van den Heuvel, W. J. A. (2007). Transfer effects of a cognitive strategy training for stroke patients with apraxia. *Journal of Clinical and Experimental Neuropsychology, 29,* 831–841.

Gillen, G. (2009). *Cognitive and perceptual rehabilitation: Optimizing function.* St. Louis: Elsevier/Mosby.

Gillen, G. (2011). Trunk control: Supporting functional independence. In G. Gillen (Ed.), *Stroke rehabilitation: A function-based approach.* St. Louis: Elsevier/Mosby.

Gillen, G., Boiangiu, C., Neuman, M., Reinstein, R., & Schaap, Y. (2007). Trunk posture affects upper extremity function of adults. *Perceptual Motor Skills, 104,* 371–380.

Giuffrida, C. G., Demery, J. A., Reyes, L. R., Lebowitz, B. K., & Hanlon, R. E. (2009). Functional skill learning in men with traumatic brain injury. *American Journal of Occupational Therapy, 63*(4), 398–407.

Giuffrida, C. G., Shea, J. B., & Fairbrother, J. T. (2002). Differential transfer benefits of increased practice for constant, blocked, and serial practice schedules. *Journal of Motor Behavior, 34,* 353–365.

Goldenberg, G., Daumuller, M., & Hagmann, S. (2001). Assessment and therapy of complex activities of daily living in apraxia. *Neuropsychological Rehabilitation, 11,* 147–169.

Goldenberg, G., & Hagmann, S. (1998). Therapy of activities of daily living in patients with apraxia. *Neuropsychological Rehabilitation, 8,* 123–141.

Grabiner, M. D., Bareither, M. L., Gatts, S., Marone, J., & Troy, K. L. (2012). Task-specific training reduces trip-related fall risk in women. *Medicine and Science in Sports and Exercise, 44*(12), 2410–2414.

Hall, L. M., Brauer, S., Horak, F., & Hodges, P. W. (2010). Adaptive changes in anticipatory postural adjustments with novel and familiar postural supports. *Journal of Neurophysiology, 103,* 968–976.

Hardwick, D. D., & Lang, C. E. (2011). Scapular and humeral movement patterns of people with stroke during range-of-motion exercises. *Journal of Neurological Physical Therapy, 35,* 18–25.

Hayner, K., Gibson, G., & Giles, G. M. (2010). Comparison of constraint-induced movement therapy and bilateral treatment of equal intensity in people with chronic upper-extremity dysfunction after cerebrovascular accident. *American Journal of Occupational Therapy, 64,* 528–539.

Hesse, S., Werner, C., Pohl, M., Rueckriem, S., Mehrholz, J., & Lingnau, M. L. (2005). Computerized arm training improves the motor control of the severely affected arm after stroke: A single-blinded randomized trial in two centers. *Stroke, 36,* 1960–1966.

Hirsch, M. W., Smale, S., & Devaney, R. L. (2004). *Differential equations, dynamical systems and an introduction to chaos* (2nd ed.). San Diego: Academic Press/Elsevier.

Hoare, B., Imms, C., Carey, L., & Wasiak, J. (2007). Constraint-induced movement therapy in the treatment of the upper limb in children with hemiplegic cerebral palsy: A Cochrane systematic review. *Clinical Rehabilitation, 21,* 675–685.

Hoffman, A. N., Malena, R. R., Westergom, B. P., Luthra, P., Cheng, J. P., Aslam, H. A., Zafonte, R. D., & Kline, A. E. (2008). Environmental enrichment-mediated functional improvement after experimental traumatic brain injury is contingent on task-specific neurobehavioral experience. *Neuroscience Letters, 431,* 226–230.

Hogan, N., Krebs, H. I., Rohrer, B., Palazzolo, J. J., Dipietro, L., Fasoli, S. E., Stein, J., Hughes, R., Frontera, W. R., Lynch, D., & Volpe, B. T. (2006). Motions or muscles? Some behavioral factors underlying robotic assistance of motor recovery. *Journal of Rehabilitation Research and Development, 43,* 605–618.

Hosomi, M., Koyama, T., Takebayashi, T., Terayama, S., Kodama, N., Matsumoto, K., & Domen, K. (2012). A modified method for constraint-induced movement therapy: A supervised self-training protocol. *Journal of Stroke and Cerebrovascular Diseases, 21,* 767-775.

Howle, J. M. (2002). *Neuro-developmental treatment approach: Theoretical foundations and principles of clinical practice.* Laguna Beach, CA: North American Neuro-Developmental Treatment Association.

Hubbard, I. J., Parsons, M. W., Neilson, C., & Carey, L. M. (2009). Task-specific training: Evidence for and translation to clinical practice. *Occupational Therapy International, 16,* 175-189.

Ivanhoe, C. B., Francisco, G. E., McGuire, J. R., Subramanian, T., & Grissom, S. P. (2006). Intrathecal baclofen management of post-stroke spastic hypertonia: Implications for function and quality of life. *Archives of Physical Medicine and Rehabilitation, 87,* 1509-1515.

Jain, S., Janssen, K., & DeCelle, S. (2004). Alexander technique and Feldenkrais method: A critical overview. *Physical Medicine and Rehabilitation Clinics of North America, 15,* 811-825.

Janssen, W., Bussmann, J., Selles, R., Koudstaal, P., Ribbers, G., & Stam, H. (2010). Recovery of the sit-to-stand movement after stroke: A longitudinal study. *Neurorehabilitation and Neural Repair, 24*(8), 763-769.

Jaraczewska, E., & Long, C. (2006). Kinesio® taping in stroke: Improving functional use of the upper extremity in hemiplegia. *Topics in Stroke Rehabilitation, 13,* 31-42.

Jeannerod, M., Arbib, M. A., Rizzolatti, G., & Sakata, H. (1995). Grasping objects: The cortical mechanisms of visuomotor transformation. *Trends in Neuroscience, 18,* 314-320.

Kane, L. A., & Buckley, K. A. (2011). Functional mobility. In G. Gillen (Ed.), *Stroke rehabilitation: A function-based approach* (pp. 350-388). St. Louis: Elsevier/Mosby.

Kantak, S. S., Sullivan, K. J., Fisher, B. E., Knowlton, B. J., & Winstein, C. J. (2010). Neural substrates of motor memory consolidation depend on practice structure. *Nature Neuroscience, 13,* 923-925.

Katalinic, O. M., Harvey, L. A., & Herbert, R. D. (2011). Effectiveness of stretch for the treatment and prevention of contractures in people with neurological conditions: A systematic review. *Physical Therapy, 91,* 11-24.

Kim, Y. H., You, S. H., Ko, M. H., Park, J. W., Lee, K. H., Jang, S. H., Yoo, W. K., & Hallett, M. (2006). Repetitive transcranial magnetic stimulation-induced corticomotor excitability and associated motor skill acquisition in chronic stroke. *Stroke, 37,* 1471-1476.

Kimberley, T. J., Samargia, S., Moore, L. G., Shakya, J. K., & Lang, C. E. (2010). Comparison of amounts and types of practice during rehabilitation for traumatic brain injury and stroke. *Journal of Rehabilitation Research and Development, 47,* 851-862.

Kloubec, J. A. (2010). Pilates for improvement of muscle endurance, flexibility, balance, and posture. *Journal of Strength and Conditioning Research, 24,* 661-667.

Kollen, B. J., Lennon, S., Lyons, B., Wheatley-Smith, L., Scheper, M., Buurke, J. H., Halfens, J., Geurts, A. C., & Kwakkel, G. (2009). The effectiveness of the Bobath concept in stroke rehabilitation: What is the evidence? *Stroke, 40,* e89-e97.

Krakauer, J. W., & Shadmehr, R. (2006). Consolidation of motor memory. *Trends in Neurosciences, 29,* 58-64.

Krebs, H. I., Volpe, B., & Hogan, N. (2009). A working model of stroke recovery from rehabilitation robotics practitioners. *Journal of Neuro-Engineering and Rehabilitation, 6,* 1-8.

Kumar, R., Metter, E. J., Mehta, A. J., & Chew, T. (1990). Shoulder pain in hemiplagia: The role of exercise. *American Journal of Physical Medicine and Rehabilitation, 69,* 205-208.

Kwakkel, G., Kollen, B. J., van der Grond, J., & Prevo, A. J. (2003). Probability of regaining dexterity in the flaccid upper limb: Impact of severity of paresis and time since onset in acute stroke. *Stroke, 34,* 2181-2186.

Laufer, Y., Hausdorff, J. M., & Ring, H. (2009). Effects of a foot drop neuro-prosthesis on functional abilities, social participation, and gait velocity. *American Journal of Physical Medicine and Rehabilitation, 88,* 14-20.

Laufer, Y., Ring, H., Sprecher, E., & Hausdorff, J. M. (2009). Gait in individuals with chronic hemiparesis: One-year follow-up of the effects of a neuroprosthesis that amelioriates foot drop. *Journal of Neurological Physical Therapy, 33,* 104-110.

Law, M., Cooper, B., Strong, S., Stewart, D., Rigby, P., & Letts, L. (1996). The person-environment-occupation model: A transactive approach to occupational performance. *Canadian Journal of Occupational Therapy, 63,* 9-23.

Layne, C. S., & Spooner, B. S. (1992). Effects of postural set on anticipatory muscle activation prior to rapid arm flexion. *Research Quarterly for Exercise and Sport, 63,* 196-199.

Levine, P., & Page, S. J. (2004). Modified constraint-induced therapy: A promising restorative outpatient therapy. *Topics in Stroke Rehabilitation, 11,* 1-10.

Liepert, J. (2006). Motor cortex excitability in stroke before and after constraint-induced movement therapy. *Cognitive and Behavioral Neurology, 19,* 41-47.

Lin, K. C., Chang, Y. F., Wu, C. Y., & Chen, Y. A. (2009). Effects of constraint-induced therapy versus bilateral arm training on motor performance, daily functions, and quality of life in stroke survivors. *Neurorehabilitation and Neural Repair, 23,* 441-448.

Lin, K. C., Chen, Y. A., Chen, C. L., Wu, C. Y., & Chang, Y. F. (2010). The effects of bilateral arm training on motor control and functional performance in chronic stroke: A randomized controlled study. *Neurorehabilitation and Neural Repair, 24,* 42-51.

Lin, K. C., Chung, H. Y., Wu, C. Y., Liu, H. L., Hsieh, Y. W., Chen, I. H., Chen, C. L., Chuang, L. L., Liu, J. S., & Wai, Y. Y. (2010). Constraint-induced therapy versus control intervention in patients with stroke: A functional magnetic resonance imaging study. *American Journal of Physical Medicine and Rehabilitation, 89,* 177-185.

Lin, K. C., Wu, C. Y., Chen, C. L., Chern, J. S., & Jong, W. H. (2007). Effects of object use on reaching a postural balance: A comparison of patients with unilateral stroke and healthy controls. *American Journal of Physical Medicine and Rehabilitation, 86,* 791-799.

Lo, A. C., Guarino, P. D., Richards, L. G., Haselkorn, J. K., Wittenberg, G. F., Federman, D. G., Ringer, R. J., Wagner, T. H., Krebs, H. I., Volpe, B. T., Bever, C. T., Bravata, D. M., Duncan, P. W., Corn, B. H., Maffucci, A. D., Nadeau, S. E., Conroy, S. S., Powell, J. M., Huang, G. D., & Pedruzzi, P. (2010). Robot-assisted therapy for long-term upper-limb impairment after stroke. *New England Journal of Medicine, 362,* 1772-1783.

Ma, H. I., & Trombly, C. A. (2004). Effects of task complexity on reaction time and movement kinematics in elderly people. *American Journal of Occupational Therapy, 58,* 150-158.

Massie, C., Malcolm, M. P., Greene, D., & Thaut, M. (2009). The effects of constraint-induced therapy on kinematic outcomes and compensatory movement patterns: An exploratory study. *Archives of Physical Medicine and Rehabilitation, 90,* 571-579.

Mastos, M., Miller, K., Eliasson, A. C., & Imms, C. (2007). Goal-directed training: Linking theories of treatment to clinical practice for improved functional activities in daily life. *Clinical Rehabilitation, 21,* 47-55.

Mathiowetz, V., & Bass-Haugen, J. (1994). Motor behavior research: Implications for therapeutic approaches to CNS dysfunction. *American Journal of Occupational Therapy, 48,* 733-745.

Michaelsen, S. M., Dannenbaum, R., & Levin, M. F. (2006). Task-specific training with trunk restraint on arm recovery in stroke: Randomized control trial. *Stroke, 37,* 186-192.

Michelon, P., Vettel, J. M., & Zacks, J. M. (2006). Lateral somatotopic organization during imagined and prepared movements. *Journal of Neurophysiology, 95,* 811-822.

Morris, D. M., Taub, E., Macrina, D. M., Cook, E. W., & Geiger, B. F. (2009). A method for standardizing procedures in rehabilitation: Use in the extremity constraint induced therapy evaluation multisite randomized controlled trial. *Archives of Physical Medicine and Rehabilitation, 90,* 663-668.

Murayama, T., Numata, K., Kawakami, T., Tosaka, T., Oga, M., Oka, N., Katano, M., Takasugi, J., & Shimizu, E. (2011). Changes in the brain activation balance in motor-related areas after constraint-induced movement therapy: A longitudinal fMRI study. *Brain Injury, 25,* 1047–1057.

Murphy, T. H., & Corbett, D. (2009). Plasticity during stroke recovery: From synapse to behavior. *Nature Reviews: Neuroscience, 10,* 861–872.

Murtha, P. K., Sainburg, R. L., & Haaland, K. Y. (2010). Coordination deficits in ideomotor apraxia during visually targeted reaching reflect impaired visuomotor transformations. *Neuropsychologia, 48,* 3855–3867.

Neumann, D. A. (2010). *Kinesiology of the musculoskeletal system: Foundations for rehabilitation* (2nd ed.). St. Louis: Mosby/Elsevier.

Nilsen, D. M., Gillen, G., & Gordon, A. M. (2010). Use of mental practice to improve upper-limb recovery after stroke: A systematic review. *American Journal of Occupational Therapy, 64,* 695–708.

Page, S. J., & Levine, P. (2006). Back from the brink: Electromyography-triggered stimulation combined with modified constraint-induced movement therapy in chronic stroke. *Archives of Physical Medicine and Rehabilitation, 87,* 27–31.

Page, S. J., Levine, P., Leonard, A., Szaflarski, J. P., & Kissela, B. M. (2008). Modified constraint-induced therapy in chronic stroke: Results of a single-blinded randomized controlled trial. *Physical Therapy, 88,* 333–340.

Page, S. J., Maslyn, S., Hermann, V. H., Wu, A., Dunning, K., & Levine, P. G. (2009). Activity-based electrical stimulation training in a stroke patient with minimal movement in the paretic upper extremity. *Neurorehabilitation and Neural Repair, 23,* 595–599.

Page, S. J., Sisto, S. A., Levine, P., Johnston, M. V., & Hughes, M. (2001). Modified constraint induced therapy: A randomized feasibility and efficacy study. *Journal of Rehabilitation Research and Development, 38,* 583–590.

Park, S. W., Wolf, S. L., Blanton, S., Winstein, C., & Nichols-Larsen, D. S. (2008). The EXCITE trial: Predicting a clinically meaningful motor activity log outcome. *Neurorehabilitation and Neural Repair, 22,* 486–493.

Paulignan, Y., Frak, V. G., Toni, I., & Jeannerod, M. (1997). Influence of object position and size on human prehension movements. *Experimental Brain Research, 114,* 226–234.

Ploughman, M., Shears, J., Hutchings, L., & Osmond, M. (2008). Constraint-induced movement therapy for severe upper extremity impairment after stroke in an outpatient rehabilitation setting: A case report. *Physiotherapy Canada, 60,* 161–170.

Popović, D. B., Sinkaer, T., & Popović, M. B. (2009). Electrical stimulation as a means for achieving recovery of function in stroke patients. *NeuroRehabilitation, 25,* 45–58.

Pound, P., Bury, M., & Ebrahim, S. (1997). From apoplexy to stroke. *Age and Ageing, 26,* 331–337.

Raghavan, P. (2007). The nature of hand motor impairment after stroke and its treatment. *Current Treatment Options in Cardiovascular Medicine, 9,* 221–228.

Ramachandran, V. S., & Altschuler, E. L. (2009). The use of visual feedback, in particular mirror visual feedback, in restoring brain function. *Brain, 132,* 1693–1710.

Ring, H., Treger, I., Gruendlinger, L., & Hausdorff, J. M. (2009). Neuroprosthesis for footdrop compared with an ankle-foot orthosis: Effects on postural control during walking. *Journal of Stroke and Cerebrovascular Disease, 18,* 41–47.

Rowe, V. T., Blanton, S., & Wolf, S. L. (2009). Long-term follow-up after constraint-induced therapy: A case report of a chronic stroke survivor. *American Journal of Occupational Therapy, 63,* 317–322.

Ryerson, S., & Levit, K. (1997). *Functional movement reeducation.* New York: Churchill Livingstone.

Sabari, J. (2008). *Occupational therapy practice guidelines for adults with stroke.* Bethesda, MD: American Occupational Therapy Association.

Schlinger, M. (2006). Feldenkrais method, Alexander technique, and yoga-body awareness therapy in the performing arts. *Physical Medicine and Rehabilitation Clinics of North America, 17,* 865–875.

Schmidt, R., & Lee, T. (2011). *Motor control and learning: A behavioral emphasis* (5th ed.). Champaign, IL: Human Kinetics.

Seitz, R. J., Azari, N. P., Knorr, U., Binkofski, F., Herzog, H., & Freund, H. J. (1999). The role of diaschisis in stroke recovery. *Stroke, 30,* 1844–1850.

Shi, Y. X., Tian, J. H., Yang, K. H., & Zhao, Y. (2011). Modified constraint-induced movement therapy versus traditional rehabilitation in patients with upper-extremity dysfunction after stroke: A systematic review and meta-analysis. *Archives of Physical Medicine and Rehabilitation, 92,* 972–982.

Shumway-Cook, A., & Woollacott, M. H. (2012). *Motor control: Translating research into clinical practice* (4th ed.). Philadelphia: Lippincott Williams & Wilkins.

Sirtori, V., Corbetta, D., Moja, L., & Gatti, R. (2009). Constraint-induced movement therapy for upper extremities in stroke patients. *Cochrane Database of Systematic Reviews,* (7), CD004433.

Smania, N., Agloti, S. M., Girardi, F., Tinazzi, M., Fiaschi, A., Cosentino, A., & Corato, E. (2006). Rehabilitation of limb apraxia improves daily life activities in patients with stroke. *Neurology, 67,* 2050–2052.

Smania, N., Girardi, F., Domenicali, C., Lora, E., & Aglioti, S. (2000). The rehabilitation of limb apraxia: A study in left brain-damaged patients. *Archives of Physical Medicine and Rehabilitation, 81,* 379–388.

Stevens, J. A., & Stoykov, M. E. (2004). Simulation of bilateral movement training through mirror reflection: A case report demonstrating an occupational therapy technique for hemiparesis. *Topics in Stroke Rehabilitation, 11,* 59–66.

Stinear, C. M., Barber, A., Coxon, J. P., Fleming, M. K., & Byblow, W. D. (2008). Priming the motor system enhances the effects of upper limb therapy in chronic stroke. *Brain, 131,* 1381–1390.

Stoykov, M. E., Lewis, G. N., & Corcos, D. M. (2009). Comparison of bilateral and unilateral training for upper extremity hemiparesis in stroke. *Neurorehabilitation and Neural Repair, 9,* 945–953.

Stroke Unit Trialists' Collaboration. (2007). Organised inpatient (stroke unit) care for stroke. *Cochrane Database of Systematic Reviews,* (4), CD000197.

Sullivan, K. J., Brown, D. A., Klassen, T., Mulroy, S., Ge, T., Azen, S. P., & Winstein, C. J. (2007). Effects of task-specific locomotor and strength training in adults who were ambulatory after stroke: Results of the STEPS randomized clinical trial. *Physical Therapy, 87*(12), 1580–1602.

Surburg, P. R. (1997). Proprioceptive neuromuscular facilitation techniques in sports medicine: A reassessment. *Journal of Athletic Training, 32,* 34–39.

Taub, E. (1976). Movement in nonhuman primates deprived of somatosensory feedback. *Exercise & Sport Science Review, 4,* 335–374.

Taub, E., Uswatte, G., Mark, V. W., & Morris, D. M. (2006). The learned nonuse phenomenon: Implications for rehabilitation. *Europa Medicophysica, 42,* 241–256.

Teasell, R., Foley, N., Salter, K., Bhogal, S., Jutai, J., & Speechley, M. (2012). Evidence-based review of stroke rehabilitation (15th Ed.). Retrieved on July 20, 2013 from http://www.ebrsr.com/reviews_list.php.

Thelen, E. (1989). Self-organization in developmental processes: Can systems approaches work? In M. R. Gunnar & E. Thelen (Eds.), *Systems and development* (pp. 77–117). Hillsdale, NJ: Lawrence Erlbaum.

Tung, F. L., Yang, Y. R., Lee, C. C., & Wang, R. Y. (2010). Balance outcomes after additional sit-to-stand training in subjects with stroke: A randomized controlled trial. *Clinical Rehabilitation, 24,* 533–542.

Twitchell, T. E. (1951). The restoration of motor function following hemiplegia in man. *Brain, 74,* 443–480.

van Heugten, C. M., Dekker, J., Deelman, B. G., Stehmann-Saris, J. C., & Kinebanian, A. (2000). Rehabilitation of stroke patients with apraxia: The role of additional cognitive and motor impairments. *Disability and Rehabilitation, 22,* 547–554.

van Heugten, C. M., Dekker, J., Deelman, B. G., van Dijk, A. J., Stehmann-Saris, J. C., & Kinebanian, A. (1998). Outcome of strategy training in stroke patients with apraxia: A phase II study. *Clinical Rehabilitation, 12,* 294–303.

Wardlaw, J. M., del Zoppo, G. J., Yamaguchi, T., & Berge, E. (2003). Thrombolysis for acute ischaemic stroke. *Cochrane Database of Systematic Reviews,* (3), CD000213.

Whitall, J., Waller, S. M., Sorkin, J. D., Forrester, L. W., Macko, R. F., Hanley, D. F., Goldberg, A. P., & Luft, A. (2011). Bilateral and unilateral arm training improve motor function through differing neuroplastic mechanisms: A single-blinded randomized controlled trial. *Neurorehabilitation and Neural Repair, 25,* 118–129.

Winstein, C. J., & Knecht, H. G. (1990). Movement science and its relevance to physical therapy. *Physical Therapy, 70,* 759–762.

Winstein, C. J., Miller, J. P., Blanton, S., Taub, E., Uswatte, G., Morris, D., Nichols, D., & Wolf, S. (2003). Methods for a multisite randomized trial to investigate the effect of constraint-induced movement therapy in improving upper extremity function among adults recovering from a cerebrovascular stroke. *Neurorehabilitation and Neural Repair, 17,* 137–152.

Wolf, S. L. (2007). Revisiting constraint-induced movement therapy: Are we too smitten with the mitten? Is all nonuse "learned"? and other quandaries. *Physical Therapy, 87,* 1212–1223.

Wolf, S. L., Lecraw, D. E., Barton, L. A., & Jann, B. B. (1989). Forced use of hemiplegic upper extremities to reverse the effect of learned nonuse among chronic stroke and head injured patients. *Experimental Neurology, 104,* 125–132.

Wolf, S. L., Thompson, P. A., Winstein, C. J., Miller, J. P., Blanton, S. R., Nichols-Larsen, D. S., Morris, D. M., Uswatte, G., Taub, E., Light, K. E., & Sawaki, L. (2010). The EXCITE stroke trial: Comparing early and delayed constraint-induced movement therapy. *Stroke, 41,* 2309–2315.

Wolf, S. L., Winstein, C. J., Miller, J. P., Blanton, S., Clark, P. C., & Nichols-Larsen, D. (2007). Looking in the rear view mirror when conversing with back seat drivers: The EXCITE trial revisited. *Neurorehabilitation and Neural Repair, 21,* 379–387.

Wolf, S., Winstein, C. J., Miller, J. P., Taub, E., Uswatte, G., Morris, D., Giuliani, C., Light, K. E., Nichols-Larsen, D., & EXCITE Investigators. (2006). Effect of constraint-induced movement therapy on upper extremity function 3 to 9 months after stroke: The EXCITE randomized clinical trial. *Journal of the American Medical Association, 296,* 2095–2104.

Wolf, S. L., Winstein, C. J., Miller, J. P., Thompson, P. A., Taub, E., Uswatte, G., Morris D., Blanton, S., Nichols-Larsen, D., & Clark, P. C. (2008). Retention of upper limb function in stroke survivors who have received constraint-induced movement therapy: The EXCITE randomized trial. *Lancet Neurology, 7,* 33–40.

Woodbury, M. L., Howland, D. R., McGuirk, T. E., Davis, S. B., Senesac, C. R., Kautz, S., & Richards, L. G. (2009). Effects of trunk restraint combined with intensive task practice on poststroke upper extremity reach and function: A pilot study. *Neurorehabilitation and Neural Repair, 23,* 78–91.

Wu, C. Y., Chen, C. L., Tang, S. F., Lin, K. C., & Huang, Y. Y. (2007). Kinematic and clinical analyses of upper extremity movements after constraint-induced movement therapy in patients with stroke: A randomized controlled trial. *Archives of Physical Medicine and Rehabilitation, 88,* 964–970.

Wu, C. Y., Chen, Y. A., Chen, H. C., Lin, K. C., & Yeh, I. L. (2012). Pilot trial of distributed constraint-induced therapy with trunk restraint to improve poststroke reach to grasp and trunk kinematics. *Neurorehabilitation and Neural Repair, 26,* 247–255.

Wu, C. Y., Chuang, L. L., Lin, K. C., Chen, H. C., & Tsay, P. K. (2011). Randomized trial of distributed constraint-induced therapy versus bilateral arm training for the rehabilitation of upper-limb motor control and function after stroke. *Neurorehabilitation and Neural Repair, 25,* 130–139.

Wu, C. Y., Lin, K. C., Chen, H. C., Chen, I. H., & Hong, W. H. (2007). Effects of modified constraint-induced movement therapy on movement kinematics and daily function in patients with stroke: A kinematic study of motor control mechanisms. *Neurorehabilitation and Neural Repair, 21,* 460–466.

Wu, C., Trombly, C. A., Lin, K., & Tickle-Degnen, L. (1998). Effects of object affordances on reaching performance in persons with and without cerebrovascular accident. *American Journal of Occupational Therapy, 52,* 447–456.

Yavuzer, G., Selles, R., Sezer, N., Sütbeyaz, S., Bussmann, J. B., Köseoğlu, F., Atay, M. B., & Stam, H. J. (2008). Mirror therapy improves hand function in subacute stroke: A randomized controlled trial. *Archives of Physical Medicine and Rehabilitation, 89,* 393–398.

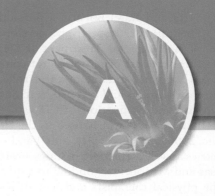

Optimizing Motor Behavior Using the Bobath Approach

Kathryn Levit

Learning Objectives

After studying this chapter, the reader will be able to do the following:

1. Identify the major problems that result from stroke according to Bobath and Bobath.
2. Describe the major principles underlying the Neuro-Developmental Treatment (NDT)/Bobath approach to stroke rehabilitation.
3. Discuss the role of muscle tone and postural control in the production of normal movement, and describe how problems in these areas contribute to impaired occupational functioning.
4. Integrate NDT/Bobath concepts and techniques with the Occupational Functioning Model.
5. Develop an occupational therapy treatment plan for a patient with acute stroke using NDT/Bobath principles and techniques.

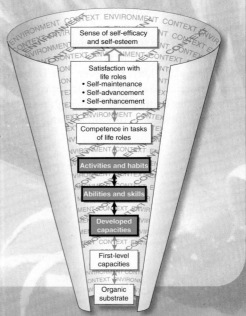

Berta and Karel Bobath, a physiotherapist and a neurologist, respectively, developed the Neuro-Developmental Treatment (NDT) approach to reduce impairments of sensorimotor control of children with cerebral palsy and adults with stroke. They founded a center in London and traveled, teaching their method to physical and occupational therapists. As a result, the Bobath approach is widely used in the United Kingdom (Raine, 2006; Tyson & Selley, 2007) and other European countries as well as the United States. Of 107 therapists in Kansas and Missouri responding to a questionnaire, 93% of the physical therapists and 85% of the occupational therapists reported using either the Bobath or Brunnstrom approaches (Natarajan et al., 2008).

Bobath practitioners elicit and reestablish movement patterns through therapist-controlled sensorimotor experiences within the context of task accomplishment (Levin & Panturin, 2011). The therapist inhibits synergistic movements and abnormal tone and facilitates normal movement through handling techniques (Teasell et al., 2008). The therapist assists and/or guides normal movement patterns to accomplish functional tasks until no guidance is necessary (Tyson & Selley, 2007).

The Bobath approach has been researched more than any of the other neurophysiologically based approaches. The online chapter mentions some of the studies. Since that was written, several other studies have been reported. One study compared the Bobath approach to the Motor Relearning Programme (MRP) of Carr and Shepherd (2003) and found that the task-oriented exercises of the MRP resulted in significantly better quality of movement in acute rehabilitation of patients with stroke (Langhammer & Stanghelle, 2011). Another study found the two approaches equally effective for improving movement ability and functional independence (Van Vliet, Lincoln, & Foxall, 2005). A systematic review of randomized, controlled trials designed to evaluate the effectiveness of the Bobath concept in stroke rehabilitation (16 studies involving 813 patients) concluded that the Bobath concept is not superior to other approaches (Kollen et al., 2009). However, the Bobath approach was found superior to an orthopedic approach of strengthening weak muscles using passive through resistive movement for improving functional mobility (Wang et al., 2005).

Bobath instructors continue to publish (Gjelsvik, 2007) and offer courses in this method, which continues to develop as therapists' understanding of movement science broadens (Raine, 2006). Worldwide course locations and schedules are available from the NDT Association, which is listed in the Resources Box of the online chapter.

This chapter is available online at http://thepoint.lww.com/Radomski7e.

References

Carr, J. H., & Shepherd, R. B. (2003). *Stroke rehabilitation: Guidelines for exercise and training to optimize motor skill.* London, United Kingdom: Butterworth-Heinemann.

Gjelsvik, B. E. B. (2007). *The Bobath concept in adult neurology.* Stuttgart, Germany: Thieme Medical Publishers, Inc.

Kollen, B. J., Lennon, S., Lyons, B., Wheatley-Smith, L., Scheper, M., Buurke, J. H., Halfens, J., Geurts, A. C. H., & Kwakkel, G. (2009). The effectiveness of the Bobath concept in stroke rehabilitation: What is the evidence? *Stroke, 40,* e89–e97.

Langhammer, B., & Stanghelle, J. K. (2011). Can physiotherapy after stroke based on the Bobath concept result in improved quality of movement compared to the Motor Relearning Programme. *Physiotherapy Research International, 16,* 69–80.

Levin, M. F., & Panturin, E. (2011). Sensorimotor integration for functional recovery and the Bobath approach. *Motor Control, 15,* 285–301.

Natarajan, P., Oelschlager, A., Agah, A., Pohl, P. S., Ahmad, S. O., & Liu, W. (2008). Current clinical practices in stroke rehabilitation: Regional pilot survey. *Journal of Rehabilitation Research & Development, 45,* 841–850.

Raine, S. (2006). Defining the Bobath concept using the Delphi technique. *Physiotherapy Research International, 11,* 4–13.

Teasell, R. W., Foley, N. C., Salter, K. L., & Jutai, J. W. (2008). A blueprint for transforming stroke rehabilitation care in Canada: The case for change. *Archives of Physical Medicine and Rehabilitation, 89,* 575–578.

Tyson, S. F., & Selley, A. B. (2007). The effect of perceived adherence to the Bobath concept on physiotherapists' choice of intervention to treat postural control after stroke. *Disability and Rehabilitation, 29,* 395–401.

van Vliet, P. M., Lincoln, N. B., & Foxall, A. (2005). Comparison of Bobath based and movement science based treatment for stroke: A randomized controlled trial. *Journal of Neurology, Neurosurgery, and Psychiatry, 76,* 503–508.

Wang, R.-Y., Chen, H.-I., Chen, C.-Y., & Yang, Y.-R. (2005). Efficacy of Bobath versus orthopaedic approach on impairment and function at different motor recovery stages after stroke: A randomized controlled study. *Clinical Rehabilitation, 19,* 155–164.

Optimizing Motor Behavior Using the Brunnstrom Movement Therapy Approach

Catherine A. Trombly Latham

Learning Objectives

After studying this chapter, the reader will be able to do the following:

1. State the assumptions that underlie the Brunnstrom Movement Therapy approach.
2. List the six stages of recovery for the upper extremity and for the hand.
3. State the treatment principles of this approach.
4. Describe the treatment procedures to facilitate movement control in the trunk and upper extremity of patients with hemiparesis following stroke using this approach.
5. Suggest functional activities suitable to encourage practice of movement behavior at various stages of recovery.

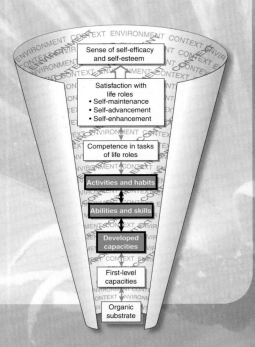

sing the literature of the time and through reflective practice, Signe Brunnstrom, a physical therapist, devised a program of therapy aimed at recovering movement and therefore function in the paretic trunks, arms, and legs of people who had suffered stroke (Brunnstrom, 1970; Sawner & LaVigne, 1992). The program was designed for patients at any level of recovery, from flaccid to synergistic movement to beginning voluntary movement. To move the patient in the flaccid stage of recovery from preserved organic substrate to first-level capacities (reflexive movement), Brunnstrom used sensory stimulation. Once reflexive movement was evoked, she advocated attention to movement (willed movement to gain control over synergistic movement patterns) and functional, repetitive use of the movement in everyday activities to move the patient to developed capacities (voluntary movement). Ms. Brunnstrom practiced at a time when demonstration of the method and its effects by her or other skilled therapists was enough evidence for other therapists to adopt the method. There has been no formal research on the effectiveness of this approach, and therefore it lacks an evidence base.

From observation of patients recovering from stroke and prior work of Twitchell (1951), Brunnstrom developed what has come to be known as the Brunnstrom Stages of Recovery, still commonly in use and verified to be valid (Naghdi et al., 2010). That classification system was further refined and quantified by Fugl-Meyer et al. (1975) into what is now called the Fugl-Meyer Motor Assessment (FMA), a widely used tool in research as well as clinical evaluation. It has been found to be a valid and reliable assessment tool (Duncan, Propst, & Nelson, 1983; Gladstone, Danells, & Black, 2002). There is an example of it in the online chapter.

This chapter is available online at http://thepoint.lww.com/Radomski7e.

References

Brunnstrom, S. (1970). *Movement therapy in hemiplegia*. New York: Harper & Row.

Duncan, P. W., Propst, M., & Nelson, S. G. (1983). Reliability of the Fugl-Meyer Assessment of sensorimotor recovery following cerebrovascular accident. *Physical Therapy, 63,* 1606–1610.

Fugl-Meyer, A. R., Jaasko, L., Leyman, L., Olsson, S., & Steglind, S. (1975). The post-stroke hemiplegic patient: I. A method for evaluation of physical performance. *Scandinavian Journal of Rehabilitation Medicine, 7,* 13–31.

Gladstone, D. J., Danells, C. J., & Black, S. E. (2002). The Fugl-Meyer Assessment of motor recovery after stroke: A critical review of its measurement properties. *Neurorehabilitation and Neural Repair, 16,* 232–240.

Naghdi, S., Ansar, N. N., Mansouri, K., & Hasson, S. (2010). A neurophysiological and clinical study of Brunnstrom recovery stages in the upper limb following stroke. *Brain Injury, 24,* 1372–1378.

Sawner, K. A., & LaVigne, J. M. (1992). *Brunnstrom's movement therapy in hemiplegia* (2nd ed.). Philadelphia: J. B. Lippincott Co.

Twitchell, T. E. (1951). The restoration of motor function following hemiplegia in man. *Brain, 74,* 443–480.

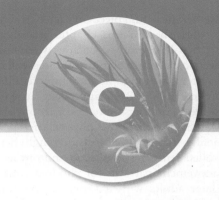

Managing Deficit of First-Level Motor Control Capacities Using Rood and Proprioceptive Neuromuscular Facilitation Techniques

Kathy Longenecker Rust

Learning Objectives

After studying this chapter, the reader will be able to do the following:

1. Use knowledge of controlled sensory input to reduce first-order motor impairments and prepare patients with orthopedic and central nervous system conditions for successful participation in occupational performance.
2. Delineate treatment strategies for improving mobility and stability.
3. Analyze the diagonal components of functional activities, and use this knowledge to incorporate optimal movement patterns and positions in treatment.
4. Perform the proprioceptive neuromuscular facilitation (PNF) diagonal patterns of the head, neck, trunk, and upper extremities.

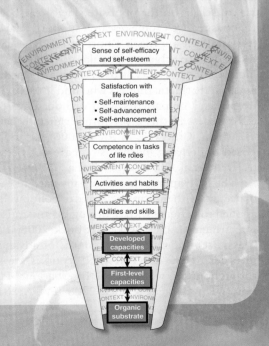

Therapists find pieces of each of the two approaches described in this chapter useful in remediating first-level motor capacities when muscular activity has been lost because of injury or disease of the central nervous system, although neither approach has been validly researched *in toto*. Both approaches used Sherrington's (1910, 1947) findings on reflex neurophysiology.

Margaret Rood, both a physical therapist and an occupational therapist, developed and taught her procedures of controlled sensory stimulation and ontogenetic postures and movement patterns for children with cerebral palsy and later adults with a variety of neurological impairments (Rood, 1956). The Rood approach was later further explicated by Stockmeyer (1967). No study examines both aspects of her approach, but a few studies have examined the sensory stimulation aspect, which has been found to be effective in activating muscular response when there appears to be none, although, without specific training, the elicited response does not carry over to functional movement (Carey, 1990; Feys et al., 1998; Kawahira et al., 2010).

Margaret Knott, a physical therapist, and Dr. Herman Kabat, a clinical neurophysiologist, developed the philosophy and practices of proprioceptive neuromuscular facilitation (PNF) in the 1940s (Adler, Beckers, & Buck, 2008; International PNF Association [IPNFA], 2011). Kabat, Knott, and later Voss identified spiral and diagonal patterns of movement as being basic to functional movement. They looked for a balance of agonists and antagonists and facilitated the inclusion of all the muscles involved in a movement through sensory stimulation (resistance) to movement (Voss, 1967; Voss, Ionta, & Myers, 1985). Resistance to movement was believed to cause not only recruitment of muscles in the limb being worked on but also cross-education, that is, activation of the comparable muscle(s) on the opposite side of the body, a notion that has received some research support (Arai et al., 2001). As part of the approach, Knott and Voss developed several techniques to achieve particular goals. One of those techniques, contract-relax, is used frequently by physical therapists and athletic trainers who find it useful in limbering up athletes or patients with orthopedic problems. The effectiveness of this procedure is generally acknowledged (Sharman, Cresswell, & Riek, 2006), although the proposed underlying mechanisms have not been supported (Azevedo et al., 2011; Mitchell et al., 2009).

The PNF approach was initially used in the treatment of persons with multiple sclerosis or poliomyelitis and later applied to patients with neurological and musculoskeletal impairments (Adler, Beckers, & Buck, 2008; IPNFA, 2011). Therapists underwent 3–6 months of advanced training in order to practice PNF. PNF courses are still offered throughout the world by the International PNF Association (Adler, Beckers, & Buck, 2008: IPNFA, 2011).

Both approaches focused the treatment of neuromuscular impairments on remediation of the impaired underlying neuromuscular substrate at a time when treatment was otherwise focused on adaptation. Successful demonstrations by the developers and skilled practitioners of these approaches provide the only testament to their effectiveness.

This chapter is available online at http://thepoint.lww.com/Radomski7e.

References

Adler, S. S., Beckers, D., & Buck, M. (2008). *PNF in practice: An illustrated guide* (3rd ed.). Heidelberg: Springer Medizin Verlag.

Arai, M., Shimizu, H., Shimizu, M. E., Tanaka, Y., & Yanagisawa, K. (2001). Effects of the use of cross-education to the affected side through various resistive exercises of the sound side and settings of the length of the affected muscles. *Hiroshima Journal of Medical Sciences, 50*, 65–73.

Azevedo, D. C., Melo, R. M., Alves Corrêa, R. V., & Chalmers, G. (2011). Uninvolved versus target muscle contraction during contract-relax proprioceptive neuromuscular facilitation stretching. *Physical Therapy in Sport, 12*, 117–121.

Carey, J. R. (1990). Manual stretch: Effect on finger movement control and force control in stroke subjects with spastic extrinsic finger flexor muscles. *Archives of Physical Medicine and Rehabilitation, 71*, 888–894.

Feys, H. M., De Weerdt, W. J., Selz, B. E., Cox Steck, G. A., Spichiger, R., Vereeck, L. E., Putman, K. D., & Hoydonck, G. A. (1998). Effect of a therapeutic intervention for the hemiplegic upper limb in the acute phase after stroke: A single-blinded, randomized, controlled multicenter trial. *Stroke, 29*, 785–792.

International PNF Association. (2011). What is the IPNFA? Retrieved August 19, 2011 from www.ipnfa.org/index.php?id=115.

Kawahira, K., Shimodozono, M., Etoh, S., Kamanda, K., Noma, T., & Tanaka, N. (2010). Effects of intensive repetition of a new facilitation technique on motor functional recovery of the hemiplegic upper limb and hand. *Brain Injury, 24*, 1202–1213.

Mitchell, U. H., Myrer, J. W., Hopkins, J. T., Hunter, I., Feland, J. B., & Hilton, S. C. (2009). Neurophysiological reflex mechanisms' lack of contribution to the success of PNF stretches. *Journal of Sport Rehabilitation, 18*, 343–357.

Rood, M. S. (1956). Neurophysiological mechanisms utilized in the treatment of neuromuscular dysfunction. *American Journal of Occupational Therapy, 10*, 220–225.

Sharman, M. J., Cresswell, A. G., & Riek, S. (2006). Proprioceptive neuromuscular facilitation stretching: Mechanisms and clinical implications. *Sports Medicine (Auckland, NZ), 36*, 929–939.

Sherrington, C. S. (1910). Flexion reflex of the limb, crossed extension reflex and reflex stepping in standing. *Journal of Physiology, 40*, 28–121.

Sherrington, C. S. (1947). *The integrative action of the nervous system* (2nd ed.). New Haven: Yale University Press.

Stockmeyer, S. A. (1967). An interpretation of the approach of Rood to the treatment of neuromuscular dysfunction. *American Journal of Physical Medicine, 46*, 900–956.

Voss, D. E. (1967). Proprioceptive neuromuscular facilitation. *American Journal of Physical Medicine, 46*, 838–898.

Voss, D. E., Ionta, M. K., & Myers, B. J. (1985). *Proprioceptive neuromuscular facilitation: Patterns and techniques* (3rd ed.). New York: Harper & Row.

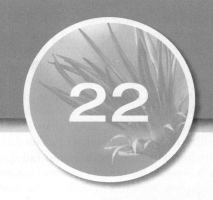

Optimizing Sensory Abilities and Capacities

Catherine Trombly Latham and Karen Bentzel

Learning Objectives

After studying this chapter, the reader will be able to do the following:

1. Select appropriate sensory treatment for a patient.
2. Explain the rationale for sensory reeducation and desensitization.
3. Demonstrate a variety of sensory reeducation and desensitization strategies for patients following peripheral nerve injury or repair.
4. Name several mechanisms of damage to areas of skin that result in diminished protective sensation and describe related compensatory strategies to prevent injury.
5. Demonstrate a variety of passive sensory training and active sensory training strategies for patients with sensory impairment following stroke.

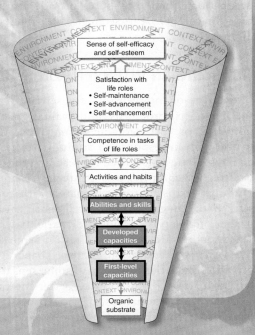

The extent and number of difficulties resulting from loss of tactile and proprioceptive information are difficult to comprehend. The story of Ian Waterman (Cole, 1991), who lost all tactile and proprioceptive sensations from the neck down as a result of a rare neurological illness, can help us understand the disability. When Waterman tried to explain to others what was wrong with him, he found that they could not begin to realize the severe difficulties he faced as a result of his sensory loss. His family and friends failed to find the connection between his sensory loss and his inability to move and complete activities of daily living. Even those in the medical community did not comprehend the extent of his difficulties. Cole provides a detailed account of Waterman's struggle to compensate for his lost sensation in the book *Pride and a Daily Marathon*.

Touch is a developed capacity that supports abilities and skills such as grasping and releasing objects (Duff & Estilow, 2010). These abilities and skills are necessary for competence in self-maintenance, self-enhancement, and self-advancement. Handling and manipulating objects enhances learning and helps human beings appreciate the world. Touch is also a means of communication and a source of pleasure (Lundborg & Rosén, 2007; Rosén & Lundborg, 2010).

Without sensation in the hand, there is a greater risk of injury to the hand and decreased ability to manipulate small objects. There is also a tendency not to use the hand in functional activities, which adds to the phenomenon of learned nonuse, loss of function that results from not using the hand (Carr & Shepherd, 2010; Lundborg & Rosén, 2007; Oud et al., 2007). Because of the role of tactile sensation in learning, exploring, and communicating and because loss of hand sensation is particularly disabling, occupational therapists should provide treatment or education in compensatory strategies for patients with lost or diminished sensation.

CHOOSING AN INTERVENTION STRATEGY

The choice of interventions for sensation is based on the diagnosis, prognosis, and evaluation findings. Diminished or lost protective sensation, the inability to feel pain in response to stimuli that are potentially damaging, suggests a need for teaching the patient and/or caregiver compensatory strategies to prevent injury. Findings of discomfort associated with touch (hypersensitivity) suggest a need for desensitization. Passive sensory training is provided for patients who have lost sensation but are expected to regain some sensory ability. Sensory reeducation (active sensory training) is provided for patients who have some sensation and potential for better sensation or better interpretation of sensory information. Most of the sensory interventions described in this chapter are learning experiences for the patient. Strategies of learning (see Chapter 13) should be applied including practice within the natural context of activities.

COMPENSATION FOR IMPAIRED OR ABSENT PROTECTIVE SENSATION

Protective sensations are sensations of pain and temperature extremes that signal the threat of tissue damage. When the brain receives this message, the normal response is to move the body part away from the source of the stimulus. Without this message, tissue damage can quickly occur. The goal of treatment for the patient with diminished or absent protective sensation is to avoid injury. Treatment consists of teaching the patient and/or the caregiver precautions necessary to prevent injury to any body part with compromised protective sensations. The loss of sensation could be due to diagnoses such as stroke, head injury, spinal cord injury, peripheral nerve injury, or nerve reconstruction.

Rationale for Compensation

In a classic 1969 article in the *American Journal of Occupational Therapy*, Helen Wood described the role of the occupational therapist in preventing injury and deformity in hands that lacked sensitivity. She stated that when hands are used in activities without protective sensory feedback, there is a high frequency of burns, cuts, lacerations, and bruises. Damage or injury to an insensitive limb is the result of external forces that are normally avoided by people who are able to feel pain, which acts as a warning mechanism. Sensations of pain warn us when we are gripping an item too tightly or sitting in one position for too long. Therefore, pain has been considered the most valuable sensation that humans have (Brand, 1979).

Brand (1979) described five mechanisms of damage to insensitive limbs: continuous low pressure, concentrated high pressure, excessive heat or cold, repetitive mechanical stress, and pressure on infected tissue (Definition 22-1). Prevention principles evolve from an understanding of these mechanisms of damage.

Compensation Techniques

Brand et al. (1999) recommend the following content for patient education sessions, based on the five mechanisms of damage to insensitive skin. Skin areas over bony prominences are particularly prone to pressure ulcers because the cutaneous tissue is trapped between the unyielding bone and the external pressure. Frequent position changes are necessary for patients with decreased or absent protective sensation to avoid damage caused by **continuous low pressure**. Cushions for seating and shoe insoles help to distribute forces over larger areas.

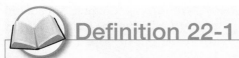

Definition 22-1

Mechanisms of Damage Secondary to Loss of Protective Sensation

- Continuous low pressure: With sustained pressure as light as 1 pound per square inch, capillary flow is blocked; this can cause tissue necrosis, leading to pressure sores (decubitus ulcers).
- Concentrated high pressure: Sudden high force that is accidental and/or a high force applied over a very small area, so that the force is inadequately distributed. This may result in tearing of skin and/or soft tissue or tissue necrosis as a result of insufficient blood supply.
- Excessive heat or cold: Temperature extremes that lead to burn or frostbite injuries.
- Repetitive mechanical stress: Repetitive motions or shearing of skin against clothing or objects that causes inflammation of the tendons or skin. Blistering of skin can also occur.
- Pressure on infected tissue: Continued use and pressure on infected tissue can hinder or prevent the natural healing process.

Adapted from Brand, P. (1979). Management of the insensitive limb. *Physical Therapy, 59*, 8–12.

Instruct patients to avoid **concentrated high pressure** by careful handling of sharp tools and by using enlarged handles on suitcases, drawers, tools, and keys. Patients may need to become consciously aware to use only as much force as necessary to grasp objects. Excessive pressure can also result from splint straps that are too narrow and splints that are too tight; therefore, therapists must carefully construct splints to prevent injury.

Teach patients to increase their awareness of potential sources of **extreme heat or cold** and to protect themselves from contact with them. Insulated coffee mugs are recommended. Oven mitts or quality pot holders are necessary for cooking. Utensils with wooden or plastic handles are better than metal ones. Patients using wheelchairs should insulate exposed hot water pipes under sinks. In cold weather, gloves or mittens are necessary protection for insensate hands.

Instruct patients to avoid **repetitive motions and excessive friction** between skin and objects. Decrease repetitions by working for shorter periods, resting, using a variety of tools, or alternating hands or type of grip. Methods to reduce friction include wearing well-fitting gloves and using enlarged or padded handles on tools.

Educate patients who have lost protective sensation regarding special care for blisters, cuts, and bruises necessary to avoid infection. If infection occurs, in conjunction with treatment for the infection, the **infected part** should be completely rested to keep it **free from pressure** and overuse, allowing healing to occur.

Additional techniques of compensating for absent sensation incorporate reliance on other senses. For example, vision may be used to prevent contact with sharp objects. Using a body part with intact sensation to test water temperature before immersion of any body part without sensation is recommended. Auditory cues may also help to prevent injury. For instance, a person with paraplegia might hear the rubbing of the wheelchair caster against the foot if it slips from its proper position on the leg rest.

Finally, patients should be instructed in good skin care. Applying lotion or oil daily enhances skin hydration. Well-hydrated skin is more elastic and pliant and less prone to injury. Skin needs to be visually inspected daily. A warm or reddened area indicates a possible site of tissue breakdown, which will lead to a decubitus ulcer, and extreme care must be taken to relieve pressure totally from this area until the color returns to normal. *Safety Message: If the time for the skin to recover its normal color exceeds 20 minutes, it is absolutely essential to discover the cause of the skin irritation and correct it. Modification of position, schedule, procedure, equipment, or orthotics is necessary.* If the patient cannot inspect and care for the skin properly, instruct a care provider to perform these tasks every day.

Effectiveness of Compensatory Techniques

A review of the literature reveals no research studies that confirm the effectiveness of instructing patients to avoid injury. These compensatory techniques have face validity in that they evolved out of evidence that patients lacking protective sensation had incurred injuries, many of which could have been prevented. Anecdotal evidence of effectiveness includes Wood's (1969) description of a patient who had a series of hand injuries prior to occupational therapy and none following instruction and fitting of gloves to be worn in his electronics repair work.

Widespread acceptance of compensatory techniques is further evidence of reliance on their assumed effectiveness. The American Diabetes Association (2004) recommends sensory testing of the feet of all people with diabetes so that foot ulcers and amputations can be prevented in those with sensory loss. Techniques of testing and education for patients with diabetes appear in the nursing and physical therapy literature (e.g., Thompson, Medley, & Motts, 2002).

DESENSITIZATION

Desensitization is chosen when the sensory evaluation reveals an area of hypersensitivity, in which ordinary stimuli produce exaggerated or unpleasant sensations (Pillet, Didierjean-Pillet, & Holcombe, 2010). The term hypersensitivity includes allodynia, which is the perception of pain as a result of a nonpainful stimulus, and hyperesthesia, which is a heightened sensitivity to tactile stimuli. Desensitization is an intervention designed to decrease the discomfort associated with touch in the hypersensitive area. A program of desensitization generally includes repetitive stimulation of the hypersensitive skin with items that provide a variety of sensory experiences, such as textures ranging from soft to coarse.

Rationale for Desensitization

Hypersensitivity is observed in some but not all patients following nerve trauma, soft tissue injuries, burns, and amputation. Patients with hypersensitivity tend to avoid using the affected part in functional activities and typically hold the affected part protectively (Hardy, Moran, & Merritt, 1982). Hypersensitivity can lead to disability through nonuse of the involved body part (Robinson & McPhee, 1986).

Desensitization is based on the idea that progressive stimulation will allow progressive tolerance. The origin of the concept of desensitization is unknown. Civil War veterans with amputations were known to tap silver spoons on their residual limbs to improve their tolerance of artificial limbs, which, in those days, were constructed from wood (Hardy et al., 1982). Desensitization can be considered relearning to interpret sensory stimuli as nonnoxious (Dellon, 2000; Jerosch-Herold, 2011), and therefore learning principles and methods apply, including structured practice within the context of functional activities.

Desensitization Techniques

Initially, a patient may have to compensate for hypersensitivity by wearing a splint or padding over the affected area but is gradually weaned from the protective device as improvement occurs. In the treatment program, the patient develops progressive tolerance to a hierarchy of sensory stimuli. Several different hierarchies of desensitization materials exist. The hierarchy described by Hardy, Moran, and Merritt (1982) includes five levels:

- Level 1. Tuning fork, paraffin, massage
- Level 2. Battery-operated vibrator (Fig. 22-1), deep massage, touch pressure with pencil eraser
- Level 3. Electric vibrator, texture identification
- Level 4. Electric vibrator, object identification
- Level 5. Work and daily activities

Desensitization begins outside the area of hypersensitivity and progresses toward the area of greatest sensitivity. Constant contact of the stimulus is preferable to intermittent contact, which may be harmful (Walsh, 2010). Patients advance to the next level after they demonstrate tolerance of the current level without signs of irritation.

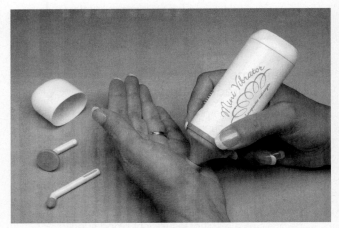

Figure 22-1 The small head of this battery-powered vibrator is useful for desensitization of specific areas of the hand. (Photo courtesy of North Coast Medical, Inc., Gilroy, CA.)

McCabe (2011) suggests use of mirror visual feedback (MVF) in conjunction with a desensitization program. In MVF, the mirror is positioned at the patient's midsagittal plane so that the affected arm is hidden from view behind the mirror and the reflected image of the unaffected limb is in the perceived position of the affected one, thereby giving the impression of the patient having two "normal" limbs. The patient observes the unaffected limb in the mirror as it is touched with various textures. The touch is perceived to be applied to the affected limb and found tolerable. Then the mirror is removed, and the affected limb is actually touched. This procedure has anecdotal clinical support but no research support (McCabe, 2011).

Table 22-1 shows the Downey Hand Center hierarchy of textures and vibration (Barber, 1990/2010; Yerxa et al., 1983). Commercial dowel and immersion textures (Resource 22-1) are similar to this hierarchy. Patients arrange the dowel textures and immersion textures (Fig. 22-2) according to their own perception, in the order of least to most irritating. They select the dowel texture, immersion texture, and vibration level that are uncomfortable but tolerable for 10 minutes three or four times daily. Advancing to the next level of treatment depends on tolerance of lower levels. Documentation should include the patient's initial hierarchy and progress for each of the three modalities (dowel texture, immersion texture, and vibration level).

Other interventions thought to decrease hypersensitivity include weight-bearing pressure, twice daily massage of a surgical scar less than 6 months old with steroid-containing cream, transcutaneous nerve stimulation (TENS), fluidotherapy, and home shower-massager (Dellon, 2000). Use of the affected body part in leisure, work, and daily occupations is believed to facilitate desensitization; the activities must be tailored to the patient's interests and occupations to promote compliance.

Table 22-1 Hierarchy of Texture and Vibration Used in Desensitization

Level	Dowel Textures	Immersion Textures	Vibration
1	Moleskin	Cotton	83 cps near area
2	Felt	Terry cloth pieces	83 cps near area, 23 cps intermittent
3	QuickStick[a]	Dry rice	83 cps near area, 23 cps intermittent
4	Velvet	Popcorn	83 cps intermittent, 23 cps intermittent
5	Semirough cloth	Pinto beans	83 cps intermittent, 23 cps continuous
6	Velcro loop	Macaroni	83 cps continuous, 53 cps intermittent
7	Hard foam	Plastic wire insulation pieces	100 cps intermittent, 53 cps intermittent
8	Burlap	Small BBs, buckshot	100 cps intermittent, 53 cps continuous
9	Rug back	Large BBs, buckshot	100 cps continuous, 53 cps continuous
10	Velcro hook	Plastic squares	No problem with vibration

[a]A closed-cell, firm splint padding material.
Adapted from Barber, L. (1990/2010). Desensitization of the traumatized hand. In J. Hunter, L. Schneider, E. Mackin, & A. Callahan (Eds.), *Rehabilitation of the hand* (3rd ed., pp. 721–730). St. Louis: Mosby. Archived online in T. M. Skirven, A. L. Osterman, J. M. Fedorczyk, & P. C. Amadio (Eds.). (2010). *Rehabilitation of the hand and upper extremity* (6th ed.). Philadelphia: Mosby, Inc./Elsevier.

Effectiveness of Desensitization

Evidence of the effectiveness of desensitization techniques in therapy is limited to a small number of studies. Barber (1990/2010) completed a chart review with descriptive statistics and reported the effectiveness of a graded program. Additional evidence of the success of desensitization includes a narrative single-case study (Robinson & McPhee, 1986) and a small-sample, nonrandomized trial (Hardy, Moran, & Merritt, 1982).

Despite the lack of evidence, desensitization techniques are generally accepted as effective in clinical practice. Experts in the field of hand therapy describe patient improvement and promote use of desensitization techniques (Dellon, 2000; Porretto-Loehrke & Soika, 2010; Walsh, 2010). In a large study of hand therapy practice, all of the therapists surveyed used desensitization techniques on at least some of their patients, and more than half of the therapists elected to use the techniques for 26%–50%

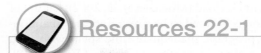

Resources 22-1

Medex Supply

(Sammons-Preston tactile activity kit)
Phone: 888-433-2300
www.medexsupply.com

North Coast Medical

(three-phase desensitization kit, vibrators, stereognosis kit)
Phone: 800-821-9319
www.ncmedical.com

Patterson Medical (formerly Sammons-Preston-Roylan)

(Roylan multi-phase desensitization kit, stereognosis kit)
1000 Remington Boulevard, Suite 210
Bolingbrook, IL 60440-5117
Phone: 800-323-5547; 630-378-6000
Fax: 630-378-6010
www.pattersonmedical.com

Rehabmart

(three-phase desensitization kit)
Phone: 800-827-8283
www.rehabmart.com

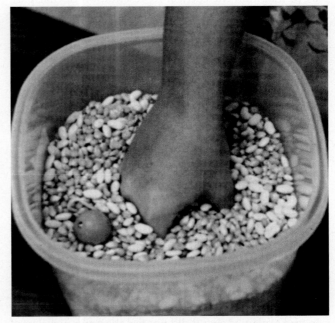

Figure 22-2 Immersion of the hand into a container filled with popcorn kernels and pinto beans facilitates desensitization. Patients use touch to find objects hidden in the immersion particles.

of their patient caseload (Muenzen et al., 2002). Failure of desensitization is believed to be a result of early abandonment of the program, inadequate time spent with each modality, or inappropriate stimulus choice (Walsh, 2010).

SENSORY TRAINING

Because of the newer research evidence concerning brain reorganization in response to lack of stimuli, to repetitive stimuli, and to problem solving, sensory training currently consists of two approaches: passive sensory training and active sensory training. Sensory training may be passive, for those with and without any sensation, or active, for those with beginning return of sensation.

Ninety-nine percent of hand therapists in the United States (Muenzen et al., 2002) and 90% of 70 therapists in 10 European-member countries (Jerosch-Herold, 2011) surveys reported using classical and newer sensory reeducation techniques. Sensory reeducation is an appropriate and commonly used treatment for patients with a variety of peripheral nerve injuries, including nerve lacerations and neural compressions and injuries resulting in replantation, toe-to-thumb grafting, and skin grafting (Dellon, 2000). Sensory reeducation is also used for patients who have diminished or distorted sensation secondary to cerebral vascular accident.

The goals of sensory training are to maintain or restore the cortical hand representation and to regain the use of sensation of the hand (Lundborg & Rosén, 2007; Rosén & Lundborg, 2010). Therefore, treatment must address both the brain and the peripheral nerve. Passive sensory training involves use of repetitive stimulation of the denervated part to maintain the cortical representation of that part. Passive sensory training requires no attention on the part of the patient but improves sensation through long-term highly repetitive stimulation of the patient's skin.

Active sensory training, or sensory reeducation, combines techniques of attention, learning, repeated practice, and use of alternative senses such as vision or hearing to help the patient learn to reinterpret sensation (Dellon, 2000; Jerosch-Herold, 2011; Rosén & Lundborg, 2007, 2010). Dellon (2000), a hand surgeon, related his experience in the 1970s with nerve-injured patients who could feel fingertip stroking, pinprick, and pressure but could not correctly identify a nickel and a quarter using only touch sensation. These patients could feel a difference between the coins, but they could not identify them because the coins did not feel the same as before the injury. Dellon concluded that the sensibility was recovered but that there was a mismatch of the new sensory profile with past profiles in the association cortex. Within a few minutes, he could train patients to tell the difference between the two coins. With the patient's vision shielded, he placed a nickel in the hand, said what it was, and explained that it did not feel the way a nickel used to feel but that what the patient was feeling should thereafter be called a nickel. After repeating the process with a

quarter, the patient could correctly identify both coins. The sensation had been reeducated. Dellon (2000) described sensory retraining strategies based on learning principles. His recommendations included this advice: tailor training and training materials to the interest and ability of the patient, grade the activity so that the patient can meet the expectations for improved performance, and be sure that the patient attends to the stimuli and information provided and perceives them as important and relevant.

Rationale for Sensory Reeducation after Peripheral Nerve Injury or Repair

Cortical hand representation has been found to change immediately as a result of peripheral nerve injuries (Lundborg & Rosén, 2007; Merzenich & Jenkins, 1993). After nerve repair, the corresponding area of the somatosensory cortex reorganizes (Dellon, 2000; Merzenich & Jenkins, 1993). In children, this reorganization is sufficient for return of normal sensory interpretation without sensory retraining. In adults, the neural reorganization requires sensory reeducation (Dellon, 2000; Rosén & Lundborg, 2010; Rosén et al., 1994).

The return of sensation following hand injury is an extremely complex process. Recovery is not just a process of altering the cortical representation; it also depends on reinnervation. Following nerve laceration and surgical repair, some sensory fibers, given sufficient time, regenerate. Peripheral nerve regenerates at a rate of 1 mm per day or 1 inch per month (Dellon, 2000). No surgical repair technique can ensure recovery of tactile discrimination after nerve damage in adults (Lundborg & Rosén, 2007). Sensory return is limited by malalignment of axonal sheaths that allows misdirection of regrowing fibers, meaning that fibers do not usually regrow to innervate the same sensory receptors that they innervated before the injury (Callahan, 1995/2010; Rosén & Lundborg, 2010). Return of sensation is further limited by scar tissue that blocks sensory fiber regrowth and atrophy of sensory receptors prior to reinnervation.

As a result of scar tissue, atrophy of sensory receptors, and the misdirection of fibers, there is an inevitable change in the profile of neural impulses reaching the sensory cortex. A previously well-known stimulus initiates a different set of neural impulses from that elicited by the same stimulus before the injury. When this altered profile reaches the sensory cortex, the patient cannot match it with patterns previously encountered and remembered (Callahan, 1995/2010; Dellon, 2000) and hence cannot identify or recognize the stimulus. According to Rosén and Lundborg (2010), "The hand speaks a new distorted language to the brain" (p. 637). The purpose of active sensory reeducation in patients with peripheral injuries is to help them learn to recognize the new sensory patterns from the hand and associate the new sensation to current movements or tactile experiences (Lundborg & Rosén, 2007).

Sensory Reeducation Techniques after Peripheral Nerve Injury or Repair

In the past, sensory reeducation after peripheral nerve injury or repair was delayed until adequate axonal regeneration and reinnervation of the hand had occurred (Lundborg & Rosén, 2007). However, a newer approach, based on current knowledge of brain plasticity, is to begin phase 1 of sensory reeducation immediately after nerve repair to preserve the cortical representation of the dener-vated part (Lundborg & Rosén, 2007; Rosén & Lundborg, 2010) and has been found effective in improving tactile gnosis (Rosén & Lundborg, 2007). Phase 2 of sensory reeducation begins when the patient first can appreciate deep, moving touch. At first, in phase 2 of reeducation, the patient concentrates on learning to match the sensory perception of stimuli with the visual or auditory perception. The alternative sense, vision or hearing, is used to train the new sensation and thereby improve tactile discrimination (Lundborg & Rosén, 2007). After time, when reinnervation allows for perception of light nonmoving touch with good touch localization, the focus of intervention changes to more functional tasks, such as object identification through touch (Fig. 22-3) (Dellon, 2000).

Phase 1 Techniques

Phase 1 is the period following nerve injury or repair and before the start of reinnervation. During phase 1, the formerly innervated part is without sensation, and cortical representation is undergoing rapid remodeling. Treatment techniques used in phase 1 have the goal of maintaining the cortical hand representation (Lundborg & Rosen, 2007).

Alternative Sensation Techniques. The somatosensory cortex is activated by visual observation of touch (visuotactile interaction) or by listening to the sounds of

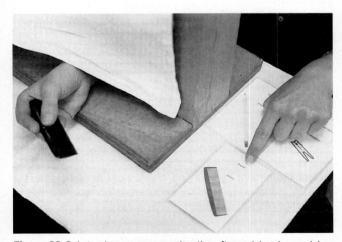

Figure 22-3 Late-phase sensory reeducation after peripheral nerve injury includes identification of various objects by touch.

touching (e.g., a hand touching various textures) (audiotactile interaction) (Lundborg & Rosén, 2007; Rosén & Lundborg, 2007). Visuotactile techniques include direct observation of the part being touched by the therapist and use of a mirror.

One Form of Visuotactile Interaction Therapy: Mirror Therapy or Mirror Visual Feedback Therapy. Mirror therapy was first proposed as a means to relieve amputee phantom limb pain in the 1990s. Therapists have increasingly tried it to treat a range of other chronic pain conditions and as a means to reeducate sensorimotor abilities and capacities in persons with peripheral and central nerve injury (McCabe, 2011). Mirror visual feedback therapy is thought to work by improving sensory perception of the affected limb via false but congruent visual feedback of the unaffected limb, thereby restoring the normal sensory feedback–motor intention linkage (McCabe, 2011). A mirror is placed in front of the patient so that the sensory-deprived hand is hidden behind the mirror and the healthy hand is visible in the mirror and appears as if it were the affected hand. Touching the healthy hand gives the illusion of touching the affected hand. Using a different protocol, Moseley and Wiech (2009) reported that looking towards the reflected hand while the sensory stimulation was applied to the affected hand, hidden behind the mirror, improved two-point discrimination in the affected limb of patients with complex regional pain syndrome and that improvement lasted at least until the 2-day follow-up reevaluation.

Audiotactile Interaction Therapy. Audiotactile interaction techniques can range from simple (listening and identifying sounds of the healthy hand touching various textures) to complex (Sensor Glove System mechanism with microphones and ear phones that allows the patient to listen intently to what the hand feels) (Rosén & Lundborg, 2007).

Deficient Sensation Techniques: Selective Cutaneous Anesthesia. Deafferentation of a specific cortical area, such as that serving the shoulder and elbow, allows expansion of adjacent cortical representation areas, such as the hand (Björkman, Rosén, & Lundborg, 2004; Lundborg & Rosén, 2007). Therefore, cutaneous deafferentation of the forearm of the affected hand should result in expansion of the adjacent hand representation (Rosén, Björkman, & Lundborg, 2006). Cutaneous deafferentation of the forearm is accomplished using a topical anesthetic cream (2.5% lidocaine and 2.5% prilocaine) applied for 1 hour twice a week for 2 weeks in conjunction with classical sensory retraining (Lundborg & Rosén, 2007; Rosén, Björkman, & Lundborg, 2006). This procedure was found to be significantly effective in two small samples of persons with ulnar or median nerve repair in improving perception of touch/pressure, tactile gnosis, and two-point discrimination as compared with the control/placebo groups (Hassan-Zadeh et al., 2009; Rosén, Björkman, & Lundborg, 2006).

Phase 2 Techniques

Phase 2, active sensory reeducation, begins with the start of reinnervation of the hand. Sensory reeducation protocols differ among facilities, even those treating patients with similar diagnoses. A summary of the protocol Dellon (2000) presented from the Raymond M. Curtis Hand Center of Union Memorial Hospital, which is based on his earlier work, is given in Procedures for Practice 22-1. Others describe similar procedures. They begin each moving and constant touch sequence with eyes closed, followed by eyes open, and concluding with eyes closed. They recommend using a smaller and lighter stimulus as the patient

improves, with a goal of localization of a touch that is near the light-touch threshold. Touch localization continues throughout the sensory reeducation process, and more tasks are added to the training program. Discrimination of similar and different textures using sandpaper, fabrics, and edges of coins are introduced early. Patients practice identification of shape or letter blocks and graphesthesia, which is the ability to identify a letter or number drawn on the skin. In the later stages of training, patients feel for objects from containers filled with sand or rice and identify them by feel before looking at them for feedback. They progress to practicing identification of common objects. A variety of activities, including games or puzzles, are more engaging and therefore may be more beneficial than simply practicing with various objects. Finally, patients practice daily living activities, especially those in which the hand is out of the line of vision.

 Procedures for Practice 22-1

Phase 2 Sensory Reeducation

Sensory Reeducation Principles

- Choose a quiet environment that will maximize concentration.
- Sessions in the clinic should be brief, approximately 5–15 minutes, two or three times a week.
- Because in-clinic training is brief, homework practice sessions are important. Three or four 5-minute sessions per day are recommended.
- Instruct the patient and/or family in techniques to be used during practice.
- Monitor patient's home program and progress during therapy sessions.
- Allow frequent rest breaks during which the patient can open his eyes. This reduces feelings of disorientation and anxiety.

Prerequisites for Early-Phase 2 Sensory Reeducation

- Patient must be able to perceive 30 cycles per second vibration and moving touch in the area.
- Patient must be motivated and able to follow through with the program.

Techniques for Early-Phase 2 Sensory Reeducation

- Use the eraser end of a pencil.
- Apply moving strokes to the area.
- Use enough pressure for the patient to perceive the stimulus but not so much that it causes pain.
- Ask the patient to observe what is happening first and then to close the eyes and concentrate on what is being felt.

- Instruct the patient to put into words (silently) what is being felt.
- Instruct the patient to observe the stimulus again to confirm the sensory experience with the perception.
- When perception of constant touch returns to the area, use a similar process for constant touch stimuli.
- Test the patient by requiring localization of moving and constant touch without seeing the stimulus.

Prerequisites for Late-Phase 2 Sensory Reeducation

- Patient must be able to perceive constant and moving touch at the fingertips.
- Patient must demonstrate good localization of touch.

Techniques for Late-Phase 2 Sensory Reeducation

- Use a collection of common objects that differ in size and shape.
- Instruct the patient to grasp and manipulate each item with eyes open, then with eyes closed, and then with eyes open for reinforcement.
- The patient should concentrate on the tactile perception.
- Grade the practice by starting with large familiar objects with great differences in size, shape, and texture. Further grade practice by introducing objects of similar sizes but different textures and then small objects that vary in size and shape but are similar in texture.
- Test the patient by counting the number of objects correctly identified or the time required to correctly identify each object without vision.

Adapted from Dellon, A. L. (2000). *Somatosensory testing and rehabilitation*. Baltimore: The Institute for Peripheral Nerve Surgery.

Nakada and Uchida (1997) described a five-stage sensory reeducation program that was useful for a patient with very limited sensation in her left hand as a result of peripheral neuropathy secondary to leprosy (Hansen's disease). She also had total impairment of vision, so that sensory feedback was critical to occupational performance. Following reeducation, the patient regained hand function for activities of daily living such as drying dishes, putting on socks, and holding dentures while brushing them. The reeducation program included the following five stages:

- Stage 1. Object recognition using feature detection strategies. Objects that varied greatly in shape, material, and weight were used. The patient was encouraged to handle each object, pay attention to the object, and identify the characteristics of the object.
- Stage 2. Prehension of various objects with refinement of prehension patterns. In this stage, grasping objects that varied in size and shape was emphasized. The patient needed to maximize the contact between the object and the hand to develop the ability of the hand to closely contour to objects, which is seen in normal grasp.
- Stage 3. Control of prehension force while holding objects. Feedback regarding excessive force that was used to maintain grasp was provided through the use of a strain gauge and therapy putty.
- Stage 4. Maintenance of prehension force during transport of objects. While holding an object, the patient moved the shoulder, elbow, and wrist into varying positions of flexion and extension.
- Stage 5. Object manipulation. The patient practiced grasp and release of objects and moved objects in the hand into various positions.

Appropriate grading of sensory reeducation activities is important to optimize patient motivation and progress. Choose activities that provide a challenge but allow for success. During stimulus localization tasks, progress from firm pressure to lighter pressure. When working with objects, progress from larger items to smaller items and from dissimilar items to more similar items. Progress from differentiation of a few objects to selecting, sequencing, or organizing many objects.

Because daily training is necessary for successful sensory reeducation, teach patients techniques appropriate for after-therapy practice. Patients can be involved in assembling their own collection of objects for use in their program. Include objects with varying size, shape, texture, weight, and temperature (Fess, 2002/2010). Development of a new set of stimulus-response associations has been shown to require thousands of trials (Lewis et al., 2009). Recovery from peripheral nerve injury can take years and is often incomplete with ongoing discomfort and poor tactile gnosis (Jerosch-Herold, 2011).

Effectiveness of Sensory Reeducation after Peripheral Nerve Injury or Repair

To evaluate the effectiveness of sensory reeducation following peripheral nerve injury, Oud et al. (2007) reviewed the 7 out of 760 identified studies that met inclusion criteria. Five of those were characterized by poor methodological quality; the methodology of the two others was adequate to high quality. They concluded that there was positive but limited evidence for the effectiveness of sensory reeducation. This review represents the best evidence in the therapy literature for the effectiveness of sensory reeducation to date. Further evidence is described in Evidence Table 22-1. Sensory reeducation effectiveness following digital replantation and revascularization has also been demonstrated in a small, randomized controlled trial (Shieh et al., 1995).

Rationale for Sensory Treatment after Cerebral Vascular Accident

Loss of sensation impairs a person's ability to explore the immediate environment and execute everyday tasks and therefore affects quality of life and personal safety (Carey, Macdonell, & Matyas, 2011; Smith et al., 2009). Sensory dysfunction following stroke involves tactile discrimination and proprioceptive senses more than pain or temperature senses (Carr & Shepherd, 2010). This loss significantly limits the use of the upper limb (Doyle et al. 2010). Functional use of the arm and hand with reduced sensation is possible, but spontaneous use is limited. Without training, there is a tendency not to use the extremity, and learned nonuse leads to further loss of sensory and motor abilities (Dannenbaum & Dykes, 1988; Sabari & Lieberman, 2008). Therapists may alter the cortical map by directing the sensory experiences of the patient. Increased cerebral blood flow and changed cerebral activation in the somatosensory cortex following proprioceptive stimulation has been demonstrated experimentally (Nelles et al., 1999).

Studies of both passive and active therapeutic interventions have shown improvements in use of the extremity. Passive sensory training is based on evidence of cortical reorganization in response to repetitive stimulation. Passive sensory training procedures involve extensive repetitive stimulation applied to the impoverished part and do not require participation by the patient. Carr and Shepherd (2010), in their review of the scientific evidence for the ability of the brain to reorganize following brain lesions, stated that reorganization seems to be related to frequency of use.

Active sensory training after cerebral vascular accident (CVA) is based on the concepts of neural plasticity and learning. Carr and Shepherd (2010) suggested that enlargement of sensory receptive areas within the cortex is a result of increased participation of the body part in activities requiring

Evidence Table 22-1		Best Evidence for Occupational Therapy Practice Regarding Sensory Reeducation				

Intervention	Description of Intervention Tested	Participants	Dosage	Type of Best Evidence and Level of Evidence	Benefit	Statistical Probability and Effect Size of Outcome	Reference
Early tactile stimulation for digital nerve injuries	In-clinic stimulation of digital sensation by pressing injured finger against rotating disc with raised and lowered segments; home program of rubbing finger over rows of raised staples on a plastic card	Forty-nine subjects with a total of 65 digital nerve injuries following surgical repair	Clinical program required 20 minutes twice weekly; home program completed daily, as much as patient desired; clinic program averaged 11 weeks in duration; home program averaged 16 weeks	Randomized controlled trial, using ordinal measures and nonparametric statistics; Level: IB2a	More participants in the experimental group recovered touch threshold measuring 0.217 g or less, and static and moving two-point discrimination of 6 mm or less.	$p = 0.097$, $r = 0.22$ for touch threshold; $p = 0.0023$, $r = 0.48$ for static two-point discrimination; and $p = 0.0144$, $r = 0.36$ for moving two-point discrimination	Cheng, 2000; Cheng et al., 2001
Temporary anesthesia in combination with sensory reeducation	Experimental: Anesthetic cream (Lidocaine-PTC) applied to the flexor aspect of the affected arm (from wrist to 15 cm of forearm) under occlusive bandage; sensory reeducation not described; Control: Placebo + sensory reeducation	Thirteen patients with median ($n = 7$) or ulnar ($n = 6$) nerve repair at wrist level; age range 20–43 years; range of time since surgery 5–38 months; randomly assigned to experimental or control groups	One hour, two times per week, for 2 weeks + reeducation time	Randomized controlled trial; Level: IC2b	Yes. Perception of touch (Semmes–Weinstein monofilaments) improved significantly immediately and at 4-week follow-up in the experimental vs. control group. Two-point discrimination (Disk-Criminator) improved significantly immediately and at 4-week follow-up in the experimental vs. control group. Effects were large for all comparisons.	Differences between groups: touch perception, $p = 0.025$, $r = 0.56$ for post treatment and $p = 0.003$, $r = 0.76$ for 4-week follow-up; two-point discrimination, $p = 0.000$, $r = 0.97$ for post treatment and $p = 0.001$, $r = 0.85$ for 4-week follow-up	Hassan-Zadeh et al., 2009

Perceptual learning-based sensory discrimination to improve lost abilities of texture discrimination, limb position sense, tactile object recognition	Experimental: Graded progression of discrimination from easy to difficult; attentive exploration with vision occluded, anticipation trials, cross-modal calibration via vision, feedback on sensation and method of exploration, intermittent feedback and self-checking of accuracy, feedback on ability to identify distinctive features in novel stimuli (shape, size, weight, texture, hardness, temperature), summary feedback, and intensive training; Control: grasping of various objects and passive movements of the limb	Fifty subjects with impaired tactile discrimination, limb position sense, and/ or tactile object recognition at least 6 weeks poststroke. Randomized to experimental and control groups, with attrition of 3; mean age = 61 years; 29 left and 21 right hemispheric lesions; Median time poststroke = 48.14 weeks	Trained on each sensory task in random sequence for 15–20 minutes at a time. Ten total treatment sessions of 60-minute duration, 3 times/week	Randomized controlled trial with blinding of subjects, assessors, and data analysts; Level: IA1a	Yes. Sensory retraining is effective in improving sensory discrimination in stroke survivors in the chronic phase of recovery. Thirty-six percent of subjects had a reduction of deficit of at least 50%, 24% performed in the normal range, and only 2 did not show improvement. There were no adverse effects. Improvement lasted at 6-week and 6-month follow-ups. Effects transferred to novel stimuli not trained.	Sensory discrimination of the experimental group improved 19.1 points on the composite standardized somatosensory deficit index as compared with 8.0 points by the control group ($t_{47} = 2.75$, $p = 0.004$, $r = 0.38$).	Carey, Macdonell, & Matyas, 2011

tactile sensations. Therefore, the goal of both passive and active sensory treatment after CVA is to gain a larger cortical representation for the areas of skin from which sensory feedback is crucial to performance of daily tasks.

Sensory Therapeutic Techniques after Cerebral Vascular Accident

Cerebrovascular accident often disrupts the sensory–motor relationship of the affected side, resulting in paralysis or weakness, sensory loss or distortion, and subsequent loss of spontaneous usage and occupational performance. Therapy to recover motor behavior was discussed in the previous chapter, and therapy to recover occupational performance is discussed in the chapter on stroke (Chapter 33). Here, therapy to improve sensory awareness and discrimination of the affected limb is described.

Passive Sensory Training

Passive sensory training or tactile coactivation via electrical stimulation or repetitive mechanical stimulation is applied to the patient and does not require the patient's active attention. The following studies provide guidelines for application of these types of interventions, although no standard protocol has been established.

In a study of passive tactile coactivation to improve sensorimotor functions in healthy elderly, Kalisch, Tegenthoff, and Dinse (2008) demonstrated significant improvement in tactile acuity (two-point discrimination), haptic object recognition, and fine motor object manipulation skills as compared with a sham control group. The tactile coactivation was administered via 8-mm solenoid devices attached to each finger of the dominant hand. These devices tapped the fingertips to deliver stimuli to the dermal mechanoreceptors in the fingertip skin. The taps of approximately 100 microns for 10 milliseconds with a variable interstimulus interval of 100–300 milliseconds were delivered for 3 hours, during which the subject could move and pay attention to other activities such as watching TV or reading. The sham group participated in the same setup but did not receive tactile coactivation via the taps. Touch thresholds did not change significantly in either group. Two-point discrimination thresholds were significantly ($p \leq 0.007$) and strongly ($r = 0.52$) lowered (improved) in the coactivation group. Time to complete ($p = 0.004; r = 0.56$) haptic object recognition and number of errors ($p = 0.019; r = 0.58$) reduced significantly in the experimental group. Manipulation of fine objects improved significantly in the experimental group as compared with the sham group ($p \leq 0.001; r = 0.65$). The researchers suggest this treatment as potentially useful in improving sensorimotor functions in patients.

Smith et al. (2009) conducted a preexperimental study of the effects of tactile coactivation via electrical impulses on four persons with a Fugl-Meyer Motor Assessment upper extremity subtest score of 56–60 and loss of sensory abilities more than 6 months poststroke. The fingers of the involved hand were electrically stimulated (20-Hz single pulses of 5–50 mA current range in bursts of 1 second with a 5-second interburst interval) for 90 minutes, 4 days a week for 6 weeks. There was improvement in sensory discrimination and motor task performance in all four subjects, and the results held over the 4-week follow-up period, although no statistical analysis was reported. There were no adverse reactions.

In another, more controlled study of 36 patients in the acute stage of recovery post-CVA, the results were equivocal between two groups receiving Bobath neurodevelopmental treatment or Bobath neurodevelopmental treatment plus electrical stimulation of the wrist and finger extensors. That is, both groups improved in kinesthetic sense and proprioception, as well as hand movement (Yozbatiran et al., 2006). The results cannot be appreciated separately from ongoing recovery that occurs during the acute stage. Although the use of passive interventions makes sense on the basis of documented effects of repetitive peripheral stimulation on brain reorganization (Jenkins, Merzenich, & Ochs, 1990), the evidence to date is insufficient to recommend a particular protocol.

Active Sensory Training

Sensory reeducation after CVA is less well defined than the protocols described for peripheral injuries. Carr and Shepherd, in their book *Neurological Rehabilitation* (2010), emphasize task-specific sensory training in which learning occurs concurrently with motor learning. They advocate the use of meaningful and relevant sensory and motor experiences very early in rehabilitation. Use of the more involved hand in bimanual tasks such as opening jars and using eating utensils is advocated. They suggest that the patient be cued to attend to the goal of the task and the tactile aspects of the objects involved in the task.

Dannenbaum and Jones (1993) gave detailed goals and proposed methodology for sensory intervention following CVA. According to them, appreciation of some form of tactile stimulation and some basic motor skills are prerequisite to success in sensory reeducation. To establish that a patient with severe sensory loss can perceive some stimuli, they recommend testing and early training using 100-Hz electrical stimulation. Patients identify which finger was stimulated, first with vision and then with eyes closed. Patients with better sensation perform a similar task, first with textured moving stimuli followed by nonmoving stimuli. In addition, they suggested early incorporation of the hand into functional activities and prevention of abnormal patterns of grasp and movement. Further suggestions are to add textures to handle surfaces to increase the friction and support weak grasping ability, to enlarge or modify handles to facilitate both tactile contact and tactile feedback, and to have patients practice modulation of grip forces in response to various objects and maintenance of appropriate grip force during forearm movements.

Yekutiel and Guttman's (1993) research protocol included the following sensory reeducation activities, all completed with vision occluded:

- Identification of the number of touches
- Identification of numbers or letters drawn on the arm or hand (graphesthesia tests)
- "Find your thumb" without looking
- Discrimination of shape, weight, and texture of objects or materials placed in the hand
- Passive drawing and writing: patient identification of a letter, number, or drawing made by the therapist passively moving the patient's hand while it holds a pencil

They started and ended each session with sensory tasks the person could do.

Mirror Therapy

Mirror therapy is reported to elicit cortical activation (Dohle et al., 2009) and restore sensorimotor linkage (McCabe, 2011) in patients post-CVA. The mirror is placed so that the unaffected arm appears to be in the position of the affected arm. The patient is asked to move both limbs into a variety of gradually more difficult postures. One protocol for mirror visual feedback is outlined in Procedures for Practice 22-2.

A secondary finding in a study of mirror therapy used in combination with standard therapy to improve motor recovery in severely affected patients after initial ischemic stroke was a significant ($p = 0.009$) and strong effect ($\eta = 0.57$) on light touch, as measured by the sensory subscale of the Fugl-Meyer Motor Assessment, compared with a control condition of viewing the affected extremity (Dohle et al., 2009). In this study, the mirror was placed in the participant's midsagittal plane, presenting the mirror image of the nonaffected arm as if it were the affected one. The therapy protocol for both the experimental and control groups required execution of arm, hand, and finger postures in response to verbal instruction. Both groups were told to move the affected limb as well as possible. Neither the side nor site of the lesion were related to outcome.

These sensory treatment activities are just a few examples of a wide variety of techniques that can be used in clinical treatment for patients after CVA. Therapists working with this population use creativity, patients' interests, and theoretical understanding to develop programs of sensory intervention because no one protocol has been widely accepted or thoroughly researched.

Effectiveness of Sensory Reeducation after Cerebral Vascular Accident

Multiple interventions for upper limb sensory impairment after stroke are described in the literature, but Doyle et al. (2010) concluded from their review of 13 studies out of a pool of 662 possible studies that there is insufficient evidence to support or refute their effectiveness in improving sensory

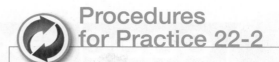

Procedures for Practice 22-2

One Protocol of Mirror Visual Feedback Therapy in Sensory Reeducation

1. Remove all jewelry that could interfere with imagining the reflected limb as the affected limb.
2. Position the patient comfortably so that the mirror is easily accommodated between the upper limbs and the patient can visualize the reflected unaffected limb. The mirror should be large enough to hide the affected limb and to show the entire reflected limb while the patient performs a range of bilateral movements.
3. Ask the patient to look at the reflected limb, without movement, and to try to believe that it is his affected limb.
4. Once the patient feels engaged with the mirrored limb, have him perform slow, easy-to-achieve bilateral movements while looking at the reflected image.
5. Check behind the mirror to see that the affected arm is moving, moving synchronously, and not stopping after initial movement. For those for whom movement is impossible, they should simply look at the reflected image until they are able to progress to moving.
6. To fully believe in the illusion requires concentration; therefore, the technique should be used often, but for short periods (five or six times per day until concentration is lost, but no longer than 5 minutes). Patients are advised to practice this therapy in a quiet area, without distraction, so that concentration can be at the optimum.
7. If adverse effects are observed (e.g., dystonia, tremor, increased pain levels), therapy should be stopped immediately. Otherwise, the patient is advised to carry out the therapy as long as he perceives it to be helpful.
8. Contraindications to mirror visual feedback therapy are motor extinction, increased pain, exacerbation of movement disorders, and inability to believe in the illusion.

Adapted from McCabe, C. (2011). Mirror visual feedback therapy. A practical approach. *Journal of Hand Therapy, 24,* 170–179.

impairment. This review included only studies that used the randomized controlled trial design. Three of the 13 studies examined active sensory training, and the remainder studied passive sensory training. Schabrun and Hillier (2009) concluded from their systematic review of 14 studies that met their inclusion criteria, involving 199 subjects, that there is some evidence to support use of passive sensory training on patients poststroke, but at this time data are insufficient to determine the effectiveness of active sensory training. The best evidence of effectiveness of active sensory reeducation following CVA is the study by Carey, Macdonell, and Matyas (2011), published after the above-mentioned reviews were completed and described in Evidence Table 22-1. That carefully controlled study of 50 subjects showed significant and large improvement using a systematic program that heavily incorporated principles of learning.

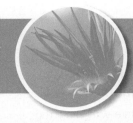

case example
Mr. T.: Sensory Remediation after Median Nerve Laceration

Occupational Therapy Intervention Process	Clinical Reasoning Process	
	Objectives	Examples of Therapist's Internal Dialogue
Patient Information	Appreciate the context	(See Chapter 9 for description of the assessment process and patient's background.)
Mr. T., a 25-year-old appliance repairman with a laceration of the median nerve, was reassessed approximately 6 weeks after his injury. The outpatient occupational therapy reassessment identified the following sensory problems:	Develop intervention hypotheses	"Although a good bit of time in therapy will be spent on Mr. T.'s motor deficits, I know that good sensation is needed for hand coordination and for return to full function at work."
• Absent and decreased protective sensation in the thumb, index and middle fingers, and radial palm • Mislocalization of touch sensations in the radial portion of the palm • Hypersensitivity in the area of the scar • Decreased ability to pick up and manipulate objects • Decreased use of the right hand in functional activities	Select an intervention approach	"Because Mr. T. has multiple sensory issues, he will need multiple approaches. A compensatory approach will be needed for lost protective sensation, and a remedial approach will be needed to decrease hypersensitivity and relearn touch localization and object identification."
	Reflect on competence	"As I work with Mr. T., I may need to discuss ideas with a colleague, particularly for creative sensory retraining strategies to increase the variety of activities."
Recommendations	Consider the patient's appraisal of performance	"Mr. T. has demonstrated quick learning of therapy instructions so far. He does not seem to fully understand the connection between sensation exercises and his eventual hand function, so I may need to give him more examples of how he uses sensory feedback in his work and daily activities."
The occupational therapist recommended outpatient occupational therapy twice a week for 6 weeks followed by reassessment, with reduction to one session per week likely at that time. Mr. T. has demonstrated quick learning of therapy instructions and will be responsible for an intensive home program. Because recovery of the ability to differentiate small objects at the fingertips will probably not occur until 10–12 months after the nerve repair, therapy would ideally continue for that length of time. In collaboration with Mr. T., the occupational therapist established the following long-term goals for sensory intervention:	Consider what will occur in therapy, how often, and for how long	"During therapy, I will definitely need to focus on teaching Mr. T. what he needs to do at home. Experts in the field of hand therapy suggest that the home program should be completed three to four times daily. The various aspects of the program should not require more than 10 minutes at a time to facilitate compliance. During therapy sessions, I will need to provide evaluation of progress, grading of sensory activities for the home program, and motivational strategies."
• Mr. T. will correctly interpret sensory stimuli throughout the right hand, as demonstrated by correct tactile identification of objects. • Mr. T. will demonstrate good use of the right hand in work simulation activities that rely on touch sensation.	Ascertain the patient's endorsement of plan	"Mr. T. seems eager to complete therapy tasks right now, and if he follows through with his home program, that should further indicate his agreement with the plan of care."

Summary of Short-Term Goals and Progress

1. Mr. T. will avoid injury to the right hand by demonstrating compensatory protective strategies during functional activities. The therapist instructed Mr. T. about risk of injury from sharp and hot objects and gripping forces. Mr. T. and the therapist discussed an appropriate routine for skin care and implementation of precautions in his daily routine. By the end of the second session, Mr. T. demonstrated good understanding of these techniques during home and simple work simulation activities.

2. Mr. T. will tolerate touch of all textures over and around his scar area so that hypersensitivity does not interfere with functional hand use. Mr. T. ranked the 10 dowel textures from least to most irritating. At that time, he easily tolerated the first four textures as they were rubbed by the therapist over the scar area. He disliked touch from the fifth texture and was unable to tolerate textures 6–10. The therapist provided textures for a home desensitization program, beginning with textures 5 and 6. Mr. T. used these textures three or four times a day for scar desensitization. During therapy sessions, massage and vibration were provided around and over the scar area. At the end of 3 weeks, Mr. T. tolerated all textures and no longer reported discomfort from sleeve cuffs or inadvertent touch during functional activities.

3. Mr. T. will demonstrate touch localization below 10 mm in the right palm to improve interpretation of tactile sensations during work activities. The therapist initiated a sensory reeducation program for touch localization using moving and static touch stimuli in the palm. Instructions were provided, and Mr. T. faithfully followed through with this program at home, four sessions per day. At the end of 3 weeks, localization in the palm measured 12–14 mm. The therapist initiated graphesthesia and texture discrimination activities in the palmar area. After 6 weeks of sensory reeducation, localization measured 9–10 mm, and Mr. T. could identify 50% of the letters and shapes drawn in his palm and 40% of the textures.

Next Steps

Revised Short-Term Goals (1 month):
To improve interpretation of tactile sensations during work activities, Mr. T. will demonstrate:

- 100% correct graphesthesia and texture identification in his right palm
- touch localization below 10 mm in the proximal phalanges of the right thumb, index, and middle fingers

Assess the patient's comprehension	"Mr. T. not only understands his home program but is also learning when to progress to the next dowel texture without me needing to tell him."
Understand what he is doing	
Compare actual to expected performance	"Mr. T. is progressing even faster than I expected he would in his desensitization program. His sensory reeducation is proceeding at the expected rate, consistent with the typical rate of neural regrowth."
Know the person	"Mr. T. demonstrated such good learning of techniques that, after these first 3 weeks, I could consider decreasing the frequency of therapy for his sensory deficits to once weekly. He will need to continue his home program at the same intensity of three to four sessions daily. Whether or not to decrease frequency of therapy will also depend on how his motor recovery is progressing."
Appreciate the context	
Anticipate present and future patient concerns	"Mr. T. has made exceptional progress over the past 6 weeks and is eager to return to work, which will make attendance at therapy and completion of his home exercise program more difficult."
Analyze patient's comprehension	"Mr. T. continues to need extensive home program activities to improve his sensation. He has learned his home program well and knows how to advance it."
Decide if the patient should continue or discontinue therapy and/ or return in the future	"Because recovery of the ability to differentiate small objects at the fingertips will probably not occur until 10–12 months after the nerve repair, he will require ongoing sensory reeducation for at least a year or more. It would be advisable to follow up with reassessment and program revision every 2–3 months during that time period. This will also help Mr. T. to be more motivated to continue his home program throughout this long time period."

Clinical Reasoning in Occupational Therapy Practice

Transition of Sensory Reeducation Program from Early Phase to Late Phase

Mr. T. will begin the second phase of sensory reeducation at the fingertips approximately 6–8 months after his surgery to repair the median nerve. What reassessment findings will indicate the appropriate time for Mr. T. to begin late-phase sensory reeducation? What treatment activities and home program activities would be appropriate for Mr. T. as he begins this phase? What work simulation activities could be incorporated into his therapy program during sensory reeducation?

Clinical Reasoning in Occupational Therapy Practice

Facilitating the Effects of Desensitization and Sensory Reeducation through Mirror Therapy

Mr. T. read about mirror therapy in the popular press. He asked his therapist about incorporating mirror therapy into his program. The therapist has heard about the use of mirror therapy for patients with amputation and stroke, but not for improving sensory abilities and capacities. Instead of immediately agreeing or disagreeing to this request, how should the therapist proceed? How will the therapist and Mr. T. use it as part of the desensitization program? The reeducation program? What recommendations does the therapist make regarding incorporating mirror therapy into Mr. T.'s home program?

Summary Review Questions

1. What are the rationales for sensory reeducation after peripheral nerve injury or repair and CVA?
2. What are the differences and similarities between early-phase 2 and late-phase 2 sensory reeducation for patients with peripheral nerve injury or repair?
3. Describe or demonstrate intervention techniques for a patient with hypersensitivity after a fingertip amputation.
4. List five mechanisms of injury for skin areas with absent or diminished protective sensation. For each of the five mechanisms of injury, describe appropriate preventive education and/or adaptive strategies.
5. What should be done if a patient with sensory loss develops an area of skin redness?
6. Describe the procedure for mirror therapy to reeducate sensory perception.

Glossary

Active sensory training—The patient is actively involved in the reeducation process. Sensory retraining is based on learning principles.

Allodynia—Condition in which nonpainful stimuli produce painful sensations.

Decubitus ulcer—Open sore caused by pressure, friction, and moisture. These factors lead to reduced blood flow to the area and consequent tissue death. The most common sites for decubitus ulcers are over bony prominences.

Graphesthesia—The ability to identify numbers or letters traced on the skin.

Hyperesthesia—Condition in which there is increased sensitivity to somatosensory stimuli.

Hypersensitivity—Condition in which ordinary stimuli produce an exaggerated or unpleasant sensation.

Learned nonuse—Loss of capacity in an impaired extremity because of a tendency to avoid using that extremity and to use other body parts instead.

Motor extinction—Motor neglect; underutilization of one side, without defects of strength, reflexes, or sensibility (McCabe, 2011).

Passive sensory training—Stimulation applied to the patient who is not required to pay attention (Kalisch, Tegenthoff, & Dinse, 2008). Sensory training is delivered via high-repetition modalities, e.g., mechanical tapping, electrical stimulation, passive rubbing of the skin surface over highly textured materials.

Protective sensation—Painful sensation evoked by potentially damaging sensory stimuli, such as excessive temperature, pressure, or tissue stress.

Tactile gnosis—Functional tactile perception; ability to complete functional tasks through the use of sensory feedback.

References

American Diabetes Association. (2004). Position statement: Preventive foot care in diabetes. *Diabetes Care, 27,* S63–S64.

Barber, L. (1990/2010). Desensitization of the traumatized hand. In J. Hunter, L. Schneider, E. Mackin, & A. Callahan (Eds.), *Rehabilitation of the hand* (3rd ed., pp. 721–730). St. Louis: Mosby, Inc.. Archived online in T. M. Skirven, A. L. Osterman, J. M. Fedorczyk, & P. C. Amadio (Eds.). (2010). *Rehabilitation of the hand and upper extremity* (6th ed.). Philadelphia: Mosby, Inc./Elsevier.

Björkman, A., Rosén, B., & Lundborg, G. (2004). Acute improvement of hand sensibility after selective ipsilateral cutaneous forearm anesthesia. *European Journal of Neuroscience, 20,* 2733–2736.

Brand, P. (1979). Management of the insensitive limb. *Physical Therapy, 59,* 8–12.

Brand, P. W., Hollister, A. M., Giurintano, D., & Thompson, D. E. (1999). External stress: Effect at the surface. In P. W. Brand & A. M. Hollister (Eds.), *Clinical mechanics of the hand* (3rd ed., pp. 215–232). St. Louis: Mosby.

Callahan, A. D. (1995/2010). Methods of compensation and reeducation for sensory dysfunction. In J. M. Hunter, E. J. Mackin, & A. D. Callahan (Eds.). *Rehabilitation of the hand: Surgery and therapy* (4th ed., pp. 701–713). St. Louis: Mosby. Archived online in T. M. Skirven, A. L. Osterman, J. M. Fedorczyk, & P. C. Amadio (Eds.). (2010). *Rehabilitation of the hand and upper extremity* (6th ed.). Philadelphia: Mosby, Inc./Elsevier.

Carey, L., Macdonell, R., & Matyas, T. A. (2011). SENSe: Study of the effectiveness of neurorehabilitation on sensation: A randomized controlled trial. *Neurorehabilitation and Neural Repair, 25,* 304–313.

Carr, J. H., & Shepherd, R. B. (2010). *Neurological rehabilitation: Optimizing motor performance* (2nd ed.). London: Churchill Livingstone/Elsevier.

Cheng, A. S. (2000). Use of early tactile stimulation in rehabilitation of digital nerve injuries. *American Journal of Occupational Therapy, 54,* 159–165.

Cheng, A. S., Hung, L., Wong, J. M., Lau, H., & Chan, J. (2001). A prospective study of early tactile stimulation after digital nerve repair. *Clinical Orthopedics and Related Research, 384,* 169–175.

Cole, J. (1991). *Pride and a daily marathon.* Cambridge, MA: MIT.

Dannenbaum, R. M., & Dykes, R. (1988). Sensory loss in the hand after sensory stroke: Therapeutic rationale. *Archives of Physical Medicine and Rehabilitation, 69,* 833–839.

Dannenbaum, R. M., & Jones, L. A. (1993). The assessment and treatment of patients who have sensory loss following cortical lesions. *Journal of Hand Therapy, 6,* 130–138.

Dellon, A. L. (2000). *Somatosensory testing and rehabilitation.* Baltimore: The Institute for Peripheral Nerve Surgery.

Dohle, C., Püllen, Nakaten, A., Küst, J., Rietz, C., & Karbe, H. (2009). Mirror therapy promotes recovery from severe hemiparesis: A randomized controlled trial. *Neurorehabilitation and Neural Repair, 23,* 209–217.

Doyle, S., Bennett, S., Fasoli, S. E., & McKenna, K. T. (2010). Interventions for sensory impairment in the upper limb after stroke. *Cochrane Database of Systematic Reviews,* Issue 6, Art No. CD006331, DOI: 10:1002/14651858.CD006331.pub2.

Duff, S. V., & Estilow, T. (2010). Therapist's management of peripheral nerve injury. In T. M. Skirven, A. L. Osterman, J. M. Fedorczyk, & P. C. Amadio (Eds.), *Rehabilitation of the hand and upper extremity* (6th ed., pp. 619–633). Philadelphia: Mosby, Inc./Elsevier.

Fess, E. E. (2002/2010). Sensory reeducation. In E. J. Mackin, A. D. Callahan, T. M. Skirven, L. H. Schneider, A. L. Osterman, & J. M. Hunter (Eds.), *Rehabilitation the hand and upper extremity* (5th ed., pp. 635–639). St. Louis: Mosby. Archived online in T. M. Skirven, A. L. Osterman, J. M. Fedorczyk, & P. C. Amadio (Eds.). (2010). *Rehabilitation of the Hand and Upper Extremity* (6th ed.). Philadelphia: Mosby, Inc./Elsevier.

Hardy, M., Moran, C., & Merritt, W. (1982). Desensitization of the traumatized hand. *Virginia Medical Journal, 109,* 134–137.

Hassan-Zadeh, R., Lajevardi, L., Esfahani, A. R., & Kamali, M. (2009). Improvement of hand sensibility after selective temporary anaesthesia in combination with sensory re-education. *Neurorehabilitation, 24,* 383–386.

Jenkins, W. M., Merzenich, M. M., & Ochs, M. T. (1990). Functional reorganization of primary somatosensory cortex in adult owl monkeys after behaviorally controlled tactile stimulation. *Journal of Neurophysiology, 63,* 82–104.

Jerosch-Herold, C. (2011). Sensory relearning in peripheral nerve disorders of the hand: A web-based survey and Delphi consensus method. *Journal of Hand Therapy: Official Journal of the American Society of Hand Therapists, 24,* 292–298.

Kalisch, T., Tegenthoff, M., & Dinse, H. R. (2008). Improvement of sensorimotor functions in old age by passive sensory stimulation. *Clinical Interventions in Aging, 3,* 673–690.

Lewis, C. M., Baldassarre, A., Committeri, G., Romani, G. L., & Corbetta, M. (2009). Learning sculpts the spontaneous activity of the resting human brain. *Proceedings of the National Academy of Sciences U.S.A., 106,* 17558–17563.

Lundborg, G., & Rosén, B. (2007). Hand function after nerve repair. *Acta Physiologica, 189,* 207–217.

McCabe, C. (2011). Mirror visual feedback therapy: A practical approach. *Journal of Hand Therapy, 24,* 170–179.

Merzenich, M. M., & Jenkins, W. M. (1993). Reorganization of cortical representations of the hand following alterations of skin inputs induced by nerve injury, skin island transfers, and experience. *Journal of Hand Therapy, 6,* 89–104.

Moseley, G. L., & Wiech, K. (2009). The effect of tactile discrimination training is enhanced when patients watch the reflected image of their unaffected limb during training. *Pain, 144,* 314–319.

Muenzen, P. A., Kasch, M. C., Greenberg, S., Fullenwider, L., Taylor, P. A., & Dimick, M. P. (2002). A new practice analysis of hand therapy. *Journal of Hand Therapy, 15,* 215–225.

Nakada, M., & Uchida, H. (1997). Case study of a five-stage sensory reeducation program. *Journal of Hand Therapy, 10,* 232–239.

Nelles, G., Spiekermann, G., Jueptner, M., Leonhardt, G., Muller, S., Gerhard, H., & Diener, C. (1999). Reorganization of sensory and motor systems in hemiplegic stroke patients: A positron emission tomography study. *Stroke, 30,* 1510–1516.

Oud, T., Beelan, A., Eijffinger, E., & Nollet, F. (2007). Sensory re-education after nerve injury of the upper limb: A systematic review. *Clinical Rehabilitation, 21,* 483–494.

Pillet, J., Didierjean-Pillet, A., & Holcombe, L. K. (2010). Aesthetic hand prosthesis: Its psychological and functional potential. In T. M. Skirven, A. L. Osterman, J. M. Fedorczyk, & P. C. Amadio (Eds.). *Rehabilitation of the hand and upper extremity* (6th ed., pp. 1282–1292). Philadelphia: Mosby, Inc./Elsevier.

Porretto-Loehrke, A., & Soika, E. (2010). Therapist's management of other nerve compressions about the elbow and wrist. In T. M. Skirven, A. L. Osterman, J. M. Fedorczyk, & P. C. Amadio (Eds.). *Rehabilitation of the hand and upper extremity* (6th ed., pp. 1695–709). Philadelphia: Mosby, Inc./Elsevier.

Robinson, S., & McPhee, S. (1986). Case report: Treating the patient with digital hypersensitivity. *American Journal of Occupational Therapy, 40,* 285–287.

Rosén, B., Björkman, A., & Lundborg, G. (2006). Improved sensory relearning after nerve repair induced by selective temporary anesthesia: A new concept in hand rehabilitation. *Journal of Hand Surgery (British and European), 31B,* 126–132.

Rosén, B., & Lundborg, G. (2007). Enhanced sensory recovery after median nerve repair using cortical audio-tactile interaction. A randomised multicentre study. *Journal of Hand Surgery (European), 32E,* 31–37.

Rosén, B., & Lundborg, G. (2010). Sensory reeducation. In T. M. Skirven, A. L. Osterman, J. M. Fedorczyk, & P. C. Amadio (Eds.). *Rehabilitation of the hand and upper extremity* (6th ed., pp. 634–645). Philadelphia: Mosby, Inc./Elsevier.

Rosén, B., Lundborg, G., Dahlin, L. B., Holmberg, J., & Karlson, B. (1994). Nerve repair: Correlation of restitution of functional sensibility with specific cognitive capacities. *Journal of Hand Surgery (British), 19B,* 452–458.

Sabari, J. S., & Lieberman, D. (2008). *Occupational therapy practice guidelines for adults with stroke.* Bethesda, MD: American Occupational Therapy Association Press.

Schabrun, S. M., & Hillier, S. (2009). Evidence for the retraining of sensation after stroke: A systematic review. *Clinical Rehabilitation, 23,* 27–39.

Shieh, S. J., Chiu, H. Y., Lee, J. W., & Hsu, H. Y. (1995). Evaluation of the effectiveness of sensory reeducation following digital replantation and revascularization. *Microsurgery, 16,* 578–582.

Smith, P. S., Dinse, H. R., Kalisch, T., Johnson, M., & Walker-Batson, D. (2009). Effects of repetitive electrical stimulation to treat sensory loss in persons poststroke. *Archives of Physical Medicine and Rehabilitation, 90,* 2108–2111.

Thompson, M., Medley, A., & Motts, S. (2002). Foot sensations measured by Semmes-Weinstein monofilaments in persons newly diagnosed with diabetes. *Journal of Geriatric Physical Therapy, 25,* 42.

Walsh, M. T. (2010). Therapist's management of complex regional pain syndrome. In T. M. Skirven, A. L. Osterman, J. M. Fedorczyk, & P. C. Amadio (Eds.), *Rehabilitation of the hand and upper extremity* (6th ed., pp. 1479–1492). Philadelphia: Mosby, Inc./Elsevier.

Wood, H. (1969). Prevention of deformity in the insensitive hand: The role of the therapist. *American Journal of Occupational Therapy, 23,* 488–489.

Yekutiel, M., & Guttman, E. (1993). A controlled trial of the retraining of the sensory function of the hand in stroke patients. *Journal of Neurology, Neurosurgery, and Psychiatry, 56,* 241–244.

Yerxa, E., Barber, L., Diaz, O., Black, W., & Azen, S. (1983). Development of a hand sensitivity test for the hypersensitive hand. *American Journal of Occupational Therapy, 37,* 176–181.

Yozbatiran, N., Donmez, B., Kayak, N., & Bozan, O. (2006). Electrical stimulation of wrist and fingers for sensory and functional recovery in acute hemiplegia. *Clinical Rehabilitation, 20,* 4–11.

Acknowledgment

Paul Petersen and Melanie Seltzer assisted with the photography for this chapter.

Optimizing Vision and Visual Processing

Jennifer Kaldenberg

Learning Objectives

After studying this chapter, the reader will be able to do the following:

1. Identify and describe specific treatments for low vision and oculomotor dysfunction.
2. Identify and describe treatment approaches for visual field defects and unilateral neglect.
3. Describe the similarities and differences between low vision diagnoses and visual deficits resulting from neurological insult.
4. Apply understanding of best intervention strategies with accompanying case examples.

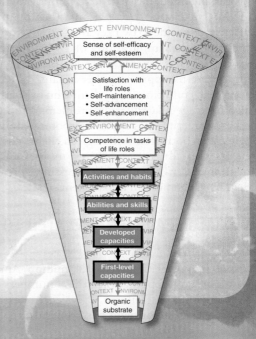

INTRODUCTION

Occupational therapy practitioners working with adults often address the impact of visual impairment on occupational performance as a result of neurological insult or age-related eye disease. Occupational therapy practitioners should understand the impact of visual impairment on occupational performance and be prepared to provide clients with appropriate intervention to maximize independence and safety in desired occupations.

Although the literature on the identification and evaluation of visual and perceptual dysfunction is extensive, information on the effectiveness of treatment is limited. In addition, much of the research in the area of vision impairment and low vision (LV) has been carried out by ophthalmology and optometry, even though the compensatory techniques for adapting to vision impairment are carried out by a variety of practitioners including occupational therapy, ophthalmology, optometry, LV therapy, rehabilitation teachers, or orientation and mobility specialists. Unfortunately, occupational therapy practitioners, who see first hand the deleterious effects of visual and perceptual dysfunction on a person's daily living skills, have been slow to generate research that supports this type of intervention.

Warren (1993a) developed a hierarchy of visual perception (see Fig. 5-1 in Chapter 5), which emphasizes the importance of intervention for visual foundation skills including acuity, visual fields (VFs), and oculomotor function before addressing higher level perceptual skills. Therefore, rather than focus on high-level perceptual skills, this chapter discusses specific treatment options for visual foundation skills including LV, ocular motor dysfunction, and homonymous hemianopsia (also called hemianopia as termed in Chapter 5) and for the visual processing or cognitive deficit of unilateral neglect (UN).

In this chapter, occupational therapy intervention is discussed specific to two key areas: intervention to address the functional implications of LV and intervention for vision issues associated with neurologic conditions. It is important to appreciate this because clients may have comorbid conditions (e.g., client who has had a stroke may also have age-related vision problems), and occupational therapy practitioners often incorporate intervention strategies from both areas with a given client. The chapter concludes with a discussion of intervention for UN, which is a neurologically based visual processing or cognitive disorder rather than vision impairment.

VISUAL IMPAIRMENT RELATED TO LOW VISION AND AGING

Visual impairment affects 3.4 million Americans, and with our aging populations, these numbers are expected to increase (Eye Disease Prevalence Research Group, 2004). Visual impairment has been linked to falls, deficits in activities of daily living (ADL) and instrumental activities of daily living (IADL) performance, as well as increased secondary health conditions (Campbell et al., 1999; Congdon, 2004). Although many older adults equate vision loss to normal aging, some age-related visual changes occur (such as yellowing of the lens or smaller pupil size) that do not result in vision impairment. Four of the five major causes of visual impairment are directly related to the aging process: age-related macular degeneration, diabetic retinopathy, glaucoma, and cataracts (Table 23-1). Uncorrected refractive errors is the fifth leading cause of vision impairment; however, in many cases this can be addressed through education and improved access to health care (Coleman et al., 2006).

Low Vision

LV is defined as a bilateral visual impairment that cannot be corrected by corrective lenses, medication, or surgery (Freeman et al., 2007). For reimbursement purposes, a visual impairment diagnosis is based on visual acuity and VF measurement, and ranges from 20/70 visual acuity to total blindness, or a VF constriction of 20° or less, central scotoma, or homonymous or heteronomous bilateral VF defect (Colenbrander & Fletcher, 1995; Social Security Administration, 2011) (discussed further in Chapter 5; see Table 5-1).

Most occupational therapists do not specialize in vision rehabilitation but, instead, encounter LV as a complication in clients with other functional impairments and medical conditions (Weisser-Pike & Kaldenberg, 2010). Because of our education and expertise, occupational therapists are in a unique position to collaborate with LV specialists (see Definitions 5-1 in Chapter 5) by providing input on the client's functional impairment and how this may affect the selection and use of assistive devices. For example, an individual with tremors may not benefit from a handheld magnifier or may require certain positioning before using the device. Occupational therapy input is necessary for the most informed recommendations for assistive devices and the parameters for their use. Occupational therapists should have supervision and/or specialized training to recommend and train clients in the use of their prescribed LV aides.

Occupational Therapy for Low Vision

The goal of occupational therapy in working with individuals with visual impairment is to maximize the individual's use of his or her remaining vision in order to be able to complete occupations of choice. Many basic ADL tasks can be completed with minimal vision. However, individuals with LV often struggle to complete tasks that require reading such as meal preparation, financial management, and social participation. When considering intervention, occupational therapy practitioners need to consider the

| Table 23-1 | **Age-Related Changes in Vision** | | |

Condition	Definition and Functional Complaint	Simulation	Medical Treatment and Occupational Therapy (OT) Interventions
Cataracts	Opacity or clouding of the crystalline lens of the eye Functional Complaint: decreased visual acuity, decreased contrast sensitivity, difficulty with night driving, and diplopia	 **Figure 23-1A** Courtesy: National Eye Institute, National Institutes of Health.	Medical: surgery OT: color and contrast enhancement, magnification, management of lighting, sensory substitution, organizational strategies
Glaucoma	Damage to the optic nerve caused by increased intraocular pressure results in decreased peripheral vision; in end stages impacts central visual acuity. Functional Complaint: difficulty with night vision, mobility impairment, in end stages deficits in central visual field (reading, facial recognition)	 **Figure 23-1B** Courtesy: National Eye Institute, National Institutes of Health.	Medical: medications, surgery OT: color and contrast enhancement, glare control, field enhancement, sensory substitution, visual skills training, organizational strategies, and in end stages magnification for central field loss, mobility training (may benefit from Orientation and Mobility [OM] referral)
Diabetic retinopathy	Affects nearly 40% of all individuals with diabetes (Kempen et al., 2004). Diabetes affects the small blood vessels in the retina, causing swelling or bleeding, which can lead to serious vision loss. Functional Complaint: Diabetes can impact all aspects of visual function. A person can develop scotomas, decreased contrast and color discrimination, decreased night vision, and fluctuations in vision.	 **Figure 23-1C** Courtesy: National Eye Institute, National Institutes of Health.	Medical: surgery, laser treatments, vitrectomy OT: color and contrast enhancement, glare control, magnification, lighting, visual skills training, sensory substitution, organizational strategies mobility training (may benefit from O&M referral)
Age-related macular degeneration	A progressive and irreversible loss of central vision caused by fibrous scarring or atrophy of the macula. Two types: wet and dry Functional Complaint: decreased visual acuity, central scotoma, decreased contrast sensitivity, difficulty with facial recognition, and reading	 **Figure 23-1D** Courtesy: National Eye Institute, National Institutes of Health.	Medical: for dry, vitamins and antioxidants, implantable miniature telescope (IMT); for wet, laser surgery OT: color and contrast enhancement, magnification, management of lighting, visual skills training, sensory substitution, and organizational strategies

goals of the client and the individual client factors, activity demands, performance skills, performance patterns, and contexts and environments that either support or inhibit participation in desired occupations. Occupational therapy intervention often includes visual skills training, environmental adaptation (lighting and contrast), magnification, compensatory techniques (sensory substitution-auditory and tactile strategies), organizational strategies, and client/family education (refer to Table 23-2).

Visual Skills Training

Individuals with peripheral or central VF defects often can learn new visual skills to maximize their awareness and functional use of their available VF. Use of scanning and/or eccentric viewing can be effective strategies for ADL and IADL tasks, work, education, play, leisure and social participation.

Visual scanning is the ability to locate a target using an organized visual search pattern (Pambakian, Currie, & Kennard, 2005). Teaching a systematic method of scanning can assist an individual in moving through their environment safely and independently. Central field impairments (such as macular degeneration with a central scotoma) have a significant impact on reading, writing and facial recognition and affect 83% of individuals with visual impairment (Colenbrander & Fletcher, 1995). A central scotoma may cause a blurring, distortion, or absence of part or all of an image. Individuals may be aware of their central scotoma or may require education to locate it. For instance, when looking in a certain direction, he or she may notice that things appear clearer, but when turning to look at the object face on, the blur or distortion returns. To use their residual vision, individuals with central field impairment must learn to move the scotoma out of the way and use their peripheral retina as central (macula) retina through eccentric viewing training (EV). Individuals can be taught to use their peripheral vision as an alternate viewing area or preferred retinal locus (PRL) to maximize the use of their remaining vision. This new PRL can be used for near and distance tasks and can be used independently or with LV aids. EV can be a very successful strategy, but it takes patience and hard work (Wright & Watson, 1995). Some individuals with central scotoma can locate their PRL independently, whereas others need training to do so. However, even if an individual is able to locate a PRL, it may not be the best viewing area. Instead, the patient may benefit from developing another area or trained retinal locus (Nilsson, Frennesson, & Nilsson, 2003; Stelmack, Massof, & Stelmack, 2004). Virtually all clients require training to develop the ability to efficiently and effectively use this new PRL (Crossland, Culham, & Rubin, 2005; Schuchard, 2005). Development of oculomotor skills, fixation stability, and the ability to refixate on an object is essential in order to return to reading and independence in all areas of occupation (Crossland, Culham, & Rubin, 2005; Fletcher, Schuchard, & Watson, 999; Markowitz, 2006;

Schuchard, 2005; Wright & Watson, 1995) (refer to Procedures for Practice 23-1).

Environmental Adaptations

Environmental adaptations are often necessary to maximize independence and safety. Managing lighting, glare and contrast for individuals with LV and neurological visual impairments is important. Increased lighting is needed for all older adults, because of age-related eye changes; those with vision loss often require even greater levels of lighting. Increased lighting has been shown to increase independence, safety, and quality of life (Brunnstrom et al., 2004; Duffy, 2002; Figueiro, 2001). Lighting should be tailored to the individual and the specific task (see Procedures for Practice 23-2).

As with the need for increased lighting, there is also an increased need for higher contrast as one ages. Improving contrast can increase safety and support safe navigation of the environment. For example, clients with poor contrast sensitivity require increased contrast and lighting and may have difficulty identifying curbs, stairs, and finding objects in low light, whereas a person with VF loss may have more difficulty in a busy, moving environment.

Environmental factors can be adapted to improve the person's ability to perform a task. For example, an individual experiencing difficulty with meal preparation may benefit from changing the lighting, marking the oven controls with contrasting colors, using high–color-contrast utensils, using proper positioning, and avoiding glare from windows or surfaces. All of these adaptations may assist clients in meeting their desired goals. For additional examples of environmental factors, refer to Table 23-2.

Magnification

Most older adults with LV will benefit from some form of magnification. Magnification is a fundamental means of improving vision by making an object larger and thus more visible (Nowakowski, 2000). For some, use of large-print items can be helpful to complete desired activities. There are now many commercially available large-print items, such as clocks, checks, books, newspapers, telephones, remotes, and bingo cards. (Patients may also choose to adjust computer screens for greater contrast, brightness, and magnification. For other individuals, optical devices may be required.) A variety of optical devices are available including spectacles (microscopes), stand magnifiers, hand magnifiers, telescopes, and electronic magnification. When working with optical devices for magnification, it is important to assess monocular and binocular function in order to determine eye dominance and the potential for eye rivalry. For example, if the dominant eye is no longer the better seeing eye, it may interfere with binocular function and may require occlusion (Markowitz, 2006). There are benefits and challenges to all devices, and these factors must be considered to determine best fit (refer to Table 23-2). Further,

Table 23-2 | **Low Vision Interventions**

Intervention Approach	Methods	Description
Visual skills	Scanning	Use with peripheral or central visual field defects
		Simplest to learn
		No needed equipment
		Improves safety and independence
	Eccentric viewing training	Use with central visual field defects
		Train to use an alternate viewing area or preferred retinal locus (PRL) to maximize the use of his or her remaining vision
		Can be used for both distance and near tasks, such as facial recognition or reading
		Requires patience and hard work
		(Mogk & Mogk, 2003; Warren, 1996; Watson et al., 1996)
Environmental adaptation	Lighting Figure 23-2A	All older adults regardless of visual impairment
		Should be tailored to activities regularly performed
		Consider natural, ambient, and task lighting
		Even lighting transitions, avoid dark and bright
		Task lighting—use of a gooseneck lamp is optimal for task lighting and can be adjusted so that light is directed onto the task rather than on the person. For writing, the lamp can be positioned on the side opposite the dominant hand to avoid shadows.
	Contrast Figure 23-2B	Increasing contrast between objects and their backgrounds is a simple and effective way to improve visual function, such as high contrast black numbers on a silver mailbox or a black light switch cover on a white wall.
	Filters Figure 23-2C	Filters can be used for glare control, contrast enhancement, retinal adaptation, and eye protection. Filters absorb certain portions of the light spectrum, heat energy, and harmful light rays and can assist with light scatter. Filters can improve comfort, increase visual acuity and contrast sensitivity, and assist with light/dark adaptation. Filters come in a variety of colors, levels of light transmission, styles, and costs.

(continued)

| Table 23-2 | Low Vision Interventions (continued) |
| | |

Intervention Approach	Methods	Description
Sensory substitution	Tactile strategies 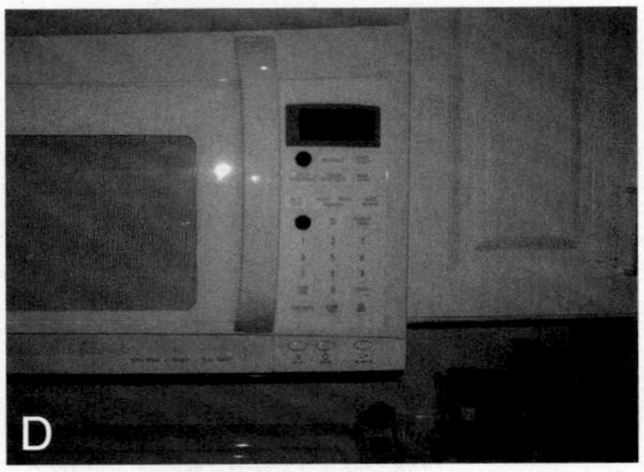 **Figure 23-2D**	Cost effective, commercially available Bump dots on appliances to mark settings, i.e., 350° on the oven or one-minute button on the microwave Puff paint, safety pins, rubber band, Braille markings
	Auditory strategies 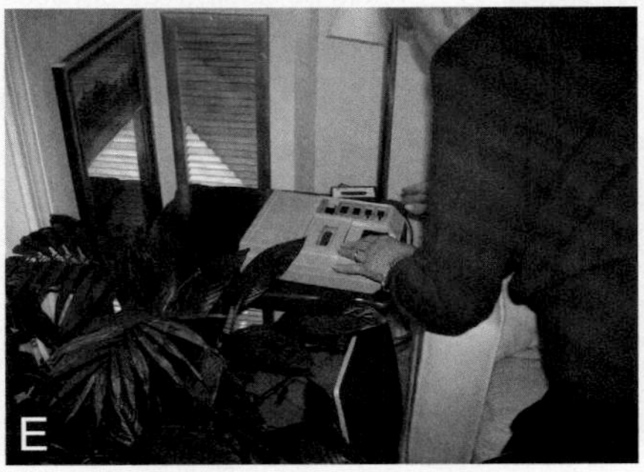 **Figure 23-2E**	Commercially available audio books are a simple and accessible resource for many individuals with visual impairment; occupational therapists can register a client to receive this service. Other available talking items: "say when" device, talking scales, talking glucometers, medication reminders, and organizers
Magnification *Safety Message: Optical devices are generally prescribed by an optometrist or ophthalmologist.*	General principles	Does not necessarily make vision clearer; it enlarges the object of regard, which is then more recognizable. The stronger the magnification, the smaller the field of view and the closer the magnifier is held to the eye.
	Relative size magnification	Increasing the size of the object: large print
	Relative distance magnification	Moving closer to an object makes it relatively larger, for instance, holding a book closer to the face.
	Large print 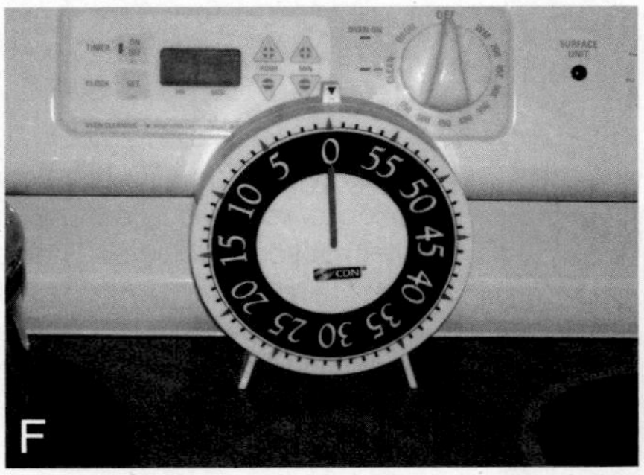 **Figure 23-2F**	Simple, commercially available Limitations in power/size Examples: books, address books, bill statements can be requested from companies, and checks and check registers can be requested from banks

Table 23-2 | **Low Vision Interventions** *(continued)*

Intervention Approach	Methods	Description
	Spectacles **Figure 23-2G**	Most individuals with visual impairment would like to get a pair of glasses that improve their vision and magnify the image; however, often individuals require greater powers that result in decreased focal distances, which are not acceptable to the individual. **Range of power:** binocular +1.00 diopter (D) to +14 D; or monocular up to 64 D (A diopter is a unit of power of the lens.) **Pros:** Common, in lower powers allow for greatest field of view, portable, relatively inexpensive **Cons:** Reduced focal distance
	Stand magnifiers **Figure 23-2H**	Stand magnifiers consist of a convex lens in a housing that is held flat onto the material. Clients should wear their own eyeglasses while using the optical device unless instructed otherwise by the doctor. The stand housing sets the focal distance. Devices can come illuminated or nonilluminated. **Range of power:** 6-50D **Pros:** Common, allows for increased working distance, relatively inexpensive, does not have to be held, less grasp required **Cons:** Portability and size, less light because of housing in nonilluminated forms
	Hand magnifiers **Figure 23-2I**	Hand magnifiers consist of a convex lens with a handle. Devices can come illuminated or nonilluminated and in many styles, i.e., folding, pocket, etc. **Range of power:** 2-60 D: variety of powers similar to stand magnifiers **Pros:** Because it does not have a housing that sets the focal distance, the individual must hold the magnifier at the focal distance to have a clear magnified image. There is greater flexibility with hand magnifiers for spot reading tasks. **Cons:** Must maintain focal distance, which would be difficult for extended reading tasks
	Telescopes **Figure 23-2J**	Telescopes can come in a variety of styles—handheld or spectacle mounted, monocular or binocular, Galilean or Keplarian. In a reverse position a telescope can be used for field enhancement. **Range of power:** 2–14× **Pros:** Great for brief spotting tasks, can be modified for near tasks **Cons:** Reduced visual field, limited depth of focus

(continued)

Table 23-2	Low Vision Interventions *(continued)*	
Intervention Approach	**Methods**	**Description**
	Electronic magnification **Figure 23-2K**	Comes in variety of formats; in general, used for long-term reading or distance spotting. Most typical form is closed-circuit television (CCTV): portable or table top versions. Portable camera-based magnifiers are also available. **Range of power:** up to 70× magnification **Pros:** Can be used for reading, writing, and leisure activities. It has its own light source and brightness controls, the contrast can be enhanced through reversing the polarity, and it allows for a wide field of view, especially in lower magnifications. It allows for greater working distance and allows the individual to comfortably read for extended periods. **Cons:** Cost, portability, requires coordination and eye–hand coordination
Organizational strategies	Effective organizational strategies **Figure 23-2L**	Avoid clutter Establish regular schedules for cleaning Create consistent locations for common items: keys, low vision devices

training in proper care and use of LV devices is also required for device acceptance and functional use (Fok et al., 2011).

Sensory Substitution

Many people who cannot use residual vision to safely complete a task use tactile or auditory strategies. Tactile strategies are cost effective and easy to incorporate into many daily activities. For instance, older adults often have difficulty distinguishing blues and blacks, thus making identification of clothing difficult. A tactile strategy, such as placing rust-proof safety pins in the label of the clothing can aid in color identification (one safety pin for black, two for blue). Tactile strategies can also facilitate safe use of appliances, such as demarcating 350° on the oven dial with a high contrast bump dot or pouring salt into the palm of the hand prior to adding it to food to avoid over seasoning.

Someone with peripheral neuropathy who cannot safely rely on tactile sensation may use auditory strategies. There are many commercially available talking products, such as audiobooks, computer screen readers, talking watches, or talking thermostats. To that end, it is important to consider the type of voice that is used, because some pitches or sounds are easier to comprehend than others. As with any condition, it is important to look at an individual's abilities and limitations, in order to determine the best interventions strategies.

Organizational Strategies

Using good organizational strategies is important for individuals with visual impairment. General considerations include

- **C**onsistency: keep walkways clear from clutter and place items in a consistent location

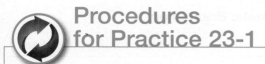

Procedures
for Practice 23-1

Eccentric Viewing Progression

1. Educate client on the presence of the scotoma.
2. Identification of scotoma.
3. Identification of the preferred retinal locus (PRL).
4. Client learns to move in and out of scotoma, looking at an object, bring the object in and out of focus using the new PRL.
5. Begin with large, simple, static targets (identify distance or near single targets).
6. Use steady eye technique or scrolling technique; maintain a fixed gaze and physically move the object or text into the best area of vision (rather than using saccadic eye movements to scan across the page of text).
7. Progress to complex, small, dynamic targets (words, sentences, saccades).

- **O**rder items: keep address books, phone books, or money in a wallet alphabetized or sorted by denomination
- **P**air like items: put shoes, socks, or outfits together
- **E**stablish routines: such as cleaning

These strategies can decrease frustration and potential for injury for those with visual impairment. In addition, it is important when working with family and caregivers to ensure that systems of organization are maintained. For example, caregivers or those providing housekeeping assistance must be consistent about object and furniture placement after cleaning so that the client knows where things will be. If a

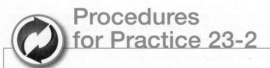

Procedures
for Practice 23-2

Principles for Managing Lighting

- General ambient lighting is important for safe mobility.
- When addressing task lighting, it is important to consider safety as well as brightness of light. Often, a gooseneck lamp is recommended for reading and writing tasks. Note, these lamps often come with metal shades and when used with an incandescent bulb can create a lot of heat. Use of a compact fluorescent lightbulb can reduce the risk of injury.
- The closer the light is to the task, the brighter the illumination. Therefore, you can use a lower wattage bulb if you can manipulate the distance from the light.
- When increasing light, it is important to remember the negative influences of glare on performance. Glare from light sources or a reflected source can cause discomfort, as well as functional impairment. Use of filters, visors, or polarized lenses can assist in decreasing glare discomfort.

caregiver neglects to place a low-lying footrest back under the coffee table, the client with LV could trip and fall.

Client/Family Education

Education to the client and family on the ocular condition, prognosis, and functional implications of the visual impairment is essential. Review of recommendations for environmental adaptations/modifications, psychological consequences, and need for support, as well as available support and social services can ease adjustment to visual loss. Family and caregiver education can assist with carryover of information taught, as well as assist in the individual's ability to transfer the techniques to new situations or changes as they arise.

VISUAL IMPAIRMENT AS A RESULT OF NEUROLOGICAL CONDITIONS

Many people with neurological conditions also present with vision-related difficulties. Some of the performance problems can be attributed to difficulty coordinating eye movements, such as ocular motor dysfunction, whereas others are the result of brain damage that interferes with the interpretation or processing of visual stimuli, such as VF deficits and UN. As visual deficits are identified, it is important that an optometrist or ophthalmologist be consulted or an appropriate referral is made in order to maximize the individual's rehabilitation potential.

Clients who have had a cerebrovascular accident (CVA) may experience a variety of vision-related problems. VF impairments associated with CVA or traumatic brain injury (TBI) include hemianopsia or quadrantanopsia. There is reported VF loss in 36% of those with right (R) stroke and 25% of people with left (L) stroke and visual inattention impairment in 82% of R stroke and 65% of L stroke (Wolter & Preda, 2006). The VF impairment (nasal, temporal, superior, inferior) is specific to the area of the brain that is involved. The patient may also experience diplopia caused by cranial nerve palsy or oculomotor dysfunction; sensitivity to light; VF impairments; and/or UN (Rowe et al., 2009).

Similarly, Suchoff et al. (2008) found that 39% of individuals with TBI experienced VF defects. Many service members from Operation Enduring Freedom and Operation Iraqi Freedom have survived blast injuries resulting in TBI and eye injuries. It has been estimated that up to 18% of returning troops have mild TBI, and 75% of those individuals report visual deficits (Hoge et al., 2008; Stelmack et al., 2009). Brain injury may result in acuity loss, VF defects, ocular motor dysfunction, and binocular vision dysfunction (Ciuffreda, Ludlam, & Kapoor, 2009; Stelmack et al., 2009) (refer to Table 23-3).

In addition, individuals with visual deficits occurring as a result of neurological conditions often demonstrate symptoms similar to those of individuals with more typical LV diagnoses. Photosensitivity or light sensitivity;

Table 23-3 **Visual Complications Associated with Traumatic Brain Injury**

Visual Complication	Rates	Definition	Functional Implications
Convergence insufficiency	40%–56%	Inability of the eyes to turn in enough to allow for fusion during near tasks	Reading deficits Diplopia Blurred vision
Accommodative deficits	21%–56%	Inability of the eyes to adjust focal power for distance and near tasks	Reading deficits Diplopia Blurred vision
Pursuits and saccades deficits	25%–59%	Pursuits: inability of the eyes to follow a moving target Saccades: inability to accurately and efficiently refixate from one point to another	Reading deficits Visual motor deficits Balance and vestibular deficits Blurred vision
Fixation instability	5%–13%	Inability of the eyes to maintain gaze so that the image falls on the macula	Reading deficits Visual motor deficits Blurred vision
Strabismus	11%–32%	Misalignment of the eyes	Binocular vision deficits Depth perception deficits Potential visual field deficits Eye movement deficits Double vision Balance deficits
Diplopia	19%	Double vision	Blurred vision Balance and vestibular deficits Nausea Reading deficits Visual motor deficits

From Brahm, K. D., Wilgenburg, H. M., Kirby, J., Ingalla, S., Chang, C. Y., & Goodrich, G. L. (2009). Visual impairment and dysfunction in combat-related military personnel: A population study. *Optometry and Vision Science, 86*, 817–825; Ciuffreda, K. J., Ludlam, D. P., & Kapoor, N. (2009). Clinical oculomotor training in traumatic brain injury. *Optometry & Vision Development, 40*, 16–23; Cockerham, G. C., Goodrich, G. L., Weichel, E. D., Orcutt, J. C., Rizzo, J. F., Bower, K. S., & Schuchard, R. A. (2009). Eye and visual function in traumatic brain injury. *Journal of Rehabilitation Research & Development, 46*, 811–818; Stelmack, J. A., Frith, T., Van Koevering, D., Rinee, S., & Stelmack, T. (2009). Visual function in patients followed at a veterans affairs polytrauma network site: An electronic medical records review. *Optometry, 80*, 419–424.

difficulty with light/dark adaptation; deficits in scanning, saccades, and pursuits; difficulty tolerating complex visual environments; deficits in depth perception; and eye strain are all visual complaints associated with LV and neurological visual diagnoses (Chang, Ciuffreda, & Kapoor, 2007; Roth et al., 2009; Schrupp, Ciuffreda, & Kapoor, 2009). In terms of treatment, the occupational therapist should consider the functional complaint and develop appropriate intervention strategies. For example, when an individual with homonymous hemianopsia complains of glare discomfort, the occupational therapist should consider lighting and glare control and perhaps use filters to manage the photosensitivity.

In this section, interventions for three categories of neuro-related vision dysfunction are presented: VF deficits, ocular motor dysfunction, and UN.

Intervention for Visual Field Deficits

As part of their intervention, occupational therapy practitioners teach clients to use scanning techniques and compensatory strategies, as well as train and assist the individual in adapting to the use of prisms (Fresnel, Yoked, Peli prism, or visual awareness systems) as prescribed by optometry or ophthalmology (see Evidence Table 23-1).

Scanning

Visual scanning, the most common intervention for field loss, is the ability to use an organized visual search of the task or environment (left to right, top to bottom). If an individual has awareness of his or her impairment, visual scanning training can be done simply with no special equipment, and family can be easily instructed to facilitate carryover of

| Evidence Table 23-1 | | Best Evidence for Vision Intervention | | | | | |

Intervention	Description of Intervention Tested	Participants	Dosage	Types of Best evidence and Level of Evidence	Benefit	Statistical probability and effect size of outcome	Reference
Prism (UN)	Effectiveness of prisms creating a 10° deviation to the right to ameliorate neglect symptoms	Twenty patients with stroke, mean age = 62 years, mean time post stroke = 10 months	Ten daily sessions over 2 weeks with 90 pointing tasks throughout the visual field, while wearing prismatic goggles deviating the visual field 10° toward the right	Randomized controlled trial Level: IB1a	Yes. Sustained improvements in visuospatial abilities and reading performance	Long-term effects: Behavioral Inattention Test $p < 0.00001$, $\eta = 0.81$; cancellation scores $p < 0.0001$, $\eta = 0.75$; reading accuracy $p < 0.0003$, $\eta = 0.61$	Serino et al. (2009)
Prisms (hemianopsia)	Adaptation to a 40D prism for mobility and obstacle avoidance	Forty-three patients with homonymous hemianopsia; mean age = 63 years	Patients were fitted with a 40D Fresnel prism, followed by an office interview	One-group, pre-post design Level: IIIB2b	Yes. Improved awareness of visual field and improvements in mobility and obstacle avoidance	Seventy-four percent of patients continued to wear the prism, patients rated the prism as very helpful and reported significant benefit for mobility and obstacle avoidance: $p < 0.001$	Bowers, Keeney, & Peli (2008)
Scanning	Examined restoration of visual field, visual search/scanning strategies, and transfer of scanning skills to activities of daily living (ADL) performance, especially reading	Fourteen studies included in review	Systematic review of interventions: restoration visual field, visual search/ scanning strategies, and transfer of scanning skills to ADL performance, especially reading	Level: I	Yes. Improved attention to the side of visual loss or inattention and improved reading performance	With scanning training, improvements were noted in reading time and reading errors; improved scanning up to a 30° visual search field; unclear findings with restoration therapy; recommendation for further study	Bouwmeester, Heutink, & Lucas (2006)
Patching	Patching interventions: hemifield and full-field patching	Twenty-two RCVA patients with left unilateral spatial neglect	Patching 1. Half visual field patching 2. Complete visual field patching 3. Control, no patching	Randomized controlled trial Level: IB2b	Yes. Improved awareness of left, improved scanning, and improved ADL performance	Improvements noted with half visual field patching; improved Functional Independence Measure (FIM) scores $p = 0.01$; scanning (left reference zone) $p = 0.02$ (data not available to calculate effect size)	Beis et al. (1999)

(continued)

| Evidence Table 23-1 | Best Evidence for Vision Intervention *(continued)* |

Intervention	Description of Intervention Tested	Participants	Dosage	Types of Best evidence and Level of Evidence	Benefit	Statistical probability and effect size of outcome	Reference
Visuomotor feedback training	Exercises included visual scanning, reading, and copying	Fifty-nine patients with right brain damage (RBD), 12 received training for neglect, 36 had no neglect	Visual scanning training, specific training for five 1-hour sessions per week for 8 weeks, altered cognitive stimulation three times per week for 8 weeks; all training done in conjunction with physical rehabilitation	Random assignment to intervention groups; cross-over design with repeated measures Level: IC2b	Yes. Functional and motor improvements as well as improved scanning	Improvements were noted in intervention group of motor skills and function; Rivermead mobility, $p < 0.05$, $r = 0.367$; Barthel Index, $p < 0.05$, $r = 0.373$; letter cancellation, $p < 0.01$, $r = 0.484$	Paolucci et al. (1996)
Limb activation	1. Lateralized task approach 2. Controlled sensory stimulation 3. Limb activation	Forty-seven patients with cerebrovascular accident (CVA) and visual neglect without hemianopsia	Reviewed studies related to three approaches to addressing visual neglect: 9 group studies, 22 single-subject design studies	Meta-analysis Level: I	Improved body image and visual awareness with limb activation	Unilateral neglect appears to be amenable to change by way of activation of the right hemisphere (group designs $r = 0.77$ and single subject designs $r = 0.89$); line bisection tests, cancellation tests, copying tasks, reading tests	Lin (1996)

See other important intervention studies (Fortis et al., 2010; Pisella et al., 2006; Scheiman, Gwiazda, & Li, 2011; Shiraishi et al., 2010; Ting et al., 2011).

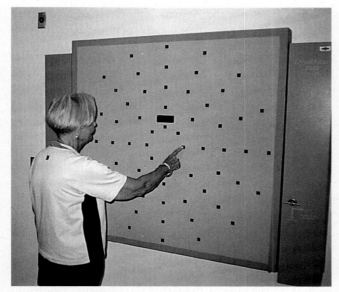

Figure 23-3 Dynavision.

training. Training can include paper and pencil tasks; computer programs; scanning in a functional setting, such as a grocery store; and use of the Dynavision (Fig. 23-3) (Suchoff & Ciuffreda, 2004). Research supports improvement on visual perceptual tasks, reading, and academic work with this type of training but found it does not generalize to gross motor tasks (Pollock et al., 2011). The literature indicates that the effects of scanning training are contextual, that is, specific to the situation. If the goal is to improve the client's ability to read or scan at tabletop, tabletop scanning training is appropriate. However, if the therapist wants to

improve a client's ability to scan in the community, practice in the community is needed. Warren (1993b) provided guidelines for the selection of treatment activities for clients with deficits in visual attention and visual scanning (Table 23-4). Visual scanning training, including mental imagery, pencil-paper tasks, computerized visual scanning, and functional scanning tasks, has been shown to improve attention in individuals with VF defects as well as UN (Bouwmeester, Heutink, & Lucas, 2006; Niemeier, Cifu, & Kishore, 2001).

Clients being trained to scan must learn to synthesize information in an organized manner, such as left to right or through use of anchoring (supplying a cue on the impaired side to indicate starting position). This assists the client in focusing attention back to the side of VF loss or neglect (Table 23-5). In order to develop an organized

Table 23-4 | **Training Guidelines for Visual Attention and Visual Scanning**

Train client to use scanning strategy.	Use anchoring techniques; reorganize scanning strategies (Weinberg et al., 1979).
Broaden visual field which requires that client must scan.	Use activities that the client is required to turn the head or change body positions to complete the task (e.g., scanning items on a kitchen shelf).
Reinforce visual experience with sensorimotor experiences.	Use activities in which the client is required to manipulate what is seen (e.g., reach for or touch items scanned).
Emphasize conscious attention to detail and careful inspection of objects.	Use matching tasks in which the client may be encouraged to slow down and double-check interpretation of what is seen.
Practice the skill in context to ensure carryover.	Treatment may begin in the clinic, but strategies must be practiced in a variety of real-life situations.

From Warren, M. (1993b). A hierarchical model for evaluation and treatment of visual perceptual dysfunction in adult acquired brain injury, part 2. *American Journal of Occupational Therapy, 47,* 55–66.

Table 23-5 | **Anchoring Technique**

Sequence of Cueing	Task Demand
1. A vertical anchoring line is used on the left side; the beginning and ending of the line are sequentially numbered.	Client uses the vertical line to find the beginning and the numbers to avoid skipping lines.

Example: 1   The law was passed to allow the   1
            2   state to conduct a national FBI   2
            3   criminal records check before   3
            4 certifying teachers. 4	

2. A vertical anchoring line is used on the left side; only the beginning of the line is sequentially numbered.	Client uses the vertical line and numbers on the left; the number cue on the right has been eliminated.

Example: 1   Family members, followed by
            2   coworkers, are the most
            3   frequent targets of
            4 anger.	

3. A vertical anchoring line is used on the left side.	Client uses only the vertical line to find left side.

Example: Environmental groups hope to
            minimize the divisiveness and
            avoid mistakes made in the
            Pacific Northwest.	

4. No cues are provided.	Client must read without any cues.

Example: The state distributes its
            lottery proceeds without
            regard to which communities
            generate the revenue.	

From Quintana, L. A. (1995). Remediating perceptual impairments. In C. A. Trombly (Ed.), *Occupational therapy for physical dysfunction* (4th ed., pp. 529–537). Philadelphia: Williams & Wilkins.

search, it is helpful to begin scanning training with cancellation tasks, a structured array (symbols arranged in neat, straight rows across the page), or computer-based programs (Suchoff & Ciuffreda, 2004). This array can be made increasingly more complex by instructing the patient to scan for two target letters, decreasing the spacing between letters, or decreasing the size of the letters as the client progresses (Cooke, 1992).

Compensatory Strategies

Individuals with homonymous hemianopsia or quadrantanopsia often have difficulty with reading tasks. Individuals with right VF impairment must look into their field impairment as they read across the line. They may lose their place reading along or have difficulty identifying the end of the line. They may also have errors in word identification, such as with compound words; they may read foot when the word is football. Individuals with left VF impairment may have difficulty finding the beginning of the reading materials. Use of anchoring, cueing techniques, and reorientation of the reading materials can be effective techniques for reading tasks (Pambakian, Currie, & Kennard, 2005) (see Fig. 23-4).

Prism

A prism is a type of lens that is thicker on one side than the other. Its purpose is to bend the light coming into the eye, moving the image onto the fovea. In the case of hemianopsia, prisms are often used to shift an image from the nonseeing area into the seeing area. Current prism interventions look to improve VF awareness (Gottlieb, Freeman, & William, 1992; Peli, 2000, 2001) versus shifting the VF (yoked or sector prism). Prisms may be a permanent part of the client's prescription or they may be temporary. For example, a Fresnel prism, is a flexible plastic sheet with small ridges that can be cut to shape and adhered to the client's glasses. The Fresnel prism is advantageous because it is inexpensive and temporary and can be easily applied and removed. The

disadvantages are that it may distort visual acuity and tends to cloud and increase distortion (Gianutsos & Suchoff, 2002).

Prisms appear to improve VFs through a number of mechanisms. For example, Gottlieb, Freeman, and Williams (1992) developed a button-type prism (a round, base out prism) that is placed in the peripheral field of the individual's glasses. As the individual shifts gaze, the prism shifts the image from the nonseeing area into the seeing area. This shift creates improved VF awareness and is referred to as a visual awareness system. Peli (2000) introduced another method of field expansion using Fresnel prisms. The 40D monocular prisms are initially placed in the superior VF, with the prism's base positioned toward the side of the VF defect, in the peripheral field. It is placed along the entire length of the glasses so that the prism creates peripheral diplopia, while allowing for clear central vision. This diplopia acts as a cue to look to the side of the visual impairment. Traditionally, prisms were used in the hemianopic field when the individual is in primary gaze, only creating a shift in the image when the individual switched their gaze. The Peli prism placement, created a constant peripheral diplopia, providing a field expansion of about 20°, in standard perimetry testing (Bowers, Keeney & Peli, 2008; Giorgi, Woods, & Peli, 2009). The advantages of using prisms include effects can be obtained within a short period of time, they do not require voluntary orientation of attention to the involved side, and they are noninvasive and can be used anywhere (Frassinetti et al., 2002). Occupational therapists work with vision specialists (such as optometrists) when incorporating prisms into intervention (see Fig. 23-5).

Ocular Motor Dysfunction

Ocular motility refers to the ability of the eyes to move smoothly and with coordination through full range of motion. Ocular motor dysfunction includes problems with binocular vision, accommodation, scanning, and

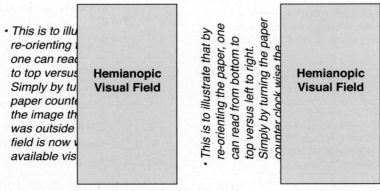

Figure 23-4 Impact of reorienting reading material.

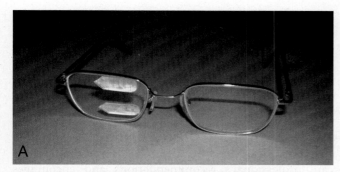

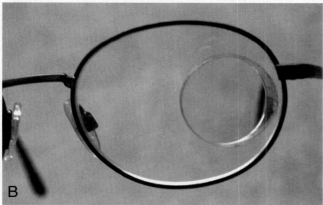

Figure 23-5 **A, B.** Peli prism placement. (Printed with permission from Eli Peli Schepens Eye Research Institute, Boston, MA.)

saccades. Problems with binocular vision typically result in diplopia or double vision, deficits in reading, and other functional tasks. Intervention for oculomotor dysfunction may include lenses, prisms, occlusion, and/or vision therapy.

Vision Therapy

Vision therapy (VT), or orthoptic training, "is an organized regime used to treat a number of neuromuscular, neurophysiological, and neurosensory conditions that interfere with visual function" (Scheiman, 2002, p. 129). VT can range from the use of an eye patch to more complex treatment involving instrumentation and computers. It is generally used to treat disorders of binocular vision, accommodation, ocular motility, strabismus, and visual information processing (Scheiman, 2002). Some of the training provided in VT such as saccades, pursuits, and ocular motility exercises are often incorporated into typical occupational therapy intervention, whereas others, such as base-in and base-out stereograms, pencil push-ups, Brock String exercises, jump-ductions, prisms, and use of lenses, are more typically carried out by optometrists or an occupational therapist under the supervision of the vision specialist (refer to Table 23-6).

Lavrich (2010) and the Convergence Insufficiency Treatment Trial Study Group (2008) found that an intensive VT program appears to be the most effective

Table 23-6	Vision Therapy	
Intervention	**Description**	**Deficits**
Base in and base out stereograms	Pair of images that are viewed through lenses to facilitate binocular vision (try viewing training on YouTube)	Binocular vision deficits Eye teaming and fusion
Pencil push ups	Hold a pencil out at arm's length in front of you. Focus on the tip of the pencil. Slowly bring the pencil in toward your nose. Bring it in until you are no longer able to see just one pencil tip. At that point, hold the pencil and try to refocus on the tip (hold 10 seconds). Slowly return to the starting position. (try viewing training on YouTube; convergence insufficiency exercises)	Binocular vision deficits Convergence insufficiency
Brock string exercises	Place three beads (one red, one yellow, and one green) on 4 feet of string. Hold one end of the string against the bridge of your nose. Place the red bead at about 60 cm from the nose, yellow at 40 cm, and the green at about 20 cm. Look at the green bead, what do you see? You should see one green, two yellow, and two red beads. Now, look at the red bead. You should now see one red bead and two yellow and two green beads. (try viewing training on YouTube)	Binocular vision deficits Convergence and divergence
Jump vergences	Alternating viewing from near to distance objects.	Binocular vision deficits Convergence and divergence

From National Eye Institute. (2008). More effective treatment identified for common childhood vision disorder. Retrieved january 12, 2012 from http://www.nei.nih.gov/news/pressreleases/101308.asp; Scheiman, M., Mitchell, G. L., Cotter, S., Copper, J., Kulp, M., Rouse, M., Borsting, E., London, R., & Wensveen, J. (2005). A randomized clinical trial of treatments for convergence insufficiency in children. *Archives of Ophthalmology, 123,* 14–24.

intervention for convergence insufficiency. However, it was unclear whether the duration or intensity of programming impacted the effectiveness. Pencil push-ups and prism glasses, especially in the presbyopic population, had the most positive outcomes.

The occupational therapy practitioners addressing and training clients with lenses, prisms, and occlusion should always be supervised by an eye care professional (Hellerstein & Fishman, 1999). The occupational therapist can (1) provide the optometrist with critical observations of the client and his or her function; (2) assist with compliance of wearing schedules of prisms, patches, and/or glasses; (3) report on improvements in function or complaints/symptoms; and (4) integrate oculomotor activities, eye exercises, saccades, and pursuits into interventions. It is important to work closely with the eye care professional to provide input as to the client's functional needs and situation and then follow through with training that is set up by the eye care professional.

Lenses and Prisms

Lenses are used to treat a variety of refractive, accommodative, and binocular disorders. In most cases, they are used as a means of compensation to allow the person to function despite any disorder (Suchoff, Ciuffreda, & Kapoor, 2001). The purpose of prisms in the treatment of oculomotor dysfunction is to bend the light entering the eye, allowing the image from each eye to converge onto the fovea, allowing for single vision. Lenses and prisms are recommended by the eye care professional, who is responsible for the strength of the lenses and prisms and any vision exercise programs recommended. The occupational therapist assists the client with follow-through of the eye care professional's recommendations and encourages compliance with the wearing schedule.

Occlusion

Occlusion should be carried out in consultation with the eye care professional. It may be either total or partial and helps minimize the impact of diplopia by forcing the patient to primarily rely on monocular vision. Total occlusion is achieved by means of a patch or opaque tape on the client's glasses (Fig. 23-6). Compliance with this method is often poor because (1) total occlusion can cause clients to feel off balance because of loss of peripheral and central vision input to the central nervous system,

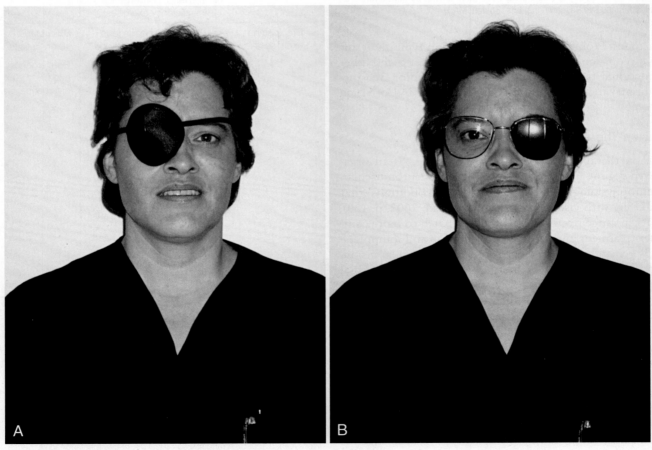

Figure 23-6 Total occlusion. **A.** Pirate patch. **B.** Opaque material covering lens of glasses.

and reduced depth perception; and (2) monocularity can cause discomfort, especially when the dominant eye is occluded (Warren, 1993). The recommendation is to avoid total occlusion if at all possible (Hellerstein & Fishman, 1999) and, if necessary, to alternate occlusion between the eyes every hour (Warren, 1993).

Partial occlusion appears to have better compliance (Rucker & Tomsak, 2005). With partial occlusion, an opaque material added to the client's glasses blocks input to the central VF, leaving the peripheral field unobstructed (Fig. 23-7). Partial occlusion can result in single vision while preserving the greatest amount of peripheral field. Two types of spot patching can be used: (1) a round disk of tape is placed in the individual's line of sight; or (2) the tape is placed in the nasal portion of the individual's glasses (nasal occlusion) allowing for maximal single vision. Because diplopia in the central VF is the most bothersome, the tape is applied to the nasal portion of the

glasses of the nondominant eye (Warren, 1993). As the client focuses on a target, the tape is applied as far centrally as the client reports diplopia. As the muscles get stronger, the occluded area is decreased. When using occlusion, the client should do prescribed range-of-motion exercises to the unaffected eye to prevent contractures. Warren (1999) recommends that exercises first be done with the unaffected eye covered and then with both eyes together.

Unilateral Neglect

UN is referred to by a variety of names, including hemi-inattention, hemispatial neglect, and unilateral spatial agnosia, and is reported in approximately 23% of individuals with CVA (Marshall, 2009). It is manifested by a failure to respond or orient to stimuli presented contralateral to a brain lesion (Hillis, 2006). It is observed functionally in the client who eats the food on only half of the plate, shaves only one side of the face, and walks into objects on the side contralateral to the brain lesion. It has been suggested that there are two types of neglect: motor or output neglect (impaired initiation or execution of movement into contralateral hemispace by either limb) and sensory or input neglect (awareness of stimuli on one side of the body or one side of space) (Pierce & Buxbaum, 2002; Plummer, Morris, & Dunai, 2003). The presence of UN negatively impacts rehabilitation and functional outcomes of clients with right brain damage (RBD) (Cumming et al., 2009; DiMonaco et al., 2011; Gillen, Tennen, & McKee, 2005). As discussed in Chapter 5, UN is not related to eye function but is a processing problem associated with brain damage.

Intervention Approaches for Unilateral Neglect

Intervention for UN can be approached in a variety of ways. First, the client must be aware of the problem. If aware that they have a problem, many clients can voluntarily orient, even though they have difficulty doing so automatically (Ladavas, Carletti, & Gori, 1994). If they are unaware and unable to orient voluntarily or automatically, the only recourse is to modify and simplify the environment (Warren, 1993).

Some of the early research on the treatment of neglect was done by Weinberg et al. (1977), who developed a training program that included reading, writing, and calculation. It was expanded to include sensory awareness and spatial organization and tasks to increase complex visual perception (Weinberg et al., 1979, 1982). Unfortunately, although improvements were seen, they tended to be task specific, with little generalization to other tasks or areas of self-care. Therefore, it is important to train persons in a functional setting using objects readily available in the environment.

The results of a systematic review by Riggs et al. (2007) suggested that the most effective interventions for unilateral inattention or neglect were prisms, scanning, visuomotor feedback training, and patching intervention.

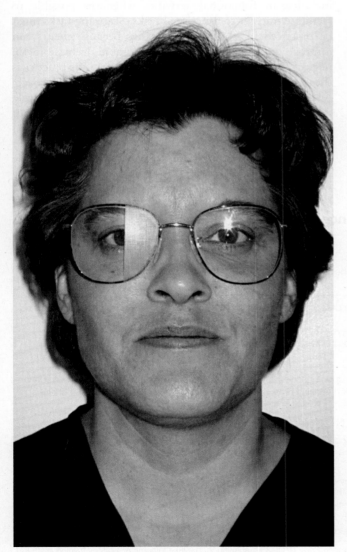

Figure 23-7 A method of partial occlusion to alleviate diplopia.

However, much of the current literature relies on paper and pencil tasks as outcome measures rather than measures of functional abilities.

Attention Training. One theory of UN is that the problem is due to an attention deficit. If this is the case, a treatment program aimed at increasing attention and general level of alertness should improve UN. Robertson et al. (1995) trained clients with RBD and UN to self-alert during activities. With 5 hours of training, they could mentally alert themselves during tasks. Improvement in UN and sustained attention lasted 1–14 days.

In another study, Robertson et al. (1998) found that providing a warning tone as a means of alerting the client that something was going to happen prior to a task increased perceptual processing and shifting of spatial attention to the left. This system was further expanded by a limb-activation device that can be attached to the affected shoulder, arm, or leg (Robertson et al., 2002) that is programmed to emit a tone if there is no movement within a set period of time (2–120 seconds). The researchers found a significant effect on motor function of the arm and leg, which persisted for 18–24 months.

Another method of self-activation is the client's use of the contralateral extremity as a cue to attend to the neglected side (e.g., to mark the left side of the page while reading or to move the extremity while walking to increase attention to that side). Robertson and North (1994) found that clients who moved their contralateral hand when walking through a doorway exhibited a decrease in neglect.

Scanning. Similar to visual scanning training for individuals with VF defects, individuals with UN may benefit from mental imagery, computerized visual scanning, and functional scanning tasks. Mental imagery can be used to self-direct environmental or task scanning in an organized manner. Niemeier (1998) and Niemeier, Cifu, and Kishore (2001) developed a visual imagery technique called the lighthouse strategy in which clients are taught to visualize themselves as a lighthouse and use the eyes to sweep the environment. This method was found to increase attention to the neglected side of space. Paolucci et al. (1996, 2001) used a training program for neglect that included scanning, copying, and description of scenes in addition to a traditional rehabilitation approach and found that there was an improvement not only on tests of neglect but also in function. On the other hand, although Bailey, Riddoch, and Crome (2002) found an improvement with scanning and cueing, no generalization to functional activity was present.

It seems that scanning tasks and cueing should be included in functional activities whenever possible to facilitate transfer to functional tasks. Scanning tasks must be practiced in a variety of settings because clients can improve on a task without a measurable decrease in VF neglect. An excellent therapeutic model to guide practice is the use of Toglia's (1991) multicontext treatment approach. An example of levels of transfer for a letter cancellation task, consisting of crossing out a specific letter on a page of four rows of random letters, can be seen in Table 23-7.

Patching. Eye patching techniques for UN include single-eye patching (see Fig. 23-6) and half-field patching

---

Table 23-7 **Levels of Transfer for a Letter Cancellation Task**

Transfer Distance	Task
Near	Client is instructed to cross out the number 5 on a worksheet comprised of rows of numbers (number cancellation task).
Intermediate	Four horizontal rows of various coins are presented. Client is instructed to place a marker over all the nickels (tabletop task).
Far	Client is presented with a spice rack and is asked to pick out all of the jars that need to be refilled (standing and reaching at kitchen cabinets).
Very far	Client is evaluated on the ability to initiate spontaneously left-to-right scanning in the context of simple, everyday life tasks (reading four lines in a large-print magazine or locating an item in the medicine cabinet or on a shelf).
Feedback	• Verbal feedback: ○ In terms of the result ○ To encourage the client to consciously evaluate the results (see, hear, feel, smell, taste) • Physical feedback as to: ○ Posture of the client ○ Support of the limbs ○ Pointing or handing the object to the client • Verbal and physical feedback to assist client's knowledge of performance: ○ Place a mirror in front of the client ○ Video record performance and then review together

Adapted from van Heugten, C. M., Dekker, J., Deelman, B. G., van Dijk, A. J., Stehmann-Saris, J. C., & Kinebanian, A. (1998). Outcome of strategy training in stroke patients with apraxia: A phase II study. *Clinical Rehabilitation, 12,* 294–303.

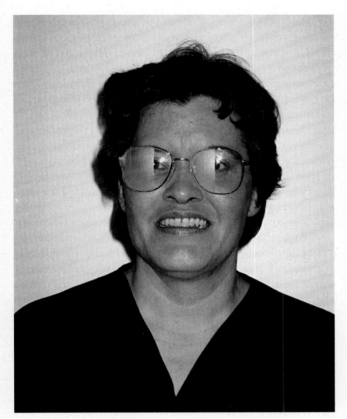

Figure 23-8 Right hemifield patching for left visual neglect.

(Fig. 23-8). For the client with neglect, either the entire eye ipsilateral to the lesion is covered, or the hemifield of both eyes is covered. For example, in the case of left UN, the right eye or right hemifields of both eyes is patched.

Patching one eye is believed to influence the central nervous system by way of the superior colliculus (Posner & Rafal, 1987), increasing eye movements to the contralateral side and decreasing neglect. Patching the ipsilateral hemifield is thought to increase activation of the involved hemisphere, resulting in increased attention to the contralateral side. Butter and Kirsch (1992) found that patching the right eye of clients with left neglect decreased the clients' left neglect score. When lateralized visual stimulation was added, the relative benefits were larger. The beneficial effects, however, were present only when the eye patch was on, and the study did not include generalization to functional tasks.

Beis et al. (1999) followed 22 clients with UN: 7 wore glasses with patches covering the right eye, 7 wore glasses with right half-field patches, and 8 controls had no patching. The patches were worn up to 12 hours a day for 3 months. The results of the clients with the right half-field glasses were significantly better from those of the controls, with the right half-field clients exhibiting an increase in total Functional Independence

Measure (FIM™) score (Uniform Data System for Medical Rehabilitation, 1997) and increased time looking to the left. Similarly, Zeloni, Farne, and Baccini (2002) looked at continuous wear of hemi blinding goggles for 1 week and found improvements that continued over the 3-week testing. Arai et al. (1997) also looked at the effects of half-field patching with 10 RBD clients. They found a decrease in neglect, improvement on pencil and paper tasks, and good functional return in one client. Harrell, Kramer-Stutts, and Zolten (1995) also reported an improvement of neglect in clients wearing goggles with half-field glasses. Riggs et al. (2007) and Jutai et al. (2003) completed an analysis of the evidence, 27 studies and 32 studies, respectively, on the effectiveness of UN interventions and found that hemifield patching showed moderate improvements on standard neglect tests.

Patching has many benefits. It may be used throughout the day during a variety of functional activities and does not rely on memory and training. Patching is simple, inexpensive, and carried out by a variety of disciplines.

Prisms. Prisms are also used in the treatment of UN, in which the image from the neglected area is shifted into the non-neglected area. Gianutsos and Suchoff (2002) recommended the use of the Fresnel prisms as a temporary or diagnostic device. Unlike the use of Fresnel prisms with individuals with VF defects, these were not as beneficial as yoked prisms ground into the client's prescription for individuals with UN. The strongest evidence shows that full-field yoked prisms are most beneficial for individuals with UN because they do not require the individual to shift gaze into the prism to elicit the VF shift (Rossetti et al., 1998). This prism does not require effort of the individual to shift focus into the prism; the image is shifted in the direction of the apex of the prism. Nys et al. (2008) and Serino et al. (2009) studied the use of prism goggles with 10° rightward deviation while engaged in pointing tasks to improve greater VF awareness. These randomized controlled trials found significant improvement in standard neglect tests at the end of the study and 1 month follow-up.

Rossetti et al. (1998) used prisms to shift the VF to the right in 16 RBD clients with left UN. Initially, the clients exhibited a shift to the left when pointing straight ahead. Following adaptation, clients were given tasks including line bisection, line cancellation, copying, drawing from memory, and reading. Clients in the experimental group exhibited an improvement in neglect, which was maintained for 2 hours. Frassinetti et al. (2002) expanded this and found that the prism adaptation was maintained for at least 5 weeks and, for some subjects, was maintained for up to 17 weeks.

Spatiomotor Cuing. It has been suggested that there are two types of neglect (Bisiach et al., 1990; Coslett et al.,

1990; Tegner & Levander, 1991), and therefore, it is reasonable to expect that each has its own form of intervention. For a client with primarily a motor or output neglect, encouragement of left-hand activation may reduce neglect to a greater extent than visual perceptual cuing. An example might be having the client move the left hand (or use whatever movement is available) while performing a scanning task, instead of using a visual anchoring technique such as supplying a visual cue on the impaired side to indicate starting position. Robertson and North (1992) found that left motor activation in left hemispace reduced neglect more than did left motor activation in right hemispace, right motor activation in left hemispace, or visual cuing. They further reported that (1) left lower extremity activation reduced neglect, (2) passive movement of the left extremity had no effect on neglect, (3) bilateral movements produced no effect, and (4) there was no effect if the movement became automatic. In a further study, Robertson and North (1994) found that simultaneous activation of right and left hands produces a phenomenon similar to extinction, such that the advantage gained by activating the left hand is lost. Only single left-hand movement produced a large reduction in neglect. This could have implications for use of bilateral activities, such as those used in the Bobath techniques. Opportunity for unilateral activation of the hemiplegic arm as well as bilateral activation should be provided (Robertson & North, 1994). Lin (1996) completed a meta-analysis looking at three approaches to UN in right CVA: lateralized task approach, controlled sensory stimulation, and limb activation and found that there was reduction in neglect symptoms with hemispheric activation.

If the client demonstrates a sensory or input neglect, he may benefit from visual cuing such as anchoring (Table 23-5) or reminders to look to the left. Training the client to use the left upper extremity as an anchor during functional activities provides both a perceptual anchor and a means of left-limb activation (Robertson, North, &

Geggie, 1992). Kalra et al. (1997) found that spatial cueing with motor or functional activity improved neglect symptoms, improved body image, and decreased length of stay.

Compensatory Techniques. Compensatory techniques can be environmental or cognitive. Adaptation of the environment includes such things as arranging the client's bed so that the involved side is toward the activity in the room and always interacting with the client on the involved side. If the client has a left visual neglect, the bed should be arranged so that the client must turn to look to the left to see people enter the room or watch television, thus allowing for constant cueing to look to the left.

Cognitive compensation includes metacognitive training (Toglia, 1991), use of video feedback (Soderback et al., 1992), and teaching clients a routine to complete a specific activity like donning a shirt while self-cueing themselves through each step. What is most important is that clients must be aware that there is a problem before they can successfully use compensatory techniques (Crosson et al., 1989; Tham, Borell, & Gustavsson, 2000). These techniques must be practiced, and eventually, if the client becomes an active problem solver, the techniques can be generalized to new situations involving visual challenges.

SUMMARY

Our population is aging, and as a result occupational therapy practitioners are often faced with addressing multiple conditions as a result of aging, disease, or injury, including vision impairment. It is important that occupational therapists have the skills and knowledge to be able to provide appropriate, evidenced-based interventions, including visual skills training, environmental adaptation (lighting & contrast), magnification, compensatory techniques (sensory substitution—talking and tactile strategies), organizational strategies, and client/family education to maximize their client's occupational performance.

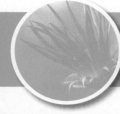

case example

Mrs. F.: Occupational Therapy Intervention to Address Problems with Reading

Occupational Therapy Intervention Process	Clinical Reasoning Process	
	Objectives	Examples of Therapist's Internal Dialogue

Client Information

Mrs. F. is a 78-year-old female who was admitted for rehabilitation following a hip fracture, past medical history included osteoarthritis, hypertension, and macular degeneration. She participated in an inpatient occupational therapy (OT) assessment, and the following problems were identified: (1) decreased awareness and acceptance of her ocular condition, (2) decreased awareness of how her visual impairment will impact the rehabilitative process, (3) difficulty recognizing people's faces, (4) difficulty reading standard newsprint, and (5) difficulty comprehending reading materials.

Appreciate the context

See Chapter 5 for description of the assessment process and client's background.

Develop intervention hypotheses

"I believe that Mrs. F.'s visual skills are limiting her ability to read and participate in the rehabilitative process. These abilities may be further limited by her depression. She is motivated to return home."

Select an intervention approach

"I think that Mrs. F. would benefit from large print, increased contrast, and improved lighting, which, according to the research, is successful although task specific. She will probably need to learn compensatory techniques that she can apply to various functional situations."

"I'm afraid that Mrs. F. is going to continue to require support and increased time for task completion and acceptance of compensatory strategies because of her probable depression and lack of acceptance of her visual impairment."

Recommendations

In collaboration with Mrs. F., the occupational therapist established the following long-term goals:

1. In 2 weeks, Mrs. F. will be independent in her home exercise program with 100% accuracy.
2. In 2 weeks, Mrs. F. will be independent in activities of daily living (ADL) and instrumental activities of daily living (IADL) tasks using compensatory and visual strategies.
3. In 2 weeks, Mrs. F. will verbalize awareness of her ocular disease and its impact on occupational performance and will make an appointment for outpatient OT to continue to address visual skills, psychosocial adjustment, and functional implications of vision loss.

Consider what will occur in therapy, how often, and for how long

"I know Mrs. F.'s goal is to return home. In order to do this, she will need to address not only her hip fracture but also her vision loss. She will need to be able to accept the permanence of her visual impairment and accept recommendations to compensate. Her family or personal care attendant will be instrumental in assisting her to follow through with recommendations and compensatory techniques. Hopefully, she and her family will be accepting of recommendations for a low vision assessment and outpatient vision rehabilitation services."

Summary of Short-Term Goals and Progress

1. Mrs. F. demonstrated improved use of compensatory strategies (large print, increased contrast, and improved lighting) such that she was able to read her exercise program with 80% accuracy.
2. Mrs. F. is having difficulty with lower extremity (LE) dressing using long-handled reacher, sock aid, and shoe horn. The task was adapted by use of high-contrast tape to increase contrast between clothing, floor, and adaptive devices. With increased contrast, Mrs. F. was able to don her pants with stand-by assistance.
3. Mrs. F. was having difficulties with ADL task completion. It was decided to continue to address necessary ADL and IADL tasks for discharge home. Because Mrs. F. was unable to read her menus or home program, it was probable that she would be unable to read labels, medicine bottles, or the mail. It was determined a home evaluation would be needed prior to discharge home.

Assess the client's comprehension

Understand what she is doing

Compare actual to expected performance

"When she first started, Mrs. F. had difficulty because she did not accept the need for modifications. We spent some time working on visual skills, and she was able to see the benefit of the strategies. I am encouraged this has worked for her."

"Mrs. F. is making progress on LE dressing with use of compensatory strategies."

"I hope Mrs. F. will be accepting of a home assessment."

Next Steps

Revised short-term goals (1 week):

1. In 1 week, Mrs. F. will independently complete her home program using compensatory and visual strategies with 100% accuracy.
2. In 1 week, Mrs. F. will be independent in dressing using high-contrast adaptive devices.
3. Mrs. F. will make an appointment with outpatient OT services to continue to address visual skills, psychosocial adjustment, and functional implications of vision loss by discharge.

Anticipate present and future client concerns	"Mrs. F. has made progress on established goals. Her accuracy and use of compensatory strategies have improved but would benefit from continued outpatient treatment. She is also managing her ADL, but will require continued treatment to address IADL tasks (i.e., money management, medication management, home management)."
Decide whether the client should continue or discontinue therapy and/ or return in the future	"I feel Mrs. F. is progressing and will benefit from outpatient occupational therapy one to two times per week for 6 weeks."

 ## Clinical Reasoning in Occupational Therapy Practice

Effects of Low Vision on a Functional Task

Based on an optometrist's report for the client, Mrs. F., after her discharge from rehab, her best corrected acuity is 20/80 at distance. She was able to read standard large-print materials; however, her speed was slow. She has macular degeneration in both eyes and a history of a hip fracture following a fall. She lives alone in a single-family home with limited family support. She has recently lost her husband. She is a retired teacher, and her primary leisure pursuits are reading and cross-stitch.

You have received a referral to see Mrs. F. because of her visual impairment. The home assessment from the rehabilitation facility found a cluttered environment and decreased lighting throughout.

What modifications could be made to her environment to support engagement in occupations of choice?

Summary Review Questions

1. List three compensatory techniques for use with clients with low vision, and give two examples of each.
2. You have a client with diabetic retinopathy. What might you need to consider when deciding on treatment options?
3. You have a client with macular degeneration and mild cognitive decline whose goal is to be able to read. What potential intervention strategies may be difficult? What intervention strategies would you use?
4. You have a client with double vision. What should you do first?
5. Based on an optometrist's report, your client's best corrected acuity is 20/160. He has a cataract in the right eye and glaucoma in both eyes, for which he is receiving medication. How might his low vision affect his ability to do self-care, meal preparation, and money management?
6. Summarize the guidelines for visual scanning training.
7. How does the use of occlusion for diplopia differ from that used for unilateral neglect?
8. Your client has a left visual field defect and is struggling with reading. What would you expect to be difficult, and what compensatory strategies would you implement?
9. Your client with left unilateral neglect is having difficulty finding things in the kitchen cabinets during meal preparation. What activities might you plan for your therapy session?
10. Why is it important for occupational therapists to become involved in research?

Glossary

Anchoring—Method of providing a cue on the side contralateral to the brain damage, in the presence of unilateral neglect.

Extinction—Phenomenon of neglect that occurs when stimuli are presented in both visual fields or both sides of space at one time and only one stimulus is reported, whereas if presented to either side individually, the client reports the stimulus.

Fresnel prism—A prism that is applied to glasses to shift an image from the nonseeing area into the seeing area, typically used with individuals with hemianopsia or unilateral neglect

Low vision—A bilateral visual impairment that cannot be corrected by corrective lenses, medication, or surgery that impairs an individual's ability to complete occupations of choice.

Occlusion—Covering part or all of the visual field of the eye.

Prism—A type of lens that is thicker on one side (base) than the other (apex); the purpose is to bend the light and shift the image from the base of the prism to the apex.

Vision rehabilitation—The process of providing education and treatment to individuals with visual impairment that aims to maximize the individual's awareness of their visual impairment, optimize their adjustment, and facilitate participation in occupations of choice.

Vision therapy—An organized regimen used to treat a number of neuromuscular, neurophysiological, and neurosensory conditions that interfere with visual function carried out typically by eye care professionals or by occupational therapists with additional training and under the supervision of the prescribing eye care practitioner.

References

Arai, T., Ohi, H., Sasaki, H., Nobuto, H., & Tanaka, H. (1997). Hemispatial sunglasses: Effect on unilateral spatial neglect. *Archives of Physical Medicine and Rehabilitation, 78,* 230–232.

Bailey, M., Riddoch, M. J., & Crome, P. (2002). Treatment of visual neglect in elderly patient with stroke: A single-subject series using either a scanning and cueing strategy or a left-limb activation strategy. *Physical Therapy, 82,* 782–797.

Beis, J.-M., Andre, J.-M., Baumgarten, A., & Challier, B. (1999). Eye patching in unilateral spatial neglect: Efficacy of two methods. *Archives of Physical Medicine and Rehabilitation, 80,* 71–76.

Bisiach, E., Geminiani, G., Berti, A., & Rusconi, M. L. (1990). Perceptual and premotor factors of unilateral neglect. *Neurology, 40,* 1278–1281.

Bouwmeester, L., Heutink, J., & Lucas, C. (2006). The effect of visual training for patients with visual field defects due to brain damage: A systematic review. *Journal of Neurology, Neurosurgery & Psychiatry, 78,* 555–564.

Bowers, A. R., Keeney, K., & Peli, E. (2008). Community-based trial of a peripheral prism visual field expansion device for hemianopia. *Archives of Ophthalmology, 126,* 657–664.

Brahm, K. D., Wilgenburg, H. M., Kirby, J., Ingalla, S., Chang, C.-Y., & Goodrich, G. L. (2009). Visual impairment and dysfunction in combat-injured military personnel: A population study. *Optometry and Vision Science, 86,* 817–825.

Brunnstrom, G., Sorensen, S., Alsterstad, K., & Sjostrand, J. (2004). Quality of light and quality of life-the effect of lighting adaptation among people with low vision. *Ophthalmic and Physiological Optics, 24,* 274–280.

Butter, C. M., & Kirsch, N. (1992). Combined and separate effects of eye patching and visual stimulation on unilateral neglect following stroke. *Archives of Physical Medicine and Rehabilitation, 73,* 1133–1139.

Campbell, V. A., Crews, J. E., Moriarty, D. G., Zach, M. M., & Blackman, D. K. (1999). Surveillance for sensory impairment, activity limitation, and health related quality of life among older adults—United States, 1993–1997. *Centers for Disease Control Surveillance Studies: Morbidity and Mortality Weekly Report, 48,* 131–156.

Chang, T. T., Ciuffreda, K. J., & Kapoor, N. (2007). Critical flicker frequency and related symptoms in mild traumatic brain injury. *Brain Injury, 21,* 1055–1062.

Ciuffreda, K. J., Ludlam, D. P., & Kapoor, N. (2009). Clinical oculomotor training in traumatic brain injury. *Optometry & Vision Development, 40,* 16–23.

Cockerham, G. C., Goodrich, G. L., Weichel, E. D., Orcutt, J. C., Rizzo, J. F., Bower, K. S., & Schuchard, R. A. (2009). Eye and visual function in traumatic brain injury. *Journal of Rehabilitation Research & Development, 46,* 811–818.

Coleman, A. L., Yu, F., Keeler, E., & Mangione, C. M. (2006). Treatment of uncorrected refractive error improves vision specific quality of life. *Journal of the American Geriatric Society, 54,* 883–990.

Colenbrander, A., & Fletcher, D. C. (1995). Basic concepts and terms for low vision rehabilitation. *American Journal of Occupational Therapy, 49,* 865–869.

Congdon, N. (2004). Causes and prevalence of visual impairment among adults in the United States. *Archives of Ophthalmology, 122,* 477–485.

Convergence Insufficiency Treatment Trial Study Group. (2008). Randomized clinical trial of treatments for symptomatic convergence insufficiency in children. *Archives of Ophthalmology, 126,* 1336–1349.

Cooke, D. (1992). Remediation of unilateral neglect: What do we know? *Australian Occupational Therapy Journal, 39,* 19–25.

Coslett, H. B., Bowers, D., Fitzpatrick, E., Haws, B., & Heilman, K. M. (1990). Directional hypokinesia and hemispatial inattention in neglect. *Brain, 113,* 475–486.

Crossland, M., Culham, L., & Rubin, G. (2005). Predicting reading fluency in patients with macular disease. *Optometry and Vision Sciences, 82,* 11–17.

Crosson, B., Barco, P. P., Velozo, C. A., Bolesta, M. M., Cooper, P. V., Werts, D., & Brobeck, T. C. (1989). Awareness and compensation in post-acute head injury rehabilitation. *Journal of Head Trauma Rehabilitation, 4,* 46–54.

Cumming, T. B., Plummer-D'Amato, P., Linden, T., & Bernhardt, J. (2009). Hemispatial neglect and rehabilitation in acute stroke. *Archives of Physical Medicine & Rehabilitation, 90,* 1931–1936.

DiMonaco, M., Schintu, S., Dotta, M., Barba, S., Tappero, R., & Gindri, P. (2011). Severity of unilateral spatial neglect is an independent predictor of functional outcome of the acute inpatient rehabilitation in individuals with right hemispheric stroke. *Archives of Physical Medicine & Rehabilitation, 92,* 1250–1256.

Duffy, M. A. (2002). *Making life more livable: Simple adaptations for living at home after vision loss.* New York: AFB Press.

Eye Disease Prevalence Research Group. (2004). Causes and prevalence of visual impairment in the United States. *Archives of Ophthalmology, 122,* 477–485.

Figueiro, M. G. (2001). *Lighting the way: A key to independence.* Troy, NY: Rensselear Polytechnic Institute.

Fletcher, D., Schuchard, R., & Watson, G. (1999). Relative locations of macular scotomas near the PRL: Effect on low vision reading. *Journal of Rehabilitation, Research and Development, 36,* 356–364.

Fok, D., Polgar, J. M., Shaw, L., & Jutai, J. W. (2011). Low vision assistive technology device usage and importance in daily occupations. *Work: A Journal of Prevention, Assessment and Rehabilitation, 39,* 37–48.

Fortis, P., Ronchi, R., Senna, I., Perucca, L., Posteraro, L., Maravita, A., Gallucci, M., Grassi, E., Olgiati, E., Banco, E., Tesio, L., & Vallar, G. (2010). Rehabilitating patients with left spatial neglect by prism exposure during a visuomotor activity. *Neuropsychology, 24,* 681–697.

Frassinetti, F., Angeli, V., Meneghello, F., Avanzi, S., & Ladavas, E. (2002). Long-lasting amelioration of visuospatial neglect by prism adaptation. *Brain, 125,* 608–623.

Freeman, K. F., Cole, R. G., Faye, E. E., Freeman, P. B., Goodrich, G. L., & Stemlack, J. A. (2007). *Optometric clinical practice guidelines: Care of the patient with visual impairment.* St. Louis: American Optometric Association.

Gianutsos, R., & Suchoff, I. B. (2002). Visual fields after brain injury: Management issues for the occupational therapist. In M. Scheiman (Ed.), *Understanding and managing vision deficits: A guide for occupational therapists* (2nd ed., pp. 247–263). Thorofare, NJ: Slack.

Gillen, R., Tennen, H., & McKee, T. (2005). Unilateral spatial neglect: Relation to rehabilitation outcomes in patients with right hemisphere stroke. *Archives of Physical Medicine and Rehabilitation, 86,* 763–767.

Giorgi, R. G., Woods, R. L., & Peli, E. (2009). Clinical and laboratory evaluation of peripheral glasses for hemianopia. *Optometry & Vision Science, 86,* 492–502.

Gottlieb, D. D., Freeman, P., & Williams, M. (1992). Clinical research and statistical analysis of a visual field awareness system. *Journal of the American Optometric Association, 63,* 581–588.

Harrell, E. H., Kramer-Stutts, T., & Zolten, A. J. (1995). Performance of subjects with left visual neglect after removal of the right visual field using hemifield goggles. *Journal of Rehabilitation, 61,* 46–49.

Hellerstein, L. F., & Fishman, B. I. (1999). Collaboration between occupational therapists and optometrists. *Journal of Behavioral Optometry, 10,* 147–152.

Hillis, A. E. (2006). Neurobiology of unilateral spatial neglect. *Neuroscientist, 12,* 153–163.

Hoge, C. W., McGurk, D., Thomas, J. L., Cox, A. L., Engel, C. C., & Castro, C. A. (2008). Mild traumatic brain injury in U.S. soldiers returning from Iraq. *New England Journal of Medicine, 358,* 453–463.

Jutai, J. W., Bhogal, S. K., Foley, N. C., Bayley, M., Teasell, R. W., & Speechley, M. R. (2003). Treatment of visual perceptual disorders post stroke. *Topics in Stroke Rehabilitation, 10,* 77–106.

Kalra, L., Perez, I., Gupta, S., & Wittink, M. (1997). The influence of visual neglect on stroke rehabilitation. *Stroke, 28,* 1386–1391.

Kempen, J. H., O'Colmain, B. J., Leske, M. C., Haffner, S. M., Klein, R., Moss, S. E., Taylor, H. R., Hamman, R. F., West, S. K., Wang, J. J., Congdon, N. G., & Friedman, D. S. (2004). The Eye Diseases Prevalence Research Group. The prevalence of diabetic retinopathy among adults in the United States. *Archives of Ophthalmology, 122,* 552–563.

Ladavas, E., Carletti, M., & Gori, G. (1994). Automatic and voluntary orientating of attention in patients with visual neglect: Horizontal and vertical dimensions. *Neuropsychologia, 32,* 1195–1208.

Lavrich, J.B. (2010). Convergence insufficiency and its current treatment. *Current Opinion in Ophthalmology, 21,* 356–360.

Lin, K. (1996). Right-hemisphere activation approaches to neglect rehabilitation post stroke. *American Journal of Occupational Therapy, 50,* 504–515.

Markowitz, S. N. (2006). Principles of modern low vision rehabilitation. *Canadian Journal of Ophthalmology, 41,* 289–312.

Marshall, R. S. (2009). Rehabilitation Approaches to Hemi neglect. *Neurologist, 15,* 185–192.

Mogk, L. G., & Mogk, M. (2003). *Macular degeneration: The complete guide to saving and maximizing your sight.* New York: Ballantine Books.

National Eye Institute. (2008). More effective treatment identified for common childhood vision disorder. Retrieved January 12, 2012 from http://www.nei.nih.gov/news/pressreleases/101308.asp.

Niemeier, J. P. (1998). The lighthouse strategy: Use of a visual imagery technique to treat visual inattention in stroke patients. *Brain Injury, 12,* 399–406.

Niemeier, J. P., Cifu, D. X., & Kishore, R. (2001). The lighthouse strategy: Improving the functional status of patients with unilateral neglect after stroke and brain injury using a visual imagery intervention. *Topics in Stroke Rehabilitation, 8,* 10–18.

Nilsson, U. L., Frennesson, C., & Nilsson, S. E. (2003). Patients with AMD and a large absolute central scotoma can be trained successfully to use eccentric viewing, as demonstrated in a scanning laser ophthalmoscope, *Vision Research, 43,* 1777–1787.

Nowakowski, R. W. (2000). Basic optics and optical devices. In M. Warren (Ed.), *Low vision: Occupational therapy intervention with the older adult* (Lesson 4). Bethesda, MD: American Occupational Therapy Association.

Nys, G. M. S., de Haan, E. H. F., Kunnerman, A., de Kort, P. L. M., & Dijkerman, H. C. (2008). Acute neglect rehabilitation using repetitive prism adaptation: A randomized placebo-controlled trial. *Restorative Neurology and Neuroscience, 26,* 1–12.

Pambakian, A., Currie, J., & Kennard, C. (2005). Rehabilitation strategies for patients with homonymous visual field defects. *Journal of Neuro-Ophthalmology, 25,* 136–142.

Paolucci, S., Antonucci, G., Grasso, M. G., & Pizzamiglio, L. (2001). The role of unilateral spatial neglect in rehabilitation of right brain-damaged ischemic stroke patients: A matched comparison. *Archives of Physical Medicine and Rehabilitation, 82,* 743–749.

Paolucci, S., Antonucci, G., Guariglia, C., Magnotti, L., Pizzamiglio, L., & Zoccolotti, P. (1996). Facilitatory effect of neglect rehabilitation on the recovery of left hemiplegic stroke patients: A cross-over study. *Journal of Neurology, 243,* 308–314.

Peli, E. (2000). Field expansion for homonymous hemianopsia by optically induced peripheral exotropia. *Optometry and Vision Science, 77,* 453–464.

Peli, E. (2001). Vision multiplexing: An engineering approach to vision rehabilitation device development. *Optometry and Vision Science, 78,* 304–315.

Pierce, S. R., & Buxbaum, L. J. (2002). Treatments of unilateral neglect: A review. *Archives of Physical Medicine and Rehabilitation, 83,* 256–268.

Pisella, L., Rode, G., Farne, A., Tilikete, C., & Rossetti, Y. (2006). Prism adaptation in the rehabilitation of patients with visuo-spatial cognitive disorders. *Current Opinion in Neurology, 19,* 534–542.

Plummer, P., Morris, M. E., & Dunai, J. (2003). Assessment of unilateral neglect. *Physical Therapy, 83,* 732–740.

Pollock, A., Hazelton, C., Henderson, C. A., Angilley, J., Dhillon, B., Langhorne, P., Livingstone, K., Munro, F. A., Orr, H., Rowe, F. J., & Shahani, U. (2011). Interventions for visual field defects in patients with stroke. *Cochrane Database of Systematic Reviews, 10,* CD008388.

Posner, M. I., & Rafal, R. D. (1987). Cognitive theories of attention and the rehabilitation of attentional deficits. In M. J. Meier, A. L. Benton, & L. Diller (Eds.), *Neuropsychological rehabilitation after brain injury* (pp. 182–201). New York: Churchill Livingston.

Quintana, L. A. (1995). Remediating perceptual impairments. In C. A. Trombly (Ed.), *Occupational therapy for physical dysfunction* (4th ed., pp. 529–537). Philadelphia: Williams & Wilkins.

Riggs, R. V., Andres, K., Roberts, P., & Gilewski, M. (2007). Visual deficit interventions in adult stroke and brain injury. *American Journal of Physical Medicine & Rehabilitation, 86,* 853–860.

Robertson, I. H., Mattingley, J. B., Rorden, C., & Driver, J. (1998). Phasic alerting of neglect patients overcomes their spatial deficit in visual awareness. *Nature, 395,* 169–172.

Robertson, I. H., McMillan, T., MacLeod, E., Edgeworth, J., & Brock, D. (2002). Rehabilitation by limb activation training reduces left-sided motor impairment in unilateral neglect patients: A single-blind randomized control trial. *Neuropsychological Rehabilitation, 12,* 439–454.

Robertson, I. H., & North, N. (1992). Spatio-motor cueing in unilateral left neglect: The role of hemi space, hand and motor activation. *Neuropsychologia, 30,* 553–563.

Robertson, I. H., & North, N. T. (1994). One hand is better than two: Motor extinction of left hand advantage in unilateral neglect. *Neuropsychologia, 32,* 1–11.

Robertson, I. H., North, N. T., & Geggie, C. (1992). Spatiomotor cueing in unilateral left neglect: Three case studies of its therapeutic effects. *Journal of Neurology, Neurosurgery, and Psychiatry, 55,* 799–805.

Robertson, I. H., Tegner, R., Tham, K., Lo, A., & Nimmo-Smith, I. (1995). Sustained attention training for unilateral neglect: Theoretical and rehabilitation implications. *Journal of Clinical and Experimental Neuropsychology, 17,* 416–430.

Rossetti, Y., Rode, G., Pisella, L., Farne, A., Li, L., Boisson, D., & Perenin, M. T. (1998). Prism adaptation to a rightward optical deviation rehabilitates left hemispatial neglect. *Nature, 395,* 166–169.

Roth, T., Sokolov, A. N., Messias, A., Roth, P., Weller, M., & Trauzettel-Klosinski, S. (2009). Comparing explorative saccades and flicker training in hemianopsia: A randomized controlled study. *Neurology, 72,* 324–331.

Rowe, F., Brand, D., Jackson, C. A., Price, A., Walker, L., Harrison, S., Eccleston, C., Scott, C., Akerman, N., Dodridge, C., Howard, C., Shipman, T., Sperring, U., MacDiarmid, S., & Freeman, C. (2009). Visual impairment following stroke: Do stroke patients require vision assessment? *Age and Ageing, 38,* 188–193.

Rucker, J. C., & Tomsak, R. L. (2005). Binocular diplopia: A practical approach. *Neurologist, 11,* 98–110.

Scheiman, M. (2002). Management of refractive, visual efficiency and visual information processing disorders. In M. Scheiman (Ed.), *Understanding and managing vision deficits: A guide for occupational therapists* (2nd ed., pp. 117–162). Thorofare, NJ: Slack.

Scheiman, M., Gwiazda, J., & Li, T. (2011). Non-surgical interventions for convergence insufficiency. *Cochrane Database of Systematic Reviews, 3,* CD006768.

Scheiman, M., Mitchell, G. L., Cotter, S., Cooper, J., Kulp, M., Rouse, M., Borsting, E., London, R., & Wensveen, J. (2005). A randomized clinical trial of treatments for convergence insufficiency in children. *Archives of Ophthalmology, 123,* 14–24

Schrupp, L. E., Ciuffreda, K. J., & Kapoor, N. (2009). Foveal versus eccentric retinal critical flicker frequency in mild traumatic brain injury. *Optometry, 80,* 642–650.

Schuchard, R. A. (2005). Preferred retinal loci and macular scotoma characteristics in patients with age-related macular degeneration. *Canadian Journal of Ophthalmology, 40,* 303–312.

Serino, A., Barbiani, M., Rinaldesi, M. L., & Landavas, E. (2009). Effectiveness of prism adaptation in neglect rehabilitation: A controlled trial study. *Stroke, 40,* 1–7.

Shiraishi, H., Muraki, T., Itou, Y. S. A., & Hirayama, K. (2010). Prism intervention helped sustainability of effects and ADL performances in chronic neglect: A follow up study. *NeuroRehabilitation, 27,* 165–172.

Social Security Administration. (2011). Disability Programs: Disability evaluation under social security. Retrieved January 12, 2011 from http://www.ssa.gov/disability/professionals/bluebook/2.00-Special SensesandSpeech-Adult.htm.

Soderback, I., Begtsson, I., Ginsburg, E., & Eleholm, J. (1992). Video feedback in occupational therapy: Its effect in patients with neglect syndrome. *Archives of Physical Medicine and Rehabilitation, 73,* 1140–1146.

Stelmack, J. A., Frith, T., Van Koevering, D., Rinee, S., & Stelmack, T. (2009). Visual function in patients followed at a veterans affairs polytrauma network site: An electronic medical records review. *Optometry, 80,* 419–424.

Stelmack, J. A., Massof, R. W., & Stemlack, T. R. (2004). Is there a standard of care for eccentric viewing training? *Journal of Rehabilitation Research & Development, 41,* 729–738.

Suchoff, I. B., & Ciuffreda, K. J. (2004). A primer for the optometric management of unilateral spatial inattention. *Optometry, 75,* 305–318.

Suchoff, I.B., Ciuffreda, K.J., & Kapoor, N. (2001). An overview of acquired brain injury and optometric implications. In I.B. Suchoff, K.J. Ciuffreda, & N. Kapoor (Eds.), *Visual & Vestibular Consequences of Acquired Brain Injury* (pp. 1–9). Santa Ana, CA: Optometric Extension Program Foundation, Inc.

Tegner, R., & Levander, M. (1991). Through a looking glass. A new technique to demonstrate directional hypokinesia in unilateral neglect. *Brain, 114,* 1943–1951.

Tham, K., Borell, L., & Gustavsson, A. (2000). The discovery of disability: A phenomenological study of unilateral neglect. *American Journal of Occupational Therapy, 54,* 398–405.

Ting, D. S. J., Pollock, A., Dutton, G. N., Doubal, F. N., Ting, D. S. W., Thompson, M., & Dhillon, B. (2011). Visual neglect following stroke: Current concepts and future focus. *Survey of Ophthalmology, 56,* 114–134.

Toglia, J. P. (1991). Generalization of treatment: A multicontext approach to cognitive perceptual impairment in adults with brain injury. *American Journal of Occupational Therapy, 45,* 505–516.

Uniform Data System for Medical Rehabilitation. (1997). *Guide for the uniform data set for medical rehabilitation.* Buffalo, NY: State University of New York.

van Heugten, C. M., Dekker, J., Deelman, B. G., van Dijk, A. J., Stehmann-Saris, J. C., & Kinebanian, A. (1998). Outcome of strategy training in stroke patients with apraxia: A phase II study. *Clinical Rehabilitation, 12,* 294–303.

Warren, M. (1993a). A hierarchical model for evaluation and treatment of visual perceptual dysfunction in adult acquired brain injury, part 1. *American Journal of Occupational Therapy, 47,* 42–54.

Warren, M. (1993b). A hierarchical model for evaluation and treatment of visual perceptual dysfunction in adult acquired brain injury, part 2. *American Journal of Occupational Therapy, 47,* 55–66.

Warren, M. (1996). Providing low vision rehabilitation services with occupational therapy and ophthalmology: A program description. *American Journal of Occupational Therapy, 49,* 877–883.

Warren, M. (1993). A hierarchical model for evaluation and treatment of visual perceptual dysfunction in adult acquired brain injury, Part 1. *American Journal of Occupational Therapy, 47,* 42–54.

Watson, G. R., Wright, V., De l'Aune, W., & Long, S. (1996). The development and evaluation of a low vision reading comprehension test. *Journal of Visual Impairment & Blindness, 90,* 480–484.

Weinberg, J., Diller, L., Gordon, W. A., Gerstman, L. J., Liberman, A., Lakin, P., Hodges, G., & Ezrachi, O. (1977). Visual scanning training effect on reading-related tasks in acquired right brain damage. *Archives of Physical Medicine and Rehabilitation, 58,* 479–486.

Weinberg, J., Diller, L., Gordon, W. A., Gerstman, L. J., Liberman, A., Lakin, P., Hodges, G., & Ezrachi, O. (1979). Training sensory awareness and spatial organization in people with right brain damage. *Archives of Physical Medicine and Rehabilitation, 60,* 491–496.

Weinberg, J., Pcasetsky, E., Diller, L., & Gordon, W. (1982). Treating perceptual organization deficits in non-neglecting RBD stroke patients. *Journal of Clinical Psychology, 4,* 59–75.

Weisser-Pike, O., & Kaldenberg, J. (2010). Occupational therapy approaches to facilitate productive aging for individuals with low vision. *OT Practice, 15,* CE1–CE7.

Wolter, M., & Preda, S. (2006). Visual deficits following stroke: Maximizing participation in rehabiliation. *Topics in Stroke Rehabilitation, 13,* 12–21.

Wright, V., & Watson, G. R. (1995). Learn to use your vision for reading (LUV reading series). Lilburn, GA: Bear Consultants

Zeloni, G., Farne, A., & Baccini, M. (2002). Viewing with less to see better. *Journal of Neurology, Neurosurgery, and Psychiatry, 73,* 195–198.

Acknowledgements

Thanks to Lee Ann Quintana for her preparation of the previous edition of this chapter and thanks to Amy Wagenfeld, Karen Jacobs, and Sue Berger for their thoughtful review and feedback.

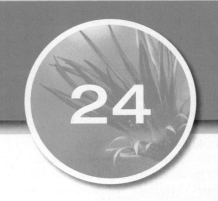

24

Optimizing Cognitive Performance

Mary Vining Radomski and Gordon Muir Giles

Learning Objectives

After studying this chapter, the reader will be able to do the following:

1. Discuss the field of cognitive rehabilitation in general.
2. Distinguish cognitive rehabilitation approaches used by occupational therapists from those provided by other disciplines.
3. Describe theoretical approaches to occupational therapy cognitive intervention for persons with physical disabilities and/or who are aging.
4. Employ specific clinical interventions that are supported by theory and research.

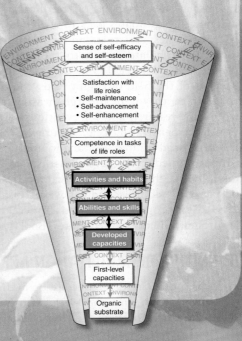

Many people who are referred for occupational therapy experience cognitive dysfunction associated with injury, illness, pain, emotional distress, and/or aging. Because a person's ability to concentrate, remember, and solve problems is central to fulfilling the valued life roles described in Chapter 1 (self-maintenance, self-advancement, and self-enhancement), cognitive dysfunction is often the primary focus of occupational therapy intervention.

The central aim of this chapter is to advance evidence-informed cognitive intervention that reflects occupational therapists' focus on occupational performance. To that end, we first highlight milestones in the history of the cognitive rehabilitation field and then describe both theory and practices associated with occupation-oriented cognitive rehabilitation.

COGNITIVE REHABILITATION

Although definitions vary, the term cognitive rehabilitation generally describes a multidisciplinary field and the application of "therapeutic interventions designed to improve cognitive functioning and participation in activities that may be affected by difficulties in one or more cognitive domains" (Brain Injury Association of America, n.d., p. 1). Many rehabilitation disciplines, including occupational therapy, speech-language pathology, special education, and neuropsychology, attempt to help patients optimize cognitive abilities, with occupational therapy and speech therapists most often providing cognitive rehabilitation services (Stringer, 2003).

Historical Perspectives

Interest in the possibility of "reeducating" persons with a damaged brain dates back to the 1800s (Finger, 1994), with the earliest efforts stemming from Broca's work that localized articulate speech to the frontal brain region (Boake, 1991; Finger, 1994). Concurrent with the development of the field of cognitive psychology, the wars of the 20th century were, in large measure, the impetus for worldwide research and interventions to improve cognition after penetrating brain injuries. Most notably, the needs of head-injured veterans injured in the 1973 Yom Kippur war led to the development of an intensive, interdisciplinary rehabilitation program in Israel that focused on patients' cognitive and behavioral disabilities (Boake, 1989). This program influenced the development of similar programs in the United States (Boake, 1989).

COGNITIVE REHABILITATION APPROACHES

There has been considerable evolution in the field of cognitive rehabilitation since the 1970s, with continued debate about the extent to which the aims of intervention should be restitution (or recovery) of lost brain functions or compensation (the development of new ways to circumvent or "get around" the problem) (Institute of Medicine [IOM], 2011). Within these two broad aims, this chapter reviews five approaches to cognitive rehabilitation: skill-task-habit training, strategy training, task-environment modification, cognitive stimulation therapy (CST), and process-specific training. Because there is no agreement regarding the labeling and composition of cognitive rehabilitation approaches, readers will likely find approaches otherwise labeled as they continue to expand their reading on this topic. Best evidence for each approach is described in Evidence Table 24-1. Evidence suggests that the first three approaches (skill-task-habit training, strategy training, and task-environment modification) can result in improved occupational performance and as such are especially important to cognitive rehabilitation as practiced by occupational therapists. The effectiveness of these three approaches is linked to the teaching-learning concepts and methods employed in therapy, some of which are described in Definition 24-1. Readers are also referred to Chapter 13 of this text.

Skill-Task-Habit Training

It is widely accepted that human beings have two systems for the control and execution of behavior: a conscious, controlled, slow, effortful, and deliberative cognitive system used when people are engaged in problem solving, and a rapid, relatively effortless, habitual, or automatic system that supports frequently performed skills, tasks, and habits (Schneider, Dumais, & Shiffrin, 1984). These two systems may be seen as paralleling the implicit and explicit memory systems described in Chapter 13. Solving novel problems constitutes a relatively small part of people's days, and most of human behavior is automatic (Muraven, Tice, & Baumeister, 1998). Automatic habits and routines enable people to perform complex skills and carry out everyday tasks with little or no mental energy, freeing people to think and react to new events in the environment (Jog et al., 1999). For example, most people employ relatively consistent procedures for daily activities such as showering, brushing teeth, crossing the street, and getting to work. These activities are engaged in effortlessly, and mental resources are deployed to review unrelated upcoming events as a function of automaticity (the ability to perform tasks with little or no contribution from the conscious mind). The automatic activities only enter conscious awareness if there is a problem that the automatic system cannot manage. In fact, many people are somewhat disturbed by this ability when they find that they have driven to school or work and have no recollection of the process of doing so because they relied almost entirely on automatic skills.

Helping patients develop new habits and routines that improve specific skills/behaviors (sometimes called specific

Evidence Table 24-1 Best Evidence for Occupational Therapy Practice Regarding Cognitive Intervention

Intervention	Description of Intervention Tested	Participants	Dosage	Type of Best Evidence and Level of Evidence	Benefit	Statistical Probability and Effect Size of Outcome	Reference
Skill-habit training	Cognitive-didactic versus functional-experiential rehabilitation therapy (neurofunctional approach [NFA]) integrated into interdisciplinary acute inpatient programs with another 2–2.5 hours daily of standard occupational and physical therapy	Adult veterans or active-duty military service members (n = 360) with moderate to severe traumatic brain injury (TBI)	1.5–2.5 hours of protocol-specific intervention provided for 20–60 days as needed	Level IA2b Single-blind, multicenter randomized controlled trial	No significant difference overall between the two groups in outcome measures Post hoc exploratory analyses suggested that the younger group (<30 years) and those with less education who participated in the cognitive intervention had better work-related outcomes at 1 year follow up than the NFA group. Also, the older group (>30 years) and those with more education who participated in the NFA intervention had better independent living outcomes at 1-year follow-up than the cognitive group.	Primary outcome measures showed no between group difference for the two experimental treatments at 1-year follow-up	Vanderploeg et al. (2008)
Metacognitive strategy instruction (MSI)	Instruction in use of metastrategy such as time pressure management or goal management training Examples of control intervention included concentration training and motor skills training.	One hundred sixty-five participants in the five synthesized studies; subjects varied in injury severity (mild to severe impairment)	Intensity and duration of intervention varied across the five studies, ranging from a single 3–4-hour intervention to 2–3 hours of weekly treatment for 24 weeks.	Level I Meta-analysis involving 15 studies, 5 of which were randomized controlled trials of step-by-step MSI. The results of the 5 studies were synthesized and are reported here.	Effect sizes (ESs) from immediate activity-participation outcomes were significantly larger for MSI than the control intervention. ESs from immediate impairment outcomes after MSI and the control intervention were similar (both significantly greater than chance).	*Activity and participation outcomes:* p < 0.05; mean ES = 0.57	Kennedy et al. (2008)

(continued)

Evidence Table 24-1	Best Evidence for Occupational Therapy Practice Regarding Cognitive Intervention (*continued*)					
Intervention	Description of Intervention Tested	Participants	Dosage	Type of Best Evidence and Level of Evidence	Benefit	Statistical Probability and Effect Size of Outcome	Reference
Task-environment modification training	Home-based family caregiver education and physical and social environmental modifications provided by an occupational therapist. Control condition: unspecified usual care	Two hundred two family caregivers (171 at posttest) living with a person with Alzheimer's disease (AD) or similar condition 66.1% (113) of the caregivers in posttest analyses were female.	Five 90-minute sessions every other week over 3 months	Level IA2a No control for therapist time and attention; unblinded evaluation	Yes. At 3-month posttest, persons with AD whose caregiver received intervention had fewer declines in instrumental activities of daily living (IADL) compared to controls. Interaction effects between sex of caregiver and intervention. Female caregivers who received intervention reported reduced upset and improved ability to manage behavior and functional dependency.	$p = 0.030$; $r = 0.21$ Reduced patient upset ($p = 0.049$); managing behaviors ($p = 0.038$); managing functional dependence of loved one ($p = 0.049$) (data not available to calculate effect sizes)	Gitlin et al. (2001)
Cognitive stimulation therapy	Intervention incorporated Reality Orientation and Reminiscence Therapy. It was composed of four phases: the senses (involving multisensory stimulation), remembering the past (reminiscence), recognizing people and objects, and general orientation (recognizing money, knowing way around) (see Spector et al. [2001] for more details).	Two hundred one people with dementia who were recruited from 23 day centers and nursing homes (intervention group 115, control group 86)	Fourteen 45-minute group sessions provided twice weekly for 7 weeks	Level IA2b Single-blind, multicenter randomized controlled trial	Yes. At follow-up, those who received intervention showed statistically significant differences in cognition and quality of life as compared to controls.	Mini-Mental Status Exam ($p = 0.044$; $r = 0.156$), Alzheimer's Disease Assessment Scale–Cognition ($p = 0.014$; $r = 0.19$) Quality of Life–Alzheimer's Disease scales ($p = 0.028$; $r = 0.171$)	Spector et al. (2003)
Process-specific training	Three intervention groups + one no treatment group: Memory training Reasoning training Speed of processing training (SOPT)	2,832 persons aged 65–94 years who were living independently with good functional and cognitive status	Intervention was provided during ten 60–75-minute sessions over a 5–6-week period in small group setting. Eleven months after the initial training, booster training was provided to a subset of subjects in each group (four sessions over 2–3 weeks)	Level IA1b Randomized, controlled, single-blind four-group design (one no-contact group)	Yes. Participants who received process-specific training demonstrated statistically significant improvements in the respective domain of training at 1 and 2 years posttest. No statistically significant changes in everyday functioning for any group at 1 or 2 years posttest; significant improvement for posttest only for SOPT group.	$p < 0.001$ for all groups in their respective domains at 1 or 2 years posttest (effect size data unavailable) $p = 0.02$ for SOPT at posttest on measure of everyday speed of processing (data not available to calculate effect sizes) Booster training had no impact on everyday functioning	Ball et al. (2002)

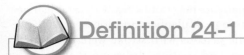

Definition 24-1

Concepts and Methods Central to Teaching-Learning in Cognitive Rehabilitation

Errorless Learning

When errorless learning is employed during the teaching-learning process, the therapist orchestrates the training and practice process so that the patient consistently performs the desired behavior or strategy correctly. In trial-and-error learning, errors are corrected; in errorless learning, errors are prevented. The therapist provides sufficient support (i.e., cueing, environmental physical and verbal, implicit guidance) to prevent the propagation of errors; cues are faded as learning occurs. See Procedures for Practice 24-1 for more details on graded cueing.

The errorless learning method has been established as a viable intervention across populations (e.g., healthy adults, older adults, and persons with mild and major neurocognitive disorder) (Kessels & de Haan, 2003; Kessels & Olde Hensken, 2009), age groups (Kessels & de Haan, 2003), and types of material to be learned (e.g., word list learning, face-name association, procedural skills) (Kessels & de Haan, 2003; Kessels & Olde Hensken, 2009). Errorless learning is recommended as the "foundation for all information to be presented to patients with severe memory impairment" (Haskins, 2011, p. 48) in part because these individuals may not recognize when they make errors and/or get "stuck" with early response errors (Baddeley & Wilson, 1994). As a practical matter, it may be difficult to completely prevent all errors, but errors can be kept to a minimum. Giles et al.'s (1997) report of washing and dressing training are examples of errorless learning techniques applied to clinical practice, which may be used as an intervention guide. A review of the available literature suggests that the techniques are effective (Ehlhardt et al., 2008). Errorless learning is particularly important in the skill, task, and habit training approach in cognitive rehabilitation.

Spaced Retrieval

Spaced retrieval involves asking the patient to recall information for progressively longer periods of time and is used to maximize the recall of relatively limited amounts of information in people with severe memory disorder (Cermak et al., 1996;

Davis, Massman, & Doody, 2001). The technique has been used primarily with face-name recognition training because this aspect of memory impairment may be particularly disturbing to people and improvement can have positive effects on self-esteem (Davis, Massman, & Doody, 2001).

Here is an example of how spaced retrieval might be used to help a client learn the name of a friend whom he met at a day program. The memory failure is important to the client because he is embarrassed that he cannot recall his friend's name each day when they meet at the center. The therapist might show the client a photograph of the person whose name is to be learned, saying, "This is Mary. What is her name?" After a 15-second delay, the client is again asked the friend's name. If the patient correctly states the friend's name, the therapist builds in a progressively longer delay, 15 seconds and then 30 seconds, 45 seconds, 2 minutes, 5 minutes, and so on. Failure leads to going back to the beginning and starting the process again. The effectiveness of the technique has been demonstrated in people with TBI, stroke, and Alzheimer's disease (Clare et al., 2000; Davis, Massman, & Doody, 2001; Thivierge et al., 2008). These techniques are not used to retrain memory in the abstract sense but rather to facilitate memorization of specific information in which the client is trained. Spaced retrieval may be used during the acquisition phase of strategy training.

Multicontext Approach

Toglia's (2011) Dynamic Interactional Model of Cognition posits that cognition is a product of the dynamic interaction between the person (his or her capacities, self-awareness, and personal context), the activity at hand, the strategies used, and the environment in which the activity occurs. Cognitive dysfunction is viewed as a mismatch among personal (such as cognitive capacities), task, strategy, and environmental variables. This approach emphasizes the establishment of transfer criteria and practice in the context of varied activities and environments (Table 24-1). Client-specific processing strategies are selected or designed and then practiced in a variety of graded tasks and settings. The therapist guides the transfer of learning by asking the client to employ the new skill or strategy first on similar tasks and then in the context of those that are increasingly dissimilar (Toglia, 1991).

skill or task-specific training) (Mastos et al., 2007) is a potentially potent means of advancing occupational performance (Giles, 2011; Spikeman & van Zomeren, 2010). Skill-task-habit training addresses the disruption in long-standing habits and routines that may accompany disability, aging, and life changes (Dyck, 2002; Wallenbert & Jonsson, 2005). Previously automatic skills and tasks can require conscious control and become effortful and time

consuming. The loss of effortless predictability in an individual's own performance has a profound impact on that individual's energy level and sense of continuity, competence, and self (Charmaz, 2002).

Therapists use different methods to teach patients to use new cognitive strategies (discussed in the next sections) than those used to teach new skills-tasks-habits. Strategy training, which relies more on the conscious control

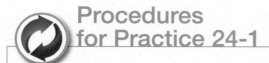

Procedures for Practice 24-1

Graded Cues

Graded or vanishing cues are used in cognitive rehabilitation to enable the patient to perform tasks with the least amount of cueing (Dougherty & Radomski, 1993). The following terms (from Sohlberg & Mateer [1989]) are useful when writing goals and documenting progress.

- A **general or nonspecific cue** alerts the patient to monitor performance. It usually takes the form of a statement such as, "You'll need to make sure you remember to do this before our next session." The therapist or family offers a general cue if the patient fails to recognize situational or environmental conditions that might otherwise prompt use of a compensatory strategy or behavior.
- A **specific cue**, which is presented if the patient does not respond to a general cue, reminds the patient he or she must act. It often takes the form of a question such as, "What do you need to do to make sure you remember to do your homework before our next session?"
- An **explicit instruction**, the most directive of the graded cues, is sometimes provided if the patient does not initiate the desired strategy or behavior upon first receiving a general cue and then a specific cue. For example, the patient may be asked to take out the planner and record the assignment to ensure follow-through before the next session.

system, is typically applied to persons with mild to moderate impairment and relatively intact self-awareness. Skill-task-habit training, which relies on procedural and errorless learning, is often used with persons with severe impairment or impaired self-awareness (Giles, 2011) and/or those who have problems with activities of daily living (ADL) or instrumental activities of daily living (IADL) (Giles, 2010). However, skill-task-habit training is not reserved for those with disabilities. This cognitive rehabilitation approach may benefit anyone interested in making a complex skill automatic (e.g., a golf swing) or adding a new health behavior (e.g., daily exercise program) (see Duhigg [2012]).

Clinical Example(s) of This Approach

Numerous case examples and single-subject research studies in the rehabilitation literature describe the use of applied behavioral analysis to establish or reestablish self-care and/or home-management routines and habit sequences for persons with cognitive impairment (Giles & Clark-Wilson, 1988; Giles et al., 1997; Giles & Shore, 1989; Schwartz, 1995; Zanetti et al., 2001). The following principles of applied behavioral analysis frame occupational therapy intervention to establish routines and habit sequences. However, therapists should be sensitive to the fact that some patients may not be ready to establish new ways of doing things. Wallenbert and Jonsson (2005) reported that some persons with stroke were reluctant to create new habits and routines, believing that doing so could interfere with their physical recovery. Therefore, the development of new habits and routines are presented as a key method for advancing recovery from illness or injury.

- Guided by the client (and caregiver where appropriate), the therapist selects a key behavioral sequence that becomes the target of intervention (Giles, 1998; Parish & Oddy, 2007). Giles emphasized the importance of working with the client to select behaviors and prospective routines that clients regard as having clinical and personal significance.
- The therapist analyzes the physical and social context in which the routine or sequence is expected to occur to identify environmentally available cues or determine where to create new cues (Schwartz, 1995). Because routines and habit sequences are thought to be context specific, training is most effective if it occurs in the environment in which the routines will ultimately be performed (Giles, 1998).
- A task analysis is performed on the target behavioral routine or sequence (Giles, 1998; Parish & Oddy, 2007). Task analysis involves examining each step of the task as well as the setting, stimulus events, and consequences (Gelfand & Hartmann, 1984). (See further discussion of activity analysis in Chapter 12 of this book.)
- The therapist and client decide on an optimal sequence of steps and use chaining, prompting, and reinforcement each time the sequence is performed (Giles et al., 1997). Giles et al. (1997) suggested that "[routine] tasks can be thought of as complex-stimulus-response chains in which the completion of each activity acts as the stimulus for the next step in the chain" (p. 257). They also recommended the use of the whole-task method, in which each step of the chain is trained on each presentation. The therapist often creates a checklist that outlines each component of the task so that the desired sequence of steps remains invariant (Davis & Radomski, 1989) (Fig. 24-1).

For some clients, prompts and reinforcers are established. The checklist itself may be both a prompt (if placed in an obtrusive location) and a reinforcer as the patient checks each completed step. Technology may also be employed. Schwartz (1995) reported use of a daily tape-recorded message activated by an automatic timer that prompted initiation of a self-care routine. In addition, NeuroPage™, a time- and task-specific vibrating paging system, was used to facilitate establishing routines related to taking medications and using checklists (Wilson et al., 2001; Wilson et al., 2003). Family members may also be enlisted to provide prompts and reinforcement, typically social praise.

The therapist facilitates consistent repetition of the behavioral routine or sequence beyond mastery to

Table 24-1 Components of the Multicontext Treatment Approach

Component	Definition	Example
Consideration of personal context	Gaining understanding of the client's premorbid personality characteristics, beliefs, valued occupations, and previous lifestyle	Interviewing the client about his or her premorbid everyday routines and exploring how those routines have changed after injury or illness and using this information to inform occupational therapy assessment and intervention
Enhancing self-monitoring and self-awareness	Methods designed to enhance the client's understanding of his or her strengths and limitations that are incorporated into every treatment session	• Asking the client to anticipate and identify specific challenges or obstacles that might occur in performance of a therapy task • Instructing the client to watch the therapist perform a task during which client-relevant errors are demonstrated (such as distractibility). Asking the client to identify problems and recommend strategies
Strategy training	Small units of behavior that reflect internal or external cognitive techniques that contribute to the effectiveness of performance	• Mental repetition, visual imagery (i.e., internal processing strategies) • Memory notebooks, alarm cueing devices, use of checklists (i.e., external processing strategies)
Activity analysis	Identifying, manipulating, and/or stabilizing salient activity parameters (e.g., physical features, number of items, number of steps or choices involved in the task)	As part of her therapy, a homemaker who has difficulty attending to visual details locates the soup spoons in a drawer of unsorted spoons, forks, and knives. As she progresses, she will locate a set of soup spoons in a drawer of unsorted spoons of different sizes (teaspoons, soup spoons, serving spoons). Note how differentiating between spoons of different sizes requires greater visual attention than differentiating between spoons, forks, and knives.
Establishment of criteria for transfer	Identify series of tasks that decrease in degrees of physical and conceptual similarity to the original task	Task: Donning a pullover T-shirt in the therapy area
	Near transfer: only one or two surface characteristics changed	Donning a pullover sweater (color and texture different from T-shirt)
	Intermediate transfer: three to six surface characteristics change; tasks share some physical similarities	Donning a button-down cotton shirt in the client's room (type of clothing, color and texture, fine motor requirements, and environment changed)
	Far transfer: tasks are conceptually similar; surface characteristics are different or only one surface characteristic is similar	Donning outerwear (coat, jacket), pajamas, undershirt or camisole (different types of upper body clothing)
	Very far transfer: generalization, spontaneous application of what is learned to everyday life	Donning pants (strategy of dressing affected side first remains the same for lower body dressing)
Practice in multiple environments	Strategies are used in a variety of situations (e.g., tasks and locations) to demonstrate their applicability and use to the client	The strategy of left-to-right scanning is practiced on letter cancellation tasks and then used to locate items in a medicine cabinet or to count books on a shelf.

From Toglia, J. P. (1991). Generalization of treatment: A multi-contextual approach to cognitive perceptual impairment in the brain-injured adult. *American Journal of Occupational Therapy, 45*, 505–516; Toglia, J. P. (2011). The dynamic interactional model of cognition in cognitive rehabilitation. In N. Katz (Ed.), *Cognition and occupation across the life span* (pp. 161–201). Bethesda, MD: American Occupational Therapy Association.

promote overlearning (Parish & Oddy, 2007). Patients with neurological impairment typically need to perform as many practice trials to truly consolidate learning (and maximize resistance to skill loss) as it took to be able to reliably perform the skill in the first place (Driskell, Willis, & Copper, 1992). As the patient frequently and consistently performs the behavioral sequence and learning occurs, steps begin to "chunk" together so that gradually prompts can be combined and the program shortened (Giles, 2011). The therapist tracks ongoing compliance with the target behavioral sequence; monitors the patient's perceptions of ease, accuracy, and speed (evidence of increasing automaticity); and, with the patient, determines when applied behavioral analysis methods should be employed to make another important task routine.

Morning planning checklist

Directions: Check-off each step after it is completed.

	M	T	W	Th	F	Sa	Su
1) After breakfast, open planner to yesterday's page.							
2) Check off all of the tasks you completed yesterday.							
3) Draw an arrow in front of undone or incomplete tasks							
4) Re-write these tasks on today's page.							
5) Move the bookmark to today's planner page.							
6) Review your schedule.							
7) Ask your wife if there are any tasks or appointments that you should write down for today.							
8) Write down at least 3 tasks you intend to complete today.							

Wind-down routine

Directions: Check-off each step after it is completed.

	M	T	W	Th	F	Sa	Su
1) When your MotivAider vibrates at 9:00 p.m, discontinue your current activity.							
2) Make notes where you left off on your project.							
3) Put on your pajamas.							
4) Brush your teeth.							
5) Wash your face.							
6) Gather your magazines and go to your recliner.							
7) Set the MotivAider for 30 minutes and peruse your reading material.							
8) When cued by the MotivAider, retire to bed.							

Figure 24-1 Checklists like these are used to help patients reestablish routines and habit sequences.

Presumed Mechanisms

Although the exact mechanisms are not known, automaticity is believed to occur as the brain becomes increasingly efficient in processing specific stimulus encoding, storage, and retrieval sequences (Logan, 1988a, 1988b; Logan, Taylor, & Etherton, 1999). Practice progressively strengthens automaticity by virtue of additional representations in memory; thus, performance may be more automatic after 100 repetitions than after 50. Practice increases the availability of target responses, such that conscious decision making is replaced by the implementation of automatic action sequences (Kramer, Strayer, & Buckley, 1990). When a skill becomes automatic, it becomes the easiest behavior to initiate from an array of possible behaviors, reduces interference error, and is experienced by the individual as effortless. Automatization, then, is a relative phenomenon in that, although it may occur after only a few trials, it may never be complete (Logan, 1988b).

Expectations for Transfer-Generalization

Implicit memory refers to an unconscious change in behavior that results from previous experience (Eldridge, Masterman, & Knowlton, 2002) and is closely tied to the original learning situation and hence is less flexibly applied to novel contexts (Reber, Knowlton, & Squire, 1996). Habit learning is a form of implicit learning (Squire, Knowlton, & Musen, 1993) and so generalization of skills to new stimulus conditions may be problematic.

In order for generalization to occur, the stimulus conditions in which the skills are exercised have to be varied. Random practice schedules, in which many different tasks are interspersed in a practice schedule, may also facilitate transfer of skills (Giuffrida et al., 2009). (See Chapter 13 for further discussion.) For example, a client had a severe traumatic brain injury (TBI) and is working to independently and safely cross the street. In occupational therapy, she has learned a set of skills composed of finding the crosswalk, pressing the button on the stoplight, and stepping off the curb only after "walk" is displayed on the light and traffic has stopped. She receives supervision and cueing as she practices crossing a wide range of different streets. Ultimately after much repetition, she automatically classifies the stimulus characteristics of a wide range of streets that she routinely encounters and her street-crossing skill is elicited. Tasks undertaken frequently, on a daily basis or more, are likely to be self-maintaining once competency has been achieved (e.g., washing and dressing). Tasks that are engaged in less frequently will be learned more slowly and will be less stable and are more likely to be extinguished.

Alignment with Occupational Therapy Theory and Objectives

Skill-task-habit training reflects a recommended, occupation-oriented approach to cognitive rehabilitation. However, cognitive interventions have historically been preferred to functional interventions for people with neurological impairments based on the erroneous assumption that "fixing" cognition will automatically lead to improved function (Giles, 2010; Vanderploeg et al., 2008). According to this logic, treatment of occupational performance deficits would be unnecessary if cognitive functioning could be adequately remediated: cognitive rehabilitation would "automatically" result in improved functional behaviors (Giles, 2010). For this reason, the direct approach to occupational performance problems offered by skill-task-habit training has unfortunately often been undervalued by occupational therapists despite its alignment with occupational therapy theory and goals. Therapist concerns regarding having adequate patient contact time for skill-task-habit training and/or generalization may be addressed by using family members and technology as "therapy extenders."

Strategy Training

In the context of cognitive rehabilitation, compensatory cognitive strategies refer to an array of tactics that are intentionally employed in order to optimize performance despite a cognitive limitation. Cognitive strategies take many forms: using a global metacognitive strategy or rubric to organize a project to manage executive dysfunction, using a device (e.g., diary or smartphone) to keep track of information that might be otherwise forgotten, employing a task-specific strategy such as setting alarms on a cell phone as a reminder to return from morning and afternoon breaks at work, and selecting a workspace with minimal noise and visual distractions to best manage problems with attention. Although expectations for strategy transfer and generalization will vary for each patient's situation, the effectiveness of compensatory strategy training often depends on the patient's ability to transfer what is learned in the clinical setting to everyday activities. Currently, there is considerable interest in training clients in metacognitive strategies so that they can develop their own methods to overcome ADL or IADL problems rather than retrain these skills directly. Strategy training is not aimed at relearning specific tasks, but at teaching patients new ways to handle problems resulting from cognitive impairment.

Cognitive strategy training is organized around three training phases: acquisition, application, and adaptation (Haskins, 2011; Sohlberg & Mateer, 2001). Because clients must have some degree of insight into the skill deficit for which they need to compensate, intervention also typically addresses self-awareness (see Procedures for Practice 24-2).

- Acquisition—Through drill and practice exercises, clients learn the mechanics of using the compensatory tool or strategy. For example, with coaching and written

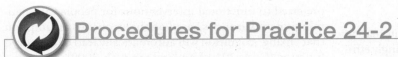

Procedures for Practice 24-2

Helping Patients Improve Self-Awareness

Occupational therapists use a variety of techniques to help patients become more aware of their cognitive strengths and weaknesses:

- Appreciate the differences between organically based unawareness and adjustment-based denial. Anticipate that sometimes, as patients become more aware of impairments, they may feel emotional distress, including depression and anxiety (Fleming & Strong, 1995).
- Recognize levels of awareness and focus intervention on helping the patient move up the awareness hierarchy (see Chapter 6). For example, therapists try to help patients who are unaware of their cognitive impairments first to develop intellectual awareness of the problem and then to progress toward emergent or anticipatory awareness (Crosson et al., 1989).
- Create opportunities for the patient to monitor and judge his or her own performance, analyze the results, and determine what to continue or do differently next time. Dougherty and Radomski (1993) recommended a graded approach to performance analysis that consisted of three levels: (1) using an answer key to self-correct; (2) answering multiple choice questions about various aspects of performance after performing the task; and (3) making predictions about performance ahead of time, comparing actual performance to predictions, and determining how to modify performance in the future.
- Introduce therapeutic structured failure when appropriate. That is, do not interfere with the natural consequences of the cognitive impairment during selected supervised activities. For example, if the patient fails to initiate a cognitive compensatory strategy in response to general or specific cues, do not provide further instruction, but rather create an opportunity for the patient to observe what happens when the strategy is not used.
- Collaborate with family members to provide feedback. In some cases, family members should focus on maintaining harmony in the household and appropriately prefer that the therapist assume the responsibility of providing any negative feedback to the patient. In other cases, family members or coworkers are so afraid of offending or discouraging the patient that they insulate the patient from any and all challenges or avoid mentioning errors and, as a result, deprive him or her of information that might improve self-awareness.
- Respect the patient's readiness to participate in therapy. Avoid badgering the patient into improved awareness of deficits by maintaining a therapeutic partnership so that he or she will want to return for services in the future.

---

instructions from the therapist, clients rehearse setting their alarm watches or practice filing and finding information in function-specific sections of their day planners.

- Application—Clients use the compensatory strategy during clinic-based simulated work tasks. These tasks are designed to require use of the targeted strategy and may include clerical or clinic maintenance projects or crafts. With guidance from the therapist, clients also directly apply the compensatory strategy to real-life problems at home or work.
- Adaptation—Once the client has experience with the strategy in simulations and real-life tasks, the strategy may be further adapted to the client's personal preferences and the demands of additional areas of application in daily life.

As indicated earlier, patients may improve occupational performance by learning to use attention-management strategies, executive functioning strategies, memory strategies, and metacognitive strategies. (See Haskins [2011] for a detailed discussion of all of these.) An exhaustive review of all possible methods to circumvent cognitive impairments or inefficiencies is beyond the scope of this chapter. Instead, we provide an overview of two categories of cognitive strategies: memory-related strategies and metacognitive strategies.

Presumed Mechanism

Cognitive strategy training is based on the premise that given cognitive processes are no longer able to support independent functioning and that the original cognitive processes cannot be restored. Learning is hypothesized to be top-down (i.e., learning based on explicit knowledge structures that may or may not become implicit with practice) (Geusgens et al., 2007).

Memory Strategies

Occupational therapists consider the client's degree of memory impairment, his or her specific needs and preferences, past memory strategy or technology use, recovery status, expectations, and goals in planning intervention for memory-related problems. The intervention approach will be informed, in part, by whether the patient is anticipated to be a passive user or active initiator of the memory compensation strategy (Radomski et al., 2004). *Passive memory strategy users* are typically individuals with severe memory impairment whose carers set up and maintain the external memory strategy/system. In this situation, for example, the goal of therapy may be to teach the patient's wife to fill out a daily timetable or task list and the patient to perform listed tasks when prompted by an alarm (also set by the patient's wife). (The next section describes this approach in greater detail.) *Active initiators* are aware of their problems with forgetting and would be expected to learn to recognize situations in which to use the memory strategy and then correctly perform the strategy—possibly associated with a variety of tasks and contexts.

In this section, we discuss the use of internal and external memory strategies to advance occupational performance. *Note that there is general agreement in the cognitive rehabilitation literature that direct attempts to improve memory through drill and practice of remembering are ineffective (Robertson, 1999).*

Internal Memory Strategies. Internal strategies are methods of mentally manipulating information so as to increase its likelihood of later recall. Association techniques and organizational techniques are two categories of internal memory strategies (Haskins, 2011) (see Table 24-2 for examples). These strategies received a great deal of attention in the late 1970s and early 1980s. Although some people with left-hemisphere stroke showed greater retention of material by using visual association techniques when tested in a laboratory situation (e.g., visualizing items in conjunction with absurd images [Gasparrini & Satz, 1979]), most studies failed to show transfer of the techniques to novel or everyday situations (Crovitz, 1979). Organizational techniques may involve using first letter mnemonics to form a single word or pseudo-word, which simplifies the storage and retrieval of the to-be-remembered information (Haskins, 2011). For example, the PQRST method (Preview, Question, Read, State, Test) can be used in academic contexts for recall of more complex verbal and written information (Haskins, 2011); it has been applied successfully in TBI and cerebrovascular accident (CVA) (Wilson & Moffat, 1984).

Although a recent study demonstrated positive outcomes of teaching internal memory strategies to patients with TBI who were already using external memory strategies (O'Neil-Pirozzi et al., 2010), internal memory strategies are considered effortful to learn and employ and may be best used as a complement to external strategies for memory tasks that cannot be practically managed by jotting or inputting a note (such as remembering name-face associations).

External Memory Strategies. People who are not neurologically impaired use external strategies for remembering more often than they use internal strategies (Harris, 1980). Examples of commonly used external strategies include having someone else provide a reminder to do a task, leaving objects in places so that they will be encountered when needed (e.g., placing things to take with you the next day by the front door), setting an alarm on a cell phone, smartphone, or personal digital assistant (PDA) in order to remember an appointment. Low-tech memory aids (such as notes or calendars) are the most widely used among persons with TBI (Evans et al., 2003), but this may change with the ease of use of smartphones, availability of relevant apps, and benefits of "availability at the point of need" (Gillespie, Best, & O'Neill, 2012, p. 14). Although many different types of external aids are useful to people with memory impairment, here we briefly mention checklists, timetables, memory books, day planners/organizers, and assistive technologies for cognition (ATC). Note that checklists, timetables, and memory books are often most appropriate for passive strategy users, whereas day planners and ATC are typically used by active initiators.

Checklists. A client who is memory impaired may not remember performing a task or the sequence for doing so, resulting in either a repeat of the activity or nonengagement

Table 24-2 Examples of Internal Compensatory Strategies

Technique	Description
Rehearsal	Patient repeats the information to be remembered out loud or to self.
Visual imagery	Patient consolidates information to be remembered by making a mental picture that includes the information (e.g., to remember the name *Barbara*, the patient pictures a barber holding the letter A).
Semantic elaboration	Patient consolidates information by making up a simple story (e.g., patient who has to remember the words *lawyer*, *game*, and *hat* develops a sentence such as "The lawyer wore a hat to the game").
First-letter mnemonics	Parenté's NAME mnemonic adds rules to observing features and drawing associations when remembering names: **N**otice the person with whom you speak. **A**sk the person to repeat his or her name. **M**ention the name in conversation. **E**xaggerate some special feature.

Information from Malec, J., & Questad, K. (1983). Rehabilitation of memory after craniocerebral trauma: Case report. *Archives of Physical Medicine and Rehabilitation, 64*, 436–438; Milton, S. B. (1985). Compensatory memory strategy training: A practical approach for managing persistent memory problems. *Cognitive Rehabilitation, 3*, 8–15; Wilson, B. A. (1982). Success and failure in memory training following a cerebral vascular accident. *Cortex, 18*, 581–594; Parenté, R., & Herrmann, D. (2002). *Retraining cognition: techniques and applications* (2nd ed.). Austin, TX: Pro-ed.

in the activity in the mistaken belief that it has already been performed. Being taught to mark off each instruction or activity on a checklist as it is performed may assist some clients. Some people can be taught to follow checklists as a "meta" procedure; whatever they need to learn can be designed as a checklist.

Timetables. A timetable is a simplified version of a personal calendar (diary). Most institutions have a routine that can be presented in the form of a timetable. Caregivers for people with TBI, stroke, or major neurocognitive disorder can be taught to use a timetable with regular activities throughout the day. The timetable may include wake-up time, an appropriate time to wash and dress, lunch, dinner, laundry time, and regularly scheduled individual and group therapy times. For people with major neurocognitive disorder (formerly referred to as dementia; see Definition 24-2), a timetable may provide a good means of managing repetitive questioning (Bourgeois et al., 1997). For people recovering from TBI, a timetable can be a method for gradually training self-management skills.

Memory Books. A memory book may be used at many stages of recovery from acquired brain injury (ABI) or at

certain stages of progressive neurocognitive disorders. The book—usually a loose-leaf notebook with function-specific sections—is typically composed of orientation information (e.g., a page with information about where the patient is and why) and daily log sheets, on which the patient, family, or staff write down what occurs on an hour-by-hour basis. Memory books are advantageous when new learning is very difficult. Early in recovery, the memory book is most useful in encouraging staff to interact with the client around orienting information. The client should be cued repeatedly to look up information in the memory book. As clients recover, it becomes possible for them to review the book spontaneously and make entries about ongoing events and/or progress to using a day planner/organizer.

Day Planners/Organizers and Assistive Technologies for Cognition. Individuals with mild cognitive inefficiencies (such as those with concussion/mild TBI) or neurodegenerative conditions such as multiple sclerosis (MS) and those who are recovering from moderate to severe TBI are often taught to use a day planner or ATC as a "memory prosthesis" to improve their functioning in daily life (Gentry, 2008; Gentry et al., 2008; Schmitter-Edgecombe et al., 1995). To do this successfully, clients (active initiators) are taught to recognize the type of information that is pertinent for them in real time, initiate entry of the material into the planner or device (and perform procedures for doing so), take or input notes accurately, and establish daily procedures and/or employ alarm prompts for referring to needed information in a timely fashion.

Some clients are able to manage memory problems by using day-at-a-glance organizers or day planners, which are commercially available in a variety of formats and sizes (see Fig. 24-2). As with memory books, many day planners have function-specific sections that may include a daily

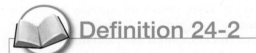

Definition 24-2

Mild Neurocognitive Disorder and Major Neurocognitive Disorder

The fifth edition of the Diagnostic and Statistical Manual of Mental Disorders (DSM-5) proposes to replace the terms mild cognitive disorder and dementia (the latter is now considered pejorative or stigmatizing) with mild neurocognitive disorder and major neurocognitive disorder, respectively (American Psychiatric Association, 2012). Readers are referred to the DSM-5 manual (published in 2013) for a full discussion of symptomatology and diagnostic criteria; general descriptions of these terms are provided below.

Mild neurocognitive disorder refers to a modest cognitive decline as evidenced by testing and/or report of the patient or an informant. The individual remains independent in instrumental activities of daily living but greater effort, compensatory strategies, and/or accommodations are required.

Major neurocognitive disorder refers to a substantial cognitive decline as evidenced by testing and/or by report of patient or informant. Cognitive deficits interfere with independence in instrumental activities of daily living, and the individual requires assistance with complex tasks such as paying bills or managing medication.

Note that both types of neurocognitive disorders must be distinguished from delirium and cognitive decline from other conditions (e.g., major depression).

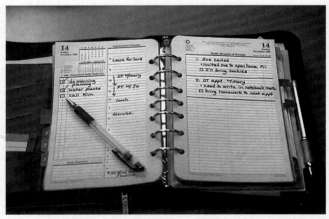

Figure 24-2 Use of function-specific portions of the planner page helps the patient organize notes about the day.

schedule/to-do lists; checklists pertaining to frequently performed procedures, notes about projects in-process, reference information about medical providers or family members, and contact information.

Clients may need or prefer to use some form of ATC as either a replacement for or complement to a planner/organizer. Evans et al. (2003) interviewed 101 people who reported memory problems from brain injury and their carers. External aids such as calendars and wall charts (72%) and notebooks (64%) were the most commonly used memory aids. Electronic organizers, pagers, or mobile phones were used as memory aids by only 16% of people, although this may have changed since the study was published. In another consumer survey of 80 persons with moderate to severe TBI (a median of 3.7 years postinjury), less than a third of those interviewed used PDAs, and of these, 75% of interviewees showed interest in their use (Hart, Buchhofer, & Vaccaro, 2004). Electronic memory aids and paging systems offer advantages, particularly in regard to prospective memory (Wilson et al., 2001; Wilson et al., 1997). Some examples of ATC are described below.

- Specialized pagers. NeuroPage™ uses radio paging or SMS (text messaging) technology to send reminders of things to do to people with significant memory impairment. It is operated out of the Oliver Zangwill Centre for Neuropsychological Rehabilitation (United Kingdom). The client wears an ordinary pager or mobile phone. He or she provides Neuropage™ operators with a list of required date/time-specific prompts, and then the system automatically sends out reminders for things like task initiation, taking medications, and sending birthday cards. Neuropage™ has been studied extensively and shown to improve day-to-day functioning in the postacute period after TBI (Wilson et al., 2005) and in other conditions (Wilson et al., 2001).

  Similarly, preprogrammed electronic memory aids have also been demonstrated to help outpatients with neurocognitive disorder remember to do time-specific tasks, significantly more so than use of written lists or trying to recall without any memory aid (Oriani et al., 2003).
- PDAs. Commercially-available PDAs provide time-specific alarms and reminders to help people with memory impairment complete intended tasks. Gentry reported statistically significant improvements in task performance for those with TBI and those with MS who were trained to use PDAs (Gentry, 2008; Gentry et al., 2008).
- Smartphones/mobile apps and other devices. The burgeoning of mobile technologies has expanded the array of consumer products that may help people compensate for cognitive problems. However, there is little research at present to demonstrate efficacy or effectiveness for individuals with cognitive impairment. Furthermore, smartphones tend to have smaller buttons and screens as compared with PDAs, possibly

making them more difficult to use after TBI (de Joode et al., 2010). Voice organizers, which can be set up to provide time-specific audio prompts and instructions, and smart pens, which audio record information as the user takes notes, are examples of other options that may solve client memory-related problems but for which there is no evidence at present.

Expectations for Training and Transfer-Generalization

Teaching clients to be active initiators of memory strategies should follow the three-stage progression described earlier (acquisition, application, and adaptation stages), and this may be time consuming, depending on client factors and outcome goals. For example, Schmitter-Edgecombe et al. (1995) described an 8-week protocol of 16 sessions, and Donaghy and Williams (1998) used a 9-week protocol of 27 sessions for patients with TBI to learn to use memory aids of this nature. The I-MEMS protocol (internal memory strategy instruction for persons with TBI) involved 12 group sessions of 90 minutes over 6 weeks (O'Neil-Pirozzi et al., 2010). Gentry's instructional protocol for PDA use by persons with TBI and MS required just two home-based sessions to learn to input appointments and to-dos (Gentry, 2008; Gentry et al., 2008).

The generalization of the use of internal visualization of verbal elaboration strategies with persons with significant memory impairments who are in the postacute phase of recovery has either not been evaluated or is disappointing (Harris, 1980). There is a limited literature that suggests that clients who learn to use external memory strategies are able to independently apply those same strategies to new situations (Kim et al., 2000). Additionally, clients do appear to use the newly learned material (e.g., face-name associations) in their daily lives (i.e., they generalize to the real world) (Clare et al., 2000). External strategies such as using a calendar have not been found to be effective in accelerating the return of orientation in people in the acute stage of recovery from brain injury (i.e., those in PTA) (Watanabe et al., 1998).

Alignment with Occupational Therapy Theory and Objectives

Intervention to help patients use memory strategies to improve everyday functioning is considered consistent with occupational therapy theory and objectives. Evidence suggests that persons with neurologically based cognitive impairment often do continue to use memory strategies in their daily life after intervention. Kim et al. (2000) described the experience of 12 participants exposed to the use of PDAs: 9 of the 12 found the PDA useful and 7 of these participants continued use of the PDA when followed up between 2 months and 4 years after initial exposure to the device. Based on their evidence review, the

Institute of Medicine (IOM) (2011) concluded that there are long-term benefits of teaching persons with mild TBI to use internal strategies and that individuals with moderate to severe brain injury often use external memory strategies months after treatment ends.

Metacognitive Strategies

Metacognition refers to thinking about thinking or the higher order self-awareness and monitoring of a person's own cognitive processes. It is possible to think of a hierarchy of cognitive processes with metacognition and self-awareness at the top, executive functions such as planning, organizations skills, and reasoning in an intermediate position, and basic cognitive processes (e.g., memory) at the lowest level (Stuss, 1991). Metacognitive strategy training involves teaching clients how to identify problems and develop their own methods to overcome these problems and to implement and evaluate the solutions (Polatajko & Mandich, 2004; Polatajko, Mandich, & McEwen, 2011; Toglia et al., 2010). One such approach in the occupational therapy literature is Cognitive Orientation to Daily Occupations.

Cognitive Orientation to Daily Occupations. The Cognitive Orientation to Daily Occupational Performance (CO-OP) approach teaches a global strategy (goal, plan, do, check), derived from the work of Meichenbaum (1977). This global strategy is used in a process of "guided discovery" so that clients can develop their own domain-specific strategies to solve personally relevant specific performance problems. Most of the research into the application of the CO-OP approach has centered on its use with children with developmental coordination disorder (Polatajko, Mandich, & McEwen, 2011). More recently, CO-OP has been applied to adults with TBI and stroke, and some positive results of single cases and small series have been reported (Dawson et al., 2009; McEwen et al., 2009).

The main goal of CO-OP is skill acquisition in functional everyday tasks. However, the process of therapist-guided skill acquisition is also intended to help the client learn a general approach to problem solving that he or she can apply to new performance problems and use to independently develop new domain-specific strategies (Polatajko, Mandich, & McEwen, 2011). Because a goal of CO-OP is for clients to be able to apply the global strategy beyond treatment sessions and to new issues (i.e., generalization), the process itself is a specific focus of the approach (Polatajko, Mandich, & McEwen, 2011), as illustrated next.

1. The client sets the goals that he or she wishes to work on, and then the therapist teaches the global strategy of Goal, Plan, Do, Check.
2. The client is guided in dynamic performance analysis in which he or she identifies the performance problems that interfere with goal achievement.

3. The client is further guided to identify potential strategies that may solve his or her problems. The client then implements the strategy to solve the real world functional problem and checks to see whether it worked. The implementation of the domain-specific strategy may or may not be done in the presence of the therapist, depending on the treatment context, stage of training, and other factors.

The process of guided discovery in which the client learns how to solve performance problems is central to the approach. Therefore, how the therapist interacts with the client during CO-OP is important, which the authors of the approach have distilled into key features: "One thing at a time"; "Ask, don't tell"; "Coach, don't adjust"; and "Make it obvious" (Polatajko, Mandich, & McEwen, 2011).

Expectations for Transfer-Generalization

The goal of metacognitive strategy training is for the client to independently apply newly learned strategies in novel circumstances. As such, transfer and generalization are central to this intervention approach. Metacognitive strategy training in adults with neurological impairment is a relatively new area of study for occupational therapists, and data are limited but encouraging (McEwen et al., 2010). Geusgens et al. (2007) conducted a systematic review of transfer in cognitive strategy training pertaining to information processing, problem solving/executive functioning, memory/attention, language, neglect, apraxia, and daily activities. Transfer outcomes were classified into three groups: nontrained items, standardized daily tasks, and daily life. Most studies reported at least one type of transfer; however, the methodological quality of the studies was low, and the authors concluded that further study is indicated (Geusgens et al., 2007).

Alignment with Occupational Therapy Theory and Objectives

Metacognitive strategy approaches are almost by necessity client centered and, as described here, focused on real-life problems. Practiced in this way, metacognitive strategy training is well aligned with the overarching concerns of occupational therapists. In occupational therapy practice, strategies are not taught in the abstract and are always taught within the context of an occupational performance goal. Global strategy training, rather than teaching a solution to a specific problem, attempts to equip the client to solve novel problems in the future. There are reasons to believe that metacognitive strategy training may be limited to clients with mild to moderate levels of impairment (Giles, 2010), but currently the evidence is encouraging, and further research is warranted.

Task and/or Environmental Modification Training

Patients may demonstrate improved occupational performance when caregivers are trained to make task or environmental changes that lower the cognitive demands placed on the patient (see examples in Procedures for Practice 24-3). Caregivers are trained to use new ways of interacting with the patient; the patient is not expected to learn or change, but the press of the task, social dynamics, and/or environment are lessened. (See Fig. 24-3, A & B for an example of how environmental modifications may lower press.) This approach is particularly appropriate for persons with major neurocognitive disorder or severe neurocognitive deficits from other causes (e.g., TBI, encephalitis, and anoxia).

Clinical Example of this Approach

The work of Gitlin and colleagues with individuals with dementia and their caregivers exemplify and evidence the impact of this type of approach. In an evaluation of a home-based environmental intervention, 171 caregivers

Procedures for Practice 24-3

Strategies to Decrease Cognitive Demands and Increase Occupational Performance

Mr. J. is a 74-year-old man with major neurocognitive disorder caused by Alzheimer's disease (AD) who lives in a suburban home with his wife of 50 years. He used to be impeccably groomed and dressed but now resists any articles of clothing perceived as unfamiliar. He was a master gardener and delighted in preparing food with ingredients from his garden. He no longer has the cognitive or physical capacities for managing the garden or preparing food independently. Mrs. J. worked with an occupational therapist to identify strategies that would enable Mr. J. to participate in activities in ways that were enjoyable to them both. Principles of lowering cognitive demand and examples are described below.

Modify the Environment

- Reduce visual and auditory clutter. *Mrs. J. set up Mr. J.'s workstation at the kitchen table before they started their task. She removed the lunch dishes, mail, and newspaper and set out only the items needed for the task at hand: first just the towel for drying the basil, then a bowl for the basil leaves and a small container for trash.*
- Provide assistive devices to optimize safety. *Mrs. J. had grab bars installed near the toilet and bath tub. Her son also installed a motion detector near the front door so that Mrs. J. could prevent Mr. J. from wandering outdoors. She had a StoveGuard installed with a 30-minute delay. The stove then automatically turns off after 30 minutes, decreasing the risk that Mr. J. will turn on and then forget to turn off a burner.*
- Use visuals to provide orientation and instructions. *Mrs. J. modified the telephone so there are pictures of family members beside their speed dial buttons. She also posted a 1-day calendar near Mr. J.'s favorite chair.*
- Organize so that the right items are easily located. *Mrs. J.'s daughter helped her remove everything from the countertop in the bathroom, leaving only a plastic basket containing Mr. J.'s toothbrush, toothpaste, and comb.*

Simplify the Task

- Break down a task into small steps. Decide what steps the client can do, what steps the clinician or caregiver will do,

and what steps might be eliminated. *Mr. and Mrs. J. prepared pesto together, using basil from their garden. Some of the steps included picking the basil from the garden; sorting, washing, and drying the basil leaves; toasting pine nuts; chopping garlic; and combining in a food processor.*
- Select tasks (or steps) for the patient that are familiar and repetitive, if possible. *With supervision, Mr. J. picked basil from the garden. Mrs. J. washed the basil leaves in the sink, and while seated at the table, Mr. J. dried the basil leaves with a towel and separated the leaves from the stems.*
- Simplify objects involved in the task. *Mrs. J. purchased duplicates of Mr. J.'s favorite sweaters and underwear so that he did not notice that he was putting on different (clean) clothes each day. She also set his clothing out each day on the bed in the order he was to put it on.*

Routinize the Day

- Establish a consistent daily schedule of activities. *Mrs. J. created a daily schedule, which she set by his calendar and newspaper. The schedule includes frequently performed activities such as meals/meal times, their afternoon walk, favorite TV show, and bedtime activities.*

Simplify Communication

- Simplify verbal instructions (one-step instructions using as few words as possible); avoid lengthy explanations. *Mrs. J. used simple instructions like "pick the basil now" and "dry off the basil now." Mrs. J. avoided making conversation when Mr. J. was involved in picking the basil because she understood that too much stimulation made the task more difficult.*
- Celebrate participation by relaxing rules and requirements. *Mrs. J. noticed that Mr. J. missed a few basil stems here and there, but she did not correct him.*

From Corcoran, M. A. (2003). Practical skills training for family caregivers. San Francisco: Family Caregiving Alliance. Retrieved August 19, 2012 from http://www.caregiver.org/caregiver/jsp/content_node.jsp?nodeid=954; Corcoran, M. A. (n.d.a). Environmental modification strategies: Customized toolkit of information and practical solutions (C-TIPS). Retrieved August 19, 2012 from http://www.c-tips.com/la_tools/modifying_the_environment.pdf; Corcoran, M. A. (n.d.b). Task breakdown strategies. Customized toolkit of information and practical solutions (C-TIPS). Retrieved August 19, 2012 from http://www.c-tips.com/la_tools/task_breakdown_strategies.pdf.

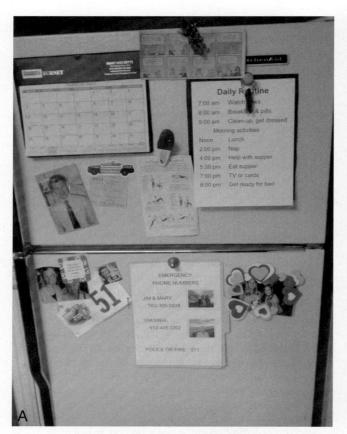 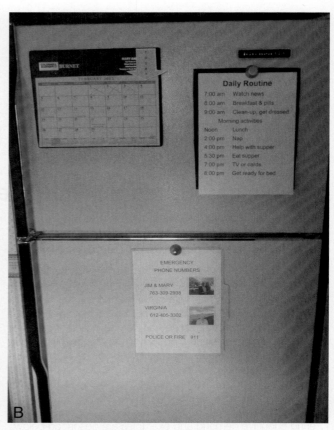

Figure 24-3 A, B. Simple changes in the kitchen lower the cognitive demands, making it easier for a person with cognitive limitations to find relevant information.

were randomized to usual care or a series of five 90-minute home visits with an occupational therapist (Gitlin et al., 2001). Caregivers received education about the impact of the environment on dementia-related behaviors, instruction related to functional concerns, and guidance to implement environmental and task simplification strategies. (See further information in Evidence Table 24-1.) More recently, Gitlin et al. (2008; 2009) developed and evaluated a tailored activity program (TAP) for those with major neurocognitive disorder and their families. TAP is an eight-session home-based occupational therapy intervention that occurred over 4 months. It involved the following: neuropsychological and functional testing; identification of the patient's preserved capabilities, habits, and interests; therapist selection and customization of activities to match patient capabilities based on testing; and training family members in how to use these activities with their loved ones. A total of 170 activities were prescribed during the study (e.g., cutting out coupons, wiping silverware, playing a matching card game, doing chair aerobics, and watching birds at a bird feeder); 81.5% were used by families (Gitlin et al., 2009). Patient-caregivers receiving TAP reported significantly fewer problem behaviors and greater activity engagement than did the

caregivers of control patients at 4 months posttest (Gitlin et al., 2008).

Presumed Mechanism

This approach is informed by the competence-environmental press framework (Lawton & Nahemow, 1973). This framework suggests that the patient's negative behaviors and/or excess disability is caused by the misalignment between the patient's declining cognitive ability and the unchanged demands of the physical and social environment. The patient's functional performance and behavioral control may be optimized as task and environmental demands are matched to the patient's capacities (Gitlin et al., 2001).

Expectations for Transfer-Generalization

Research has not been conducted on the extent to which caregivers who receive training to match cognitive demands to patients' capabilities are able to transfer or generalize this training to new problems or situations. However, it appears that the effects of this training are maintained for at least 6–12 months (Gitlin et al., 2005).

Alignment with Occupational Therapy Theory and Objectives

This approach, which emphasizes improved occupational performance, is well-aligned with occupational therapy theory and practice. In addition to education of caregivers of individuals with dementia, modification of the environment and task have also been recommended for persons with visual neglect and problems with prospective memory (Gillen, 2009). However, caregiver training protocols with these populations have not yet been formalized.

Cognitive Stimulation Therapy

In the 1970s and 1980s, general stimulation approaches to cognitive rehabilitation were applied to persons with both stroke and TBI in the acute recovery period. General stimulation was believed to facilitate the normal process of recovery from the neurological impairment by challenging the patient's deficits and/or weakened cognitive process, thereby strengthening them so that the person demonstrates gains in functional performance (Soderback & Normell, 1986a, 1986b). By the 1990s, these approaches had largely been abandoned as ineffective in regard to persons with stroke and TBI in favor of process-specific or milieu-oriented approach (Cicerone et al., 2011). During this same period, a new approach called CST emerged for people with mild and major neurocognitive impairment as a cross-pollination of reality orientation (RO) and reminiscence therapy (RT). RO is provided in a group format for 45 minutes a number of times per week or continuously (24-hour RO) and was introduced as a means to address confusion and disorientation in "geriatric" or "psycho geriatric" patients and to provide nursing staff with a positive way to interact with patients with dementia (Clare & Woods, 2004; Moniz-Cook, 2006). The approach was noted to reduce patient hopelessness; improve cognitive function and social behaviors; and provide a format for positive engagement of nursing staff with confused patients, thereby improving staff morale (Moniz-Cook, 2006). RT is usually provided at least once a week in a group context and involves the discussion of past activities, events, and experiences. Familiar music, photographs, or objects such as household items from the individuals' lives are often used as prompts. RT may also include an individual life review, in which the person is guided chronologically through life experiences, is encouraged to evaluate them, and may produce a biography (Spector et al., 2009).

Presumed Mechanism

When applied to persons with neurocognitive disorders in home or institutional settings, CST often additionally involves positive social interactions and/or deliberate attempts to improve the 24-hour stimulation in an otherwise understimulating environment. In the presence of neurocognitive impairment, a general cognitive stimulation approach presumes to address the multiple areas of cognitive decline on the premise that real-life activity requires the integration of cognitive skills rather than their use in isolation (Clare & Woods, 2004; Moniz-Cook, 2006).

Expectations for Transfer-Generalization

Woods et al. (2012) conducted a systematic review of CST including RO for people with major neurocognitive disorder. Interventions took place in various settings and were of varying duration and intensity. Data for 718 participants (407 receiving CST, 311 in control groups) were included in the meta-analyses. In the primary analysis, Woods et al. found a consistent benefit on cognitive function, and the benefit was maintained up to 3 months after treatment. In secondary analyses with smaller total sample sizes, benefits were also noted on self-reported quality of life and well-being and on staff ratings of social interaction and communication. No effects on ADL, mood (self-report or staff-rated), or behavior problems were noted. This latter finding of no impact on ADL or IADL in general stimulation approaches is the most frequent finding across studies (Woods et al., 2012).

Alignment with Occupational Therapy Theory and Objectives

Although occupational therapists have a specific focus on occupational engagement, occupational therapists also recognize the importance of other outcomes such as reducing distress in both clients and their caregivers. Therefore, the incorporation of CST programs in populations with neurocognitive disorders may be appropriate for occupational therapists.

Process-Specific Training

Process-specific training involves use of cognitive exercises to remediate or improve specific cognitive systems (Sohlberg & Mateer, 2001). Cognitive exercises, typically pencil and paper, tabletop, or computer-based, are designed to stimulate the deficient cognitive capacity but may have little inherent value in and of themselves (Sohlberg & Mateer, 1989). Functional activities are typically multifaceted, require activation of many different cognitive processes, and can often be performed in many different ways. Therefore, they are not employed in process-specific training (Sohlberg & Mateer, 2001). In this section, process-specific training for attention and speed of processing are presented as examples of this approach.

Process-Specific Training: Attention

As discussed in Chapter 6, many recipients of occupational therapy services have problems with attention, including persons who have had a stroke or TBI. Attention is thought to underlie all effortful cognitive activity (Shiffrin & Schneider, 1977); involve many dimensions such as maintaining vigilance, managing distractions, and deploying resources in complex tasks (Gray et al., 1992); and play a central role in learning (Robertson et al., 2002). Attention process training (APT) (Sohlberg & Mateer, 1987) and limb activation therapy (LAT) (Robertson, Hogg, & McMillan, 1998) are examples of process training specific to attention-related impairments.

Attention Process Training. APT was originally developed for adults with attention deficits caused by TBI. APT employs hierarchically organized tasks (pencil and paper, audio recordings, and computer) intended to challenge specific aspects of attention (sustained, selective, alternating, and divided) (Sohlberg & Mateer, 1987; Sohlberg et al., 2000). The patient performs exercises specific to his or her problematic attentional process, and the clinician or computer collects data on performance. As the patient meets criterion levels, the therapist raises the complexity or difficulty of the cognitive exercises, maintaining challenge to the original weakened process or capacity (Sohlberg & Mateer, 1989). This progression culminates with rehearsal of a naturalistic activity supported by the previously weakened cognitive capacity (Haskins, 2011; Sohlberg & Mateer, 2001).

Intensive practice of hierarchical attention tasks, such as APT, appears to have a positive impact on psychometric measures of attention (Gray et al., 1992; Sohlberg et al., 2000) and on self- and informant-reported daily performance (Sohlberg et al., 2000). The IOM (2011) and the Brain Injury Special Interest Group of the American Congress of Rehabilitation Medicine (Cicerone et al., 2011) suggest this type of intervention may be appropriate in the subacute and/or chronic phases of recovery from TBI, especially when combined with strategy training (Cicerone et al., 2000, 2005, 2011), but not appropriate during the acute phase. *Sole reliance on computer-based exercises for attention training without involvement of a therapist is not recommended (Cicerone et al., 2000, 2005, 2011).*

Limb Activation Therapy. As discussed in Chapters 5 and 23, unilateral neglect (UN) is "the failure to report, respond, or orient to novel or meaningful stimuli presented to the side opposite a brain lesion, when this failure cannot be attributed to either sensory or motor defects" (Maddicks, Marzillier, & Parker, 2003, p. 391). UN is a common consequence of right-hemisphere stroke and thought to be an attentional disorder that operates in three distinct areas of space (personal [body], peripersonal [reaching], and locomotor [far]) (Maddicks, Marzillier, & Parker, 2003) (see Fig. 24-4). Those who have UN appear to have poorer rehabilitation outcomes, possibly because decreased attention to the neglected hemispace interferes

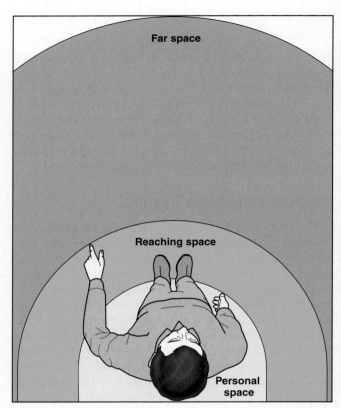

Figure 24-4 Three distinct areas of space in which unilateral neglect interferes with occupational performance: personal (body), peripersonal (reaching), and locomotor (far).

with learning that is critical in rehabilitation (Robertson et al., 2002).

Robertson and North (1992) and Robertson, Hogg, and McMillan (1998) developed a process-specific intervention approach called limb activation therapy. It is based on the hypothesis that when tasks are performed using the contralesional limb in the contralesion hemispace (i.e., using the left hand or leg in the left half of space when the lesion is in the right brain), the motor circuits of the damaged hemisphere are activated, which then reduces neglect (Maddicks, Marzillier, & Parker, 2003). In LAT, the patient moves the left limb in the left hemispace when prompted by an alarm-type device at randomly occurring points during daily sessions (i.e., upon hearing a buzzer, the patient presses a switch with the left hand or foot) (Robertson & North, 1992; Robertson, Hogg, & McMillan, 1998). In some studies, LAT is incorporated into traditional occupational therapy sessions or perceptual training (Bailey, Riddoch, & Crome, 2002; Robertson et al., 1998). Most studies in this area involve multiple baseline, single subject research designs. For example, a patient who was 18 months post stroke demonstrated improvement in treatment tasks as a result of LAT added to traditional occupational therapy, with some evidence of retained gains in terms of peripersonal space but not in personal and locomotor space (Robertson et al., 1998). In a similar study, Maddicks, Marzillier, and Parker (2003) found a treatment effect during the first phase of treatment on peripersonal and locomotor space but no long-term impact on daily life tasks. Other versions of LAT have been evaluated. Bailey, Riddoch, and Crome (2002) compared visual scanning/cueing training with a version of limb activation training in which subjects with stroke-related UN performed functional activities with the left upper extremity; patients demonstrated improvement on posttest measures with both interventions. Others have examined the impact of adding functional electrical stimulation as a means of cueing left limb movement to visual scanning training (Eskes et al., 2003), with improvements noted in visual scanning post-treatment. It is important to note that although all of the aforementioned studies demonstrated post-treatment improvements in some measures of UN, there is no clear evidence at present that results of this intervention generalize to occupational performance (Bailey, Riddoch, & Crome, 2002; Eskes et al., 2003; Maddicks, Marzillier, & Parker, 2003; Robertson, Hogg, & McMillan, 1998; Robertson et al., 2002).

Process-Specific Training: Speed of Information Processing Training

Age-related declines in speed of information processing and other cognitive capacities are considered a normal part of the aging process, but there is evidence suggesting that the cognitive abilities of older adults may be enhanced through process-specific training (Ball et al., 2002). Speed of information processing has to do with how quickly someone perceives, analyzes, and responds to sensory input. Proficiency in this cognitive capacity, as determined by a computerized measure of visual processing speed for attentional tasks called the Useful Field of View (UFOV) test (Visual Resources, Inc., Bowling Green, KY), appears to be linked with driving ability for healthy elders (Edwards et al., 2009) and individuals with TBI (Novack et al., 2006).

Speed of information processing training (SOPT) is a computerized set of cognitive exercises that involve identifying and localizing visual targets at rapid display speeds (16–500 milliseconds) that are designed to improve UFOV (O'Connor, Hudak, & Edwards, 2011). Visual stimuli in SOPT are presented in the context of a driving task. SOPT has evolved into commercial products: Road Tour and DriveSharp (see Resources 24-1).

The results of multiple, large-scale, randomized controlled studies of SOPT suggest that training may be beneficial for healthy elders. It may improve visual processing speed (as measured by the UFOV) (Ball et al., 2002; Ball, Edwards, & Ross, 2007; Wolinsky et al., 2011) and protect against driving mobility declines and incidence of at-fault motor vehicle crashes among seniors (Ball et al., 2010; Edwards et al., 2009).

Presumed Mechanism

Process-specific training is premised on the assumption that one cognitive capacity may be treated in isolation from other dimensions of cognition. It is believed to repeatedly activate and stimulate a specific cognitive system, which presumably facilitates change in cognitive capacity (Sohlberg & Mateer, 2001; Wolinsky et al., 2011). However, this assumption does not yet have empirical support. Current evidence suggests that engagement in process-specific training often improves cognitive performance on neuropsychological tests. A small but potentially important group of studies suggests that process-specific training may improve everyday performance when certain cognitive functions are targeted (most notably, speed of information processing). Even so, it may be difficult to differentiate the impact of this approach on neuroplasticity, as suggested above, from the implicit development of cognition-related skills or strategies.

Alignment with Occupational Therapy Theory and Outcomes

There are no occupational therapy cognitive models, theories, or frameworks that are directly related to process-specific training in cognitive rehabilitation. Process-specific training does not incorporate chosen occupations or occupational performance into the treatment regimen. For patients with ABI, process-specific training alone does not appear to generalize to everyday functioning, whereas SOPT for healthy elders may extend their ability to drive. Given the above, process-specific training may be appropriate in occupational therapy intervention after ABI only as an adjunct to other approaches that appear to have greater potential to impact occupational functioning.

CLINICAL REASONING IN COGNITIVE INTERVENTION

In everyday practice, occupational therapists often use multiple approaches to help patients optimize cognitive performance. For example, consider a client who is learning to use a day planner to compensate for memory impairment. Although the primary treatment approach centers on strategy training, successful outcome depends on teaching the individual's family to provide the right prompts and reinforcement (task-environment modification) and creating a daily planning routine in which the person reviews and adds notes to the planner (skill-task-habit training). Furthermore, it is possible that the learning process challenges the attentional and memory systems in such a way as to stimulate neuroanatomical and physiological changes (cognitive stimulation).

In designing a cognitive intervention plan to address a given patient's problems, clinicians must consider the

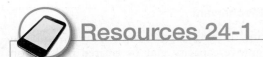

Resources 24-1

Optimizing Cognitive Performance

Skill-Task-Habit Training: Prompting Devices and Clinician-Generated Checklists

MotivAider®

http://habitchange.com/motivaider.php
MotivAider® is a vibrating timing device that is worn on a belt or in a pocket. At preset intervals (determined by the user), it emits scheduled or randomly generated silent pulsing signals to prompt specified actions (also as determined by the user).

NeuroPage™

http://www.neuropage.nhs.uk/

Compensatory Strategy Training

Cognitive Orientation to Daily Occupational Performance
http://www.ot.utoronto.ca/coop/about.htm

Day Planners (essential features are predated pages and defined notebook sections)
FranklinCovey
www.franklincovey.com
DayTimer
www.daytimer.com

Electronic devices that support scheduling and time management
Alarm watches, alarms on cell phones and smartphones
Also see MotivAider® and NeuroPage™ above

Information about using PDAs and other electronic aids in therapy
http://www.brainline.org/content/2008/11/pda-intervention-plan-implementing-electronic-memory-and-organization-aids.html

Assistive Technology for Cognition by Mackay Sohlberg
http://www.asha.org/Publications/leader/2011/110215/Assistive-Technology-for-Cognition.htm

Task-Environment Modification Training

Dementia Care and the Built Environment

Alzheimer's Australia
http://www.fightdementia.org.au/common/files/NAT/20040600_Nat_NP_3DemCareBuiltEnv.pdf

Corcoran, M. A. (2003). *Practical skills training for family caregivers*. San Francisco: Family Caregiving Alliance. Retrieved August 19, 2012 from http://www.caregiver.org/caregiver/jsp/content_node.jsp?nodeid=954.

Corcoran, M. A. (n.d.a). *Environmental modification strategies: Customized toolkit of information and practical solutions (C-TIPS)*. Retrieved August 19, 2012 from http://www.c-tips.com/la_tools/modifying_the_environment.pdf.

Corcoran, M. A. (n.d.b). *Task breakdown strategies: Customized toolkit of information and practical solutions (C-TIPS)*. Retrieved August 19, 2012 from http://www.c-tips.com/la_tools/task_breakdown_strategies.pdf.

Automatic appliance shut-off devices
StoveGuard
http://stoveguard.ca/

Exit alarms and patient wandering devices
AbleData
http://abledata.com

Process-Specific Training

Attention Process Training-II
http://www.pearsonassessments.com/HAIWEB/Cultures/en-us/Productdetail.htm?Pid=015-8010-086

DriveSharp
Interactive SOPT software package that includes Jewel Diver, Road Tour, and Sweep Seeker; available to AAA members. http://drivesharp.positscience.com/?CJAID=10685832&CJPID=3529639

Road Tour interactive SOPT software package http://brainreview.info/positscienceproductdetails/

Clinician Websites

Brainline.org
http://www.brainline.org/
Brain Injury Association of America
http://www.biausa.org/
The Society for Cognitive Rehabilitation
http://www.societyforcognitiverehab.org/

Institute of Medicine, *Cognitive Rehabilitation Therapy for Traumatic Brain Injury: Evaluating the Evidence*. (2011). Retrieved from http://www.iom.edu/Reports/2011/Cognitive-Rehabilitation-Therapy-for-Traumatic-Brain-Injury-Evaluating-the-Evidence.aspx.

American Occupational Therapy Association Statement on Cognition

American Occupational Therapy Association (2012). *Cognition, Cognitive Rehabilitation, and Occupational Performance*. Retrieved July 21, 2013 from http://www.aota.org/~/media/Corporate/Files/AboutAOTA/OfficialDocs/Statements/Cognition%20Cognitive%20Rehabilitation%20and%20Occupational%20Performance.ashx.

interplay between client and family factors; outcome expectations, setting, and time frame; and alignment with scope of practice, clinician competence, and interdisciplinary team.

Client and Family Factors

The occupational therapist makes decisions regarding who is the primary recipient of services—the patient, caregiver, or both. In general, care partners must be involved in intervention for patients with severe cognitive impairments because these patients are not likely to be able to independently practice or transfer what they learn in clinical sessions to the home setting. Individuals with more mild cognitive problems will be better able to apply therapy recommendations in their daily lives with only the support of the therapist. In addition, the therapist considers the nature of the underlying condition that is causing the client's cognitive problems. For example, are the client's problems attributed to organic impairments in primary cognitive abilities or characterized as a shorter term cognitive inefficiency caused by transient stressors or circumstances? Is the client in the process of recovering, or is his or her condition likely to result in progressive deterioration? How are other systems, such as motor, visual, and perceptual systems, functioning (Schwartz, 1995)? To what extent is the client aware of the cognitive problems and motivated to improve function in this area? In general, patients must have some degree of awareness and motivation to benefit from strategy training, whereas even those with severe cognitive deficits have the potential to benefit from skill-task-habit training or changes to tasks and environments to match current capabilities.

Outcome Expectations, Setting, and Anticipated Contact Time

Where the patients are in their injury or illness trajectories will influence the overall outcome expectations of therapy and the amount of time available for patient–therapist contact—all of which should be carefully considered in developing the cognitive intervention plan.

During acute medical care, occupational therapists may only have a limited number of sessions with the patient; discharge planning is typically the focus. Inpatient rehabilitation may extend for a week to a month or so and focuses on impairment remediation and assuring competence in basic ADL. Patients typically receive an hour and a half of occupational therapy per day during this phase. Outpatient rehabilitation is often provided two to three times per week, and this may continue for weeks to months, depending on patient needs, goals, and insurance coverage.

It is imperative that clinicians are well versed in published cognitive rehabilitation guidelines and evidence-based reviews (Cicerone et al., 2000, 2005, 2011; Haskins, 2011; IOM, 2011) so that the most promising interventions are matched to patients' needs and goals at various points in the continuum of care. For example, a patient with a new stroke demonstrates forgetfulness during his kitchen evaluation immediately prior to discharge home from an acute medical setting. He would be best served if the therapist focused on task-environment modification (provision of recommendations to the patient and wife that the patient perform cooking tasks only when supervised by his wife). Broader memory concerns could be addressed by memory strategy training when he returns to occupational therapy as an outpatient.

Alignment with Scope of Practice, Clinician Competence, and Interdisciplinary Team

As introduced earlier, cognitive rehabilitation is an interdisciplinary enterprise. This means that there is the potential for complementary, overlapping, or conflicting roles with other disciplines. Often, the expertise of the clinicians at a given site will determine whether, for example, memory strategy training is provided by an occupational therapist or a speech language pathologist. Occupational therapists have the education and training to provide cognitive intervention and are accountable to their patients and the profession to employ occupation-focused, evidence-based cognitive intervention and to invest in ongoing learning in this important area of rehabilitation.

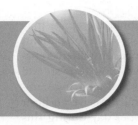

case example

D.B.: Using Multiple Approaches to Optimize Cognitive Functioning after Traumatic Brain Injury

Occupational Therapy Intervention Process	Clinical Reasoning Process	
	Objectives	**Examples of Therapist's Internal Dialogue**
Patient Information	Appreciate the context	See Chapter 6 for description of the assessment process and client's background.
D.B., a 26-year-old man who is 3 months post traumatic brain injury, participated in an outpatient occupational therapy assessment, and the following problems were identified: (1) decreased initiation of activities of daily living (ADL) and instrumental activities of daily living (IADL), (2) decreased productivity because of poor stamina and limited repertoire of appropriate avocational outlets, (3) memory inefficiency and inadequate repertoire of memory compensation strategies, and (4) decreased awareness of cognitive deficits interfering with compensatory strategy use.	Develop intervention hypotheses	"I believe that D.B.'s cognitive problems are the most salient barriers to his occupational functioning at present, specifically his limited awareness of his cognitive deficits. I think that he could better adapt to his physical limitations if he employed an array of strategies to compensate for his cognitive limitations. His motivation and family support are real facilitators of his occupational functioning and recovery."
	Select an intervention approach	"I will develop an intervention plan that emphasizes compensation for deficits, because given the severity of his brain injury, D.B. will likely have long-term cognitive challenges (*strategy instruction*). D.B. will no longer need assistance from his brother if I help him reestablish an ADL routine (*skill-habit training*). I know that I will also want to work with D.B.'s family to change the social context so that they are not providing him more cues and assistance than is really necessary (*task-environment modification*). I will suggest some computer games that place demands on attention and memory that D.B. might enjoy during some of his free time (*cognitive stimulation*). I know that these games won't 'fix' his brain, but they may help him gain insight about his cognitive functioning, especially if I provide some guided reflection questions for him to complete afterward."
	Consider the evidence	"A recent systematic review (Cicerone et al., 2011) indicates that evidence supports helping patients with traumatic brain injury (TBI) learn to use compensatory strategies for memory and attention problems but that there is no empirical support for patient exposure to computer-based exercises, without a therapist. The literature also suggests that habit training results in improved independence, even with people who have more severe TBI (Giles & Clark-Wilson, 1988; Giles et al., 1997)."
	Reflect on competence	"D.B. reminds me of three or four other clients I've worked with in recent years. I'm a little concerned that I may not be able to satisfactorily address emotional or adjustment issues that might emerge as he gains insight, and so I need to start thinking about a counselor I might refer him to later."

Recommendations

The occupational therapist recommended two or three treatment sessions each week for 8 weeks. In collaboration with D.B. and his brother, the occupational therapist established the following long-term treatment goals: (1) D.B. will independently initiate and carry out all self-care and selected light housekeeping tasks (through use of external memory aids), (2) D.B. will increase his level of productive activity at home such that he initiates avocational activities at least three times per week, and (3) D.B. will follow through on intended tasks at least 85% of the time through use of external memory aids and strategies. D.B.'s brother indicated a willingness to provide transportation to appointments and to attend at least weekly.

Consider what will occur in therapy, how often, and for how long	"I think that a fairly intensive outpatient program is warranted because of the scope of our goals and D.B.'s motivation and potential to make progress. I have real hope for D.B.'s recovery for many reasons, including his level of cooperation, his cognitive strengths, and his brother's commitment to the therapy process. D.B. seems agreeable to the plan, but I really don't know how much he truly understood what I'm proposing and why."
Ascertain the client's endorsement of plan	

Summary of Short-Term Goals and Progress

1. *D.B. will independently initiate note-taking when presented with occupational therapy homework (at least 60% of the time) and thereby improve his follow-through on intended tasks.*

   The therapist ascertained that D.B. would be most likely to carry a memory aid if it was highly portable. Therefore, she assisted D.B. in selecting a commercially available, pocket-sized week-at-glance planner. The therapist created opportunities for D.B. to practice filing and locating information in function-specific planner sections. The therapist used an event record to log each of the three to four homework assignments she presented to D.B. during all treatment sessions, taking note of the extent to which D.B. required cues to initiate note-taking. Any level of note-taking initiation was verbally reinforced. Progress in this realm was reviewed at each session, graphing both note-taking initiation and homework completion as reinforcement and to improve insight. During the last week of this period, D.B. averaged a 65% independent note-taking rate and a 70% homework completion rate.

2. *D.B. will initiate and employ consistent routines for self-care tasks (including medication management) through use of checklists and alarm cueing devices.*

   Based on the therapist's recommendation, D.B. purchased a container for medications taken each week as well as an alarm watch. The therapist set the alarm to sound at 5:00 pm as a prompt to refer to his medication checklist and take medications. D.B. required cueing and supervision with this system for 2 weeks, but by the end of the month, he took medications on schedule, once his brother filled the medication container. A "morning checklist" (D.B.'s hygiene sequence) was posted in D.B.'s bathroom, and after 1 month, he progressed to the point that he required his brother's cueing to initiate these activities only one or two times per week.

3. *D.B. will improve his attention to detail such that he has an error rate of less than 10% on pencil-paper tasks.*

   D.B. was highly motivated to "fix" his memory and eager to carry out any exercises that might help. To that end, he agreed to work on various attention-concentration worksheets as part of his homework while experimenting with various strategies that might help him focus on the task. For example, he tracked and compared his performance under various conditions: while watching television versus sitting in a quiet room; in the morning when rested versus after dinner; working in a space crowded with many papers and belongings versus a corner of his bedroom from which his "stuff" was not visible.

Assess the client's comprehension Understand what he is doing Appreciate the context	"At first when I started giving D.B. homework, he simply sat and nodded his head as if to confirm that he understood and would remember. It was hard for me to say nothing and 'let the chips fall where they may.' It was uncomfortable for a while when he would argue with me at our next session, telling me that I had never assigned him anything, but as I showed him my log and how to use his planner, he seemed to realize that it's o.k. to write things down rather than trying to memorize everything. I'm seeing progress." "I am so glad that D.B.'s brother is part of the team. Ordinarily, I like to allow patients to go ahead and make forgetting errors as a means of helping them improve awareness, but I simply can't allow that when it comes to remembering to take medications on schedule."
Know the person	"D.B. would rather 'fix' his memory than learn to compensate for memory problems, but the research evidence just doesn't support the notion that repetitive cognitive exercises lead to functional changes. I don't want to create any false hope but have tried to both give him some activities to fill his time at home and create a structure in which he can think about his thinking. He still needs a lot of help to understand the circumstances under which he performs at his best, but he seems to feel that these activities give him something important to do during his days off from therapy."

Next Steps

Revised short-term goals (1 month):

1. D.B. will use his daily planner and planning checklists in order to schedule and carry out at least two housekeeping tasks and three avocational activities each week.
2. D.B. will be able to use compensatory strategies to independently take medications on schedule (once his brother sets up the medication box each week).
3. D.B. will demonstrate improved awareness of his current problems with memory by independently initiating note-taking to the presentation of homework at least 85% of the time and at least 75% of the time when his brother provides instructions.

Anticipate present and future client concerns

Decide whether he or she should continue or discontinue therapy and/ or return in the future

"D.B. has made great progress over the past month but is not yet ready to be living on his own, which remains his primary goal. He really needs to be able to handle self-care tasks (including medications) and perform critical household tasks in order to do so. I would like to help D.B. prepare himself to do some sort of volunteer work within the next couple of months, and he has indicated at least preliminary interest in doing so. He'll need to be quite proficient with his planner to be a successful volunteer."

 Clinical Reasoning in Occupational Therapy Practice

Incorporating Task-Environment Modification Training into Occupational Therapy Intervention

D.B.'s brother was an important member of the rehabilitation team. Because D.B. had significant problems with memory and self-awareness, D.B.'s brother assumed central responsibility for trying to transfer and apply therapy recommendations in the home setting. Based on D.B.'s long-term goals, what information do you think that the occupational therapist should specifically teach D.B.'s brother? Provide some examples regarding how that teaching might take place.

Summary Review Questions

1. Describe the characteristics of the two systems people use for the control and execution of behavior. Keep a notebook with you for a day and write down the minutes that you spend in controlled effortful processing. How do you think this might differ it you are engaged in usual activities or in a new activity such as starting a new work environment?
2. How would your efforts to optimize cognitive function be different for a person with Alzheimer's disease compared with a patient in acute recovery from a traumatic brain injury?
3. Describe the pros and cons of process-specific training. Describe ways that this approach could be appropriately incorporated into an occupational therapy intervention plan.
4. Write down the steps to one of your daily routines or habit sequences. Now change the order of steps and, next time, try to follow this revised sequence. How do these changes affect your speed of performance and the attentional demands of the task? What does this experience teach you about helping patients establish daily routines?
5. Describe three changes you could make to your own living environment to decrease its cognitive demands.
6. Explain the ways in which metacognitive strategy training such as CO-OP is both similar to and different from external memory strategy training.
7. Consider practices or habits that optimize your memory performance and ability to concentrate, plan, and problem solve. How might these same strategies be used by an individual with cognitive impairment?

Glossary

Automaticity—The ability to perform activities or behaviors with little or no contribution from the conscious mind. Automaticity occurs as a result of practice of the behavior or skill.

Chaining—A task analysis breaks down complex tasks into a series steps or subtasks. In forward chaining, the client is taught to complete the first action in the task sequence; once mastery is achieved, the client is taught the first and second tasks and so on until all of the steps in the chain have been mastered and the complete task can be performed.

Cognitive rehabilitation—Multidisciplinary field and a broad category of intervention methods aimed at improving cognitive function.

Compensatory cognitive strategies—An array of tactics that are intentionally employed in order to optimize performance despite a cognitive limitation, such as using a metacognitive strategy to organize a project despite executive dysfunction or using an alarm watch to monitor the passage of time despite attentional problems.

Domain-specific strategies—Strategies people use to assist them to manage occupational performance problems related to a specific area of functioning (e.g., the person who has a tendency to leave needed items at home adopts the strategy of setting items he needs to take to work by the door).

Habits—The continuum of automatic physical, emotional, and social behaviors that become increasingly effortless with repetition within the same context.

Metacognitive strategies—Global tactics that people use to guide their approach to occupational performance problems. These strategies can be applied to a variety of problems and are applicable to many domains of functioning.

Press—Aspects of the person's physical or social environment that influence the challenge of an activity (activity demand). Reducing the press can make an activity easier to perform.

Routines—Semiautomatic sequences of activities that are prompted by physical context and are fairly consistent for each individual on a day-to-day basis (e.g., a person's morning ADL routine).

References

American Psychiatric Association. (2012). DSM-5 Development–Neurocognitive disorders. Retrieved July 20, 2013 from http://www.dsm5.org/Pages/RecentUpdates.aspx.

Baddeley, A., & Wilson, B. A. (1994). When implicit learning fails: Amnesia and the problem of error elimination. *Neuropsychologia, 32,* 53–68.

Bailey, M. J., Riddoch, M. J., & Crome, P. (2002). Treatment of visual neglect in elderly patients with stroke: A single-subject series using either a scanning and cueing strategy or a left-limb activation strategy. *Physical Therapy, 82,* 782–797.

Ball, K., Berch, D. B., Helmers, K. F., Jobe, J. B., Leveck, M. D., Marsiske, M., Morris, J. N., Rebok, G. W., Smith, D. M., Tennstedt, S. L., Unverzagt, F. W., & Willis, S. L. (2002). Effects of cognitive training interventions with older adults: A randomized controlled trial. *Journal of the American Medical Association, 288,* 2271–2281.

Ball, K., Edwards, J. D., & Ross, L. A. (2007). The impact of speed of processing training on cognitive and everyday functions. *Journals of Gerontology, 62B,* 19–31.

Ball, K., Edwards, J. D., Ross, L. A., & McGwin, G. (2010). Cognitive training decreases motor vehicle collision involvement of older drivers. *Journal of the American Geriatric Society, 58,* 2107–2113.

Boake, C. (1989). A history of cognitive rehabilitation of head-injured patients, 1915 to 1980. *Journal of Head Trauma Rehabilitation, 4,* 1–8.

Boake, C. (1991). History of cognitve rehabiliation following head injury. In J. S. Kreutzer & P. H. Wehman (Eds.), *Cognitve rehabiliation for persons with traumatic brain injury: A functional approach.* Baltimore, MD: Paul H. Brookes.

Bourgeois, M., Burgio, L., Schulz, R., Beach, S., & Palmer, B. (1997). Modifying repetitive verbalization of community dwelling patients with AD. *Gerontologist, 37,* 30–39.

Brain Injury Association of America. (n.d.). Definition and practice of cognitive rehabilitation. Retrieved October 12, 2012 from www.biausa.org/LiteratureRetrieve.aspx?ID=43818.

Cermak, L. S., Verfaellie, M., Lanzoni, S., Mather, M., & Chase, K. A. (1996). Effects of spaced repetitions on amnesia patients' recall and recognition performance. *Neuropsychology, 10,* 219–227.

Charmaz, K. (2002). The self as habit: The reconstruction of self in chronic illness. *Occupational Therapy Journal of Research, 22(Suppl. 1),* 31S–41S.

Cicerone, K. D., Dahlberg, C., Kalmar, K., Langenbahn, D. M., Malec, J. F., Bergquist, T. F., Felicetti, T., Giacino, J. T., Preston Harley, J., Harrington, D. E., Herzog, J., Kneipp, S., Laatsch, L., & Morse, P. A. (2000). Evidence-based cognitive rehabilitation: Recommendations for clinical practice. *Archives of Physical Medicine and Rehabilitation, 81,* 1596–1615.

Cicerone, K. D., Dahlberg, C., Malec, J. F., Langenbahn, D. M., Felicetti, T., Kneipp, S., Ellmo, W., Kalmar, K., Giacino, J. T., Preston Harley, J., Laatsch, L., Morse, P. A., & Catanese, J. (2005). Evidence-based cognitive rehabilitation: Updated review of the literature from 1998 through 2002. *Archives of Physical Medicine and Rehabilitation, 86,* 1681–1692.

Cicerone, K. D., Langenbahn, D. M., Braden, C., Malec, J. F., Kalmar, K., Fraas, M., Felicetti, T., Laatsch, L., Harley, J. P., Bergquist, T., Azulay, J., Cantor, J., & Ashman, T. (2011). Evidence-based cognitive rehabilitation: Updated review of the literature from 2003 through 2008. *Archives of Physical Medicine and Rehabilitation, 92,* 519–530.

Clare, L., Wilson, B. A., Carter, G., Breen, K., Gosses, A., & Hodges, J. R. (2000). Intervening with everyday memory problems in dementia of Alzheimer's type: An errorless learning approach. *Journal of Clinical and Experimental Neuropsychology, 22,* 132–146.

Clare, L., & Woods, R. T. (2004). Cognitive training and cognitive rehabilitation for people with early stage Alzheimer's disease: A review. *Neuropsychological Rehabilitation, 14,* 385–401.

Corcoran, M. A. (2003). Practical skills training for family caregivers. San Francisco: Family Caregiving Alliance. Retrieved August 19, 2012 from http://www.caregiver.org/caregiver/jsp/content_node.jsp?nodeid=954.

Corcoran, M. A. (n.d.a). Environmental modification strategies: Customized toolkit of information and practical solutions (C-TIPS). Retrieved August 19, 2012 from http://www.c-tips.com/la_tools/modifying_the_environment.pdf.

Corcoran, M. A. (n.d.b). Task breakdown strategies. Customized toolkit of information and practical solutions (C-TIPS). Retrieved August 19, 2012 from http://www.c-tips.com/la_tools/task_breakdown_strategies.pdf

Crosson, B., Barco, P. P., Velozo, C. A., Bolesta, M. M., Cooper, P. V., Werts, D., & Brobeck, T. C. (1989). Awareness and compensation in postacute head injury rehabilitation. *Journal of Head Trauma Rehabilitation, 4,* 46–54.

Crovitz, H. F. (1979). Memory rehabilitation in brain damaged patients: The airplane list. *Cortex, 15,* 131–134.

Davis, R. N., Massman, P. J., & Doody, R. S. (2001). Cognitive intervention in Alzheimer disease: A randomized placebo-controlled study. *Alzheimer Disease and Associated Disorders, 15,* 1–9.

Davis, E. S., & Radomski, M. V. (1989). Domain-specific training to reinstate habit sequences. *Occupational Therapy Practice, 1,* 79–88.

Dawson, D. R., Gaya, A., Hunt, A., Levine, B., Lemsky, C., & Polatajko, H. J. (2009). Using the cognitive orientation to occupational performance (CO-OP) approach with adults with executive dysfunction. *Canadian Journal of Occupational Therapy, 76,* 115–127.

de Joode, E., van Heugten, C., Verhey, F., & van Boxtel, M. (2010). Efficacy and usability of assistive technology for patients with cognitive deficits: A systematic review. *Clinical Rehabilitation, 24,* 701–714.

Donaghy, S., & Williams, W. (1998). A new protocol for training severely impaired patients in the usage of memory journals. *Brain Injury, 12,* 1061–1076.

Dougherty, P. M., & Radomski, M. V. (1993). *The cognitive rehabilitation workbook* (2nd ed.). Gaithersburg, MD: Aspen.

Driskell, J. E., Willis, R. P., & Copper, C. (1992). Effect of overlearning on retention. *Journal of Applied Psychology, 77,* 615–622.

Duhigg, C. (2012). *The power of habit: Why we do what we do in life and business.* New York: Random House.

Dyck, I. (2002). Beyond the clinic: Restructuring the environment in chronic illness experience. *Occupational Therapy Journal of Research, 22* (Suppl. 1), 52S–60S.

Edwards, J. D., Myers, C., Ross, L. A., Roenker, D. L., Cissell, G. M., McLaughlin, A. M., & Ball, K. K. (2009). The longitudinal impact of cognitive speed of processing training on driving mobility. *Gerontologist, 49,* 485–494.

Ehlhardt, L. A., Sohlberg, M. M., Kennedy, M., Coelho, C., Ylvisaker, M., Turkstra, L., & Yorkston, K. (2008). Evidence-based practice guidelines for instructing individuals with neurogenic memory impairments: What have we learned in the past 20 years? *Neuropsychological Rehabilitation, 18,* 300–342.

Eldridge, L. L., Masterman, D., & Knowlton, B. J. (2002). Intact implicit habit learning in Alzheimer's disease. *Behavioral Neuroscience, 116,* 722–726.

Eskes, G. A., Butler, B., McDonald, A., Harrison, E. R., & Phillips, S. J. (2003). Limb activation effects in hemispatial neglect. *Archives of Physical Medicine and Rehabilitation, 84,* 323–328.

Evans, J. J., Wilson, B. A., Needham, P., & Brentnall, S. (2003). Who makes good use of memory aids? Results of a survey of people with acquired brain. *Journal of the International Neuropsychological Society, 9,* 925–935.

Finger, S. (1994). *Origins of neuroscience: A history of explorations into brain function.* New York: Oxford University Press.

Fleming, J., & Strong, J. (1995). Self-awareness of deficits following acquired brain injury: Considerations for rehabilitation. *British Journal of Occupational Therapy, 58,* 55–60.

Gasparrini, B., & Satz, P. (1979). A treatment for memory problems in left hemisphere CVA patients. *Journal of Clinical Neuropsychology, 1,* 137–150.

Gelfand, D. M., & Hartmann, D. P. (1984). *Child behavioral analysis and therapy.* Needham Heights, MA: Allyn & Bacon.

Gentry, T. (2008). PDAs as cognitive aids for people with multiple sclerosis. *American Journal of Occupational Therapy, 62,* 18–27.

Gentry, T., Wallace, J., Kvarfordt, C., & Lynch, K. B. (2008). Personal digital assistants as cognitive aids for individuals with severe traumatic brain injury: A community-based trial. *Brain Injury, 22,* 19–24.

Geusgens, C. A. V., Winkens, L., van Heugten, C. M., Jolles, J., & van den Heuvel, W. J. A. (2007). Occurrence and measurement of transfer in cognitive rehabilitation: A critical review. *Journal of Rehabilitation Medicine, 39,* 425–439.

Giles, G. M. (1998). A neurofunctional approach to rehabilitation following severe brain injury. In N. Katz (Ed.), *Cognition and occupation in rehabilitation* (pp. 125–147). Bethesda, MD: American Occupational Therapy Association.

Giles, G. M. (2010). Cognitive versus functional approaches to rehabilitation after traumatic brain injury: Commentary on a randomized controlled trial. *American Journal of Occupational Therapy, 64,* 182–185.

Giles, G. M. (2011). A neurofunctional approach to rehabilitation following brain injury. In N. Katz (Ed.), *Cognition, occupation and participation across the life span* (3rd ed., pp. 351–381). Bethesda, MD: AOTA Press.

Giles, G. M., & Clark-Wilson, J. (1988). The use of behavioral techniques in functional skills training after severe brain injury. *American Journal of Occupational Therapy, 42,* 658–665.

Giles, G. M., Ridley, J. E., Dill, A., & Frye, S. (1997). A consecutive series of adults with brain injury treated with a washing and dressing retraining program. *American Journal of Occupational Therapy, 51,* 256–266.

Giles, G. M., & Shore, M. (1989). A rapid method for teaching severely brain injured adults how to wash and dress. *Archives of Physical Medicine and Rehabilitation, 70,* 156–158.

Gillen, G. (2009). *Cognitive and perceptual rehabilitation: Optimizing function.* St. Louis: Mosby.

Gillespie, A., Best, C., & O'Neill, B. (2012). Cognitive function and assistive technology for cognition: A systematic review. *Journal of the International Neuropsychological Society, 18,* 1–19.

Gitlin, L. N., Corcoran, M., Winter, L., Boyce, A., & Hauck, W. W. (2001). A randomized, controlled trial of a home environmental intervention: Effect on efficacy and upset in caregivers and on daily function of persons with dementia. *Gerontologist, 41,* 4–14.

Gitlin, L. N., Hauck, W. W., Dennis, M. P., & Winter, L. (2005). Maintenance of effects of the home environmental skill-building program for family caregivers and individuals with Alzheimer's disease and related disorders. *Journal of Gerontology Series A: Biological Sciences and Medical Sciences, 60,* 368–374.

Gitlin, L. N., Winter, L., Burke, J., Chernett, N., Dennis, M. P., & Hauck, W. W. (2008). Tailored activities to manage neuropsychiatric behaviors in persons with dementia and reduce caregiver burden: A randomized pilot study. *American Journal of Geriatric Psychiatry, 16,* 229–239.

Gitlin, L. N., Winter, L., Vause Earland, T., Adel Herge, E., Chernett, N. L., Piersol, C. V., & Burke, J. P. (2009). The Tailored Activity Program to reduce behavioral symptoms in individuals with dementia: Feasibility, acceptability, and replication potential. *Gerontologist, 49,* 428–439.

Giuffrida, C. G., Demery, J. A., Reyes, L. R., Lebowitz, B. K., & Hanlon, R. E. (2009). Functional skill learning in men with traumatic brain injury. *American Journal of Occupational Therapy, 63,* 398–407.

Gray, J. M., Robertson, I., Pentland, B., & Anderson, S. (1992). Microcomputer-based attentional retraining after brain damage: A randomized group controlled trial. *Neuropsychological Rehabilitation, 2,* 97–115.

Harris, J. E. (1980). Memory aids people use: Two interview studies. *Memory and cognition, 8,* 31–38.

Hart, T., Buchhofer, R., & Vaccaro, M. (2004). Portable electronic devices as memory and organizational aids after traumatic brain injury: A consumer survey study. *Journal of Head Trauma Rehabilitation, 19,* 351–365.

Haskins, E. C. (2011). *Cognitive rehabilitation manual: Translating evidence-based recommendations into practice.* Reston, VA: American Congress of Rehabilitation Medicine.

Institute of Medicine. (2011). *Cognitive rehabilitation therapy for traumatic brain injury: Evaluating the evidence.* Washington DC: National Academies Press.

Jog, M. S., Kubota, Y., Connolly, C. I., Hillegaart, V., & Graybiel, A. M. (1999). Building neural representations of habits. *Science, 286,* 1745–1749.

Kennedy, M. R. T., Coelho, C., Turkstra, L., Ylvisaker, M., Sohlberg, M. M., Yorkston, K., Chiou, H.-H., & Kan, P.-F. (2008). Intervention for executive functions after traumatic brain injury: A systematic review, meta-analysis and clinical recommendations. *Neuropsychological Rehabilitation, 18,* 257–299.

Kessels, R. P. C., & de Haan, E. H. F. (2003). Mnemonic strategies in older people: A comparison of errorless and errorful learning. *Age and Ageing, 32,* 529–533.

Kessels, R. P. C., & Olde Hensken, L. M. G. (2009). Effects of errorless skill learning in people with mild-to-moderate or severe dementia: A randomized controlled pilot study. *NeuroRehabilitation, 25,* 307–312.

Kim, H. J., Burke, D. T., Dowds, M. M., Boone, K. A., & Park, G. J. (2000). Electronic memory aids for outpatient brain injury: Follow-up findings. *Brain Injury, 14,* 187–196.

Kramer, A. F., Strayer, D. L., & Buckley, J. (1990). Development and transfer of automatic processing. *Journal of Experimental Psychology: Human Learning and Memory, 16,* 505–522.

Lawton, M. P., & Nahemow, L. E. (1973). Ecology and the aging process. In C. Eisdorfer & M. P. Lawton (Eds.), *The psychology of adult development and aging* (pp. 619–674). Washington DC: American Psychological Association.

Logan, G. D. (1988a). Automaticity, resources, and memory: Theoretical controversies and practical implications. *Human Factors, 30,* 538–598.

Logan, G. D. (1988b). Toward an instance theory of automaticity. *Psychological Reviews, 95,* 492–527.

Logan, G. D., Taylor, S. E., & Etherton, J. L. (1999). Attention and automaticity: Toward a theoretical integration. *Psychological Research, 62,* 165–181.

Maddicks, R., Marzillier, S. L., & Parker, G. (2003). Rehabilitation of unilateral neglect in the acute recovery stage: The efficacy of limb activation therapy. *Neuropsychological Rehabilitation, 13,* 391–408.

Malec, J., & Questad, K. (1983). Rehabilitation of memory after craniocerebral trauma: Case report. *Archives of Physical Medicine and Rehabilitation, 64,* 436–438.

Mastos, M., Miller, K., Eliasson, A. C., & Imms, C. (2007). Goal-directed training: Linking theories of treatment to clinical practice for improved functional activities in daily life. *Clinical Rehabilitation, 21,* 47–55.

McEwen, S. E., Politajko, H. J., Huijbregts, M. P., & Ryan, J. D. (2009). Exploring a cognitive-based treatment approach to improve motor-based skill performance in chronic stroke: Results of three single case experiments. *Brain Injury, 23,* 1041–1053.

McEwen, S. E., Polatajko, H. J., Huijbregts, M. P., & Ryan, J. D. (2010). Inter-task transfer of meaningful, functional skills following a cognitive-based treatment: Results of three multiple baseline design experiments in adults with chronic stroke. *Neuropsychological Rehabilitation, 20,* 541–561.

Meichenbaum, D. (1977). *Cognitive-behavior modification: An integrative approach.* New York: Plenum Press.

Milton, S. B. (1985). Compensatory memory strategy training: A practical approach for managing persistent memory problems. *Cognitive Rehabilitation, 3,* 8–15.

Moniz-Cook, E. (2006). Cognitive stimulation and dementia. *Aging and Mental Health, 10,* 207–210.

Muraven, M., Tice, D. M., & Baumeister, R. F. (1998). Self-control as limited resource: Regulatory depletion patterns. *Journal of Personality and Social Psychology, 74,* 774–789.

Novack, T. A., Baños, J. H., Alderson, A. L., Schneider, J. J., Weed, W., Blankenship, J., & Salisbury, D. (2006). UFOV performance and driving ability following traumatic brain injury. *Brain Injury, 20,* 455–461.

O'Connor, M. L., Hudak, E. M., & Edwards, J. D. (2011). Cognitive speed of processing training can promote community mobility among older adults: A brief review. *Journal of Aging Research, vol. 2011,* 4 pages. doi: 10.4061/2011/430802.

O'Neil-Pirozzi, T. M., Stangman, G. E., Goldstein, R., Katz, D. I., Savage, C. R., Kelkar, K., Supelana, C., Burke, D., Rauch, S. L., & Glenn, M. B. (2010). A controlled treatment study of internal memory strategies (I-MES) following traumatic brain injury. *Journal of Head Trauma Rehabilitation, 25,* 43–51.

Oriani, M., Moniz-Cook, E., Binetti, G., Zanieri, G., Frisoni, G. B., Geroldi, C., De Vreese, L. P., & Zanetti, O. (2003). An electronic memory aid to support prospective memory in patients in early stages of Alzheimer's disease: A pilot study. *Aging and Mental Health, 7,* 22–27.

Parenté, R., & Herrmann, D. (2002) *Retraining cognition: Techniques and applications* (2nd ed.). Austin, TX: Pro-ed.

Parish, L., & Oddy, M. (2007). Efficacy of rehabilitation for functional skills more than 10 years after extremely severe brain injury. *Neuropsychological Rehabilitation, 17,* 230–243.

Polatajko, H. J., & Mandich, A. (2004). *Enabling occupation in children: The cognitive orientation to daily occupational performance.* Ottawa, Canada: CAOT Publications.

Polatajko, H. J., Mandich, A., & McEwen, S. (2011). Cognitive oreintation to daily occupational performance (CO-OP): A cognitive-based intervention for children and adults. In N. Katz (Ed.), *Cognition and occupation across the life span* (pp. 299–321). Bethesda, MD: AOTA Press.

Radomski, M. V., Davis, E. S., Newman, S., & White, M. (2004). Everyday evidence: Using research and stakeholder input to inform use of high tech memory aids. Minneapolis, MN: Workshop presented for the American Occupational Therapy Association Annual Conference.

Reber, P. J., Knowlton, B. J., & Squire, L. R. (1996). Dissociable properties of memory systems: Differences in the flexibility of declarative and nondeclarative knowledge. *Behavioral Neuroscience, 110,* 861–871.

Robertson, I. H. (1999). Setting goals for rehabilitation. *Current Opinions in Neurology, 12,* 703–708.

Robertson, I. H., Hogg, K., & McMillan, T. M. (1998). Rehabilitation of unilateral neglect: Improving function by contralesional limb activation. *Neuropsychological Rehabilitation, 8,* 19–29.

Robertson, I. H., McMillan, T. M., MacLeod, E., Edgeworth, J., & Brock, D. (2002). Rehabilitation by limb activation reduces left-sided motor impairment in unilateral neglect patients: A single-blind randomized control trial. *Neuropsychological Rehabilitation, 12,* 439–454.

Robertson, I. H., & North, N. (1992). Spatio-motor cueing in unilateral neglect: The role of hemisphere, hand and motor activation. *Neuropsychologia, 30,* 553–563.

Schmitter-Edgecombe, M., Fahy, J. F., Whelan, J. P., & Long, C. J. (1995). Memory remediation after severe closed head injury: Notebook training over supportive therapy. *Journal of Consulting and Clinical Psychology, 63,* 484–489

Schneider, W., Dumais, S. T., & Shiffrin, R. M. (1984). Automatic and control processing and attention. In R. Parasuraman & D. R. Davis (Eds.), *Varieties of attention* (pp. 1–27). London: Academic Press.

Schwartz, S. M. (1995). Adults with traumatic brain injury: Three case studies of cognitive rehabilitation in the home setting. *American Journal of Occupational Therapy, 49,* 655–667.

Shiffrin, R. M., & Schneider, W. (1977). Controlled and automatic information processing: II. Perceptual learning, automatic attending, and a general theory. *Psychological Review, 84,* 127–190.

Soderback, I., & Normell, L. A. (1986a). Intellectual function training in adults with acquired brain damage: An occupational therapy method. *Scandinavian Journal of Rehabilitation Medicine, 18,* 139–146.

Soderback, I., & Normell, L. A. (1986b). Intellectual function training in adults with acquired brain damage: Evaluation. *Scandinavian Journal of Rehabilitation Medicine, 18,* 147–153.

Sohlberg, M. M., & Mateer, C. A. (1987). *APT: Attention process training manual.* Puyallup, WA: Association for neuropsychological research and development.

Sohlberg, M. M., & Mateer, C. A. (1989). *Introduction to cognitive rehabilitation.* New York: Guilford Press.

Sohlberg, M. M., & Mateer, C. A. (2001). *Cognitive rehabilitation.* New York: Guilford Press.

Sohlberg, M. M., McLaughlin, K. A., Pavese, A., Heidrich, A., Posner, M. I. (2000). Evaluation of attention process training and brain injury education in persons with acquired brain injury. *Journal of Clinical and Experimental Neuropsychology, 22,* 656–676.

Spector, A., Orrell, M., Davies, S., & Woods, R. T. (2001). Can reality orientation be rehabilitated? Development and piloting of an evidence-based programme of cognition-based therapies for people with dementia. *Neuropsychological Rehabilitation, 11,* 377–397.

Spector, A., Orrell, M., Davies, S., & Woods, R. T. (2009). Reminiscence therapy for dementia. *Cochrane Database of Systematic Review, (4),* CD001120.

Spector, A., Thorgrimsen, L., Woods, B., Royan, L., Davies, S., Butterworth, M., & Orrell, M. (2003). Efficacy of an evidence-based cognitive stimulation therapy programme for people with dementia. *British Journal of Psychiatry, 183,* 248–254.

Spikeman, J., & van Zomeren, E. (2010). Assessment of attention. In J. M. Gurd, U. Kischka, & J. C. Marshall (Eds.), *The handbook of clinical neuropsychology* (pp. 81–96). Oxford: Oxford University Press.

Squire, L. R., Knowlton, B. J., & Musen, G. (1993). The structure and organization of memory. *Annual Review of Psychology, 44,* 453–495.

Stringer, A. Y. (2003). Cognitive rehabilitation practice patterns: A survey of American Hospital Association Rehabilitation Programs. *Clinical Neuropsychologist, 17,* 34–44.

Stuss, D. T. (1991). Self-awareness and the frontal lobes: A neuropsychological perspective. In J. Strauss & G. R. Goethals (Eds.), *The self: Interdisciplinary approaches* (pp. 255–278). New York: Springer-Verlag.

Thivierge, S., Simard, M., Jean, L., & Grandmaison, E. (2008). Errorless learning and spaced retrieval techniques to relearn instrumental activities of daily living in mild Alzheimer's disease: A case report study. *Neuropsychiatric Disease and Treatment, 4,* 987–999.

Toglia, J. P. (1991). Generalization of treatment: A multi-contextual approach to cognitive perceptual impairment in the brain injured adult. *American Journal of Occupational Therapy, 45,* 505–516.

Toglia, J. P. (2011). The dynamic interactional model of cognition in cognitive rehabilitation. In N. Katz (Ed.), *Cognition and occupational across the life span* (pp. 161–201). Bethesda, MD: American Occupational Therapy Association.

Toglia, J. P., Johnston, M. V., Goverover, Y., & Dain, B. (2010). A multicontext approach to promoting transfer of strategy use and self regulation after brain injury: An exploratory study. *Brain Injury, 24,* 664–677.

Vanderploeg, R. D., Schwab, K., Walker, W. C., Fraser, J. A., Sigford, B. J., Date, E. S., Scott, S. G., Curtiss, G., Salazar, A. M., & Warden, D. L. (2008). Rehabilitation of traumatic brain injury in active duty military personnel and veterans: Defense and veterans brain injury center randomized controlled trial of two rehabilitation approaches. *Archives of Physical Medicine and Rehabilitation, 89,* 2227–2238.

Wallenbert, I., & Jonsson, H. (2005). Waiting to get better: A dilemma regarding habits and daily occupations after stroke. *American Journal of Occupational Therapy, 59,* 218–224.

Watanabe, T. K., Black, K. L., Zafonte, R. D., Millis, S. R., & Mann, N. R. (1998). Do calendars enhance posttraumatic temporal orientation?: A pilot study. *Brain Injury, 12,* 81–85.

Wilson, B. A. (1982). Success and failure in memory training following a cerebral vascular accident. *Cortex, 18,* 581–594.

Wilson, B. A., Emslie, H., Quirk, K., & Evans, J. J. (2001). Reducing everyday memory and planning problems by means of a paging system: A randomized controlled crossover study. *Journal of Neurology, Neurosurgery, and Psychiatry, 70,* 477–482.

Wilson, B. A., Emslie, H., Quirk, K., Evans, J., & Watson, P. (2005). A randomized control trial to evaluate a paging system for people with traumatic brain injury. *Brain Injury, 19,* 891–894.

Wilson, B. A., Evans, J. J., Emslie, H., & Malinek, V. (1997). Evaluation of NeuroPage: A new memory aid. *Journal of Neurology, Neurosurgery, and Psychiatry, 63,* 113–115.

Wilson, B. A., & Moffat, N. (1984). *Clinical management of memory problems.* London: Croom Helm.

Wilson, B. A., Scott, H., Evans, J., & Emslie, H. (2003). Preliminary report of a NeuroPage service within a health care system. *Neurorehabilitation, 18,* 3–8.

Wolinsky, F. D., Vander Weg, M. W., Howren, M. B., Jones, M. P., Martin, R., Luger, T. M., Duff, K., & Dotson, M. M. (2011). Interim analyses from a randomized controlled trial to improve visual processing speed in older adults: The Iowa Healthy and Active Minds study. *British Medical Journal Open, 1,* e000225.

Wolinsky, F. D., Vander Weg, M. W., Howren, M. B., Jones, M. P., Martin, R., Luger, T. M., Duff, K., Goerdt, C., Wolfe, S., & Dotson, M. M. (2011). Protocol for a randomized controlled trial to improve visual processing speed in older adults: The Iowa Healthy and Active Minds study. *British Medical Journal Open, 2,* e000218.

Woods, B., Aguirre, E., Spector, A. E., & Orrell, M. (2012). Cognitive stimulation to improve cognitive functioning in people with dementia. *Cochrane Database of Systematic Review, (2),* CD005562.

Zanetti, O., Zanieri, G., Giovanni, G. D., de Vreese, L. P., Pezzini, A., Metitieri, T., Trabucchi, M. (2001). Effectiveness of procedural memory stimulation in mild Alzheimer's disease patients: A controlled study. *Neuropsychological Rehabilitation, 11,* 263–272.

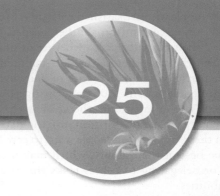

25

Restoring the Role of Independent Person

Anne Birge James

Learning Objectives

After studying this chapter, the reader will be able to do the following:

1. Describe the use of occupation-as-end as a therapeutic medium.
2. Distinguish between activities of daily living (ADL) and instrumental activities of daily living (IADL).
3. State principles to restore adapted function to persons with varied impairments and activity limitations.
4. Modify tasks and the environment to promote participation in ADL and IADL for people with varied impairments and activity limitations.
5. Prescribe and evaluate the use of assistive devices to promote safe independence in ADL and IADL.
6. Articulate the clinical reasoning and demonstrate the implementation of solutions to unique situations for persons with a variety of impairments and activity limitations.
7. Develop appropriate teaching strategies for persons with varied impairments to maximize progress toward occupation-based goals.

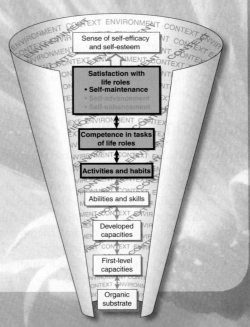

People who are satisfied with their life roles have the resources and capabilities needed to accomplish their everyday tasks, whether or not they actually perform the task themselves. Self-maintenance roles include participation in activities of daily living (ADL) and instrumental activities of daily living (IADL) (Latham, 2008a). The occupational therapist is the rehabilitation specialist responsible for teaching the patient to accomplish these tasks. Most people want to care for themselves to the best of their ability, which may include directing and/or delegating to others tasks that are beyond their capabilities.

The term *activities of daily living* is synonymous with self-care. ADL include feeding, grooming, dressing, bathing, toileting, bowel and bladder management, personal device care, sexual activity, functional mobility, sleep/rest, and eating (chewing and swallowing) (American Occupational Therapy Association [AOTA], 2008). The first eight ADL are included in this chapter. Functional mobility, including bed mobility, transfers, and wheelchair mobility, is addressed in Chapter 26, and chewing and swallowing are addressed in Chapter 43. Although every human engages in most or all ADL to some degree, the way that each is done and the importance attached to each differ culturally. ADL are the focus of most insurance coverage for rehabilitation. Baseline measures and examination of progress is documented by such evaluative measures as the Functional Independence Measure (FIM™) (see Chapter 4).

Suggesting that people are independent in self-maintenance if they can complete their ADL gives a false impression of independence. True independence also requires participation in *instrumental activities of daily living*, including but not limited to management of one's own medications, food, shelter, and finances; caring for other people or pets; communication device use; and community mobility (AOTA, 2008). IADL include a range of diverse tasks that often require greater interaction with the physical and social environments and may have more demanding physical and/or cognitive demands than ADL (James, 2014).

OCCUPATION-AS-END

When remedial therapy can correct performance skills/patterns or client factors that interfere with ADL, patients are often able to resume meaningful tasks and activities as they become able. Intervention that targets ADL directly is necessary for those who do not regain full capabilities, prefer not to engage in remedial therapy, or require interim strategies to enable participation in ADL and IADL as they regain required capacities. Occupation-as-end is an intervention focused on learning how to accomplish the activities and tasks that constitute roles in an adapted way (Latham, 2008b). The therapist employs a modification approach that enables patients to accomplish activities by changing the task and/or environment and providing appropriate patient and/or caregiver education (AOTA, 2008). The modifications recommended by the therapist may be aimed at the patient and/or the caregiver (Chen et al., 2000). Intervention is frequently aimed at improving independence in ADL and IADL, that is, the person's ability to complete the task without assistance from others. However, intervention may also be used to address other important task parameters, including safety and adequacy conditions, such as perceived difficulty or ease of performance, pain, fatigue, or dyspnea precipitated by activities, length of time to complete a task, and the ability to complete tasks in a way that meets personal and societal expectations (Rogers & Holm, 2009). For example, a person with rheumatoid arthritis may be independent in cooking, but experience significant pain that makes her unwilling to engage in the task. The therapist may instruct her in the use of adapted methods of cooking that protect painful joints to help her cook both independently and without pain.

The extent and focus of services for a particular patient depends on the person's needs and the level of independence required in the anticipated context. Patients' perceptions of ADL capabilities may differ from others' perceptions or even actual performance (Goverover et al., 2009), affecting their investment in treatment. Therefore, identification of patients' perceptions, values, and goals is a crucial part of the evaluation process that can be done informally or via standardized assessments, such as the Canadian Occupational Performance Measure (COPM; Law et al., 2005) or the Melville-Nelson Self-Identified Goals Assessment (Melville et al., 2002) available at http://www.utoledo.edu/eduhshs/depts/rehab_sciences/ot/melville.html. Involving patients in setting goals not only supports the therapist's ability to develop an appropriate treatment plan, but patients tend to have better outcomes (Kristensen et al., 2011).

Independence in ADL may be sufficient for a person returning to a supportive living situation in which IADL needs are few and willingly assumed by others, but it is never enough for a person who expects to reintegrate into community life. This person not only must master ADL and common IADL tasks but also must learn to solve problems that interfere with performing new tasks. For some patients, however, independence in only one or a few activities, such as transferring and toileting, may determine whether discharge is to home or an institution. Therefore, full effort should concentrate on achievement of critical goal(s), and additional goals may be determined and addressed, as possible, at a later time.

Intervention by occupation-as-end, then, is a modify approach (AOTA, 2008) that uses education of adapted methods, assistive technology, and adaptation of physical and/or social contexts to enable people to participate in desired roles with a permanent or temporary disability.

EDUCATION

In the modify approach, the therapist and patient engage in a collaborative learning process. Although the therapist is the teacher and the patient and caregivers are the learners in this relationship, sometimes roles are reversed when engaged in a collaborative relationship. Both teaching and learning are active processes (Dreeben, 2010). The patient must be both ready and able to learn. Assessing a client's readiness to learn can help the therapist select appropriate tasks and educational methods to maximize client outcomes.

Readiness to Learn

Patients' self-efficacy can have a significant impact on learning and can be evaluated and addressed in the context of ADL intervention. Self-efficacy is defined as the judgments people have of their capabilities to do or learn a task (Bandura, 1977, 1997; Sanford et al., 2006). Self-efficacy is positively related to actual performance and helps people to persist in tasks, even when faced with tasks that are difficult or new (Dreeben, 2010; Sanford et al., 2006). Persons with a new disability may have low self-efficacy for engaging in ADL because they lack experience with their limitations in the context of familiar tasks. Self-efficacy can be measured by asking patients to predict their performance on a given task using a Likert-type scale (e.g., 1 = very unlikely to learn this task, 5 = very likely to learn this task). A baseline self-efficacy measure can be used to determine the need for intervention to address self-efficacy along with the ADL skills training to enhance goal achievement.

Depression is another factor that can impede learning and occurs concurrently with a wide variety of physical disabilities. Depression has been demonstrated to have a negative relationship with functional outcomes for persons with varied physical disabilities, e.g., stroke (Pohjasvaara et al., 2001) and Parkinson's disease (Weintraub et al., 2004). Depression may impact functional outcomes by reducing self-efficacy needed for learning. Identifying depression in patients and referring them to physicians for prescription of antidepressant medications may reduce depressive symptoms, enhancing functional performance (Chemerinski, Robinson, & Kosier, 2001; Lin et al., 2003). In addition, occupational therapy that directly addresses the patient's depression can enhance outcomes, e.g., providing structure that promotes initiation in ADL and selecting tasks that provide the patient with successes will increase self-efficacy for future performance.

Other factors may interfere with patient learning, such as cognitive deficits (see Chapters 6 and 24). Persons with severe cognitive deficits may not be candidates for ADL training. Instead, the caregiver should be taught appropriate methods for assisting the patient and told to seek reevaluation if the patient's cognitive status improves.

Patients with cognitive disabilities who have the capacity to learn often have limited insight into their ADL or IADL impairments. This may interfere with treatment because patients see little reason to work on tasks they believe they can do. Integrating self-awareness training into occupation-as-end–focused treatment can improve functional outcomes for patients with limited self-awareness, compared to treatment focused simply on skill acquisition (Goverover et al., 2007). Pain may interfere with attention and learning and should be addressed directly or by selecting adaptive methods that minimize pain.

Patients with receptive aphasia or who speak a different language from the therapist have communication limitations that may impact learning. Therapists should use demonstration for patients who do not understand verbal instructions. A translator can be used to support learning for patients who speak another language. Patients with low literacy will not be able to use written materials to supplement learning, so other methods must be explored that support carryover of new skills outside of therapy. Chapters 3 and 13 describe ways to accommodate low literacy.

Clients may require adaptive equipment to maximize independence in ADL; however, attitudes toward adaptive equipment can impede learning and performance. Persons with disabilities have reported that assistive devices have both positive and negative connotations (Skymne et al., 2012). People value a device if the task is important and cannot be done any other way (Wielandt & Strong, 2000), but they dislike the stigma associated with device use. Disabled persons reported that they not only had to learn to use the device, but they had to learn to go out in public with it (McMillen & Söderberg, 2002). Assessing a patient's "gadget tolerance" can help therapists tailor their approach when presenting adaptive equipment as an option. Patients with a low tolerance for "gadgets" may need more trust in their therapist before considering equipment. Building this trust may become an important component of the therapeutic intervention for maximizing independence (See chapter 14).

Finally, the motivation to learn is influenced by the learner's values, which guide actions and effort (Dreeben, 2010; Falvo, 2011). Therefore, therapists must collaborate with patients to identify those tasks that will be within their capabilities and are also consistent with their values and goals. Attending to the many factors that may impact a patient's ability to learn helps the therapist select the most appropriate teaching strategies to enhance patient performance of ADL.

Teaching Strategies for Effective Learning

This section will address points of effective teaching, which are also summarized in Procedures for Practice 25-1. Throughout the teaching and learning process,

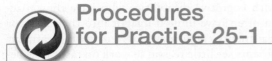

Procedures for Practice 25-1

Effective Teaching

1. Identify the patient's goals and learning needs.
2. Determine what the learner knows.
3. Use active learning strategies.
4. Engage the patient and/or caregivers in a collaborative learning process.
5. Select learning activities that present the "just-right challenge."
6. Adapt the presentation to the learner's capabilities.
7. Provide opportunities for practice, considering context and schedule.
8. Facilitate the learner's use of internal feedback and provide appropriate external feedback.
9. Test the learner in the appropriate context(s) to confirm that learning has occurred.
10. Discuss progress toward goals with the patient and revise teaching–learning strategies, as indicated.

occupational therapists should look for and address potential barriers for learning. Some barriers that are intrinsic to the patient were discussed when considering readiness to learn, such as self-efficacy, depression, pain, and gadget tolerance. External barriers to learning related to the physical and social environment may also exist. Occupational therapists' skills in analyzing tasks in context and adapting environments can be applied to removing barriers to learning in the treatment environment (Smith & Gutman, 2011). Examples of barriers and how to minimize them are included in the teaching strategies below:

1. Identify patients' goals and what they must learn to reach their goals (James, 2014). These become learning objectives or goals expressed in behavioral terms, such as "The patient will brush his teeth independently in less than 5 minutes." Although patients' needs vary, toileting is often a priority (Clark & Rugg, 2005). Identifying realistic goals may be difficult, particularly for patients with a sudden-onset disability, e.g., a stroke or spinal cord injury, because they have not had time to experiment with solutions to functional problems. Setting goals supports the learning process, and patient goals that are poorly defined or unrealistic may present a barrier to learning. Occupational therapists can help patients identify goals by sharing their vision of what is possible or by helping patients see how smaller, more realistic goals serve as important stepping stones to goals that are unrealistic or require a long time frame.

2. Determine what routines and skills patients have retained and whether they do them safely, including the ability to figure out adapted methods independently. Embedding the learning in context facilitates retention of new information and skills.

3. Present the material in a way that requires patients to be active in the learning process (Dreeben, 2010). Verbal or written instructions and demonstration are passive learning strategies and are often insufficient for mastering a new task. Active learning requires learners to apply new knowledge to real-life problems. For example, patients learning energy conservation can be asked to describe a typical day, identify ways they could conserve energy, and then practice strategies in an actual task, e.g., cooking. Active learning is vital when the patient is learning a motor task, such as putting on a shirt with one paralyzed arm, and should be guided by motor learning principles (see Chapter 13).

4. Use a collaborative approach, recognizing that each participant in the learning process (therapist, patient, and/or caregiver) has experience and expertise to contribute to the learning task. Engaging patients and caregivers in the intervention process enhances problem-solving skills, increases "ownership" of functional gains, and enhances self-efficacy (Jack & Estes, 2010). Allowing patients to participate in the selection of equipment appears to have a positive influence on adherence (Wielandt & Strong, 2000). Peer learning can also be effective by providing psychosocial support, promoting self-management, and improving patient's self-efficacy (Packer et al., 2009).

5. Select the "just-right challenge." A "just-right challenge" is one that is within the outside limits of the patient's ability, ensuring success, but requiring effort. Initially, keep the challenge low to enhance self-efficacy by reducing anxiety and promoting success (Falvo, 2011). For example, if the patient is learning to eat with adapted utensils, begin with sticky foods that stay on the spoon and progress to more difficult foods, such as spaghetti and peas. Scaffolding is the technique of providing just the amount of assistance the person needs and then gradually removing assistance as the person can do more of the task (Thomas, 2012). The form of assistance can vary, including setup, verbal cues, or physical assistance (James, 2014).

6. Adapt the presentation of new information to the particular learner, given his or her abilities and deficits. For patients without brain damage and with average intelligence and literacy, teaching methods can include discussion, demonstration, and written instructions (Falvo, 2011). Printed materials and verbal instructions should be simple and direct, as almost half of the population in the United States has low health literacy, that is, their comprehension and ability to act on health-related information is inadequate (Smith & Gutman, 2011).

The availability of high-quality, online educational media is increasing rapidly. Libin et al. (2011) reported that social media, such as YouTube, provide a virtual context for sharing ideas for disability self-management in a forum that is increasingly accessible to people with disabilities. Occupational therapists can access a number of "how to" videos, produced by the National Rehabilitation Hospital for persons with spinal cord injuries at http://www.youtube.com/user/HealthyTomorrow. Not all information on YouTube or other nonprofessional sites is correct, therefore note the credentials of the source before adopting any method from these sites.

ADL and IADL training for persons with intact cognition should occur in varied contexts so they become independent problem solvers. Effective problem solvers have an accurate awareness of their abilities and limitations and the ability to identify and define problems. They can select appropriate solutions to a problem from past experience or create a new solution when prior strategies are inadequate. Finally, effective problem solvers assess the outcome of the problem solving, which helps them organize the learning experience so that it is accessible for solving problems in the future.

Patients with brain damage require a different approach to the teaching–learning process. If patients cannot do previously familiar tasks automatically using old habit programs, they are learning a new skill. Several learning approaches may be considered for patients with cognitive deficits. Impairment in self-awareness of abilities and limitations may need to be addressed, because patients are not likely to value or engage in learning for ADL or IADL they perceive themselves to be competent in. Self-awareness training in the context of ADL and IADL tasks can help patients identify performance errors and initiate self-correction strategies (Gillen, 2009). Consistent and systematic use of cueing may be effective in helping patients focus on relevant task cues to support performance (Wesolowski et al., 2005). Errorless learning is a teaching method in which the learner is prevented from making errors by the therapist. For example, providing step-by-step verbal cues during ADL training or handing patients the necessary adaptive equipment rather than allowing them to choose. Research on the effectiveness of errorless learning has been mixed and may reflect its application to different types of learning deficits. For example, errorless learning was effective for people with acquired brain injury in learning to use electronic aids to daily living (EADL) (Boman et al., 2007); however, Mount et al. (2007) found no difference between errorless learning and trial-and-error learning of ADL in people post stroke. Monitoring response to treatment can help the occupational therapist determine whether errorless learning is effective for a given patient.

Patients with acquired brain injury often have difficulty processing abstract information or large chunks of information at a time, so instructions should be reduced to one- or two-word concrete cues. Given consistently, these key word cues help the patient chain the task from beginning to end. For tasks that can be easily broken into isolated subtasks, it may be helpful for the patient to practice one step at a time, combining steps as learning progresses, e.g., begin brushing teeth with the toothpaste already on the brush. For some tasks and some patients, however, performance of the whole task will enhance learning (see Chapter 13). If the task will occur in different places, the patient must practice each task until it is learned within all the contexts in which it will be required.

Progress in learning ADL for those with brain damage may be slow (Boman et al., 2007). Given the economic constraints, it is unrealistic to expect to teach such patients in the brief period of treatment authorized. The therapist should teach the caregiver how to help the patient learn some ADL skills at home.

Patients with damage to their dominant hemispheres usually have difficulty processing verbal or written language but may benefit from demonstrated or pictorial instruction. Those with damage to their nondominant hemisphere may have difficulty with spatial relationships that make it difficult to interpret pictures and demonstrations but may be able to process step-by-step verbal instruction.

7. Arrange appropriate practice schedules. Motor skills are learned only through practice. Multiple studies have shown that motor skills were better retained when participants without neurological impairment practiced with contextual interference (random practice) rather than repetitive drill (blocked practice) (Lin et al., 2009). However, for patients with movement disorders, response to practice schedules may vary, and alternatives may need to be considered (Lin et al., 2007). Chapter 13 has a discussion of practice schedules.

8. Provide opportunities for internal feedback and use appropriate external feedback. External feedback comes from outside the patient, typically the therapist, and can be provided in many forms. Motivational feedback ("Looks good!" or "Keep trying!") has some benefit, but specific feedback about what was correct and what was not correct has more definitive benefit. Persons who are not aware of the outcome of their efforts benefit from external feedback so that they gain knowledge of the results of their efforts, a requirement for learning (Schmidt & Lee, 2011). Although external feedback from the therapist is an effective teaching method, patients must eventually respond to internal and task feedback, that is, feedback from their own sensory system or the outcome of task performance ("My pants are on, but twisted and uncomfortable"). Asking patients to articulate internal feedback before providing external feedback can support their ability to rely on internal feedback when faced with novel tasks outside of therapy.

9. Test whether the learner has acquired the knowledge or skill by requiring that it be done independently at the appropriate time and place.

10. Discuss progress toward goals and revise teaching strategy or goal as indicated. Gagné and Hoppes (2003) found that patients in a rehabilitation center who regularly discussed and updated their goals with their therapists made greater gains in ADL than patients whose treatment did not emphasize goal attainment.

ADAPTATION AND MODIFYING APPROACHES TO INTERVENTION

Adaptation is the process by which people change their approach to a task when faced with an occupational challenge (AOTA, 2008). It is a cumulative process that evolves over time. Older people therefore have a rich repertoire of adaptive strategies based on personal experience that may be helpful in dealing with disability.

A modifying approach to occupational therapy intervention means adapting the method of accomplishing the task and/or the environment to promote independence in occupational functioning by compensating for impairments (AOTA, 2008). Examples of modifying the task are to switch to loafers instead of tie shoes or to order from catalogs instead of going to the shops. Adapted methods of dressing for persons with loss of the use of one side of the body or weakness of all four extremities (discussed later) are examples of modifying the method of accomplishing a task. Installation of grab bars in the bathroom to enable safe transfers and storing often-used items within easy reach are examples of modifying the physical environment. Teaching wheelchair users ways of interacting with individuals who are not disabled so that they present themselves as self-assured, capable people is an example of adapting the social environment.

Prescription of and training in the use of assistive devices or adapted tools and utensils to enable occupational performance by persons who are physically disabled is a primary function of occupational therapy. Examples are adding extensions to keys and door handles to extend the force arm and reduce the force required to turn the key or knob (Fig. 25-1) and use of a button hook to button a shirt (Fig. 25-2). Grasp, a problem for many patients, can be helped by using enlarged handles and ergonomic designs that put the hand and wrist in optimal biomechanical alignment (Figs. 25-2 and 25-3). A therapist may experiment with adaptations to utensils by wrapping a washcloth, foam rubber, or other material around the handle and securing it with a rubber band. If enlarging the handle improves performance, permanent adaptation is prescribed and purchased or, if necessary, custom built. Low-temperature thermoplastic materials that bond to themselves can be used for this purpose (see Chapter 16), or thermoplastic pellets can be heated and shaped into handles.

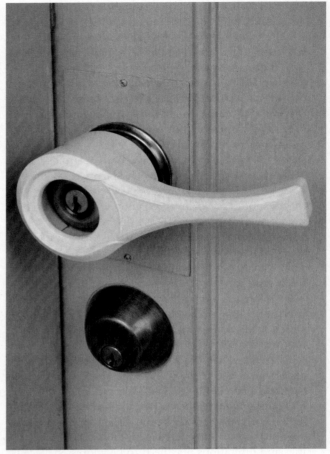

Figure 25-1 Doorknob extension.

Adaptation entails the following seven aspects, summarized in Procedures for Practice 25-2:

1. Analyze the activity. Determine the essential demands of the activity. The activity demands are a combination of the performance requirements of a task, such as

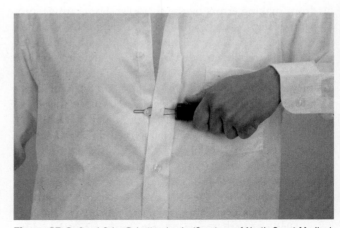

Figure 25-2 Good Grips® button hook. (Courtesy of North Coast Medical, www.ncmedical.com.)

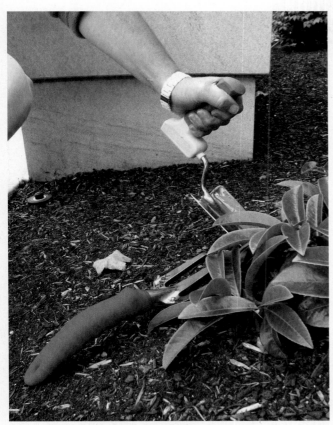

Figure 25-3 Garden tools with ergonomic handles keep the joints and musculotendinous units in optimal alignment, optimizing strength and protecting joints.

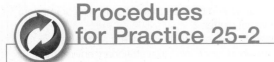

Procedures
for Practice 25-2

Adaptation Process

1. Analyze activity demands, including performance and contextual requirements.
2. Identify the problem: what performance and/or contextual requirements prevent the person from accomplishing the task?
3. Know principles of compensation for the given limitation.
4. Creatively apply principles of compensation to solve the problem.
5. Select appropriate adapted methods and assistive devices, and specify environmental adaptations to implement the solution.
6. Check out all modifications to verify that they solve the problem.
7. Train in safe use of the assistive devices or modified environment.

lifting, reaching, and manipulating, and the contextual demands. Contextual demands include the physical environment, such as counter height or location of faucets in the bathtub, as well as social demands, such as the ability to communicate with others, and temporal demands such as the need to complete a morning care routine within 45 minutes in order to get to work on time. Performance requirements must be quantified: What is the weight to be lifted? How high must it be lifted? and so on. Examination of these objective dimensions of the activities suggests how the environment and equipment can be adapted to meet the capabilities of the person (Thomas, 2012). Studies have examined specific performance components of particular tasks, such as the minimal wrist ranges of motion needed to accomplish ADL (Ryu et al., 1991), pinch and grasp strength requirements for varied tasks (Rice, Leonard, & Carter, 1998; Smaby et al., 2004), effect of object width on hand muscle activation and grip force (Vigouroux, Domalain, & Berton, 2011), differences in cardiovascular demands of carrying a bag at the side versus against the chest (Irion et al., 2010), and the effect of reacher length on muscle strength needed to lift objects (Pinkston, Boersma, & Spaulding, 2005). Such studies can help occupational therapists set realistic goals and identify the need for adaptations more quickly and accurately.

2. Identify the problem. Why can't the person do what the task demands? It is helpful to consider the problem from two perspectives: patient limitations and contextual features. For example, the patient is unable use the left hand, but toothpaste with a screw cap requires the use of two hands. Or the patient has precautions against bending over so pots needed for cooking stored in low cabinets cannot be reached. Linking the performance limitations with contextual features helps the therapist identify appropriate solutions.

3. Know the principles of compensation. Principles of compensation for common functional limitations are presented in Procedures for Practice 25-3.

4. Propose solutions. Consider creative ways that the principles of compensation can be applied to a specific task to enable the particular person to do it. Collaboration with the patient or a group of similarly involved patients often generates solutions and increases compliance with assistive devices (Wielandt et al., 2001).

5. Know the resources for implementing the solution. For example, it is important to know what reliable and safe equipment is available to solve the problem. Sources of equipment are rehabilitation supply stores, web-based businesses, and gadget stores (see Resources 25-1). The occupational therapist needs to know and evaluate each piece of equipment being recommended. The fact that a piece of equipment is sold does not mean that it is

(text continued on page 12)

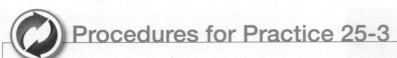

Procedures for Practice 25-3

Compensation Principles for Particular Impairments

Weakness

- Use lightweight objects, utensils, and tools.
- Let gravity assist.
- Provide external support, e.g., sit if trunk or lower extremities are weak, use a mobile arm support for proximal upper extremity weakness, or splint a weak wrist.
- Use assistive devices or methods to stabilize objects and replace lost functions such as grasp.
- Use power tools and utensils.
- Use biomechanical principles of levers (e.g., lengthen the force arm in relation to the resistance arm) and friction (e.g., increase friction to decrease power required for pinch or grasp).
- Use two hands for tasks ordinarily done one-handed.

Low Endurance and/or Fatigue

- Use energy conservation methods (see Procedures for Practice 25-4).
- Pace work to prevent fatigue.
- Use principles listed for weakness that reduce workload, such as lightweight utensils and power equipment.
- Match activity demands to ability.
- Avoid stressful positions and environmental stressors.
- Coordinate optimal breathing patterns with movement during activities to maximize oxygen exchange.

Limited Range of Motion

- Use long-handled tools and utensils to increase reach and/or eliminate the need for bending over.
- Build up handles to compensate for limited finger flexion range of motion.
- Store frequently used things closer to reduce reach.
- Use joint protection techniques for rheumatoid arthritis (see Chapter 39).

Incoordination

- Stabilize the object being worked on, including use of assistive devices that reduce slipperiness.
- Stabilize proximal body parts to reduce degrees of freedom, improving control of distal body parts.
- Use heavy utensils, cooking equipment, tools, and so on.
- Use adaptations that reduce or eliminate the need for fine motor skill (e.g., replace buttons with Velcro™).

Loss of the Use of One Side

- Provide assistive devices that substitute for the stabilizing or holding function of the involved upper extremity.

- Teach one-handed methods for activities ordinarily done two-handed.
- Provide assistive devices that change bilateral tasks into unilateral tasks.
- Improve dexterity of the uninvolved upper extremity if use of the dominant arm is impaired.

Limited Vision

Blindness

- Organize living space and stress the importance of putting everything in its place after use (e.g., in the pantry cabinets, on refrigerator shelves, and in the medicine cabinet).
- Use Braille labels or optical scanners to distinguish canned goods, medications, clothing colors, etc.
- Use devices that operate through voice commands.
- Use assistive devices that provide auditory, tactile, or kinesthetic feedback to compensate for low vision and blindness.
- Eliminate environmental clutter.
- Expect tasks to require extra time.

Low Vision

Some of the above principles are useful for those with low vision. Some others are:
- Provide high color contrast (e.g., white mug for coffee, colored towels in a white bathroom)
- Increase the light on a task by bringing the light closer, increasing wattage, or changing the background to increase contrast.
- Use techniques and devices that magnify type or images.
- Reduce visual clutter.
- Use organized scanning techniques (e.g., left to right or top to bottom) when functioning in a stationary environment.

Decreased or Absent Sensation

- Protect the anesthetic part from abrasions, bruises, cuts, burns, and decubiti.
- Develop habit of using areas with intact cutaneous sensation to test temperature, e.g., test bath water temperature with the forearm if finger sensation is impaired.
- Substitute vision for poor awareness of limb position and limb movement or to detect texture.
- Develop habits of directing attention to the affected part.
- Incorporate visual skin inspection into daily ADL routine.

Poor Memory and/or Executive Skills

- Use assistive devices that substitute for memory or poor organizational skills (e.g., pill minders, day books, sticky notes, or watches/phones/tablets with programmable alarms or reminder apps).

Procedures for Practice 25-3 *(continued)*

- Teach strategies such as writing memos to self, making to-do and other lists, and placing objects together at the point needed ahead of time.
- Develop habits regarding time use and how activities are to be accomplished.
- Teach self-awareness strategies to improve carryover of adapted methods or devices.

Low Back Pain and Post Back Surgery

- Teach body mechanics for moving and lifting (e.g., hold objects close to the body and squat to lower the body rather than bending over).
- Use long-handled or bent-handled equipment or sit to substitute for bending over.
- Change position frequently.

- When standing, put one foot up on a step to rotate the pelvis.
- Rest before fatigue results in awkward, careless movements.
- Avoid twisting the trunk, especially when lifting.

Obesity

- Ensure that adaptive equipment will accommodate the person's size (e.g., sock aids) and that durable medical equipment has been approved for the patient's weight.
- Use long-handled equipment to reach feet and perineum.
- Use compensation principles for decreased endurance and/or weakness, as appropriate.

Resources 25-1

The Internet has supported an explosion of online resources for persons with disabilities and the professionals who work with them. This section is organized by topic area. Books that are included in this section can all be purchased through an online book vendor, such as www.amazon.com or www.barnesandnoble.com.

General Online Resources

AbleData

www.abledata.com
Database sponsored by the U.S. Department of Education National Institute on Disability and Rehabilitation Research. It has information on almost 40,000 products including manufactured items, customized devices, and noncommercial prototypes.

The Boulevard

www.blvd.com/accent
Quarterly online magazine (previously *Accent on Living*) that addresses all aspects of living a full life with a disability and makes good suggestions for solving problems of persons with physical disabilities.

disABILITY Information and Resources

http://www.makoa.org/index.htm
Offers a wide range of links to information, vendors, and services. Maintained by Jim Lubin, a man with C2 quadriplegia.

NARIC (National Rehabilitation Information Center)

http://www.naric.com
1010 Wayne Ave., Suite 800, Silver Spring, MD 20910.
800-34-NARIC.
A bibliographical database of documents on rehabilitation that includes journals, unpublished documents, audiovisual materials, commercial publications, and government reports.

American Occupational Therapy Association

www.aota.org
AOTA's Occupational Therapy Buyer's Guide, a yearly supplement in *OTPractice*. Note: Access granted to AOTA members only.

Environmental Adaptations: Equipment, Modification, Installation Resources

The following sources focus on bathrooms, kitchens, and wheelchair lifts.

Accessible Environments, Inc.

http://www.acessinc.com/index.htm

Accessibility Professionals

http://www.ada-handicapped-showers.com/about_us.htm

(continued)

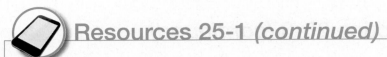

Resources 25-1 *(continued)*

Barrier Free Architecturals, Inc.

http://www.barrierfree.org/

Online Vendors for Adaptive Equipment for Persons with Disabilities

Most vendors offer a wide array of products. Specialty vendors are indicated below, some with a brief description.

Active Forever

http://www.activeforever.com

AliMed, Inc.

http://alimed.com

Andicap

http://www.andicap.com

Be Adaptive Equipment LLC

http://www.beadaptive.com/
Adaptive equipment for hunting and fishing.

Dynamic Living.

http://www.dynamic-living.com
A range of daily living needs for people with varied disabilities and needs.

EnableMart

http://www.enablemart.com

Invacare

http://www.invacare.com/cgi-bin/imhqprd/index.jsp
Also a source for bathroom and other equipment for people weighing over 200 pounds.

North Coast Medical, Inc.

www.ncmedical.com

Patterson Medical
(formerly Sammons Preston Royalan)

http://www.pattersonmedical.com

Self-Wipe Toilet Aids

http://www.selfwipe.com
Sells a toilet aid for limited reach and grasp.

Online Vendors with Devices for the General Public

Several vendors are selling items aimed at making life easier for the general population. These products tend to be more "transparent" than those sold by medical vendors, and they are often less expensive because they cater to a much larger population.

Oxo International

http://www.oxo.com
Maker of Good Grips™ and many other products.

The Wright Stuff

http://www.wrightstuff.biz/

Comfort House

http://www.comforthouse.com/sicroomsup1.html

Carol Wright Gifts

http://www.carolwrightgifts.com

Dynamic Living

http://www.dynamic-living.com

Adaptations and Specialized Equipment for Activities of Daily Living for Specific Limitations

Resources and Products for Persons with Low Vision

Access-USA

http://www.access-usa.com
Supplier of Braille stickers (salt, pepper, food, beverage, and spice tags) and other Braille products, such as menus and maps.

Optelec

www.optelec.com
On-screen magnifier for low vision.

Lighthouse International

www.lighthouse.org

Independent Living Aids, Inc.

http://www.independentliving.com

Sight Connection

http://www.sightconnection.com

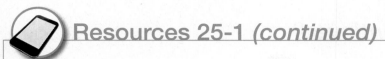
Resources 25-1 *(continued)*

En-Vision America

http://www.envisionamerica.com/

Resources and Products for Persons Doing Activities of Daily Living One-Handed

Mayer, T.-K. (2000). *One-handed in a two-handed world* (2nd ed.). Boston: Prince-Gallison, P.O. Box 23, Hanover Station, Boston, MA 02113-0001.

One-handed typing app

http://www.onehandkeyboard.org/

The Left-Hand Store

http://www.leftyslefthanded.com/

Resources for People of Exceptional Size

See also companies that provide durable medical equipment as they often carry a line of products for bariatric care.

Amplestuff

http://www.amplestuff.com

Bariatric hospital beds

http://bariatricbeds.com/

Dynamic Living

http://www.dynamic-living.com
Has a section for the "generously sized."

Seatbelt extenders

www.extend-its.com

Management of Personal Care Assistants

Center for Personal Assistance Services

http://www.pascenter.org/home/index.php

Making the move to managing your own personal assistance service (PAS): A toolkit for youth with disabilities transitioning to adulthood
http://www.ncwd-youth.info/PAS-Toolkit
Although developed for youth, much of the information in this extensive packet is appropriate for adults with newly acquired disabilities.

Personal care assistants: How to find, hire, and keep them.
http://www.craighospital.org/repository/documents/HeathInfo/PDFs/713.PCAHowtoFindHireKeep.NOD.pdf
Educational brochure from Craig Rehabilitation Hospital.

Personal care assistance: How much help should I hire?
http://www.craighospital.org/repository/documents/HeathInfo/PDFs/715.PCAHowMuchHelp.NOD.pdf
Educational brochure from Craig Rehabilitation Hospital.

Resources on Sexuality and Disability

Brackett, N. L., Ibrahim, E., & Lynne, C. M. (2010). *Male fertility following spinal cord injury: A guide for patients* (2nd ed.). Miami Project to Cure Paralysis. University of Miami. Available via link to pdf file at: http://www.themiamiproject.org/document.doc?id=247

Disabilities-R-Us

http://www.disabilities-r-us.com/
Has resources, products, and chat room/forums related to sexuality.

Sexuality and Disability

Specifically for women with disabilities, addressing sexuality, intimate relationships, and reproduction.
http://www.sexualityanddisability.org

Facing Disability

http://www.facingdisability.com/spinal-cord-injury-videos/social-life-and-sex
For families facing spinal cord injury. For information specific to sexuality and SCI.

Service Dogs

Canine Companions for Independence

www.cci.org
There are six regional centers in the United States that train and supply service dogs.

NEADS: National Education for Assistance Dog Services

http://www.neads.org/

Pet Partners (formerly Delta Society)

www.petpartners.org
A non-profit organization committed to promoting the human-animal health connection, with a wide range of resources on service animals.

(continued)

Resources 25-1 *(continued)*

Organizations for Persons with a Specific Diagnosis

These organizations provide information for the professional and consumer for regaining independence and offer support groups and free brochures.

American Foundation for the Blind

www.afb.org

American Heart Association

www.americanheart.org

American Stroke Association

www.strokeassociation.org

Arthritis Foundation

www.arthritis.org

Brain Injury Association of America

www.biausa.org

National Multiple Sclerosis Society

www.nmss.org

National Parkinson Foundation, Inc.

www.parkinson.org

National Spinal Cord Injury Association

www.spinalcord.org

National Stroke Association.

www.stroke.org

---

effective or safe. The therapist must know construction techniques needed to implement the solution when environmental modification is needed (e.g., anchor grab bars in studs) and should be familiar with local contractors who provide quality home modifications.

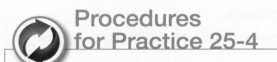

Procedures for Practice 25-4

Energy Conservation Methods (Carson, Gaya, & Milantoni, 2008; Matuska, Mathiowetz, & Finlayson, 2007)

- Rest.
  - Balance work and rest, including alternating heavy and light tasks.
  - Rest before fatiguing.
- Examine and modify standards and priorities.
  - Eliminate unnecessary tasks.
  - Combine or delegate tasks to reduce work.
- Reduce task demands.
  - Use good body mechanics.
  - Sit to work when possible.
  - Plan ahead. Organize work.
  - Use electrical appliances to conserve personal energy.
  - Use lightweight utensils and tools and assistive technologies.
  - Work with gravity assisting, not resisting.

6. Check it out. The assistive device or environmental modification should be checked out for reliability (always works as it should), durability (can withstand repeated use at the force levels the person will apply to it), safety, effectiveness, and patient satisfaction.

7. Train the person. The person must understand and be able to implement the safe use of the assistive device, environment, or method. Gitlin and Burgh (1995) suggested five aspects to device training: develop an activity in which to introduce the device, choose a site for instruction, determine the best time in the rehabilitation process to introduce the device, provide instruction that meets the patient's needs, and reinforce device use with the patient and caregivers. Guidetti and Tham (2002) reported that therapists also use important overarching strategies, such as building trust and motivating their clients, collaborating on goals, and selecting training methods uniquely suited to each client.

It is important to some people that assistive devices be transparent, that is, not call attention to the person as disabled or reveal the extent of disability. Use of conventional devices or gadgets that are sold to the general public qualify as transparent. Examples are felt-tipped pens, slip-on shoes, lightweight pots and pans, kitchen tools with large, grippy handles, and magnifying makeup mirrors. They become adaptive because of their specific application. This perception of transparency and its importance are unique to the individual. Transparency is becoming easier because the principles of universal design focus on designing environments and products that are inclusive of the needs of all (Iwarsson & Stahl, 2003).

ACTIVITIES OF DAILY LIVING

This chapter describes methods and devices suggested by occupational therapy practitioners and former patients to enable independence in ADL and IADL. These suggestions are presented according to typical problems. Many patients have more than one problem. For example, persons with rheumatoid arthritis have weakness as well as limited range of motion. Persons with spinal cord injury have decreased sensation as well as weakness. The therapist will have to use information from pertinent sections for a patient with particular combinations of impairments. Procedures to enable ADL are presented. The need to do these activities and the task demands of each are fairly universal. However, because each person has unique constellations of IADL that describe their roles (James, 2014; Latham, 2008a), only representative IADL can be included as examples of solutions for particular problems.

All tasks that the patient expects to perform independently after discharge must be practiced as they will be done. For example, if a patient will bathe in a tub at home, it is inadequate to practice only sponge bathing while he or she is hospitalized. It is also crucial to address the more intermittent activities inherent in ADL, such as nail care, ear care, and menstrual care, and those ADL that are not universally engaged in, such as managing contact lenses, handling catheters, or flossing teeth. Do not assume that all self-care tasks that a particular person may need to learn are listed on an evaluation checklist.

Techniques and equipment for self-care presented in this chapter are not the only methods of accomplishing these particular tasks. This presentation is meant to provide the student or novice therapist with a repertoire of basic skills with which to approach patients with confidence. The principles of compensation for each problem are key pieces of information that allow the developing therapist to brainstorm a range of techniques or equipment that might meet the needs of a particular patient. For many tasks not mentioned here, either no adaptation is required or the adaptation can be extrapolated from the examples cited.

As each task is taught, all equipment should be close at hand. For early training in dressing, clothing that is a size too large should be used, because it can be managed more easily. The patient's attention should be called to design details of clothing, because persons with certain disabilities find some styles and/or fabrics easier to don. The details to be considered are the cut of the garment, sleeve style, type of fabric, and type of closure or fasteners (Dallas & White, 1982). Clothing especially designed for people with disabilities is now commercially available (see Resources 25-1).

Weakness

For other information and suggestions, see Chapters 12, 18, 26, 35, and 38 (see also Procedures for Practice 25-3).

Suggestions for Activities of Daily Living

When muscle weakness affects all four extremities and the trunk, the techniques and devices are extensive; therefore, this section focuses on compensation for whole body weakness. If the patient has lower extremity paralysis but has normal upper extremities, many of the techniques or devices are unnecessary. Often, compensation for trunk weakness is in the form of support to compensate for poor balance in sitting, standing, or both. Some of the principles described below apply as well to limited weakness, such as weak pinch secondary to osteoarthritis of the carpometacarpal joint.

When paralysis is extensive, a personal care assistant is needed to carry out ADL. The patient must learn to hire, supervise, instruct, compensate, set limits for, and terminate personnel (see "Management of Personal Care Assistants" in Resources 25-1).

Feeding. The problem with feeding is the inability to grasp and/or bring the hand to the mouth. A universal cuff can be used to hold the utensil if grasp is absent (Fig. 25-4). This cuff fits around the palm and has a pocket for insertion of the handle of a utensil for feeding, although it can also be used for other devices, as shown. Some universal cuffs include a wrist support if wrist extensors are weak. Alternatively, the utensil handle can be woven through the fingers, that is, index and ring fingers on top and middle and little fingers under, and held in place passively. A spork, a utensil that combines the bowl of a spoon with the tines of a fork (Fig. 25-5), can be used with the cuff to eliminate the need to change utensils. Some of these have a swivel feature to substitute for the inability to supinate. Gravity and the weight of the food keep the bowl level on the way to the mouth. If the patient has weak grasp, lightweight enlarged handles can be used. The patient may use a wrist-driven wrist–hand orthosis to increase the strength of palmar pinch (see Chapter 15), or an alternative design that was found to be effective in increasing lateral pinch strength and independence in a range of ADL (King et al., 2009). For cutting, a sharp serrated knife is used, because less force is needed, and it is less likely to slip. L-shaped rocker knives enable patients with weak grasp to apply force for cutting with stronger, larger proximal muscles.

An attachable open-bottomed handle can be added to a glass or soft drink can to permit picking it up in the absence of grasp. A mug with a T-shaped handle or a handle that allows all four fingers to be inserted (Fig. 25-6) provides leverage and stabilizes the fingers around the mug, allowing pick-up with a tenodesis grasp. A foam can insulator can be

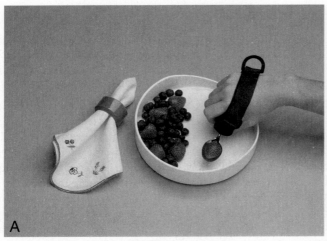 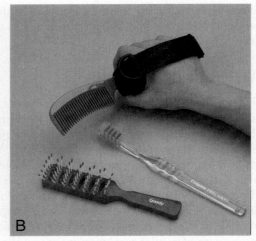

Figure 25-4 **A.** Universal cuffs can be used to hold feeding utensils. **B.** They can also be used for many other items, such as grooming tools. (Both photos courtesy of North Coast Medical, www.ncmedical.com.)

used for a glass to provide friction to assist weak grasp. A long straw can be used to eliminate the need for lifting the cup to the mouth for drinking. *Safety Message: Using a cup with a lid, such as a commuter mug, minimizes the risk of spills in the event that the cup slips, reducing the risk of mess or injury for people with weak grasp, especially when drinking hot liquids.* Commuter mugs have the added benefit of being a transparent device.

A mobile arm support or suspension sling (see Chapter 15) may be required to enable patients with very weak proximal upper extremities to feed themselves. A table placed at axilla height offers support for the arm and eliminates the pull of gravity, allowing the patient with elbow flexors graded 3 or 3+ to bring the food to the mouth. As strength increases, the surface can be lowered. For patients who lack active upper extremity movement, powered feeders are available that are operated with a

head or sip-and-puff switch (search "powered feeders" on AbleData's website, listed in Resources 25-1).

Grooming. Weakness in grasp and pinch are the most common barriers to grooming. Adaptations for makeup jars, tubes, and applicators have been suggested (Hage, 1988). Jar openers can be used to open twist-off caps, or products can be selected that open more easily, given the patient's capabilities, for example proximal muscles can be used to dispense toothpaste in a pump container. A universal cuff or a splint can be used to hold a rattail comb, toothbrush, lipstick tube, or safety razor if grasp is absent. A handcuff can be constructed to hold an electric razor. If grasp is weak, lightweight enlarged handles may be enough. Applying friction material to the utensil or tool can reduce force needed for maintaining a firm grasp and may be especially helpful for people with nerve

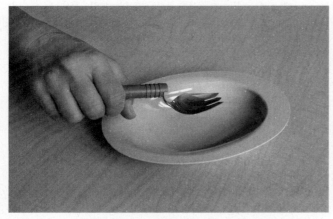

Figure 25-5 Spork (combination fork and spoon). This one also swivels to prevent loss of food when the patient cannot supinate.

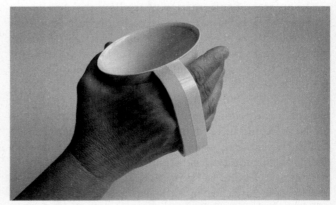

Figure 25-6 Cup with large D-shaped handle assists drinking when grasp is weak. This cup has an oval shape that compensates for weakness or impaired motor control in directing liquid into the mouth.

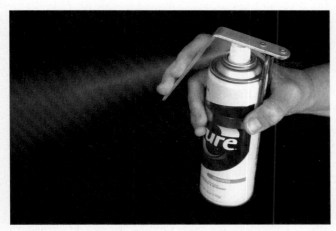

Figure 25-7   Aerosol-can adapter that reduces the force needed to operate the spray.

injuries that also reduce sweating and limit the normal friction between the hand and task objects (Smaby et al., 2004). A small plastic brush with a cuff attachment may be used to assist in shampooing hair. Lengthening the force arm relative to the resistance arm may allow use of spray deodorant (Fig. 25-7) or nail care (Fig. 25-8, A & B).

Toileting. Transfers, proximal stability and balance while raising and lowering clothing, and weak pinch and grasp are common problems for people with significant weakness. Wheelchair users often require adaptations for the toilet, such as a raised toilet seat and toilet armrests. Alternatively, a commode can be used over the toilet, which both raises the height of the seat and provides armrests. People using a sliding board for transfers or who need to reach behind for toilet hygiene can use a drop-arm commode (Fig. 25-9). Commodes also offer flexibility; for example, they can be moved to the bedside to minimize transfers for people with mobility limitations who need to use the bathroom at night.

For people with spinal cord injury, concomitant loss of bowel and bladder control requires special procedures, including bladder irrigation, use of a catheter, or intermittent catheterization (Medline Plus, 2010a, 2010b). Generally, the person can push down the pants while in the wheelchair by leaning from side to side. If the person cannot stand or has precarious standing balance, it is necessary to transfer back to the wheelchair before raising the clothing after toileting. If the person uses an indwelling catheter or external drainage device, the collection bag can be emptied into the toilet without transfer or removal

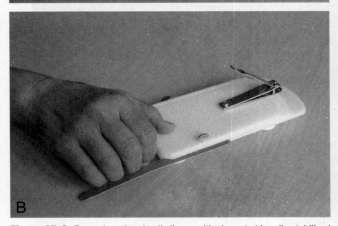

Figure 25-8   Emery board and nail clipper with elongated handle stabilized to reduce force required (**A**) and for one-handed use (**B**).

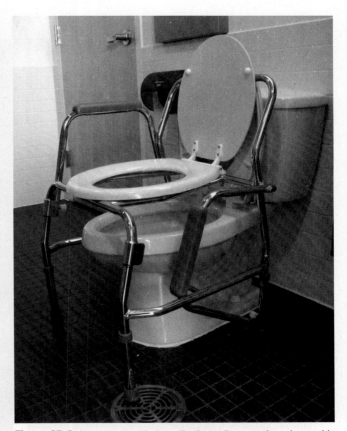

Figure 25-9   A commode with the collection pail removed can be used in place of a raised toilet seat with toilet armrests. This commode has a "drop-arm" feature, which improves access for transferring and toilet hygiene.

of clothing. Usually, nurses or enterostomal therapists teach clean intermittent self-catheterization, but the occupational therapist should be aware of the process of this ADL:

1. Assemble the equipment.
2. Wash hands and penis or vulva and urethral opening. Clean gloves may be used, if desired.
3. Lubricate the catheter tip with water-soluble lubricant. Males hold penis at sides, and insert catheter with firm, gentle pressure. Females separate labia, palpate meatus or use a mirror, and insert catheter into the bladder.
4. Push catheter in until urine starts to flow.
5. Allow urine to flow until it stops, gently pressing on abdomen or bearing down to empty bladder.
6. Slowly remove the catheter, holding catheter tip as it is removed to prevent spilling.
7. Discard disposable catheters, or clean reusable catheters with soap and water, rinse, dry, and store in a plastic bag.
8. Wash hands with soap and water (Medline Plus, 2010a, 2010b).

Knee spreaders with a mirror help hold weak or paralyzed lower extremities in abduction and enable people with limited trunk control to see the urethral opening.

People on a bowel program may use suppositories or digital stimulation to initiate a bowel movement. Suppositories may be inserted while the person is in the bed or on the toilet. When people use digital stimulation or insert suppositories while on the toilet, a raised toilet seat with a space between the seat and toilet bowl rim is needed to allow them to reach the rectum. Suppository inserters for those with weak or absent pinch are commercially available and can be adapted with cuffs for patients who lack grasp. Some inserters have a spring ejector that releases the suppository after it is properly positioned in the rectum. An inspection mirror is needed if the patient lacks anal sensation. Bowel stimulators are available for patients who lack adequate digit control. People with weak grasp and pinch can wrap toilet tissue around the hand for use. For people with very limited hand function, bidets can be fit to the toilet to clean and dry the perineal area. Menstrual needs can be met by adaptations to positioning, pants, pad versus tampons, and aids such as mirrors and knee spreaders (Duckworth, 1986).

Bathing. The problems with bathing include the transfer, dynamic sitting balance, lack of lower extremity movement, and lack of pinch and grasp. Transfer tub seats (Fig. 25-10A), which have two legs in the tub and two legs

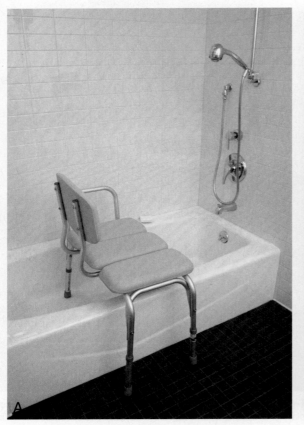
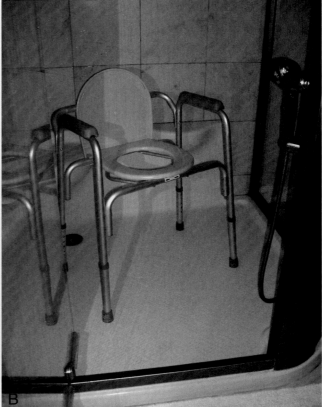

Figure 25-10 **A.** Transfer tub bench. **B.** For patients with a walk-in shower, a commode with the pail removed can double as a shower chair.

outside the tub, provide a safe means to transfer from the wheelchair to tub. For persons with a walk-in shower in their home environment, a commode with the pail removed can be used in the shower, eliminating the need for a separate piece of equipment (Fig. 25-10B). *Safety Message: Individuals who are prone to pressure ulcers need to use padded seats. Each person's requirements should be evaluated and a seat selected to fit him or her.* Users of tub seats (both patients and caregivers) have reported that safety, adequate support, stability of equipment, and comfort are some of the most important considerations in selecting appropriate equipment (Pain & McLellan, 2003). The tub seat must be placed so that the faucets are within reach. Grab bars help during the transfer and while the person is seated (Procedures for Practice 25-5). Nonslip material is used in the bottom of the tub. The faucets must have lever handles for ease in tapping them off and on with the fist or foot. A handheld shower that is adapted with a hook handle is used. *Safety Message: No-scald faucets and shower heads should be used, but if they are unavailable, water temperature should be regulated by turning on the cold water first and then adding the hot, which prevents scalding desensitized skin.* Soap on a string or in a wall-mounted dispenser is helpful. A bath mitt is used if grasp is weak or absent. The person dries off before transferring back to the wheelchair. A towel placed in the wheelchair seat will dry the perineal area and can be removed when the person transfers to the bed for dressing. Alternatively, some people don a terry cloth robe, which absorbs water without having to reach all areas. Bathing and drying the feet and legs are particular problems for people with poor trunk balance, and they may prefer to do foot hygiene while in bed (Shillam, Beeman, & Loshin, 1983).

A custom-made shower stall and shower wheelchair provide the easiest bathing solution for a person with tetraplegia, however, it typically requires an expensive home modification. The shower area should have a raised slope to prevent the water from running out but allow the person to enter the shower on a shower wheelchair. Prefabricated bath enclosures and remodeling designs are listed under "Environmental Adaptations: Equipment, Modification, Installation Resources" on Resources 25-1. Shower wheelchairs have commode seats and can be positioned over the toilet for bowel programs, reducing the number of transfers required for morning care. For people who prefer a bath, a number of electronic bath lifts are available that enable them to transfer onto a seat and then be lowered into the tub for independent or assisted bathing, depending on their needs.

Dressing. Dressing ability for persons with tetraplegia varies in both level of independence and time required. Individuals who are independent but require extensive additional time must decide whether this time requirement is acceptable or whether a personal care assistant is a better option. Problems with dressing include moving the paralyzed limbs to dress them, decreased sitting balance, and the need to compensate for the lack of pinch and grasp. Rudhe and van Hedel (2009) found moderate to strong correlations between dressing ability and both upper extremity strength and hand function. While in bed, people with spinal cord injuries at C6 and below can pull their knees up to dress the lower extremities by using their wrist extensors and elbow flexors. Loops of twill tape can be added to the cuffs of socks to facilitate pulling them on by hooking the thumb in the loop when pinch is absent.

A buttonhook attached to a cuff or with a built-up handle is used when fingers are unable to manipulate buttons (Fig. 25-2). The hook is inserted through the buttonhole to hook the button and pull it through the buttonhole. The other hand is used to hold the garment near the buttonhole. A loop of string or leather lacing may be attached to the zipper pull of pants or other garments so that in the absence of pinch, the thumb can be hooked in the loop to close the zipper. Alternatively, a zipper hook can also be used.

Adaptation of clothes should also be considered to facilitate dressing, undressing, and toileting; to regulate temperature; to increase comfort; and to increase feelings of self-confidence (Kratz et al., 1997; see Resources 25-1). For business people who are wheelchair users, suit jackets, pants, and skirts tailored to accommodate the sitting position look better than off-the-rack suits.

Initially, the occupational therapist may use the following adapted dressing techniques for persons with tetraplegia (Runge, 1967). Demonstrations of persons with spinal cord injury dressing, produced by the International Spinal Cord Society and Livability (2012), can also be viewed on the Internet, providing additional examples that underscore the need for an individualized approach to modifying self-care activities (see http://www.elearnsci.org/). You will need to establish a free account, which will give you access to many training videos embedded in educational modules for occupational therapists, including many on dressing.

Pants and Underwear

1. Have the patient sit in bed with the back against the head of an elevated hospital bed or against the wall. Pants are positioned with the front up and pant legs over the bottom of the bed.
2. The patient lifts one of his legs by hooking the opposite wrist or forearm under the knee, and puts the foot into the pants leg. The thumb of the other hand hooks a belt loop or pocket to hold the pants open. Working in a cross-body position aids stability for those with poor balance.
3. The other foot is inserted.
4. The palms of the hands are used to pat and slide the pants onto the calves and to get the trouser cuffs over the feet. The wrist or wrists are hooked under the waistband or in the pockets to pull the pants up over the knees.

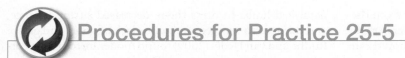

Procedures for Practice 25-5

Grab Bars and Safety Rails for the Bathroom

Selection

Grab bars can be used in both the tub area and near the toilet, if it is close to a wall. Grab bars can be purchased from rehabilitation product vendors and many plumbing or home improvement stores. *Safety Message: Towel bars are NOT safe for use as a grab bar.* Grab bars must be able to support the person's weight, so recommendations should take the weight of the person into account. Grab bar specifications will include a weight limit.

Horizontal bars are for pushing up; vertical bars are for pulling up. An L-shaped grab bar that includes both vertical and horizontal legs is a good choice for the bathtub or shower enclosure. Clamp-on bathtub safety rails fix onto the edge of the tub, providing a secure handhold for stepping in and out of the tub; however, they cannot be used on fiberglass tubs because these tubs cannot withstand the stress.

The optimum diameter for grab bars is 1.25–1.5 inches for adults. The distance between the wall and the bar should be 1.5 inches (U.S. Access Board, 2004). A wider space is dangerous because if the arm slips, it may get caught between the wall and the bar and/or the person may fall.

Toilet armrests can provide the necessary support for using the upper extremities to transfer on and off the toilet. Some models are incorporated directly into a raised seat (Fig. 25-11), whereas other models bolt onto the toilet, providing more security for people with balance impairments who may weight the seat unevenly. Toilet armrests are easier to secure than wall-mounted grab bars and are typically better positioned than a wall-mounted bar, which may be too far away or available only on one side.

Placement

Locate bathtub grab bars where a person may be off balance, such as going into or out of the tub, turning in the tub or shower, or standing up from or sitting down on a bench or seat. One vertical bar outside the tub and one horizontal or diagonal bar on the wall along the length of the tub is recommended as a basic installation. An L-shaped bar can be substituted for the bar on the wall along the length of the tub. If an L-shaped bar is used, locate the horizontal bar 16 inches above the tub rim and the vertical bar approximately 32 inches from the corner of the tub or as the placement suits the height and transfer and bathing process of the user.

Installation

Grab bars must be mounted to the wall with 2-inch stainless steel screws driven into the wall studs. Use a stud finder to locate the studs. It may be necessary to locate the studs from the other side of the wall if the bathroom walls are tiled. The typical mounting flange has three holes for three screws. Drill a small pilot hole before drilling holes in ceramic tile, using an

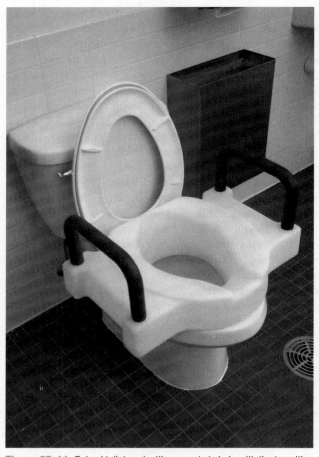

Figure 25-11 Raised toilet seat with armrests to help with the transition to and from sitting.

eighth-inch masonry bit to drill three holes for the mounting screws. Only two screws will actually fit into the stud. Therefore, use a toggle bolt for the third screw. The length of horizontal bars must be the same as the stud spacing. Alternatively, existing walls can be cut into to add a horizontal 2 × 4 and then replace the wallboard in order to securely place a horizontal bar.

In new construction or during a renovation, double the studs where grab bars are to be fastened so there will be a 3-inch place to fasten the screws rather than the 1.5 inches offered by only one stud. For horizontal bars, add a 2 × 4 between the studs as a screwing surface or back a large area with plywood, which enables bars to be mounted in any place or desired orientation.

Suction grab bars are available for areas where it is not possible to secure a bar to the studs or a solid wall backing. These bars should be used with caution as weight capacity varies with security of the mounting surface and the direction of force on the grab bar. Suction grab bars are not ADA approved.

Toilet armrests attach using the bolts that hold the toilet seat in place. No alteration of the fixture itself is required.

5. The patient continues to pull on the waistband or pockets while returning to supine position to pull the pants up onto the thighs. This may have to be repeated. Hooking the wrist or thumbs in the crotch helps pull up the pants.
6. In a side-lying position, the thumb of the top arm is hooked in the back belt loop, and the pants are pulled over the buttocks. Then the patient rolls to the other side and repeats the process until the pants are on.
7. In a supine position, the pants can be fastened using a zipper pull loop and Velcro™ tab closing or buttonhook.
8. The pants are removed by reversing the procedures and pushing the pants off.

An alternative method for getting the pant legs over the feet may be useful for patients with limited forward reach. The pants are positioned parallel to the patient's legs. The first leg is lifted and crossed over the other leg so the pant leg can be slid all the way over the foot, up to the knee. The leg is uncrossed and the second leg is slid in (Regional Spinal Cord Injury Center of Delaware Valley, 2001). To pull the pants over the hips, use the method described above.

Socks. Socks with tight elastic should be avoided. While sitting in the wheelchair or bed, the patient crosses one leg over the other and uses tenodesis grasp to put on the sock and the palms of the hands to help pull it on. If the patient cannot cross his or her legs, the foot can be placed on a stool or chair. Socks are removed by pushing them off with a dressing stick, long shoehorn, or the thumb hooked over the sock edge.

Shoes. Loafers that are a half to one size larger are most practical for people who cannot walk. Shoes are put on by crossing one leg at a time as for putting on socks. The shoe is pulled onto the foot by balancing the sole of the shoe in the palm of the hand. Then with the foot on the floor or on the foot pedal of the wheelchair, the foot is pushed down into the shoe by pushing on the knee. A long shoehorn may be helpful for getting the heel into the shoe. Shoes can be removed by pushing them off with the shoehorn.

Cardigan Garments: Shirts and Blouses

1. Shirts may be donned in either the wheelchair or bed. The shirt is positioned with the brand label of the shirt facing down and the collar toward the knees.
2. The patient puts his or her arms under the shirt and into the sleeves and pushes them up over the elbows.
4. The shirt is gathered up by using wrist extension and by hooking the thumbs under the shirt back.
5. The shirt is placed over the head.

6. The patient shrugs to get the shirt down across the shoulders and hooks the wrists into the sleeves to free the axillae.
7. The patient leans forward and reaches back with one hand to rub on the shirt back to pull it down.
8. The shirt fronts are lined up, and buttoning begins from the bottom button up, using a buttonhook. Alternatively, shirts can be adapted with Velcro™ fasteners.

A cardigan garment is removed by pushing first one side and then the other off the shoulders and then alternately elevating and depressing the shoulders to allow gravity to assist in lowering the shirt down the arms. Then one thumb is hooked into the opposite sleeve to pull the shirt over the elbow, and the arm is removed from the shirt.

With the exception of buttons, an overhead garment is put on in a similar manner and removed by hooking one thumb in the back of the neckline and pulling the shirt over the head. The sleeves are pushed off each arm.

Bra. Either a front- or back-closure bra can be used. Velcro™ can replace hooks for fastening, but some patients can manage the standard hook fastener if it is hooked in front at waist level. After the bra is hooked, it is positioned with the cups in front, and the arms are placed through the shoulder straps. Then, by hooking the opposite thumb under a strap, one strap at a time is pulled over the shoulder.

Sexual Activities. Many persons with disabilities have concerns about their sexuality and challenges to resuming sexual expression. Depending on the extent of weakness, patients may need help identifying positions that best support engagement in sexual expression. Much of the literature on sexuality and disability has focused on people with spinal cord injury and resulting impairment in sensorimotor function, including sexual function. Although they may not be ready to learn about the particulars of resuming sexual activities or procreation early in the rehabilitation process, knowing that they may have concerns about sexual expression and that there are a variety of sources of information for them when they are ready (McAlonan, 1996) should be discussed. Fisher et al. (2002) conducted a longitudinal study of people post-spinal cord injury that examined a range of issues, including the optimal timing of interventions addressing sexuality. Their findings suggest that people post-spinal cord injury are most interested in receiving information regarding sexuality in the 6 months following discharge from rehabilitation, suggesting that discussion during outpatient therapy or at follow-up appointments might be most appropriate for this population.

In a pioneering book, *Sexual Options for Paraplegics and Quadriplegics*, Mooney, Cole, and Chilgren (1975) explicitly described methods of sexual expression for persons with spinal cord injury. They pictured the process of getting ready for sex (emptying the bladder, washing). They addressed how to handle a catheter that is left in place during sex (bend the catheter and fold it over along the shaft of the penis where it will be out of the way, but do not anchor it until the erection has taken place to avoid pulling out the balloon of the Foley catheter; be sure the tubing and collection bag are not leaned on to prevent the flow of urine). They presented positions for genital and orogenital sexual expression, alternative means of sexual expression (vibrators, touch, or talking), and how to achieve and maintain a reflex erection of the penis. They discussed fertility of men: ability to ejaculate depends on the level of the lesion, and production of sperm depends on healthy testicles. They pointed out that women remain fertile and therefore pregnancy is as possible as for able-bodied women. Although this book is out of print, it is available in many university libraries, and used copies are available through online booksellers, such as amazon.com and barnesandnoble.com.

Suggestions for Selected Instrumental Activities of Daily Living

For the persons with severe paralysis, high-tech adaptations as described in Chapter 18 offer opportunities to engage in communication, leisure, and work activities. Some low-tech adaptations are suggested here.

Handling a Book. The person with tetraplegia encounters problems with holding a book and turning the pages, with writing or recording notes in business or school, and possibly in telephoning. Some book holders support a book on a table, whereas others are designed to hold a book when reading supine in bed. If a person is reading while supine, and the book is not held directly above, prism glasses are needed to direct the vision to a 90° angle so that the book may be seen.

To turn pages, some solutions are as follows:

1. When wearing a splint, the person can use a rubber thimble or finger cot on the posted thumb.
2. A pencil with the eraser end down can be used in a universal cuff (typing stick) or hand splint.
3. Electric page turners automatically turn pages when activated by a microswitch or other means of control.
4. A mouthstick with a friction tip end may be useful. Mouthsticks may have flat mouthpieces or custom-molded mouthpieces that conform to the person's dentition. The mouthpiece has a lightweight plastic or aluminum rod to which an eraser or other type of end piece, such as pencil, pen, or paintbrush, can be added. AbleData has information on a wide range of mouthsticks (www.abledata.com).

An alternative is books that have been audio-recorded on tape, CD, or digital platforms, which can be obtained from libraries and bookstores. The Library of Congress has a large collection of tapes, including many current issues of magazines, and tape players that are available to the blind and the physically disabled for no charge through the National Library Service for the Blind and Physically Handicapped. Information about this service and a link to the catalog can be found at: http://www.loc.gov/nls/. Depending on a patient's limitations, an electronic reader may be easier to hold and manipulate than printed books. Some have a text-to-speech output feature that will read books for people and may be useful for those with severe weakness who are unable to lift and hold books or turn pages.

Writing. Extensive writing is usually done with computerized word processing. Keyboarding can be done with typing sticks or a mouthstick for hitting the keys. Voice recognition software is a better option for people who need to regularly create large amounts of text. If speed is important, as in taking notes in the classroom or in business, a tape recorder can be used.

Handwriting is important for legal documents and personalizing cards and typed notes. Splints that provide pinch can be used to hold a writing instrument. If pinch is absent, and the patient does not use a splint, a pencil holder (Fig. 25-12) that encircles the pencil, thumb, and index finger can be made of thermoplastic materials. Pens with textured grips provide friction to make a weak grip more effective. Felt-tipped pens require little pressure and are therefore easier to use than other types of pens. If the arms cannot be used, with practice a mouthstick with pencil attached can become an effective writing tool.

Opening Containers. Jar openers, including rubber sheets, clamp style, and mounted style, or pliers can be used to open jars, bottles, and pill bottles. In one study, a pop-off lid was found to require approximately 13 pounds of force to open, and medicine bottles required 2–6 pounds

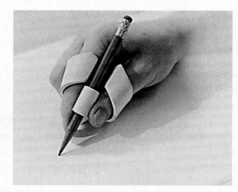

Figure 25-12 Pencil holder made of thermoplastic material.

(Rice, Leonard, & Carter, 1998). If childproof containers are not necessary in a person's home environment, he or she can ask the pharmacist to use easy-open rather than childproof containers. Many over-the-counter medications and supplements can also be selected with easy-open caps.

Telephoning. As phone technology advances at a rapid pace, the occupational therapist exploring telephone options with persons with significant upper extremity weakness will need to identify what type of telephone is needed or desired. Home telephones frequently include a speaker feature, which eliminates the need to lift and hold the receiver. Buttons may be pushed with the eraser end of a pencil in a universal cuff or with a mouthstick. Speed dial options reduce the complexity of calls to commonly dialed numbers. Many mobile phones have voice-recognition features that enable the caller to dial through voice commands provided the person can activate the phone. Finally, voice-over-Internet calling provides another communication option for people who have accessible computers.

Turning Electrical Appliances On and Off. The expansive field of EADL, formerly known as environmental control units, includes remote control devices for TV, entertainment centers, VCR and DVD players, computers, cell phones, electronic tablets, lights, door openers, electric beds, and appliances. Voice-activated remote controls are available in specialty stores for operating the TV, VCR, and DVD player. See Chapter 18 for a discussion of high-tech assistive devices that are useful for persons with severe weakness or paralysis resulting from a spinal cord injury or degenerative disease such as amyotrophic lateral sclerosis. Many consumer electronics, such as tablets and mobile phones, offer features that enable access to people with a range of abilities, for example, many functions can be accessed through voice commands, making them accessible to people with limited hand function.

Low Endurance and Fatigue

For other information and suggestions, see Chapter 42. See also Procedures for Practice 25-3.

Suggestions for Activities of Daily Living

Endurance, a physiological characteristic, is the ability to sustain activity over time. General endurance is primarily a reflection of cardiopulmonary function and overall level of fitness. Fatigue is not simply low endurance, but a subjective experience of feeling tired or exhausted (Stout & Finlayson, 2011). Fatigue is multidimensional and includes cognitive, behavioral, and emotional components (Matuska, Mathiowetz, & Finlayson, 2007), as well as

physical factors. Patients of various diagnoses and circumstances (e.g., extended time in bed because of illness or injury) have low endurance and/or fatigue, which may be temporary or chronic. Many disorders cause a more or less permanent reduction of endurance to which patients must adapt, e.g., cardiac and pulmonary disease, or recurrent fatigue, e.g., multiple sclerosis, rheumatoid arthritis, and chronic fatigue syndrome. Patients with low endurance and/or fatigue may also have higher level cognitive impairments that impact learning. Fatigue can directly affect patients' memory, attention, and ability to process new information, whereas patients with severe cardiac and pulmonary disorders have reduced ability to use oxygen needed for muscle, including cardiac muscle, and brain functions. If oxygen deprivation is severe enough, neuro-psychological changes involving memory, perception, and information processing may occur.

Adaptations for ADL and IADL for people with low endurance and/or fatigue involve education and training in self-management (Migliore, 2004; Taylor, 2004). People with low endurance learn to work within limits of cardiac and pulmonary capacity by reducing the energy demands of tasks and routines and by maximizing pulmonary function during ADL and IADL. *Safety Message: Cardiac patients are cautioned to stop activity when they have angina or shortness of breath (SOB). Patients with pulmonary disease may need to have blood oxygen saturation levels monitored with a pulse oximeter (see Chapter 42) during initial ADL training to establish levels of activity that do not reduce blood oxygen to harmfully low levels.* People who experience fatigue learn to monitor bodily signals to manage activity tolerance and to identify and manage cognitive-affective triggers of fatigue (Taylor, 2004).

Some activities require higher levels of energy than do others. One way to guide activity selection is to use metabolic equivalent (MET) tables. Most self-care activities require less than 3 METs. Ainsworth et al. (2011) have been compiling and revising a Compendium of Physical Activities since 1993 and now maintain a website with MET values for a wide range of activities at http://sites.google.com/site/compendiumofphysicalactivities/home. It should be remembered that MET charts are averages, do not account for particular circumstances, and therefore cannot be used without also monitoring the patient's breathing, heart rate, blood pressure, oxygen saturation levels, cognitive demands, or affective components. Dyspnea (SOB) is a signal for people with low endurance that the activity is beyond their cardiopulmonary capacity. Angina or excessive increase in heart rate (20 beats over resting rate) signals patients with a cardiac condition that they have reached their limit. Activity restrictions and precautions vary depending on the nature and severity of the cardiac disorder (Goodman & Smirnova, 2009). Adapted methods may be used to compensate for activity restrictions, e.g., prolonged bending over may be avoided with long-handled utensils (described in this chapter in the section on limited range of motion). Patients with chronic obstructive pulmonary disease should learn to modify ADL methods to coordinate diaphragmatic and pursed lip breathing into activity routines to minimize dyspnea (Migliore, 2004).

Energy conservation is a primary intervention approach for patients with low endurance or fatigue. All patients with fatigue or reduced endurance are taught to take rest periods throughout the day and use other energy-conserving techniques. Principles of energy conservation are listed in Procedures for Practice 25-4 and elaborated on in Chapter 27. The principles themselves are relatively straightforward; however, they require people to change habits, which can be difficult to do but may be supported by having them set goals, monitor progress, and develop problem-solving strategies to promote goal attainment. In addition, adaptive methods, e.g., keeping frequently used items in the kitchen within easy reach, or adaptive equipment, e.g., using a long-handled sponge to eliminate bending in the shower, can support energy conservation strategies.

People with low endurance and fatigue should attend to getting sufficient sleep. Fatigue and sleep disturbances often coexist, creating a downward spiral of sleep deprivation and increasing fatigue. Sleep is identified as an area of occupational performance in the Occupational Therapy Practice Framework II (AOTA, 2008). Occupational therapists possess the skills needed for helping patients identify effective sleep hygiene, that is, habits that promote quality sleep. Strategies for the patient who is having trouble sleeping include developing a bedtime routine and schedule; avoiding consumption of alcohol, tobacco, and caffeine within 4 hours of bedtime; avoiding upsetting, important (e.g., paying bills), or stimulating activities (e.g., playing video games or answering e-mail) just before bedtime; and having a comfortable environment in which to sleep (Mastin, Bryson, & Corwyn, 2006).

Sexual Activities. The American Heart Association (2012) online article *Sex and Heart Disease* discusses the cardiovascular changes that occur during sexual intercourse, when the patient can resume sex after myocardial infarction or heart surgery, how other factors affect sex interest and capacity, guidelines for resuming sex, what to do if symptoms arise during sex, Viagra, and myths and misconceptions. The booklet can be helpful to both the patient and the health professional and can be ordered online at www.americanheart.org. Diaphragmatic breathing is facilitated in supine (Migliore, 2004), so individuals with pulmonary conditions may find dyspnea is easier to manage when lying supine during sexual activities. People with fatigue may need to plan sexual activities for a time of day or day of the week when energy levels are highest.

Limited or Restricted Range of Motion

For other information and suggestions see Chapters 36, 37, 39, and 40. See also Procedures for Practice 25-3.

Suggestions for Activities of Daily Living

Feeding. The most common problems with feeding that occur with limited range of motion are the inability to close the hand enough to grasp the utensil or inability to bring the hand to the mouth. Enlarged or elongated handles can be added to spoons or forks. Elongated handles may need to be angled to enable patients to reach their mouths. Remember that the longer the handle (resistance arm), the heavier and less stable the device; therefore, the handle should be only as long as is necessary and made of lightweight material.

A universal cuff, or utensil holder, can be used when grasp is not possible (Fig. 25-4). For some people, such as those with arthrogryposis, independent eating may only be possible with electric feeders. However, the device must be set up and cleaned up by an assistant, and some insurance carriers will not pay for both device and assistant. Another factor to be considered when prescribing this device: for an institutionalized person, being fed by another may be an opportunity for social contact that the device would eliminate (Hermann et al., 1999).

Grooming. The problems with grooming are the same as for feeding. Enlarged or extended handles can be attached to a comb (Fig. 25-13), brush, toothbrush, shampoo brush,

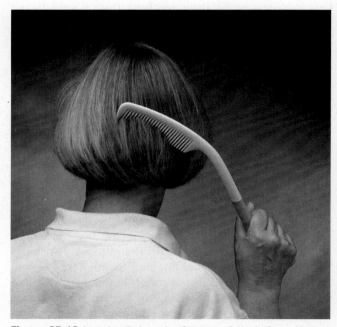

Figure 25-13 Long-handled comb. (Courtesy of North Coast Medical, www.ncmedical.com.)

lipstick tube, or safety razor. Aerosol deodorant, hair spray, powder, and perfume can be used by those with limited range. An assistant may be needed to wash and style hair if the person cannot reach the head to do it independently. A simple hairstyle may eliminate the need for blow-drying and styling.

Toileting. The problem with toileting is the inability to reach. The toilet tissue dispenser should be within reach. Wiping tongs can extend reach when using toilet tissue. If grasp is poor, the tissue can be wrapped around the hand, or wiping tongs with a cuff-shaped handle can be used. A bidet or personal cleansing system eliminates the need for wiping by hand. Gravity assists in pulling clothes down; loose clothes slide off easily. A dressing stick can be used to pull up the clothing (Fig. 25-14). Sanitary napkins with adhesive strips can be used more easily than tampons; the protective wrapper can be removed with the teeth. If limited range or movement precautions prevent the person from using a low toilet, a raised toilet seat may solve the problem (Fig. 25-11).

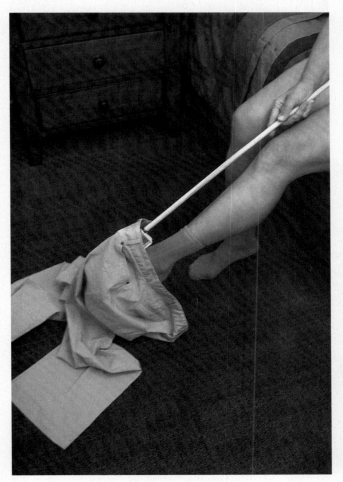

Figure 25-14 A dressing stick used to pull clothing up or around the body when reach is not permitted or possible.

Bathing. *Safety Message: Tub transfers are facilitated by grab bars. Nonslip material should be placed on the bottom of the tub.* A tub seat is used when a person is unable or not allowed to get down into the tub or up from the bottom of the tub (Mann et al., 1996). Different heights and styles of tub benches are available (Fig. 25-10A), and it is important to select the right one for each patient in terms of stability, ease of transfer, need for padding or back support, access to perineal area, and position of hips and knees. A handheld shower hose is used for rinsing if a tub seat is required; adding a strap can enable use by those with limited finger range of motion (Procedures for Practice 25-5). Alternatively, walk-in bathtubs have built-in seats and could be an option for people who prefer bathing to showering but are unable to get down into a standard tub. Whether using a tub seat or walk-in tub, it is essential to provide practice of strategies to bathe the back, feet, and perineal area when seated, especially if the patient also has impaired sitting balance. Lever handles on faucets are recommended because they do not require grasp and they allow better leverage for turning on and off. *Safety Message: For patients with hip precautions, it is important to position the tub seat so that faucets can be reached without excessive hip flexion.* It is helpful if the soap is on a string or to use soap and shampoo dispensers that can be fixed to the wall within easy reach. When grasp is limited, a sponge or terry cloth bath mitt works well. A long-handled bath sponge can be used to reach the feet or back; some are designed to hold the soap inside the sponge and others are designed especially for cleaning feet. A terry cloth bathrobe is effective for drying.

The following procedure is used for patients who cannot step over the edge of the tub and who require a transfer tub seat (Fig. 25-10A).

1   The patient walks to the side of the tub using assistive devices and weight-bearing precautions, as prescribed, and turns to face away from the tub.
2.   The patient reaches for the back of the tub bench with one hand and the edge of the tub seat with the other.
3.   The patient sits down on the tub bench and lifts both legs into the tub, turning to face the faucet, being careful to adhere to range of motion precautions for the leg(s), as appropriate.

Dressing. Lack of ability to reach and grasp, as well as restricted shoulder, back, hip, or knee range of motion, are limitations that cause problems in dressing. *Safety Message: Many patients post-total hip replacement will need to follow movement precautions for 2 months. A posterolateral surgical approach is commonly used, and while patients can typically bear weight as tolerated, they must avoid flexing the hip past 90°, adducting the leg past midline, or externally* *rotating the leg)* (van Stralen, Struben, & van Loon, 2003). Other surgical techniques or complications may necessitate different precautions, so therapists must always confirm activity precautions prior to treatment (see also Chapter 36).

Reaching clothes from closets and dressers and dressing the lower extremities are common problems for people who cannot reach their feet or who are not allowed to flex the hip. A dressing stick can be used to pull clothing over the feet (Fig. 25-14) or to reach hangers in the closet. Reachers can be used to remove clothes from shelves, to start clothes over parts of the body, and to pick up objects from the floor (Fig. 25-15, A & B). People can don socks using a sock or stocking aid and use a dressing stick to remove socks (Fig. 25-16, A & B). To use a stocking aid, the trough is inserted into the foot of the stocking; the top of the stocking is pushed down below the top edge of the trough. While the strings are held, the stocking aid with stocking in place is placed on the ground, and the person's foot is moved into the trough until the toes reach the tip of the stocking. The aid is then removed by pulling the strings, bringing it out of the stocking behind the heel. This brings the stocking within reach so it can be pulled up the leg. Patients with a temporary range-of-motion restriction, such as those post-total hip replacement, may opt to go without socks for that time period. A long shoehorn assists in putting on shoes when the feet cannot be reached. Some long shoehorns have a hook on the opposite end that may be used as a dressing stick. *Safety Message: Positioning the shoehorn between the legs, rather than on the lateral aspect of the foot,*

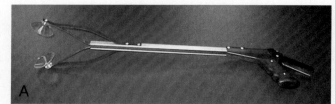

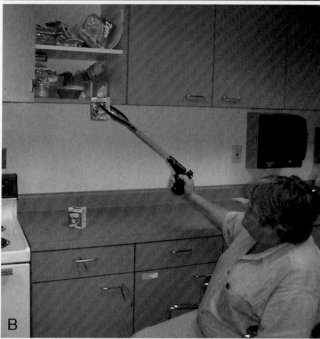

Figure 25-15 **A.** Reacher with a pistol grip and suction cup tips. **B.** Reacher in use.

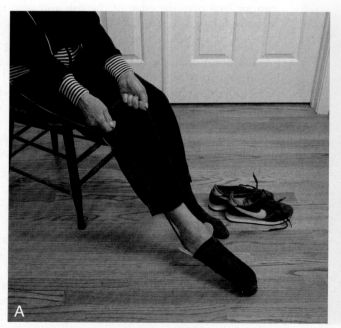

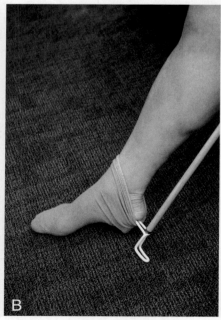

Figure 25-16 **A.** Stocking aid in use. (Courtesy of North Coast Medical, www.ncmedical.com). **B.** Socks are removed using the inverted hook on a dressing stick.

reduces the chance that the patient will move the hip into internal rotation when donning shoes. Slip-on shoes and elastic shoelaces avoid the need to tie shoelaces. Collaborating with patients to select the equipment they view as most helpful and providing adequate training with opportunity to practice increase the likelihood that patients will use the adaptive equipment effectively after discharge (Kraskowsky & Finlayson, 2001).

Dressing the upper body with limited upper extremity range of motion is easier when using button- or zipper-front garments rather than over-the-head garments. A dressing stick or reacher is used to bring the garment around the shoulders. Fasteners are particularly difficult, especially if limitation in the range of motion is accompanied by weakness. A study that examined the ability of 97 women with arthritis to manage clothing fasteners found that zippers were the easiest to use, especially easy-sliding, large-toothed plastic type. Snaps and buttons were rated as difficult, although vertical buttonholes made buttoning easier (Dallas & White, 1982). Velcro™ tabs can replace buttons, snaps, or hooks if limited mobility in the fingers prevents buttoning or fastening. Because few clothes come with this type of fastener, the patient's clothing must be adapted. To preserve the look of a buttoned garment, the buttonhole is sewn closed and the button is attached over the hole. The hook and pile Velcro™ tabs are sewn to replace the buttons.

Sexual Activities. If a person's range of motion limitations are accompanied by pain and stiffness (e.g., with rheumatoid arthritis), the person should time pain relief medication so its effects are greatest during sexual activities. A warm bath may reduce joint stiffness as well as serve as a part of foreplay. Satisfying sex includes romance and intimacy even though engaging in intercourse may be too difficult or painful soon after injury or during a flare-up of arthritis. People should explore options for skin-to-skin contact that do not cause pain. The occupational therapist and patient can problem solve together to identify new, comfortable, and biomechanically safe positions for intercourse and other forms of sexual expression. For example, both partners may lie on their sides with a man entering from behind for a partner with hip problems; both partners may lie on their sides facing each other with one person providing most of the hip movement, for a partner with back problems (American College of Rheumatology, 2012).

Sexual activities such as touching, holding hands, and caressing can be resumed immediately after total hip joint replacement, but patients should follow their surgeon's guidelines for resuming intercourse. Positions during all sexual activities should be consistent with hip precautions. A booklet, *Sex after Joint Replacement,* is available for a nominal fee at http://mediapartnersinc.com/products/catalog/cat_JSEXBK.htm.

Suggestions for Selected Instrumental Activities of Daily Living

Writing. If finger range of motion is limited, the size of the writing instrument can be increased by using cylindrical foam, passing the instrument through the holes in a practice golf ball, using commercially available grips that slip on the instrument, or using a comfort-grip pen.

Telephoning. Cordless or mobile phones can be positioned near the person to reduce the reaching distance required. People who cannot grasp the phone or lift it to their ear may benefit from a phone with a speaker feature or from a hands-free device.

Shopping. Online shopping is common, convenient, and economical. People who need to access shops can enlist the help of clerks. Many grocery stores offer this service to people with disabilities to help them get out-of-reach items too heavy to be obtained by use of a reacher (Fig. 25-15B). Shopping during the off hours might increase the likelihood that clerks are available to assist.

Gardening. Strategies that reduce range of reach include the use of raised beds, wearing a carpenter's apron with pockets to keep tools in easy reach, and minimizing planting and weeding, for example, the use of low-maintenance perennial plants. Use tools with ergonomic grips (Fig. 25-3). Use of a rolling or stationary stool to sit while working reduces the range of motion in trunk and lower extremities required to work at the ground level.

Incoordination and Poor Dexterity

For more information and suggestions, see Chapter 35. See also Procedures for Practice 25-3.

Suggestions for Activities of Daily Living

Teach patients to use the body in as stable a posture as is possible, to sit when possible, and to stabilize the upper extremities by bearing weight on them against a surface or by holding the upper arms close to the body, or both (Gillen, 2000). Stabilizing the head may improve a person's ability to control the upper extremities. Friction surfaces, weighted utensils, or weighted cuffs (Fig. 12-14) added to the distal segments of the extremities, and the use of larger and/or less precise fasteners all contribute to increasing independence by lessening the effects of the incoordination (McGruder et al., 2003). For involuntary movements, for example, intention tremors or ataxia, splints may be used to stabilize selected joints, reducing the degrees of freedom that must be controlled by an individual during an activity (Gillen, 2000).

Feeding. The plate can be stabilized on a friction surface, such as a damp towel or nonskid mat. A plate guard or scoop dish can be used to prevent the food from being pushed off the plate. The utensil may be weighted for stability, have an enlarged handle to facilitate grasp, and/or be plastic coated to protect the person's teeth. Sharp utensils should be avoided. A weight cuff on the wrist is often chosen rather than a weighted utensil because the cuff can be heavier; also the cuff makes it unnecessary to weight each item that the patient will use. Weighted cuffs may improve food-to-mouth time, decrease spills, and diminish tremor during eating (McGruder et al., 2003), compared to feeding with no weight. A person may successfully drink from a covered glass or cup with a sipping spout or opening. Some may use a long plastic straw that is held to the side of the cup or glass by a straw holder attachment; the person moves the head to the straw but does not touch it or the cup or glass with the hand. People with incoordination may consider food choices that minimize spilling or staining (e.g., avoiding soups and foods with sauces), particularly when dining outside of the home. In the home, protecting the clothes with a cloth or bib may be desired to minimize soiling clothes and increase satisfaction with the feeding experience.

Grooming. Weighted cuffs on the wrists may help some patients gain greater accuracy while grooming. Standing in a corner enables people with incoordination to stabilize their trunk and head on the wall to the side, and their forearms on the wall in front for activities involving the face, such as brushing teeth, shaving, applying make-up (Gillen, 2000). Large lipstick tubes are easier to use than small ones. The arms must be stabilized to use lipstick. A simple hairstyle is the best choice. For a person who has difficulty holding a large-handled comb, a brush without a handle and with a strap attached across the back of it can be used. Stick deodorant is preferred to spray because it eliminates the risk of accidentally spraying the eyes. *Safety Message: An electric razor is preferred to a safety razor both because it is more easily held and because a safety razor can cut if it is moved sideways over the skin.* People with fairly good head control improve their accuracy shaving by holding the electric razor steady and moving the face over the cutting surface. An electric toothbrush is also useful both because it is heavier and because it can be held steady while the head is moved. This same principle can be employed when filing the nails: fasten the emery board to a flat surface and move each nail over the emery board. Cutting the nails may be unsafe for incoordinated patients, so filing is recommended.

Toileting. The principles described above can be applied to toileting. People with incoordination who require self-catheterization may have difficulty inserting the catheter into the urinary meatus. For women, the Asta-Cath female catheter guide (available online through many sources) helps spread the labia and guide the catheter accurately into the urinary meatus (Ryan & Sullivan, 2011). Sanitary napkins with adhesive strips to hold them in place may be easier to use than tampons.

Dressing. Clothes that facilitate independent dressing are front-opening, loosely fitting garments with large buttons, Velcro™ tape closures, or zippers. Wrinkle-resistant and stain-shedding materials enable the person to look well groomed throughout the day. To overcome difficulty with buttoning, a buttonhook with an enlarged and/or weighted handle, if necessary, can be used. A loop of ribbon, leather, or chain can be attached to the zipper pull so that the person can hook it with a finger instead of pinching the zipper pull. Velcro™ can be substituted to eliminate the need to fasten hooks on a bra. To don a bra, it is easier for the woman to put it around her waist, which is thinner and puts less tension on the garment, then fasten it in front where she can use vision to help guide movements, turn it around, put her arms in, and pull it up into place. Elastic straps or elastic inserts sewn into the straps make this relatively easy. If strength is adequate, a sports-style bra may be used, which eliminates the need for fasteners. A man who wears ties may choose to slide the knot down and pull the tie off over his head without undoing the knot.

Slip-on shoes should be worn, when possible. A shoehorn or foot funnel (available at http://www.footfunnel .com/) may be helpful, particularly for the person with lower extremity ataxia, to preserve the back of the shoe and aid in donning shoes. If tie shoes need to be worn, a variety of lacing aids are available, including elastic laces, which eliminate the need for managing any type of fastener, but create a tighter fit that may hinder slipping the shoe on and off.

Bathing. A person with incoordination may be able to shower or bathe independently but must adhere closely to safety precautions. Slipping is more likely, and often his or her ability to regain lost balance is delayed. Nonslip material should be used in the bottom of the tub, and a nonskid mat should be placed outside the tub to reduce the risk of slipping while stepping in or out of the tub. Safety grab bars should be placed where they would be most useful to the particular person's needs. A tub bench or seat can eliminate the difficulty of sitting in and getting up from the bottom of the tub or stepping over the tub to shower. Walk-in tubs are a practical, but expensive, option for people who have difficulty stepping into the tub, particularly if they desire a tub bath instead of a shower. Showering or bathing from a seated position reduces the risk of slipping and provides a stable position for people as they wash their feet. If a seat is used in the shower, a handheld shower spray is necessary.

Safety Message: Whether the person chooses to shower or bathe, the water should be turned on after the person has transferred in and is seated to reduce the risk of slipping on wet surfaces and splashing water outside of the tub area. A mixer tap is ideal, but if it is unavailable, the cool water should be turned on first and the hot water added to prevent scalding. Soap on a string keeps the soap retrievable, or a bath mitt with a pocket to hold the soap is useful. The water should be turned off and the tub drained, if taking a bath, before the person attempts to stand to transfer out of the tub. An extra large towel or large terry cloth wraparound robe facilitates drying.

Suggestions for Selected Instrumental Activities of Daily Living

Communication. Writing and speech are problems for some persons with coordination deficits. See Chapter 18 for alternative communication systems and adaptations for computers that are appropriate for these patients. If a person's speech is intelligible, the use of a large-button phone reduces the fine motor requirements of dialing the telephone, or a speaker phone with voice-activated dialing can be used.

Playing Games. Board game pieces can be weighted or turned into pegs for stability. Game boards can be reproduced to enlarge the squares. Card holders and card shufflers are useful. Computer games that use keyboarding or switches rather than a mouse or joystick are appropriate.

Loss of Use of One Side of the Body or One Upper Extremity

For other information and suggestions, see Chapters 33, 37, and 41. See also Procedures for Practice 25-3.

Suggestions for Activities of Daily Living

The methods described here pertain to the person with hemiplegia who has lost the use of one side of the body. Some patients post stroke will retain or regain some functional use of the involved upper extremity, increasing the likelihood they will regain independence in their ADL. Techniques for weakness and/or incoordination may be useful for patients who can use the affected arm. However, other patients will have deficits that preclude use of one side of the body. Additionally, they may be prevented from developing independence by cognitive-perceptual impairments, especially of the less automatic tasks, such as one-handed upper extremity dressing (Árnadóittir, 2011; Fletcher-Smith, Walker, & Drummond, 2012; Walker & Walker, 2001). Motor planning deficits, such as ideomotor apraxia, may make learning new skills more difficult; however, patients have been able to learn a new motor process, such as one-handed shoe tying (Poole, 1998).

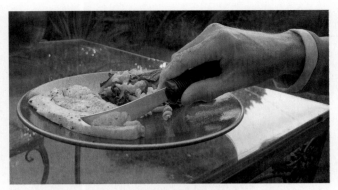

Figure 25-17 Rocker knife for one-handed cutting.

The methods and equipment described here may also be used by a person with a unilateral upper extremity amputation or temporary or permanent upper extremity limitations resulting from trauma. However, patients with upper extremity amputation or injury need fewer adaptations because they have normal trunk and lower extremity function and normal perception and cognition.

Feeding. Feeding is essentially a one-handed task, except for cutting meat and spreading condiments on bread, and these tasks can be done with assistive devices. Food can be simultaneously stabilized and cut by use of a rocker knife, a knife with a sharp curved blade that cuts when rocked over the food (Fig. 25-17). Condiments can be spread on bread if it is stabilized on a nonslip surface or trapped in the corner of a spike board (Fig. 27-2) and spread toward the corner. Soft spreads facilitate this process.

Grooming. Difficulties with grooming include care of the unaffected extremity and completing two-handed activities. Spray deodorant for the unaffected arm is easier to use than other types of applicators. Fingernails of the unaffected hand are cleaned by rubbing them on a small suction cup brush attached to the basin (Fig. 25-18). Fingernails of the affected hand can be trimmed with a stabilized nail clipper (Fig. 25-8A), and those of the unaffected hand, with an emery board fastened down to stabilize it. The fingernail is moved back and forth over the emery board (Fig. 25-8B). Toothpaste in pump bottles or a toothpaste dispenser can be used with one hand. A floss holder or disposable flossers enable patients to floss teeth one-handed.

Using another suction cup brush fastened to the inside of the basin, the person can scrub dentures by rubbing them over the brush. Partially filling the basin with water and laying a face cloth in the bottom cushions the dentures if they are dropped. Patients post stroke should use an electric razor for shaving because they are no longer able to hold the skin taut with one hand during shaving, increasing the risk of cuts.

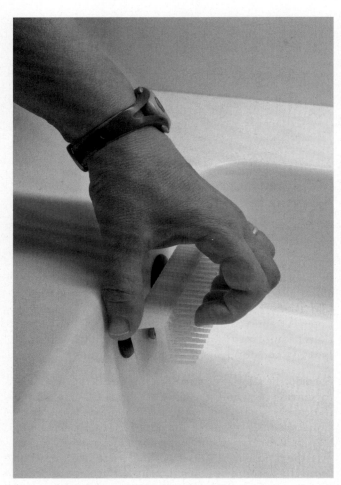

Figure 25-18 Suction cup brush for cleaning nails or dentures one-handed.

Toileting. The primary difficulty with toileting is managing clothing, which is normally done with two hands. A grab bar mounted on the wall beside the toilet and/or a frame mounted on the toilet (Fig. 25-11) will assist transfers and maintaining standing balance. Once standing, pants are unfastened, and gravity pulls them down. If the person's standing balance is impaired, pants should be unfastened before standing and the affected hand placed in the pocket, which prevents the pants from sliding below the knees where they are difficult to retrieve. A woman in a dress can raise her dress on the affected side and tuck it between her body and the affected arm. Then she lowers her underpants to knee level and pulls the dress up on the unaffected side. The toilet tissue should be mounted conveniently to the unaffected side. A woman can manage menstrual needs by use of tampons or adhesive sanitary napkins.

Bathing. The bathing arrangements described for people with incoordination also apply to people with hemiplegia who may also find a long-handled bath sponge with

a pocket to hold the soap useful to allow bathing of the unaffected upper arm and the back. The lower part of the arm of the unaffected side is bathed by putting the soapy washcloth across the knees and rubbing the arm back and forth over it, unless the patient has some return of function and can use a bath mitt on the affected hand. Pump bottles of liquid soap and shampoo are useful, as is soap on a rope. If sensory impairment exists, extra precautions should be taken to be certain of water temperature. Patients with hemiplegia should dry off as much as possible while still seated on the bath seat before transferring out of the tub.

A person with a unilateral upper extremity amputation can bathe using similar strategies. A bath bench enables individuals to place a washcloth on one leg to enable them to wash the unaffected arm without balancing on one leg, which may present a safety risk for people who lack excellent balance.

Dressing. Certain prerequisite abilities are considered important for successful dressing. These are ability to reach each foot, stand unsupported for 10 seconds, and maintain sitting balance when reaching down. The most difficult tasks for both men and women were found to be pulling pants up, putting the shoe on the affected foot, and lacing shoes (Walker & Lincoln, 1991). Many people can manage fasteners one-handed. Patients who have difficulty with one-handed fastening may prefer Velcro™ fasteners, which are easier to use.

Patients with hemiplegia should dress while seated on a stable surface with both feet on the floor to increase stability (Ryan & Sullivan, 2011). As a general rule, the affected limb is dressed first and undressed last.

Shirt or Cardigan Garment: Over-the-Shoulder Method (Ryan & Sullivan, 2011). The over-the-shoulder method is the most similar to the customary method of dressing and garments are less likely to get twisted than when using the overhead method that follows.

1. Put the shirt on the lap, label facing up, collar toward the abdomen, with the sleeve for the affected arm hanging between the knees (Fig. 25-19A)
2. Put the affected hand into the sleeve and lean forward to let gravity extend the elbow and to slide the sleeve onto the arm (Fig. 25-19B).
3. Grasp the collar at the point closest to the unaffected side (Fig. 25-19C).
4. Hold tightly to the collar, lean forward, and bring the collar and shirt around the affected side and behind the neck to the unaffected side (Fig. 25-19C).
5. Put the unaffected hand into the other armhole. Raise the arm out and up to push it through the sleeve (Fig. 25-19D).

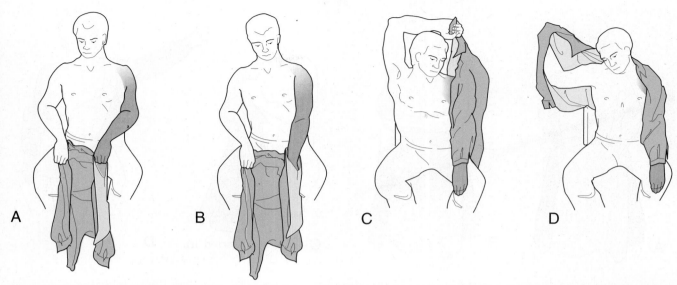

Figure 25-19 Patient with left hemiplegia putting on a shirt. **A.** Position the shirt with the collar toward the knees and the sleeve for the affected arm hanging between the legs. **B.** Guide the affected arm into the sleeve, lean forward, and pull the sleeve up to the shoulder. **C.** Hold the collar tightly. Lean forward and bring the shirt up, around, and behind toward the unaffected arm. **D.** Put the unaffected arm into the armhole. Extend the arm out and up to push it through the sleeve. Straighten the shirt and button it.

6. To straighten the shirt, lean forward, work the shirt down over the shoulders, reach back and pull the tail down, and then straighten the sleeve under the affected axilla.
7. To button, line up the shirt fronts and match each button with the correct buttonhole, starting with the bottom button.

To remove the shirt, unbutton it and use the unaffected hand to throw the shirt back off the unaffected shoulder. Work the shirt sleeve off the unaffected arm, pressing the shirt cuff against the leg to pull the arm out. Lean forward. Use the unaffected hand to pull the shirt across the back. Take the shirt off of the affected arm.

Shirt or Cardigan Garment: Overhead Method (Brett, 1960). The overhead method for putting on and removing front-opening tops may be less confusing for a patient with selected perceptual impairments or limited reach in the unaffected upper extremity. This method is not suitable for coats.

1. Put the shirt on the lap, label facing up, and the collar next to the abdomen; drape the shirttail over the knees (Fig. 25-20A).
2. Pick up the affected hand and put it into the sleeve (Fig. 25-20B).
3. Pull the sleeve up over the elbow (Fig. 25-20C). If the sleeve is not pulled past the elbow, the hand will fall out when continuing.
4. Put the unaffected hand into the armhole. Raise the arm and push it through the sleeve as far as possible (Fig. 25-20D).

5. Gather the back of the shirt from tail to collar (Fig. 25-20E).
6. Hold the gathered shirt up, lean forward, duck the head, and put the shirt over the head (Fig. 25-20F).
7. To straighten the shirt, lean forward and work the shirt down over the shoulders. Often, the shirt gets caught on the affected shoulder and must first be pushed back over the shoulder. Then reach back and pull the tail down (Fig. 25-20G).
8. To button, line up the shirt fronts and match each button with the correct buttonhole, starting with the bottom button.

To remove the shirt, the patient unbuttons it, leans forward, and uses the unaffected hand to gather the shirt up in back of the neck. He or she ducks the head, pulls the shirt over the head, and then takes the shirt off the unaffected arm first.

Pullover Garment. The following steps are used for putting on a pullover garment.

1. Position the garment on the lap, bottom toward chest and label facing down.
2. Using the unaffected hand, roll up the bottom edge of the shirt back, all the way up to the sleeve on the affected side.
3. Spread the armhole opening as large as possible. Using the unaffected hand, place the affected arm into the armhole and pull the sleeve up onto the arm past the elbow. Alternatively, the sleeve may be positioned between the legs and as described above for the cardigan over-the-shoulder method.

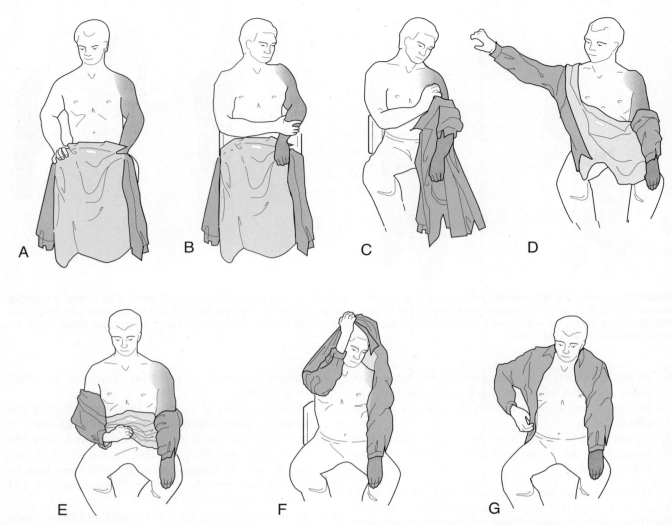

Figure 25-20 Patient with left hemiplegia putting on a shirt, overhead method. **A.** Put shirt on the lap, label facing up, collar next to abdomen, shirttail draped over knees. **B.** Pick up the affected arm and put it into the armhole. **C.** Pull the sleeve well over the elbow. **D.** Put the unaffected hand into the armhole, and raise the arm to push it through the sleeve. **E.** Gather the back of the shirt from the tail to the collar. **F.** Hold the gathered shirt up. Lean forward and duck the head to put the shirt overhead. **G.** To straighten the shirt, lean forward and work the shirt over the shoulders. Reach back and pull the tail down and the front sides forward. Button it.

4. Insert the unaffected arm into the other sleeve.
5. Gather the shirt back from bottom edge to neck, lean forward, duck the head, and pass the shirt over the head.
6. Adjust the shirt on the involved side up and onto the shoulder and remove twists.

To remove, starting at top back, gather the shirt up, lean forward, duck the head, and pull the shirt forward over the head. Remove the unaffected arm and then the affected arm.

Bra. Some patients prefer to use a jogging bra and don it using the overhead method described for a shirt. If the woman prefers to use a regular bra, it is placed around the waist and hooked in front, where she can see what she is doing. Front-fastening bras are easier, because they do not

need to be twisted around the trunk once fastened (Ryan & Sullivan, 2011). One end can be tucked into the waistband of panties or under the affected arm until the other end is brought around, if needed. It is fastened and rotated to the proper position, the affected arm is placed through the shoulder strap, and the unaffected arm is placed through the other shoulder strap. The bra is pulled up into place. It is removed by reversing the process.

A plump woman may need an adapted front-closing bra if she cannot approximate the two edges of the bra to fasten it. The bra is adapted with a D-ring on the side of the bra opening on the involved side and a pile Velcro™strap on the opposite side. After the bra is around the waist, the strap is threaded through the D-ring and pulled to bring the two ends of the bra together. Hook Velcro™ must be stitched onto the bra so the strap can be fastened.

Pants. The following steps describe how to put on pants (Ryan & Sullivan, 2011). Modifications of the following method are used for men's and women's underclothing and pantyhose.

1. Sit. If a wheelchair is used, the brakes should be locked and the footrests should be up and/or swung out of the way. Move the unaffected leg beyond the midline of the body for balance (Fig. 25-21A).
2. Grasp the ankle or calf of the affected leg. Lift and cross the affected leg over the unaffected leg (Fig. 25-21, A & B). Alternatively, cup the affected knee in clasped hands to lift and cross the leg.
3. Pull the pants onto the affected leg up to but not above the knee (Fig. 25-21C).
4. Uncross the legs.
5. Put the unaffected leg into the other pant leg.
6. Remain sitting. Pull the pants up above the knees as far as possible (Fig. 25-21D).
7. To prevent the pants from dropping when standing, put the affected hand into the pant pocket or the thumb into a belt loop (Fig. 25-21E). Alternatively, use a pant clip to attach the pants to the shirt so they do not slide down. Pants with elastic waistbands are also less likely to slide when standing up.

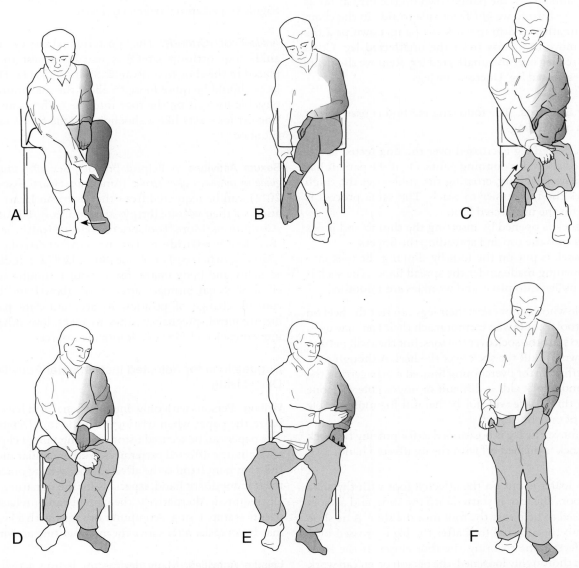

Figure 25-21 Patient with left hemiplegia putting on pants while sitting. **A.** With knees bent, move the unaffected foot across the midline of the body toward the unaffected side. **B.** Grasp the ankle of the affected leg, lift it, and cross it over the unaffected leg. **C.** Pull the pants onto the affected leg up to but not above the knee. **D.** Uncross the legs, put the unaffected leg into the pants, and pull them up above the knees. **E.** To prevent the pants from dropping when the person stands up, put the affected hand into the pocket. **F.** Stand up. Pull the pants over the hips and fasten, or sit to fasten if balance is not good enough to do it while standing.

8. Stand up. Pull the pants up over the hips (Fig. 25-21F); button and zip pants while standing. Persons with poor balance may remain seated and pull the pants up over the hips by shifting from side to side; they should button and zip the pants while seated.

To remove, unfasten the pants while sitting. Stand and let the pants drop past the knees or push down if wearing elastic-waist garment. Sit. Remove the pants from the unaffected leg. Cross the affected leg over the unaffected leg. Remove the pants from the affected leg. Uncross the legs.

Persons with poor balance should use this method: Place locked wheelchair or chair against a wall. Sit. Unfasten the pants. Work the pants down on the hips as far as possible by shifting weight from side to side in the chair. Use the unaffected arm to work the pants down past the hips. Remove the pants from the unaffected leg. Cross the affected leg over the unaffected leg. Remove the pants from the affected leg. Uncross the legs.

Socks or Stockings. The following method is used to put on socks or stockings.

1. The affected leg is crossed over the unaffected as described above for donning pants. Or, if the patient has adequate flexibility, crossing the ankle over the thigh makes the foot easier to reach. The same process is used for the unaffected foot.
2. The sock is opened by inserting the thumb and index finger into the top and spreading the fingers.
3. The sock is put on the foot by slipping the toes into the opening made under the spread hand. The sock is then pulled into place, and wrinkles are smoothed.

People who cannot cross their legs can rest the heel on a small stool. People who cannot reach their feet may use a reacher to start the sock over the toes, but they will need to reach down to pull the sock over the heel. Although sock aids are effective for overcoming limited reach, getting the sock on most sock aids is difficult or impossible with one hand, so this device will not be helpful for most people with use of only one hand.

To remove, the leg is positioned as for putting the sock on. The sock is pushed off with the unaffected hand.

Shoes. A loafer is put on the affected foot with the shoe on the floor. The foot is started into the shoe, and a shoehorn is used to help ease the foot into the shoe. A tie shoe is put onto the affected foot after the leg is crossed over the unaffected one to bring the foot closer. If the laces have been thoroughly loosened, the person often can work the shoe on while the leg is crossed over by grasping the heel of the shoe with the unaffected hand and working it back and forth over the heel until it goes on completely. Sometimes it is necessary to insert a shoehorn while the leg is crossed over and then carefully lower the foot with the shoe half on and shoehorn in the shoe and finish putting on the shoe by repeatedly pushing down on the knee and adjusting the shoehorn.

Tying the shoes is a problem. It is possible to tie a conventional bow one-handed, but it requires fine dexterity and normal perception. The person with an amputation may prefer to do this or use loafers. The person with hemiplegia can use adapted shoe closures or learn a simple, effective one-handed shoe tie as illustrated in Figure 25-22. Putting the lace through the last hole from the outside of the shoe toward the tongue lets the tension of the foot against the shoe hold the lace tight while the bow is being tied. One-handed shoe tying is difficult for patients with cognitive-perceptual deficits to learn.

Ankle–Foot Orthosis. The posterior shell or molded ankle–foot orthosis (AFO) is usually easiest to don if placed in the shoe first (Ryan & Sullivan, 2011). The shoe laces should be quite loose to allow the maximum room possible for getting the foot into the orthosis and shoe. The orthosis acts like a shoehorn, as the foot slides into the shoe.

Sexual Activities. A helpful booklet, *Sex after stroke: Our guide to intimacy after stroke* (American Heart Association, 2011), can be requested from the American Heart Association via their website (http://www.heart.org/HEARTORG /Conditions/More/ToolsForYourHeartHealth/Sex-After -Stroke-Our-Guide-to-Intimacy-After-Stroke_UCM _310558_Article.jsp) or phone (800-242-8721). It discusses sexuality and body image, fears about resuming sex, specifics of sexual intimacy after stroke (bowel and bladder control, change of position to accommodate paralysis, birth control, pregnancy, ways to make love other than intercourse), and a list of additional resources.

Suggestions for Selected Instrumental Activities of Daily Living

Writing. Persons with only one functional arm have to stabilize the paper when writing with the unaffected hand. The paper can be secured using masking tape, a clipboard, a weight, the affected extremity, or other similar means. If the dominant hand is the affected one, writing practice for the nondominant hand, especially for the signature, is usually required. Alternatively, the patient can purchase a signature stamp. Using a computer or tablet with a keyboard may be an easier alternative for many writing activities.

Leisure Activities. Many devices for leisure activities are available for people who have lost the use of one hand, including devices for knitting, crocheting, embroidery, playing cards, and fishing. The list in Resources 25-1 includes sources where devices can be explored and purchased.

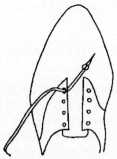

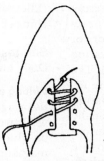

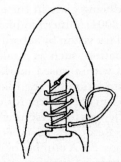

1. Tie a knot in one end of the shoelace. Thread the unknotted end up through the hole nearest the toe of the shoe on the left.

2. Take the lace across the tongue of the shoe and up under the flap on the opposite side of the shoe.

3. Continue to go across the tongue and up under the flap on the next highest hole on the opposite side until you reach the top (or go down through the last hole so the tension will be maintained for tying.)

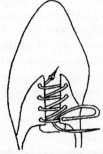

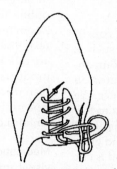

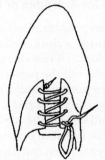

4. Circle around toward the toe of the shoe and go under the part of the lace that is going across the tongue to the last hole.

5. Circle around toward the top of the shoe. Pull free lace through the loop down toward the ankle and out to the left side.

6. Pull loop tight

Figure 25-22 One-handed shoe tie for a person with left hemiplegia. For a person with right hemiplegia, start the lace on the right side of the shoe so that the lace ends on the left side at the top.

Lower Extremity Amputation with Prosthesis

Persons with lower extremity amputations can benefit from many of the adaptations described for people with limited mobility caused by weakness or decreased range of motion; however, lower body dressing for prosthetic users presents a unique challenge not previously addressed. Prior to dressing, a person should change the shoe and/or sock on his or her prosthesis to match the day's clothing. People with a transtibial (below knee) amputation with pants wide enough to pull up to the knee should dress while seated using the following steps:

1. Place pants over unaffected leg and amputated leg, pulling pants up as far as possible.
2. Patients who are stable standing on one leg can stand to pull the pants up, then sit down to don the residual limb stocking and prosthesis, exposing the area by sliding the pant leg up over the knee.
3. Patients who are not stable standing on one leg should remain seated and don the prosthesis before standing to pull up their pants so that they have the stability of both lower extremities when standing to complete the task.

Patients with a transfemoral (above knee) amputation or those with a transtibial amputation who wish to wear fitted pants that cannot be slid up over the knee should dress as follows:

1. Slide the end of the pant leg for the amputated limb down over the top of the prosthesis so that the prosthesis is dressed first. The shoe and limited ankle mobility will prevent the pants from being slid over the prosthetic foot.
2. Don the stocking and the prosthesis.
3. Place the unaffected leg into the pants.
4. Stand to pull up and fasten the pants.

Limited Vision

The suggestions listed here pertain to blindness (20/1250 to worse than 20/2500) and to low vision (20/80 to 20/1000) (Colenbrander & Fletcher, 1995). Organization and consistency in the placement of objects is necessary for persons with visual impairment to locate things efficiently. General strategies to enhance visual performance include enlarging objects, magnification, increasing contrast through better lighting or use of color, and reducing glare in the environment (Ellexson, 2004; Smith, 2001). Other modifications eliminate or reduce the need for vision by substituting with auditory or tactile information, such as a talking clock or locating dryer settings with a raised mark (Ellexson, 2004). The American Foundation for the Blind and Lighthouse International are major sources for obtaining information and assistive devices for persons who are blind or visually impaired (see Resources 25-1). For additional information, see Chapter 23. A number of high-tech solutions are available for persons with impaired vision, particularly for computer usage (see Chapter 18; see also Procedures for Practice 25-3).

Suggestions for Activities of Daily Living

Feeding. When possible, food should be set in a consistent pattern, using a clock method of description, such as "Meat at 3 o'clock." When this is not possible, a companion or server can tell the person where food is located on the plate. When pouring liquid, the correct amount can be determined by inserting a clean finger over the rim to feel when the liquid is near the top or by using a liquid level indicator, which is placed on the rim of the cup and gives an auditory signal when the cup is nearly full. Food is cut by finding the edge of the food with the fork, moving the fork a bite-size amount onto the meat, and then cutting the food, keeping the knife in contact with the fork. For those with low vision, the plate, glass, and utensils should be a color that contrasts with both the table covering and the food.

Grooming. A major problem is identification of objects. This can be done through the use of touch (size, shape, and texture), location, and Braille or bar code labels used with a talking bar code scanner. The application of cosmetics or toiletries is another problem; fingers of the assistive (nondominant) hand can be guides, such as when shaving sideburns or applying eyebrow pencil. Aerosol sprays should be avoided as persons who have low vision cannot see the extent of the spray.

Dressing. Limited vision does not interfere with the physical aspects of dressing, but persons with impaired vision need a system to coordinate colors of clothes and compatibility of style, to determine when clothing is inside-out, and to identify spots or stains. Wrinkle-free, stain-resistant, no-iron fabrics are desirable, and clothes should be hung properly to prevent wrinkles and eliminate the need for ironing. Several adaptations, with the help of a sighted companion, can facilitate the selection of matching clothes, including storing clothes of like color together, putting matching outfits on the same hanger, or using tactile or high contrast identification tags on clothes or hangers to denote the colors

(Ellexson, 2004). Colorless wax polishes can be used to shine shoes.

Suggestions for Selected Instrumental Activities of Daily Living

Writing and Reading. Persons with visual impairment can use a signature or writing guide to stay within boundaries while writing in longhand. Using a black felt-tipped pen on white paper provides good contrast. Talking books and magazines can be used in place of written materials, and a variety of optical devices can enlarge print in newspapers, personal mail, etc. For those with moderately low vision, books, popular magazines, and *The New York Times* come in large-print versions. Many periodicals are available online and can be viewed with a screen magnifier, such as ZoomText (www.synapseadaptive.com/aisquared/zoom text_9/zoomtext_9_magnifier.htm) (Fig. 18-10). There are talking bar code scanners that can be used to identify products in the home and community and devices that scan medicine bottles and inform the person of the medicine in the bottle and the dosage schedule (www.envision-america.com).

Medication Management. Depending on the extent of visual impairment, some people may be able to manage their medications by using magnifiers or marking bottles with large, high-contrast labels or tactile identifiers. For those with significant visual loss, prescription bottle readers can be used to record information from the label. Talking blood pressure and glucose monitors are also available. The American Foundation for the Blind has ideas and resources on their website (http://www.afb.org/senior site.asp?SectionID=66&TopicID=305&Document ID=3271). Pharmacies can also organize and package medications for patients in blister packs so people with low vision can eliminate this challenging task.

Telephoning. People with very limited vision can use phones with tactile indicators on the touch pad, and those with low vision can use phones with large buttons. A phone with one-button automatic dialing is very useful, as are voice-activated phones.

Time. A person can tell time using a Braille or talking watch or clock. Many computer-based calendars and scheduling systems include alarms that can be activated to provide an audio signal when an appointment time is approaching.

Shopping. Persons with low vision may wish to shop using catalogs read by use of closed-circuit television (CCTV) or online with screen magnifiers. Portable CCTV is also available that can be taken out and used in the community. Talking barcode readers may also assist shoppers with visual impairments to identify items and prices.

Handling Money. Tactile discrimination enables the person to identify coins. Paper money can be discriminated by the way it is folded after it has been viewed by magnification or someone else has identified its denomination. Alternatively, people with blindness or low vision may prefer to use a credit card to minimize the need to identify and organize cash.

Playing Games. Braille and large print versions of popular games, such as Monopoly, Bingo, and playing cards, are available. Tactile bingo boards and markers are also available.

Decreased Sensation

For additional information, see Chapter 22. See also Procedures for Practice 25-3.

Suggestions for Activities of Daily Living

Problems of absent, decreased, or disturbed sensation affect performance of ADL and IADL because the automatic knowledge of limb movement and touch may be missing. Training and/or environmental modification to prevent injury is particularly important when interacting with hot or sharp items.

Bathing and Grooming. *Safety Message: To minimize the danger of scalding, hot water heaters should be set to a maximum of 120° Fahrenheit (49° Celsius).* Shower faucets that can be set to one temperature are also safer. When mixing hot and cold water, patients should be instructed to turn the cold water on first and then add hot water gradually. Mixer valves should be installed to compensate when decreased sensation is a permanent condition. Patients with intact areas of sensation can learn to test water temperature with those areas. Wall-mounted sinks give wheelchair users the best access. *Safety Message: but those with impaired lower extremity sensation should insulate hot water pipes and drains to prevent burns if their legs were to come in contact with the plumbing* (Fig. 25-23).

Dressing. *Safety Message: Wrinkles, seams, or bands on clothing that are sufficient to cause tissue damage may not be felt by people with impaired sensation and can cause pressure ulcers within a short time.* Clothing should be selected that is snug enough to prevent bunching, but loose enough to avoid binding or excessive pressure. Persons with insensitive skin should inspect clothing visually or with an area of intact sensation to avoid wrinkles. They must dress warmly in cold weather to prevent frostbite. Fine manipulation needed for fasteners may be affected by decreased sensation in the hand. Patients can learn to compensate visually or may benefit

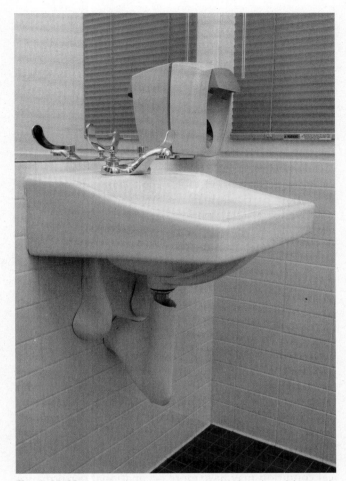

Figure 25-23 Insulating the hot water pipes and drain under a sink prevents burns to the lower extremities of wheelchair users.

from larger fasteners or adaptive devices described for people with impaired coordination, such as button hooks.

Suggestions for Selected Instrumental Activities of Daily Living

Poor sensation interferes with graduated pinch and grip on tools and utensils to meet the demands of the task (Duff, 2005). The person may grip with excessive pressure (Johansson & Westling, 1984) or inadvertently let go, when the attention is directed away from the object being held. Devices discussed earlier for poor grip may help persons with impaired sensation for activities requiring sustained grip.

Safety Message: Activities that involve using hot objects, such as a riding mower or cooking at an outdoor barbecue, pose a threat because anesthetic lower extremities can be burned if allowed to rest against the hot engine cover or bottom of the barbecue. Objects should be insulated when possible and patients trained to be extra vigilant in positioning themselves near hot items.

Cognitive-Perceptual Impairments

See Procedures for Practice 25-3 and Chapters 23 and 24 for information concerning methods to compensate for cognitive or perceptual impairments in ADL.

Pain, Including Low Back Pain

See Procedures for Practice 25-3 and Chapters 27 and 36 for information concerning body mechanics to be used during occupational functioning for persons with low back pain. Adaptations for people with limited range of motion, particularly in reaching the feet, may also be effective for people with low back pain. Adaptations for people with weakness may also increase performance for those with upper extremity pain.

Considerations in Bariatric Care

Occupational therapists are treating increasing numbers of patients who are exceptionally large. Obesity is associated with a number of health problems and is a multidimensional problem that not only impacts physical engagement in daily activities, but affects psychosocial functioning as well (Forhan et al., 2010). Persons who are exceptionally large often have movement limitations that result directly from their size, so these patients often require occupational therapy (Foti, 2005). Several considerations warrant discussion regarding adaptations for these individuals. Excessively large individuals with a medical condition may have more occupational performance deficits than are typically seen because of preexisting limitations in strength relative to body mass, limited reach, and decreased endurance. A thorough functional assessment is needed to ensure that all problems are identified (Foti & Littrell, 2004). *Safety Message: Adaptive equipment must be carefully evaluated to make sure that it has been approved to handle the patient's weight and that it is sized appropriately to meet the patient's needs.* For example, many tub seats are approved to handle up to 300 pounds and cannot be used safely by a heavier person. Traditional sock aids may be too small to accommodate the patient's foot or calf and a soft variety may need to be used (Foti, 2005). The typical home environment may present a number of obstacles for persons of exceptional size, including narrow doorways or pathways that prevent the person from entering a room, particularly those using a wider walker or wheelchair. Bathrooms are commonly too small to be functional for persons who are exceptionally large, and they may find themselves confined to one or two rooms in their homes (Foti & Littrell, 2004). Caregivers may be limited in the tasks they can assist a person with because of risk of physical injuries, so lift equipment may be required in the home. Psychosocial issues may complicate the clinical picture.

Adaptive strategies described above for persons with weakness, limited reach, and/or endurance may all be effective in treating persons of exceptional size. A number of companies have equipment especially designed for the bariatric population that can help the therapist select appropriate and safe adaptations for these patients (see Resources 25-1; also, additional resources are included in the references by Foti [2005] and Foti & Littrell [2004]).

Service Dogs: An Adaptation Option for a Range of Performance Limitations

Service dogs are specially trained to meet the needs of persons with limitations in mobility and/or ADL caused by loss of vision, hearing, and physical impairments. Service dogs are trained collaboratively with the owner so that they learn skills suited to meet the individual's unique needs. The training is extensive and, therefore, expensive, so service dogs are appropriate only for persons with permanent disabilities.

Service dogs can assist people with a variety of tasks. Dogs for people with visual impairment are primarily used for mobility by acting as a guide. Hearing dogs alert their owners to auditory stimuli that require a response, e.g., doorbells, alarm clocks, oven timers, and smoke detectors. Other physical disabilities vary significantly from person to person, and the range of activities that service dogs can assist with is very large (Rintala, Matamoros, & Seitz, 2008). Dogs at Canine Companions for Independence (see Resources 25-1) learn about 40 commands, which can be adapted to individual circumstances. For instance, the tug command is normally used on doors and drawers, but can be used to remove socks or other clothes (Fig. 25-24). The most common activities include help with wheelchair and floor transfers, mobility in home and community, carrying items, operating switches (e.g., lights and elevator buttons), retrieving and moving items, and

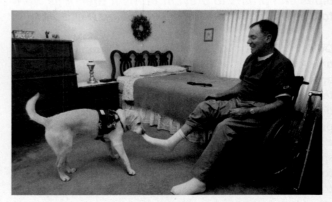

Figure 25-24 Service dog is given the "tug" command to help remove his owner's sock. (Courtesy of Canine Companions for Independence, Santa Rosa, CA.)

opening doors, drawers, and cabinets (Allen & Blascovich, 1996; Rintala, Matamoros, & Seitz, 2008).

Service dogs are an adaptive tool; however, they do not seem to carry the same stigma as assistive devices and may even support social participation. Service dog owners have reported increased interactions with friends and people out in public, increased confidence, and enhanced feelings of safety (Camp, 2001; Fairman & Huebner, 2000). Allen and Blascovich (1996) conducted a randomized controlled study to examine the impact of service dogs on a number of variables, comparing an intervention group that received a service dog and a wait-list control group with no dog. The service dog group had higher scores on psychosocial variables (including self-esteem and community integration), increased participation in school and work, and a decrease of 68% in both paid and unpaid assistance hours. The wait-list group showed a similar pattern of improvement 18 months later when they received their dogs. While the cost of training a service dog was estimated at $10,000, the researchers estimated that savings in personal care attendants would reach $60,000 after 8 years, the average working life of the dog (Allen & Blascovich, 1996). Brashear and Rintala (2007) interviewed veterans with spinal cord injury and found that about one-third had no knowledge of service dogs and 42% desired getting additional information, suggesting that occupational therapists should be knowledgeable about service dogs as an option for enhancing independence and should educate patients about the possibilities.

EFFECTIVENESS OF THERAPY TO RESTORE THE ROLE OF INDEPENDENT PERSON

Evidence from selected quantitative studies, including meta-analyses, systematic reviews, and randomized controlled trials that demonstrate occupational therapy has a positive effect on client functional outcomes in ADL and IADL is summarized in Evidence Table 25-1. Over the past several years, there has been an increase in the number of published studies that demonstrate the efficacy of occupational therapy in improving ADL and IADL. Evidence varies widely in terms of population studied, specific interventions, and outcome measures used to examine changes in ADL and IADL. Four challenges face occupational therapy practitioners searching for evidence in using a modify/adapt approach or occupation-based approach to restoring the role of the independent person, including finding studies that (1) specifically examine interventions that focus on ADL or IADL, (2) examine the practitioners' population of interest, (3) describe the nature of the intervention in sufficient detail, and (4) use relevant outcome measures.

Although many occupational therapy intervention studies include ADL or IADL outcomes, often the intervention did not focus directly on regaining occupation-based skills. For example, Hoffmann et al. (2008) focused only on research evidence related to stroke and occupational

therapy from randomized controlled trials and systematic reviews. They found 452 studies published between 1980 and 2006. Although 70% of those studies included outcome measures of ADL and/or IADL, only a small percentage of the studies were evaluating treatment specifically directed at ADL (8.4%) or assistive technology/adaptive equipment (4.0%). Many more studies examined treatment using a remediation approach, such as movement training (43.2%) or physical modalities and splinting (30.1%). Studies of interventions aimed at restoring underlying functions are important; however, direct treatment of ADL and IADL are at the core of occupational therapy practice, and more extensive evidence is needed to support practice.

The range of compensatory strategies for ADL and IADL is extensive, as is evident in the detailed descriptions in this chapter. Varied patient populations require different approaches to modifying tasks, but many research studies have focused on a single population. ADL and IADL outcomes have been extensively studied in adults post stroke, but practitioners may find limited evidence to support interventions in other populations. A few recent studies have included more heterogeneous populations (e.g., Gitlin et al., 2006), enabling practitioners to generalize results to more patient populations.

A common methodological weakness identified in several meta-analyses or systematic reviews (e.g., Legg, Drummond, & Langhorne, 2006; Steultjens et al., 2003) was that the nature of the occupational therapy was widely varied and/or poorly described, making it difficult for practitioners to apply specific interventions to practice. Variations in treatment to consider include the dosage of treatment (i.e., frequency and length of sessions, as well as overall duration), extent and type of client collaboration in goal setting and treatment planning, practice schedules, service delivery setting (e.g., home, hospital, or community), and individual versus group treatment. In many studies, variations in these approaches are not controlled for, making it difficult to identify key components of an effective intervention. Additionally, ADL and IADL outcomes are measured following multidisciplinary treatment, making it difficult to tease out the unique contributions of occupational therapy (Gitlin et al., 2006).

Finally, occupational therapists examining the evidence will find a wide array of ADL and IADL outcome measures, making comparison across studies challenging. For example, Hoffmann et al. (2008) identified 17 different ADL measures among 358 randomized controlled trials related to stroke outcomes. Different measures may conceptualize ADL in different ways, for example, the FIM™ requires the patient to gather clothing as part of dressing, whereas the Barthel Index does not.

In addition to the quantitative studies summarized in Evidence Table 25-1, qualitative studies can also provide insights that help guide occupational therapy interventions, particularly in terms of individualizing treatment

Evidence Table 25-1 | Best Evidence for Occupational Therapy Practice Regarding Activities of Daily Living

Intervention	Description of Intervention Tested	Participants	Type of Best Evidence and Level of Evidence	Benefit	Statistical Probability and Effect Size of Outcome	Reference
Task-specific practice of client-chosen activities of daily living (ADL)	Practice of specific tasks in a familiar context	Four hundred three stroke survivors (189 left cerebrovascular accident [LCVA], 194 right cerebrovascular accident [RCVA], 20 other); mean age = 72.7 years	Meta-analysis of four studies Level: I	Yes. The treated groups improved in ADL as measured by various ADL assessments.	Mean weighted effect size was $r = 0.30$, equivalent to a 30% success rate over control treatment.	Trombly & Ma (2002)
Home-based occupational therapy	In-home occupational therapy to clients with a diagnosis of stroke; "home" included own home or residential or nursing homes	Nine hundred sixty-five stroke survivors; mean age = 70.0 years	Meta-analysis of five studies Outcome measure focused on instrumental activities of daily living (IADL) Level: I	Yes. The treated group showed small improvement on the Nottingham Extended ADL Scale.	$Z = 2.97$, $p = 0.0003$, effect size $r = 0.10$.	Walker et al. (2004)
Home-based occupational therapy for people post stroke	Treatment that directly addressed ADL, common to all studies included, delivered by an occupational therapist at the patient's home	Nine studies with 1,258 participants living at home post stroke	Systematic review of randomized trials Level: I	Yes. Participants who had occupational therapy were more independent in ADL at discharge and maintained capabilities more than those who received no care or usual care.	Standardized mean difference with a random-effects model was 0.18 (95% confidence interval [CI] = 0.04–0.32), $p = 0.01$, demonstrating more independence in ADL. Odds of death or declining ADL performance were lower in the occupational therapy group (odds ratio = 60, 95% CI = 0.51–0.87, $p = 0.003$).	Legg, Drummond, & Langhorne (2006)
Use of everyday life occupations, including "adaptive or compensatory occupation"	Varied, depending on the study described, but all included direct use of occupations as a therapeutic intervention	Review of 23 studies in stroke rehabilitation, published 2000–2007	Systematic review that included two meta-analyses, seven systematic reviews, four randomized controlled trials, with additional studies at lower levels of evidence Level: I	Occupation-based interventions resulted in better outcomes in ADL, IADL, and participation.	Not reported for specific studies nor for the review overall	Kristensen et al. (2011)

Intervention	Description	Dosage/Duration	Participants	Design/Level	Benefit	Statistics	Author (year)
Occupational therapy and physical therapy at home	Problem-identification and problem-solving training, behavioral interventions (e.g., pacing), and environmental modifications	Six months, including four 90-minute occupational therapy visits, one 20-minute occupational therapy phone contact, and one 90-minute physical therapy visit	Three hundred nineteen community-dwelling adults older than 70 years of age who reported difficulties with two or more IADL and/or one ADL; 82% were female and reported a mean of seven health conditions	Prospective, two-group RCT (treatment and no treatment group) Level: IA2a	Yes. Participants with a range of chronic health conditions had better ADL and IADL performance after home intervention of occupational therapy and physical therapy (with five of six contacts conducted by occupational therapy).	There were statistically significant group differences at 6 months in ADL ($p = 0.03$) and IADL ($p = 0.04$), with biggest differences in bathing and toileting.	Gitlin et al. (2006)
Follow-up occupational therapy in the home after rehabilitation	Home occupational therapy visits for review of assistive devices for bathing introduced in hospital	Control and treatment groups got inpatient instruction; treatment group got two or three home visits	Fifty-three adults with stroke who were discharged home with bathing equipment; mean age = 72.1 years	Single-site RCT Level: IB1b	Yes. The treated group improved more in ADL as measured by the Functional Independence Measure (FIM™) than control group.	$t_{(51)} = 2.002, p = 0.051$, effect size $r = 0.27$, equivalent to a 27% success rate over control treatment	Chiu & Man (2004)
Home-based occupational therapy	Control: Conventional outpatient follow-up Treatment: Conventional plus 6 weeks of home occupational therapy	Client-centered intervention; approximately ten 30–45-minute visits over 6 weeks	One hundred thirty-eight adults with stroke	Single-site RCT Level: IA2a	Yes. Treated group reported higher performance scores on the Canadian Occupational Performance Measure (COPM).	Group differences measured with Mann Whitney $U, p = 0.0006$, $Z = 3.25$, effect size $r = 0.27$.	Gilbertson & Langhorne (2000)
Goal-specific outpatient therapy	Occupational therapy varied slightly at each site, but all included training in IADL; some also addressed ADL and work skills	Mean hours of treatment were 13, 53, and 84 hours at the three sites; mean duration ranged from 12 to 20 weeks	Thirty-one adults with TBI, Rancho Level IV or higher, receiving outpatient occupational therapy at one of three sites	Quasiexperimental pretest/posttest design with no control group Level: IIIB2a	Yes. Goal Attainment Scores (GAS) and COPM performance and satisfaction scores were higher. Gains were retained in follow-up, but no further gains were made. No change in Community Integration Questionnaire.	Improvement in treatment phase as follows: GAS, $Z = 7.52, p < 0.001$, effect size $r = 0.94$ COPM performance, $Z = 4.13, p < 0.001$, effect size $r = 0.71$ COPM satisfaction, $Z = 4.25, p < 0.001$, effect size $r = 0.76$	Trombly et al. (2002)
Inpatient rehabilitation	Occupational therapy "within nine areas of practice," delivered within a rehabilitation program; all participants received ADL training as part of their occupational therapy	Three hours of occupational therapy daily for the duration of the inpatient rehabilitation (average = 31 days)	Forty-three adults with stroke	Quasiexperimental pretest/posttest design with no control group Qualitative component to gather client perceptions of outcomes Levels: Quantitative = IIIB3a Qualitative = N	Yes. Quantitative measures demonstrated improvement in ADL and IADL from admission to discharge.	Significant improvement in ADL measured by the FIM ($t = -9.71, p = .000$) and IADL measured by the ALSAR ($t = 7.75, p = .000$). Clients also reported an improvement in ADL and IADL that they attributed to occupational therapy.	Unsworth & Cunningham (2002)

(continued)

Evidence Table 25-1 Best Evidence for Occupational Therapy Practice Regarding Activities of Daily Living (continued)

Intervention	Description of Intervention Tested	Participants	Dosage	Type of Best Evidence and Level of Evidence	Benefit	Statistical Probability and Effect Size of Outcome	Reference
Occupational therapy, primarily a compensatory approach, including adaptive equipment and energy conservation	Inpatient occupational therapy, including instruction in compensatory strategies for ADL, home management, leisure; education in managing fatigue; and treatment to increase upper extremity function	Thirty adults (27 female, 3 male) with multiple sclerosis from one inpatient unit in the Midwest United States	One week of "intensive" inpatient treatment (daily treatment dosage not indicated)	Quasiexperimental pretest/posttest design with 6-week follow-up Level: IIIB2b	Yes. There was improvement in all six ADL (tub transfers, toileting, feeding, grooming, upper body dressing, and lower body dressing) from admission to discharge and improvement continued at 6 weeks, except for feeding, which had reached maximum level.	ANOVAs for repeated measures on all six variables showed significant improvement from admission to discharge (F ranged from 12.2 to 76.8, with p values for each variable < 0.01 or 0.001). Five variables (all except feeding) showed significant improvement from discharge to 6-week follow-up (F ranged from 4.17 to 20.90, with p values ranging from < 0.05 to < 0.001)	Mathiowetz & Matuska (1998)
Joint protection educational-behavioral program	Control: Standard program, including education on joint protection Treatment: Joint protection including strategies to increase adherence	One hundred twenty-seven adults with rheumatoid arthritis <5 years since diagnosis	Both programs included four 2-hour weekly meetings	Two-site RCT Level: IA1a	Yes. At a 48-month follow-up, treated group had significantly better ADL scores compared with the control.	Group differences measured with Mann-Whitney U, $p = 0.04$, $Z = 1.75$, effect size $r = 0.15$.	Hammond & Freeman (2004)
Service dog	Control: No dog (wait list for 13 months) Treatment: Received service dog 1 month into the study	Forty-eight individuals with severe, chronic ambulatory disabilities requiring wheelchair use; mean age = 25 years	Dog training was 6–12 months; training with participants was not specified	RCT Level: IB2b	Yes. Self-reported biweekly hours of both paid and unpaid assistance were significantly less in the treatment group, suggesting more independence in ADL and IADL performance compared with the control group.	Effect of a service dog on assistance was very large, $r = 0.98$ for paid assistance and 0.96 for unpaid assistance.	Allen & Blascovich (1996)

(Kristensen et al., 2011). For example, Eklund and Ivanoff (2006) evaluated the experience of learning in participants with macular degeneration in a low-vision rehabilitation program. Results included not only participants' reported mastery of content, but which aspects of the program were most effective, such as strategy learning that can be generalized across many homemaking tasks and the value of peer mentoring. These outcomes can be helpful for clinicians in developing new programs, with the understanding that outcome measures pertinent to their own setting and population should be used to verify that the interventions transfer to their setting.

Another qualitative study that can provide valuable insight into ADL and IADL interventions was conducted by Pettersson, Appelros, and Ahlström (2007), who described the complex and, at times, contradictory perceptions individuals have related to their adaptive equipment. Understanding the dual perception patients may have that adaptive equipment supports independence while at the same time highlighting their disabilities can help occupational therapists address barriers to adaptive equipment use that may facilitate ADL or IADL independence.

Consideration of the findings of the research summarized above and in Evidence Table 25-1 may help occupational therapists develop more effective intervention and may direct occupational therapy researchers to problems that require additional study.

Environment-Client Focused Activity Analysis Case Example
Environment-Client Focused Activity Analysis: Increasing Independence in Self-Feeding

Patient Information

Mr. W. is a 20-year-old, right-handed man who sustained a traumatic brain injury 1 month ago. He was in a coma for 2 weeks and spent 3 weeks in an acute care hospital before being transferred to a rehabilitation center. Mr. W. was NPO (*nil per os*, or "nothing by mouth") until a swallowing evaluation revealed that it was safe to begin eating orally (i.e., he can swallow all foods effectively), and the occupational therapist has begun to work on self-feeding. Mr. W.'s impairments include left hemiplegia (paralysis of the left side) with poor sitting balance and mild ataxia. He has significant cognitive deficits, including poor attention span, poor short-term memory, low frustration tolerance, and very limited awareness of deficits. He is easily distracted by auditory and visual stimuli in the environment. He can follow one-step directions but is unable to follow more complex instructions. He appears to be motivated to eat, grabbing at food that is placed within his reach; however, nursing has not been able to allow him to feed himself because he does not pace himself appropriately, "shoveling" food into his mouth without chewing and swallowing between bites. Although he can swallow safely, this behavior creates a choking risk.

Task Analysis Process	Intervention Planning	Therapeutic Transactions: Preparation for and Interactions at the Occupational Therapy Session	Clinical Reasoning: Example of Therapist's Internal Dialogue
S E L E C T I O N Specify the task that the person needs or wants to perform in a given environment Specify the performance environments (environment in which the patient will perform the desired activity; environment in which the therapy session will occur)	Self-feeding is a very basic self-care skill, and Mr. W. is demonstrating motivation to feed himself by grabbing for food. When fed, he readily chews and swallows food and looks to the feeder for another bite. The therapy session will occur in Mr. W.'s room in the rehab facility. Eventually, he will need to feed himself in a variety of places, including his home, others' homes, restaurants, cafeterias, outdoors, and other possible locations, such as the car.	The occupational therapist decided to work on feeding during lunch. The nursing staff and Mr. W.'s parents have stated he is not a "morning person." The occupational therapist also consulted with Mr. W. and his family to select foods that he both liked and would meet his nutritional needs.	"Mr. W. is easily frustrated and I want to work with him at a time when he is at his best and to select foods that will be motivating for him to eat." "Being able to work with Mr. W. in his room, rather than in the patient dining area or clinic, will allow me more control over the environment, because he is very distractible. Once he is able to feed himself effectively in his room, I will make a plan to help him transition to eating in the patient dining room, which would be closer to eating with his family at home or out at a restaurant."

(continued)

| A N A L Y S I S | Evaluate the barriers or enablers to performance of this activity in this environment: 1. Task 2. Environment 3. Person | **Barriers:** 1. Some aspects of feeding require bilateral hand use, e.g., cutting food, eating sandwiches or a hamburger, and opening containers. Eating includes some safety considerations, e.g., moderating the amount of food intake to prevent choking and managing hot food and drink to prevent burns. 2. Mr. W.'s family is very involved and is usually in the room at lunchtime, presenting a distraction. His hospital bed does not enable him to sit up straight enough to get close to the table. 3. Mr. W. has no use of his left upper extremity (UE) for bilateral tasks (such as cutting meat or picking up a sandwich). His sitting balance and posture is poor. He is impulsive and does not swallow before putting more food into his mouth. **Enablers:** 1. Feeding is mostly a unilateral task, so he will be able to do most of it with his functional right UE. It is usually done seated, requiring minimal trunk control and no lower extremity function. The cognitive demands are not great. The length of the task is easily adjusted. 2. The hospital room can be modified to minimize distractions. 3. Mr. W. is right-hand dominant, so eating with the right hand will be familiar to him. Feeding is also a very well-learned task that he will likely be able to recall. | **Materials required:** • Food tray with food items placed in individual dishes, including a tuna sandwich, potato salad, applesauce, and juice (in covered cup with straw) • Wheelchair • Bedside table • Adaptive equipment: large-handled utensils, including a spoon with a small bowl, nonslip mat, covered mug • Damp towel and hospital gown **Safety precautions:** • Eliminate hot foods and the need for sharp utensils (e.g., steak knife) for initial treatment sessions • Present foods one at a time to reduce the chance of eating too fast, which could cause choking | "Before we get started, I want to optimize the environment by minimizing distractions. I explain to the family that I want to begin working with Mr. W. alone because he has a hard time focusing on eating when there are a lot of people in the room. I make sure to tell them I will invite them back at the end of the session to explain what we did and how they might be able to help Mr. W. when he is eating safely enough to do so with family, because I know they very much want to help Mr. W. but need some direction." "I make sure the TV is off and the door is closed. I help Mr. W. transfer to his wheelchair, which has been set up to provide him with good trunk stability. The wheelchair will maintain a good posture for eating and allow me to put food on the bedside table close to him. He is dressed in jeans and a t-shirt, so I put on a hospital gown to protect his clothing, and I keep a towel nearby in case of spills, which could trigger frustration." "To begin, I present only the applesauce with a spoon because (1) he is not distracted by other foods; (2) it is a limited amount, so is safer if he begins to 'shovel'; and (3) I can focus on his ability to use a spoon. I will present each food item independently and without adaptive equipment, unless I see something suggesting that the equipment might be helpful (e.g., the plate is slipping, he scoops too much onto a regular-size spoon, or he cannot control the volume of liquid when sipping through a straw). Adaptive equipment can be really helpful, but it is unfamiliar to him and I want to minimize its use." |

	Determine solutions that will enable performance: 1. Person 2. Environment 3. Task	Solutions: 1. Position upright and supported in wheelchair with table close and in front. 2. Minimize visual and auditory distractions 3. Present one food item at a time. Use softer foods to reduce choking hazard if he takes too large a bite. Have adaptive equipment available to intervene, if needed. In particular, a smaller spoon would limit how much food he could get in a single bite.		"I will not make small talk, because that would be a distraction. I will keep instructions as short and simple as I can and may need to remove the food from in front of Mr. W. when I am giving an instruction."
G R A D A T I O N	Specify task and environmental parameters to calibrate difficulty level: • Method of instruction • Nature and level of cueing • Objects and their properties (materials and equipment) • Space demands • Social demands • Sequence and timing • Required actions and performance skills • Required body functions • Familiar or novel task or environment • Known adaptations or specifics to design and build the needed adaptation	To progress Mr. W., reduce the number of verbal cues, increase the number of food items available at one time, decrease reliance on adaptive utensils (if used), and transition into more natural eating environments (e.g., the patient dining room). Feedback to increase self-awareness may be introduced, e.g., "Did you swallow the last bite before taking this one?" The family can be instructed in how to set up the environment and cue Mr. W. for safe and independent self-feeding.	Explain to Mr. W.'s family how to adapt the feeding task and environment so that he will pace self-feeding appropriately, including when and how to provide verbal, gestured, or tactile cues. Gradually increase the number of food items on the table in front of him. As Mr. W. becomes able to self-feed effectively in his room, the environmental demands can be increased, e.g., eat a meal in the dining room, gradually introducing more distractions (e.g., eat at a table at the edge of the room with one other person, then increase number of diners and/or change the placement within the room). Introduce adaptive methods for bilateral tasks (e.g., use of a rocker knife to cut meat) and/or begin to incorporate the left UE into feeding if he begins to get some active control.	"I want to provide Mr. W. with more opportunity for practice. His family really wants to help, but they do not know how to help him to avoid outbursts of frustration or control his impulsivity. Teaching them specific strategies will engage them effectively in his care. Plus they are also here for dinner, giving Mr. W. lots more practice. I will make sure to observe them to provide feedback and give them the confidence they need to carry through with this." "Right now, Mr. W. does not have the cognitive ability to problem solve, but I can start to ask questions about his self-awareness. I want to be careful not to trigger an angry response, but I want to monitor him so I can work more on that when he begins to show signs that self-awareness is emerging." "Mr. W.'s capacity for learning new tasks is limited right now, but when he shows some retention of new skills, I can teach him some news ways of doing things, such as cutting food with a rocker knife. I also want to look for any return of movement in his left UE because I can try to increase movement by having him use it in simple tasks, such as holding the dish while he eats dessert or using two hands to pick up his cup to drink."

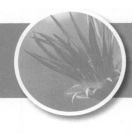

case example

Mrs. C.: Adaptation and Training for Basic Activities of Daily Living

Occupational Therapy Intervention Process	Clinical Reasoning Process	
	Objectives	Examples of Therapist's Internal Dialogue

Patient Information

Mrs. C. is a 50-year-old woman who was admitted to an inpatient rehabilitation unit 1 week after a decompression laminectomy with fusion of T5-T6 secondary to a metastatic spinal tumor with resulting paraparesis. The primary tumor was breast cancer, diagnosed and treated 3 years ago, and she was cancer free until the spinal tumor. The inpatient occupational therapy (OT) assessment revealed the following primary problems: (1) minimal to maximal assistance with bathing, dressing, toileting, bowel and bladder management, and transfers; (2) limited reach secondary to spinal orthosis, which restricts trunk and hip flexion (worn whenever upright for 8 weeks postoperatively); (3) significant trunk and lower extremity weakness (2–/5) leading to poor sitting balance; (4) persistent pain in the midthoracic area; (5) fatigue; and (6) possible depression.

Mrs. C. is in a stable and supportive marriage and has two teenage children living at home. She works as an elementary school nurse. Her husband works full time. She lives in a two-story home. All bedrooms are on the second floor. There is a half-bath on the first floor and a full bath on the second. Mrs. C. sought out both Western and complementary health care when treating her breast cancer, including acupuncture and yoga. Her immediate goal is to be able to return home without having to rely heavily on her family for assistance and to be able to cook for her family. Eventually, she wants to return to work.

Appreciate the context

"Mrs. C. has an incomplete spinal cord injury and it is hard to predict what her sensorimotor function will ultimately be. She will probably be discharged from inpatient rehabilitation within about 3 weeks, however, which means she will almost certainly still be relying on a wheelchair and will be wearing her brace for the first month she is home. Her home has some environmental barriers that will need to be looked at."

"Being diagnosed with metastatic cancer after being cancer free for 3 years must be very difficult for Mrs. C. It appears that she might have a reactive depression. I wonder if she is being treated for that. I wonder what her prognosis is. I should remember to look in her chart to find out the tumor grade and check my pathology books for a refresher on prognosis for metastatic cancer. Her active involvement in her prior treatment, such as using alternative treatments, suggests she might be anxious to work collaboratively in the rehab process."

"I wonder how her kids and husband are responding to all this. Mrs. C.'s goals suggest that she wants to return some level of 'normalcy' to their family routines as soon as possible."

Develop intervention hypotheses

"I think that the things interfering most with Mrs. C.'s ability to be independent in activities of daily living (ADL) are her limited reach (because of brace, lower extremity weakness, and impaired sitting balance), fatigue, and back pain. I am wondering if depression might be exacerbating her pain and fatigue. The home environment also presents some obstacles. Mrs. C.'s background as a nurse will support the rehabilitation process. Her prior routines that included healthy exercise (yoga) have left her with excellent upper extremity strength that she can use to compensate for her paraparesis. Her family is supportive, and her desire to return to her roles as wife and mother seems to be a powerful motivator for participation in treatment."

Select an intervention approach

"At this point, I will primarily rely on an approach that compensates for Mrs. C.'s deficits because her inpatient rehabilitation stay will be fairly short and it is important to her to minimize her dependence on her family when she returns home. Additionally, it is likely she will be using a wheelchair at discharge, and her home is not currently accessible. Modifying the physical environment will require some time and should be started right away. Although fatigue can be approached with a remediation approach to increase the physical component, I think that the level of activity required for learning compensatory strategies will be enough to increase activity tolerance without using a rote exercise program."

Reflect on competence	"I have worked with many patients who are limited by a back brace, but I have not worked with many who also have paraparesis. I'll need to think more about how to combine methods to help Mrs. C. reach her feet for dressing and bathing that will work with lower extremities that lack functional movement. I am also not sure how to address the prognosis issue. Is she worried about her life expectancy? Should I invite her to talk about this, or would that be upsetting to her?"

Recommendations

The occupational therapist will see Mrs. C. twice a day for 45-minute treatment sessions. The following long-term goals were established for Mrs. C. to reach prior to her discharge home: (1) Mrs. C. will be independent in all ADL except donning shoes and socks and washing feet; (2) Mrs. C. will be independent in sliding-board transfers, wheelchair to and from bed, upholstered chair, toilet, transfer tub seat, and car; (3) Mrs. C. will be independent in planning and preparing simple, hot meals with a maximum of a 10 on the Borg Rating of Perceived Exertion at the completion of the task; (4) Mrs. C. will be able to access necessary facilities in her home, including bed, toilet, shower, kitchen appliances, and electronics (telephone, computer, TV, etc.); and (5) Mrs. C. will be independent in wheelchair mobility on smooth level surfaces and appropriately graded ramps.

Consider the patient's appraisal of performance	"Mrs. C. seems to have a realistic view of her abilities and limitations. If anything, she seems to underestimate what she can do, for example, she feels she cannot do anything herself, but she can feed herself, complete grooming, and bathe her face, arms, and thighs."
Consider what will occur in therapy, how often, and for how long	"I'm going to bring up the issue of depression in team meeting. I think she should be evaluated because if she is clinically depressed, antidepressants might help with pain management and reducing fatigue, which would allow her to participate more actively in treatment. Right now, it is hard to make the most of the 90 minutes I have allotted for treatment each day. In the meantime, I need to make sure I use the right balance of physically challenging tasks and those that rely on more of her cognitive abilities, such as making plans to improve the accessibility of her home. That way I can use all the valuable treatment time without overtaxing her."
Ascertain the patient's endorsement of plan	"Mrs. C. strongly agrees with the goals, although she seems to doubt whether all this can be accomplished in just 3 weeks. Her sense of self-efficacy seems pretty low right now and will need to be addressed in treatment. It might help to also involve her family in this aspect of care so they can help her see her progress, no matter how small the steps seem to be at first."

Summary of Short-Term Goals and Progress

1. *Mrs. C. will require minimal assistance to don underwear and pants using adaptive equipment.*

The therapist thought that donning the elastic stockings that Mrs. C. is required to wear and donning shoes would be very difficult to master while the back brace had to be worn. The therapist explained the challenges these tasks presented, and Mrs. C. agreed that it would be all right to have her husband help with shoes and socks until the brace was removed and she could reach her feet without adaptive equipment. Mrs. C. positioned herself in long sitting, resting against the elevated hospital bed. She was able to use a dressing stick to get her pants over her feet with minimal assistance and verbal cues to increase her effectiveness with the dressing stick.

2. *Mrs. C. will be independent in self-catheterization.*

Mrs. C. could not see her urinary meatus because the back brace prevents trunk flexion. She was given a leg abductor with a mirror that enabled her to see.

Assess the patient's comprehension	"Mrs. C. follows instructions well and remembers strategies that are taught to her (for example, the steps to doing a sliding-board transfer), but she still requires help to initiate problem solving. For example, she needed prompting to come up with ways to apply energy conservation principles to a cooking task. Again, this might be related to depression. She was diagnosed with clinical depression and started on medication, but we cannot really expect to see a change for 3 weeks or so, and by that time she will be home. So I just continue to use treatment that I hope will be extra motivating. She loves to be able to transfer to the couch with her family where they can sit close on the couch and visit or watch TV without the wheelchair as a barrier between them. She said she was also glad to be able to make a snack for her kids, 'just like a mom!'"
Understand what he or she is doing	

3. *Mrs. C. will require supervision for sliding-board transfers from wheelchair to/from bed and level, firm, upholstered surfaces.*

Mrs. C. progressed quickly with sliding-board transfers because her upper extremity strength was excellent and helped her both maintain her balance and move her body along the board. The therapist now just provides supervision in case Mrs. C. loses her balance and pitches forward during the transfer. The therapist instructed Mrs. C.'s husband and children how to "guard" her during transfers, which enabled Mrs. C. to transfer onto the couch in the lounge when her family visited.

4. *Mrs. C. will prepare brownies from a box mix with verbal cues and stand-by assistance with a max of 13 on the Borg Rating of Perceived Exertion.*

Mrs. C. was instructed in energy conservation techniques prior to the cooking task and identified three strategies she could use to reduce the energy demands of the task with four verbal cues from the therapist. She used reachers, a rolling cart, and long oven mitts to complete the task. She reported her perceived exertion was a 12. She shared her brownies with her family when they came in later to visit.

5. *Mrs. C.'s husband will bring in a layout of the first floor of their home with measurements, as requested by the occupational therapist in preparation for home modifications to increase wheelchair accessibility.*

Initially, Mrs. C. and her husband preferred to wait on the home modifications, hoping that she might be able to walk with a walker upon discharge. When Mrs. C. got into her second week, they realized that significant changes needed to be made at home and the husband brought in the requested information. Mrs. C. was especially upset to learn that the bathroom door was 1 inch narrower than her wheelchair.

Next Steps

- Continue to modify short term goals to progress patient toward ADL, mobility, and cooking using adaptive equipment and methods
- Make preliminary recommendations for home assessment, collaborating with Mrs. C. and her husband to determine the "best" solution and provide a home program to support follow-through with recommendations (see Fig. 25-25)
- Complete a home visit with Mrs. C. and her husband to examine accessibility and make final recommendations
- Provide training to husband and children (as appropriate— determined collaboratively with Mrs. C.) in any areas that required assistance or supervision
- Examine options for home-based occupational therapy and write a referral

---

Compare actual to expected performance

"Mrs. C. is actually progressing a little faster than I expected with physical tasks such as transfers and lower body dressing. Maybe her experience with the difficult and controlled postures of yoga helps her adapt her movements to her 'new' body. She also is not afraid to experiment with movement and that might be why she progressed so quickly with transfers and maneuvering the dressing stick for lower body dressing. Maybe I can push her a little more with the physical activities, as long as I watch her fatigue level."

Know the person

Appreciate the context

"Funny, I did not really expect the resistance to bringing in home plans and measures. I guess those kinds of changes drive the reality of Mrs. C.'s disability home for both her and her husband. Mrs. C. seems especially upset about the bathroom. I wonder if her husband or a friend is handy enough to reframe the door so she can get to the toilet. We are also going to have to address the issue of the bed. I think she would be better off with a hospital bed until the brace is off because it helps with bed mobility and sitting balance for dressing, but this might be a 'hard sell' for both Mrs. C. and her husband."

Anticipate present and future patient concerns

"I think Mrs. C. will progress well with independence in occupational performance. I expect the home modifications will be a bigger challenge. She wants to be able to access the full bathroom and her bedroom upstairs, but this would require an expensive stair glide, which may be premature (and Mrs. C. has also said she does not want 'such an eyesore' in her house). Intellectually, I think Mrs. C. understands the problems. Emotionally, the choices are hard. The temporary 'fixes' make her feel more disabled (changing the living room to her bedroom, replacing the bathroom door with a curtain so she can get to the toilet, etc.). This is an issue that she will continue to deal with after discharge."

Decide if he or she should continue or discontinue therapy and/ or return in the future

"I think home-based therapy would be best for Mrs. C. after discharge. She certainly has a lot of skilled occupational therapy needs as we had little time to address a host of instrumental activities of daily living (IADL), as well as work and leisure tasks. She would qualify for home occupational therapy as she is home bound. Additionally, it would be helpful to work with her in her actual environment where she might feel more comfortable problem solving. Once she is out of the brace, she will become more mobile and should switch to out-patient therapy, which might include a driving evaluation and treatment and possibly return-to-work training."

Modifications for the 1st floor bathroom:

Purchase:
- Left-side toilet armrest
- Raised toilet seat
- Towel rack
- Small shelf
- Insulation for pipes under sink
- Curtain for doorway

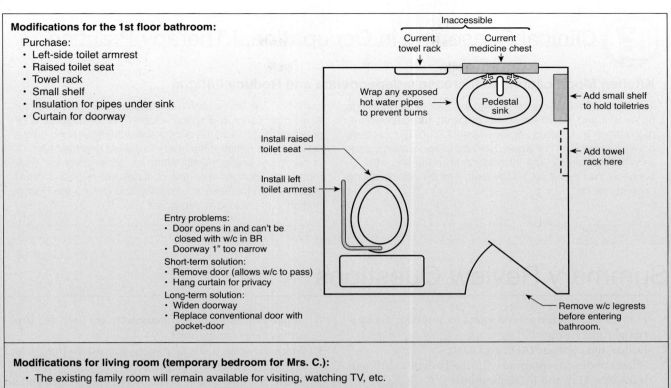

Inaccessible

Current towel rack

Current medicine chest

Wrap any exposed hot water pipes to prevent burns

Pedestal sink

→ Add small shelf to hold toiletries

→ Add towel rack here

Install raised toilet seat

Install left toilet armrest

Entry problems:
- Door opens in and can't be closed with w/c in BR
- Doorway 1" too narrow

Short-term solution:
- Remove door (allows w/c to pass)
- Hang curtain for privacy

Long-term solution:
- Widen doorway
- Replace conventional door with pocket-door

Remove w/c legrests before entering bathroom.

Modifications for living room (temporary bedroom for Mrs. C.):
- The existing family room will remain available for visiting, watching TV, etc.
- This arrangement allows Mrs. C. privacy while retaining space for quiet visiting.
- The current plan is for the arrangement to be temporary until it is possible for Mrs. C. to access the 2nd story where her bedroom and full bath is.
- Purchases and modifications:
  - 1 or 2 privacy screens to reduce visability of the bedroom portion of the living room.
  - Empty the existing bookshelf to use for everyday clothing.
  - Bring a nightstand down from the upstairs bedroom.
  - Purchase a touch-lamp for the bedside table.

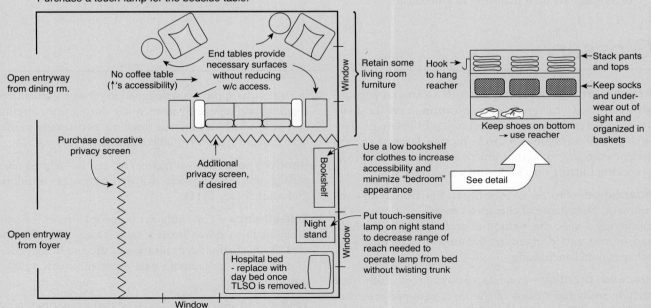

Open entryway from dining rm.

No coffee table (↑'s accessibility)

End tables provide necessary surfaces without reducing w/c access.

Window

Retain some living room furniture

Hook → to hang reacher

Stack pants and tops

Keep socks and underwear out of sight and organized in baskets

Keep shoes on bottom → use reacher

Purchase decorative privacy screen

Additional privacy screen, if desired

Bookshelf

Use a low bookshelf for clothes to increase accessibility and minimize "bedroom" appearance

See detail

Open entryway from foyer

Night stand

Window

Put touch-sensitive lamp on night stand to decrease range of reach needed to operate lamp from bed without twisting trunk

Hospital bed - replace with day bed once TLSO is removed.

Window

Figure 25-25 Home program for Mrs. C.: modifications to maximize independence in the home upon discharge.

Clinical Reasoning in Occupational Therapy Practice

Kitchen Modifications to Increase Independence and Reduce Fatigue

The occupational therapist is preparing for a predischarge home visit and would like to be prepared to make recommendations that would improve Mrs. C.'s ability to access cooking items from her wheelchair and to apply energy conservation strategies. The information from Mr. and Mrs. C. suggests that they have a fairly large kitchen with an eating nook at one end.

What are some common accessibility problems for wheelchair users in a typical kitchen? What supplies and/or equipment should the occupational therapist bring on the home visit to optimize her ability to assess and treat Mrs. C. in her home environment? What are some common environmental changes that the occupational therapist could implement to increase accessibility and reduce the energy demands of cooking in the home?

Summary Review Questions

1. How is occupation-as-end used to improve occupational functioning?
2. Define and contrast IADL and ADL.
3. What conditions interfere with the patient's ability to learn new ADL and IADL methods?
4. What principle of compensation is implemented when a patient with limited or restricted range of motion uses a sock aid?
5. What device can enable use of utensils when a patient lacks active grasp?
6. What modifications may be necessary to enable a person with C6 tetraplegia to complete the tasks required of a college student majoring in journalism?
7. What principles of compensation are used for problems of incoordination?
8. State the steps a stroke patient can use to put on and remove a cardigan-type garment.
9. Name five energy conservation techniques and give an example of each that could be used by a patient with cardiac disease for home management.
10. Identify two ways the task and/or environment can be adapted to enable a person with low vision to efficiently identify spices during cooking.

Glossary

Active learning—A process in which a learner is engaged physically and/or cognitively in a learning task. Learners are engaged in finding a solution to a problem (e.g., identifying three ways cooking can be modified to save energy) and/or engaging in actual practice of the solution (e.g., practicing putting on a sock with a sock aid).

Adaptation—Process of learning to function in an environment. Occupational therapists enable that process by modifying a task, the method of accomplishing the task, and/or the environment to promote independence in occupational functioning.

Blocked practice—Practice consisting of drills that include many repetitions of the same task performed in the same way (Schmidt & Lee, 2011).

Errorless learning—Process of learning in which the teacher structures learning activities in a way that prevents the learner from making errors. In contrast to trial-and-error

learning, this approach is designed to prevent learners from recalling and repeating errors made during prior attempts of a task, which can impede learning, particularly in those with impaired memory (Gillen, 2009).

Random practice—Practice of several related tasks within one session; sequence of tasks varies randomly (Schmidt & Lee, 2011).

Self-efficacy—The judgments people have of their capabilities to do or learn a task (Falvo, 2011; Sanford et al., 2006). Self-efficacy is task-specific and is dependent, in part, on an individual's past experience with a task or similar tasks.

Task parameter—A property or characteristic of a task that can be measured and addressed in treatment. Independence is the most commonly used, but other parameters might include duration of task, quality of performance, or level of fatigue resulting from task performance.

References

Ainsworth, B. E., Haskell, W. L., Herrmann, S. D., Meckes, N., Bassett, D. R., Tudor-Locke, C., Greer, J. L., Vezina, F., Whitt-Glover, M. C., & Leon, A. S. (2011). 2011 Compendium of physical activities: A second update of codes and MET values. *Medicine & Science in Sports & Exercise, 43,* 1575–1581.

Allen, K., & Blascovich, J. (1996). The value of service dogs for people with severe ambulatory disabilities: A randomized controlled trial. *Journal of the American Medical Association, 275,* 1001–1006.

American College of Rheumatology. (2012). *Sex and arthritis.* Retrieved June 16, 2013 from http://www.rheumatology.org/practice/clinical/patients/diseases_and_conditions/sexandarthritis.pdf.

American Heart Association. (2011). *Sex after stroke: Our guide to intimacy after stroke.* Retrieved June 16, 2013 from www.heart.org/HEARTORG/General/Sex-After-Stroke-Our-Guide-to-Intimacy-After-Stroke_UCM_310558_Article.jsp.

American Heart Association. (2012). *Sex and heart disease.* Retrieved June 16, 2013 from http://www.heart.org/HEARTORG/Conditions/More/MyHeartandStrokeNews/Sex-and-Heart-Disease_UCM_436414_Article.jsp.

American Occupational Therapy Association. (2008). Occupational therapy practice framework: Domain & process (2nd ed.). *American Journal of Occupational Therapy, 62,* 625–683.

Árnadóittir, G. (2011). Impact of neurobehavioral deficits on activities of daily living. In G. Gillen (Ed.), *Stroke rehabilitation: A function based approach* (3rd ed., pp. 456–500). St. Louis: Elsevier Mosby.

Bandura, A. (1977). Self-efficacy: Toward a unifying theory of behavior change. *Psychological Review, 84,* 191–215.

Bandura, A. (1997). Self-efficacy. New York: W. H. Freeman.

Boman, I., Tham, K., Granqvist, A., Bartfai, A., & Hemmingsson, H. (2007). Using electronic aids to daily living after acquired brain injury: A study of the learning process and the usability. *Disability & Rehabilitation: Assistive Technology, 2,* 23–33.

Brashear, T., & Rintala, D. (2007). Interest in service dogs by veterans with spinal cord injuries: A pilot study. *SCI Psychosocial Process (Online; available to subscribers), 20.*

Brett, G. (1960). Dressing techniques for the severely involved hemiplegic patient. *American Journal of Occupational Therapy, 14,* 262–264.

Camp, M. M. (2001). The use of service dogs as an adaptive strategy: A qualitative study. *American Journal of Occupational Therapy, 55,* 509–517.

Carson, D., Gaya, A., & Milantoni, C. (2008). *Energy conservation: Achieving a balance of work, rest and play.* Toronto, Canada: VHA Rehab Solutions.

Chemerinski, E., Robinson, R. G., & Kosier, J. T. (2001). Improved recovery in activities of daily living associated with remission of poststroke depression. *Stroke, 32,* 113–117.

Chen, T.-Y., Mann, W. C., Tomita, M., & Nochajski, S. (2000). Caregiver involvement in the use of assistive devices by frail older persons. *Occupational Therapy Journal of Research, 20,* 179–199.

Chiu, C. W. Y., & Man, D. W. K. (2004). The effect of training older adults with stroke to use home-based assistive devices. *OTRJ: Occupation, Participation, and Health, 24,* 113–120.

Clark, J., & Rugg, S. (2005). The importance of independence in toileting: The views of stroke survivors and their occupational therapists. *British Journal of Occupational Therapy, 68,* 165–171.

Colenbrander, A., & Fletcher, D. C. (1995). Basic concepts and terms for low vision rehabilitation. *American Journal of Occupational Therapy, 49,* 865–869.

Dallas, M. J., & White, L. W. (1982). Clothing fasteners for women with arthritis. *American Journal of Occupational Therapy, 36,* 515–518.

Dreeben, O. (2010). *Patient education in rehabilitation.* Boston, MA: Jones and Bartlett.

Duckworth, B. (1986). Overview of menstrual management for disabled women. *Canadian Journal of Occupational Therapy, 53,* 25–29. Retrieved June 16, 2013 from www.caot.ca/cjot_pdfs/cjot53/53.1Duckworth.pdf.

Duff, S. (2005). Impact of peripheral nerve injury on sensorimotor control. *Journal of Hand Therapy, 18,* 277–291.

Eklund, K., & Ivanoff, S. (2006). Health education for people with macular degeneration: Learning experiences and the effect on daily occupations. *Canadian Journal of Occupational Therapy, 73,* 272–280.

Ellexson, M. (2004). Access to participation: Occupational therapy and low vision. *Topics in Geriatric Rehabilitation, 20,* 154–172.

Fairman, S. K., & Huebner, R. A. (2000). Service dogs: A compensatory resource to improve function. *Occupational Therapy in Health Care, 13,* 41–52.

Falvo, D. R. (2011). *Effective patient education: A guide to increased adherence* (4th ed.). Boston, MA: Jones and Bartlett.

Fisher, T. L., Laud, P. W., Byfield, M. G., Brown, T. T., Hayat, M. J., & Fiedler, I. G. (2002). Sexual health after spinal cord injury: A longitudinal study. *Archives of Physical Medicine and Rehabilitation, 83,* 1043–1051.

Fletcher-Smith, J., Walker, M. F., & Drummond, A. (2012). The influence of hand use on dressing outcome in cognitively impaired stroke survivors. *British Journal of Occupational Therapy, 75,* 2–9.

Forhan, M., Bhambhani, Y., Dyer, D., Ramos-Salas, X., Ferguson-Pell, M., & Sharma, A. (2010). Rehabilitation in bariatrics: Opportunities for practice and research. *Disability & Rehabilitation, 32,* 952–959.

Foti, D. (2005). Caring for the person of size. *OT Practice,* 9–13.

Foti, D., & Littrell, E. (2004). Bariatric care: Practical problem solving and interventions. *American Occupational Therapy Association Physical Disabilities Special Interest Section Quarterly, 27,* 1–3.

Gagné, D. E., & Hoppes, S. (2003). Brief report: The effects of collaborative goal-focused occupational therapy on self-care skills: A pilot study. *American Journal of Occupational Therapy, 57,* 215–219.

Gilbertson, L., & Langhorne, P. (2000). Home-based occupational therapy: Stroke patients' satisfaction with occupational performance and service provision. *British Journal of Occupational Therapy, 63,* 464–468.

Gillen, G. (2000). Case report: Improving activities of daily living performance in an adult with ataxia. *American Journal of Occupational Therapy, 54,* 89–96.

Gillen, G. (2009). *Cognitive and perceptual rehabilitation: Optimizing function.* St. Louis: Mosby Elsevier.

Gitlin, L. N., & Burgh, D. (1995). Issuing assistive devices to older patients in rehabilitation: An exploratory study. *American Journal of Occupational Therapy, 49,* 994–1000.

Gitlin, L. N., Winter, L., Dennis, M. P., Corcoran, M., Schinfeld, S., & Hauck, W. W. (2006). A randomized trial of a multicomponent home intervention to reduce functional difficulties in older adults. *Journal of the American Geriatrics Society, 54,* 809–816.

Goodman, C. C., & Smirnova, I. V. (2009). The cardiovascular system. In C. C. Goodman & K. S. Fuller (Eds.), *Pathology: Implications for the physical therapist* (3rd ed., pp. 519–641). Philadelphia: Saunders.

Goverover, Y., Chiaravalloti, N., Gaudino-Goering, E., Moore, N., & DeLuca, J. (2009). The relationship among performance of instrumental activities of daily living, self-report of quality of life, and self-awareness of functional status in individuals with multiple sclerosis. *Rehabilitation Psychology, 54,* 60–68.

Goverover, Y., Johnston, M. V., Toglia, J., & Deluca, J. (2007). Treatment to improve self-awareness in persons with acquired brain injury. *Brain Injury, 21,* 913–923.

Guidetti, S., & Tham, K. (2002). Therapeutic strategies used by occupational therapists in self-care training: A qualitative study. *Occupational Therapy International, 9,* 257–276.

Hage, G. (1988). Makeup board for women with quadriplegia. *American Journal of Occupational Therapy, 42,* 253–255.

Hammond, A., & Freeman, K. (2004). The long-term outcomes from a randomized controlled trial of an educational-behavioural joint protection programme for people with rheumatoid arthritis. *Clinical Rehabilitation, 18,* 520–528.

Hermann, R. P., Phalangas, A. C., Mahoney, R. M., & Alexander, M. A. (1999). Powered feeding devices: An evaluation of three models. *Archives of Physical Medicine and Rehabilitation, 80,* 1237–1242.

Hoffmann, T., Bennett, S., McKenna, K., Green-Hill, J., McCluskey, A., & Tooth, L. (2008). Interventions for stroke rehabilitation: Analysis of the research contained in the OTseeker evidence database. *Topics in Stroke Rehabilitation, 15,* 341–350.

International Spinal Cord Society and Livability. (2012). *E learn SCI's videos.* Retrieved June 16, 2013 from http://vimeo.com/elearnsci/.

Irion, G., Melancon, H., Nuchereno, N., Strawbridge, B., & Young, J. (2010). Cardiovascular responses to carrying groceries in bags with and without handles. *Journal of Acute Care Physical Therapy, 1,* 64–68.

Iwarsson, S., & Stahl, A. (2003). Accessibility, usability and universal design: Positioning and definition of concepts describing person-environment relationships. *Disability and Rehabilitation, 25,* 57–66.

Jack, J., & Estes, R. I. (2010). Documenting progress: Hand therapy treatment shift from biomechanical to occupational adaptation. *American Journal of Occupational Therapy, 64,* 82–87.

James, A. B. (2014). Activities of daily living and instrumental activities of daily living. In: B. A. B. Schell, G. Gillen, & M. Scaffa (Eds.), *Willard and Spackman's Occupational Therapy* (12th ed, pp. 610–652). Philadephia: Lippincott Williams & Wilkins.

Johansson, R. S., & Westling, G. (1984). Roles of glabrous skin receptors and sensorimotor memory in automatic control of precision grip when lifting rougher or more slippery objects. *Experimental Brain Research, 56,* 550–564.

King, M. J., Verkaaik, J. K., Nicholls, A., & Collins, F. (2009). A wrist extension operated lateral key grip orthosis for people with tetraplegia. *Technology and Disability, 21,* 19–23.

Kraskowsky, L. H., & Finlayson, M. (2001). Factors affecting older adults' use of adaptive equipment: Review of the literature. *American Journal of Occupational Therapy, 55,* 303–310.

Kratz, G., Soderback, I., Guidetti, S., Hultling, C., Rykatkin, T., & Soderstrom, M. (1997). Wheelchair users' experience of non-adapted and adapted clothes during sailing, quad rugby, or wheel walking. *Disability and Rehabilitation, 19,* 26–34.

Kristensen, H. K., Persson, D., Nygren, C., Boll, M., & Matzen, P. (2011). Evaluation of evidence within occupational therapy in stroke rehabilitation. *Scandinavian Journal of Occupational Therapy, 18,* 11–25.

Latham, C. A. T. (2008a). Conceptual foundations for practice. In M. V. Radomski & C. A. T. Latham (Eds.), *Occupational therapy for physical dysfunction* (6th ed., pp. 1–20). Philadelphia: Lippincott Williams & Wilkins.

Latham, C. A. T. (2008b). Occupation: Philosophy and concepts. In M. V. Radomski & C. A. T. Latham (Eds.), *Occupational therapy for physical dysfunction* (6th ed., pp. 339–357). Philadelphia: Lippincott Williams & Wilkins.

Law, M., Baptiste, S., Carswell, A., McColl, M. A., Polatajko, H., & Pollock, N. (2005). *The Canadian Occupational Performance Measure* (4th ed.). Toronto: CAOT Publications.

Legg, L., Drummond, A., & Langhorne, P. (2006). Occupational therapy for patients with problems in activities of daily living after stroke. *Cochrane Database of Systematic Reviews 2006,* Issue 4. Art. No.: CD003585. DOI: 10.1002/14651858.CD003585.pub2.

Libin, A., Schladen, M. M., Ljungberg, I., Tsai, B., Jacobs, S., Reinauer, K., Minnick, S., Spungen, M., & Groah, S. (2011). YouTube as an on-line disability self-management tool in persons with spinal cord injury. *Topics in Spinal Cord Injury Rehabilitation, 16,* 84–92.

Lin, C., Fisher, B. E., Winstein, C. J., Wu, A. D., & Gordon, J. (2009). Contextual interference effect: Elaborative processing or forgetting-reconstruction? A post hoc analysis of transcranial magnetic stimulation-induced effects on motor learning. *Journal of Motor Behavior, 40,* 578–586.

Lin, E. H. B., Katon, W., Von Korff, M., Tang, L., Williams, J. W., Kroenke, K., Hunkeloer, E., Harpole, L., Hegel, M., Arean, P., Hoffing, M., Della Penna, R., Langston, C., & Unützer, J (2003). Effect of improving depressive care on pain and functional outcomes among older adults with arthritis: A randomized controlled study. *Journal of the American Medical Association, 290,* 2428–2434.

Lin, C., Sullivan, K., Wu, A., Kantak, S., & Winstein, C. (2007). Effect of task practice order on motor skill learning in adults with Parkinson disease: A pilot study. *Physical Therapy, 87,* 1120–1131.

Mann, W. C., Hurren, D., Tomita, M., & Charvat, B. (1996). Use of assistive devices for bathing by elderly who are not institutionalized. *Occupational Therapy Journal of Research, 16,* 261–286.

Mastin, D. F., Bryson, J., & Corwyn, R. (2006). Assessment of sleep hygiene using the Sleep Hygiene Index. *Journal of Behavioural Medicine, 29,* 223–227.

Mathiowetz, V., & Matuska, K. M. (1998). Effectiveness of inpatient rehabilitation on self-care abilities of individuals with multiple sclerosis. *NeuroRehabilitation, 11,* 141–151.

Matuska, K., Mathiowetz, V., & Finlayson, M. (2007). Use and perceived effectiveness of energy conservation strategies for managing multiple sclerosis fatigue. *American Journal of Occupational Therapy, 61,* 62–69.

McAlonan, S. (1996). Improving sexual rehabilitation services: The patient's perspective. *American Journal of Occupational Therapy, 50,* 826–834.

McGruder, J., Cors, D., Tiernan, A. M., Tomlin, G. (2003). Weighted wrist cuffs for tremor reduction during eating in adults with static brain lesions. *American Journal of Occupational Therapy, 57,* 507–516.

McMillen, A.-M., & Söderberg., S. (2002). Disabled persons' experience of dependence on assistive devices. *Scandinavian Journal of Occupational Therapy, 9,* 176–183.

Medline Plus Encyclopedia. (2010a). *Self-catheterization—Female.* Retrieved June 16, 2013 from http://www.nlm.nih.gov/medlineplus/ency /patientinstructions/000144.htm.

Medline Plus Encyclopedia. (2010b). *Self-catheterization—Male.* Retrieved June 16, 2013 from http://www.nlm.nih.gov/medlineplus/ency /patientinstructions/000143.htm.

Melville, L. L., Baltic, T. A., Bettcher, T. W., & Nelson, D. L. (2002). Patients' perspectives on the Self-Identified Goals Assessment. *American Journal of Occupational Therapy, 56,* 650–659.

Migliore, A. (2004). Management of dyspnea guidelines for practice for adults with chronic obstructive pulmonary disease. *Occupational Therapy in Health Care, 18,* 1–20.

Mooney, T. G., Cole, T. M., & Chilgren, R. A. (1975). *Sexual options for paraplegics and quadriplegics.* Boston: Little, Brown.

Mount, J., Pierce, S., Parker, J., Diegidio, R., Woessner, R., & Spiegel, L. (2007). Trial and error versus errorless learning of functional skills in patients with acute stroke. *Neurorehabilitation, 22,* 123–132.

Packer, T., Girdler, S., Boldy, D. P., Dhaliwal, S. S., & Crowley, M. (2009). Vision self-management for older adults: A pilot study. *Disability and Rehabilitation: An International, Multidisciplinary Journal, 31,* 1353–1361.

Pain, H., & McLellan, D. L. (2003). The relative importance of factors affecting the choice of bathing devices. *British Journal of Occupational Therapy, 66,* 396–401.

Pettersson, I., Appelros, P., & Ahlström, G. (2007). Lifeworld perspectives utilizing assistive devices: Individuals, lived experience following a stroke. *Canadian Journal of Occupational Therapy, 74,* 15–26.

Pinkston, N. E., Boersma, A. M., & Spaulding, S. J. (2005). The impact of reacher length on EMG activity and task. *Canadian Journal of Occupational Therapy, 72,* 89–95.

Pohjasvaara, T., Vataja, R., Leppävuori, A., Kaste, M., & Erkinjuntti, T. (2001). Depression is an independent predictor of poor long-term functional outcome post-stroke. *European Journal of Neurology, 8,* 315–319.

Poole, J. (1998). Effect of apraxia on the ability to learn one-handed shoe tying. *Occupational Therapy Journal of Research, 18,* 99–104.

Regional Spinal Cord Injury Center of Delaware Valley. (2001). *Spinal cord injury patient-family teaching manual.* Retrieved from http://www.spinalcordcenter.org/consumer/manual.html.

Rice, M. S., Leonard, C., & Carter, M. (1998). Grip strengths and required forces in accessing everyday containers in a normal population. *American Journal of Occupational Therapy, 52,* 621–626.

Rintala, D. H., Matamoros, R., & Seitz, L. L. (2008). Effects of assistance dogs on persons with mobility or hearing impairments: A pilot study. *Journal of Rehabilitation Research & Development, 45,* 489–504.

Rogers, J. C., & Holm, M. B. (2009). The occupational therapy process. In E. B. Crepeau, E. S. Cohn, & B. A. B. Schell (Eds.), *Willard and Spackman's Occupational Therapy* (11th ed., pp. 478–518). Philadelphia: Lippincott Williams & Wilkins.

Rudhe, C., & van Hedel, H. (2009). Upper extremity function in persons with tetraplegia: Relationships between strength, capacity, and the Spinal Cord Independence Measure. *Neurorehabilitation & Neural Repair, 23,* 413–421.

Runge, M. (1967). Self dressing techniques for patients with spinal cord injury. *American Journal of Occupational Therapy, 21,* 367–375.

Ryan, P. A., & Sullivan, J. W. (2011). Activities of daily living adaptations: Managing the environment with one-handed techniques. In G. Gillen (Ed.), *Stroke rehabilitation: A function based approach* (3rd ed., pp. 716–734). St. Louis: Mosby

Ryu, J., Cooney, W. P., Askew, L. J., An, K.-N., & Chao, E. Y. S. (1991). Functional ranges of motion of the wrist joint. *Journal of Hand Surgery, 16A,* 409–419.

Sanford, J. A., Griffiths, P. C., Richardson, P., Hargraves, K., Butterfield, T., & Hoenig, H. (2006). The effects of in-home rehabilitation on task self-efficacy in mobility-impaired adults: A randomized clinical trial. *Journal of the American Geriatric Society, 54,* 1641–1648.

Schmidt, R. A., & Lee, T. (2011). *Motor control and learning: A behavioral emphasis* (5th ed.). Champaign, IL: Human Kinetics.

Shillam, L. L., Beeman, C., & Loshin, P. M. (1983). Effect of occupational therapy intervention on bathing independence of disabled persons. *American Journal of Occupational Therapy, 37,* 744–748.

Skymne, C., Dahlin-Ivanoff, S., Claesson, L., & Eklund, K. (2012). Getting used to assistive devices: Ambivalent experiences by frail elderly persons. *Scandinavian Journal of Occupational Therapy, 19,* 194–203.

Smaby, N., Johanson, E., Baker, B., Kenney, D., Murray, W., & Hentz, V. (2004). Identification of key pinch forces required to complete functional tasks. *Journal of Rehabilitation Research & Development, 41,* 215–224.

Smith, B. E. (2001). Occupational therapy's role in low vision rehabilitation. *American Occupational Therapy Association Physical Disabilities Special Interest Section Quarterly, 24,* 1–3.

Smith, D. L., & Gutman, S. A. (2011). Health literacy in occupational therapy practice and research. *American Journal of Occupational Therapy, 65,* 367–369.

Steultjens, E. M. J., Dekker, J., Bouter, L. M., van de Nes, J. C. M., Cup, E. H. C., & van den Ende, C. H. M. (2003). Occupational therapy for stroke patients: A systematic review. *Stroke, 34,* 676–687.

Stout, K., & Finlayson, M. (2011). Fatigue management in chronic illness. *OT Practice, 16,* 16–19.

Taylor, R. R. (2004). Quality of life and symptom severity for individuals with chronic fatigue syndrome: Findings from a randomized clinical trial. *American Journal of Occupational Therapy, 58,* 35–43.

Thomas, H. (2012). *Occupation-based activity analysis.* Thorofare, NJ: Slack.

Trombly, C. A., & Ma, H. (2002). A synthesis of the effects of occupational therapy for persons with stroke, Part I: Restoration of roles, tasks, and activities. *American Journal of Occupational Therapy, 56,* 250–259.

Trombly, C. A., Radomski, M. V., Trexel, C., & Burnett-Smith, S. E. (2002). Occupational therapy and achievement of self-identified goals by adults with acquired brain injury: Phase II. *American Journal of Occupational Therapy, 56,* 489–498.

Unsworth, C. A., & Cunningham, D. T. (2002). Examining the evidence base for occupational therapy with clients following stroke. *British Journal of Occupational Therapy, 65,* 21–29.

U.S. Access Board. (2004). *ADA and ABA accessibility guidelines for buildings and facilities.* Retrieved June 16, 2013 from http://www.access-board.gov/adaag/html/adaag.htm#4.26.

van Stralen, G. M. J., Struben, P. J., & van Loon, C. J. M. (2003). The incidence of dislocation after primary total hip arthorplasty using posterior approach with posterior soft tissue repair. *Archives of Orthopedic Trauma Surgery, 123,* 219–222.

Vigouroux, L., Domalain, M., & Berton, E. (2011). Effect of object width on muscle and joint forces during thumb-index finger grasping. *Journal of Applied Biomechanics, 27,* 173–180.

Walker, M. F., Leonardi-Bee, J., Bath, P., Langhorne, P., Dewey, M., Corr, S., Drummond, Gilbertson, L., Gladman, J. R. F., Jongbloed, L., Logan, P., & Parker, C. (2004). Individual patient data meta-analysis of randomized controlled trials of community occupational therapy for stroke patients. *Stroke, 35,* 2226–2232.

Walker, M. F., & Lincoln, N. B. (1991). Factors influencing dressing performance after stroke. *Journal of Neurology, Neurosurgery, and Psychiatry, 54,* 699–701.

Walker, C., M., & Walker, M. F. (2001). Dressing ability after stroke: A review of the literature. *British Journal of Occupational Therapy, 64,* 449–454.

Weintraub, D., Moberg, P., Duda, M., Katz, I., & Stern, M. (2004). Effect of psychiatric and other nonmotor symptoms on disability in PD. *Journal of the American Geriatrics Society, 52,* 784–788.

Wesolowski, M. D., Zencius, A. H., McCarthy-Lydon, D., & Lydon, S. (2005). Using behavioral interventions to treat speech disorders in persons with head trauma. *Behavioral Interventions, 20,* 67–75.

Wielandt, T., McKenna, K., Tooth, L., & Strong, J. (2001). Post discharge use of equipment prescribed by occupational therapists: What lessons to be learned? *Physical & Occupational Therapy in Geriatrics, 19,* 49–65.

Wielandt, T., & Strong, J. (2000). Compliance with prescribed adaptive equipment: A literature review. *British Journal of Occupational Therapy, 63,* 65–75.

Acknowledgments

I would like to recognize Catherine Trombly Latham for her authorship of prior editions of this chapter that provided a solid foundation for this work. I also extend a special thanks to Andrew Moore, OTS, for sharing his pre-OT school expertise as a photographer in updating many of the photos in this chapter.

26

Restoring Functional and Community Mobility

Susan Lanier Pierce

Learning Objectives

After studying this chapter, the reader will be able to do the following:

1. Explain why functional mobility and community mobility are considered an activity of daily living and instrumental activity of daily living.
2. Identify mobility issues to be addressed during the occupational therapy process and the role of the occupational therapy practitioner in goal setting and intervention.
3. State the hierarchy of mobility skills used to develop an intervention plan and describe how contextual and environmental factors influence performance.
4. Plan intervention to restore mobility through therapeutic activities and use of adaptive aids, devices, or alternative options and strategies.
5. Define the various meanings of community and how to identify barriers and enhance performance for safety in community mobility.

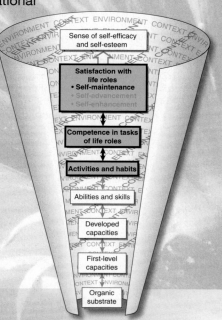

Mobility refers to moving about the home and community. Mobility is necessary for many activities and is therefore a key component of engagement in occupation. The Occupational Therapy Practice Framework (OTPF) identifies two types of mobility: functional mobility, defined as an activity of daily living, and community mobility, defined as an instrumental activity of daily living (American Occupational Therapy Association [AOTA], 2008).

Functional mobility relates to changing the position of the body, thus enabling a person to engage in chosen life occupations in the home and community. Functional mobility is defined as moving from one position or place to another during performance of everyday activities (AOTA, 2008). Functional mobility includes in-bed mobility, wheelchair or powered mobility, transfers (e.g., moving to and from wheelchair, bed, car, toilet, tub/shower, chair, floor) and ambulation while transporting task objects. Community mobility refers to moving around in the community including walking, driving, bicycling, accessing and riding buses, and using taxi cabs or other transportation systems (AOTA, 2008). Community mobility facilitates connectedness to others, to goods and services, and to the occupations of everyday life (Womack, 2012). Work, leisure, social, educational, religious, or political activities are examples of IADL that require mobility in the community. Restoring competence in functional and community mobility is a building block toward the end goal of supporting health and participation in life through engagement in occupations (AOTA, 2010). Both aspects of mobility must be addressed throughout the continuum of the occupational therapy process. Guidelines for the therapist in addressing functional and community mobility are summarized in Procedures for Practice 26-1. Evidence Table 26-1 presents the best evidence for occupational therapy practice regarding mobility.

DEVELOPMENT OF AN INTERVENTION PLAN FOR RESTORING MOBILITY

A person, whatever the age, client factor, or performance skill impairment, must be able to move about the surrounding environment to participate in the tasks and activities of the chosen life roles. Using a client-centered approach to mobility, the person and/or family contributes to goal setting and determination of successful outcomes in mobility. The therapist considers each client's individuality and personal circumstances and then customizes the therapeutic approach as necessary. The therapist must be an active listener to the client's thoughts and input during implementation of the plan and must be willing to modify techniques and strategies as needed.

During the process of obtaining an occupational profile, the therapist identifies the client's expectations for

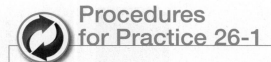

Procedures for Practice 26-1

Guidelines to Address Functional and Community Mobility

- Gather and synthesize information from the occupational profile to identify specific areas of mobility that are important and meaningful to the client and identify his or her specific contextual factors.
- Select appropriate assessments to observe, measure, and identify barriers that hinder, or supports that facilitate, occupational performance as it relates to competence in mobility.
- Interpret all data collected to develop an intervention plan for safe mobility performance using the hierarchy of skill building as a guide (See Fig. 26-1).
- Select interventions that are based on available evidence and/or are considered best practice.
- Implement interventions that include improving performance skills to meet activity demands and/or applying assistive technology, adaptive devices, or compensatory strategies.
- Collaborate with other disciplines or specialists in the total care plan for successful outcomes to meet the client's mobility goals.

functional and community mobility so that the long-term goal for successful mobility becomes part of the intervention plan. The therapist analyzes the client's occupational performance; determines his or her capacities, strengths, and resources; and considers the contextual factors unique to the person (Womack, 2012). In the process, the therapist identifies circumstances that hinder or support mobility as related to activities of daily living (ADL). As particular mobility goals are identified within the client's chosen occupations, the therapist analyzes the specific activity demands.

After the therapist evaluates the client's occupational functioning and understands his or her occupational role(s), an intervention plan is developed that reflects the client's goals and occupational needs for mobility. The intervention plan for restoring competence in mobility must be developed in a sequence to reflect the hierarchy of skills of each mobility task and their increasing complexity as shown in Figure 26-1. Mobility addressed in BADL is followed by mobility addressed in IADL. Accomplishment in each area builds a foundation of performance skills that are required for the activity demands of the next higher level of mobility.

The performance patterns for ADL and IADL such as habits, routines, and roles may need to be modified or adapted to meet the client's current level of mobility skills.

Evidence Table 26-1		Best Evidence for Occupational Therapy Practice Regarding Mobility				
Intervention	Description of Intervention Tested	Participants	Dosage	Type of Best Evidence and Level of Evidence	Benefit	Statistical Probability and Effect Size of Outcome	Reference
Review of assessment tools for predicting driving performance of persons with traumatic brain injury (TBI)	Systematic literature review of neuropsychological tests, off-road screening tests, self-reports and significant other reports, postinjury disability status, and comprehensive driving evaluation related to driving performance	Thirteen studies (5 experimental; 7 observational; 1 descriptive). Total sample size = 1,562. Exclusion criteria: published before 1995; not primary study; mainly qualitative or descriptive; if emphasized or established psychometrics; driving was not main outcome; included mixed diagnostic groups.	NA	Systematic review Level: IC2a	Recommendations based on each tool's ability to predict driving performance: Neuropsychological tests are not predictive of on-the-road performance. Simulator Testing: insufficient evidence. The Neurocognitive Driving Test (NDT), an off-road screening test: predicts on-the-road performance for people with moderate to severe TBI. Self-report and others' reports and disability status: provide low level of prediction. Comprehensive driving evaluation: insufficient evidence concerning prediction of safe driving performance.	Not reported	Classen et al. (2009)

Does Functional Capacity Evaluation, as part of a prevention program, predict at-fault crashes in older adults?	Functional Capacity Evaluation consisted of screening tools to detect loss of functional ability. The tools were: Motor-Free Visual Perception Test; visual closure subtest; Trail Making Test, part B; Delayed Recall Test; Useful Field of View Test, Subtest 2; Rapid Pace Walk Test; and Head-neck Rotation Test. First-time at-fault crashes determined from Maryland State Highway Administration data for individuals in the Maryland Pilot Older Driver Study (MaryPODS) over a 2-year period.	1,876 drivers from Maryland age 55 years and older who were randomly selected and then volunteered to participate	Volunteer participants were administered the Functional Capacity Evaluation in a one-time visit to the Motor Vehicle Administration.	One-group nonrandomized study Level: IIIA1a	Yes. Functional Capacity Screening can validly predict immediate and long-term risk of involvement in at-fault auto crashes in older drivers.	Odds ratios and chi-square tests were performed. Motor-Free visual Perceptual Test–visual closure subtest ($p < 0.001$); useful field of vision test ($p < 0.005$); rapid pace walk ($p < 0.001$); and delayed recall test ($p < 0.002$) were significantly valuable in predicting crashes shortly after the tests were administered. Delayed recall test and rapid pace walk were still predictive of crashes 1 year beyond test administration. The results indicate the need for periodic reevaluation, no more than 2 years apart.	Staplin, Gish, & Wagner (2003)
Does the environment influence walking speed and pedestrian safety in elderly people?	Participants took part in four randomly assigned trials. Two indoor trials were conducted on a level, tiled walkway and two outdoor trials were conducted on a simulated crosswalk. In one indoor and one outdoor trial, participants were told to walk a standard distance at preferred pace; in the other trials, participants were told to walk the same distance as quickly as possible.	Thirteen participants ages 77–88 years from independent-living resident facility. Exclusion criteria included deafness, history of stroke, myocardial infarction, and inflammatory arthritis.	One testing period; one trial per condition: 1. Indoor: preferred pace 2. Indoor: fast pace 3. Outdoor: preferred pace 4. Outdoor: fast pace	Randomized controlled trial Level: IC2a	For both pace conditions, significantly more time was required outdoors than indoors. Participants were significantly able to increase speed during fast-pace outdoor trial compared to the same condition indoors. The authors stated that these trials indicate that timing of crosswalk signals need adjusting to improve pedestrian safety for elders.	Not reported	Carmeli et al. (2000)

(continued)

Evidence Table 26-1 Best Evidence for Occupational Therapy Practice Regarding Mobility (*continued*)

Intervention	Description of Intervention Tested	Participants	Dosage	Type of Best Evidence and Level of Evidence	Benefit	Statistical Probability and Effect Size of Outcome	Reference
Usability of powered wheelchairs (PWCs) in home, school, or workplace, and community and outdoor environments	Assistive technology devices (includes PWCs) enable people with disabilities to function in multiple contexts and activities. The usability of such devices is indicative of the user's level of participation in multiple roles and occupations.	Seventy people of various diagnoses aged 18–65 years who used PWCs of various designs in small towns and suburbs of western New York. Exclusion: people who did not use their PWC outdoors and in the community	Each participant completed the Usability of Assistive Technology—Wheelchair Mobility (USAT-WM) questionnaire, which consists of 71 items in 7 subscales scored on a Likert scale. Participants' comments were also collected to explain ratings of ≤3 on the scales. One 45-minute interview session	Secondary analysis of data collected for psychometric evaluation of USAT-WM Level: IVA3a	Participants reported using their PWCs at home and work optimally, but issues of space and accessibility undermined their participation in these contexts. Usability issues were more apparent in community and outdoor contexts and had to do primarily with accessibility. Occupational therapists can document progress in PWC usability using the USAT-WM and can advocate for greater accessibility.	Qualitative and descriptive analysis only. Mean score for perfect usability = 5.0. PWCs were highly usable, with a mean score of 4.23 (standard deviation [SD] = 0.83) at home and 4.32 (SD = 0.59; n = 27) at workplace or school. Mean scores for the community and outdoor usability were 3.60 (SD = 0.77) and 3.74 (SD = 0.62), respectively. Mean scores for the user-wheelchair interaction subscales were high to very high at 4.25 (SD = 0.54) [ease of use], 4.36 (SD = 0.69) [seating] and 4.32 (SD = 0.56) [safety].	Arthanat et al. (2009)

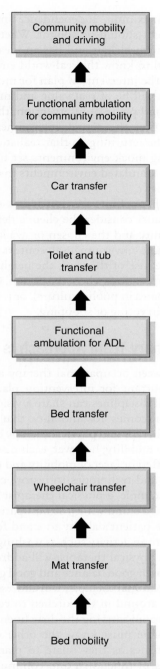

Community mobility and driving

↑

Functional ambulation for community mobility

↑

Car transfer

↑

Toilet and tub transfer

↑

Functional ambulation for ADL

↑

Bed transfer

↑

Wheelchair transfer

↑

Mat transfer

↑

Bed mobility

Figure 26-1 The hierarchy of skill building for restoring competence in mobility is based on increasing activity demands of each task and illustrates the sequence for intervention planning. ADL, activities of daily living.

The therapist will explore the client's prior methods of accomplishing a particular occupation. For example, shopping for groceries entails moving out of bed, getting dressed, and having nourishment before moving outside the home and using a safe mode of transportation to the store. Once inside the store, the person must move safely through the store to shop, push a shopping cart, stand at a cash register, pay for and transport the items outside, load them into the transportation vehicle, return home, and unload and transport the items into the house for storage. Each of these mobility tasks requires a certain level of motor skills such as strength, coordination, and range of motion, as well as visual and cognitive skills such as peripheral vision, visual acuity, problem solving, decision making, and attention. The therapist will develop a plan, along with the client, to remediate those skills that can be improved, but achievement of safe mobility may also include intervention using assistive technology and adaptive devices and/or accommodations or compensatory strategies for an identified, unremediable barrier.

A client may have more than one area of impairment in performance skills combined with one or more client or contextual factors that hinders safe mobility. A person with rheumatoid arthritis, for example, may have decreased range of motion, weakness, and low physical endurance but also may be aging poorly with obesity and diabetes. A person with a spinal cord injury may have decreased sensation and paralysis in the lower extremities as well as tall body structure and poor trunk balance. A person who had a stroke or traumatic brain injury may have motor as well as visual and cognitive impairments that all hinder safe mobility. All impairments and contextual factors must be taken into consideration in developing the intervention plan.

With inpatient rehabilitation so brief, the level of mobility a patient achieves on discharge will not be the same level that the person can achieve 6 or 8 months postdischarge. The inpatient therapist should plan long-term postdischarge goals for mobility with the patient and the family so that outpatient intervention can carry on the identified goals for maximum independence in mobility. Independence in community mobility will more than likely be achieved during or after the outpatient rehabilitation process and intervention. Educating the client and family of this fact will prevent the client from becoming discouraged and will prepare the family to provide necessary transportation until the client is ready to pursue intervention goals for restoring competence in community mobility.

Environmental or Contextual Factors Influence Mobility

To holistically evaluate the ability of a person to move about in the world requires the therapist to consider not only the person's capacity for movement but also the desired destination and the context in which the mobility will take place (Womack, 2012). Mobility may be affected differently in the various environmental contexts of the individual; therefore, the therapist must consider mobility skills in all relevant environments. For example, a client who had a stroke may require a wheelchair outside the home but be able to ambulate around the home with the assistance of an orthotic device such as a cane. Another client who had a stroke may require a wheelchair for mobility in, as well as out of, the home. For each of these clients, the wheelchair has to be considered as a necessary mobility device. Skill building strategies for mobility are listed in Procedures for Practice 26-2.

Functional mobility considers ambulation with or without an assistive device, manual wheelchair propulsion, or safe operating techniques for powered mobility. Initial mobility skill training in a controlled, therapeutic environment is the foundation for enhancing the client's safety and independent functioning eventually in the home, school, workplace, and other environments (Kirby et al., 2002). The first phase of functional mobility intervention will take place in the accessible environment of the hospital room or therapy clinic. The second phase considers the client's mobility relative to his or her actual home and chosen communities (see Chapter 10) which is crucial for discharge planning. The client's environmental context may not consist of the level floors, low-pile carpet, easy curb cuts, or nicely ramped entrances of hospitals and rehabilitation facilities. The outdoor terrain around the home may be soft dirt, sand, or thick grass. Functional ambulation with orthotic devices or mobility devices such as a wheelchair may be hindered because of a home's narrow hallways and doorways. The client may have to transfer onto a waterbed or soft mattress rather than the adjustable height surface of a firm hospital bed. There may not be a roll-in shower, so the client may have to learn to use a regular tub with a tub bench. Even if the client will be discharged to an assisted-living

environment, maximum independence in mobility for that environment should be sought. Whether the client walks or uses a wheelchair and has an ideal situation or not, it is crucial to know the real-world environment for that person so the intervention plan for mobility and the final outcomes will be of real value and meaning to the client. The second phase of intervention, therefore, takes into consideration the actual environments to which the client will be returning so that realistic training can take place using mock environments set up in the therapy clinic or in simulated environments in or around the treatment facility.

The third phase of intervention addresses community mobility and must consider the client's definition of his or her community and the chosen or available modes of travel. The whole environmental context includes exit from the house, use of the yard, the neighborhood, and the community locations where the person, works, attends school; participates in public, cultural, or religious events; or participates in voting or shopping.

Interdisciplinary Team Approach Is Important

Teamwork between occupational therapy and other disciplines is important for intervention planning in mobility so that all disciplines can share a vision of targeted intervention outcomes for mobility that are realistic. Occupational therapy and physical therapy both may have goals related to mobility; however, each discipline will be addressing a different facet of mobility and will use different modalities and techniques to restore competence in mobility. For example, a physical therapist will address a patient's ability to stand while the occupational therapist will address the patient's ability to stand for a period of time to complete an activity such as washing dishes at the kitchen sink. A physical therapist will address a patient's ability to walk with good balance and good gait technique, while the occupational therapist will address the patient's ability to walk around in the kitchen to cook a meal or into a laundry room carrying the dirty linens.

Each discipline must know the other's intervention goals and strategies as they relate to planning for targeted outcomes in functional and community mobility. Communication between team members eliminates unnecessary duplication and promotes carryover of skills. The direction the occupational therapist takes in pursuing BADL should be influenced by the patient's achievements in physical therapy with lower extremity functioning and ambulation. Conversely, independence in bed mobility achieved in occupational therapy may influence balance and transfer training in physical therapy. Achievement of physical therapy goals that are precursor skills for functional mobility intervention may take several weeks, so during this time, the occupational therapist works on BADL that do not demand a high level of lower extremity

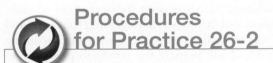
Procedures
for Practice 26-2

Skill Building for Mobility

- Moving in the immediate space, such as rolling from a supine to prone position, repositioning the trunk and extremities, or moving from a lying to seated position
- Moving in the bed for body positioning or basic ADL such as dressing or skin inspection
- Moving out of bed and into the surrounding areas such as into the bathroom for hygiene activities
- Moving around the level, accessible environment of the therapy setting for intervention of performance skills or for other ADL such as kitchen activities or feeding
- Moving on the uneven terrain of the outdoor environment
- Moving around in the client's home and neighborhood environment
- Moving about the chosen community environment(s)

strength, trunk balance, and endurance. For example, a patient who is expected to walk at discharge will initially perform grooming or kitchen tasks while seated. When the patient has achieved standing tolerance and balance in physical therapy, the occupational therapist can incorporate standing in activities such as grooming activities at a bathroom sink and washing dishes at a kitchen sink. When it is determined that the patient will be using a wheelchair when discharged from the hospital, the occupational therapist works on teaching the patient how to propel the wheelchair and perform activities from the chair, such as dressing and cooking. If the patient will be a functional, but limited, ambulator with an orthotic device, the occupational therapist must incorporate the device into the intervention goals for functional and community mobility. For example, a person who uses a cane or walker has to learn to maneuver in the kitchen with this device while cooking.

INTERVENTION FOR FUNCTIONAL MOBILITY

The OTPF suggests that functional mobility pertains to taking care of one's own body. Functional mobility tasks occur throughout a person's daily routine under varying circumstances and within changeable environments. ADL and IADL require movements with optimal motor and sensory awareness, stabilization of the body in space, and postural control with varying static and dynamic balance demands. Intervention for functional mobility begins with the basics of moving in space, and then mobility in ADL performance is considered followed by mobility for IADL performance. As successful outcomes are obtained in the basic areas, the intervention plan is reassessed to include more complex mobility skills.

Intervention plans include the type or level of assistance needed for mobility, movement patterns/techniques to control an ambulatory device or wheelchair, and types of terrain in the patient's environmental context that may hinder safe functional mobility. Intervention focuses on performance skill impairments, client factors, and contextual factors that support or impede mobility. Strategies to enhance performance skills for safe functional mobility are evaluated and continually modified to assist the person in compensating for impairments in body structure or body functions that affect movement in space. Personal factors of age, health, and well-being may influence the selection of mobility interventions. Functional mobility will be addressed at varying degrees and level depending on the time constraints and venue. For example, a practitioner seeing someone in an acute care setting may concentrate on bed mobility tasks as they relate to basic self-care activities. The practitioner within a rehabilitation setting may approach functional mobility more comprehensively in relation to the more complex ADL and IADL (Kane & Buckley, 2011). The occupational therapist must evaluate and provide intervention

if necessary for the following areas related to functional mobility:

- bed mobility
- mobility using a personal mobility device (PMD)
- transfer mobility
- functional ambulation for ADL

Implementation of intervention will initially address therapeutic goals of the client regarding functional mobility such as moving around in bed, in and out of bed, into the therapy clinic, or onto a treatment mat. For example, a patient with quadriplegia who is working toward the goal of lower extremity dressing must achieve safe bed mobility performance requirements first that involve moving and posturing the body and limbs in addition to handling task objects such as pants, socks, or leg bag. Once the basic areas of functional mobility have been achieved, intervention is modified to address functional mobility of greater complexity that is involved during the performance of specific ADL. A hierarchy of skills exists within a specific area of functional mobility. For example, a patient learns to sit on a hard surface without support, such as a mat, before sitting on a soft surface, such as a bed, in order to eventually transfer to and from the bed. The occupational therapy practitioner will determine whether functional mobility aids are needed to enhance the patient's performance or safety. The functional mobility aids to be discussed in this chapter are leg lifters, bed rope ladder, transfer boards, and PMDs such as wheelchairs, walkers, canes, and body lifting devices.

Bed Mobility

Bed mobility is the ability to move the body in bed to perform activities in the various positions of supine, prone, side lying, or sitting. Bed mobility includes all of the tasks of rolling from side to side, rolling from supine to prone and back, and sitting up. These are basic functional mobility tasks that provide the basis for initial provision of medical care in a hospital, rehabilitation center, or nursing home setting as well as to allow an individual to engage in self-care activities at home. During bed mobility maneuvers, the individual must move the trunk, head, neck, and all extremities necessary for the position change and for postural control. A person must accomplish the goal of rolling his or her body from side to side before the goal of moving the legs over the side of the bed can be accomplished in preparation for sitting on the bedside. Similarly, there are performance requirements to move the body and limbs to the side of the bed in preparation for a transfer to a wheelchair. Bed mobility is also necessary for a person to posture the body for sleep, for changing positions to shift weight or reduce pressure on bony prominences that are prone to skin breakdown, and for using a skin inspection mirror or bedpan. Basic functional mobility skills prepare for transferring out of bed. In goal setting for moving out of bed, the skills for rolling, coming to a sitting position and ability to stand up will determine whether alternative methods will be necessary for functional mobility out of the bed.

Bridging and Rolling in Bed

The first task to accomplish in bed mobility is bridging the hips. Bridging is simply lying supine on a surface and by using the back and hip extensors, the buttocks, upper legs, and lower back are lifted off of the supporting surface so that contact is only made with the upper back, shoulders, head, and feet (see Fig. 26.2). Strength in the back, quadriceps, lower abdominals, and gluteal muscles are important for this task as are ankle and knee stabilization. Bridging is a movement strategy that is taught by the occupational therapist to allow the patient to move the buttocks onto a bedpan, to pull pants over the hips, and to assist with moving the body laterally for changing bed positioning. A loss of motor or sensory function unilaterally or bilaterally will present a challenge to this task that will require the therapist to analyze the patient's impairment and enhance the bridging ability by strengthening, practicing, or learning a different technique. For example, a patient with lower extremity and abdominal/back muscle paralysis will not be able to perform bridging and will have to learn different strategies without hip bridging for donning pants. A patient with hemiplegia who is attempting to bridge the hips may cause an extension pattern in the affected extremity that does not allow for the necessary hip extension, knee flexion, or foot stabilization. The person may have to learn to compensate by bridging only with the stronger side.

The second task to accomplish in bed mobility is rolling. Rolling of the body can involve moving the body completely from a supine to a prone position or rolling onto one side. Rolling the body is vital to weight shifting, to changing postures in bed for sleep, and to pulling pants over the hips in lower extremity dressing. Rolling is also a precursor for long or short-leg sitting in bed, which in turn is a precursor for moving out of bed whether to stand or transfer onto another surface such as a wheelchair. One of the most common movement strategies used to roll from supine to prone is a lift-and-reach arm pattern (Kane & Buckley, 2011). Movement of the head and trunk is initiated by lifting the shoulder girdle and reaching with the arm and hand in the desired direction. Typically, the momentum will cause the leg on the same side to lift and follow as the body rolls.

Sitting in Bed

Long-leg sitting is the posture in which the legs are extended straight out in front of the person on a flat surface and the hips are flexed to at least 90° (Fig. 26-3C). A position greater than 90° of hip flexion must be achieved to maintain balance in a long-leg sitting position when trunk and hip musculature are weak. Long-leg sitting can permit other activities in bed such as watching TV, reading, donning a shirt, or taking medication. Short-leg sitting is the posture in which a person sits with the hips flexed at least to 90° and the knees are flexed over the edge of the surface (Fig. 26-3F). The feet may or may not touch the floor, but stability is aided if they do. Short-leg sitting allows for activities to be performed while sitting on the edge of the bed such as donning a shirt, putting on shoes, or preparing to stand or to transfer to a wheelchair. Postural stability and balance are necessary for safe short- and long-leg sitting. Trunk length, leg length, weight, abdominal circumference, muscle tone, motor strength, cognitive status, vestibular reactions, and vision must all be considered by the therapist when evaluating stability and balance for sitting.

Intervention by occupational therapy focuses first on static sitting balance and then on activities to challenge dynamic balance in a sitting position. Intervention for sitting balance would begin on a flat, hard mat and then progress onto the soft bed mattress. Throwing or catching a ball or performing dressing activities are appropriate interventions to challenge and improve a client's sitting balance. Balance improves either because weak trunk muscles get stronger or because the patient learns adaptive strategies, such as balancing by lowering the center of gravity and using the neck muscles to right the body. *Safety Message: While the person is working on improving balance on the mat or in bed, the therapist must maintain close supervision and proximity to the client and be ready to catch the person if balance is lost in any direction.*

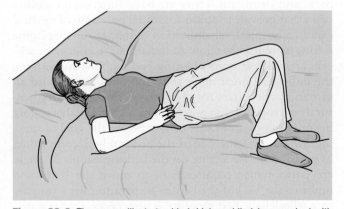

Figure 26-2 The person illustrates hip bridging while lying on a bed with hips and knees flexed and feet flat on the mattress. Using back and hip extensors, the hips are lifted off of the bed to assist in pulling pants over the hips, moving the body laterally or moving onto a bedpan.

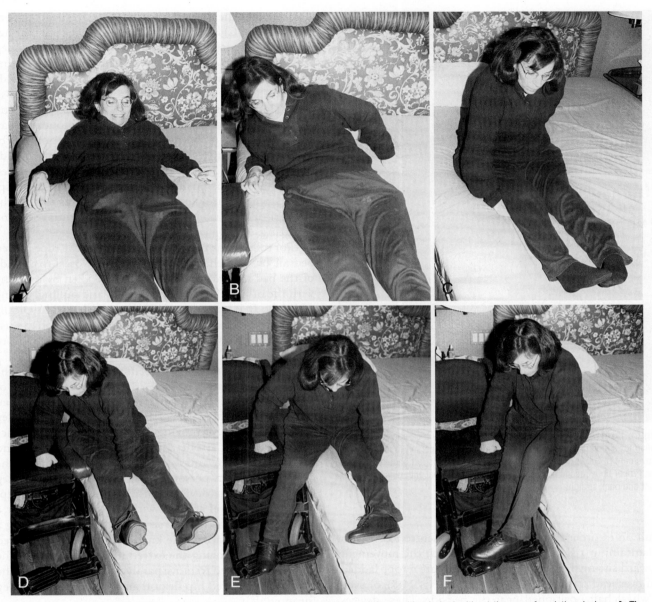

Figure 26-3 A person with C7 quadriplegia illustrates the steps for coming to a sitting position in bed without the use of assistive devices. **A.** The woman uses shoulder and scapula muscles to move to resting on elbows. **B.** Triceps and shoulder depressors in one arm are used to lift the upper trunk while balancing on the other flexed elbow. Then by straightening the bent arm, she pushes the whole trunk upright until she is in a long-leg sitting position. **C.** She can hold her balance by extending one arm behind her on the bed while using the other arm to reposition the legs as needed. **D.** Once she is close to the edge of the bed, she can lean on one arm, which is pressing into the wheelchair seat, to hold balance while she moves the outside leg off the side of the bed. **E.** She then moves the inside leg off the side of the bed. **F.** Once in a short-legged sitting position over the edge of the bed, she prepares for a sliding transfer to a wheelchair seat.

A client who does not have the ability to restore bed mobility competence will require the assistance of one or more persons to accomplish the tasks safely. One or more persons can assist with rolling the upper and lower body in the proper sequence or complete a log-roll technique that moves the entire body at once. Figure 26-4 shows a person with incomplete quadriplegia and proximal weakness in the shoulders and hips being assisted with rolling to one side. *Safety Message: The therapist must ensure that care partners learn and use good body mechanics.*

Assistive Devices for Bed Mobility

A person with motor impairment in the trunk or one or more extremities may require an assistive device to

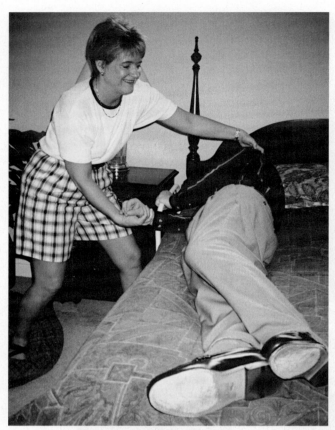

Figure 26-4 A person is assisted in bed mobility by a caregiver. In preparation for sitting up in bed, the caregiver assists the person in initiating the movement of rolling the head and trunk by pulling his left shoulder toward her. Proper body mechanics by the caregiver are crucial with hips and knees bent and back straight.

pull on in order to begin rolling and then to assist with maintaining a side-lying position or with the movement toward sitting. Devices commonly used are a rope ladder, an overhead trapeze bar, a bed rail (see Fig. 26-5), or even a wheelchair positioned near the bedside. These devices can be used to give a person something to grasp with the hand(s) or forearm(s) so that rolling can be initiated or pulling to a seated position in a long- or short-leg position in bed can be accomplished. Good scapular, shoulder, and elbow strength are the minimum requirements for using these devices. Wrist flexion and extension and hand grasping capability are helpful, but a person with weak or no grasping capability can use the same devices by hooking the forearm or the extended wrist around the device and using strong wrist extensors and/or elbow flexors for the pulling action.

The rope ladder (Fig. 26-5A) is a device having two long parallel pieces of strapping connected by "rungs." One end of the ladder is attached to the foot of the bed or over the side of the bed. The person pulls with one or both upper extremities using each rung in progression

until he is at the desired position. The overhead trapeze bar (Fig. 26-5C) is a grab handle on a stable base that has adjustable positions and flexibility in the handle angles. This device can assist a person in rolling over, lifting the hips up to move onto a bedpan, scooting the body position in bed or in obtaining a long-leg seated position. The various configurations of bedrails of long and short length, portable or permanently mounted, can assist a person in rolling over, in body positioning for sleep or obtaining a short leg seated position on the side of the bed (Fig. 26-5B). A person can also use a locked wheelchair that is positioned next to the bed. By grasping a stable secure part of the chair such as the nearby armrest or push handle, the person may initiate rolling or sitting.

For rolling, the person grabs a rung on the rope ladder, bedrail, or wheelchair part with the arm closest to the side of the bed toward which he is rolling. Then by reaching with the other arm to grab the device and pulling, rolling of the body is gained, and the hip and leg will typically follow. If the hip and leg do not follow, the person can use an extended wrist or hand to push the knee or thigh to assist in moving.

If the patient's lower extremities are paralyzed, the person must manually move the legs over the side of the bed. For the dependent person, another individual swings the person's legs off the edge of the bed. A leg lifter is a device for moving one leg at time. This device has a large loop at one end that can be placed around the foot or thigh and a smaller loop or handle at the other end that a person can grasp for lifting the leg (Fig. 26-5D). The device is offered with the strap supported by a dowel stick or without that stiffness for a flexible strap. The flexible strap is ideal when moving a leg in a small space where knee flexion may be required such as when moving the extremity into a car seat. The device can be used to move paralyzed legs in bed or if the person has limited hip flexion and cannot reach the leg for moving it.

A hospital bed with powered head and knee controls can also assist a person with bed mobility and can be helpful for lower extremity dressing in bed. By raising the head and upper trunk, both hands are freed from holding one's balance to perform the task at hand. Contextual factors may influence this choice because not every patient can afford to purchase a hospital bed or chooses to use a hospital bed once at home. The occupational therapist will analyze the individual, task, and environment to determine the best method or device for the individual to use in accomplishing safe bed mobility.

If a patient is not able to move out of bed independently, there are a variety of lifting systems that can assist the person or caregiver in moving out of bed and to multiple locations such as to a toilet or tub

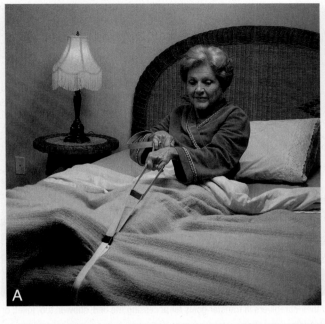

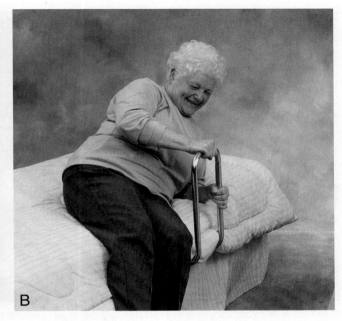

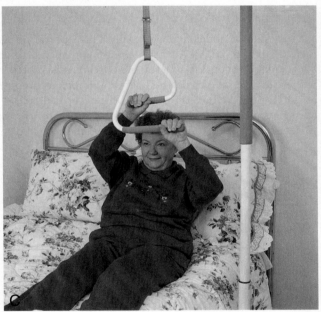

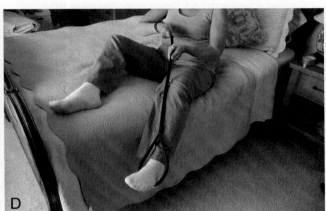

Figure 26-5 Devices that assist with bed mobility. **A.** Bed ladder pull-up. **B.** Bed rail assist. **C.** Overhead trapeze bar. **D.** Leg lifter. (Courtesy of North Coast Medical, Morgan Hill, CA.)

(see Fig. 26-6). The lifting systems can be on a movable frame, on a freestanding frame that hangs over the bed, or on a moving track that runs on the ceiling. The moveable frame lift requires one or more persons to physically move the lift with the person in it. Some lift systems can move the person from one room to another by way of ceiling tracks that run over the bed and through a doorway into the bathroom and then over the toilet, tub, and/or shower. A client who is able to attach the body support pieces of the lift and operate the remote motor control may have the capability to move independently out of bed into a wheelchair or over a toilet or into a tub. The occupational therapist must

consider client factors (such as stature, weight, and postural stability), client performance skills, where the lift will be used and for what purpose, the activity demands of the lift system to determine the safest one for the client and the operation of the remote controls. The size and configuration of the seat sling or postural support offered by the system, the location of the body support pieces, presence or absence of underarm supports, and location and type of controls vary with each make and model. *Safety Message: Intervention must include careful instruction and multiple practices during ADL with the client and family to ensure safe use and operation of the lifting system.*

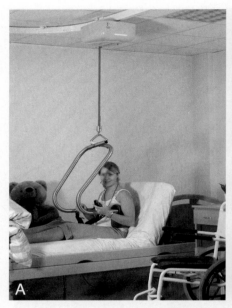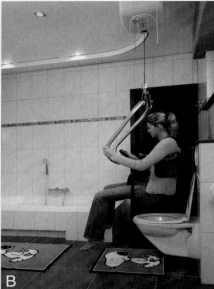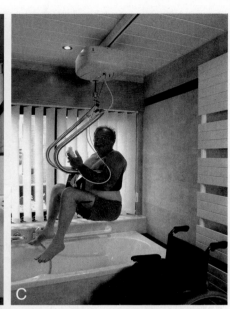

Figure 26-6 Motorized lifting systems assist physically challenged individuals or their caregivers in transfer goals for accessing the bed, shower, tub, toilet, or pool. (Courtesy of SureHands Lift & Care Systems, Pine Island, NY.)

Activities of Daily Living in Bed

Some persons may be able to, or choose to, dress while sitting on the edge of the bed or while standing. Persons with lower extremity or trunk paralysis may need to perform BADL such as dressing, skin inspection, self-catheterization, and/or a bowel program while lying in bed. Those persons that use a leg bag for urine management may need to disconnect tubing from a bed bag that collects urine during the night and reconnect the tubing to a smaller leg bag that is worn during the day. While dressing in bed, it is necessary to reach one's feet by flexing the hips and knees so that the feet are closer to the hands for preparing to don pants, socks, and/or shoes. Independence in rolling from side to side and reaching one's buttocks are important for performing manual bowel stimulation and clean up or using a long-handled mirror for skin inspection.

Bed mobility is illustrated in Figure 26-3 with a client with C7 quadriplegia who does not require the use of any assistive devices. Good strength in the deltoid, pectoralis major and minor, biceps, wrist extensors, and scapula muscles is key to support these tasks without assistive devices, so strengthening these muscle groups in therapy is preparatory to learning this technique. Even without trunk muscles, a person can perform safe bed mobility, but a sense of balance for sitting and transferring must be developed, practiced, and accomplished during intervention.

Transfers

A transfer is the means by which a person moves one's body from one surface to an adjacent surface (Definition 26-1). Therapists must consider transfers to all surfaces including the tub, shower, toilet, and eventually a transportation vehicle (Fairchild, 2013). Adaptive equipment, such as grab bars, a raised toilet seat, or a tub bench, can assist a person with easier and safer transfers. There are various techniques for safely performing a transfer, and the occupational therapist must work in conjunction with the physical therapist to determine the best method for each client.

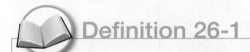

Definition 26-1

Various Types of Transfers

Dependent Transfer

Person requires maximum assistance of one or more persons using a special technique or device to assist in moving from one surface to another.

Sliding Board Transfer

Person cannot bridge the gap between two surfaces without the use of a sliding board.

Standing Pivot Transfer

Person can stand up, pivot the feet and turn the trunk, and then sit down on the transferring surface.

Independent Transfer

Person can perform all steps of a transfer with no physical assistance from another person. A device may or may not be used.

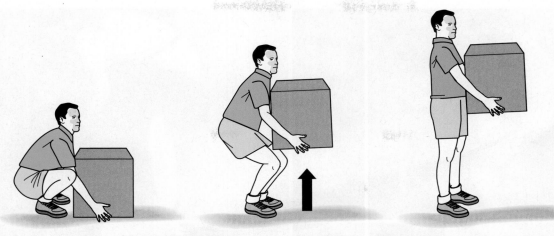

Figure 26-7 Proper body mechanics for lifting an object are illustrated. The object is maintained close to the body. The person looks straight ahead, squats by bending the hips and knees and keeping the back straight. Lifting begins by straightening the knees and hips and keeping the object close to the body.

The transfer technique can be simple or complex and the method chosen depends on the patient's client factors, upper and lower extremity strength and range of motion, physical endurance, trunk balance, body type, orthotic devices, and/or wheelchair style. Skill building for transfers is necessary as the patient progresses through the rehabilitation process. A dependent transfer may be necessary until the person can begin learning assisted or independent transfers.

The intervention must include instruction and practice in a supervised environment until the patient is safe for less supervised situations. To prevent back injuries, the therapist must know and practice proper body mechanics during lifting, bed activities, and transfers, and furthermore must instruct and ensure that the family and patient understand the concept as well (Fairchild, 2013). Figure 26-7 illustrates proper body mechanics for lifting and basic principles of good body mechanics are listed in Safety Note 26-1. Back injuries must be avoided. After the first time one injures the back, it becomes vulnerable to future injury and can alter a therapist's or family member's quality of life and even livelihood.

A client must achieve competence in basic transfer skills for moving on and off a therapy mat and bed before working on the more difficult transfers such as to a toilet, to a shower chair, and perhaps eventually into a car. Transfers from the floor to a wheelchair or into a car are the most difficult of transfers because of the height discrepancy and space gap between the two respective seat levels. In addition, during a car transfer, the patient must handle both legs through the cramped space of a car door.

Dependent Transfer

A person who is too weak to move requires assistance from another person or persons for moving his or her body from one place to another using a dependent transfer.

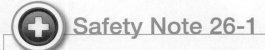

Safety Note 26-1

Principles of Good Body Mechanics

- Pause and think before lifting or moving anything. Plan the path and technique.
- Keep the load to be lifted or carried close to the body at all times and if possible at the level of the belly button.
- Maintain a good posture and keep the whole body in straight alignment throughout the activity. Keep the entire back straight with the chest out and the shoulders level and squared back (not rounded or slumped forward), looking straight ahead. The hips should be in line with the shoulders and the ankles with the hips. Avoid twisting by rotating the whole body and changing directions with the feet.
- When picking up an object, squat down, bending at the hips and knees only instead of the waist so the leg muscles are used and not the weaker back muscles. If necessary, put one knee to the floor and the other knee in front bent at a right angle in a half kneeling position. After grasping the object firmly, lift the object while keeping the back straight, tightening the abdominal muscles and slowly straightening the hips and legs (see Fig. 26-7 middle picture).
- Position the feet shoulder width apart with one foot slightly ahead of the other for a wide base of support.
- If sliding an object, such as a client in preparation for a transfer, rock back on the heels while keeping the back straight with hips/knees bent so the physical lift or rotation uses the stronger muscles of the arms and legs to carry the weight and a strain on the back muscles is avoided.

Adapted from Dartmouth-Hitchcock. (2012). *Back problems: Proper lifting.* Retrieved September 1, 2012 from http://patients.dartmouth-hitchcock.org/health_information/health_encyclopedia/sig59692.

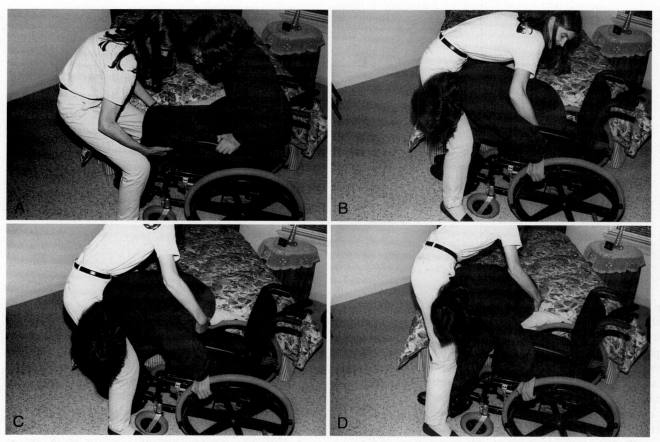

Figure 26-8 Proper body mechanics are used by a therapist during a simple and safe dependent wheelchair-to-bed transfer for a person with quadriplegia. The client must have the trunk flexibility to lean forward over the thighs, but this technique works for light to heavy weight clients. **A.** The therapist positions herself in a close proximity to the patient with feet apart, shoulders square and level, back straight, and hips and knees bent pressing around the patient's knees. The therapist slides the client's buttocks forward in the seat to eliminate proximity to the rear wheel during the transfer. **B.** The patient is leaned forward onto the therapist's outside thigh. If able, the patient can assist with balance with the left hand on the wheelchair tire. **C, D.** The therapist uses the strength in her arms and legs to rock the patient forward, placing her hands under the buttocks and lifting them off the wheelchair seat. With the patient's weight shifted forward, there is little weight to pick up, and the therapist rotates the client's buttocks onto the bed with relative ease, maintaining good body mechanics throughout the transfer.

A one-person technique entails standing in front of the patient and placing him or her in a forward flexed position with the chest lying on the thighs. This flexed position shifts the patient's body weight over the knees and ankles rather than on the buttocks, which allows the buttocks to be picked up and moved more easily. This method has proven worthy to teach family members because it enables the helper to control the movement of the patient's body while lessening the probability of hurting his or her own back (Fig. 26-8). Note that this method cannot be used for the patient with limited hip flexion, for example, those with a hip fracture or heterotopic ossificans or those who are posthip replacement surgery. For the patient with limited hip flexion, this technique is modified to sliding the buttocks toward the edge of the wheelchair (in a wheelchair to bed or toilet transfer) and placing the patient's knees between the helper's knees. Using proper body mechanics, the assistant squeezes the knees of the patient with his or her own knees while rocking the patient forward slightly and simultaneously pulling on the patient's pants or belt and rotating the hips to the surface being moved to. For a two-person dependent transfer, the first person stands behind the patient, threads his or her hands under the patient's axillae to hold onto the patient's flexed forearms, and lifts up to move the buttocks to the transfer surface while the second person moves the legs. A transfer board, sometimes called a sliding board, can be used to bridge the gap if the buttocks cannot be raised easily.

Sliding Board Transfers

A person who cannot stand but can slightly lift the buttocks off the surface by doing a push-up, can use a transfer board to slide the buttocks and bridge the gap between two transfer surfaces (Fig. 26-9). There are a wide variety of shapes, lengths, weights, and styles of transfer boards available from various manufacturers. A long transfer board may be needed for the difficult transfer into a car to bridge

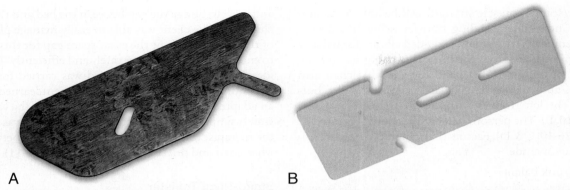

Figure 26-9 Examples of different transfer boards available through suppliers. **A.** Transfer board with hand holes and notches allows transfers from either side. **B.** Offset transfer board fits around the wheel of the wheelchair when the armrest is removed. (Courtesy of North Coast Medical, Morgan Hill, CA.)

the large gap and the seat height discrepancy between a wheelchair and a car seat (Fig. 26-10A), but a shorter board can be used for transfer to the toilet or bed because the gap is smaller. A cutout on one end of the board may be needed to allow the person with a weak grasp to pick up the board. An angled or notched board, as shown in Figure 26-9B, may be best for maneuvering around the rear wheel of the wheelchair while transferring. A board made of high-density polished plastic, shown in Figure 26-9A, provides a slippery surface for bare skin while a board with a moving center disc allows easy sliding of the body.

Most transfer boards are positioned with one end under the patient's buttocks and thighs and the other end on the surface to which the person is transferring. Level surfaces greatly aid in the transfer, although one can use gravity to assist when sliding to a lower surface. A person may require a transfer board for a car or toilet transfer but not for other transfers in the home. The client with good

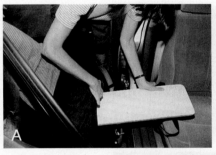

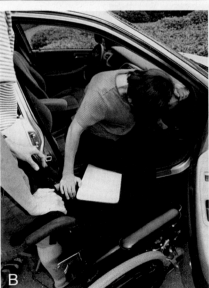

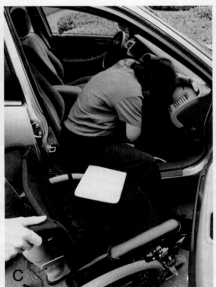

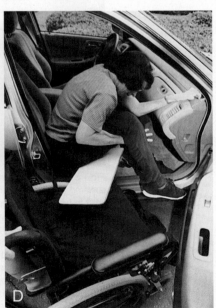

Figure 26-10 A sliding transfer with one person assist from a wheelchair to a car seat is illustrated. Assistance is required by this client for placement/removal of the transfer board as well as storing/unloading the manual wheelchair in the vehicle's trunk. **A.** The person leans to the outside of the wheelchair while the helper places the transfer board under the person's buttocks and on the car seat. The long transfer board is necessary to bridge the large gap between the wheelchair and car seat. **B.** The client extends her elbows and depresses the scapular, which lifts her weight from her buttocks and allows her to slide on the board moving sideways toward the car seat. **C.** This person found it easier to keep the legs outside the car until the transfer onto the car seat was completed. Then the left lower extremity is moved into the car with the right hand while balance is maintained by leaning against the dashboard of the car. **D.** The right leg is lifted into the car in similar manner.

shoulder/scapula muscle strength will be able to accomplish an independent sliding transfer using this device. The patient leans forward on extended elbows for balance and to shift weight from the buttocks. Using scapula depression, pushing with her hands on the wheelchair arm and seat, and maintaining balance, she slides her buttocks to the left from the wheelchair to the driver seat (Fig. 26-10, B). The person then handles both legs into the car (Fig. 26-10, C & D). Factors that can impede a safe sliding transfer include

- poor trunk balance
- spasticity
- excessive body weight or large, heavy legs
- inadequate upper extremity strength
- inability to lock elbows into extension
- joint contractures or tightness in the elbows or wrists that prevent full elbow extension and/or full wrist extension
- a low ratio of arm length to trunk length

Off-the-shelf boards do not always meet specific needs of clients, so therapists may have to custom-make or modify an off-the-shelf transfer device to meet a particular need. In Figure 26-3D, the client's occupational therapist made a custom board with plywood covered in high-density foam and vinyl to bridge the gap between the bed and the wheelchair seat. The client was able to easily manage placement of the board, and it fit the exact space gap for this transfer to enable the client to move safely and efficiently. The same idea for a custom transfer board was carried forward in community mobility goals when the client learned to drive an adapted van and needed to transfer onto the van driver seat. A similar but second custom transfer aid was made by the therapist to bridge the different space gap between the wheelchair and driver seat surface (see Fig. 26-11).

Stand-Pivot Transfer

A person with lower extremity deficits, who can support his or her weight on one or both legs, may be able to perform an independent or assisted stand-pivot transfer. An assisted stand-pivot transfer is performed with the helper standing in front of the patient and the transfer surface as close as possible. Generally, it is best to transfer the patient toward his or her stronger side. The patient should first be slid toward the edge of the surface from which the transfer is taking place, with care to protect the person from slipping off the edge completely, especially if there is lower extremity or trunk spasticity. The patient is assisted to a standing position (Fig. 26-12). The helper places his or her

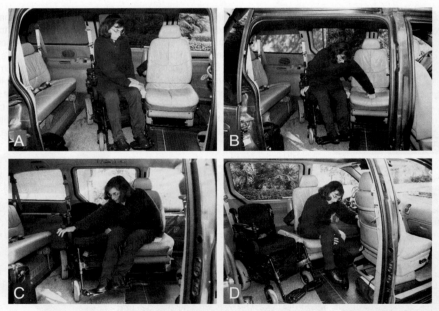

Figure 26-11 A person with C7 quadriplegia demonstrates an independent sliding transfer from a powered-base wheelchair to a van driver's seat using a custom-made transfer board made by the therapist to bridge the gap between the two seats. **A.** The person maneuvers the wheelchair into the van backward and aligns the wheelchair seat adjacent to a van seat that is powered swiveled toward the rear of the van. The transfer board is covered in vinyl and wedge shaped to fit between the wheelchair seat and the driver seat, to create a flat, smooth surface and safe bridge for the client to slide on. The special board eliminates the hard task of putting a sliding board under the buttocks pretransfer and removing it post-transfer. **B.** The person prepares to transfer by leaning slightly forward onto the left arm. By pushing down on the right hand and using shoulder depression to relieve pressure under the buttocks, she lifts and slides her buttocks to the driver seat. **C, D.** She repositions each leg from the wheelchair footrest onto the van floor. The driver seat is then swiveled to the left to allow positioning under the steering wheel.

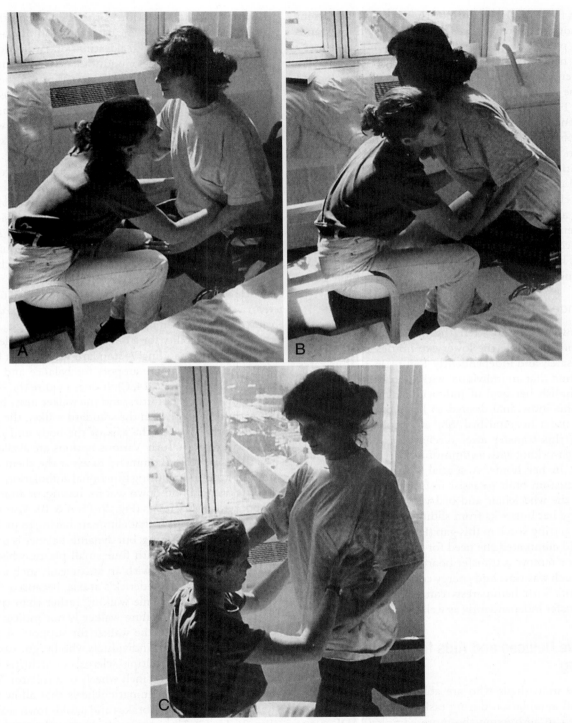

Figure 26-12 A patient with left hemiplegia is assisted to a standing position by one person. **A.** The patient places the unimpaired right hand on the therapist's shoulder for support. **B.** The therapist positions her knee in front of the patient's weak left knee to prevent the left knee from buckling as the person stands. The patient leans toward the therapist and the strong side to move the center of gravity forward. **C.** The patient uses the strength of the unimpaired side with the guidance of the therapist to extend the hips and knees to a standing position. (Reprinted with permission from Gillen, G. [2011]. *Stroke rehabilitation: A function based approach.* St. Louis: Elsevier/Mosby.)

knees in front of one or both of the knees of the patient to prevent the patient's knees from buckling upon standing. The patient wraps his or her arms around the helper's body or neck, but only for support, not to pull up. The helper bends his or her knees, keeps the back straight, and grabs the waist or belt of the patient's pants or a transfer belt. This belt with handles is wrapped snugly around the patient's waist and provides a handhold for the helper. The helper rocks the person back and forth several times and then using momentum pulls the person to a standing position. A patient can assist by using leg strength to stand or upper body strength to push off the wheelchair or chair armrest or bed rail to come to standing. By pressing against the weak knee or knees, the helper assists the patient to swivel or slide the heels toward the transfer surface while standing. The helper can then guide the patient's hips over and down to the transfer surface while again bending at the hips and knees rather than the back.

Independent Transfers

Patients with adequate strength to push up and move the trunk and to handle the lower extremities may learn to transfer safely and independently. Figure 26-13 illustrates one method that an individual with C7 quadriplegia used to accomplish her goal of independent bed transfers at home. This individual desired to live alone and did not want to use a hospital bed. She accomplished independence in this transfer after discharge as an outpatient and while working with a community-based occupational therapist in her home. A special soft-surfaced transfer aid was custom built to assist in bridging the space gap between the wheelchair and bed yet protect her skin by preventing her buttocks from sliding over the wheelchair wheel or getting stuck in this gap (Fig. 26-13, B & C). This special aid eliminated the need for the person to struggle to place or remove a transfer board from under her buttocks, which was time and energy consuming.

Patients with hemiparesis can learn to do a stand-pivot transfer independently as well.

Assistive Devices and Aids for Walking and Standing

For those individuals who are able to stand and walk, functional ambulation during task completion must be considered in addressing the more complex IADL such as caring for a child, walking a pet, home management, meal preparation and cleanup, moving about a yard for lawn care, or moving about a store for shopping. A person with balance difficulties or weakness in one or both lower extremities may require some type of orthotic mobility device to provide stability and support while ambulating. The physical therapist determines which mobility device the person should use; however, the occupational

therapist will have to address the client using the device while performing ADL. The device may only be used to assist a person in moving to a destination, or the device may be required for balance or endurance while in the process of performing the activity. The occupational therapist in collaboration with the physical therapist may need to adjust the device for the person's use such as adjusting the length of the quad cane or walker. Intervention would involve instruction and practice in the device's use during functional ambulation.

Assistive devices for ambulation come in various styles and shapes (Fig. 26-14). The type of cane chosen by the physical therapist depends on the person's balance and gripping ability, with personal preference considered. A straight cane is selected for a person with good strength, coordination, and balance who nevertheless requires a device for support. The four-prong or quad cane is chosen for a person who is weak on one or both sides, has increased muscle tone or ataxia, and needs a wider, more stable base than a straight cane provides. The hemiwalker, so called because it is often used by persons with hemiplegia, provides the greatest stability for a one-handed orthotic device and can assist with standing. A standard walker with four legs gives the user bilateral support for balance and stability while walking (Fig. 26-14, C). It does require the person to use both upper extremities, and the walker must be picked up with every step. With the standard walker, the user can simply rotate around the axis of the body and carry the walker during the turn. Various options are available that the therapist may recommend to assist the client with usability of the device during functional ambulation such as a folding frame, a fold-down seat for resting, or attached bag or pocket to carry items (Fig. 26-15, A & B). Also available are small front wheels that eliminate having to pick up the walker while ambulating, but dynamic balance is necessary.

A rolling walker with four small plastic wheels is effective for individuals with an ataxic gait, such as is seen in cerebral palsy or Frederick's ataxia, because it is easier to push the walker while walking rather than to pick it up for each step. A rolling walker is not indicated for a person who leans on the walker for support. A popular form of the walker for individuals who fatigue easily with conditions such as multiple sclerosis or arthritis is called a rolling walker with 6-inch wheels or a rollator. This device has four large pneumatic wheels that allow for easy ambulation with hand brakes and a fold-down seat to rest (Fig. 26-15, C). The user can even sit and propel it backward with stability or have someone else push them.

Some patients have the strength and balance to stand without an assistive device while performing light ADL. Patients who do not have the standing balance, strength, or endurance to stand at a work surface and use one or both hands may have to sit to perform ADL. If the activity requires the individual to carry items to various locations, then the therapist will have to consider this in addressing

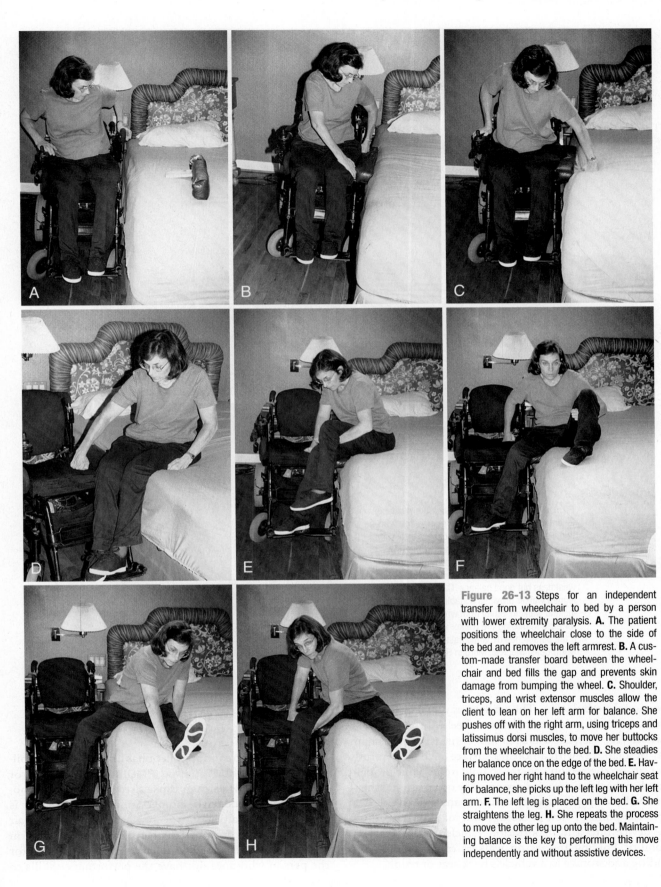

Figure 26-13 Steps for an independent transfer from wheelchair to bed by a person with lower extremity paralysis. **A.** The patient positions the wheelchair close to the side of the bed and removes the left armrest. **B.** A custom-made transfer board between the wheelchair and bed fills the gap and prevents skin damage from bumping the wheel. **C.** Shoulder, triceps, and wrist extensor muscles allow the client to lean on her left arm for balance. She pushes off with the right arm, using triceps and latissimus dorsi muscles, to move her buttocks from the wheelchair to the bed. **D.** She steadies her balance once on the edge of the bed. **E.** Having moved her right hand to the wheelchair seat for balance, she picks up the left leg with her left arm. **F.** The left leg is placed on the bed. **G.** She straightens the leg. **H.** She repeats the process to move the other leg up onto the bed. Maintaining balance is the key to performing this move independently and without assistive devices.

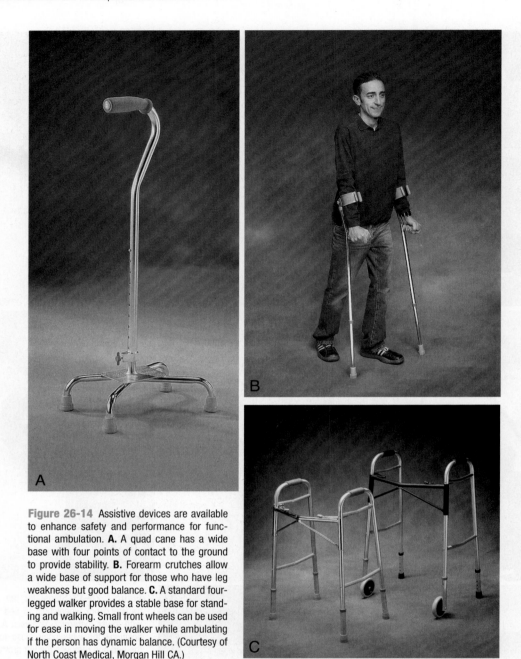

Figure 26-14 Assistive devices are available to enhance safety and performance for functional ambulation. **A.** A quad cane has a wide base with four points of contact to the ground to provide stability. **B.** Forearm crutches allow a wide base of support for those who have leg weakness but good balance. **C.** A standard four-legged walker provides a stable base for standing and walking. Small front wheels can be used for ease in moving the walker while ambulating if the person has dynamic balance. (Courtesy of North Coast Medical, Morgan Hill CA.)

functional ambulation. The walker tray or bags can be used or a small stable cart on four wheels. If the person is a wheelchair user, the therapist may consider a wheelchair tray or a lap tray with a nonslip surface such as Dycem® that sits on the person's thighs to hold items while propelling the wheelchair around a room. The occupational therapist will eventually have to consider any assistive device from the point of view of storage and loading/unloading the device into a transportation vehicle for community mobility. Folding frames on walkers can promote easy loading and storage in a vehicle's back seat or trunk.

Mobility by a Personal Mobility Device: Wheelchairs & Scooters

For a person who cannot walk or has limited walking ability, a personal mobility device (PMD) such as a manual or powered-based wheelchair can assist with functional mobility in and outside the home. A manual wheelchair is appropriate for a person who can propel the wheelchair using two arms, one arm, the feet, or a foot and an arm together. A power-based wheelchair is recommended for the person who does not have the performance skills to

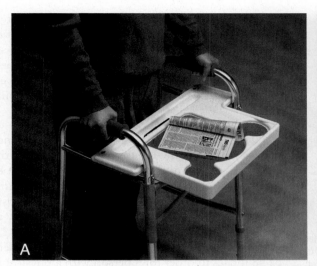

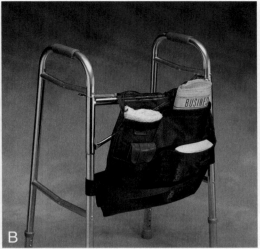

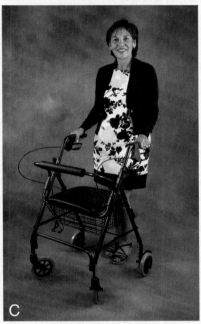

Figure 26-15 Available variations in walkers and optional features. **A** & **B**. Carrying trays and baskets on a walker. **C.** A rolling walker with 6-inch wheels is lightweight with hand brakes, a fold-down seat with curved back support and a basket. (Courtesy of North Coast Medical, Morgan Hill.)

propel a manual wheelchair. A popular PMD for those who can walk but only short distances is the three- or four-wheeled motorized scooter. The device enhances both functional and community mobility for individuals with multiple sclerosis, cerebral palsy, chronic obstructive pulmonary disease, cardiac conditions, obesity, and the elderly who have limited walking capacity. Personal requirements for a scooter are the ability to transfer, good trunk balance, and an ability to maintain an upright posture with little support. Persons who are dependent in manual wheelchair propulsion will require a manual wheelchair equipped with features to allow

another person to easily maneuver the wheelchair from behind. There are many models and styles of wheelchairs and scooters with a variety of standard and optional features (see Chapter 17).

The rehabilitation team that is prescribing a PMD for any person should *always* collaborate with all therapists and specialists to ensure that the device is suitable not only for functional mobility needs but also for community mobility needs when being transported in the chosen mode of transportation whether public or private. If a person cannot transfer from wheelchair seat to vehicle seat, a converted private or public vehicle will allow one to

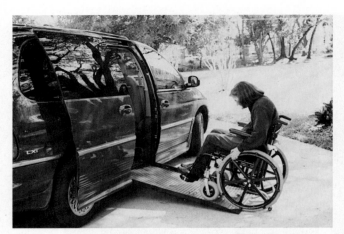

Figure 26-16 This person with quadriplegia has the skill to push her manual wheelchair up a ramp into a modified minivan to enter the interior of the vehicle. This task is easy in a power-based wheelchair but can be difficult in a manual wheelchair.

maneuver a wheelchair into the vehicle. In Figure 26-16, a person with quadriplegia demonstrates the physical abilities and balance to safely ascend a ramp through the side door of a minivan.

Intervention for Wheelchair Mobility

Environmental barriers will most likely affect a person's mobility in a PMD at some point, and he or she should be taught to deal with such barriers. When a patient receives a new PMD, intervention for indoor and outdoor mobility is important so that he or she learns to handle and maneuver the chair in whatever circumstances are encountered, such as tight spaces, a curb or ramp, and rough and uneven terrain. A program graded toward independent mobility in a PMD should be a team effort among the nursing staff and physical, occupational, and recreational therapists with the practice of skills incorporated into all rehabilitation activities.

The initial stages of PMD intervention take place inside the rehabilitation facility where the patient learns how to maneuver on a smooth, uncluttered surface. The patient learns to operate and control the PMD and all of the movable parts, as well as how to transfer in and out of the device. For those who will be independent users, a second phase of training teaches the patient to use the PMD outside on various terrains such as uneven sidewalks, gravel, and sand. The patient then learns to negotiate obstacles such as curbs and steps. Once the patient can traverse outdoor surfaces, training continues in various interior environments of public buildings such as the airport, library, or shopping mall where the person learns to operate the PMD in crowded, narrow spaces. Development of a community mobility skills course will provide a framework for the practitioner in assessment and training with mobility device skills needed in the client's natural environment (Walker et al., 2010). The

occupational therapy practitioner can incorporate wheelchair mobility goals within other ADL intervention. For example, if a patient is taken to the grocery store to shop for food in preparation for cooking a meal, there is the opportunity to explore wheelchair mobility in a public environment while also carrying items or pushing a shopping cart.

Negotiating Ramps. A ramp enables a person using a PMD to overcome steps or a height discrepancy in a doorway or entrance. Ramps are constructed with many shapes, sizes, and dimensions and can be custom built or purchased and assembled from a kit. Federal guidelines specify how ramps in public places should be constructed in terms of length, slope, and texture. For every inch of rise, the ramp must have 12 inches of length (1:12 slope). For example, a 4-inch step will require the ramp length to be 48 inches in order for a person with a physical disability to safely negotiate the ramp. A ramp in a public place must have a surface with a detectable texture for persons with visual impairments. It must have railings that are not vertical but slope at 1:10 maximum. There must be 4 feet of level landing at the top of the ramp (ADA Standards for Accessible Design, 2010).

One safe technique to use in descending a steep ramp is to orient a manual wheelchair backward and lean forward to place most of the weight over the front caster wheels as the chair slowly descends the ramp (Fig. 26-17). If the wheelchair has a tendency to tip backward easily, a helper should stand behind the wheelchair and walk with the person to catch the chair should it begin to tip backward. For a manual wheelchair user to safely use a ramp, the following are necessary:

- Upper extremity strength and coordination, including grip strength
- Trunk mobility and awareness of the balance point of the wheelchair

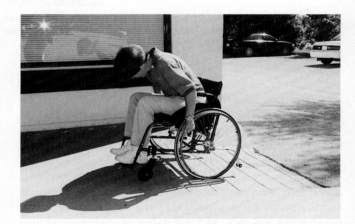

Figure 26-17 A person with good arm and trunk strength can safely negotiate a steep ramp by moving backward down the ramp. By leaning the trunk and head forward, the center of gravity is shifted, and the chair is less likely to tip backward.

- Optional anti-tipping wheels to prevent the chair from falling backwards
- Optional hill climbers or grade aids to prevent the chair from rolling backward
- Level of visual and cognitive skills to make good decisions regarding movement on the ramp and in and around environmental factors such as traffic, other pedestrians, light poles, and the pedestrian walk signage.

Wheelchair Wheelie. Advanced manual wheelchair skills are important for the client to learn to maneuver the variety of terrains typical in a community. One such skill is called a wheelchair wheelie, which allows the user to move around on uneven terrain or surfaces such as sand, rocks, pothole, curbs, steps, and high door thresholds or down a steep hill or ramp (Kirby et al., 2006). A wheelie can also be used for resting against a wall, turning in a tight space, or moving down extremely unlevel or bumpy terrains. The goal of the wheelie is to balance on the large rear tires of the wheelchair and elevate the caster wheels in the air so they are not rolling over the surface or obstacle. This allows for smoother and more efficient operation of the wheelchair (PoinTIS SCI Physical Therapy Site, 2012; Somers, 2010). For this advanced wheelchair skill, a person must have the following:

- Basic wheelchair skills
- Upper extremity strength
- Good hand function with a strong grip
- Bilateral upper extremity coordination
- Understanding of the steps to perform the task and awareness of the center balance point of the wheelchair (which varies from chair to chair)
- Ability to maintain dynamic center of balance on the back wheels

The patient must practice a wheelchair wheelie many times on level surfaces before attempting uneven surfaces or the more difficult curbs and steps. In the clinic, a mat can be placed behind the wheelchair, or the therapist can stand behind the chair ready to catch the wheelchair should it tip too far backward. *Safety Message: Because of the danger of losing balance and falling backward, the therapist must be attentive and within close proximity of the wheelchair when the patient is practicing this advanced skill. Safety rigging may be necessary for the client to practice this skill independently.* Not all wheelchair users will be able to perform this advanced skill.

To "pop a wheelie," the first step is to grasp the hand rims posteriorly and pull them forward forcefully and abruptly, throwing the head back forcefully, if needed. Once the client learns to balance in and assume a wheelie position, then intervention focuses on instruction and practice in moving forward and backward in a wheelie position. Lastly, intervention covers dynamic wheelie skills over easy and then difficult obstacles. This wheelchair skill is better understood by seeing the task demonstrated in a dynamic mode. Multiple videos of wheelies and other wheelchair skills can be viewed at http://www.wheelchairskillsprogram.ca/eng/tests_video/php. One can also search "wheelchair wheelies" on *YouTube* for demonstrations by therapists and wheelchairs users; however, the therapist should view these videos with the understanding that they are not peer-reviewed demonstrations.

Negotiating Curbs. Since the passage of the Americans with Disabilities Accessibility (ADA) Standards in 1990, curbs on sidewalks at street intersections are becoming less of a problem as curb cuts proliferate; however, at times the wheelchair user may encounter a curb. Although some power wheelchairs can negotiate curbs well, ascending and descending a curb or step in a manual wheelchair will require proficiency with a wheelchair wheelie. First, the person approaches the curb or step, facing it. Once the wheelie position has been obtained, the casters are placed on the curb. The person leans forward to redistribute the weight and propels the large rear wheels up the curb or step with a hearty push. A person must have good balance, upper extremity strength, and hand function to perform this maneuver. To go down a curb or a step, the person approaches it backward, leans forward in the chair, and rolls the rear wheels over the step or curb. An alternative method for going down a curb is to approach the curb facing it, move into the wheelie position, and roll slowly down the curb using the back wheels. The person must have an excellent sense of the balance point of the wheelchair to perform this technique safely. If a wheelchair user cannot move up or down a curb or step or roll through grass or over uneven surfaces, another person can provide assistance as in Figure 26-18.

Negotiating Steps. Ascending or descending multiple steps in a scooter or powered wheelchair is impossible. A strong manual wheelchair user may be able to descend a couple of steps safely by performing a wheelie while moving down the steps. In an emergency, a person who can perform a wheelchair-to-floor transfer can get out of the wheelchair and "bump" up or down the steps while pulling the chair along. Skin protection during this task must be understood and practiced. *Safety Message: Instruction and practice to perform this difficult task should occur before an emergency arises.*

Moving a manual wheelchair and its dependent occupant up and down steps safely requires the assistance of two people. The back of the wheelchair should be positioned facing the steps with one person standing behind the chair and the other person in front of it. The chair is tipped backward, with one person holding the push handles and the other person holding the front of the chair by

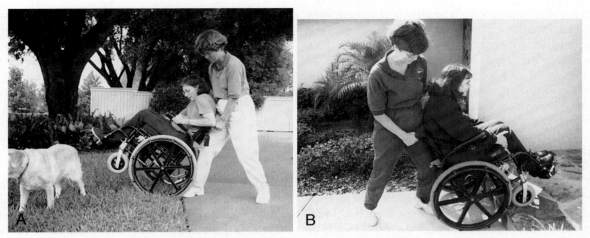

Figure 26-18 Functional mobility is enhanced by an assisted wheelchair wheelie. **A.** A therapist performs an assisted wheelchair wheelie to roll a wheelchair through grass and uneven terrain. **B.** A therapist uses an assisted wheelie to place the front castor wheels of the wheelchair on a curb so the person in the manual wheelchair can be pushed over the curb and onto the sidewalk.

its frame or leg rests. While the person in front maintains balance of the chair, the person behind pulls the chair up step by step. That person should take care to keep his or her back straight and use leg strength to move the chair. To take a person down the steps, approach the steps with the wheelchair facing forward and with it tipped backward and balanced. The procedure is reversed, with the person in front of the chair holding onto the chair while guiding and controlling the speed of the chair down each

step. Moving a power wheelchair in this manner is impossible and not safe because of the weight of the chair.

For individuals who must negotiate multiple steps in a home and are unable to ambulate or have limited ambulation, a stair lift can move a person up or down the staircase safely and efficiently. There are various configurations of stair lifts that can be installed for straight and curved stairs in a private or public location (Fig. 26-19, A & B). The person must be able to transfer onto the seat

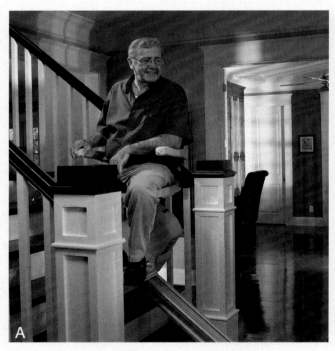

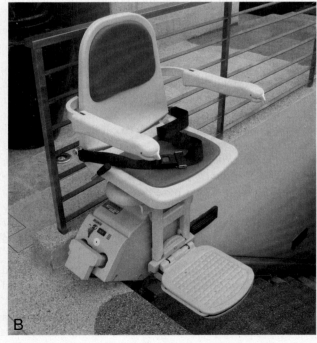

Figure 26-19 **A** & **B.** A powered stair lift allows a person to move up and down steps easy and safe on a stairway in a private residence and in a public place. (Courtesy of Acorn Stairlifts, Orlando, FL.)

surface and balance himself on the seat while the seat moves up or down the staircase. If the person cannot walk, a second wheelchair must be available at the top of the staircase for the person to transfer into. Another viable but expensive option is a small elevator, which meets the space and structural requirements, installed interiorly or exteriorly in a private or public building.

Mobility Devices to Assist with Standing or Sitting

Mobility devices are available to enable a person to perform the functional mobility tasks of standing or sitting. Some ADL requires supported standing or balance, use of two hands, and stability. Various mechanical and powered devices are available to raise a person vertically up and down. Other devices assist coming to a supported standing position or to rotate and swivel in preparation for standing/walking. Persons who have a powered up/down seat feature on a power-based wheelchair or scooter can reach work surfaces such as a sink or kitchen counter

or tall cabinets (Fig. 26-20). This feature can also allow the user to engage other people at eye level and move around in the elevated position at low speeds. Wheelchairs can have features that enhance standing, such as a mechanically operated stand-up feature on a manual wheelchair or a motorized stand-up feature on a power-based wheelchair. This feature may be important to particular people because standing can improve circulation, renal and bowel functions, reduce lower extremity spasticity, and prevent effects of prolonged immobilization. The person using a power-based chair that has a stand-up capability can even move around in the standing position at low speeds (Fig. 26-21) to meet the task demands of a job when both hands are required for tasks, such as cooking in the kitchen or working as a beautician or pharmacist. The feature can prepare a person to walk by placing him or her in the standing position so the person can then just walk out of the device.

There are portable devices to assist in standing such as a swivel disk or seat that assists a person in preparation of standing (Fig. 26-22). The powered standing lounge chair is popular for persons with a variety of disabilities because the chair raises the person totally supported to a partial standing position to allow supported standing in preparation for walking or transferring (Fig. 26-23).

COMMUNITY MOBILITY

Community mobility includes all the ways in which people move about the world in order to access goods and services and remain engaged in occupations beyond their homes (Womack, 2012). Individuals move about their world as pedestrians, drivers, or passengers in motor vehicles or on public transportation, or even as users of a wheelchair or scooter. Viewed from this perspective, community mobility is an occupation that is essential to personal health and social well-being. Restricted mobility has been linked to the onset or acceleration of physical and mental health problems (Marottoli et al., 2000). Community mobility is valuable for every person of every age group because it facilitates engagement in important areas of occupation including leisure, work, and social participation (Stav, Hunt, & Arbesman, 2006).

Today, most people travel into the community for almost everything they need, although the virtual community created by the internet and social networking has expanded a totally different avenue for seeking and playing with friends, socializing, and even shopping online for such necessities as drugs, supplies, and clothes. These resources are inaccessible to some and can be unsatisfying in terms of social human interaction. The occupational therapy practitioner can offer a range of services to a client, a client's family, a local community, or a business or agency that is concerned with participation and safety in community mobility (AOTA, 2010). Guidelines for the

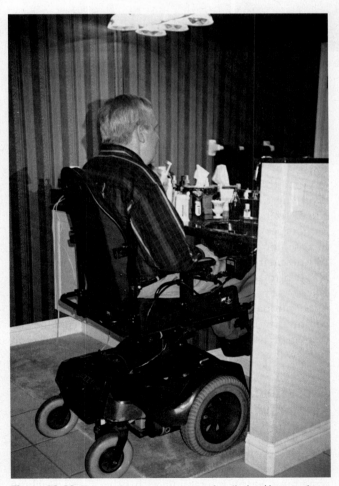

Figure 26-20 This gentleman uses a powered vertical up/down seat on a power-based wheelchair to allow better height and close approach to the sink for grooming activities.

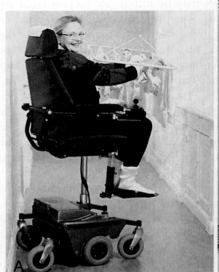

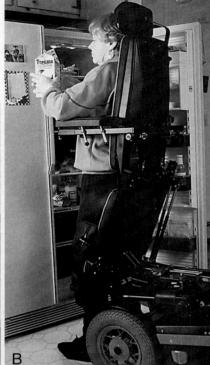

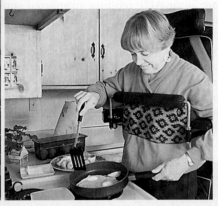

Figure 26-21 A–C. Permobil wheelchair options allow for many adjustable sitting and standing positions for activities at home and in the community. (Courtesy of Permobil Company, Woburn, MA.)

therapist in addressing community mobility are provided in Procedures for Practice 26-3.

The Meaning of Community

An occupational therapy practitioner must understand the value and need for community that exists in every person that receives occupational therapy no matter the age, cultural background, or setting in which they live. There are many ways to view "community." Merriam-Webster (2012) defines community as a "unified body of individuals" and lists various types of community as

- *family community*, which includes one's personal family members
- *neighbors*, or those that live in close proximity to an individual and collectively are called a *neighborhood*, a geographically local community
- *municipalities* or cities that consist of a collection of neighborhood communities
- *planned communities* that are developed to meet a specific need such as a retirement community

The value of feeling connected to one's environment cannot be understated. Participants in a study noted that their environment was more than just physical surroundings; it was the sense of belonging that came from doing,

being, and living in place (Vrkljan, Leuty, & Law, 2011). A sense of community requires an ability to engage and interact not only with the family but also with persons outside of the home environment. This can be as simple as going to the knitting store where mothers gather after dropping their kids off at school, the local coffeehouse where friends meet for breakfast in the mornings, the hamburger joint where the local students gather, or the local senior center for weekly social gatherings. A community destination may include the courthouse in which one is called to serve as a juror on a legal trial or the church where one gathers with others of similar religious beliefs. Occupational therapy promotes greater participation in community by identifying barriers to performance and strategizing solutions with the client to overcome the barriers (Waite, 2011).

Accessible, Safe Environments Promote Alternative Modes of Travel for Community Mobility

For persons with disabilities or for those who cannot drive, having access and use of a sidewalk network is crucial for remaining active, interacting with others, and reaching vital destinations, such as shopping and medical facilities (Kihl et al., 2005). The physical characteristics of a

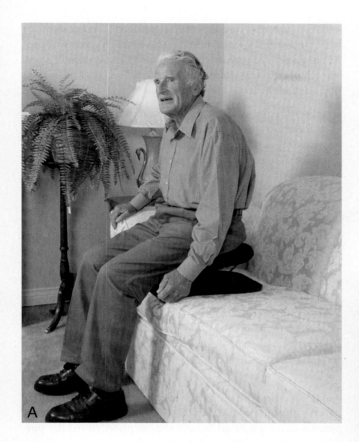

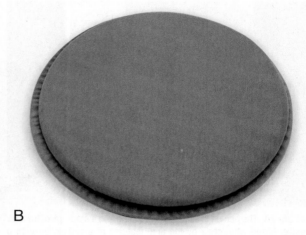

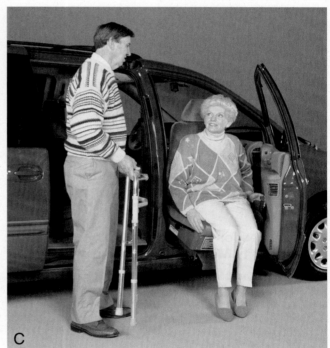

Figure 26-22 Mechanical devices to assist in standing up. **A.** Hydraulic action in this portable seat lift assists the person in rising. **B.** Portable and cushioned seat that swivels 360° and can be used in a vehicle seat or chair. **C.** A powered swivel/tilt passenger seat for a minivan. (Photos A and B courtesy of North Coast Medical, Morgan Hill, CA; Photo C courtesy of Braun Corporation, Winamac, IN.)

community often play a major role in facilitating personal independence. A safe pedestrian environment, easy access to grocery stores and other shops, a mix of housing types and nearby health centers and recreational facilities are all important elements that positively affect a client's health and well-being (National Highway Traffic Safety Administration [NHTSA], 2009). Poor community design, poorly maintained sidewalks, and physical barriers, such as busy highways and high walls, can make it difficult to remain independent and involved in the community (American Association of Retired Persons [AARP], 2005; Burkhardt, McGavock, & Nelson, 2002). AARP published a comprehensive survey entitled *Livable communities: An evaluation guide* that can identify barriers in mobility and safety in

a livable community (Kihl et al., 2005). The occupational therapy practitioner can provide consultation to a local community or municipality by using this survey as a guideline and structure.

Evaluation and Intervention for Community Mobility

The feasibility, safety, and personal control of community mobility must be explored early on in the occupational therapy process. The therapist finds out detailed information about the client's everyday routines by talking through the patient's typical day (Radomski, 2011). During the inpatient stay, the client may be allowed

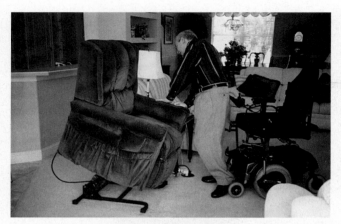

Figure 26-23 The person is assisted to standing and a stand-pivot transfer to a power-based wheelchair by the dual features of a wheelchair with a powered vertical lift feature and a lounge lift chair with a powered base that raises and tilts the seat.

home visits on the weekends in preparation for discharge. Discussing the challenges met on these visits will focus intervention on meaningful goals. Furthermore, working on community mobility while the person is still in rehabilitation will prevent feelings of isolation and lessen feelings of loss during these visits and after discharge. Exploring

Procedures for Practice 26-3

Guidelines for the Therapist in Addressing Community Mobility and Driving

- Analyze the client and the activity demands of the specific mode of travel chosen to determine whether the client is capable of returning to the chosen mode of travel or requires alternative community mobility options.
- Determine whether the client has any questionable performance skills that would impede safe driving of a personal vehicle (car or low-speed vehicle [LSV]) if that is the goal, and ensure that the client meets all state licensing requirements.
- Analyze contextual and environmental factors to identify barriers to safe community mobility.
- Evaluate to determine whether a recommendation for continued driving or no driving is appropriate or if a referral to an occupational therapy driving specialist for a comprehensive driver evaluation is necessary because of performance skill deficits that may impair driving performance or bring to question safety issues.
- If the outcome of a driver evaluation determines that the person cannot return to driving, then identify community mobility alternatives that the client has the skills to use.

where, when, and how a person desires to interact in his or her communities will guide the therapist in setting appropriate goals and making recommendations that will allow the client to participate effectively and safely. The evaluation may include

- screening for safe community wheelchair skills and safe wheelchair transportation
- assessing safe pedestrian skills for crossing a street and negotiating curbs and sidewalks
- determining readiness and skills to use paratransit
- determining driver fitness to drive (Hunt, 2010; Hunt, Carr, & Barco, 2009)
- screening a client for referral to a specialist in driving if evaluation or intervention is necessary to determine driver safety or need for adaptive driving equipment (Pierce & Schold-Davis, 2013)
- determining safe alternative travel modes available in the community for the client who is not able to drive or must retire from driving
- screening for proper child passenger safety for disabled parents who will be transporting children (Yonkman et al., 2010)

A disability or health-related change can disrupt a usual pattern of community mobility and thus challenge habits (Dickerson et al., 2007). The occupational therapy process will explore all factors that support or hinder participation in necessary, desired, and routine community mobility. After evaluating these factors and exploring the meaning of community for the person, the occupational therapist provides intervention for community mobility goals during the occupational therapy process. Because the task demands for community mobility are higher than for any other ADL or IADL, the initial intervention plan should identify community mobility goals to be implemented later in the occupational therapy process as the last IADL to be addressed. When addressing community mobility, occupational therapy practitioners must employ interventions that address

- performance skills (cognitive, visual, and motor)
- performance patterns (self-regulation and self-awareness)
- context (role of passengers and family involvement)
- activity demands (adaptive devices and strategies) (Hunt & Arbesman, 2008)

Intervention for driving skills is not relegated to just the driving specialist anymore. General practice occupational therapists use a full range of interventions to improve driving skills as well as overall community mobility (Unsworth, 2011). Practitioners must think beyond driver rehabilitation as purely recommending and training in the use of adaptive equipment and use evidence-based interventions to improve the IADL of community mobility, including driving. Interventions must address cognitive and visual function, motor function, driving skills intervention, self-regulation, and self-awareness, and the role of passenger and family involvement in the driving ability, performance, and safety of the adult (Hunt & Arbersman, 2008). The practitioner must provide intervention that addresses the impaired skills in vision, cognition, and motor function but also specific intervention that includes client education programs that aim to develop client self-awareness of driving skills (Hunt & Arbesman, 2008). Occupational therapy practitioners experienced in addressing community mobility needs recommend specific interventions be applied (Hunt & Arbesman, 2008; Pierce & Schold-Davis, 2013) such as follows:

- Provide education to develop self-awareness of driving skills.
- Provide education on the relationship between medical problems and driving.
- Use multiple training activities that excite different brain functions that are all necessary for safe driving.
- Provide education about compensatory strategies for maintaining driving skills such as changing habits and routines. For example, discuss alternative driving routes to avoid left turns, lane changing, and merging, and discuss changing habits that are known situations for frequent accidents. Discuss better times of the day to drive to avoid sun glare at dusk or dawn.
- Counsel drivers on cessation or limiting driving when it is necessary.
- Counsel families of older adult drivers on signs that indicate that driving is no longer an option.

Modes of Travel for Community Mobility

Community mobility is defined by the OTPF as "moving around in the community and using public or private transportation, such as driving, walking, bicycling, or accessing and riding buses, taxi cabs, or other transportation systems" (AOTA, 2008). Community mobility includes all of the ways in which people move about the world in order to access goods and services and remain engaged in occupation beyond their homes (Womack, 2012).

Walking

Walking enables people to get where they need to go under their own strength and energy without having to rely on another mode of travel. Whether the person walks in the community depends on specific environmental factors as well as the purpose for walking. For example, if the person needs to pick up multiple items and carry them to another location, then that activity must be considered in the mobility program. Sidewalks are the fundamental building blocks of a pedestrian network, and they allow mobility using a PMD and as such are important environmental

factors to be considered. Safety for pedestrians is enhanced by the separation of walkways from the roadway. The Federal Highway Administration provides information that includes pedestrian and bicycle safety tools (Federal Highway Adminstration, 2012). The Pedestrian and Bicycle Information Center (2012) provides planning and design tools to make roads, pedestrian crossings, trails, and separated pathways safer for pedestrians. The National Highway Traffic Safety Administration provides a booklet entitled *Stepping Out* that promotes the benefits of walking and pedestrian safety for adults aged 65 years and older, including tips for staying safe at intersections, in parking lots, in areas without sidewalks, and in bad weather (NHTSA, 2012).

Pedestrians aged 65 and older accounted for 19% of all pedestrian deaths and an estimated 11% of all pedestrians injured in 2010 (CDC, 2013). Elderly pedestrians are often hit in crosswalks or when crossing intersections and are generally hit when they have almost finished crossing. They are usually observing the law and not behaving dangerously. Many do not see the vehicle that hit them, and when they do see the vehicle, they usually believe that the driver has seen them and will avoid them. It follows that persons with walking impairments and those in wheelchairs may encounter the same dangers at intersections or crosswalks as the elderly do. Education about pedestrian safety could save lives (Classen et al., 2011). The occupational therapy practitioner can advocate for pedestrian safety by educating community planners and city leaders and encouraging changes in traffic signals at intersections, pedestrian walkways, and pedestrian warnings.

Using Nonmotorized and Motorized Personal Mobility Devices. PMDs are popular modes of travel in a neighborhood or local community as more communities are becoming accessible to bicycles, manual wheelchairs, and portable motorized chairs (three- or four-wheel scooters) or complex, power-based wheelchairs. These various nonmotorized and motorized PMDs assist a person with community mobility. If the person has the performance skills to ride a two- or three-wheel bicycle, he may be able to travel to a nearby store or facility. If the person has the strength and endurance to push a manual wheelchair for a distance and is able to handle the wheelchair in outdoor terrain, he may be able to use it to get to a local convenience store or down the street to a friend's home. If the destination does not exceed the powered device's battery charge, a person can use that device to travel to the store or visit a church in a nearby locale.

Using Personal Low-Speed Vehicles

Another type of private transportation is personal low-speed vehicles (LSVs), which are small electric or gas-powered cars designed for low-speed, local trips in areas such as planned communities, resorts, college campuses, and even large industrial parks. As an alternative mode of transportation, the low-speed "street-legal" vehicle, or golf cart, is becoming popular especially among older persons, although not all communities allow them. Older residents see the carts as a form of transportation when driving privileges are suspended but limited mobility in their community is still allowed. Many planned retirement communities in year-round mild weather states now allow mobility by way of these vehicles that are simply a golf cart or simulate a golf cart. One such community in Florida called "The Villages" brags of as many as 50,000 carts and even set the world's record in 2005 for the "largest golf cart parade with 3,321 participants" (*Orlando Sentinel*, 2011). Under Florida law, a plain golf cart can be converted into a street legal LSV with the limitations that the top speed cannot exceed 25 mph, and it cannot be operated on streets with speed limits higher than 35 mph. The law further requires the cart to have specific features such as headlamps, brake lights, turns signals, seat belts, rearview mirror, windshield wiper, and horn (*Orlando Sentinel*, 2011). A neighborhood electric vehicle is another commonly used type of LSV with the difference that it has a driving range of up to 40 miles on a single battery charge (Lynott, Poncy, & Twaddel, 2011). The client in Figure 26-24 uses a power mobility device for functional mobility and enjoys community mobility with her companion assist dog within the planned retirement community in a modified golf cart with hand controls.

The occupational therapy practitioner can use information available from multiple resources when training a person to be mobile in the community via a wheelchair, cane, scooter, golf cart, or public bus. The occupational therapy practitioner can help city planners be more sensitive to the community mobility issues of people with special needs. Occupational therapy practitioners can advocate for their clients and consumers by working with local community leaders, planners, engineers, traffic safety and enforcement professionals, public health and injury-prevention professionals, and decision makers who are seeking ideas and solutions for changes to the physical environment that improve pedestrian, bicycle, and LSV safety.

Driving a Personal Vehicle

Most adults in the U.S.A., with or without disabilities, drive a car as the primary mode of transportation. People age 65 years and older make more than 90% of community trips in cars, as either drivers or passengers (Houser, 2005). When young adults cannot drive and older adults are no longer able to drive, occupational functioning is jeopardized. An occupational therapy intervention plan therefore may include addressing the IADL of driving a personal vehicle.

Driving is the most complex IADL because it requires good physical, visual, perceptual, psychological, and cognitive skills as well as an integration of these skills (Classen, 2010). Consequently, most patients are not ready for a driving evaluation before discharge from the inpatient facility, and it should be one of the last ADL resumed during rehabilitation (Pierce, 1996). There is clear evidence that clinical and community-based practitioners must realize their role and responsibility in addressing driving. A conversation about driving is not reserved just for a driving specialist (Hunt & Arbesman, 2008). The Multifactorial Older-Driver with Dementia Evaluation Model (MODEM) will assist the practitioner's clinical reasoning about fitness-to-drive decisions (Hunt, 2010; Hunt, Carr, & Barco, 2009).

Transportation needs, particularly for the wheelchair user, may have to be addressed long before driving because the person may not be ready for a driving evaluation until 8–12 months after discharge from a hospital or inpatient rehabilitation facility. A referral to the occupational therapy specialist in driving for the sole purpose of determining transportation needs may be appropriate before discharge so that the patient, family, and funding source can be guided toward the appropriate transportation vehicle and safe wheelchair transportation modifications. If the specialist determines that the patient may be able to drive later, vehicle selection and modifications for transportation can be made with future driving needs taken into consideration.

The Role of the Occupational Therapist in Addressing Driving

The role of the occupational therapist in addressing driving has been clearly defined in the past decade (Di Stefano & Macdonald, 2005). The American Medical Association

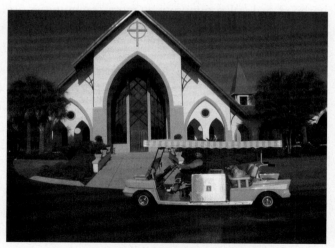

Figure 26-24 After learning to drive a personal van, Ms. S. desired community mobility via a golf cart in the planned retirement community in which she lived. The cart was specially modified to allow her to ride in a power-based wheelchair onto the golf cart, operate the cart with hand controls, and allow room for her companion assist dog.

(Carr et al., 2010) has clearly delineated occupational therapists as experts who have knowledge and skill in this area. Referral to a specialist in driving for a comprehensive driver evaluation has been the common practice in the past; however, the number and accessibility of specialists in driving are inadequate to meet all driving needs in society (Classen et al., 2010). All occupational therapists who work with adults with physical dysfunction should have the knowledge and skill to accurately determine who is a safe driver presently, who is at risk for unsafe driving, and who needs further evaluation by a specialist in driving (Dickerson et al., 2011). In situations where the client is clearly at risk for unsafe driving, the role of the occupational therapist is to explain the dangers of driving and help clients and families resolve transportation options rather than prolong driving independence (Hunt, Brown, & Gilman, 2010). Ethical decision making is crucial for the therapist in ensuring the safety of the client, families, and others on the road.

Evidence is available that indicates therapists can use clinical testing to make an informed decision regarding driving and that not all clients need the services of a driving specialist (Dickerson et al., 2011). If the results of clinical testing indicate no functional performance impairments that correlate with driving risk, then the therapist can recommend to the physician and team that the person appears capable to resume driving without a referral to a specialist in driving. On the other hand, if the client has difficulty with other complex IADL, the occupational therapist practitioner can inform the team and client that he or she would be expected to also have difficulty with driving (Dickerson et al., 2011). If the client demonstrates performance impairments that correlate with driving risk, then the therapist must recommend cessation of driving and may plan interventions to improve the client factors that prohibit driving at this time. The client can also be referred to a driving specialist for a definitive decision concerning probable driving safety (Hegberg, 2007).

If the patient drives before he or she is ready, or after being told to cease driving, the therapist has an ethical obligation to protect the public welfare by reporting the person to the appropriate licensing authority in the manner dictated by the state of residency. Every state has specific procedures for reporting an unsafe driver, and the occupational therapist should know the procedure for reporting impaired drivers in his or her state and which functions a therapist is authorized, obligated, or responsible to perform. Individual state regulations for reporting can be found in *The Physician's Guide to Assessing and Counseling Older Drivers* (Carr et al., 2010). Although it is written with older drivers in mind, the material can apply to all age and disability groups.

The American Occupational Therapy Association provides guidance concerning the IADL of driving. The association provides practitioners, other professionals, as well as the public with educational opportunities through online courses, publications, and a dedicated website with useful and timely information about the occupational therapist's role in driving, older driver safety, driver evaluation resources, and community mobility throughout the life span (Schold-Davis, 2012) (see Resources 26-1). Occupational therapists are perfect community partners

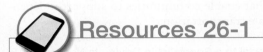

Resources 26-1

Internet Media Resources for Professional Development Regarding Community Mobility

Resources for Professional Development

Driving and community mobility for older adults: Occupational therapy roles (Revised). Presented by Susan Pierce & Elin Schold-Davis with contribution by Linda Hunt (2013). Bethesda, MD: AOTA. Retrieved September 1, 2012 from www.aota.org/older-driver (AOTA members only).

Determining capacity to drive for drivers with dementia using research, ethics, and professional reasoning: The responsibility of all occupational therapists. Presented by Linda Hunt (2010). Retrieved September 1, 2012 from www.aota.org/older-driver.

Driving rehabilitation: Analysis of occupational performance in the context of driving a vehicle. Presented by Anne Dickerson (2011). Retrieved September 1, 2012 from http://cpeprograms.ecu.edu/CourseStatus.awp?&course=DRIVER.

Driving and mobility: Driving evaluation and *Driving and mobility: Intervention.* Both retrieved September 1, 2012 from http://ceu.phhp.ufl.edu/.

Building blocks for becoming a driver rehabilitation therapist. Presented by Susan Pierce and Carol Blackburn. Retrieved September 1, 2012 from http://www.adaptive-mobility.com/therapists/.

Resources for Information Regarding Driving and Community Mobility

AAA Foundation for Traffic Safety
www.aaafoundation.org or www.seniordrivers.org

American Association for Retired Persons (AARP)
www.aarp.org

American Occupational Therapy Association (AOTA)
www.aota.org/olderdriver

National Highway Traffic Safety Administration (NHTSA)
www.nhtsa.gov

National Center on Senior Transportation
http://seniortransportation.easterseals.com

The Beverly Foundation
www.BeverlyFoundation.org

The Hartford Insurance Company
www.safedrivingforalifetime.com

to serve on city planning boards to assist in making transportation services more affordable and user friendly. Environmental factors can play a critical role in either facilitating or undermining the ability for one to move about in the community. The occupational therapist is well suited to address both the personal and environmental factors that enable communities to support independence and safe transportation.

When a Referral to a Specialist in Driving Is Necessary. If determination of driving competence requires a comprehensive and focused driving evaluation, the occupational therapy practitioner may need to consult with or refer to an occupational therapist with Specialty Certification in Driving and Community Mobility (SCDCM). These specialists may be on staff in an inpatient or outpatient facility or in a community private practice. A SCDCM is an occupational therapist with advanced knowledge and skill in evaluation and intervention specific to driving and community mobility. This specialist can provide a formal driver evaluation, driver training with specialized adaptive equipment, driver rehabilitation services for specialized driver education, or remediation for enhancing safe driving skills. The SCDCM can develop an occupational profile and perform a formal clinical and in-traffic evaluation of a person's physical, visual, perceptual, cognitive, and psychological functioning as it relates to driving, considering all contextual and environmental factors.

A fair and objective assessment by a professional is welcomed by families of older drivers or of younger potential drivers with acquired or congenital disabilities. The occupational therapy practitioner can steer the family toward the need for the driver competency evaluation and initiate the referral process to the SCDCM (Pierce & Schold-Davis, 2013). The general practitioner in occupational therapy should know the SCDCMs in the local communities, regions, and state to whom clients, patients, consumers, and agencies can be referred. A list of SCDCMs nationwide can be found on the driver safety link of www.aota.org.

The SCDCM will analyze each driving task for the person and determine the client's needs and desires and what specific aids are necessary for safe driving (Pierce & Schold-Davis, 2013). The SCDCM will take into consideration the particular contextual or environmental factors, the person's performance patterns, and the activity demands of the various driving tasks. The person's individual vehicle will be evaluated, as will the person's functional mobility in getting to and into the vehicle with any orthotic devices or mobility aids used. The client must be able to enter and exit the vehicle and store the wheelchair, scooter, or other orthotic device as needed. Figure 26-25 shows a person who accomplishes functional mobility by propelling a manual wheelchair with both feet and using an independent stand-pivot transfer into a personal vehicle she

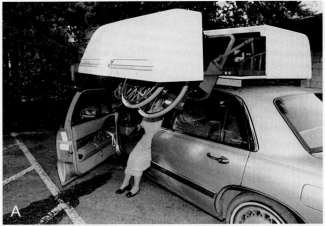

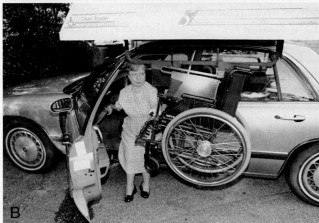

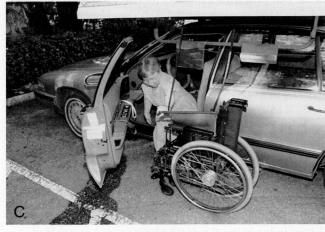

Figure 26-25 A woman with juvenile rheumatoid arthritis illustrates how a powered device assists in loading/unloading and storing her manual wheelchair on top of her personal vehicle for independence. Figures A-C show the unloading process.

drives for community mobility. A powered device assists her in loading and unloading her folding-frame manual wheelchair.

Persons with physical deficits or mobility challenges may require special driving devices or aids to assist them with particular driving tasks. Driving technology can cost

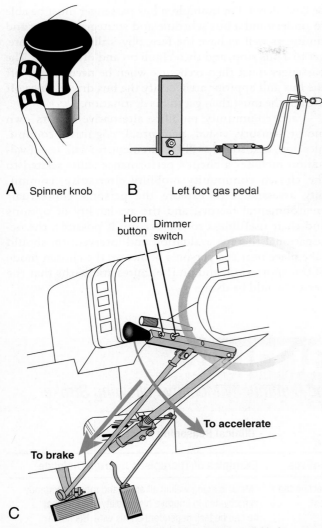

A Spinner knob   **B** Left foot gas pedal

C

Figure 26-26 Sampling of assistive driving devices available for a person to compensate for a physical disability. **A.** Spinner knob steering device. **B.** Left foot gas pedal. **C.** Mechanical hand controls.

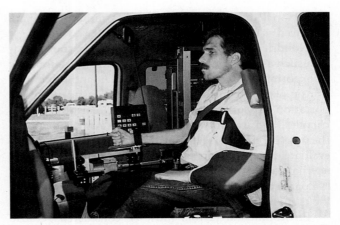

Figure 26-27 A high-technology driving system to assist a person with quadriplegia to operate the controls of a van with one arm while sitting in his wheelchair. (Courtesy of Driving Systems Inc., Van Nuys, CA.)

as little as $85 for a steering device (Fig. 26-26, A), $800 for a left-foot gas pedal (Fig. 26-26, B), or $1,200 for simple mechanical hand controls (Fig. 26-26, C). A person with no lower extremity function and minimal upper extremity function may require a specialized high-technology modified van costing upward of $100,000 (Fig. 26-27).

When a SCDCM cannot be found to assist a patient, a commercial driving school instructor who has training in driver rehabilitation services may be available. A regular driving school instructor may not have the necessary medical background to understand the client's deficits and the medical implications for the driving task. Before referring the client to a commercial driving school or driving school instructor who markets services to persons with disabilities, the therapist should investigate the instructor's background and expertise concerning the medical condition or diagnosis of the client. When using a driving

school instructor, the occupational therapy practitioner should collaborate with this person and be involved with the final outcome. The therapist completes an occupational profile and performance skill assessment and share the results with the instructor prior to the person having the road test with the driving school instructor. After the road test, the therapist and instructor collaborate on the outcome and recommendations (Pierce & Schold-Davis, 2013).

When Driving a Personal Vehicle Is Not a Viable Option. If driving is not a viable target outcome for a client, it is very important that the occupational therapy practitioner address this with the client and family and then develop a plan for accessible and safe alternative transportation options in each person's context (Hegberg, 2007; Silverstein, 2008). There is no subject more entrenched in emotion and feelings than the topic of driving. The freedom and independence that driving gives a person is so tangible that an honest conversation about driving will only occur if the person directing the conversation shows compassion, understanding, and support. Unfortunately, many older adults faced with driving retirement have made no plans for alternatives to driving. Some of those who have not thought about alternatives expect to rely on friends and family for transportation rather than use other forms of transportation. The needs of older people who depend on public transportation are not being met. Of nondrivers 75 years old and older, 75% report satisfaction with their community mobility resources; however, most of these seniors use family members and friends for transportation (NHTSA, 2006). Seniors without access to family members or those living in nonurban areas are likely to have unmet needs that are greater than those of older people who live near family members (NHTSA, 2006). If driving retirement is the recommendation, then alternatives for community mobility must be presented that are based on personal knowledge of the client's community and are perceived as real and practical by the client.

Nondriving options can include public transportation such as fixed-route rail, bus, paratransit, community transportation (e.g., community bus), demand-responsive transit (e.g., dial-a-ride), flex-route, independent transportation networks, volunteer services, taxis, bicycles or tricycles, and walking (NHTSA, 2006). An occupational therapy practitioner has the knowledge and skills to evaluate the person in using other community mobility alternatives for safe transportation. This IADL should be evaluated and treated in the same manner as the therapist looks at all other IADL (Pierce & Schold-Davis, 2013).

Environmental factors must be considered because every community has individualized resources for alternative choices for community mobility. Using public transportation may actually place more demands on the person than driving a personal vehicle. All requirements of using specific community mobility alternatives must be considered. For example, a bus passenger must be able to understand a bus schedule and strategize a route and timing as well as have the fare, physically offer the fare, get to a bus stop, and then climb on and off the bus. The passenger must then recognize when he needs to get off the bus and appropriately notify the bus driver. Once off the bus, he must then get to his destination.

Each community mobility alternative has its own motor, sensory, visual, perceptual, cognitive, communication, and social skill requirement for safe use. Evaluation includes a client's performance skills related to the chosen community mobility alternative, community assessment to explore the person's contextual/environmental factors, and the availability of options and their usefulness to the person. If possible, the occupational therapy evaluation and intervention should take place near the person's home, on the chosen mode of transportation, and on the routes and paths that the person would be using.

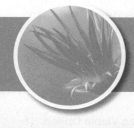

case example
Mr. J.: Restoration of Functional and Community Mobility Following Stroke

Clinical Reasoning Process

Occupational Therapy Intervention Process	Objectives	Examples of Therapist's Internal Dialogue
Patient Information Mr. J. is 69 years old with right hemiplegia and expressive aphasia from a left cerebral vascular accident (CVA). Mr. J. has a good medical history except for the CVA and has good motor functioning in the left extremities and normal visual and cognitive performance skills. He was evaluated in an outpatient rehabilitation center, and the following problems were identified by the occupational therapist:	Appreciate the context	"Mr. J. is aging well in all areas and most importantly is motivated to improve his mobility skills so that he can be less dependent on his wife. His home and community environment as well as family support will enable him to reach his chosen goals for functional and community mobility."
1. Client can roll over and sit up in bed but has difficulty moving his right leg off the bed in preparation for transferring and dressing. 2. Client cannot complete a stand-pivot transfer independently because he needs assistance coming to standing. 3. Client can propel a manual wheelchair with a one-arm drive on level surfaces but cannot negotiate a ramp or uneven terrain. 4. Client cannot perform bathroom activities at home because his bathroom is inaccessible to a wheelchair. 5. Client has not driven since the CVA but is very anxious to begin driving again. He is concerned about loading his wheelchair into a car by himself. 6. He enjoys living in a planned retirement community and has access to other modes of community mobility but has not used them in the past.	Develop intervention hypotheses	"Mr. J. has significant physical deficits that may be permanent, but with his young age and good health, I believe that his occupational performance could be enhanced greatly by improving his functional and community mobility skills."

Select an intervention approach

"I will develop an intervention plan that emphasizes functional mobility first and community mobility needs second. I know that there are precursor mobility skills that are required in the areas of bed mobility, transfers, and wheelchair mobility, so I will need to address these performance skill areas first before I address the specific tasks that he is weak in, such as handling his legs in bed or propelling his wheelchair outdoors. It will enhance my intervention if I talk with physical therapy to see if they can work on improving his leg strength and his ability to stand up independently. I will need to explain to the client and his family that we will address his driving ability as a long-term goal after we have accomplished the short-term goals in functional mobility. I will explain how the skills in functional mobility will prepare him for the driver evaluation when the time is appropriate. I will let the family know that I can research community mobility options available in their community that he may be able to use in the meantime or in case the outcome of the driver evaluation is that he is not able to return to driving."

Reflect on competence

"As an occupational therapy generalist, I am concerned that I do not know all of my responsibilities in driving and community mobility. I need to research this area before I begin addressing the topic of driving and community mobility. I also need to find resources in my state for a SCDCM so I can talk intelligently about the specialist's services and purpose to the client and family as well as make a timely referral. In the meantime, I will research options in his community and use my OT skills to consider the activity demands of each option and evaluate Mr. J.'s ability to use alternative modes of travel similar to how I evaluated his skills in the kitchen and bathroom."

Recommendations

The occupational therapist recommended two sessions per week for 8 weeks. In collaboration with the client and his wife, the occupational therapist established the following long-term intervention goals:

1. Mr. J. will be independent in bed mobility and sitting on the edge of the bed.
2. Mr. J. will be able to perform a stand-pivot transfer independently.
3. Mr. J. will improve his ability to negotiate outdoor terrain and ramps with his manual wheelchair and be advised on motorized scooters for use in independent long-distance mobility in the community.
4. In collaboration with physical therapy, Mr. J. will be instructed in using his quad cane to walk into the bathroom and perform sink activities while standing.
5. Mr. J. will be referred to SCDCM once he is able to transfer in and out of his car.

Consider what will occur in therapy, how often, and for how long

Ascertain the patient's endorsement of plan

"I do not believe that this client is aware of his potential for being more independent in functional mobility skills. Some of this may be related to his wife, who is overprotective of her husband as she is afraid that he will fall and hurt himself. She expresses concern about him driving again. I believe that he is motivated enough to be more independent and will have successful outcomes with client-focused intervention. I believe that when he sees that he can accomplish functional mobility goals and realize his potential to drive again, he will be highly motivated to work hard in occupational therapy. Mr. J. and his wife seem agreeable to the plan, and I hope that by including his wife that she will become more comfortable in letting him do tasks independently at home as he achieves each mobility skill."

Summary of Short-Term Goals and Progress

1. Mr. J. will be able to move his weak leg off the edge of a bed and come to a seated position with or without orthotic devices.

   The therapist ascertained after a week of occupational therapy that Mr. J. could move his weak leg off the bed using his stronger left leg by putting his left foot under the weak right foot and then moving both feet over the edge of the bed. She determined, however, that he would require a device to use to pull against to come to a short-leg sitting position on the edge of the bed. In the second week, various techniques and assistive devices were demonstrated to him, and it was determined that a portable half-bed rail worked best. By the fourth week, Mr. J. could come to a short-leg sitting position on the side of the bed independently. He was also shown how to use the bed rail to help him stand up and ready himself for a stand-pivot transfer.

2. Mr. J. will become independent in sink activities in the bathroom.

   The first week of therapy revealed that the client's standing tolerance and balance were not sufficient to perform sink activities while standing, even though he could walk short distances. In the second week, he was taught how to stand up from his wheelchair outside the bathroom door, walk into the bathroom using his hemiwalker and short leg brace, and sit on a tall-legged stool at the sink. The higher seat helped him come to standing when he pulled on the sink for assistance in standing up when ready to leave.

3. Mr. J. will be able to transfer into the passenger and driver side of his car independently.

   By the third week, Mr. J. could handle his leg on and off the bed and could stand up independently. In the fourth week, Mr. J. was instructed in getting in and out of the passenger side of a car. After he could perform this transfer, he was taught how to transfer into the driver's side of the car, maneuvering his legs under the steering wheel.

Next Steps: Revised Short-Term Goals (1 month)

1. Mr. J. will become independent in toilet transfers and tub transfers but will likely require some assistive technology such as elevated toilet seat, grab bars, and a tub bench.

2. Mr. J. will become independent in long-distance ambulation by using a motorized scooter but will require assistance for loading and unloading the scooter.

3. Mr. J. will be independent in driving himself to and from therapy.

In the sixth week, he was referred to a SCDCM that I found in the next town. He was instructed by this specialist to use a left-foot gas pedal and a spinner knob for driving, and the adaptive equipment was installed in his own car. In collaboration with the SCDCM, I decided that Mr. J. could not be independent in loading his wheelchair into his four-door sedan. He did not have the standing balance to use a wheelchair loader that is bumper or trunk mounted. He could, however, use a car topper that will electrically pick up, fold, and load his manual wheelchair into a box on the top of his car, all while he sits in the driver seat. By the time of his discharge, he had received all necessary in-vehicle training by the SCDCM and was beginning to drive around his own community.

Understand what he is doing

Anticipate present and future patient concerns

Decide whether the patient should continue or discontinue therapy and/ or return in the future

"It has been very helpful for Mrs. J. to attend each of Mr. J.'s treatment sessions. As she has observed his weaknesses, she has been able to encourage him to complete his home therapy exercises and activities on days that he does not come to therapy. They have learned how to use the kitchen sink for support to let him work on standing tolerance three or four times a day. Mrs. J. has indicated that he will sometimes sit outside the bathroom and appear to long to just stand up and walk in. Mr. J. knows that they cannot afford to modify the bathroom doorway, so he understands that it is very important for him to have a good outcome with standing and this goal. He keeps asking me about a driving evaluation and is beginning to show some frustration in having to wait. Mrs. J. is very understanding of why this goal has been put off to later and has assured me that she will not let him drive before he is ready."

"Mr. J. is accomplishing his goals quickly. I see him working very hard because he can tell that a driver evaluation is getting closer to becoming to reality for him. Through my contact with the occupational therapy driving specialist, I was able to discover that Mr. J. can use an adaptive equipment rebate from General Motors to help him purchase some of his driving equipment because his car was bought new 6 months ago. This will enable him to afford to buy the car topper as well as the devices he requires for driving. I introduced Mr. J. to another client of mine who also drives with adaptive equipment and went to the same occupational therapy driving specialist. This was very encouraging to Mr. J., and he actually went to see some driving equipment in this gentleman's car."

"Mr. J. has made great progress over the past month. He does not seem as depressed as when I first saw him and is coming to therapy with more and more goals that he would like to work toward. I will update the intervention plan to incorporate the new goals. I have recommended that he obtain a referral for home health occupational therapy so that he can begin working in his own home environment. The home health occupational therapist can make sure he gets the right equipment in his bathroom and give him practice with his transfers in his own environment. He is totally agreeable to this plan. It was so great to see Mr. J. come into therapy after the first session of seeing the occupational therapy driving specialist. He was so excited and could finally see that he would be able to become much less dependent upon his family now. It was nice to hear him express his appreciation for my work, and he even admitted that he was glad I did not send him for a driving evaluation sooner. He is asking if he can drive now to and from his daughter's house, which is about 45 minutes away in another small town. I have referred him back to the SCDCM to address this issue with him. Mr. J. and I decided that he no longer needs outpatient occupational therapy but can be followed for his other goals by the occupational therapy consultant in the community."

Clinical Reasoning in Occupational Therapy Practice

Environmental Contextual Factors in Mobility

Mr. J. will be returning to his home with his wife on discharge, but the environment is rural, and according to his wife the home is not wheelchair accessible. How will these environmental factors influence intervention planning for functional mobility? What will the inpatient therapist request of the community-based therapist regarding follow-up for functional and community mobility?

Clinical Reasoning in Occupational Therapy Practice

The Importance of a Client-Centered Approach

During the initial occupational therapy evaluation, Mr. J. appeared depressed and unmotivated regarding therapy and the time and effort that would be required for intervention. What factors could be contributing to his attitude? What approach should the therapist take to improve this person's motivation and participation in goal setting?

Summary Review Questions

1. Define the two areas of mobility that are within the domain of occupational therapy, and list three specific subareas to be addressed under each main area of mobility.
2. Describe the hierarchy of intervention planning for mobility and the interdependence of functional and community mobility.
3. List precursor abilities and skills that a patient with lower extremity dysfunction must possess before learning to transfer into a wheelchair and how the principles of body mechanics must be applied during the transfer.
4. List the specific outdoor mobility skills in which a therapist would instruct a patient who uses a manual wheelchair.
5. Describe the process for evaluation and intervention planning for the IADL of driving a personal vehicle.
6. State when it is appropriate to refer a client to an occupational therapy specialist in driving and why.
7. Define three modes of travel that can be used for community mobility and three transportation alternatives available when independent driving is not an option.
8. Describe how occupational therapy practitioners can become involved in functional and community mobility issues in the communities in which they practice.

Glossary

Body mechanics—The way one moves the body, spine, and extremities during every day activities to protect the body, especially the back, from pain and injury. Good body mechanics refers to proper posture and body alignment when lifting or moving.

Community—"Unified body of individuals" that includes family, neighborhood, local communities, and groups that share the same interest or goals (Merriam-Webster, 2012).

Community mobility—"Moving around in the community and using public or private transportation, such as driving, walking, bicycling, or accessing and riding buses, taxi cabs or other transportation systems" (AOTA, 2008, p. 631).

Community mobility alternatives—Various modes of transportation chosen by an individual to move about a community that can include walking, bicycling, driving a personal car, driving a powered mobility device, or using alternative modes of transportation such as private or public options of a subway, bus, or taxi.

Functional mobility—"Moving from one position or place to another (during performance of everyday activities), such as in-bed mobility, wheelchair or powered mobility, and transfers (e.g., wheelchair, bed, car, tub, toilet, tub/shower, chair, and floor). Includes functional ambulation and transporting objects" (AOTA, 2008, p. 631).

Functional mobility aids—Devices that assist a person with functional mobility such as a wheelchair, hemiwalker, leg lifter, bed rope ladder, quad cane, or transfer board.

Livable community—A community "that has affordable and appropriate housing, supportive community features and services, and adequate mobility options,

which together facilitate personal independence and the engagement of residents in civic and social life" (AARP, 2005, p. 4).

Mobility—The ability to move about the home and community.

Paratransit—An alternative mode of transportation for persons who qualify that uses taxis, minivans or small buses. It may be an on-demand, door-to-door service within a given service area or may follow a particular route. Also called community transport.

Personal mobility devices (PMDs)—Nonmotorized and motorized personal devices that assist a person with functional mobility and community mobility. Examples are a bicycle, an electric scooter, a manual or power-based wheelchair, golf cart, or low-speed vehicle.

References

Americans with Disabilities Accessibility (ADA) Standards for Accessible Design. (2010). Washington, DC: U.S. Department of Justice. Retrieved September 1, 2012 from http://www.ada.gov/2010ADA standards_index.htm.

American Association of Retired Persons. (2005). *Beyond 50:05 A report to the nation on livable communities: Creating environments for successful aging.* Washington, DC: AARP.

American Occupational Therapy Association. (2008). Occupational therapy practice framework: Domain and process. *American Journal of Occupational Therapy, 62,* 625–688.

American Occupational Therapy Association. (2010). *Statements: Driving and community mobility.* Bethesda, MD: American Occupational Therapy Association.

Arthanat, S., Nochajski, S. M., Lenker, J. A., Bauer, S. B., & Wu, Y. W. B. (2009). Measuring usability of assistive technology from a multicontextual perspective: The case of power wheelchairs. *American Journal of Occupational Therapy, 63,* 751–764.

Burkhardt, J. E., McGavock, A. T., & Nelson, C. A. (2002). *Transit Cooperative Research Program (TCRP) Report 82: Improving public transit options for older persons.* Washington, DC: Transportation Research Board.

Carmeli, E., Coleman, R., Omar, H. L., & Brown-Cross, D. (2000). Do we allow elderly pedestrians sufficient time to cross the street in safety? *Journal of Aging and Physical Activity, 8,* 51–58.

Carr, D. B., Schwartzberg, J. G., Manning, L., & Sempek, J. (2010). *Physician's guide to assessing and counseling older drivers* (2nd ed.) Washington, DC: NHTSA. Retrieved June 22, 2012 from www.ama-assn.org/go /olderdrivers.

Centers for Disease Control and Prevention [CDC]. (2013). *Pedestrian safety: Fact sheet.* Retrieved July 22, 2013 from http://www.cdc.gov /motorvehiclesafety/pedestrian_safety/factsheet.html

Classen, S. (2010). From the desk of the editor: Special issue on older driver safety and mobility. *American Journal of Occupational Therapy, 64,* 211–214.

Classen, S., Eby, D., Molnar, L. J., Dobbs, B., & Winter, S. (2011). Transportation and aging: Exploring stakeholder's perspectives on advancing safe mobility. *South African Journal of Occupational Therapy, 41,* 18–24.

Classen, S., Levy, C., McCarthy, D., Mann, W. C., Lanford, D., & Waid-Ebbs, J. K. (2009). Traumatic brain injury and driving assessment: An evidence-based literature review. *American Journal of Occupational Therapy, 63,* 580–591.

Classen, S., Winter, S. M., Velozo, C. A., Bédard, M., Lanford, D. N., Brumback, B., & Lutz, B. J. (2010). Item development and validity testing for a safe driving behavior measure. *American Journal of Occupational Therapy, 64,* 296–305.

Community. (2012). In *Merriam-Webster Online.* Retrieved June 22, 2012 from http://www.merriam-webster.com/dictionary/community

Dartmouth-Hitchcock. (2012). *Back problems: Proper lifting.* Retrieved June 22, 2012 from http://patients.dartmouth-hitchcock.org /health_information/health_encyclopedia/sig59692.

Dickerson, A. E., Molnar, L. J., Eby, D., Adler, G., Bedar, M., Berg-Weger, M., Classen, S., Foley, D., Horowitz, A., Kerschner, H., Page, O., Silverstein, N., Staplin, L., & Trujillo, L. (2007). Transportation and aging: A research agenda for advancing safe mobility. *Gerontologist, 47,* 578–590.

Dickerson, A. E., Reistetter, T., Schold-Davis, E., & Monahan, M. (2011). Evaluating driving as a valued instrumental activity of daily living. *American Journal of Occupational Therapy, 65,* 54–75.

Di Stefano, M., & Macdonald, W. (2005). On-the-road evaluation of driving performance. In J. M. Pellerito (Ed.), *Driver rehabilitation and community: Principles and practice* (pp. 255–274). St. Louis: Elsevier/Mosby.

Fairchild, S. L. (2013). *Pierson and Fairchild principles and techniques of patient care* (5th ed.). St. Louis: Elsevier/Saunders.

Federal Highway Adminstration. (2012). Pedestrian & bicycle safety. Retrieved June 22, 2012 from http://safety.fhwa.dot.gov/ped_bike.

Gillen, G. (2011). *Stroke rehabilitation: A function based approach.* St. Louis: Elsevier/Mosby.

Hegberg, A. P. (2007). *An older driver rehabilitation primer for occupational therapy professionals.* Bethesda, MD: American Occupational Therapy Association.

Houser, A. (2005). *Older drivers and automobile safety.* Washington, DC: AARP Public Policy Institute.

Hunt, L. A. (2010). *Determining capacity to drive for drivers with dementia using research, ethics and professional reasoning: The responsibility of all occupational therapists.* AOTA CEonCD Learning. Bethesda, MD: American Occupational Therapy Association.

Hunt, L. A., & Arbesman, M. (2008). Evidence-based and occupational perspective of effective interventions for older clients that remediate or support improved driving performance. *American Journal of Occupational therapy, 62,* 136–148.

Hunt, L. A., Brown, A. E., & Gilman, I. P. (2010). Drivers with dementia and outcomes of becoming lost while driving. *American Journal of Occupational Therapy, 64,* 225–232.

Hunt, L. A., Carr, D. B., & Barco, P. P. (2009). A multifactorial older-driver with dementia evaluation model (MODEM) guides fitness-to-drive decisions. Pacific University, Forest Grove, OR. Unpublished manuscript.

Kane, L. A., & Buckley, K. A. (2011). Functional mobility. In G. Gillen (Ed.), *Stroke rehabilitation: A function-based approach* (3rd ed.) St. Louis: MO: Elsevier/ Mosby.

Kihl, M., Brennan, D., Gabhawala, N., List, J., & Mittal, P. (2005). *Livable communities: An evaluation guide.* Washington, DC: AARP Public Policy Institute.

Kirby, R. L., Smith, C., Seaman, R., MacLeod, D. A., & Parker, K. (2006). The manual wheelchair wheelie: A review of our current understanding of an important motor skill. *Disability and Rehabilitation: Assistive Technology, 1,* 119–127.

Kirby, R. L., Swuste, J., Dupuis, D. J., MacLeod, D. A., & Monroe, R. (2002). The wheelchair skills test: A pilot study of a new outcome measure. *Archives of Physical Medicine and Rehabilitation, 83,* 10–18

Lynott, J., Poncy, A. T., & Twaddel, H. (2011). *Policy and design considerations for accommodating low-speed vehicles and golf carts in community transportation networks.* Washington, DC: AARP Public Policy Institute.

Marottoli, R. A., Mendes de Leon, C. F., Glass, T. A., Williams, C. S., Cooney, L. M., & Berkman, L. F. (2000). Consequences of driving cessation: Decreased out-of-home activity levels. *Journal of Gerontology, 55,* 334–340.

National Highway Traffic Safety Administration. (2006). *Community mobility and dementia* (DOT HS 810 684). Washington, DC: NHTSA.

National Highway Traffic Safety Administration. (2009). *Pedestrians* (DOT HS 811 394). Washington, DC: NHTSA.

National Highway Traffic Safety Administration. (2012) *Stepping out.* Washington, DC: U.S. Department of Transportation. Retrieved June 22, 2012 from http://www.nhtsa.gov/people/injury/olddrive/SteppingOut/.

Pedestrian and Bicycle Information Center. (2012). Designing for pedestrians with physical disabilities. Retrieved June 22, 2012 from http://www.walkinginfo.org/engineering/pedestrians.cfm.

Pierce, S. (1996). A roadmap for driver rehabilitation. *OT Practice, 10,* 30–38.

Pierce, S., & Schold-Davis, E. (2013). *Driving and community mobility for older adults: Occupational therapy roles* [Revised continuing education program (for members only). Listed in the *American Journal of Occupational Therapy, 67*(3), 372.]. Bethesda, MD: American Occupational Therapy Association. Retrievable from www.aota.org (member section).

PoinTIS SCI Physical Therapy site. (2012). *The PoinTIS SCI physical therapy SCI manual for providers: Functional rehabilitation: Wheelchair skills: Training strategies: Propel wheelchair over obstacles: Slope and wheelie strategies.* Retrieved June 23, 2012 from http://calder.med.miami.edu/providers/PHYSICAL/wheelslope.html.

Radomski, M. V. (2011). More than good intentions: Advancing adherence to therapy recommendations. *American Journal of Occupational Therapy, 65,* 471–477.

Schold-Davis, E. (2012). *The occupational therapy role in driving and community mobility across the lifespan.* Bethesda, MD: American Occupational Therapy Association.

Smith, S. C. (2011). Golf carts are hitting the streets. Orlando, FL: *Orlando Sentinel.* August 14, Section D, p. 1.

Somers, M. F. (2010). *Spinal cord injury: Functional rehabilitation* (3rd ed.). Upper Saddle River, NJ: Pearson.

Silverstein, N. M. (2008). When life exceeds safe driving expectancy: Implications for gerontology and geriatrics education. *Gerontology Journal for Geriatric Education, 29,* 305–309.

Staplin, L., Gish, K. W., & Wanger, E. K. (2003). MaryPODS revisited: Updated crash analysis and implication for screening program implementation. *Journal of Safety Research, 34,* 389–397.

Stav, W. B., Hunt, L. A., & Arbesman, M. (2006). *Occupational therapy practice guidelines for driving and community mobility for older adults.* Bethesda. MD: American Occupational Therapy Association.

Unsworth, C. (2011). Driver off-road assessment battery (OT-DORA). Bethesda, MD: American Occupational Therapy Association.

Vrkljan, B. H., Leuty, V., & Law, M. (2011). Aging-in-place: Exploring the transactional relationship between habits and participation in a community context. *Occupational Therapy Journal on Research: Occupation, Participation, and Health, 31,* 151–159.

Waite, A. (2011). Well Elderly 2 study: Evidence that occupational therapy helps prevent decline in seniors. *OT Practice, 16,* 8–10.

Walker, K. A., Morgan, K. A., Morris, C. L., DeGroot, K. K., Hollingsworth, H. H., & Gray, D. B. (2010). Development of a community mobility skills course for people who use mobility devices. *American Journal of Occupational Therapy, 64,* 547–554.

Womack, J. (2012). Continuing life on the move: Aging and community mobility. *OT Practice, 17,* CE1–CE8.

Yonkman, J., O'Neil, J., Talty, J., & Bull, M. (2010). Transporting children in wheelchairs in passenger vehicles: A comparison of best practice to observed and reported practice in a pilot sample. *American Journal of Occupational Therapy, 64,* 804–808.

Acknowledgments

I thank Carol Blackburn, OTR/L, CDRS; Brenda Johnston, OTR; Daphne Cronin; Joan Bova; Linda and Chuck Green; and Sara Castelli and Mary Nan Carroll for their assistance with the photography for this chapter. Also, appreciation to Miriam Monahan, MS, OTR/L, CDRS; Sherrilene Classen, PhD, MPH, OTR/L; and Linda A. Hunt, PhD, OTR/L, for assistance with references and the evidence table.

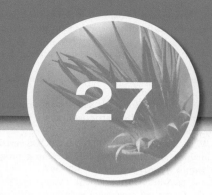

27

Restoring Competence for Homemaker and Parent Roles

Susan E. Fasoli

Learning Objectives

After studying this chapter, the reader will be able to do the following:

1. State the principles of compensation and adaptation.
2. State the principles of work simplification.
3. Identify adapted methods and equipment that enable persons with varied physical challenges and diagnoses to regain competence in homemaking roles.
4. Identify adapted methods and equipment that enable persons with varied physical challenges and diagnoses to regain competence in parenting roles.
5. Describe and teach proper body mechanics for homemaking and parenting tasks and activities.

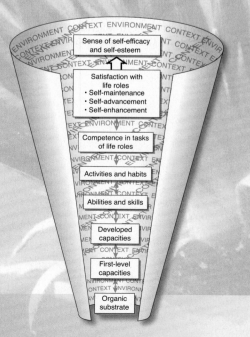

Restoring competence in homemaker and parenting roles following a disabling event can greatly enhance one's sense of efficacy and feelings of self-esteem. Therapists typically address impaired performance of these life roles after a client has regained independence in basic activities of daily living (ADL) (e.g., self-care). Home management and parenting tasks, however, can be incorporated into the rehabilitation process at any time, depending on the individual's own priorities and needs.

Homemaking and parenting tasks may be used as both occupation-as-means and occupation-as-end, depending on the client's rehabilitation potential and desired goals. This chapter focuses on the use of occupation-as-end to restore a client's competence and participation in homemaker and parent roles. This treatment approach allows for addressing significant deficits in occupational performance skills (e.g., incoordination or visual impairments) via the principles for compensation and adaptation highlighted in Procedures for Practice 27-1.

Principles of work simplification and energy conservation can be taught to clients with physical impairments who lack sufficient endurance to accomplish daily life tasks. Work simplification and energy conservation principles are common-sense ideas to improve task efficiency and reduce energy expenditure during all occupational tasks and roles, including those related to homemaking and parenting (see Procedures for Practice 27-1).

HOMEMAKER ROLES AND TASKS: TREATMENT PRINCIPLES AND METHODS

An important role of the occupational therapist is to learn what life roles and tasks are particularly meaningful to the client (i.e., to explore his or her occupational identity) and to allow him or her the opportunity to grieve for what is lost or changed (Unruh, 2004). Many factors, including psychosocial adjustment, cognitive or

---

 ## Procedures for Practice 27-1

Principles of Adaptation to Compensate for Functional Limitations

Principles for Compensation and Adaptation

- Limited range of motion (ROM): Increase the person's reach via extended handles and organize needed items within a compact work space.
- Weakness and low endurance: Use lightweight and/or powered equipment and allow gravity to assist. Employ work simplification and energy conservation techniques.
- Chronic pain: Reinforce use of proper body mechanics and pacing during physical tasks.
- Unilateral loss of motor control and limb function: Use affected limb to stabilize objects when possible. Use adapted methods and/or assistive equipment to perform bilateral activities with one hand.
- Incoordination: Stabilize at proximal joints (e.g., elbow) to reduce degrees of freedom necessary for control. Use weighted objects to minimize distal incoordination.
- Visual impairments: Use senses of smell, touch, and hearing to substitute for low vision. Enhance performance of visual tasks by improving lighting, reducing glare, or increasing contrast.
- Cognitive limitations: Employ visual and auditory aids to enhance memory and organization. Plan steps prior to beginning task. Work in familiar environment (e.g., home kitchen) to enhance cognitive performance during homemaking tasks.

Principles of Work Simplification and Energy Conservation

- Limit the amount of work. When possible, avoid overfatigue by assigning heavy homemaking tasks (e.g., vacuuming

and cleaning bathrooms) to family members or a housekeeper.
- Explore ways to reduce homemaking demands and expectations, such as using packaged mixes or frozen foods to decrease time and energy for meal preparation.
- Plan ahead. Schedule homemaking, child care tasks (e.g., changing bed linens and giving tub baths), and community outings (e.g., shopping and doctor visits) to distribute energy-demanding tasks throughout the week. Prioritize to complete important tasks before fatigue sets in.
- Use efficient methods. Organize work areas and store frequently used supplies in a convenient location. Avoid standing when it is possible to sit while doing the task (e.g., ironing). Slide objects across a counter or table rather than lift them. Identify needed items at the beginning of a task to avoid extra trips. Use a utility cart to transport items.
- Use correct equipment and techniques. Use assistive equipment (e.g., long-handled reachers) to decrease bending and stooping. Avoid prolonged holding by stabilizing items with nonskid mats. Adjust work height and use tools most appropriate for the job. When physical limitations are present, choose equipment that does not promote further deformity.
- Balance daily tasks with rest breaks. Clients are advised to perform energy-demanding tasks early in the day, when they are most rested. Encourage self-pacing of tasks ("Don't rush!") to avoid fatigue. Frequent rest periods of 5–10 minutes can greatly enhance functional endurance during homemaking and parenting tasks.

perceptual impairments, and physical limitations, can influence a client's ability to take part in homemaker roles and tasks.

Psychosocial Adjustment

When faced with the onset or progression of physical disability, a client and family may have a variety of psychological responses. These reactions may be characterized by lack of motivation and refusal to participate in therapy, expressed feelings of hopelessness or anger, and denial. For persons with chronic conditions, such as scleroderma or rheumatoid arthritis, the challenges encountered during household chores can strongly affect levels of life satisfaction and well-being (Sandqvist, Akesson, & Eklund, 2005). The family's expectations and reactions must also be considered when occupational therapists are setting intervention goals and establishing plans for treatment. These psychological reactions must be acknowledged and addressed by the occupational therapist if identified goals are to be achieved. A client-centered approach involves sensitivity and planning. These highly individualized concerns should be addressed on a timely basis that is guided by both the client's illness trajectory and psychosocial adjustment to disability. For example, a client may find it easier to tackle unfamiliar or nonpersonal tasks early in therapy because this can ease his or her confrontation with loss. By involving the client and family in the choice of activities during treatment planning, the therapist can better individualize interventions and establish rapport and trust.

Barriers to Effectiveness

The occupational therapist must identify factors, in addition to psychosocial concerns, that can interfere with the effectiveness of intervention and inhibit performance during homemaking tasks. These factors include, but are not limited to, cognitive and perceptual impairments, poor vision, and environmental constraints, including lack of family support.

Persons with cognitive impairments as a result of central nervous system disorders may have more difficulty learning compensatory techniques than persons with musculoskeletal or peripheral nervous system disorders. The client needs good memory, judgment, and problem-solving abilities to learn how an assistive device is used, when it is needed, and how it can safely enhance task performance. Cognitive demands are increased when the adapted methods greatly alter the way the task is performed (e.g., ordering groceries online or learning to use a utility cart to transport items). The occupational therapist works to educate the client's caregivers in ways to best structure tasks and provide cues to enhance performance (see Procedures for Practice 27-2). Supervision and feedback are given to reinforce use of these techniques during varied situations. Refer to Chapter 24 for other cognitive strategies that can be used during homemaking and parenting tasks.

In the absence of intact cognitive abilities, clients may be able to learn new task methods, such as how to operate a microwave oven for meal preparation, if they can follow visual cues or instructions. The occupational therapist must ensure that the client can safely perform the task

---

 Procedures for Practice 27-2

Managing Homemaker Roles with Cognitive Limitations

Clients with cognitive limitations may be unable to structure daily homemaker routines for many reasons, including impairments in attention, memory, sequencing and organization, problem solving, or executive functioning. Assessments such as the Canadian Occupational Performance Measure (COPM) (see Chapter 4) are used to identify important homemaker tasks and can assist the client and family in setting reasonable goals for intervention. The occupational therapist teaches the client and family ways to compensate for cognitive impairments while successfully returning to homemaker roles. Several examples of cognitive strategies include the following:

- Progress from gathering all needed materials and setting up tasks for the client to having him or her list and gather needed ingredients and kitchen items (e.g., cutting board, pot, utensils, etc).

- Break multistep tasks (e.g., preparing a meal) down to smaller components. Depending on the level of impairment, the family might involve client only in peeling potatoes, gather items needed for salad preparation so client can assemble salad, or assist as needed with step-by-step directions when making a casserole dish. Consider the impact of cognitive and physical limitations on the client's fatigue and motivation to participate.

- Grade difficulty of task and the amount of verbal cues and physical assist given. Preparing a peanut butter and jelly sandwich is easier than simple hot meal preparation (e.g., making scrambled eggs and toast), which is less complex than following directions to bake a cake from a prepared mix. Allow for independence, satisfaction, and success before moving on to more complex tasks.

- Set automatic timers on appliances to remind client to check cooking food or care for dishes or laundry when the cycle is complete.

with the prescribed adaptations and meet unexpected challenges encountered during task performance.

Perceptual impairments, including poor figure-ground skills, poor spatial orientation, and visual neglect, can also interfere with one's ability to manage homemaking tasks independently. Limitations in perceptual processing can interfere with one's ability to find needed items in the cupboard, decrease the safety of pouring hot coffee into a cup, and increase the likelihood of falls when vacuuming or sweeping floors. In addition, poor visual processing, such as the loss of central vision or decreased contrast sensitivity, can inhibit safety during homemaking tasks. Environmental changes, such as increasing available lighting throughout the home and enhancing contrast (e.g., pouring coffee into a light-colored mug), can improve performance.

The support of family or friends can be instrumental for carrying out recommended adaptations, reinforcing the use of assistive devices, and identifying additional concerns in need of intervention. When family assistance is not available, other support services (e.g., home health aide or companion) may be employed to ensure safety in homemaking tasks.

Preventing Decline in Homemaker Role and Tasks

Occupational therapists are often involved with preventing disability in persons who are at risk for developing impairments, activity limitations, and restrictions in the performance of life tasks and roles. Prevention programs for elderly persons include exercise classes to reduce physical limitations in balance, range of motion, and strength, in addition to group activities that exercise cognitive abilities, such as judgment and problem solving (Clark et al., 1997; Jackson et al., 1998). Homemakers may be instructed in home safety tips directed toward reducing clutter, removing loose rugs, and arranging furniture to clear walkways and allow access to electrical plugs and windows. Environmental modifications, such as the installation of grab bars and railings, can significantly decrease the occurrence of falls.

Occupational therapists can be instrumental in identifying hazards in the home and providing ideas that may enhance a person's safety and continued independence (see Resources 27-1). Many limitations encountered by well-elderly persons during homemaking tasks may be prevented or alleviated by relatively simple and inexpensive solutions.

Homemaking: Techniques and Therapeutic Aids

Competence in the role of homemaker can be attained in either of two ways, depending on the client's level of physical and cognitive ability: by managing and directing others to perform homemaking tasks or by direct participation.

Although persons with severe physical disabilities may not be able to perform many homemaking tasks without assistance, they can be effective home managers. For instance, individuals with high-level spinal cord injuries can independently manage household tasks by directing family members or paid housekeepers, managing finances, and overseeing shopping. Computerized banking systems and shopping services are accessible to those with Internet access and are relatively easy to use. Occupational therapy at this level may focus on organizing how household tasks may be scheduled, instructing the client in computer use, or identifying service resources in the community. Homemaker services, personal care assistants, and Meals on Wheels may provide the support necessary for a person with limited abilities to remain at home.

Persons who can physically participate in homemaking tasks can benefit from a variety of interventions that maximize role performance. The following sections discuss equipment and adapted methods for homemaking.

Equipment Considerations

A number of factors contribute to the selection and use of assistive devices and adapted equipment for homemaking. Simple modifications in the way a task is performed sometimes eliminate the need for an assistive device, and this is the preferable solution. When equipment is recommended, a primary concern is that the assistive device satisfies the needs of the client and enables the person to accomplish tasks that are otherwise impossible or difficult. The person must be comfortable with the idea of using an assistive device and satisfied with its appearance.

When making equipment recommendations, the occupational therapist must consider both the immediate and long-term needs of the client. Individuals with a progressive disease, such as rheumatoid arthritis or multiple sclerosis, benefit from equipment that can enhance current functional performance and provide for anticipated changes in physical status. In contrast, persons with nonprogressive conditions, such as acquired brain injury or spinal cord injury, often use fewer assistive devices as they regain physical abilities or learn alternate ways to accomplish their tasks without equipment.

Generally, assistive devices should be simple to use and maintain, as lightweight as possible, and dependable. If a client has mild cognitive impairments that interfere with equipment use, family members may be taught ways to enhance carryover at home. Insurance providers generally do not pay for assistive devices and adapted equipment. For those who cannot afford to purchase such items, loaner equipment may be available from local organizations, including disability support groups and senior citizen centers.

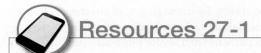 Resources 27-1

Books

Mayer, T. K. (2007). *One-handed in a two-handed world: Your personal guide to managing single handedly* (3rd ed.). Boston: Prince Gallison.

Vensand, K., Rogers, J., Tuleja, C., & DeMoss, A. (2000). *Adaptive baby care equipment: Guidelines, prototypes & resources*. Berkeley, CA: Through the Looking Glass.

Organizations, Associations, and Services

The Internet offers a wealth of information concerning resources for specific disabilities. The following are some organizations that listed information specific to home management or parenting at the time of publication:

The Arthritis Foundation

Atlanta, GA
Phone: 800-283-7800
www.arthritis.org

National Multiple Sclerosis Society

New York, NY
Phone: 800-FIGHT-MS or 800-344-4867
www.nmss.org

American Heart Association

Dallas, TX
Phone: 8000AHA-USA-1 or 800-242-8721
www.americanheart.org

American Stroke Association

Dallas, TX
Phone: 888-4-STROKE or 888-478-7653
www.strokeassociation.org

National Stroke Association

Centennial, CO
Phone: 800-STROKES or 800-787-6537
www.stroke.org

Through the Looking Glass

Berkeley, CA
Phone: 800-644-2666
www.lookingglass.org
Addresses the needs of parents with disabilities and parents of disabled children

Computerized Information Services for Persons with Disabilities

AbleData

Silver Springs, MD
Phone: 800-227-0216.
www.abledata.com

Manufacturers and Distributors of Adaptive Devices

North Coast Medical

Gilroy, CA
Phone: 800-821-9319
www.ncmedical.com

AliMed

Dedham, MA
Phone: 800-225-2610
www.alimed.com

Patterson Medical

Bolingbrook, IL
Phone: 800-323-5547
www.pattersonmedical.com

Meal Preparation, Service, and Cleanup

Efficient work areas, adapted techniques, and assistive devices can greatly enhance a client's safety and participation in meal preparation tasks.

Kitchen Storage and Work Area. Kitchens are best organized so that frequently used items are within easy reach of the place they are most often used. On average, persons who use a wheelchair can reach to retrieve items between 15 inches (low reach) and 48 inches (high reach) from the floor. Those who are ambulatory but have difficulty bending generally can reach 30 inches (low reach) to 60 inches (high reach) from the floor, depending on the person's height.

Pull-out shelves and turntables in cabinets can compensate for limited reach and maximize usable storage space. Pans, dishes, and so on may be stored vertically to alleviate the need to move unwanted items to obtain the one underneath. Pegboards with hooks can be attached to the back of closet doors to hold pots, pans, and utensils for easy access. Shelves attached to the inside of cabinet doors are handy for holding assorted wraps, canned goods, and cleaning supplies. Items that are seldom used should be removed to eliminate unnecessary clutter.

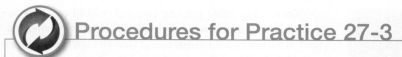

Procedures for Practice 27-3

Principles of Correct Body Mechanics

Principles of correct body mechanics that should be used during homemaking and parenting tasks include the following:

- Keep the shoulders and hips parallel and facing the task. Do not twist the trunk when lifting.
- Maintain good balance by positioning the feet shoulder distance apart with one foot forward.
- When standing for long periods, reduce pressure on the lower back by placing one foot on a low stool and changing positions frequently.
- When sitting or standing, maintain a neutral position in the lower back by tilting the pelvis slightly forward to maintain the natural curve of the spine. Use this neutral back position when lifting as well.
- Use the strongest or largest muscles and joints when lifting (e.g., use legs rather than back and palms rather than fingers).
- Keep the back upright and bend at the hips and knees rather than bending forward at the waist when reaching for low items.
- Push before pulling, and pull before lifting.
- While lifting or carrying, keep the object close to the body.
- Avoid rushing. Proper body mechanics are more effectively used when working at a comfortable pace.

Safety and independence in the kitchen can be enhanced by the availability of clear and accessible workspaces. For persons in wheelchairs, work counters should be 28–34 inches from the floor and have a depth clearance of 24 inches underneath to allow room for wheelchair leg rests. A work area that is at least 30 inches wide is recommended to provide sufficient space for needed items during meal preparation (ADA and ABA Accessibility Guidelines for Buildings and Facilities, 2004).

Gathering and Transporting Items. An important role of the occupational therapist is to help the client solve problems about gathering and transporting items at home by using work simplification principles and proper body mechanics (Procedures for Practice 27-1 and 27-3). Long-handled reachers can be helpful but should be used primarily for retrieving lightweight unbreakable items.

The wide range of assistive devices for transporting items around the home includes cup holders and walker or wheelchair bags. Homemakers who use a wheelchair may benefit from using a lap tray that easily slides on and off the wheelchair arms (Fig. 27-1). A variety of wire baskets and trays that attach to a standard walker are available for purchase, but many of these devices accommodate only a few things at a time, such as a sandwich and covered beverage. Individuals who perform homemaking tasks either from a wheelchair or ambulatory level may prefer to use a wheeled utility cart because of its larger carrying capacity. The therapist can help clients learn to maneuver the cart efficiently. Homemakers who use an assistive device or adapted methods to transport hot foods and beverages must follow strict safety precautions to avoid burns.

When limited income inhibits a client's ability to purchase assistive aids, the creative therapist can work with the client to identify inexpensive workable alternatives. No-cost solutions, such as attaching a plastic grocery bag or used bike basket to a walker, can add to independence in transporting certain items.

Food Preparation. The use of assistive devices and adapted equipment can make food preparation easier and more enjoyable. Homemakers who have lost the use of one arm following stroke or fracture find an adapted cutting board extremely useful when peeling or cutting vegetables, fruit, or meat. A raised edge along one corner of the board can stabilize a slice of bread for spreading butter or jam (Fig. 27-2).

The occupational therapist helps clients with physical limitations to solve problems such as the safest way to open cereal boxes and juice cartons. Some persons can open packaged food with one-handed techniques, while others prefer to use adapted scissors with a looped handle (Fig. 27-3). Homemakers with weakness and impaired hand function may find it easier to open plastic milk jugs than cartons. Smaller containers are generally easier to manage than large ones. Nonslip mats or suction holders may be used under jars or bottles to hold them steady for opening with one hand and to reduce sliding or turning of bowls when mixing.

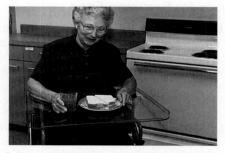

Figure 27-1 Woman eating her lunch on a clear acrylic wheelchair lap tray that allows her to observe her lower body. (Photo by Robert Littlefield.)

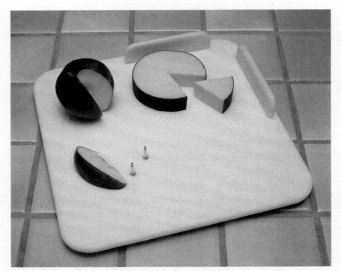

Figure 27-2 Spiked cutting board with corner guards. (Photo courtesy of North Coast Medical, Inc., Gilroy, CA.)

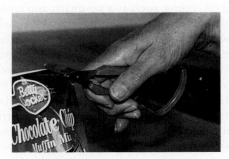

Figure 27-3 Looped scissors. (Photo by Robert Littlefield.)

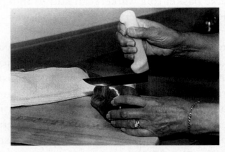

Figure 27-4 Ergonomic right-angled knife. (Photo by Robert Littlefield.)

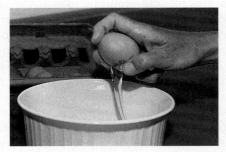

Figure 27-5 One-handed egg crack. (Photo by Robert Littlefield.)

Knives, vegetable peelers, and other kitchen tools are available in many shapes and sizes. Clients with rheumatoid arthritis benefit from using utensils with ergonomically designed handles that require less hand strength and reduce ulnar drift (Fig. 27-4). Incoordination caused by ataxia may be somewhat alleviated by the use of weighted utensils and tools. Freestanding or mounted jar openers can be helpful to persons with a variety of physical limitations. Homemakers can be taught adapted methods for cracking eggs (Fig. 27-5; Procedures for Practice 27-4).

Electric equipment, such as food processors, blenders, can openers, and electric knives, can conserve energy by reducing the physical demands and time needed for meal preparation. To be truly beneficial, this equipment must be easy to use and maintain and suited to the person's disability. For example, some one-handed cordless can openers are available only in right-handed models and therefore are not convenient for persons with significant right hemiparesis after stroke.

Homemakers with limited mobility or reach often find a side-by-side refrigerator more accessible than other models. Loops of webbing or rope can be attached to the door handles to enable clients with limited hand function to pull the doors open. Heavy items should be stored on a shelf that is level with a lapboard or wheeled cart so they can be moved in and out with minimal lifting.

Cooking. Most persons with physical impairments find lightweight nonstick pots and pans to be the easiest to handle and maintain. Ergonomically designed cookware with easy-to-grip handles can be ideal for persons with limited distal strength. The use of double-handled casserole dishes, pots, and pans can enable joint protection by evenly distributing the weight of the pan between both hands.

Ambulatory clients with back or lower extremity pain or limited endurance can save energy by sitting whenever

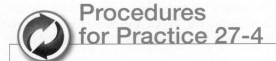

Procedures for Practice 27-4

Methods for Breaking Eggs

Individuals with weak grasp can grossly hold the egg, throw it sharply into the bottom of an empty glass or metal bowl, where it will split in two, and then remove the shell.

Clients with functional use of only one hand may prefer to use the chef's method, as follows. Place the egg in the palm with one end held by the index and middle fingers and the other end held by the thumb to form a "C" around the egg. Sharply crack the egg on the side of a bowl, and then in one motion, pull the thumb down and the fingers up to pull the two halves apart (Fig. 27-5).

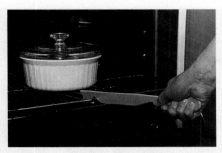

Figure 27-6 Oven push-pull stick. (Photo by Robert Littlefield.)

possible while preparing meals. Individuals who prepare food from a wheelchair can use a mirror mounted at an angle over the stove to keep an eye on cooking foods. Persons with hemiparesis may use a suction holder to stabilize pot handles while stirring. Homemakers can conserve energy when straining vegetables or pasta by placing a french-fry basket in the pot before cooking or by using a slotted spoon. This practice eliminates the need to carry a hot pot to the sink to drain it. Those who can safely transport and drain hot foods at the sink can reduce the need for lifting and holding and enhance stability by resting the pot on the sink's edge when pouring. An adjustable strainer that clamps onto the top of a pot or pan can also be used.

Homemakers who prepare meals from a wheelchair will find a self-cleaning stove with front-operated controls and a low wall oven (30–42 inches from the floor) to be the most practical to use and operate.

Individuals with limited proximal arm strength or grasp should not remove hot items from a wall oven higher than waist level without supervision because of the potential for burns caused by spilling or dropping. An oven push-pull stick may be used to manage oven racks or reposition hot dishes safely during baking (Fig. 27-6). If a client is planning to buy a new stove, the therapist may recommend a gas rather than electric range to reduce the risk of burns because the gas flames provide a visual cue that the burner is on.

Microwave ovens provide a cost-effective and safe alternative to conventional ovens and stoves. Elderly persons with arthritis, visual impairments, and limited endurance can be taught to use a microwave instead of a conventional stove to cook meals more easily and in less time.

Dishwashing. Dishwashing can be made easier for individuals in a wheelchair by placing a removable wooden rack in the bottom of a standard sink to reduce its depth to approximately 5 inches. The under-sink cabinet doors can be removed to allow persons in a wheelchair to face the sink head-on, with any exposed piping insulated to protect lower extremities from burns. A swing-away faucet with a single control lever can enhance the ability of a person with limited hand function to adjust water flow. Installing this

faucet beside rather than at the back of the sink further increases accessibility for persons in wheelchairs.

Dishwashing in a double sink should be organized to allow the person to work from one direction to the other: dirty dishes, wash water, rinse water, and drying rack. Homemakers with hemiparesis may wash dishes with greater ease when the rinse water and dish rack are on their unaffected side. Suction bottlebrushes and scrub brushes can be attached to the sink to allow for cleaning glasses or silverware with one hand. A rubber mat at the bottom of the sink prevents plates from sliding when they are washed and reduces breakage. Persons with limited grasp may prefer to use a terry cloth mitt or sponge mitt when washing dishes.

Work simplification includes air drying versus towel drying dishes and reusing them directly from the dish rack or dishwasher. Use of an electric dishwasher aids energy conservation, particularly when little prerinsing of soiled dishes is required.

Whenever possible, the homemaker can eliminate unnecessary cleaning by using oven-to-table ware or by serving directly from the pot. Pans can be lined with foil to reduce washing after baking or broiling. It is recommended that individuals clean as they prepare the meal and soak hard-to-clean dishes while eating to reduce the amount of cleanup required when the meal is over.

Grocery Shopping. Persons with physical impairments or limited endurance can more easily participate in grocery shopping with a few task modifications or assistive devices. When transportation is readily available, individuals may find that frequent visits to the market are more manageable because they can purchase and carry smaller quantities of food items at one time. Shopping at a small local market, although sometimes more expensive, can be easier and less energy consuming than shopping at a superstore. Grocery shopping can become a social event when done with a friend. Shopping together may provide an additional advantage if the friend can assist with reaching items on high and low shelves or carrying the bags.

Planning. A well-organized shopping list is necessary to make the most efficient use of time and to conserve energy at the store. Individuals should keep the list in a convenient location at home, so that needed items can easily be added between shopping trips. Store maps, available at the customer service desk of many large grocery stores, can be used to organize the list. The homemaker or occupational therapist can arrange the items on the list (e.g., produce, dairy, and meats) according to the store layout, aisle by aisle. Copies of this list can be used between store visits to record the items needed under each category.

The client should plan ahead and shop during off-peak hours, when the store is not crowded. Once at the store, he can use the grocery list and signs above the aisles to find needed items.

Carts. Ambulatory persons with mild balance impairments can use a standard grocery cart when shopping; however, they should not use it for support when bending to reach items on low shelves. Individuals who use a wheelchair may find that adapted shopping carts that attach to the wheelchair are more convenient than a standard cart; although some have found that these attached carts interfere with their ability to reach items. When this is the case, homemakers who are independent with wheelchair mobility may prefer to leave a standard cart at the end of an aisle, gather needed items in a small lap basket, and transfer them into the cart before proceeding to the next aisle.

Large stores sometimes have motorized carts for shoppers with limited endurance and mobility. These carts are handy for getting around the store, but it may be necessary to call the store in advance to reserve one. The baskets on these carts are generally small, which may be problematic if the person is planning to purchase a large order. The client may need help to figure out the safest and most effective ways to obtain items from high or low shelves from a motorized cart.

Selecting and Retrieving Items. It is wise to shop for items that are easy to open and require little preparation. Persons with limited endurance can increase the ease of meal preparation by selecting frozen rather than fresh vegetables and skinless or boneless meats.

Individuals who have limited upper extremity range of motion or who use a wheelchair find it difficult or impossible to reach items on high shelves. A reacher can be used to retrieve lightweight unbreakable items, but assistance may be needed for heavier objects. Most stores provide an employee to assist with shopping if asked. Some persons may feel comfortable asking people in the aisle for occasional help to increase opportunities for socialization.

Some individuals with traumatic brain injury or cerebrovascular accident have cognitive or visual-perceptual problems that interfere with their ability to locate items (e.g., attention, hemianopsia, or impaired figure-ground skills). These persons can be taught to find objects more easily by scanning shelves in an organized manner, top to bottom and left to right. A person with severe visual impairments needs assistance to ensure safety and effectiveness while shopping.

Transporting Items Home. Generally, plastic or reusable grocery bags are easier to manage than paper. Foam tubing can be placed around the bag handles to reduce joint stress. At the checkout counter, the client should ask the clerk to keep grocery bags as light as possible and to bag refrigerated foods separately. Several half-filled bags are easier to manage than one or two full ones. Most stores provide assistance for transferring groceries into the car,

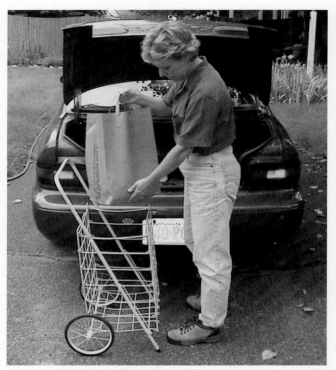

Figure 27-7 Using wheeled cart to conserve energy when transporting items.

but store workers should be instructed to place them within easy reach.

At home, a wheeled cart can be used to transport groceries into the house (Fig. 27-7). Persons with limited endurance can leave nonrefrigerated items in the car until later, when the person has rested or a family member is available to bring them into the house.

Computerized Shopping. Clients with physical limitations and limited endurance may find computer shopping to be a wonderful, energy-efficient alternative to conventional shopping. Persons with Internet access find that grocery orders can be easily placed online. Deliveries are made directly into the home, eliminating transportation and accessibility issues that may arise at the grocery store. The occupational therapist can help the client identify which method of shopping is most practical based on the individual's priorities, physical limitations, knowledge of computer use, and financial situation.

Clothing Care. When a homemaker identifies clothing care as an important goal, the occupational therapist can help the person modify the way laundry tasks are performed. Even persons with severe physical impairments can engage in some aspect of clothing care (e.g., sitting at table to fold clothes).

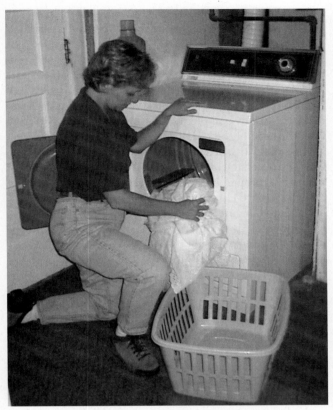

Figure 27-8 Kneeling to keep back straight when removing laundry from dryer.

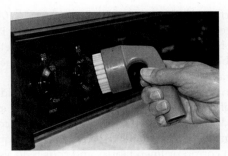

Figure 27-9 Knob turner. (Photo by Robert Littlefield.)

In-Home Appliances Versus Self-Service Commercial Laundries. Although top-loading washers decrease the amount of bending required to load and unload clothing for persons who are ambulatory, they provide an additional challenge for persons in a wheelchair. Front-loading laundry machines are easier for seated individuals to access, but persons who are ambulatory may need training in body mechanics, particularly when loading or unloading wet clothes. For example, it is recommended that ambulatory clients with low back pain kneel on one knee, bending at the hips and knees and keeping the back upright, when loading or removing clothes from a front-loading machine (Fig. 27-8). Homemakers with limited hand function caused by spinal cord injury or rheumatoid arthritis find it easier to use knob turners to set machine dials (Fig. 27-9).

Individuals who use a self-service commercial laundry for clothing care should bring needed coins and premeasured packages of soap for each load. Many laundries have rolling carts available for carrying wet clothes from washer to dryer. If possible, persons with physical impairments should choose a staffed laundry. These individuals can be called on for assistance if problems arise.

Collecting and Transporting Clothing. Ideally, the home laundry room should be on the same floor as the bedrooms to minimize the need to carry clothes up and down stairs. When this is not an option, family members can assist as needed to transport clothing to and from the laundry area.

Soiled clothing can be placed in a hamper lined with a plastic or cloth bag with handles. Seated individuals with good upper body strength can transport clothes to the washer by lifting the bag out of the hamper and either carrying it on their lap or hooking the drawstrings on the wheelchair handles. If the person is ambulatory but has difficulty bending, a clothes basket can be kept on a waist-high table or shelf to collect soiled laundry. A wheeled cart is handy for transporting clothes for persons at an ambulatory level.

Washing and Folding. Laundry detergents and bleaches should be kept within easy reach of the washing machine. Hand washing can be eliminated by laundering delicate clothing in a mesh laundry bag in the machine. Persons with visual impairments can fasten paired socks with large safety pins when they are taken off so they do not have to be sorted when clean.

A person in a wheelchair can use a handheld mirror and reacher to remove clothes from the bottom of a top-loading washer. Homemakers with very limited grasp caused by spinal cord injury have found that stubborn items can be more easily removed from the washer tub after a wet towel or shirt is put back into the washer and the spin cycle is restarted. Movement of the wet towel inside the spinning washer can loosen clothes that are stuck to the tub.

Clothes can be folded while the person sits or stands at a table. An adjustable rod 42–60 inches high is convenient for hanging permanent-press items as they are removed from the dryer. Large items, like sheets and bath towels, can be reused immediately after cleaning so they do not have to be folded. Those who choose to fold sheets may find the task easier if they use the bed as a work surface.

Ironing. One challenging task for homemakers with physical impairments is to fold and unfold an ironing board. When possible, it is best to leave the ironing board set up in a convenient, out-of-the-way place. The board surface should be at waist level for persons who stand when ironing to reinforce good posture and body mechanics. Persons who iron while seated in a wheelchair will find a work surface of 28–34 inches high comfortable (ADA and ABA Accessibility Guidelines for Buildings and Facilities, 2004). A heat-resistant pad can be placed at the end of the ironing board to eliminate the need to stand the iron up while arranging clothes on the board.

When buying a new iron, individuals should select a lightweight model with an automatic shut-off switch. A cord holder can reduce effort and keep the iron cord from getting in the way. Permanent-press clothing requires less care than cotton or linen fabrics and thus reduces ironing needs. Persons who iron only occasionally may prefer to use a small tabletop ironing board if they have sufficient upper body strength to store and retrieve it from a closet easily.

Sewing. Homemakers may enjoy sewing as a hobby or may only make occasional alterations or repairs. Persons who have hemiparesis after a stroke can still sew with an electric machine by using the unaffected leg to operate foot or knee controls. Persons who do not have use of their lower extremities can place the foot pedal of an electric sewing machine on the table and use one hand or elbow to depress it. Sewing is generally most successful when there is an adequate workspace and adapted methods to stabilize materials when cutting or stitching.

Persons with limited use of an affected arm can hand sew by using an embroidery hoop attached to the edge of a table or counter with a C-clamp (Fig. 27-10). To minimize sewing needs, sticky iron-on tape or fabric glue can be used for hems and small repairs. Rotary cutters, instead of scissors, can make cutting fabric easier.

Indoor Household Maintenance. The occupational therapist helps clients identify effective ways to do household maintenance tasks, such as bed making and floor care.

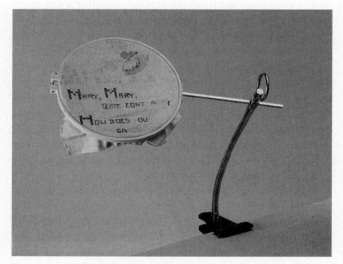

Figure 27-10 Embroidery adapted with use of a hoop that fastens to the table; requires only one hand. (Photo courtesy of Maddak, Inc.)

Adapted techniques and assistive devices can help the client to safely perform necessary chores without assistance.

Bed Making. Bed making can be simplified by straightening the sheets and blankets as much as possible before rising in the morning. Homemakers with limited mobility or impaired upper extremity function find it easier to make the bed by completing one corner at a time, starting with the head of the bed. If the individual is working from a wheelchair, the bed should be positioned so that both sides are accessible. Persons with chronic back pain must adhere to proper body mechanics when making beds, being careful to eliminate excessive forward bending.

When changing the sheets, a person can reduce extra work by carefully pulling blankets and spreads toward the foot of the bed, trying not to dislodge them from under the mattress. In this way, the person will not have to expend unnecessary energy to find and reposition the top edge of the blankets or bedspread. Although the bottom sheet should be fitted, it should also be loose enough to be easily applied.

If the client or a friend is handy at sewing, several adaptations can be made to standard sheets to increase the ease of bed making. Fitted sheets can be adapted by opening the two fitted corners at the bottom end and sewing Velcro™ straps onto each side. When fastened, these straps securely hold the bottom corners together. Persons with limited upper body strength or hemiparesis may find lightweight blankets and spreads and satin pillowcases easier to manage.

Dusting. Physically challenged homemakers can dust hard-to-reach places with assistive devices. Persons with limited upper extremity reach because of orthopedic or neurological changes can use a commercially available long-handled duster that is lightweight and easily extended to reach high places. Individuals with good hand strength may prefer to hold a dust cloth with a long-handled reacher or use a vacuum cleaner attachment to clean hard-to-reach places. Persons who cannot afford assistive devices may find that a dust cloth secured to the end of a yardstick or dowel with a rubber band meets their needs. Clients with limited grasp or fine motor control may find that an adapted spray handle (see Fig. 25-7) attached to the furniture polish can and an old sock or duster mitten significantly enhance their independence in dusting.

Floor Care. Heavy homemaking tasks, such as floor care, are often the first activities that elderly persons or individuals with physical impairments find difficult because of the amount of strength and endurance required. When the client's goal is independence in floor care, the occupational therapist must determine how this can be safely and efficiently accomplished.

Cleaning supplies can be conveniently stored and transported in a handled bin or canvas bag with a shoulder strap. When feasible, duplicate sets of equipment can be kept around the home to reduce the need to carry items. A number of lightweight, wet or dry floor-cleaning tools are commercially available and easy to use for quick cleanups. A sponge mop with the squeeze lever on the handle minimizes bending and can be used with one hand. Individuals with limited hand function but adequate proximal arm strength can use a grasping cuff to help maintain a closed fist around mop or broom handles. Persons working from a wheelchair may find it best to start at the farthest corner and work backward out of the room. Furniture should be fitted with casters or Teflon slides if moved regularly.

Lightweight upright vacuums provide a good alternative to using heavier canister-style models because they work well and are easier to manage for both those who are ambulatory and those who use wheelchairs. A lightweight carpet sweeper is another good choice because it is maneuverable, is relatively inexpensive, and does not have to be plugged into an electrical outlet. Although the carpet sweeper is easier to push, more repetitions are generally needed to clean the same area. Long-handled dustpans and brushes can ease cleanup because they eliminate the need for bending and stooping (Fig. 27-11). If the client has

good hand function, cordless handheld vacuum cleaners are handy for cleaning up small messes within easy reach.

Bathrooms. After a disabling event, a homemaker who cannot afford a housekeeper or does not have family members to assist may have to learn adapted ways to clean the bathroom. Cleaning needs can be reduced by rinsing the sink or tub immediately after use to wash away soap residue. Spray-on chemical products clean bathroom fixtures with little effort, substantially reducing physical demands. Toilet cleaning tablets can be dropped into the toilet tank to reduce the growth of bacteria between thorough cleanings. A long-handled mop with a small head is useful for cleaning inaccessible areas behind the toilet.

Many homemakers with physical impairments find that cleaning the bathtub is difficult or impossible. These suggestions may make it possible. Persons with limited endurance or balance concerns should sit to clean the tub. Cleaning sprays and foams can be easily applied and rinsed off from a seated position, particularly if a long-handled shower hose is used. A long-handled bathroom cleaner with a nonscratch scrubbing sponge can enable persons with limited reach to clean tubs and shower enclosures without assistance (Fig. 27-12). Replacing sliding doors with a plastic shower curtain can make the bathtub more accessible for bathing and cleaning. The plastic curtain can be laundered in the washing machine or inexpensively replaced when it becomes soiled.

Hard to Manage Tasks. No matter how creative the occupational therapist and client are, some household tasks may be impossible for persons with physical impairments. However, a large number of assistive devices are

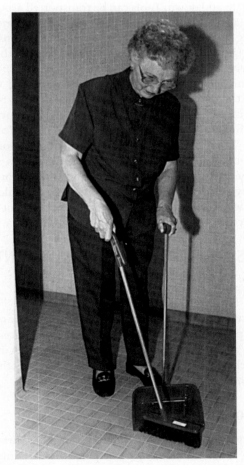

Figure 27-11   Use of a long-handled brush with dustpan. (Photo by Robert Littlefield.)

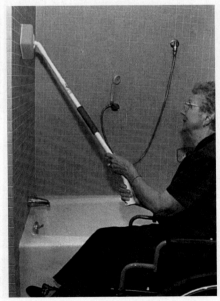

Figure 27-12   Cleaning bathroom tile using a long-handled cleaner. (Photo by Robert Littlefield.)

available to ease the physical requirements of previously difficult tasks. Electric outlet extensions can be plugged into existing baseboard outlets and secured to the wall to eliminate the need to bend when inserting or removing a plug. Devices that make it easier to replace hard to reach light bulbs are also available. The adaptive therapist is well able to analyze task demands and identify modifications or assistive devices that promote independence. When a client cannot accomplish household tasks despite adapted methods, the occupational therapist can initiate a referral to homemaker services.

Outdoor Household Maintenance. When a client's goal is to do outdoor household maintenance, such as yard work or gardening, the occupational therapist can offer suggestions to increase safety and independence.

Yard Maintenance. Persons with mild physical impairments can return to some level of outdoor home maintenance if desired. Individuals with good endurance can mow with a self-propelled lawn mower and accomplish small projects, such as maintaining a patio area. To reduce the risk of back injury when mowing, individuals should avoid stopping and turning the mower. For this reason, a lawn with rounded rather than angled corners is easier to mow (Yeomans, 1992). Rechargeable battery-operated edgers are more convenient than models that must be connected to an electric cord when operated. Numerous ergonomically designed products have been developed to reduce injury during outdoor work. For example, bent-handled shovels reduce excessive back strain and forward bending by altering the fulcrum of movement (Fig. 27-13).

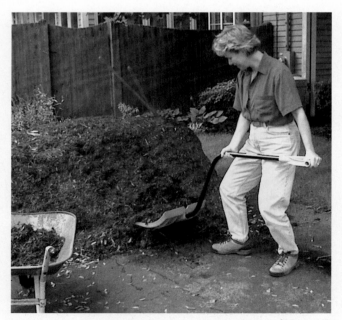

Figure 27-13 Protecting the back while shoveling by using an ergonomically designed shovel with bent handle and lifting with the legs, not the back.

Gardening. Homemakers who are physically challenged need not give up the joy of gardening. Tools can be adapted, flower and vegetable beds can be raised, and wider walkways or wheelways can be created to increase a person's access to the garden. Container gardening is also feasible for persons with limited mobility.

Gardeners with limited hand function can adapt ordinary hand tools with inexpensive foam pipe insulation, which is available at most building supply stores (Yeomans, 1992). This foam, presplit for easy application, can significantly enhance the comfort of grasping and holding the tool. In a randomized study, Tebben and Thomas (2004) reported that a garden trowel labeled as "ergonomic" did not elicit better wrist positions during use when compared to an ordinary trowel. This reinforces the need to carefully assess whether "ergonomic" garden tools truly enhance body mechanics and positioning for a given client.

Individuals who garden from a wheelchair can increase their reach by using long-handled spades, shovels, and pruners. Persons with limited trunk mobility or balance may increase their safety by sitting on a garden stool and using long-handled tools. Gardeners who are fairly mobile can use a kneeling bench, with handles that assist them in getting up and down. Tools can be transported around the yard in apron pockets, a backpack, or a child's wagon, depending on the person's needs and available options. Tools with brightly colored handles are easy to see and therefore less likely to be lost in the garden (Yeomans, 1992).

Homemakers who return to gardening need to take care of themselves while caring for their flowers. Stretching exercises before and after gardening can reduce muscle stiffness and prevent injuries (Adil, 1994; Yeomans, 1992). Work simplification, energy conservation, and proper body mechanics are essential. Gardeners should keep themselves safe by using sun and insect protection, drinking plenty of fluids, and carrying a medical-alert button or whistle around their neck in case they encounter unexpected problems when alone in the garden.

TASKS AND ACTIVITIES OF THE PARENTING ROLE: TREATMENT PRINCIPLES AND METHODS

The occupational therapist and client work closely to identify adapted methods and equipment that enhance participation and independence in parenting tasks. A holistic approach addresses parent and family needs within the home and community.

Psychosocial Adjustment

Parents whose physical limitations are due to an acute event, such as spinal cord injury or acquired brain injury, may initially lack a sense of competence, not only in their ability to care for themselves but also in their ability to care for their children. The impact of the client's impairments on family responsibilities and expectations must be considered when establishing a treatment plan (see Procedures for Practice 27-5). The occupational therapist also must be sensitive to the client's psychosocial concerns about changes in family relationships and roles. Restoration of parenting roles can be challenging for the client, the family, and the therapist.

Parents with diminished physical abilities following an acute event (e.g., spinal cord injury) are likely to have different intervention needs than parents with a chronic or progressive disease or disorder (e.g., rheumatoid arthritis or multiple sclerosis). Persons subjected to the acute onset of physical or cognitive impairments are confronted by sudden and sometimes drastic changes in the ways they can participate in important life roles and tasks. In contrast, individuals with progressive conditions and their families can gradually learn adapted ways to cope with changing abilities and levels of role participation over time. The child's age and developmental stage will greatly impact parent/child relationships in both acute and chronic situations. It is important to recognize that parenting needs and concerns evolve as the child grows and as the parent's disability changes. Even small changes in physical status (e.g., transition from use of a walker to scooter for a mother with multiple sclerosis) can have significant effects on all family members. Children who were accepting of a parent's physical disability at a younger age may become more sensitive to peer pressures and their parent being "different" as they approach teen years.

During the evaluation, the occupational therapist asks clients to list their concerns and identify which parenting tasks they highly value, as well as which tasks are necessary for them to resume their parenting role. The client should then prioritize parenting goals in a way that addresses both valued and necessary tasks in a balanced way.

Barriers to Effectiveness

Barriers to a client's ability to return to parenting tasks and roles are similar to those for homemaker responsibilities. A client's child care needs within home and community environments must be identified and addressed. Factors such as the child's age, activity level, and behavior greatly influence the challenges encountered by the parent with physical impairments. The occupational therapist works to identify the barriers that interfere with a client's ability to accomplish important parenting tasks, devises adapted methods that reduce or remove these constraints, and assists the individual in regaining competence in his or her parenting role by addressing physical, cognitive, and psychosocial needs.

Child Care: Techniques and Therapeutic Aids

Caring for young children under the age of 4 years is physically demanding and can contribute to musculoskeletal pain, even in parents without physical disabilities (Sanders & Morse, 2005). Parents with rheumatoid arthritis, spinal cord injury, and stroke find that child care tasks that require lifting and carrying are the most challenging, followed by tasks that demand fine motor dexterity and/or grip strength. A national survey of parents with physical disabilities revealed that parenting tasks such as traveling outside the home with a child, recreational activities, and chasing and retrieving children require the greatest assistance from others (Barker & Maralani, 1997). Although researchers have shown that adaptive baby care equipment can reduce fatigue and increase parent satisfaction (Vensand et al., 2000), funding for adapted parenting equipment and

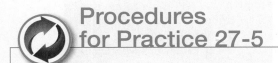

Procedures for Practice 27-5

Managing Parenting Roles with Cognitive Limitations: Structuring Age-Appropriate Play Experiences

Positive play experiences are key to parent/child bonding and facilitating child development. The therapist can use Internet resources and parenting texts to help the client with cognitive impairments choose age-appropriate activities for the child. Activities should allow for gross and fine motor play, creativity, and cognitive exploration through varied sensory modalities (visual, auditory, and tactile).

- Help parent to recognize and respond to the child's needs and interests. Being attuned to the child's energy level and interests will help the parent choose appropriate play activities (e.g., bean bag toss or push toys when active; manipulatives, puzzles, or story time when calm or tired).
- The client's physical and cognitive challenges must be considered when planning play time activities. For example, ball toss with a toddler can be frustrating when the parent lacks the physical ability to catch or retrieve stray balls. Kid-sized basketball or bean bag toss games may be more satisfying, particularly when the child's job is to gather balls for the next round of play.
- Various card and board games involve sustained attention, memory, or use of strategies and problem solving, so are good therapeutic activities for the parent facing cognitive challenges. Select games carefully, so they are fun and engaging to both the child and parent while providing the "just-right challenge" in light of the parent's cognitive impairments.
- Trips to the playground are among the most challenging for parents with physical and cognitive impairments. Small play groups with friends, or offered through community education programs, can provide great opportunities for socialization and support, physical assistance when needed, and modeling of appropriate parenting behavior.

personal assistance services to help with child care is extremely limited. Therefore, the parent and therapist must work together to identify adapted methods and inexpensive solutions that best address parenting needs.

Equipment Considerations

The occupational therapist and client should initially explore whether simple adaptations to the way child care tasks are performed can enhance performance. When these simple solutions do not work, the client and therapist should evaluate whether commercially available child care equipment can feasibly meet the needs of the parent and child. If not, more creative solutions and adaptations must be devised.

The occupational therapist should consider the cost of the adapted equipment and whether it is acceptable to the client in terms of appearance and ease of use. In addition, the therapist must understand that the appropriateness of any equipment changes over time as the child grows and develops (Vensand et al., 2000).

Transitional Tasks

When working with parents of infants, the occupational therapist must first address transitional tasks that occur before or between baby care activities such as feeding or dressing. These transitional tasks are holding, carrying and moving, transfers, and positional changes. The occupational therapist works with the parent to identify the safest methods for managing these transitions, including use of proper positioning techniques and holding devices such as wedge pillows or slings, alternate means for carrying that may include securing infant seats to rollator walkers, or emphasizing good body mechanics and use of lifting slings or harnesses during transfers and positional changes (Rogers & Kirshbaum, 2011).

Adapted equipment that provides alternative ways of carrying the infant or young child or reduces the need for multiple transfers can greatly enhance the parent's satisfaction and ability to care for the child. Parents with distal weakness and pain, as seen with rheumatoid arthritis, benefit from wearing wrist supports to reduce joint stress when lifting and carrying their child (Nordenskiold, Grimby, & Dahlin-Ivanoff, 1998). Many clients prefer to practice lifting and carrying techniques with a weighted doll before trying to manage an active child.

A variety of cloth infant carriers and child front packs are available. Although these carriers allow the parent to transport a small child while leaving hands free, they may be contraindicated for persons with chronic back pain because the shoulders and back carry the weight of the child. Individuals who use wheelchairs may find child front packs handy for holding the infant while performing other homemaking tasks. Ease of use is important: adaptations may be needed to enable the parent with physical impairments to get the baby into and out of the infant carrier. The straps can be modified to reduce the parent's coordination needs

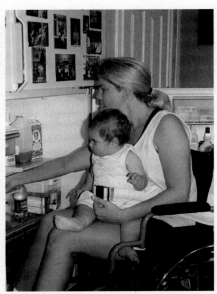

Figure 27-14 A mother confined to a wheelchair using a safety strap for an older baby while gathering items from the refrigerator.

(Vensand et al., 2000). Older babies with good neck and trunk control can safely ride on their parent's lap with only a safety belt attached to the wheelchair (Fig. 27-14).

Bathing

Parents need to be sure that all necessary equipment and clothes have been gathered and are within easy reach before they begin bathing their infant or young child. A terry cloth apron worn during bathing can protect clothing and dry the baby after the bath. Persons who are ambulatory may find that bathing the infant in a portable plastic tub in or near the kitchen sink is a good option because the height of the sink or counter minimizes bending and the tub can be easily filled and drained at the sink. Parents who use wheelchairs, however, may find this arrangement inconvenient because it is too high for safely lifting the baby in and out of the tub. Persons in wheelchairs also find it difficult to bathe the infant if the baby tub is in a regular bathtub because it is too low (Vensand et al., 2000). An alternative is to secure the baby bathtub to a sturdy table or computer table placed near a sink. A portable hose can be connected to the sink faucet for filling the tub, and a separate hose can be used to drain the bath water (Vensand et al., 2000). It may be easier for the parent to use this arrangement to bathe the older infant until the child is mobile enough to help with getting in and out of a regular bathtub. This diminishes the parent's need to lift a wet, slippery child from a low tub.

Diapering and Dressing

Commercially available changing tables are usually inaccessible for persons who use a wheelchair because the wheelchair does not fit under the table for diapering or dressing the child. In addition, the surface may be too high for a seated parent to lift and transfer the baby safely, particularly as the infant grows (Vensand et al., 2000). The client and therapist should work together to determine the changing surface that most effectively and safely meets the individual's needs. Concave diapering pads that keep the baby from rolling off the changing surface can be adapted and safely attached to a computer table or dining room table to allow better wheelchair access (Rogers & Kirshbaum, 2011).

Safety straps should always be used to secure the active baby to prevent falls. These straps are particularly helpful when the parent needs extra time to manipulate diaper or clothing fasteners because of diminished fine motor control. A mobile attached to the changing surface and assorted toys can keep the baby distracted during changing.

Although adapted fasteners for diapers and baby clothing can require initial assistance from family or friends, they can greatly enhance one's independence in child care during the day. For example, Velcro™ attachments on diaper wraps that hold either cloth or disposable diapers can be adapted by attaching metal or plastic key rings that are more easily managed by parents with limited hand function. In addition, many disposable diapers now have Velcro™ fasteners which, unlike tape closures, allow for easier repositioning and handling. Small pieces of Velcro™ can also be sewn onto a variety of infant and baby clothes. Ideally, clothing should have full-length openings with closures that the parent can manage. When a zipper pull is used, zippers are easier to manipulate than snaps. Many caregiver techniques that emphasize baby collaboration with the parent can be explored. For example, simple physical cues such as gently pushing on the baby's elbow can facilitate arm extension into the sleeve during dressing (Rogers & Kirshbaum, 2011).

Feeding

Mothers with physical challenges may choose to nurse or bottle-feed their baby. After an initial adjustment period, breast-feeding can be easier than bottle-feeding because it eliminates formula preparation. If the mother is taking medications, it is important that she check with her physician before deciding to breast-feed to be sure that the medication will not harm the nursing infant. The mother should sit in a relaxed, comfortable position, using pillows to support the holding arm and baby while nursing. Pillows that are specifically designed to support the nursing infant are commercially available. When needed, wheelchair lap trays with foam padding can be fabricated to assist with infant positioning while nursing.

Some parents find bottle-feeding easier and more convenient with the older infant in a child seat, although others prefer to hold the child close to them when feeding (Fig. 27-15). Individuals with limited grasp may be able to hold a bottle and feed their infant after slipping their hand

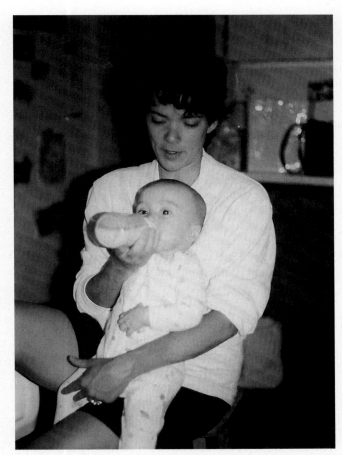

Figure 27-15 Alternative feeding position for mother with mild left hemiparesis following cerebrovascular accident.

through a loop of webbing material attached to the bottle (Vensand et al., 2000). Many different types of bottle holders are available on the internet. Lightweight plastic bottles with screw-on lids are recommended over glass bottles.

Older babies can be spoon-fed by a person with tetraplegia when the parent's wrist cock-up splint is adapted by attaching a Velcro™ loop to the palmar surface. The spoon is inserted into a utensil pocket made of Velcro™ hook and attached to the splint at the best angle for feeding (Vensand et al., 2000). An insulated baby dish can be used to keep food warm throughout the meal. Spoons should be rubber coated to protect the baby's gums and teeth if bumped while feeding.

Parents with impaired grasp and arm strength may not be able to attach or remove the tray on commercial high chairs (Vensand et al., 2000). In addition, it may be difficult for the parent to lift the child in and out of a standard high chair. Options to make high chairs more accessible for parents with physical limitations include altering the chair height, designing swing-away trays, and adding a climbing ladder to encourage the older infant to climb into the seat with supervision only (Vensand et al., 2000).

Play

Parents with physical impairments may find that their ability to play with their young children is hindered because they cannot sit on the floor or bend to reach into standard playpens. Although infants can be entertained while they are sitting in a bouncy seat, older babies need a larger safe play area to develop gross motor skills. If cost is not an issue, a play care center, essentially a raised playpen that allows wheelchair access, can be built in the corner of a room (Vensand et al., 2000). If the center is equipped with swing-away or sliding doors, the parent can wheel up to the play center and easily reach into it to play with the baby. This play area can also be used for the child's naps during the day, eliminating extra transfers in and out of the crib (Vensand et al., 2000). Walking toddlers and their parents may find that a child's table approximately 18 inches high is a convenient place to play while the parent is sitting in a wheelchair or standard chair.

Cribs

Standard cribs are inaccessible for parents who use wheelchairs, and they require ambulatory parents to bend forward when putting the baby in or out of bed. A standard drop-side crib can be adapted in several ways, depending on the parent's physical needs.

Persons who are ambulatory but have difficulty bending because of chronic back pain can raise the crib by inserting leg extenders or blocks of wood under the crib legs. The crib mattress can also be raised to the highest setting but should not remain in this position once the baby is old enough to sit or to climb over the crib rail.

Parents who use a wheelchair will find it easier to transfer the baby in and out of the crib if the rail is adapted. One suggestion involves extending the legs of the crib to allow wheelchair access under the mattress in its lowest position. The drop-down rail is cut to form two gates that open at each end of the crib. Hinges for the gates are attached to a center post that is connected to two horizontal bars that run between the head and foot of the crib. Latches that are inaccessible to the child secure the gate when the baby is sleeping (see http://www.disabled parents.net/?page_id=95). Another option is to adapt the crib rail so that it slides along a horizontal channel (Dunn, 1978; Versand et al., 2000). Whatever crib design is used, the release mechanism for the crib rail must be child resistant yet manageable for the parent to manipulate with one hand or with limited coordination and dexterity. When planning adaptations, the structural integrity of the crib and baby safety during transfers are major considerations. For example, babies who are mobile are at a greater risk for falling when a parent backs away from the crib to open a gate that swings outward. Horizontal bars that add structural support above the crib rail may pose a bumping hazard for older babies who pull up to stand before transferring out of the crib. Adapted cribs should be checked frequently to assure that they safely meet needs of both parent and child (Rogers & Kirshbaum, 2011).

EFFICACY AND OUTCOMES RESEARCH

Although the number of studies on occupational therapy outcomes continues to grow, there continues to be little evidence concerning specific effects of occupation-as-end on homemaking and parenting abilities. Much of the research describes interventions that either combine occupation-as-means (task-specific training in ADL or meal preparation) with occupation-as-end (task adaptation or environmental modification) (e.g., Clarke et al., 2009), or reports effects of a multidisciplinary approach in which the impact of occupational therapy cannot be distinguished from that of physical therapy (Gitlin et al., 2006; Ziden, Frandin, & Kreuter, 2008). An American Occupational Therapy Association (AOTA) critically appraised topic (CAT) paper on the effect of occupation and activity-based interventions on instrumental activities of daily living (IADL) in community dwelling older adults highlighted the need for stronger evidence of best practice. This is a challenging issue that must take into account the client's performance skills and patterns, the activity demands of the task at hand, and the complexities of context and environment (AOTA, 2010). Although one cannot expect to find a "one size fits all" intervention to improve IADL performance in clients with physical and/or cognitive impairments, it is important to identify which therapy approach is most effective based on the client's personal situation and needs. This CAT reported limited evidence to support the use of a compensatory approach to improve IADL in frail community dwelling adults and highlighted the need for more specific and sensitive outcome instruments to better assess IADL performance and change (AOTA, 2010).

Generally, occupational therapy outcomes are based on more global measures of ADL or IADL, such as the Frenchay Activity Index or the Nottingham Extended Activities of Daily Living Scale. As can be seen from the studies described in the best evidence table, the effects of occupational therapy intervention on homemaking, meal preparation, or household management abilities are often embedded within these broader IADL scales, making it challenging to discern specific changes in task performance. In addition, two of the three studies in Evidence Table 27-1 combined treatment approaches (occupation-as-means and occupation-as-end) or therapy disciplines (occupational therapy and physical therapy), making it difficult to interpret research findings.

Research is needed to further examine the degree to which adapted methods and equipment (i.e., occupation-as-end) contribute to one's satisfaction and competence in homemaker and parenting roles after a disabling event. Empirical support for the cost effectiveness of adapted equipment and supportive services may lead to improved reimbursement from third-party payers.

Evidence Table 27-1 | Best Evidence for Occupational Therapy to Restore Competence for Homemaker and Parenting Roles

Intervention	Description of Intervention Tested	Participants	Dosage	Type of Best Evidence and Level of Evidence	Benefit	Statistical Probability and Effect Size of Outcome	Reference
Home-based, client-centered occupational therapy targeting limitations in ADL & IADL, mobility, and home safety	Occupational therapy methods included task-specific practice, reducing task complexity or demands, and/or altering environment through adaptive aids. Control group received occupational therapy after completion of trial.	Parkinson's disease, $n = 39$; mean age = 73 years	Six 45-minute sessions of occupational therapy over 2 months	Randomized controlled trial (RCT) pilot study with cross-over design Level: IC2b (small group sizes; blinding not reported; unclear whether sample was representative of Parkinson's disease population and what theoretical support was for intervention)	Yes. Mean group difference in Nottingham Extended ADL Scale at 8 months was 3.5 (95% confidence interval = 3.2–10.2) favoring the intervention group. Strong correlations were found between PDQ-39 and other measures.	Formal statistical analysis not completed because of small sample size.	Clarke et al. (2009)
Home-based, client-centered occupational therapy/physical therapy intervention to reduce functional difficulties	Treatment group: occupational therapy focus on training of cognitive and behavioral strategies for problem solving/pacing and environmental modifications. Physical therapy intervention was one visit (90 minutes) that addressed balance, strengthening and fall-recovery techniques. Control group did not receive intervention.	Adults aged 70 years and older, $n = 319$, reporting difficulty with two IADL or one or more ADL	Over a 6-month period, treatment group received four 90-minute occupational therapy visits and one 20-minute phone call in addition to one 90-minute physical therapy visit. During the 6 months that followed treatment, three follow-up phone calls were made to reinforce use of strategies and a final home visit was conducted for closure.	RCT, prospective two-group trial Level: IA1a	Yes. At 6 months, the intervention group was significantly better than control in IADL, with fewer home hazards, increased use of adaptive strategies, and better self-efficacy (confidence in managing ADL) as compared to control group. Benefits sustained for most outcomes at 12 months.	At 6 months, change in IADL scores were significantly better in treatment group ($p = 0.04$); unable to calculate effect size from study report.	Gitlin et al. (2006)

(continued)

Evidence Table 27-1	Best Evidence for Occupational Therapy to Restore Competence for Homemaker and Parenting Roles *(continued)*

Intervention	Description of Intervention Tested	Participants	Dosage	Type of Best Evidence and Level of Evidence	Benefit	Statistical Probability and Effect Size of Outcome	Reference
Community-based energy conservation course	Energy conservation course for adults with fatigue caused by chronic illness; lectures, goal setting, and assignments applicable to everyday tasks. Control group received delayed intervention.	Multiple sclerosis, $n = 169$; of these, $n = 131$ compliant participants (attended at least five of six sessions)	Six sessions over a 6-week period	RCT, cross-over design Level: IA2a (study evaluators not blinded)	Beneficial effects of energy conservation training were maintained 1 year postcourse.	Intention to treat analysis showed significant benefits for training group on Fatigue Impact Scale ($p = 0.05$) and SF-36® ($p = 0.02$); unable to calculate effect size from study report. Benefits were maintained at 12 months.	Mathiowetz et al. (2007)

ADL, activities of daily living; IADL, instrumental activities of daily living; OT, occupational therapy; PDQ-39, Parkinson's Disease Questionnaire; RCT, randomized controlled trial; SF-36®, Short Form-36 Health Survey.

Activity-Focused Analysis
Baking Chocolate Chip Cookies

Task Analysis Process			Example
Describe the task demands	Objects used	Properties of the utensils, tools, materials and their locations relative to the person	Ingredients as listed on recipe (including flour, baking soda, sugar, eggs, and chocolate chips) Measuring cups and spoons Mixing bowls, spoons for mixing and placing dough on baking sheet Electric mixer Baking sheet, spatula, cooling rack, and timer
	Environmental demands	Characteristics of the environment in which the activity usually is carried out, including possible environmental barriers and enablers	Clinic kitchen in rehabilitation facility or client's own kitchen at home Familiarity with location of needed items in kitchen cabinets; kitchen size and distance items will be transported
	Social demands	Nature of and extent to which the activity involves others and/or holds particular meaning associated with social roles	May be performed alone or with family/child participation; may hold personal meaning when preparing warm cookies for friends or loved ones
	Contextual demands	Nature of and extent to which the activity or the way it is carried out holds particular meaning to certain cultures or age groups	Appropriate for a wide range of ages; type of cookie may be adapted to cultural backgrounds and likes
	Sequencing and timing	Monological task (requiring a singular sequence in order to be performed correctly) or a multilogical task in which a variety of sequences will work Extent to which the task involves temporal requirements or timing requirements	Monological: combining ingredients and baking cookies allow for little variation in sequencing of task Small batches of cookies can be prepared within one therapy session. Baking time must be closely monitored.
	Required actions	Steps that comprise the activity	1. Preheat oven. 2. Gather all needed ingredients and kitchen items (bowls, measuring cups/spoons) for mixing dough, baking, and cooling cookies. 3. Measure and combine dry ingredients in a small bowl. 4. Use electric mixer to combine butter, sugar, vanilla, and eggs. 5. Gradually add and beat in flour mixture with wet ingredients. Add chocolate chips. 6. Drop by rounded tablespoons onto ungreased baking sheets. 7. Bake until golden brown (9–11 minutes). 8. Cool on wire racks and eat! 9. Clean up work space.

(continued)

	Prerequisite capacities, abilities, and skills necessary to successful task performance	Sensorimotor: range of motion, strength, motor control, postural control, endurance, coordination/dexterity	Volitional functioning of at least one upper extremity; shoulder flexion, abduction; elbow flexion/extension; forearm supination/pronation; wrist flexion/extension; grasp/release
		Vision-perceptual: visual acuity, visual scanning, visual perception, awareness of extrapersonal space	Visual acuity for reading directions; visual scanning to locate needed items, spatial awareness when placing uncooked batter on cookie sheets
		Cognitive: attention, memory, executive functioning, problem solving, self-awareness	Ability to follow step by step directions and sustain attention for 20–30 minutes; ability to sequence task and detect errors/omissions of ingredients and self-correct; demonstrates divided attention when baking multiple batches of cookies
		Emotional, relational	Varied; can be completed in isolation or with others. Although baking cookies with others will increase interaction and socialization, the client may be distracted and require additional cues/support.
	Safety precautions	Nature of safety considerations if performed in a therapy context	Clients who perform task in standing may need supervision related to balance and/or endurance; closely monitor safety when using oven and hot baking sheet
Identify the primary therapeutic aspect of the task; adapt task demands to align with therapy goals	Sensorimotor	Range of motion	Ingredients are located in overhead cabinets to encourage reaching
		Strength, motor control	Heavier objects (canisters of flour, sugar, large mixing bowl) are carried from cabinet to work surface.
		Postural control, endurance	Client uses postural control and weight shifting when reaching for ingredients that are located on the counter/table.
			Client is required to stand for increasingly longer times between seated rests.
			Client has to bend to reach oven racks/door.
		Coordination, dexterity	Use teaspoons versus tablespoons to increase number of repetitions when scooping and dropping cookie batter onto baking sheet.
	Vision-perceptual	Visual scanning	Client needs to locate needed ingredients and supplies within kitchen space. Increased number of distracters (e.g., needing to find needed items on crowded shelf) requires greater figure ground/perceptual processing.
		Visual perception, extrapersonal space	
	Cognition	Attention, memory	To reduce attention/memory demands, instructions can be written out and checked off when each step is completed.
			Client may be asked to retrieve two or more ingredients at a time to increase memory demands.
			Client is challenged to work in an increasingly distracting or noisy kitchen.
			Therapist may interrupt client to determine whether he or she is able to return to task efficiently.
			Increase needs for divided attention by asking client to keep track of when baking cookies will be done while preparing the next batch for the oven.

		Executive functioning, problem solving, awareness	Client is given general cues to monitor performance and check for errors (missed ingredients, sequence of steps, etc).
			Client predicts what task components will be most challenging and then assesses performance after task to check predictions and identify ways to optimize performance during future cooking activities.
	Emotional-relational	Mood, engagement, interactions with others	Client performs task with others, working in parallel or cooperatively to reach task goal.
Modify task demands to calibrate difficulty level	Objects used		Use of prepared mix or unbaked, packaged cookies versus recipe from scratch reduces number of ingredients and steps involved.
			Location of items (within reach, fewer visual distractions).
			Have adaptive equipment available for clients with physical challenges (e.g., oven pull, dycem to stabilize bowl when mixing, etc.).
	Space demands		Quiet versus busy kitchen environment
	Social demands		Working alone or with others; may involve family/caregivers
	Contextual demands		Working in clinic versus home kitchen.
			Preparing cookies for family or friends may increase personal meaning and motivation.
	Sequencing and timing		Reduce task complexity by providing initial setup (e.g., gather needed ingredients for client)
			Prepare only one batch to reduce attentional demands

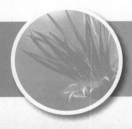

case example

Mrs. B: Treatment to Improve Homemaking and Child Care Abilities

		Clinical Reasoning Process
Occupational Therapy Intervention Process	**Objectives**	**Examples of Therapist's Internal Dialogue**
Patient Information Mrs. B. is a 54-year-old widow referred for a home occupational therapy (OT) assessment following recent exacerbation of rheumatoid arthritis (RA). She lives alone in a ranch house and ordinarily cares for her 6-month-old granddaughter 3 days a week while her daughter works. Prior to her exacerbation, she was fairly active and able to manage all household and child care tasks independently with the exception of yard work. An avid gardener, she spent a good deal of time in her greenhouse prior to her exacerbation. She is able to use joint protection principles (e.g., avoiding positions of deformity, such as ulnar deviation) during functional tasks.	Appreciate the context	"Mrs. B. is ordinarily a fairly active woman who has been caring for her 6-month-old granddaughter since she was a month old. She truly values the time she spends with the baby and is frustrated and somewhat depressed by her present limitations. Although her daughter has offered to find another child care provider while her mother recovers, this has been difficult to arrange in their small community. Mrs. B.'s prior level of independence, combined with a strong desire to help her daughter and care for the infant, have motivated occupational therapy goals to optimize homemaking and child care abilities."

As a result of this exacerbation, she has decreased strength and dexterity in her hands and wrists, increased pain during activity, and a significant decrease in overall endurance. The OT evaluation identified the following problems: (1) moderately decreased ability to perform the household management tasks needed to maintain her independence at home, with fatigue after 30 minutes of activity; (2) moderate impairments in her ability to care for her granddaughter secondary to decreased strength and pain during resistive activities, such as opening baby food jars and attempting to lift the child; and (3) poor use of body mechanics and a tendency to rush through tasks when fatigued.

Recommendations

The occupational therapist recommended three treatment sessions each week for 4 weeks. In collaboration with Mrs. B. and her daughter, the therapist established the following long-term treatment goals: (1) Mrs. B. will independently perform all indoor homemaking tasks, except floor care, with only occasional complaints of fatigue, using energy conservation and work simplification techniques; (2) Mrs. B. will independently care for her granddaughter for 4-hour periods with only occasional complaints of pain, demonstrating appropriate use of assistive devices to protect joints during resistive activities; and (3) Mrs. B. will use proper body mechanics when lifting and carrying her granddaughter and performing household tasks, such as meal preparation and laundry (see Home Program in Procedures for Practice 27-6).

Develop intervention hypotheses	"I think that Mrs. B.'s weakness, pain, and reduced endurance are the biggest barriers to her independence right now. Although she can tell me how to protect her joints during homemaking tasks, her pain and resulting fatigue are causing her not to use proper techniques. She tends to hurry through tasks so she can rest, and I'm concerned about her safety. I expect that, as her pain lessens, she'll do much better overall."
Select an intervention approach	"I will develop an intervention plan that emphasizes compensation for deficits; this will help to protect her from injury long term. By engaging her in important home and child care tasks, we will use occupation-as-means to improve her physical abilities as well."
Reflect on competence	"Mrs. B. reminds me of a couple of other clients I've worked with in home care. It will be really important to involve her in problem solving of ways to best accomplish important tasks. This way she'll gain skills in handling unexpected situations outside of therapy."
Consider what will occur in therapy, how often, and for how long

Ascertain the patient's endorsement of plan | "I think that occupational therapy in the home will be the most effective means of addressing Mrs. B.'s current needs, especially because she is highly motivated to make changes that will optimize her home and child care abilities. Her house is pretty accessible, and I think small changes will really help improve her independence and safety. We should be able to accomplish a lot in the next 4 weeks." |

 Procedures for Practice 27-6

Home Program for Body Mechanics

Mrs. B., please focus on using proper body mechanics during all of your daily tasks. Below are specific ideas for you to incorporate every day:

- Be sure to have a broad base of support when lifting your granddaughter. Keep feet shoulder distance apart, and place one foot forward of the other to help with balance.
- Face the task you're doing, and don't twist your trunk when lifting.
- When doing tasks around the house that take a while (like feeding your granddaughter or repotting small plants) sit instead of standing to conserve energy. Sit up straight, and think about keeping a neutral position in your lower back by tilting the pelvis slightly forward.
- When doing laundry, use your rolling basket to help transport clothes. When you do need to lift clothes, use your strongest muscles (legs versus back) and bend at your hips and knees to avoid straining your back.
- Don't rush! It's best to take rests before you feel tired, and it's much easier to use good body mechanics when working at a comfortable pace!

Summary of Short-Term Goals and Progress

1. Mrs. B. will independently and safely prepare a light meal for herself without complaints of fatigue, using work simplification and energy conservation principles after initial instruction.

   The therapist and Mrs. B. first reviewed work simplification principles in the context of preparing a hot beverage, taking the opportunity to organize work areas in the kitchen so frequently used items were easily accessible. They identified ways Mrs. B. could conserve energy during meal preparation, such as by retrieving all items needed at one location (e.g., refrigerator) before moving on to the next and sitting when possible to prepare foods. After instruction in self-pacing, Mrs. B. was more willing to take brief rests during meal preparation before fatigue or pain began to worsen. After practicing proper body mechanics, she was better able to obtain and carry items safely around the kitchen without increasing pain. In addition, use of a jar opener significantly reduced the discomfort in her hands. To reduce preparation time and effort, Mrs. B. decided to use frozen rather than fresh vegetables until her endurance improved. Mrs. B. found that these strategies greatly reduced her level of fatigue during meal preparation, and she began to apply these techniques to other tasks around the house.

2. Mrs. B. will safely and independently transfer her granddaughter from the infant seat to changing pad on the kitchen table with good body mechanics and safety and no complaints of discomfort.

   Mrs. B., her daughter, and the occupational therapist determined that the need for lifting and carrying the infant could be minimized by organizing essential child care materials, such as the infant seat, changing pad with straps, diapers, and toys, on one side of the oversized kitchen table and nearby hutch. Mrs. B. found that bilateral wrist supports greatly reduced pain in her wrists when she lifted the baby.

   Proper body mechanics were reinforced and practiced, such as standing close to the child with feet staggered and placed shoulder distance apart and using stronger muscles (legs rather than back) when lifting. Mrs. B. progressed from requiring minimal assistance to lift and transfer the baby safely to performing the task independently. As she gained confidence in her abilities, her body mechanics improved and complaints of discomfort decreased.

Assess the patient's comprehension	"Mrs. B. has cognitive strengths that I expect will help her to readily integrate new techniques with her current knowledge of joint protection."
Understand what she is doing	"I was a bit concerned about her rushing through tasks when we first started therapy, but I think that was partly related to her desire to show us that she 'could do it.' I see that, as we gain rapport, she is becoming more comfortable with voicing her concerns about the long-term changes she is experiencing from her arthritis and her fears about losing independence."
Compare actual to expected performance	
Know the person	"Mrs. B. is lucky to have such a supportive daughter; she has helped to identify creative ways for her mother to manage the baby's care. I sense that she is concerned about her mother's chronic RA and the physical changes that Mrs. B. is facing now. I wonder what their long-term plans will be regarding living arrangements, etc."
Appreciate the context	

Next Steps

Revised goals include the following: (1) Mrs. B. will use work simplification techniques and proper body mechanics to do laundry independently, and (2) Mrs. B. will safely and independently lift and transfer her granddaughter from a stroller to the infant seat with good body mechanics and will prepare and feed the child a warm meal without assistance.

Anticipate present and future patient concerns	"Mrs. B. has been very responsive to therapy and has made great gains over the past couple of weeks. She is much more confident in her abilities, and her pain is being better managed through medication and the compensatory strategies she has learned to use. She is now ready to practice work simplification techniques during more physically challenging tasks. With a bit more therapy, she will be able to care for her granddaughter independently once again."
Decide if the patient should continue or discontinue therapy and/ or return in the future	

Clinical Reasoning in Occupational Therapy Practice

Effects of Fatigue on Upper Extremity Functioning and Instrumental Activities of Daily Living

Since her recent RA exacerbation, Mrs. B. reported that end-of-day fatigue is more significantly impacting her arm and hand strength and coordination. She reports that it is more difficult to complete needed tasks, such as cleaning up after dinner, transferring laundry from washer to dryer, or holding her pen well when paying bills or writing cards to friends.

What further adaptations may be made to improve her ability to manage these daily tasks? How might you help her to prioritize and best manage her time for needed tasks throughout the week?

Summary Review Questions

1. Describe how work simplification and energy conservation techniques can help persons with low endurance and shortness of breath caused by chronic obstructive pulmonary disease with meal preparation and household maintenance tasks.

2. Identify at least three principles of correct body mechanics that a person with chronic back pain should use when doing laundry and transporting groceries from the store.

3. Describe how a homemaker who has pain and weakness in her hands and wrists caused by rheumatoid arthritis can use adapted methods or assistive equipment when preparing brownies from a mix.

4. Using the principles of compensation and adaptation, what recommendations would you make to a client with limited upper extremity coordination and strength caused by multiple sclerosis when

gathering the items needed to prepare breakfast from a wheelchair?

5. Give two examples of adaptations that may assist a paraplegic parent with spinal cord injury at T4 (see Chapter 38) to lift and carry an 11-month-old infant from the crib to the changing area.

6. Describe how a mother with upper extremity weakness and limited hand function in her right arm after a stroke can use one-handed techniques and assistive equipment to prepare a bottle and feed her 5-month-old infant.

7. How would you recommend that a parent set up a baby bathtub and needed supplies to bathe a 2-month-old infant from a wheelchair?

8. Discuss proper body mechanics for a person with general pain related to fibromyalgia who is playing with a 10-month-old baby and putting the baby to bed.

References

ADA and ABA Accessibility Guidelines for Buildings and Facilities. (2004). Retrieved May 10, 2012 from http://www.access-board.gov/ada-aba/final.htm.

Adil, J. R. (1994). *Accessible gardening for people with physical disabilities: A guide to methods, tools, and plants.* Bethesda, MD: Woodbine House.

American Occupational Therapy Association. (2010). AOTA Critically Appraised Topics and Papers Series: Occupation and activity-based interventions. Retrieved February 1, 2012 from www.aota.org/CCL/Occupation/IADL.aspx. Access only to AOTA members.

Barker, L. T., & Maralani, V. (1997). *Challenges and strategies of disabled parents: Findings from a national survey of parents with disabilities: Final report.* Oakland, CA: Berkeley Planning Associates.

Clark, F., Azen, S. P., Zemke, R., Jackson, J., Carlson, M., Mandel, D., Hay, J., Josephson, K., Cherry, B., Hessel, C., Palmer, J., & Lipson, L. (1997). Occupational therapy for independent-living older adults: A randomized controlled trial. *Journal of the American Medical Association, 278,* 1321–1326.

Clarke, C. E., Furmston, A., Morgan, E., Patel, S., Sackley, C., Walker, M., Bryan, S., & Wheatley, K. (2009). Pilot randomised controlled trial of occupational therapy to optimise independence in Parkinson's disease: The PD OT trial. *Journal of Neurology, Neurosurgery & Psychiatry, 80,* 976–978.

Dunn, V. M. (1978). Tips on raising children from a wheelchair. *Accent on Living, 22,* 78–83.

Gitlin, L. N., Winter, L., Dennis, M. P., Corcoran, M., Schinfeld, S., & Hauck, W. W. (2006). A randomized trial of a multicomponent home intervention to reduce functional difficulties in older adults. *Journal of the American Geriatrics Society, 54,* 809–816.

Jackson, J., Carlson, M., Mandel, D., Zemke, R., & Clark, F. (1998). Occupational lifestyle redesign: The well-elderly study occupational therapy program. *American Journal of Occupational Therapy, 52,* 326–336.

Mathiowetz, V. G., Matuska, K. M., Finlayson, M. L., Luo, P., & Chen, H. Y. (2007). One-year follow-up to a randomized controlled trial of an energy conservation course for persons with multiple sclerosis. *International Journal of Rehabilitation Research, 30,* 305–313.

Nordenskiold, U., Grimby, G., & Dahlin-Ivanoff, S. (1998). Questionnaire to evaluate the effects of assistive devices and altered working methods in women with rheumatoid arthritis. *Clinical Rheumatology, 17,* 6-16.

Rogers, J., & Kirshbaum, M. (2011). Parenting after stroke. In G. Gillen (Ed.), *Stroke Rehabilitation: A function-based approach* (pp. 583-597). St. Louis: Elsevier Mosby.

Sanders, M. J., & Morse, T. (2005). The ergonomics of caring for children: An exploratory study. *American Journal of Occupational Therapy, 59,* 285-295.

Sandqvist, G., Akesson, A., & Eklund, M. (2005). Daily occupations and well-being in women with limited cutaneous systemic sclerosis. *American Journal of Occupational Therapy, 59,* 390-397.

Tebben, A. B., & Thomas, J. J. (2004). Trowels labeled ergonomic versus standard design: Preferences and effects on wrist range of motion during a gardening occupation. *American Journal of Occupational Therapy, 58,* 317-323.

Unruh, A. M. (2004). Reflections on: "So…what do you do?" Occupation and the construction of identity. *Canadian Journal of Occupational Therapy, 71,* 290-295.

Vensand, K., Rogers, J., Tuleja, C., & DeMoss, A. (2000). *Adaptive baby care equipment: Guidelines, prototypes & resources.* Berkeley, CA: Through the Looking Glass.

Yeomans, K. (1992). *The able gardener: Overcoming barriers of age and physical limitations.* Pownal, VT: Storey.

Ziden, L., Frandin, K., & Kreuter, M. (2008). Home rehabilitation after hip fracture. A randomized controlled study on balance confidence, physical function and everyday activities. *Clinical Rehabilitation, 22,* 1019-1033.

ACKNOWLEDGMENT

Many thanks to Robert Littlefield, photographer, and to Patterson Medical for the assistive devices pictured in this chapter. Special thanks to the individuals who shared their ideas about adapted techniques with me, based on their personal experiences with physical challenges.

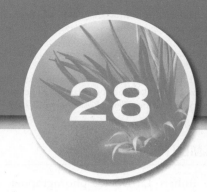

28

Restoring Competence for the Worker Role

Valerie J. Rice

Learning Objectives

After studying this chapter, the reader will be able to do the following:

1. Understand and articulate the reasons people work.
2. Recognize and verbalize the unique role of occupational therapy in the return-to-work process.
3. Describe job analysis and how it is used in the return-to-work process, and identify other possible applications for the results of job analysis.
4. Describe functional capacity evaluations and considerations in selecting appropriate evaluations for clients.
5. Recognize how return-to-work evaluation tools can be used as treatment tools.

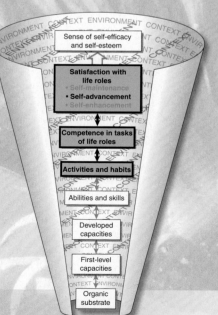

Two people meet for the first time at a social event. After introducing themselves, the inevitable question is asked: "What do you do?"

The focus of this chapter is on returning a worker who has been incapacitated in some way to the workforce. The intervention begins after an individual has been identified as being unable to meet the requirements of his or her job. Thus, the primary roles for the clinician are *evaluating* the individual's functional performance, strengths, and impairments as compared with the job requirements; *treating* the client; *matching* the client-worker with the job (enabling and integration process); and *reevaluation*. To understand the progression, it is first necessary to understand why people work, recognize how occupational therapists view work and their role in work rehabilitation, understand how the work role can be interrupted, and become acquainted with a few work-related assessments. An extensive explanation of the evaluation process is provided to enable a thorough understanding of the process and permit tailoring of the intervention to both the individual and the context in which the individual will work. With this knowledge, the occupational therapy process can be understood and implemented within the appropriate context.

WHAT IS WORK?

"He who complains against his work knoweth not life; work is an uplifting force by which all things may be moved. Repose is death, and work is life!" (Jastrzebowski, 1857/1997, p. 1)

Although we may not all agree with Jastrzebowski's enthusiastic assertion that work is uplifting and *life itself*, there is some merit in his declaration. Used in the broadest sense of the term, everyone must work. It is part of life. Work, as seen in the first definition in Definition 28-1, consists of any physical or mental effort or activity directed toward the purposeful production or accomplishment of something. This means that work occurs in the home, in schools, as part of one's employment, during volunteer work, and as part of one's leisure. To work is *to do*, to accomplish. With this definition, returning the worker to work encompasses occupational therapy as a whole, as clinicians assist their clients to achieve their fullest capacity in all aspects of life. In this chapter, however, returning the worker to work refers to helping a client reenter the workforce, go to a place of employment or job (including volunteer positions), and/or develop a means to earn a livelihood.

MOTIVATIONS FOR WORK

Why would an individual want to reenter the labor force? Why do people work in the first place? For most

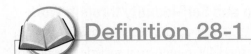

Definition 28-1

Work-Related Definitions

Work (noun)

1. Physical or mental effort or activity directed toward the purposeful production or accomplishment of something: labor. **2.** Employment: job. **3.** The means by which one earns one's livelihood. **4.**a. Something that one is doing, making, or performing, especially as part of one's occupation: a duty or task. b. The amount of effort required or done.

Work (verb)

1. To exert one's efforts for the purpose of doing or making something: labor. **2.** To be employed. **3.** To perform a function or act: operate.

Work (synonyms)

Business, employment, job, occupation. Core meaning: what one does to earn a living. Work, the most general of these terms, can refer to the mere fact of employment or to a specific activity.

Career

1. Chosen profession or occupation. **2.** The general progression of one's life, especially in one's profession.

Job

1. An action that needs to be done: task. **2.** An activity performed regularly for payment, especially a trade, occupation, or profession. **3.** A specific piece of work to be done for a set fee. **4.** A position in which one is employed.

Occupation

Any activity or task with which one occupies oneself, usually specifically the productive activity, service, trade, or craft for which one is regularly paid.

Vocation

A regular occupation or profession, especially one for which an individual is particularly suited or qualified.

people, work is an economic necessity. In earlier times, people traded their wares and their abilities to attain the goods they needed by bartering. Although this practice still exists in some communities, most residents of industrialized countries have distinct employment and pay for their goods and services with money earned at their jobs.

Self-Creation and Self-Identity through Work

We work to finance lives, homes, families, education, and fun. However, especially in industrial societies, we do not have to work from dawn to dusk to earn a living, and we are also not required to enter jobs dictated by our birth or heritage. For the most part, we have choices. We can choose our line of work according to our own values. Occupations are key, not just to being a person, but to being a particular person and to creating and maintaining an identity (Matuska & Christiansen, 2009; Unruh, 2004). The use of one's time during the day provides a sense of purpose and structure, as well as building an identity. We create ourselves through our actions. Although we may define ourselves daily through our work, we may also fulfill other needs. Our values and the meaning of our lives arise from (and are seen in) our work and how we spend our leisure, home, self-care, and family time.

Work can fulfill our primary motivations (needs), as defined by some of the great psychologists and psychiatrists of our time. Work can fulfill the need to find meaning in life as asserted by Frankl's (1984) logotherapy. Work can fulfill the need to find pleasure, on which Freudian psychology is based. Work can also fulfill the need for power or striving for superiority stressed by Adlerian psychology (Stein, 2002). The point is that work can meet a number of needs. For some, work meets multiple needs of financial achievement, a sense of accomplishment and competence, socialization and status within society, pleasure and gratification, a sense of meaning and purpose, self-respect, and an identity. For others, work answers a singular need, leaving them to meet other needs elsewhere in their lives.

Matching Personal Values with Work Requirements

If our work forces us to behave in ways that directly conflict with our view of ourselves, we feel discomfort and are motivated to change our line of work. This is because people try to maintain positive views of themselves and refute or avoid feedback that is negative or disagrees with their ideal self (Alicke & Sedikides, 2009; Swann, Chang-Schneider, & Larsen, 2007). As an example, Enid DuBois worked as a telephone solicitor for a newspaper. Often, the solicitors were told to tell the potential customers that a portion of their money would go to a particular cause to encourage people to subscribe. "After a while, I didn't care. Surely I could have fast-talked people. Just to continually lie to them. But it just wasn't in me. The disgust was growing in me every minute. I would pray and pray to hold on a little longer" (Terkel, 1974, pp. 94–97).

We have seen a change in the desires of the workforce. In addition to the emphasis on pay and security, workers value and expect their work to be psychologically meaningful. They expect to participate in decisions that affect their work lives (Hendrick & Kleiner, 2009). The current, better-educated workforce in industrialized nations seeks challenges, advancement, and a voice in their work lives.

Balance is particularly important to the younger generation entering today's workforce. Occupational balance refers to the integrating of one's work, home, and leisure activities (Anaby, Backman, & Jarus, 2010; Matuska & Christiansen, 2009). Other work-related values of younger persons in today's workforce include independence, autonomy, self-expression, recognition for their work, and continual learning (Chester, 2005; DuToit & Coetzee, 2012). Younger workers need to feel valued and prefer work environments where they are mentored, treated with respect, and allowed to try some of their own ideas (even if they fail occasionally). More than past generations, they need to understand why things need to be done in a particular way, and they need to believe in and value the product, service, or mission they help to deliver (Chester, 2005; DuToit & Coetzee, 2012). They value their social interactions at work as well as their own perception of the importance of the product created by their work (Murphy & Patrick, 2007; Polanyi & Tompa, 2004).

Employers are recognizing the importance of meaningful work, because the psychological well-being of workers is enhanced when they are engaged in work considered meaningful to them (Arnold et al., 2007; Cheney et al., 2008). In fact, meaningful work is associated with personal hardiness and people often derive personal benefits from even difficult work situations, such as military deployments (Bartone et al., 2008).

The importance of occupational involvement and the characteristics of work most valued differ according to one's culture (Kuchinke et al., 2009) and personal values. In fact, the importance of work within a single culture and perhaps within an individual can vary over time. As discussed earlier, some researchers note that work alone is considered as a declining value, replaced by a high value of success in both personal and professional life and valuing leisure, friends and family, especially among the younger generation (Buddeberg-Fischer et al., 2008; Klaghofer et al., 2011). Similarly, people's values change over time, and their view of work can change accordingly. Thus, in rehabilitation, the therapist and the patient/client must explore the perceptions and values of the client, discover the client's occupational identity, and create an appropriate occupational balance intervention (Anaby, Backman, & Jarus, 2010; Matuska & Christiansen, 2008).

INTERRUPTIONS IN THE ABILITY TO WORK

People's ability to work may be interrupted by changes in physical, psychological and behavioral, or socioeconomic status.

Physical Status

Mr. L. worked in a collision repair shop. His brother was fond of saying that he "banged on cars" for a living. The job required him to stand and manually remove the dents from car fenders using specialized tools. He was physically strong because his job demanded it. He wasn't prepared for what happened after he broke his leg. It never seemed to heal correctly. He developed what they called reflex sympathetic dystrophy. The term didn't matter. All he knew was it hurt all the time and he couldn't stand or even sit for long periods. He received workers compensation and wondered if he'd ever work again (D. Rice, personal communication, 2000).

Injury or illness may result in permanent or temporary inability to resume work activities because the worker cannot fulfill the physical, cognitive, or emotional demands of the job. This mismatch between requirements and performance has been traditionally addressed by retraining the individual. The focus was on improving the deficits; thus the therapist worked to diminish individual shortfalls in strength, dexterity, coordination, range of motion, endurance, or cognitive functioning. Whatever interrupted the client's ability to resume normal activities was addressed. More recently, the focus has broadened to include altering or redesigning the job to realign its requirements to the individual's residual abilities through ergonomic intervention.

Not all injuries or illnesses that disrupt the ability to work are the result of a sudden injury or illness. Nontraumatic injuries may also interfere with a person's ability to work. Nontraumatic injuries thought to be related to workplace demands include work-related musculoskeletal disorders (WRMDs). These injuries are typically thought of as transient, although they can result in permanent disability. WRMDs include a wide range of health problems arising from repeated stress to the body encountered in the workplace. These health problems, which may affect the musculoskeletal, nervous, and neurovascular systems, include the various occupation-induced cumulative trauma disorders, cumulative stress injuries, and repetitive motion disorders. Examples include damage to tendons and tendon sheaths and synovial lubrication of the tendon sheaths, bones, muscles, and nerves of the hands, wrists, elbows, shoulders, neck, back, and legs. Specific diagnoses include chronic back pain, carpal tunnel syndrome, de Quervain's disease, epicondylitis (tennis elbow), Raynaud's syndrome (white finger), synovitis, stenosing tenosynovitis crepitans (trigger finger), tendinitis, and tenosynovitis. (For additional information on WRMDs, see Barbe & Barr [2006] and Koh & Takahashi [2011]; for WRMD low back pain, see Pransky, Buchbinder, & Hayden [2010]; for upper extremity injuries, see Roquelaure et al. [2009] and Sommerich, Marras, & Karwowski [2006]).

Traumatic injury, aging, or progressive disability may also alter self-perception and personal identity. When a person loses his or her sense of identity, life becomes less meaningful, which may lead to depression so severe that it can interfere with a person's ability to carry out daily work (Bender & Farvolden, 2008). Thus, it is not always the initial injury that prevents a return to work; the resulting psychological adjustments can also interfere (Iles, Davidson, & Taylor, 2008; Sullivan, Simmonds, & Velly, 2011). For example, recovery expectations and fear avoidance can be predictive of failure to return to work (Iles, Davidson, & Taylor, 2008). Unless both the physical and psychological problems are addressed, the individual may not develop the skills needed to return to work (Snodgrass, 2011).

Cognitive Status

People's cognitive abilities directly influence their ability to do a job and the type of job they can assume. For example, individuals who have had a brain injury (including mild to moderate traumatic brain injuries and strokes) can have difficulties with memory, concentration, sustained attention, decision making, and reasoning and may also experience changes in their sensory processing and/or communication skills. After injury, they may suffer from depression, anxiety, or personality changes. All of these symptoms can interfere with return to work (Bender & Farvolden, 2008; Shames et al., 2007).

Adults who have attention deficit hyperactivity disorder (ADHD) also experience thought and behavior patterns that contribute to reduced work quantity and quality (deGraaf et al., 2008). The association between adult ADHD symptoms and functional impairments is quite high (0.83–0.85) (Mannuzza et al., 2011). A therapist who specializes in working with adults who have ADHD in the workforce can help them recognize their strengths and the types of jobs or job structure that will take advantage of their skills and give them a good chance of success. For example, many adults with ADHD are innovative, energetic risk takers who can do well in jobs that permit multitasking, self-determination of scheduling, physical action, and outsourcing of time-intensive detailed tasks.

Psychological and Behavioral Status

Psychosocial events may interrupt a person's ability to work, either temporarily or permanently. Divorce, severe illness, death of a family member, or change in job status sometimes triggers underlying psychopathology such as a mood or anxiety disorder. The disruption may be due not to underlying psychopathology but to the expression or manifestation of a normal reaction to a difficult situation. Each individual reacts differently to life situations, and adaptation may come more quickly for some than for others. Examples of an individual's inability to meet work requirements include disruptions in the ability to concentrate and follow complex directions, react quickly to emergencies (psychomotor retardation), attend to detail, or handle the pressures and anxieties associated with the work environment. Although there is less information on individuals returning to work after a psychological disorder compared with after physical injuries/illnesses, this is no less a problem than is a physical injury. In fact, it may be more difficult to return to work because of the attitudes and lack of knowledge and empathy of employers and coworkers, in addition to the fears and concerns of the workers themselves.

Depression is predicted to be one of the fastest growing maladies of the 21st century and is often associated with physical injury or loss of work. Although treatment for depression and other psychological and emotional disturbances has vastly improved, there are definite implications for the individual's ability to work (Sullivan, Simmonds, & Velly, 2011). Work seems to mitigate the rate of mental health deterioration, with employment status being more important for men than women (Llena-Nozal, Lindeboom, & Portrait, 2004). In addition, Schene et al. (2007) found the addition of occupational therapy intervention in the treatment of depression accelerated and increased clients' return to work. Finally, adding a work-focus to cognitive behavioral therapy increased full return to work by 65 days and partial return to work by 12 days, compared with cognitive behavioral therapy only, saving approximately estimated at $5,275 U.S. dollars per individual (Lagerveld, et al., 2012).

Even when a physical injury or illness is the primary reason for ceasing work or ones' inability to return to work, there are typically associated psychosocial aspects that need to be addressed. For example, targeting psychosocial risk factors while providing physical rehabilitation increased return to work likelihood after whiplash (75% versus 50%) (Sullivan et al., 2006), and incorporating psychosocial interventions along with physical treatments decreased disability among back pain patients (Sullivan & Adams, 2010).

Socioeconomic Factors for Individuals with Disabilities

One reason that individuals with disabilities may choose not to work is their fear of losing their government-funded health coverage, i.e., Medicare and Medicaid benefits. In the United States and other countries, fewer than 1% of those who receive government disability ever leave that system, and few who receive a temporary disability pension ever return to work (Ahlgren et al., 2005). Many long-term sick-listed individuals (46%) move from vocational rehabilitation to permanent pensions rather than returning to work (Ahlgren et al., 2005). However, in the United States, disabled Americans are guaranteed the ability to keep their government-funded health coverage when they accept a paying job because of the Ticket to Work and Work Incentives Improvement Act of 1999 (http://www.chooseworkttw.net/). The Ticket to Work program underwent a major overhaul in 2008, with new regulations revising employment networks so beneficiaries receive more money as they make progress toward employment. Whereas personal stories of success are noted on the Social Security website (http://www.choosework.net/index.html), criticisms of the program have also been raised, especially regarding the cost of the program. According to one news story (Adams, 2011), beneficiaries doubled under the program between 2007 and 2010, employment network approvals increased by nearly 100%, and costs increased from $3.8 million to $13 million. One might imagine this is good news for the beneficiaries but a concern to the taxpayers who foot the bill.

Aging and age discrimination may also prevent workers from continuing to work or from returning to work following physical or psychological problems or following a downsizing. This problem may become more evident as the proportion of older workers increases, because Americans aged 65 years and older will comprise approximately 20% of the population by 2030 (Centers for Disease Control and Prevention, 2007).

WORK AND AGING

Society is challenged to consider three questions regarding older workers: (1) Can our nation "afford" older individuals who do not work? (2) Do older workers stand in the way of younger workers? (3) Are older workers less productive, slower, harder to supervise, less cognitively aware, and less physically able to do a job?

Today's workforce is multigenerational (Pitt-Catsouphes & Smyer, 2007), as well as older (Gibbs, 2011; Pitt-Catsouphes & Smyer, 2007). Strategic planners in varying industries, governments, and rehabilitation services are investigating plans to counter the impending shortage of workers as the current graying workforce retires, including consultant roles and part-time positions for older workers and mentoring programs to assist older workers with transferring their knowledge to younger workers (Bazley, 2012; Sanders, 2012). In fact, in the United States, those aged 55 years and older have increased their employment by more than 14% between December 2007 and April 2012, perhaps because of the increase in the population of persons in that age range (Rix, 2012). Despite the fact that an increasing number of older people remain in the workforce, barriers stand in the way of their working. There are concerns about the safety of both older workers and their colleagues, their ability to learn and retain information, and the quality of their work, all of which sometimes leads to age discrimination (Johnson, 2007). Also, although older workers are not laid off more often than younger workers, once laid off, it takes older workers longer to find a job compared with their younger counterparts (35 weeks versus 26 weeks) (U.S. Government Accounting Office, 2012). In recent years, job seekers of age 55 years and older comprised 16.2% of the unemployed, accounting for approximately 2 million individuals (Rix, 2012).

Who Are Our Older Workers and Why Do They Work?

The proportion of the population that works decreases with age. However, the most recent data suggest that more older individuals are working than ever (Tables 28-1 and 28-2). The retirement patterns among older workers appear to be changing, with 60% moving to short-duration or part-time employment (bridge jobs) before leaving the labor force entirely (Giandrea, Cahill, & Quinn, 2008). Also, a number of older workers leave and reenter the labor force (approximately 15%) (Cahill, Giandrea, & Quinn, 2011; Maestas, 2010).

Although some older workers choose to work in order to remain active and productive, to do something fun, and for access to money and health care (American Association of Retired Persons [AARP], 2006), others do so out of economic necessity (Rix, 2012). At the beginning of the recession of 2008 in the United States, 826,000 individuals aged 55 years and older reported wanting a job; that number had grown to 1.2 million by June 2009 (Rix, 2012). Those who would like to work but cannot find a job report believing that work is not available, those hiring would consider them too old, they lack necessary training, or they are experiencing discrimination (Rix, 2012).

McLaughlin, Jette, and Connell (2012) found that only 3.3% of those in their study could be considered as "aging successfully" according to the following definitions provided by Rowe and Kahn (1999): (1) being free of disease, risk factors for disease, and disability; (2) having high physical and cognitive functioning; and (3) being socially and productively engaged. They suggested lowering the criteria, such as eliminating active engagement and risk factors for chronic conditions, which can increase the prevalence of those experiencing healthy aging from 3.3% to 35.5%. However, healthy aging is a multidimensional and complex concept, with both cultural and individual influences, and active engagement can be an integral part of one's life satisfaction. If, indeed, active engagement (such as having close

Table 28-1 | **The Aging U.S. Workforce (Selden, 2008)**

Year	Average Working Age
1980	35 years
2008	41 years
2015	One in five workers will be 55 years or older

Impact:
- Fewer available workers
- Need to reduce staff turnover
- Need to keep older workers engaged/employed

Table 28-2 | **Expected Years of Retirement for Men**

Country	Years of Retirement
France	24
Italy	21.7
Spain	20.9
Germany	19.8
United States	17.6

Data from National Institutes of Health, National Institute on Aging. (2011). Global health and aging. Retrieved August 8, 2012 from http://www.nia.nih.gov/research/publication/global-health-and-aging.

personal relationships or pursuing activities of meaning) is an important component of healthy aging, then continuing to work may lead to greater satisfaction with life and perhaps even a longer life of higher quality. In fact, Hao (2008) found that productive activities, in the form of full-time and low-level volunteering, had protective effects against decreases in self-reported psychological well-being.

Paid Employment, Volunteer Work, and Occupation of Time

It is intuitive to expect that an individual's occupational identity and the meeting of his or her needs and values (mentioned earlier) can be met through paid employment, volunteer work, or meaningful activities that occupy time, but few researchers have investigated this concept. However, both Hao (2008) and Schwingel (2009) found that seniors who work or volunteer maintain a higher (and healthier) state of mental health compared with those who do not work or volunteer. Those who continued to work or volunteer demonstrated better cognitive performance, fewer symptoms of depression, and higher self-satisfaction ratings than those who neither worked nor volunteered (Schwingel, 2009).

WORK AND OCCUPATIONAL THERAPY

Adolph Meyer (1922) advocated a "freer conception of work, a concept of free and pleasant and profitable occupation including recreation and any form of helpful enjoyment as the leading principle." He said the "whole of human organization has its shape in a kind of rhythm," and through structured use of time, people could achieve well-being (pp. 1–2). By assisting the client to achieve a balanced lifestyle in work, play, rest, and sleep, early occupational therapists helped clients achieve a sense of homeostasis and health. Meyer broadly defined the term *occupation* as purposeful activity within the full spectrum of a person's life.

Occupational therapy, based on the concept of returning the injured worker to work, was founded on the belief that merely eliminating the disease or providing immediate treatment for traumatic injury was insufficient for full recovery and ability to assume life roles. Instead, a client should be guided through a strengthening and training process, both physically and mentally, to prepare him or her to resume occupational status in society (Committee on Installations and Advice, 1928; Rice, 2007). Therapists used "crafts" in their treatment. What were once called crafts are today considered jobs. The term *craft* included activities such as carpentry, metal work, and bookbinding, all of which were full-time vocations. Initially, a wide variety of crafts or jobs were used in occupational therapy clinics. Occupational therapists believed, however, that carefully chosen occupation-based activities resulted in a transfer of training to almost any occupation the recovered client chose to pursue. This is opposite the current trend of work hardening, which simulates specific job tasks that will be required of the client upon return to work. The latter certainly has greater face validity, but to date, no published outcome research clearly supports one approach as superior to the other. Occupational therapy as a treatment intervention has been shown to be effective in assisting with a successful return to work process, but the components of the therapeutic programs vary, which makes comparisons difficult (Désiron et al., 2011).

Occupational Therapists' Unique Contributions

Occupational therapists, with their solid background in the full spectrum of human performance (physiological, biomechanical, psychosocial, and behavioral), are uniquely qualified to help clients return to work. A fundamental goal of occupational therapy is to facilitate the client's highest level of functional status in all occupations and contexts of life, including physical, emotional, social, cognitive, and communicative dimensions. Occupational therapists recognize that successful return to work is likely to depend on adequate function in many aspects of life, not solely task performance at a work site. Occupational therapists apply their knowledge of human performance and the human mind to determine whether the impediments to returning to work are physical, psychosocial, or both and to integrate appropriate interventions.

The application of the full spectrum of human performance elucidates the unique contributions of occupational therapists in returning the injured worker to the workforce. This holistic approach is instrumental in a successful return to work process (Désiron et al., 2011). Indeed, a systems approach integrating aspects of biomedical, psychosocial, and economic models may be the most effective (Schultz et al., 2007).

Burwash Model

There are a number of models depicting the return to work process (Schultz et al., 2007), but few that focus specifically on occupational therapy. However, one overarching model is shown in Figure 28-1. A more specific model, which focuses on occupational therapy intervention, is presented by Burwash (1999) and is shown in Figure 28-2 and further described in Table 28-3. Although this is an older model, it is clear, concise, and easy for therapists and for clients to understand. Returning to work is seen as one of the triangles representing concerns of clients. To facilitate a return to work, however, the therapist may be involved in each of the eight areas. For example, the client may be leaving one line of work because of disease or disability and need to reevaluate his or her values to explore and choose another career. While building the requisite physical and cognitive skills for the chosen job or career field, the client may also need to develop skills in searching for work along with the work habits needed to sustain a successful career.

The therapist must understand the client's value of work and self-perception as related to work (such as self-definition and self-esteem), so as to design the rehabilitation process and identify short-term goals and techniques to motivate the client. This client-centered approach to evaluation and treatment involves joint identification of goals and priorities by the therapist and the client. For example, therapists can help clients ascertain whether they want their work to be a job rather than a career (see Definition 28-1) by examining where they fulfill their social, emotional, and achievement needs.

THE RETURN-TO-WORK PROCESS

Returning to work entails three main procedures: evaluation, intervention, and reevaluation.

Functional Work Assessments

Functional work assessments include evaluation of both the individual client and the work requirements the client will encounter. Individual evaluations incorporate the standard occupational therapy assessment, a delineation of the conditions preventing the client from returning to work, and a functional capacity evaluation (FCE). The evaluation of the work requirements is often referred to as a functional job analysis, or simply job analysis.

Job Analysis

A job analysis is a systematic evaluation of the job that identifies its physical, cognitive, social, and psychological requirements. Conducting a job analysis entails going to the job site, observing workers performing their tasks, measuring equipment and equipment placement, and

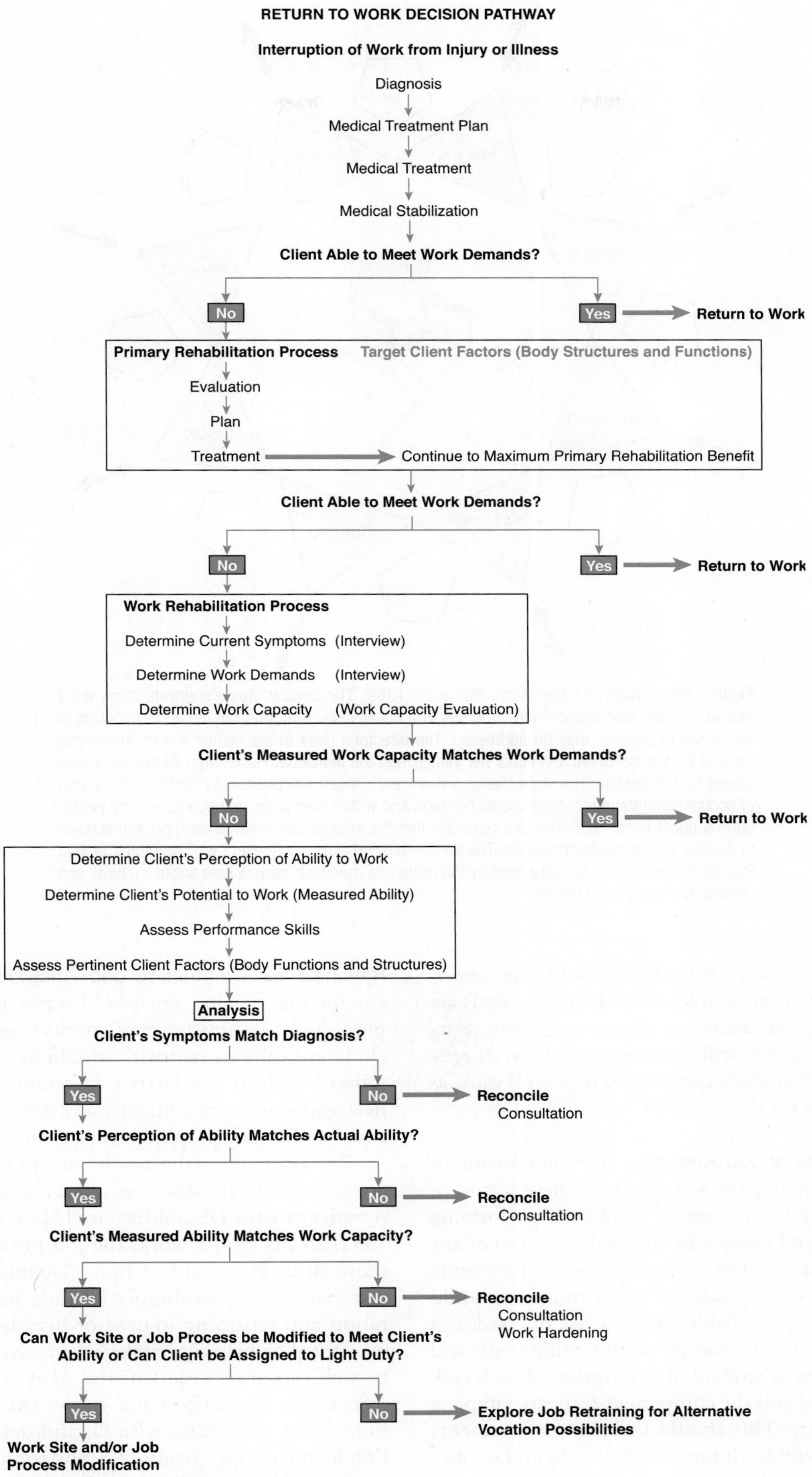

RETURN TO WORK DECISION PATHWAY

Interruption of Work from Injury or Illness

Diagnosis

Medical Treatment Plan

Medical Treatment

Medical Stabilization

Client Able to Meet Work Demands?

No → **Primary Rehabilitation Process**   Target Client Factors (Body Structures and Functions)

Yes → **Return to Work**

Evaluation

Plan

Treatment ⟶ Continue to Maximum Primary Rehabilitation Benefit

Client Able to Meet Work Demands?

No → **Work Rehabilitation Process**

Yes → **Return to Work**

Determine Current Symptoms (Interview)

Determine Work Demands   (Interview)

Determine Work Capacity   (Work Capacity Evaluation)

Client's Measured Work Capacity Matches Work Demands?

No

Yes → **Return to Work**

Determine Client's Perception of Ability to Work

Determine Client's Potential to Work (Measured Ability)

Assess Performance Skills

Assess Pertinent Client Factors (Body Functions and Structures)

Analysis

Client's Symptoms Match Diagnosis?

Yes

No → **Reconcile**
Consultation

Client's Perception of Ability Matches Actual Ability?

Yes

No → **Reconcile**
Consultation

Client's Measured Ability Matches Work Capacity?

Yes

No → **Reconcile**
Consultation
Work Hardening

Can Work Site or Job Process be Modified to Meet Client's Ability or Can Client be Assigned to Light Duty?

Yes

No → **Explore Job Retraining for Alternative Vocation Possibilities**

Work Site and/or Job Process Modification

Figure 28-1 Return-to-duty decision pathway.

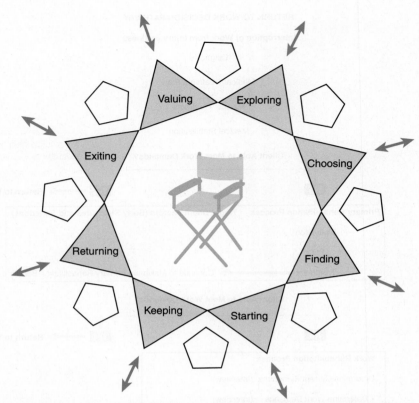

Figure 28-2 Work Practice Model (Burwash, 1999). The circular shape suggests many entry and exit points; intervention may progress in a linear fashion around the circle; or only one or two areas of concern may be addressed. The director's chair in the center is a reminder that focus is on the individual and his or her values, and the individual, rather than diagnosis or age, should be the director. The eight triangles represent concerns expressed by clients and are part of occupational therapy's professional heritage and within therapists' competencies. The pentagons suggest artists' palettes as a reminder that the intervention requires both art and science in dealing with productivity issues. The double-headed arrows represent environmental factors that influence and can be influenced by the client and therapist; they include social, cultural, and political factors, among others.

interviewing those who perform the job and their supervisors. Some of the tools employed in the job analysis are video cameras, tape measures, scales, goniometers, stopwatches, dynamometers, still cameras, and strain gauges. The results of a job analysis can be used in several ways, as seen in Procedures for Practice 28-1.

Basic Components of Job Analysis. The components of any job analysis include the job title, basic description or objectives of the job, number of employees performing the job, the work and break schedule, a description of any rotation or enrichment program, and output requirements for the workers. A description of the environment should include temperature, available space, a list of fixed and movable equipment, personal protective equipment, and a sketch of the area. A sequential description of each task (essential function) and the component steps to complete it are also necessary. This should include measurements such as heights, weights, durations, distances, and so on.

Rationale for Conducting Job Analysis. The reason for conducting the job analysis dictates its questions and procedures. The purposes of conducting a job analysis include returning a person with a disability to work, identifying musculoskeletal risk factors, matching a rehabilitated or new worker with job demands, and developing assessments such as FCEs and preplacement screening tests.

For example, if the results are to be used to return an individual classified as disabled according to the Americans with Disabilities Act (ADA) (Federal Register, 1991) to his or her work, the job must be described in terms of its essential functions (Definition 28-2). Therapists whose responsibilities include industrial rehabilitation and returning injured or disabled workers to the workforce or helping employers to advertise jobs should be well versed in Title I of the ADA. Therapists should refer to the regulations and guides (ADA Title I Regulations, 1991; Americans with Disabilities Act, 1990; Equal Employment Opportunity Commission, 1992). The U.S.

Table 28-3   **Examples Using the Burwash Model (1999)**

Model Segment	Client Concerns	Therapist Resources: Assessment Tools, Techniques, and Programs	Environmental Considerations
Valuing	"Why work?" "How does work fit into my life?" "What are my personal values and what types of work fit?" "Why am I not happy in this work?" "Is working worth it?"	Work Values Inventory, Life Roles Inventory, work values auction, a spirituality of work questionnaire, Occupational Performance History Interview	Family and social group attitudes toward work; economic considerations for persons on disability pensions; religious beliefs about work; work and gender issues
Exploring	"I don't know what I'm physically capable of." "Are there any occupations that match my interests?" "What am I good at?"	Functional Capacity Evaluation, Self-Directed Search, work samples, computerized career exploration systems	Role definition of occupational therapy versus other team members (career counselors, vocational rehabilitation counselor, or teachers); family expectations
Keeping	"How is this health problem going to affect my work?" "I hurt so much after a day at work!" "I'm about to take stress leave; all of these changes are really getting to me." "I can't figure out how to get ahead at work; I'm really feeling stuck."	Ergonomic interventions, stress management and relaxation techniques, energy conservation and work simplification techniques, goal setting, injury prevention and health promotion programs, advocacy	Family and friends' expectations; public laws on disability and workplace ergonomic standards; employer, coworker, and public attitudes toward persons with disabilities; client's support system; funding issues; job market; physical accessibility; access to transportation
Returning	"Will I be able to work again?" "How do I prevent reinjury?" "How do I deal with coworkers' comments about my illness?" "If I'm hurting at work, how do I cope with the pain?"	Work Environment Impact Scale, Worker Role Interview, graduated return-to-work programs, work hardening and chronic pain programs, assertiveness skills, Loma Linda Activity Sort, other resources as noted in the Exploring row above	Laws on injured workers and employers' responsibilities to them, job market, funding for retraining, family responsibilities, possible financial settlements, advice from lawyers and others, employer–employee relations

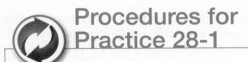

Procedures for Practice 28-1

Ways to Use Job Analysis Data

- Develop FCE
- Match injured workers' capabilities to job task requirements
- Place workers on light duty
- Return previously injured workers to work
- Identify risk factors associated with work-related musculoskeletal disorders
- Develop preplacement, postjob offer screenings which enable companies to place new hires in positions that minimize potential future injuries
- Write job description (possibly using ADA terminology)
- Describe and advertise jobs

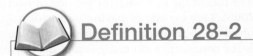

Definition 28-2

Essential Functions

Fundamental, Not Marginal, Job Duties

Some considerations in determining whether a function is essential include

- whether the position exists to perform that function
- the number of other employees available to perform the function or among whom the function can be distributed
- the degree of expertise required
- whether past and/or present employees in the job have performed the function
- the time spent performing the function
- the consequences of not performing the function

Reasonable Accommodations

Modifications of the work environment include job restructuring and providing adaptive or adaptable equipment and similar modifications to enable equal opportunities for employment by individuals with disabilities.

government maintains an excellent website, with guidance, suggestions, and publications available and updated regularly (http://www.ada.gov/). Another useful website is http://www.disabilityrightsca.org/pubs/506801.htm).

If the reason for performing the job analysis is to identify risk factors that may predispose a person to musculoskeletal disorders, listing the essential functions is not compulsory. A job analysis primarily geared to injury prevention, such as WRMDs, should include descriptions of observed risk factors, such as repetitive motions, force, static postures, awkward postures, mechanical compressions, vibration, and the acceleration and velocity of dynamic motions, noted for each body part and quantified. For example, the duration of static hold using a pinch grip is noted in seconds. Literature on job analysis related to injury prevention can be found in several excellent sources (Brannick, Levine, & Morgeson, 2007; Cronin et al., 2011; Lysaght & Shaw, 2011; Singh, 2008).

For matching workers' capabilities with the job requirements, placing workers on light duty, or returning previously injured workers to work, tasks (i.e., essential functions) are broken into their component steps and quantitatively described in enough detail to permit them to be matched with the worker's residual capabilities (Procedures for Practice 28-2). The therapist who only occasionally participates in returning injured workers to the workforce may prepare a unique job analysis for each client using various tools (Brannick, Levine, & Morgeson, 2007), whereas those who work full time in industrial rehabilitation generally keep a file of job descriptions that lets them quickly determine whether a client can return by comparing the results of the FCE with the job description (Isernhagen, 2006). One benefit of having occupational therapists involved in job analysis is the ability to combine these purposes for conducting job analysis and developing a comprehensive database for an industry's use.

Use of Job Analysis in Developing and Selecting a Functional Capacity Evaluation. A job analysis should be conducted *prior to development or selection of an FCE.* An FCE consists of two parts: a general evaluation of physical abilities and a job-specific evaluation. Before one can decide whether to use solely the general evaluation versus the job-specific evaluation, the therapist must know whether the client intends to return to a specific job or type of job. If so, the information from the job analysis can be used to develop one of two types of FCE using criterion-referenced tasks. The first uses task components, whereas the second uses work simulations (both discussed later in the chapter). In both cases, the initial information is gathered during the job analysis.

Predicting Work Performance. Although general tasks such as lifting (Gouttebarge et al., 2009) or general mental ability (Lang et al., 2010) can be predictive of return to work, the fidelity of the prediction is enhanced when multiple constructs

are used (Lang et al., 2010). During a well-constructed job analysis, job tasks are broken into component parts, often by construct. (An example of component tests and a work simulation can be seen in Procedures for Practice 28-3.) Successful predictions also tend to use multiple assessment techniques, such as interviews with ratings of key tasks for frequency, duration, and difficulty; direct observation; videotaping; measurements of masses moved and forces exerted; and identification of pace and frequency.

Job Analysis Conclusion. The ability to conduct a thorough job analysis is an essential skill for an occupational therapist working in an industrial setting. In other practice settings, the prudent therapist conducts a similarly comprehensive analysis of the job of a homemaker, athlete, or child. The instruction in task analysis (activity analysis) received during entry-level training for occupational therapy provides an excellent basis for building expertise in job analysis. However, job analysis for guidance in the cognitive, psychological, and social requirements of work is neither well-defined nor illustrated by a large number of case studies.

One important concept is that, although the job analysis is part of the evaluation, the results are used to develop the treatment intervention and establish the end goals. In traditional occupational therapy, the treatment intervention and goals are based solely on the evaluation of the client and his or her desires, not on evaluation of the work site and the job demands.

Functional Capacity Evaluations

A variety of assessments are available for evaluating work performance, with the majority coming under the classification of an FCE. An FCE is a systematic process designed to assess a client's physical capacities and functional abilities. Identification of an individual's capabilities also reveals his or her limitations. The FCE uses information available from traditional occupational therapy and medical evaluations along with performance-based evaluations.

The information gained from an FCE can be used in a number of ways: (1) to match the individual's residual capacities with the demands of a specific job as a basis for establishing work or work site modifications or accommodations, (2) as evidence in the determination of disability or compensation status, and (3) as a baseline for noting the physical capabilities of new employees. FCEs can be used in a variety of circumstances, including in industrial settings for preemployment and postoffer screenings, in clinical settings for setting goal and treatment regimens, and for determining a worker's ability to resume his or her job duties. Although an FCE can be used in determining whether a claimant is eligible for Social Security disability benefits, the results of an FCE are based on many factors including the therapists' expertise and the clients'

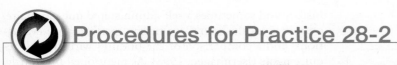

Procedures for Practice 28-2

Matching Job Analysis with Functional Capacity Evaluation

Job Title: Meat Grinder (ground beef, chicken, pork, turkey)

Job Analysis

Tasks	Physical Requirements
1. Load grinder	Standing, walking, climbing stairs, carrying, lifting, stooping, handling, reaching, grasping
2. Grind and load meat tubs	

Steps for Task 1	Physical Requirements for Task 1
Remove top from tub of meat	Lift 0.5 pound
Place top of tub to the side	Lift, hold, turn, and place 0.5 pound
Lift tub from stack	Lift 70 pounds
Carry tub up stairs	Carry 70 pounds 5 feet, climb three stairs
Empty meat from tub into grinder	Lift 70 pounds to height of 4.5 feet
Walk down stairs	Climb down three stairs carrying empty tub, 1.5 pounds
Place empty tub on stack	Walk 3 feet behind grinder, stack tub
Steps for Task 2	**Physical Requirements for Task 2**
Retrieve empty tub	Walk 6 feet, lift weight 1.5 pounds
Place tub beneath grinder spigot	Stoop, place 1.5 pounds beneath spigot
Turn on grinder	Turn handle, 0.8-pound resistance
Visually supervise grinding	Stand
Guide beef from spigot	Use handle of large metal spoon
Spread beef in tub	Use handle of large metal spoon
Turn off grinder	Turn handle, 0.8 pound resistance
Lift tub	Lift five full tubs, 28 pounds each
Carry tub(s) either up the stairs to reload grinder (repeat steps 4–6 for task 1) or to packaging area	See steps 4–6 Carry five tubs at 28 pounds each a distance of 15 feet

Functional Capacity Evaluation Results	FCE Results Match Job Requirements
No limitations standing, walking, climbing, and descending stairs	Yes
Vision: 20/20 with glasses	Yes
Upper extremity reach and manual dexterity within normal limits as measured by Purdue pegboard	Yes
Grasp: 50 pounds	Yes
Lifts	
Single lift of 29 kg to height of 4 feet	Yes
Repetitive lift to height of 4 feet	Yes
One lift of 20 kg every 8 minutes	Yes

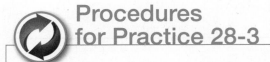

Procedures for Practice 28-3

Example of Component Tests and Work Simulation for Military Medic Task: Stretcher Carrying

Job Title: Military Medic

Task

Carrying stretcher containing a wounded soldier to and from medical transport vehicles as part of a two-person team

Task Description

Maximal height a stretcher must be lifted is 135 cm, based on ground and air ambulance loading platform heights. Literature review revealed weight of 50th percentile male U.S. Army soldier as 84.2 kg (Paquette, Gordon, & Brandtmiller, 2009). The stretcher weighs 6.8 kg. When unloading air ambulances, patients must be carried to a ground ambulance, typically approximately 50 m.

Task Components for Functional Capacity Evaluation

1. Lift and lower a box approximately 91 kg to and from a 135-cm height.
2. Perform isometric grip strength test.
3. Run 1 mile in 10 minutes or perform aerobic treadmill testing.
4. Carry handheld weights approximately 35.5 kg for 50 m.

Work Simulation for Functional Capacity Evaluation

Soldier walks or runs 50 m on treadmill carrying a stretcher holding an 88.6-kg mannequin. Soldier dismounts treadmill and walks or runs 5 m to a weight stack machine adjacent to treadmill and lifts weight equal to the patient's load to 135 cm to simulate loading patient into ground or air ambulance. Soldier gets back on treadmill and walks or runs 50 m to retrieve next patient. Treadmill speed is self-paced using toggle switch attached to stretcher handle.

motivation and perceptions (Chen, 2007). FCEs based on the specific job requirements themselves may be more advantageous for determining current capabilities and future work sustainment, because FCEs with predetermined lifts (not related to the specific job) generally have low to moderate predictive ability (Gouttebarge et al., 2009). For example, some FCEs use a lift from ground level to 4 feet, with no twisting, to determine lifting ability, but the job may require a lift from a height of 2 feet, a partial turn, with placement at 4 feet. The closer the evaluation can replicate the task, the more accurate the assessment.

Most FCEs include a review of the client's medical record, an interview that includes a work and educational history and sometimes a self-administered questionnaire, a basic musculoskeletal evaluation, performance evaluations, and a comparison of the findings with the job requirements (Isernhagen, 1995). As mentioned previously, the two performance categories are a general evaluation of physical abilities and a set of job-specific evaluations. Some therapists include psychosocial aspects; however, this remains more of an exception than the rule unless the individual has specific mental health or neurological concerns. Both the psychosocial and cognitive aspects of FCEs are ripe for exploration, implementation, and research.

General Evaluation of Physical and Cognitive Abilities. Physical and cognitive abilities are evaluated to examine basic functional abilities thought to be common to a number of jobs. The evaluation is conducted to give baseline information and is a special concern when the job to which the individual will return is unknown. The general evaluation of physical abilities may include measures of flexibility, strength, balance, coordination, cardiovascular condition, and body mechanics. It should also include the individual's ability to sit, stand, walk, lift, carry, bend, squat, crawl, climb, reach, stoop, and kneel and any limitations with those activities. WRMDs have become prevalent; therefore, the individual's ability to do particular types of repetitive motions should also be noted. Documentation should specify weight limits, duration of activity tolerance, unambiguous environmental restrictions, and the exact side effects of medications. Subjective findings, such as reported degree and frequency of pain, along with any observations (grimacing), should be noted.

Job-Specific Evaluations. The second part of an FCE is job specific. This means that specific work tasks are designed to simulate the critical tasks associated with a specific job or set of jobs (described previously in the Job Analysis section as either task components or simulations). For example, the International Association of Fire Fighters uses a two-part system, the "Wellness/Fitness Initiative" and a "Candidate Physical Ability Test Program." The former uses peer fitness trainers to enhance cardiovascular respiratory fitness, muscular endurance, and flexibility. The latter is a preemployment test composed of job-specific tasks, including a stair climb, ladder raise and extension, hose drag, equipment carry, forcible entry, search (searching for victims while crawling through dark spaces), rescue drag, and a ceiling pull (to simulate locating fire and checking for fire extension) (International Association of Fire Fighters, 2012).

Identifying Task Components. Task component testing means that the most difficult and important functions of the job are identified, and an evaluation or treatment plan is developed using the task components. An example of selecting the most difficult essential task is when a person must lift tools weighing 10 pounds and a 50-pound toolbox. The criterion task includes the more difficult of the two tasks on the assumption that a worker who can accomplish the more difficult task is also competent for the lesser one. The criterion tasks, in the form of task components or work simulations, are used because they are believed to predict job performance. It is assumed that testing applicants on single aspects of job performance that are critical to job success is a valid approach to determining work performance, as the content requirements are used. Often, several criterion referenced tasks are used in the assessment. For example, an assembly job might require perceptual-motor performance for fitting pieces together, balance as one reaches for parts, and upper body strength to tighten components; therefore validated assessments of perceptual-motor abilities, balance, and grip strength might be used as criterion tasks. An example of the development of criterion-referenced tasks using both the task component and work simulation techniques can be seen in Procedures for Practice 28-3.

Work Simulations. Work simulations differ from task components in that they replicate essential series of tasks required on a job. For example, a firefighter's task of removing a hose, attaching it to a nozzle, and holding the hose during spraying is one task simulation. The same task series analyzed according to its task components might include only two portions: lifting an item that weighs the same as the hose and pushing a sled whose weight equals the amount of hose pressure. Work simulations frequently combine multiple constructs, such as strength, balance, and agility, and they have greater face validity.

Psychosocial Behaviors. Some evaluations include the individual's psychosocial behaviors as they apply to work habits and motivation; however, this is not consistently part of the process. This part of the FCE should describe the client's limitations in comprehension, recall, and ability to follow instructions. Other psychosocial issues, such as the ability to handle work pressures, respond to supervision, and relate to coworkers or customers, should also be noted.

Many FCEs use an evaluation called the detection of sincerity of effort, which is said to be an indication of a client's motivation to perform optimally during an FCE. Although it is suspected that a client who is not sincere will have a different recovery pattern and perhaps even receive unwarranted disability payments, the ability to detect insincerity of effort remains elusive. In a review on assessment of effort, response bias, and malingering, neuropsychologists offered little to uphold such claims and instead encouraged continued research on the topic, admonishing researchers to adhere to recommended procedures and statistical evaluations (Heilbronner et al., 2010).

Because alterations in mood and affect commonly coexist with and exacerbate physical problems, these issues should be included in the assessment. A brief screening tool can be used in conjunction with clinical observations to determine the influence of any psychosocial problems.

The Generalized Contentment Scale is a quick 25-item paper and pencil measure of nonpsychotic depression that is useful in determining the extent of mood alterations associated with loss of the work role (Hudson, 1982). Other mood scales are also available (Heuchert & McNair, 2012), and therapists should select the appropriate scale for the client and the circumstances. If significant test results are obtained, assistance from psychological services may be indicated. Therapists should select the type of assessment(s) that best suit the client and the situation, for example targeting anxiety, depression, general health attitudes, etc.

Selecting a Functional Capacity Evaluation. More than 55 FCEs are available, and selection of an appropriate one can be difficult. They differ in the physical and psychological factors they assess and the way the measures are administered. They also differ in the training required for competency in administration and interpretation. Some use a battery of tests that may or may not be based on a specific task analysis of the job in question. Such a battery may include strength, flexibility, and endurance tests. Others use actual simulations of the tasks required of the job. Although test–retest reliability can be high (Brouwer et al., 2003; Gibson et al., 2010), few FCEs have undergone rigorous examination to determine whether the evaluation predicts actual job performance (Chen, 2007).

Cheng and Cheng (2011) found that job-specific FCEs demonstrated superior predictive value, when used with specific injuries, such as distal radius fractures, than when used with less specific injuries. They also found that job-specific FCEs were of benefit in evaluating the employment status of individuals with nonspecific, chronic low back pain (Cheng & Cheng, 2010).

The Isernhagen work system was the only FCE found showing good predictive validity in the systematic review by Gouttebarge et al. (2004) of the four most used FCEs: the Blankenship system, Ergos work simulator, Ergo-Kit, and the Isernhagen work system. Although some systems appear to show promise (Lechner, Page, & Sheffield, 2008), others fall short of expectations (Gouttebarge et al., 2009). Although it may seem easy to select an FCE based on the availability of workshops and related products, the decision-making process should be performed carefully, with a thorough knowledge of the current research literature.

Payment

In general, functional capacity assessments and work hardening are paid for by worker's compensation insurance, individual insurance, or managed care plans, state or local agencies, or private pay (American Occupational Therapy Association [AOTA], 2012). In general, such assessments and training must be medically necessary and meet certain medical criteria, delineated by insurance company policy statements. Precertification of the service and fee verification are advised (AOTA, 2012).

Functional Work Assessments Conclusion

Knowledge of the two primary means of assessment in industrial rehabilitation, job analysis and functional capacity assessment, sets the stage for intervention. Individual clients' goals, work site design alterations, and bringing the capabilities of the worker closer into alignment with the demands of the job are all built on a well-performed set of assessments. The practitioner must integrate into the intervention process the detail the assessments provide, and the results of the FCE should be used to indicate a client's potential to work. This information should be clearly communicated to the employer and to the client. The bottom line is this: The best "evaluation" is one that is holistic; it examines the work, the work environment, and the workers needs, interests, desires (motivations), behaviors (habits and lifestyle), and personal characteristics. Additional research is needed to demonstrate the success of FCEs in returning injured workers to work, and predicting their success. At this time, keeping one's own records about the predictive success (or failure) of FCE interventions may be the best method to demonstrate potential effectiveness to clients.

Intervention

Intervention that is specific for returning the individual to the workforce builds on traditional occupational therapy intervention, taking it a few steps further into the daily work requirements of the client. Throughout intervention, the therapist should maintain communication with the client's work supervisor and iteratively determine the potential for work site modification to match the levels of performance being discovered during the evaluation. These modifications may continue throughout the process, permitting the client to return to a work setting much earlier and encouraging personal identification as a contributing, competent worker.

Work Conditioning

Work conditioning generally follows acute care and precedes work hardening. Like traditional occupational therapy intervention, work conditioning focuses on remediation of underlying physical or cognitive deficits to improve function. The difference between traditional rehabilitation and work conditioning is that the intervention is focused on functional requirements of a job or employment setting rather than on life skills required at home or for recreational activities. Restoration of flexibility, strength, coordination, and endurance may be addressed. Work conditioning should increase physical abilities, engineer successful performance, and provide realistic feedback regarding the client's capabilities (Fig. 28-3). The client's day may include a regimen of warm-up exercises tailored to the activities planned for the day, conditioning exercises based on job requirements, and job-related tasks using work samples that replicate essential task components of a job. A program

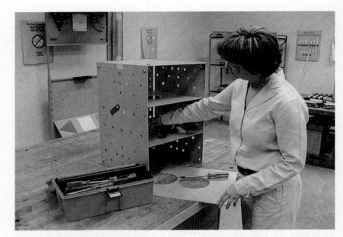

Figure 28-3 Work conditioning using a simulated work task. This is an initial simulation, because the requirements for bending and stooping have not yet been added.

may begin with sessions of an hour or two and progress as the client-worker's condition improves to 8 hours per day.

Work Hardening

Work hardening is a multidisciplinary structured treatment designed to maximize a client's ability to return to employment. Work hardening includes all aspects required for the client to return to full employment function, such as psychosocial, communication, physical, and vocational needs. Although general physical abilities are addressed in work conditioning, work hardening is aimed more specifically at a particular job or classification of jobs and therefore tends to involve work simulation. Considerations added during work hardening include productivity (speed, accuracy, and efficiency), safety (ability to adhere to safety principles and use of safety equipment and algorithms), physical tolerances for specific tasks (endurance and ability to carry out the repetitive task requirements), organizational skills, and decision making. Work hardening differs from work conditioning in the following ways: use of real or simulated work activities in a graded fashion, building to work over periods comparable with those in actual work settings, the full spectrum of work-related intervention, and involvement of a multidisciplinary approach (Isernhagen, 1988). Disciplines included in work-hardening programs can include occupational and physical therapy, psychology, vocational rehabilitation, social work, and social services. Other professionals participate full time or as needed including drug and alcohol counselors, nutritionists, and educators (special education or educational evaluators).

Work hardening environments should replicate the workplace as closely as possible. Sufficient space is needed for both traditional equipment for work conditioning and specialized equipment that may be brought from a job site. Also, the behaviors and interactions required of the clients should replicate a work setting, such as arriving and leaving on a set schedule, working with fixed breaks, having supervisors who give positive and negative feedback on performance, performance standards, and so on. Returning a client to a part-time or full-time light-duty assignment during rehabilitation may help the client feel like part of the team. It may also assist employers by building their confidence in the process and by letting them observe firsthand the capabilities of the client-worker.

All involved parties should be kept informed of the process. This includes employers, supervisors, insurance representatives, occupational health nurses, and the physician.

Reevaluation of the Client and Program Evaluation

Two types of intertwined evaluations should be conducted. Individual clients should be reevaluated, and the program as a whole should be evaluated. Monitoring clients' progress and annotating whether they have achieved functional goals should occur as in traditional occupational therapy during clinic-based treatment. Follow-up evaluations with the client and the client's supervisor are suggested so that, in case of a problem, the therapist can intervene before reinjury or exacerbation of the injury occurs. In addition, it is important to combine this information (having removed individual identifiers) with that of other clients to determine whether overall program goals are being met. It is important to know whether the program is meeting the needs of individual clients as well as those of the referral sources (employers). Tracking information such as the rate of successful return to work, the length of limited-duty time, and the subjective responses of past clients and their supervisors enables the therapist to improve the program. This information is important for showing the cost-benefit value of the services and should be available if reimbursement questions arise. The same information can be used in marketing strategies.

A CLINICAL IMPLEMENTATION OF THE RETURN-TO-WORK PROCESS

This chapter contains basic information about work-related assessment, intervention through work conditioning and work hardening, and reevaluation of both the individual and the program, along with background information on work motivation, interruption of work, and ways occupational therapists can intervene. Still, the application of this knowledge can be confusing without a framework. Therefore, this section describes a decision pathway and an example of an FCE (Fig. 28-4). The interventions identified in this decision pathway are closely aligned with the interventions articulated in the second edition of the Occupational Therapy Practice Framework: Domain and Process (American Occupational Therapy Association, 2008). These interventions are therapeutic use of self, education, consultation, and therapeutic use of occupations (occupation-based activity).

These interventions are broad based, and it is probably beyond the scope of this chapter to present a meaningful discussion of their merits or limitations.

The return-to-work decision pathway shown in Figure 28-1 presents work rehabilitation processes in the larger context of injury, medical management, and acute rehabilitation. Because cost containment is a paramount issue in any health care organization, the decision pathway encourages a logical process to return the client to the workforce in a time-efficient manner. The decision pathway begins with an interruption of the work process, includes medical and rehabilitative intervention, incorporates the return-to-work process of evaluation and intervention, and offers several junctures at which the client may return to work.

The FCE in Figure 28-4 is composed of measures that are routinely available in most clinical settings (Resources 28-1). Additional tests can be added as available and desired. The many available off-the-shelf FCEs all have some limitations as well as merits, and therapists should be broad minded in their selection of tools for the FCE. It may be most efficacious for therapists first to develop an understanding of the return-to-work evaluation and intervention process and then to develop a structured evaluation system composed of available components that are specific to individual patients and the specific environmental context to which they must return.

The first page of information seen on the FCE contains the evaluation of the findings, an explanation of the discrepancies between the job requirements and work performance, and recommendations. This arrangement seems to put the end (the results) at the beginning before permitting the reader to follow and understand the evaluative process. The format is designed so the "bottom line" is immediately available for the employer and/or client to read. Background information in the form of the evaluative process is then provided as substantiation of the findings. Each section of the decision pathway and FCE is explained in the next section. Also refer to the Case Example, which further demonstrates the use of the FCE.

Medical Management and Acute Rehabilitation

The return-to-work process begins as soon as a patient enters the medical system for treatment. Medical management concerns the use of medical and surgical treatment to control and remedy acute medical problems that have interrupted the work role. Acute rehabilitation naturally follows medical management when medical problems and their treatments have caused physical debilitation, muscle weakness, impaired joint motion, decreased flexibility and/or coordination, or other limitations. Acute rehabilitation for physical injuries can involve the use of physical agents,

(text continued on page 895)

Work Capacity Evaluation

Occupational Therapy Service

Note: Patient has been medically evaluated and cleared for Functional/Work Capacity

Evaluation by _____, MD

—Evaluation completed by _____(occupational therapist)

Client Name _____ Date _____

Assessment of Evaluation Findings

____**Incomplete and/or invalid evaluation**

☐ Insufficient information to determine physical and/or work capacity

☐ Client refused to participate or complete evaluation process

☐ Client's symptoms prevented active participation in evaluation process

____**Successful demonstration of work performance**

Department of Labor Physical Demands of Work Level

Job Requirement	Client's Demonstrated Performance
☐ **Less than Sedentary**—Infrequent lifting <2 pounds, minimal walking, no carrying	☐
☐ **Sedentary**—Infrequent lifting of 10 pounds or less, no sustained walking or carrying	☐
☐ **Sedentary-Light**—Infrequent lifting of 15 pounds; frequent lifting of 10 pounds or less; intermittent, self-paced, no-load walking	☐
☐ **Light**—Infrequent lifting of 20 pounds; frequent lifting of 10 pounds or less no-grade, slow-speed, 10-pound load carry/walking	☐
☐ **Light-Medium**—Infrequent lifting of 35 pounds; frequent lifting of 20 pound or less; no-grade, slow-speed, 20-pound load carry/walking	☐
☐ **Medium**—Infrequent lifting of 50 pounds; frequent lifting of 25 pound or less; no-grade, slow-speed, 25-pound load carry/walking	☐
☐ **Medium-Heavy**—Infrequent lifting of 75 pounds; frequent lifting of 35 pound or less; no-grade, slow-speed, 35-pound load carry/walking	☐
☐ **Heavy**—Infrequent lifting of 100 pounds; frequent lifting of 50 pound or less; ☐slow-speed, 50-pound load carry/walking	☐
☐ **Very Heavy**—Infrequent lifting in excess of 100 pounds; frequent lifting of 50 to 100 pounds; slow-speed, 50-pound load carry/walking	☐

Factors Explaining Discrepancies between Job Requirements and Work Performance

☐ Suboptimal voluntary effort in testing

☐ Discrepancies between diagnosis and symptoms presented

☐ Discrepancies between client's perception of ability & actual ability

☐ Limited physical abilities

    ☐ Joint motion/flexibility

    ☐ Strength

    ☐ Physical endurance

    ☐ Sensation

    ☐ Hand dexterity

☐ Limited psychosocial abilities

    ☐ Mood/affect

    ☐ Cognition

    ☐ Pain tolerance/behavior

Figure 28-4 Functional capacity evaluation. *(continued)*

Recommendations

☐ Demonstrated work capacity matches job requirements

☐ Perform target job at full capacity

☐ Full time

☐ Part time _____ hr/day _____ days/week

☐ Demonstrated work capacity approximates job requirements and demonstrates client's potential to return to work.

☐ Perform target job with limits or light duty

"Safe" performance recommendations are calculated as maximum infrequent exertion/movement/lift (<1/hr in optimal position/conditions) calculated at 60% of measured maximum demonstration where applicable.

☐ Two-hand floor to thigh level lift   # _____

☐ Two-hand thigh to shoulder lift   # _____

☐ Two-hand shoulder to overhead lift   # _____

☐ Push (waist level)   # _____

☐ Pull (waist level)   # _____

☐ Overhead pull to shoulder level   # _____

☐ Sit   ☐ Unlimited ☐ Limit to _____

☐ Stand   ☐ Unlimited ☐ Limit to _____

☐ Walk   ☐ Unlimited ☐ Limit to _____

☐ Bend/stoop   ☐ Unlimited ☐ Limit to _____

☐ Reach overhead   ☐ Unlimited ☐ Limit to _____

☐ Precision tool use   ☐ Unlimited ☐ Limit to _____

☐ Hand/power tool use   ☐ Unlimited ☐ Limit to _____

☐ **Work Site Modification**
Ergonomic work site evaluation with recommendations for job pace/process or equipment modifications

☐ **Work Conditioning**
Structured, supervised work activity to physically and psychologically condition client for return to work

☐ **Retest Functional Capacity**
Following resolution of psychosocial and or physical issues

Background Information

Age ___ Sex ___ Hand Dominance ___

Current Employment ___ Full time ___ Part time ___ Days/week ___Hrs/day ___ Full Duty

___ Light Duty ___ Not employed

Job Title _____

Essential tasks of current or target job

Key physical and cognitive tasks required by job

_____

‒ _____

_____

‒ _____

_____

Figure 28-4 *(continued)*

Select the "Best Fit" rating of current job physical demands

☐ **Less than Sedentary**—Infrequent lifting <2 pounds, minimal walking, no carrying

☐ **Sedentary**—Infrequent lifting of 10 pounds or less, no sustained walking or carrying

☐ **Sedentary-Light**—Infrequent lifting of 15 pounds, frequent lifting of 10 pounds or less, intermittent self paced no load walking

☐ **Light**—Infrequent lifting of 20 pounds, frequent lifting of 10 pound or less, no grade slow speed 10 pound load carry/walking

☐ **Light-Medium**—Infrequent lifting of 35 pounds, frequent lifting of 20 pound or less, no grade slow speed 20 pounds load carry/walking

☐ **Medium**—Infrequent lifting of 50 pounds, frequent lifting of 25 pound or less, no grade slow speed 25 pound load carry/walking

☐ **Medium-Heavy**—Infrequent lifting of 75 pounds, frequent lifting of 35 pound or less, no grade slow speed 35 pound load carry/walking

☐ **Heavy**—Infrequent lifting of 100 pounds, frequent lifting of 50 pound or less, slow speed 50 pound load carry/walking

☐ **Very-Heavy**—Infrequent lifting in excess of 100 pounds, frequent lifting of 50 to 100 pounds, slow speed 50 pound load carry/walking

Medical Condition

Diagnosis related to work deficit _____

_____

_____

Concurrent medical conditions _____

_____

_____

Time off work _____

Surgery and medical treatment _____

_____

Current Symptoms Relating to Work Situation

Symptom	Location	Intensity				
		Mild		**Mod**		**Severe**
Pain		•	•	•	•	•
Numbness		•	•	•	•	•
Weakness		•	•	•	•	•
Clumsiness		•	•	•	•	•
Fatigue		•	•	•	•	•
Anxiousness		•	•	•	•	•

Figure 28-4 *(continued)*

Evaluation Data Demonstrated Work Capacity using Selected Work Samples

Valpar Standardized Work Samples Rate quality of work performance (1 poor. . . to 5 excellent) during testing situation	Time in Seconds	MTM Rate
1 Small Tools 1 2 3 4 5 Follows instructions 1 2 3 4 5 Maintains physical stamina 1 2 3 4 5 Maintains motivation 1 2 3 4 5 Communicates 1 2 3 4 5 Shows self-confidence		
4 Upper Extremity Range of Motion 1 2 3 4 5 Follows instructions 1 2 3 4 5 Maintains physical stamina 1 2 3 4 5 Maintains motivation 1 2 3 4 5 Communicates 1 2 3 4 5 Shows self-confidence		
9 Whole-Body Range of Motion and Endurance 1 2 3 4 5 Follows instructions 1 2 3 4 5 Maintains physical stamina 1 2 3 4 5 Maintains motivation 1 2 3 4 5 Communicates 1 2 3 4 5 Shows self-confidence		
15 Electrical Circuitry and Print Reading 1 2 3 4 5 Follows instructions 1 2 3 4 5 Maintains physical stamina 1 2 3 4 5 Maintains motivation 1 2 3 4 5 Communicates 1 2 3 4 5 Shows self-confidence		
19 Dynamic Physical capacity (Endurance test at PDC level set by BTE strength testing and actual job demand) P DC Test level _____ 1 2 3 4 5 Follows instructions 1 2 3 4 5 Maintains motivation 1 2 3 4 5 Communicates 1 2 3 4 5 Shows self-confidence	Number of completed tasks	

Figure 28-4 *(continued)*

Perception of Ability to Perform Work
EPIC Hand Function (HFS) and Spinal Function Sorts (SFS)

	Sedentary		Light	
	HFS % of total	SFS % of total	HFS % of total	SFS % of total
Able				
Slightly Restricted				
Moderately Restricted				
Very Restricted				
Unable				
Don't Know				
	Medium		**Heavy**	
	HFS % of total	SFS % of total	HFS % of total	SFS % of total
Able				
Slightly Restricted				
Moderately Restricted				
Very Restricted				
Unable				
Don't Know				

Client Description of Role Demands and Perceived Performance

	Required	Perform Well	Perform Poorly	Unable
Standing 50% of work day				
Sitting 50% of work day				
Frequent walking 30 min/hr				
Frequent/prolonged bending or stooping				
Occasional (1⁻2/day) max lift				
Circle "best fit" 100# 50# 20# 10# Frequent (1/hour) lift/carry				
Circle "best fit" 50# 20# 10# ,10#				
Frequent overhead reach 10 times/hr				
Frequent/prolonged computer use 45 min/hr				

Figure 28-4 *(continued)*

Frequent/prolonged use of hand tools				
Frequent/prolonged use of vibrating power tools				
Frequent/prolonged use of precision instruments				
Analytical decision making				
Personnel supervision				

Abilities (Potential to Work) Work-Related Body Motion						
	Right			Left		
	Normal	**Impaired**	**Unable**	**Normal**	**Impaired**	**Unable**
Raise arm over head						
Touch hand to back of neck						
Touch hand to middle of back						
Touch hand to opposite shoulder						
Elbow bend— palm up and down						
Wrist flex and extend						
Gross hand grasp and release						
Bend— stoop to touch floor						
Kneel (one knee) on floor						
Crawl (10 feet)						

Static Postures (time in minutes maintaining posture before onset of symptoms)

Sitting _____   Standing _____   Reaching above shoulder level _____

Figure 28-4 *(continued)*

Hand Sensation

(Moving two-point discrimination at digit tips)

	Thumb	Index	Middle	Ring	Small
Right Hand					
Left Hand					

Hand Dexterity   **Jebsen-Taylor Hand Function Test**

(Time in seconds) (Benchmark score = 2 SD below mean)

Item	Writing Cards	Turning Small	Pick Up Objects	Feeding	Placing Checkers	Stacking Light	Stacking Heavy
Raw score, Right hand							
Raw score, Left hand							
Male, Dom hand	19.2	5.8	7.9	8.2	4.7	3.8	4
Male, Non-dom hand	55.9	6.3	8	10.5	5	4.4	3.9
Female, Dom hand	15.9	7.1	7.1	8.9	4.5	4.1	4.2
Female, Non-dom hand	47.4	7	8	11.2	5.2	4.5	4.3

Static Isometric Strength BTE/Primus Work Simulator Testing

	Right			Left		
	In #	Percentile rank	CV	In #	Percentile rank	CV
Grip						
3 Jaw Pinch						
Wrist Extension						
Forearm Supination						
Elbow Flexion						
Shoulder Flexion						
	Pre-Test		Post-Test			
Pulse						
Blood Pressure						

Figure 28-4 *(continued)*

Dynamic Isotonic Lifting, Pushing, and Pulling (BTE/Primus Testing)

Perform to fatigue, initial onset of symptoms or evidence of deteriorating technique

	Tool	Weight Lifted/Pulled	Percentile Rank
Floor to Knuckle	191		
Knuckle to Shoulder	191		
Shoulder to Overhead	191		
Push (Waist Level)	191		
Pull (Waist Level)	191		
Overhead Pull	191		

	Pre-Test	Post-Test
Pulse		
Blood Pressure		

Physical Endurance

(Tuxworth Step Test) 5 min (25 steps/min rate) 16″ (40 cm) step

Formula = cumulative resting heart rates (HR)/body weight

HR 0.5 min—1 min ×2 ___ + HR 1.5 min—2 min ×2 ___ + HR 2.5 min—3 min ×2 ___

Body weight ___ Kg (1 Kg = 2.2 lb)

Mean = 5.40 SD = 1.145   Z score =

Cognitive/Behavioral

Generalized Contentment Scale _____

(Range 25–125) Lower scores suggest greater life contentment

Decision-Making Test (record percentile ranking) _____

Mini Mental Status Exam (MMSE) _____

Range 0–30

Score <24 suggests need for detailed testing

Figure 28-4 *(continued)*

Summary of Findings

Patient's description/perception of job requirements

Less than sedentary Sedentary   Sedentary-Light   Light Light-Medium

Medium   Medium-Heavy   Heavy   Very Heavy

Client's Perception of Performance Ability

Cognition/Behavior

Body Range of Motion

Static Standing and Sitting and Reaching Tolerance

Upper Body Strength, Lifting/Pushing/Pulling, and Consistency of Effort

Physical Endurance

Hand Sensation and Dexterity

	Work Performance	**Worker Qualification Profile Valpar Work Samples** **Indicate level based on MTM percent rate of work**
Valpar 1	Small Tools (hand tool use in awkward and confined space)	Not tested Exceeds work standard Meets work standard Does not meet work standard (good potential to meet standard) Does not meet work standard (minimal potential to meet standard)
Valpar 4	Upper Extremity ROM in function (finger/hand dexterity in awkward and confined space)	Not tested Exceeds work standard Meets work standard Does not meet work standard (good potential to meet standard) Does not meet work standard (minimal potential to meet standard)
Valpar 9	Whole-Body ROM (hand function in combination with reaching and bending)	Not tested Exceeds work standard Meets work standard Does not meet work standard (good potential to meet standard) Does not meet work standard (minimal potential to meet standard)
Valpar 15	Electrical Circuitry and Print Reading (attention, memory, new learning, finger dexterity)	Not tested Exceeds work standard Meets work standard Does not meet work standard (good potential to meet standard) Does not meet work standard (minimal potential to meet standard)
Valpar 19	Dynamic Physical Capacity (manual materials handling)	Not tested Exceeds work standard Meets work standard Does not meet work standard (good potential to meet standard) Does not meet work standard (minimal potential to meet standard)

Figure 28-4 *(continued)*

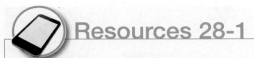

Resources 28-1

Work Evaluation Equipment

A number of companies sell work evaluation equipment, some more complex than others. The two listed below incorporate a number of parts that can be configured for multiple uses. Inclusion in this list does not constitute endorsement.

Baltimore Therapeutic Equipment Co.

Corporate & Products Group
7455-L New Ridge Road
Hanover, MD 21076
Phone: 410-850-0333/Toll Free: 800-331-8845
www.btetech.com

ValparWork Sample Product Line is available from:

BASES of VA, LLC
7010 Colgate Drive
Alexandria, VA 22307
Phone Toll Free: 888-823-8251
www.basesofva.com

exercise, and education to restore abilities impaired by injury, illness, surgery, or enforced inactivity. Both medical management and acute rehabilitation entail evaluation, diagnosis, and procedures to remedy pathological conditions. At the end of each of these processes, a decision as to the potential for the client to return to work must be made. If the client is able and willing to return to work at these junctures, intervention is discontinued. Many clients with minimal residue of injury or illness and high internal motivation return to work without further intervention.

Work Rehabilitation

If medical management and acute rehabilitation do not result in a return-to-work status, efforts focus on the feasibility of returning the client to work. The method to determine return-to-work feasibility is the functional work assessment, which includes general medical information, a job analysis (if the job or type of job is known), an FCE, and an assessment of the client's perceptions of his or her abilities.

In addition to being evaluative, the functional work assessment forms the framework within which the therapist builds intervention strategies to bring about the return to work. The FCE used here can be carried out in seven steps.

Step 1: Preevaluation Information

As indicated in Figure 28-4, information is recorded about the client's job, along with demographics and information

regarding the client's medical condition and symptoms. Details about the job can be obtained through the client's self-report, a written job description, interviews with the employer, and/or an on-site job analysis.

Job Demands. The evaluator seeks to determine the specifics of the job in terms of physical, cognitive, and social demands. Careful review of the job description and interviews with client and supervisor allow the therapist to form a picture of the demands of the job. The therapist may also choose to conduct a job-site analysis so that objective measurements and observations can further elucidate the demands. These job demands are key in setting up work samples later in the evaluation.

Medical History and Current Symptoms. In addition to a complete review of the medical record, the client is asked to describe his or her medical history, including medical treatment, surgery, rehabilitation, and time off work. Information about the client's current symptoms is gathered. The Current Symptoms Relating to Work Situation grid on the FCE allows the client to describe symptoms and rate them on intensity. Clients are encouraged to state their desired resolutions to the current work/disability situation so as to enable the therapist and client to establish goals jointly. Even though the evaluation is in the early stages at this point, there is usually sufficient information to initiate treatment that can coincide with the continuing evaluation.

The therapist should determine whether the cluster of symptoms presented by the client matches those usually associated with the diagnosis or disorder. Significant variances between diagnosis and expected symptoms can be a sign of a client being overwhelmed by the situation or an early indication of symptom magnification. At this point in the FCE, the process may change from evaluation to intervention. The therapist may now choose to use a consultation intervention in which the client is assisted in explaining the discrepancies between conflicting findings. Although the client may not be intentionally misrepresenting symptoms or diagnosis, conflicting findings should be addressed at once. During this intervention, it is appropriate to provide the client with additional information about the medical condition and its usual presentation and course in rehabilitation. It is important to allow the client a face-saving way out, such as the opportunity to restate or discuss symptoms. The purpose of the consultation process is to help the client to either clarify information or adjust behavior according to new information presented by the therapist. Alignment of symptoms may also help to delineate those who have a well-defined WRMD versus those who may have signs and symptoms of overuse that are not yet at a stage of clinical diagnosis. This process may also assist the client to accept and understand his or her symptoms.

Step 2: Work Performance Measurement

In accordance with the job demands identified in step 1, the therapist determines which of the available work performance measures best simulates the demands of the current or target job. Although testing of ability components can be fairly general and applied to many jobs and tasks, if the job to which the client will return is known, the evaluation should be tailored to it. Figure 28-4 has a reporting format for selected work performance measures, including the following:

- Valpar 1: Small tools; fine motor dexterity
- Valpar 4: Upper extremity range of motion; prolonged use of both hands in confined space with awkward angles (Fig. 28-5)
- Valpar 9: Whole-body range of motion; reaching, bending, and stooping while using hands
- Valpar 15: Electrical circuitry and print reading requiring attention, memory, new learning, and hand dexterity (Fig. 28-6)
- Valpar 19: Dynamic physical capacities; reaching, lifting, reading, decision making, and following directions (Fig. 28-7)

Methods Time Measurement (MTM) scoring criteria are used with all of these work performance measurements (Valpar International Corp., 1992). MTM compares work sample performance with a standard that relates to competitive performance rather than to normative data. The standards were developed by an engineering company and are designed to mimic the real pace of work rather than the burst activity common to clinical testing. MTM grades performance in a percent rate of work from 0% to 150%. The percent rate of work is scaled against the following competitive work standards:

- Performance exceeding work standards
- Performance meeting work standards
- Performance below work standards with potential to meet standard

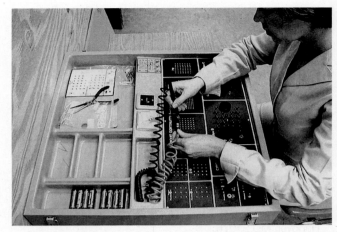

Figure 28-6 Valpar Work Sample 15: Electricity circuitry and print reading.

- Performance below work standard with minimal potential to reach standard

MTM can, at first, be confusing to clinicians accustomed to using only standard normative data, but it is essential for the therapist to understand it for proper analysis of work performance measurement data and to explain the results to the client and employer.

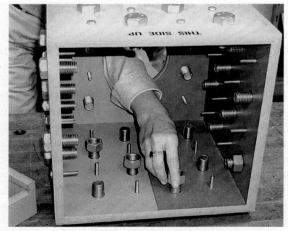

Figure 28-5 Valpar Work Sample 4: Upper extremity range-of-motion work sample.

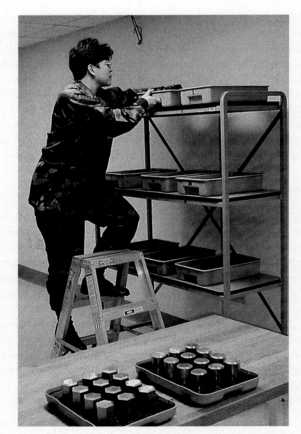

Figure 28-7 Valpar Work Sample 19: Work dynamic physical capacities.

In the event that the client's work sample performance falls below competitive standards, steps 3 and 4 of the evaluation are used to discover the deficits responsible for the impaired work performance. Deficient work performance is generally the result of disconnects between job demands, internal motivation based on perception of ability, and/or performance and ability levels. If, however, demonstrated work performance on job-specific work samples meets the competitive standards, steps 3 and 4 can be omitted, and the therapist can proceed to data analysis and recommendations.

Step 3: Client's Perception of Ability to Work

Figure 28-4 shows two methods for gathering information regarding clients' perception of their abilities. The Employment Potential Improvement Corporation (EPIC) Hand Function Sort (HFS) and the Spinal Function Sort (SFS) (Fig. 28-8) are ratings of perceived capacity. These sorts require the client to view pictures of work situations (62 for the HFS and 50 for the SFS) and then sort them into four categories based on his or her perception of ability to perform the task within the situation. The categories include "able," "slightly restricted," "moderately restricted," and "unable."

The picture sort results can be analyzed in depth with the data compared with normative standards. The results can also be recorded in the format illustrated in Figure 28-4 as to the client's reported ability within each of the four physical demand characteristics categories of sedentary, light, medium, and heavy work. The second method of gaining the client's perception of ability is a self-rating of performance on a variety of common work tasks. Careful analysis of picture sort results and self-reports of ability give important information about the client's perception of his or her ability in relation to the diagnosis, presented symptoms, and the measures of ability that follow.

Step 4: Ability Measurement

Figure 28-4 incorporates tests and measures of ability, including body range of motion; static posture tolerance; hand sensation and dexterity; extremity strength; lifting, pushing, and pulling strength; physical endurance; mood and affect; and cognitive problem solving. These are measures of performance skills and client factors that may affect an individual's capabilities at a number of jobs rather than being tailored to any particular job or set of tasks. Examples include the following:

- Body range of motion, assessed by observing functional movements of the trunk and extremities to include reaching, touching hands to back of neck and middle of back, and bending or stooping toward the floor.
- Tolerance to the static postures of sitting and standing, observed and documented as the client performs other components of testing that require sitting or standing for extended periods.
- Physical strength, documented using both static strength and dynamic lift tests. A device such as the work simulator (Baltimore Therapeutic Equipment Co., 1999) can accomplish both static and dynamic lifting tests and allow comparison of strength between body sides and comparison against normative standards (Fig. 28-9).
- Physical endurance, using either a step test (Tuxworth & Shanawaz, 1977) or treadmill testing if available. *Safety Message: Before any strength or physical endurance testing, it is essential to ensure that the patient's medical record has been reviewed and that the referring physician has given clearance for physical testing.*
- Hand dexterity and function, using any of a number of tests. The Jebsen-Taylor Hand Function Test is a standard in most clinical settings and can rapidly gather information on hand function using common objects rather than pegs or pins (Jebsen et al., 1969).

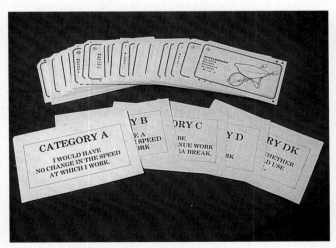

Figure 28-8 EPIC Hand Function Sort and Spinal Function Sort. Patients sort cards based on their perceptions of ability to perform work tasks.

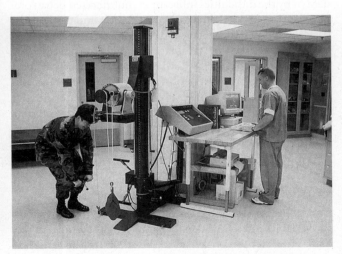

Figure 28-9 BTE Work Simulator used for dynamic strength testing.

- Mood and affect; alterations can exacerbate physical problems. This aspect of function should therefore be included in the assessment. A brief screening tool can be used in conjunction with clinical observations to determine any potential psychosocial problems. (See previous discussion of the Generalized Contentment Scale.) If significant findings are obtained, referral to psychological services may be indicated.
- Cognition should be tested to determine whether difficulties with attention, memory, vision, reading skills, and problem solving are contributing to work deficits. The Mini Mental Status Exam (Folstein, Folstein, & McHugh, 1975) is a brief paper-and-pencil test that can give the clinician a quick look at the client's cognitive functioning. A score of less than 24 without obvious external confounding factors would strongly suggest the need for more formal cognitive testing before proceeding on in the evaluation. In addition, the PSI Decision Making Test is a 5-minute standardized paper-and-pencil test measuring attention, immediate memory, reading, and judgment (Ruch et al., 1981). Either or both of these tests can give the evaluator a general idea of cognitive function and help in determining whether further specialized testing is indicated. Still a third alternative is the Barrow Neurological Institute Screen for Higher Cerebral Functions (BNIS). The BNIS is a screening method developed for identifying cognitive dysfunction. The BNIS has been shown to be related to activities of daily living abilities for patients who have experienced a stroke or anoxic brain injury, as well as to return to work (Hofgren, 2009).

Step 5: Summarize Test Data

The complexity of work demands and human behavior requires that therapists approach evaluation and intervention in a structured manner. If a structured approach is not used, there is a risk of being overwhelmed by the sheer amount of data or by the difficulties inherent in multifaceted behavioral interventions. To help manage information and use it as the basis for analysis, treatment, and recommendations, the sample FCE uses grids for summarizing and recording perception of ability, actual ability, and performance and work data. The evaluator summarizes observations from the tests and converts raw data to standard scores using either normative or MTM criteria. Completion of this section begins to paint a comprehensive picture of the patient's perceptions, abilities, and demonstrated performance in sample work situations. This information is the basis for the analysis in step 6.

Step 6: Analyze Findings

Under Assessment of Evaluation Findings, Figure 28-4 shows the variables to be considered in analyzing the results of test data. The first opinion relates to the quality of the FCE. Was this an incomplete or invalid evaluation, and if so, why did the therapist perceive it as such? The therapist annotates the

client's demonstrated work performance to the job requirements on the Department of Labor Physical Demands of Work Level chart (U.S. Employment Service, 2011). If work performance in sample testing does not meet competitive standards of job requirements, the therapist explains the difference in terms of the client's abilities and/or motivation. In essence, this is a return-to-work equation involving several variables. The therapist must look for matches and disconnects in the data collected during the evaluation to present a meaningful analysis and recommendations.

1. The first match is between the diagnosis and the symptoms. A given diagnosis usually results in a constellation of symptoms. The therapist must decide whether the symptoms match the diagnosis.
2. The next match is the agreement between the symptoms and the client's perception of his or her ability to work as expressed in the picture sort. An example of a disconnect is for the client to report hand paresthesias but not to indicate problems with precision tools on the card sort.
3. Next is assessment of the degree of agreement between the client's perception of ability to work and his or her demonstrated physical and cognitive abilities (potential to work). Examples of disconnects include the client who indicates an inability to use heavy tools on the card sort but shows above-normal strength and endurance during physical testing.
4. The therapist compares the client's physical and cognitive abilities (potential to work) with actual work performance demonstrated during work simulations or task component testing to determine the level of agreement. Demonstrated physical and cognitive abilities should be close to those demonstrated during performance of work samples.

The analysis in this section is the basis for flowing the evaluation process seamlessly into treatment. Problems in incorrect perception can be addressed and reconciled through consultation and education about the pathophysiological aspects of the injury or disorder and expected course of recovery. Education in techniques such as joint protection, energy conservation, and body mechanics can increase the client's ability to deal with symptoms and limitations. Instruction in movement and stretching exercises can provide further skills for managing symptoms and limitations. Work conditioning can be initiated. Work conditioning using work samples can increase physical abilities, engineer successful performance, help the client to recognize his or her abilities, and assist the client to develop realistic goals.

Step 7: Recommendations

Figure 28-4 incorporates recommendation statements that can be supported from the information gathered in steps 1–4, summarized in step 5, and analyzed in step 6. The first section of recommendations concerns the client who can return to either full duty or limited or light duty. The referring physician may well use evaluation recommendations to determine the parameters of light duty, so it is important to base the definition of the limits of light duty on the results of test data and to include what the individual can do as well as what he or she cannot do. The recommendations section also addresses clients who are not ready to return to work but who may be brought to work standards with interventions such as education or work conditioning and hardening. Finally, for clients who do not appear to have the potential to return to target-level work or the preinjury job, the practitioner may recommend prevocational testing and vocational exploration of jobs within the client's physical demand capability.

SPECIALIZED OCCUPATIONAL THERAPY PRACTICE

Return-to-work evaluation and therapeutic intervention are complicated yet fascinating and rewarding. Work-oriented therapy, also known as industrial therapy, pushes the envelope of professional practice by demanding the blending of expert skill in assessment and data gathering with clinical reasoning and behavioral treatment. Applying occupational therapy skills and knowledge to the process is equally challenging because of the necessity of using physical and biomechanical knowledge along with cognitive and psychosocial knowledge. One particular benefit of practicing in the return-to-work field is being able to see the results of therapeutic efforts beyond those seen when practicing exclusively within the confines of a clinic.

Although the core of occupational therapy practice can be used as a basis for work rehabilitation and following step-by-step procedures should greatly increase the probability of seamlessly moving clients through the return-to-work process, this is considered to be a practice area that requires specialization. Therapists who specialize in return-to-work rehabilitation must develop observational and communication skills that are clearly understood by the client-worker, the work supervisor and/or the occupational health physician at the work site, the insurance representative, and medical professionals within the health care setting. Therapists must become comfortable in the work settings of their clients, just as they are comfortable in clinic settings. Occupational therapists specializing in this area have the potential to contribute to the growth of empirical evidence regarding outcomes of work-related interventions.

Désiron et al. (2011) conducted a literature review in which publications on the effectiveness of multidisciplinary return-to-work programs were evaluated. Their criteria were specific, requiring that the intervention programs evaluated include occupational therapy and be conducted between 1980 and 2010, that the studies be randomized, controlled trials or cohort studies, and that work-related outcome measures be used. Only six studies met the criteria. Although all six studies demonstrated a positive effect on return to work, comparisons were difficult because of differing interventions, patients, follow-up periods, and

definitions. Also, the contribution of individual professions could not be delineated. Although their review concluded that multidisciplinary return-to-work programs that include occupational therapy improved return to work, they also strongly suggested the need for additional research that includes uniform terminology and specific descriptions of therapeutic contributions (Désiron et al., 2011).

Snodgrass (2011) examined interventions for individuals with work-related low back pain and illnesses. Seven studies examined therapeutic exercise as an intervention, concluding that insufficient evidence exists to support or to refute the effectiveness of therapeutic exercise or other conservative treatments for subacute or chronic low back injury. The author recommended occupational therapists' use of multiple intervention strategies, and a holistic, client-centered, biopsychosocial approach in which psychological, social, and physical impairments and interruptions to function are considered (Snodgrass, 2011).

Briand et al. (2007) adapted a return-to-work rehabilitation program designed for use with individuals with musculoskeletal injuries for use with clients with mental health problems. Although they did not report on the effectiveness of the program, they delineated and described the elements from the musculoskeletal program that appeared to be relevant for mental health patients, such as psychological, work-environment, and stakeholder involvement. Using the approach with eight workers, they retrospectively documented their pathway through the program, providing rich information on program content. Four primary steps and their associated objectives and clinical activities were identified: evaluate the work disability situation, increase the readiness to return to work, support commitment (mobilization) to return to work, and maintain work (once the client is back in the workforce). The associated tasks are very similar to those described in this chapter including exploration of obstacles, perceptions, physical and mental conditioning, meeting with stakeholders (supervisors, occupational health practitioners), cooperative planning and goal setting, ergonomic evaluation and fit, etc.

The dynamic interplay between evaluation, intervention, and maintenance; the complexity of the return-to-work process; and the multiple professionals involved may explain the relatively weak body of evidence regarding return-to-work programs. Evaluating the effectiveness of such a program can be a challenge! Evidence Table 28-1 showing such results can be seen at the end of the chapter.

Most important to remember is that return-to-work rehabilitation programs using a comprehensive, multidisciplinary approach provide improved service to clients, guiding clients through the medical and rehabilitation processes without abandoning them along the way to fend for themselves in their quest to return to meaningful employment. The needs of both client and employer are addressed, one by one, until the client is a client no more, having once again become a worker and a valued contributing member of the workforce and of society.

Evidence Table 28-1 | Best Evidence for Occupational Therapy Practice Regarding Efficacy of Return-to-Work Programs Including Occupational Therapy

Intervention	Description of Intervention Tested	Participants	Dose	Type of Best Evidence and Level of Evidence	Benefit	Statistical Probability and Effect Size of Outcome	Reference
Care as usual (CAU) versus integrated care. Integrated care included participatory ergonomics, graded activity, and occupational therapy (OT). Those receiving care as usual were seen by physician and/or allied health professionals.	Occupational therapy contribution: functional capacity assessment, workplace intervention, graded activity, and input during monthly team meetings; also contributed to participatory ergonomics	One hundred thirty-four adults aged 18–65 years sick listed with low back pain for ≥12 weeks	Occupational therapy: assessment, workplace intervention, 26 graded activity sessions, monthly input. Measures taken at baseline and 3, 6, 9, and 12 months	Level: IA2b Randomized controlled trial, unblinded	• Integrated care reduced time off work (disability): 88 days compared with 208 days in CAU group • Integrated care effective in return to work • After 12 months, clients in integrated care improved more on functional status • No difference in pain	$p = 0.003$ $p = 0.004$ $p = 0.01$ $p > 0.05$	Lambeek et al. (2010)
Multidisciplinary return-to-work program including OT (two groups: treatment as usual (TAU) and TAU + OT)	Occupational therapy contribution: multidisciplinary team member. Assessment: occupational history, videotape of a role-play work situation, contact with work site occupational health physician with joint reintegration plan	Sixty-two adults with major depressive disorder and history of absenteeism (mean absenteeism = 242 days)	Diagnostic: five contacts (occupational history, video observation, contact with employer occupational physician, and work reintegration) Therapeutic: 24 group sessions and 12 individual sessions. Follow-up: individual visits (three). Measures taken at baseline and 3, 6, 12, and 42 months	Level: IB2a Randomized controlled trial	For those who did not work at baseline: reduced time between baseline and resuming work for those who participated in OT at 18 months, but effect disappeared over follow-up to 42 months. The addition of OT to TAU had a 75.5% probability of being more cost effective than TAU alone. Addition of OT did not affect depression or increase work stress.	$p < 0.05$ $p > 0.05$	Schene et al. (2007)

| Compared multidisciplinary return-to-work programs | Cognitive-didactic versus functional-experiential rehabilitation therapy integrated into inpatient traumatic brain injury programs

Occupational therapy contribution: multidisciplinary team member (no specifics mentioned) | Adult veterans or active duty military personnel with moderate to severe traumatic brain injury ($n = 360$) | Participants in both groups received 1.5–2.5 hours of protocol-specific cognitive-didactic versus functional-experiential rehabilitation therapy in addition to usual care.

Measures taken via telephone calls at 1, 6, 12, and 24 months | Level: IA2b
Randomized controlled trial; single blinded | No difference between groups on global outcome measures at 1 year.

Cognitive-didactic participants improved more in immediate posttreatment

Exploratory subgroup analyses suggested that at 1 year post, younger participants in the cognitive group had higher rates of return to work or school than those in functional group, whereas those age 30 years or more with more education in functional group had higher levels of independent living than those in cognitive group. | $p > 0.05$

$p = 0.01$ | Vanderploeg (2008) |

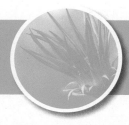

case example
Mr. B.: Return to Work after Hand Surgery

Occupational Therapy Intervention Process	Clinical Reasoning Process	
	Objectives	Examples of Therapist's Internal Dialogue

Patient Information

Mr. B. is a 37-year-old married civil service employee. He works as an audiovisual support assistant and has a 2-year history of right dominant radial wrist pain. Mr. B. was intermittently treated for stenosing tenosynovitis of the first dorsal wrist compartment (de Quervain's disease) during the previous year. Conservative treatment, including activity limitations, limiting wrist motion with a thermoplastic thumb spica-type splint, superficial heat and cold, deep heat using ultrasound, and trials of transcutaneous and percutaneous corticosteroid medication via phonophoresis, iontophoresis, and injection, did not relieve symptoms to a level allowing Mr. B. to work at full capacity. About 10 weeks prior to referral for functional capacity evaluation (FCE), Mr. B. underwent a surgical procedure to release the right first dorsal wrist compartment. The surgery and postoperative recovery period were unremarkable. By postoperative week 10, however, Mr. B. could not return to work because of continued pain in the radial wrist during job-specific tasks. His supervisor referred Mr. B. to occupational health services, and Mr. B. was subsequently referred to occupational therapy for FCE and recommendations for return to duty.

A review of Mr. B.'s medical record and results of an initial interview revealed that he was in reasonable health and, excluding de Quervain's tendonitis, was without significant pathological medical history. Mr. B. had not been working for a total of 10 weeks, including the postoperative phase of his treatment. He was now back to work and on unofficial light-duty status administered by the good graces of his supervisor.

Appreciate the context

"I believe that Mr. B. has received a reasonable standard of treatment for the diagnosed condition. He has progressed through an expected treatment regimen with invasive (surgical) treatment initiated only when conservative had failed."

"Mr. B. seems to have a good working relationship with his supervisor as evidenced by the allowance of nonmedically directed light duty."

Description of Assessment

Mr. B. gave the therapist a specific listing of job tasks that included infrequent lifting and carrying of 50-pound items and fairly frequent lifting of approximately 25-pound objects. As part of his additional duties, Mr. B. was required to lift with one hand and carry a flagpole base weighing 17 pounds. The lift and carry were usually done with the right wrist slightly flexed and in radial deviation. Aspects of Mr. B.'s job description were verified by review of his written job description, an interview with his supervisor, and on-site observation.

Mr. B. stated that any use of his right hand caused wrist pain. He could perform all basic and instrumental activities of daily living but could not perform his job except for answering the phone and doing paperwork. He stated that it had taken "the doctors" 2 years to figure out his problem and that the surgery had not fixed it. When asked about his desired outcome, he replied that he needed either to be trained for another kind of job or receive disability for this work-related injury.

Based on his job demands, the occupational therapist decided to use the Valpar 1 (small tools), Valpar 9 (whole-body range of motion), and Valpar 19 (dynamic physical capacity) to sample Mr. B.'s actual work performance. Mr. B. performed at the Methods Time Measurement (MTM) rate of 95% on the Valpar 1, 90% on the Valpar 9, and 78% on the Valpar 19. Work performance on the Valpar 1 and 9 met competitive work standards; performance on the Valpar 19 was below competitive work standards.

Planning the evaluation

"My task is to try to discover the reason this medical condition continued to limit Mr. B.'s successful return to work despite successful surgical treatment and hand rehabilitation. I will need to consider his medical history in light of the job demands and try to determine his motivations regarding recovery and return to work. I will need to assess his ability to perform work tasks to see whether he is actually 'work ready.' If he is not able to perform at job standards, then I will need to assess his physical, cognitive, and behavioral potentials to try to understand the 'why' of his work inability."

Interpret observations

"The severity level of Mr. B.'s symptoms does not seem to match the expected response to surgical treatment and recovery for de Quervain's disease. Mr. B.'s perception of his performance ability does not match the severity of his reported symptoms either but does match measurement of physical and cognitive abilities. Work sample performance was greater than I expected from the evaluation of his physical abilities. Finally, I don't think that the sample work performance fully met target job requirements."

The therapist gathered subjective and objective data about Mr. B.'s abilities to examine the possible causes of the discrepancy between his abilities and the test and job demands. The EPIC Hand Functions Sort and the Spinal Function Sort allowed Mr. B. to express his perceptions of his ability to perform common work and leisure tasks. The results of these two sorts revealed that he perceived he could perform 80.5% of the tasks at normal or subnormal rates and intensity (categories A, B, and C); 19.5% of the tasks were rated as unable to perform in his present condition. Many of the tasks in both categories that were reported as not performable did not fall into the work domains usually associated with hand and wrist pain.

Measurement of physical abilities revealed body range of motion, ability to maintain static postures, and hand sensation as within normal range. Three of the seven subtests on the Jebsen-Taylor Hand Function Test were significantly below the mean. Static isometric strength testing using the BTE Work Simulator indicated that the right arm was below the 1st percentile, whereas the left arm showed average strength ratings at the 60th percentile. Lifting, pushing, and pulling ability of both arms using the BTE dynamic lift tests was below the 1st percentile. The general contentment scale score was 62. Cognitive performance under time pressure (decision-making test) was at the 45th percentile. Physical endurance using the step test was three standard deviations below the mean for age group.

"In general, I am seeing mismatches between diagnosis and symptoms, symptoms and abilities, and abilities and performance. I believe that this fits a pattern of psychological overlay that limits the application of ability to work performance. Combined with this situation, there is a general physical debilitation from several months of inactivity. The duration of his symptoms and perceived slow postoperative recovery are no doubt influencing symptom intensity and may be limiting his willingness to exert full effort during ability testing. At this time, he does not appear ready or willing to return to full duty."

"At no time during the evaluation did Mr. B. appear to be exerting himself to the full extent of his ability, as would be evidenced in concentrated facial expression, sweating, or grimacing with effort. At no time did he express pain or appear to be in pain."

Recommendations

The occupational therapist interpreted Mr. B.'s potential for return to work as moderate and recommended that Mr. B. participate in a work rehabilitation program. Skillful application of physical and psychosocial therapeutic interventions would be required to meet the long-term goal of return to full-time work. Mr. B.'s perceptions regarding his ability and performance would probably have to change to restore Mr. B.'s work role competency.

Consider the patient's appraisal of performance

"Before we started treatment, I thought it would be important to review the results of the test data with Mr. B. and encourage him to explore and explain the variances in the data. Selective retesting (requested by Mr. B. and agreed upon by the therapist) allowed Mr. B. to clarify conflicts in data and demonstrate higher performance levels."

Consider what will occur in therapy, how often, and for how long

"I am recommending that Mr. B. participates in daily work rehabilitation sessions for 1 month, with each session lasting 1–2 hours initially and increasing until he can tolerate a full 8 hours (as is required at his job)."

Ascertain the patient's endorsement of plan

"Mr. B. readily agreed with my recommendations, and I am pleased, because this appears to signify a real engagement in this process."

Summary of Short-Term Goals and Progress

In 1 month, Mr. B. will be able to do the following:

1. Use principles of body mechanics, energy conservation, and work simplification to perform work simulations
2. Improve his endurance and work tolerance so that he can use his right hand and wrist during work activities
3. Problem solve with the therapist regarding necessary adaptations to work tasks and work area

Here is a summary of Mr. B.'s formal work rehabilitation. The therapist provided several lessons on anatomy, pathophysiology, and wound healing, which related to Mr. B.'s surgical procedure. A focal point was that wound healing is a multiple-month process and that some pain during that process is normal.

Based on recommendations from the FCE, the referring physician assigned Mr. B. to an official light-duty status that specified physical demand limitations, with Mr. B. participating in work in accordance with FCE results.

Assess the patient's comprehension

Understand what he is doing

Compare actual to expected performance

Know the person

Appreciate the context

"The plan and goals were devised in conjunction with Mr. B. so as to increase his compliance. The goals specifically avoided the psychosocial issues and focused on tangible items such as knowledge of the healing process, body mechanics, and increasing endurance. I wanted Mr. B. to have the opportunity to change his perceptions about his work ability by experiencing successful activity rather than psychological analysis."

"Analysis of the job tasks indicated that there were tasks that could cause a reoccurrence of wrist symptoms. I felt that it was important that Mr. B. know that the problem was not just related to his physical abilities but also to the job demands and that those job demands could be modified by changing the pace of work and by using adapted equipment."

Mr. B. participated in daily 90-minute work conditioning treatment activities with emphasis on regaining physical endurance and progressive use of the right hand and wrist during work activities. A secondary purpose was to arrange for progressive successful work experiences, so Mr. B. would begin to habituate a positive work role.

Mr. B. was provided training in body mechanics, energy conservation, and work simplification, especially as they related to his FCE results and the demands of his job.

A formal work site and job analysis provided the work site supervisor with sufficient information to modify task and pace to match Mr. B.'s abilities.

The occupational therapist fabricated an ergonomic tool adaptation to correct the identified injury-producing task. This modification corrected the extreme hand posture of radial deviation, allowing a more neutral posture. The device was adopted shopwide in Mr. B.'s work area.

Next Steps

Following 1 month of work conditioning, Mr. B. completed a partial FCE. Testing with the Valpar work samples indicated ability to work at target job standards. Mr. B. subsequently returned to full duty.

Anticipate present and future patient concerns	"I am pleased as to how Mr. B. responded to intervention. We succeed in helping, in part, because at no time during the evaluation or intervention phases of Mr. B.'s participation in the return-to-work process was there any attempt to confront, catch, or expose his psychological issues. I was careful to remain neutral and request only that he try to explain the variances in the data. Mr. B. was always given "wiggle room" and face-saving avenues in all interactions. Over the course of the rehabilitation, the combination of education, nonjudgmental interactions, and successful repetitive work experience encouraged Mr. B. to choose to alter his perceptions of ability and performance and regain work role competency."
Analyze patient's comprehension	
Decide if the patient should continue or discontinue therapy and/ or return in the future	

Clinical Reasoning in Occupational Therapy Practice

Work Rehabilitation

Right dominant radial wrist pain was the central feature in Mr. B.'s inability to return to work. At the time of the evaluation, Mr. B. had been out of work for 10 weeks following minimally invasive wrist surgery. He returned to work but reported continued pain with work-related activities that have not resolved. His supervisor permitted unofficial light duty. He voiced feelings of disappointment and discouragement. He did not attend therapy during his initial recovery period. How should the therapist interpret Mr. B.'s emphasis on his wrist pain? Is it "real" or enhanced? Should Mr. B. have been given a longer period of protection from physical work stressors following surgery? What are the possible consequences of an extended recuperation period? What other psychosocial interventions might therapists have considered, given the possibility of a psychological component to his inability to return to full duty?

Summary Review Questions

1. List four reasons people work, and explain how each might affect their ability to return to work.
2. List four reasons older persons choose to work, along with four methods of attracting older workers to continue working.
3. Describe the unique contributions of occupational therapy to the return-to-work process.
4. Describe how job analysis is used in both the evaluation and treatment phases of the return-to-work process.
5. Describe other potential uses for the results gained from a job analysis.
6. Compare and contrast the two types of performance evaluation suggested in an FCE.
7. Using the job of grocery store clerk and scanning, keying, and bagging as the essential tasks, write a brief description of a treatment program based on task components and a description of a treatment program based on work simulation.
8. Use the return-to-work decision pathway to develop an evaluation plan for a 42-year-old diabetic who has intermittent retinal bleeding (loss of sight) and who has recently lost his job as a computer systems analyst.

Glossary

Functional capacity evaluation (FCE)—Systematic process designed to assess a client's functional abilities. Functional abilities may include all physical and psychosocial abilities required in a work setting, such as musculoskeletal (strength, range of motion, etc.), cognitive, emotional, and communication abilities. The two performance categories include a general evaluation of physical abilities and an evaluation of job-specific capabilities.

Functional work assessment—Entire return-to-work evaluation process, including evaluations of (1) the individual client (traditional occupational therapy and FCEs) and (2) the requirements of the job or potential jobs (job analysis).

Job analysis—Systematic evaluation of a job; a physical evaluation of the job site, observing workers performing their tasks, conducting a task analysis of the criterion tasks, measuring equipment and equipment placement, reviewing work-related documents such as job descriptions, and interviewing those who perform the job and their supervisors.

Task component testing—Functional capacity testing that identifies criterion tasks based on the most difficult, essential components of a job and develops specific evaluations or training programs based on those components. It is assumed that evaluating or training using task

components critical to job success is a valid approach to determining work performance, because the content requirements of the job are used to develop the evaluation or training.

Work conditioning—Treatment program focused on functional requirements of a job or employment setting; incorporates basic physical conditioning such as restoration of flexibility, strength, coordination, and endurance. Work conditioning is conducted after completion of acute care and before work hardening.

Work hardening—Multidisciplinary structured, graded return-to-work treatment program that progressively introduces greater rehabilitation requirements on the client-worker to achieve full capability of the worker to meet the demands of a job. Work hardening includes all aspects required for the client to return to full function in employment, such as psychosocial, communication, physical, and vocational needs, and typically incorporates work simulation as part of the treatment process.

Work-related musculoskeletal disorder (WRMD)—Wide range of health problems arising from repeated stress to the body encountered in the workplace; may affect the musculoskeletal, nervous, and neurovascular systems and include the various occupationally induced cumulative trauma disorders, cumulative stress injuries, and repetitive motion disorders.

References

Adams, L. (2011). Social Security Administration "Ticket to Work" program costs tripled from 2007 to 2010. *iWatch News*. Retrieved July 18, 2013 from http://www.publicintegrity.org/2011/06/06/4820/social-security-administration-ticket-work-program-costs-tripled-2007-2010-0.

Ahlgren, A., Broman, L., Bergroth, A., & Ekholm, J. (2005). Disability pension despite vocational rehabilitation? A study from six social insurance offices of a county. *International Journal of Rehabilitation Research, 28,* 33–42.

Alicke, M. D., & Sedikides, C. (2009). Self-enhancement and self-protection: What they are and what they do. *European Review of Social Psychology, 20,* 1–48.

American Association of Retired Persons. (2006). The state of 50+ America 2006. Retrieved July 13, 2013 from http://www.aarp.org/money/budgeting-saving/info-2006/fifty_plus_2006.html.

American Occupational Therapy Association. (2008). *Occupational therapy practice framework: Domain and process* (2nd ed.). Retrieved from the American Occupational Therapy Association at http://www.aota.org/.

American Occupational Therapy Association. (2012). *Functional capacity evaluation*. Retrieved July 13, 2013 at http://www.aota.org/en/About-Occupational-Therapy/Professionals/WI/Facts/Capacity-Eval.aspx.

Americans with Disabilities Act. (1990). *Public Law 101-336, 42 U.S.C. 12101.* Washington, DC: U.S. Department of Justice. Retrieved March 11, 2005 from http://www.usdoj.gov/crt/ ada/adahom1.htm.

Americans with Disabilities Act Title I Regulations. (1991). 29 CFR '1630.01 et seq. and appendix.

Anaby, D. R., Backman, C. L., & Jarus, T. (2010). Measuring occupational balance: A theoretical exploration of two approaches. *Canadian Journal of Occupational Therapy, 77,* 280–288.

Arnold, K. A., Turner, N., Barling, J., Kelloway, E. K., & McKee, M. C. (2007). Transformational leadership and psychological well-being: The mediating role of meaningful work. *Journal of Occupational Health Psychology, 12,* 193–203.

Baltimore Therapeutic Equipment Co. (1999). *BTE Work Simulator operator's manual*. Hanover, MD: Baltimore Therapeutic Equipment Co.

Barbe, M. F., & Barr, A. E. (2006). Inflammation and the pathophysiology of work-related musculoskeletal disorders. *Brain, Behavior, and Immunity, 20,* 423–429.

Bartone, P. T., Roland, R. R., Picano, J. J., & Williams, T. J. (2008). Psychological Hardiness Predicts Success in US Army Special Forces Candidates. *International Journal of Selection and Assessment, 16,* 78–81.

Bazley, C. (2012). Challenges for the nuclear workforce: Ageing and knowledge transfer. Presented at the *Applied Human Factors & Ergonomics Conference*, San Francisco, CA.

Bender, A., & Farvolden, P. (2008). Depression and the workplace: A progress report. *Current Psychiatry Reports, 10,* 73–79.

Brannick, M. T., Levine, E. L., & Morgeson, F. P. (2007). Job analysis: Methods, research, and applications for human resource management (2nd ed.). Thousand Oaks, CA: Sage Publications.

Briand, C., Durand, M., St-Arnaud, L., & Corbiére, M. (2007). Work and mental health: Learning from return-to-work rehabilitation programs designed for workers with musculoskeletal disorders. *International Journal of Law and Psychiatry, 30,* 444–457.

Brouwer, S., Reneman, M. F., Dijkstra, P. U., Groothoff, J. W., Schellenkens, J. M. H., & Göeken, L. N. (2003). Test-retest reliability of the Isernhagen Work Systems Functional Capacity Evaluation in patients with chronic low back pain. *Journal of Occupational Rehabilitation, 13,* 207–218.

Buddeberg-Fischer, B., Stamm, M., Buddeberg, C., & Klaghofer, R. (2008). The new generation of family physicians, career motivation, life goals, and work-life balance. *Swiss Medical Weekly, 138,* 305–312.

Burwash, S. C. (1999). A teaching model for work practice in occupational therapy. *Work, 12,* 133–137.

Centers for Disease Control and Prevention. (2007). The state of aging and health in America. Retrieved February 7, 2012 from www.cdc.gov/aging and www.merck.com/cr.

Cahill, K. E., Giandrea, M. D., & Quinn, J. F. (2011). *Reentering the Labor Force after Retirement, Monthly Labor Review,* 34–42. Retrieved July 13, 2013 from http://www.bls.gov/opub/mlr/2011/06/art2full.pdf.

Chen, J. J. (2007). Functional capacity evaluation and disability. *The Iowa Orthopaedic Journal, 27,* 212–127.

Cheney, G., Zorn, T. E., Planalp, S., & Zair, D. J. (2008). Meaningful work as personal/social well-being: Organizational communication engages the meanings of work. In C. S. Beck (Ed.), *Communication yearbook* (pp. 137–186). New York: Routledge.

Cheng, A. S., & Cheng, S. W. (2010). The predictive validity of job-specific functional capacity evaluation on the employment status of patients with nonspecific low back pain. *Journal of Occupational and Environmental Medicine, 52,* 719–724.

Cheng, A. S., & Cheng, S. W. (2011). Use of job-specific functional capacity evaluation to predict the return to work of patients with a distal radius fracture. *American Journal of Occupational Therapy, 65,* 445–452.

Chester, E. (2005). *Getting them to give a damn: How to get your front line to care about the bottom line.* Chicago: Dearborn Trade Publishing, Kaplan.

Committee on Installations and Advice. (1928). Analysis of crafts. *Archives of Occupational Therapy, 6,* 417–421.

Cronin, B., Heinen, B., Jenkins, J., Anderson, L., Fien-Helfman, D., Cook, A., Matheson, L., Davis, P., & Chapman-Day, K. (2011). *Final Report on the Review and Evaluation of Job Analysis Practices.* Call Order 0001: Job Analysis, Submitted to the Social Security Administration. Retrieved July 13, 2013 from www.ssa.gov.

deGraaf, R., Kessler, R. C., Fayyad, J., ten Have, M., Alonso, J., Angermeyer, M., Borges, G., Demyttenaere, K., Gasquet, I., Girolama, G., Haro, J. M., Jin, R., Karam, E. G., Ormel, J., & Posada-Villa, J. (2008). The prevalence and effects of adult attention-deficit/hyperactivity disorder (ADHD) on the performance of workers: Results from the WHO World Mental Health Survey Initiative. *Occupational and Environmental Medicine, 65,* 835–842.

Désiron, H. A. M., de Rijk, A., Van Hoof, E., & Donceel, P. (2011). Occupational therapy and return to work: A systematic literature review. *Biomed Central Public Health, 11,* 615–629.

DuToit, M. D., & Coetzee, M. (2012). Archetypal values of science and engineering staff in relation to their career orientations. *South African Journal of Industrial Psychology, 38,* 955–969.

Equal Employment Opportunity Commission. (1992). *A technical assistance manual on the employment provisions (Title I) of the Americans with Disabilities Act.* Washington, DC: Equal Employment Opportunity Commission.

Federal Register (1991). Part V: Equal Employment Opportunity Commission 29 CFR part 1630, *Equal Employment Opportunity for Individuals with Disabilities*; Final Rule.

Folstein, M. F., Folstein, S. E., & McHugh, P. R. (1975). Mini-Mental State: A practical method for grading the state of patients for the clinician. *Journal of Psychiatric Research, 12,* 189–198.

Frankl, V. (1984). *Man's search for meaning.* New York: Touchstone.

Giandrea, M. D., Cahill, K. E., & Quinn, J. F. (2008). *Self-employment transitions among older American workers with career jobs.* Working Paper Series WP-418 (U.S. Bureau of Labor Statistics). Retrieved July 13, 2013 from http://www.bls.gov/osmr/abstract/ec/ec080040.htm.

Gibbs, L. I. (2011). Keynote for Preparing for an Aging Workforce. 2011 Workforce Symposium, New York Academy of Medicine, New York. May 4, 2011.

Gibson, L. A., Dang, M., Strong, J., & Khan, A. (2010). Test-retest reliability of the GAPP functional capacity evaluation in healthy adults. *Canadian Journal of Occupational Therapy, 77,* 38–47.

Gouttebarge, V., Kuijer, P. P., Wind, H., van Duivenbooden, C., Sluiter, J. K., & Frings-Dresen, M. H. (2009). Criterion-related validity of functional capacity evaluation lifting tests on future work disability risk and return to work in the construction industry. *Occupational and Environmental Medicine, 66,* 657–663.

Gouttebarge V., Wind, H., Kuijer, P. P. F. M., & Frings-Dresen, M. H. W. (2004). Reliability and validity of functional capacity evaluation methods: A systematic review with reference to Blankenship system, Ergos work simulator, Ergo-Kit and Isernhagen work system. *International Archives of Occupational and Environmental Health, 77,* 527–537.

Hao, Y. (2008). Productive activities and psychological well-being among older adults. *Journal of Gerontology, Series B: Psychological Sciences and Social Sciences, 63,* S64–S72.

Heilbronner, R. L., Sweet, J. J., Morgan, J. E., Larrabee, G. J., Millis, S. R., & conference participants. (2010). American Academy of Clinical Neuropsychology Consensus Conference Statement on the Neuropsychological Assessment of Effort, Response Bias, and Malingering. *The Clinical Neuropsychologist, 23,* 1093–1129.

Hendrick, H. W., & Kleiner, B. (2009). *Macroergonomics: Theory, methods, and applications.* Taylor & Francis e-library.

Heuchert, J. P., & NcNair, D. M. (2012). Profile of Mood States (2nd ed.). Multi-Health Systems Inc. Retrieved July 13, 2013 from http://www.mhs.com.

Hofgren, C. (2009). *Screening of cognitive functions: Evaluation of methods and their applicability in neurological rehabilitation.* Institute of Neuroscience and Physiology, the Sahlgrenska Academy at the University of Gothenburg, Göteborg, Sweden. Retrieved February 24, 2012 from http://gupea.ub.gu.se/bitstream/2077/20294/4/gupea_2077_20294_4.pdf.

Hudson, W. W. (1982). The Generalized Contentment Scale. In *The clinical measurement package.* Homewood, IL: Dorsey Press.

International Association of Fire Fighters. (2012). Health, Safety, & Medicine. Retrieved July 13, 2013 from http://www.iaff.org/HS/CPAT/cpat_index.html.

Iles, R. A., Davidson, M., & Taylor, N. F. (2008). Psychosocial predictors of failure to return to work in non-chronic non-specific low back pain: A systematic review. *Occupational and Environmental Medicine, 65,* 507–517.

Isernhagen, S. J. (1988). *Work Injury Management and Prevention.* Rockville, MD: Aspen.

Isernhagen, S. J. (1995). Job analysis. In S. J. Isernhagen (Ed.), *The comprehensive guide to work injury management* (pp. 70–85). Gaithersburg, MD: Aspen.

Isernhagen, S. J. (2006). Job matching and return to work: Occupational rehabilitation as the link. *Work, 26,* 237–242.

Jastrzebowski, W. (1857/1997). *An outline of ergonomics, or the science of work based upon the truths drawn from the science of nature* (T. Baluk-Ulewiczowa, trans.). Warsaw: Central Institute for Labor Protection.

Jebsen, R. H., Taylor, N., Trotter, M. J., & Howard, L. A. (1969). An objective and standardized test of hand function. *Archives of Physical Medicine and Rehabilitation, 50,* 311.

Johnson, R. W. (2007). *Managerial attitudes toward older workers: A review of the evidence.* Washington, DC: The Urban Institute. Retrieved July 13, 2013 from http://www.urban.org.

Klaghofer, R., Stamm, M., Buddeberg, C., Bauer, G., Hammig, O., Knecht, M., & Buddeberg-Fischer, B. (2011). Development of life satisfaction in young physicians: Results of the prospective SwissMedCareer Study. *International Archives of Occupational and Environmental Health, 84,* 159–166.

Koh, D., & Takahashi, K. (2011). *Occupational medicine practice* (3rd ed.). Hackensack, N J: World Scientific.

Kuchinke, K. P., Ardichvili, A., Borchert, M., & Rozanski, A. (2009). The meaning of working among professional employees in Germany, Poland and Russia. *Journal of European Industrial Training, 33,* 104–124.

Lagerveld, S. E., Blonk, R. W. B., Brenninkmeijer, V., Wijngaards-de Meij, L., & Schaufeli, W. B. (2012). Work-focused treatment of common mental disorders and return to work: A comparative outcome study. *Journal of Occupational Health Psychology, 17,* 220–234.

Lambeek, L. C., van Mechelen, W., Knol, D. L., Loisel, P., & Anema, J. R. (2010). Randomised controlled trial of integrated care to reduce disability from chronic low back pain in working and private life. *British Medical Journal, 340,* 779.

Lang, J. W. B., Kersting, M., Hülshenger, U. R., & Lang, J. (2010). General mental ability, narrower cognitive abilities, and job performance: The perspective of the nested factors model of cognitive abilities. *Personal Psychology, 63,* 595–640.

Lechner, D. E., Page, J. J., & Sheffield, G. (2008). Predictive validity of a functional capacity evaluation: The physical work performance evaluation. *Work: A Journal of Prevention, Assessment and Rehabilitation, 31,* 21–25.

Llena-Nozal, A., Lindeboom, M., & Portrait, F. (2004). The effect of work on mental health: Does occupation matter? *Health Economics, 13,* 1045–1062.

Lysaght, R., & Shaw, L. (2011). Job analysis (what it is and how it is used). In J. H. Stone & M. Blouin (Eds.), *International Encyclopedia of Rehabilitation.* Retrieved July 13, 2013 from http://cirrie.buffalo.edu/encyclopedia/en/article/268/.

Maestas, N. (2010). Back to work: Expectations and realizations of work after retirement. *Journal of Human Resources, 45,* 719–748.

Mannuzza, S., Castellanos, F. X., Roizen, E. R., Hutchison, J. A., Lashua, E. C., & Klein, R. G. (2011). Impact of the impairment criterion in the diagnosis of adult ADHD: 33-year follow-up study of boys with ADHD. *Journal of Attention Disorders, 15,* 122–129.

Matuska, K., & Christiansen, C. (2008). A proposed model of lifestyle balance. *Journal of Occupational Science, 15,* 9–19.

Matuska, K., & Christiansen, C. (Eds.). (2009) *Life balance: Multidisciplinary theories and research.* Washington, DC: Slack, Inc. and AOTA Press.

McLaughlin, S. J., Jette, A. M., & Connell, C. M. (2012). An examination of healthy aging across a conceptual continuum: Prevalence estimates, demographic patterns, and validity. *Journal of Gerontology: Biological Sciences, Medical Sciences, 67,* 783–789.

Meyer, A. (1922). The philosophy of occupational therapy. *Archives of Occupational Therapy, 1,* 1–10.

Murphy, F., & Patrick, K. (2007). Employee experiences of effort, reward and change: Themes from a regional Australian energy company. *Rural Society, 17,* 165–182.

National Institutes of Health, National Institute on Aging. (2011). Global health and aging. Retrieved August 8, 2012 from http://www.nia.nih.gov/research/publication/global-health-and-aging.

Paquette, S., Gordon, C. C., & Brandtwiller, B. (2009). *Anthropomentric Survey II Pilot Study: Methods and summary statistics.* Natick, MA: U.S. Army Natick RD & E Center.

Pitt-Catsouphes, M., & Smyer, M. A. (2007). The 21st century multigenerational workplace. The Center on Aging and Work. Retrieved July 13, 2013 from http://www.agingsociety.org/.

Polanyi, M., & Tompa, E. (2004). Rethinking work-health models for the new global economy: A qualitative analysis of emerging dimensions of work. *Work, 23,* 3–18.

Pransky, G., Buchbinder, R., & Hayden, J. (2010). Contemporary low back pain research—and implications for practice, best practice and research, *Clinical Rheumatology, 24,* 291–298.

Rice, V. J. (2007). Ergonomics: An introduction. In K. Jacobs & C. Bettencourt (Eds.), *Ergonomics for therapists* (pp. 3–12). New York: Andover Press.

Rix, S. (2012). The Employment Situation, April 2012: Little Encouraging News for Older Worker. AARP Public Policy Institute. Retrieved from http://star.aarp.org/

Roquelaure, Y., Ha, C., Rouillon, C., Fouquet, N., Leclerc, A., Descatha, A., Touranchet, A., Goldberg, M., & Imbernon, E. (2009). Risk factors for upper-extremity musculoskeletal disorders in the working population. *Arthritis Care and Research, 61,* 1425–1434.

Rowe, J. W., & Kahn, R. L. (1999). *Successful aging.* New York: Random House.

Ruch, W. W., Shub, S. M., Moinat, S. M., & Dye, D. A. (1981) *PSI basic skills tests for business, industry and government.* Glendale, CA: Psychological Services.

Sanders, M. (2012). Optimizing job design for older adult workers. Presented at the Applied Ergonomics & Human Factors Conference, San Francisco, CA. July 21–25, 2012: Santa Monica, CA

Schene, A. H., Koeter, M. W. J., Kikkert, M. J., Swinkels, J. A., & McCrone, P. (2007). Adjuvant occupational therapy for work-related major depression works: Randomized trial including economic evaluation. *Psychological Medicine, 37,* 351–362.

Schultz, I. Z., Stowell, A. W., Feuerstein, M., & Gatchel, R. J. (2007). Models of return to work for musculoskeletal disorders. *Journal of Occupational Rehabilitation, 17,* 327–352.

Schwingel, A., Niti, M. M., Tang, C., & Ng T. P. (2009). Continued work employment and volunteerism and mental well-being of older adults: Singapore longitudinal ageing studies. *Age and Ageing, 38,* 531–537.

Selden, B. (2008). The aging workforce: A disappearing asset? *Management Issues.* Retrieved February 24, 2012 from http://www.management-issues.com/2008/3/21/opinion/the-aging-workforce-%E2%80%93-a-disappearing-asset.asp.

Shames, J., Treger, I., Ring, H., & Giaquinto, S. (2007). Return to work following traumatic brain injury: Trends and challenges. *Disability and Rehabilitation, 29,* 1387–1395.

Singh, P. (2008). Job analysis for a changing workplace. *Human Resource Management Review, 18,* 87–99.

Snodgrass, J. (2011). Effective occupational therapy interventions in the rehabilitation of individuals with work-related low back injuries and illnesses: A systematic review. *American Journal of Occupational Therapy, 65,* 37–43.

Sommerich, C. M., Marras, W. S., & Karwowski, W. (2006). Work-related upper extremity musculoskeletal disorders. In G. Salvendy (Ed.), *Handbook of human factors* (pp. 855–888). Hoboken, NJ: Wiley and Sons.

Stein, H. T. (2002). *The collected clinical works of Alfred Adler.* Bellingham, WA: Alfred Adler Institutes of San Francisco and Northwestern Washington.

Sullivan, M. J. L., & Adams, H. (2010). Psychosocial treatment techniques to augment the impact of physical therapy interventions for low back pain. *Physiotherapy Canada, 62,* 180–189.

Sullivan, M. J. L., Adams, H., Rhodenizer, T., & Stanish, W. (2006). A psychosocial risk factor targeted intervention for the prevention of chronic pain and disability following whiplash injury. *Physical Therapy, 86,* 8–18.

Sullivan, M. L., Simmonds, M., & Velly, A. (2011). *Pain, depression, disability and rehabilitation outcomes.* Occupational Rehabilitation Report R-675, Bibliothèque et Archives Nationales du Québec. Retrieved February 8, 2012 from http://www.irsst.qc.ca/media/documents/PubIRSST/R-675.pdf.

Swann, W. B., Chang-Schneider, C., & Larsen, K. (2007). Do people's self-views matter? Self-concept and self-esteem in everyday life. *American Psychologist, 62,* 84–94.

Terkel, S. (1974). *Working: People talk about what they do all day and how they feel about what they do.* New York: Pantheon.

Tuxworth, W., & Shanawaz, H. (1977). The design and evaluation of a step test for the rapid prediction of physical work capacity in an unsophisticated industrial work force. *Ergonomics, 20,* 181–191.

Unruh, A. M. (2004). Reflections on: "So . . . what do you do?" Occupation and the construction of identity. *Canadian Journal of Occupational Therapy, 71,* 290–295.

U.S. Employment Service (2011). Dictionary of Occupational Titles. Retrieved July 18, 2013 from http://www.occupationalinfo.org/.

U.S. Government Accounting Office (2012). Unemployed older workers: Many experience challenges regaining employment and face reduced retirement security. GAO 12-455. Retrieved July 13, 2013 from http://www.gao.gov/assets/600/590408.pdf.

Valpar International Corp. (1992). *Valpar work sample administration manual* (pp. 2–3). Retrieved July 13, 2013 from BASES of Virginia, LLC, http://www.basesofva.com.

van Selm, M., & Dittmann-Kohli, F. (1998). Meaninglessness in the second half of life: The development of a construct. *International Journal of Aging and Human Development, 47,* 81–104.

Vanderploeg, R. D. (2008). Rehabilitation of traumatic brain injury in active duty military personnel and veterans: Defense and Veterans Brain Injury Center randomized controlled trial of two rehabilitation approaches. *Archives of Physical Medicine, 89,* 2227–2238.

Wigdor, A. K., & Green, B. F. (1991). *Performance assessment for the workplace.* Washington, DC: National Academy.

Willert, M. V., Thulstrup, A. M., & Bonde, J. P. (2011). Effects of a stress management intervention on absenteeism and return to work: Results from a randomized wait-list controlled trial. *Scandinavian Journal of Work Environment & Health, 37,* 186–195.

Acknowledgements

With gratitude and love to a wonderful man, a consummate professional, a friend, and former coauthor, Stephen Luster. May the force continue to be with you, even in the world that follows this one.

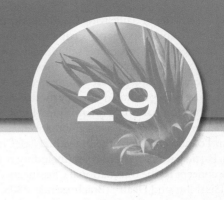

Restoring Competence in Leisure Pursuits

Carolyn Schmidt Hanson

Learning Objectives

After studying this chapter, the reader will be able to do the following:

1. Define leisure in a conceptual and pragmatic fashion.
2. List physiological and psychological benefits of engagement in active and quiet leisure.
3. Describe how leisure can be integrated into occupational therapy practice.
4. Identify various leisure assessments, and describe how they are used.
5. Discuss barriers and challenges for clients and therapists engaging in leisure activities.

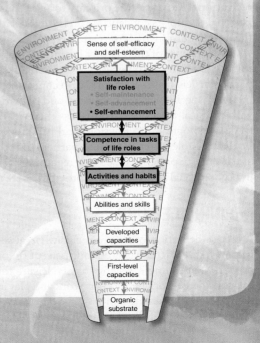

Activities of daily living (ADL), work, and play/leisure are core aspects of occupational therapy intervention that promote self-efficacy and self-esteem. Although information concerning the use of play/leisure in occupational therapy is scarce compared to ADL and work, play/leisure is incorporated into key models that inform practice. In the Occupational Functioning Model, engagement in play/leisure is categorized as a self-enhancement role under the control of and chosen by the individual (see Chapter 1 of this text). Participation in social roles (including that of leisure) is a key concept in the International Classification of Functioning, Disability and Health (Brachtesende, 2005; World Health Organization, 2002), and the Occupational Therapy Practice Framework (American Occupational Therapy Association [AOTA], 2008) endorses participation in leisure activities as a legitimate goal in occupational therapy treatment.

Terms such as play, leisure, and recreation are often used interchangeably. Leisure can be viewed as the adult version of play, because many similarities are present. Also, leisure is viewed as a more encompassing concept than play or recreation and is the term most frequently used in the occupational therapy literature. Recreation is often used to describe how we occupy time that is not devoted to work or self-care. Therapeutic recreation specialists, professionals who are trained to use recreational activities to improve the quality of life for patients, have played a major role in developing leisure programs in medical settings. The profession of therapeutic recreation (TR) gained prominence and became more formalized after World War II, as recreational activities were used in the treatment of disabled war veterans. The history of TR is similar to the history of occupational therapy because our profession was launched after working with veterans from World War I. The distinguishing difference between the two professions is that treatment protocols for TR always use recreational activity as the primary form of treatment. Occupational therapists concentrate on the overall functioning of the individual, of which recreation is only one component.

The purpose of this chapter is multifold: to briefly review the use of leisure with persons with disabilities, to highlight particular leisure assessments, to recommend the development of specific leisure programs and activities for adults with physical disabilities, to discuss the evidence regarding the psychological and physiological benefits of leisure (see Evidence Table 29-1), to discuss barriers for both therapists and clients, to present a case study regarding the use of leisure in occupational therapy, and to provide leisure resources.

DEFINING LEISURE

A precise definition of leisure is elusive because our attitude toward a given activity shapes our perception of it as leisure or work. For example, sewing may be leisure for one person but considered work by another. Work and play are not always dichotomous experiences, however. Sometimes they become blended, and hopefully they are balanced. The Life Balance

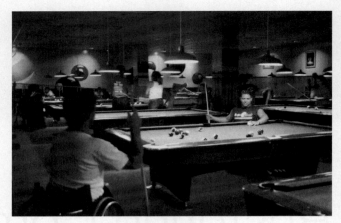

Figure 29-1 Recreational activity: billiards.

Model explains the essential nature of everyday activities (see Chapter 4 for specifics). Balancing work and leisure is crucial for mental and physical health. When balance occurs, life is viewed as less stressful and more satisfying. However, excessive time spent in work at the expense of leisure or vice versa may lead to occupational imbalance, which may aggravate health and quality of life, resulting in injury or illness (Wilcock, 1998).

Law et al. (1994) have partitioned leisure into three major categories: active leisure, which consists of recreational activities incorporating physical exertion such as wheelchair sports and travel; quiet leisure, which incorporates activities such as watching television, reading the newspaper, and crafts; and socialization, which consists of visiting, correspondence, and Internet communication. Both quiet and active leisure activities appear to contribute to occupational balance, self-esteem, and wellness for persons with disabilities (Fig. 29-1).

Quiet Leisure

Generally, adults with physical disabilities tend to engage in quiet and passive activities (Law, 2002), such as needlecrafts, reading, video games, and playing cards (Fig. 29-2).

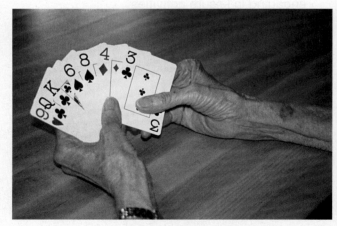

Figure 29-2 Large-print playing cards typify leisure adaptations available to elders. (Photo by Laurie Manuel.)

Evidence Table 29-1	Best Evidence for Leisure					
Intervention	Description of Intervention Tested	Participants	Dosage	Type of Best Evidence and Level of Evidence	Benefit	Statistical Probability and Effect Size of Outcome	Reference
Leisure versus home visit	Leisure education program (experimental) versus a friendly home visit (control)	Sixty-two stroke survivors: 33 in experimental group, 29 in control group	Once a week for ~60 minutes for 8–12 weeks	Randomized controlled trial Level: 1A1a	Leisure program members spent more time recreating and engaging in more activities according to Leisure Satisfaction Scale and Individual Leisure Profile; reported less depression	Statistical significance between groups. Improved participation in leisure and satisfaction with leisure and reduced depression for experimental group	Desrosiers et al. (2007)
Leisure rehab versus instrumental activities of daily living (IADL) treatment	Leisure group: sports and games, gardening, and entertainment IADL group: mobility, transfer training, dressing, cooking, and bathing	Three hundred nine stroke survivors	Median number of sessions = 10; median duration of sessions = 55 minutes	Randomized, controlled trial Level: 1A1a	No difference between leisure rehab group and IADL group on outcome measures of leisure participation or functional training	No statistically significant differences between groups; no improvement in outcome in either group	Logan et al. (2003)
Intensive Tai Chi versus wellness education for fall prevention	Discussion of wellness strategies versus active participation in Tai Chi	Two hundred ninety-one women and 20 men residing in congregate living facilities; ages 70–97 years	Wellness group, 1 hour per week; Tai Chi group, 2 days per week; sessions were between 60 and 90 minutes for 48 weeks and then a year later follow-up testing session	Randomized, controlled trial Level: 1A1b	No significant difference in number of falls sustained by either group	Overall, no statistical differences. However, during 4–12 months, Tai Chi group showed early significant lower risk of falls, but wellness group showed steady decrease over the 2-year study.	Wolf et al. (2003)
Leisure activity; in-home treatment	Leisure activity training versus leisure discussion about effects of stroke	Forty stroke survivors (20 per group); mean age = 69.6 years	Sixty-minute sessions once a week for 5 weeks	Randomized controlled trial Level: IB2b	No. Leisure activities training group did not have significantly increased scores on Katz Adjustment Index. The conclusion was that low dose of therapy is ineffective.	No significant differences between groups on activity level and satisfaction with free-time activity	Jungbloed & Morgan (1991)

Another type of quiet leisure, horticulture therapy (HT), refers to gardening for therapeutic reasons. Occupational therapists have traditionally used HT to facilitate leisure and occupational skills in diverse populations. Gardening assists in enhancing the emotional well-being of patients by affirming life and establishing a sense of peace in addition to improving range of motion and endurance (Harnish, 2001). Raised flower boxes enable wheelchair users to employ gardening skills while improving functional, emotional, cognitive, and physical skills. Various tools are designed to allow people with arthritis and upper extremity weakness to garden (Resources 29-1).

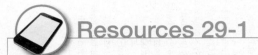# Resources 29-1

Organizations, Social Networking, and Equipment for Leisure Pursuits

Sport Organizations

Disabled Sports USA
http://www.dsusa.org
Provides sports opportunities to people with disabilities. Listing of summer and winter sports and equipment for these sports; methods to contact existing chapters.

National Wheelchair Basketball Association
www.nwba.org
Provides rules, team registration, divisions of wheelchair basketball, and listing of basketball camps. Additional links.

Paralyzed Veterans of America (PVA)
http://www.pva.org/
Research and education, sports and recreation, resources for professionals, publications, and products. Includes events, news and listing of PVA chapters.

National Center on Physical Activity and Disability
http://www.ncpad.org/
Offers training, nutrition tips, sports resources, blogs, discussion groups, newsletter subscription.

National Sports Center for Disabled
http://www.nscd.org
Over 20 sport programs/resources listed under fall/winter/summer headings.

Wheelchair Sports USA
http://www.wsusa.org/
Qualifying standards and rules for sports. Links to various organizations and sporting events.

National Veterans Wheelchair Games (Department of Veterans Affairs/PVA)
http: www.wheelchairgames.va.gov and http://www.va.gov/adaptivesports
Open to veterans receiving care at a Veterans Affairs facility who use a wheelchair for competition because of amputation, spinal cord injury, or other neurological problems. The annual week-long event consists of 17 different events such as swimming, basketball, archery, etc.

Ride2Recovery
http://www.ride2recovery.com
Cycling events across the United States for wounded veterans who have physical and psychological disabilities. Opportunities for volunteers to assist.

Specific Leisure Activities

Gardening
American Horticulture Therapy Association
www.ahta.org/
Membership information, conferences and educational opportunities, publications and information packets, accessible gardening and other.

Travel
http://www.accessable.com/
http://www.disabilitytravel.com/
World travel options focusing on accessible services and transportation. Includes review of cruise ship accessibility. Excellent source of links to sports and other disability sources.

http://www.gimponthego.com
Travel tips and resources recommended by editor who has quadriplegia.

Video Games
http://alteraeon.com
http://www.sryth.com
Video games online for the visually impaired.

http://www.gameaccessibility.com
http://www.ics.forth.gr/hci/ua-games/games.html
Accessible games for those with disabilities

Social Networking

Blue Redefined, Inc.
http://www.blueredefined.org
Nonprofit group dedicated to creating social and entertainment opportunities for those who have disabilities, are hospitalized, or are residing in assistive living environments.

Dating Disabled
http://www.datingdisabled.net
Dating site for people with disabilities. Requests information on what you are seeking, your health condition, and type of relationship desired (pen pal to marriage partner).

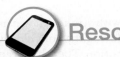

Resources 29-1 (continued)

Disabled Online
http://www.disabledonline.com
Entertainment site featuring live chats, blogs, arcade
games, music, etc. Touted as the Internet portal for people
with disabilities. Has specific page for disabled singles
interested in dating.

Disabled United
http://www.disabledunited.com
United Kingdom site featuring chat room, travel, dating, job
seeking, and health issues.

Equipment

Haverich
http://www.haverich.com
Cycles for the physically challenged: hand cycles, tandem
tricycles, tandem bicycles, seats, backrests, footrests, and
accessories.

TRS, Inc.
http://www.oandp.com/trs
Prosthetic hands for sports and other leisure activities, such
as photography and playing musical instruments. Highlights
adult, children, and infant technology.

KY Enterprises
http://www.quadcontrol.com
Adaptive recreational equipment and controllers for video
games for those with limited use or no use of their hands;
head and mouth devices.

Miscellaneous
Adaptive recreation and sporting equipment for people
with disabilities and the aged. Leisure activities range
from crafts and gardening to motorcycling and sailing
and skiing.

Achievable Concepts Pty Ltd.
http://www.achievableconcepts.com.au/

Access to Recreation, Inc.
http://www.accesstr.com/

Spokes 'n Motion
http://www.spokesnmotion.com
Various programs as well as equipment offered.

Fishing Has No Boundaries, Inc.
http://www.fhnbinc.org
Gear and programs for everyone.

Active Leisure

People with chronic musculoskeletal diseases may be
afraid to engage in activities that require physical exertion and believe that their leisure options are limited to
quiet activities. Occupational therapists may inadvertently contribute to this misperception. Therapists may
not introduce active leisure to clients because exercise
recommendation guidelines have not been fully developed
for people with physical disabilities. Sports for those with
disabilities, however, have been connected to rehabilitation efforts since the 1940s when archery was used as therapy for paraplegic war veterans. Wheelchair sports now
include wheelchair basketball, tennis, and quad rugby as a
few of the better established popular activities (Fig. 29-3).
In fact, people with physical disabilities are engaging in
vigorous and demanding sports such as marathons, rock
climbing, and downhill skiing. As you will see, evidence
demonstrates that strenuous physical activity is not only
well tolerated by those with disabilities, but it has beneficial effects.

ACTIVE LEISURE AND HEALTH FOR PEOPLE WITH DISABILITIES

Developing active leisure outlets is important to health and
wellness for all people, including those with disabilities

(Buchholz et al., 2009). Active leisure minimizes the consequences of a sedentary lifestyle and advances health and
wellness in a number of ways.

Consequences of a Sedentary Life

Despite the increased growth of wheelchair sports and
opportunities for engagement in various leisure activities
of all types, many people with disabilities lead sedentary

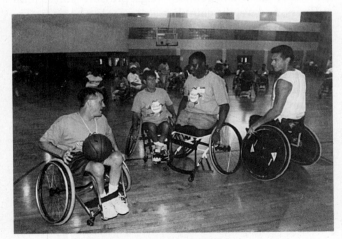

Figure 29-3 Active leisure: wheelchair basketball.

lives. Motl and McAuley (2010) stated that "there is an alarming rate of physical inactivity among older adults, particularly those aging with a disability" (p. 299). Research has shown that cardiovascular disease is the leading cause of death for people with spinal cord injuries (SCI) as well as the able-bodied, although people with SCI are affected at a younger age (Warburton et al., 2010). Participation in regular daily living activities alone is insufficient in promoting health and warding off cardiovascular disease (Warburton et al., 2010). Exercise and active leisure have been relatively unexplored methods of reducing the decline and deconditioning that most people with physical disabilities experience (White & Dressendorfer, 2004). To combat this spiral of physical decline, Painter (2003) emphasized that physicians play a role in encouraging their patients with chronic diseases to become physically active to improve function and quality of life. Occupational therapists can certainly encourage clients to improve their health by providing active leisure experiences, recommending adaptive techniques/equipment, and connecting people to existing activity programs.

Health Benefits of Active Leisure after Physical Disability

Evidence suggests that active leisure (such as sports and exercise) has many potential benefits for people with disabilities. In fact, there is beginning consensus concerning the imperative need for exercise and active leisure for people with physical disabilities in order to improve mental and physical health. It could be said that people with a disability have more to lose if they do not maintain a suitable level of fitness.

White and Dressendorfer (2004) advocated for exercise programs that focus on increasing cardiorespiratory fitness, muscular strength, and mobility for people with multiple sclerosis (MS). They discovered that not only are secondary disorders reduced (e.g., pressure sores, joint stiffness, and weight gain) but also people who engage in aquatic exercise and other aerobic activity attest to better quality of life and improved lifestyle. Exercisers with MS and other disabilities commonly mention the psychological benefits inherent in activity participation. Disabled veterans in a wheelchair games event testified that sports participation enhanced their disability acceptance, improved their mobility skills and added greatly to their life (Sporner et al., 2009).

In the Northern Manhattan Stroke study of 1,000 elders, those who engaged in physically active leisure were found to have a decreased incidence of ischemic stroke (Sacco et al., 1998). Researchers of this study stressed that physically active leisure should be emphasized in stroke prevention campaigns. Tai Chi, which is available in many communities, is an example of active leisure that has

health benefits for elders and those with stroke. Known as a soft martial art, Tai Chi involves moving the body slowly and smoothly through its range of motion. There has been an exponential increase in randomized controlled trials on the effects of practicing Tai Chi. In a meta-analysis performed by Klein and Adams (2004), 17 clinical trial studies were critically reviewed with all showing statistical significance in at least one outcome measure. Typical outcome measures included the positive effects Tai Chi had on quality of life and physical function. In addition, Tai Chi was credited in improving pain management and balance. People with stroke who practiced Tai Chi for several months had less depression than a control group (Desrosiers et al., 2007), and Tai Chi has been associated with better balance, lower blood pressure, and improved mood (Taylor-Piliae & Haskell, 2007).

Not only does active leisure such as exercise offer specific physiologic and psychological benefits, improved fitness may enable other aspects of active participation in life. Adults with SCI who enrolled in a 12-week fitness and weight management class reported that they hoped that losing weight and becoming more fit would enable them to more safely and frequently engage in leisure pursuits that required improved strength and stamina (Radomski et al., 2011). Many participants limited their leisure activities, such as travel, for fear of encountering an unexpected barrier that they did not have the capacity to manage. It was found that the same weight loss strategies used by people without disabilities, such as exercise, good nutrition, and behavioral techniques, benefitted individuals with SCI, who have a higher than average rate of developing heart disease.

In summary, engagement in leisure activities is essential to health and wellness for all people. Therefore, occupational therapists incorporate this area of functioning into the assessment and intervention process.

ASSESSMENT TOOLS

Before recommending specific leisure activities or using leisure as an intervention, one should assess the patient's interest in leisure. The following are instruments that identify the types of activities that are meaningful to clients. Although this is not an exhaustive list of the leisure assessments available in the fields of occupational therapy and TR, the following sections present some of the better known instruments.

The Canadian Occupational Performance Measure

Designed by occupational therapists, the Canadian Occupational Performance Measure (COPM) detects self-perceived change in occupational performance over time

(Law et al., 1994). The COPM contains three sections: self-care, productivity, and leisure. The leisure section is divided into quiet recreation, such as hobbies, crafts, and reading; active recreation, such as sports, outings, and travel; and socialization, such as visiting, phone calls, and correspondence. Individuals are requested to identify any problems in the three sections and to rate the importance of each activity on a scale of 1 to 10. Then five of the most important problems are identified, and individuals rate their performance and satisfaction with performance on these five problems.

Interest Checklists

Occupational therapists have developed and used many interest checklists. The Nottingham Leisure Questionnaire, developed in England for stroke patients, is a 38-item list of activities ranging from watching television to doing sporting activities (Drummond & Walker, 1994). A 5-point scale is used to describe frequency of doing the activity, ranging from regularly (every day) to never. In obtaining test–retest reliability scores, 21 subjects completed the same questionnaire on two occasions within a 2-week period. Based on Cohen's kappa coefficient, reliability was determined to be excellent (0.75–1.00) and good (0.60–0.74) for 23 of the 38 items and fair (0.40–0.59) for another 6 items. Inter-rater reliability was tested using the ratings of two occupational therapists and showed excellent agreement on 40 items and good agreement on 1 item; the total was more than 38 items because of write-ins of other activities not specified in the questionnaire (Drummond & Walker, 1994).

The Interest Checklist (Matsutsuyu, 1967) consists of 80 items grouped into the following categories: ADL, manual skills, cultural-educational, physical sports, and social recreation. The rating given to each item ranges from no interest to casual interest to strong interest.

Kautzmann (1984) developed an interest checklist for persons with arthritis that uses similar categories, as well as games, organizational activities, and entertainment. This instrument consists of 64 items rated according to their importance, ranging from none to high, and their relevance to the person with arthritis (importance of activity and whether there is a priority for further development) (Kautzmann, 1984).

Finally, the Lin Interest Check List (LICL), developed in 1991, contains 151 interests and activities within six categories: sports, physical activities, and nature; crafts; games; sociocultural and entertainment activities; community and education; and hobbies and miscellaneous. The level of interest, frequency, and history of participation are to be identified for each item. The LICL has high content validity and good test–retest reliability (Lin, 1991).

Occupational Therapy Assessment of Leisure Time

The Occupational Therapy Assessment of Leisure Time (OTALT) was based on a review of the leisure literature in occupational therapy and provides a frame of reference specifically for leisure (Soderback & Hammarlund, 1993). The purpose of the OTALT is to enable the client to use leisure time more effectively and to improve satisfaction with leisure activities. Using open-ended questions, the therapist interviews the client on the dimensional concepts of time, intrinsic motivation, and free choice of leisure activity; capability; structure of social and cultural environment; engagement in leisure activity; pleasure for pleasure's sake; goal self-fulfillment, goal diversion, recreation, and relaxation; leisure role; leisure behavior; and influence on his or her leisure role and leisure behavior. Although multiple questions are provided for each dimension, therapists are encouraged to structure the interview the best way they see fit.

Leisure Questionnaires from Therapeutic Recreation

Beard and Ragheb (1980) have developed four leisure questionnaires that are commonly used by TR specialists in medical settings. The Leisure Satisfaction Measure contains 51 statements about how patients perceive their needs being met through leisure. The Leisure Attitude Measurement contains 36 items that quantify the patient's attitude in three areas: cognitive, affective, and behavioral (Ragheb & Beard, 1982). The Leisure Interest Measure identifies patients' interest in the following eight domains: physical, outdoor, mechanical, artistic, service, social, cultural, and reading (Beard & Ragheb, 1990). The Leisure Motivation Scale contains 48 items regarding motivation to engage in leisure activities and reflects four areas: intellectual, social, competence-mastery, and stimulus avoidance (Beard & Ragheb, 1983). As a whole, reliability and validity are good for these measures because items and domains have been analyzed extensively according to the test manuals for the four aforementioned assessments.

Physical Activity Scale for Individuals with Physical Disabilities

The Physical Activity Scale for Individuals with Physical Disabilities (PASIPD) was developed to obtain information on the physical activity habits of people with physical disabilities. The PASIPD was based on and then modified from the Physical Activity Scale for the Elderly (PASE), a 10-item instrument administered in person or via the phone. Using the PASE as a starting point, qualitative interviews were conducted with 15 people with disabilities along with four rehabilitation professionals. Goals for the new instrument included a brief time to complete, administered by self or interview, and targeted quantitative areas previously unexplored in the disabled population (Washburn et al., 2002).

Three hundred seventy-two people completed the PASIPD to determine its construct validity and represented the following conditions: postpolio, quadriplegia, cerebral palsy, and other locomotor impairments (Washburn et al., 2002). Descriptive characteristics of this sample population revealed an average age of 50 years, well educated, Caucasian, and a moderately high annual income—not necessarily representative of people with disabilities. However, information gleaned from this sample revealed that younger respondents reported higher levels of activity (the exception being questions regarding home and garden maintenance) than older respondents. Individuals who rated their health as "excellent/very good" reported significantly higher total activity scores than those individuals who rated their health as "good" or "fair/poor."

The resulting brief scale consists of 13 items representing five distinct categories: home repair/lawn and garden work, housework, vigorous sport and recreation, moderate sport and recreation, and occupation/transportation. Respondents are provided with four options to indicate how many days and hours per session they engage in the aforementioned activities. Based on the option selected, a specific multiplier related to energy expenditure is used to determine a value for each of the 12 questions. The first question is not scored because it taps sedentary activity and is meant to familiarize the person to the survey format. All of the values are summed for a total activity score with the highest being a maximum of 199.5.

OCCUPATIONAL THERAPY INTERVENTION TO RESTORE COMPETENCE IN LEISURE PURSUITS

Based on the results of the occupational therapy assessment, occupational therapists help clients resume premorbid leisure interests and explore new options (see Procedures for Practice 29-1). Social networking, in particular, is a quiet leisure outlet that is of increasing interest to those with disabilities.

Computers can provide extensive leisure outlets for people with disabilities from video and online arcade gaming to dating and blogging. Popular YouTube, Google, and Facebook platforms have allowed people to easily communicate with others globally and to learn instantaneously about events taking place in another hemisphere. Individuals with physical disabilities can form friendships with people who are simply online but may live thousands of miles away. Several websites specialize in matching people with disabilities who are interested in

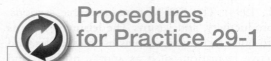

Procedures for Practice 29-1

Strategies to Promote Leisure

- Elicit enthusiasm and support from health professionals through in-service education that links leisure, health, and quality of life.
- Elicit support from family and friends.
- Identify interest and enjoyment in activity via leisure assessments and interviewing techniques.
- Evaluate for special needs and assist in choosing an appropriate activity based on current abilities.
- Provide exposure to activity and establish a schedule to learn.
- Set basic goals for activity that can be mastered early, and establish more challenging goals with progress.
- Follow up to evaluate success and to make possible adjustments.
- Create opportunities to reinforce engaging in activity that may be extrinsically or intrinsically motivating (longer lasting effect).

dating and in offering entertainment opportunities (see Resources 29-1). Although distinctly having many advantages, computers may encourage individuals to be sedentary and remain in one position for extended periods. As with any activity, moderation is the key. Frequent breaks and repositioning are crucial.

As described earlier, moderate to strenuous activity may reduce functional decline, improve cardiorespiratory function and possibly decrease depression and fatigue for people with disability. A greater amount of time spent in physically active leisure pursuits has been associated with lower chronic disease risk (Buchholz et al., 2009). Therefore, this section focuses on helping people with disability engage in active leisure.

Guidelines for Exercise Regimens

Research data on the activity patterns of those with disabilities are scarce; insufficient evidence is available to determine exactly what activity is best for an adult with a physical disability based on safety, effectiveness, and outcome measures. Using the research on the ablebodied, we know that a properly designed physical activity program includes aerobic, flexibility, and strength components (Durstine et al., 2000). The exercise dosage (intensity, frequency, and duration of the physical activity) may need to be modified for persons with disabilities to maintain a training effect that does not cause abnormal clinical symptoms/signs or injury. For example, it is recommended that adults with physical disabilities lower the intensity of the exercise but increase the duration and the frequency of the activity (Durstine et al., 2000). Exercise guidelines have recently been proffered for elders by Elsawy and Higgins (2010).

Active Leisure Options for Various Diagnostic Groups

Research of the past 15 years provides ideas regarding activities that may be appropriate for certain patient populations. As can be imagined, this area of research is lacking and is a fertile field for those interested in contributing to the leisure literature.

Persons with Spinal Cord Injury

Researchers surveyed 160 persons with SCI regarding their postdischarge activities (Hoffmann et al., 1995). On the basis of their activity level, respondents were placed in an active or an inactive group. Over a 1-year period, the active individuals spent, on average, 3.2 days in the hospital compared with 10.7 days for the inactive individuals. Inactive individuals were more than 2.5 times as likely to have pressure sores as the active ones. The results of this study underscore the cost-saving benefits of being physically active.

One hundred forty-three individuals with SCI from 18 to 55 years of age were surveyed regarding their engagement in physical activity before and after their injury (Wu & Williams, 2000). Individuals who participated in sports such as wheelchair basketball, rugby, and tennis were shown to have less depression, improved social interaction, and less incidence of rehospitalization. The participants in this study reported that they engaged in sport because it was fun and provided a means to be fit and healthy and a means to interact with a variety of people. Peers with disabilities, as opposed to therapists, were invaluable in introducing newly injured people to wheelchair sports. Wu and Williams (2000) emphasized that therapists should take a more active role in educating clients about sports training and leisure activities (see the Case Example about K.J.).

Persons with Joint Replacements

Individuals with modern joint replacement can expect to have their joints last at least 10–15 years. This does not apply to people with hip and knee joint replacements who regularly jog or hike because this type of activity may endanger the integrity of the prosthetic components (Kuster, 2002). Because there are no prospective, randomized studies on physical activities after total joint replacement, the conservative opinions of orthopedic surgeons have guided current recommendations on suitable leisure activities. In general, speed,

prior sport experience, and joint impact are factors when considering load or joint stress. High-impact activities requiring speed, such as football, soccer, and handball, are discouraged, whereas low-impact activities, such as swimming, cycling, and walking, are encouraged. Technically demanding sports (snow skiing, mountain biking) are not suggested for those individuals who have never engaged in these activities prior to their joint replacement. The rationale is that the learning curve for technical sports is too demanding on the replaced joints (Kuster, 2002).

Persons with Rheumatoid Arthritis and Osteoarthritis

Three hundred nine individuals with rheumatoid arthritis (RA) enrolled in a randomized controlled trial and participated for 2 years in either an exercise program of high intensity or usual care (standard physical therapy) (de Jong et al., 2003). The high-intensity exercise program was more effective at improving functional ability in this population. In addition, it also demonstrated that exercise did not increase radiographic damage of the large joints. Bulthuis et al. (2007) found that short-term exercise immediately after hospital discharge of RA and osteoarthritis (OA) patients had results of improved function. Aerobic exercise (particularly swimming) and strengthening regimens are viewed as being beneficial for people with joint problems (Esser & Bailey, 2011). In an older but still relevant publication, Minor and Lane (1996) noted that people with RA are prescribed rest and medication for their condition, which is appropriate for the acute condition but harmful in the chronic state. People with RA and OA often stop engaging in leisure and recreational activities. Unfortunately, inactivity produces the same symptoms as the rheumatoid disease process: muscle weakness, decreased flexibility, fatigue, incoordination, depression, and lowered pain threshold. People with RA who do engage in aerobic exercise may experience a significant reduction in swelling, which is attributed to increased synovial blood flow. Minor and Lane (1996) emphasized that vigorous activity is only supported in people with no joint inflammation; otherwise, joint damage may ensue. Developing strong muscles by engaging in mild resistance training may also take pressure off of joints.

Persons with Multiple Sclerosis

Prescribed exercise does not appear to increase or exacerbate the condition of MS. Aquatic exercise, especially, may decrease the incidence of obesity, heart disease, and diabetes—all leading problems associated with inactivity. Salem et al. (2011) found that a 5-week community-based aquatic program augmented rehabilitation efforts and was beneficial for people with

MS. Yoga is also deemed an appropriate activity because it assists in improving range of motion and balance. In dealing with this condition, it is essential to alternate periods of rest and activity and to monitor heat tolerance. People with MS commonly have more energy in the morning, so activity may be better tolerated earlier in the day before fatigue occurs.

Elders

In addition to a variety of sports, physically active leisure, such as walking, armchair or wheelchair aerobics (exercising the upper extremities while seated), swimming, and weight training (using light weights or machines; using resistive bands), is ideal for increasing endurance and tone in elders. As elders constitute more of our population, it behooves us to create and promote leisure and socialization opportunities in assisted-living facilities and retirement homes.

Sports Camps/Specific Sports Clinics

Camps have been developed to introduce sports and leisure activities to people with disabilities and to facilitate engagement in physically active leisure and to promote health (Hanson, 1998). Focus may be on one particular sport, such as with wheelchair tennis camp, or an introduction to a variety of sports. Some camps or clinics are specialized for individuals with particular diagnoses; others include anyone with a mental or physical disability. Because of the focused nature of the camp or clinics and the time invested (from several days to several weeks), participants have the chance to socialize and learn specific sport skills. In addition, camp participants often learn techniques and obtain tips from each other on daily living skills such as transferring and catheterization. Affiliation with others is a strong motivating factor in promoting leisure activities.

Ride2Recovery is an example of a cycling group for wounded U.S. veterans and active service members. Founded in 2008, this nonprofit group puts on cycling events around the country to enable military personnel with all sorts of physical and psychological issues to ride together over a period of days. The primary purpose is to help veterans heal and to socialize with others. Riders who have participated in the events have testified to the healing quality of biking as an outlet for stress, a way to become fit and a source of enjoyment from the camaraderie that occurs during the trips. Although only veterans can participate in the ride, volunteers are needed to help with the cycling events in their hometowns and to sponsor riders. Many opportunities are available for nonveterans to be a part of this active group. Other well-orchestrated clinics involving multiple sports and leisure activities have been developed for veterans as well (see Resources 29-1).

Occupational therapists realize the many benefits of directing a camp or being involved with specific sports

events or clinics, which range from raising the awareness of the able-bodied to providing the disabled with opportunities to explore sport. Additional benefits may include training for students and staff who serve as camp or clinic volunteers. Volunteers assist in monitoring participants for heat exhaustion and any untoward effects of exercise (Safety Note 29-1) and assist with coaching. Directing a camp takes time, energy, and funding. Only therapists who are passionate about sport would be willing to expand their duties by being a camp director or

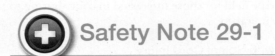

Safety Note 29-1

Safety Considerations during Active Leisure

Spinal Cord Injury and Autonomic Dysreflexia (T6 and above)

Risk factors

- Being overheated
- Having an obstructed fecal mass
- Having a kink in a catheter tube
- Pain

Symptoms and signs

- Hypertension
- Pounding headache
- Profuse sweating
- Flushing
- Pupil constriction
- Nasal congestion

Occupational therapy assistance

- Obtain medical help: this is a MEDICAL EMERGENCY.
- Remove restrictive binders or clothing.
- Elevate head.
- Check leg bag for obstruction.
- Monitor blood pressure.

Guidelines for monitoring during active leisure pursuits

- Terminate activity if safety is questionable.
- Supervise closely the person with a recent disability.
- Consider extreme environmental conditions.
- Monitor body temperature.
- Monitor sweating and color of skin.
- Encourage fluid intake.
- Observe for signs of fatigue.
- Check for incontinence.
- Encourage skin inspection/recommend pressure relief.
- Evaluate positioning, cushioning, and strapping during activity.
- Consider special training for activity.

offering organized physical activity on a consistent basis. A more efficient method to educate clients about sport opportunities is being aware of clinics for people with disabilities in your city and encouraging participation in these events.

BARRIERS TO LEISURE ENGAGEMENT

A number of factors interfere with ensuring that persons with disabilities ultimately can engage in leisure activities that maintain a satisfactory occupational balance. Some factors stem from contemporary trends in occupational therapy; other interfering factors have to do with client access.

Barriers for Therapists

Occupational therapists often have limited time to work with clients and may feel they lack adequate knowledge about leisure activities and resources, but this is a crucial area for intervention. Asking about leisure interests and desires allows occupational therapists to provide exploratory experiences in a monitored and controlled setting and offer the "just-right challenge" to their clients. Moreover, we can follow up by forging relationships with community and recreational centers to encourage continued participation upon discharge (Procedures for Practice 29-1).

Barriers for Clients

Access to recreational and leisure pursuits may be difficult for persons with disabilities. Personal, environmental, and societal factors may all limit leisure participation. Personal factors may include fatigue, pain, depression, comorbid illness, and medical condition. Activity safety and weather conditions may impact participation as well (Mallinson et al., 2005). Environmental barriers such as poorly designed parking lots and sidewalks without curb cuts may prevent access. A recreational facility may have outdated, inaccessible bathrooms. Transportation to a facility or center may also pose problems, as may the financial requirements for specialized equipment such as wheelchairs designed for specific sports and adapted sports equipment. It may be difficult to find coaches and other personnel who understand the needs of those with disabilities and challenging to find a training partner. Despite these possible barriers, it is vital that people with disabilities have support and encouragement from their family and friends to participate in leisure activities that interest them and are within their capabilities.

Attitudinal barriers in our society are often more disabling than personal and environmental barriers. Individuals with disabilities such as tetraplegia and bilateral upper or lower extremity amputations may not be-

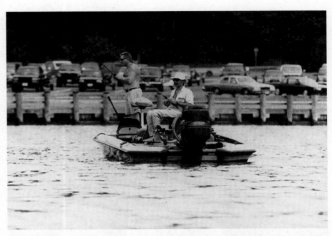

Figure 29-4 Technology to allow independent fishing from a wheelchair. (Photo by Gary Rudolph.)

lieve that they are capable of participating in a variety of activities because of the attitudes of others. Advances in technology and changes in attitudes have allowed people with spinal cord injury and neuromuscular diseases to water ski using a sit ski, people with hand amputations can windsurf using sport-specific prostheses, wheelchair users can rock climb with special equipment, fishermen can fish (Fig. 29-4), and individuals with lower extremity amputations can play tennis (Fig. 29-5). Self-defense classes have been formed for community dwellers with visual impairments (Fig. 29-6). Wheelchairs designed specifically for use on the beach have been developed in addition to numerous models for various sports. With developing technology, opportunities to engage in numerous activities are possible if there is interest and motivation on the part of the therapist and the individual (Fig. 29-7).

In conclusion, human occupation is commonly taken for granted, and its health benefits are not acknowledged

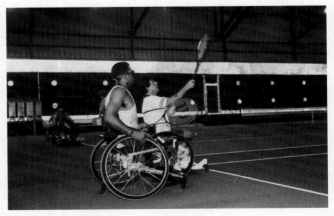

Figure 29-5 Active leisure: wheelchair tennis.

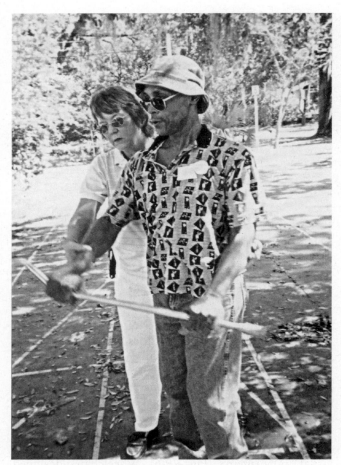

Figure 29-6 Self-defense training with the visually impaired.

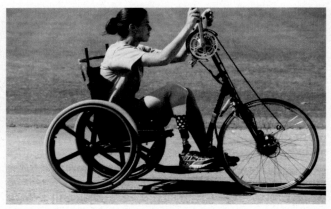

Figure 29-7 Independent or group activity: hand-crank three-wheeled bicycle.

(Wilcock, 1998). This is even more pronounced in leisure. Engagement in leisure promotes health and decreases medical costs. Efforts to provide leisure opportunities for adults with disabilities are gradually increasing as we shift from hospital- to community-based treatment. Our renewed interest in community-based intervention supports our efforts to encourage leisure exploration and develop leisure programs for *all* people. Occupational therapists can become more aware of existing leisure opportunities and integrate leisure activities into assessment and treatment. By forming partnerships to develop and promote leisure options in new areas for people with disabilities, we can improve quality of life.

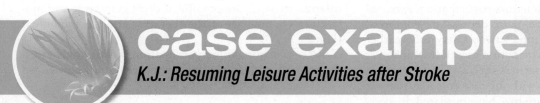

case example

K.J.: Resuming Leisure Activities after Stroke

Occupational Therapy Intervention Process	Clinical Reasoning Process	
	Objectives	Examples of Therapist's Internal Dialogue
Patient Information K.J. is a 42-year-old woman who sustained a left cerebrovascular accident (LCVA) resulting in right-sided paresis. She has good return of right upper extremity muscles but lacks coordination. Muscles of right lower extremity are spastic, and K.J. cannot safely ambulate, so she is learning to use a wheelchair. K.J. feels sad and helpless at times, although she is making steady gains in feeding, dressing, and transferring. Previous leisure interests include playing basketball and driving her sports car.	Appreciate the context	"K.J.'s past lifestyle was active, and she valued mobility. I will bring up leisure adaptations when she is receptive. I will want to encourage gains in self-care activities and help her see how this success can transfer over into engaging in leisure pursuits. It will be important for me to listen to K.J.'s concerns and fears. I will provide examples of disabled athletes and information on wheelchair sports. Maybe I'll show a video of wheelchair athletes playing basketball."

Select an intervention approach	"I will address attitudinal barriers regarding belief in self by structuring successful activities of daily living (ADL) sessions. A visit with a wheelchair basketball player may motivate K.J. to work harder and feel better about the rehab process. I will find a car with hand controls because this may also facilitate interest in driving again."
	"I will strengthen K.J.'s upper extremities by having her engage in ADL tasks as well as using light weights and resistive bands. It makes sense to work on gross and fine motor coordination tasks. I will introduce adaptive equipment and sports chairs for wheelchair basketball and discuss driver training programs. I will remediate skills when possible (strength and coordination) and compensate when necessary (wheelchair for mobility and hand controls for driving)."
Reflect on competence	"I will address ADL tasks and equipment, but I may need to refer K.J. to a wheelchair specialist to prescribe a custom chair. Local wheelchair sports camp (offering basketball and other sports) is available in the summer. I will provide contact info and website addresses regarding sports chairs and the rules of wheelchair basketball. I will identify driver training programs in the area and refer her to a driving specialist."

Recommendations

I will involve K.J. in treatment by making tasks relevant and meaningful. K.J. has begun to realize that basic ADL skills are needed to be able to leave the house. Leisure activities of playing basketball and driving a sports car may motivate her to make the most of her time in therapy. I will provide information on wheelchair basketball rules and sports chairs or refer to the Internet for specifics. I will contact an athlete with a disability (preferably a wheelchair basketball player) to demonstrate that K.J. can still be active even though she has had a stroke. This athlete (former patient) may most likely have a modified car or van if he is a wheelchair user. Having someone with a disability who is also an athlete will serve as an excellent role model for K.J., who is unsure about her abilities.

Consider what will occur in therapy, how often, and for how long	"When K.J. can dress and groom independently (with or without devices), transfer safely from a variety of surfaces, and obtain and maneuver the wheelchair efficiently for 30 minutes, she will be able to physically begin playing basketball with a local group of wheelchair players who practice weekly at the community college. I believe that playing basketball will motivate K.J. to gain strength.
Ascertain the patient's endorsement of plan	My therapy sessions will consist of grooming and dressing with adaptive equipment, increasing upper extremity strength by one muscle grade, increasing tolerance to activity, and practicing transfers from all surfaces and planes. I will expose K.J. to driving equipment and sports chairs. I'll conduct daily therapy sessions for 30 minutes for 2–3 weeks. I want to arrange for a wheelchair basketball athlete to visit K.J. (who may also have car controls on a modified vehicle). Because K.J. is anxious to return to past activities, she is looking forward to meeting the wheelchair player and inspecting a car with hand controls. She is beginning to ask me for info on wheelchair basketball rules and specifics about team practices."
	"I want K.J. to understand the importance of doing daily self-care activities to be independent as well as use muscles on a continuous basis. She told me that she feels better about herself now that she can do more and depend less on others."

"I have seen K.J. improve dramatically; she has been less tearful and more motivated to try activities. The visit with the disabled athlete really helped in introducing her to life in a new but satisfying way. She established an easy rapport with him and shared some of her frustrations and fears. K.J. told her family that she is excited about playing basketball again even though she is in a wheelchair."

Summary of Short-Term Goals and Progress		
1. Dresses and grooms self independently and uses assistive devices for lower extremity dressing (long-handled shoe horn, sock aid, elastic shoelaces). 2. Upper extremity strength has improved by one grade (from 3/5 to 4/5 on Manual muscle testing). 3. Transfers from a variety of surfaces and planes. Able to perform car transfers and is practicing placing wheelchair in back of driver's seat independently. 4. Referred to a driving specialist. Appointment to be made when patient is ready. 5. Wheelchair athlete visited facility and played a one-on-one makeshift game with patient.	Compare actual to expected performance Know the person Appreciate the context	"K.J. has met and surpassed all my short-term goals. Although hesitant about using adaptive equipment, she has learned how to use devices well. I think that she will continue to work on perfecting her turning skills in a wheelchair (for tight turns in basketball practices). I have noticed that K.J. has had a brighter affect since the visit with the wheelchair athlete. I think she finally realizes that she can still engage in her prestroke preferred leisure activities. I know that K.J.'s motivation has made a big difference in her therapy outcomes. K.J. enjoyed her active lifestyle before her stroke and thought that it was all over for her after the LCVA. With encouragement and support from the wheelchair athlete and me, she was able to see that life would be slightly different but she could still engage in these favorite activities."

Next Steps		
1. Prepare patient for discharge by providing specifics on driver training programs (in case identified specialist is not available in the area), sports equipment, and stroke information. 2. Make sure that patient has all equipment (self-care, customized wheelchair) or knows about what equipment would be most beneficial to obtain (e.g., basketball chair). 3. Encourage patient to contact therapist if any problems or questions arise.	Anticipate present and future patient concerns	"I want to make sure K.J. understands how to manage paralysis as well as signs of stroke. I will review stroke risk factors and how to prevent stroke as well as review info on driver training programs."
	Analyze patient's comprehension	"I will ask K.J. to identify ways to minimize stroke. I will have her list strategies she will use at home to take care of daily tasks. Then I'll evaluate her competence in using assistive devices."
	Decide if the patient should continue or discontinue therapy and/or return in the future	"When K.J. is able to take care of all self-care skills and can use her wheelchair effectively, she is ready for discharge. I will make sure that she has all the necessary resources so that she can obtain info or items if she has not been issued them already."

Clinical Reasoning in Occupational Therapy Practice

Promotion of Leisure Exploration

K.J.'s goal of playing wheelchair basketball after sustaining a stroke may take a while to achieve. What are some preparatory leisure activities she could do before engaging in this sport?

Summary Review Questions

1. How would you define leisure to a patient?
2. What are the benefits of engaging in quiet leisure? Active leisure? Socialization?
3. How might leisure goals be different for someone with a stroke? Spinal cord injury? Lower extremity amputation?
4. Describe specific ways that occupational therapists can integrate leisure into evaluation and treatment.
5. What kinds of barriers limit leisure introduction and exploration? How would you remove those barriers in your own practice?
6. Describe the ways in which leisure activities enhance health and wellness for all people, including individuals with disabilities.
7. Discuss the advantages and disadvantages of the various types of leisure assessments described in this chapter.
8. What leisure activities would you recommend for people with no lower extremity use? No use of one side of the body? Overall general weakness?

Glossary

Horticulture therapy—Gardening as a therapeutic intervention.

Leisure—Freely chosen activity that requires control and commitment. Active leisure involves mental and physical exertion (e.g., wheelchair sports), whereas quiet leisure involves activities, such as reading and crafts, that require less physical effort. Socialization entails contact with others via telecommunication, computer, and/or in person.

Occupational imbalance—Excessive time spent in one area, usually work, at the expense of another, usually leisure. May aggravate health and quality of life.

Recreation—Time that is not spent in work or self-care and may or may not result in observable activity; similar to free time.

Therapeutic recreation—Professional use of recreational activities as primary form of treatment with patients; sometimes called recreational therapy.

Therapeutic recreation specialist—Trained professional who uses recreational activities as a therapeutic intervention with patients.

References

American Occupational Therapy Association. (2008). Occupational therapy practice framework: Domain and process (2nd ed.) *American Journal of Occupational Therapy, 62,* 625–683.

Beard, J. G., & Ragheb, M. G. (1980). Measuring leisure satisfaction. *Journal of Leisure Research, 12,* 20–33.

Beard, J. G., & Ragheb, M. G. (1983). Measuring leisure motivation. *Journal of Leisure Research, 15,* 219–228.

Beard, J. G., & Ragheb, M. G. (1990). Leisure Interest Measure. Paper presented at the meeting of the National Recreation and Park Association Symposium on Leisure Research, Phoenix, AZ. October 12-15, 1990 in Arizona. Publisher: National Recreation and Park Association, Alexandria, VA.

Brachtesende, A. (2005). ICF: The universal translator. *OT Practice, 10,* 14–17.

Buchholz, A. C., Martin Ginis, K. A., Bray, S. R., Craven, B. C., Hicks, A. L., Hayes, K. C., Latimer, A. E., McColl, M. A., Potter, P. J., & Wolfe, D. L. (2009). Greater daily leisure time physical activity is associated with lower chronic disease risk in adults with spinal cord injury. *Applied Physiology, Nutrition and Metabolism, 34,* 640–647.

Bulthuis, Y., Drossaers-Bakker, K. W., Taal. E., Rasker, J., Oostveen, J., van't Pad Bosch, P., Oosterveld, F., & van de Laar, M. (2007). Arthritis patients show long-term benefits from 3 weeks intensive exercise training directly following hospital discharge. *Rheumatology, 46,* 1712–1717.

de Jong, Z., Munneke, M., Zwinderman, A. H., Kroon, H. M., Jansen, A., Ronday, K. H., van Schaardenburg, D., Dijkmans, B. A., Van den Ende, C. H., Breedveld, F. C., Vliet Vlieland, T. P., & Hazes, J. M. (2003). Is a long-term high-intensity exercise program effective and safe in patients with rheumatoid arthritis? Results of a randomized controlled trial. *Arthritis and Rheumatology, 48,* 2415–2424.

Desrosiers, J., Noreau, L., Rochette, A., Carbonneau, H., Fontaine, L., Viscogliosi, C., & Bravo, G. (2007). Effect of a home leisure education program after stroke: A randomized control trial. *Archives of Physical Medicine and Rehabilitation, 88,* 1095–1100.

Drummond, A., & Walker, M. (1994). The Nottingham Leisure Questionnaire for stroke patients. *British Journal of Occupational Therapy, 57,* 414–418.

Durstine, J. L., Painter, P., Franklin, B. A., Morgan, D., Pitetti, K. H., & Roberts, S. O. (2000). Physical activity for the chronically ill and disabled. *Sports Medicine, 30,* 207–219.

Elsawy, B., & Higgins, K. E. (2010). Physical activity guidelines for older adults. *American Family Physician, 81,* 55–59.

Esser, S., & Bailey, A. (2011). Effects of exercise and physical activity on knee osteoarthritis. *Current Pain and Headache Reports, 15,* 423–430.

Hanson, C. (1998). A sports exploration camp for adults with disabilities. *OT Practice, 3,* 35–38.

Harnish, S. (2001). Gardening for life- adaptive techniques and tools. *OT Practice, 6,* 12–15.

Hoffmann, L., Williford, R., Mooney, B., Brown, C., & Davis, C. (1995). Leisure activities provide rehab potential. *Case Management Advisor, 6,* 71.

Jungbloed, L., & Morgan, D. (1991). An investigation of involvement in leisure activities after stroke. *American Journal of Occupational Therapy, 45,* 420–427.

Kautzmann, L. (1984). Identifying leisure interests: A self-assessment approach for adults with arthritis. *Occupational Therapy in Health Care, 2,* 45–51.

Klein, P. J., & Adams, W. D. (2004). Comprehensive therapeutic benefits of taiji: A critical review. *American Journal of Physical Medicine, 83,* 735–745.

Kuster, M. S. (2002). Exercise recommendations after total joint replacement. *Sports Medicine, 32,* 433–445.

Law, M. (2002). Participation in the occupations of everyday life. *American Journal of Occupational Therapy, 56,* 640–649.

Law, M., Polatajko, H., Pollock, N., McColl, M. A., Carswell, A., & Baptiste, S. (1994). Pilot testing of the Canadian Occupational Performance Measure: Clinical and measurement issues. *Canadian Journal of Occupational Therapy, 61,* 191–197.

Lin, S. (1991). Content validity and test-retest reliability of the Lin Interest Check List. Unpublished thesis. Richmond: Virginia Commonwealth University.

Logan, P. A., Gladman, J. R. F., Drummond, A. E. R., & Radford, K. A. (2003). A study of interventions and related outcomes in a randomized controlled trial of occupational therapy and leisure therapy for community stroke patients. *Clinical Rehabilitation, 17,* 249–255.

Mallinson, T., Waldinger, H., Semanik, P., Lyons, J., Feinglass, J., & Chang, R. W. (2005). Promoting physical activity in persons with arthritis. *OT Practice, 10,* 10–14.

Matsutsuyu, J. (1967). The Interest Checklist. *American Journal of Occupational Therapy, 11,* 170–181.

Minor, M. A., & Lane, N. E. (1996). Recreational exercise in arthritis. *Rheumatic Disease Clinics of North America, 22,* 563–577.

Motl, R. W., & McAuley, E. (2010). Physical activity, disability, and quality of life in older adults. *Physical Medicine Rehabilitation Clinics North America, 21,* 299–308.

Painter, P. (2003). Exercise for patients with chronic disease: Physician responsibility. *Current Sports Medicine Report, 2,* 173–180.

Radomski, M. V., Finkelstein, M., Hagel, S., Masemer, S., Theis, J., & Thompson, M. (2011). A pilot wellness and weight management program for individuals with spinal cord injury: Participant's goals and outcomes. *Topics in Spinal Cord Injury Rehabilitation, 17,* 59–69.

Ragheb, M. G., & Beard, J. G. (1982). Measuring leisure attitude. *Journal of Leisure Research, 14,* 155–167.

Sacco, R. L., Gan, R., Boden-Albala, B., Lin, I. F., Kargman, D. E, Hauser, W. A., Shea, S., & Paik, M. C. (1998). Leisure-time physical activity and ischemic stroke risk: The Northern Manhattan Stroke Study. *Stroke, 29,* 380–387.

Salem, Y., Scott, A. H., Karpatkin, H., Concert, G., Haller, L., Kaminsky, E., Weisbrot, R., & Spatz, E. (2011). Community-based group aquatic programme for individuals with multiple sclerosis: A pilot study. *Disability and Rehabilitation, 33,* 720–728.

Soderback, I., & Hammarlund, C. (1993). A leisure-time frame of reference based on a literature analysis. *Occupational Therapy in Health Care, 8,* 105–133.

Sporner, M. L., Fitzgerald, S. G., Dicianno, B. E., Collins, D., Teodorski, E., Pasquina, P. F., & Cooper, R. A. (2009). Psychosocial impact of participation in National Wheelchair Games and Winter Sports Clinic. *Disability Rehabilitation, 31,* 410–418.

Taylor-Piliae, R. E., & Haskell, W. L. (2007). Tai Chi and stroke rehabilitation. *Topics in Stroke Rehabilitation, 14,* 9–22.

Warburton, D. E. R., Sproule, S., Krassioukov, A., & Eng, J. J. (2010). Cardiovascular health and exercise following spinal cord injury. In J. J. Eng, R. W. Teasell, W. C. Miller, D. L. Wolfe, A. F. Townson, J. T. C. Hsieh, S. J. Connolly, S. Mehta, & B. M. Sakakibara (Eds.), *Spinal Cord Injury Rehabilitation Evidence,* Version 3.0 (pp. 1–38). Vancouver, British Columbia and London, Ontario.

Washburn, R. A., Zhu, W., McAuley, E., Frogley, M., & Figoni, S. F. (2002). The physical activity scale for individuals with physical disabilities: Development and evaluation. *Archives of Physical Medicine and Rehabilitation, 83,* 193–200.

White, L. J., & Dressendorfer, R. H. (2004). Exercise and multiple sclerosis. *Sports Medicine, 34,* 1077–1100.

Wilcock, A. A. (1998). Occupation for health. *British Journal of Occupational Therapy, 61,* 340–345.

Wolf, S. L., Sattin, R. W., Kutner, M., O'Grady, M., Greenspan, A. I., & Gregor, R. J. (2003). Intense Tai Chi exercise training and fall occurrence in older transitionally frail adults: A randomized controlled trial. *Journal of the American Geriatrics Society, 51,* 1693–1701.

World Health Organization. (2002). *International Classification of Functioning. Disability and Health (ICF).* Geneva, Switzerland: World Health Organization.

Wu, S. K., & Williams, T. (2000). Factors influencing sport participation among athletes with spinal cord injury. *Medicine and Science in Sports and Exercise, 33,* 177–182.

Acknowledgements

We thank Pat Dasler for her case study contribution and Laurie Manuel and Gary Rudolph for the photographs.

Optimizing Personal and Social Adaptation

Jo M. Solet

Learning Objectives

After studying this chapter, the reader will be able to do the following:

1. Integrate the psychosocial perspective in formulating a rehabilitation program.
2. Consider alternative practice models and value their application within the therapeutic relationship.
3. Place patients within life-cycle and family contexts and recognize the implications of this placement for occupations and life roles.
4. Understand the impact of history and course of disability on psychosocial adaptation.
5. Appreciate existential issues raised by illness, injury, and disability; describe ways individuals construct meaning from these experiences.
6. Be alert for psychiatric complications and recognize indications for referral.

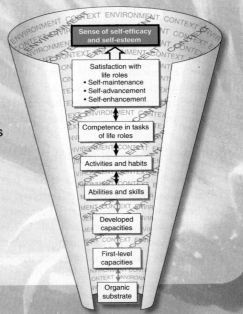

Man's origin is dust and his end is dust. He spends his life earning bread. He is a clay vessel, easily broken, like withering grass, a fading flower, a passing shadow, a fugitive cloud, a fleeting breeze, a scattering dust, a vanishing dream. (Mazor for Rosh Hashanah and Yom Kippur: A Prayer Book for the Days of Awe, 1972)

The immediate change in physical functioning that an individual undergoes as a result of illness or injury is not alone a sufficient predictor of the capacity to benefit from treatment or of the future quality of life. Although the adaptation process may follow a general outline of stages, it is unique for each person and is influenced by the circumstances of onset and course, by age and place in the life cycle, and by the specific personality with characteristic ways of coping. This chapter begins by introducing practice models and treatment structures that address the psychosocial perspective and then guides the reader through life contexts, psychological, and social factors, which must be considered in individualizing occupational therapy (OT) treatment for physical disabilities.

PRACTICE MODELS

Each practice model uses its own theoretical framework to interpret clinical observations, guide treatment planning, and promote recovery. Many occupational therapists use components of more than one of these models; this can lead to rich, empathic, creative treatment, and fruitful participation with the treatment team.

Psychodynamic Model

The psychodynamic practice model, which had its origin in Freud's theories, emphasizes the relationship with the therapist as providing a safe, empathic, and consistent environment in which healing may take place (Rowe & MacIsaac, 1991). It considers patients' internal experiences; conscious and unconscious longings for wholeness, love, and protection; and conflicts about dependency and helplessness. Motivation is conceived as the critical element for successful rehabilitation. The psychodynamic model both values the symbolic nature of activities and mandates that they be selected for intrinsic meaning and relevance for the patient.

Cognitive-Behavioral Model

The cognitive-behavioral practice model focuses therapeutic efforts on the development of patterns of thinking and specific behaviors (Burns, 1990). Therapists who incorporate cognitive-behavioral treatment (CBT) become careful observers and recorders, examining patients' reactions to their experiences and the interactions among their ways of thinking and ways of behaving. These therapists reward successive graded goals shaping thoughts and behaviors that indicate successful adaptation. They point out patterns in client narratives that suggest helplessness or negative projections about the future, helping to substitute more positive thoughts and self-statements. Treatment programs reinforce adherence and good self-care, such as wearing a splint or taking medication, and work to extinguish damaging habits, such as smoking, and socially isolating behaviors, such as aggressive outbursts. CBT treatment components may be designed for individual or group work directed toward specific symptoms including pain, depression, or insomnia (Perlis et al., 2008). Skills for self-regulation, including assertive communication and practicing the relaxation response (RR), may also be components of cognitive-behavioral treatment (Benson & Proctor, 2010).

Relaxation Response

As a component of treatment, the RR bridges conceptual models and is frequently applied in CBT and the Wellness Model (below) (Hamilton, Kitzman, & Guyotte, 2006). The RR is a natural physiological state of deep rest that counteracts stress by lowering heart rate, blood pressure, respiratory rate, and muscle tension. Because the RR and meditative techniques are often sought by patients coping with medical and psychological problems, current evidence related to safety and efficacy continues to receive careful review (Arias et al., 2006; Ospina et al., 2007). Research supports the benefits including decreased emotional distress and improved autonomic and psychoimmune responses (Benson & Proctor, 2010; Kiecolt-Glaser et al., 2010); brain changes related to enhancement of learning and memory, and perspective taking (e.g., empathy, compassion, self-awareness) (Holzel et al., 2011); and even gene expression changes associated with positive physiological outcomes (Dusek et al., 2008).

The RR can be elicited by a number of techniques involving mental focusing through repetition of a word, sound, phrase, prayer, image, or physical activity in the context of passive disregard of ongoing thoughts (Benson, 1993). Techniques include progressive muscle relaxation (PMR), diaphragmatic breathing, and practices such as mindfulness, meditation, Tai Chi, and yoga. As a foundation structure of the RR, focus on the breath is a powerful and ancient tool with a history in various religious and spiritual traditions (see Procedures for Practice 30-1 for basic RR directions). Breathing is a process that is automatic yet also available to personal control and observation through which both physiological state and parallel state of mind may be altered. Nonevaluative attention to in-and-out breaths is undertaken to bring a present-centered mindfulness and compassionate nonattachment to the ebb and flow of inner life. When taught in therapeutic settings, these practices are directed at symptoms such as anxiety, pain, depression, and insomnia. Mindfulness can be practiced in sitting meditation as well as with any occupation: walking, eating, bathing, or stroking a pet.

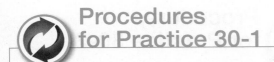

Procedures for Practice 30-1

Directions for Use in Eliciting the Relaxation Response

- Pick a focus word, short phrase, or prayer that is firmly rooted in your belief system, such as "one," "peace," "The Lord is my shepherd," "Hail Mary, full of grace," or "shalom."
- Sit quietly in a comfortable position.
- Close your eyes.
- Relax your muscles, progressing from your feet to your calves, thighs, abdomen, shoulders, head, and neck.
- Breathe slowly and naturally, and as you do, say your focus word, sound, phrase, or prayer silently to yourself as you exhale.
- Assume a passive attitude. Don't worry about how well you're doing. When other thoughts come to mind, simply say to yourself, "Oh well," and gently return to your repetition.
- Continue for 10–20 minutes.
- Do not stand immediately. Continue sitting quietly for a minute or so, allowing other thoughts to return. Then open your eyes and sit for another minute before rising.
- Practice the technique once or twice daily. Good times to do so are before breakfast and before dinner.

From Benson-Henry Institute for Mind Body Medicine, Massachusetts General Hospital. (2013). *Eliciting the relaxation response.* Retrieved from http://www.massgeneral.org/bhi/basics/eliciting_rr.aspx

With the development of a mindful focus, proponents believe that daily experience need not be held hostage to regret or fear of the future (Chodron, 1997). Through release from old habits of thought and feeling, mindfulness and other meditative practices are believed to generate novel and creative responses that support psychological resilience. Along with benefits, adverse effects from meditation practices, including psychosis, have also been documented (Arias et al., 2006). In taking patients' occupational history, the culturally aware therapist reviews current and past use of meditation and other spiritual practices, including prayer, yoga, Tai Chi, and Qi Gong. Occupational therapists interested in incorporating RR practices as part of their treatment model seek special training and supervision to adapt programs. For example, Stoller et al. (2012) adapted a yoga program through sensory enhancements to address combat stress in military personnel.

Wellness Model

Research over the past decade confirms that we function as integrated organisms, with changes in one bodily system felt throughout. Separation of the mind from the body is an academic exercise rather than a true reflection of the functioning of the human organism. Mainstream medicine now recognizes important relationships between immune functioning and psychological health first proposed in the early 1980s (Ader, 1981). Psychological states such as depression (Denollet, 1998) and anxiety (Kubzansky et al., 1998) are now routinely assessed as risk factors for heart disease, not just as reactions to it. In addition, the growing preventive perspective in health care has begun to define the behaviors and habits related to sleep (Chien et al., 2010), nutrition (Buning, 1999), and exercise (Ratey & Hagerman, 2009) that, through multiple interconnected channels, are likely to extend life and lead to greater physical and psychological well-being.

Health behaviors may be difficult to address, and psychological well-being may be difficult to achieve in the face of the stresses such as pain and limited mobility, compromised social integration, and altered sleep and appetite. The occupational therapist works with other members of the clinical team to ensure that treatment addresses a foundation of health-promoting behaviors to support maintenance of function and reserve capacity of organ systems in those with chronic disabling conditions.

Model of Human Occupation

Although the cognitive-behavioral and psychodynamic models are also applied by psychologists, social workers, and psychiatrists, the Model of Human Occupation (Kielhofner, 1992) evolved in the context of OT. This model focuses on engagement in the experience of living. The client is recognized as "an occupational being for whom access and participation in meaningful and productive activities is central to health and well-being" (American Occupational Therapy Association [AOTA], 2002, p. 613). Human activities are defined as multidimensional: physical, social, spiritual, and symbolic, and as embedded within each individual's specific psychological, and cultural contexts (AOTA, 2008). Evaluation in this model considers strengths and difficulties in occupational behaviors that are necessary to the fulfillment of life roles such as worker, parent, or friend. Treatment seeks to develop, remediate, or enhance performance and support occupational balance (Anaby, 2010). Success in occupational performance is inherently organizing to the personality and is importantly related to feelings of mastery, competence, group acceptance, and sense of identity (AOTA, 1995a, 1995b).

PRACTICE STRUCTURES

Practice structures associated with service delivery influence efforts to optimize patient personal and social adaptation. Occupational therapists work with patients individually and in groups. Group participation is often an adjunct to or follow-up for individual treatment.

Individual Treatment

Individual treatment is framed by the therapeutic relationship, the alliance between a patient and therapist, which begins during the evaluation period (see Chapter 14 for an in-depth discussion of therapeutic rapport). As the relationship develops, the occupational therapist learns not only about the physical capacities of the patient, such as strength and range of motion, but also about the type and degree of explanation the patient will find helpful during the course of treatment.

Patients who retain the capacity may wish to tell their story, describing to the occupational therapist how the illness or injury came to pass, their reactions to it, their losses, and their expectations of recovery. Listening attentively to patients' stories, even when their histories are available in some form in the medical record, develops trust and tells patients that they are unique and their feelings and experiences are valued. Listening also supplies important information about interaction and communication ability, mood states such as depression or anxiety, ways of coping, and family and cultural contexts. All of these are critical to formulating social and psychological goals as part of intervention planning.

Group Treatment

Group treatment supplies a practice environment for patients' social participation, a therapeutic envelope or safe holding environment that is broader than that of individual treatment. Groups have a developmental progression over time depending on the chosen activities and capacities of participants: from parallel activity, through brief interactions, to mature camaraderie and supportive cooperation (Donohue, Hanif, & Berns, 2011). Group treatment interrupts isolation and provides a context within which to identify and solve common problems. Groups may be organized to address goals related to specific disabilities, to promote mastery of skills, to practice leisure or creative activities, or to facilitate transitions. Multiple family groups may be organized to help members socialize and adapt to caregiving roles (Rodgers et al., 2007). Although the primary focus of any specific group may not be to address psychological or social needs, treatment components influence participants' total well-being and provide a shared space for creating dignity, responsibility, meaning, and pleasure (Ziegler, 1999).

As groups evolve beyond parallel participation into interaction among members, participants support and learn from each other and begin to value themselves more highly. A group can also serve as a magnifying glass in which difficult behavior can be brought under the observation of others. When supportive confrontation is used to address and modify this behavior, it improves an individual's opportunities outside the treatment setting. When group discussions deepen, they provide for disclosure of grief and fears, for voicing existential concerns, for organizing personal

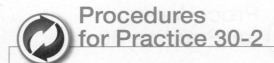

Procedures for Practice 30-2

Planning Group Treatment

Choosing Goals for Group Participation

- Practicing social behaviors
- Following rules and recognizing group needs
- Identifying and solving common problems
- Learning specific skills and activities
- Accepting supportive confrontation and modifying behavior
- Disclosing feelings, existential concerns, and shared hopes
- Enhancing self-esteem through supporting others

Considerations for Choosing Group Members

- Cognitive and social capacities
- Readiness for broader interaction
- Congruence with other members
- Attention and memory
- Psychosis and dangerousness
- Communication ability
- Cultural background
- Energy limits

narratives, and for engendering shared hopes (Alonso & Swiller, 1993). Occupational therapists include these social and psychological goals in all group planning, treatment, and documentation (Procedures for Practice 30-2).

THE ADAPTATION PROCESS

Substantial individual variations in psychological and social adaptation to disability are related to many factors including the onset, course, and severity of the disability; the patient's age and place in the life cycle; and individual differences in personality, ways of coping, and attributing meaning to experience. In addition, access to quality care, accessible housing, barrier-free public transportation, and consistent social and community connection support occupational participation and the adaptation process (Crawford et al., 2008; Jenkins, 2011). Some illnesses and disabilities that limit occupational participation are "visible" to the layman and may affect the way individuals are treated in the social and vocational contexts. Other "invisible" disabilities require patients to make choices about disclosure and the need to seek special accommodations. As part of therapeutic support for adaptation, occupational therapists address patients' experiences in social and vocational arenas by engaging with them about disability disclosure issues related to employment barriers, adaptive technology, and housing (Griffin, 2011).

Stage Theories

Viewing adaptation to disability as a natural course of stages, such as denial, resistance, affirmation and integration or shock, denial, anger, depression, and acceptance (Miner, 1999), can be a useful way to conceptualize the psychological reorganization. In reality, these stages may flow together and even be reexperienced as new challenges arise (Dewar & Lee, 2000). Conflicts and unmet needs in love and work, unresolved before illness or injury, may assume greater proportions. Clinicians may unconsciously protect themselves from recognizing the realities of living with a disability by assuming that all patients are passing through a natural series of stages that will lead to a satisfying outcome. Adaptation to mild disability may be substantial by 3 years. However, even at 4 years, the process is likely to be less complete following severe disability, as measured by satisfaction with income, social life, and leisure activities (Powdthavee, 2009).

The four phases from acute injury through rehabilitation described by Morse and O'Brien (1995) constitute a template that may help therapists to recognize changing psychological states and anticipate the needs of their patients. The empirical study of traumatic injury and hospitalization upon which the stages are based demonstrates the special challenges of traumatic onset and offers illustrations of each stage using the language of patients' own recollections.

The first phase, "vigilance: becoming engulfed," encompasses the overwhelming physiological insult in which extraordinary cognitive efforts and heightened senses are recruited to preserve life. During this period immediately following traumatic injury, some patients in the study recalled detachment, a sense of being both observer and participant, as they began to direct the helpers who had arrived to care for them.

The second phase, "disruption: taking time out," begins when the individual relinquishes responsibility to caregivers or becomes unconscious. Patients remembered this part of their experience as a fog in which they were lost between nightmares and intolerable wakefulness. Patients in critical condition could not distinguish reality or focus beyond themselves. They were disoriented, heavily sedated, and not in control of their reactions. Patients at this stage sometimes perceived their caregivers as dangerous and the environment as hostile. Recognizing that during this stage many patients are afraid to be alone, the occupational therapist in the acute setting may facilitate the continuous presence of friends and family members, enlisting their help in orienting the patient.

The third phase, "enduring the self: confronting and regrouping," starts as the patient becomes more aware of his or her surroundings and begins to recognize the extent of the injuries. This is a time of focus on the present in which the conscious decision to carry on and rejoin the world must be made, even as growing awareness intensifies the psychological pain. Patients in the study described fear, panic over complete dependence, dread of painful treatments, and desperate efforts at control. During this stage, patients expressed shock at the loss of their former selves and began to anchor to staff and others for support and assistance. Some expressed an idealized view of their past selves as competent and attractive and their lives before the disablement as fully satisfying. Often, they believed full recovery would occur in weeks or months, even with severe spinal cord injuries; the smallest gains were very important.

This is a time when the sensitivity of caregivers is critical for supporting hope. The therapist avoids making predictions and promises about the expected degree of recovery, because these may later prove unattainable, compromising the therapeutic relationship and leaving the patient feeling cheated, angry, resentful, and depressed (Davidhizer, 1997). Although hopes are often initially focused on full recovery, such as "walking again" after spinal cord injury, over time with successful adaptation, hopes are likely to evolve toward the development of life quality and satisfaction (Dorset, 2010). An early intervention for certain patients during this stage is training in diaphragmatic breathing to induce the RR. As described earlier, breathing may provide the first avenue for perceived self-control.

The last stage, "striving to regain the self: merging the old and new reality," is the period of physical and psychological challenge in which active rehabilitation takes place. Goals include making sense of the experience, getting to know the altered body, and accepting the consequences, including the possibility of continued dependency. This is the stage during which patients may begin to revise and reformulate expectations. The OT treatment plan integrates these psychological demands and addresses them in concert with activities of daily living, strengthening, endurance, mobility, and prevocational training. As preparation for the social situations that may be encountered after discharge from the protective rehabilitation environment, treatment anticipates and addresses fears of inadequacy and of rejection by others (Gardner, 1999). Participation in group treatment, including role-playing specific situations, such as facing direct questions about the disability or about altered appearance, may be a component of this social preparation.

Onset and Course

The circumstances of onset and the course of the specific disability are important factors influencing the adaptation process.

Early Onset

When an individual is born with a disability such as spina bifida or has an injury in early childhood, the sense of self develops continuously with the disability, typically within the framework of the family and often with the support of therapy mandated through school programs. The challenge for the individual born with a disability or disabled in early childhood is to grow into each life stage encountering new developmental expectations—physical, psychological, and social. A disability that does not have major effects in childhood may later become significant as cognitive, emotional, and behavioral demands change and expectations for independence increase (Simkins, 1999). A significant proportion of individuals with early disabilities later develop new medical, functional, and support needs as they reach their forties and fifties (Kemp, 2005). Through a series of interviews with adults disabled as children, King et al. (1993) identified three pathways—belonging, doing, and understanding—through which challenges were met at these life "turning points." Successful adaptation came through social support, described as feeling "believed in"; through determination and the conviction that challenges could be met; and through realization, by changing beliefs and expectations.

Degenerative Illness

When disability has a slow onset and course, as is the case with degenerative illnesses such as rheumatoid arthritis and multiple sclerosis, increasing disability is expected. Degenerative illnesses are not fully predictable; the course may be slow or rapid, complicating efforts to retain control over the life course. Each loss can feel like a reminder, a new insult. In multiple sclerosis, for example, there may be plateaus or even periods when symptoms remit but later recur (Hwang et al., 2011). Postpoliomyelitis syndrome occurs in a different pattern. Seventy percent of individuals who had a primary polio infection years before develop new symptoms, such as fatigue, pain, and atrophy, that require them to revisit struggles from their past (Thoren-Jonsson, 2001). Some with degenerative illnesses may stretch to the limits of their physical capacity in an effort to maintain occupations intrinsic to their life roles and to remain connected to valued peer groups. Ideally, as symptoms progress, processes of realization and reorganization bring with them adaptation and an acceptable compromise including altered patterns and balance of daily occupations (Jonsson, Moller, & Grimby, 1998). Maintenance of a hopeful attitude is more difficult when stabilization or improvement in quality of life cannot be anticipated (Dorset, 2010). The challenges of degenerative illness are to adjust self-concept, continually adapt to reorganized life roles, maintain internal resources, and evolve concrete supports in the face of impending decline (Boeije et al., 2002).

Traumatic Injury and Illness of Rapid Onset

Traumatic injuries, such as spinal cord injury, and disease processes with extremely rapid onset, such as Guillain-Barré syndrome, do not allow for psychological preparation (Ville et al., 2001). The dramatic nature of the onset may quickly exhaust the reserves of friends and family. Affected individuals may undergo not only an immediate change in ability to function but also a discontinuity in time and sense of self, a loss of personal identity, and a shift in confidence about the world as safe and just (Morse & O'Brien, 1995). The individual is also at risk for development of post-traumatic stress disorder (PTSD), characterized by hyperarousal and reexperience of the trauma known as flashbacks (Champagne, Koomar, & Olsen, 2010).

Late Effects of Traumatic Injury

Decisions made earlier in life can have serious consequences for later abilities. Evidence of the long-term effects of repetitive head trauma leading to chronic traumatic encephalopathy (CTE) has now been conclusively linked to participation in contact sports such as football, boxing, wrestling, and soccer (Stern et al., 2011). Efforts are underway to document the mechanisms and relate function to extent of the damage. This is needed to better inform policy for the protection of millions of school and professional athletes. Military personnel are also at risk from blast effects and from accumulated concussive injuries, with full consequences potentially manifesting years after service. Individuals at risk or already showing effects are challenged to reorganize their plans around uncertainty and the possibility of progressive decline. Cognitive, mood, and behavioral symptoms such as memory changes, depression, emotional instability, and poor impulse control may compromise coping strategies and undermine important supporting relationships (Stern et al., 2011). An added burden for some affected individuals is the recognition that their progressive disability may have been preventable. Attention to the neurodegenerative effects of repetitive head trauma is decades overdue.

Disability and the Life Cycle

The developmental tasks of each period of life are biologically, socially, and culturally determined and build upon those that have preceded them (Franz & White, 1985). Therefore, the point in a person's life at which he or she becomes disabled, together with the trajectory and severity of the disability, helps to determine what will be entailed in the long-term process of adaptation. The occupational therapist holds in mind the developmental demands of a patient's place in the life cycle and addresses ways in which these demands may be met even within the context of disability.

Adolescence

Currently, 90% of those born in the United States with a disability live to at least age 20 years (Schultz & Liptak, 1998). Along with the usual challenges of young adulthood,

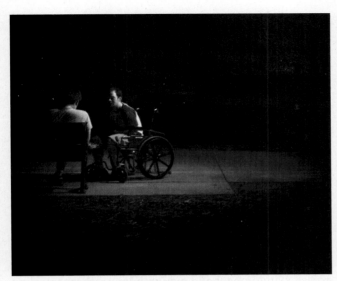

Figure 30-1 Running partners. (Black and white photo by Paul Solet, Los Angeles, CA; see paulsolet.com.)

including transition from school to work and from parents and family to the broader community, those disabled at birth or in childhood must negotiate the change from child to adult health care. This can include losing long-term supportive relationships and taking increased responsibility for care coordination and decision making (Schultz & Liptak, 1998). When adolescents or young adults who have already acquired some independence from their parents become disabled, they may find being thrown back into childhood dependence especially painful. Psychological distress in adult rehabilitation inpatients has been reported to be greatest among these younger patients (Laatsch & Shahani, 1996).

The emphasis on peer acceptance, athletic ability, physical appearance, and emerging sexuality at this time of life puts the disabled young adult at special risk for rejection and social isolation; development of social competence is an especially important contributor to successful adaptation (King et al., 1993) (Fig. 30-1). In addition, as they reach the age that society presumes coincides with independence, young adults may no longer qualify for the instruction and therapy available through many public schools and mandated by law when they were younger. Research confirms the need for community-based transition services to support adolescents with disabilities in "building bridges" to the adult world (Stewart et al., 2001).

Adulthood

The developmental tasks of adulthood may include confirming career choice, finding a partner, and parenting children. When an adult at this point in the life cycle becomes disabled, plans and conceptions about the future, which may already have been the focus of substantial effort, require reorganizing. Adapting to disability occurring at this stage may require altering vocational course, finding different leisure activities,

redesigning an intimate partnership, and rebalancing parenting roles, just when some sense of competence and direction has been won (Rena, Moshe, & Abraham, 1996).

Midlife

A disability that strikes in midlife may find the individual at the peak of his or her career mastery and earning capacity, sometimes with adolescent children or aging parents as dependents. Although a history of successful coping with multiple life roles may already exist, this may be a difficult time to accommodate change and reorganize responsibilities (Quigly, 1995). Available resources may be limited, especially when the disabled person has been serving as the financial head of the household. Historically, disabled workers age 18–60 years have been shown to have substantially lower adjusted family incomes than others in the same age brackets and to be twice as likely to live in poverty (Social Security Administration, n.d.). A person disabled at midlife may feel prematurely aged, deprived of the anticipated leisure activity of healthy retirement and the hard-earned relief that follows discharge of career and parenting duties. In addition, marriage or intimate partnership may be at risk, because some nondisabled partners choose to avoid additional demands or find that the now-disabled partner seems no longer to be the same person they married.

Later Life

The rising wave of aging "baby boomers" will provide a special challenge to health care resources in the next decades. Disability in later life, even at a time when health decline may be anticipated, threatens the individual's ability to participate in the community in which he or she may have a long history and feel an important identification. Isolation is common. The elderly person may be realistically worried about losing his or her home or may already be institutionalized. He or she may be concerned about being a financial or care burden to an aging partner or to children who are stressed by their own responsibilities. Many caregivers of individuals older than 65 years are themselves older and in fair to poor health. Anticipated generative roles such as grandparent or mentor, with the opportunity to offer wisdom and nurturance, may be short-circuited. An elderly disabled person may already have lost his or her social cohort and main supporting relationships. Interests and leisure activities developed over a lifetime may have to be abandoned and efforts made to find other satisfactions (Hasselkus, 1991). Furthermore, the devaluation of the elderly in our society, commonly combined with limited financial resources, can compromise care and undermine motivation (Kemp, 1993). The experience of overwhelming loss without hope for the future can lead to despair. Just as when working with younger patients, the occupational therapist models a problem-solving mindset with realistic expectations, reconciling capacities and marshalling patient strengths toward a sense of fulfillment (Bontje et al., 2004). When remaining time before death is limited, some elderly people feel an urgent need to undertake a life review, drawing together the strands of meaning from their past. The occupational therapist recognizes the privilege of participating in this life-review process (Frank, 1996).

Individual Differences

Patients come to treatment with formed personalities and ways of interacting with the world that may or may not have been healthy or effective even before the injury or illness. Patients may regress during hospitalization when deprived of occupations, relationships, and areas of control that supported their personal and cultural identities. Some must deal with lost bowel or bladder function or inability to walk, capacities that they developed as babies. Others may have cognitive or memory changes that diminish their ability to make plans or follow directions. Those hospitalized for medical problems are known to suffer more psychiatric illness than their healthy peers, especially depression (Joseph, 2005). Some patients seem easy to treat; others are recalcitrant, uncooperative, or resistant. Some become increasingly demanding, ask for special treatment, break rules, and exhaust all efforts (Main, 1957). Some appeal to the therapist's wishes to rescue them; others, in their failure to improve, stir feelings of disappointment, shame, and helplessness in the therapist (Groves, 1978; Kahana & Bibring, 1964). It is some comfort for the new occupational therapist to recognize that these feelings are all part of the normal experience of being a clinician. Collegial support and knowledgeable supervision can help with the treatment of difficult patients and the management of the therapist's own feelings.

Personality

Individual differences in personality, along with variations in cultural context and personal history, contribute to the uniqueness of responses to illness and injury. It is often said about head injury: "It is not just the injury, but the head that matters." Serious stresses may intensify normal fears, longings, and relationship demands. Ongoing pain, with the attendant loss of sleep and degraded sense of mastery, can further alter functioning. Psychiatric illness and character problems can be exacerbated by threats to physical health and the integrity of the body (Zegans, 1991). The occupational therapist treats each individual as unique and addresses distinctions among an array of personality styles (Kahana & Bibring, 1964) and ways of coping (Solet, 1991).

Personality characteristics that have driven an individual's career choices and have helped define relationships may be a mismatch for the requirements of hospitalization. Patients who are orderly, punctual, and conscientious may find that perceived loss of control distorts their self-esteem. They may react by becoming demanding, inflexible, and obstinate; if they become openly angry, they may feel ashamed (Kahana & Bibring, 1964). A clinical approach that is congenial, efficient, predictable, and routine and that includes explanations and appropriate inclusion in decision making is most reassuring for these individuals. The occupational therapist takes special care in pacing and grading challenges to provide for and recognize periods of control and success.

Patients who have a history of loss, helplessness, abuse, or abandonment may react to illness or injury with fears that no one will take care of them. They may make intense, urgent demands and seem overly dependent, angry if disappointed, occasionally impulsive, and insatiable in their need for reassurance. Some, feeling unlovable, may expect abandonment and may withdraw rather than cling (Kahana & Bibring, 1964). A successful clinical approach for these individuals includes readiness to give care and to show concern, along with setting limits that are consistent and not punitive. Good coordination between caregivers is especially important for these patients, who sometimes compare team members or complain about one team member to another.

Some individuals act guarded or suspicious when hospitalized (Kahana & Bibring, 1964). These characteristics may be an intensified part of their usual personality but may also arise from the disorientation and lost sense of continuity that can accompany illness or injury. Neurological and sensory changes can make relatively ordinary events difficult for patients to interpret; a right-hemisphere lesion or even the loss of eyeglasses or a hearing aid may have important ramifications. The occupational therapist is alert to the variety of conditions and diagnoses that may relate to such behavior. Wary, suspicious patients may need continual orienting and often benefit from the reassurance and company of friends or family. The occupational therapist uses language patients can understand to acknowledge their worries, answer questions, and address complaints without arguing or reinforcing false observations. Especially if suspiciousness evolves or becomes more elaborate, the occupational therapist seeks neurological or psychiatric consultation.

Patients may react to their helpless state by asserting their importance, being smug or grandiose, or demanding that only the most esteemed clinicians be involved in their care. When they are deprived of the surroundings, belongings, and roles from which they derive identity, dignity, and status, patients need confirmation that these things are recognized. The occupational therapist uses history taking as a time to begin offering this recognition and acknowledgment. Repeatedly feeling forced to confront their impairments can provoke some patients to make compensatory claims of superiority. The therapist resists the urge to put these difficult patients in their place because such expressions of entitlement are often a sign of deep vulnerability (Groves, 1978). The occupational therapist is compassionate and points out areas of strength and strategies for ongoing effort (Keith, 1999).

Some patients seem to reject caregivers' efforts to reduce their suffering. They may appear self-sacrificing, have a history of bad luck, or even seem to revel in their misery (Kahana & Bibring, 1964). When patients do not seem to wish to recover, their symptoms may be serving a hidden purpose, such as penance or atonement (Solet, 1991). The occupational therapist may have to refer a patient who appears excessively guilt ridden for psychotherapy. Alternatively, illness or injury sometimes returns isolated or lonely people to a caring social environment from which they do not wish to be separated by recovery. Treatment planning should recognize needs for social stimulation and companionship. In collaboration with the patient, the occupational therapist organizes in advance for appropriate social contact after discharge.

Ways of Coping

Coping can be defined broadly as the cognitive, emotional, and behavioral efforts individuals make to manage external and internal challenges that tax their ordinary resources. Coping includes what people think, feel, and do in response to stress. Ways of coping can be understood as organized between three sets of poles: seeking versus withdrawing from social connections, seeking versus avoiding information and control, and expressing or repressing emotional reactions. Coping efforts contribute to health because they help define capacity for perceiving and reporting symptoms, for decision making, for complying with treatment demands, and for accepting comforting and support, all of which affect physiological processes and the sense of well-being (Stone & Porter, 1995).

Although individuals may have characteristic ways of coping that align with their personalities, the demands of any particular situation, including the length of time the challenge has lasted, are also important in determining ways of coping. For example, the period before surgery that provides the opportunity for active coping by seeking information and making decisions is very different from the postsurgical period, in which little control can be exercised and detachment or distraction may be most useful. In parallel fashion, coping with an acute health crisis may draw on different coping capacities from a patient and family than those required by an ongoing disability. As coping requirements change or awareness increases, the patient and family may reappraise their situation, recognizing new possibilities and drawing on additional resources.

In the clinical setting, ways of coping are assessed by self-report questionnaires, clinical observation checklists, and interviewing (Lazarus & Folkman, 1984; Solet, 1991).

As part of evaluation, the occupational therapist asks the patient and family members about prior challenges or crises and the coping efforts that were made. Treatment then draws on successful coping, such as securing arrangements for continued religious participation during hospitalization when this has proven to be an important source of strength in the past (Larson & Milano, 1995). Treatment may include active teaching to enlarge the patient's universe of coping alternatives. Examples include keeping a journal to encourage emotional expression (Pennebaker, 1995); participating in a specialized group to enhance social connection (Weber, 1993); gaining companionship, comfort, or direct help from a pet or companion animal assistant (Gal, 1999); practicing the RR to decrease perceived pain and anxiety (Benson & Proctor, 2010); and learning assertive communication to feel more confident about asking questions, identifying goals, and collaborating in treatment decisions. No particular way of coping is in itself good or bad; it must suit the individual in his or her specific circumstances. For example, coping by wishful thinking, denial, and withdrawal may serve important protective purposes early after an injury, when recognition of the extent of losses could overwhelm the individual. Because successful adaptation can involve cycles of approach and avoidance, occupational therapists are cautious about fracturing patients' protective ways of coping; they are aware of possible reactions including anxiety, shame, and resentment. An avoidant coping strategy when it lasts over an extended period can prevent full participation in treatment and limit needed emotional expression, knowledge acquisition, and social reintegration. Lasting avoidance, denial, or withdrawal may indicate overwhelming fears, guilt, or self-loathing or signal cognitive impairments and is cause for seeking psychiatric or neurological consultation.

THE SEARCH FOR MEANING

Occupational therapists are confronted daily with illness and injury. We grapple with ways to continually affirm our profession and to make sense of the suffering we witness (Peloquin, 2002). Our patients, facing these same questions of meaning, look to us not just for help in physical recovery but for our vision to guide them in interpreting their experiences. Their confrontation with the fragile nature of life may bring their deepest longings to the surface; they wish for vanished loved ones, protection, belonging, vigor, significance, and relief (Brendel et al., 2001).

Existential Questions

What is really important for a life to be worth living? What is it others will say about me when I die? What will my life say? Those are the kinds of questions my brain was filled with after the accident. It's no wonder I couldn't focus on details when the questions of life were asking to be answered. (Lowenstein, 1999)

Our patients ask us to recognize and acknowledge these questions and longings. They offer us the privilege of helping them to reclaim personal continuity and to create meaningful life narratives, which integrate their experiences of illness or injury (Charon, 2005, 2006). They challenge us to seek and reinforce their motivation to heal and to nurture their well-being at critical turning points and in the face of what for some will be lasting physical compromise (Pande & Tewari, 2011). They need us to join with them in celebrating the presence of interior life, personal connection, and the mystery of existence, despite ambiguity, painful loss, and the final certainty of death (Fig. 30-2).

Attributions

Meaning and belief systems are fundamentally woven into the human mind and society. The way we make sense of experience not only describes but actually affects our reality (Kleinman, 1988; Peloquin, 2002). Many people with an illness, injury, or traumatic life event eventually ask "Why me?" and try to make an attribution about or create an explanation for their experience. Clinical research has demonstrated the range and nature of these attributions (Solet, 1991) (Table 30-1).

Retribution

Some individuals see their illness or injury as a punishment, penance, or retribution. As children, we are taught that when we break rules, we will be punished; thus, it may be natural on some deep level to believe that

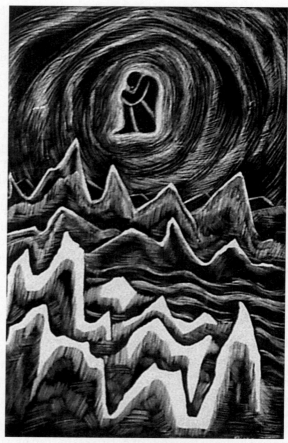

Figure 30-2 The self in danger. (Pen and ink by Margaret Rusciano Tolksdorf, Pelham, NY; see virtualeasel.com.)

Table 30-1	Patient Attributions

Type of Attribution	Description of Individual and Situation	Quotation Showing Explanation for Illness or Injury
Retribution	Salesman drinking and driving, now a paraplegic following an accident	"I don't believe God could be persuaded to forgive me for killing a child in the accident."
Faith	Computer expert, mother, hit by an electronic garage door when dropping off her car for repair	"I have learned to live one level higher. Life requires a leap of faith when you no longer understand or validate in the same way. The intuitive comes to the forefront; before it stood behind."
Personal responsibility	Poet, mother, rode as a passenger on an icy day in a car she knew to be in poor repair	"I never thought about what I was doing then, but because I'm responsible for my injury, I think about that choice all the time."
Victimization	College student, former swimming champ, attacked when skinny dipping by hoods offended by his exposure in front of their girlfriends	"I am afraid the possibilities for my future are diminished. It is so hard to see friends and younger sibs going through school, finishing, moving on with their lives. I am NOT an evil guy; what is this for? When this happened, I was sure I had died and gone to purgatory."
Acceptance	Biochemist hit by a bus crossing the street	"Is there any reason the owl eats the bunny and not the other way around? Injury and death are part of all nature. I am different now: I have lost my arrogance."
Chance	Engaged woman following an accident that disabled her and killed her fiancé	"People like to take credit for the good things and blame others for the bad things, but really, an awful lot happens by chance. The important thing is to be ready for the good things—and I am ready."

a painful event indicates badness or unworthiness deserving of punishment. In actuality, no realistic connection may be present between patients' behavior and their injuries, or they may be accurate in describing a connection, such as a history of drunk driving or unsafe sexual practices. In either case, attributions of retribution can render individuals immobilized by guilt and shame, unable to seek information or emotional support or to participate actively in their own recovery (Solet, 1991). They may require support to forgive themselves; some also need to focus on altering their dangerous behaviors. The opportunity to be heard and the reality of being accepted by the occupational therapist can help them begin to value themselves, feel worthy of treatment, and invest in the future.

Victimization

Again, either through a realistic analysis or based on deep feelings alone, some patients see themselves as victims. Especially when facts support the construction, such as after an assault, or serious medical error, where injury seems to have been personally directed or avoidable through reasonable diligence, the occupational therapist validates the attribution and acknowledges the loss of trust that follows from such an experience. The risk for patients who make attributions of victimization is that they may take on the role of victim more broadly as a lasting self-characterization. They may be unable, because of fear, anger, or sense of helplessness, to see the world as a safe place safe to rejoin. Some may react by withdrawing; others may misdirect their anger, potentially alienating caregivers. The occupational therapist helps by showing the realistic boundaries of these beliefs, by being a reliable and trustworthy caregiver, and by offering activities that help generate tolerance.

Chance

Chance or luck may sometimes be invoked by patients to explain illness or injury. Such an arbitrary universe as these patients perceive may be seen as dangerous and out of control, a form of impersonal victimization. Alternatively, an arbitrary universe may be benign and open to individual willingness to accept not just loss, but opportunity. The occupational therapist encourages patients who endorse chance to see hopeful possibilities.

Faith

Many patients demonstrate faith that their experience of illness or injury will, in the end, have meaning and purpose. These attributions based on faith need not exist only within the context of formal religion to engender optimism and encourage adaptation (Benson, 1995). Some hold a deep conviction that there is a plan for the universe in which good will ultimately prevail, a plan beyond ordinary human understanding (Rankin, 1985). Attributions of faith may be especially poignant for those who are isolated and have few

relationships because of their disability, allowing them to feel deeply valued beyond their difficult individual circumstances (Solet, 1991). Recent research points to the healing nature of deep self-disclosure such as may take place in prayer (Pennebaker, 1995). Occupational therapists are open to hearing about patients' spiritual lives and practices as elements of culture and daily life that can support healing.

Narratives and Metaphors

Patients want to tell their stories, and they need to be heard. The process of constructing and sharing a narrative of illness or injury organizes experience, shapes continuing perceptions, and breaks isolation. Through narrative, patients connect the present to the past, forming continuity in their lives and identities (Charon, 2005, 2006).

Increasingly, patients are turning to the Internet, especially to disease- or disability-specific sites to exchange narratives of their experiences and to offer support and treatment information. Analyses of some virtual communities has shown the information offered can be accurate and sophisticated, with patients helping each other and family members to become more aware of treatment possibilities and more ready to be active partners in decision making (Hoch & Ferguson, 2005). Occupational therapists may help patients identify virtual communities connected to reputable sources and may serve as translators and interpreters when relevant materials are complicated or raise questions about care and prognosis.

Occupational therapists use specific structures to collaborate with patients in interpreting their lives, including life charts, assisted autobiographies, and occupational storytelling (Frank, 1996). Through attentive listening, occupational therapists not only validate patients' experiences but also enhance their own clinical reasoning, tailoring empathic language and treatment activities to match patients' individual needs and motivations (Kautzman, 1992).

A common characteristic of these narratives is the use of certain metaphors that connect individuals' experiences to universal themes of culture and help to place their suffering in meaningful contexts. Hawkins (1993) described five metaphors that frequently serve as frames for interpreting illness or injury; each can be understood as coordinating with role expectations for the therapist and with specific risks for patient adaptation (Solet, 1991).

Rebirth

The metaphor of rebirth is a central religious and mythological theme. Through it, illness, injury, and the closeness of death are seen as transformative and regenerative (Hawkins, 1993). It is common for patients to reevaluate their lives around their illness or injury and to describe a profound altering of values and priorities. The old self dies, and a new and different self is born through suffering. The change brought about through this confrontation can be experienced like a religious conversion; wisdom and spiritual renewal can become the gift and compensation for suffering. Part of the role of the occupational therapist is to bear witness to these changes. Sometimes the illness is equated with a life of sinfulness: drugs, unsafe sex, smoking, bad diet, and aggressive treatment of others. The patient may wish the therapist to grant absolution and confirm worthiness for care. The risk to patients using this metaphor is its association with passivity and attributions of deserved punishment, rendering them unable to mobilize for the rigors of treatment (Solet, 1991).

Battle

The metaphor of battle is very common and is the most congruent with the Western system of medical care (Hawkins, 1993). It is frequently used by clinicians and even politicians. We hear often of "the war on cancer" and "the war on drugs." In this metaphor, the patient becomes the hero doing battle with a monstrous foe; the therapist is the ally in "fighting disease." The illness or disease is seen as exogenous, from the outside, and a crusade is launched to attack it. This metaphor combines aggression with social optimism and dignifies the active, courageous stance known colloquially as "fighting spirit" (Walker, 1999). Although some patients may relate easily to this aggressive position; others, by personality or beliefs, find the metaphor disturbing. The battle metaphor of attack may not be fully suitable for some illnesses. Cancer cells are, in fact, not an external threat, like plague or tuberculosis, but parts of the self turned unruly (Mukherjee, 2010). Pain can also be difficult to conceptualize as an invading adversary with which to do battle, because it may be experienced as coming from within by the patient. In treating rheumatoid arthritis and other autoimmune diseases, the goal is quite the contrary: to help the patient's body to stop fighting itself.

Athlete

Somewhat related to the battle metaphor is that of the athlete. The patient deals with illness as a game or sport in which the central issues are courage, stamina, and endurance (Hawkins, 1993). The therapist is the coach; the patient is in training; new skills are learned through practice. This is particularly effective for individuals who have a history of sports participation or are sports fans. The risk to patients with this metaphor is in its implications regarding performance. There is an audience in sports; there are rules and standards that must be followed, and trespass may lead to shame, as if the game were lost. The requirement to be courageous and strong throughout the ordeal so as not to lose or disappoint may prevent real communion with others over the reality of suffering and the inevitability of death. It may be helpful to emphasize that patients, caregivers, and family are all part of the team.

Journey

Illness as journey is a common metaphor found in narratives in which the patient travels to the kingdom of the sick, returning with the gift of wisdom. Susan Sontag (1988), writing about cancer, described the disease as granting "a more onerous citizenship" (p. 3). Within this metaphor, the therapist serves as a guide, having accompanied others in this same land. The journey of illness or injury may be a rite of passage involving degradation, humiliation, and depersonalization (Hawkins, 1993). This metaphor fits especially well with the loss of vision or with traumatic brain injury and the period of rehabilitation. The individual leaves the world of ordinary sensations and consciousness and finds that expectations must be redefined; roles and relationships are changed, and activities that were once taken for granted must be relearned or abandoned.

One risk to patients with the journey metaphor is that it can lead to a perception of exile as injury, illness, and disability can be isolating, sometimes permanently. In a very real sense, withdrawal from society may result when the individual cannot cope because of alterations in appearance, personality, mastery, or ability to communicate. Lack of accessibility and actual physical barriers may prevent return to the community (Jenkins, 2011). Historically, exile has been forced when behavior or appearances ranged far from society's accepted norms or when the spread of infectious diseases threatened others, as with acquired immune deficiency syndrome (AIDS) or leprosy. Group participation with other "travelers" may help limit isolation.

Nature

In contrast to the four metaphors described earlier, the New Age metaphor places faith in the healing powers of nature, especially the efficacy of positive emotions. This metaphor may be construed as a reaction to aspects of modern medical care, which has been faulted for defining the patient as the passive focus of technology, subject to external treatment forces, rather than as a vessel filled with self-healing resources. The therapist's role here is as caring partner. The disease or injury may be described as presenting an opportunity to alter values or to recognize and integrate hidden powers of the self. The risk to patients is the sense of bafflement, failure, and shame they may feel if conscientious efforts are not rewarded with health. This construction emphasizes the requirement to be "positive." Individuals may construe normal feelings of grief, fear, or anger as hindering their own recovery. They may be unable to accept ownership of authentic feelings. This metaphor works best when the occupational therapist demonstrates belief in the goodness of the full spectrum of human feelings and in the whole cycle of nature, which includes not only spring but also winter.

Pathography

Occupational therapists may prepare themselves to respond with empathy to their patients' narratives by exploring published accounts of illness or injury known as pathographies (see Resources 30-1). Authors have many

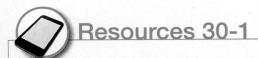 Resources 30-1

Supplemental Readings: Pathographies

Ackerman, D. (2011). *One hundred names of love: A stroke, a marriage and the language of healing.* New York: W. W. Norton. Video of the author and her husband available at http://www.powells.com /biblio/62-9780393072419-0.

Bauby, J. (1997). *The diving bell and the butterfly.* New York: Random House.

Broyard, A. (1992). *Intoxicated by my illness.* New York: Fawcett Columbine.

Hull, J. (1990). *Touching the rock: An experience of blindness.* New York: Pantheon.

Interlandi, J. (2011). Waking Chris: Consciousness returns after vegetative state. *New York Tiimes Magazine,* December 4, pp. 42–47.

Jamison, K. R. (1996). *An unquiet mind.* New York: Random House.

Kerpelman, L. C. (2011). *Pieces missing: A family's journey of recovery from traumatic brain injury.* Minneapolis, MN: Two Harbors Press.

Linton, S. (2006). *My body politic: A memoir.* Ann Arbor, MI: University of Michigan Press.

Luria, A. R. (1968). *The mind of a mnemonist.* Cambridge, MA: Harvard University.

Luria, A. R. (1972). *The man with a shattered world.* Cambridge, MA: Harvard University.

Mairs, N. (1996). *Waist high in the world.* Boston: Beacon.

Mukherjee, S. (2010). *The emperor of all maladies.* New York: Scribner.

Pierce, C. P. (2011). Rebuilding Ryan: Red Sox top prospect returns to minor leagues to try to relearn game after brain surgery. *Boston Globe Magazine,* March 20, 15–19.

Rogers, A. G. (1995). *A shining affliction.* New York: Viking.

Sacks, O. (1985). *The man who mistook his wife for a hat.* New York: Simon & Schuster.

Wakefield, D. (2005). *I remember running: The year I got everything I wanted and ALS.* New York: Marlowe.

Wiltshire, S. F. (1994). *Seasons of grief and grace: A sister's story of AIDS.* Nashville: Vanderbilt University.

Supplemental Readings: Adaptation

Chodron, P. (1997). *When things fall apart: Heart advice for difficult times.* Boston: Shambala.

Dalai Lama, & Cutler, H. C. (1998). *The art of happiness: A handbook for living.* New York: Riverhead Books.

Flach, F. (2004). *Resilience.* New York: Hatherleigh Press.

Sacks, O. (2008). *Musicophilia: Tales of music and the brain.* New York: Random House.

Sadler, B., & Ridenour, A. (2009). *Transforming the healthcare experience through the arts.* San Diego, CA: Aesthetics, Inc. (See www.artinhealthcare.com.)

Weber, R. J. (2000). *The created self: Reinventing body, persona, and spirit.* New York: Norton.

Website Resources

Benson-Henry Institute for Mind Body Medicine at Mass General Hospital
http://www.massgeneral.org/bhi/basics/eliciting_rr.aspx

Division of Sleep Medicine at Harvard Medical School and WGBH Educational Foundation
http://healthysleep.med.harvard.edu/healthy/

Sleep Education
http://www.sleepcenters.org

Center for Health Design
http://www.healthdesign.org/chd/research/validating -acoustic-guidelines-healthcare-facilities

Research report on sleep and noise in hospitals (Solet et al., 2010).

(continued)

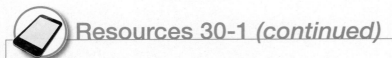

Resources 30-1 *(continued)*

Suggested Films for Viewing and Discussion

A Beautiful Mind (2002)	My Left Foot (1989)	Shooting Beauty (2009)
Awakening (1990)	Memento (2000)	Station Agent (2003)
Born on the Fourth of July (1989)	Marwencol (2010)	Temple Grandin (2010)
Children of a Lesser God (2000)	Murderball (2005)	The Best Years of Our Lives (1946)
Edward Scissorhands (1990)	Rainman (1988)	The Diving Bell and the Butterfly (2007)
Emmanuel's Gift (2005)	Ray (2004)	The Elephant Man (1989)
Indigo Factory (2010)	Regarding Henry (1996)	The Men (1950)
Iris (2001)	Scent of a Woman (1993)	Waterdance (1992)
		When Billy Broke His Head (1995)

For movie summaries, see the Internet Movie Database, www.imdb.com/find.

motivations, including trying to find meaning in their own experiences, consolidating changed identities, breaking isolation, validating others, offering hope or counsel, exposing inhumane care, and giving specific information about treatment alternatives. Some pathographies are inspiring tales of recovery or of transcendence over pain or disability, even over imminent death. Some are offered by family members as a testimonial to a loved one or a journal of the shared ordeal; others aim to elevate natural healing capacities and transform our health care system. Numerous popular films also depict disabled characters, their struggles and ways of coping (see Resources 30-1). Such films, even when their stories are fictional, help us understand views of illness and disability in our culture. For some patients or their families, the occupational therapist selects readings or films as an educational component of treatment. For patients who are able, journaling, writing, or visual arts are therapeutic, support hope, and document improvement; this is one of the founding principles of our field.

THE HEALING CONTEXT

Although health care policy makers assume families will provide a healing context for their disabled members, very little formal structure is in place to support their efforts (Levine, 1999). As the population ages and advances in medical technology extend lives, the burden on family members continues to grow. Idealizing or romanticizing the position of disabled individuals and their families avoids confronting the real deprivations many suffer and camouflages important ethical questions regarding responsibility for the allocation of societal resources (Saetersdal, 1997).

Family Caregiving

In the United States, 52 million unpaid informal caregivers provide care to individuals age 18 years and older who cannot perform necessary activities on their own; the overwhelming majority of these caregivers are family members (Coughlin, 2010; Institute of Medicine, 2008). Caring for a spouse continues to be the most commonly reported caregiving situation for those older than 75 years (Wagner & Takagi, 2010). The proportion of individuals older than 65 years in the United States is growing and will in 2030 be more than double what it was at the turn of this century. The level of stress on partners and family members suggests some carry a degree of responsibility that can damage their own health and well-being.

Loss of disabled persons' income often places families in financial jeopardy. Although government expenditures on health care for the disabled have risen rapidly, spending on education, training, and employment has been declining (Taylor, 2011). Analysis of census supplementary survey data showed that for men and women at least 55 years of age, the presence of long-lasting conditions that substantially limit one or more basic physical activity is inversely related to social class (Minkler, Fuller-Thompson, & Guralnik, 2006).

Family Reorganization and Identity

Families with a newly disabled member or one who is losing functional capacity through the common pattern of accelerated aging, experience grief and changes in routines, roles, and expectations, often compounded by expanded financial burdens (Lynch, Kaplan, & Shema, 1997). These additional stresses may exacerbate preexisting marital discord or substance abuse. Family reorganization requires learning and concrete problem solving, as well as transformation within the family unit, parallel to that of the disabled person. Partners and families struggle to forge new identities among themselves and for integration within their communities.

Engaging with Family Members

The occupational therapist, often working in concert with a nurse or social worker, may be the major preparatory interface with the formal health care system for a family planning to receive a disabled member at home. To initiate collaboration with the family, the occupational therapist assesses readiness and does not force premature instruction that could frighten, anger, or alienate the family (Levine, 1999). In all contacts with the family, the occupational therapist remains aware and respectful of the rights (see the discussion in Chapter 2 regarding the Health Insurance Portability and Accountability Act [HIPAA]) and wishes of the patient with regard to privacy and confidentiality (Procedures for Practice 30-3).

Important differences between what occupational therapists and family members value as treatment and support have been documented. Hasselkus (1991, 1994) found that occupational therapists focused treatment planning on disabled individuals' level of independence. Family members, however, were more likely to express concern that their returning member will be safely cared for with a sense of maintained identity. Ongoing life satisfaction and dignity, rather than level of self-care, are becoming recognized as the most valuable measures of rehabilitation success and may be most congruent with patient and family hopes and expectations (Dorset, 2010; Wadensten & Ahlstrom, 2009).

If the patient is to be discharged home, the occupational therapist ideally accompanies the patient on a predischarge visit to assess home safety, to plan for installation of assistive devices, and to organize the sleep environment. This is a good time to facilitate social participation by helping the patient (and family) become aware of community resources and barrier-free opportunities. Community connection is especially important to those living independently with a disability. The occupational therapist also offers information to the patient and family related to specific support and advocacy groups through which they may share problem solving, feel a sense of camaraderie, and be empowered if they choose to work to improve the system for themselves and others.

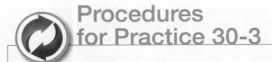

Procedures for Practice 30-3

Engaging with Family Members

Goals of Interaction with Patients' Families

- Seeking information about family medical and social history
- Offering specific information about disability and treatment
- Collaborating and fostering inclusion in decision making
- Validating feelings
- Acknowledging experiences
- Fostering hope and successful coping
- Guiding reconnection with patient
- Instructing in issues of patient care and safety, including home visits and use of assistive devices
- Facilitating use of community resources, including barrier-free opportunities and support groups

Considering the Family Context

Try to answer the following questions when assessing a patient's family context:

- Where is the patient in the life cycle, and what have been the patient's roles and responsibilities?
- How have the roles, responsibilities, and expectations of family members now been altered?
- Is there lost income and/or added medical and caregiving expense?
- What family problems may be exacerbated by this crisis?
- How has the family coped with crises in the past?
- How will the likely course of the disability affect the family?
- How is the family making sense of the experience? Do they have a specific cultural perspective or religious beliefs?
- To what communities do they belong that may be a source of help or strength?
- Do they need referral for family counseling?

Some patients are discharged to separate quarters or to institutional settings. Discharge of a family member to a long-term care facility can involve wrenching decisions, especially in families in which traditional culture and values include loyalty and strong bonds among members (Banks, 2003). This is true even when it seems clear to the clinical community that taking the individual home would seriously overtake the resources of the family. The occupational therapist acknowledges these feelings and helps organize ways to maintain family relationships when the disabled member will not be returning home.

In certain cases, family stress may be extreme, communication difficult, and reactions overwhelming. Family members may disagree over what care is appropriate for individuals who are not legally competent to make decisions about their own care. In nontraditional family constructions and partnerships, additional stresses may result from lack of legal recognition of couple and parenting commitments with the associated rights to direct and oversee care and to qualify for certain health insurance coverage. In the United States, many states grant marriage licenses to same-sex couples; same-sex marriage is legally recognized throughout Canada. The occupational therapist makes sure to be aware of whom the patient considers "family."

Although most people fail to prepare legally for sudden illness or disability, when decline can be anticipated, as with degenerative illness, individual wishes about palliative care can be discussed, powers of attorney can be organized, and health care proxies completed. When an illness has been shown to have possible genetic links, additional questions arise, including whether other family members should undertake testing and what the implications might be for pregnancy. Specially trained genetic counselors can clarify the ethics and science, supporting informed decision making (Patenaude, 2005). The occupational therapist is alert to the possible necessity of specialized referrals.

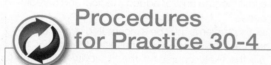

Procedures for Practice 30-4

Addressing Substance Abuse

- Take an occupational history. Was the patient functioning in work or school? Was the patient maintaining relationships?
- Are any family members likely to be helpful in describing the patient's history?
- Is there any evidence that substance abuse was a primary cause of the condition?
- Might the condition have provoked substance abuse?
- Are there predisposing factors such as depression, trauma, family history, or membership in a marginalized group?
- Does evidence support need for referral?

Treatment Goals for Substance Abuse

- Improve health habits and self-care
- Develop skills in self-regulation and impulse control
- Experience group participation, learn to communicate needs, learn to give and receive support
- Prepare for constructive vocational role
- Value a clean and sober identity
- Connect with community resources such as Alcoholics Anonymous to maintain sobriety

Partnership and Sexuality

The unique role of occupational therapists in addressing both activity and meaning places them in an ideal position to include sexual well-being among treatment goals. Sexual well-being correlates with adjustment and satisfaction in other areas of life and is an important component of the partnership bond (Woods, 1984). As one of the activities of daily living, sexual activity merits an accepting, problem-solving focus.

To acknowledge and accept the sexual identity of their patients, occupational therapists become aware of their own beliefs and values and suspend judgment when these values differ from those of their patients. Even when the primary sexual counseling is done by another team member, occupational therapists are prepared to recognize intimate needs within different stages of the life cycle and sexual orientation and to initiate discussion of sexual activity, including birth control and safe practices, while maintaining clinically appropriate boundaries. Embarrassment or a sense of undesirability may prevent patients from raising sexual concerns themselves. The occupational therapist acquires sufficient medical and psychological background to anticipate patients' needs and questions. Desire, sexual responsiveness, sensory channels, and mobility may be altered by disability (Basson, 1998; Hulter & Lundberg, 1995). The occupational therapist explicitly helps the disabled person by encouraging him or her to reconceptualize sexuality and sexual activity more broadly and to explore new possibilities for sexual expression. When the disabled individual has a consistent sexual partner, the therapist may offer the opportunity to include him or her in teaching or treatment sessions. A satisfying sexual relationship is learned; it is based on more than simple instinct or appetite and does not have to be unplanned or spontaneous to be fulfilling (Woods, 1984). The disabled person and his or her sexual partner may learn to adapt to periods of fatigue, continence timing, or requirements for special positioning.

Fears may contribute to the disabled person's hesitancy about sexual activity. Fear of rejection may be based on altered appearance or on perceptions of the social acceptance of the needs and desires of disabled people. Patients with certain diagnoses may have been warned about the danger of overexertion and may harbor fears about heart attacks or strokes. Some patients fear being injured by sexual activity or anticipate increases in their pain. Here a physician knowledgeable in sexual medicine can be a critical resource. Informed and sensitive medical management, sometimes including medications, can help disabled individuals claim their sexual selves.

In some settings, disabled individuals are vulnerable to sexual exploitation or abuse, especially when cognitive or verbal limitations prevent them from reporting their experiences or serving as reliable witnesses in a court of law. Occupational therapists who work with such patients are aware and alert to these possibilities and meet legal and ethical requirements for reporting concerns.

COMPLICATING FACTORS

Disruption and reintegration are natural to the life course; the capacity to adapt to disruption with new integration is described as resilience (Flach, 2004). The occupational therapist recognizes that positive change and reorganization may also be part of the portrait of illness and disability (Schroevers, Kraaij, & Garnefski, 2011). However, a trajectory of resilient adaptation can be compromised, especially when multiple serious stressors come together or when loss is a result of victimization (Quale & Schanke, 2010). Substance abuse, pain, depression, PTSD, and disrupted sleep are among complications of illness and injury that hinder adaptation and mandate specific treatment.

Substance Abuse

Social isolation, losses producing painful feeling states, and traumatic experiences related to injury confer special vulnerability putting disabled individuals at higher than normal risk for substance abuse (Moore & Li, 1994). Alcohol and drug use have been implicated not just as reactions to but also as causative agents in disability, most notably in relation to auto accidents. Evidence points to alcohol playing a role in a significant number of spinal cord injuries (Heinemann, Mamott, & Schnoll, 1990). Beyond health complications such as malnutrition and liver disease, which may affect all abusers, disabled abusers may be at increased risk for adverse drug interactions, falls caused by balance or mobility impairments, and sores and gastrointestinal bleeding that can go undetected because of sensory losses (Yarkony, 1993).

In studying users' history of drug choice, Khantzian (1990), who posited a self-medication theory of substance abuse, found that individuals experiment with various classes of drugs and settle on those that offer a specific needed relief. For example, individuals used stimulants to relieve depression and hyperactivity, opioids to mute psychologically disorganizing feelings such as rage and aggression, and alcohol to break emotional constriction and allow for release or social connection. Primary causes for substance abuse, he concluded, are difficulties in managing feelings, low self-esteem, lack of supporting relationships, and poor self-care, which are particularly common among individuals with abusive or traumatic histories or living in under-resourced circumstances. Use of drugs and alcohol is associated with depression and anxiety after traumatic head injury (Anson

& Ponsford, 2006). Meyer (1999) studied not only the neurobiology of addiction but its sociology as well. He concluded that for some individuals, drug use becomes a main source of activity and occupation, especially when no compelling or achievable alternative future can be perceived or undertaken. As members of the treatment team, occupational therapists are alert to the possibility of substance abuse (see discussion in Chapter 3), prepared to make appropriate referrals, and able to participate in humane, respectful care (Procedures for Practice 30-4). Well-designed substance abuse treatment addresses appropriate stages of recovery; is sensitive to ethnic, cultural, and linguistic differences; and is responsive to patients' particular needs (Cambridge Health Alliance, 1995). Community-based 12-step programs such as Alcoholics Anonymous offer a philosophy for living a fulfilling life and provide an opportunity not only to receive sponsorship support but to provide service to others as well. Suggested treatment goals for substance abuse are listed in Procedures for Practice 30-2.

Pain

Although not a diagnosis in itself, pain accompanies many illnesses, injuries, and disabilities including spinal cord injury, acquired amputation, cerebral palsy, multiple sclerosis, postpolio syndrome, and many developmental disabilities (Ehde et al., 2003; Engel, 2011). The experience of pain is directly related to well-being and is an impediment to resilience. More than a simple sensation, pain is a perception that emerges at the intersection of body, mind, and culture. Pain is an ineffable private experience that each individual must learn to interpret, but it is also a universal phenomenon with broad influence on society at large, in terms of lost workdays and use of health care resources. According to a 2011 Institute of Medicine report, 116 million Americans suffer from chronic pain, with many partially or fully disabled; arthritis, headaches, and back pain are among the largest contributors.

The Personal Experience of Pain

The daily reality of the individual in pain often includes sleeping difficulties, problems concentrating, and decreased mobility, all of which may limit occupational performance. Altered moods, especially agitation or lethargy with depression, are common among those who experience pain over an extended period, especially after multiple treatments without relief. Grief over lost mastery and diminished life roles with feelings of rage, helplessness, victimization, and defectiveness can lead to social withdrawal. Prompt and preemptive treatment of pain is a strong priority, ideally before roles, relationships, and even identity become irretrievably eroded (Harris, Morley, & Barton, 2003).

Pain Treatment

A full pain treatment program includes educational, physical, psychological, and pharmacological components and is administered through a team of clinicians that includes an occupational therapist (Robinson, Kennedy, & Harmon, 2011). Group and individual treatments are often combined. Education that presents a mind–body pain model gives recognition to both the stress and distress that accompany pain, breaks down the mysteries of the pain experience, and supports the efficacy of several avenues of treatment (Caudill, 1995; Solet, 1995). Recognition and validation are crucial elements because patients with pain may feel that no one understands the extent of their suffering (Main & Spanswick, 1991).

The mind–body model encourages patients to view their pain not as a simple response to tissue damage but as a complex experience that can be affected by many factors, such as positioning for activities, sufficient sleep, and emotional reactions (Jenkins, 2011). Diary keeping (self-monitoring) provides information about which specific factors affect an individual's pain experience; this is vital for collaboration in treatment planning. Diary keeping also documents evidence of improvement, which bolsters motivation and supports treatment adherence.

The various components of a pain treatment program can include instruction in pacing and body mechanics, stretching, strengthening, low-impact aerobic exercise, massage, acupuncture, as well as RR training, biofeedback, CBT affect management (control of emotional reactions), and practice in assertive communication (Rochman & Kennedy-Spain, 2007). Each of these treatment components properly chosen and applied may help patients manage their pain, even when complete relief is out of reach (Persson, Andersson, & Eklund, 2011).

Depression

Theoretical debate and research over the etiology of depression continues, with exploration including reactions to loss, neurobiological mechanisms, and genetic predispositions. These explanations need not be mutually exclusive because the brain is the substrate for interpretation of personal experience. Clinicians sometimes mistakenly assume that depression is simply a stage or normal reaction to a disabling illness or injury and that it will remit if left untreated. With periods of hospitalization so short in the current health-care environment, those with lasting depression are in danger of being lost to follow-up.

Among medically ill older adults, major depression is experienced by an estimated 20%, and minor depression is experienced by an additional 20%–30% (Koenig & George, 1998). Personal or family histories of depression constitute special risk factors following the onset of illness or injury. In some cases, depression is part of a larger picture that includes swings in energy level and emotions, called bipolar disorder or manic depression. Depression, whatever the cause or pattern, can undermine all areas of functioning and, when severe, is life-threatening. The presence of depression mandates referral for assessment, including for risk of suicide. As many as 15% of those who suffer from depression or bipolar disorder commit suicide each year. Suicide is the ninth leading cause of death in the United States (Nemeroff, 1998).

Diagnosis and Treatment of Depression

Coping styles characterized by avoidance, wishful thinking, self-blame, and use of drugs and alcohol are associated with higher levels of depression, anxiety, and poorer psychosocial functioning (Anson & Ponsford, 2006). Patients whose motivation to participate in treatment is sapped by significant or unrelenting depression not only lose a critical opportunity to reorganize life skills and identity in a protected setting but also fare poorly if depression remains untreated after discharge. Depression is a confirmed risk factor for future heart disease (Denollet, 1998) and increases the risk of dying after a heart attack or stroke (Nemeroff, 1998).

Making a diagnosis of depression in cases of ill, injured, or disabled patients can be complicated; symptoms customarily associated with depression, such as sleep or appetite changes, can be directly related to the primary conditions for which some disabled patients are seeking care. In addition, brain damage also alters neurobiology.

Because occupational therapists often have a close and continuous relationship with their patients, careful observation and documentation of behaviors, feelings, and ways of thinking contribute important information to diagnosis. The occupational therapist looks not only for somatic or bodily symptoms but also for cognitive and emotional signs of depression. These include indecisiveness, inability to concentrate, diminished interest or loss of pleasure in formerly enjoyable activities, feelings of worthlessness or excessive guilt, and recurrent thoughts of death or suicide (Nemeroff, 1998).

Patients with bipolar disorder commonly receive diagnostic attention during a depressive phase; the full scope of their illness is at first not always clear. Because the implications for treatment are different, especially for medications, it is important when considering depression also to look for any personal or family history of mania. Symptoms include very high energy, sleeplessness, pressured speech, grandiose thinking, unbridled spending, and even delusions (Ghaemi & Sachs, 1999). Patients' lack of insight into and inability to report their own psychological state during manic periods is the rule.

The occupational therapist documents concerns about depression or mania in the medical record, including supporting observations, and brings this information

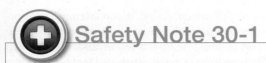

Safety Note 30-1

Indications for Psychiatric Referral

- Inability or unwillingness to comply with treatment
- Substance abuse
- Uncontrolled pain
- Traumatic flashbacks or dissociation
- Depression with suicidal tendency
- Mania
- Hostility, agitation
- Paranoia, unwarranted fears
- Hearing voices, delusions
- Social isolation or withdrawal
- Extended denial
- Unresolved religious or existential crisis
- Overwhelming guilt
- Family upheaval

to the attention of the treating physician or team to facilitate referral for psychiatric evaluation (Safety Note 30-1). Assessment for antidepressant and/or mood-stabilizing medications and psychotherapy is a high priority. Components of OT treatment for depression include restoring self-care and appetites, improving feelings of mastery through meaningful goal-directed activities, reframing self-defeating cognitions, and encouraging social integration.

Post-Traumatic Stress Disorder

Individuals injured or disabled through war, natural disaster, accident, abuse, or violent crime are at special risk for the symptom complex called post-traumatic stress disorder. Symptoms can include hyperarousal (vigilance), nervousness, fearfulness, nightmares, flashbacks (spontaneous reexperiencing), ruminations, emotional numbing, and mental absence or dissociation (Champagne, Koomar, & Olsen, 2010). For some patients, the resulting disability may constitute life-long physical evidence of the traumatic experience, even serving as a proprioceptive cue or trigger for PTSD symptoms and continuing stress reactions.

Individuals showing symptoms of PTSD require immediate referral to be evaluated for specialized psychotherapy and possible medication. Coordination between caregivers is critical to a positive outcome for these patients, who need a safe, predictable environment in which they can make sense of their experiences. Occupational therapists help individuals with PTSD to organize daily life structure and to enhance their ability to feel safe while participating in meaningful roles and activities (Champagne, Koomar, & Olsen, 2010). Listening to their

narratives can be disturbing, so strong team support and supervision become important for all involved caregivers, including occupational therapists.

Limited Sleep

The ordeal of injury or illness can be exhausting in itself, fraught with layers of uncertainty and challenges to managing care in our often-difficult health-care system. Beyond this, patients may be not be getting sufficient quality sleep. There are multiple routes through which sleep affects adaptation and the ability to benefit from treatment. Deficient sleep affects attention, memory consolidation, and even tolerance of frustration. Because occupational therapists typically meet with patients several times a week and have the opportunity to evaluate sleep environments, they are in a good position to screen for sleep problems.

A complex, dynamic state, critical to growth and development, sleep changes through the life cycle, typically becoming shorter and lighter with aging (Ohayon & Vecchierini, 2005). The Occupational Therapy Practice Framework (AOTA, 2008) recognizes sleep as an occupation. Along with nutrition, exercise, and social connection, sleep is one of the pillars of health and well-being.

Two processes interact to determine our drive for sleep: the homeostatic drive increases with accumulated time awake, and the circadian biological clock organizes a physiological cycle of body temperature and hormone release, regulating the variability of sleepiness and wakefulness throughout the night and day. Sleep is characterized by patterns of changing brain waves that present in cycles of about 90 minutes each, throughout the night. Within these cycles, different stages of sleep are identified by the frequency and amplitude of the brain waves. The stages of sleep fall into two categories, non-rapid eye movement (NREM or non-REM) sleep, which indicates progressively deeper stages and predominates in the earlier cycles of the night in adults, and rapid eye movement (REM) sleep, in which most dreaming occurs and which predominates closer to morning (Kryger, Roth, & Dement, 2011). Clinical research in sleep medicine includes exploration of the roles of NREM and REM sleep stages in contributing to specific functions, including emotional regulation, cognition, learning, and memory consolidation.

Even healthy adults, when deprived of sleep, will show deterioration in performance (Cohen et al., 2010). Adequate sleep is necessary for restoration of mind and body and for successful occupational balance (Anaby, 2010). Disordered sleep is a major public health concern affecting both genders, all races, and all socioeconomic levels (Hale, 2005). Research and clinical evidence confirm the impact of lack of sleep on safety, learning and memory, cognitive performance (Durmer & Dinges, 2005; Poe, Walsh, & Bjorness, 2010), and even immune function (Irwin et al., 2008).

Insufficient sleep is negatively associated with psychological well-being: lowered mood, irritability, aggressiveness, and psychosocial difficulties (Haack & Mullington, 2005). The range of health effects that may result from insufficient or disordered sleep includes elevated stress hormones and inflammatory markers, impaired glucose tolerance, diabetes (Zizi et al., 2011), obesity (Flier & Elmquist, 2004; Patel & Hu, 2008), hypertension (O'Connor, Caffo, & Newman, 2009; Redline, 2009), and cardiovascular disease and stroke (Buxton et al., 2012). However, assessment of sleep is still not routine in primary care (Sorscher, 2008). Insufficient or disordered sleep may be implicated as a causal factor or resulting complications for many patients treated by occupational therapists (Stroe et al., 2010; Zee & Turek, 2006).

In addition, pain, depression, substance abuse, and PTSD may have negative reciprocal interactions with sleep; they disturb sleep, and then disturbed sleep can make them worse. Conditions that may compromise sleep include acute and chronic pain (Hamilton, Karlson, & Catley, 2007; Roehrs et al., 2006), head injury (Parcell et al., 2008), spinal cord injury (Epstein & Brown, 2010), Parkinson's disease (Sixel-Doring et al., 2011), multiple sclerosis (Braley & Chervin, 2010), stroke (Coelho et al., 2010; Johnson & Johnson, 2010; Watson, 2010), rheumatoid arthritis (Luyster et al., 2011), chronic fatigue syndrome (Burton et al., 2010), Alzheimer's disease (Hwang et al., 2011), and heart disease (Chandola et al., 2010), as well as disorders of breathing, anxiety disorders including PTSD, and major mental illness.

Because excessive sleepiness has been repeatedly implicated in auto, truck, and major industrial accidents (Drake et al., 2010), when injury is known to be accident related, a red flag for sleep screening should be raised. No prior sleep assessment is currently required federally or shared by individual states to secure a commercial driver's license.

Assessing Sleep

Questionnaires and self-reports can be useful for screening or initial assessment of some patients. However, some sleep problems, even when severe, can be outside patient awareness; some patients may report unexplained excessive daytime sleepiness. Especially when greater than expected impairments in occupational and social functioning are seen during evaluations, sleep problems may be implicated. Although diagnosis of deficient sleep is outside the professional expertise of occupational therapists, they may provide initial screening through questionnaires such as the Epworth Sleepiness Scale (Johns, 1991) and may document partner or family reports leading to referral. Full sleep assessment includes a polysomnogram, composed of electroencephalogram, electrooculogram for eye motion, and electromyogram for muscle activity. The "sleep study" is used to differentiate the stages of sleep; to indicate time to fall asleep, called "sleep latency"; proportion of time in bed actually spent sleeping, called "sleep efficiency"; and to indicate how often arousals from sleep occur and for how long (Kryger, Roth, & Dement, 2011).

Sleep Disorders and Treatments

Although sleep difficulties are secondary to many illnesses and injuries, they may also occur as primary disorders. A summary of some common barriers to sleep with related OT treatment contributions follows.

Sleep Environments. Hospitals and long-term care facilities too often fail to provide adequate sleep environments (Buxton et al., 2012); hospital noise levels have been rising for decades (Busch-Vishniac, 2005), compromising healing and adaptation. Night noise is among the most common complaints on patient quality-of-care surveys. Critical care units are particularly difficult for patient sleep, in part because of monitor alarms, a large proportion of which may not be clinically relevant (Solet & Barach, 2012). Multistep programs have been designed and tested to improve night noise and light exposure, timing of medications, and night care routines. The Somerville Protocol is an evidence-based night care program that can be implemented by staff to improve quality of care and better preserve patient sleep (Bartick et al., 2010).

Sleep Hygiene. Sleep hygiene is characterized as a sleep-friendly environment together with specific behaviors. For patients who will be discharged home, the home visit checklist should include examination of sleep quarters that should be rendered *quiet*, *dark*, *cool*, *comfortable*, *clean*, and *safe*. Because light counteracts the hormone melatonin that initiates sleep, "black-out" window shades or eye masks can be used to block ambient light. Light sources within the room such as bright digital clocks should be dimmed or removed, and lighted screens on TVs and computers should ideally be kept out of bedrooms or at least shut down at night. Because body temperature drops as part of initiating sleep, a cool bedroom (mid to high 60s) should be maintained as most conducive to sleep. Cords, equipment, and obstructing furniture should be removed to prevent falls during night awakenings. Commitments from partners, roommates, or family members should be solicited to ensure sufficient nighttime quiet, to keep pets under control, and to facilitate a consistent sleep schedule. For those with very limited resources, availability of a safe place for sleep should be understood as an occupational justice issue, because it is a determinant of health (Blakeney & Marshall, 2009).

Along with a sleep-friendly environment, specific behaviors support health. These include exposure to sunlight, especially in the morning, to increase alertness and reinforce normal circadian rhythms; sufficient time in bed; and a relatively consistent natural sleep-wake schedule.

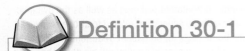

Definition 30-1

Sleep Disorders

Insomnia refers to repeated difficulty with sleep initiation, duration, consolidation, or quality that occurs despite adequate time and opportunity for sleep, resulting in some form of daytime impairment. Insomnia with short sleep duration is associated with increased mortality (Vgontzas et al., 2010). Occupational therapy interventions include: relaxation response, cognitive behavioral therapy (especially addressing sleep-related anxieties) (Haynes, 2009), exercise (Passos et al., 2010), modifying sleep environments, and limiting caffeine and alcohol (Roehrs & Roth, 2011).

Obstructive sleep apnea (OSA) is caused by partial or complete blockage of airway passages during sleep. Snoring is a common sign. Repeated awakenings, typically not remembered, driven by decreased oxygen saturation affecting the brain, occur dozens or even hundreds of times a night. These can lead to excessive daytime sleepiness and cognitive impairments, as well as diabetes, cardiovascular disease, stroke, and even increased cancer risk. Treatments include continuous positive airway pressure (CPAP), a system that pushes air through the nose via a face mask (Tomfour et al., 2011), sleep positioning to side-lying, dental devices, corrective surgery (Verse & Hormann, 2011), and weight loss (Vasquez et al., 2008). The occupational therapist may be enlisted to help with treatment adherence and weight loss programs.

REM Sleep Behavior Disorder (RBD) results when the normal muscle paralysis or atonia that occurs during rapid eye movement (REM) sleep fails, and the affected individual moves as if acting out a dream. Most common in men older than 50 years, there is research documentation that RBD may be a precursor to dementias or Parkinson's disease (Sixel-Doring et al., 2011).

Restless Leg Syndrome (RLS) is a sleep disorder in which there is an urge to move the legs in order to stop unpleasant leg sensations that may be described as "crawling" or "tingling" especially during the evening. During sleep, involuntary leg movements occur and can lead to repeated arousals that are not remembered (Bayard, Avonda, & Wadzinski, 2008; Kushida, 2007). Risk factors include peripheral neuropathy, chronic kidney disease, iron deficiency, Parkinson's disease, and medication side effects. There is also higher prevalence among clients with a history of stroke (Coelho et al., 2010) and fibromyalgia (Viola-Saltzman et al., 2010). The occupational therapist may provide recommendations for exercise, stretching, massage, and warm baths to bring symptomatic relief.

The occupational therapist addresses issues of inconsistent or limited sleep time as a result of poor lifestyle choices, management of multiple roles and responsibilities, or difficult shift-work requirements. Better choices, prophylactic napping, limitations on alcohol and caffeine, and contracts with family members with regard to sleep needs and timing are options for improving sleep hygiene. Many patients will be cared for at home by family members; education for caregivers about their own sleep needs and optimal sleep environments can be valuable. When well rested, caregivers are more able to offer attentive and compassionate care.

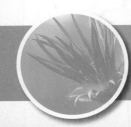

case example

Mr. D.: Adaptation after Stroke

I felt a cleaving in my mind
As if my brain had split;
I tried to match it, seam by seam,
But could not make them fit.

The thought behind I strove to join
Unto the thought before,
But sequence ravelled out of reach
Like balls upon a floor.

Emily Dickinson (1830–1886)

This case study follows the structure introduced in this chapter for integrating psychosocial components in treatment planning as well as the dynamic interactional approach described by Toglia (2005). The internal dialogue in the Case Example emphasizes these aspects as related to stroke recovery. The patient described, Mr. D., was in active inpatient rehabilitation for 3 months, followed by periodic home visits for outpatient treatment. Medical complications contributed to his unusually long length of stay. During the period following his stroke and after a second stroke until his death, he continued to correspond with this author, his occupational therapist. He expressed the wish that his experiences be used to help others. He often quoted the Emily Dickinson poem above. The accompanying series of drawings demonstrate his growing awareness during his inpatient stay (Fig. 30-3).

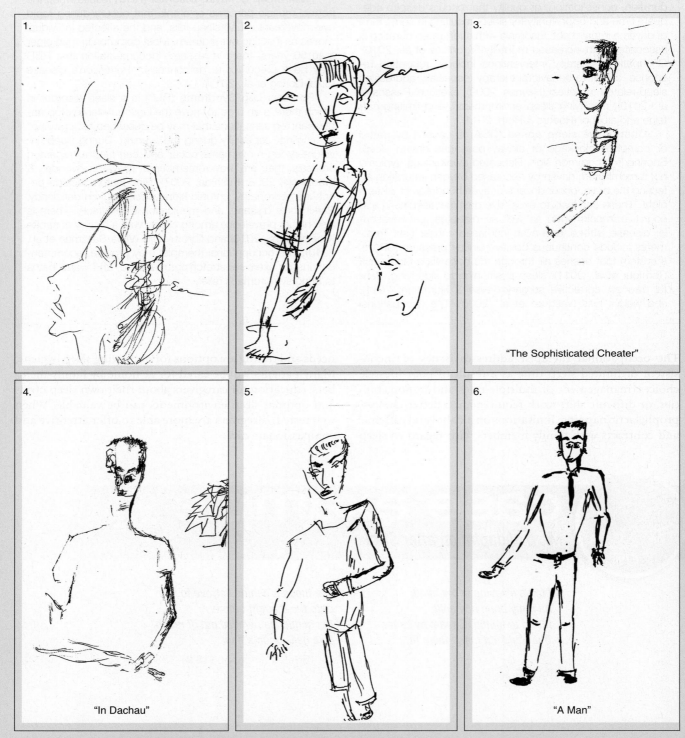

1.

2.

3. "The Sophisticated Cheater"

4. "In Dachau"

5.

6. "A Man"

Figure 30-3 Six serial self-portraits drawn by Mr. D. during months 3, 4, and 5 after right-hemisphere stroke.

Clinical Reasoning Process

Occupational Therapy Intervention Process	Objectives	Examples of Therapist's Internal Dialogue
Patient Information Mr. D. was a 53-year-old right-handed white man who suffered a severe right thalamic hemorrhage with rapid onset and steady improvement. His presenting problems at inpatient occupational therapy assessment included left hemiparesis; left homonymous hemianopsia; left neglect and anosognosia; disorientation to time and place; deficits in perception, attention, memory, and visuospatial processing; and complete dependence in activities of daily living. Mr. D. retained superior verbal ability, had an advanced education, strong family support, and adequate health insurance. He was a husband, father, and former university dean and public administrator and was his family's primary breadwinner.	Appreciate the context Understand premorbid circumstances and characteristics	"Mr. D. was obviously in the prime of his career at the time of his stroke; it must have come as such a shock to him and his family. His vocational background suggests that he is used to being highly respected and in charge. He has been directing others, not accepting direction. I imagine that it will be particularly difficult for him to adjust to a dependent role of any duration. I will want to think of as many ways that he can be in control as possible and support his family in recognizing his needs in this regard." "With high school–aged children and a spouse who has not been working outside the home, financial pressures may add to the stress. I wonder if his wife may need to seek employment and may not be available as a caregiver for him when he returns home." "Mr. D.'s denial of the severity of his disability is a major obstacle to recognizing the need for and committing to occupational therapy treatment."
	Select an intervention approach	"I know it will be important that I show respect for his history of life roles by prioritizing occupational therapy goals related to intellectual and social skills and beginning with activities that emphasize **compensation** through his most preserved areas of function. This strategy should help increase his motivation and sense of personal continuity." "Mr. D.'s preserved verbal strengths will help in building our therapeutic alliance."
Recommendations Related to Personal and Social Adaptation The following goals were set for inpatient treatment (5 days/week for 3 months) and outpatient follow-up: (1) foster therapeutic alliance; (2) identify/enlist motivating strategies; (3) consider past occupational roles and future adaptation; (4) encourage partnership in setting priorities for goals; (5) develop sense of mastery and control through specific skill development and relearning—reading, self-care, and mobility; and (6) guide the search for meaning.	Consider the patient's appraisal of performance Consider what will occur in therapy, how often, and for how long Solicit the patient's modifications and endorsement of plan	"Trust will be critical in countering neurologically based denial. I must help him to believe there are good reasons for what I am asking of him. As his denial begins to break, the increased awareness of his losses will be painful; questions of meaning are likely to arise. I will try to help him find his own best way of making sense of his experiences. I will have to examine my own feelings about what has happened to him, a robust and gifted man at the height of his career." "I think that it is important to integrate safety and self-care goals into treatment if he is to return home without requiring a full-time aide. Continued dialogue will be needed to negotiate for attention to these goals and to address issues of physical dependency, which at present do not appear relevant to him."
Interventions Related to Personal and Social Adaptation • Improve orientation to time and place. • Solicit narrative of his experiences related to the stroke. • Compensate for left visual field deficits and denial using cues from occupational therapist. • Improve awareness/positioning and range of motion in left upper and lower extremities.	Assess the patient's comprehension and processing strategies	"I need to continually orient Mr. D. to his surroundings and circumstances and, later, to the occupational therapy role. Other staff and team members can be enlisted to help so that Mr. D. is getting a consistent message. Staff and team should be made aware of the effects of his neurological deficits on his reasoning and tendency to confabulate."

- Maneuver the wheelchair for short distances.
- Practice supervised self-care.
- Attempt reading and writing.
- Address existential questions.
- Open lines of communication with family.

Organize cues, structure

Compare actual to expected performance

Know the person

"Sometimes he sounds almost psychotic, but I appreciate that actually he is trying to make narrative sense of what he experiences through a limited field of vision and with a damaged perceptual framework normally supported by the right hemisphere."

"With his denial breaking, I believe that it is crucial to avoid flooding Mr. D. with failures in these areas. Time must be allocated in occupational therapy to enjoy relative successes before new demands are added. With growing awareness of losses, periods of despair or depression may emerge."

"I can see our alliance is deepened when I identify and name his feelings and reflect back what I have heard. Mr. D.'s drawings convey a great deal about his changing body image and sense of self."

"His stories help me understand and guide the developing ways in which he is trying to make sense of what has happened to him."

Appreciate the context and cognitive strategies in use

"I need to keep in mind how much Mr. D.'s life has changed. He was accustomed to giving orders, delegating authority, and having his decisions respected. How can I help him find some sense of mastery outside those roles that have been so much of his identity? What are his family members expecting? What additional relationships, institutional, and community supports are in place that can help Mr. D.'s world work for him when he is discharged? Friends? Church?"

Next Steps

As an outpatient, Mr. D. worked toward being able to (1) compensate for neglect and visual field deficits in the context of reading and writing tasks, (2) initiate social interaction including telephone management skills, (3) monitor moods, (4) walk short distances with an assistive device, (5) carry out exercises to maintain left arm range of motion, (6) continue drawings and narrative, (7) explore vocational requirements and expectations, and (8) participate in a home visit for assessment of safety and equipment.

Anticipate present and future patient concerns

Recognize that which has brought meaning and purpose to his life in the past

Assess patient's comprehension and changing awareness of deficits and the related implications for adaptation.

Engage family and other caregivers to recognize needed resources for safety, daily structure, cueing, and social support

Plan for discharge and outpatient follow-up

"As Mr. D. continues to adjust to what has happened to him, I anticipate that he will have concerns with his level of dependency. He was the breadwinner; he is not likely to return to a high-paying position. He took care of his wife and family. Will they now have to take care of him? There is a risk of repeat stroke; ongoing medical management is critical. Does he have fears about this? What fears and questions might his family have?"

"So far, no signs of a plateau in improvement have been seen. Mr. D. wants to continue occupational therapy after discharge, and I agree that he should. Coming home will be hard. He has been in a supportive environment with much interaction where his safety has been assured. His family has been attentive, but they have not had primary responsibility for his care. Outpatient therapy will maintain alliance during this critical transition and continue building competence. Family expectations must be explored; they will require transitional support as he returns home."

Clinical Reasoning in Occupational Therapy Practice

Cognitions Associated with Pain

Chronic pain is commonly associated with certain elements of self-narrative. As part of effective pain treatment, the individual must learn to become aware of and change thoughts or cognitions that are undermining function and self-esteem (Gallagher, 1997). The statements that follow might be uncovered through monitoring or in dialogue. Using Helplessness and Dependency as examples, write positive alternative statements for the examples of Rumination and Retribution, Punishment in the spaces provided below.

Helplessness: The pain prevents me from doing all the things I want to do. The pain makes me bad at everything I used to be good at. Why try?

Alternatives: When I pace myself, I get things accomplished. It is harder to do some things, but I can still do many things well.

Dependency: I can't be expected to do anything when I feel like this. Others should take over for me.

Alternative: Some things are harder to accomplish, but I can still do them. I will ask for help when I truly need it.

Rumination: I think about the pain every minute to be sure it is not getting worse.

Alternative _____
_____
_____

Retribution, Punishment: I must have done something to deserve this.

Alternative _____
_____
_____

 ## Clinical Reasoning in Occupational Therapy Practice

Mr. D. Sleeps Poorly

The wife of Mr. D. reports that he was "never a good sleeper" and now continues to snore loudly at night. Could a sleep disorder have contributed to his stroke risk? How might poor sleep compromise Mr. D.'s adaptation and ability to benefit from therapy? How might the occupational therapist respond to this new information?

Summary Review Questions

1. Write a letter from the rehabilitation hospital to a close friend or family member describing your feelings and efforts to cope following a disabling accident.

2. Generate five short hypotheses through which to understand why a patient might seem unmotivated in treatment. Considering your hypotheses, what components would you expect interventions for pain and depression to have in common. Why?

3. Present briefly the four stages from injury to rehabilitation as described by Morse and O'Brien (1995). In what ways are stage theories helpful? What wrong assumptions can they produce?

4. What stresses might disabled patients' families or partners experience? What are three ways occupational therapists ease those stresses?

5. Explore an Internet site serving a virtual community of ill or disabled individuals. Give examples of support and information that you find being exchanged. What criteria would you use to evaluate this connection and information for participants? In what ways might the interchange be like group treatment? In what ways might it be different?

6. Respond to this patient's question: "Why go on living with a severe disability?" What feelings or reactions in yourself over such a question would lead you to seek extra support or supervision?

7. List four indications that would cause you to seek psychiatric consultation or referral for the patient in Question 6.

8. Describe three ways in which disordered sleep might compromise patient adaptation. List the parallel

occupational therapy interventions that could support improved patient sleep.

9. View one or more of the films that portray a disabled person. What strategies for coping are depicted in the film(s)? What is demonstrated about the close relationships and occupations of disabled individuals? How might the film(s) influence the audience's understanding of living with a disability?

10. Examine a pathography by a patient or a patient's family member. In what ways are the experiences portrayed useful to you? Might they be helpful to patients?

Glossary

Adaptation—Alteration or adjustment by which an individual or species improves its condition in relation to its situation or environment.

Attribution—The process by which an individual assigns causality.

Cognitive-behavioral therapy (CBT)—A systematic form of talk therapy that emphasizes the impact of thoughts on emotions and behaviors.

Coping—Cognitive, emotional, and behavioral efforts individuals undertake to manage external and internal challenges that tax their ordinary resources.

Existential—Description of a perspective that emphasizes the human condition, including the recognition of mortality and the felt necessity to create meaning.

Mindfulness—Maintaining a calm and nonjudgmental awareness of consciousness in the present moment.

Obstructive sleep apnea (OSA)—Partial or complete blockage of airway passages during sleep leading to repeated awakenings driven by decreased oxygen saturation.

Post-traumatic stress disorder (PTSD)—Lasting psychological response to witnessing or experiencing traumatic events, especially when helpless to prevent them.

Relaxation response (RR)—A physiological state characterized by slowed brain waves, lowered heart and respiratory rates, and lowered blood pressure that is believed to enhance health and well-being.

Resilience—The psychological capacity to respond to disruption with a new integration.

References

Ader, R. (1981). *Psychoneuroimmunology*. Orlando, FL: Academic.

Alonso, A., & Swiller, H. (1993). *Group therapy in clinical practice*. Washington, DC: American Psychiatric Association.

American Occupational Therapy Association. (1995a). Position paper: Occupational performance: Occupational therapy's definition of function. *American Journal of Occupational Therapy, 49*, 1019–1020.

American Occupational Therapy Association. (1995b). Position paper: The psychosocial core of occupational therapy. *American Journal of Occupational Therapy, 49*, 1021–1022.

American Occupational Therapy Association. (2002). Occupational therapy practice framework: Domain and process. *American Journal of Occupational Therapy, 56*, 609–639.

American Occupational Therapy Association. (2008). Occupational therapy practice framework: Domain and process (2nd ed.). *American Journal of Occupational Therapy, 62*, 625–683.

Anaby, D. R. (2010). Theoretical exploration of two approaches to occupational balance. *The Canadian Journal of Occupational Therapy, 77*, 280–288.

Anson, K., & Ponsford, J. (2006). Coping style and emotional adjustment following traumatic brain injury. *Journal of Head Trauma Rehabilitation, 21*, 248–259.

Arias, A. J., Steinberg, K., Banga, A., & Trestman, R. A. (2006). Systematic review of the efficacy of meditation techniques as treatments for medical illness. *Journal of Alternative and Complementary Medicine, 12*, 817–832.

Banks, M. E. (2003). Disability in the family: A life span perspective. *Cultural Diversity and Ethnic Minor Psychology, 9*, 367–384.

Bartick, M. C., Thai, X., Schmidt, T., Altaye, A., & Solet, J. M. (2009). Decrease in as-needed sedative use by limiting nighttime sleep disruptions from hospital staff. *Journal of Hospital Medicine, September 18, 5*(3), E20–E24.

Basson, R. (1998). Sexual health of women with disabilities. *Canadian Medical Association Journal, 159*, 359–362.

Bayard, M., Avonda, T., & Wadzinski, J. (2008). Restless legs syndrome. *American Family Physician, 78*, 235–240.

Benson, H. (1993). The relaxation response. In D. Goleman & J. Gurin (Eds.), *Mind-body medicine: How to use your mind for better health* (pp. 233–258). New York: Consumer Reports Books.

Benson, H. (1995). Commentary: Religion, belief and healing. *Mind/Body Medicine, 1*, 158.

Benson, H., & Proctor, W. (2010). *Relaxation revolution: Enhancing your personal health through the science and genetics of mind body healing*. New York: Scribner.

Bhogal, S. K., Teasell, R. W., Foley, N. C., & Speechley, M. R. (2003). Community reintegration after stroke. *Topics in Stroke Rehabilitation, Summer, 10*(2), 107–129.

Blakeney, A., & Marshall, A. (2009). Water quality, health, and human occupations. *American Journal of Occupational Therapy, 63*, 46–57.

Boeije, H. R., Duijnstee, M. S., Grypdonck, M. H., & Pool, A. (2002). Encountering the downward phase: Biographical work in people with multiple sclerosis living at home. *Social Science Medicine, 55*, 881–893.

Bontje, P., Kinebanian, A., Josephsson, S., & Tamuura, Y. (2004). Occupational adaptation: The experience of older persons with physical disabilities. *American Journal of Occupational Therapy, 58*, 140–149.

Braley, T. J., & Chervin, R. D. (2010). Fatigue in multiple sclerosis: Mechanisms, evaluation and treatment. *Sleep, 33*, 1061–1067.

Brendel, D. H., Florman, J., Roberts, S., & Solet, J. M. (2001). "In sleep I almost never grope": Blindness, neuropsychiatric deficits, and a chaotic upbringing. *Harvard Review of Psychiatry, 9,* 178–188.

Buning, M. E. (1999). Fitness for persons with disabilities: A call to action. *OT Practice, 8,* 27–32.

Burns, D. (1990). *The feeling good handbook.* New York: Plume.

Burton, A. R., Rahman, K., Kadota, Y., Lloyd, A., & Vollmer-Conna, U. (2010). Reduced heart rate variability predicts poor sleep quality in a case-control study of chronic fatigue syndrome. *Experimental Brain Research, 204,* 71–78.

Busch-Vishniac, I. J., West, J. E., Barnhill, C., Hunter, T., Orellana, D., & Chivukula, R. (2005). Noise levels in Johns Hopkins Hospital. *Journal of the Acoustic Society of America, 118,* 3629–3645.

Buxton, O. M., Ellenbogen, J. M., Wang, W., Carballeira, A., O'Connor, S., Cooper, B. S., McKinney, S. M., & Solet, J. M. (2012). Sleep disruption due to hospital noises. *Annals of Internal Medicine, 157,* 170–179.

Cambridge Health Alliance. (1995). *Mental health and addictions.* Unpublished training document.

Caudill, M. A. (1995). *Managing pain before it manages you.* New York: Guilford.

Champagne, T., Koomar, J., & Olsen, L. (2010). Occupational therapy's role with post-traumatic stress disorder. Retrieved July 4, 2013 from http://www.aota.org/Consumers/Professionals/WhatIsOT/MH/Facts/PTSD.aspx.

Chandola, T., Ferrie, J. E., Perski, A., Akbaraly, T., & Marmor, M. G. (2010). The effect of short sleep duration on coronary heart disease risk is greatest among those with sleep disturbance: A prospective study from Whitehall II cohort. *Sleep, 33,* 739–744.

Charon, R. (2005). Narrative medicine: Attention, representation, affiliation. *Narrative, 13,* 261–270.

Charon, R. (2006). *Narrative medicine: Honoring the stories of illness.* New York: Oxford University Press.

Chien, K., Chen, P., Hsu, H., Sung, F., Chen, M., & Lee Y. (2010). Habitual sleep duration and insomnia and the risk of cardiovascular events and all cause death: Report from an community-based cohort. *Sleep, 33,* 177–184.

Chodron, P. (1997). *When things fall apart: Heart advice for difficult times.* Boston: Shambala.

Coelho, F. M. S., Georgsson, H., Narayansingh, M., Swartz, R. H., & Murray, B. J. (2010). Higher prevalence of periodic limb movements of sleep in patients with history of stroke. *Journal of Clinical Sleep Medicine, 6,* 428–431.

Cohen, D. A., Wang, W., Wyatt, J. K., Konuer, R. E., Dijk, D.-J., Czeisler, C. A., & Klerman, E. B. (2010). Uncovering residual effects of chronic sleep loss on human performance. *Science Translational Medicine, 2,* 14ra3.

Coughlin, J. (2010). Estimating the impact of care-giving and employment on well-being. *Outcomes & Insights in Health Management, 2,* 1–7.

Crawford, A., Hollingsworth, H. H., Morgan, K., & Gray, D. B. (2008). People with mobility impairments: Physical activity and quality of participation. *Disability and Health Journal, 1,* 7–13.

Davidhizer, R. (1997). Disability does not have to be the grief that never ends: Helping patients adjust. *Rehabilitation Nursing, 22,* 32–35.

Denollet, J. (1998). Personality and coronary heart disease: The type-D scale-16. *Annals of Behavioral Medicine, 20,* 209–226.

Dewar, A. L., & Lee, E. A. (2000). Bearing illness and injury. *Western Journal of Nursing Research, 22,* 912–926.

Dickinson, E. (1999). I felt a cleaving in my mind. In R. W. Franklin (Ed.), *The poems of Emily Dickinson.* Cambridge, MA: Belknap.

Donohue, M. V., Hanif, H., & Berns, L. W. (2011). An exploratory study of social participation in occupational therapy groups. *Special Interest Section Quarterly, Mental Health, 34,* 1–3.

Dorset, P. (2010). The importance of hope in coping with severe acquired disability. *Australian Social Work, 63,* 83–102.

Drake, C., Roehrs, T., Breslau, N., Johnson, E., Jefferson, C., Scofield, H., & Roth, T. (2010). The 10-year risk of verified motor vehicle crashes in relation to physiologic sleepiness. *Sleep, 33,* 745–752.

Durmer, J. S., & Dinges, D. F. (2005). Neuro-cognitive consequences of sleep deprivation. *Seminars in Neurology, 25,* 117–129.

Dusek, J. A., Out, H. H., Wohluerter, A. L., Bhasin, M., Zerbini, L. F., Joseph, M. G., Benson, H., & Libermann, T. A. (2008). Genomic counter-stress changes induced by relaxation response. *PLoS One, 3,* e2576.

Ehde, D. M., Jensen, M. P., Engel, J. M., Turner, J. A., Hoffman, A. J., & Cardenas, D. D. (2003). Chronic pain secondary to disability: A review. *Clinical Journal of Pain, 19,* 3–17.

Engel, J. M. (2011). Pain in persons with developmental disabilities. *OT Practice, 16,* CE-1-8.

Epstein, J. E., & Brown, R. (2010). Sleep disorders in spinal cord injury. In V. W. Lin (Ed.), *Spinal cord medicine: Principles and practice* (2nd ed., pp. 230–240). New York: Demos.

Flach, F. (2004). *Resilience.* New York: Hatherleigh Press.

Flier, J., & Elmquist, J. K. (2004). A good night's sleep: Future antidote to the obesity epidemic? *Annals of Internal Medicine, 141,* 885–886.

Frank, G. (1996). Life histories in occupational therapy clinical practice. *American Journal of Occupational Therapy, 50,* 251–264.

Franz, C. E., & White, K. M. (1985). Individuation and attachment in personality development: Extending Erikson's theory. *Journal of Personality, 53,* 224–256.

Gal, B. (1999). Veterinary update: Pets keep people healthy. *Veterinary Economics, Summer,* 3–4.

Gallagher, R. M. (1997). Behavioral and bio-behavioral treatment in chronic pain: Perspectives on effectiveness. *Mind/Body Medicine, 2,* 176–186.

Gardner, D. (1999). The protective barrier in brain injury. *TBI Challenge, April/May,* 8–12.

Ghaemi, S. N., & Sachs, G. (1999, April 10). Practical psychiatric update: Improving assessment and treatment of the bipolar spectrum. *American Occupational Therapy Association Conference Proceedings,* Boston.

Gilbertson, L., Langhorne, P., Walker, A., Allen, A., & Murray, G. D. (2000). Domiciliary occupational therapy for patients with stroke discharged from hospital: Randomised controlled trial. *British Medical Journal, 320,* 603–606.

Griffin, C. (2011). *Adaptation to disability in the workplace.* Unpublished presentation. Cambridge, MA: Cambridge Commission for Persons with Disabilities.

Groves, J. E. (1978). Taking care of the hateful patient. *New England Journal of Medicine, 298,* 883–887.

Haack, G., & Mullington, J. M. (2005). Sustained sleep restriction reduces emotional and physical well-being. *Pain, 119,* 56–64.

Hale, L. (2005). Who has time to sleep? *Journal of Public Health, 27,* 205–211.

Hamilton, N. A., Karlson, C., & Catley, D. (2007). Sleep and affective response to stress and pain. *Health Psychology, 26,* 288–295.

Hamilton, N. A., Kitzman, H., & Guyotte, S. (2006). Enhancing health and emotion: Mindfulness as a missing link between cognitive therapy and positive psychology. *Journal of Cognitive Psychotherapy, 20,* 123–134.

Harris, S., Morley, S., & Barton, S. B. (2003). Role loss and adjustment in chronic pain. *Pain, 105,* 363–370.

Hasselkus, B. R. (1991). Ethical dilemmas in family caregiving for the elderly: Implications for occupational therapy. *American Journal of Occupational Therapy, 45,* 206–212.

Hasselkus, B. R. (1994). Working with family caregivers: A therapeutic alliance. In B. R. Bonder & M. B. Wagner (Eds.), *Functional performance in older adults* (pp. 339–351). Philadelphia: F.A. Davis.

Hawkins, A. H. (1993). *Reconstructing illness: Studies in pathography.* West Lafayette, IN: Purdue University.

Haynes, P. L. (2009). Is CBT-1 effective for pain? Commentary on: Cognitive behavioral therapy for insomnia improves sleep and decreases pain in older adults with co-morbid insomnia and osteoarthritis. *Journal of Clinical Sleep Medicine, 5,* 355–362 and 363–364.

Heinemann, A. W., Mamott, B., & Schnoll, S. (1990). Substance abuse by persons with recent spinal cord injuries. *Rehabilitation Psychology, 35,* 217–228.

Hoch, D., & Ferguson, T. (2005). What I have learned from E-patients. *PLoS Medicine, 2,* e206.

Holzel, B. K., Carmody, J., Vangel, M., Congleton, C., Yerramsetti, S. M., Gard, T., & Lazar, S. W. (2011). Mindfulness practice leads to increase in regional gray matter density. *Psychiatry Research: Neuroimaging, 191,* 36–43.

Hulter, B. M., & Lundberg, P. O. (1995). Sexual function in women with advanced multiple sclerosis. *Journal of Neurology, Neurosurgery, and Psychiatry, 59,* 83–86.

Hwang, J. E., Cvitanovich, D. C., Doroski, E. K., & Vajarakitiongse, J. G. (2011). Correlations between quality of life and adaptation factors among people with multiple sclerosis. *American Journal of Occupational Therapy, 65,* 661–669.

Irwin, M., Wang, M., Ribeiro, D., Jin Cho, H., Olmstead, R., Breen, E., & Cole, S. (2008). Sleep loss activates cellular inflammatory signaling. *Bio-psychiatry, 64,* 538–554.

Institute of Medicine. (2008). *Retooling for an aging America: Building the health care workforce.* National Academies Press.

Institute of Medicine. (2011). *Relieving pain in America: A blueprint for transforming care, education, and research.* Washington DC: National Academies Press.

Jenkins, G. R. (2011). The challenges of characterizing people with disabilities in the built environment. *OT Practice, 9,* CE1–CE7.

Johns, M. W. (1991). A new method for measuring daytime sleepiness: The Epworth Sleepiness Scale. *Sleep, 14,* 540–545.

Johnson, K. G., & Johnson, C. D. (2010). Frequency of sleep apnea in stroke and TIA patients: A meta-analysis. *Journal of Clinical Sleep Medicine, 6,* 131–137.

Jonsson, A. T., Moller, A., & Grimby, G. (1998). Managing occupations in everyday life to achieve adaptation. *American Journal of Occupational Therapy, 53,* 353–362.

Joseph, R. (2005). *Integrated healthcare and disease management.* Unpublished presentation. Cambridge, MA: Cambridge Health Alliance.

Kahana, J. R., & Bibring, G. (1964). Personality types in medical management. In N. Zinberg (Ed.), *Psychiatry and medical practice in a general hospital* (pp. 108–123). New York: International Universities.

Katz, N., Hartman-Maeir, A., Ring, H., & Soroker, N. (2000). Relationship of cognitive performance and daily function of clients following right hemisphere stroke: Predictive and ecological validity of the LOTCA Battery. *Occupational Therapy Journal of Research, 20,* 3–16.

Kautzman, L. N. (1992). Linking patient and family stories to caregivers' use of clinical reasoning. *American Journal of Occupational Therapy, 47,* 169–173.

Keith, B. (1999). *Psychological aspects of recovery from brain surgery.* Unpublished manuscript.

Kemp, B. J. (2005). What the rehabilitation professional and consumer need to know. *Physical Medicine and Rehabilitation Clinics of North America, 16,* 1–18.

Kemp, J. K. (1993). Psychological care of the older rehabilitation patient. *Geriatric Rehabilitation, 9,* 841–857.

Khantzian, E. J. (1990). Self-regulation and self-medication factors in alcoholism and the addictions. In M. Galanter (Ed.), *Recent developments in alcoholism* (Volume 8, pp. 255–271). New York: Plenum.

Kiecolt-Glaser, J., Christian, L., Preston, H., Houts, C., Malarkey, W., Emery, C., & Glaser, R. (2010). Stress, inflammation, and yoga practice. *Psychosomatic Medicine, 72,* 113–121.

Kielhofner, G. (1992). *Conceptual foundations of occupational therapy.* Philadelphia: F.A. Davis.

King, G. A., Shultz, I. Z., Steel, K., Gilpin, M., & Cathers, T. (1993). Self-evaluation and self-concept of adolescents with physical disabilities. *American Journal of Occupational Therapy, 47,* 132–140.

Kleinman, A. (1988). *The illness narratives: Suffering, healing, and the human condition.* New York: Basic.

Koenig, H. G., & George, L. K. (1998). Depression and physical disability outcomes in depressed medically ill hospitalized older adults. *American Journal of Geriatric Psychiatry, 6,* 230–247.

Kryger, M. H., Roth, T., & Dement, W. C. (2011). *Principles and practice of sleep medicine* (5th ed.). Philadelphia: Elsevier Saunders.

Kubzansky, L. D., Kawachi, I., Weiss, S. T., & Sparrow, D. (1998). Anxiety and coronary heart disease: A synthesis of epidemiological, psychological, and experimental evidence. *Annals of Behavioral Medicine, 20,* 47–58.

Kushida, C. A. (2007). Clinical presentation, diagnosis, and quality of life issues in restless legs syndrome. *American Journal of Medicine, 120,* S4–S12.

Laatsch, L., & Shahani, B. T. (1996). The relationship between age, gender and psychological distress in rehabilitation inpatients. *Disability and Rehabilitation, 18,* 604–608.

Larson, D. B., & Milano, M. A. G. (1995). Are religion and spirituality clinically relevant in health care? *Mind/Body Medicine, 1,* 147–158.

Lazarus, R. S., & Folkman, S. (1984). *Stress, appraisal, and coping.* New York: Springer.

Levine, C. (1999). The loneliness of the long-term care-giver. *New England Journal of Medicine, 340,* 1587–1590.

Lowenstein, A. (1999). *Alice's story: Notes from the rehabilitation center.* Unpublished manuscript.

Luyster, F. S., Chasens, E. R., Wasko, M. C. M., & Dunbar-Jacob, J. (2011). Sleep quality and functional disability in patients with rheumatoid arthritis. *Journal of Clinical Sleep Medicine, 7,* 49–55.

Lynch, J. W., Kaplan, G. A., & Shema, S. J. (1997). Cumulative impact of sustained economic hardship on the physical, cognitive, psychological and social functioning. *New England Journal of Medicine, 337,* 1889–1895.

Main, C. J., & Spanswick, C. C. (1991). Pain: Psychological and psychiatric factors. *British Medical Bulletin, 47,* 732–742.

Main, T. F. (1957). The ailment. *British Journal of Medical Psychology, 30,* 129–217.

Mazor for Rosh Hashanah and Yom Kippur: A prayer book for the days of awe. (1972). New York: Rabbinical Assembly.

Meyer, R. (1999). *Our models of addiction: Their promise and their problems.* Unpublished presentation. Psychiatry Grand Rounds, June 16, Cambridge Health Alliance.

Miner, L. (1999, March 25). The psychosocial impact of limb or digit amputation. *Occupational Therapy Week,* 10–11.

Minkler, M., Fuller-Thompson, E., & Guralnik, J. M. (2006). Gradient of disability across socioeconomic spectrum in the United States. *New England Journal of Medicine, 355,* 695–704.

Moore, D., & Li, L. (1994). Substance abuse among applicants for vocational rehabilitation services. *Journal of Rehabilitation, 60,* 48–53.

Morse, J. M., & O'Brien, B. (1995). Preserving self: From victim, to patient, to disabled person. *Journal of Advanced Nursing, 21,* 88–896.

Mukherjee, S. (2010). *The emperor of all maladies.* New York: Scribner.

Nemeroff, C. B. (1998, June). The neurobiology of depression. *Scientific American, 278,* 42–49.

O'Connor, G. T., Caffo, B., & Newman, A. B. (2009). Prospective study of sleep disordered breathing and hypertension: The Sleep Heart Health Study. *American Journal of Respiratory Critical Care Medicine, 179,* 1159–1164.

Ohayon, N. M., & Vecchierini, M. F. (2005). Normative sleep data, cognitive function and daily living activities in older adults in the community. *Sleep, 28,* 981–989.

Ospina, M. B., Bond, K., Karkhanah, M., Tjosvold, L., Vandermeer, B., Lang, Y., Bialy, L., Hooton, N., Buscemi, N., Dryden, D. M., & Klassen, T. P. (2007). *Meditation practices for health: State of the research* (AHRQ Publication No. 07-E010). Rockville, MD: Agency of Healthcare Research and Quality.

Pande, N., & Tewari, S. (2011). Understanding coping with distress due to physical disability. *Psychology and Developing Societies, 23,* 177–209.

Parcell, D. L., Ponsford, J. L., Redman, J. R., & Rajaratnam, S. W. M. (2008). Poor sleep quality and changes in objectively-recorded sleep after traumatic brain injury: A preliminary study. *Archives of Physical Medicine and Rehabilitation, 89,* 843–850.

Passos, G. S., Poyares, D., Santana, M. G., Garbuio, S., Tufik, S., & Mello, M. T. (2010). Effect of acute physical exercise on patients with chronic primary insomnia. *Journal of Clinical Sleep Medicine, 6,* 270–275

Patel, S. R., & Hu, F. B. (2008). Short sleep duration and weight gain: A systematic review. *Obesity, 16,* 643–653.

Patenaude, A. F. (2005). *Genetic testing for cancer: Psychological approaches for helping patients and families.* Washington, DC: American Psychological Association.

Peloquin, S. M. (2002). Reclaiming the vision of reaching heart as well as hands. *American Journal of Occupational Therapy, 56,* 517–526.

Perlis, M. L., Jungquist, C., Smith, M. T., & Posner, D. (2008). *Cognitive behavioral treatment of insomnia: A session by session guide.* New York: Springer.

Persson, D., Andersson, I., & Eklund, M. (2011). Defying aches and reevaluating daily doing: Occupational perspectives on adjusting to chronic pain. *Scandinavian Journal of Occupational Therapy, 18,* 188–197.

Pennebaker, J. W. (1995). *Emotion, disclosure, and health.* Washington, DC: American Psychological Association.

Poe, G., Walsh, C. M., & Bjorness, T. E. (2010). Both duration and timing of sleep are important to memory consolidation. *Sleep, 33,* 1277–1280.

Powdthavee, N. (2009). What happens to people before and after disability? Focusing effects, lead effects, and adaptation in different areas of life. *Social Science and Medicine, 69,* 1834–1844.

Quale, A. J., & Schanke, A.-K. (2010). Resilience in the face of coping with a severe personal injury: A study of trajectories of adjustment in a rehabilitation setting. *Rehabilitation Psychology, 55,* 12–22.

Quigly, M. C. (1995). Impact of spinal cord injury on the life roles of women. *American Journal of Occupational Therapy, 49,* 780–786.

Rankin, W. (1985). A theologian's perspective on illness and the human spirit. *Linacre Quarterly, November,* 329–334.

Ratey, J., & Hagerman, E. (2009). *Spark: The revolutionary new science of exercise and the brain.* New York: Little, Brown, and Company.

Redline, S. (2009). Does sleep disordered breathing increase hypertension risk? A practical perspective on interpreting the evidence. *Journal of Clinical Sleep Medicine, 5,* 406–408.

Rena, F., Moshe, S., & Abraham, O. (1996). Couple's adjustment to one partner's disability: The relationship between sense of coherence and adjustment. *Social Science Medicine, 43,* 163–171.

Robinson, K., Kennedy, N., & Harmon, D. (2011). Is occupational therapy adequately meeting the needs of people with chronic pain? *American Journal of Occupational Therapy, 65,* 106–113.

Rochman, D., & Kennedy-Spain, E. (2007). Chronic pain management: Approaches and tools for occupational therapy. *OT Practice, 12,* 9–15.

Rodgers, M. L., Strode, A. D., Norell, D. M., Short, R. A., Dyck, D. G., & Becker, B. (2007). Adapting multiple-family group treatment for brain and spinal cord injury intervention development and preliminary outcomes. *American Journal of Physical Medicine and Rehabilitation, 86,* 482–492.

Roehrs, T., Hyde, M., Blaisdell, B., Greenwald, M., & Roth, T. (2006). Sleep loss and REM sleep loss are hyperalgesic. *Sleep, 29,* 145–151.

Roehrs, T., & Roth, T. (2011). Sleep, sleepiness, and alcohol use. National Institute of Alcohol Abuse and Alcoholism website. Retrieved July 4, 2013 from pubs.niaaa.nih.gov/publications/arh25-2/101-109.htm.

Rowe, C. E., & MacIsaac, D. S. (1991). *Empathic attunement: The technique of psychoanalytic self psychology.* Northvale, NJ: Jason Aronson.

Saetersdal, B. (1997). Forbidden suffering: The Pollyanna syndrome of the disabled and their families. *Family Process, 36,* 431–435.

Schultz, A. W., & Liptak, G. S. (1998). Helping adolescents who have disabilities negotiate transitions to adulthood. *Issues in Comprehensive Pediatric Nursing, 21,* 187–201.

Schroevers, M. J., Kraaij, V., & Garnefski, N. (2011). Cancer patient's experience of positive and negative changes due to illness: Relationships with psychological well-being, coping, and goal reengagement. *Psycho-Oncology, 20,* 165–172.

Simkins, C. N. (1999). Pediatric brain injury may last a lifetime. *TBI Challenge, April/May,* 4–5.

Sixel-Doring, F., Schweitzer, M., Mollenhauer, B., & Trenkwalder, C. (2011). Intra-individual variability of REM sleep behavior disorder in Parkinson's disease: A comparative assessment using a new REM Sleep Behavior Disorder Severity Scale (RBDSS) for clinical routine. *Journal of Clinical Sleep Medicine, 7,* 75–80.

Social Security Administration. (n.d.). *Income of disabled-worker beneficiaries.* Retrieved July 4, 2013 from http://www.ssa.gov/policy/docs/chartbooks/income_workers/di_chart.pdf.

Solet, J. M. (1991). *Coping and injury attribution in head-injured adults.* Unpublished doctoral dissertation. Boston: Boston University.

Solet, J. M. (1995). Educating patients about pain. *Occupational Therapy Week, August 17,* 3–4.

Solet, J. M., & Barach, P. (2012). Managing alarm fatigue in cardiac care. *Progress in Pediatric Cardiology* (in press).

Solet, J. M., Buxton, O. M., Ellenbogen, J. M., Wang, W., & Carballiera, A. (2010). Validating Acoustic Guidelines for Healthcare Facilities - Evidence-based design meets evidence-based medicine: The sound sleep study. The Center for Health Design Research Coalition. Retrieved July 4, 2013 from http://www.brikbase.org/sites/default/files/CHP_SoundSleepStudy.pdf

Sontag, S. (1988). *Illness as metaphor and AIDS and its metaphors.* New York: Anchor.

Sorscher, A. J. (2008). How is your sleep? A neglected topic for health care screening. *Journal of the American Board of Family Medicine, 21,* 141–148.

Stewart, D. A., Law, M. C., Rosenbaum, P., & Williams, D. G. (2001). A qualitative study of transition to adulthood for youth with physical disabilities. *Physical and Occupational Therapy Pediatrics, 21,* 3–21.

Stern, R. A., Riley, D. O., Daneshvar, D. H., Nowinski, C. J., Canfu, R. C., & McKee, A. C. (2011). Long-term consequences of repetitive brain trauma: Chronic traumatic encephalopathy (concussion supplement). *Physical Medicine and Rehabilitation, 3,* 460–467.

Stoller, C. C., Gruel, J. H., Cimini, L. S., Fowler, M. S., & Koomar, A. A. (2012). Effects of sensory-enhanced yoga on symptoms of combat stress in deployed military personnel. *American Journal of Occupational Therapy, 66,* 59–68.

Stone, A. A., & Porter, M. A. (1995). Psychological coping: Its importance for treating medical problems. *Mind/Body Medicine, 1,* 46–54.

Stroe, A. F., Roth, T., Jefferson, C., Hudgel, D. W., Roehrs, T., Moss, K., & Drake, C. L. (2010). Comparative levels of excessive daytime sleepiness in common medical disorders. *Sleep Medicine, 11,* 890–896.

Taylor, D. (2011). Health costs of working age disabled adults. *The Incidental Economist.* Retrieved July 4, 2013 from http://theincidental economist.com/wordpress/health-costs-of-working-age-disabled-adults/.

Thoren-Jonsson, A. L. (2001). Coming to terms with the shift in one's capabilities: A study of adaptation to poliomyelitis sequelae. *Disability Rehabilitation, 23,* 341–351.

Toglia, J. P. (2005). A dynamic interactional approach to cognitive rehabilitation. In N. Katz (Ed.), *Cognition and occupation across the lifespan: Models for intervention in occupational therapy* (pp. 29–72). Bethesda, MD: American Occupational Therapy Association.

Tomfour, L. M., Ancoli-Isreal, S., Loredo, J. S., & Dimsdale, J. E. (2011). Effects of continuous positive airway pressure on fatigue and sleepiness in patients with obstructive sleep apnea: Data from a randomized controlled trial. *Sleep, 34,* 121–126.

Trombly, C. A., & Ma, H. (2002). A synthesis of the effects of occupational therapy for persons with stroke: Part l. Restoration of roles, tasks, and activities. *American Journal of Occupational Therapy, 56,* 250–259.

Vasquez, M. M., Goodwin, J. L., Drescher, A. A., Smith, T. W., & Quan, S. F. (2008). Associations of dietary intake and physical activity with sleep disordered breathing in the Apnea Positive Pressure Long-term Efficacy Study (APPLES). *Journal of Clinical Sleep Medicine, 4,* 411–418.

Verse, T., & Hormann, K. (2011). The surgical treatment of sleep related upper airway obstruction. *Sleep Diagnosis and Therapy, 6,* 55–59.

Vgontzas, A. N., Liao, D., Pejovic, S., Calhoun, S., Karataraki, M., Basta, M., Fernandez-Mendoza, J., & Bixler, E. O. (2010). Insomnia with short sleep duration and mortality: The Penn state cohort. *Sleep, 33,* 1159–1164.

Ville, I., Ravaud, J. F., & Tetrafigap Group. (2001). Subjective well-being and severe motor impairments: The Tetrafigap survey on the long-term outcome of tetraplegic spinal cord injured persons. *Social Science Medicine, 52,* 369–384.

Viola-Saltzman, M., Watson, N. F., Bogart, A., Goldberg, J., & Buchwald, D. (2010). High prevalence of restless legs syndrome among patients with fibromyalgia: A controlled cross sectional study. *Journal of Clinical Sleep Medicine, 6,* 423–427.

Wadensten, B., & Ahlstrom, G. (2009). The struggle for dignity by people with severe functional disabilities. *Nursing Ethics, 16,* 453–465.

Wagner, D., & Takagi, E. (2010). Informal care-giving by and for older adults. *Health Affairs Blog.* Retrieved July 4, 2013 from http://healthaffairs.org/blog/2010/02/16/informal-caregiving-by-and-for-older-adults/.

Walker, L. G. (1999). Psychological intervention, host defenses, and survival. *Advances in Mind-Body Medicine, 15,* 273–281.

Watson, N. (2010). Stroke and sleep specialists: An opportunity to intervene? *Journal of Clinical Sleep Medicine, 6,* 138–9.

Weber, R. L. (1993). *Group therapy training materials.* Unpublished documents. Cambridge, MA: Cambridge Health Alliance and Harvard Medical School.

Woods, F. W. (1984). *Human sexuality in health and illness.* St. Louis: Mosby.

Yarkony, G. M. (1993). *Medical complications in rehabilitation.* New York: Hawor.

Zee, P. C., & Turek, F. W. (2006). Sleep and health: Everywhere and in both directions. *Archives of Internal Medicine, 166,* 1686–1688.

Zegans, L. (1991). The embodied self: Integration in health and illness. *Advances: Journal of the Institute for the Advancement of Health, 7,* 29–45.

Ziegler, R. G. (1999). *Individual and group psychotherapy: Principles for an epilepsy practice.* Unpublished manuscript. Boston: Seizure Unit, Children's Hospital.

Zizi, F., Jean-Louis, G., Brown, C. D., Ogebde, G., Boutin-Foster, C., & McFarlane, S. I. (2011). Sleep duration and risk of diabetes mellitus: Epidemiologic evidence and pathophysiologic insights. *Sleep Diagnosis and Therapy, 6,* 30–33.

Acknowledgements

I would like to thank the patients who have been my teachers for the more than 40 years I have been an occupational therapist; Jenny Lee Olsen, recently retired Director of Library Services at Cambridge Health Alliance for her generous help and guidance in the literature search; and editors Mary Radomski and Catherine Trombly Latham for their continued confidence in my contribution.

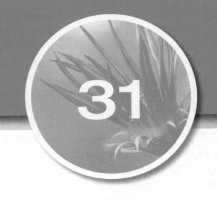

31

Optimizing Access to Home, Community, and Work Environments

Dory Sabata

Learning Objectives

After studying this chapter, the reader will be able to do the following:

1. Understand key historical events and policies that influence accessibility of home, work, and communities.
2. Explore occupation-based interventions to maximize access to participation at home, in the workplace, and in communities.
3. Recognize examples of products, design features, and other contextual factors that interact with each unique client's ability to perform occupations.
4. Summarize current evidence that considers how to reduce environmental demands and facilitate access to home, work-place, and community.
5. Identify occupational outcomes when creating a fit between environmental demands and the individual's capacities.

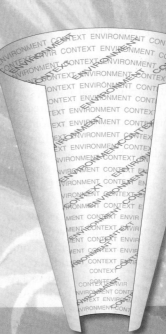

The focus of this chapter is on optimizing accessibility as an avenue for improving occupational performance for adults with physical dysfunction. The physical environment and technology are primary factors to consider relative to accessibility. Two overarching approaches are described in this chapter to address the barriers and strategies for optimizing access to home, work, and community: (1) changing policy and (2) changing the physical environment through environmental modifications and technology. Research demonstrating efficacy for these types of interventions will also be described in terms of client outcomes.

HISTORICAL PERSPECTIVES AND POLICIES AFFECTING ACCESS

Political advocacy and legislation influence current occupational therapy practices for optimizing environmental access worldwide. This section summarizes key public policies and legislation that supports increased access to home, community, and workplace in the United States and other nations. In the last 20 years, many countries have expanded their public policies promoting accessible design standards in the home and community. International policy changes were evident in the early 1990s with the United Nations General Assembly approval of Standard Rules on the Equalization of Opportunities for Persons with Disabilities (1993).

Legislative Movement toward Accessibility

A number of key legislative initiatives in the United States paved the way for increasing access for people with disabilities to community, job, and residential environments (Procedures for Practice 31-1). The following historical review highlights the impact of advocacy efforts over the past 50 years.

In 1954, the Hill-Burton Act, Pub. L. No. 83-565 addressed construction and design in federally funded hospitals. The Architectural Barriers Act of 1968, Pub. L. No. 90-480 (1968) created the United States Architectural and Transportation Barriers Compliance Board (ATBCB), which was authorized to study architectural design and develop standards for the construction of accessible buildings. Their findings are reported in the Minimum Guidelines for Accessible Design (MGRAD) (ATBCB, 1982). The Rehabilitation Act of 1973, Pub. L. No. 93-112 (1973) expanded the powers of the ATBCB or Access Board, which was then authorized to enforce federal accessibility requirements in federally funded buildings, federally funded programs, subsidized and public housing, and transportation facilities. These standards, called the Uniform Federal Accessibility Standards (UFAS), are based on MGRAD and guidelines of the American National Standards Institute (ANSI). Services to increase quality of life for people with disabilities were

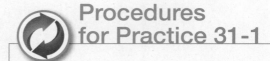

Procedures for Practice 31-1

U.S. Guidelines, Standards, and Regulations of Accessible Design

Occupational therapists who work with contractors and designers familiarize themselves with the following standards, guidelines, and legislation that affect accessibility and the physical environment.

- Americans with Disabilities Act of 1990 (ADA), Amended 2008
  - Americans with Disabilities Act Accessibility Guidelines (ADAAG)
  - Americans with Disabilities Act Accessibility Standards
  - Olmstead Decision of 1999
- American National Standards Institute (ANSI)
  - Minimum Guidelines for Accessible Design (MGRAD)
- Architectural Barriers Act of 1968 (Public Law 90-480)
  - Architectural and Transportation Barriers Compliance Board (ATBCB)
- Fair Housing Amendments Act of 1988 (FHAA)
  - Fair Housing Act Accessibility Guidelines (FHAAG)
- Hill-Burton Act (Public Law 83-565)
- Rehabilitation Act of 1973 (Public Law 93-112)
  - Section 504 of the Rehabilitation Act
- Uniform Federal Accessibility Standards (UFAS)

established in accordance with the Comprehensive Rehabilitation Services Amendment of the Rehabilitation Act of 1973. Activists led the movement for independent living and civil rights among people with disabilities (Ainsworth, de Jonge, & Sanford, 2011).

Grassroots advocacy for civil rights have led to federal policy changes affecting access for people with disabilities in the United States. Additionally, state governments in Australia and New Zealand have adopted policies addressing civil rights of people with disabilities. However, other countries, including Canada and the United Kingdom, have not shared a civil rights perspective in affecting policies at a state or federal level. In Canada, various principalities have adopted their own standards and principles for public accessibility for people with disabilities, but the standards and principles lack consistency. In the United Kingdom, social policies have also begun to address accessibility for people with disabilities (Ainsworth, de Jonge, & Sanford, 2011).

Housing Accessibility Policies

This section discusses public policies affecting accessibility in Japan, Australia, European Countries, Canada, and the US. Japan is perhaps on the leading edge of accessibility in private housing implementing universal design in new construction. Denmark requires minimum standards for wheelchair accessibility in single family homes. Norway, Sweden, and select parts of Australia have basic accessibility regulations for multifamily homes as well (Ainsworth, de Jonge, & Sanford, 2011).

Although the United States may be considered a leader in federal policies for public accessibility, it falls short in terms of policies for private housing accessibility. At present, housing is rarely built to adapt over time to owners' changing needs. The only housing policies in the United States pertain to public housing.

The Fair Housing Amendments Act (FHAA) of 1988 established the Fair Housing Act Accessibility Guidelines (FHAAG) for multifamily housing of four units or more and civil rights housing protection for people with disabilities. The FHAA mandates accessibility compliance and civil rights protection in private housing. People with disabilities are provided equal access to housing and a mechanism for filing complaints when their civil rights are violated. According to this law, the resident cannot be denied the opportunity to modify the rented home to meet individual needs for accessibility. The cost of the modification, however, is the responsibility of the renter. The landlord may require that the work be done by an approved professional, and an escrow account may be established in which the tenant must place funds for returning the residence to its original state.

Additional advocacy efforts have slowly begun to affect practices in housing construction at local levels. Eleanor Smith of Concrete Change coined the concept of visitability and suggests that all home environments be designed so that people can visit one another. Visitability considers three basic features of homes that make them accessible to visitors who use wheelchairs: a no-step entrance, wide doorways (32 inches), and access to a first floor bathroom. In some communities, builders now offer these features as an option in new home construction. All of these efforts laid the groundwork for current practices for optimizing physical accessibility of homes.

Contemporary Policies Affecting Public Accessibility for People with Disabilities

In 1990, with Congressional approval, the Americans with Disabilities Act (ADA) was enacted to protect the civil rights of Americas with disabilities by extension of equal rights protection established by the Civil Rights Act of 1964. Part of the ADA stipulated that state and local accessibility regulations must be considered in the design or modification of public spaces including businesses, schools, parks, and other recreational facilities, state and local government buildings, and public transportation. The ATBCB used both the Uniform Federal Accessibility Standards (UFAS) and FHAAG standards to create the Americans with Disabilities Act Accessibility Guidelines

(ADAAG) in 2004. Even with the implementation of this policy and associated practices, challenges to accessing home, work, and community persist.

A group of people with disabilities advocated for access to the community and challenged current practices under the ADA. That led to a pivotal U.S. Supreme Court decision: the Olmstead Decision (1999), which upheld the rights of persons with disabilities under the ADA and led to increased opportunities for people with disabilities to live in the community and receive services.

ADAAG was developed to offer some specifications for designing more accessible public spaces. However, ADAAG was based primarily on the needs of younger adults with disabilities and was not designed to meet the needs of older adults (Sanford, 2001). ADAAG was replaced in 2010 with Accessibility Standards that consider some of the needs of older adults and serve as a starting point to improving access to public places for employment and community activities in the United States. The U.S. Accessibility Standards have applied since March 15, 2012 (see Table 31-1).

Grab-bar configuration is one notable change from the former guidelines to the current standards. The Accessibility Standards considered that older people often need to use grab bars in public toilets. Previously, the Accessibility Guidelines indicated that toilets have two horizontal grab bars on a side wall and one on the wall behind the commode. These bars were intended to support an upper body transfer for someone with lower extremity amputations. However, the current standards now take into account that many older people need support for a standing transfer. Therefore, an option for grab bars on either side was included as a current alternative to the bar behind the toilet.

The Accessibility for Ontarians with Disabilities Act (AODA) in Canada (AODA, 2012) is similar to the ADA. Both policies have corresponding design specifications for each locality. Table 31-1 compares some of the accessible features in the United States and Ontario, Canada laws. Moreover, the Ontario Government has a greater goal to create a barrier-free community by 2025. A series of standards are currently under development to improve accessibility in Ontario. Policy changes can occur at the local level through grassroots efforts or can take years to decades to change at a federal level. Therefore, occupational therapists typically make more of a difference by changing the physical environment whether for a population or for an individual. The next section will explore the process by which occupational therapists plan and implement interventions to the physical environment to optimize access.

CHANGES TO THE PHYSICAL ENVIRONMENT

To develop an intervention plan that optimizes access, occupational therapy practitioners need to consider policies and laws affecting accessibility (described

Table 31-1	Select Accessibility Standards in the United States and Ontario	
Public Space Measurement	**U.S. Accessible Design Standard**	**Ontario Accessible Design Standard**
Accessible entrance	At least one	50%, at least one
Minimum clear width of an accessible route	Clear opening 32 inches (815 mm)	900 cm (35 inches)
Thresholds	1/2 inch maximum, 3/4 inch maximum on existing doors, beveled maximum slope 1:2	13 mm (0.5 inches) maximum, beveled maximum slope 1:2
Unobstructed reach range for placing controls	Adults: high forward reach 48 inches (1220 mm) maximum and the low forward reach 15 inches (380 mm) minimum above	For adults, controls not mounted above 1200 mm (47 inches) or below 400 mm (16 inches)
Stairs	Rise: 4–7 inches (100–180 mm) high, run: 11 inches (280 mm) deep minimum	Rise 125–175 mm (5–7 inches); run 280–355 mm (11–14 inches)
Ramp	Ramps cannot be higher (rise more) than 30 inches (760 mm) from the ground; ramps can be steeper for historic buildings than the minimum 1:12 rise to run (length); less steep ramps (1:18 run to rise) are recommended where space permits; standards include considerations for cross slope, edge rails, handrails.	Clear width 1100 mm (43 inches), slope no steeper than 1:15; considerations for cross slope, edge rails, handrails

Comparison of select accessibility standards under the Americans with Disabilities Act (ADA), amended 2008, and Integrated Accessibility Regulation under the Accessibility for Ontarians with Disabilities Act (AODA) of 2008.

earlier), theoretical underpinnings of how the environment affects occupation, and assessment tools and approaches described in Chapter 10. That information contributes to activity analysis and professional reasoning which results in an intervention plan. As we analyze an activity, we consider the context in which the activity occurs. This includes the space and object demands, as well as social and cultural expectations (American Occupational Therapy Association [AOTA], 2008).

Role of Occupational Therapy in Environmental Modifications

Occupational therapists analyze the physical environment as it relates to human performance, determine specific functional and environmental demands, and negotiate intervention options in collaboration with the client and support network. Strategies for reducing environmental demands in relation to specific performance skills are outlined in Procedures for Practice 31-2.

The generalist practitioner understands that the environment can be changed to decrease demands or to maximize abilities to facilitate performance. Specialists in accessibility and environmental modifications also understand the range of possible interventions and are conversant in the language needed to communicate effectively with building professionals in addition to their clients. Other specialist competencies have been identified by the AOTA for the Specialty Certification in Environmental Modifications (AOTA, 2009).

Occupational therapy practitioners who are generalists or specialists both have skills to optimize accessibility. Occupational therapists evaluate the occupational functioning of their clients in the physical context and make recommendations for changes to the environment to optimize accessibility. A client-centered approach to service delivery empowers the client to advocate for his or her own needs with knowledge and a wide array of resources (see Resources 31-1).

Intervention Strategies to Optimize Accessibility

Through activity analysis, occupational therapists can identify the barriers in the physical environment that may contribute to further disabling a person with functional limitations (see Procedures for Practice 31-2). Four intervention strategies will be introduced that optimize access and promote participation in the home, workplace, or community.

1. Inclusive and universal design
2. Environmental modifications
3. Assistive technology
4. Task simplification strategies

Inclusive and Universal Design

Occupational therapists understand the needs of people with a variety of health conditions; occupational therapists can contribute to increasing accessibility of spaces

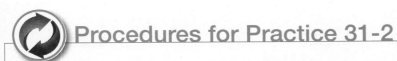

Procedures for Practice 31-2

Selected Limitations in Performance Skills and Sample Environmental Interventions to Reduce Activity Demands

Performance Skills					Environmental Intervention to Reduce Activity Demands
Visual	Hearing	Motor	Attention	Communication	
X					Tactile indicators, raised labels, task lighting
	X				Closed caption features on television and videos
X		X			Grab bars, bath bench; low-glare lighting
X		X	X		Automated medication management
		X	X	X	Preprogrammed telephone numbers
X	X				Vibrating devices/alarms, amplification device
X		X			Paths free of obstacles, no-step entrance
X			X		High contrast, few busy patterns
X				X	Furniture arranged so people sit facing each other
X		X			Angled mirror over the stove
	X		X		Minimize background noises
	X			X	Paper and pen
		X	X	X	Personal emergency response system
		X		X	Environmental control unit
			X	X	Visual schedule

and products that are used by many people. Inclusive design of objects and spaces takes into account the needs of people with disabilities, whereas universal design considers all possible users of the space or object. These two related design approaches address the extremes rather than simply the means or average features of a population. Because of these approaches, a broader range of people can better access products and spaces.

Products that are designed for use by everyone should use universal design principles (see Procedures for Practice 31-3). One example is the use of an automatic opening door. Automatic doors decrease the need for strength, motor skills, and cognitive skills. In addition to being useful to people with these types of functional limitations, automatic doors can be helpful to any worker who is carrying packages through the doorway. A no-step entrance and a curbless shower are examples of universal design features in the home.

Use of various readily available applications for computers for a variety of input and output such as voice recognition, screen reading, and other augmentative communication features are examples of inclusive design in the workplace (Definition 31-1). Schools and other community environments where learning occurs also need to consider the design of learning materials and whether or not they are accessible to a wide range of users.

The original principle of universal design considered products and spaces. Later, a set of universal design learning principles (CAST, 2011) were developed with the intent of increasing access to education (see Procedures for Practice 31-4).

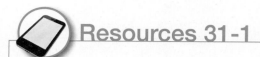

Resources 31-1

Optimizing Access to Home, Community, and Work Environments

Training Programs and Designations in Housing Accessibility and Modification

AOTA Continuing Education

http://www.aota.org/Practitioners/ProfDev/CE.aspx

Abilities O.T. Services Inc.

3309 W. Strathmore Avenue
Baltimore, MD 21215-3718
Phone: 410-358-7269
Fax: 410-358-6454
E-mail: shoshamberg@yahoo.com

CEAC (administered by Accessible Home Improvement of America)

http://www.accesshomeamerica.com/

Lifease, Inc.

Margaret Christenson, MPH, OTR, FAOTA
Phone: 800-961-3273

RESNA Assistive Technology Practitioner (ATP) and Assistive Technology Supplier (ATS) Credentialing Program

RESNA
1700 N. Moore Street, Suite 1540
Arlington, VA 22209-1903
Phone: 703-524-6686 (voice), 703-524-6639 (TTY), or 703-524-6630 (TTY)
http://www.resna.org

National Association of Home Builders (NAHB) Certified Aging in Place Specialist (CAPS)

1201 15th Street, NW
Washington, DC 20005
Phone: 800-368-5242
Fax: 202-266-8400
http://www.nahb.org

National Resource Center on Supportive Housing and Home Modification

University of Southern California
Andrus Gerontology Center
3715 McClintock Avenue
Los Angeles, CA 90089-0191
Phone: 213-740-1364
Fax: 213-740-7069
http://www.homemods.org

Technical Assistance and Organizations

AbleData

Phone: 800-227-0216
www.abledata.com

Accessible Space, Inc.

2550 University Avenue, Suite 330 N.
St. Paul, MN 55114
Phone: 800-466-7722
http://www.accessiblespace.org

AARP

601 E. Street, NW
Washington, DC 20049
Phone: 202-434-6120
http://www.aarp.org

American National Standards Institute (ANSI)

Phone: 212-868-1220

American Occupational Therapy Association (AOTA)

4720 Montgomery Avenue
P.O. Box 31220
Bethesda, MD 20814-1220
Phone: 800-SAY-AOTA
http://www.aota.org

Center for Universal Design

North Carolina State University
School of Design
Box 8613
Raleigh, NC 27695-8613
www.ncsu.edu/ncsu/design/cud

Concrete Change

600 Dancing Fox Road
Decatur, GA 30032
Phone: 404-378-7455
http://concretechange.org/

Easter Seals

http://www.easterseals.com/

Fall Prevention Center of Excellence

http://www.stopfalls.org

(continued)

Resources 31-1 *(continued)*

Future Home Foundation Inc.

Att: Dave Ward, curator
12900 Jarrettsville Pike
Phoenix, MD 21131
Phone: 410-666-0086
E-mail: cdavidward@aol.com

Habitat for Humanity International (HFHI)

1 Habitat Street
Americus, GA 31709-3498
Phone: 800-422-4828 (800-HABITAT) or 912-924-6935
http://www.habitat.org

Independent Living Centers

For a listing of local centers, call the national office at
314-531-3055.

IDeA Center for Inclusive Design and Environmental Access

School of Architecture and Planning
State University of New York at Buffalo
Buffalo, NY 14214-3087
Phone: 716-829-3485
Fax: 716-829-3256
http://www.ap.buffalo.edu/idea/

Industrial Design Society of America

IDSA-UD Special Interest Section
1141 Walker Road
Great Falls, VA 22066
Phone: 703-759-0100
Fax: 703-759-7679
http://www.idsa.org

Institute for Human Centered Design

http://www.humancentereddesign.org/

Leading Age

http://www.leadingage.org/

Lighthouse International

http://www.lighthouse.org/

National Association of Home Builders

http://www.nahb.org

National Association of the Remodeling Industry (NARI)

4900 Seminary Road, Suite 320
Alexandria, VA 22311
Phone: 800-966-7601 or 703-575-1100
Fax: 703-575-1121
http://www.nari.org

National Kitchen & Bath Association (NKBA)

687 Willow Grove Street
Hackettstown, NJ 07840
Phone: 800-367-6522 or 800-843-6522
Fax: 908-852-1695
http://www.nkba.org

Paralyzed Veterans of America (PVA)

801-18th Street, NW
Washington, DC 20008
Phone: 800-424-8200 (voice) or 800-795-4327 (TTY)
Fax: 202-785-4452
http://www.pva.org

Rebuilding Together

1536 Sixteenth Street, NW
Washington, DC 20036-1402
Phone: 800-4-REHAB-9
Fax: 202-483-9081
http://www.rebuildingtogether.org

Technical Assistance Collaborative, Inc.

One Center Plaza, Suite 310
Boston, MA 02108
Phone: 617-742-5657
Fax: 617-742-0509
www.tacinc.org

TRACE Research and Development Center

University of Wisconsin at Madison
5901 Research Park Boulevard
Madison, WI 53719-1252
Phone: 608-262-6966
www.trace.wisc.edu

Universal Designers & Consultants, Inc. (UDC)

6 Grant Avenue
Takoma Park, MD 20912
Phone: 301-270-2470 (voice and TTY)
Fax: 301-270-8199
http://www.UniversalDesign.com

U.S. Access Board (ATBCB)

Phone: 800-872-2253
www.access-board.gov

U.S. Department of Housing and Urban Development (HUD)

Phone: 800-827-5005
www.hud.gov

Volunteers for Medical Engineering

Baltimore, MD
Phone: 410-455-6395

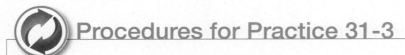

Procedures for Practice 31-3

Principles of Universal Design

When designing a space or product to be used by all potential users, consider the following principles.

Equitable Use: The design is useful and marketable to people with diverse abilities.

Guidelines

- Provide the same means of use for all users: identical whenever possible; equivalent when not.
- Avoid segregating or stigmatizing any users.
- Provisions for privacy, security, and safety should be equally available to all users.
- Make the design appealing to all users.

Flexible in Use: The design accommodates a wide range of individual preferences and abilities.

Guidelines

- Provide choice in methods of use.
- Accommodate right- or left-handed access and use.
- Facilitate the user's accuracy and precision.
- Provide adaptability to the user's pace.

Simple and Intuitive: Use of the design is easy to understand, regardless of the user's experience, knowledge, language skills, or current concentration level.

Guidelines

- Eliminate unnecessary complexity.
- Be consistent with user expectations and intuition.
- Accommodate a wide range of literacy and language skills.
- Arrange information consistent with its importance.
- Provide effective prompting and feedback during and after task completion.

Perceptible Information: The design communicates necessary information effectively to the user, regardless of ambient conditions or the user's sensory abilities.

Guidelines

- Use different modes (pictorial, verbal, and tactile) for redundant presentation of essential information.
- Provide adequate contrast between essential information and its surroundings.

- Maximize "legibility" of essential information.
- Differentiate elements in ways that can be described (i.e., make it easy to give instructions or directions).
- Provide compatibility with a variety of techniques or devices used by people with sensory limitations.

Tolerance for Error: The design minimizes hazards and the adverse consequences of accidental or unintended actions.

Guidelines

- Arrange elements to minimize hazards and errors: the most used elements should be most accessible; hazardous elements should be eliminated, isolated, or shielded.
- Provide warnings of hazards and errors.
- Provide fail-safe features.
- Discourage unconscious action in tasks that require vigilance.

Low Physical Effort: The design can be used efficiently and comfortably and with a minimum of fatigue.

Guidelines

- Allow user to maintain a neutral body position.
- Use reasonable operating forces.
- Minimize repetitive actions.
- Minimize sustained physical effort.

Size and Space for Approach and Use: Appropriate size and space is provided for approach, reach, manipulation, and use regardless of user's body size, posture, or mobility.

Guidelines

- Provide a clear line of sight to important elements for any seated or standing user.
- Make reach to all components comfortable for any seated or standing user.
- Accommodate variations in hand and grip size.
- Provide adequate space for the use of assistive devices or personal assistance.

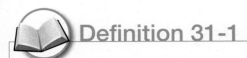

Definition 31-1

Assistive Technology for Communication

- Augmentative and alternative communication
- Speech recognition
- Voice recognition
- Personal e-communication system
- Closed captioning
- Open captioning

Environmental Modifications

Most existing environments have not been built with universal design features in mind, and therefore, environmental modifications are needed to increase accessibility. Environmental modifications are changes made to the current physical environment. Occupational therapy practitioners collaborate with the client and with other team members (such as design, construction, and other building professionals) to develop a plan for reducing environmental barriers.

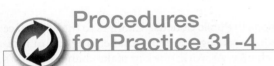

Procedures for Practice 31-4

Universal Design Learning Principles

Principle I. Provide Multiple Means of Representation

Guideline 1: Provide options for perception
Guideline 2: Provide options for language, mathematical expressions, and symbols
Guideline 3: Provide options for comprehension

Principle II. Provide Multiple Means of Action and Expression

Guideline 4: Provide options for physical action
Guideline 5: Provide options for expression and communication
Guideline 6: Provide options for executive functions

Principle III. Provide Multiple Means of Engagement

Guideline 7: Provide options for recruiting interest
Guideline 8: Provide options for sustaining effort and persistence
Guideline 9: Provide options for self-regulation

CAST. (2011). *Universal design for learning guidelines* (version 2.0). Wakefield, MA: Author.

Home Modifications. Modifications can be made to any physical environment. Individuals have more control over changes to their own homes, and they often spend a great deal of time in their homes. Therefore, when changing the physical environment, the home is most likely to be addressed. Evidence suggests that home environment interventions are most effective when they consider the needs of the individual client (Stark et al., 2009; Velligan et al., 2009).

A home bathroom in the United States is not typically built to accommodate someone who uses a wheelchair. Therefore, a bathroom in the home may need to be remodeled or modified to provide the resident access to the bathroom. One modification might be replacing a bathtub with a curbless shower to facilitate bathing in a wheelchair or adding grab bars near a toilet (Figs. 31-1 and 31-2).

Even the bathroom entrance may not be designed for a wheelchair. The Accessibility Standards outline the turning radius needed for a standard wheelchair to be able to enter and exit a room, such as a bathroom (Fig. 31-3). This standard only applies to public spaces but is often used as a guide for remodelers designing bathroom modifications for a wheelchair user.

A systematic review suggests that home modifications contribute to fall risk reduction and lessen the effects of functional decline. Outcomes were particularly strong when home modifications addressing the environment

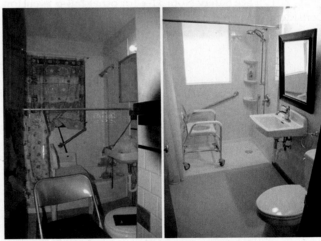

Figure 31-1 The photo on the left is a typical bathroom with sink, toilet, and shower. A grab bar and a tub transfer bench are in the shower to assist with transfers. The wall-hung sink without a cabinet is accessible to roll under. The pipe is insulated to prevent leg burns. The transfer bench prohibits the shower curtain from fully closing and water gets on the floor. The lighting is poor and the space is cluttered. The photo on the right has been modified and has a curbless shower with a handheld shower head. The rolling bath seat allows for transfer prior to reaching the shower. The cutout in the seat allows for washing without having to stand. The lighting is improved with access to natural lighting as well as ambient lighting. Clutter has been removed. (Photos courtesy of Lifewise Renovations, Prairie Village, KS.)

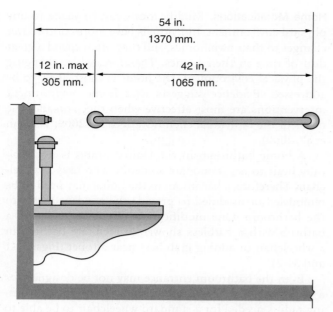

Figure 31-2 This illustration provides information about the placement of a side-wall grab bar near a public toilet according to the ADA Standards for Accessible Design. The grab bar in this position needs to be at least 42 inches (1065 mm) and must be placed no more than 12 inches (305 mm) away from the rear wall. (This figure is in the public domain and is not copyrighted.)

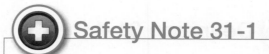

Safety Note 31-1

Safety Considerations to Reduce Fall Risk

Falls can cause injury and even fatality. A multifactorial approach can help reduce the risk of falls among people at greatest risk of falls and fall-related injuries. However, all of us are susceptible to falls. Some strategies can contribute to safety and minimize environmental fall risk factors.

- Exercise regularly. Engage in balance and mobility activities such as walking or Tai Chi.
- Manage medications, particularly if taking multiple medications.
- Discuss fall risk factors and assessment with your medical provider.
- Reduce clutter in your path.
- Have adequate, low-glare lighting for work.
- Use readily available mobility supports (grocery cart, handrails, seating to rest).
- Get sufficient sleep.
- Reduce cognitive demands or limit multitasking while moving around.
- Select useful and fitting mobility devices (cane, walker, and wheelchair) when needed.

were combined with other interventions addressing the person's capacities. For instance, physical activity such as strength training combined with environmental modifications has greater impact on reducing fall risk (Chase et al., 2012). See Safety Note 31-1 for other fall-prevention considerations.

Modifications to Public Spaces. Changes to the workplace or community settings are more challenging for an individual to change. At work, one can make changes to one's own workstation more than one is able to change the larger workplace. Evidence suggests that people are more likely

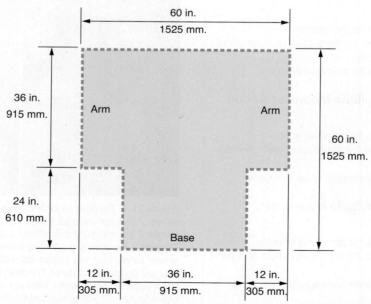

Figure 31-3 This diagram indicates the dimensions required according to ADA Standards for Accessible Design for the turning radius of a standard wheelchair in entering and exiting a doorway, including a bathroom stall. (This figure is in the public domain and is not copyrighted.)

to have accommodations at their workstation to optimize their access at work than in the general workplace (Sabata et al., 2008). In broader community environments, any modifications or accessibility features are typically the result of advocacy for a population and changes in policies but are even less likely to have changes to the physical environment to meet specific individual needs.

Assistive Technology

The Assistive Technology Act of 1998 defines assistive technology as "any item, piece of equipment, or product system, whether acquired commercially off the shelf, modified, or customized, that is used to increase, maintain, or improve functional capabilities of individuals with disabilities." Assistive technology can be added to the physical environment (p. 6). Some examples of assistive technology in the bathroom can range from a long-handled sponge for bathing to digital motion sensors to detect a fall.

Task Simplification Strategies

Design features, modifications, and assistive technology are used to decrease environmental demands and to reduce barriers. Task simplification minimizes the steps or demands of the procedure for completing a task (Procedures for Practice 31-5). Occupational therapists provide

training to clients who need to learn how to do a task in a different way.

One way in which a task can be simplified is by teaching a client to perform a task from a different position, such as seated rather than standing. Sitting to complete an activity can reduce physical demands and free up the person to focus on other skills needed to complete an activity. For instance, people typically shower while standing. For someone fearful of falling, sitting during a shower still engages the person in self-care. The addition of a shower chair along with learning to bathe from a seated position provides the person with access to activities of daily living (ADL) at home.

Another way to simplify the demands of tasks is to plan for high- and low-energy activities. Moving around the community can use more energy than moving around one's home. A person who fatigues easily may need to plan for manageable community outings followed by periods of restful activities. Also, by recognizing their peak energy times (whether morning or afternoon), clients can plan and prioritize their schedules to best meet their needs.

Individuals may be able to make changes to decrease activity demands. However, some activities may require a community effort to make a community environment more accessible. For example, places of worship may need to consider inclusive designs to optimize participation in spiritual or religious practices, particularly as part of a church community. In one study, researchers found that spiritual leaders were often willing to make changes but needed to be made aware of strategies to create a more inclusive environment (Griffin et al., 2012).

Occupation-Based Interventions to Optimize Access

Contractors, designers, policy advocates, and other health providers may all be concerned about accessibility. However, occupational therapy specifically addresses the occupations of a person's life within the context of where those occupations are performed. Many leisure activities, instrumental activities of daily living (IADL), and some ADL are performed in community spaces. At work, occupational therapy is often focused on access to the work site and accommodations to complete the job tasks. Additionally, other activities such as socializing with coworkers, lunchtime, and accessing the restrooms need to be considered.

In these public spaces, government regulations can affect current accessibility features (see Procedures for Practice 31-1). Public spaces allow for less individualization and instead attempt to meet the needs of a broad population. However, these mandates often fall short of universal design. Advocacy may be needed to improve current standards for access to public spaces for a heterogeneous population.

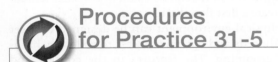

Procedures for Practice 31-5

Therapeutic Intervention to Promote Safety and Independence: Principles of Task Simplification

- Use both hands to work with symmetrical motions when possible.
- Organize work supplies within reach.
- Slide heavy objects rather than lifting and carrying. For example, slide pots from sink to range. Use a wheeled cart.
- Stabilize tools to work surface, so both hands are free to work.
- Let gravity work for you (e.g., refuse chute, gravity-fed bins, or a pan below the level of a cutting board).
- Create efficient, visible storage (e.g., wall mount with hooks, magnetic racks for knife and utensil storage, and vertical storage racks).
- Place controls and switches within reach, or automate.
- Consider body mechanics, seating, and surface height in design of individual workstations.
- Provide sufficient lighting and ventilation.
- Create pleasant working conditions to minimize stress and strain

In the home, interventions can be more tailored to individual needs. In this setting, people engage in ADL such as bathing, dressing, eating, and moving around their home. Cooking, cleaning, and caring for others are IADL commonly performed at home. Interventions directed at the environment may be just as important as those that address a person's abilities. The American Occupational Therapy Association has developed practice guidelines on home modifications (Siebert, 2005). The original version is currently under revision to better identify and demonstrate current evidence-based practices in home modifications.

Occupational therapy recognizes that each individual has varying skills, each home has unique features, and the occupations of daily life may be performed differently by different people. Therefore, interventions addressing the environment must also consider how an occupation is performed and what skills the person has to be able to perform each activity.

Home and Community Mobility

When moving around the house or walking around the community, steps can pose a challenge to some. Steps require a person to manage a change in balance and in elevation. For people who are ambulatory but unsteady, a solution may be adding secure handrails to support the body. Handrails can be a low-cost modification initially used to support older people as they are trying to use the steps. People who use mobility devices (e.g., walkers and wheelchairs) may need more extensive modifications to the environment such as a ramp or lift.

Ramps are one option to creating a no-step entrance. The slope of a ramp must address the trade-off between human endurance and strength. A steeper ramp can be a shorter distance, while a less steep ramp will be longer. Figure 31-4 demonstrates the rise to run ratio or ramp slope as indicated in the Accessibility Standards. Although these standards are not applied to personal homes, many builders use these standards as their guide for residential ramps as well.

When the entrance to a home is very steep or the yard space required to build a ramp is insufficient, lifts may be another alternative. An often aesthetically pleasing option is to use soil and ground covering to create a gradual sloping feature called an earth berm.

Additionally, policies designed to create equal access for people with disabilities can result in design that promotes movement in and around the workplace. For example, heavy doors can be challenging to open. The U.S. Accessibility Standards indicate that doors should open with 5 pounds or less of pressure or with electronic controls. This standard applies to public spaces such as workplaces.

An increasingly obese population adds to the need for more accessible home and public environments. Now employers are taking steps to modify physical demands in the workplace in order to promote more healthy movement while at work. For instance, some employers have used the workplace environment to promote healthy lifestyle choices and have had some success in influencing healthy behaviors (Brehm et al., 2011; DeJoy et al., 2011).

Toileting, Bathing, and Grooming

Toileting, bathing, and grooming are typically performed in the bathroom. When bathrooms are not accessible, people may perform these activities in other locations. For instance, some people use a bedside commode in a bedroom or living room instead of the toilet in the bathroom. People who cannot access their second-floor bathroom may sponge bathe in the kitchen sink or consider remodeling to create a first floor bath.

The physical environment can be designed to meet individual needs and optimize access to toileting, bathing, and grooming. The features in the context and environment must be considered in relation to the person's performance skills and the activity demands (AOTA, 2008). Squatting down to sit on the toilet and standing up when finished require leg strength and range of motion. However, the demands can be reduced by raising the height of the toilet to better fit one's body to reduce the amount of squatting needed to get on and off the toilet. Other people need upper body support to balance or push up when shifting from sit to stand, so grab bars may be installed. The interventions in the environment need to consider both the person and the

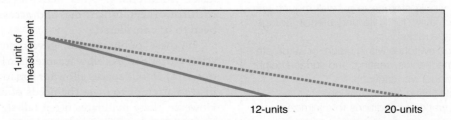

Figure 31-4 The solid line depicts a ramp slope of 1:12 (rise:run). This ramp is steeper and shorter. The dotted line depicts a longer less steep slope of 1:20 (rise:run).

activity demands. Figure 31-1 shows some features that offer different options for creating a more accessible bathroom.

Workplace restrooms and break rooms at work often are subject to accessibility standards. Toileting is not part of a job task but is still a necessary occupation at work. Therefore, occupational therapists need to understand how to optimize access to bathrooms for clients in the workplace.

As is clear from the previous discussion, occupational therapists can help clients optimize access to home and work in many ways. The interactions of the person's abilities and the environment are key in determining which interventions will best facilitate occupational performance. Specific environmental modifications can help to minimize activity demands for specific performance skills.

FROM PLAN TO IMPLEMENTATION: ENVIRONMENTAL INTERVENTIONS

Occupational therapy practitioners work with clients to make them aware of the ways in which environmental interventions can decrease activity demands. Clients can often identify the occupational areas that are difficult for them, but they may not realize that the environment presents barriers to their occupational functioning. Occupational therapy practitioners identify the demands and barriers presented in the environment and help clients address these accessibility issues in treatment plans.

The goal of environmental interventions is to optimize accessibility to facilitate performance in occupations. Some common challenges to environmental interventions include the client's awareness of resources, funding availability, and interdisciplinary communication.

Awareness of Resources

Occupational therapy practitioners can help families identify needed home modifications and access services. Home modifications are often pieced together through a variety of service providers. In the United States, Area Agencies on Aging and Centers for Independent Living are federally supported social service organizations that vary by location as to whether they offer home modification services. Rebuilding Together is a national nonprofit provider of home modifications and home repair with local chapters across the United States. The variability across geographic locations can be challenging in finding service providers who assist with creating accessible home environments.

Vocational rehabilitation services often assist with workplace accommodations for people with disabilities. Some workplaces have ergonomic consultants or departments that help create workplace environments that reduce the risk of injuries while optimizing work productivity. The needs of aging workers is a new challenge for many workplaces to begin to address.

Accessibility of public spaces is regulated by the ADA. Many buildings and spaces, however, were built prior to 1990 (when the ADA took effect). Older buildings continue to contain many accessibility barriers. New construction in the United States is subject to meeting the ADA Accessibility Standards. Occupational therapists can serve not only as consultants to projects aimed at increasing community accessibility but also as advocates raising awareness of the barriers to community participation.

Community coalitions, local building codes, and local services available can all affect community accessibility. Interested individuals and organizations may form local coalitions to promote changes in building codes or to better coordinate the delivery of services. Since the information age, virtual communities also exist through the internet. Occupational therapy practitioners can assist with gaining access to electronic and information technology for people with disabilities. This can be achieved by understanding the various formats, software programs, and interfaces with the technology needed by people with disabilities.

Funding Issues

One of the major barriers to home, workplace, and community access is finding funding for the changes. Universal design is a relatively recent concept and is not yet a standard practice in the design of new building and construction of homes, workplaces, and communities. New construction with accessibility features costs less than retrofitting existing structures.

Funding must be pieced together from a variety of sources. Individuals pay out of pocket. Employers may assist with funding workplace accommodations. Some insurance companies may pay for home and/or workplace accommodations. Community organizations with grant funds may pay for services that improve community accessibility and home accessibility. Funding options vary greatly by location, organization, and reason for the intervention.

Communication and the Interprofessional Team

As in other areas of practice, occupational therapy practitioners work in collaboration with other professionals who have different perspectives and terminology. Building professionals, such as contractors, designers, architects, and building code officials, are not part of a typical health care team but can be part of the team providing environmental interventions to promote accessibility. Interprofessional teams need to develop a method of communication that promotes collaborative problem solving.

Evidence Table 31-1 | Best Evidence for Occupational Therapy Practice Regarding Home Modification Interventions

Intervention	Description of Intervention Tested	Participants	Dosage	Type of Best Evidence and Level of Evidence	Benefit	Statistical Probability and Effect Size of Outcome	Reference
Assistive technology (AT) and environmental interventions (EIs)	Occupational therapy (OT) visit with recommendations, implementation of AT and EI	Frail elderly adults in New York (N = 104; treatment, n = 52; controls, n = 52).	For treatment group, mean AT devices received, n = 15; mean EI, n = 1.44; mean visits from OT, n = 8.9; and mean visits from technician, n = 2.4. Those in control received usual care (e.g., nursing visits).	Randomized, controlled study; Level: IA2a	Significant difference in number of AT devices received Significant difference in number of EIs received Cost-effective alternative to long-term care	AT devices: t = 6.57, p < 0.001, r = 0.297 EIs received: t = 4.1, p < 0.001 r = 0.14 Lower mean total costs for those in treatment group ($14,173) compared to controls ($31,610); effect size, d = 0.56	Mann et al. (1999)
Home intervention to reduce functional difficulties	OT and physical therapy (PT) home visits including home modifications, education about cognitive and behavioral strategies, balance-related exercises	Community-dwelling older adults who had difficulty performing daily activities (N = 319; controls, n = 159; intervention, n = 160)	Intervention group: five 90-minute OT visits plus one 20-minute phone follow-up and one 90-minute PT visit Control group did not receive any intervention (received safety book after posttest)	Randomized, controlled block design; Level: IA1b	Significantly less difficulty with bathing and toileting compared with control group	Intervention participants had less difficulty with instrumental activities of daily living (IADL) than controls p = 0.04, confidence interval (CI) = −0.28–0.00; similar with ADL (P = 0.03, 95% CI = −0.24 to −0.01)	Gitlin et al. (2006)
Comparison of environmental assessment and modification provided by an occupational therapist versus an unqualified trained assessor	Westmead Home Safety Assessment and strategies to address hazards	Community-dwelling adults age 70 years and older with a recent history of falls (controls, n = 78; OT assessor, n = 87; trained assessor, n = 73)	1.5–2-hour home assessment and two follow-up phone calls	Randomized controlled trial Level: IA1a	Participants in the OT group had significantly fewer falls at 12-month follow-up; no change in fall rate for those in trained assessor group (controls)	OT group: Incident rate ratio (IRR) = 0.54; CI = 0.36–0.83, p = 0.005 Trained assessor group: IRR = 0.78 CI = 0.51–1.12, p = 0.34	Pighills et al. (2011)

Occupational therapy recommendations that address client's occupational functioning are made in collaboration with the contractor who understands structural and construction issues. As with any type of team, all members need to have a similar understanding of the goal to effectively achieve the desired outcome.

EFFICACY AND OUTCOMES

The ultimate goal of optimizing accessibility is to maximize occupational functioning and social participation. People with disabilities, older adults, caregivers, personal assistants, and potentially anyone who is part of a particular environment can all benefit from the outcomes of environmental interventions.

As a person ages, changes with aging may be modulated by reducing participation in activities rather than in changing the environment. Unknowingly, by limiting activities, the older person may contribute to further declines in physical functioning. However, researchers have demonstrated that home modifications and assistive technology can actually reduce the risk of functional decline among people as they age (Gitlin et al., 2009; Gitlin et al., 2006; Wilson et al., 2009). A growing body of evidence (see Evidence Table 31-1) supports the notion that home environment interventions can optimize access. Even as a person ages, the environment can play a significant role in the person's access to ongoing participation (Petersson et al., 2009; Yen et al., 2012).

Individualized interventions, often in the home, help meet the specific needs of a person. Ongoing public policies that promote accessibility and inclusive design help to make community spaces and activities available to a wide range of people. Advocacy efforts along with individualized interventions are both needed to continue to improve the access to home, work, and community.

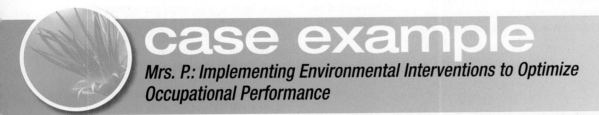

case example
Mrs. P.: Implementing Environmental Interventions to Optimize Occupational Performance

Occupational Therapy Intervention Process	Clinical Reasoning Process	
	Objectives	Examples of Therapist's Internal Dialogue
Patient Information	Appreciate the context	(See related assessment chapter, Chapter 10, for description of the assessment process and patient's background.)
Mrs. P. is an 85-year-old woman who sustained a right-sided cerebrovascular accident 2 months ago resulting in left-sided hemiparesis. She was recently discharged from the rehabilitation center to an apartment that she has shared with her husband for more than 30 years. Mr. P. would like to hire an attendant a few hours a day to assist with Mrs. P.'s personal care and to help with the housekeeping, but financial constraints do not allow for this. Both Mr. P. and their daughter carry out most of the household tasks and have reported becoming increasingly frustrated and fatigued. They both say that they do not believe that they can leave Mrs. P. alone because of their concerns about her safety and independence. Prior to her stroke, Mrs. P. prided herself on her ability to care for her husband and her home. Mrs. P. has been referred to the community occupational therapist to address concerns about her independence and safety in her home environment.		"Mrs. P. is returning home where she lives with her husband. She needs assistance with personal care and housekeeping. Her husband wants help but cannot financially afford to hire an assistant for his wife. Their daughter lives nearby and helps when she can."
	Select an intervention approach	"I anticipate that Mrs. P. will be able to safely engage in some self-care and housekeeping activities. I may be able to help her delay further decline or even delay institutionalization by implementing environmental interventions and helping her acquire assistive technology that promotes accessibility and optimizes her occupational performance."
		"I will focus on environmental modifications and assistive technology and determine how to decrease demands in the home environment to increase occupational performance."

| Reflect on competence | "I have worked with several clients with unilateral hemiparesis resulting from a stroke who were discharged home. I am knowledgeable about various tools and databases (such as AbleData) and am confident that I will be able to offer some options of products that may be useful to the needs of my client. I will work with another therapist who is knowledgeable in other techniques for stroke recovery that focus more on remediation such as constraint-induced movement therapy. I will also make referrals to social work for assistance with finding funding sources and locating caregiver support for the family members." |

Recommendations

The occupational therapist recommended three to five visits to negotiate environmental modifications and assistive technology. In collaboration with Mrs. P., her husband, and her daughter, the occupational therapist established the following long-term treatment goals: (1) following bathroom modifications, Mrs. P. will safely complete bathing activities with minimal supervision and prompting; (2) after instruction on task modification, Mrs. P. will engage in light housekeeping tasks with minimal assistance from family; (3) Mrs. P. will complete dressing and grooming tasks with the use of assistive devices and verbal prompting; and (4) Mrs. P. will participate in activities at a senior center two or three times a week.

Consider the patient's appraisal of performance	"Mrs. P. lacks awareness of safety risks. I suspect that she may have attention deficits or executive function disorder, and further assessment is needed. This might explain why she does not demonstrate any memory deficit but does seem to have difficulty with initiation and sequencing. She is aware of changes in her abilities to perform meaningful activities."
Consider what will occur in therapy, how often, and for how long	"Mrs. P. will have home modifications made to her bathroom including replacing the tub with a shower, placing nonskid strips on the shower floor, and installing grab bars. Here is how I plan to approach Mrs. P.'s other needs: provide Mrs. P. and her family members with training on safety issues and how to protect and care for her paralyzed side, which is likely to be neglected; use task modification strategies to engage Mrs. P. in meaningful housekeeping tasks; provide visual and verbal cues to encourage visual scanning to the affected side and to avoid injury; and provide assistive devices to assist with dressing, grooming, and meal preparation activities."
Ascertain the patient's endorsement of plan	"Mrs. P. is motivated to engage in housekeeping tasks, which are important to her. She is agreeable to the plan and understands that her family will feel more secure if she follows through with the recommended safety features."

Summary of Short-Term Goals and Progress

1. Mrs. P. will complete dressing and grooming tasks daily with the use of assistive devices.
2. Mrs. P. will complete at least two instrumental activities of daily living (IADL) with task modification strategies, assistive devices, and setup from family.

The occupational therapist introduced task modification strategies and assistive devices that facilitate access to participation in self-care and household activities. The therapist recognized that Mrs. P. was motivated to contribute to her family and her household.

The occupational therapist recognized that Mrs. P. liked gadgets and that she was open to trying assistive devices that reduced physical barriers. The therapist assisted Mrs. P. and her family in selecting several assistive devices to increase activities of daily living (ADL) and IADL performance and then trained Mrs. P. to use them. Mrs. P.'s family reported that Mrs. P. was less dependent on them for self-care activities.

Assess the patient's comprehension	"I could see that Mrs. P. became frustrated with learning to use a button hook for dressing. We discussed other alternatives, and eventually, she preferred to have Velcro® fasteners on her clothes to replace buttons."
Compare actual to expected performance	"Mrs. P. was able to use a spiked cutting board while seated at the kitchen table. Her family assisted with setup, but otherwise, she was able to complete most meal preparation."
Know the person	
Appreciate the context	"I anticipated that Mrs. P. would improve her participation in activities with the strategies and devices. She was highly motivated. We did have to try some different strategies to get the expected outcome. An additional outcome was that her family caregivers felt less burdened."

Next Steps

Revised short-term goals (1 month):

Following bathroom modifications and training with assistive devices, Mrs. P. will complete bathing with minimal supervision two times per week.

> Decide whether the patient should continue or discontinue therapy and/or return in the future

"Mrs. P. does not want to be dependent on her husband to assist her with bathing. She is waiting for assistance from Rebuilding Together to provide a roll-in shower in place of her tub."

"I am concerned about Mrs. P.'s visual left neglect. She does not seem to be aware of the deficit, and she is resistant to strategies for visual scanning to the left. Also, she has fallen a couple times in the past month. Her visual and sensory perception is impaired, and she has difficulty when getting up from a chair. I wonder if she is experiencing orthostatic hypotension, which is contributing to her fall risk. I have referred her to a physical therapist. Following her bathroom modifications, I will visit her again and provide training."

Clinical Reasoning in Occupational Therapy Practice

Mr. P.: Determining Environmental Interventions to Optimize Access to Community

Mr. P. had a rough night and did not get much sleep. He got up early to take his wife to a doctor appointment. He took a shower, and on his way out he fell on the tile floor. He was very sore and developed bruising but did not have any serious injury or breaks. However, since then he has become fearful of falling again. Although he used to bathe nearly every day, now he is bathing once a week. He meets up with his friends or leaves the house only on days that he bathes. This has significantly changed his outings in the community. He has a combination shower/tub and has to enter the tub to take a shower. The bathroom lighting is over the sink. The shower is poorly lit, once the shower curtain is pulled.

What factors in the environment might have contributed to the fall? What environmental interventions might support his bathing and therefore support his participation in activities with his friends?

Summary Review Questions

1. What historical events and policies affect current practices and trends in accessibility of homes, workplaces, and communities? Why is knowledge of these important to the occupational therapy practitioner who consults on accessibility?
2. What are some examples of how each of the four intervention strategies presented could be applied in the home, workplace, or community?
3. What are some of the design and product solutions that help to reduce activity demands at home, at work, or in the community?
4. How do the types of occupations performed at home, in the workplace, and in the community affect the types of environmental interventions selected?
5. What resources are available to occupational therapists and families to help them implement environmental modification interventions?
6. What does evidence suggest are some of the key benefits to clients who use environmental interventions?

Glossary

Activity demands—The objects, space, skills, and abilities required to complete a series of tasks.

Context—The social, physical, cultural, and temporal factors external to a person.

Environmental demands—External factors that interact with a person's capacity.

Environmental modifications—Changes to the physical environment, with the intent of improving safety and occupational performance.

Inclusive design—Design that takes into account the needs of people with disabilities.

Performance skills—The actions of a person based on abilities.

Physical environment—Features of a person's surroundings that are built or exist in nature.

Space and object demands—The room required and tools needed for a specific occupation.

Universal design—Concept that products and spaces are designed to meet the needs of all possible users.

Visitability—Concept that homes can be accessible for a person in a wheelchair to visit.

References

Accessibility for Ontarians with Disabilities Act. (2005). Integrated Accessibility Standards, Ontario Regulation 191/11. Retrieved June 16, 2012 from http://www.e-laws.gov.on.ca/html/source/regs/english/2011/elaws_src_regs_r11191_e.htm.

Ainsworth, E., de Jonge, D., & Sanford, J. (2011). Legislation, regulations, codes and standards influencing home modification practice. In E. Ainsworth & D. de Jonge (Eds.), *An occupational therapist's guide to home modification practice* (pp. 49-66). Thorofare, NJ: SLACK Inc.

American Occupational Therapy Association. (2008). Occupational therapy practice framework: Domain & process (2nd ed.). *American Journal of Occupational Therapy, 62,* 625-683.

American Occupational Therapy Association. (2013). AOTA Certification: Update on Changes. Retrieved July 10, 2013 from: http://www.aota.org/Practitioners/ProfDev/Certification.aspx

Americans with Disabilities Act of 1990, 42 U.S.C. § 12101 *et seq.* (2008).

Architectural Barriers Act of 1968, 20 U.S.C. § 1132D-11 *et seq.* (1968).

Assistive Technology Act of 1998, 29 U.S.C. § 3001 *et seq.* (1998).

Brehm, B. J., Gates, D. M., Singler, M., Succop, P. A., & D'Alessio, D. A. (2011). Environmental changes to control obesity: A randomized controlled trial in manufacturing companies. *American Journal of Health Promotion, 25,* 334-340.

CAST. (2011). Universal design for learning guidelines (version 2.0). Wakefield, MA: CAST.

Center for Universal Design. (1997). The principles of universal design. Retrieved June 16, 2012 from http://www.ncsu.edu/project/design-projects/udi/center-for-universal-design/the-principles-of-universal-design/.

Chase, C. A., Mann, K., Wasek, S., & Arbesman, M. (2012). Systematic review of the effect of home modification and fall prevention programs on falls and the performance of community-dwelling older adults. *American Journal of Occupational Therapy, 66,* 284-291.

DeJoy, D. M., Parker, K. M., Padilla, H. M., Wilson, M. G., Roemer, E. C., & Goetzel, R. Z. (2011). Combining environmental and individual weight management interventions in a work setting: Results from the Dow chemical study. *Journal of Occupational and Environmental Medicine, 53,* 245-252.

Fair Housing Act, 42 U.S.C. § 3601-3619 *et seq.* (1988).

Gitlin, L. N., Hauck, W. W., Dennis, M. P., Winter, L., Hodgson, N., & Schinfeld, S. (2009). Long-term effect on mortality of a home intervention that reduces functional difficulties in older adults: Results from a randomized trial. *Journal of the American Geriatrics Society, 57,* 476-481.

Gitlin, L. N., Winter, L., Dennis, M. P., Corocan, M., Schinfeld, S., & Hauck, W. W. (2006). A randomized trial of a multicomponent home intervention to reduce functional difficulties in older adults. *Journal of the American Geriatrics Society, 54,* 809-816.

Griffin, M. M., Kane, L. W., Taylor, C., Francis, S. H., & Hodapp, R. M. (2012). Characteristics of inclusive faith communities: A preliminary survey of inclusive practices in the United States. *Journal of Applied Research in Intellectual Disabilities, 25* (4), 383-391.

Hill-Burton Act, 42 U.S.C. § 291c(e) (1976).

Mann, W. C., Ottenbacher, K. J., Fraas, L., Tomita, M., & Granger, C. V. (1999). Effectiveness of assistive technology and environmental interventions in maintaining independence and reducing home care costs for the frail elderly: A randomized controlled trial. *Archives of Family Medicine, 8,* 210-217.

Architectural and Transportation Barriers Compliance Board. (1982). Minimum guidelines and requirements for accessible design. Final rule. 150 Fed. Reg. 33862.

Olmstead v. L. C. (1999). 527 U.S. 581 (98-536).

Petersson, I., Kottorp, A., Bergstrom, J., & Lilja, M. (2009). Longitudinal changes in everyday life after home modifications for people aging with disabilities. *Scandinavian Journal of Occupational Therapy, 16,* 78-87.

Pighills, A. C., Torgerson, D. J., Sheldon, T. A., Drummond, A. E., & Bland, J. M. (2011). Environmental assessment and modification to prevent falls in older people. *Journal of the American Geriatrics Society, 59,* 26-33.

Rehabilitation Act of 1973, 29 U.S.C. § 701 *et seq.* (1973).

Sabata, D., Williams, M., Milchus, K., Baker, P., & Sanford, J. A. (2008). A retrospective analysis of recommendations for workplace accommodations for persons with mobility and sensory limitations. *Assistive Technology, 20,* 28-35.

Sanford, J. (2001). Best practices in the design of toileting and bathing facilities for assisted transfers. Report for the U.S. Access Board. Retrieved November 20, 2006 from http://www.access-board.gov/research/Toilet-Bath/report.htm.

Siebert, C. (2005). *Occupational therapy practice guidelines for home modifications*. Bethesda, MD: American Occupational Therapy Association Press.

Stark, S., Landsbaum, A., Palmer, J. L., Somerville, E. K., & Morris, J. C. (2009). Client-centered home modifications improve daily activity performance of older adults. *Canadian Journal of Occupational Therapy, 76,* 235–245.

United Nations. (1993). The standard rules on the equalization of opportunities for persons with disabilities. Retrieved May 30, 2012 from http://www.un.org/esa/socdev/enable/dissre00.htm.

Velligan, D. I., Diamond, P., Mueller, J., Li, X., Maples, N., Wang, M., and Miller, A. L. (2009). The short-term impact of generic versus individualized environmental supports on functional outcome sand target behaviors in schizophrenia. *Psychiatry Research, 168,* 94–101.

Wilson, D. J., Mitchell, J. M., Kemp, B. J., Adkins, R. H., & Mann, W. (2009). Effects of assistive technology on functional decline in people aging with a disability. *Assistive Technology, 21,* 208–217.

Yen, I. H., Shim, J. K., Martinez, A. D., & Barker, J. C. (2012). Older people and social connectedness: How place and activities keep people engaged. *Journal of Aging Research.* Retrieved June 15, 2012 from http://downloads.hindawi.com/journals/jar/2012/139523.pdf.

Acknowledgements

Thanks to Shoshana Shamberg and Michael Williams for their contributions to previous iterations of this chapter.

32

Preventing Occupational Dysfunction Secondary to Aging

Glenn D. Goodman and Bette R. Bonder

Learning Objectives

After studying this chapter, the reader will be able to:

1. Describe normal age-related changes as they relate to areas of occupation, performance skills, performance patterns, and client factors (body functions and body structures).
2. Discuss activity patterns of older adults as related to activities of daily living, instrumental activities of daily living, education, work, play, leisure, and social participation.
3. Describe considerations in assessing the function of older adults.
4. Discuss occupational therapy interventions that facilitate function in older adults.
5. Describe the factors that make intervention following illness or injury for older adults different from that of younger adults.

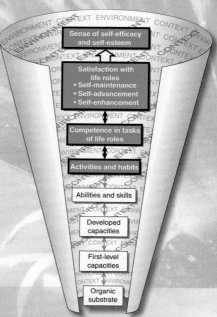

The older population (persons 65 years or older) was 39.6 million in 2009 (Administration on Aging, 2013). They represented 12.9% of the U.S. population, about one in every eight Americans. By 2030, there will be about 72.1 million older persons, more than twice the number in 2000. People age 65 years and older represented 12.4% of the population in the year 2000 but are expected to grow to be 19% of the population by 2030 (Administration on Aging, 2013).

Minority populations are projected to have increased from 5.7 million in 2000 (16.3% of the elderly population) to 8.0 million in 2010 (20.1% of the elderly) and then to 12.9 million in 2020 (23.6% of the elderly). Between 2010 and 2030, the white population of those age 65 years and older is projected to increase by 59% compared with 160% for older minorities, including Hispanics (202%), African Americans (114%), American Indians, Eskimos and Aleuts (145%), and Asians and Pacific Islanders (145%) (Administration on Aging, 2011). As the older population increases, more services will be required for the treatment and management of chronic and acute health conditions. Providing health care services for Americans of all ages will be a major challenge in the 21st century (Administration on Aging, 2011).

These figures have considerable import for health care providers, particularly occupational therapists. Enhancing functional performance of older adults can have economic, social, and personal benefits for these individuals, their families, and society as a whole.

The emphasis in this chapter is on the normal aging process. Older adults are, of course, subject to all of the illnesses and injuries that affect younger people, as well as some that are far more likely to occur in older individuals, such as cerebrovascular accidents, dementing illnesses, and cancer. Other chapters in this volume address mechanisms by which therapists can provide effective intervention for these conditions. When illness or injury occurs, however, the therapist must put the consequences in the context of the individual's life stage, which makes understanding normal aging essential. Special considerations in intervening with older adults are also discussed in this chapter.

NORMAL AGING

Many theories are applied in the study of successful aging. Theories related to aging include biological (genetic/cellular, evolutionary), neuropsychological, psychological (life span/developmental, selective optimization with compensation, cognitive and personality theories), and sociological theories (life course, social exchange, and critical perspectives of aging (Bengston & Bonder, 2009).

Changes that accompany normal aging occur in every sphere. At an individual level, normal aging affects the organic substrate, first-level capacities, developed capacities, abilities and skills, activities and habits, competence and satisfaction of life roles, and self-efficacy/self-esteem. It is essential to remember, however, the wide variation among individuals. Many individuals at age 80 years have a vigorous stride and engage in activities that would exhaust many a younger person.

Age-related changes occur to varying degrees among older adults, with varying effects on performance. The existence of a physical change does not necessarily lead to a commensurate decrement in function. Many studies identify multiple factors related to successful aging. Some of these factors include genetics (Glatt et al., 2007), level of education (Depp & Jeste, 2006), marital status, family status (e.g., families with and without children), working for pay, volunteering, practicing healthy behaviors, having adequate social supports, and maintaining strong religious beliefs (Pruchno et al., 2010).

ORGANIC SUBSTRATE AND FIRST LEVEL CAPACITIES

This section summarizes age-related changes in the sensory, neuromuscular, cardiovascular, and cognitive systems. These organic substrate and first-level capacities are client factors and performance skills as described in the Occupational Therapy Practice Framework (American Occupational Therapy Association [AOTA], 2008).

Sensory Changes

Some sensory changes normally occur with aging; others result from disease processes common among older adults (Hooper & Dal Bello-Haas, 2009). One role of the occupational therapist is to evaluate the level of dysfunction caused by changes in sensation and in the process skills that allow individuals to interpret sensory input. Therapists then can determine strategies to compensate for problems that interfere with abilities, activities, tasks, and engaging in life roles.

Changes typically occur in all sensory spheres, including vision, hearing, gustation, olfaction, touch, and vestibular sensation. Changes in multiple sensory channels require careful intervention to optimize function. Furthermore, decrements may occur at the level of reception, interpretation, or integration, that is, either peripherally or centrally in the nervous system (Bottomly & Lewis, 2007). Sensory loss can severely impair the older person's ability to communicate; the psychosocial consequences can be devastating (Brennan & Bally, 2007).

Vision

Of older adults, 18% experience deficits in vision. Among people age 85 years and older, 28% reported trouble seeing (Federal Interagency Forum on Aging-Related Statistics, 2010).

Primary age-related changes in visual function include loss of subcutaneous fat around the eye; decreased tissue elasticity and tone; decreased strength of eye muscles; decreased corneal transparency; degeneration of sclera, pupil, and iris; increase in density and rigidity of the lens; disease processes such as diabetes; and slowing of central nervous system processing (Hooper & Dal Bello-Haas, 2009).

Deterioration of near vision, called presbyopia, begins to affect most people when they are about age 40 years (American Optometric Association, n.d.). The lens loses its elasticity and becomes less able to focus because of weakness in the ciliary body (Lewis, 2003). Presbyopia is easily accommodated through the use of a well-known assistive device: eyeglasses.

Another common change is development of degenerative opacities (cataracts) of the lenses, which lead to decreased sensitivity to colors, increased sensitivity to glare, and diminished acuity (Hooper & Dal Bello-Haas, 2009). Additionally, musculature that controls eye movement tends to lose strength and tone (Tideiksaar, 2009). Tear secretion may be reduced, and degenerative changes may occur in the sclera, pupil, and iris (Bottomly & Lewis, 2007). Such changes can result in excessive dryness, loss of light/dark accommodation, and poor night vision. Finally, decreased color vision and changes in the vitreous body that affect retinal function occur with aging (Bottomly & Lewis, 2007).

The effects of diseases like diabetic retinopathy and retinitis pigmentosa, both of which may lead to total blindness, are most pronounced in the elderly population because both are progressive and degenerative (Hooper & Dal Bello-Haas, 2009). Macular degeneration, a disorder causing loss of central vision as the macula deteriorates, is most common among older individuals. Most older individuals with macular degeneration retain sufficient peripheral vision to assist in mobility but not enough for activities such as reading or watching television (Perski, n.d.).

Hearing

In 2008, 42% of older men and 30% of older women reported trouble hearing (Federal Interagency Forum on Aging-Related Statistics, 2010). The percentage was higher for people age 85 years and older (60%) than for people age 65–74 years (28%). Conductive hearing loss may be the result of problems in the external or middle ear, such as wax buildup, eustachian tube blockage, or stiffness of the ossicles and membranes (Lewis, 2003). Age-related sensorineural hearing loss, known as presbycusis, results from dysfunction of the sensory hair cells of the cochlea, neural connections from the cochlea to the cerebral cortex and brainstem, or vascular changes in the auditory system (Lewis, 2003). Tinnitus, a buzzing or ringing sensation, is experienced by 2–3 million Americans and increases with age (Hooper & Dal Bello-Haas, 2009). Functional consequences of these changes include difficulty hearing high-frequency sounds and speech, problems filtering background noise during conversation, an increase in auditory reaction time, and challenges to balance caused by inner ear changes (Hooper & Dal Bello-Haas, 2009).

Taste and Smell

Thresholds for taste and smell increase with age (Hooper & Dal Bello-Haas, 2009). The inability to detect aromas may cause food to seem tasteless, possibly resulting in secondary nutritional disorders. Individuals may not be able to detect harmful odors such as natural gas, spoiled food, or smoke (Hooper & Dal Bello-Haas, 2009). Smoking or environmental exposures may exacerbate age-related changes in taste and olfaction (Bottomly & Lewis, 2007).

Tactile Changes

Changes in the number and sensitivity of touch and pressure receptors have been reported (Hooper & Dal Bello-Haas, 2009). A decreased response to tactile stimuli, higher touch thresholds, and a decrease in the ability to detect touch and pressure can result but are highly variable. Tactile sensation can be preserved and improved with therapeutic interventions (Hooper & Dal Bello-Haas, 2009). Some literature suggests there are structural and biochemical changes in nerve fibers that occur in older adults related to perception of pain and temperature (Caprio & Williams, 2007).

Proprioceptive and Kinesthetic Changes

Documentation of changes in proprioception or kinesthesia that are purely related to aging is scant. Changes in proprioception secondary to loss of vision, peripheral vascular disease, arthritis, cardiovascular disorders, stroke, disorders of the inner ear, and diabetes have been reported (Bottomly & Lewis, 2007).

Vestibular Function

Vestibular changes are particularly significant because of the importance of falls as a health risk for older adults. Approximately 33% of older adults fall each year, and 15% of these individuals experience serious health consequences, such as broken hips and traumatic brain injury. Falls are the leading cause of death caused by accidents in persons age 65 years or older (Tideiksaar, 2009).

Vestibular righting response diminishes with age, which can lead to problems in maintaining balance. Age-related changes in static balance, dynamic balance, and gait appear to increase the probability of falls (Bottomly & Lewis, 2007; Tideiksaar, 2009).

Central Nervous System

With age, the cerebrum atrophies (Bottomly & Lewis, 2007), and cerebrospinal fluid space increases. Neurons are lost or atrophy, particularly in the precentral gyrus, postcentral gyrus, superior temporal gyrus, and Purkinje cells of the cerebellum (Bottomly & Lewis, 2007). The number of synapses decreases, and neurotransmitter systems change (Dal Bello-Haas, 2009). In addition, plaques, fibrillary tangles, and other cellular abnormalities have been found in the brains of functionally normal older adults (Lewis, 2003). Responses to stimuli as measured by electroencephalogram also slow down.

Peripheral Nervous System

Among the changes in the peripheral nervous system seen in aging are loss of neurons and both myelinated and unmyelinated nerve fibers, decrease in myelin, axonal atrophy, and slowed nerve conduction velocity (Dal Bello-Haas, 2009). Variation among individuals makes functional and structural generalizations problematic.

Musculoskeletal System

The normal change in the musculoskeletal system can have consequences for mobility and function. The following sections describe the normal aging process as it affects muscles and bone, as well as the impact of various diseases on the musculoskeletal system.

Muscles

Changes in muscles that are attributed to aging include a decline in the number and size of muscle fibers, decreased muscle mass, an increase in fatty and connective tissue, decreased metabolism of protein, increased muscle fatigue, and a reduction in the number of motor neurons (Dal Bello-Haas, 2009), resulting in loss of muscle strength, decreased endurance, and slower walking and rising times.

Joints

Joint function declines steadily after age 20 years. Ligaments and tendons become less resilient and more prone to injury (Bottomly & Lewis, 2007). The quantity and viscosity of synovial fluid decrease with aging. Cartilage becomes opaque, with an increase in cracks and fraying (Bottomly & Lewis, 2007), which can be reduced with preventive intervention or may require corrective surgery. The effects of weight bearing and stress on joints and the effects of diseases, such as the various kinds of arthritis, make the rate and nature of cartilage deterioration highly variable.

Bones

Bone loss of up to 1% a year occurs until age 50 years for men and women (Dal Bello-Haas, 2009). Women older than age 50 years have a rate of bone loss double that of men. By age 65 years, at least 50% of women have developed some form of osteoporosis. The rate of degeneration slows by age 70 years (Lewis, 2003). The rate of bone loss continues to increase similarly in men and women after age 80 years (Dal Bello-Haas, 2009).

Effect of Disease on the Musculoskeletal System

Arthritis, osteoporosis, connective tissue diseases, orthopedic injuries from falls and trauma, and repetitive motion disorders are most prevalent in elderly individuals (Tideiksaar, 2009). Almost 50% of men and women have some form of arthritis by age 65 years (Federal Interagency Forum on Aging-Related Statistics, 2010). Approximately 332,000 hip fractures occur annually in the United States, primarily in individuals age 65 years and older. Almost 25% of older adults who fracture a hip die within 1 year (Tideiskaar, 2009).

Cardiovascular Changes

The cardiovascular system loses efficiency with age, which is the result of changes in the frequency and regularity of the conduction system; a reduction in pacemaker cells (Bottomly & Lewis, 2007); alterations in blood pressure (Federal Interagency Forum on Aging-Related Statistics, 2010); changes in the elasticity, length, and thickness of the arteries (Bottomly & Lewis, 2007); a decrease in heart rate and stroke volume; and a general thickening of specific heart tissues, such as the atria and valves (Bottomly & Lewis, 2007).

Elastic tissues decrease and fibrous tissues increase, affecting the medium and small airways constructed of smooth muscle. The joints of the chest wall stiffen, the muscles of the diaphragm flatten, and the chest wall becomes more barrel shaped and less compliant (Dean & De Andrade, 2009). Approximately 50% of individuals older than age 65 years have hypertension (Federal Interagency Forum on Aging-Related Statistics, 2010). However, conditioning training can elicit the same physiological benefits to older adults as in younger people (Dean & De Andrade, 2009).

Cognitive Changes

Age-related changes occur in some aspects of intelligence, problem solving, abstract reasoning, memory, memory processing, and attention. Changes are most noticeable after age 70 years, although gradual decline occurs when individuals reach the age of 30 years (Anstey & Low, 2004). As measured by the Wechsler Adult Intelligence Scale, the intelligence quotient decreases with advancing age, largely the result of decreases in the performance rather than verbal subscales

(Miller et al., 2009). Performance subscales may depend on fluid intelligence (the ability to use new information), whereas verbal subscales may use crystallized intelligence (recall of stored memories) (Anstey & Low, 2004). In particular, flexibility in reasoning tasks seems to decline (Miller et al., 2009), although older adults show wide individual variation in these cognitive capacities. Some kinds of problem-solving skills also seem to become less efficient (Anstey & Low, 2004), although older adults show actual improvement in solving interpersonal or emotionally salient problems (Blanchard-Fields, Mienaltowski, & Seay, 2007).

In general, well older adults do not have problems with processing and short-term storage of information, although some have difficulty encoding large amounts of information at once (Anstey & Low, 2004). Decrements in long-term memory and encoding are noticeable (Anstey & Low, 2004). Older adults have more trouble recalling information than do younger ones. An older person may remember the face and personality of an acquaintance but have difficulty retrieving the name. This difficulty is much less pronounced when the information has practical significance. Everyday or practical memory may be of considerable salience for elders (Riley, 2009).

When cognitive changes begin to interfere with function, the decline is labeled mild cognitive impairment (MCI) (National Library of Medicine, 2007). MCI is characterized by changes in memory. Unlike dementia, other cognitive functions are relatively spared. There is ongoing research to understand whether MCI is a precursor to Alzheimer's disease (AD). It is estimated that roughly 25% of individuals with MCI develop AD within a year (Petersen et al., 1999). For some individuals, memory training has helped minimize associated functional decrements (Riley, 2009). One challenge in examining cognitive change in older adults is the clear association between sensory decline and cognition (Valentin et al., 2005), because visual or hearing deficits may reduce the individual's ability to respond accurately to questions or to follow instructions.

A Special Note about Dementia

Dementing illnesses are common among older adults. Dementia, which is characterized by forgetfulness, difficulty finding words, and other cognitive loss, is not a normal condition of aging. Rather, it is a symptom of any of several disease processes (Riley, 2009). Some, such as depression, sensory deprivation, malnutrition, and drug toxicity, are reversible; others are not. AD, the most common form of dementia, is a progressive disorder that eventually leads to total disability and death. In its later stages, AD causes motor impairment as well as personality change, and individuals with AD will have difficulty participating in prevention or rehabilitation for other conditions. Of particular concern are catastrophic reactions, severe emotional

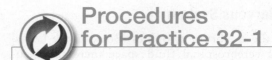

Procedures for Practice 32-1

Strategies for Working with Individuals with Dementia

- Place items used frequently in visible locations.
- Use simple, one-step instructions.
- Maintain habitual activities as much as possible; simplify as needed.
- Obtain a bracelet identifying the person as memory impaired in case of wandering.
- Encourage physical activity during the day to improve nighttime sleep.
- Provide activities that stimulate memory (e.g., baking or music that the person used to enjoy).
- Include activities that enrich life; access procedural memory to support participation.
- Avoid excessively crowded or unfamiliar surroundings that might lead to catastrophic reactions.
- Contact the local Alzheimer's Association for resource lists and support groups.

outbursts that typify the middle stages of AD associated with confusing or overwhelming situations.

It is beyond the scope of this chapter to deal with the methods for intervening with individuals with dementing disorders. A few suggested intervention strategies are included in Procedures for Practice 32-1 and in Chapter 24 of this book. Health care professionals should be familiar with the early symptoms of cognitive disorder, such as difficulty finding words, forgetfulness about everyday events, and a lack of recollection of familiar individuals. When noted, these symptoms should be carefully evaluated by a geriatrician, a physician trained to work with older individuals. Reversible causes may be treated relatively easily. If the individual has an irreversible dementing illness, a variety of management strategies can help caregivers to cope with resulting problems. This enhances quality of life for both the ill person and the caregivers.

DEVELOPED CAPACITIES: CHANGES IN VOLUNTARY RESPONSES

Changes in organic substrates and first-level capacities may impair such voluntary responses as rising from a chair and gait speed. Weakness in ankle dorsiflexion and knee extension has been correlated with falls in older individuals (Tideiksaar, 2009).

Loss of dexterity and coordination are common with aging (Dal Bello-Haas, 2009). Scores on dexterity tests (Jebsen et al., 1969; Mathiowetz et al., 1985a, 1985b) decline with age.

ABILITIES AND SKILLS: PHYSICAL CAPACITY

The following changes in physical capacity typify skills and abilities that are affected by normal aging: postural alignment, sway, and instability with postural changes (Tideiksaar, 2009), gross motor coordination (Bottomly & Lewis, 2007), fine motor coordination and dexterity, strength and endurance (Bottomly & Lewis, 2007), walking speed, step length, and step height (Bottomly & Lewis, 2007; Tideiksaar, 2009), and reaction time (Bottomly & Lewis, 2007).

ACTIVITIES, HABITS, AND ROLES

Elders have greater personal choice in determining their tasks and life roles than do younger individuals. Although some individuals must continue to work to support themselves, particularly in challenging economic times, many have the option of retiring from paid employment. Those who have children typically have finished rearing them. Because living in certain school districts is no longer an issue, some elders opt to sell their home and move to an apartment or to new community. For others, aging in place is a significant issue (Rantz et al., 2011). Occupational therapists can assist in this by evaluating for safety in the home environment, recommending modifications that improve access, and assisting with community mobility to facilitate both daily living needs and access to meaningful tasks and life roles.

As with physiological changes, activity patterns are highly individual (Gauthier & Smeeding, 2003). Some older adults engage in many activities; others focus on one or two. Changes in habits include different time use; more time is spent in leisure and less in paid employment. There are gender and cultural differences in activities such as housework and social activities (Gauthier & Smeeding, 2003). The development of useful, dominating, or impoverished habits (AOTA, 2008) can impact an older adult's health and longevity.

Most older adults accommodate to age-related changes well by modifying routines or finding and accepting assistance. This is especially true when the activity is one for which it is socially acceptable to receive help. Help with driving, cooking, or managing finances is often acceptable. Some older adults are determined to do for themselves, whereas others are accepting, even relieved, when they can rely on others to take care of them.

Self-Care

Independence in self-care is a significant issue for older adults. In 2007, 42% of individuals older than age 65 years reported difficulty with activities of daily living (ADL) and instrumental activities of daily living (IADL). Of institutionalized older Americans, 83% report difficulties in ADL (Administration on Aging, 2011). Heavy housework, such as mopping floors and washing windows, is difficult for many individuals and may be hired out or done by family members. In addition, most elders spend more time on self-care activities than they did when younger (Christiansen, Haertl, & Robinson, 2009). Issues of time can be significant when self-care consumes such a large proportion of the day that other desired activities cannot be pursued.

Substantial disability in self-care is most likely to be perceived when there is a sudden change because of illness or change in social circumstances rather than the gradual ones that affect most well elders. If the change is loss related, emotional reactions that typically accompany loss must be addressed. Changes perceived as positive, however, such as a move to a long-desired retirement location, can also cause unanticipated emotional difficulties.

Urinary Incontinence

Urinary incontinence affects more than 25 million Americans. Of homebound older adults, 53% are incontinent (National Association for Continence, 2008). The inability to bathe and urinary and bowel incontinence are issues that can influence life-altering decisions for elders. Those who are unable to bathe or who are incontinent are most likely to be placed in institutional settings, which is an event that most elders wish to avoid. Interventions for urinary/bowel incontinence include surgery, medications, and behavioral treatment. Occupational therapists provide behavioral interventions that may include regular scheduling of toileting, pelvic muscle reeducation (Kegel exercises), biofeedback, bladder training, urge inhibition, bowel management, and dietary and fluid modifications (Dumoulin, Korner-Bitensky, & Tannenbaum, 2007).

Work

Emerging patterns in work and retirement reflect increasing diversity in the older population (Sterns, Lax, & Chang, 2009). Many older adults are making choices that differ from those of previous generations. Although there is a trend toward earlier retirement compared with previous generations, there is also a trend toward continued paid employment, albeit in new work circumstances (Bambrick & Bonder, 2005). Elders describe multiple reasons for wanting to continue to work, including issues of independence, sense of self-worth, and a wish to continue to contribute to society. Elders remain capable of work far beyond the traditional retirement age of 65 years (Sterns, Lax, & Chang, 2009). The work force is changing rapidly, with an increase in the number of female workers and an increase in the percentage of workers age 55 years and older being major trends (Sterns, Lax, & Chang, 2009).

Historical discrimination against older workers is being addressed through policy initiatives such as the Age Discrimination in Employment Act and the Americans with Disabilities Act (Sterns, Lax, & Chang, 2009). Changing demographics require fundamental reconsideration of policies designed to either encourage or discourage elders' choices about paid employment.

Older workers require slightly more time to learn new skills. They respond best to learning that is based on practical examples. They also complete less work than younger workers but with an equivalent error rate. Given appropriate accommodations, however, older workers can continue to be productive and valuable workers far into later life. Age has not been found to be related to work performance, and other characteristics such as personality, essential job functions, and motivation are more important in matching an individual to any given work situation (Sterns, Lax, & Chang, 2009) (Fig. 32-1). Many older workers continue in jobs requiring high levels of physical function.

Retirement

Substantial evidence exists that voluntary retirement is not viewed as a negative event (Bambrick & Bonder, 2005). When retirement is involuntary, however, either as a result of a personal situation such as failing health or external events such as layoffs, individuals are likely to be dissatisfied with retirement (Sterns, Lax, & Chang, 2009). Retirement often does not mean the cessation of productive activity (Bambrick & Bonder, 2005). Individuals who engage in volunteer work, child care, or other forms of unpaid service report that these have value both to them and to others. Bambrick and Bonder (2005) found that older adults value this kind of work for contributing to self-concept, giving back to the community, and staying

engaged. Key elements in addressing adjustment to retirement include time use, meaningful occupations, self-worth, and health maintenance or wellness.

Leisure

Leisure provides a sense of identity and life satisfaction for individuals who are no longer working and appears to delay onset of some disabling conditions. Furthermore, it offers opportunities for expression of important personal meanings. For older adults, the line between leisure and work may be indistinct, with activities providing both a sense of usefulness to others and satisfaction of personal need for engagement and challenge (Bambrick & Bonder, 2005) (Fig. 32-2). Older adults can derive great satisfaction from meaningful leisure activities.

Bundy and Clemson (2009) identify three elements that contribute to the leisure experience of older adults: control, motivation, and freedom from constraints of real life. Occupational therapists should identify the amount of involvement, flow, and commitment (engagement) in activities and help older adults to identify these activities, manage them, adapt them, and enjoy them. Other important concepts to consider when addressing leisure with older adults include personal characteristics or preferences (e.g., social participation versus isolation), self-perception ("If I can't golf the regular way, golfing is meaningless to me"), physical, cognitive, and social skills, and context and environment.

Driving

According to the Insurance Institute for Highway Safety (2011), in 2009, 61% of the deaths in crashes involving drivers age 70 years and older were the older drivers themselves, and 16% were their passengers. In contrast, in

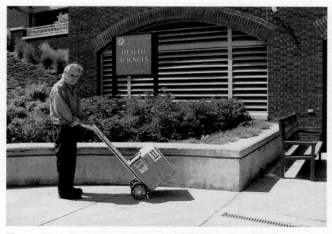

Figure 32-1 The gentleman pictured is still on the job, despite the physical demands of his work in delivering supplies around his organization.

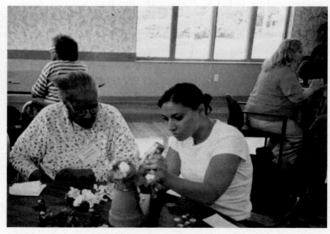

Figure 32-2 Even elders with substantial impairments derive great satisfaction from meaningful leisure activities.

crashes involving at least one driver younger than 30 years of age, 42% of the deaths were the drivers younger than age 30 years; 24% were their passengers. However, since 1997, deaths of older passenger vehicle occupants have declined 33%, whereas deaths of older pedestrians have declined 38% (Insurance Institute for Highway Safety, 2011).

AOTA is an excellent resource for materials related to driving safety for all persons with special assistance for working with older drivers (http://www.aota.org/Older-Driver.aspx). One example of an AOTA collaborative program with AAA and AARP is Car Fit (http://www.car-fit.org/). This educational program helps older drivers assess the fit of their personal vehicles. Model driving evaluation and rehabilitation programs for the older driver include measuring driver potential before on-road evaluation; measuring and improving driver performance with on-road testing and intervention; proper documentation of fitness to drive; environmental and ergonomic factors impacting drivers, passengers, and pedestrians; and communication with all of the stakeholders in making a decision about the safe performance of an older driver (Ekelman et al., 2009; Pellerito, 2006).

Sexuality

Miracle and Miracle (2009) identify three myths about sex and older adults.

- Older adults do not have sex.
- New drugs have greatly enhanced sex lives of older adults.
- People find each other less physically attractive over time.

The opportunity to develop and maintain intimacy in later life is challenging. Factors that affect this include a disproportionate number of females because they live longer than males; older adults living in institutions where opportunities may be limited by policies and environmental factors, declining health; increased incidence of diseases that affect physical and psychological function; and impoverished habits such as smoking and alcohol (Miracle & Miracle, 2009). Occupational therapists should recognize this as a valued activity for some older adults and provide interventions to support sexual activity as appropriate.

Sexuality is frequently ignored in studies examining quality of life. One study reported a strong relationship between the amount of sexual activity and measures of intimacy and satisfaction with personal relationships (Robinson & Molzahn, 2007). One major concern that is frequently cited is the unwillingness of health care providers to address sexuality with clients old or young (Miracle & Miracle, 2009; Robinson & Molzahn, 2007). Barriers and factors that are important to address regarding sexuality in older adults include the loss of a life partner and the ability or interest to "date" again; knowledge and understanding of sexuality; family values and contexts; acquisition of privacy; patient safety; physiological issues; effects of disease;

medications; pain with intercourse; cognitive, physical, psychological, and social skills; and the effects of alcohol and smoking (Miracle & Miracle, 2009).

Satisfaction of Emerging Personal Needs and Meanings

Researchers and practitioners have made increasing attempts to understand the occupations of older adults (Bambrick & Bonder, 2005; Nilsson et al., 2007; Windsor, 2009). In particular, researchers are interested in knowing what is important to elders and how their occupations contribute to quality of life.

Physical health is not, in and of itself, sufficient to ensure good quality of life (Lent, 2004). Occupational therapy reflects a belief that individuals are most satisfied with their lives when they engage in a variety of occupations that balance self-care, work, and leisure (AOTA, 2008). Research suggests that this is true for older adults as well as younger individuals (Nilsson et al., 2007; Rowe & Kahn, 1998; Windsor, 2009).

Elimination or Alteration of Roles

Elders can make choices about adding roles, but far less choice is involved in loss of social roles. Death of a spouse or loss of physical capacity dramatically shifts occupational tasks. As an example, one woman who had made her living as a weaver found that she could no longer sit at a floor loom. She chose to weave at a small table loom (Bonder, 2009b). The salient issue seems to be finding outlets for expression of personal meaning (Menec, 2003; Morrow-Howell et al., 2003).

Additional Roles

Elders not only lose or choose to end previous roles; they also add roles. An elder who stops paid employment becomes a retiree and may become a volunteer. A parent whose children are grown may become a grandparent. In some instances, even roles that are not chosen may be satisfying. For example, some elders become not only grandparents but surrogate parents for their grandchildren. As many as 10% of elders are custodial grandparents (Hayslip & Kaminski, 2005). Although this may be perceived by some as a burden, many grandparents express great satisfaction with this role.

COMPETENCE AND SELF-ESTEEM: PSYCHOSOCIAL

Psychosocial status may be the most significant predictor of occupational function. Motivated, enthusiastic individuals tend to fare well, often despite what appear to be substantial physical limitations (Chappell, 2008). Practitioners must attend to situations in which the individual, following an injury or illness, becomes depressed, loses motivation, and becomes increasingly disabled.

Self-esteem drops sharply in later life (Robins & Trzesniewski, 2005). Protective factors include strong coping skills (Moyle et al., 2010). In particular, keeping active, maintaining relationships and community connections, and spirituality contribute to a sense of well-being in later life.

Changes in psychosocial status must be separated into those that are psychological and those that are social. For a well older adult, the former relate to developmental tasks of later life. The latter relate to external factors, including major life changes such as retirement and the loss of social contacts through residential relocation, retirement, or death of peers.

A number of theorists have attempted to identify the normal psychological processes that accompany aging. Among the theories are disengagement, activity, continuity, and life span models. The principal characteristics of these theories are noted in Table 32-1. Although each theory has appeal, each also has limitations in explaining the psychological functioning of older individuals.

It is well established that older individuals have significant losses of social contacts (Bonder, 2009a). There is,

Table 32-1 **Summary of Theories Related to Occupational Therapy for Older Adults**

Theories/Category	Constructs
Genetic theories/biological (Slagboom et al., 2010)	1. Particular genes can predict longevity or susceptibility to disease. 2. Mutation of genes could extend longevity. 3. Familial studies may identify longevity genes in families where there is a history of long life.
Activity theory/psychological (Havighurst, 1963; Longino & Kart, 1982)	1. Elderly strive to maintain activity. 2. High levels of activity correlate with well-being.
Continuity theory/psychological (Atchley, 1989)	1. Elderly attempt to continue activities that were always important to them. 2. Elderly perceive activities as continuous. 3. Elderly adapt activity to compensate for change. 4. Successful aging is characterized by degree of continuity achieved.
Life span theories/psychological (Erikson, 1963; Levinson, 1986; Neugarten, 1975)	1. Old age is continuation of the developmental process, representing a new developmental stage. 2. Tasks specific to the stage can be identified. 3. Successful aging results from accomplishing tasks.
Selective optimization with compensation/psychological (Baltes & Baltes, 1990).	Elders cope with changing function by: 1. selecting activites they can maintain 2. optimizing those they choose to continue 3. compensating for those they give up
Neurodegenerative change theories/ Neuropsychological (Woodruff-Pak & Papka, 1999)	1. Age-linked neuropathological changes occur in some diseases (Alzheimer's and Parkinson's) that produce changes in cognitive function. 2. No one theory adequately explains these observed phenomena. 3. Activities such as cognitive exercises and diet changes may stave off or reverse these changes.
Social constructionist theory/ sociological (Bengston, Burgess, & Parrott, 1997)	1. Individual processes of aging are influenced by social definitions and structures. 2. Each individual constructs meanings from his or her own experiences. 3. Qualitative research is emphasized.
Person-environment-occupation/ occupational therapy (Christiansen & Baum, 1997)	1. Successful occupational engagement results from an interaction of the person, the environment, and the occupation. 2. Intervention can occur in any of these three elements to enhance performance.

Adapted from Bengston, V. L., & Bonder, B. (2009). Theories of aging: A multidisciplinary review of occupational and physical therapists. In B. R. Bonder & V. Dal Bello-Haas (Eds.), *Functional performance in older adults* (3rd ed., pp. 28–44). Philadelphia: F. A. Davis.

however, great variability in how individuals cope with such losses. For example, loss of a spouse is devastating for most older individuals (McGarry & Schoeni, 2005). Some individuals compensate within a year or so, whereas others never recover. Higher socioeconomic status and social and spiritual resources seem to predict better long-term adjustment to loss of a spouse. Some elders are open to and actively seek new social relationships, whereas others become increasingly isolated. Because social relationships are so closely linked to well-being in later life (Park, 2009), therapy can be beneficial if it focuses on supporting strategies to build social networks.

IMPEDIMENTS TO OCCUPATIONAL FUNCTION

We review two categories of barriers to occupational function: disease and environmental factors.

Impact of Disease

Almost all older adults eventually fall ill or have an injury that may call for secondary or tertiary preventive interventions, that is, minimizing consequences early in treatment or enhancing rehabilitation once severe disability has occurred. The following special characteristics of older adults must be considered in planning intervention.

Differential Severity of Condition

Some conditions that are relatively innocuous in younger individuals, influenza, for example, can have severe consequences for older individuals (Dal Bello-Haas, 2009). On the other hand, cancers that may be terminal in younger adults are often quite slow growing in older individuals.

Multiple Health Problems

Otherwise well older adults are likely to have two or three chronic health problems (Administration on Aging, 2013); for example, rheumatoid arthritis and osteoporosis, each of which may require a different intervention. Although moderately strenuous weight-bearing exercise may be the treatment of choice to prevent bone loss, such activity may exacerbate the arthritis.

Duration of Recuperation

Older adults generally recuperate more slowly than younger ones, even if the eventual outcome is every bit as good. Treatment often ends too soon for older individuals.

Consequences of Dysfunction

Most elders prefer to live independently or "age in place" (Bonder, 2009a). It is their wish to remain in the living situation to which they have grown accustomed. Illness and dysfunction, however, can lead to a decision to institutionalize. Functional abilities are central to such decisions. In particular, bathing and toileting abilities influence family decisions. For this reason, occupational therapists often find that elders want to emphasize these abilities in treatment.

Environmental Factors

As with all clients, environmental factors, both physical and social, can have a profound influence on function. Issues described in Chapters 3 and 10 of this text should be carefully considered during interaction with elderly clients, because changes to the personal, social, cultural, and environmental context can greatly facilitate personal abilities.

Depression and Other Mental Health Concerns

As is true for all age groups, older adults may experience a number of significant psychiatric disorders. Dementia, which was discussed above, is listed in the *Diagnostic and Statistical Manual of Mental Disorders* (American Psychiatric Association [APA], 2000) and is one of the few psychiatric disorders that affects primarily older adults. The most common disorders among older adults are anxiety disorders and depression (Meeks et al., 2009).

Depression may be a continuation of a lifelong mood disorder. However, depression can also be linked to physical illnesses such as heart disease (Ai, Rollman, & Berger, 2010; Mast, 2010), stroke, or hip fracture (Meeks et al., 2009). Depression also presents somewhat differently in older adults as compared with younger individuals. Older adults are likely to have more somatic complaints, social withdrawal, and lethargy, often without reported depressed mood. In addition, depression in older adults may present as dementia (Meeks et al., 2009). Depressive dementia is characterized by poverty of response and apathy and is reversible if the depression is successfully treated.

Older adults, especially older men, have high rates of suicide as compared with younger populations (Szanto et al., 2002). Clinicians should be alert to signs of suicidal ideation and should ensure that appropriate intervention is provided when risk is suspected.

Depression is one of the more treatable psychiatric disorders. Among the potentially effective interventions are specific kinds of reminiscence focused on life review and on building relationships (Cappeliez, O'Rourke, & Chaudhury, 2005). Another strategy that has beneficial impact, not only for treating depression but also for supporting mental health well-being more generally, is intervention to enhance resilience (Moyle et al., 2010).

Elder Abuse

It is an unfortunate reality that a significant proportion of older adults experience some form of abuse (Anetzberger, 2009). Prevalence is estimated at 1%–10% of the older population. Elder abuse takes many forms, including physical or sexual abuse, neglect, and financial abuse (Anetzberger, 2009). Physical abuse involves active physical violence against the elder. Sexual abuse involves varying forms of sexual imposition. Neglect is characterized by failure to provide adequate care. Financial abuse is characterized by misappropriation of funds. Abuse may be perpetrated by informal caregivers (family members or friends) or by formal care providers (home health aides, therapists, or financial planners).

Clinicians have a responsibility to screen for abuse and are required to report suspected abuse to adult protective services. There are a number of screening instruments (Fulmer et al., 2004), although when the elder has dementia, self-report may not be accurate. Even elders who are cognitively intact may not report accurately, perhaps because they fear retribution or loss of independence. Thus, although screening assessments can be helpful, clinicians should attend to other signs of abuse, including weight loss, unexplained bruises, and unexplained changes in checking accounts. A very helpful checklist for occupational therapists has been developed by Lafata and Helfrich (2001).

FACILITATORS OF OCCUPATIONAL FUNCTION

Clinicians consider each patient's age as they plan assessment and interventions to optimize occupational function.

Evaluation

Careful evaluation is vital to successful intervention focused on supporting functional performance of older adults. Perhaps the most attention has been given to assessment of self-care (Wilkins, Law, & Letts, 2009). In assessing older adults, however, it is important to be cognizant of the goals of the individual (Canadian Association of Occupational Therapists, 2002). Assessment should focus on the individual's goals and proceed to determination of factors that support or impede those goals. The Occupational Therapy Practice Framework (AOTA, 2008) recommends completing an occupational profile and an analysis of occupational performance. The two combined provide information about what the individual needs and wants to do and what factors limit ability to accomplish those tasks.

Several instruments may be helpful in determining those goals. The Canadian Occupational Performance Measure (Law et al., 2005) involves interview of the client and joint identification of goals for therapy. These goals then become the measures of outcome. Other helpful assessments include the Melville/Nelson Evaluation System (Melville & Nelson, n.d.), the Assessment of Motor and Process Skills (Fisher, 1995), the Arnadottir OT-ADL Neurobehavioral Evaluation (A-ONE) (Arnadottir, 1990), and the Activity Card Sort (Baum & Edwards, n.d.).

Legislation, particularly the Omnibus Budget Reconciliation Act (OBRA) (Glantz & Richman, 1991), requires that people in nursing homes have an environmental assessment, but such assessment should be done in community settings as well. A number of good environmental assessment instruments are available including the SAFER-HOME (Chiu & Oliver, 2006; Mann & Hicks, 2009; Tideiksaar, 2009) (see Chapter 10).

Instruments are also being developed to assess driving ability (Pellerito, 2006). In addition, it is important to evaluate risk for falls (Tideiksaar, 2009) for the reasons discussed above. It is important to evaluate both the physical and the social environment as well.

Some assessment is mandated by third-party payers. For example, the U.S. government has implemented a minimum data set (MDS) (Centers for Medicare and Medicaid Services, n.d.[a]) for residents of nursing homes, and the Outcomes Assessment Information (OASIS) (Centers for Medicare and Medicaid Services, n.d.[b]) for home health.

Intervention

An important role for occupational therapists working with older adults is prevention or remediation of functional disability (AOTA, 2008). Intervention may include prevention, ongoing screening for previously unidentified issues or concerns, environmental modifications, modification or substitution of activities, educational interventions, and collaboration with older adults and their families to individualize care plans (client-centered care). Evidence Table 32-1 lists studies proving the benefits of occupational therapy for older adults.

Screening

During the course of all intervention activities, occupational therapists should be alert to potential problems (Wilkins, Law, & Letts, 2009). If individuals who are nutritionally compromised or who have recently had a life-changing loss receive early intervention, disability may be minimized or avoided. For example, if a client becomes unable to drive because of increasing visual impairment, the therapist may acquaint him or her with community transit services or help make contact with friends and relatives who can provide occasional transportation. Such an intervention helps reduce the likelihood of social isolation, which can lead to depression and perhaps to significant disability. Screening should include record review, consultation with the client, family, and other professionals, and considerations for ultimate living

Evidence Table 32-1		Best Evidence for Occupational Therapy Practice for Older Adults				
Intervention	Description of Intervention Tested	Participants	Dosage	Type of Best Evidence and Level of Evidence	Benefit	Statistical Probability and Effect Size of Outcome	Reference
Independent living for community-dwelling elderly people	Assistive devices, skills training, evaluation of home hazards, comprehensive occupational therapy interventions	Over 3,800 participants represented in the studies reviewed		Systematic literature review of 17 studies	Strong evidence for the efficacy of advising on assistive devices as part of a home-hazard assessment	Two randomized controlled trials reported statistically significant effect sizes (odds ratios = 0.39 and 0.97) for training in assistive devices	Steultjens et al. (2004)
Environmental interventions for prevention of falls	Home assessment interventions	Over 3,200 participants represented in the studies reviewed		Meta-analysis of six clinical trials	The highest effects are with interventions conducted with high-risk groups	Pooled analysis of six trials ($n = 3,298$) demonstrated a 21% reduction in falls risk (relative risk)	Clemson et al. (2008)
Community-based occupational therapy for older adults with dementia	Cognitive and behavioral interventions to train patients in the use of aids to compensate for cognitive decline and to train caregivers in coping behaviors and supervision	One hundred thirty-five participants with moderate to mild dementia	Ten sessions were provided over a 5-week period	Randomized controlled trial and cost-effectiveness study Level: IA1a	Mean costs lower in the intervention group; significant difference in proportions of successful treatments at 3 months	Average total cost savings of $2,641 per couple receiving occupational therapy $p < 0.05$	Graff et al. (2008)
Lifestyle redesign program	Small group sessions with modular content areas led by an occupational therapist; community outings	Four hundred sixty older adults (well elderly)	Up to 10 individual 1-hour sessions, as well as the group sessions	Randomized controlled trial Level: IA1a	Intervention group showed positive change scores in bodily pain, vitality, social functioning, mental health, mental functioning, life satisfaction depressive symptomatology and quality-adjusted life years	$p < 0.05$ for all variables mentioned; effect sizes ranged from 0.14 to 0.23	Clark et al. (2011)
Review of research evidence on productive aging	Review of 14 articles published in *American Journal of Occupational Therapy* 2008–2009			Four systematic reviews, one instrument development, seven basic research articles, one effectiveness study, and one link between occupational engagement and health	Strongest evidence found in area of driving		Murphy (2010)

situation such as PACE Programs (www.medicare.gov /Nursing/Alternatives/PACE.asp) designed to keep older adults in their homes.

Environmental Modifications

Another highly effective intervention is to reduce some demands through alteration of the environment (Procedures for Practice 32-2).

Technological Aids to Function

Numerous technological assists can maximize function (Procedures for Practice 32-3). Some are simple, such as an alarm on the doorknob to warn family members that a person is wandering away or automatic off-switches on stoves to reduce fire hazard. Others, such as the computer-operated Smart House, are highly sophisticated and expensive.

 Procedures for Practice 32-2

Environmental Modifications for Elderly Individuals

Cognitive Problems

- Reduce clutter.
- Label drawers and cabinets by their contents; for individuals who have dementia or other serious cognitive deficits, pictures may be easier to understand than words.
- Use color, texture, and lighting changes to provide location cues, such as changes from carpet to tile signaling the move from dining area to hallway.
- Use timers as reminders for specific functions.
- Put safety off-switches on stoves and furnaces.

Visual Problems

- Use high tone colors and low gloss finishes to improve visual acuity and depth perception (Tideiksaar, 2009).
- Encourage use of other sensory systems such as touch and hearing.
- Maintain a consistent environment for individuals with visual impairments.
- Reduce clutter, simplify, and reorganize the environment to establish routines.
- Write with felt-tipped pens and in bold print to help improve visibility (Mann & Hicks, 2009).
- Access optometrists, ophthalmologists, and staff at sight centers or the Society for the Blind.
- Provide high-intensity, low-glare light; avoid fluorescent lights; and put glare-reducing screens over televisions and windows (Tideiksaar, 2009).
- Teach compensatory techniques to individuals with visual field deficits (Lewis, 2003).
- Consider assistive technologies such as portable magnifiers, computer-screen readers, electronic books with speech function, talking wrist watches, devices to assist with pouring liquids, and tactile maps.

Hearing and Communication Problems

- Refer for a thorough evaluation from a speech pathologist, audiologist, or otolaryngologist.

- Speak slowly and clearly and use a deep voice with someone who has high-frequency loss.
- Make sure the individual can see you when you speak (Hooper & Dal Bello-Haas, 2009).
- Write messages if necessary.
- Modify the environment to improve acoustics and reduce ambient noise.
- Select activities for which verbal interaction may not be essential.
- Check that hearing aids are fitted and used properly and that batteries are fresh; remember that these aids do not restore normal hearing and may not help everyone with hearing impairment.
- Use visual cues, such as flashing lights, to get the client's attention. Address safety needs.
- Consult with other professionals and implement assistive technologies such as iPad, alternative communication strategies with assistive devices, or textual and pictorial communication. See further discussion in Chapter 18.

Neuromuscular, Motor, or Mobility Problems

- Make sure the environment is free of hazards such as slippery floors and architectural barriers.
- Adjust the height of chairs, beds, dressers, and toilet seats; provide a bath chair and grab bars.
- Provide task-oriented treatment in the individual's environment with numerous repetitions.
- In institutional settings, keep in mind OBRA regulations that mandate reduced use of restraints.
- Use alternative furniture or technologies such as floor-level bed and alarm systems.

Self-Care: Toileting and Continence Problems

- Make sure that the bathroom is physically accessible. Add grab bars and nonskid mats.
- Mark the bathroom clearly. Use large, clear words, pictures, and color code if necessary.
- Reduce liquid intake prior to bedtime.
- Institute regular reminders to use the bathroom.
- Institute timed voiding (regularly scheduled toileting) and prompted voiding (caregiver reminders) (Wiatrowski, Riccio, & Scheer, 2008)

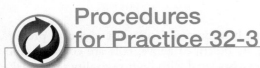

Procedures for Practice 32-3

Assistive Technology for Problems Associated with Aging

- Telephones with amplifiers, large-print numbers, one-touch dialing and memory features; cordless, cellular, or digital phones; external speakers
- "Smart" technologies such as sensors in automobiles to facilitate parking; door answering systems; and sensors in the home to detect motion, falls, and intrusions
- Overhead track systems, stair glides, ramps, elevators, and other devices to assist with mobility
- Screen magnification, print enhancements, and voice synthesizers for computer-screen reading
- Assistive listening devices, telecommunication devices (TDDs) or computer software; closed captioning for television; and devices to convert auditory output to flashing lights for smoke detectors, telephones, and doorbells
- Life call systems that provide a link with emergency services
- Advances in technology for mobility, such as wheelchair seating systems, power carts, wheeled walkers with wheel locks and built-in seating systems, and adaptive controls for cars.

Sources for Specific Devices

AbleData
http://www.abledata.com/abledata.cfm?pageid=19327&
    ksectionid=19327

RESNA Directories and Databases
http://www.resna.org/resources/at_and_re_info.dot

Assistive Technology Disability Resources
http://www.disabilityresources.org/AT.html

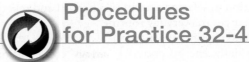

Procedures for Practice 32-4

Promoting Activity Choice for Intervention with Elders

- Link older adults with activities that express important personal meanings, especially connectedness with others, spirituality, service to others, and self-expression (Bonder, 2009b).
- Recognize individual variability in selection of activities that express personal meanings.
- Find out what specific self-care activities are perceived as vital to elders who are concerned about remaining in their homes.
- Employ reminiscence as a means to establish and maintain connections with others.
- Use activity inventories to stimulate an older client to think about what he or she values.
- Adapt the activity or help the client identify an activity that meets similar needs when preferred activities become too difficult for a client. Ascertain what component of the activity is meaningful.

Maintaining Wellness

The wellness movement (Gallup, 1999) is based on the principle of maximizing health and performance. Activities focused on stress management, exercise, nutrition, driving training, and safety are associated with this model (Bonder, 2009a). Wellness programs tailored for older adults focus on seven dimensions: physical, social, emotional, spiritual, professional/vocational, cognitive/intellectual, and environmental (International Council on Active Aging, n.d.).

Lifestyle Redesign

Lifestyle redesign is an approach that focuses on "health through occupation" (Clark et al., 1997). Participants are encouraged to recognize that meaningful occupation is important to both health and satisfaction. Small healthy lifestyle changes coupled with engagement in meaningful activities are critical to healthy aging (Clark et al., 1997; Waite, 2011). This model program consisted of weekly 2-hour small group sessions led by a licensed occupational therapist. Some examples of session modules include

- identification and implementation of feasible and sustainable activity-relevant changes
- development of plans to overcome mundane obstacles to enacting activity-relevant changes (e.g, bodily aches or transportation limitations)

There are limits to the application of technology with older clients. Some clients may resist learning to use the new technologies. Devices can break down and may be expensive to repair. Acquiring the devices may be expensive and not covered by insurance. Sometimes, a new and better device appears on the market as soon as a client has purchased an expensive piece of equipment. Many older adults, however, enjoy technological devices and gain considerable independence with them (Mann & Hicks, 2009).

Modification and Substitution of Activity

Activity analysis, a cornerstone of occupational therapy, can be particularly helpful in assisting older clients. The process involves matching present skills, interests, and motivation with activities that are stimulating, challenging, enjoyable, goal-directed, and purposeful. Some specific suggestions are presented in Procedures for Practice 32-4.

- participation in selected activities; rehearsal and repetition of changes to everyday routine
- time use and energy conservation
- assessing daily energy patterns; energy conservation and joint protection; adapting activities and daily routines
- home and community safety

Studies of this approach have established evidence that preventive and wellness care for older people must be a key element in health care provision (Clark et al., 1997, 2003, 2011). Interventions in the lifestyle redesign program were found to be cost effective and to improve vitality, social function, mental health, and overall life satisfaction. There was a decrease in body pain and depression in the program participants.

Cognitive Exercises

An emerging strategy for prevention of dementia is cognitive exercise (Clare et al., 2003). This is an intervention using structured practice on standardized tasks intended to maintain cognitive ability (primary prevention) or minimize cognitive loss (secondary prevention). The outcomes of CE have been studied through both correlational and experimental strategies (Hogan, 2005). Both approaches have limitations, and a recent review of the literature (Gates & Valenzuela, 2010) found that it is difficult to be certain about the impact of the intervention because of the wide variability in approaches to studying outcomes. Nevertheless, a significant body of research suggests that such CE may well be beneficial not only for preventing dementia but also for minimizing dysfunction (Gates & Valenzuela, 2010). CE has no identified risks, and there is evidence that participation in activities of any kind can enhance well-being (Kaminsky, 2010).

In prevention programs, occupational therapists work with other health care providers to maximize the individual's physical and functional well-being. The occupational therapist may emphasize socialization and physical fitness, modification of the environment to reduce the possibility of accidents, and identification of roles and activities that are satisfying to the individual.

Falls

One particularly important issue with regard to prevention is falls. As described above, falls are common and cause injuries associated with high mortality rates, making falls a serious concern for older adults. In addition, because they are aware of the potential for falls, many older adults have considerable fear of falling (Lach, 2005). Some older adults curtail their activities because of this fear; their accomplishment of desired occupations suffers even in the absence of a physical injury.

Falls are multifactorial in nature. Among the contributing factors are changes in sensation necessary to avoid falls (Tideiksaar, 2009), changes in musculoskeletal and vestibular function that compromise balance and gait (Nitz & Choy, 2004; Waddington & Adams, 2004), and environmental hazards such as wet or uneven surfaces (Tideiksaar, 2009). Risk factors include a previous fall, mobility limitations, polypharmacy, dizziness or orthostasis, and confusion or cognitive impairment. The risk of falling also increases as the number of risk factors increase (Tinetti & Kumar, 2010).

Recent outcomes research is mixed in reporting the most effective interventions for fall reductions. Home modifications, vitamin D, and Tai Chi were found to be cost effective in one study (Frick et al., 2010). A systematic review reported physical therapy, home modifications, and vitamin D to reduce falls with a more limited effect found for comprehensive management programs (Michael et al., 2010). Other studies show incorporation of exercise and strategies to improve balance during ADL to be effective in reducing falls (Clemson et al., 2010; Pai et al., 2010).

In conclusion, intervention with older adults requires understanding of the normal developmental processes that affect performance as well as the special life circumstances of older adults. To be most effective, intervention must address all spheres of function. The special factors that alter intervention with older adults must be taken into account. New model programs should be developed to address individual needs of communities and older adults (Kaminsky, 2010). With older adults, the goal of good quality of life as measured by engagement in satisfying activities is within reach for many elders. Thoughtful intervention by occupational therapists can ensure it.

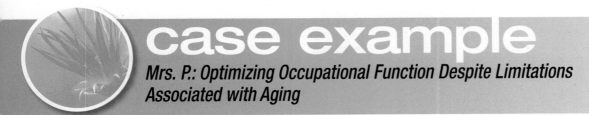

case example

Mrs. P.: Optimizing Occupational Function Despite Limitations Associated with Aging

Occupational Therapy Intervention Process	Clinical Reasoning Process	
	Objectives	Examples of Therapist's Internal Dialogue

Patient Information

Mrs. P. is a 73-year-old woman who lives alone in a ranch-style house in a small town. Her grown daughter visits about four times a year, and her son visits once a year. Mrs. P. was divorced 12 years ago and never remarried. Mrs. P. worked as a nurse for more than 20 years at a large university hospital. Now she works 2 days a week at a nursing home three blocks from her house, where she reviews charts for quality assurance. Mrs. P. has always enjoyed work and feels that the staff are close friends. Other than her income from the job, Mrs. P.'s only source of funds is Social Security.

Throughout her adult life, Mrs. P. has been in a sorority consisting of about a dozen women who have been friends since they were young women. They live nearby. For many years, she was a member of a women's group that raised funds for the ballet in the nearby city. When she is at home, Mrs. P. enjoys working on a dollhouse that she built.

Mrs. P. has a long history of health problems. She survived breast cancer when she was in her 40s, and 3 years ago she had surgery to remove a cancerous tumor from her colon. She has high blood pressure, controlled with medication. She also has a significant hearing loss that is gradually worsening.

Appreciate the context

"Mrs. P. strikes me as a very independent woman—someone who is used to calling the shots. I will want to be very careful to respect that in her throughout this process."

"Clearly, Mrs. P. has a strong social network. It impresses me that she has maintained strong connections with both her friends from work and her sorority sisters. I wonder if she would consider allowing these lifelong friends to help her out now."

Reason for Referral to Occupational Therapy

Recently, Mrs. P.'s sorority sisters noted changes in her social behavior (missing meetings, not answering her phone, refusing social invitations) and contacted her son with their concerns. He urged his mother to make an appointment with her family physician, her primary care provider for the past 30 years. During the visit, the physician discovered that her high blood pressure has worsened, as has her hearing. She also reported being very tired and having difficulty managing around the house. The physician ordered a series of medical tests and asked a home health agency to send an occupational therapist to evaluate the home and Mrs. P.'s function. He assured her that her son agreed to pay for this evaluation.

"It's important for me to get a sense of how Mrs. P. is functioning in her own environment, and I am pleased that a home visit was ordered. She will likely be most comfortable here and I'll be able to get a clearer sense of what the barriers are to her occupational functioning."

Results of Occupational Therapy Assessment

Mrs. P. agreed to a home visit by the occupational therapist. The therapist decided to evaluate Mrs. P.'s home and her performance of basic self-care and instrumental activities of daily living. The therapist used the Check It Out Check-List (Pynoos & Cohen, 1990), the Interest Checklist, and the Self Assessment of Occupational Functioning. She also asked Mrs. P. to give her a tour of the house and to describe problems encountered in daily tasks.

"I decided to use these instruments because they will help identify areas of occupation that are most important to Mrs. P. as we collaborate to develop an intervention plan, and they apply a theoretical model of practice (the Model of Human Occupation)."

	Develop intervention hypotheses	"I have a number of core hypotheses as I approach this consultation:
		1. Return to work is feasible and valued by employer and client
		2. Consultation with physical therapy, physician, audiology, and social work is feasible.
		3. Client's reasons for social withdrawal need further assessment.
		4. Client continues to have interests in current occupations.
		5. Client may be interested in alternative occupations to replace current work and leisure activities if these are not feasible."
	Select an intervention approach	"Consultative, adaptive, collaborative, client-centered, and rehabilitative approaches could all possibly be implemented."
	Reflect on competence	"I have knowledge and skills that I believe can help Mrs. P. Occupational therapy has strengths in energy conservation, adaptation of work and home for safety, meaningful occupations, and social skills. Physical therapy, audiology, physician, and social work could provide assistance with hearing, hypertension, financial, and social problems."

Recommendations

1. Develop an intervention plan in consultation with client, family, employer, and sorority sisters if appropriate.
2. Recommend consultation with physical therapy, social work, physician, and audiology.
3. Prioritize goals with interventions that are financially and functionally feasible in consultation with all stakeholders.

	Consider the patient's appraisal of performance	"Mrs. P. seems to want help to improve her functioning, but I do feel that I am somewhat limited as to how much I can do for her in just one session. I will want to make sure that I am addressing her priorities, and if she is interested, I am willing to work with her to explore availability of alternative resources to fund care."
	Consider what will occur in therapy, how often, and for how long	"I find myself wondering about whether or not other stakeholders are invested in the client over the long term. What are they willing and able to provide in support?"
	Ascertain the patient's endorsement of plan	

Problem List and Solutions

The therapist and Mrs. P. discussed these concerns and worked jointly toward identifying potential solutions. Because the therapist was asked to do an evaluation, not to provide long-term intervention, she must provide Mrs. P. with sufficient information to address her concerns.

Home safety
Mrs. P. acknowledged that the house was cluttered with old papers, knickknacks, and clothes. She was reluctant to throw anything away but agreed to have her daughter store some of the items for her. Mrs. P. also indicated that she had no funds to replace the worn carpet, although both agreed that worn spots and loose edges contribute to falls. She and the therapist identified several possible sources of funds and discussed the possibility of taking the carpet up entirely.

	Assess the patient's comprehension	"Mrs. P. was very forthright about her concerns and could readily agree with some of my observations about the potential safety hazards related to all of her clutter. I can't tell whether her reluctance to get rid of things reflected difficulty with decision making or perhaps, her overall fatigue and deconditioning."
	Understand what she is doing	"Mrs. P. is remarkably insightful. She realizes that falling at home or at work could have serious health consequences, but she may be self-limiting her activities more than is necessary. She seemed very receptive to my suggestions regarding how she could safely increase her activity level."

Physical deconditioning

Mrs. P. indicated that she had much less energy than she used to, quickly becoming short of breath when walking around the house. She agreed to begin a gradual plan of physical activity, starting with a stroll around the block each day.

Social isolation

Mrs. P.'s hearing loss was quite noticeable. The therapist encouraged her to see an audiologist to have her hearing evaluated. Mrs. P. expressed concern about paying for a hearing aid but agreed to ask her son for help.

Mrs. P. indicated that her friends were all in poor health and "no fun" anymore. She also said she was worried about falling at work. She was unwilling to discuss any alternatives for maintaining ties with her friends but agreed that she could discuss her concerns about work with her supervisor.

Next Steps

1. Client will consult with physician to address hypertension and fatigue.
2. Client will consult with physical therapy to address lack of endurance.
3. Client will consult with audiologist to address hearing loss.
4. Client will return to work.
5. Client will employ methods of energy conservation to work, self-care, and home maintenance tasks and will report ability to complete these tasks with fewer incidence and severity of fatigue symptoms.
6. Client will address safety hazards in the home such as clutter and unsafe flooring by removing these dangerous barriers.
7. Client will engage in activities with sorority sisters twice a week.

Mrs. P. and her occupational therapist developed a time line for Mrs. P. to call her doctor, her daughter, her son, and her boss, and Mrs. P. and her therapist agree that the therapist will make a follow-up call to check on her progress in 2 weeks. On follow-up, the therapist learned that Mrs. P. had accomplished a great deal. Mrs. P.'s physician determined that she had pernicious anemia and instituted monthly injections of vitamin B_{12}. Mrs. P. reported that she already felt more energetic.

Mrs. P. was now walking around her yard twice a day. Her daughter came to visit and helped her organize the house. Her son sent a check for a new hearing aid. Mrs. P. had not yet talked with her boss and was worried about doing it. She and the therapist practiced the conversation to provide Mrs. P. with a strategy. A week later, Mrs. P. called the therapist to tell her she was back at work.

Analysis of Reasoning

The therapist's initial task was to gather the information needed to clearly identify the problem. As the therapist secured information, it became evident that both Mrs. P. and her family needed to be consulted. Goals were identified based on their input. In this case, the occupational therapist provided an assessment and recommendations but left implementation of the plan to this capable client and family.

Anticipate present and future patient concerns	"I wonder if the employer is satisfied with Mrs. P.'s work performance. Is Mrs. P. enjoying her work?"

Anticipate present and future patient concerns

Analyze patient's comprehension

Decide whether he or she should continue or discontinue therapy and/or return in the future

"I wonder if the employer is satisfied with Mrs. P.'s work performance. Is Mrs. P. enjoying her work?"

"I should ask Mrs. P. about her interactions with the sorority sisters and her family. Are there more frequent interactions? What is the quality of those interactions?"

"Is Mrs. P. falling at home or at work and how frequently? How could I best evaluate for this? How about incidence of shortness of breath? I should consider these factors before deciding to discontinue intervention. Is the client able to manage daily activities, including work, without a worsening of hypertension or fatigue?"

"If I am only able to intervene for one session, how could I most effectively address these complex issues using consultation, advocacy, and ethical/professional behavior? Can communication with the physician, the family, and other professionals involved address this concern adequately?"

Clinical Reasoning in Occupational Therapy Practice

Intervention to Prevent Performance Decrements

If clutter in Mrs. P.'s home is not reduced despite recommendations by the therapist to make this a top priority, what are some next steps that the therapist might consider to address this problem?

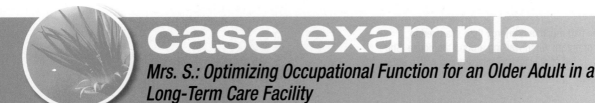

case example

Mrs. S.: Optimizing Occupational Function for an Older Adult in a Long-Term Care Facility

Occupational Therapy Intervention Process	Clinical Reasoning Process	
	Objectives	**Examples of Therapist's Internal Dialogue**

Patient Information

Mrs. S., an 80-year-old nursing home resident, has five children. Four of them live within 50 miles. Mrs. S. worked as the personal secretary for the provost of a small college for 20 years. She had a variety of interests, including reading, cooking, baking, participating in church and local theater, and gardening.

Mrs. S. faced a number of challenges in her life, including the early death of her father, the Great Depression, her husband's absence for 3 years of service in World War II, raising a child with schizophrenia, the early and sudden death of her husband (she was 51 years old when he died), and adjusting to a move from her home to an apartment and now to a nursing home.

Mrs. S.'s medical history is fairly typical for a person her age. She developed osteoarthritis in both knees, resulting in several arthroscopic surgeries and two total knee replacements. She was hospitalized for a brief bout of depression secondary to menopause. She has both near and far vision loss that are well corrected with eyeglasses. She has severe hearing loss in both ears that is partially corrected with hearing aids.

She also had a series of strokes that began when she was 70 years old. The strokes left her with mild spasticity, about 50% of proximal upper extremity active range of motion, and only a mass grasp in her left hand. She had full use of lower extremities except for a loss of about 15° of right active knee flexion and mild spasticity and weakness in the left lower extremity. She lost approximately 25% of the visual field on the left side to hemianopsia but can accommodate for this by turning her head. Mrs. S. also had mild dysarthria and dysphagia. She dribbled urine because of changes in bladder function and weak sphincter musculature. She wore a small protective pad and took medication to control this. She was hospitalized a year ago for an attempted suicide and major depression as a result of the breaking of her knee replacement and difficulty adjusting to the idea of another major surgery. She received psychiatric services and a long rehabilitation stay after she agreed to have the knee replacement. Her recovery from the knee replacement was very good except for her complaint of chronic pain in the knee that has not responded to medication.

Prior to the failure of her first knee replacement, she was totally independent in all basic activities of daily living (ADL). After her knee replacement and rehabilitation stay, a trial in her assisted living facility became problematic because of her declining ability to walk and transfer to the bathroom and her inability to do her own personal care. She and her family decided that Mrs. S. should be admitted to a nursing home, where she would receive closer supervision and assistance for her personal care.

Appreciate the context

"I should focus on past and current occupations and performance in areas of occupation. I want to take note of the current status of body functions and structures and how these may influence performance in the areas of occupation. It is important that I identify performance patterns, habits, and routines and try to make sense of all that relative to the cultural, spiritual, physical, social, personal, temporal, and virtual contexts of Mrs. S.'s past and current environment. For example, I wonder if possible changes in these factors have influenced her occupations, and what areas of occupation may be compromised by these changes?"

Reason for Referral to Occupational Therapy

Nursing home staff was concerned about Mrs. S.'s safety and social withdrawal. Mrs. S. was still using a wheeled walker but found placing her left hand on the walker handle difficult. She was able to move from her bed to the bathroom independently but had several recent falls. She dressed independently if her clothes were placed on a chair beside her bed. However, she displayed poor judgment in activities such as bending too far over the edge of the bed and dangerously reaching for things she dropped on the floor. She also tripped over things while walking. She used a wheelchair on outings with her family and with the activities program at the nursing home. Mrs. S. rarely smiles, and nursing staff reports difficulty getting her to participate in group activities or outings, even though she was physically able to do so. Her family was supportive. Her oldest daughter had power of attorney and durable medical power of attorney. Mrs. S. paid privately for nursing home care and had funds remaining to cover about 2 more months of care. She was willing to pay privately for brief occupational therapy (OT) intervention.

Results of Occupational Therapy Assessment

After reviewing the medical records, the occupational therapist evaluated Mrs. S.'s life roles, tasks, activities, skills, abilities, and developed capacities. Mrs. S. was interviewed along with her oldest daughter and primary nurse. Some of the critical questions raised during the interviews:

- What safety issues are you most concerned about?
- What is your level of satisfaction with life right now? What do you think could be done to improve it?
- What things do you like to do right now? What things irritate you?
- If you could change five things around here to make things better for yourself, what would you change?
- What worries you most? What makes you happiest?
- Do you have any goals to improve yourself, your environment, or your living situation?

"Are there standardized or nonstandardized assessments that could be used to address the above issues?"

Develop intervention hypotheses	"I have a number of core hypotheses as I approach intervention planning:
	1. The client is motivated to improve.
	2. The caregivers are motivated to collaborate on the established goals.
	3. The family is supportive and motivated to assist in achieving the goals.
	4. Direct intervention as well as consultation and collaboration are necessary to achieve the goals.
	5. The client has the potential to achieve the goals.
	6. The other stakeholders have the resources to collaborate in accomplishing the agreed upon goals.
	7. It is financially possible to consult other professionals such as physical therapy, urology, orthopedic surgery, pain management specialist, audiology, social work."
Select an intervention approach	"Rehabilitative, client-centered, consultative, adaptive, and collaborative therapy approaches may all apply to this client."
Reflect on competence	"Skills from other professionals will be needed to address many of the issues. Occupational therapy has strengths in the areas of safety, urinary incontinence, meaningful occupations, functional mobility, ADL, and psychosocial issues.

Recommendations

1. Interview client, family, caregivers, and nursing home staff to identify problems that are of highest priority for each stakeholder.
2. Further assess safety and performance of ADL.
3. Recommend consultation with physical therapy, social work, audiology, psychiatry, and urology.
4. Develop plan of care in consultation with all stakeholders.

Consider the patient's appraisal of performance

Consider what will occur in therapy, how often, and for how long

Ascertain the patient's endorsement of plan

"I need to address issues that are most important to the client, the family, and the caregivers. I wonder if there is consensus among all stakeholders about these issues and their relative importance. I will need to consider what can be done in the way of consultation, direct occupational therapy intervention, and collaboration with others considering the client's strengths and weaknesses, the motivation of all stakeholders, and the context. Who will be responsible for goal achievement using which model of team intervention?"

Summary of Short-Term Goals and Progress

The interviews and evaluation revealed the following problems:

- Mrs. S. tends to get upset and take things into her own hands when she has to wait for assistance. This results in unsafe or dangerous behavior and activities.
- Mrs. S. gets depressed and does not feel like socializing with others, especially residents with problems similar to hers or worse.
- Mrs. S. needs some meaningful activities to replace the wide variety of activities that formerly gave her pleasure.
- Mrs. S. needs some modifications to her environment to increase safety and orientation to reality and current events.
- Mrs. S. is easily embarrassed and has difficulty asking for personal assistance, especially with urination and personal hygiene.
- Mrs. S. would like more interaction and visits from her family.

Assess the patient's comprehension

Understand what she is doing

Compare actual to expected performance

Know the person

"How can I and the team best monitor falls, frequency of urinary incontinence, quality and quantity of participation in mandatory or optional leisure activities, and list of positive and negative feelings?"

"What can be done to assess motivation of client, staff, and family in monitoring follow-through with recommendations, and do I need to adjust instructions and goals depending on progress or lack of progress achieved?"

"I should consider standardized assessments of depression, occupational function, cognition/judgment, and ADL function."

Occupational Therapy Goals

The following goals were agreed upon by Mrs. S., her family, and the nursing staff:

1. Mrs. S. will request and wait for assistance or supervision for trips to the bathroom or will use a female urinal at bedside.
2. Mrs. S. will call for assistance should she drop any item on the floor that is not within easy reach of her long-handled reacher. Otherwise, she will continue to dress herself independently with setup at bed or chair level.
3. Mrs. S. will attend at least two outings per week with family or with the nursing home activities program. She will provide constructive criticism to the staff as to how the activity could be improved.
4. Mrs. S. will learn to propel her wheelchair so that she can safely navigate throughout the building without falling. She will be supervised for walks to the bathroom or in the hall.
5. Mrs. S. will choose and successfully complete three leisure activities within a month using adaptive equipment or techniques recommended by the occupational therapist.
6. Mrs. S. will complete a list of things that she is unhappy with as well as a list of things she is grateful for and review them with her daughter at least once a week to encourage her to express her feelings appropriately.

Next Steps

The occupational therapist decided to see Mrs. S. once or twice a week for a month to achieve these goals. Mrs. S. agreed to pay for the therapy because she did not qualify for skilled services under Medicare regulations.

Direct intervention

1. Instruction in safety for mobility within her room.
2. Adjustment of call signal button and chairs and removal of throw rugs and other barriers to safe mobility in the room.
3. Provision of long-handled reachers and instruction in use of them.
4. A session to assess safety issues during dressing and hygiene activities.
5. Suggestions for adaptive equipment for playing cards, reading, and plant care.
6. A daily calendar and structured time to read the paper or watch the news on television for current events.
7. A meeting with Mrs. S. and her family at the end of the month to review progress on goals and to make decisions about continuance of therapy or discharge.

The occupational therapist suggested referrals to physical therapy for a program to maintain or enhance mobility and physical conditioning, speech pathology to review issues related to dysphagia and dysarthria, and social work to help Mrs. S. and her family apply for Medicaid or other support, because financial concerns were becoming an issue. The therapist consulted the nursing and activities staff and provided written copies of suggestions for the staff to facilitate accomplishment of the therapy goals. Suggestions were also made to Mrs. S. and her family to explore a visit to a chronic pain specialist for the knee pain and to a urologist for follow-up on bladder control issues.

Anticipate present and future patient concerns

Analyze patient's comprehension

Decide whether he or she should continue or discontinue therapy and/or return in the future

"Are the goals being met? Why or why not? Did the other consultants contribute to the interventions and what were the outcomes? How are the client, caregivers, and family responding? What barriers could be further addressed to more effectively address the problems and goals? Is additional support needed to ensure safety? Has the client reached maximum potential to achieve the goals based on progress notes and consultation with all stakeholders? What progress can be documented? Do all stakeholders agree that further therapy would be beneficial in reaching particular goals? Which particular goals?"

Clinical Reasoning in Occupational Therapy Practice

Intervention Despite Age-Related Deterioration

1. Therapy for Mrs. S. focused on ADL and safety. It was clear that she also needed to find activities that were meaningful to her. The therapist was able to make some suggestions. What else might have been helpful in addressing this aspect of Mrs. S.'s occupational performance?

2. What additional strategies might be employed to ensure that Mrs. S. remembers the safety precautions she has been taught?

Summary Review Questions

1. In a well elderly individual, what are the most typical changes in sensation? How can they affect function?

2. How do normal neuromuscular changes that accompany aging affect mobility? How can these changes ultimately affect occupational function?

3. What are some key differences in the cognitive complaints of adults with age-associated memory impairment versus AD? Describe ways the therapeutic response to these complaints may differ.

4. In general, what adjustments do older adults face in transitioning to retirement?

5. What is the first step an occupational therapist should take in assessing the status of an older individual?
6. What factors are important in selecting substitute activities for an older adult?
7. In deciding about technological interventions, what factors must be considered to ensure acceptance of the device?
8. What factors complicate intervention with an older adult who falls ill or is injured?
9. What are some myths about sexuality and older adults?
10. What evidence exists to support interventions for incontinence, fall prevention, and wellness/lifestyle redesign?

Glossary

Aging in place—Remaining in the home and community in which one has lived as a younger adult.

Catastrophic reaction—Emotional outburst characteristic of the middle stage of Alzheimer's disease, often as a consequence of excessive and confusing environmental stimuli.

Crystallized intelligence—Ability to use stored or previously learned information.

Dementia—Symptom caused by a number of conditions and characterized by loss of memory, language functions, ability to think abstractly, and ability to care for oneself.

Fluid intelligence—Ability to use new information.

Presbycusis—Age-related sensorineural hearing loss, especially for high-frequency sounds.

Practical memory—Ability to remember routines, schedules, important phone numbers, appointments, or other practical information needed to carry out every day activities.

Presbyopia—Age-related vision change caused by loss of flexibility of the lens, which leads to poor near vision.

References

Administration on Aging. (2011). A profile of older americans 2010. Retrieved August 10, 2011 from http://www.aoa.gov/AoARoot/Aging_Statistics/Profile/2010/4.aspx.

Administration on Aging. (2013). Aging statistics. Retrieved August 10, 2011 from http://www.aoa.gov/AoARoot/Aging_Statistics/index.5aspx.

Ai, A. L., Rollman, B. L., & Berger, C. S. (2010). Comorbid mental health symptoms and heart diseases: Can health care and mental health care professionals collaboratively improve the assessment and management? *Health & Social Work, 35,* 27–38.

American Occupational Therapy Association. (2008). Occupational Therapy Practice Framework: Domain and process (2nd ed.). *American Journal of Occupational Therapy, 62,* 625–683.

American Optometric Association. (n.d.). Presbyopia. Retrieved August 10, 2011 from http://www.aoa.org/x4697.xml.

American Psychiatric Association. (2000). *Diagnostic and Statistical Manual of Mental Disorders* (4th ed.). Washington, DC: Author.

Anetzberger, G. (2009). Elder abuse. In B. R. Bonder & V. Dal Bello-Haas (Eds.), *Functional performance in older adults* (3rd ed., pp. 609–632). Philadelphia: F.A. Davis.

Anstey, K. J., & Low, L. (2004). Normal cognitive changes in aging. *Australian Family Physician, 33,* 783–787.

Arnadottir, G. (1990). *The brain and behavior: Assessing cortical dysfunction through activities of daily living.* St. Louis: Mosby.

Atchley, R. C. (1989). Continuity theory of normal aging. *Gerontologist, 29,* 183–190.

Baltes, P. B., & Baltes, M. M. (1990). Psychological perspectives on successful aging: The theory of selective optimization with compensation. In P. B. Baltes & M. M. Baltes (Eds.), *Successful aging: Perspectives from the behavioral sciences* (pp. 1–35). Cambridge, UK: University of Cambridge Press.

Bambrick, P., & Bonder, B. (2005). Older adults' perception of work. *Work: A Journal of Prevention, Assessment, and Rehabilitation, 24,* 77–84.

Baum, C., & Edwards, C. (n.d.). Activity Card Sort (2nd ed.). Retrieved from http://myaota.aota.org/shop_aota/prodview.aspx?TYPE=D&PID=763&SKU=1247.

Bengston, V. L., & Bonder, B. (2009). Theories of aging: A multidisciplinary review for occupational and physical therapists. In B. R. Bonder & V. Dal Bello-Haas (Eds.), *Functional performance in older adults* (3rd ed., pp. 28–44). Philadelphia: F. A. Davis.

Bengston, V. L., Burgess, E. O., & Parrott, T. M. (1997). Theory, explanation, and a third generation of theoretical development in social gerontology. *Journal of Gerontology, Social Sciences, 52b,* 572–588.

Blanchard-Fields, F., Mienaltowski A., & Seay RB. (2007). Age differences in everyday problem solving effectiveness: Older adults select more effective strategies for interpersonal problems. *Journals of Gerontology Series B: Psychological Sciences & Social Sciences, 2007, 62B,* 61–64.

Bonder, B. R. (2009a). Interactions and relationships. In B. R. Bonder & V. Dal Bello-Haas (Eds.), *Functional performance in older adults* (3rd ed., pp. 386–408). Philadelphia: F.A. Davis.

Bonder, B. R. (2009b). Meaningful occupation in later life. In B. R. Bonder & V. Dal Bello-Haas (Eds.), *Functional performance in older adults* (3rd ed., pp. 45–62). Philadelphia: F.A. Davis

Bottomly, J. M., & Lewis, C. B. (2007). *Geriatric rehabilitation: A clinical approach* (3rd ed.). Upper Saddle River, NJ: Prentice Hall.

Brennan, M., & Bally, S. J. (2007). Psychosocial adaptations to dual sensory loss in middle and late adulthood. *Trends in Amplification, 11,* 281–300.

Bundy, A., & Clemson, L. (2009). Leisure. In B. R. Bonder & V. Dal Bello-Haas (Eds.). *Functional performance in older adults* (3rd ed., pp. 290–310). Philadelphia: F.A. Davis.

Canadian Association of Occupational Therapists. (2002). *Enabling occupation: An occupational therapy perspective* (Rev. ed.). Ottawa, Canada: Author.

Cappeliez, P., O'Rourke, N., & Chaudhury, H. (2005). Functions of reminiscence and mental health in later life. *Aging & Mental Health, 9,* 295–301.

Caprio, T. V., & Williams, T. F. (2007). Comprehensive geriatric assessment. In E. H. Duthie, P. R. Katz, & M. L. Malone (Eds.), *Practice of Geriatrics* (4th ed.). Philadelphia: Saunders Elsevier. Retrieved August 10, 2011 from http://www.mdconsult.com/books/page.do?eid=4-u1.0-B978-1-4160-2261-9..50007-0&isbn=978-1-4160-2261-9&sid=1198639207&uniqId=277039270-571#4-u1.0-B978-1-4160-2261-9.50007-0.

Centers for Medicare and Medicaid Services. (n.d.[a]). MDS 3.0 for nursing homes. Retrieved August 10, 2011 from https://www.cms.gov/nursinghome qualityinits/25_nhqimds30.asp.

Centers for Medicare and Medicaid Services. (n.d.[b]). OASIS Overview. Retrieved August 10, 2011 from https://www.cms.gov/OASIS/01_Overview.asp.

Chappell, N. L. (2008). Aging and mental health. *Social Work in Mental Health, 7,* 133–138.

Chiu, T., & Oliver, R. (2006). Factor analysis and construct validity of the SAFER-HOME. *OTJR: Occupation, Participation, and Health, 26,* 132–142.

Christiansen, C., & Baum, C. (1997). Person-environment occupational performance: A conceptual model for practice. In C. Christiansen & C. Baum (Eds.), *Occupational therapy: Enabling function and well-being* (2nd ed.). Thorofare, NJ: Slack.

Christiansen, C., Haertl, K., & Robinson, L. (2009). Self care. In B. R. Bonder & V. Dal Bello-Haas (Eds.). *Functional performance in older adults* (3rd ed., pp. 267–289). Philadelphia: F.A. Davis.

Clare, L., Woods. R. T., Moniz Cook, E. D., Orrell, M., & Spector, A. (2003). Cognitive rehabilitation and cognitive training for early-stage Alzheimer's disease and vascular dementia. *Cochrane Database of Systematic Reviews,* (4), CD003260.

Clark, F., Azen, S. P., Zemke, R., Jackson, J., Carlson, M., Mandel, D., Hay, J., Josephson, K., Cherry, B., Hessel, C., Palmer, J., & Lipson, L. (1997). Occupational therapy for independent-living older adults: A randomized controlled trial. *Journal of the American Medical Association, 278,* 1321–1326.

Clark, F. A., Carlson, M., Jackson, J., & Mandel, D. (2003). Lifestyle redeisgn improves health and is cost-effective. *OT Practice, 8*(2) 9–13.

Clark, F., Jackson, J., Carlson, M., Chou, C. P., Cherry, B. J., Jordan-Marsh, M., Knight, B.G. Mandel, D., Blanchard, J., Granger, D.A., Wilcox, R.R., Lai, M. L., White, B., Hay, J. Lam, C., Marterella, A., & Azen, S. P. (2012). Effectiveness of a lifestyle intervention in promoting the well-being of independently living older people: Results of the Well Elderly 2 Randomised Controlled Trial. *Journal of Epidemiology and Community Health, 66*(9), 782–790.

Clemson, L., Fiatarone Singh, M., Bundy, A., Cumming, R. G., Weissel, E., Munroe, J., Manollaras, K., & Black, D. (2010). LiFE Pilot Study: A randomized trial of balance and strength training embedded in daily life activity to reduce falls in older adults. *Australian Journal of Occupational Therapy, 57,* 42–50.

Clemson, L., Mackenzie, L., Ballinger, C., Close, J. C. T., & Cumming, R. B. G. (2008). Environmental interventions to prevent falls in community-dwelling older people: A meta-analysis of randomized trials. *Journal of Aging and Health, 20,* 954–971.

Dal Bello-Haas, V. (2009). Neuromusculoskeletal and Movement Function. In B. R. Bonder & V. Dal Bello-Haas (Eds.), *Functional performance in older adults* (3rd ed., pp. 130–176). Philadelphia: F.A. Davis

Dean, E., & De Andrade, A. D. (2009). Cardiovascular and pulmonary function. In B. R. Bonder & V. Dal Bello-Haas (Eds.), *Functional performance in older adults* (3rd ed. pp. 65–100). Philadelphia: F.A. Davis.

Depp, C. A., & Jeste, D. V. (2006). Definitions and predictors of successful aging: A comprehensive review of larger quantitative studies. *American Journal of Geriatric Psychiatry, 14,* 6–20.

Dumoulin, C., Korner-Bitensky, N., & Tannenbaum, C. (2007). Urinary incontinence after stroke: Identification, assessment, and intervention. *Stroke, 38,* 2745–2751.

Ekelman, B., Stav, W., Baker, P., O'Dell-Rossi, P., & Mitchell, S. (2009). Community mobility. In B. R. Bonder & V. Dal Bello-Haas (Eds.), *Functional performance in older adults* (3rd ed., pp. 332–385). Philadelphia: F.A. Davis.

Federal Interagency Forum on Aging-Related Statistics. (2010). *Older Americans: Key indicators of well-being.* Retrieved August 10, 2011 from http://www.agingstats.gov/agingstatsdotnet/Main_Site/Data/2010_Documents/Docs/OA_2010.pdf.

Fisher, A. G. (1995). *The assessment of motor and process skills.* Fort Collins, CO: Third Star Press.

Erikson, E. (1963). *Childhood and society.* New York: Norton Publications.

Frick, K. D., Kung, J. Y., Parrish, J. M., & Narrett, M. J. (2010). Evaluating the cost-effectiveness of fall prevention programs that reduce fall-related hip fractures in older adults. *Journal of the American Geriatrics Society, 58,* 136–141.

Fulmer, T., Guadagno, L., Dyer, C. B., & Connolly, M. T. (2004). Progress in elder abuse screening and assessment instruments. *Journal of the American Geriatrics Society, 52,* 297–304.

Gallup, J. W. (1999). *Wellness centers: A guide for the design professional.* New York: Wiley.

Gates, N., & Valenzuela, M. (2010). Cognitive exercise and its role in cognitive function in older adults. *Current Psychiatry Report, 12,* 20–27.

Gauthier, A. H., & Smeeding, T. M. (2003). Time use in older ages: Cross cultural differences. *Research on Aging, 25,* 247–274.

Glantz, C., & Richman, N. (1991). *Occupational therapy: A vital link to implementation of OBRA.* Rockville, MD: American Occupational Therapy Association.

Glatt, S. J., Chayavichitsilp, P., Depp, C., Shork, N. J., & Jeste, D. V. (2007) Successful aging: From phenotype to genotype. *Biological Psychiatry, 62,* 282–293.

Graff, M. J. L., Adang, E. M. M.,Vernooij-Dassen, M. J. M., Dekker, J., Jönsson, L., Thijssen, M., Hoefnagels, W. H. L., & Rikkert, M. G. M. O. (2008). Community occupational therapy for older patients with dementia and their care givers: Cost effectiveness study. *British Medical Journal, 336,* 134.

Havighurst, R. J. (1963). Successful aging. In R. H. Williams, C. Tibbitts, & W. Donahue (Eds.), *Processes of aging* (Vol. 1, pp. 299–320). New York: Atherton.

Hayslip, B., & Kaminski, P. L. (2005). Grandparents raising their grandchildren: A review of the literature and suggestions for practice. *The Gerontologist, 45,* 262–269.

Hogan, M. (2005). Physical and cognitive activity and exercise for older adults: A review. International *Journal of Aging and Human Development, 60,* 95–126.

Hooper, C. R., & Dal Bello-Haas, V. (2009). Sensory function. In B. R. Bonder & V. Dal Bello-Haas (Eds.), *Functional performance in older adults* (3rd ed., pp. 101–129). Philadelphia: F.A. Davis.

Insurance Institute for Highway Safety. (2011). *Older drivers.* Retrieved August 10, 2011 from http://www.iihs.org/research/fatality.aspx?topicName=Older-people&year=2009.

International Council on Active Aging. (n.d.). Wellness programs. Retrieved August 10, 2011 from http://www.icaa.cc/activeaging andwellness/wellness.htm.

Jebsen, R., Taylor, N., Trieschmann, R., Trotter, M., & Howard, L. (1969). An objective and standardized test of hand function. *Archives of Physical Medicine and Rehabilitation, 50,* 311–319.

Kaminsky, T. (2010,). The role of occupational therapy in successful aging. *OT Practice, 15*(6), 11–14.

Lach, H. W. (2005). Incidence and risk factors for developing fear of falling in older adults. *Public Health Nursing, 22,* 45–52.

Lafata, M. J., & Helfrich, C. A. (2001). The occupational therapy elder abuse checklist. *Occupational Therapy in Mental Health, 16,* 141–161.

Law, M., Baptiste, S., Carswell, A., McColl, M. A., Polatajko, H., & Pollock, N. (2005). *Canadian Occupational Performance Measure* (4th ed.). Ottawa, Canada: Canadian Occupational Therapy Association.

Lent, R. W. (2004). Toward a unifying theoretical and practical perspective on well-being and psychosocial adjustment. *Journal of Counseling Psychology, 51,* 482–509.

Levinson, D. J. (1986). A conception of adult development. *American Psychologist, 49,* 3–13.

Lewis, S. C. (2003). *Elder care in occupational therapy* (2nd ed.). Thorofare, NJ: Slack.

Longino, C. F., & Kart, C. S. (1982). Explicating activity theory: A formal replication. *Journal of Gerontology, 37,* 713–722.

Mann, W. C., & Hicks, E. E. (2009). Products and technology. In B. R. Bonder & V. Dal Bello-Haas (Eds.). *Functional performance in older adults* (3rd ed., pp. 591–608). Philadelphia: F. A. Davis

Mast, B. T. (2010). Vascular depression: Cardiovascular implications for mental health. *Annual Review of Gerontology and Geriatrics, 30,* 135–154.

Mathiowetz, V., Volland, G., Kashman, N., & Weber K. (1985a). Adult norms for the Box and Block Test of manual dexterity. *American Journal of Occupational Therapy, 39,* 386–391.

Mathiowetz, V., Weber, K., Kashman, N., & Volland G. (1985b). Adult norms for the Nine Hole Peg Test of finger dexterity. *Occupational Therapy Journal of Research, 5,* 24–38.

McGarry, K., & Schoeni, R. F. (2005). Widow(er) poverty and out-of-pocket medical expenditures near the end of life. *Journal of Gerontology: Social Sciences, 60B,* S160–S168.

Meeks, T. W., Lanounette, N., Vahia, I., Dawes, S., Jeste, D. V., & Lebowitz, B. (2009). Psychiatric assessment and diagnosis in older adults. *Focus, 7,* 3–16.

Melville, L. L., & Nelson D. L. (n.d.). Melville/Nelson Evaluation System. Retrieved May 13, 2013 from http://www.utoledo.edu/eduhshs/depts/rehab_sciences/ot/melville.html.

Menec, V. H. (2003). The relation between everyday activities and successful aging: A 6-year longitudinal study. *Journal of Gerontology: Social Sciences, 58B,* S74–S82.

Michael, Y. L., Whitlock, E. P., Lin, J. S., Fu, R., O'Connor, E. A., & Gold, R. (2010). Primary care–relevant interventions to prevent falling in older adults: A systematic evidence review for the U.S. preventive services task force. *Annals of Internal Medicine, 153,* 515–525.

Miller, L. J., Myers, A., Prinzi, L., & Mittenberg, W. (2009). Changes in intellectual functioning associated with normal aging. *Archives of Clinical Neuropsychology, 24,* 681–688.

Miracle, A. W., & Miracle, T. S. (2009). Sexuality in late adulthood. In B. R. Bonder & V. Dal Bello-Haas (Eds.), *Functional performance in older adults* (3rd ed., pp. 409–426). Philadelphia: F.A. Davis.

Morrow-Howell, N., Hinterlong, J., Rozario, P. A., & Tang, F. (2003). Effects of volunteering on the well-being of older adults. *Journal of Gerontology: Social Sciences, 58B,* S137–S145.

Moyle, W., Clarke, C., Gracia, N., Reed, J., Cook, G., Klein, B., Marais, S., & Richardson, E. (2010). Older people maintaining mental health well-being through resilience: An appreciative inquiry study in four countries. *Journal of Nursing and Healthcare of Chronic Illness, 2,* 113–121.

Murphy, S. L. (2010). Geriatric research. *American Journal of Occupational Therapy, 64,* 172–181.

National Association for Continence. (2008). Urinary incontinence. Retrieved August 10, 2011 from http://www.nafc.org/index.php?page=facts-statistics.

National Library of Medicine. (2007). 8 Areas of Age-Related Change: 1. Brain: Memory and Alzheimer's disease (AD). Retrieved from http://www.nlm.nih.gov/medlineplus/magazine/issues/winter07/articles/winter07pg10-13.html.

Neugarten, B. L. (1975). *Middle age and aging.* Chicago: University of Chicago.

Nilsson, I., Bernspang, B., Fisher, A. G., Gustafson, Y., & Löfgren, G. (2007). Occupational engagement and life satisfaction in the oldest-old: The Umeå 85+ study. *OTJR: Occupation, Participation, and Health, 27,* 131–139.

Nitz, J. C., & Choy, N. L. (2004). The relationship between ankle dorsiflexion range, falls, and activity level in women aged 40–80 years. *New Zealand Journal of Physiotherapy, 32,* 121–125.

Pai, Y., Bhatt, T., Wang, E., Espy, D. D., &, Pavol, M. J. (2010). Inoculation against falls: Rapid adaptation by young and older adults to slips during daily activities. *Archives of Physical Medicine and Rehabilitation, 66,* 782–90.

Park, N. S. (2009). The relationship of social engagement to psychological well-being of older adults in assisted living facilities. *Journal of Applied Gerontology August, 28,* 461–481.

Pellerito, J. M. (2006). *Driver rehabilitation and community mobility.* St. Louis: Mosby.

Perski, T. (n.d.). Watching TV with low vision. Macular Degeneration International website. Retrieved August 10, 2011 from http://www.maculardegeneration.org/large/biglvarticle2.htm.

Petersen, R. C., Smith, G. E., Waring, S. C., Ivnik, R. J., Tangalos, E. G., & Kokmen, E. (1999). Mild cognitive impairment: Clinical characterization and outcome. *Archives of Neurology, 56,* 303–308.

Pruchno, R. A., Wilson-Genderson, M., Rose, M., & Cartwright, F. (2010). Successful aging: Early influences and contemporary characteristics. *Gerontologist, 50,* 821–833.

Pynoos, J., & Cohen, E. (1990). *Home safety guide for older people: Check it out, fix it up.* Washington, DC: Serif.

Rantz, M. J., Phillips, L., Aud, M., Popejoy, L., Marek, K. D., Hicks, L. L., Zaniletti, I., & Miller, S. J. (2011). Evaluation of aging in place model with home care services and registered nurse care coordination in senior housing. *Nursing Outlook, 59,* 37–46.

Riley, K. P. (2009). Mental function. In B. R. Bonder & V. Dal Bello-Haas (Eds.), *Functional performance in older adults* (3rd ed., pp. 177–182). Philadelphia: F.A. Davis.

Robins, R. W., & Trzesniewski, K. H. (2005). Self-esteem development across the lifespan. *Current Directions in Psychological Science, 14,* 158–162.

Robinson, J. G., & Molzahn, A. E. (2007). Sexuality and quality of life. *Journal of Gerontological Nursing, 33,* 19–27.

Rowe, J., & Kahn, R. (1998). *Successful aging: The MacArthur Foundation study.* New York: Pantheon.

Slagboom, P. E., Beekman, M., Passtoors, W. M., Deelen, J., Vaarhorst, A. M., Boer, E. B., . . . Westendorp, R. G. (2010). Genomics of human longevity. *Philosophical Transactions of the Royal Society of Biological Science, 366,* 35–42.

Sterns, H., Lax, G. A., & Chang, B. (2009). Work and retirement. In B. R. Bonder & V. Dal Bello-Haas (Eds.), *Functional performance in older adults* (3rd ed., pp. 311–331). Philadelphia: F.A. Davis.

Steultjens, E. M. J., Dekker, J., Bouter, L. M., Jellema, S., Bakker, E. B., & van den Ende, C. H. M. (2004). Occupational therapy for community dwelling elderly people: A systematic review. *Age and Ageing, 33,* 453–460.

Szanto, K., Gildengers, A., Mulsant, B. H., Brown, G., Alexopoulos, G. S., & Reynolds, C. F., III. (2002). Identification of suicidal ideation and prevention of suicidal behaviour in the elderly. *Drugs & Aging, 19,* 11–24.

Tideiksaar, R. (2009). Falls. In B. R. Bonder & V. Dal Bello-Haas (Eds.), *Functional performance of older adults* (3rd ed., pp. 193–214). Philadelphia: F.A. Davis.

Tinetti, M. E., & Kumar, C. (2010). The patient who falls: "It's always a trade-off." *Journal of the American Medical Association, 303,* 258–266.

Valentin, S. A., van Boxtel, M. P., van Hooren, S. A., Bosma, H., Beckers, H. J., Ponds, R. W., & Jolles, J. (2005). Change in sensory functioning predicts change in cognitive functioning: Results from a 6-year follow-up in the Maastricht aging study. *Journal of the American Geriatrics Society, 53,* 374–380.

Waddington, G. S., & Adams, R. D. (2004). The effect of a 5-week wobble-board exercise intervention on ability to discriminate different degrees of ankle inversion, barefoot and wearing shoes. A study in healthy elderly. *Journal of the American Geriatrics Society, 52,* 573–576.

Waite, A. (2011). Well Elderly 2 Study. *OT Practice, 16*(13), 8–10.

Wiatrowski, N. L., Riccio, L., & Scheer, J. (2008).Using evidence to inform practice for urinary incontinence. *Gerontology Special Interest Section Quarterly Newsletter, 31,* 2–4.

Wilkins, S., Law, M., & Letts, L. (2009). Evaluation of functional performance. In B. R. Bonder & V. Dal Bello-Haas (Eds.), *Functional performance in older adults* (3rd ed., pp. 429–448). Philadelphia: F.A. Davis.

Windsor, T. D. (2009). Persistence in goal striving and positive reappraisal as psychosocial resources for ageing well: A dyadic analysis. *Aging & Mental Health, 13,* 874–884.

Woodruff-Pak, D. S., & Papka, M. (1999). Theories of neuropsychology and aging. In V. L. Bengston & K. W. Schaie (Eds.), *Handbook of theories of aging* (pp. 113–132). New York: Springer

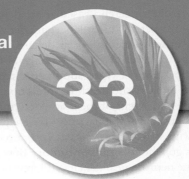

Stroke

Anne M. Woodson

Learning Objectives

After studying this chapter, the reader will be able to do the following:

1. Define stroke, or cerebrovascular accident, and briefly describe the causes, incidence, and impairments and disabilities that can result from stroke.
2. Describe the continuum of care for individuals recovering from stroke, including the interdisciplinary team, the various settings for care, and the phases of recovery and intervention.
3. Describe methods for evaluating areas of occupation, performance skills and client factors of patients recovering from stroke.
4. Suggest goals and methods for treatment to improve the occupational performance and performance skills and client factors of patients recovering from stroke.
5. Analyze the effectiveness of occupational therapy intervention in improving a patient's quality of life and adjustment to life with stroke.

S troke, or cerebrovascular accident (CVA), describes a variety of disorders characterized by the sudden onset of neurological deficits caused by vascular injury to the brain. Vascular damage in the brain disrupts blood flow, limits oxygen supply to surrounding cells, and leads to brain tissue death or infarction. The mechanism, location, and extent of the lesion determine the symptoms and prognosis for the patient. This chapter focuses on patients with stroke, but nonvascular brain trauma or disease, such as gunshot wounds or tumors, may manifest many of the same neurological deficits and may be treated similarly.

CAUSATION

Strokes are usually classified by the mechanism and location of the vascular damage. The two broad causes are ischemia and hemorrhage. Ischemic strokes result from a blockage of a cerebral vessel and can further be categorized as caused by thrombosis or embolism. Thrombosis is the stenosis or occlusion of a vessel, usually as a result of atherosclerosis. This occlusion is typically a gradual process, often with preceding warning signs, such as transient ischemic attack (TIA). An embolism is dislodged platelets, cholesterol, or other material that forms at another location, travels in the bloodstream, and blocks a cerebral vessel. Ischemic strokes are the most common type, accounting for about 87% of strokes (American Stroke Association, 2011).

Hemorrhagic strokes result from a rupture of a weakened cerebral blood vessel. In such strokes, blood accumulates outside of the vascular space and compresses surrounding brain tissue. Hemorrhagic strokes are either intracerebral (bleeding into the brain itself) or subarachnoid (bleeding into an area surrounding the brain). Aneurysms and arteriovenous malformations are the most common types of weakened blood vessels causing hemorrhagic strokes (American Stroke Association, 2011). Hemorrhagic strokes are less common (an estimated 13% of strokes), but they result in a higher mortality rate than ischemic strokes (Roger et al., 2011).

Location of Involvement

Most lesions are either anterior circulation strokes, which present signs and symptoms of hemispheric dysfunction, or posterior circulation strokes, which display signs and symptoms of brainstem involvement (Simon, Greenberg, & Aminoff, 2009). Another distinction related to location of CVA is whether the lesion results from large-vessel or small-vessel disease. Thrombosis occurs most often in the large cerebral blood vessels. Small-vessel, or lacunar, strokes are very small infarctions that occur only where small arterioles branch off the larger vessels (National Institutes of Health, 2011).

INCIDENCE

Stroke is the third leading cause of death in the United States and a leading cause of chronic disability among adults. Of the estimated 795,000 persons who have first or recurrent

CVAs in the United States each year, approximately two-thirds survive, bringing the number of stroke survivors in the U.S. population at any one time to over nine million (American Stroke Association, 2011). Stroke is the most common neurological diagnostic category among patients seen by occupational therapists (National Board for Certification in Occupational Therapy, 2008). The projected aging of the U.S. population is expected to raise the incidence of stroke, because about two-thirds of all strokes occur in those older than age 65 years (National Institutes of Health, 2011).

MEDICAL MANAGEMENT

Acute stroke care focuses on determining the cause and site of the stroke, preventing progression of the lesion, reducing cerebral edema, preventing secondary medical complications, and treating acute neurological symptoms (Bartels, 2011). Techniques of diagnostic imaging, including computed tomography (CT) and magnetic resonance imaging (MRI), can distinguish ischemic from hemorrhagic lesions and define their location, size, and vascular territory (National Institutes of Health, 2011).

In acute ischemic stroke, treatment concerns include restoration of blood flow and limitation of neuronal damage. Medications, including antithrombotics and thrombolytics, are the most common medical intervention for stroke (National Institutes of Health, 2011). Antithrombotics include antiplatelet drugs (such as aspirin) and anticoagulation drugs (such as heparin) and are used to prevent further clotting or thrombosis. After stroke, physicians mainly prescribe antithrombotics for prevention, because first time stroke survivors are at a high risk for recurrent strokes (National Institutes of Health, 2011). Thrombolytic drugs, such as tissue plasminogen activator (tPA), help reestablish blood flow to the brain by dissolving clots in cerebral vessels. A 5-year trial conducted by the National Institute of Neurological Disorders and Stroke found that appropriately selected subjects treated with tPA within 3 hours of onset of stroke symptoms were at least 33% more likely than patients given a placebo to recover from their stroke with little or no disability (National Stroke Association, 2011). The use of thrombolytics is limited, however, by the associated increased risk of hemorrhage and the fact that they must be administered within a 3-hour window after stroke onset for effectiveness. It is estimated that only 3%–5% of persons suffering a stroke will seek medical attention in time for possible tPA treatment (American Stroke Association, 2011). With hemorrhagic stroke, acute treatment includes control of intracranial pressure, prevention of rebleeding, maintenance of cerebral perfusion, and control of vasospasm. Surgery or endovascular procedures are often recommended to limit damage (National Stroke Association, 2011).

RECOVERY FROM STROKE

The specific abilities lost or affected by stroke and the degree and time course of recovery from stroke vary with the location, type, and extent of the initial injury, and treatment provided (National Stroke Association, 2011). Early initial improvement or spontaneous recovery occurs because pathologic processes in the brain resolve, and neurotransmission resumes near and remote from an infarct or hemorrhage (Dobkin, 2005). Later, ongoing improvement occurs with structural and functional reorganization within the brain, or neuroplasticity; the term neuroplasticity refers to transiently achieved functional changes in the context of learning and recovery, as well as structural changes on the cellular level. Neuroplasticity includes greater excitability and recruitment of intact neurons in both hemispheres of the brain as a response to stimulation, participation, training, and experience (Albert & Kesselring, 2011). Langton Hewer (1990) described a model of stroke recovery that includes both intrinsic neurological and compensatory adaptive recovery.

Intrinsic recovery refers to the remediation of neurological impairments, such as return of movement to a paralyzed limb. Adaptive recovery entails regaining the ability to perform meaningful activities, tasks, and roles without full restoration of neurological function, such as using the unaffected hand for dressing or walking with a cane or walker. Most patients gain some degree of both intrinsic (neurological) and adaptive (compensatory) recovery. Rehabilitation, including occupational therapy (OT), is designed to facilitate both processes to maximize an individual's function and participation after stroke.

Neurological Impairments and Recovery

Each survivor of a CVA has a unique combination of deficits determined by the location and severity of the lesion. Definition 33-1 lists the most commonly encountered

 Definition 33-1

Neurological Impairments Following Stroke

Neurological Deficit	Possible Effect on Occupational Function
Hemiplegia, hemiparesis	Impaired postural adaptation, bilateral integration
	Impaired mobility
	Decreased independence in any or all basic activities of daily living (BADL) and instrumental activities of daily living (IADL)
Hemianopsia, other visual deficits	Decreased awareness of environment, decreased ability to adapt to environment
	Impaired ability to read, write, navigate during mobility, recognize people and places, drive; can affect all BADL and IADL
Aphasia	Impaired speech and comprehension of verbal or written language; inability to communicate, read, or comprehend signs or directions
	Decreased social, community involvement; isolation
Dysarthria	Slurred speech, difficulty with oral motor functions such as eating, altered facial expressions
Somatosensory deficits	Increased risk of injury to insensitive areas
	Impairment of coordinated, dexterous movement
Incontinence	Loss of independence in toileting
	Increased risk of skin breakdown
	Decreased social, community involvement
Dysphagia	At risk for aspiration
	Impaired ability to eat or drink by mouth
Apraxia	Decreased independence in any motor activity (ADL, speech, mobility), decreased ability to learn new tasks or skills
Cognitive deficits	Decreased independence in BADL and IADL, decreased ability to learn new techniques, decreased social interactions
Depression	Decreased motivation, participation in activity; decreased social interaction

neurological impairments following stroke and describes the possible effects of each on occupational functioning. The most typical manifestation of CVA is hemiparesis or hemiplegia, ranging from mild weakness to complete paralysis on the side of the body opposite the site of the CVA. About 80% of people who have had a stroke have some degree of hemiparesis (National Stroke Association, 2011), although the rate of physical impairment usually decreases after the first 3–6 months poststroke (Roger et al., 2011).

Certain impairments are associated with lesions in a particular hemisphere. For example, left CVA may cause right hemiparesis, aphasia or other communication deficits, and/or apraxia or motor planning deficits. Right CVA may result in left hemiparesis, visual field deficits (VFDs) or spatial neglect, poor insight and judgment, and/or impulsive behavior (American Stroke Association, 2011).

Many patients do not regain full movement or function of the upper extremity. Studies report that 65% of individuals after stroke are unable to incorporate their hemiparetic upper extremity into daily function (Lum et al., 2009). Historically, motor recovery in the patient with hemiparesis was described as progressing from proximal to distal movement and from mass, patterned, undifferentiated movement to selective, coordinated movement (Brunnstrom, 1970; Fugl-Meyer et al., 1975). Therapists now rarely see such a distinct progression of motor recovery in patients, partly because thrombolytic agents limit brain damage and partly because insurance restrictions limit long-term rehabilitation services.

Functional Recovery

Much attention is given to the functional outcomes of patients surviving stroke. Although residual neurological deficits can lead to permanent impairments, activity limitations, and participation restrictions, impairments alone do not predict levels of disability or occupational functioning (Kelly-Hayes et al., 2003). Important aspects of functional recovery include the amount of assistance required to carry out daily living tasks and whether a stroke survivor can resume function at home. The National Stroke Association (2011) estimates that 10% of persons surviving stroke recover almost complete function, 25% recover with minor impairments, 40% experience moderate to severe impairments requiring special care, 10% require care in a nursing home or other long-term care facility, and 15% die shortly after the stroke. Studies indicate that independence in activities of daily living (ADL) improves with time after an acute stroke, although a large community-based study found that among persons 65 years of age or older who survived an ischemic stroke, 26% were dependent in ADL, and 30% were unable to walk without some assistance 6 months after stroke (Kelly-Hayes et al., 2003).

Few studies have addressed the recovery of instrumental activities of daily living (IADL), such as home management, work, leisure, or community skills. One study analyzing stroke survivors' functional status found that the majority of participants were able to perform basic activities of daily living (BADL) 3 months after acute care but had difficulties in performing more complex IADL, which play a key role in enabling full participation in home and community life (Shih et al., 2009). Most persons surviving stroke report decreased levels of activity, socialization, and overall quality of life, with only an estimated 25% returning to the level of everyday participation of community-matched persons who have not had a stroke (Lai et al., 2002).

Factors Influencing Recovery

Research in stroke outcomes has sought to identify characteristics and indicators that predict survival rate, degree of disability, and functional status. No simple predictors have been identified from numerous prospective studies. Applying the Occupational Therapy Practice Framework (American Occupational Therapy Association [AOTA], 2008) to individuals poststroke illustrates the complexity and wide variability of factors influencing each stroke survivor. Body structures such as the type, size, and site of the brain lesion and body functions such as presence and severity of hemiparesis or aphasia influence the extent and course of recovery. In addition, the context of personal factors such as advanced age and the presence and severity of coexisting disease, such as diabetes, heart disease, and peripheral vascular disease, can impede optimal functional recovery. The effect of age may partly explain more frequent coimpairments, such as arthritis or dementia; many elderly patients with poor outcomes following a stroke had reduced function prior to the stroke (Stein & Brandstater, 2010). Environmental factors, such as access to acute stroke units and rehabilitation services, help from family members, can also enhance or inhibit recovery.

Occupational performance, particularly in BADL, is often used to predict long-term recovery because ADL measures are relatively objective, simple to use, and very relevant to quality of life (Shih et al., 2009). A study of patients with severe strokes, however, found that ADL status at discharge from a stroke center was not accurate for predicting recovery, suggesting that longer periods of time were needed to predict outcome in this group of patients (Kashihara et al., 2011).

Factors associated with poor functional outcomes include severe initial motor deficits, poor sitting balance, dependence in BADL, prior stroke, persistent bowel and urinary incontinence, severe visuospatial deficits, severe cognitive impairments, depression, severe aphasia, altered level of consciousness, and poor social supports (e.g., living alone). Factors that may predict good quality of life after stroke include family support, independence in BADL, and access to continued services (Stein & Brandstater, 2010).

Time Frame for Recovery

Summarizing stroke literature, the largest percentage of motor and functional recovery occurs in the first month after stroke. Improvement after 6 months poststroke can be expected but is limited (Verheyden et al., 2008). Plateaus in recovery may reflect the insensitivity of measurement scales to incremental improvements rather than a patient's reduced potential for learning new tasks or gaining skills (Dobkin, 2005). Lack of rehabilitation continuity or less intensive treatment over time may also explain plateaus (Verheyden et al., 2008). Studies examining recovery status tend to focus on limited factors (motor or BADL improvements) rather than on levels of activity or participation. Multiple studies have shown that patients more than 1 year poststroke can exhibit substantial motor and functional improvement after participation in novel rehabilitation protocols (Page, Gater, & Bach-y-Rita, 2004). Individual stroke survivors who have successfully resumed life roles or taken on new ones report the process of recovery as continuing years after onset of stroke, with gains reported both in component skills and occupational performance (Matola, 2001).

Stages of Recovery

A person's stage of stroke recovery, as well as setting for treatment and extent of impairment, will influence a therapist's selection of assessments and interventions. In this chapter, the description of OT services for stroke patients is divided into three stages: the acute phase immediately following stroke, the rehabilitation phase, and reentry to the community or stage of continuing adjustment (Sabari & Lieberman, 2008). For most patients, progression of recovery and provision of services are not this clear-cut. For a variety of reasons, many patients do not have access to the full spectrum of services with smooth continuity of care. Any evaluation or treatment described, therefore, may apply to any or all other stages for a particular patient and should be viewed as part of a continuum of care adapted to meet changing needs over time. Coordination of services and ongoing communication among patients, families, and care providers at each step of rehabilitation is mandatory for optimum outcomes.

ASSESSMENT

Numerous evaluations exist to identify stroke impairments and disability. Assessment practices vary greatly among therapists caring for individuals poststroke, and no single test is universally accepted (Gresham et al., 1995). To help in the selection and ordering of assessment tools, therapists are guided by models of practice and evidence-based practice guidelines. The OT assessment of a patient poststroke includes both determination of the occupational profile (the roles, tasks, and activities important to that individual) and analysis of the individual's occupational performance (his or her competence in performing these valued roles, tasks, and activities). Therapists consider each individual and the individual's stage of recovery when determining whether to follow a bottom-up or a top-down approach to client evaluation. During the acute stage, assessments of client factors and performance skills are most critical in determining immediate posthospital placement. During the rehabilitation and community-reentry stages, therapists must also consider activity demands, contexts, patterns of performance, and integration of skills in order to help clients reach goals for quality of life and participation in meaningful roles (Sabari & Lieberman, 2008).

Therapists can use available practice guidelines to assist in the selection of assessment tools. Recommended guidelines are the American Occupational Therapy Association's Occupational Therapy Practice Guidelines for Adults with Stroke (Sabari & Lieberman, 2008) and Appendix D of the American Heart Association/American Stroke Association's (AHA/ASA) Management of Adult Stroke Rehabilitation Care: A Clinical Practice Guideline (Duncan et al., 2005). The AOTA guideline lists both standardized assessments and observationally based assessments commonly used by occupational therapists with stroke survivors. The AHA/ASA guideline lists recommended well-validated standardized measures for all disciplines and stages of stroke care. The use of standardized evaluation tools helps ensure reliable documentation, achieve consistency of treatment decisions, facilitate team communication, and monitor progress for each survivor (Duncan et al., 2005). Often, multiple assessment instruments must be used because of the wide variation in individual stroke manifestations and the patient's changing needs over the course of recovery.

Therapists should be familiar with commonly used standardized stroke deficit scales because they are frequently used as an interdisciplinary summary of baseline function and as indicators of recovery or treatment outcomes. The National Institutes of Health Stroke Scale (NIHSS) (Brott et al., 1989) is a brief, well-validated tool that can be administered by physicians, nurses, or therapists. Items scored include consciousness, vision, extraocular movements, facial palsy, limb strength, ataxia, sensation, speech, and language. Although no single measure can fully describe or predict the diverse picture of stroke disability and recovery, the NIHSS is widely used as an initial assessment tool and for planning discharge disposition (Kasner, 2006).

Assessment of Areas of Occupation

The patient's ability to perform the self-care, leisure, vocational, home, and community tasks that he or she hopes to continue is evaluated by observation rather than report because there can be a difference between what a patient can do and actually does. Evaluation to determine a patient's level of occupational functioning is administered early to predict answers to the following questions (Wade, 1992): (1) Where will the patient live, and what physical adaptations will be necessary? (2) How much and what type of assistance will the patient need? (3) What roles will the patient be able to fulfill, and how will he or she spend his or her time?

A patient's ADL performance in a structured clinical setting may not indicate performance at home. For example, patients who can put on and remove clothing during therapy sessions may not be able to find and retrieve their clothes in a cluttered closet, select clothing appropriate for the weather, or initiate the dressing routine without prompting (Campbell et al., 1991). Conversely, a patient may be unable to master simple meal preparation in the unfamiliar environment of a clinic kitchen but may re-adapt easily to this task upon returning home. A home evaluation can help determine what resources and means a patient has to achieve independence in areas of occupation as well as assessing safety and accessibility (see Chapter 10).

Self-Care

Methods for assessing self-care, or BADL, and examples of evaluation tools are discussed in Chapter 4. Measures of disability in ADL recommended by the AHA/ASA guideline (Duncan et al., 2005) are the Barthel Index (Mahoney & Barthel, 1965) and the Functional Independence Measure (FIM) (Keith et al., 1987). These interdisciplinary measures are well known and widely used in stroke research; the FIM is reported to be the most commonly used functional measure in rehabilitation hospitals. Their use can strengthen the team approach to stroke, with occupational therapists typically completing the self-care portions of these assessments and practitioners of other disciplines completing portions pertaining to bowel and bladder control, mobility, communication, cognition, and social interaction. These functional scales tend to have ceiling effects and are limited in their ability to measure higher levels of function or quality of life (Duncan et al., 2005; Wolf, Baum, & Connor, 2009).

Instrumental Activities of Daily Living

A patient's goals and probable discharge situation may direct a therapist to evaluate more complex areas of occupational performance. The AHA/ASA guideline recommends that "all patients planning to return to independent community living be assessed for IADL before discharge" and recommends that "minimal IADL skills required to stay at home alone include the ability to (1) prepare or retrieve a simple meal, (2) use safety precautions and exhibit good judgement, (3) take medication, and (4) get emergency aid, if needed" (Duncan et al., 2005, p. e120). Measures of IADL recommended by this guideline include the Frenchay Activities Index (Holbrook & Skilbeck, 1983) and the Philadelphia Geriatric Center Instrumental Activities of Daily Living Scale (IADL Scale) (Lawton, 1988). The Frenchay Activities Index

is a self-report tool developed specifically for patients with stroke that compares how frequently a patient engaged in activities, such as washing clothes, going on social outings, and gardening, prior to a stroke with frequency of participation in the same activities afterward. The stated purposes of this evaluation are to record changes in patterns of activity after stroke and to reflect quality of life rather than to measure performance in survival skills. The IADL Scale, on the other hand, is an observed measure that ranks quality of performance of activities such as using a telephone, managing medications, and handling finances. Additional measures recommended by the AOTA Practice Guideline include the Canadian Occupational Performance Measure (Law et al., 2005), the Assessment of Motor and Process Skills (Fisher, 1995) (see Chapter 4), and the Stroke Impact Scale (Duncan et al., 1999). The Stroke Impact Scale was developed to be a more comprehensive measure of outcomes for stroke survivors (Lai et al., 2002). The scale is a self-report interviewer-administered measure with questions pertaining to higher level functions of affected limbs, memory and thinking, mood and emotions, communication skills, home and community mobility, typical daily activities, and participation in meaningful life roles. Items included in this scale were derived from feedback of stroke patients and their caregivers who identified the persistent consequences of stroke that interfered the most with quality of life.

When appropriate, potential for driving and return to work may be evaluated by an occupational therapist or other specialist trained in these areas. A patient's ability to resume driving and/or vocational tasks is discussed later in this chapter (see also Chapters 26 and 28).

Assessment of Performance Skills and Client Factors

Observation of a patient's occupational performance suggests to the therapist specific performance skills and client factors that can enhance or impair the client's desired functional outcome. Assessment of performance skills helps to determine motor and cognitive abilities available to an individual in order to resume valued tasks and roles. Assessment of client factors, including primary and secondary impairments associated with stroke, helps determine potential for improvement in skills and occupational performance (Sabari & Lieberman, 2008). These skills and factors can be measured directly by administration of selected tests. Areas to be evaluated include postural adaptation, specific components of upper extremity function, and motor learning ability.

Postural Adaptation

Postural adaptation, or postural control, refers to the individual's ongoing ability to achieve, maintain, or restore an upright position against gravity (balance) for stability during activities or changes in body position (Pollock et al., 2000). The recognition and treatment of deficits in postural adaptation constitute an important aspect of therapy for stroke patients because so many daily living tasks (e.g., putting on socks, getting in and out of a bathtub, housework, and participating in sports) depend on this skill. Evaluation and treatment limited to a patient securely supported in bed or in a wheelchair fail to address most usual daily tasks that require dealing with gravity. A person with hemiplegia typically has decreased motor control, poor bilateral and sensory integration, and impaired automatic postural responses (Oliveira et al., 2008). As a result, the patient must devote increased effort to remaining upright, with decreased ability to focus on purposeful tasks. When engaging in a challenging activity, the hemiplegic patient often resorts to compensatory strategies to help maintain stability, such as using upper extremities for support (Oliveira et al., 2008).

Postural adaptation factors and skills can best be observed during the performance of meaningful functional activities, although the Berg Balance Scale (Berg et al., 1989) is listed as a recommended tool in both the AHA/ASA clinical guideline and the AOTA practice guideline. The Functional Reach Test (Duncan et al., 1990) is another measure of balance recommended by the AOTA guideline. Determining status of a patient's trunk control after stroke is an important starting point for assessing motor capacities or skills because poor trunk control can lead to dysfunctional limb control, increased risk of falls, contracture and deformity, diminished sitting and standing endurance, decreased visual feedback and swallowing effectiveness secondary to head and neck malalignment, and impaired ability to interact with the environment (Gillen, 2011a). A patient's posture and balance, both static and dynamic, can be observed and noted while the patient is seated and standing and during self-care tasks such as dressing, transfers, and bathing. Definition 33-2 compares functional seated posture with the dysfunctional positioning typically observed in patients recovering from stroke.

 Definition 33-2

Common Impairments in Sitting Posture Seen after Stroke

Body Part	Normal Sitting Posture Ready for Function	Abnormal Sitting Posture Typical of Stroke
Head, neck	Neutral	Forward Flexed to weak side Rotated away from weak side
Shoulders	Symmetrical height Aligned over pelvis	Uneven height Involved shoulder retracted
Spine, trunk	Straight from posterior view Appropriate lateral curves Lateral trunk muscle lengths equal bilaterally	Curved from posterior view Thoracic kyphosis Shortened lateral trunk muscles on one side, elongation on opposite side
Arms	Not used to maintain static upright posture Relaxed	Use of stronger arm to maintain upright posture Increased or decreased muscle tone in involved arm
Pelvis	Symmetrical weight bearing through both ischial tuberosities Neutral to slight anterior pelvic tilt Neutral rotation	Asymmetrical weight bearing Posterior pelvic tilt One hip angled forward
Legs	Hips at 90° flexion Knees aligned with hips; hips in neutral adduction or abduction and internal or external rotation Feet under knees Feet flat on floor, able to bear weight	Hips in more extension Hips adducted so that knees touch or involved hip externally rotated so that knees wide apart Feet in front of knees Feet not flat on floor, unable to bear weight

Adapted from Gillen, G. (2011a). Trunk control: Supporting functional independence. In G. Gillen (Ed.), *Stroke rehabilitation: A function-based approach* (3rd ed., pp. 156–188). St. Louis: Mosby.

Upper Extremity Function

Occupational therapists are the clinicians most often involved with the evaluation and treatment of motor deficits in the hemiplegic or hemiparetic upper extremity. Achievement of skilled arm and hand function is a complex, often difficult process following stroke and involves interaction of several body functions and structures. Evaluation of the involved upper extremity should address sensation; the mechanical and physiological deterrents to movement; the presence and degree of active or voluntary movement; the quality of this movement, including strength, endurance, and coordination; and the extent of function resulting from movement.

Somatosensory Assessment. During evaluation of sensory deficits in the person with stroke, it is important to remember that sensation is a component of function that is only a focus for treatment when it relates to the ability to perform usual daily living tasks. When somatosensory disturbances are present, they usually accompany motor impairment in the same anatomic distribution (Stein & Brandstater, 2010).

Most tests of sensation require attention, recognition, and response to multiple stimuli; therefore, sensory testing is difficult in patients with aphasia, confusion, and other cognitive deficits. It is often necessary to determine the patient's level of comprehension and communication, including yes/no reliability. An expressively aphasic patient can nod, gesture, point to written or pictured cues, or select a stimulus object from an array of objects. When testing with standard procedures is not possible, information may still be gained from observing a patient's reactions to the testing. The presence of gross protective sensation (flinching when pricked with a sharp pin) can be documented even if discriminatory perception cannot be determined.

Patients who have had mild CVAs and who have intact primary sensory awareness may need to be tested for more subtle discriminatory problems using two-point discrimination testing or the Moberg Pick-up Test (Dellon, 1981). Such testing is indicated when motor return is good, but hand dexterity remains impaired. Chapter 9 provides details of sensory assessment.

Mechanical and Physiological Components. Factors that can interfere with movement and function of the hemiplegic upper extremity include limitations in PROM, joint malalignment, abnormal muscle tone, and pain. Interview and medical records can help determine whether these conditions resulted from the stroke or were present prior to onset. Passive movement restrictions in the joints and soft tissues of the extremity may result from an individual's anatomy and lifestyle or from premorbid conditions such as arthritis or injury. Limitations may result more directly from the stroke, with sudden and

prolonged immobilization of joints caused by weakness or spasticity in muscles. Persistent stereotyped positioning of joints without counteracting movement results in the shortening and eventual contracture of muscles, tendons, and ligaments. Edema secondary to reduced circulation and loss of muscle action can further limit passive joint motion, particularly in the hand. Goniometric measurement of passive range of motion (PROM) is usually not indicated unless treatment is specifically aimed at increasing passive motion, such as when trying to eliminate an elbow flexion contracture. More useful in assessing patients with stroke is a comparison of the involved to the uninvolved arm to determine probable baseline joint motion.

Shoulder subluxation, or malalignment of the glenohumeral joint, occurs in approximately 50% of stroke patients (Yu, 2009). This condition is probably caused by the weight of the arm pulling down the humerus when the supraspinatus and deltoid muscles are weak and by weakness of scapular muscles that allows the glenoid cavity to rotate downward (Stein & Brandstater, 2010). Shoulder subluxation can be identified by palpation: the seated patient's arm hangs freely with trunk stabilized while the examiner palpates the subacromial space for the separation between the acromion and the head of the humerus. The distance separating the two is measured in finger widths, that is, the number of fingers that can be inserted in the space (Yu, 2009). The role of subluxation in the painful shoulder is controversial; in the shoulder, adhesive capsulitis, tendonitis, bursitis, rotator cuff tear, traction/compression neuropathy, and complex regional pain syndrome (CRPS) are common complications of hemiparesis, and all can result in pain and limited range of motion (ROM) (Duncan et al., 2005).

Spasticity, defined as velocity-dependent hyperactivity of tonic stretch reflexes, can result in ROM limitations and pain, often leading to contractures and functional impairments. The Ashworth Scale/Modified Ashworth Scale (Bohannon & Smith, 1987) is included in the AOTA practice guideline as a recommended assessment of spasticity (see Chapter 8; see Chapter 3 for descriptions of pain evaluation).

Voluntary Movement. Determining the amount and quality of voluntary movement a patient can produce is one of the first steps in assessing movement potential (Warren, 1991). The patterns of motion available are different for each stroke patient. Movement can change dramatically or subtly with time; hence, it requires careful reassessment throughout recovery. Factors to consider when evaluating motor control of the involved upper extremity include the following:

- Can the patient perform reflexive but not voluntary movement? Example: Patient demonstrates active elbow extension in the involved arm when balance is disturbed (equilibrium reaction) or flexes the hemiparetic elbow while yawning (associated reaction) but cannot perform these movements on request.

- Do proximal segments (neck, trunk, shoulder, hip) stabilize as needed to provide firm support for movement of the distal parts, or do they substitute for distal movement? Example: A patient can raise his hemiparetic arm only with pronounced lateral bending of the trunk and excessive elevation of the shoulder girdle.
- Can voluntary movement be performed unassisted against gravity, or is it possible only with assistance in the form of positioning, support, or facilitation? Example: A patient can bring her hand to her mouth only by flexing her elbow in a horizontal plane with gravity eliminated.
- Can voluntary movement be performed in an isolated fashion or only in a synergistic pattern? Example: A patient can reach for an object on a table only with a pattern of shoulder abduction, elbow flexion, and trunk flexion rather than with the more efficient pattern of shoulder flexion and elbow extension.
- Can reciprocal movement (the ability to perform agonist/antagonist motion in succession in an individual joint) be performed with practical speed and precision? Examples: A patient cannot produce a smooth pattern of elbow extension-flexion-extension needed to grasp a glass, take a drink, and set it back on the table but can perform each movement separately. A patient cannot perform the rapid alternating movements necessary to brush teeth.

One of the major movement difficulties following stroke is attaining the capacity and ability to isolate and control single muscle actions and combine them in a pattern appropriate for the task at hand. In motor patterns typical in hemiplegia, movement initiated in one joint results in automatic contraction of other muscles linked in synergy with that movement. This results in limited, stereotyped movement patterns rather than adaptive, selective motions. In Brunnstrom's theory of hemiplegic limb synergies (Brunnstrom, 1970), typical stereotyped patterns are described as flexor or extensor synergy patterns according to the motion at the elbow. The flexor synergy presents with scapular retraction and/or elevation, shoulder abduction and external rotation, elbow flexion, and forearm pronation. The extensor synergy presents with scapular protraction, shoulder horizontal adduction and internal rotation, elbow extension, and forearm pronation. Wrist and hand position varies (Brunnstrom, 1970). There is considerable variation in synergistic patterning, and other causes of abnormal stereotyped patterns include compensatory movements, unnecessary movement, muscle tension resulting from exertion or stress, and movement in response to gravity (e.g., pronation). According to Brunnstrom (1970), movement recovery after stroke is determined by an individual's ability to move independently of synergies. More contemporary clinical studies suggest that in addition to pathological limb synergies, loss of strength or centrally mediated impaired interjoint coordination can contribute to

movement disturbances and impaired function (Welmer, Holmqvist, & Sommerfeld, 2006). A study designed to look at the extent abnormal limb synergies influence voluntary movements of hemiparetic patients with first-time stroke found that 3 months after stroke, 13% of all subjects moved within synergies (Welmer, Holmqvist, & Sommerfeld, 2006).

Several methods for evaluating voluntary movement poststroke are described in Chapter 8 and online Chapters A, B, and C. Valid and reliable tools for evaluating voluntary movement poststroke recommended by both the AHA/ASA clinical guideline and the AOTA practice guideline are the Fugl-Meyer Assessment of Motor Function (Fugl-Meyer et al., 1975) and the Motor Assessment Scale (Carr et al., 1985). The Fugl-Meyer Assessment is an adaptation of Brunnstrom's original Hemiplegia Classification and Progress Record (Brunnstrom, 1970) and incorporates Brunnstrom's six stages of motor recovery with an underlying predicted sequence of recovery. The Fugl-Meyer Assessment of the Upper Extremity (FMA-UE) is the most commonly used research assessment to describe upper extremity motor impairment and evaluate the success of new interventions, but its focus on synergy patterns no longer forms the basis for newer function-oriented treatments (Woodbury et al., 2007). After investigating the dimensionality and construct validity of the FMA-UE, researchers suggest that assessment of reflexes in the FMA-UE gives little information about volitional movement. They also challenge the stepwise orderly sequence of motor recovery described by Brunnstrom and Fugl-Meyer and suggest instead that "UE motor behavior during recovery may be a dynamic interaction of neural factors with the task-specific difficulty of a movement" (Woodbury et al., 2007, p. 720).

Strength and Endurance. Muscle weakness ranging from slightly less than normal strength to total inability to activate muscles has been recognized as a limiting factor in the occupation and participation of patients with hemiplegia (Harris & Eng, 2007). The measurement of muscle strength to monitor recovery after stroke has been controversial because traditional neurological rehabilitation frameworks link muscle resistance to increased upper extremity tone and pain (Bobath, 1990). A meta-analysis of randomized controlled trials examining the evidence for strength training of the paretic upper extremity found evidence that strengthening can improve upper limb strength and function without increasing tone or pain in individuals with stroke (Harris & Eng, 2010). Methods used to quantify muscle strength after stroke include assessments of motor performance (e.g., Fugl-Meyer), manual muscle testing, dynamometry to measure grip strength, and measurements of active range of motion (Bohannon, 2007; Wagner et al., 2007). The motor assessment evaluations mentioned in this chapter and techniques described in Chapter 7 are recommended to establish baseline levels of muscle strength. It is important to consider that studies have also demonstrated muscle weakness in nonparetic limbs and trunk muscles of patients after stroke (Bohannon, 2007).

Reduced endurance, seen as a decrease in the ability to sustain movement or activity for practical amounts of time, is an important limiting factor in the motor performance of stroke patients because it affects the patient's ability to participate fully in rehabilitation and occupation (deGroot, Phillips, & Eskes, 2003) (Research Note 33-1). Decreased endurance can be the result of physical and/or mental fatigue caused by the exertion required to move weakened limbs or the result of comorbid cardiac or respiratory conditions (see Chapter 7).

Functional Performance. Assessing functional use of a hemiparetic arm poststroke is problematic, because although occupational performance evaluations identify deficits in ADL and IADL, they do not accurately reflect a patient's ability to use the affected arm for tasks. As observed in a population-based study, recovery of function in more

than half of patients with significant upper extremity paresis was achieved only with compensatory use of the unaffected arm (Nakayama et al., 1994). Similarly, evaluations of client factors and motor or process skills may predict a patient's potential for functional use of a hemiparetic arm but are not measures of occupational performance. Studies have suggested that "performance of a functional movement can be normal or near-normal despite the presence of underlying sensorimotor impairments" (Wagner et al., 2007, p. 762). Reimbursement trends in fact encourage focus on a client's ability to perform daily self-care activities after stroke rather than performance skills of the hemiparetic arm (Sabari & Lieberman, 2008). Further, many tests described in the literature as useful for evaluating function of the involved upper extremity can be categorized as task-oriented evaluations, with portions or simulations of familiar activities rather than relevant real-life activities (Okkema & Culler, 1998).

One difficulty in measuring function after stroke results from the normal differences in performance ability between dominant and nondominant arms. Eating with utensils, combing hair, and writing, for example, are

---

Research Note 33-1

Schepers, V. P., Visser-Meily, A. M., Ketelaar, M., & Lindeman, E. (2006). Poststroke fatigue: Course and its relation to personal and stroke-related factors. *Archives of Physical Medicine and Rehabilitation, 87,* 184–188.

Abstract

The objective was to describe the course of fatigue during the first year poststroke and to determine the relation between fatigue at 1 year poststroke and personal characteristics, stroke characteristics, and poststroke impairments. Participants included 167 patients with a first-ever stroke admitted for inpatient rehabilitation; mean age was 56.4 years, and 73.7% of participants lived with a spouse or partner. The main outcome measure was the Fatigue Severity Scale, a self-report assessment of the impact of fatigue on daily life, measured at admission to rehabilitation, 6 months poststroke, and 1 year poststroke. Results showed that the frequency of self-reported fatigue among patients was greater at 6 months and 1 year poststroke (64.1% and 69.5% of the patients, respectively) than at admission (51.5% of patients). Fatigue impact 1 year poststroke ($p < 0.1$) was greater among subjects with symptoms of depression, higher age, female sex, and those who perceived that their health-related outcomes were controlled more by powerful others (e.g., physicians) than by their own behavior. Of the subjects reporting fatigue 1 year poststroke, 29.3% were also depressed, supporting earlier studies. These four determinants explained 20% of the variance of fatigue impact scores; therefore, the majority of fatigue impact could not be attributed to specific factors. Other factors analyzed and found to not be significant in this study included marital status, type of stroke, extent of physical recovery (patients with both good and poor motor recovery reported fatigue impact), global cognitive impairments, and presence of sleeping disorders. Suggestions for further research on the impact of fatigue would be to analyze factors such as level of physical fitness, medication side effects, use of coping strategies, and higher level cognitive skills.

Implications for Practice

- Fatigue is expected to be a problem soon after stroke but is not always considered a deterrent to functional capacity or occupational therapy treatment several months or years poststroke. The impact of fatigue can become more pronounced as clients try to resume work or social roles. Therapists should recognize the long-term effect of fatigue symptoms when planning therapy in community or home programs.
- Patient education regarding poststroke fatigue should be routinely provided to patients and their families to increase recognition of the problem and decrease distress. Training in energy conservation and work simplification techniques, including pacing and balancing of rest with activity, is appropriate for patients with stroke, as are mind–body wellness interventions to improve perceptions of self-control over health.
- Although depression and fatigue are separate poststroke consequences, depression is an important focus for poststroke fatigue intervention. Therapists should be attuned to patients' symptoms of depression and refer patients and families to appropriate professionals.

normally performed by the dominant arm; testing the ability of a hemiparetic nondominant arm to perform these tasks is not relevant or useful to a patient. The arm has a wide range of functions, and any single test assesses only a portion of the actual possible functions. Therapists must choose tests that seem best suited for the individual patient.

Functional tests listed in AOTA's Practice Guideline for Adults with Stroke include the Functional Test for the Hemiplegic/Paretic Upper Extremity (Wilson, Baker, & Craddock, 1984a, 1984b), the Arm Motor Ability Test

(Kopp et al., 1997), and the Wolf Motor Function Test (Wolf et al., 2001).

The Functional Test for the Hemiplegic/Paretic Upper Extremity is a standardized test developed by occupational therapists specifically to evaluate patients' ability to use the hemiplegic upper extremity for purposeful tasks. This test consists of 17 tasks divided into seven functional levels that range from absence of voluntary movement to selective and coordinated movement (Figs. 33-1 and 33-2). The tasks follow a pattern of increasing difficulty and complexity

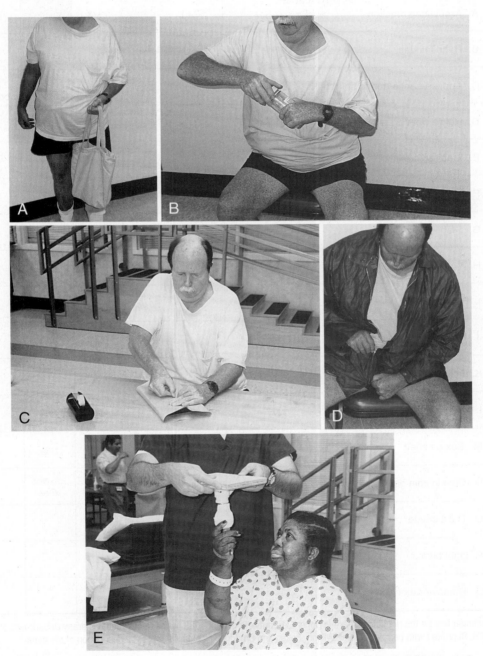

Figure 33-1 Functional Test for the Hemiplegic/Paretic Upper Extremity, sample tasks. **A.** Holding a pouch with a 1-pound weight. **B.** Stabilizing a jar while removing lid. **C.** Stabilizing a package while wrapping. **D.** Hooking and zipping a zipper. **E.** Putting in a light bulb.

FUNCTIONAL TEST FOR THE HEMIPLEGIC/PARETIC UPPER EXTREMITY

Patient Name _E.G. (L CUA)_

LEVEL	TASK	DATE: 6-17-13 EXAMINER: AMW GRADE	TIME	DATE: 7-13-13 EXAMINER: AMW GRADE	TIME	DATE: 8-12-13 EXAMINER: AMW GRADE	TIME
1	Patient is unable to complete higher level tasks						
2	A. Associated reaction	(NA)		(NA)		(NA)	
	B. Hand into lap	+	2 sec	+	2 sec	+	2 sec
3	C. Arm clearance during shirt tuck	+	5 sec	+	5 sec	+	3 sec
	D. Hold a pouch	+	15 sec	+	15 sec	+	15 sec
	E. Stabilize a pillow	+	25 sec	+	14 sec	+	8 sec
4	F. Stabilize a jar	+	12 sec	+	8 sec	+	5 sec
	G. Stabilize a package	+	75 sec	+	66 sec	+	40 sec
	H. Wringing a rag	+	32 sec	+	15 sec	+	10 sec
5	I. Hold a pan lid	+	20 sec	+	20 sec	+	19 sec
	J. Hook and zip a zipper	+	55 sec	+	22 sec	+	15 sec
	K. Fold a sheet	−	>3 min	+	90 sec	+	50 sec
6	L. Blocks and box	+	35 sec	+	20 sec	+	18 sec
	M. Box on shelf	−	helped w/ L hand	+	15 sec	+	7 sec
	N. Coin in coin gauge	−	unable to pick up dime	−	dropped dime	+	15 sec
7	O. Cat's cradle			−		+	45 sec
	P. Light bulb			−		+	30 sec (difficult)
	Q. Remove rubber band					+	15 sec

Figure 33-2 Functional Test for the Hemiplegic/Paretic Upper Extremity. (Copyright 1980 by the Occupational Therapy Department, Rancho Los Amigos Hospital, Downey, CA. Reprinted with permission. See Wilson, Baker, and Craddock [1984a, 1984b] for a description of the items.)

and reflect Brunnstrom's hierarchy of motor recovery in hemiplegia. This test was found to be valid because scores strongly correlated to scores on the Fugl-Meyer Assessment of Motor Function (Filiatrault et al., 1991). It is reported to have interrater reliability, but psychometric data are not presented (Wilson, Baker, & Craddock, 1984a). The Functional Test for the Hemiplegic/Paretic Upper Extremity is dominance neutral in that most items are activities normally performed by either arm or bilaterally. Disadvantages of this test are that it does not provide specific information about why a patient has failed a task (Wilson, Baker, & Craddock, 1984a), and it uses pass/fail scoring rather than an ordinal scale, making it difficult to use for documenting partial progress. For descriptions of the Arm Motor Ability Test and the Wolf Motor Function Test, refer to Chapter 8.

Motor Learning Ability

Motor learning refers to an individual's acquisition of strategies for solving movement challenges in changing contexts, enabling one to adapt to his or her environment (Bass-Haugen, Mathiowetz, & Flinn, 2008). Successful motor learning after stroke requires regaining an adequate person-environment-occupation fit for optimal occupational function. In this context, therapists should assess factors that can affect a patient's ability to learn or relearn, including visual function, speech and language disorders, motor planning ability, cognitive disorders, and psychosocial adjustments. Although discussed as separate categories, these factors operate as parts of an integrated system. It is often difficult to discern or separate, for example, cognitive functioning from visual-perceptual or speech-language skills. Does a patient fail to respond to a request to brush his teeth because he cannot locate the toothbrush in his visual field, because he has forgotten how to sequence this task, because he cannot understand the verbal request, or because he is not motivated to perform grooming tasks? These classifications are meant to assist the therapist in recognizing the components of learning impairments that follow stroke.

Visual Function. The visual system is a complex of many parts of the central and peripheral nervous system; therefore, any type or degree of brain damage is expected to have some effect on the function of the visual system (Warren, 1999). Chapter 5 describes assessments of vision and visual perception.

VFD is the most common visual disturbance associated with stroke, and homonymous hemianopsia is the type of VFD occurring most often. Hemianopsia affects half of the visual field. Homonymous means the deficit involves both eyes. A patient with left homonymous hemianopsia has decreased or absent vision in the nasal field of the right eye and the temporal field of the left eye. Deficits in visual attention in stroke patients are hemi-inattention and hemi-neglect or unilateral neglect. Hemiinattention describes a patient's tendency to ignore objects on one side of the visual field and can occur with or without a measureable VFD (Khan, Leung, & Jay, 2008). Similarly, patients can have hemianopsia without hemiinattention or neglect. Neglect, a complex deficit that can affect personal (body) perception as well as near or far extrapersonal space (Albert & Kesselring, 2011), is almost always associated with right parietal lobe damage (Shinsha & Ishigami, 1999) and is highly predictive of poor functional recovery (Khan, Leung, & Jay, 2008). Patients with VFD only will usually learn that there are objects in the area of loss and adapt their head and eye movements in order to complete tasks. For the patient with neglect, however, objects in the area of loss simply do not exist, and adaptation is difficult if not impossible (Khan, Leung, & Jay, 2008).

Because visual deficits are disabling to the degree that they prevent completion of necessary ADL, observation of the patient's occupational performance provides the most valuable information concerning the visual system (Warren, 1999, 2009). A pilot study investigating the impact of VFD on ADL performance by adults with acquired brain injury (Warren, 2009) found that people with VFD were impaired in their ability to use environmental context to inform and assist performance. Evaluation of patients with visual deficits therefore should focus on this capability and assess the space demands of ADL as well as the patient's ability to locate and discern features of objects necessary to complete tasks effectively and safely. The study identified personal hygiene-grooming and feeding as the BADL most difficult for patients with VFD (e.g., behaviors such as not noticing food on the left side of the tray, shaving only the right side of the face). The most challenging IADL were driving, shopping, financial management, and meal preparation, all requiring one or more of the performance skills of mobility, reading, or writing (Warren, 2009).

Speech and Language. Disturbances in the ability to communicate or to comprehend oral or written information can significantly affect the ability to resume or relearn usual activities. The speech and language disorders associated with stroke include aphasia, dysarthria, and apraxia of speech. Aphasia is an acquired multimodality disorder that can result in impaired understanding or input (listening, reading) and/or impaired expression or output (speaking, writing, using gestures) (Cherney & Small, 2009). Stroke is the leading cause of aphasia, with damage to the left cerebral hemisphere the usual origin. Systems for classifying and diagnosing the various types of aphasia have evolved and remain controversial, but a simplified clinical classification of aphasia recognizes fluent and nonfluent aphasias based on the patient's ability to produce speech (Goodglass, 1993). Other considerations in classification include auditory comprehension, repetition, and word retrieval (Cherney & Small, 2009). In the fluent aphasias, patients can easily produce spontaneous speech, but auditory comprehension and understanding of language is limited. The most common type of fluent aphasia is Wernicke's aphasia, or "receptive aphasia," characterized by the smooth articulation of speech but marked by incorrect word or sound substitutions and the inability to name objects, repeat phrases, or follow commands. Nonfluent aphasia is speech output that is difficult to produce and is characterized by slow, awkward articulation with limited vocabulary and grammar usage in the presence of relatively well-preserved auditory comprehension. An example is Broca's aphasia, or "expressive aphasia," in which the patient can follow commands but cannot name objects, repeat phrases, or convey ideas. A patient with large or multiple lesions in the left hemisphere may exhibit "global aphasia," with all language modalities severely impaired. Most individuals with aphasia demonstrate reading and writing difficulties (Cherney & Small, 2009). It is important to remember that speech and language disorders are complex, highly individualized, and rarely seen in pure forms of the types just described (Stewart & Riedel, 2011).

Dysarthria is a speech disorder caused by paralysis, weakness, or incoordination of speech musculature resulting in problems in speech production (poor articulation, poor phonation, poor voice quality) as well as drooling or decreased facial expression. Apraxia of speech is a communication problem in which the patient has difficulty initiating and sequencing the movements necessary to produce speech (Cherney & Small, 2009).

The occupational therapist needs to work collaboratively with the speech-language pathologist to learn the results of a patient's communication evaluation, support the patient's language goals, and request suggestions for communication strategies with patients in order to enhance their participation poststroke (Stewart & Riedel, 2011).

Motor Planning. Motor planning deficits, or apraxia, are deficits of skilled, organized, purposeful movement sequences used to achieve a goal. Apraxia cannot be explained by motor or sensory impairments or inability to follow a command (West et al., 2008). These deficits are best identified during performance of daily living tasks. Clinical manifestations of motor planning difficulties include the following (Warren, 1991):

- Failure to orient the head or body correctly to a task, such as a patient attempting a toilet transfer who tries to sit on the toilet before correctly positioning the body in front of it.
- Failure to orient the hand properly to objects and/or poor tool use, such as a patient who has to be reminded of the correct way to hold a pen when writing with the uninvolved hand.

- Difficulty initiating or carrying out a sequence of movements, such as a patient with nearly normal motor performance who cannot put on a shirt without step-by-step verbal and physical cueing.
- Movements characterized by hesitations and perseveration, such as a patient who, after brushing his teeth, is handed a razor and asked to shave. After a delay, the patient brings the razor to his mouth and tries to brush his teeth with it.
- Movements that can be performed only in context or in the presence of a familiar object or situation, such as a patient who does not follow a command to move hand to mouth unless given something to eat or drink.

These deficits are most pronounced during learning sessions, such as when training in wheelchair propulsion or one-handed buttoning, and in activities with multiple steps, such as making a sandwich.

Cognition. Disorders in cognitive functioning, including problems with attention, orientation, memory, and executive functioning, are common after stroke (Duncan et al., 2005). Higher level executive abilities allow individuals to form goals, plan how to achieve them, and complete the plans effectively in order to perform an array of complex ADL necessary for independent living (Baum et al., 2008). Patients impaired in these abilities may have decreased safety awareness and difficulty learning new techniques for performing tasks. Wolf, Baum, and Connor (2009), while analyzing a large population of individuals after stroke, found that increasing percentages of patients who have mild to moderate severity of stroke at a younger age (<65 years old), are discharged directly home, and although they may have received rehabilitation services including OT, are unable to resume IADL requiring complex cognitive behavioral strategies. This suggests a need for greater focus by therapists on the subtle deficits in executive functioning that interfere with family and community participation. Although mental status screening tests such as the Mini-Mental State Examination (Folstein, Folstein, & McHugh, 1975) are often used during the acute phase after stroke, occupational performance-based assessments focusing on the adaptive abilities of planning, initiation, organization, sequencing, judgment, and problem solving are more predictive of real-world ability (Baum et al., 2008). Chapter 6 describes specific cognitive assessment techniques. See also assessments recommended in the AOTA Practice Guidelines for Adults with Stroke (Sabari & Lieberman, 2008). Therapists must be careful to differentiate between cognitive deficits and communication difficulties common to stroke (Gresham et al., 1995).

Psychosocial Aspects. Adjustment to disability is a critical component of rehabilitation, although effective measures of adjustment have not been described. Most patients have natural emotional reactions to their stroke, including denial, anxiety, anger, and depression (Falk-Kessler, 2011). Poststroke depression is the most frequently reported reaction, affecting 25%–40% of patients within the first year after a stroke (Eriksson et al., 2004). Depression in stroke is both a physiological result of biochemical changes in the brain and a reaction to the personal losses of patients who realize, with time, that they will not fully recover (Eriksson et al., 2004). Although poststroke depression has been found to have a negative effect on recovery and independence for patients with stroke, assessment is difficult: there is no universally accepted assessment tool for poststroke depression, and cognitive and language deficits can make assessment difficult (Duncan et al., 2005).

Other common psychological manifestations poststroke include anxiety and emotionalism. Anxiety disorders have been found to frequently coexist with depression in individuals with stroke and can create feelings of worry or fear as well as physical symptoms that can decrease participation in rehabilitation or family/community roles (Duncan et al., 2005). For individuals poststroke, emotional responses to situations are expected. For many stroke survivors, however, a more extreme form of emotional reaction occurs, referred to as emotional lability. This is an involuntary emotional response, such as uncontrollable laughing or crying, that is disproportionate to the emotional stimulus (Falk-Kessler, 2011). A patient may, for example, cry whenever seeing a family member or when asked about a valued activity.

Emotional reactions, compounded by cognitive, perceptual, and language impairments, may lead to behavioral outcomes including denial, frustration, anger, impatience, irritability, overdependence, apathy, aggression, insensitivity to others, and rigid thinking (Falk-Kessler, 2011). These responses can further result in impaired personal interactions, decreased social participation, and eventual isolation. Evaluation of the patient's and family's adjustments to the stroke, to rehabilitation, and to the prospect of living with the aftermath of the stroke can be done through interview and observation and by sharing information with other members of the rehabilitation team.

TREATMENT

A careful interpretation of evaluation results helps determine a patient's assets and deficits in areas of occupational functioning. General goals of OT intervention with stroke survivors are to prevent secondary impairments, restore performance skills, modify activity demands and contexts as necessary, promote a healthy and satisfying lifestyle, and maintain available performance and health (Sabari & Lieberman, 2008). Intervention is always a collaborative process between therapist and client/family or caregiver. Possible goals for individuals recovering from stroke include the following:

- The patient will gain competence in valued and necessary BADL and IADL in order to perform at the highest level of independence possible in the desired postdischarge setting.
- The patient will improve postural control in order to perform daily living tasks requiring balance and changes in body position.
- The patient will gain increased somatosensory perception and/or will employ compensatory strategies in order to perform ADL safely.
- The patient and/or caregiver will demonstrate appropriate management techniques for the hemiparetic upper extremity to prevent pain and other secondary mechanical or physiological movement restrictions.
- The patient will gain the necessary strength, endurance, and control of movement of the involved upper extremity in order to use the involved upper extremity spontaneously during the performance of ADL.
- The patient will gain visual function or will employ compensatory strategies in order to safely resume previously performed ADL.
- The patient will improve motor planning ability in order to relearn old methods or learn new methods of performing ADL.
- The patient and/or caregiver will demonstrate appropriate strategies for improving or compensating for cognitive deficits during the performance of ADL.
- The patient and/or caregiver will be able to verbalize the reality and impact of emotional reactions to stroke and identify coping strategies or resources to help adjust to living with a stroke.
- The caregiver will demonstrate appropriate methods and problem-solving strategies for assisting the patient with ADL and with home activities to improve/preserve performance skills.
- The patient will gain competence in tasks and activities necessary to resume valued roles or to assume new meaningful roles in the community.

Intervention will vary with the patient's stage of recovery, intervention setting, living environment, extent of impairment, and personal goals and preferences (Sabari & Lieberman, 2008). Safety of the patient, during and after treatment, is a concern during all phases (Safety Note 33-1).

Acute Phase

Stroke rehabilitation begins "as soon as the diagnosis of stroke is established and life-threatening problems are under control" (Duncan et al., 2005, p. e104). Length of stay in acute hospital beds is typically just long enough for necessary diagnostic tests, for initiation of appropriate

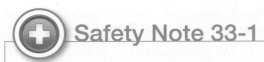

Safety Note 33-1

Precautions with Stroke Patients

- In the acute period after stroke, ascertain the patient's medical status and stability daily before treatment. Know the symptoms of progressing or recurrent stroke.
- In the acute-care setting, know how to read ICU monitors and handle drains and lines as necessary (e.g., vital sign monitors, Foley catheters, IV lines, feeding tubes).
- Determine whether cardiac or respiratory precautions apply for a particular patient and monitor accordingly, watching for signs of cardiac distress and blood pressure changes, including dizziness, breathing difficulties, chest pain, excessive fatigue, and altered heart rate or rhythm.
- Guard against falls by providing appropriate supervision and assistance during transfers and other transitional movements.
- To avoid shoulder injury or pain, never pull or lift a patient by or under the weak arm during transfers or other transitional movements.
- Use appropriate precautions in the presence of skin with diminished sensation, particularly if a patient also has visual field deficits and/or unilateral neglect.
- Ascertain a patient's ability to swallow and follow recommended management techniques during feeding.
- Provide appropriate supervision for patients who demonstrate impulsive behavior and/or poor safety awareness.
- Teach the patient, family members, and other health care workers about safety concerns for an individual patient.

medical treatment, and for making decisions and arrangements for the next phase of rehabilitation. Priorities during this early period are to prevent recurrent stroke and complications, mobilize the patient as soon as possible, encourage performance of self-care activities, and provide emotional support to patient and family (Duncan et al., 2005). Patients who have just had a stroke may need to be seen bedside because of precautions, monitoring, and varying levels of consciousness. During this phase, the patient must adjust to the sudden, unexpected shift from usual life roles to the role of patient.

Early Mobilization and Return to Self-Care

The patient with acute stroke should be mobilized and encouraged to perform self-care as soon after admission as is medically feasible. The early introduction of BADL, such as rolling in bed, sitting on the side of the bed, transferring to a wheelchair or commode, self-feeding, grooming, and dressing, helps the patient reestablish

some control over the environment and begin to improve occupational functioning and component abilities and capacities (Gresham et al., 1995). Even at this early stage, the occupational therapist's assessment of a patient can help determine the most appropriate setting for rehabilitation and discharge. The goals of discharge planning during the acute phase are to determine the need for postacute rehabilitation, arrange the best possible living environment, and ensure continuity of care after discharge (Gresham et al., 1995).

Lowering Risk for Secondary Complications

As part of the stroke care team, the occupational therapist should practice methods to prevent or lessen complications resulting from stroke.

Skin Care. It is estimated that up to 21% of patients with stroke develop pressure sores (Langhorne et al., 2000). Those who are comatose, malnourished, or incontinent or who have diabetes, peripheral vascular disease, abnormal sensation, severe paralysis, or muscle spasticity are at greatest risk (Duncan et al., 2005). The occupational therapist helps patients maintain skin integrity by doing the following:

- Using proper transfer and mobility techniques to avoid undue skin friction
- Recommending appropriate bed and seated positioning and participating in scheduled position changes as needed
- Assisting with wheelchair and seating selection and adaptation
- Teaching patient and caregiver precautions to avoid injury to insensitive skin and involved side of body
- Watching for signs of skin pressure or breakdown on a patient (bruising, redness, blisters, abrasions, ulceration), especially over bony areas, and alerting nursing or medical staff as appropriate

Maintaining Soft-Tissue Length. Contractures, or shortening of skin, tendons, ligaments, muscles, and/or joint capsules, may result from the immobilization following stroke. Risk factors include muscle paralysis, spasticity, and imbalance between agonist and antagonist muscle groups. Contractures restrict movement, may be painful, and may limit functional recovery (Gillen, 2011b). The appropriate management is therefore a preventive program of proper positioning and soft tissue and joint mobilization. Suggested bed positioning for patients with stroke, based on a literature review (Carr & Kenney, 1992), is summarized in Procedures for Practice 33-1. However, bed positioning, like any treatment, must be adapted to meet the individual needs of the patient. Care must be taken to protect the weak upper extremity during

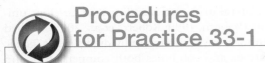

treatment because improper handling, positioning, and transferring techniques can exert great stress on the vulnerable shoulder early after stroke (Walsh, 2001). Specific techniques for supporting the hemiparetic shoulder are discussed later in this chapter. Resting hand splints are often applied to prevent soft tissue shortening, but their use has not been found to significantly prevent or reverse contracture of wrist and finger flexor muscles (Lannin et al., 2007).

Controlled and frequent soft tissue and joint mobilization is the preferred method to prevent contractures (Gillen, 2011b). When a patient cannot use the involved side to engage in meaningful activities, therapists should initiate supervised active or active-assistive movement activities. When active movement is not possible, therapists

should see that immobile body parts go through PROM at least once daily. If performing PROM on the involved arm, ensure mobility of the scapula on the thoracic wall before elevation of the arm and manually assist upward rotation of the scapula if needed. *Safety Message: Do not attempt overhead ranges unless the scapula glides freely in upward rotation.* The humerus should be externally rotated during abduction to prevent impingement of the supraspinatus between the greater tubercle of the humerus and the acromion process (Gillen, 2011b). As soon as possible, patients should learn strategies for safe ROM activities they can perform independently or with assistance of caregivers.

Fall Prevention. For patients hospitalized with stroke, falls are the most common cause of injury (Gresham et al., 1995). Factors that increase the risk of falls include advanced age, confusion, comorbidity, impulsive behavior, mobility deficits, poor balance or coordination, visual impairments or neglect, and communication deficits that interfere with a patient's ability to request assistance in a timely manner. Treatment that helps to prevent falls includes detecting and removing environmental hazards, scheduled routine toileting, optimizing motor control, recommending appropriate adaptive devices, and teaching safety measures to the patient and family.

Patient and Family Education. Early in recovery, support for patients who have had strokes and their families may best be provided in the form of education to promote a realistic understanding of the causes and consequences of stroke and the process, goals, and prognosis of rehabilitation (Duncan et al., 2005). In a systematic review, Forster et al. (2001) found evidence that passive education alone, such as providing written handouts, is not as effective as a combination of passive and interactive education, such as classes or training sessions. All aspects of OT assessment and treatment for survivors of stroke should be considered opportunities for education: to engage cooperation and participation in the identification of meaningful treatment goals, to highlight residual abilities as well as disabilities, and to promote carryover of treatment gains. Because the period after stroke is stressful, emotional, and tiring for both the patient and family, education sessions provided during the acute phase should be brief, simple, and reinforced as needed with repetition or appropriate learning aids (see Chapter 13).

Rehabilitation Phase

Part of discharge planning during the acute phase of stroke is screening for rehabilitation services. The AHA/ASA guideline recommends that "patients who have sustained an acute stroke should receive rehabilitation services if their poststroke functional status is below their prestroke status, and if there is a potential for improvement" (Duncan et al., 2005, p. e118). Rehabilitation choices depend on a patient's condition, the social support system, and the resources available in a community. To qualify for further treatment in an inpatient rehabilitation facility, a patient must require active and ongoing intervention of multiple therapy disciplines, require an intensive rehabilitation therapy program (generally consisting of at least 3 hours of therapy per day at least 5 days per week), and reasonably be expected to actively participate in and significantly benefit from the rehabilitation program (U.S. Department of Health and Human Services, 2011). Patients who do not qualify for this level of rehabilitation may receive multidisciplinary rehabilitation services at a skilled nursing facility or long-term care facility or treatment by one or more disciplines in home care or in an outpatient clinic.

During this phase of recovery, the patient and family are focused on getting better and are usually more concerned with recovering lost function than on adapting to a life of chronic disability (Sabari, 1998). Successful OT intervention coordinates a patient's striving for restoration of function with the potential for compensation and alternative occupational roles.

Treatment to Improve Performance of Occupational Tasks

The occupational therapist's primary role in stroke rehabilitation is to enhance clients' participation and quality of life through occupation. Interventions to improve performance of BADL is a major component of therapy for people who have had a stroke. Indeed, levels of independence in BADL are used to measure the success of rehabilitation (Stroke Unit Trialists' Collaboration, 2001), serve as outcomes in stroke research trials (Sulter, Steen, & De Keyser, 1999), and, in current U.S. trends, determine reimbursement for services (Sabari & Lieberman, 2008). A systematic review of nine randomized controlled trials (Legg et al., 2007) found that OT focused on improving BADL after stroke can improve performance and reduce the risk of deterioration of these skills.

It is accepted practice to teach patients with significant performance skills deficits compensatory methods for performing important tasks and activities, using the affected limb when possible and, when not, the unaffected limb (Gresham et al., 1995). Many consider that early ADL training focusing on modifying activity demands, contexts, and performance patterns (compensatory techniques) results in faster success and is therefore more cost effective and more satisfying to the patient, who again feels competent (Nakayama et al., 1994). Others contend that, when ADL training focuses on one-handed techniques and use of devices or modifications without working to restore performance skills, the patient fails

to relearn bilateral movements and instead develops unilateral habits (Bobath, 1990; Roberts et al., 2005). Skilled OT intervention considers each individual's needs, goals, and motivations and combines both compensatory and remedial treatment strategies and attempts to improve both areas of occupation and performance skills by engaging the patient in meaningful activities. Putting on a front-buttoning shirt, for example, besides helping a patient gain independence in the task of dressing, addresses the following component abilities, capacities, and conditions:

- Joint and soft-tissue integrity (self-stretching or relaxation techniques for involved arm in preparation for dressing, positioning of arm on a surface to prevent stretching of weak shoulder structures)
- Voluntary movement and function of involved upper extremity (abducting shoulder to put on a sleeve, extending elbow to push the hand through the sleeve, pinching one side of the shirt to stabilize while buttoning)
- Somatosensory perception (the texture of the shirt, the position of the affected arm)
- Postural adaptations (anterior pelvic tilt, trunk rotation, sitting/standing balance, weight shifting)
- Visual-perceptual skills (finding the shirt in the visual field, distinguishing top from bottom, finding the sleeve opening)
- Cognitive skills and emotional reactions (sequencing, attention span, frustration tolerance, motivation)

ADL training with stroke patients begins with simple tasks and gradually increases in difficulty as a patient gains competency (Gresham et al., 1995). Several studies discerned a hierarchy of achievement of self-care skills. Results of one study showed that bathing, dressing, and climbing stairs were the activities for which stroke survivors most often required assistance, with 32% of patients needing help with bathing, 25.5% needing help with dressing, and 32% requiring assistance with stairs 12 months poststroke (Carod-Artal et al., 2002). Aspects of dressing that are particularly difficult for stroke patients are putting a sock and shoe on the affected foot, lacing shoes, and pulling up trousers or pants (Walker & Lincoln, 1990). A study that investigated the relationship between dressing abilities and cognitive, perceptual, and physical deficits found that, in general, lower extremity dressing correlates more with motor performance, and upper extremity dressing correlates more with cognitive or perceptual performance (Walker & Lincoln, 1991). Adaptive devices should be considered if they increase simplicity, independence, and safety for the patient or caregiver.

As the patient progresses, occupational performance tasks other than basic self-care should be addressed, particularly if the patient expects to return to independent community living (Duncan et al., 2005). IADL tasks such as homemaking, home management, and community mobility involve greater interaction with the physical and social environment and require higher level problem-solving and social skills than BADL tasks (Carod-Artal et al., 2002). Chapter 25 discusses specific techniques for regaining independence in BADL/IADL for those with loss of the use of one side of the body. Avocational interests, including adapted methods of continuing familiar hobbies, are an important area of treatment. Many stroke survivors are faced with increases in leisure time because of the inability to go back to work; however, a reduction in social and leisure participation commonly occurs after stroke (Lai et al., 2002).

Treatment to Improve Performance Skills and Client Factors

Performance-component goals are based on the impairments associated with an individual's stroke and are directly linked to occupational performance goals. The goals and modalities used to address these component deficits must be purposeful and meaningful from the patient's point of view (Trombly, 1995/2011). Therapists use occupation-based interventions, purposeful activity, and preparatory methods to help patients achieve long-term occupational goals (AOTA, 2008). Thus, in addition to direct practice of dressing and grooming activities, a patient may be engaged in a floor game to improve sitting balance needed to don socks, or use therapy putty for resistive grasp activities to strengthen muscles needed to squeeze a tube of toothpaste. Treatments for stroke deficits are described individually in the following sections, but most patients in rehabilitation programs have multiple interacting problems requiring efficient, integrated intervention plans that simultaneously address several deficit areas.

Postural Adaptation. The ability to make automatic postural adjustments, including trunk control and the maintenance of balance, is a prerequisite for successful performance of occupational tasks. A systematic review of recent evidence related to the effect of balance training on balance performance among individuals poststroke supports the use of balance training for individuals with moderately severe stroke (Lubetzky-Vilnai & Kartin, 2010). Part of the occupational therapist's role in training a patient with stroke in ADL independence poststroke is in understanding each patient's particular strengths and weaknesses regarding stability and mobility. For example, some clients may be challenged in maintaining sitting balance on the side of a bed for the duration of eating an entire meal, whereas others may be ready to improve dynamic standing balance in order to cast a fishing line or play golf. Therapists should teach patients the safest, most effective and efficient "ready" position for engaging in activities (see Definition 33-2) as well as strategies for adapting to changes in body position.

Suggested techniques to enhance postural control during task performance include the following:

- Provide feedback to help the patient feel the difference between an aligned and misaligned posture (Gillen, 2011a) (patient views self in mirror or tries to copy therapist's positions/movements).
- Use varying postures and incorporate transitional movements into activities (standing rather than sitting to perform grooming; putting away groceries by reaching for items in bag on floor while sitting, then standing and placing on overhead shelf).
- Grade reaching activities to elicit various trunk movements and weight shifts (place clothing needed for dressing in locations requiring forward flexion or trunk rotation; locate items needed for cooking task in upper and lower shelves).
- Use bilateral upper extremity activities to improve sitting or standing balance without arm support (folding towels; grating cheese at counter using involved hand to stabilize grater).

A particularly challenging and poorly understood impairment of postural control is pusher behavior. Pusher behavior is clinically defined to describe hemiplegic patients who actively push away from their nonparalyzed side with their stronger limbs and resist attempts to make them more upright (Davies, 2000). A pilot study by Perennou et al. (2002) concluded that pusher behavior does not result from disrupted processing of vestibular information but from a higher order disruption in the processing of somesthetic information from the left side of the body, possibly an extinction or neglect phenomenon. Because patients with pusher behavior resist hands-on attempts to correct their alignment, therapists should select treatment that manipulates the environment (reaching for objects to encourage weight shift to the strong side) and provides external cues ("bring your right shoulder toward the wall") (Gillen, 2011a) (see Definition 33-2).

Upper Extremity Function. Bilateral use of the upper extremities is crucial to efficient and effective occupational performance. Patients recovering from stroke usually place a high priority on regaining function in the involved arm. The occupational therapist must determine which deficits most affect a patient's upper extremity performance and plan realistic multilevel, task-oriented treatment to restore function or promote adaptation to the loss of function.

Somatosensory Deficits. It is estimated that 60% of individuals present with some form of sensory deficit poststroke (Winward, Halligan, & Wade, 1999). Decreased sensory awareness in the hemiparetic side can result in safety concerns, impaired grasp and manipulation skills in the affected hand, reduced ability to regain skilled movements necessary for ADL, and impaired spontaneous use of the affected hand, frequently leading to learned nonuse (Schabrun & Hillier, 2009). In spite of this, there is little evidence to support treatment for sensory impairment poststroke.

Compensatory treatment entails substituting intact senses (e.g., vision) for those lost or dysfunctional and is usually included as safety education during occupational tasks. An example of remedial treatment is the protocol described by Yekutiel and Guttman (1993). Their sensory reeducation program included exploring with each patient the nature and extent of sensory loss, selecting sensory tasks of interest to the patient that promoted learning, and practicing detection, localization, and discrimination. Another proposed method of increasing sensory input to the affected hand is repeated nonspecific exposure to sensory stimuli via passive movements and grasp (Schabrun & Hillier, 2009). The patient is encouraged to use the involved hand in ADL as soon as possible and use different textures (e.g., foam, terry cloth, and Velcro®) on weight-bearing surfaces or on the holding surfaces of commonly used utensils, such as cups, forks, and pens.

Therapists must determine the appropriateness of each type of treatment for individual patients. For example, sensory retraining is unrealistic for patients with minimal voluntary movement, visual field neglect, or poor cognitive skills.

Schabrun and Hillier (2009) examined the volume and quality of evidence available on the retraining of sensory function following stroke and found some support for the effectiveness of passive sensory training (application of electrical stimulation to produce activation of cutaneous nerves in the absence of muscle contraction). Although some individual studies report positive effects on function following sensory discrimination training (Carey, Macdonell, & Matyas, 2011), Schabrun and Hillier (2009) found evidence for active sensory training limited by small sample sizes, subject heterogeneity, and unreliable outcome measures. Treatment to restore tactile awareness and teach compensation for sensory loss is discussed in Chapter 22.

Mechanical and Physiological Components of Movement. Techniques for maintaining soft-tissue length and avoiding pain in the involved upper extremity initiated during the acute phase of stroke recovery should be continued and adapted in response to changes in the patient's movement or muscle tone. As the patient in a rehabilitation program gains in mobility, measures should be taken to protect weak upper extremity structures from stretching or injury caused by the effects of gravity and improper movement. Procedures for Practice 33-2 summarizes handling techniques for an affected upper extremity.

Treatment of problems related to the hemiplegic shoulder centers on prevention and management of symptoms and underlying causes. The use of supportive devices such as slings, orthoses, and wheelchair attachments as a

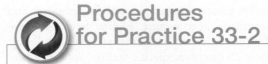

Procedures for Practice 33-2

Proper Handling of the Hemiparetic Upper Extremity

- Teach the patient as early as possible to be responsible for the positioning of the arm during transfers, bed mobility, and other activities involving change of position.
- Use gait belts or draw sheets, rather than the affected arm, to assist the patient in moving his or her body.
- Avoid shoulder range of motion beyond 90° of flexion and abduction unless there is upward rotation of the scapula and external rotation of the humerus (Gresham et al., 1995).
- Avoid overhead pulley exercises, because they appear to increase the frequency of pain in the shoulder because neither scapular nor humeral rotation occurs, and the force may be excessive (Kumar et al., 1990).

prevention or treatment for subluxation or to decrease pain of the hemiplegic shoulder is not supported by empirical research (Ada, Foongchomcheay, & Canning, 2009). Reasons for using slings are to reduce the subluxation of the glenohumeral joint, provide support for the arm, protect against trauma, and prevent or reduce pain. Zorowitz et al. (1995) studied radiographs of hemiplegic shoulders in four types of slings and reported that the slings did not eliminate the asymmetry of subluxation. Further, these supports have not been found to improve trunk or scapular alignment (Gillen, 2011b). Pain control is a valid reason for use of a positioning device; however, the relation between subluxation and shoulder pain is unclear. A review of literature concerning hemiplegic shoulder pain and the association between shoulder pain and subluxation shows contradictory opinions (Gillen, 2011b), with most studies finding a low correlation between shoulder pain after stroke and subluxation and others finding a high correlation between shoulder pain and limited passive shoulder external rotation (Zorowitz et al., 1996). These studies support a general recommendation that the hemiplegic arm should be appropriately supported but that shoulder supports should not be issued uniformly to all patients with shoulder subluxation. If considering a sling, therapists should address the following questions (Gillen, 2011b; Ridgway & Byrne, 1999). A positive response to the following questions might indicate a sling:

- Does pain or edema increase when the arm hangs down?
- Is the patient's balance and performance during standing, walking, or transfers improved by the use of a sling?
- Is the patient unable to attend to and protect the arm during movement?

- Can the patient or caretaker independently put on and take off a sling correctly?

A positive response to the following questions might contraindicate a sling:

- Would the sling prevent or hinder active movement or function in the arm?
- Would a sufficiently supportive sling impair circulation or cause excessive pressure on the neck?
- Would the sling put the patient at risk for contracture as a result of immobilization?
- Would a sling decrease sensory input and promote unilateral disregard?

Alternative positioning methods and devices for shoulder support include taping of the shoulder and scapula (Ridgway & Byrne, 1999), wheelchair lapboards and armrest troughs, use of a table while seated or standing, putting the hand in a pocket or under a belt, and using an over-the-shoulder bag while standing (Gillen, 2011b) (Fig. 33-3). Functional electrical stimulation (FES) has been used to prevent or improve shoulder subluxation, decrease pain, and improve ROM. Studies evaluating the effectiveness of FES showed benefits during treatment but reduction of gains after treatment was discontinued (Walsh, 2001). Any patient with shoulder pain that persists and consistently interferes with function or progress in therapy should be referred to specialists best qualified to diagnose and treat specific shoulder problems.

Along with protection, patients learning to manage their involved arm should know techniques of active, active-assistive, or passive movement designed to maintain ROM, stretch tight tissues, or relax hypertonicity.

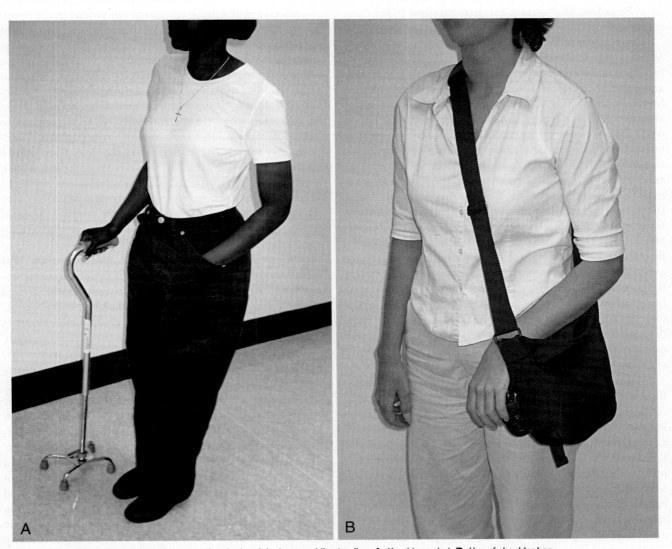

Figure 33-3 Alternative methods for supporting the hemiplegic arm while standing. **A.** Hand in pocket. **B.** Use of shoulder bag.

The combination of positioning for comfort and muscle imbalances brought on by spasticity and weakness can lead to the development of stereotyped nonfunctional positioning of the hemiplegic upper extremity with shoulder retraction, adduction, and internal rotation, elbow flexion, forearm pronation, and wrist and finger flexion. Therapists should emphasize frequent changes of position to prevent contractures and pain and recognize that if a patient is only moving his affected arm during therapy sessions, then therapy alone may not provide sufficient soft-tissue lengthening to maintain full ROM (Ada et al., 2005). In a prospective randomized control trial of 36 subjects with recent strokes, the experimental group received two daily 30-minute sessions of positioning of the affected arm in maximum comfortable shoulder external rotation in addition to shoulder exercise and standard upper limb care, whereas the control group received only exercise and standard care. At the end of 4 weeks, the experimental group had significantly less loss of shoulder external rotation ROM than the control group (Ada et al., 2005).

Even in the absence of motor recovery, passive and assisted active movement of the affected arm can be incorporated into activities, with the patient experiencing and concentrating on movement in a functional context. Methods of teaching self-managed ROM include bilateral activities such as having the patient clasp his or her hands while leaning forward to reach for the floor or pushing both hands forward with arms supported on a towel on a table (Gillen, 2011b). The advantages of these activities are that they can easily be given a functional context, such as picking up objects off the floor or dusting a table, and the patient can monitor his or her own pain threshold and is therefore not apprehensive about movement of the arm. Nelson et al. (1996), in a study of persons with hemiplegia, found that using a simple dice game to achieve bilaterally assisted forearm supination brought better results (more ROM, more repetitions) than use of a rote exercise routine. Self-management of ROM should be closely supervised and may not be appropriate for patients who have decreased awareness of the involved side, who move too quickly, who do not respect pain, or who lack a mobile scapula.

Hand edema is a frequent complication of hemiplegia. Edema control techniques include elevation of the hand, retrograde massage, and use of pressure gloves and sleeves. Patients with minimal voluntary movement should avoid allowing the hand and arm to hang down for long periods. Prolonged hand edema can lead to limited passive movement, pain, and soft-tissue contractures. Edema combined with severe pain, hypersensitivity, and vasomotor disturbances of the hand are signs of shoulder–hand syndrome, often referred to as CRPS and should be addressed vigorously to prevent further loss of functional potential (Gillen, 2011b) (see Chapter 37).

Voluntary Movement and Function. Chapter 21 and Web Chapters A, B, and C describe various treatment approaches to promote motor abilities and capacities in the patient recovering from stroke. Therapists usually employ a variety of techniques in response to the complex multiple factors that interfere with upper extremity use in an individual patient. Studies examining the components of occupational therapy intervention for inpatient stroke rehabilitation found that occupational therapists provide a combination of impairment-focused and function-focused activities tailored to an individual patient's disabililty (Richards et al., 2005) and that occupational therapists use preparatory methods aimed at improving performance skills and body structures more than occupation-based interventions (Smallfield & Karges, 2009). Gillen (2011b) suggests that "the complex problems that interfere with upper extremity function may require an integrated treatment approach that uses functional tasks as the intervention foundation" (p. 219) and preparatory, remediative methods as adjuncts.

Success in restoring voluntary movement in the hemiplegic upper extremity and incorporating that movement into ADL performance has been limited, perhaps because investigation of factors enhancing or impeding motor skills and processes following stroke is limited (Winstein et al., 2004). Lum et al. (2009) defined recovery of functional voluntary movement as including normalization of movement smoothness, interjoint coordination, active range of motion, and muscle activation patterns. Compensatory movement is defined as the use of alternative degrees of freedom and/or muscles to complete a task (such as using increased trunk movement during a reaching task). Interventions that promote compensation may lead to short-term functional gains but inhibit long-term motor recovery (Lum et al., 2009). Many recent studies have used kinematic and electromyographic (EMG) analysis to identify qualitative features (such as speed, accuracy, and efficiency) of voluntary movement of the hemiparetic upper extremity during components of arm function, such as reach or grasp of an object (Lum et al., 2009; Wagner et al., 2007). These and other studies have supported findings that negative neurological symptoms (decreased strength, impaired coordination) may contribute more to the loss of functional movement than positive neurological symptoms (spasticity and hyperactive reflexes) (Gillen, 2011b).

Although more studies are needed to determine the effectiveness of specific clinical strengthening methods in improving upper limb function and occupational performance of stroke patients, carefully selected resistive activities have been shown to improve performance as measured by motor function tests (Kluding & Billinger, 2005). In their meta-analysis involving 517 patients, Harris and Eng (2010) found significant effect for strength training increasing grip strength and function of the hemiparetic arm but found no treatment effect for strength training on ADL measures. The authors suggest that because ADL are composed of complex combinations of strength, ROM, and coordination, practice of all components is required for improvement of occupational performance, and it may be difficult to isolate the effect of one component.

Decreased physical and mental endurance resulting from stroke can limit participation and performance in therapy; treatment should therefore be carefully graded to compensate for and improve reduced endurance. Length of treatment sessions, energy requirements, and need for rest periods should be monitored to meet patients' needs.

Coordinated movement is the product of successful control of the strength, range, speed, direction, and timing of movement. Because almost all purposeful activity requires coordination, encouraging use of the affected extremities in BADL or IADL is an appropriate way to improve coordination. Treatment should progress from unilateral activities, in which the patient can concentrate fully on control of the hemiparetic arm, to bilateral simultaneous activities, in which both arms perform the same movement together (such as lifting and carrying a box and catching and throwing a large ball), to bilateral alternating activities, in which the two arms perform different movements at the same time (such as sorting and assembling nuts and bolts). Grading fine motor activities entails progressing from gross to precise manipulation tasks and attempting more difficult patterns of grasp and pinch. Because hand and arm control for patients with hemiplegia becomes more difficult as the arm moves away from the body, the placement of activities should be varied. Writing is a highly coordinated task that is frequently a goal for stroke patients who need at least to be able to sign documents. Training in writing may be necessary if a patient plans to use the hemiparetic hand or the uninvolved nondominant hand.

Task-Specific and Task-Oriented Interventions. In light of the range and complexity of possible motor impairments and the myriad of treatment strategies available, the occupational therapist should design treatment to fit the patient's level and interests. There is growing evidence that intervention strategies providing context-relevant, meaningful engagement in activities are more beneficial for skill acquisition than rote exercise or passive modalities (Winstein et al., 2004). Task-specific training is aimed at improving component skills of selected tasks through goal-directed practice and repetition, such as using hand muscles to practice gripping a fork for feeding. An example of task-oriented training is a patient simulating a useful or familiar activity such as using a spoon to transfer dried beans from one container to another. Occupational engagement, such as a patient using a hemiparetic arm to eat a meal at home, involves the greatest degree of patient self-choice, motivation, and meaning (AOTA, 2008), although therapists must judge adaptations necessary to allow patients to succeed. Trombly and Wu (1999) found that

providing a meaningful object within a functional context during treatment (e.g., reaching for food on a plate) leads to improved performance over exercise or reaching for a neutral target. Similarly, Fasoli et al. (2002) found that, during functional reaching tasks, instructions focused on specific movements (e.g., "straighten your elbow") resulted in slower, less forceful reach than instructions focused on the task (e.g., "think about the size, shape, and weight of the water bottle you are reaching for") in samples of adults with and without CVA.

Therapists should review the wide range of possible functions of the upper extremity to select activities patients can succeed in. Patients who have limited arm movement or no voluntary hand movement can practice nonmanipulatory activities such as actively positioning the weaker arm for safety, bed mobility, or self-care and weight bearing on forearm or hand for support or to stabilize objects. If minimal hand movement is available, patients can hold objects in a static grasp (such as holding a washrag to wash the unaffected arm) and, as able, attempt varying reach-grasp-carry-release activities, graded for different positions of shoulder, elbow, and forearm and for different grasp and pinch patterns. Some patients may be able to work toward isolated finger movements and advanced manipulative skills, such as dialing a touch tone phone or keyboarding.

Constraint-Induced Movement Therapy. It is important to promote functional use of the involved upper extremity early and consistently because patients tend to have difficulty translating limited upper extremity movement into functional use. They often report that their arm is "dead" or "useless" despite sufficient arm movement for simple activities. Movement may return spontaneously, but it appears that function or purposeful use of the arm is enhanced with therapeutic intervention and practice (Blanton & Wolf, 1999). Based on studies involving both animal and human subjects, Taub et al. (1993) described the phenomenon of learned nonuse: the person with hemiparesis notices negative consequences of efforts to use the affected limb that are reinforced by successful compensatory use of the unaffected limb (Blanton & Wolf, 1999). Constraint-induced movement therapy (CIMT), is a well-studied and evidence-based intervention developed to counteract the effects of learned nonuse in stroke survivors who exhibit specific motor criteria (Fig. 33-4). In a comparative clinical study, Taub et al. (1993) restrained the unaffected upper extremity of chronic stroke patients (at least 1 year postonset) in a sling during waking hours for 2 weeks. This group also participated in sessions of intensive practice of functional tasks with the impaired arm. A comparison group was given activities designed to encourage use of the impaired arm but without practice and without restraint of the unimpaired arm. The restraint subjects showed greater improvement on measurements

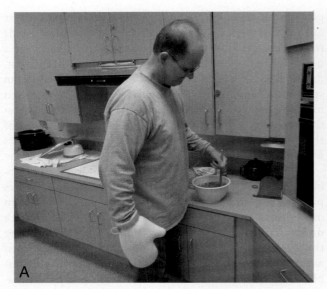 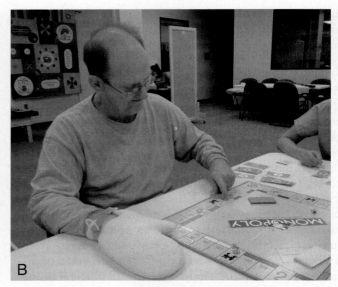

Figure 33-4 Constraint-induced movement therapy. **A.** Stirring brownie mix. **B.** Playing a board game with involved upper extremity while noninvolved hand is restrained.

of motor function than the control group and showed carryover of this function to life tasks and maintenance of gains during a 2-year follow-up period. Dromerick, Edwards, and Hahn (2000) found that CIMT could be implemented during acute rehabilitation (1–2 weeks after stroke) with resulting improvement in involved arm function at the end of 14 days of treatment. This study suggests that preventing or minimizing learned nonuse with early intervention is preferable to extinguishing learned behaviors. The Extremity Constraint-Induced Therapy Evaluation (EXCITE) trials, a series of multisite, randomized, prospective, single-blind clinical studies including 222 poststroke subjects who met standard CIMT criteria, have strengthened the evidence that this intervention is effective in improving arm and hand function in stroke survivors 3–9 months poststroke (Wolf et al., 2006), that achievements gained from CIMT are maintained 2 years after intervention (Wolf, et al., 2008), and that CIMT is effective for chronic stroke in individuals 15–21 months poststroke (Wolf et al., 2010).

In order to participate in standard CIMT protocols, patients must meet minimal voluntary movement requirements, including the ability to initiate 20° or more of wrist extension and 10° or more of finger extension. As a result, benefits from this treatment are limited to those with less severe motor involvement, or approximately 20%–25% of patients with chronic stroke (Blanton & Wolf, 1999). CIMT is difficult to implement in clinical practice because the standard protocol includes 6-hour sessions of functionally oriented task practice with the paretic arm and hand for 5 days a week for 2 weeks. In addition, the uninvolved arm is physically restrained in a sling or hand mitt during 90% of waking hours. Other problems

limiting the application of CIMT techniques include poor compliance with patient restraint schedules, concerns over safety and limitations on independence caused by the restrictive device, lack of facility resources to provide intensive training sessions, and concerns about reimbursement (Page et al., 2008). In response to these limitations, Page et al. (2004) described a modified constraint-induced movement therapy (mCIMT) for outpatients that combines involving the affected arm in functional tasks during structured 30-minute sessions three times a week with restraint of the unaffected arm every weekday for 5 hours. Subsequent studies have indicated that mCIMT is as effective as CIMT in increasing hemiparetic arm use and function (Page et al., 2008)

Although "the collective body of research about CIMT and its various adaptations provides direct support for the essential OT tenet that opportunities for practice within the natural context of activity engagement are critical and necessary for improving motor skill" (Sabari & Lieberman, 2008, p. 55), more research is needed to identify the most beneficial factors of treatment, dose-response relationships, and kinematic outcomes. Studies of CIMT efficacy have included other commonly used OT interventions, such as massed practice, shaping, functional activities, client-centered approach, home programs, and preparatory modalities without determining the separate effects of each (Hayner, Gibson, & Giles, 2010). Some studies have concluded that treatment intensity rather than constraint of the less involved extremity may account for improved outcomes (Dobkin, 2007; Uswatte et al., 2006). Massie et al. (2009) suggest that CIMT may encourage patients to rely on common compensatory and/or synergy-dominated movement rather than promote more normal movement patterns.

Emerging Techniques and Technologies. The proliferation of novel stroke rehabilitation treatment techniques and technologies in recent years has resulted from growing evidence of neuroplasticity in response to movement therapy, and efforts to improve functional outcomes in the face of increased health care costs and decreased access to rehabilitation services (Fasoli, 2011). Clinicians should explore new approaches and adopt interventions that show evidence of enhancing patients' occupation and participation in more efficient, economical ways. Some of these interventions are used clinically to assist those patients with moderate to severe motor impairments who would not be able to participate in repetitive task-specific or task-oriented therapies, such as CIMT. Others are used to increase the opportunities for repetitive task training in the face of reduced therapy allowances.

- Neuromuscular Electrical Stimulation (NMES)—NMES has been used as an adjunct to poststroke upper extremity rehabilitation to reduce shoulder subluxation and pain, and improve movement and function of the arm. Hsu et al. (2010) found that both higher and lower doses of NMES combined with standard inpatient stroke rehabilitation improved motor recovery for subjects with severe motor deficits of the upper extremity. A systematic review of interventions for upper extremity hemiparesis (Urton et al., 2007) concluded that NMES can be used to improve outcomes of patients with moderate to severe arm deficits and is feasible for home-based use (see Chapter 18).

- Mental Practice/Imagery—Mental practice is a training method increasingly examined as an adjunct for use in stroke rehabilitation that involves the use of motor imagery to rehearse a motor skill without actual physical movement (Nilsen, Gillen, & Gordon, 2010). Page, Levine, and Hill (2007) have suggested that mental practice can be an effective pathway whereby patients with upper extremity hemiparesis can qualify for mCIMT and achieve increased functional gains. A systematic review concluded that mental practice in poststroke rehabilitation appears promising, but more research is required to guide therapists in its use to improve occupational performance (Nilsen, Gillen, & Gordon, 2010).

- Robot-assisted therapy—Many robotic devices for use in neurorehabilitation have been developed in both laboratory and clinical settings. In general, a patient's hemiparetic arm is placed on a handle or support that allows passive, assisted, or graded task-oriented movement. Although currently cost-prohibitive in most clinical settings, robot-assisted therapy allows patients who are unable to independently perform task-specific or task-oriented movements the benefits of intense, repetitive practice greater than possible with one-on-one therapy (Sabari & Lieberman, 2008). A systematic review of the effects of robot-assisted therapy on upper limb recovery after stroke (Kwakkel et al., 2008) found marked variability in studies between distal and proximal arm robotics, although subsequent sensitivity analysis showed significant improvement in upper arm motor function. Future research is needed to better define the effects of robotics on functional outcomes. For more information, see Fasoli (2011) and Pignolo (2009).

- Virtual reality (VR)—The use of computer technology and "off-the-shelf" gaming consoles (such as Nintendo Wii) to simulate real-world activities and objects is a recent approach to enhance the effects of repetitive task training on stroke upper extremity rehabilitation. VR has the advantage of offering an interactive, highly motivating intervention that can be individualized to offer practice of functional tasks at a greater intensity than traditional therapy. Research is limited, but preliminary studies suggest that VR has promise as an additional tool for improving upper extremity movement and function poststroke (Joo et al., 2010; Saposnik et al., 2010).

- Mirror therapy—In this form of visual feedback, a mirror is placed vertically close to the midline of a patient seated at a table. As the involved arm is placed behind the mirror and the noninvolved arm is positioned in front of the mirror, the patient is instructed to watch the noninvolved arm in the mirror while attempting movements with both arms. The patient thereby receives the visual impression that the affected limb (the limb in the mirror) is functioning normally (Albert & Kesselring, 2011). Although data are limited, two randomized trials have found improved hemiparetic hand function in subjects receiving mirror therapy (Dohle et al., 2009; Yavuzer et al., 2008).

- Orthotic-aided therapy—Two examples of commercial orthotics used for upper extremity neurorehabilitation in OT clinics are a neuroprosthetic device and a dynamic spring-loaded orthosis. The neuroprosthetic device (Bioness H-200: Bioness Inc., Valencia, CA) is a forearm-hand molded orthosis providing functional electrical stimulation for muscle retraining, specifically to elicit active grasp and release in the hemiparetic hand. Although the high cost of this device limits its use, an advantage is that it allows arm support and facilitation without a therapist's physical assistance. Two studies (Alon, Levitt, & McCarthy, 2008; Hill-Hermann et al., 2008) have reported clinically meaningful outcomes in patients participating in this technique. The SaeboFlex (Saebo, Inc., Charlotte, NC) is a mechanical dynamic orthosis that positions the hemiparetic hand so that active finger flexion can be used for grasp and then assists release. A preliminary study on the clinical effectiveness of this device (Farrell et al., 2007) suggests that the SaeboFlex may be an affordable tool for repetitive motor training for individuals with moderate arm movement impairment after stroke who may not be eligible for other treatments such as CIMT (Fasoli, 2011).

Motor Learning Ability. Because occupational therapists mainly teach skills, they must address the learning process to help patients improve occupational performance and participation. Even the most familiar tasks, such as dressing, require adapting to a variety of circumstances or contexts. Therapists can best assist patients with stroke by helping them develop their own problem-solving techniques and strategies to deal with their environment.

Visual Dysfunction. Chapter 23 describes treatment for patients with visual deficits. In general, therapists can employ either of two basic intervention approaches for patients with visual problems following stroke, determined by the extent of visual impairment and a patient's intact capabilities: (1) establish or restore the person's performance skills or (2) modify the context of the activity and/or environment (Warren, 2009). With the first approach, the goal of therapy might be to improve a patient's visual scanning ability using functional activities to increase the speed and accuracy of visual search to the area of the VFD or by training in the compensatory skill of turning the head to the left. Examples of the second approach include simplifying activity demands, such as locating all items needed for grooming in one drawer; simplifying task sequence, such as installing a speed dial feature on a phone; or altering the built environment to eliminate clutter and obstacles (Warren, 2009).

Although research is limited, there is evidence for using visual scanning interventions to improve the efficiency and effectiveness of visual search in clients with VFDs (Pambakian et al., 2004). This study and others suggest that visual-perceptual deficits following stroke must be confronted, and patients must be taught to recognize their deficits for treatment to be effective. Sharing results of objective evaluations with the patient and family, giving feedback on the effects of visual deficits on functional performance, and teaching patients to recognize and correct errors in performance have been suggested as techniques for increasing a patient's awareness of his or her deficits.

Studies of the effects of visual training skills on unilateral neglect (Cherney, Halper, & Papachronis, 2003; Tham et al., 2001) indicate that treatment involving forced awareness of neglected space, task-specific practice, and use of consistent strategies to accomplish functional activities improve cognitive-perceptual abilities after stroke. To ensure transfer of training, Toglia (1991) recommended a multicontext approach of practicing strategies in multiple environments with varied tasks and component demands. Therapists, for example, can provide a stronger learning event by reinforcing a visual searching task (finding all the forks in a dishwasher bin) with touching and moving the targets (picking up the forks and putting them in the correct space in a drawer). Training must be specific to the individual's deficits and goals for occupational

functioning; a patient with hemianopsia and/or unilateral visual neglect with a goal of achieving safe wheelchair propulsion will benefit more from specific environmental scanning activities in a wheelchair (obstacle courses or grocery shopping) than from paper and pencil or computer activities.

Speech and Language Disorders. Occupational therapists should work closely with speech-language pathologists to contribute to a patient's improvement in speech and language functioning. Therapists can promote proper posture to aid respiration and eye contact important to speech. Therapy sessions also provide a social context supportive of communication and opportunities for practice of speech/language skills. Whenever possible, therapists should incorporate speech and language goals into their treatment sessions, such as requiring verbal responses (counting repetitions of an activity or naming objects used) or addressing functional reading and writing tasks (reading signs and recipes or writing checks). Occupational therapists can assist in selecting and adapting a nonverbal form of communication for a patient, such as writing, drawing, use of a communication board, and gestures. Suggestions for working with patients with aphasia and their families include the following (American Heart Association, 1994):

- Avoid unnecessary noise: turn off the television, find a quiet space.
- Do not speak to the patient or request speech when he or she is engaged in a physical activity.
- Allow enough time for the patient to respond; do not rush or force communication; do not switch topics quickly.
- Never assume that the person with aphasia cannot understand what is being said; never allow others to ignore the person with aphasia.
- Speak slowly and clearly using simple, concise language; do not speak loudly unless hearing is impaired; do not talk down as if to a child.
- Use demonstration, visual cues, and gestures as needed to help with comprehension.

Motor Planning Deficits. Motor planning deficits, or apraxia, are serious learning disorders and among the most difficult to rehabilitate. The emphasis of treatment is on teaching compensatory skills during ADL with focus on which stage(s) of motor planning present the most difficulty for a client: initiation of a task, execution of the plan, or control of activity to achieve adequate result (van Heugten et al., 1998). Suggestions for treatment include strategy training for specific ADL, sensory/proprioceptive stimulation, manually guided movement, cueing and prompting, repetitive graded use of objects and contexts to evoke more automatic responses, forward or backward chaining, and practicing activities as closely as possible to the patient's usual context or routine (West et al., 2008). A Cochrane Collaboration study (West et al., 2008) reviewed the few randomized controlled trials of therapeutic intervention for motor apraxia in stroke and found small short-term clinical effects in two studies.

Cognitive Deficits. Treatment to optimize cognitive abilities is discussed in Chapter 24. As in other areas of dysfunction, treatment for cognitive problems after stroke can include retraining of specific component skills, teaching compensation techniques or substitution of intact abilities, and adaptation of the environment. Examples of treatment techniques include using prompts or cues to shape desired behavior; providing feedback on performance with suggestions and strategies for improvement; providing visual aids, such as memory logs, checklists, maps, or diagrams for deficits of memory, sequencing, or organization; and simplifying the environment and grading tasks for patients with attention deficits. Caregivers must be educated regarding recommended adaptations, safety precautions, and the need for supervision (refer to Safety Note 33-1).

Interventions aimed at the role performance/participation level appear to have a greater impact on an individual's quality of life than approaches stressing only impairment or activity restriction (Gillen & Rubio, 2011). A comprehensive review of evidence-based literature on cognitive remediation for stroke (Cicerone et al., 2000) reveals limited support for remediation of attention and memory deficits and executive function and problem-solving difficulties in stroke patients. Henshaw et al. (2011) have begun preliminary investigation of a cognitive task-specific training program to improve participation after stroke.

Psychosocial Adjustment. Patients and families usually need assistance in making healthy emotional adjustments after stroke. It may be unreasonable to expect full participation in treatment programs when patients and their families are coping poorly with the losses associated with stroke. Patients typically employ hope and determination to cope with hospitalization, the hard work of rehabilitation, and changes in body image, but many cling to the belief that they will be "normal" again (Sabari, 1998). Therapists should reinforce the efforts of the rehabilitation team and encourage patients and families to talk about their reactions to stroke and their comprehension of its progression and prognosis. In light of the shortening time frames for rehabilitation, therapists should make sure patients and families understand that recovery from stroke does not end with discharge from a hospital or rehabilitation program. Therapists should also help patients and families to realize that the ultimate goal of rehabilitation is not complete recovery from physical and intellectual impairments but the ability to resume valued life roles.

Therapists should recognize the signs and symptoms of depression and inform appropriate team members if treatment has not been initiated. For the patient with emotional lability, both patient and family need to be reassured that lability is a symptom of the stroke. Helping patients and families develop coping strategies, including problem-solving strategies, social support, information seeking, and engagement in activities, helps decrease the impact of psychological distress (Falk-Kessler, 2011). Because community support is reported to buffer the effects of disability on stroke survivors and their caregivers (Duncan et al., 2005), therapists should strive to provide opportunities for patients to participate in the community. Group activities, social interactions, and community outings are important methods for allowing a patient to practice roles from before the stroke and to realize that the patient role is a temporary transition to getting on with life despite residual impairments.

Transition to the Community

"Living with disabilities after a stroke is a lifelong challenge during which people continue to seek and find ways to compensate for or adapt to persisting neurological deficits. For many stroke survivors and their families, the real work of recovery begins after formal rehabilitation" (Duncan et al., 2005, p. 135).

Discharge Planning

Discharge planning takes place throughout the rehabilitation phase. Successful planning allows the patient and family to feel comfortable with the decisions made for discharge, feel capable of maintaining gains and continuing progress without the intense level of support provided by rehabilitation specialists, and feel able to monitor for changes requiring adjustments or further intervention. Occupational therapists assist in identifying the most appropriate discharge setting; training the patient, family, and caregiver in essential skills; and arranging for continuity of care with community services. Factors determining discharge setting include patient's and family's preferences, level of patient's disabilities, level of caregiver's support, and safety and accessibility of the home (Gresham et al., 1995). Often, a patient with a fairly high level of physical functioning cannot return home because there is no caregiver or the residence is unsafe or inaccessible, whereas a more disabled patient can return home because a healthy spouse is willing to assume the role of caregiver and the residence is safe and accessible. Therapists perform a major role by participating with patients and families in home visits and safety assessments and recommending necessary home alterations or adaptive equipment.

Patient, Family, and Caregiver Education

Ideally, every treatment session is an opportunity to teach the patient, family, or caregiver techniques and problem-solving strategies for use after rehabilitation. Because learning styles vary and repetition is important for learning, patients and their families are best served by a combination of demonstration, experiential sessions, and written instructions. Caregivers should demonstrate, rather than simply verbalize, their ability to assist the patient safely and independently. At the time of discharge from a rehabilitation program, patients and their families are often overwhelmed with information from several disciplines that they must try to assimilate. After formal therapy sessions have ended, many patients and caregivers report good intentions of following home programs as prescribed but admit that the routine of daily activity leaves little time or energy for carrying out therapeutic recommendations at home. The most effective home programs therefore are those that incorporate treatment for impairments into self-care, IADL, and leisure routines. For example: "Before bathing or dressing, briefly perform the following stretching movements to get the best posture and arm movement for these tasks" is more likely to be continued at home than: "Perform the following exercises, 10 repetitions each, at least twice a day." Home programs should, of course, be individualized and should remind the patient of skills already mastered, of skills the patient can reasonably expect to gain, and of possible problems common to stroke. Patients and families should be well informed of sources for information or assistance as new capabilities or problems evolve. Fall prevention is a necessary component of the home program and should encourage greater independence in mobility while identifying and reducing the risks of falls (Gresham et al., 1995).

Resuming Valued Roles and Tasks

Although most individuals who have had stroke regain functional abilities such as walking and self-care, this does not always mean that an individual will be able to successfully participate in the community (Beckley, 2006). A study of long-term occupational engagement of community-dwelling stroke survivors (White et al., 2008) found that altered occupation and role loss persisted up to 5 years after stroke, regardless of disability levels. These findings support other studies that suggest the need for occupational therapists to expand rehabilitation services into the community and to look beyond an emphasis on basic self-care skills to more complex occupations necessary for resuming or adapting work, family, and community roles (White et al., 2008; Wolf, Baum, & Connor, 2009).

Work. For patients who expect to resume working, prevocational or vocational evaluation and appropriate work-readiness training should be encouraged (see Chapter 28).

Although this area is not emphasized in most stroke rehabilitation programs (Wolf, Baum, & Connor, 2009), return to paid employment is a significant indicator of recovery for many following stroke, especially considering over one-third of stroke survivors are under the age of 65 years, and greater numbers of Americans are working beyond retirement age (Hartke, Trierweiler, & Bode, 2011). A literature review (Treger et al., 2007) examining return to work following stroke found that between 19% and 73% of the patients were able to return to work. The wide variability seen in return to work is explained by the diversity of sample populations and differences in defining work. A smaller percentage of patients were able to resume full-time competitive employment, and a greater percentage returned to part-time or home-based work. Those able to return to work reported significantly higher levels of subjective life satisfaction (Vestling, Tufvesson, & Iwarsson, 2003). The factors generally found to relate positively to return to work included independence in self-care, ability to walk, younger age, high educational and occupational levels, stable marital status, and preserved language and cognitive capacities, whereas the most significant negative predictor is greater severity of stroke (Treger et al., 2007; Vestling, Tufvesson, & Iwarsson, 2003). Treger et al. (2007) noted that the results of this quantitative research have done little to inform us about effective interventions for assisting poststroke clients resume employment. In their qualitative study, Hartke, Trierweiler, and Bode (2011) suggest that interventions to address return to work must focus on the individual (e.g., adjustment to disability), work (physical and psychological demands of a client's job), and community (e.g., access to transportation)—emphasizing the person-environment-occupation fit rather than impairments after stroke.

Leisure and Recreation. Throughout rehabilitation, valued leisure activities should be identified, encouraged, and enabled. Leisure participation has increasingly been included as an important factor in preventing health decline and isolation poststroke (Bhogal et al., 2003). Effective therapy incorporates leisure interests into treatment so that the patient recovering from stroke can begin to analyze the effects of impairments on valued activities and anticipate strategies for return to these activities. A study of 40 individuals discharged from rehabilitation programs poststroke found factors influencing leisure participation include family and social support, transportation or financial barriers, attitudes toward altered leisure performance, amount of free time available and number of leisure interests (Jongbloed & Morgan, 1991). Many patients following stroke report decreased energy, motivation, or time for leisure pursuits because of fatigue, depression, and/or the increased demands of self-care. Many do not accept performance of a valued activity at a lower standard; for example, a patient with hemiparesis may give up golf rather than play at a reduced level of performance. Many patients, particularly those who were working at the time of their stroke, do not have established leisure roles or do not admit to any leisure interests. A randomized controlled trial by Desrosiers et al. (2007) evaluated the effect of a home-based leisure education program following stroke that included leisure awareness and self-awareness (exploration of new leisure activities suitable for a patient's interests and abilities) and competency development (finding ways to overcome physical barriers in the home or community in order to adapt or adopt a valued activity). The study found positive effects for leisure participation, leisure satisfaction, and reduced depression.

Sexuality. Surveys of patients and their spouses show that typical effects of stroke on sexuality include decreased libido, impaired erectile functioning in men, decreased vaginal lubrication in women, and decreased frequency of sexual activity (National Stroke Association, 2006). Causes may be physiological (decreased motor, sensory, or cognitive functioning; dependency in ADL; decreased endurance; incontinence; coexisting disease; or side effects of medications) or psychosocial (poor self-image, depression, role changes, impaired communication ability, fear of impotence, or fear of recurring stroke) (Farman & Friedman, 2011; National Stroke Association, 2006).

To assist with sexual expression, all therapists can impart the message that patients are permitted to have concerns and seek information about sexual problems after stroke. Therapists should reassure their clients that these problems are common and that sexual activity after stroke is not contraindicated (Duncan et al., 2005). Other possible interventions include providing or referring to resources to increase the patient's knowledge, encouraging open communication between partners, suggesting adaptations such as changes in positioning or timing, and referring to a qualified specialist (Duncan et al., 2005; Farman & Friedman, 2011).

Driving. Nearly all adults in the United States drive (Warren, 1999), so the ability to resume driving is a high priority for most individuals with stroke and is seen as a way to continue community independence and avoid isolation. Improved survival rates and longevity after stroke increase the need for health professionals to make recommendations regarding a patient's ability to drive (Korner-Bitensky et al., 2006). Because of its complexity and danger, driving after stroke is usually not addressed until a patient has returned home and gained a satisfactory level of independence with self-care, IADL, and short-distance mobility. It has been reported that only 30% of those who drove before stroke are able to resume driving, and 87% of those who drove before stroke did not receive any form of driving evaluation (Fisk, Owsley,

& Pulley, 1997). Although it is not known with certainty which factors are associated with return to driving, earlier studies identify younger age, higher functional status, and higher scores on visual attention tasks as predictive of ability to resume driving, whereas a recent multicenter cohort study suggests that clients with ischemic strokes versus hemorrhagic stroke and those with higher levels of strength, motor activity, and cognition at 3 months poststroke are more likely to be able to resume driving at 1 year poststroke (Perrier, Korner-Bitensky, & Mayo, 2010). Hemiparesis alone does not appear to prevent a return to driving because vehicles or techniques can be adapted to compensate for most motor deficits seen poststroke. A study by Elgin et al. (2010) found that some clients with hemianopsia (without neglect) given a standardized on-road evaluation demonstrated performance ratings similar to those of persons with normal visual fields. There are no standard evaluation procedures for determining the ability of cerebrally injured patients to return to driving, but consistent practices include (1) a predriving evaluation battery to test for visual scanning, visual attention, higher level visual-cognitive skills, distractibility, mental slowness, problem solving, and ability to follow directions; (2) a driving simulator evaluation; and (3) a road test, both on a protected course and in traffic (Korner-Bitensky et al., 2006). Studies have failed to establish evidence of the accuracy of various components of predriving assessment in predicting on-road driving performance.

Few studies have substantiated the effectiveness of rehabilitation to assist patients return to driving, but two approaches used include treatment to remediate underlying impairments through retraining visual and cognitive skills and a functional approach using simulators and on-road driving lessons. Two small randomized controlled trials (Crotty & George, 2009; Devos et al., 2009) found greater improvement in the behind-the-wheel driving performance of poststroke subjects when a more contextual, functional treatment approach was taken. Crotty and George (2009), examined remediation training using the Dynavision, a device designed to address underlying motor and visual deficits such as visual scanning, peripheral visual awareness, visual attention, and visual-motor reaction time. They were unable to find an effect of this training on on-road driving perfomance. Devos et al. (2009) found that subjects who received driver simulator training showed better performance on overall on-road driving when compared with subjects in a cognitive training program. Therapists must remember that the decision to allow a person who has had a stroke to resume driving rests with the state licensing bureau (see Chapter 26).

Community Support and Resources. Methods to reintegrate the patient into the community (e.g., transportation options, dealing with architectural barriers, assistance from family or friends, and access to senior citizen centers)

should be addressed throughout rehabilitation because failure to resume premorbid community activities has been significantly correlated with isolation and depression in stroke patients (Logan, Dyas, & Gladman, 2004). Reintegration into the community, according to individuals who have had strokes, can take years rather than months (White et al., 2008), continuing after a patient has ended regular contact with rehabilitation specialists. The AHA/ASA clinical practice guidelines recommend that acute-care hospitals and rehabilitation facilities maintain current inventories of community resources, provide this information to stroke survivors and their caregivers, and offer assistance in obtaining needed services (Duncan et al., 2005). In general, supports for patients and their families include educational, instrumental, and emotional supports (Duncan et al., 2005). Educational resources are available through organizations (Resources 33-1) that offer direct audiotaped, videotaped, printed, and/or online information specific to stroke. Instrumental supports are physical assistance programs such as personal provider services, Meals on Wheels, and volunteer groups who can build wheelchair ramps. Emotional support can come from family, friends, mental health professionals, and other survivors of stroke.

Support for long-term caregivers is especially important because caregivers appear to be at substantial risk for burnout, depression, isolation, and general health problems (Duncan et al., 2005). Therapists can encourage and suggest sources for respite care, support groups, or counseling. Many communities, unfortunately, are limited in resources for the patient and family. Therapists can be advocates and consultants for the development of community programs; this can range from referring patients and families to others in the community living with stroke, to organizing a stroke club, to identifying opportunities for volunteer jobs for patients.

Postdischarge Continuity of Care. The trends toward decreasing age of people who have had stroke, greater numbers of mild to moderate severity strokes, and earlier discharges from acute centers and rehabilitation programs challenge occupational therapists to expand beyond traditional clinical management of stroke to practices that facilitate community participation. "Stroke is no longer considered an acute episode but rather a chronic condition that requires behavioral and health changes" (Wolf, Baum, & Connor, 2009, p. 625). Sabari and Lieberman (2008) refer to the long-term period after discharge from a rehabilitation program as the "stage of continuing adjustment" when stroke survivors strive to resume activity and role participation in their homes or in a supported environment such as long-term or assisted living facilities. Recommended rehabilitation practices include follow-up visits to monitor a stroke survivor's progress within 1 month of return to the community and

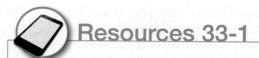

Resources 33-1

American Stroke Association (division of American Heart Association)

7272 Greenville Avenue
Dallas, TX 75231
Phone: 888-4STROKE (888-478-7653)
www.strokeassociation.org
www.heart.org

Internet Stroke Center

University of Texas Southwestern Medical Center
Department of Neurology and Neurotherapeutics
5323 Harry Hines Boulevard
Dallas, TX 75390
Phone: 214-648-3111
www.strokecenter.org

National Aphasia Association

350 Seventh Avenue, Suite 902
New York, NY 10001
Phone: 800-922-4622
www.aphasia.org

National Institute of Neurological Disorders and Stroke
National Institutes of Health Neurological Institute

P.O. Box 5801
Bethesda, MD 20824
Phone: 800-352-9424, 301-496-5751
www.ninds.nih.gov

National Stroke Association

9707 East Easter Lane, Suite B
Centennial, CO 80112
Phone: 303-649-9299; 800-STROKES (800-787-6537)
www.stroke.org

StrokEngine

McGill University
Canadian Stroke Network
http://strokengine.ca

Stroke Support Groups

Obtain listings of local stroke clubs from above websites or organizations.

at regular intervals for at least 12 months (Gresham et al., 1995). Sabari and Lieberman suggest that clients and their families may require intermittent OT services at various times after the formal stage of rehabilitation: referrals may be indicated for a home assessment after a change of living environment, for consultation after placement in a long-term care facility, for assessment/treatment for specific activity or role participation (such as return to work or driving a car), and for evidence of improvements or decreases in motor functioning that might have an impact on occupational performance.

Managed health care programs tend to focus resources on the most acute patients and on the outcomes of independence in BADL and return to home. As life expectancies increase after stroke, occupational therapists should seek improved methods of providing cost-effective community-based services to meet the continuing needs of stroke survivors to remain active and independent in their communities, to reduce the risk of secondary complications, and to enhance quality of life (Sabari & Lieberman, 2008). For example, therapists can investigate with stroke survivors alternative community resources to help promote/maintain health, such as water aerobics (Mehrholz, Kugler, & Pohl, 2011), yoga (Lynton, Kligler, & Shiflett, 2007), and Tai Chi (Taylor-Piliae & Haskell, 2007).

EFFECTIVENESS OF TREATMENT

The Occupational Therapy Practice Guidelines for Adults with Stroke (Sabari & Lieberman, 2008) stresses the importance of using scientific literature to justify the value of interventions provided to patients with stroke. This guideline states that "occupational therapy practice has expanded to unite clinical reasoning with evidence from scientific literature and client characteristics and preferences" (Sabari & Lieberman, 2008, p. 39). The guideline summarizes evidence for the efficacy of OT interventions with stroke survivors to the following broad categories:

- Neural plasticity is possible after brain lesions and is positively influenced by task-based environmental challenges.
- OT interventions are effective in remediating motor and process skills poststroke as seen by functional improvements.
- OT interventions effectively improve activity and role performance, which often leads to perceived improvement in quality of life.

Therapists have a responsibility to use this scientific evidence base when selecting evaluations and interventions rather than relying on dated professional training or clinical resources (Doucet, 2012). For example, see Evidence Table 33-1, as well as the studies cited in this chapter. Basing treatment on scientific evidence often involves giving up traditionally used methods that are not scientifically supported or adopting new evidence-based techniques. Developing evidence-based best practices for the treatment of individuals with stroke is a dynamic, ongoing process: as the body of professional literature grows and more therapists implement evidence-based practice, more data can be collected and assessed so that new practice-based evidence may emerge.

Evidence Table 33-1		Best Evidence for Occupational Therapy Practice Regarding Stroke				
Intervention	Description of Intervention Tested	Participants	Type of Best Evidence and Level of Evidence	Dosage	Benefit	Statistical Probability and Effect Size of Outcome	Reference
Task-specific practice of client-chosen BADL or IADL	Practice of specific tasks in a familiar context	Three hundred twenty-three acute stroke survivors (147 left cerebrovascular accident [LCVA], 156 right cerebrovascular accident [RCVA]); mean age = 72.5 years	Meta-analysis of two studies Level: I	Ranged from 1 to 15 visits over a period of 6 weeks to 5 months	Yes. The treated groups improved in BADL as measured by Barthel Index, and improved in IADL as measured by Nottingham EADL Scale.	Mean weighted effect size was r = 0.16, equivalent to a 16% success rate over control treatment.	Trombly & Ma (2002)
Use of cueing strategies to improve scanning function in unilateral neglect	Practice of scanning tasks with visual or motor cues	Thirteen acute stroke survivors (0 with LCVA, 13 with RCVA); mean age = 57.5 years	Randomized controlled study Level: IC1b	Twenty-one trials/day for 4 consecutive days. Order of condition randomized.	Yes. Bias Index of Line Bisection improved in all cued conditions compared with controls (strongest effect with motor cueing).	Mean effect size was r = 0.87, equivalent to a 87% success rate over control treatment.	Lin et al. (1996)
Practice of goal-directed tasks to increase voluntary active range of motion	Experimental group: use of exercise apparatus and game to increase forearm supination. Control: use of same apparatus without game	Thirty acute stroke survivors (11 with LCVA, 15 with RCVA, 4 with other); mean age = 68.4 years	Randomized controlled study Level: IC2c	Two sets of 10 trials for each condition; different days	Yes. Mean gain of 13.4° more supination (handle rotation) in experimental group.	Effect size was r = 0.42, equivalent to a 42% success rate over control treatment.	Nelson et al. (1996)
Use of goal-directed object-present activity to enhance quality of movement	Practice of reaching movement with object present or to accomplish functional goal versus reaching without object or without functional goal	Twenty-eight chronic stroke survivors (17 with LCVA, 9 with RCVA, 2 with other); mean age = 63.4 years	Meta-analysis of two studies Level I	10 trials/condition within 1 day	Yes. Better organization of reaching movement for functional goal as described by kinematic variables for speed, smoothness, strategy used, and force.	Combined effect size was r = 0.62, equivalent to a 62% success rate over control treatment.	Ma & Trombly (2002)
Use of modified constraint-induced movement therapy to reduce disability and improve use of paretic arm	Experimental groups: modified CIMT with repetitive task training; ADL tasks; constraint of nonparetic arm Control groups: traditional rehabilitation treatments included NDT, PNF, ADL compensatory techniques, task training, strengthening	Two hundred seventy-eight patients poststroke with clinical diagnosis of UE hemiparesis; mean age = 57 years; time of onset since stroke ranged from 2 days to 60 months	Meta-analysis of 13 randomized controlled trials Level I	Ranged from 30 minutes to 3 hours/day for 3–5 days/week for a total of 2 to 10 weeks For mCIMT group, restraint time of nonparetic arm ranged from 5 to 6 hours/day	Yes. mCIMT groups showed higher scores on Fugl Meyer Assessment, FIM, and Motor Activity Log than patients in traditional rehabilitation group.	For Fugl Meyer Assessment: mean difference (MD) = 7.8; (95% confidence interval [CI], 4.21–11.38; p < 0.001); r_w = 0.40.[1] For FIM: MD 57 (95% CI, 0.75–13.26; p = 0.03); r_w = 0.45.[2] For Motor Activity Log: Amount of use: MD = 1.09, 95% CI, 0.26–1.91; p = 0.01; r_w = 0.64.[3]	Shi et al. (2011)

[1]Average weighted effect size, r, based on two studies (n = 73) that reported effect size; indicates 40% greater improvement rate in motor control of the upper extremity because of CIMT as compared to traditional therapy.
[2]Average weighted effect size, r, based on all three studies (n = 88) using the FIM assessment; indicates a 45% greater improvement rate in basic ADL because of CIMT as compared to traditional therapy.
[3]Average weighted effect size, r, based on four studies (n = 135) that reported effect size; indicates a 64% greater improvement rate in use of affected upper extremity because of CIMT as compared to traditional therapy.
ADL, activities of daily living; BADL, basic activities of daily living; CIMT, constraint-induced movement therapy; FIM, functional independence measure; IADL, instrumental activities of daily living; mCIMT, modified constraint-induced movement therapy; NDT, neurodevelopmental therapy; PNF, Proprioceptive neuromuscular facilitation (See online chapter A); UE, upper extremity.

case example

Mrs. H.: Right Cerebrovascular Accident

Occupational Therapy Process	Clinical Reasoning Process	
	Objectives	**Examples of Therapist's Internal Dialogue**

Patient Information

Mrs. H. is an 82-year-old widow who lived alone, independent in activities of daily living (ADL) and instrumental activities of daily living (IADL) except for community transportation. She was found unresponsive at home by a neighbor and diagnosed with a large right middle cerebral artery infarction.

During her acute hospital stay, an occupational therapist evaluated Mrs. H. and reported inconsistent levels of awareness, no spontaneous movement on the left side, and signs of left hemianopsia and spatial neglect. Treatment consisted of involving the patient in simple self-care tasks and initiating a bed positioning and mobility program in conjunction with nursing and physical therapy to prevent secondary complications. Ten days poststroke, Mrs. H. was able to sit in a wheelchair for 1-hour periods, follow one-step commands consistently, and perform simple grooming and bed mobility tasks with minimal assistance. She was transferred to an inpatient rehabilitation unit for more intensive treatment. At the time of discharge from acute care, Mrs. H. was incontinent of bowel and bladder and had a small area of skin breakdown over her coccyx. The social worker reported that Mrs. H. had led a sedentary life and enjoyed going to church, visiting with neighbors and family, reading her Bible, and watching television. Staff reported her verbal skills, comprehension, and memory to be good, although Mrs. H. expressed frustration at her continued hospitalization and stated that she expected a full recovery and return home. Mrs. H.'s family consisted of four adult grandchildren and their families, who were unable to change their work or living situations to care full time for Mrs. H. The family was supportive and hopeful that Mrs. H. could return home with a hired care provider, although they were willing to consider skilled nursing home placement if Mrs. H. did not gain sufficient functioning to return home.

Objectives: Understand the patient's diagnosis or condition

"The large size of Mrs. H.'s lesion, persistent altered levels of consciousness, initial severe ADL dependence and motor deficits, visuospatial deficits, and incontinence all predict poor functional outcomes and lengthy recovery period. In her favor, Mrs. H. was able to live alone at home and has no significant prior medical history."

Objectives: Know the person

"Mrs. H. seems to have limited knowledge and understanding of the nature of her stroke and resulting impairments. She appears to be someone with limited experience living in a dependent role. Because she had not been a physically active person, she may fatigue easily during an intense rehabilitation program. It would not be difficult for her, however, to resume valued roles and activities from a wheelchair level, especially with supportive friends and family. The fact that her thinking skills appear intact will help Mrs. H. achieve her rehabilitation goals, but her visual-perceptual impairments will hinder learning new techniques."

Reason for Referral to Occupational Therapy

Mrs. H. was referred to occupational therapy (OT) to increase self-care independence, increase awareness of left visual spatial field, recommend proper management of the left arm, and assist in determination of optimum discharge plans. She will also be seen daily by physical therapy and periodically by speech-language pathology, social work, psychology, and therapeutic recreation.

Objectives: Appreciate the context

Develop provisional hypotheses

"I will coordinate my services closely with other disciplines to avoid patient fatigue and develop consistent strategies. I will involve family in therapy early because it seems likely that Mrs. H. will need moderate to maximum skilled care upon discharge."

Assessment Process and Results

The rehabilitation team completed the Functional Independence Measure (FIM) (Keith et al., 1987) for Mrs. H. as part of the standard care process for the unit. Mrs. H. scored a 28 (out of a possible 91) on the FIM motor score, and 30 (out of a possible 35) on the cognitive score. In areas assessed by OT, Mrs. H. required minimal (25%) assistance with eating, grooming, and upper body dressing; maximum (75%) assistance with bed bathing and toilet transfers; and total (more than 75%) assistance for lower body dressing, toileting, and tub transfers. During interview/observation of leisure skills, Mrs. H. described difficulty reading ("I think I need new glasses") and watching TV ("The picture isn't very good"). Mrs. H. was observed consistently keeping her head turned to the right and having difficulty finding or concentrating on people or objects in her left visual field.

OT assessment of component abilities and capacities revealed impaired sensation in the left arm; inconsistent minimal movement in left pectorals, internal rotators, and biceps only; and mild shoulder pain with movement above shoulder level. In addition, a screen of visual field function found significant loss of left peripheral field perception.

The speech-language pathologist reported swallowing difficulties and recommended a pureed diet with no thin liquids. Physical therapy described Mrs. H. as requiring maximum (75%) assistance to perform a scooting transfer and unable to sit unsupported, stand, or propel a wheelchair.

Consider evaluation approach and methods	"From the physical therapy assessment, I learned of Mrs. H.'s postural control deficits. It was important to observe her performance in self-care rather than rely on self-report because she seems to have limited insight into her disabilities. Although observation of ADL gave me information about her visual field and inattention problems, I will consider more in-depth testing of her visual function, perhaps portions of the Brain Injury Vision Assessment Battery for Adults (Warren, 1996) because of her desire to resume reading."
Interpret observations	"I can observe that Mrs. H.'s limited ability in lower extremity dressing, bathing, and transfers are due to her poor sitting balance and lack of mobility. Her difficulties with upper extremity dressing, grooming, and feeding are a result of decreased attention to left visual space and the left side of body. Her left side somatosensory and motor deficits and her lack of awareness of her visual problems add to her left inattention."

Occupational Therapy Problem List

- Loss of independence in basic activities of daily living (BADL)
- Loss of independence in IADL and leisure activities
- At risk for injury or complications in left arm because of lack of voluntary movement, decreased sensation, and visual-spatial neglect
- Limited insight into impairments and disabilities resulting from stroke and the predicted course of recovery

Synthesize results	"Mrs. H.'s stroke has severely reduced her ability to live independently in her home, although returning home is her discharge goal. Her degree of hemiparesis, postural instability, and neglect, along with her lack of awareness, increases her risk for secondary complications."

Occupational Therapy Goal List

Patient will be able to do the following:

- Perform feeding, grooming, and upper body dressing with supervision and minimal cueing
- Perform lower body dressing, toilet transfers, and bathing on a tub bench with moderate (50%) assistance
- Independently operate television by remote control and tape recorder for books on tape
- Maintain sitting balance on the side of bed for at least 2 minutes while engaged in upper body activity
- Properly position left arm during change of position in bed and while seated in wheelchair
- Independently perform stretching and range-of-motion activities for left hand, wrist, forearm, and elbow; perform stretching and range-of-motion activities for shoulder with moderate assistance
- Demonstrate proper techniques for positioning
- Assist with left arm mobility
- Pay attention to left visual field at least 50% of time

Develop intervention hypotheses	"I do not think Mrs. H. will be able to return to independent living, but improving basic capacities (balance, visual attention) would allow her to succeed in simple meaningful activities. Education will assist with continuity of care in a new setting and allow the patient and family to feel they can contribute to the recovery process."
Select an intervention approach	"Occupational therapy intervention will include restoration, compensation, and prevention approaches."
Consider what will occur in therapy, how often, and for how long	"I predict that Mrs. H. will progress slowly in therapy but will benefit from multidisciplinary treatment. She will need at least 2 weeks of inpatient rehabilitation. She will be seen daily in OT, twice a day for shorter periods (30 minutes) to allow rest between sessions."

Intervention

The treatment program during Mrs. H.'s 2-week inpatient rehabilitation stay consisted of (1) an activity program emphasizing BADL and IADL training to address sitting balance, transitional movements, management of left upper extremity, and attention to and scanning of the left visual field and (2) patient and family education regarding the consequences and course of recovery of stroke, safety awareness and prevention of secondary impairments, and compensatory techniques and adaptations to promote functional independence.

At discharge, Mrs. H. was able to feed herself, perform simple grooming activities, and use her television and tape recorder with setup and supervision. Status in all other ADL remained unchanged. Sitting balance remained poor, and left spatial neglect remained pronounced. Mrs. H. required maximum assistance with protection and mobilization of her left arm.

Mrs. H.'s family attended family training sessions prior to discharge and was provided with written instructions of material covered in training.

Assess the patient's comprehension	"Mrs. H. had difficulty learning new techniques for familiar activities, so she required repeated practice and reinforcement from nursing and other disciplines. Because Mrs. H. could not recognize or monitor her visual or balance impairments, interventions to improve these capacities had to rely more on external rather than internal adjustments. Mrs. H. was always pleasant and cooperative and continued to feel that soon she would get better and go home. It was disappointing that she did not gain more independence, but I feel the family understands the impact of Mrs. H.'s stroke and the probability of a lengthy recovery period."
Understand what she is doing	
Compare actual to expected performance	
Know the person	
Appreciate the context	

Next Steps

Mrs. H. was transferred to a skilled nursing facility, where she will continue occupational and physical therapy. Copies of all therapy documentation were forwarded to the center, and information was shared through phone calls.

During a conference prior to discharge, the family was informed of possible future settings for continuing care for Mrs. H. and provided with a list of home health agencies, outpatient services, and provider services.

Anticipate present and future patient concerns	"I felt it was important to talk directly to the therapists at the skilled nursing facility to discuss Mrs. H.'s unique problems. It has been less than a month since the onset of her stroke, which is too soon to determine the extent of her recovery. I have emphasized to the patient and family that transfer from the rehabilitation unit does not mean her recovery is over, but it is merely moving to a different stage. I have tried to give the patient and family as much information as possible to help them recognize signs of progress or regression so that they can be advocates to ensure that Mrs. H. receives the proper type of therapy at the proper time."
Analyze patient's comprehension	
Decide whether the patient should continue or discontinue therapy and/ or return in the future	

 Clinical Reasoning in Occupational Therapy Practice

Preventing Secondary Complications

Mrs. H. has many impairments resulting from her stroke that put her at risk for developing secondary complications. Name these impairments and possible resulting complications. Which impairments increase Mrs. H's risk of falls?

What specific therapy interventions could therapists employ to help prevent these complications? What instructions could therapists give to the patient and family to prevent complications and to prevent falls?

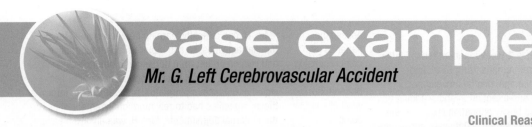

case example
Mr. G. Left Cerebrovascular Accident

Clinical Reasoning Process

Occupational Therapy Process	Objectives	Examples of Internal Dialogue
Patient Information Mr. G. is a 38-year-old man with a history of hypertension who had abrupt onset of right-sided weakness and loss of speech. He was hospitalized quickly and diagnosed with a left subarachnoid hemorrhage. He spent 9 days in acute care and 2 weeks on an inpatient rehabilitation unit before being discharged home to live with his wife and two children aged 10 and 12 years. During his hospitalization, Mr. G. made rapid progress and regained most of his speech and movement on the right side. Upon discharge, Mr. G. could perform self-care tasks, simple meal preparation, and household walking using a straight cane with supervision for increasing amounts of time. He had mild apraxia resulting in delays initiating and sequencing multistep tasks. He had decreased control of his right arm, particularly when he tried to raise it above shoulder level or attempted fine motor activities. Before his stroke, Mr. G. worked in the parts department of an automobile dealership. His job included inventory, ordering, stocking, and pickup and delivery of parts. His wife was a teacher who was home for the summer but planned to return to work when school started in 2 months.	Understand the patient's diagnosis or condition Know the person	"Mr. G.'s rapid recovery and young age predict good functional recovery. He should continue to gain independence in basic self-care, but persisting problems with higher level right arm and leg function, with higher level cognitive and communication skills, and with skilled motor planning may interfere with his participation in desired life roles." "Mr. G. was quite successful in achieving inpatient rehabilitation goals and will probably expect similar rapid progress after he returns home. He and his wife will be anxious for him to gain higher levels of function within 2 months. The early months after discharge home can be stressful and frustrating as patients encounter difficulty resuming previous roles."
Reason for Referral to Occupational Therapy Mr. G. was referred to outpatient occupational therapy to continue progress in activities of daily living (ADL) and instrumental activities of daily living (IADL) independence and to assist with resuming community roles. He was also referred for outpatient physical therapy to work on improving balance and upgrading gait and for speech therapy to improve word retrieval and higher level reading and math skills.	Appreciate the context Develop provisional hypotheses	"Home is the best place for Mr. G. to practice and refine his ADL/IADL skills. As he gains confidence at home and competence in performance skills, he will look more to resuming community roles, especially his worker/provider role."
Assessment Process and Results Mr. G.'s goals for occupational therapy were to function safely alone at home after his wife returned to work, to regain normal function of his right dominant arm, and to return to work as soon as possible. Initial outpatient assessments included the Stroke Impact Scale (Duncan et al., 1999), which allowed Mr. G. to rate how various impairments and disabilities caused by his stroke affected his quality of life. Responses to this scale and further interview revealed that Mr. G. is concerned about the continuing difficulty in using his right arm; worries about being a burden on his family and returning to work; feels foolish and inadequate because of frequent mistakes in speech, reading, writing, and math; admits that he is very slow with his daily care routine and household tasks and depends on his wife for help more than he would like; tires easily; and feels unable to participate in most previous leisure or social activities. A home assessment was completed to observe Mr. G. perform his morning bathing/dressing/grooming tasks and to assess safety risks. He took almost 2 hours to complete these tasks, needed occasional rest breaks, needed occasional physical assistance for balance, and verbal cueing for sequencing, and had difficulty with fine motor tasks such as buttoning. The Functional Test for the Hemiplegic/Paretic Upper Extremity (Wilson, Baker, & Craddock, 1984a, 1984b) was administered to determine level of functional use of his right arm (see Fig. 33-3).	Consider evaluation approach and methods Interpret observations	"I like using the Stroke Impact Scale and Functional Test for the Hemiplegic/Hemiparetic Upper Extremity because they are specific to stroke and help patients focus on functional results and appreciate that their problems are typical. These assessments are both useful for tracking progress over a long period of time." "Mr. G. is at a stage where he is beginning to experience and realize the effects of his stroke on his unique life roles. He shows good insight into his problems, and that will help him achieve or adapt his goals. His ADL deficits are due to a combination of dynamic balance problems, delays in initiation, fatigue, and decreased coordination of his right arm. He is able to use his right arm effectively as a stabilizing assist and for simple grasp and release, but he has difficulty with activities involving moving the arm above shoulder level or right-hand fine motor prehension or manipulation."

Occupational Therapy Problem List

- Requires supervision and extended time to complete bathing, grooming, and dressing
- Requires supervision and/or increased time to perform home IADL tasks (writing checks, preparing meals)
- Unable to perform tasks required for job, including using computer, lifting heavy boxes, and driving
- Unable to resume leisure activities, including bowling and coaching son's baseball team
- Difficulty using right arm for activities above shoulder level
- Unable to use right hand for fine motor prehension or manipulation tasks
- Depressed, anxious over loss of independence and role functioning and financial uncertainties

Synthesize results

"Mr. G. has shown good functional recovery in a short period of time and is working hard to readapt to his home environment. However, his deficits in higher level areas of occupation and performance skills hinder his role competence."

Occupational Therapy Goal List

- Perform morning self-care independently in 45 minutes or less
- Assume partial meal preparation and laundry tasks
- Use right arm to comb hair and to place and retrieve objects on shelf at eye level
- Use right hand to tie shoelaces, manipulate coins, sign name, and perform simple computer functions
- Participate in gross motor recreational activities with children (swimming, table tennis)
- Perform job simulation activities for 2 hours without rest break
- Complete predriving evaluation
- Be able to use community transportation independently

Develop intervention hypotheses

"I think Mr. G. will gain independence in basic activities of daily living (BADL) and limited IADL. I think he will make substantial progress in resuming valued roles, but this may take a long time, and he may need to accept modified roles."

Select an intervention approach

"Occupational therapy intervention will primarily be restorative and maintaining, with compensation/adaptation intervention used as needed."

Consider what will occur in therapy, how often, and for how long

"Because Mr. G. has a time goal (his wife's return to work), I will see him three times a week for 1 month, and then two times a week for a month."

Intervention

Treatment consisted of the following:

1. Task-specific training in ADL, IADL, and job activities. Activities were adapted, graded, and expanded as Mr. G. gained competency.
2. Repetitive task-oriented program to improve motor planning, postural adaptation, and right arm strength and control. This program was designed to be carried over to home.
3. Education concerning safety issues, home and activity adaptations, social supports, and available community resources.

Mr. G.'s wife and children attended therapy sessions at least once a week and provided valuable suggestions and encouragement for carryover of therapy in the home.

All goals were achieved at the end of 2 months. He scored significant improvements on both the Functional Test for the Hemiplegic/Paretic Upper Extremity and the Stroke Impact Scale. Mr. G. was able to demonstrate independence with written home programs addressing component skills and was able to verbalize appropriate safety precautions.

Assess the patient's comprehension

Understand what he is doing

Compare actual to expected performance

Know the person

Appreciate the context

"Mr. G. was highly motivated for therapy and was relieved to see incremental improvements. He had problems that seemed to respond best to familiar, meaningful, repetitive treatment activities. Treatment was designed to provide structure to substitute for his loss of employment, to allow him to resume alternative roles at home, and to allow him to explore the feasibility of returning to his previous job."

Next Steps

Mr. G. was scheduled for follow-up visits with his neurologist in the outpatient stroke clinic every 3 months for a year poststroke, which allowed OT a chance to contact him and monitor his progress. He was referred for behind-the-wheel driving assessment and training. He initiated application procedures for his state's vocational rehabilitation financial aid and training services. He and his wife were given the names of counseling resources to help them deal with the stresses of his continued recovery.

Anticipate present and future patient concerns	"I anticipate that Mr. G. will continue to gain competence in component skills and occupational functioning but that his rate of recovery will slow down. I am glad I will have a chance to check with him periodically to alter his home program if necessary and to determine whether he will benefit from additional therapy. Depending on the results of vocational screening, he may decide to pursue different employment that might require specific job training. Both he and his wife seem to understand that depression and fatigue are common complications of stroke."
Analyze patient's comprehension	
Decide whether the patient should continue or discontinue therapy and/ or return in the future	

Clinical Reasoning in Occupational Therapy Practice

Addressing the effects of cognitive impairments on community reintegration

Mr. G. was successful in regaining sufficient physical functioning to allow BADL skills and independence within the home but was less successful in regaining independence in IADL requiring higher level cognitive functions.

What particular cognitive deficits would interfere with Mr. G.'s ability to return to work and to resume his previous community roles? Name interventions that could address these deficits.

Summary Review Questions

1. Name the two main categories of stroke and the subtypes and causes of each.
2. Name six neurological deficits that can result from stroke and describe how each may interfere with the task of dressing.
3. What is the difference between neurological recovery and functional recovery after stroke? How might OT facilitate both types of recovery in a patient?
4. Name five settings where occupational therapists work with patients recovering from stroke, and describe the characteristics of a patient who might be treated in each setting.
5. Define postural adaptation, and name three ways impairments in this area affect occupational performance. Describe treatment methods to improve postural control.

6. What mechanical and physiological components of movement should be evaluated in the hemiplegic upper extremity? What methods can be used to prevent development of a painful shoulder?
7. What variables should be considered during evaluation for voluntary movement in the hemiplegic upper extremity?
8. What factors can affect a stroke patient's ability to learn and organize movement? Describe how deficits in each of these areas affect self-care.
9. Select a treatment activity for a patient recovering from stroke, and describe how this activity can both increase ADL independence (reduce disability) and improve component abilities and capacities (reduce impairment).
10. Describe methods to assist a poststroke patient resume valued home and community roles after discharge from rehabilitation services.

Glossary

Aphasia—Language disorder caused by brain damage that affects production and/or comprehension of written or spoken language.

Apraxia—Impairment of organized, controlled movement or motor planning not explained by motor or sensory impairment.

Hemiparesis—Weakness or partial paralysis on one side of the body caused by brain damage.

Hemiplegia—Paralysis on one side of the body caused by brain damage.

Hemorrhage—Bleeding resulting from the rupture of a blood vessel.

Homonymous hemianopsia—Visual field deficit caused by brain damage in which the patient cannot perceive half of visual field of each eye.

Ischemia—Loss of blood flow through a vessel resulting in an insufficient supply of blood and oxygen to surrounding tissues, as when a blood clot blocks a cerebral artery.

Learned nonuse—Phenomenon observed in patients with hemiparesis in which patient avoids functional use of involved arm after failed attempts to use it and successful attempts to use uninvolved arm.

Postural adaptation—Ability of body to maintain balance automatically and remain upright during alterations in position and challenges to stability.

Shoulder subluxation—Incomplete dislocation of humerus out of glenohumeral joint caused by weakness, stretch, or abnormal tone in the scapulohumeral and/or scapular muscles.

Unilateral neglect—Disturbance in the ability to notice, orient, or respond to stimuli in space on side of body opposite site of brain damage.

References

Ada, L., Foongchomcheay, A., & Canning, C. G. (2009). Supportive devices for preventing and treating subluxation of the shoulder after stroke. *Cochrane Database of Systematic Reviews,* (1), CD003863.

Ada, L., Goddard, E., McCully, J., Stavrinos, T., & Bampton, J. (2005). Thirty minutes of positioning reduces the development of shoulder external rotation contracture after stroke: A randomized controlled trial. *Archives of Physical Medicine and Rehabilitation, 86,* 230–234.

Albert, S. J., & Kesselring, J. (2011). Neurorehabilitation of stroke. *Journal of Neurology, Online First,* 1 October 2011. doi: 10.1007/s00415-011-6247-y.

Alon, G., Levitt, A. F., & McCarthy, P. A. (2008). Functional electrical stimulation (FES) may modify the poor prognosis of stroke survivors with severe motor loss of the upper extremity: A preliminary study. *American Journal of Physical Medicine and Rehabilitation, 87,* 627–636.

American Heart Association. (1994). *Caring for the person with aphasia.* Dallas: American Heart Association.

American Occupational Therapy Association. (2008). Occupational therapy practice framework: Domain and process (2nd ed.). *American Journal of Occupational Therapy, 62,* 625–683.

American Stroke Association, American Heart Association. (2011). About stroke: What are the types of stroke? Retrieved September 27, 2011 from www.strokeassociation.org/STROKEORG/AboutStroke/AboutStroke_UCM_308529_SubHomePage.jsp.

Bartels, M. N. (2011). Pathophysiology and medical management of stroke. In G. Gillen (Ed.), *Stroke rehabilitation: A function-based approach* (3rd ed., pp. 1–48). St. Louis: Mosby.

Bass-Haugen, J., Mathiowetz, V., & Flinn, N. (2008). Optimizing motor behavior using the occupational therapy task-oriented approach. In M. V. Radomski & C. A. Trombly Latham (Eds.), *Occupational therapy for physical dysfunction* (6th ed., pp. 598–617). Baltimore: Lippincott Williams & Wilkins.

Baum, C. M., Connor, L. T., Morrison, T., Hahn, M., Dromerick, A. W., & Edwards, D. F. (2008). Reliability, validity, and clinical utility of the Executive Function Performance Test: A measure of executive function in a sample of people with stroke. *American Journal of Occupational Therapy, 62,* 446–455.

Beckley, M. N. (2006). Community participation following cerebrovascular accident: Impact of the buffering model of social support. *American Journal of Occupational Therapy, 60,* 129–135.

Berg, K., Wood-Dauphinee, S., Williams, J. I., & Gayton, D. (1989). Measuring balance in the elderly: Preliminary development of an instrument. *Physiotherapy Canada, 41,* 304–311.

Bhogal, S. K., Teasell, R. W., Foley, N. C., & Speechley, M. R. (2003). Community integration after stroke. *Topics in Stroke Rehabilitation, 10,* 107–130.

Blanton, S., & Wolf, S. L. (1999). An application of upper-extremity constraint-induced movement therapy in a patient with subacute stroke. *Physical Therapy, 79,* 847–853.

Bobath, B. (1990). *Adult hemiplegia: Evaluation and treatment* (3rd ed.). London: Heinemann Medical.

Bohannon, R. W. (2007). Muscle strength and muscle training after stroke. *Journal of Rehabilitation Medicine, 39,* 14–20.

Bohannon, R. W., & Smith, M. B. (1987). Interrater reliability of a modified Ashworth scale of muscle spasticity. *Physical Therapy, 67,* 206–207.

Brott, T., Adams, H. P., Olinger, C. P., Marler, J. R., Barsan, W. G., Biller, J. Spilker, J., Holleran, R., Eberle, R., & Walker, M. (1989). Measurements of acute cerebral infarction: A clinical examination scale. *Stroke, 20,* 864–870.

Brunnstrom, S. (1970). *Movement therapy in hemiplegia.* New York: Harper & Row.

Campbell, A., Brown, A., Schildroth, C., Hastings, A., Ford-Booker, P., Lewis-Jack, O., Adams, C., Gadling, A., Ellis, R., & Wood, D. (1991). The relationship between neuropsychological measures and self-care skills in patients with cerebrovascular lesions. *Journal of the National Medical Association, 83,* 321–324.

Carey, L., Macdonell, R., & Matyas, T. A. (2011). SENSe: Study of the effectiveness of neurorehabilitation on sensation: A randomized controlled trial. *Neurorehabilitation and Neural Repair, 4,* 304–313.

Carod-Artal, F. J., Gonzales-Gutierrez, J. L., Herrero, J. A. E., Horan, T., & deSeijas, E. V. (2002). Functional recovery and instrumental activities of daily living: Follow-up 1 year after treatment in a stroke unit. *Brain Injury, 16,* 207–216.

Carr, E. K., & Kenney, F. D. (1992). Positioning of the stroke patient: A review of the literature. *International Journal of Nursing Studies, 29,* 355–369.

Carr, J. H., Shepherd, R. B., Nordholm, L., & Lynne, D. (1985). Investigation of a new motor assessment scale for stroke patients. *Physical Therapy, 65,* 175–180.

Cherney, L. R., Halper, A. S., & Papachronis, D. (2003). Two approaches to treating unilateral neglect after right hemisphere stroke: A preliminary investigation. *Topics in Stroke Rehabilitation, 9,* 22–33.

Cherney, L. R., & Small, S. L. (2009). Aphasia, apraxia of speech, and dysarthria. In J. Stein, R. L. Henry, R. F. Macko, C. J. Winstein, & R. D. Zorowitz (Eds.), *Stroke recovery and rehabilitation* (pp. 155–181). New York: Demos Medical.

Cicerone, K. D., Dahlberg, C., Kalmar, K., Langenbahn, D. M., Malec, J., F., Bergquist, T. F., Felicetti, T., Giacino, J. T., Harley, J. P., Harrington, D. E., Herzog, J., Kneipp, S., Laatsch, L., & Morse, P. A. (2000). Evidence-based cognitive rehabilitation: Recommendations for clinical practice. *Archives of Physical Medicine and Rehabilitation, 81,* 1596–1615.

Crotty, M., & George, S. (2009). Retraining visual processing skills to improve driving ability after stroke. *Archives of Physical Medicine and Rehabilitation, 90,* 2096–2102.

Davies, P. M. (2000). *Steps to follow: A guide to the treatment of adult hemiplegia* (2nd ed.). Berlin: Springer-Verlag.

deGroot, M. H., Phillips, S. J., & Eskes, G. A. (2003). Fatigue associated with stroke and other neurologic conditions: Implications for stroke rehabilitation. *Archives of Physical Medicine and Rehabilitation, 84,* 1714–1720.

Dellon, A. (1981). *Evaluation of sensibility and re-education of sensation in the hand.* Baltimore: Williams & Wilkins.

Desrosiers, J., Noreau, L., Rochette, A., Carbonneau, H., Fontaine, L., Viscogliosi, C., & Bravo, G. (2007). Effect of a home leisure education program after stroke: A randomized controlled trial. *Archives of Physical Medicine and Rehabilitation, 88,* 1095–1100.

Devos, H., Akinwuntan, A. E., Nieuwboer, A., Tant, M., Truijen, S., De Wit, L., Kiekens, C., & De Weerdt, W. (2009). Comparison of the effect of two driving retraining programs on on-road performance after stroke. *Neurorehabilitation and Neural Repair, 23,* 699–705.

Dobkin, B. H. (2005). Rehabilitation after stroke. *New England Journal of Medicine, 352,* 1677–1684.

Dobkin, B. H. (2007). Confounders in rehabilitation trials of task-oriented training: Lessons from the designs of the EXCITE and SCILT multicenter trials. *Neurorehabilitation and Neural Repair, 21,* 3–13.

Dohle, C., Pullen, J., Nakaten, A., Kust, J., Rietz, C., & Karbe, H. (2009). Mirror therapy promotes recovery from severe hemiparesis: A randomized controlled trial. *Neurorehabilitation and Neural Repair, 23,* 209–217.

Doucet, B. M. (2012). The issue is . . . Neurorehabilitation: Are we doing all that we can? *American Journal of Occupational Therapy, 66,* 488–493.

Dromerick, A. W., Edwards, D. F., & Hahn, M. (2000). Does the application of constraint-induced movement therapy during acute rehabilitation reduce arm impairment after ischemic stroke? *Stroke, 31,* 2984–2988.

Duncan, P. W., Wallace, D., Lai, S. M., Johnson, D., Embretson, S., & Laster, L. (1999). The Stroke Impact Scale Version 2.0: Evaluation of reliability, validity, and sensitivity to change. *Stroke, 30,* 2131–2140.

Duncan, P. W., Weiner, D., Chandler, J., & Studenski, S. (1990). Functional reach: A new clinical measure of balance. *Journal of Gerontology: Medical Sciences, 45,* M192–M197.

Duncan, P. W., Zorowitz, R., Bates B., Choi, J. Y., Glasberg, J. J., Graham, G. D., Katz, R. C., Lamberty, K., & Reker, D. (2005). Management of adult stroke rehabilitation care: A clinical practice guideline. *Stroke, 36,* 100–143.

Elgin, J., McGwin, G., Wood, J. M., Vaphiades, M. S., Braswell, R. A., DeCarlo, D. K., Kline, L.B., & Owsley, C. (2010). Evaluation of on-road driving in people with hemianopia and quadrantanopia. *American Journal of Occupational Therapy, 64,* 268–278.

Eriksson, M., Asplund, M. D., Glader, E. L., Norrving, B., Stegmayr, B., Terent, A., Asberg, K. H., & Wester, P. O. (2004). Self-reported depression and use of antidepressants after stroke: A national survey. *Stroke, 35,* 936–941.

Falk-Kessler, J. (2011). Psychological aspects of stroke rehabilitation. In G. Gillen (Ed.), *Stroke rehabilitation: A function-based approach* (3rd ed., pp. 49–65). St. Louis: Mosby.

Farman, J., & Friedman, J. D. (2011). Sexual function and intimacy. In G. Gillen (Ed.), *Stroke rehabilitation: A function-based approach* (3rd ed., pp. 648–664). St. Louis: Mosby.

Farrell, J. F., Hoffman, H. B., Snyder, J. L., Giuliani, C. A., & Bohannon, R. W. (2007). Orthotic aided training of the paretic upper limb in chronic stroke: Results of a phase 1 trial. *NeuroRehabilitation, 22,* 99–103.

Fasoli, S. E. (2011). Rehabilitation technologies to promote upper limb recovery after stroke. In G. Gillen (Ed.), *Stroke rehabilitation: A function-based approach* (3rd ed., pp. 280–306). St. Louis: Mosby.

Fasoli, S. E., Trombly, C. A., Tickle-Degnen, L., & Verfaellie, M. H. (2002). Effect of instructions on functional reach in persons with and without cerebrovascular accident. *American Journal of Occupational Therapy, 56,* 380–390.

Filiatrault, J., Arsenault, A. B., Dutil, E., & Bourbonnais, D. (1991). Motor function and activities of daily living assessments: A study of three tests for persons with hemiplegia. *American Journal of Occupational Therapy, 45,* 806–810.

Fisher, A. G. (1995). *Assessment of motor and process skills.* Fort Collins, CO: Three Star Press.

Fisk, F. D., Owsley, C., & Pulley, L. V. (1997). Driving after stroke: Driving exposure, advice and evaluations. *Archives of Physical Medicine and Rehabilitation, 78,* 1338–1345.

Folstein, M. F., Folstein, S. E., & McHugh, P. R. (1975). Mini-mental State: A practical method for grading the cognitive state of patients for the clinician. *Journal of Psychiatric Research, 12,* 189–198.

Forster, A., Smith, J., Young, J., Knapp, P., House, A., & Wright, J. (2001). Information provision for stroke patients and their caregivers. *Cochrane Database of Systematic Reviews, (3),* CD001919.

Fugl-Meyer, A. R., Jaasko, L., Leyman, I., Olsson, S., & Steglind, S. (1975). The post-stroke hemiplegic patient: I. A method for evaluation of physical performance. *Scandinavian Journal of Rehabilitation Medicine, 7,* 13–31.

Gillen, G. (2011a). Trunk control: Supporting functional independence. In G. Gillen (Ed.), *Stroke rehabilitation: A function-based approach* (3rd ed., pp. 156–188). St. Louis: Mosby.

Gillen, G. (2011b). Upper extremity function and management. In G. Gillen (Ed.), *Stroke rehabilitation: A function-based approach* (3rd ed., pp. 218–279). St. Louis: Mosby.

Gillen, G., & Rubio, K. B. (2011). Treatment of cognitive-perceptual deficits: A function-based approach. In G. Gillen (Ed.), *Stroke rehabilitation: A function-based approach* (3rd ed., pp. 501–533). St. Louis: Mosby.

Goodglass, H. (1993). *Understanding aphasia.* San Diego: Academic Press, Inc.

Gresham, G. E., Duncan, P. E., Stason, W. B., Adams, H. P., Adelman, A. M., Alexander, D. N., Bishop, D. S., Diller, L., Donaldson, N. E., Granger, C. V., Holland, A. L., Kelly-Hayes, M., McDowell, F. H., Myers, L., Phipps, M. A., Roth, E. J., Siebens, H. C., Tarvin, G. A., & Trombly, C. A. (1995). *Post-stroke rehabilitation. Clinical Practice Guideline 16* (AHCPR Publication 95-0662). Rockville, MD: U.S. Agency for Health Care Policy and Research.

Harris, J. E., & Eng, J. J. (2007). Paretic upper-limb strength best explains arm activity in people with stroke. *Physical Therapy, 87,* 88–97.

Harris, J. E., & Eng, J. J. (2010). Strength training improves upper-limb function in individuals with stroke. *Stroke, 41,* 136–140.

Hartke, R. J., Trierweiler, R., & Bode, R. (2011). Critical factors related to return to work after stroke: A qualitative study. *Topics in Stroke Rehabilitation, 14,* 341–351.

Hayner, K., Gibson, G., & Giles, G. M. (2010). Research Scholars Initiative: Comparison of constraint-induced movement therapy and bilateral treatment of equal intensity in people with chronic upper-extremity dysfunction after cerebrovascular accident. *American Journal of Occupational Therapy, 64,* 528–539.

Henshaw, E., Polatajko, H., McEwen, S., Ryan, J. D., & Baum, C. (2011). Cognitive approach to improving participation after stroke: Two case studies. *American Journal of Occupational Therapy, 65,* 55–63.

Hill-Hermann, V., Strasser, A., Albers, B., Schofield, K., Dunning, K., Levine, P., & Page, S. J. (2008). Task-specific, patient-driven neuro-prosthesis training in chronic stroke: Results of a 3-week clinical study. *American Journal of Occupational Therapy, 62,* 466–472.

Holbrook, M., & Skilbeck, C. E. (1983). An activities index for use with stroke patients. *Age and Ageing, 12,* 166–170.

Hsu, S. S., Hu, M. H., Wang, Y. H., Yip, P. K., Chiu, J. W., & Hsieh, C. L. (2010). Dose-response relation between neuromuscular electrical stimulation and upper-extremity function in patients with stroke. *Stroke, 41,* 821–824.

Jongbloed, L., & Morgan, D. (1991). An investigation of involvement in leisure activities after a stroke. *American Journal of Occupational Therapy, 45,* 420–427.

Joo, L. Y., Yin, T. S., Xu, D., Thia, E., Chia, P. F., Kuah, C. W., & Kong, K.-H. (2010). A feasibility study using interactive commercial off-the-shelf computer gaming in upper limb rehabilitation in patients after stroke. *Journal of Rehabilitation Medicine, 42,* 437–441.

Kashihara, L., Nakao, S., Kawasaki, J., Takata, S., Nagahiro, S., Kaji, R., & Yasui, N. (2011). Long-term outcome of severe stroke patients: Is the ADL status at discharge from a stroke center indicative of the long-term outcome? *Journal of Medical Investigation, 58,* 227–234.

Kasner, S. E. (2006). Clinical interpretation and use of stroke scales. *Lancet Neurology, 5,* 603–612.

Keith, R. A., Granger, C. V., Hamilton, B. B., & Sherwin, F. S. (1987). The Functional Independence Measure: A new tool for rehabilitation. In M. G. Eisenberg & R. C. Grzesiak (Eds.), *Advances in clinical rehabilitation* (Vol. 2, pp. 6–18). New York: Springer.

Kelly-Hayes, M., Beiser, A., Kase, C. S., Scaramucci, A., D'Agostino, R. B., & Wolf, P. A. (2003). The influence of gender and age on disability following ischemic stroke: The Framingham study. *Journal of Stroke and Cerebrovascular Diseases, 12,* 119–126.

Khan, S., Leung, E., & Jay, W. M. (2008). Stroke and visual rehabilitation. *Topics in Stroke Rehabilitation, 15,* 27–36.

Kluding, P., & Billinger, S. A. (2005). Exercise-induced changes of the upper extremity in chronic stroke. *Topics in Stroke Rehabilitation, 12,* 58–69.

Kopp, B., Kunkel, A., Flor, H., Platz, T., Rose, U., Maurtiz, K. H., Gresser, K., McCulloch, K. L., & Taub, E. (1997). The Arm Motor Ability Test: Reliability, validity, and sensitivity to change of an instrument for assessing disabilities in activities of daily living. *Archives of Physical Medicine and Rehabilitation, 78,* 615–620.

Korner-Bitensky, N., Bitensky, J., Sofer, S., Man-Son-Hing, M., & Gelinas, I. (2006). Driving evaluation practices of clinicians working in the United States and Canada. *American Journal of Occupational Therapy, 60,* 428–434.

Kumar, R., Metter, E. J., Mehta, A. J., & Chew, T. (1990). Shoulder pain in hemiplegia: The role of exercise. *American Journal of Physical Medicine and Rehabilitation, 69,* 205–208.

Kwakkel, G., Boudewijn, J., Kollen, B. J., & Krebs, H. I. (2008). Effects of robot-assisted therapy on upper limb recovery after stroke: A systematic review. *Neurorehabilitation and Neural Repair, 22,* 111–122.

Lai, S.-M., Studenski, S., Duncan, P. W., & Perera, S. (2002). Persisting consequences of stroke measured by the Stroke Impact Scale. *Stroke, 33,* 1840–1844.

Langhorne, P., Stott, D. J., Robertson, L., MacDonald, J., Jones, L., McAlpine, C., Dick, F., Taylor, G. S., & Murray, G. (2000). Medical complications after stroke: A multicenter study. *Stroke, 31,* 1223–1229.

Langton Hewer, R. (1990). Rehabilitation after stroke. *Quarterly Journal of Medicine, 76,* 659–674.

Lannin, N. A., Cusick, A., McCluskey, A., & Herbert, R. D. (2007). Effects of splinting on wrist contracture after stroke: A randomized controlled trial. *Stroke, 38,* 111–116.

Law, M., Baptiste, S., Carswell, A., McColl, M., Polatajko, H., & Pollock, N. (2005). *Canadian Occupational Performance Measure manual* (4th ed.). Ottawa, Canada: CAOT Publications.

Lawton, M. P. (1988). Instrumental activities of daily living (IADL) scale: Original observer-rated version. *Psychopharmacology Bulletin, 24,* 785–787.

Legg, L., Drummond, A., Leonardi-Bee, J., Gladman, J. R. F., Corr, S., Donkervoort, M., Edmans, J., Gibertson, L., Jongbloed, L., Logan, P., Sackley, C., Walker, M., & Langhorne, P. (2007). Occupational therapy for patients with problems in personal activities of daily living after stroke: Systematic review of randomized trials. *British Medical Journal/Online First, 335,* doi:10.1136/bmj.39343.466863.55.

Lin, K.-C., Cermak, S. A., Kinsbourne, M., & Trombly, C. A. (1996). Effects of left-sided movements on line bisection in unilateral neglect. *Journal of the International Neuropsychological Society, 2,* 404–411.

Logan, P. A., Dyas, J., & Gladman, J. R. F. (2004). Using an interview study of transport use by people who have had a stroke to inform rehabilitation. *Clinical Rehabilitation, 18,* 703–708.

Lubetzky-Vilnai, A., & Kartin, D. (2010). The effect of balance training on balance performance in individuals poststroke: A systematic review. *Journal of Neurologic Physical Therapy, 34,* 127–137.

Lum, P. S., Mulroy, S., Amdur, R. L., Requejo, P., Prilutsky, B. I., & Dromerick, A. W. (2009). Gains in upper extremity function after stroke via recovery or compensation: Potential differential effects on amount of real-world limb use. *Topics in Stroke Rehabilitation, 16,* 237–254.

Lynton, H., Kligler, B., & Shiflett, S. (2007). Yoga in stroke rehabilitation: A systematic review and results of a pilot study. *Topics in Stroke Rehabilitation, 14,* 1–8.

Ma, H., & Trombly, C. A. (2002). A synthesis of the effects of occupational therapy for persons with stroke: Part II. Remediation of impairments. *American Journal of Occupational Therapy, 56,* 260–274.

Mahoney, F. I., & Barthel, D. W. (1965). Functional evaluation: The Barthel Index. *Maryland State Medical Journal, 14,* 61–65.

Massie, C., Malcolm, M. P., Greene, D., & Thaut, M. (2009). The effects of constraint-induced therapy on kinematic outcomes and compensatory movement patterns: An exploratory study. *Archives of Physical Medicine and Rehabilitation, 90,* 571–579.

Matola, T. (2001). Stroke: A bird's eye view. *Topics in Stroke Rehabilitation, 7,* 61–63.

Mehrholz, J., Kugler, J., & Pohl, M. (2011). Water-based exercises for improving activities of daily living after stroke. *Cochrane Database of Systematic Reviews, (1),* CD008186.

Nakayama, H., Jorgenson, H. S., Raaschou, H. O., & Olsen, T. (1994). Compensation in recovery of upper extremity function after stroke: The Copenhagen study. *Archives of Physical Medicine and Rehabilitation, 75,* 852–857.

National Board for Certification in Occupational Therapy. (2008). Executive summary of the practice analysis study for the occupational therapist registered OTR. Retrieved November 8, 2011 from www.nbcot.org

National Institutes of Health, National Institute of Neurological Disorders and Stroke. (2011). *Stroke: Hope through research.* Retrieved September 29, 2011 from www.ninds.nih.gov/disorders/stroke/detail_stroke.htm.

National Stroke Association. (2006). Recovery after stroke: Redefining sexuality. Retrieved December 7, 2011 from http://www.stroke.org/site/PageServer?pagename=Recov_factsheets.

National Stroke Association. (2011). Stroke treatment. Retrieved October 7, 2011 from www.stroke.org/site/PageServer?pagename=treatment.

Nelson, D. L., Konosky, K., Fleharty, K., Webb, R., Newer, K., Hazboun, V. P., Fontane, C., & Licht, B. C. (1996). The effects of an occupationally embedded exercise on bilaterally assisted supination in persons with hemiplegia. *American Journal of Occupational Therapy, 50,* 639–646.

Nilsen, D. M., Gillen, G., & Gordon, A. M. (2010). Use of mental practice to improve upper-limb recovery after stroke: A systematic review. *American Journal of Occupational Therapy, 64,* 695–708.

Okkema, K., & Culler, K. (1998). Functional evaluation of upper extremity use following stroke: A literature review. *Topics in Stroke Rehabilitation, 4,* 54–75.

Oliveira, C. B., Medeiros, I. R. T., Frota, N. A. F., Greters, M. E., & Conforto, A. B. (2008). Balance control in hemiparetic stroke patients: Main tools for evaluation. *Journal of Rehabilitation Research & Development, 45,* 1215–1226.

Page, S. J., Gater, D. R., & Bach-y-Rita, P. (2004). Reconsidering the motor recovery plateau in stroke rehabilitation. *Archives of Physical Medicine and Rehabilitation, 85,* 1377–1381.

Page, S. J., Levine, P., & Hill, V. (2007). Mental practice as a gateway to modified constraint-induced movement therapy: A promising combination to improve function. *American Journal of Occupational Therapy, 61,* 321–327

Page, S. J., Levine, A., Leonard, A., Szaflarski, J. P., & Kissela, B. M. (2008). Modified constraint-induced therapy in chronic stroke: Results of a single-blinded randomized controlled trial. *Physical Therapy, 88,* 333–340.

Page, S. J., Sisto, S., Levine, P., & McGrath, R. E. (2004). Efficacy of modified constraint-induced movement therapy in chronic stroke: A single-blinded randomized controlled trial. *Archives of Physical Medicine and Rehabilitation, 85,* 14–18.

Pambakian, A. L. M., Mannan, S. K., Hodgson, T. L., & Kennard, C. (2004). Saccadic visual search training: A treatment for patients with homonymous hemianopsia. *Journal of Neurology, Neurosurgery, and Psychiatry, 75,* 1443–1448.

Perennou, D. A., Amblard, B., Laassel, E. M., Benaim, C., Herisson, C., & Pelissier, J. (2002). Understanding the pusher behavior of some stroke patients with spatial deficits: A pilot study. *Archives of Physical Medicine and Rehabilitation, 83,* 570–575.

Perrier, M.-J., Korner-Bitensky, N., & Mayo, N. E. (2010). Patient factors associated with return to driving poststroke: Findings from a multicenter cohort study. *Archives of Physical Medicine and Rehabilitation, 91,* 868–873.

Pignolo, L. (2009). Robotics in neuro-rehabilitation. *Journal of Rehabilitation Medicine, 41,* 955–960.

Pollock, A. S., Durward, B. R., Rowe, P. J., & Paul, J. P. (2000). What is balance? *Clinical Rehabilitation, 14,* 402–406.

Richards, L. G., Latham, N. K., Jette, D. U., Rosenberg, L., Smout, R. J., & De Jong, G. (2005). Characterizing occupational therapy practice in stroke rehabilitation. *Archives of Physical Medicine and Rehabilitation, 86* (Suppl. 2), 51–60.

Ridgway, E. M., & Byrne, D. P. (1999). To sling or not to sling? *OT Practice, 4,* 38–42.

Roberts, P. S., Vegher, J. A., Gilewski, M., Bender, A., & Riggs, R. V. (2005). Client-centered occupational therapy using constraint-induced therapy. *Journal of Stroke and Cerebrovascular Diseases, 14,* 115–121.

Roger, V. L., Go, A. S., Lloyd-Jones, D. M., Adams, R. J., Berry, J. D., Brown, T. M., Carnethon, M. R., Dai, S., diSimone, G., Ford, E. S., Fox, C. S., Fullerton, C. G., Greenlund, K. J., Hailpern, S. M., Heit, J.A., Ho, P. M., Howard, V. J., Kissels, B. M., Kittner, S. J., Lackland, D. T., Lichtman, J. H., Lisabeth, L. D., Makuc, D. M., Marcus, G. M., Marelli, A., Matchar, M. M., McDermott, M. M., Meigs, J. B., Moy, C. S., Mozaffarian, D., Mussolino, M. E., Nichol, G., Paynter, N. P., Rosamond, W. D., Sorlie, P. D., Stafford, R. S., Turan, T. N., Turner, M. B., Wong, N. D., & Wylie-Rosett, J. (2011). Heart disease and stroke statistics—2011 Update: A report from the American Heart Association. *Circulation, 123,* 18–209.

Sabari, J. S. (1998). Occupational therapy after stroke: Are we providing the right services at the right time? *American Journal of Occupational Therapy, 52,* 299–302.

Sabari, J. S., & Lieberman, D. (2008). *Occupational therapy practice guidelines for adults with stroke.* Bethesda, MD: American Occupational Therapy Association, Inc.

Saposnik, G., Teasell, R., Mamdani, M., Hall, J., McIlroy, W., Cheung, D., Thorpe, K. E., Cohen, L. G., & Bayley, M. (2010). Effectiveness of virtual reality using Wii gaming technology in stroke rehabilitation: A pilot randomized clinical trial and proof of principle. *Stroke, 41,* 1477–1484.

Schabrun, S. M., & Hillier, S. (2009). Evidence for the retraining of sensation after stroke: A systematic review. *Clinical Rehabilitation, 23,* 27–39.

Schepers, V. P., Visser-Meily, A. M., Ketelaar, M., & Lindeman, E. (2006). Poststroke fatigue: Course and its relation to personal and stroke-related factors. *Archives of Physical Medicine and Rehabilitation, 87,* 184–188.

Shi, Y. X., Tian, J. H., Yang, K. H., & Zhau, Y. (2011). Modified constraint-induced movement therapy versus traditional rehabilitation in patients with upper-extremity dysfunction after stroke: A systematic review and meta-analysis. *Archives of Physical Medicine and Rehabilitation, 92,* 972–982.

Shih, M.-M., Rogers, J. C., Skidmore, E. R., Irrgang, J. J., & Holm, M. B. (2009). Measuring stroke survivors' functional status independence: Five perspectives. *American Journal of Occupational Therapy, 64,* 600–608.

Shinsha, N., & Ishigami, S. (1999). Rehabilitation approach to patients with unilateral spatial neglect. *Topics in Stroke Rehabilitation, 6,* 1–14.

Simon, R. P., Greenberg, D. A., & Aminoff, M. J. (2009). *Clinical neurology* (7th ed.). New York: Lange Medical Books/McGraw-Hill.

Smallfield, S., & Karges, J. (2009). Classification of occupational therapy intervention for inpatient stroke rehabilitation. *American Journal of Occupational Therapy, 63,* 408–413.

Stein, J., & Brandstater, M. E. (2010). Stroke rehabilitation. In W. R. Frontera, J. A. DeLisa, B. M. Gans, N. E. Walsh, L. R. Robinson, J. Basford, W. Bockenek, G. Carter, J. Chae, L. H. Gerber, A. Jette, T. P. Stitik, G. Stucki, & R. Zafonte (Eds.), *Physical medicine and rehabilitation principles and practice* (5th ed., pp. 551–574). Philadelphia: Lippincott Williams & Wilkins.

Stewart, C., & Riedel, K. (2011). Managing speech and language deficits after stroke. In G. Gillen (Ed.), *Stroke rehabilitation: A function-based approach* (3rd ed., pp. 534–552). St. Louis: Mosby.

Stroke Unit Trialists' Collaboration. (2001). Organised inpatient (stroke unit) care for stroke. *Cochrane Database of Systematic Reviews,* (3), CD000197.

Sulter, G., Steen, C., & De Keyser, J. (1999). Use of Barthel index and modified Rankin scale in acute stroke trials. *Stroke, 30,* 1538–1541.

Taub, E., Miller, N. E., Novack, T. A., Cook, E. W., III, Fleming, W. C., Nepomuceno, C. S., Connell, J. S., & Crago, J. E. (1993). Technique to improve chronic motor deficit after stroke. *Archives of Physical Medicine and Rehabilitation, 74,* 347–354.

Taylor-Piliae, R. E., & Haskell, W. L. (2007). Tai Chi exercise and stroke rehabilitation. *Topics in Stroke Rehabilitation, 14,* 9–22.

Tham, K., Ginsburg, E., Fisher, A. G., & Tegner, R. (2001). Training to improve awareness of disabilities in clients with unilateral neglect. *American Journal of Occupational Therapy, 55,* 46–54.

Toglia, J. P. (1991). Generalization of treatment: A multicontext approach to cognitive perceptual impairment in adults with brain injury. *American Journal of Occupational Therapy, 45,* 505–516.

Treger, I., Shames, J., Giaquinto, S., & Ring, H. (2007). Return to work in stroke patients. *Disability and Rehabilitation, 29,* 1397–1403.

Trombly, C. A. (1995/2011). Occupation: Purposefulness and meaningfulness as therapeutic mechanisms. *American Journal of Occupational Therapy, 49,* 960–972. Reprinted in Padilla, R., & Griffiths, Y. (Eds.). (2011). *A professional legacy: The Eleanor Clarke Slagle lectures in occupational therapy, 1955–2010* (3rd ed.). Bethesda, MD: AOTA Press.

Trombly, C. A., & Ma, H. (2002). A synthesis of the effects of occupational therapy for persons with stroke, Part I: Remediation of roles, tasks, and activities. *American Journal of Occupational Therapy, 56,* 250–259.

Trombly, C. A., & Wu, C.-Y. (1999). Effect of rehabilitation tasks on organization of movement after stroke. *American Journal of Occupational Therapy, 53,* 333–344.

Urton, M. L., Kohia, M., Davis, J., & Neill, M. R. (2007). Systematic literature review of treatment interventions for upper extremity hemiparesis following stroke. *Occupational Therapy International, 14,* 11–27.

U.S. Department of Health and Human Services. (2011). Inpatient rehabilitation therapy services: Complying with documentation requirements. Retrieved April 21, 2012 from www.cms.hhs.gov/Outreach-and-Education/Medicare-Learning-Network-MLN/MLNProducts/Downloads/Inpatient_Rehab_Fact_Sheet_ICN905643.pdf.

Uswatte, G., Taub, E., Morris, D., Barman, J., & Crago, J. (2006). Contribution of the shaping and restraint components of constraint-induced movement therapy to treatment outcome. *NeuroRehabilitation, 21,* 147–156.

van Heugten, C. M., Dekker, J., Deelman, B. G., van Dijk, A. J., Stehmann-Saris, J. C., & Kinebanian, A. (1998). Outcome of strategy training in stroke patients with apraxia: A phase II study. *Clinical Rehabilitation, 12,* 294–303.

Verheyden, G., Nieuwboer, A., De Wit, L., Thijs, V., Dobbelaere, J., Devos, H., Severijns, D., Vanbeveren, S., & De Weerdt, W. (2008). Time course of trunk, arm, leg, and functional recovery after ischemic stroke (Clinical report). *Neurorehabilitation and Neural Repair, 22,* 173–180.

Vestling, M., Tufvesson, B., & Iwarsson, S. (2003). Indicators for return to work after stroke and the importance of work for subjective well-being and life satisfaction. *Journal of Rehabilitation Medicine, 35,* 127–131.

Wade, D. T. (1992). Stroke: Rehabilitation and long term care. *Lancet, 339,* 791–793.

Wagner, J. M., Lang, C. E., Sahrmann, S. A., Edwards, D. F., & Dromerick, A. W. (2007). Sensorimotor impairments and reaching performance in subjects with poststroke hemiparesis during the first few month of recovery. *Physical Therapy, 87,* 751–765.

Walker, M. F., & Lincoln, N. B. (1990). Reacquisition of dressing skills after stroke. *International Disability Studies, 12,* 41–43.

Walker, M. F., & Lincoln, N. B. (1991). Factors influencing dressing performance after stroke. *Journal of Neurology, Neurosurgery and Psychiatry, 54,* 699–701.

Walsh, K. (2001). Management of shoulder pain in patients with stroke. *Postgraduate Medical Journal, 77,* 645–649.

Warren, M. (1991). Strategies for sensory and neuromotor remediation. In C. Christensen & C. Baum (Eds.), *Occupational therapy: Overcoming human performance deficits* (pp. 632–662). Thorofare, NJ: Slack.

Warren, M. (1996). *Brain injury vision assessment battery for adults.* Birmingham, AL: visABILITIES Rehabilitation.

Warren, M. (1999). *Evaluation and treatment of visual perceptual dysfunction in adult brain injury* (Part I). Birmingham, AL: visABILITIES Rehabilitation.

Warren, M. (2009). Pilot study on activities of daily living limitations in adults with hemianopsia. *American Journal of Occupational Therapy, 63,* 626–633.

Welmer, A. K., Holmqvist, L., & Sommerfeld, D. K. (2006). Hemiplegic limb synergies in stroke patients. *American Journal of Physical Medicine & Rehabilitation, 85,* 112–119.

West, C., Bowen, A., Hesketh, A., & Vail, A. (2008) Interventions for motor apraxia following stroke. *Cochrane Database of Systematic Reviews.* doi: 10.1002/14651858.CD004132.pub2.

White, J. H., MacKenzie, L., Magin, P., & Pollack, M. R. P. (2008). The occupational experience of stroke survivors in a community setting. *Occupational Therapy Journal of Research: Occupation, Participation and Health, 28,* 160–167.

Wilson, D. J., Baker, L. L., & Craddock, J. A. (1984a). Functional test for the hemiparetic upper extremity. *American Journal of Occupational Therapy, 38,* 159–164.

Wilson, D. J., Baker, L. L., & Craddock, J. A. (1984b). Protocol: Functional test for the hemiplegic/paretic upper extremity. Unpublished manuscript. Downey, CA: County Rehabilitation Center, Rancho Los Amigos, Occupational Therapy Department.

Winstein, C. J., Rose, D. K., Tan, S. M., Lewthwaite, R., Chui, H. C., & Azen, S. P. (2004). A randomized controlled comparison of upper-extremity rehabilitation strategies in acute stroke: A pilot study of immediate and long-term outcomes. *Archives of Physical Medicine and Rehabilitation, 85,* 620–628.

Winward, C. E., Halligan, P. W., & Wade, D. T. (1999). Current practice and clinical relevance of somatosensory assessment after stroke. *Clinical Rehabilitation, 13,* 48–55.

Wolf, T. J., Baum, C., & Connor, L. T. (2009). Changing face of stroke: Implications for occupational therapy practice. *American Journal of Occupational Therapy, 63,* 621–625.

Wolf, S. L., Catlin, P. A., Ellis, M., Link Archer, A., Morgan B., & Piacentino, A. (2001). Assessing Wolf Motor Function Test as outcome measure for research inpatients after stroke. *Stroke, 32,* 1635–1639.

Wolf, S. L., Thompson, P. A., Winstein, C. J., Miller, J. P., Blanton, S. R., Nichols-Larsen, D. S., Morris, D. M., Uswatte, G., Taub, E., Light, K. E., & Sawaki, L. (2010). The EXCITE stroke trial: Comparing early and delayed constraint-induced movement therapy. *Stroke, 41,* 2309–2315.

Wolf, S. L., Winstein, C. J., Miller, J. P., Taub, E., Uswatte, G., Morris, D., Giuliani, C., Light, K. E., & Nichols-Larsen, D. (2006). Effect of constraint-induced movement therapy on upper extremity function 3 to 9 months after stroke: The EXCITE randomized clinical trial. *Journal of the American Medical Association, 296,* 2095–2104.

Wolf, S. L., Winstein, C. J., Miller, J. P., Thompson, P. A., Taub, E., Uswatte, G., Morris, D., Blanton, S., Nichols-Larsen, D., & Clark, P. C. (2008). Retention of upper limb function in stroke survivors who have received constraint-induced movement therapy: The EXCITE randomised trial. *The Lancet Neurology, 7,* 33–40.

Woodbury, M. L., Velozo, C. A., Richards, L. G., Duncan, P. W., Studenski, S., & Lai, S. M. (2007). Dimensionality and construct validity of the Fugl-Meyer Assessment of the Upper Extremity. *Archives of Physical Medicine and Rehabilitation, 88,* 715–723.

Yavuzer, G., Selles, R., Sezer, N., Sutbeyaz, S., Bussmann, J. B., Koseoglu, F., & Stam, H. J. (2008). Mirror therapy improves hand function in subacute stroke: A randomized controlled trial. *Archives of Physical Medicine and Rehabilitation, 89,* 393–398.

Yekutiel, M., & Guttman, E. A. (1993). A controlled trial of the retraining of the sensory function of the hand in stroke patients. *Journal of Neurology, Neurosurgery and Psychiatry, 56,* 241–244.

Yu, D. T. (2009). Shoulder pain and other musculoskeletal complications. In J. Stein, R. L. Henry, R. F. Macko, C. J. Winstein, & R. D. Zorowitz (Eds.), *Stroke recovery and rehabilitation* (pp. 437–451). New York: Demos Medical.

Zorowitz, R. D., Hughes, M. B., Idank, D., Ikai, T., & Johnston, M. V. (1996). Shoulder pain and subluxation after stroke: Correlation or coincidence? *American Journal of Occupational Therapy, 50,* 194–201.

Zorowitz, R. D., Idank, D., Ikai, T., Hughes, M. B., & Johnston, M. V. (1995). Shoulder subluxation after stroke: A comparison of four supports. *Archives of Physical Medicine and Rehabilitation, 76,* 763–771.

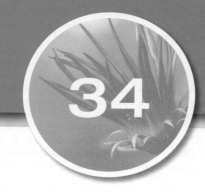

34

Traumatic Brain Injury

Janet M. Powell

Learning Objectives

After studying this chapter, the reader will be able to do the following:

1. Describe the similarities and differences in the typical course of recovery for persons with severe, moderate, and mild traumatic brain injury.
2. Select appropriate assessment tools and strategies for persons with traumatic brain injury during acute medical management and inpatient and postacute rehabilitation.
3. Apply information from related chapters of this text to the treatment of motor, cognitive, behavioral, and emotional aspects of traumatic brain injury.
4. Analyze how needs of family members change during recovery and adaptation, and determine how to meet their needs in occupational therapy.
5. Anticipate possible roles for occupational therapists in addressing long-term needs of survivors of traumatic brain injury.

People who have had a traumatic brain injury (TBI) with alteration in brain function as a result of some external force often undergo changes in their ability to carry out valued roles, tasks, and activities as a result of impairments in cognitive, behavioral, emotional, and/or physical functioning. In fact, moderate to severe brain injury affects virtually every area of life for the survivor and his or her family (Pagulayan et al., 2006). For the many individuals who are young adults at the time of injury, changes in capacities and abilities may affect their occupational functioning for months, years, or decades. The complex interaction of factors associated with impairment, context, and environment require a multidisciplinary approach to treatment. Therefore, occupational therapists who work with patients with TBI must appreciate the contributions and expertise of other team members as they offer the patient what is unique to occupational therapy.

To enable the reader to appreciate the effect of TBI on society, this chapter begins with a discussion of its incidence and causes. Next, mechanisms of injury are explained. A review of the typical clinical course of recovery from severe TBI emphasizes how occupational therapy contributes to remediation of impairments and adaptation to deficits throughout the continuum of care. The unique needs of persons with mild traumatic brain injury, the least severe type of brain injury, and those with combat-related TBI are also highlighted, but it is hoped that readers can determine appropriate evaluation and treatment approaches for persons with moderate TBI based on descriptions of the two extremes of severity of injury. Because brain injury rehabilitation requires an integration of many aspects of occupational therapy evaluation and treatment, the reader will frequently be referred to other chapters of this text. Evidence Table 34-1 presents evidence for occupational therapy interventions after severe brain injury.

INCIDENCE, PREVALENCE, AND CAUSATION

As noted above, TBI is defined as an alteration in brain function, or other evidence of brain pathology, caused by an external force. Alteration in brain function is determined by (1) any loss of or decrease in the level of consciousness; (2) any loss of memory for events immediately before or after the injury (i.e., post-traumatic amnesia [PTA]); (3) a neurological deficit such as weakness, paralysis, loss of balance, change in vision, sensory loss, or aphasia; (4) any change in mental state at the time of the injury such as confusion, disorientation, or slowed thinking; and/or (5) visual, neuroradiologic, or laboratory evidence of damage to the brain (Menon et al., 2010). External forces causing a TBI can include (1) the head being struck by or striking an object, (2) the brain undergoing an acceleration/deceleration movement without direct external trauma to the head, (3) a foreign body penetrating the brain, and (4) forces generated from events such as a blast or explosion.

Each year, approximately 1.7 million civilians in the United States sustain a TBI (Faul et al., 2010). Of these, 3% (52,000) die, 16% (275,000) are hospitalized, and 80% (1.4 million) are treated in an emergency department and released. In addition, there are an unknown number of individuals with TBI who are not included in these estimates because they are seen in an emergency department but discharged without a diagnosis of TBI (Powell et al., 2008), are seen outside an emergency department or hospital, or do not seek care (Faul et al., 2010). Approximately 80,000–90,000 Americans experience a new onset of disability resulting from TBI each year (Langlois, Rutland-Brown, & Thomas, 2004) with an estimated 3.1 million children and adults in the United States living with a lifelong TBI-related disability. After children ages 0–4 years, older adolescents aged 15–19 years have the highest rates of TBI-related emergency department visits in the United States (2002–2006 data), whereas adults aged 75 years and older have the highest rates of TBI-related hospitalization and death (Faul et al., 2010). Regardless of age, the rates for TBI are higher for males than for females.

Between 2002 and 2006, falls were the leading cause of TBI among all age groups in the United States (35%), followed by motor vehicle-traffic incidents (17%), striking against or being struck by an object (17%), and assault (10%) (Faul et al., 2010). Across all age groups, fall-related TBIs resulted in the greatest number of emergency department visits and hospitalizations, whereas TBIs from motor vehicle-traffic incidents were the leading cause of TBI-related death. Falls accounted for 61% of TBIs among adults age 65 years and older with the rates of fall-related TBIs even higher for adults age 75 years and older. The rates of TBIs from motor vehicle or traffic incidents and assault were highest among adults aged 20–24 years with only 1% of TBIs in adults age 65 years and older resulting from an assault.

Alcohol use is a contributing factor to many events that result in a TBI, with estimates that one-third to one-half of people who sustain a TBI were intoxicated at the time of injury (Corrigan, 1995). Preinjury alcohol use has implications for outcome, treatment, and long-term adjustment to TBI. Patients who were intoxicated when injured reportedly have a longer hospitalization, longer duration of excesses in behavior related to agitation, and lower cognitive status at discharge than those who were not intoxicated (Kelly et al., 1997; Sparadeo & Gill, 1989). Furthermore, a history of TBI increases a person's risk of TBI. After one TBI, the risk of a second may be up to three times greater than for those who have never sustained a TBI, and, after a second TBI, the risk of a third injury may be up to eight times greater (Annegers et al., 1980).

Finally, it is important to appreciate the incidence of TBI based on severity. TBI is typically characterized as mild, moderate, or severe. Severity categorization schemes vary but are most often based on depth of coma as measured by the Glasgow Coma Scale (GCS) (Teasdale & Jennett, 1974)

Evidence Table 34-1		Best Evidence for Interventions Used in Occupational Therapy after Severe Brain Injury				
Intervention	Description of Intervention Tested	Participants	Dose	Type of Best Evidence and Level of Evidence	Benefit	Statistical Probability	Reference
Cognitive rehabilitation	Various cognitive rehabilitation approaches	Participants (number not specified) with TBI or stroke from 112 studies	Varied by study	Systematic review Level: I	Recommendations based on review: Practice standard for attention remediation in postacute rehab, metacognitive strategy training; practice guidelines for use of memory compensations in severe TBI	Not calculated	Cicerone et al. (2011)
Errorless learning	Learning tasks such as word lists, word-pair associations	One hundred sixty-eight with severe memory impairment (number with TBI not specified)	Varied by study	Meta-analysis of eight studies Level: I	Yes. Errorless learning was more effective than trial-and-error learning.	Effect size = 0.87 $p = 0.008$	Kessles & de Haan (2003)
Self-care skills training	Subjects received a washing and dressing protocol that involved behavioral methods	Four patients in a residential setting (three with TBI) at least 7 months postinjury, severe physical and cognitive impairments	Daily ADL retraining with fading physical assistance and cueing	Four single-subject studies Level: IV C 2 b	Three of four subjects achieved independence in washing and dressing (in 20, 37, and 11 days, respectively); one of four did not.	No formal statistical tests reported	Giles et al. (1997)

ADL, activities of daily living; TBI, traumatic brain injury.

| Table 34-1 | **Glasgow Coma Scale** | |

Table 34-1	**Glasgow Coma Scale**	
Eye opening (*E*)	Spontaneous	4
	To speech	3
	To pain	2
	Nil	1
Best motor response (*M*)	Obeys	6
	Localizes	5
	Withdraws	4
	Abnormal flexion	3
	Extensor response	2
	Nil	1
Verbal response (*V*)	Oriented	5
	Confused Conversation	4
	Inappropriate words	3
	Incomprehensible sounds	2
	Nil	1

Coma score = (*E* + *M* + *V*) = 3–15

Reprinted with permission from Jennett, B., & Teasdale, G. (1981). *Management of head injuries*. Philadelphia: F. A. Davis.

(Table 34-1), length of loss of consciousness, and/or length of PTA (Institute of Medicine [IOM], 2011). Most people who sustain a TBI have a relatively mild injury (at least 75% of all TBIs in the United States) (Faul et al., 2010).

MECHANISMS OF INJURY AND CLINICAL IMPLICATIONS

A TBI can be classified as either open or closed based on the biomechanics of the injury (IOM, 2009). In an open brain injury, an object, such as a bullet, enters the cranial cavity. Some classification systems categorize all open injuries as penetrating injuries (Mass et al., 2010). Other systems differentiate between penetrating and perforating injuries depending on whether the object remains lodged within the cranial cravity (penetrating) or passes through and exits the cranial cravity (perforating). In an open brain injury, the extent of the damage depends on the shape, mass, direction, and velocity of the object (IOM, 2009).

A TBI that results from a direct or indirect impact, without penetration of the brain tissue, is classified as a closed brain injury. Closed head injuries can result from dynamic or static loading (IOM, 2009). A dynamic loading injury occurs when there is rapid acceleration and deceleration of the brain. A static loading injury, also termed crush injury (Mass et al., 2010), occurs

when a slow mechanical force is applied to the brain, for example, if the head were trapped for an extended time under heavy debris after an earthquake. This type of injury is uncommon. The damage from a closed brain injury is directly related to the type (e.g,. shear, tensile) and amount of forces generated during the traumatic event (Katz, 1992). In the case of crush injuries, there tends to be more damage to the skull than the brain (Mass et al., 2010).

Blast injuries have recently been recognized as a specific type of TBI (Mass et al., 2010). A blast injury results from any type of blast explosion, including improvised explosive devices (IEDs). A blast injury can occur in conjuction with an open or closed brain injury.

Focal versus Diffuse Injuries

Brain injuries can also be categorized into focal or diffuse injuries based on the extent of the pathology. Focal injuries result from brain contusions, lacerations, and masses of blood called hematomas (Duff, 2001). Focal lesions are usually seen at the anterior poles and inferior surfaces of the frontal and temporal lobes. They occur when the brain hits the skull and scrapes over the irregular bony structures at these locations (Katz, 1992). The occipital and parietal lobes, which have smooth surfaces, are less likely to incur damage. Focal lesions to the prefrontal and anterior temporal areas interrupt connections to subcortical limbic structures and affect modulation of memory, emotion, and drive (Katz, 1992). Damage to the orbitofrontal areas generally results in impulsivity that is greater than with diffuse damage, whereas damage to the frontolateral cortex results in hemiparesis, impulsivity, and attentional impairments as well as decreased mental flexibility (Trexler & Zappala, 1988).

Diffuse injuries typically occur in motor-vehicle crashes where there is rapid movement of the head (Smith, Meaney, & Shull, 2003). Traumatic axonal injury (TAI), previously termed diffuse axonal injury (DAI), is a type of diffuse injury that results when the brain accelerates, decelerates, and rotates inside the skull. The brainstem is more stable than the cerebrum, which rotates around the brainstem during impact. The rotation places a stretch or shear force on the long axons that transmit information throughout the brain and brainstem (Leech & Shuman, 1982). Although the mechanisms for TAI are not completely understood, contributing factors include altered permeability of the axonal cell membrane, which impedes axonal transport. This results in focal swelling of the axon and, ultimately, detachment of the axon at the point of the swelling (Povlishock & Katz, 2005). These injuries are likely to result in coma (Duff, 2001).

Coma caused by axonal injuries may quickly reverse if the axonal damage was mild or may continue as a vegetative state if axons were ruptured. Recovery from coma progresses to a period of confusion with impaired attention and PTA. When confusion clears, any cognitive impairments become more evident. Impairments may include diminished mental processing speed and efficiency and difficulty with divided-attention tasks, which require the patient to respond simultaneously to two sources of information. There is a reduced capacity for higher level cognitive functions, including abstract reasoning, planning, and problem solving. Typical behavioral outcomes range from impulsivity, irritability, and exaggerated premorbid traits to apathy and poor initiative (Katz, 1992). Diffuse injuries often include damage to the brainstem and cerebellar pathways, resulting in ataxia, diplopia, and dysarthria (Trexler & Zappala, 1988). It is common to find both focal and diffuse damage with a TBI, especially in more severe cases. In both types of injuries, secondary pathogenic events at the cellular, biochemical, and molecular levels contribute to widespread damage beyond the effect of the primary insult (IOM,2009).

Cranial Nerve Damage Associated with Traumatic Brain Injury

Cranial nerves can be torn, stretched, or contused. The olfactory nerve (I) is often abraded or torn when the frontal lobes scrape across the orbital surface of the skull (Leech & Shuman, 1982). The optic nerve (II) may be damaged directly, or vision can be compromised by injury to the eye, the optic tracts, or the visual cortex (Brandstater et al., 1991). Cranial nerves III, IV, and VI, which control eye movements, are all vulnerable to injury (Brandstater et al., 1991; Leech & Shuman, 1982). The oculomotor nerve (III) can be stretched when edema or bleeding expands the contents of the skull, causing the uncus of the temporal lobe to herniate into the foramen magnum and compress the brainstem (Leech & Shuman, 1982). The abducens nerve (VI) is very long and consequently vulnerable to injury. The facial and vestibulocochlear nerves (VII and VIII, respectively) may be damaged if the temporal bone is fractured at the base of the skull (Brandstater et al., 1991; Leech & Shuman, 1982). Cranial nerves V and IX–XII are rarely damaged (Leech & Shuman, 1982).

Fractures and Other Cooccuring Medical Conditions Associated with Traumatic Brain Injury

The skull may fracture from the force of the blow in the area of or at a distance from the actual impact site. The patient with a brain injury from a motor vehicle crash or a fall may have other systemic trauma, such as fractures of the extremities, shoulder girdle, pelvis, or face; cervical fractures with possible spinal cord injury; abdominal trauma; and pneumothorax or other chest cavity trauma.

Second Insults and Secondary Effects

Hypoxia, hypotension, hypothermia, and hyperthermia are the most common systemic second insults that occur following TBI (Mass et al., 2010). Medical personnel in the field and the hospital setting strive to avoid or minimize the occurrence of these additional insults because they can exacerbate secondary processes that can cause additional damage to the brain beyond the primary injury (Mass et al., 2010). The secondary effects can occur immediately or develop within hours or days of the injury (Jennett & Teasdale, 1981). Trauma can abolish or disrupt autoregulation of cerebral blood flow, the blood–brain barrier, and vasomotor functions, resulting in disordered cerebral energy metabolism, intracranial hypotension, cerebral vasospasm, and increases in intracranial pressure (ICP) and cerebral edema (Duff, 2001; Jennett & Teasdale, 1981). Other secondary effects of brain trauma include intracranial hemorrhage, uncal herniation resulting in brainstem compression, seizures, electrolyte abnormalities, altered respiratory regulation, intracranial infection, and abnormal autonomic nervous system responses (Lillehei & Hoff, 1985). Usually by the time the patient is stabilized and occupational therapy is ordered, the secondary effects of brain trauma are present, influencing the patient's ability to respond to therapy.

FOUR PHASES OF LIFE FOR THE SURVIVOR OF TRAUMATIC BRAIN INJURY

Based on their review of the literature, authors of the Agency for Health Care Policy and Research Evidence Report on the effectiveness of rehabilitation for persons with TBI described four phases of life for the adult survivor of moderate to severe TBI: preinjury, medical treatment, rehabilitation, and survivorship (Fig. 34-1) (Chestnut et al., 1999). Although management of TBI is typically a multidisciplinary enterprise, the following description of each phase is based on a typical recovery from severe TBI with emphasis on occupational therapy evaluation and treatment. Note how the role of occupational therapy changes with each phase, increasingly focusing on occupational functioning the further the patient progresses in recovery.

Preinjury Phase

In Chris's first 17 years she became used to being called "outstanding." She usually was one of the top students in every honors class. . . . Chris was a fairly good organist and gymnast too. In her first 17 years, outstanding was normal. Outstanding was easy. (Rain, 2000, p. 6)

Occupational therapists always appreciate the person as distinct from his or her condition, impairment, or disability. People who sustain a TBI bring their personal, social,

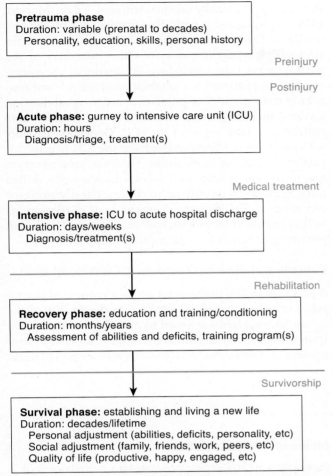

Pretrauma phase
Duration: variable (prenatal to decades)
   Personality, education, skills, personal history

Preinjury

Postinjury

Acute phase: gurney to intensive care unit (ICU)
Duration: hours
   Diagnosis/triage, treatment(s)

Medical treatment

Intensive phase: ICU to acute hospital discharge
Duration: days/weeks
   Diagnosis/treatment(s)

Rehabilitation

Recovery phase: education and training/conditioning
Duration: months/years
   Assessment of abilities and deficits, training program(s)

Survivorship

Survival phase: establishing and living a new life
Duration: decades/lifetime
   Personal adjustment (abilities, deficits, personality, etc)
   Social adjustment (family, friends, work, peers, etc)
   Quality of life (productive, happy, engaged, etc)

Figure 34-1 Four phases of life of the TBI survivor. (Reprinted with permission from Chestnut, R. M., Carney, N., Maynard, H., Mann, N. C., Patterson, P., & Helfand, M. [1999]. Summary report: Evidence for the effectiveness of rehabilitation for persons with traumatic brain injury. *Journal of Head Trauma Rehabilitation, 14,* 176–188.)

and cultural backgrounds to recovery (see Chapter 3). Chestnut et al. (1999) suggested that, although standard treatments are appropriate for the acute medical treatment phase of TBI, consideration of individual differences becomes increasingly important as patients progress through recovery and adaptation.

Rosenthal and Bond (1990) summarized the importance of understanding premorbid factors that may affect the patient's recovery. They reported that researchers have noted a high frequency of preinjury learning disabilities and behavior disorders in persons with TBI. They suggested finding out about the patient's premorbid cognitive strengths and weaknesses through school records or family interviews and investigating any preexisting neurological conditions. Eames, Haffey, and Cope (1990) further recommended asking family members how the patient previously reacted to frustration so as to recognize and avoid stress-provoking situations.

Medical Treatment of Traumatic Brain Injury

As I gradually regain consciousness in the hospital, I imagine I am having a nightmare. . . . As I open my eyes and stare around the room at the monitors and plugs and dripping IV bottles, I hope this nightmare will end quickly. (Rain, 2000, p. 6)

The primary goals of this phase of recovery center on surviving, achieving medical stability, and preventing or minimizing the impact of second insults and secondary effects on the injured central nervous system (Hartl & Ghajar, 2005).

Emergency Medical Treatment

Emergency Medical Services (EMS) personnel are typically the first medical specialists to respond to the needs of a person with severe TBI. The paramedics' first priority is rapid restoration of physiological homeostasis with stabilization of the airway, breathing, and circulation (Hartl & Ghajar, 2005). Because secondary hypoxia and arterial hypotension are associated with greater mortality and morbidity (Baron & Jallo, 2007), supplemental oxygen or endotracheal intubation may be used to maintain oxygen saturation, and intravenous fluids may be administered to help maintain systolic blood pressure (Brain Trauma Foundation, 2007).

Recommendations for neurological assessment in the field include determination of an initial GCS score (Teasdale & Jennett, 1974) and a pupillary exam. The GCS provides an assessment of brain injury severity using a 15-point system to assess depth of coma through motor, eye-opening, and verbal capabilities (Table 34-1). A GCS score of 13–15 indicates a mild brain injury, a score of 9–12 indicates a brain injury of moderate severity, and a score of 8 or below indicates a severe injury. In some cases, alcohol or other drug intoxication, sedation administered by EMS personnel, and/or intubation prevent assessment of all three areas (Marion, 1996). Whenever possible, patients are transported to the closest facility where computed tomography (CT) scanning, neurosurgical expertise, and ICP monitoring are available. EMS personnel routinely immobilize the injured person's spine using a rigid backboard with the neck in a rigid cervical collar because cervical spinal injury is associated with 4%–8% of TBIs (Baron & Jallo, 2007). Oxygen saturation and blood pressure are monitored en route to the trauma center, and any deterioration is addressed immediately (Brain Trauma Foundation, 2007).

Once in the emergency department, the medical team continues to ensure protection of the airway and adequacy of breathing and blood pressure (Baron & Jallo, 2007). The primary goals at this stage are to avoid further neurological damage and to stabilize critical extracranial injuries to the thorax, abdomen, face, and extremities. The medical team performs a general assessment of other injuries and repeats the GCS and pupillary exam to assess neurological function. Chest and cervical spine x-rays are taken. A CT scan of the head is performed soon after arrival to assess intracranial injury and identify structural lesions such as hematomas and contusions (Baron & Jallo, 2007).

A hematoma is a mass of blood confined to an organ or space and caused by a broken blood vessel (Scott & Dow, 1995). Acute subdural hematomas are located between the dura and the arachnoid and epidural hematomas between the dura and the skull. With the exception of small lesions in patients with stable neurological signs, hematomas must be surgically evacuated as soon as possible to optimize chances for survival and recovery. Contusions, i.e., bruising of the brain, result in a collection of blood and necrotic tissue. More severe intracerebral contusions may also be treated surgically to reduce ICP (Baron & Jallo, 2007).

Intensive Medical Management

After appropriate evaluation and treatment for life-threatening injuries, the patient with a severe TBI is taken to the intensive care unit (ICU). Medical treatment in the ICU aims to optimize cerebral perfusion and brain tissue oxygenation, minimize brain swelling, and maintain all other physiological variables within the normal range (Marion, 1996). The length of stay in the ICU is primarily determined by the ability to manage the patient's brain

swelling, which usually subsides within 4–5 days (Marion, 1996). A physiatrist is typically consulted within the first few days of admisssion to the ICU to make decisions for appropriate rehabilitative care. Other members of the rehabilitation team, including occupational therapists, often see the patient for a rehabilitation consult and contribute their input. The physiatrist orders rehabilitation services, including occupational therapy, for the coma patient that may begin in the ICU. Generally, patients with more severe injuries move from the ICU to acute inpatient rehabilitation facilities. However, rehabilitation may also occur in acute medical or subacute units, skilled nursing facilities, or outpatient clinics. The decisions for care are made based on the degree and rate of recovery, as well as logistical factors such as insurance coverage and proximity of facilities to the patient's support system.

Patients with Severe Disorders in Consciousness

A person with TBI may exhibit any of a number of altered states of consciousness, depending on the severity of the injury. Various terms are used to describe the continuum from complete consciousness to complete absence of consciousness (Definition 34-1). Patients with severe TBI begin

---

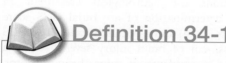

Definition 34-1

Definitions of Severe Disorders of Consciousness

Coma

Coma denotes unarousability with the absence of sleep-wake cycles on an electroencephalogram (EEG) and loss of capacity for environmental interaction. Neurobehavioral criteria include (American Congress of Rehabilitation Medicine, 1995):

- Patient's eyes do not open either spontaneously or to external stimulation.
- Patient does not follow commands.
- Patient does not mouth or speak recognizable words.
- The patient does not demonstrate intentional movement (may show reflexive movement such as posturing, withdrawal from pain, or involuntary smiling).
- Patient cannot sustain visual pursuits through a 45° arc in any direction when the eyes are held open manually.
- These criteria cannot be attributed to use of paralytic agents.

Vegetative State

Vegetative state indicates complete unawareness of the self or the environment. Patients in a vegetative state have cyclical patterns of sleeping and waking with periodic opening of the eyes, but no evidence of nonreflexive "sustained, reproducible, purposeful, or voluntary behavioral responses to visual, auditory, tactile, or noxious stimuli" (Multi-Society Task Force on PVS, 1994, p. 1500).

Minimally Conscious State

Patients in a minimally conscious state have some conscious awareness. They demonstate observable behaviors that are not purely reflexive and that show some awareness of the self or the environment (Giacino et al., 2002). Diagnostic criteria consist of reproducible or sustained demonstration of one or more of the following behaviors:

- Following simple commands
- Gestural or verbal yes/no responses (regardless of accuracy)
- Intelligible verbalization
- Purposeful behaviors in response to relevant environmental stimuli such as (1) reaching for objects in a way that demonstrates a clear relationship between object location and direction of reach, (2) shaping the hand to hold an object in response to the object's size and shape, and (3) smiling or crying appropriately in response to emotional topics or stimuli

For a patient to be characterized as having emerged from a minimally conscious state, he or she must demonstrate the ability for functional communicaton and object use (Giacino et al., 2002). Functional communciation is defined for this purpose as accurate yes/no responses to six out of six basic situational orientation questions (e.g., "Are you sitting down?") on two consecutive evaluations. Demonstration of functional object use is based on appropriate use of at least two different objects on two consecutive evaluations (e.g., bringing a comb to the head).

in coma. Some patients gradually or abruptly recover consciousness directly from coma, whereas others shift more gradually over 2–4 weeks into a vegetative state (Duff, 2001). Vegetative patients may still recover consciousness, but they do so gradually, spending long periods in a minimally conscious state in which there is verifiable evidence of conscious processing (Phipps et al., 1997). The ability to sustain visual pursuit eye movement seems to be one of the first signs of the transition out of vegetative state (Giacino & Kalmar, 1997) and is an early indicator of possible readiness for rehabilitation (Ansell, 1993).

Assessment. Diagnosis of specific disorders of consciousness and prognostic decisions must be reserved for physicians and other professionals with experience in neurological assessment of patients with impaired consciousness (American Congress of Rehabilitation Medicine, 1995). The rehabilitation team, however, including occupational therapists, uses a number of objective assessments to monitor changes in function and response to pharmacological, environmental, and behavioral interventions and for early detection of neuromedical complications.

Rancho Los Amigos Levels of Cognitive Functioning Scale. The Rancho Los Amigos Levels of Cognitive Functioning Scale uses behavioral observations to categorize a patient's level of cognitive function (Table 34-2) (Hagen, 1998; Hagen, Malkmus, & Durham, 1979). It helps clinicians to communicate about a patient's level of cognitive function among themselves and with families and to develop appropriate rehabilitation strategies. The first three levels of the Rancho Los Amigos Levels of Cognitive Functioning Scale describe the response to stimulation and the environment of patients emerging from coma.

Behavior-Based Assessment Instruments. In addition to the GCS, the instruments described in Table 34-3 are all brief assessments that occupational therapists and other rehabilitation team members can use at bedside to evaluate patients with severe alterations in consciousness.

Use of Single-Subject Experimental Methodology. DiPasquale and Whyte (1996) proposed that clinicians use single-subject experimental methodology as a means of answering individualized questions about responsiveness. They described how these methods were used to determine whether or not a patient with a brain injury was able to follow a verbal command to squeeze her hand. The protocol began with the therapist performing passive range of motion (PROM) to the patient's right hand, placing the patient's hand in hers, and then waiting 1 minute. There were three conditions: (1) correct command ("Squeeze my hand"), (2) incorrect command ("Tie your shoes"), and (3) observation period (equal duration, but no command given). Six trials were performed in random order with the therapist waiting 5 seconds to observe the patient's response. If the patient did not respond in 5 seconds, the command was given again. If again, there was no response in 5 seconds, the trial was recorded as no response.

Table 34-2 Rancho Los Amigos Levels of Cognitive Functioning

Level	Description
I	No response: unresponsive to stimuli
II	Generalized response: nonspecific, inconsistent, and nonpurposeful reaction to stimuli
III	Localized response: response directly related to type of stimulus but still inconsistent or delayed
IV	Confused—agitated: response heightened, severely confused, may be aggressive
V	Confused—inappropriate: some response to simple commands, but confusion with more complex commands; high level of distractibility
VI	Confused—appropriate: response more goal directed but cues necessary
VII	Automatic—appropriate: response robot-like, judgment and problem solving lacking
VIII	Purposeful—appropriate (*with standby assistance*): response adequate *to familiar tasks, subtle impairments require standby assistance with acknowledging other people's needs and perspectives, modifying plans*
IX	*Purposeful—appropriate (with standby assistance on request): responds effectively to familiar situations but generally needs cues to anticipate problems and adjust performance; low frustration tolerance possible*
X	*Purposeful and appropriate (modified independent): responds adequately to multiple tasks but may need more time or periodic breaks; independently employs cognitive compensatory strategies and adjusts tasks as needed*

Rancho levels I–VIII are widely used in brain injury rehabilitation. The addition of levels IX and X in 1998 (revisions italicized) describe higher level cognitive, behavioral, and emotional barriers to optimal functioning (Hagen, 1998; Hagen, Malkmus, Durnham, 1979).

| Table 34-3 | Behavior-Based Assessment Tools for Altered States of Consciousness |

Agitated Behavior Scale[a] (Corrigan, 1989)	Measure of agitation that can be used to measure changes in agitation level over time (Center for Outcome Measurement in Brain Injury [COMBI], 2011). Consists of 14 items. Total score reflects overall agitation, with subscales specific to disinhibition, aggression, and lability.
Disability Rating Scale[a] (Rappaport et al., 1982)	Provides quantitative information on recovery from severe traumatic brain injury (TBI) from coma to community (COMBI, 2011). Consists of eight items in four categories: arousal and awareness; cognitive ability to handle self-care functions; physical dependence on others; and psychosocial adaptability for work, housework, or school.
JFK Coma Recovery Scale-Revised (CRS-R)[a] (Kalmar & Giacino, 2005)	Detects subtle changes in neurobehavioral status to differentiate between vegetative and minimally conscious states and identifies emergence from minimally conscious state (COMBI, 2011). Twenty-three items in six areas: auditory, visual, motor, oromotor-verbal, communication, and arousal. Specific stimuli are administered to elicit specific responses with responses criterion referenced.
Western NeuroSensory Stimulation Profile (Ansell & Keenan, 1989)	Assesses cognitive function in severely impaired adults (Rancho levels II–IV) and monitors change in noncomatose patients who are slow to recover. Battery consists of 32 items related to arousal, attention, response to stimuli, and expressive communication and results in a profile of six subscales that summarize individual patterns of responses.

[a]From Centers for Outcome Measurement in Brain Injury. (2011). COMBI: featured scales. Retrieved from http://www.tbims.org/combi/list.html.

The results of assessment using this approach allowed for objective assessment of volitional responses and helped inform team/family planning. They describe a similar methodology to assessing vision in minimally responsive patients (Whyte & DiPasquale, 1995).

Prognosis and Outcome. Early prediction of outcome presumably helps direct expensive medical treatment or rehabilitation to patients who have the best chance for survival with fewer residual impairments and enables the family to make informed, realistic decisions on immediate and long-term care (Jennett & Teasdale, 1981). Many researchers have attempted to assess the predictive power of age; clinical observations such as the GCS, duration of unconsciousness, and length of PTA; and neuroimaging evidence of structural damage (Healey et al., 2003; Nakase-Richardson et al., 2011). Even with sophisticated clinical and radiological techniques, during the first days after injury, it is not possible to predict outcome with sufficient accuracy to guide early treatment or justify withholding treatment (Marion, 1996). Repeated observations of neurological recovery over weeks or months remain the best means to predict complete or nearly complete recovery (Marion, 1996).

Outcome scales have been developed to allow physicians to correlate "final" recovery levels to early treatment and prognostic indicators. The Glasgow Outcome Scale (Extended) (GOS-E) (Wilson, Pettigrew, & Teasdale, 1998) is one of the most commonly used global outcome measures. The GOS-E uses a structured interview with questions relating to conciousness, independence inside and outside the home, work, social and leisure activities, family and friendships, and return to normal life. For individuals who have survived, outcome is categorized as vegetative state, lower severe disability, upper severe disability, upper moderate disability, lower good recovery, or upper good recovery.

The therapist is not required to predict but should consider predictive factors when deciding on treatment goals or length of rehabilitation efforts. Cognition, personality, and motivation, all of which may substantially affect quality of survival (Jennett et al., 1981), should also be considered in determining treatment goals. However, outcome predictions are based on groups of patients, not on individuals who may recover more completely than anticipated given the severity of the injury.

Intervention for Patients with Severe Disorders of Consciousness. Rehabilitation for patients with severe disorders of consciousness should include both preventative and restorative strategies (Hirschberg & Giacino, 2011). Patients in a vegetative or minimally conscious state are at risk for complications associated with prolonged immobilization, and preventive measures should be taken to minimize or avoid pulmonary and urinary tract infections; skin breakdowns; and muscle, tendon, and soft-tissue contractures (Hirschberg & Giacino, 2011; Mysiw, Fugate, & Clinchot, 1996). Restorative strategies are aimed at fostering alertness and goal-directed behavioral responsiveness and may include pharmacotherapy with centrally activating medications, thalamic deep brain stimulation, and sensory stimulation procedures (Hirschberg & Giacino, 2011). Early intervention is believed to result in shorter rehabilitation stays and higher Rancho levels at discharge (Lippert-Grüner, Wedekind, & Klug, 2003). With contradictory evidence regarding its effectiveness, however, sensory stimulation programs aimed at facilitating coma arousal remain particularly controversial (Giacino et al., 1997; Golisz, 2009). Giacino et al. (1997) recommended that, at a minimum, patients with disorders of consciousness receive intervention that includes range-of-motion exercise, positioning protocols, and tone alteration methods. They suggested that the additional provision of sensory stimulation trials be considered on a case-by-case basis, appreciating that it is often difficult to distinguish between brain recovery and an intervention effect. Golisz (2009) noted that although existing evidence is not sufficient to determine whether a sensory stimulation program can facilitate return to consciousness, such programs do help the rehabilitation team identify emergence from coma and give therapists a systematic way of reinforcing the patient's purposeful responses to environmental stimuli. Reducing possible agitation (Eames, Haffey, & Cope, 1990) and supporting and educating overwhelmed family members are critical aspects of rehabilitation at this phase (Phipps et al., 1997).

For patients at this phase of recovery, intervention typically addresses impairments in body functions to lay the foundation for later focus on activities, tasks, and roles (Procedures for Practice 34-1). Because of the medical acuity of many of these patients, occupational therapists attend to the safety precautions summarized in Safety Note 34-1.

Positioning. Occupational therapists collaborate with other members of the rehabilitation team to optimize positioning to normalize muscle tone and minimize the development of contractures and atypical postures associated with more severe injuries that can ultimately affect motor performance (Rinehart, 1990). The patient's position must be reevaluated frequently with close monitoring of his or her reactions, including facial expression, changes in muscle tone, and vocalizations. Minor adjustments can make a difference between comfort and discomfort. Assistive positioning supports are removed as the patient's neuromuscular status improves. The nursing staff and the patient's family must be made aware of the desired bed and wheelchair positioning and of the wearing schedule for any splints.

Side-lying or semiprone in bed, if permitted, with good body alignment is preferable to supine if the patient has abnormal posture (Carr & Shepherd, 1980). Lying supine triggers an extensor response. In side-lying, the head, resting on a small pillow, should be in neutral alignment with the trunk; the bottom upper extremity should be in moderate scapular protraction and humeral external rotation; the top upper extremity should be in scapular protraction, slight shoulder flexion, and resting on a pillow to avoid horizontal adduction; the bottom elbow should be flexed; the top elbow should be extended; wrists should be in extension; and cones should be placed in the hands to decrease spasticity and maintain thumb web spaces. Attention should be paid to ensure that the mobility in the thumb comes from the first carpometacarpal (CMC) joint and not compensatory hyperextension in the first metacarpophalangeal joint. A pillow between the knees decreases hip internal rotation and adduction. The lower leg also may need pillow support to align it with the thigh. The foot should not be placed higher than the knee and hip as this can result in torque on the knee and cause the hip to go into internal rotation. The hip and knee are flexed only slightly. If necessary, a firm pillow filling

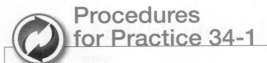

Procedures for Practice 34-1

Goal Setting for and with Persons with Traumatic Brain Injury

Occupational therapy treatment goals address changing aspects of occupational functioning as patients with severe traumatic brain injury (TBI) progress through recovery and adaptation. Here are some examples based on the phases of recovery and adaptation as described by Chestnut et al. (1999).

Medical Treatment Phase: Treatment Focuses on Body Functions

- In 3 weeks, the patient will make localized responses in less than 15 seconds after the presentation of tactile, olfactory, auditory, or visual stimuli at least 75% of the time to lay the foundation for using a communication board.
- In 3 weeks, the patient will independently reach out to hold a hairbrush in her hand and bring to her hair in four out of five trials.

Rehabilitation Phase: Treatment Primarily Focuses on Abilities and Skills, Activities and Habits, and Task Competency

- In 2 weeks, the patient will follow a checklist to carry out personal hygiene tasks with no more than two specific cues per session.
- In 2 weeks, the patient will independently locate and follow a daily schedule in his planner.
- In 2 weeks, the patient will be able to carry out his upper extremity range of motion exercises without assistance following written and pictorial instructions.

Survivor Phase: Treatment Primarily Focuses on Habits, Competency in Tasks, and Satisfaction with Life Roles

- In 4 weeks, the client will structure 100% of her children's after school activities (scheduling and making transportation arrangements) using compensatory cognitive strategies.
- In 4 weeks, the client will arrive on time to 100% of work meetings using an alarm cueing device.

the space between the thigh and calf can prevent excessive knee flexion. Elongation of the lower side of the trunk between the shoulder and pelvis is desirable. A side-lying trunk position may have to be maintained by a pillow or sandbag behind the back and shoulder. A pillow tucked in front of the trunk can also assist in maintaining the alignment. If a long body pillow is used, it can often be positioned to maintain some abduction in the lower extremities and support the calf and foot of the upper leg. Footboards should be avoided because they elicit extensor thrust. Splints or special shoes that are cut to avoid pressure to the ball of the foot,

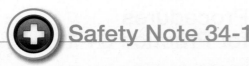

Safety Note 34-1

Safety Precautions for Treating Patients with Disorders of Consciousness

The patient with a severe traumatic brain injury (TBI) may be referred for occupational therapy before he or she is completely medically stable. Precautions may be numerous because of systemic injuries, secondary effects of the brain injury itself, disturbance of basic body regulatory systems, and the life support equipment used to treat the patient; such precautions must be heeded by the therapist. Typical precautions are described here; other precautions may also be necessary and should be ascertained from the nurse, physician, or patient's chart before the evaluation begins.

- A major concern with acute brain trauma is control of intracranial pressure (ICP). Sustained increased ICP can be fatal (Jennett & Teasdale, 1981). The patient with an ICP monitor can be readily checked during treatment sessions. The therapist must closely observe patients who are not on a monitor for pupil changes; decreased neurological responses; abnormal brainstem reflexes; flaccidity; behavioral changes; vomiting; and changes in pulse rate, blood pressure, and respiration rate. Fluids may be restricted, or the patient's head may be positioned in neutral at 30° of elevation in an attempt to regulate ICP. Turning the patient's head to one side may obstruct the internal jugular vein and result in a sudden increase of ICP (Boortz-Marx, 1985). The neck should be neither flexed nor extended but kept in neutral for maximum venous drainage and decreased ICP. The presence of a family member, gentle touching, quiet talking, and stroking the face have been found to decrease ICP in adults (Mitchell, 1986). Side-lying with the head of the bed elevated is the most desirable position. Supported sitting at 90° is used as soon as tolerated to help breathing, to provide symmetrical body alignment, and to increase awareness of surroundings (Palmer & Wyness, 1988).
- Early (i.e., within the first 7 days) post-traumatic seizures occur in 5% of patients with brain injuries, and late post-traumatic seizures occur in 20% of those with prolonged unconsciousness, depressed skull fracture, or intracranial

hematoma (Jennett & Teasdale, 1981; Schaffer, Kranzler, & Siqueira, 1985). Current recommendations are to provide pharmacological seizure prophylaxis for the first week after injury. To reduce the chance of a seizure during treatment, begin tactile stimulation and range of motion slowly to assess the patient's physiological response. Monitor the heart rate, blood pressure, and facial color and any autonomic changes, such as sudden perspiration or increased restlessness. As the therapist becomes more familiar with the patient's responses, he or she gradually increases intensity of stimulation. Use seizure precautions: avoid rapid, repetitive stimuli, such as vibration, flickering lights, and an oscillating fan. If a seizure does occur, ensure that the airway is open, position the patient on his or her side to prevent aspiration of stomach contents, and summon medical assistance (Greenberg, Aminoff, & Simon, 1993). The patient's limbs should not be restrained during a seizure.
- If the patient has had a craniotomy for evacuation of a hematoma, the bone flap may be left off, and the brain may be covered only by scalp to allow the brain to expand. Direct pressure to this site must be avoided, and the patient should wear a helmet at all times when out of bed until the bone flap is replaced. This generally occurs within 6 weeks, providing that the edema has resolved and there is no other infection.
- The patient may have a tear in the dura and cerebrospinal fluid leak. In this case, the patient initially is treated with head elevation, antibiotics, and precautions against nose blowing (Jennett & Teasdale, 1981; Schaffer, Kranzler, & Siqueira, 1985).
- If the patient has other systemic trauma, such as fractures or chest cavity trauma, appropriate precautions must be taken when he or she is stimulated or moved. Care must also be taken to avoid disturbing intravenous lines, tracheostomy, nasogastric tube, endotracheal or respirator tubes, and traction for extremity fractures. If the patient has a nasogastric tube, caution must be taken that the patient's head remains above the level of his or her stomach to avoid regurgitation and aspiration.

but still maintain ankle flexion to 90° and reduce foot drop, may be used to avoid stimulating an extensor thrust.

If the patient must be supine, a small pillow under the head is used, with small rolled pillows under that pillow to keep the head in midline if the patient cannot do so. Furthermore, small pillows are placed under the scapulae to protract them slightly, shoulders are positioned in slight abduction and external rotation, elbows are extended, and cones or finger spreaders position the fingers (Charness, 1986). If the pelvis is retracted on one side, a small folded towel is placed behind it, and that leg is positioned in neutral rotation. Some knee flexion should be encouraged by

a small towel roll placed under the distal thigh just above the knee, although care should be taken to avoid a knee flexion contracture. A semirecumbent bed position with head-of-bed angle maintained at 45° is recommended for patients on mechanical ventilators to minimize risk of aspiration and pneumonia (Helman et al., 2003).

Early and correct upright positioning in a wheelchair helps to facilitate arousal by stimulating the visual and vestibular systems, inhibiting abnormal tone, providing normal proprioceptive input, and reducing the likelihood and/or extent of contractures and complications from prolonged bed rest. The pelvis must be positioned correctly before other areas can be addressed. The pelvis should be in a neutral position or have a slight anterior tilt if needed to decrease extensor thrust. The pelvis should be symmetrical, without one side retracted or elevated. Solid seat and back inserts are used along with other inserts, pads, and cushions to gain optimal alignment.

Because the spine and rib cage are the essential connecting parts between the shoulders and the pelvis, it is important to obtain optimal alignment in these structures to facilitate optimal alignment of the shoulders. The trunk should be symmetrical and in midline with shoulders over pelvis in sagittal, frontal, and horizontal planes. Lateral trunk supports can be used to decrease lateral trunk flexion. Experimentation with the positioning is essential because trunk control varies among patients. The therapist must not provide too much trunk support, only enough to facilitate the patient's normal movement and control. With a solid seat and back, the patient may not require additional trunk support, whereas in other instances, a harness, shoulder straps, or a chest strap may be necessary to prevent forward trunk flexion.

Knees and ankles are flexed to 90°, heels are slightly behind the knees in sitting, feet are in neutral pronation-supination and inversion-eversion. The footplate should be large enough to support the whole foot. A foot wedge, heel loops, an insert behind the foot, special shoes, toe guards, or a combination of these may be helpful in decreasing abnormal tone and in achieving weight bearing on the heels.

The ideal upper extremity position is neutral scapular elevation or depression with the scapulae in slight protraction, slight shoulder external rotation, and slight flexion and abduction. Elbows are in comfortable flexion, and the forearm is in partial pronation. The wrists are in neutral flexion-extension and neutral ulnar-radial deviation, the fingers are relaxed, and the thumb is radially abducted with the mobility coming from the first CMC. Reclining the seat unit and/or positioning of shoulder straps, chest straps, and/or lateral trunk supports may help to obtain adequate shoulder position. In addition, a lapboard may be used to allow for upper extremity weight bearing. Note that while positioning recommendations often emphasize scapular protracton, scapular retraction and neutral scapular position are also critical.

Ideally, the head should be in midline with cervical elongation posteriorly and the chin tucked in slightly. It is important that positioning eliminate chin jutting and neck hyperextension. The position of the patient's pelvis, trunk, and shoulders all influence head position. See Chapter 17 for further discussion of wheelchair and seating system selection and positioning.

Passive Range of Motion. PROM programs are used in conjunction with positioning to minimize the development of contractures from abnormal tone and static postures. PROM can be difficult when muscle tone is increased. Inhibitory movements opposite the abnormal tone are performed slowly, holding the stretch until muscles relax. Sudden stretch and inappropriate stimulation and handling should be avoided. Scapular mobility should be addressed before upper extremity PROM to free the scapula and facilitate normal scapular and humeral movement during the rest of PROM (Palmer & Wyness, 1988). PROM within the limits of pain and positioning helps to minimize contractures from heterotopic ossification (Citta-Pietrolungo, Alexander, & Steg, 1992). See Chapter 20 for a complete discussion of exercise to improve range of motion.

Splinting and Casting. The goals of splinting and casting are to decrease abnormal tone and increase the patient's functional movement. Although it appears that serial casting may be more effective in treating range of motion limitations in the lower extremity (Golisz, 2009), plaster or fiberglass serial casting may be indicated when there is severe spasticity in the elbow and/or wrist (Mortenson & Eng, 2003). Dropout casts, which leave a portion of the limb free to relax out of a tightly contracted position; bivalve casts, which are split in two, with moleskin protecting the edges so they can be removed during therapy and nursing procedures; and weight-bearing inhibitory casts, which are fabricated to approximate the ideal weight-bearing posture of the foot or hand, can also be used (Carr & Shepherd, 1980). Casting is contraindicated with uncontrolled hypertension, major open wounds, unhealed fracture, impaired circulation, acute inflammation, a recent episode of autonomic dysreflexia, or if professionals need access to the extremity for lines or monitoring of vital signs (Stoeckmann, 2001).

Sensory Stimulation. The goals of a sensory stimulation program are to promote arousal from coma, appropriate patterns of movement, and interaction with the environment (Rinehart, 1990). Sensory stimulation programs are individualized to the patient's physical and cognitive functioning, but they always include multiple periods of observation and careful data collection (Mysiw, Fugate, & Clinchot, 1996). Clinicians use consistent protocols to standardize the administration of stimuli and data sheets to record observations regarding rate of response and changes in respiration, pulse, blood pressure, head movements, eye opening, eye movements, eye fixations, mimic responses, aimed and nonaimed motor reactions, and articulations (Lippert-Grüner & Terhaag, 2000) in response to tactile, vestibular, olfactory, kinesthetic, proprioceptive, auditory, and visual stimuli. Gustatory stimulation may be used if the patient's oral motor status permits. Pleasant and unpleasant and familiar and unfamiliar stimuli are used. Responses are measured at the beginning and end of every session and as each sense is stimulated. The patient's response to stimulation may be quite slow because central nervous system processing is slowed or prevented by the damage. Stimuli with emotional significance to the patient may be most likely to elicit a response. The therapist should wait for a response to the stimulation and, if necessary, repeat the stimulus.

(Refer back to the earlier discussion of using single-subject experimental methodology [DiPasquale & Whyte, 1996].) Clinicians monitor observation records in the hopes of seeing patterns of increasingly specific responses to stimuli, signifying improved responsiveness. Patients at Rancho level II often demonstrate nonspecific responses, such as motor restlessness in response to auditory stimuli. As the patient moves to level III, the responses become more stimulus specific. For example, with oral motor stimulation, one expects a motor response such as lip closure.

Management of Agitation. Once patients begin localizing stimuli, they may become quite agitated and restless (Scott & Dow, 1995). Post-traumatic agitation is reported to occur in the acute setting in 33%–50% of patients with TBI (Sandel, Bell, & Michaud, 1998) and may last for days or weeks. Agitation is a subtype of delirium in the coma-emerging patient that is associated with frontotemporal injury, disorientation, comorbid medical complications, and/or use of anticonvulsant medication (Kim, 2002). Agitation causes excesses of behavior that include some combination of aggression, akathisia (motor restlessness or a sense of inner restlessness [Ivanhoe & Bontke, 1996]), disinhibition, and emotional lability (Sandel, Bell, & Michaud, 1998). Eames, Haffey, and Cope (1990) suggested that efforts to manage behavior be preceded by a contextual assessment in which clinicians

attempt to determine what factors are contributing to the problem. Clinicians examine the following variables:

- Client factors—Extent and location of brain damage; state of bodily dysfunction, including pain; and premorbid factors such as intellect, personality traits, and coping style
- Social context and environment—Persons present during maladaptive behavior; reinforcers
- Physical environment—Properties of the environment in which problematic behavior occurs

During the period of medical instability, patients may exhibit agitation that stems from post-traumatic confusion and inability to process information (Eames, Haffey, & Cope, 1990). Patients may demonstrate apparently non–goal-directed body movements, such as thrashing; goal-directed behaviors, such as trying to remove life-sustaining tubes or get out of bed; screaming, moaning, or bizarre verbalizations; and disinhibited behavior, such as uncontrolled laughter or inappropriate sexual behavior (Eames, Haffey, & Cope, 1990). The primary aim of behavior management at this phase is to avoid inadvertent reinforcement of undesirable behaviors while ensuring the continuation of medically necessary treatment and doing as little as possible to impede the natural course of recovery (Eames, Haffey, & Cope, 1990). Procedures for Practice 34-2

 Procedures for Practice 34-2

Managing Agitation: Rancho Level IV

During this stage of recovery, occupational therapists primarily seek to decrease the patient's agitation by attempting to structure tasks and the environment to minimize overstimulation, confusion, and frustration and employing appropriate physical management methods that allow the patient to move and release energy without jeopardizing safety (Eames, Haffey, & Cope, 1990; Golisz, 2009). Remember that the patient is not accountable for the agitation, hostility, or aggressiveness. He or she is responding to internal confusion, not specifically to you as a person or professional. At the same time, you must structure your interactions to protect the patient and yourself.

Strategies to Normalize the Environment

- Ask family members to bring in familiar objects (photographs or belongings) and position them so they are visible to the patient (Eames, Haffey, & Cope, 1990).
- Work in a quiet environment with minimal distracters.
- Provide orientation information and maintain a predictable daily structure and routine.
- Introduce yourself at each session, telling the patient where he or she is and what you are going to do (Eames, Haffey, & Cope, 1990). Minimize asking orientation and other questions when it is unlikely that the patient knows the answer.

Strategies for Physical Management

- Use equipment and devices that maximize freedom of movement along with safety. Mittens without separations for the thumb may keep patients from pulling out tubes. A floor bed (a mattress on the floor that is surrounded by portable walls lined with therapy mats) allows the patient to move freely in bed without risk of falling. Extensions to the wheelchair so that it can neither tip over backward nor fit through doorways also allow for safe mobility (Eames, Haffey, & Cope, 1990).
- Engage the patient in gross motor activities such as face washing, catching a ball, hitting a balloon, and putting on simple clothing, if he or she is able. Physical activity, walking, or even being wheeled in the wheelchair may help decrease agitation.
- Be prepared to change activity or take a break at the first sign that the patient is becoming restless or agitated. Consider moving to another environment or offering a drink or snack if the patient has normal oral motor activity. Avoid responding to obscenities or bizarre verbalizations; simply view them as cues to distract the patient with another activity.
- Exude calm, confidence, and acceptance. The patient needs you to provide consistency and predictability that counters his or her confusion.

has specific suggestions regarding management of agitation during occupational therapy sessions.

Family Support and Education. TBI has almost as many implications for family members as it does for the patient. After an individual sustains a severe TBI, family members are typically relieved that the patient has survived but have little experience to help them understand the situation or what lies ahead (Phipps et al., 1997). Television portrayals of people who abruptly "wake" from coma with no apparent deficits may lead families to expect full recovery, and they may have difficulty processing information that is inconsistent with that hope (Phipps et al., 1997).

Families often see a level of responsiveness that is not verifiable by staff, and early in recovery, they tend to interpret unresponsiveness in ways other than as a reflection of cognitive status, such as deafness, lack of interest, or laziness (Phipps et al., 1997). Because the patient's level of responsiveness often drives decisions about what services are appropriate, how long they will be provided, and whether the patient is making progress, tension between the overwhelmed family and rehabilitation team is fairly common (Phipps et al., 1997). By providing the family with clear and concise information that matches their most immediate concerns, therapists can help families begin to understand what has happened in ways that neither inflame expectations nor squelch hope.

Holland and Shigaki (1998) proposed a three-phase model for educating families and caregivers of persons with TBI. They suggested that families benefit from information that is relevant to the patient's stage of recovery and their own stage of adjustment. They recommended that during the first phase (ICU through acute hospitalization), family education should focus on providing basic orientation to help the family decipher what is unfolding and to clarify terms and procedures associated with trauma care and TBI. Family members also need help to understand the disordered and occasionally bizarre behavior associated with agitation and to appreciate it as a natural part of recovery (Eames, Haffey, & Cope, 1990). Finally, conversations and instructions have to be repeated frequently, because the family is under considerable stress and flux. To provide right-timed education at the appropriate level, clinicians should also try to learn about patient and family background including such matters as family structure, family routines and activities, and experiences with service providers (Sohlberg et al., 2001). (See Resources 34-1 for materials that could be used in family education.)

Rehabilitation

My occupational therapist (OT) has promised to take me to the hospital chapel to play the organ. My mom brought my organ books to the hospital. . . . Now I can show the therapists that I don't need their exercises . . .[and] don't belong here in the hospital. (Rain, 2000, p. 6)

Rehabilitation occurs in inpatient, outpatient, and residential settings. In general, the primary goals of inpatient rehabilitation are medical stability, reduction of physical impairments, and acquisition of basic self-care skills. Postacute rehabilitation emphasizes reducing the obstacles of community integration posed by cognitive and behavioral impairments (Malec et al., 2000). It may take weeks, months, or years until goals are achieved and/or the patient no longer appears to benefit from intervention. Decreases in lengths of stay, however, result in many patients being discharged from inpatient rehabilitation settings without realizing their potential to recover capacities and basic skills. Rehabilitation efforts outside the inpatient setting increasingly address medical needs, fundamental capacities, and basic skill acquisition before or instead of community reentry.

Inpatient Rehabilitation

Although referral patterns vary, patients can generally participate in intensive inpatient rehabilitation when they demonstrate stimulus-specific responses and when post-traumatic confusion and agitation either resolve or do not present a barrier to participation in intensive therapies, such as Rancho levels V and VI. At level V, patients are still disoriented and confused but increasingly goal directed (Heinemann et al., 1990) and capable of teaching–learning interactions (Abreu & Toglia, 1987). They cannot process information at a normal rate or produce an appropriate response to all environmental situations. A patient at this level may require maximum assistance for independent living skills, exhibit significant neuromuscular impairments, need maximum cueing for orientation, display severe memory impairment, possibly show confused verbal and mental processes, and have little carryover of new learning. As patients progress to Rancho level VI, they remain inconsistently oriented but begin to be aware of appropriate responses to staff and family and demonstrate carryover for relearned, familiar tasks (Hagen, 1998).

Assessment: Inpatient Rehabilitation. Patients with TBI who are in rehabilitation can participate in formal assessment. Occupational therapists often begin by screening vision, visual perception, and cognition. Chapters 5 and 6 detail numerous assessment tools and methods appropriate for persons at this phase of recovery from TBI. Clinicians must determine the extent to which patients can scan, attend, follow, and retain instructions to interpret performance on other traditional assessments, including upper extremity strength and function and activities of daily living (ADL). A number of tools developed specifically to assess patients with TBI are used in a variety of rehabilitation disciplines, including occupational therapy (Table 34-4). Assessment tools are also detailed in the Occupational Therapy Practice Guidelines for Adults with Traumatic Brain Injury (Golisz, 2009) and at the Center of

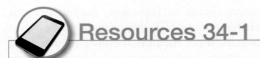

Resources 34-1

American Occupational Therapy Association

Brain injury evidence briefs and structured abstracts of traumatic brain injury (TBI)-related research.
www.aota.org (members only)

Be Smart. Be Well.

Brief educational videos by brain-injury experts and real-life accounts from people living with brain injury.
http://besmartbewell.com/index.htm

Brain Injury Association of America (BIAA)

National brain injury advocacy organization providing information on brain injury, including resources for survivors, families, professionals, and on state brain injury associations (BIAs). Resources include the "The Road to Rehabilitation" series, which are articles written for laypersons on an array of relevant topics that can be downloaded for free.
http://www.biausa.org

BrainLine.org and BrainLineMilitary.org

This multimedia website funded by the Defense and Veterans Brain Injury Center provides videos, personal stories, research briefs, and current news related to brain injury symptoms, treatment, and family issues. Some information available in Spanish. Military-specific information and resources are available at BrainLineMilitary.org.
http://www.brainline.org/
http://www.brainlinemilitary.org/

Center for Outcomes Measurement in Brain Injury (COMBI)

Assessment tools used in brain injury rehabilitation.
http://www.tbims.org/combi/

Family Caregiver Alliance

Provides resources for caregivers of individuals with chronic conditions including TBI. Fact sheets available in Spanish and Chinese.
http://caregiver.org

Living with Traumatic Brain Injury

Downloadable 30-minute documentary featuring four first-person accounts from people living with TBI and TBI experts sharing information about the effects of brain injury. A 5-minute version suitable for advocacy purposes is also available.
http://www.brainline.org/content/multimedia.php?id=957

Model Systems Knowledge Translation Center (MSKTC)

Provides consumer information resources relating to living with TBI, systematic reviews of TBI-related research, and summaries of research conducted by the TBI Model System centers funded by the National Institute on Disability and Rehabilitation Research (NIDRR).
http://www.msktc.org

National Institute of Neurological Disorders and Stroke.

National Institutes of Health. (2002). *Traumatic brain injury: Hope through research.* (NIH Publication No. 02-158). Bethesda, MD: National Institutes of Health.
http://www.ninds.nih.gov/disorders/tbi/detail_tbi.htm

National Resource Center for Traumatic Brain Injury

The mission of this center is to provide practical, relevant information to professionals, persons with brain injury, and family members. Materials available for purchase include workbooks, survivor and caregiver guides, intervention workbooks, and assessment kits, many of which were developed as part of the Virgina TBI Model System project.
http://www.tbinrc.com/

Outcome Measurement in Brain Injury (COMBI) website (www.tbims.org/combi).

Treatment: Inpatient Rehabilitation. Occupational therapy during inpatient rehabilitation is aimed at optimizing motor, visual-perceptual, and cognitive functions; restoring competence in fundamental self-maintenance tasks; contributing to the patient's continuing behavioral and emotional adaptation; and supporting the patient's family as they prepare for discharge.

Optimizing Motor Function. Therapists initially help patients with more severe cognitive impairments optimize their motor function by engaging them in gross motor activities that they can perform almost automatically, such as playing catch or hitting a punching bag (Fig. 34-2). Such activities minimize the demands on weakened cognitive functions, such as attention, concentration, and memory. Intervention increasingly focuses on refining motor functions as the patient's motor and cognitive recovery progress. Patients perform traditional exercise regimens as well

| Table 34-4 | Assessment and Outcomes Tools for Traumatic Brain Injury Patients in Rehabilitation |

Instrument	Brief Description
Mayo-Portland Adaptability Inventory[a] (Malec & Thompson, 1994)	Designed for interdisciplinary postacute rehabilitation; covers broad range of observable attributes, such as physical function, cognitive capacity, emotional status, social behavior, self-care, work, and driving (Center for Outcome Measurement in Brain Injury [COMBI], 2011). Patient's status on 30 items is rated on a four-category scale: no impairment, impairment on clinical examination but does not interfere with everyday function, impairment does interfere with everyday function, or complete or nearly complete loss of function.
Moss Attention Rating Scale (MARS)[a] (Whyte et al., 2003)	Twenty-two–item observational scale of attention-related behavior following TBI (COMBI, 2011). Items, which include behaviors indicative of good as well as impaired attention, are rated on a 5-point Likert-type scale.
Neurobehavioral Rating Scale (Levin et al., 1987)	Twenty-seven–item clinical rating scale measures common cognitive, behavioral, and emotional disturbances associated with TBI; used to track neurobehavioral recovery and measure behavioral change in response to intervention.
Patient Competency Rating Scale (PCRS)[a] (Leathem, Murphy, & Flett, 1998)	Thirty-item self-report measure to evaluate self-awareness following TBI (COMBI, 2011). The patient's responses are compared to the ratings of a relative or therapist to identify discrepancies indicating overestimation of abilities. Domains include activities of daily living, behavioral and emotional function, cognitive abilities, and physical function.
Participation Objective, Participation Subjective (POPS)[a] (Brown et al., 2004)	Twenty-six–item measure of participation in five categories: (1) domestic life; (2) major life activities; (3) transportation; (4) interpersonal interactions and relationships; and (5) community, recreational, and civic life (COMBI, 2011). For each item, the person is asked about level of participation (objective), satisfaction with that level of participation (subjective), and how important that particular activity is to satisfaction with life (subjective). Objective and subjective responses contribute to total score.

[a]Available online at http://www.tbims.org/combi. Psychometric data on these instruments, including reliability, are found at the COMBI site.

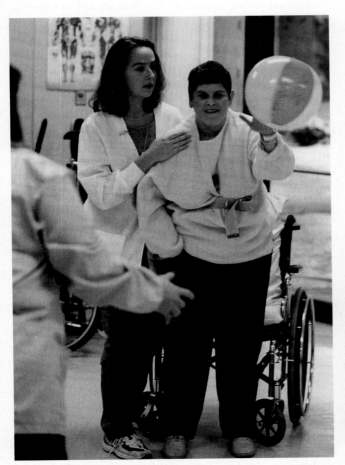

Figure 34-2 Early efforts to optimize motor function focus on eliciting automatic movement.

as exercise and activity delivered by virtual reality to improve strength and balance (Holden, 2005; Thorton et al., 2005) (Fig. 34-3). Occupational therapists use approaches that best match therapy goals and the patient's abilities, as detailed in Chapters 20 and 21.

Optimizing Visual and Visual-Perceptual Function. TBI frequently results in foundational visual and/or visual-perceptual disturbances that impair occupational function (Bouska & Gallaway, 1991). Transient changes in refractive error, impaired accomodative (i.e., focusing) function, and impaired convergence of the eyes are common

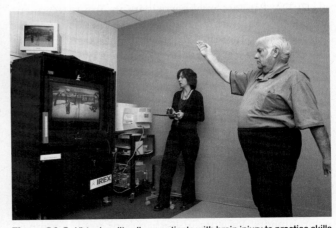

Figure 34-3 Virtual reality allows patients with brain injury to practice skills while participating in interesting and motivating activities that might otherwise be unsafe or unavailable to them.

(Suter, 2004). Visual field loss is often in the superior fields, and the oculomotor system is frequently impaired, with poor fixation, deviation of the eyes resulting in diplopia, and difficulty in visual scanning (Scott & Dow, 1995). Limitations in complex visual processing become evident during perceptual evaluation (Warren, 1993). It is important to identify possible visual impairments as early as possible so that appropriate patients are referred for specialized optometry and/or ophthalmology assessments, and therapists can make an effort to circumvent the influence of visual impairments on performance. Chapter 5 details specific assessments that may be applicable to patients with TBI. As Kaldenberg recommends in Chapter 23, intervention for primary visual deficits emphasizes environmental adaptation, compensatory techniques, assistive devices, and patient and family education. The efficacy of perceptual remediation is controversial. Based on her review of research on remedial perceptual retraining, Neistadt (1994b) was pessimistic about its appropriateness for TBI patients: "Far and very far transfer from remedial to functional tasks will not occur for clients with diffuse brain injuries and severe cognitive deficits, in either early or late stages of recovery, even with a variety of training tasks and up to 6 weeks of training" (p. 232).

Optimizing Cognitive Function. Chapter 24 presents occupational therapy approaches for optimizing cognitive function, all of which may be appropriate for persons with TBI. Inpatients with TBI are typically in a period of relatively rapid improvement, so therapists provide cognitive remediation activities and exercises to challenge and stimulate primary cognitive domains (attention, memory, and executive function) in the hope that natural recovery will be enhanced and accelerated. Card or board games, puzzles, and paper-and-pencil tasks such as word recognition or letter or number cancellation drills, and computer programs may be used. However, sole reliance on repeated exposure to and practice of computer-based tasks devoid of clinician involvement is not recommended (Cicerone et al., 2011). Patients may participate in group treatment, such as an orientation group in which they rehearse and reinforce awareness of time, place, and circumstances.

Vanderploeg et al. (2008) compared two of the primary inpatient rehabilitation approaches to treating TBI-related cognitive impairments in a military and veteran sample with moderate to severe brain injury. The cognitive-didactive approach emphasized trial-and-error learning and building self-awareness with targeted 1:1 remedial training for the various cognitive domains. The functional-experiential approach focused on developing functional abilities or skills using errorless learning techniques, environmental management, and compensatory strategies primarily in group sessions in real-life environments. Patients in both groups used a compensatory memory notebook. In addition to 1.5–2.5 hours

each day of protocol-specific treatment, patients received an additional 2–2.5 hours of occupational and physical therapy daily following the designated approach for each patient. At 1 year postinjury, 56% of the cognitive treatment group and 62% of the functional treament group were living independently, and 39% of the cognitive group and 35% of the functional group had returned to work or school. Although the differences in the primary outcomes between the two intervention groups were not statistically significant, it is not possible to know how people who did not receive either intervention would have fared, as the study did not include a nontreatment group for ethical reasons. Vanderploeg et al. concluded that the relatively high rate of independent living and return to work or school in a sample with 90% severe TBIs was evidence of the potential benefit of both of the two approaches.

The Cognitive Rehabilitatation Task Force of the American Congress of Rehabilitation Medicine Brain Injury Interdisciplinary Special Interest Group conducted three systematic reviews of studies of cognitive rehabilitation, which led to more specific practice recommendations for TBI (Cicerone et al., 2000, 2005, 2011). There was insufficient evidence to determine whether improvements seen in attention during acute rehabilitation are a result of directed attention training, other cognitive interventions, or spontaneous recovery. However, there was substantial evidence to support the use of direct attention training and metacognitive training for the remediation of attention deficits during postacute rehabilitation after TBI. Memory strategy training including internalized strategies such as visual imagery and external memory compensations such as day planners and memory books was recommended for people with mild memory deficits. They recommended the use of external memory compensations directly related to functional activities for people with severe memory impairments. They further recommended metacognitive strategy training to address impairments in executive functioning.

An evidence review by the Institute of Medicine (2011) was more conservative in its recommendations, finding limited to modest support for cognitive rehabilitation therapy (CRT) in TBI with efficacy varying across cognitive domains, injury severity, and time since injury. The committee clarified that the lack of more definite clinical recommendations for CRT was primarily due to limitations in the existing research, which should not preclude the ongoing clinical use of cognitive rehabilitation for individuals with TBI (IOM, 2011).

In conjunction with the approaches described above, occupational therapists often use a dynamic investigative approach (Toglia, 1989) in which cognitive retraining activities become opportunities for assessing performance under a variety of circumstances. Careful activity analysis and logging of observations and environmental variables informs discharge recommendations to families regarding the circumstances in which their loved one is best able to function. Such information is invaluable to families as they assume day-to-day responsibility for structuring the patient's time and activities.

Occupational therapists also use the physical environment to optimize patients' cognitive capacities and abilities during this phase of recovery. Specialized brain injury units typically incorporate signage and physical landmarks that enhance orientation and technology, such as monitoring systems, that allow the patient to move even though he or she may be confused and disoriented. Occupational therapists also strategically place familiar pictures and objects, calendars, and clocks in the patient's room to optimize orientation.

Restoring Competence in Self-Maintenance Tasks. As previously mentioned, inpatient rehabilitation usually focuses on helping patients reacquire basic self-care skills, such as bathing, dressing, hygiene, and eating. In general, a given self-care task is simplified until the patient is consistently successful in performing it, and then the complexity is gradually increased while the externally provided structure is gradually decreased. Environmental distractions are kept to a minimum. The therapist structures the task, gathers the items to be used, and sequences the task by providing the patient with the appropriate item and instructions, one step at a time. For example, in dressing, the therapist first hands the patient his undershorts and then gives simple verbal instructions and physical assistance as necessary to have the patient put the shorts over his legs and pull them up. The therapist does not present the patient's tee shirt until the shorts are on. Initially, the therapist selects solid colors with minimal fastenings to decrease perceptual confusion. The therapist may also choose to limit the task by having the patient do only one or two steps of the entire task (e.g., put on tee shirt only) if the patient has very low endurance, low frustration tolerance, or limited motor skills. Selection of the position of the patient (i.e., dressing in bed, sitting in the wheelchair, or sitting on the edge of the bed) and the method of dressing is based on the patient's neuromuscular function. Gradually, as the patient becomes more successful in dressing, the therapist decreases verbal and physical cueing, using checklists and/or graded cues (see Chapter 24). Bathing, hygiene training, feeding, and wheelchair transfer training are structured in the same fashion. Occupational therapists can help set the stage for establishing consistent and automatic self-care routines at home by outlining the sequence of steps in which the patient is most successful.

During inpatient rehabilitation, occupational therapists assess the patient's ability to handle more complex ADL, such as meal preparation and cleanup, laundry, and using the telephone (Fig. 34-4). Therapists take into

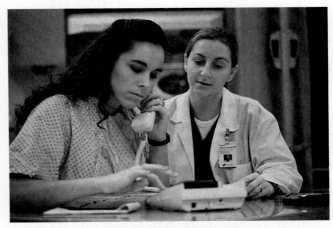

Figure 34-4 Occupational therapists often simulate real-life activities, such as gathering information over the telephone.

consideration the client's prior familiarity with a task to determine whether the client will be reestablishing familiar habits and routines or learning new, or relatively unfamiliar, skills (Powell et al., 2007). Again, a dynamic investigative approach is employed to determine under what circumstances the patient can safely and competently carry out these activities and the most effective intervention strategies.

Contributing to Behavioral and Emotional Adaptation. Behavioral sequelae may intermittently influence the patient's ability to participate in therapy at this stage. Brain damage itself may cause psychosocial changes, such as irritability, aggressiveness, or apathy (Prigatano, 1992). As the patient becomes more alert, his or her awareness of the situation may increase irritability, uncooperativeness, or mood fluctuations. Patients who lack awareness of deficits may also become frustrated with staff and family who limit their activities. Furthermore, patients who repeatedly fail on a variety of tasks may become depressed or anxious (Prigatano, 1992). It is important for occupational therapists to appreciate the state of internal chaos and vulnerability of many patients with TBI at this phase of recovery (Groswasser & Stern, 1998). Without the anchor of intact memory to make connections between experiences, "life is downgraded to a collection of unrelated, disjointed, and sporadic episodes" (Groswasser & Stern, 1998, p. 73). Rather than force confrontation of deficits early on, therapists avoid placing patients in situations that are fraught with frustration and failure and instead structure experiences that reinforce patients' confidence that they still have the potential to accomplish things (Groswasser & Stern, 1998). Doing so establishes therapeutic trust, the foundation for later phases of recovery, when patients are better able to compare premorbid and current capabilities. See Chapter 14 for guidelines to establish a therapeutic relationship.

When behavioral sequelae associated with brain injury interfere with progress and the potential for community reintegration, the rehabilitation team establishes an interdisciplinary plan to minimize or eliminate socially unacceptable behavior and promote prosocial, adaptive behavior. Eames, Haffey, and Cope (1990) pointed out, "Since the primary aim of rehabilitation is a return to the community, simple containment or toleration of disordered behavior within the rehabilitation setting is inadequate because the community at large will not adopt a lenient attitude toward such behavior" (p. 420). Ylvisaker, Jacobs, and Feeney (2003) recommend focusing on antecedents associated with positive behavior and less on consequences related to problems. The following are examples of strategies that contribute to patients' ability to learn effective behaviors during inpatient rehabilitation and beyond:

- Redesign the environment (Ylvisaker, Jacobs, & Feeney, 2003). For example, if noise and distractions seem to contribute to a patient's irritability and aggressiveness, provide treatment and care in areas that are calm and quiet.
- Capitalize on the superiority of procedural over declarative memory after brain injury by helping patients learn context-sensitive routines rather than broader transfer-dependent strategies (Ylvisaker, Jacobs, & Feeney, 2003).
- Identify positive competing behavior and, as a team, consistently and frequently reward all instances of adaptive behavior (Eames, Haffey, & Cope, 1990).
- Withhold all rewards that maintain maladaptive behavior. Use time-outs in a calm, mechanical manner that does not reward the patient with increased social contact (Eames, Haffey, & Cope, 1990).
- Help the patient to learn new skills and to experience success to reduce frustration-induced maladaptive behavior.

Supporting the Patient's Family. Patients' families continue to require information and support to understand the recovery and rehabilitation process and to inform their decision making and discharge planning. Holland and Shigaki (1998) recommended that the rehabilitation team provide the family with information about (1) the full spectrum of possible TBI outcomes to enhance realistic expectations; (2) the effects of TBI on family systems and possible alterations in family dynamics post discharge; (3) the benefits, challenges, and responsibilities of caretaking and supervision post discharge; and (4) resources available for postacute rehabilitation. Participation in inpatient rehabilitation sessions can help family members learn about the patient's strengths and weaknesses, techniques for helping him or her optimize performance, and help minimize expectations of an abrupt recovery to the "same person" the patient was before the injury (Phipps et al., 1997).

Postacute Rehabilitation

Malec and Basford (1996) described the array of postacute rehabilitation programs in the literature and possibly available to clients with TBI. (The transition to references to the "client" rather than "patient" signifies the increasingly collaborative therapeutic relationship between therapist and TBI survivor during postacute rehabilitation and survivor phases.) Occupational therapists are typically involved in all of these options, including the following:

- Home-based therapy provides a single-discipline or interdisciplinary intervention for clients who are unable to get to clinic-based services or who would benefit from context-specific training within the home environment.
- Residential neurobehavioral programs provide intensive treatment for clients with severe behavioral disturbances.
- Residential community reintegration programs provide integrated cognitive, emotional, behavioral, physical, and vocational rehabilitation to clients who cannot participate in outpatient programs because of severe cognitive and behavioral impairments or lack of availability of outpatient options.
- Comprehensive (holistic) day treatment programs provide integrated, multidisciplinary rehabilitation that emphasizes self-awareness, social skills, and cognitive compensation.
- Outpatient community reentry programs provide specific rehabilitation therapies as well as vocational services.

In their review article comparing outcomes of postacute brain injury rehabilitation with natural recovery after TBI, Malec and Basford (1996) concluded, "Although generally uncontrolled, the studies reviewed document benefits for many individuals with brain injury, including increased independence and a rate of return to independent work or training that exceeds 50% and may reach 60% to 80% for intensive comprehensive (holistic) day treatment programs" (p. 198). Postacute rehabilitation typically is not a continuous sequence of rehabilitation services but, more often, a time-limited, goal-specific series of rehabilitation episodes.

In general, the aim of postacute rehabilitation is to prepare the client to reenter the community, although some programs also offer specialized tracks or pathways that focus on prerequisite physical, behavioral, cognitive, or self-care skills (Abreu et al., 1996). Although the occupational therapist's roles and responsibilities vary with the type and even location of the program, this section of the chapter reviews areas that are typically addressed. This section also discusses mild TBI, because these survivors rarely receive inpatient rehabilitation services.

Occupational Therapy Assessment: Postacute Rehabilitation. Occupational therapists continue to use many of the instruments and methods described earlier in this chapter (see Table 34-4) and text. As clients have more real-world experiences and their self-awareness continues to improve, tools like the Canadian Occupational Performance Measure (COPM) (Law et al., 1994) become appropriate for identifying treatment goals that are important to the client. This instrument, however, is not useful for clients with significant problems with insight and self-awareness, because these individuals are unlikely to view themselves as having problems that can be addressed in therapy. Furthermore, improved accuracy of self-appraisal can result in a self-rated decrease in performance and satisfaction at follow-up despite actual gains.

Treatment: Postacute Rehabilitation. After discharge from acute rehabilitation, many clients require occupational therapy treatment aimed at teaching them to compensate for residual cognitive and visual-perceptual impairments so that they may resume self-maintenance, self-advancement, and self-enhancement roles.

Optimizing Cognitive Function. In postacute rehabilitation, clients (usually in Rancho level VII or VIII) may continue to demonstrate specific impairments in short- and long-term memory, reasoning, conceptualization, comprehension, abstract thinking, information-processing speed, organization of information, simplification of problems, judgment, and problem solving (Dikmen, Reitan, & Temkin, 1983). They may display decreased attention during attempts to store information, inability to determine the salient or relevant details of what they hear or read, decreased ability to structure or associate incoming information appropriately, and decreased cognitive flexibility (Scherzer, 1986). Especially if the client also has decreased self-awareness, these impairments will affect his or her ability to make coherent decisions and plan for the future.

Occupational therapists continue to help clients and their families to change the physical and social contexts and environment to optimize occupational functioning. This may include decreasing distracting stimuli and increasing important visual cues at the home and work site to optimize cognitive function. Home and work site visits allow therapists to identify opportunities for these modifications. Also, because clients in postacute rehabilitation typically have a more stable living situation than they did as inpatients, their occupational therapists can capitalize on consistency of clients' environments and daily activities to help them create routines and habits that minimize the demands of information processing with frequently performed tasks. Occupational therapists also use a variety of activities and exercises, such as computer games, worksheets, crafts and projects, and simulated home and work tasks, to help clients improve their awareness of strengths and weaknesses. As clients appreciate the significance of residual cognitive impairments for resumption of roles, occupational therapists teach them to use compensatory cognitive strategies, such as paper or electronic calendars/organizers, cueing devices, smart phones, and problem-solving schemata, in the context of personally relevant real-world tasks (see Chapter 24).

Optimizing Visual and Visual-Perceptual Function. Similarly, occupational therapists continue to help clients make changes in environment and strategy to circumvent the influence of visual and visual-perceptual impairments. For example, Williams (1995) described occupational therapy intervention for problems with reading and writing of a woman who was more than 12 months post-TBI. A comprehensive vision evaluation performed by an ophthalmologist and occupational therapist revealed adequate central visual acuity, slightly reduced contrast sensitivity, an inferior visual field cut in both eyes, and a dense scotoma bordering the fovea in both eyes. Intervention, which consisted of changes in lighting for reading and writing, oculomotor exercises, and strategy training, ultimately allowed her to resume these valued activities.

Restoring Competence in Self-maintenance Roles. Clients who have not achieved independence in basic self-care and homemaking tasks continue to work toward those goals in postacute rehabilitation. Giles et al. (1997) used behavioral training to help TBI clients in a transitional living center develop independence in dressing and washing skills in a relatively short period (11–37 days) of treatment. Even clients with proficient self-care skills benefit from treatment that links individual skills to automatic routines (see Chapter 24). Based on performance on the Rabideau Kitchen Evaluation–Revised (Neistadt, 1992), Neistadt (1994a) used a meal preparation protocol to help outpatients with TBI learn to prepare a hot beverage and snack. After three 30-minute sessions per week for 6 weeks, participants made gains in independence and decreased their performance times. Interventions in self-care and homemaking always involve input from family and/or caregivers and measures to ensure transfer of newly acquired skills to the client's living environment.

When client and family are satisfied with the client's ability to perform daily living skills and homemaking tasks, such as cleaning, meal preparation, and laundry, occupational therapy addresses community reentry skills. Many clients rely on occupational therapy to help them learn or relearn to manage money, go shopping, use the bank, and use public transportation. To do so, clinicians again adapt the environment, help clients acquire behavioral routines, and teach clients to use compensatory strategies. The therapist must carefully assess the amount of supervision and structuring necessary because of impaired judgment and problem-solving ability, as well as any physical limitations.

Almost as soon as they are discharged from the hospital, many survivors of TBI inquire about their readiness to drive. The client's residual physical, cognitive, perceptual, and visual dysfunction must be thoroughly assessed to determine his or her ability to drive safely. The client's psychosocial status, including self-control, impulse control, and frustration tolerance, must be also carefully considered. A car can be adapted to compensate for some physical problems (see Chapter 26) and measures such as turning off the radio can be taken to reduce distracting stimuli while driving; however, no compensation can be made for slowed reaction to emergencies, lack of judgment or problem-solving ability, spatial or directional confusion on the road, or impairment in depth perception (Jones, Giddens, & Croft, 1983).

Restoring Competence in Leisure and Social Participation. Occupational therapy plays an important role on the postacute rehabilitation team by helping the client resume previous leisure activities or determine new leisure outlets that are more in line with current abilities. Many survivors of TBI have to change not only what they do for fun but also where and with whom they do it. Leisure activities post-TBI tend to be sedentary, home-based, and socially isolated (Wise et al., 2010). Few friendships withstand the cognitive, behavioral, and emotional upheaval that comes with TBI. Changes in the types of activities (e.g., fewer alcohol-related activities), also contribute to less contact with preinjury friends (Wise et al., 2010). Occupational therapy intervention may focus on helping the client initiate new social contacts, participate in support groups, and reestablish the social skills necessary for maintaining and building a social network. Social skills retraining following severe head injury develops skill in social behaviors and facilitates successful social interactions. In general, behavioral learning methods are the most effective for training severely brain-injured individuals to overcome social skill impairments (Giles & Clark-Wilson, 1993). Treatment typically entails instruction and modeling of the social skill, practicing the skill with feedback, and shaping the skill until it is used correctly (Yuen, 1997).

Restoring Competence in Work. After clients reestablish their competence in self-maintenance roles, they are ready to explore return to work. Postacute occupational therapy facilitates that process with prevocational programs that focus on work behaviors and habits, such as punctuality, thoroughness, response to feedback, and ability to take and use notes. Occupational therapists may also link clients with appropriate volunteer jobs where they can employ newly learned compensatory cognitive strategies and build their endurance and work tolerance.

Contributing to Behavioral and Emotional Adaptation. As clients attempt to resume familiar activities, they cannot escape the awareness that they have changed in some manner

(Groswasser & Stern, 1998). Emotional and behavioral difficulties can be attributed to premorbid personality and coping style, cognitive consequences of TBI, and/or grief associated with injury-related losses (Hanks et al., 1999). These emotional and behavioral changes may include social or sexual disinhibition, low tolerance for frustration or stress, reduced insight or judgment, labile affect, irritability, impulsivity, and depression. In the extreme, the patient may experience psychiatric disorders such as paranoia, phobias, confusion, or delusional ideation (Ashman et al., 2004; Benton, 1979). Regardless of the specific goals of therapy, occupational therapists support and guide clients with TBI as the clients confront and address impairments and inefficiencies that interfere with performance. They provide sensitive and timely feedback regarding behaviors that could otherwise result in rejection and social isolation in the community. Because depression negatively influences psychosocial functioning after TBI (Hibbard et al., 2004), occupational therapists also respond to indicators that clients may be in need of psychological or psychiatric intervention and make referrals as needed (see Chapters 3 and 30; see also Research Note 34-1).

Supporting the Client's Family. In most cases, the client's family ultimately provides long-term assistance and support for the survivor. Caregivers of persons with moderate to severe TBI report a mix of positive and negative caregiving experiences with negative experiences associated with more severe injuries, worse neuropsychological functioning, and increased dependence (Machamer, Temkin, & Dikmen, 2002). As time passes and the implications of the injury become clearer, family members may undergo mourning that is intense, disorganized, and prolonged (Muir, Rosenthal, & Diehl, 1990). Occupational therapists continue to support families in this stage by providing education. Holland and Shigaki (1998) recommended emphasis on the following topics in family education at this phase of recovery and adaptation: (1) the protracted nature of TBI recovery, (2) the experience of recovery from the patient's perspective, (3) adjustment to and possible management of behavioral and personality changes, (4) sexuality issues, (5) community resources, and (6) home adaptation.

Survivorship

I have been living with multiple effects of a severe TBI for 23 years. . . . Many of these years were spent in lonely isolation, wondering when the nightmare would end. . . . Now, I am focusing my energy on reaching out as well as within to live this life. (Rain, 2000, p. 6)

The medical treatment and rehabilitation phases of life for the survivor are relatively brief compared to the years during which he or she will continue to live with the consequences of TBI. Most survivors ultimately achieve independence in self-care skills and recover motor function,

Research Note 34-1

Bombardier, C. H., Fann, J. R., Temkin, N. R., Esselman, P. C., Barber, J., & Dikmen, S. S. (2010). Rates of major depressive disorder and clinical outcomes following traumatic brain injury. *Journal of the American Medical Association, 303,* 1938–1945.

Abstract

The purpose of this study was to describe the rates, predictors, outcomes, and treatment of major depressive disorder (MDD) for people with traumatic brain injury (TBI) during the first year postinjury. Researchers contacted 559 consecutively hospitalized adults with complicated mild to severe TBI monthly for the first 6 months postinjury and then at 8, 10, and 12 months. At each follow-up, study personnel administered the Patient Health Questionnaire (PHQ) depression and anxiety modules. Over one-half (53.1%) of participants met the criteria for MDD at least once during the follow-up, substantially more than the expected rate of 6.7% in the general population, with about half of those identified by 3 months. The risk for developing MDD postinjury was higher for those with a history of MDD prior to the time of injury, MDD at the time of injury, and lifelong alcohol dependence. Those with MDD had higher rates of co-occurring anxiety disorders and reported lower quality of life, but only 44% had received antidepressants or counseling.

Implications for Practice

- MDD following TBI is underrecognized and undertreated. Occupational therapists should be aware of the risk factors for MDD and realize that people without full awareness of their limitations can experience a depressive reaction. Occupational therapists should participate with other team members throughout the continuum of care in screening TBI survivors for depressive symptoms and referring for diagnosis and treatment.
- The efficacy of antidepressants in people with TBI may be limited by co-occurring substance abuse and/or anxiety disorders. Individuals with TBI have been found to favor counseling and exercise over other treatment modalities. Occupational therapists can assist TBI survivors in identifying and participating in pleasurable activities and healthy routines, including exercise, using compensatory strategies and devices as needed.

---

but cognitive, behavioral, and emotional problems are long-term barriers to good quality of life (IOM, 2009). Dikmen et al. (2003) found that personal care and ambulation were least affected at 3–5 years after a moderate to severe TBI, with approximately 65% and 50%, respectively, of survivors having recovered to preinjury levels. However, about 60% experienced cognitive problems in performing their daily activites, 60% were not performing their major role activity at preinjury levels, and approximately 25% were completely dependent on others financially. In comparison with preinjury levels, approximately 60% had more limitations in leisure and recreation, 45% more limitations in social integration, and 40% more limitations in home management.

TBI also affects people's ability to work. Moderate to severe TBI in individuals who were workers preinjury increases the probability of unemployment postinjury and decreases the likelihood of returning to the same position for those who do return to work (IOM, 2009). Individuals with TBI take longer to return to work than people with non-brain trauma with poor employment outcomes associated with injury severity and postinjury neuropsychological impairments (IOM, 2009). Decreased ability to successfully return to work is of particular concern, because employment appears to be linked to quality of life after TBI (O'Neill et al., 1998). O'Neill et al. (1998) found that being employed part or full time contributed to survivors' sense of well-being, social integration, and pursuit of meaningful home activities.

These long-term and often unmet needs underscore the importance of intermittent long-term rehabilitation services and community resources for persons with TBI. Unfortunately, most rehabilitation services remain medically oriented, often focusing heavily on intervention for physical impairments.

The contrast between need and service availability is particularly disturbing to occupational therapists who have the education and skills to make a difference in the lives of survivors of TBI. For example, Nelson and Lenhart (1996) described a case in which weekly outpatient occupational therapy sessions over 5 months helped a woman who was 5 years post-TBI to improve her ability to handle school, household, and social responsibilities. Trombly, Radomski, and Davis (1998) and Trombly et al. (2002) found that adults with TBI, many of whom were more than 2 years postinjury, met self-identified goals in outpatient occupational therapy.

The survivorship phase of life for persons with TBI presents opportunities for clinicians to employ all that is truly unique to occupational therapy, synthesizing the totality of our education, philosophy, and values to enhance occupational functioning in society. Readers are challenged to consider the following ways to poise themselves for action:

- Recommend that a life care plan be prepared for survivors of moderate to severe TBI (Sherer, Madison, & Hannay, 2000). A life care plan delineates the services and items required for the current and long-term care of the survivor as well as the costs of these services. A life care plan can be used clinically to plan appropriate long-term care, including intermittent follow-up, and for forensic purposes, such as determination of an appropriate settlement that will provide for the lifetime needs of the injured person (Sherer, Madison, & Hannay, 2000). Pursue credentialing to prepare life care plans as part of your role as an occupational therapist.

- Promote to possible referral sources what you are able to do to enhance community integration and quality of life for persons with TBI. Join your local brain injury association, connect with your state's vocational rehabilitation division, familiarize yourself with key personnel supporting disabled students at local colleges and universities.

- Establish the kind of therapeutic relationship with clients and family members that will make them want to return to you for help. Respecting the client's readiness for treatment means sometimes not intervening, but making sure that he or she knows that your door is open in the future.

- Make sure that the discharge from outpatient occupational therapy incorporates plans for follow-up and clear information regarding possible circumstances in the future when further occupational therapy services may be helpful. Provide information to the survivor and his or her family regarding mechanisms to reinstate services. Remember that the nature of TBI interferes with survivors' ability to advocate for themselves (e.g., lack of initiation, impaired memory), and so you must build in opportunities to discern and respond to their needs.

MILD TRAUMATIC BRAIN INJURY

A mild TBI, or concussion, is characterized by a shorter and less severe disruption of brain functioning than with a more severe injury. It is estimated that, each year, more than 1.1 million people in the United States experience a mild TBI (National Center for Injury Prevention and Control, 2003). There is some variation in the specifics of how mild TBI is defined. One of the most commonly used definitions states that mild TBI is an impact to or forceful movement of the head resulting in a brief alteration of mental status, such as confusion or disorentation, loss of memory lasting 24 hours or less, loss of consciousness lasting 30 minutes or less, and/or an acute seizure after injury to the head (National Center for Injury Prevention and Control, 2003). Symptoms of mild TBI may include headache, dizziness, nausea, irritability, fatigue, and cognitive deficits such as impaired concentration, information processing speed, and memory (National Center for Injury Prevention and Control, 2003). Most people with a mild TBI return to normal functioning within 1–3 months, although approximately 10% of patients continue to have problems a year after injury (Ruff, Camenzuli, & Mueller, 1996).

Experts disagree about the persistence and cause of cognitive problems after mild TBI (Dikmen, Machamer, &

Temkin, 2001). Some link cognitive inefficiencies to acute stress disorder (Bryant et al., 2003), whereas others attribute disability to brain damage (DeKruijk, Twijnstra, & Leffers, 2001). Montgomery (1995) described a multifactor explanation for disability after mild TBI. He suggested that personal factors (perfectionism or tendency toward negative thinking) interact with transient sequelae of mild brain injury, such as headache and mental inefficiency, that lead to short-term decrements in performance. Premature resumption of normal activities places an undue load on information-processing capacities that leads to errors and slowness of performance. Over time, the individual begins to make misattributions of causation and starts questioning his or her fundamental competence and even sanity (Montgomery, 1995). These individuals profit from outpatient rehabilitation services that address residual physical symptoms, provide information and support, and teach them to use cognitive compensatory strategies that decrease the demands on working memory. By normalizing and explaining cognitive inefficiencies, helping reestablish routines, and teaching use of memory backups, occupational therapists can play a pivotal role in helping these clients resume premorbid tasks and roles. There is some evidence that it may be possible to minimize the development and subsequent impact of symptoms following mild TBI. Bell et al. (2008) provided a brief program (four or five sessions) of proactive telephone-based counseling to individuals beginning shortly after the onset of mild TBI. The sessions focused on education, symptom management, and encouragement to gradually resume everyday activities. At 6 months after injury, those who received the counseling intervention reported fewer symptoms and less effect of symptoms on everyday function.

Clinicians need to appreciate that persons with mild TBI who find their way to rehabilitation professionals represent a fraction of the cases with mild TBI and that cognitive problems may be observed for a variety of reasons that have nothing to do with brain injury (artifacts from testing, preexisting conditions, litigation, or emotional problems) (Dikmen, Machamer, & Temkin, 2001). Given the disagreement regarding the mechanism underlying cognitive problems after mild TBI, it is not surprising that there is little consensus about the best intervention. At present, there is little in the literature to guide occupational therapists looking for an evidence-based approach to intervention, which is why there is no evidence table to accompany the mild TBI case example in this chapter.

Combat-Related Traumatic Brain Injury

From 2000 to 2012, over 267,000 service members (SMs) sustained a TBI with approximately 20% deployment-related (Defense and Veterans Brain Injury Center, 2013). Combat-related TBI can occur via several mechanisms, the most common being a concussive blast. Powerful blast waves produced by IEDs or "roadside bombs" can cause damage to the brain in the form of TAI, edema, or hemorrhage (Taber, Warden, & Hurley, 2006). Those injuries resulting from the blast itself are considered primary. A secondary type of blast injury is caused when overpressure from the blast propels debris and shrapnel away from the detonation site causing penetrating injuries to the brain and body. A tertiary form of blast injury occurs when individuals in close proximity to the blast are thrown in the air or against stationary objects causing acceleration/deceleration injuries. Quaternary blast injuries include other related injuries such as burns, respiratory problems from inhaling toxic gases, and blood loss from traumatic amputation (DePalma et al., 2005). TBIs in the military can also result from gunshot wounds to the head or face, training activities, and non–combat-related causes as in the civilian population.

SMs who sustain a moderate or severe TBI in combat are medically evacuated from the war zone and treated at a military medical treatment facility or a Veterans Affairs (VA) Polytrauma Rehabilitation Center. SMs receive treatment in inpatient, outpatient, and community reentry settings. Occupational therapy focuses on resuming independence with ADL, instrumental activities of daily living (IADL), and social and community activities. Through Department of Defense and VA programs, wounded SMs are eligible to receive adaptive equipment for cognition, communication, sensory loss, mobility, and environmental control. Vocational rehabilitation and home modification services are also available.

SMs who sustain a mild TBI in combat experience an alternate course of treatment and recovery. According to civilian estimates, approximately 75%–90% of individuals with a mild TBI experience a full recovery within minutes to weeks of the incident (Levin, Goldstein, & MacKenzie, 1997). SMs exposed to a blast receive evaluation and treatment during the acute stages of injury by military medical professionals. Often, they are able to return to duty after a brief rest period of 3–10 days. In some cases, symptoms persist beyond the anticipated recovery period. Recovery may be mediated by several factors. The presence of concomitant post-traumatic stress disorder (PTSD) and other mental health conditions are associated with persistent mild TBI symptoms and related physical health problems (Bryant & Harvey, 1998; Hoge et al., 2008). Polytrauma injuries, including amputation, burns, and vision and hearing loss may also impact recovery.

Returning to duty is the primary goal for many wounded SMs because of a strong desire to support their battle comrades and use their carefully honed skills. Occupational therapists should be aware that, in some cases, SMs may underreport symptoms in order to be cleared for duty. Careful evaluation and clinical observation is necessary to identify any barriers to function. When injuries render an SM unfit for duty, he or she may reclass into a new military role or transition into the civilian workforce. This can be a challenging process. Occupational therapy interventions such as vocational interest inventories and job-acquisition skills training are valuable tools to assist veterans in making smooth transitions out of the military. Considerations for working with SMs are discussed in Procedures for Practice 34-3.

 Procedures for Practice 34-3

Considerations for Working with Service Members

- Observe for symptoms of undiagnosed mild traumatic brain injury (TBI) and make medical referrals as appropriate:
  - Headache
  - Difficulty sleeping
  - Problems with memory and concentration
  - Dizziness and imbalance
  - Light sensitivity
  - Increased irritability
- Become familiar with military terminology and acronyms. Service members (SMs) are often guarded and may be more willing to open up to individuals who they feel understand the military experience and culture.
- When possible, address active duty SMs by their ranks and last names.
- Be mindful of the treatment environment in light of the presence of postcombat stress:
  - Select a private or semiprivate location with limited auditory and visual distractions.
  - Allow SMs to sit where they can see the door.
  - Reduce the use of bright, fluorescent light.
  - Explain the source of unanticipated noises from nearby construction work, lawn care, alarm testing, etc.
  - If there is a television in the waiting room, consider positive, uplifting programming versus news of violence or combat.
- Provide patient and family education to explain and normalize symptoms and functional changes.
- Set a positive expectation for recovery.
- Consider group intervention in addition to one-on-one treatment. SMs are trained to operate in small teams or squads and are often motivated and encouraged by working with their comrades.
- Be knowledgeable regarding available community, Veterans Affairs, and Department of Defense resources.
- Make appropriate referrals for comorbid mental health dysfunction.

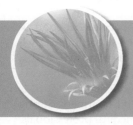

case example

K.R.: Occupational Therapy during Acute and Rehabilitation Phases of Recovery from Severe Traumatic Brain Injury

Occupational Therapy Intervention Process	Clinical Reasoning Process	
	Objectives	**Examples of Therapist's Internal Dialogue**

Patient Information

K.R. is a 20-year-old college student who sustained a traumatic brain injury (TBI) in a motor vehicle accident. Prior to the accident, K.R. was a physics major described by family as dependable and hardworking, with a 3.8 grade point average during his first 2 years of college.

Examination in the emergency department revealed a laceration over his forehead and right pneumothorax. His blood alcohol level was 0.226 (more than twice the legal limit). He had an initial Glasgow Coma Scale score of 3. Intracranial pressure was elevated. He sustained facial fractures. Serial computed tomography demonstrated traumatic axonal injury, edema, and right posterior temporoparietal intraparenchymal hemorrhage. Within the first week after the injury, a tracheostomy and feeding tube were inserted, and shortly thereafter, K.R. underwent open reduction and internal fixation of the right zygomatic maxillary complex fracture.

Occupational and physical therapy were initiated 10 days post-injury, with orders for range of motion, positioning, and assessment of response to sensory stimuli. At the time he was first seen in occupational therapy just before his transfer from intensive care unit (ICU) to the medical unit, his passive range of motion (PROM) was within normal limits for all extremities with mild spasticity in the right elbow and wrist flexors. K.R. did not speak or follow commands consistently. He was frequently observed to thrash around, primarily moving his left side, and at times, his movement appeared purposeful (pulling at tubes, seeming to scratch his right leg with his left foot). He appeared to track objects with his left eye inconsistently. His initial total score on the Western Neuro Sensory Stimulation Profile was 23, and he was believed to be functioning at a Rancho levels II–III (increasingly responsive to specific stimuli).

Objectives

Understand the patient's diagnosis or condition

Know the person

Examples of Therapist's Internal Dialogue

"K.R.'s recent medical history suggests that he had a severe brain injury and will likely require occupational therapy services and other rehabilitation services throughout the continuum of care (acute medical, inpatient, outpatient, and follow-up)."

"From what his parents tell me, K.R. sounds like a really hardworking guy. Apparently, in addition to his course work, K.R. worked 16 hours a week as a dishwasher in his dormitory. It sounds like K.R. tends to be quiet and soft-spoken but enjoys the company of a small circle of friends. I found out that his leisure interests include golf, cross-country skiing, and playing piano. It was really worth the time it took to talk with K.R.'s parents. I can tell that I will like working with them, and the information they provided me with will help me as I try to make therapy interesting and engaging for K.R."

Reason for Referral to Occupational Therapy

After less than a week on the medical unit, K.R. was transferred to the inpatient brain injury rehabilitation unit and was again referred to occupational therapy and to physical therapy, speech-language pathology, and neuropsychology (he was 3 weeks postinjury). He was referred to occupational therapy to assess responsiveness to stimuli, positioning, and activities of daily living (ADL) training as appropriate. Consistent with his acute hospitalization, a family member (typically his mother) was present at most therapy sessions.

Appreciate the context

Develop provisional hypotheses

"The transfer from the medical unit to the rehabilitation unit represents a significant change in K.R.'s care. There is much more stimulation on the rehabilitation unit, and the overall emphasis of care changes from one of medical survival to recovery and adaptation."

"I anticipate that, by putting in place formal interventions and observational protocols, we will be able to maximize K.R.'s responsiveness to stimuli and ultimately his ability to benefit from rehabilitation. It will be important to involve his family for their sake as much as for his."

Assessment Process and Results

The Western Neuro Sensory Stimulation Profile was readministered, and K.R. obtained scores ranging from 54 to 80, with notable improvements in auditory comprehension, visual tracking, object manipulation, and arousal and attention.

On the Galveston Orientation and Amnesia Test, K.R. was oriented to person, but not to place or time, and was unable to describe events before or after his injury.

During assessment, K.R. sustained eye contact less than 25% of the time and was awake for approximately 20 minutes of each session. He horizontally tracked across midline with both eyes approximately 50% of the time and tracked vertically in one direction somewhat less. He generally followed gross motor commands approximately 25% of the time.

Minimal formal assessment of K.R.'s right upper extremity function was performed, but he was observed to not use or move it. He did not appear to have any limitations in range of motion in either upper extremity.

During assessment, K.R. did not contribute to any aspect of ADL.

Consider evaluation approach and methods	"I need to primarily rely on observational methods during assessment and carefully document what I am seeing so that I will be able to detect changes in responsiveness and function."
Interpret observations	"I am finding that my assessment sessions really blur with treatment; it seems I am doing both at all times. I am encouraged that K.R. is demonstrating more specificity in his overall responses. Although his speech is not intelligible, he seems to be making more frequent verbalizations. Since he came to the rehab unit, I am noticing that he can participate for longer periods of time, and that is encouraging as well."

Occupational Therapy Problem List

- Decreased arousal and attention
- Impaired memory
- Decreased and inconsistent visual tracking
- Inability to follow commands consistently
- Decreased right upper extremity function
- Dependence in ADL

Synthesize results	"K.R.'s overall responsiveness appears to be steadily improving based on records of his status on the acute medical unit. I am going to use my interventions related to ADL and upper extremity function as vehicles to improve arousal and attention."

Initial Occupational Therapy Goal List

Because it was difficult to predict the patient's rate of recovery or response to therapy, the team set goals for 2-week intervals, with the understanding that the patient's length of stay on the rehabilitation unit would be dictated by his apparent ability to profit from intervention. Meanwhile, the patient's family was exploring possible discharge options to home for continued home-based services or to a subacute rehabilitation facility.

K.R. will stay awake for three 30-minute sessions per day, demonstrating sensory-specific responses to visual and auditory stimuli at least 75% of the time.

K.R. will respond to one-step commands during simple grooming activities at least 50% of the time.

K.R. will complete upper body dressing with step-by-step verbal cueing and moderate assistance.

Develop intervention hypotheses	"My underlying assumption is that, as we provide that 'just-right' amount of stimulation and structure, K.R. will become increasingly aroused and attentive, which is necessary for him to be truly engaged in the rehabilitation process. Daily training in performing familiar basic ADL will facilitate independence in daily activities while providing an opportunity for K.R. to improve his ability to follow simple motor commands."
Consider the evidence	"The evidence-based review by Cicerone et al., (2011) recommended the use of errorless learning techniques to teach specific skills to patients with severe memory impairments after TBI."
Select an intervention approach	"At this point, my approach to intervention will involve both remedial and compensatory approaches."
Consider what will occur in therapy, how often, and for how long	"K.R. is at the beginning of what will likely be a long course of rehabilitation, and it is impossible to come up with firm projections as to how long that process might be. Based on my experience, I expect that it may be a matter of a couple of weeks before K.R. can consistently follow instructions and truly participate in therapy. I will be seeing him at least three times per day throughout his inpatient rehabilitation stay, which could be 3–4 weeks. I am always reluctant to talk about specifics at this point, especially to family members, because it really is hard to project the outcome with any certainty."

Intervention

K.R. was seen three times daily, twice in the therapy clinic, with sessions lasting 20–30 minutes as tolerated. He participated in daily light hygiene and dressing activities in which, for example, he was instructed to turn on the faucet and was handed a wet washcloth and asked to wash his face. As recommended by the therapist, K.R.'s parents brought in pictures of friends and family and posted them in his room. PROM for the right upper extremity was incorporated into his sensory stimulation program, and efforts were made to elicit automatic upper extremity movement by, for example, challenging K.R. to catch or hit a balloon. He made steady gains in all areas, so that within 3 weeks of his admission to rehabilitation, he followed one-step commands approximately 70% of the time and participated in morning hygiene activities for 25-minute intervals with ongoing verbal and tactile cues. He was able to feed himself with the utensil in his right hand once the therapist scooped the food. K.R. started speaking in short phrases approximately 6 weeks after onset and progressed rapidly to whole sentences, indicating, for example, when he had to go to the bathroom. As K.R.'s cognitive recovery progressed, the occupational therapist helped him to become more independent in dressing, grooming, and his upper extremity exercise program and to increase his orientation and attention span. He was able to use a memory log (with entries recorded by others) to answer questions about his daily activities.

At the time of discharge, K.R. needed supervision with grooming and upper extremity dressing and moderate assistance with lower extremity dressing and bathing. K.R.'s mother was taught methods to assist him at home. He was able to walk with a quad cane and moderate assistance; he needed contact guard assistance with standing balance. At discharge, he was oriented to person, place, and time, scoring in the normal range on the Galveston Orientation and Amnesia Test, and demonstrated at least some degree of session-to-session carryover. The therapist recommended 24-hour supervision because of continued impairments in memory, problem solving, and judgment. He was discharged to his parents' home 2 months post-TBI with plans to return for daily therapy in the day hospital program (supervised all-day multidisciplinary therapies with return home each evening).

Next Steps

The occupational therapy intervention plan during K.R.'s 3 weeks in the day hospital focused on use of a memory aid and reestablishing competence in IADLs including light meal preparation, laundry, checkbook management, and bill paying. His living situation contributed to motivation and improved insight more than the insulated experience of the rehabilitation unit. When he no longer required all-day supervision, he was discharged from the day hospital but continued outpatient occupational therapy three times a week.

Assess the patient's comprehension	"At the time of his transfer to the rehabilitation unit and referral to occupational therapy, K.R.'s cognitive status posed the primary barrier to his functioning, specifically his low levels of arousal and attention."
Understand what he is doing	"Motor activities and ADL are means by which I can try to promote arousal, tracking K.R.'s, responsiveness, and ability to follow commands."
Compare actual to expected performance	"K.R. continues to require cueing to perform basic ADL. I can begin to provide more of an active learning-based intervention when K.R. begins to show within-session carryover."
Know the person	"I am beginning to see glimpses of K.R.'s personality and so are his family members. Even though he is disoriented and quite unaware of his circumstances, he can be easily engaged in therapy tasks, especially if he views them as competitive."
Appreciate the context	"K.R. was discharged home before he was fully competent in ADL because his parents were able to provide assistance and supervision and because intensive outpatient services were available."
Anticipate present and future patient concerns	"I feel good about the fact that we can offer K.R. and his family comprehensive and long-term rehabilitation services. They will need us off and on as they face new milestones over the next year such as driving, return to independent living, and return to school and work. His parents have joined a support group and are working closely with our staff to carry over what he is working on in therapy."
Analyze patient's comprehension	"K.R.'s attention and awareness have improved to the level where he could benefit from more active learning-based interventions such as cognitive-didactive treatment and strategy training."
Decide whether he should continue or discontinue therapy and/or return in the future	K.R. is continuing to make gains and would benefit from continued therapy on an outpatient basis."

Clinical Reasoning in Occupational Therapy Practice

Occupational Therapy Intervention in the Acute Phase of Recovery

Just prior to K.R.'s transfer to the inpatient rehabilitation unit, his family excitedly reported that he was blinking his eyes when asked almost 100% of the time. Your assessment shows that he is following simple motor commands less than 20% of the time. What are some possible explanations for this discrepancy? How can you help his family better assess his ability to respond?

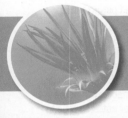

case example

Dr. N.: Occupational Therapy after Mild Traumatic Brain Injury

Occupational Therapy Intervention Process	Clinical Reasoning Process	
	Objectives	**Examples of Therapist's Internal Dialogue**
Patient Information	Understand the patient's diagnosis or condition	"Given her GCS score and the fact that she did not lose consciousness, I can assume that her TBI was not severe and that she has a good prognosis for a full recovery."
Dr. N. is a 29-year-old single woman who sustained a mild traumatic brain injury (TBI) when she fell off her bicycle. She was not wearing a helmet. She reports that she did not lose consciousness, and her Glasgow Coma Scale (GCS) score in the emergency department was 13. Dr. N. returned to work 2 days after her hospital discharge despite moderately severe headaches and balance and memory problems.		
	Know the person	"My guess is that Dr. N. is used to pushing herself, as evidenced by a rather speedy return to work after her hospitalization. Clearly, Dr. N. is a bright woman and has high expectations of herself. The cognitive inefficiencies since her injury must be frightening and confusing for her. I am glad that she appears to have social support."
Dr. N. has a degree in biochemistry and works as a postdoctoral fellow at a university. Her parents and four siblings reside in another state, and she lives with her significant other of 4 years.		
Dr. N. participated in neuropsychological assessment approximately 6 months postinjury because cognitive inefficiencies continued to interfere with her function, especially at work. Findings suggested mild impairment for recent verbal and nonverbal memory and subtle impairment for executive function abilities. These cognitive changes contributed to decreased efficiency at work (slowness in problem solving, needing to reread professional literature, disorganized note-taking, and difficulty keeping track of her schedule and work tasks). Furthermore, Dr. N. was anxious and depressed. She reported difficulty falling asleep despite overwhelming fatigue. She worried about whether or not she had completed intended tasks, checking and double-checking herself throughout the day. She described herself as easily frustrated, lacking confidence, and more dependent than usual on her significant other. She continued to have headaches approximately 4 days a week. The neuropsychologist expected Dr. N. to maintain her job successfully and pursue premorbid career goals with assistance in adjusting self-expectations and information-processing habits.		

Reason for Referral to Occupational Therapy

Dr. N. was referred to occupational therapy for assistance in developing compensatory cognitive strategies and behavioral routines that would improve her efficiency at home and work. She was also referred to a psychologist for support and biofeedback to help her manage her headaches.

Appreciate the context	"Dr. N. was referred to an outpatient brain injury clinic that has expertise in serving people with mild TBI."
Develop provisional hypotheses	"The literature suggests that clients with mild TBI are best served if the staff avoids overemphasizing concerns about permanent cognitive impairment and encourages clients to reinterpret symptoms as short term and manageable."

Assessment Process and Results

- Interview and self-report questionnaire related to client's problems, inefficiencies, and concerns and how Dr. N. manages information at present
- Interview regarding "typical day"
- Observations of response and follow-through to orally presented homework.

Consider evaluation approach and methods	"Because I have reviewed Dr. N.'s neuropsychological evaluation results, it is not necessary or appropriate to reassess cognition. In fact, repeated assessment of similar domains might be detrimental, potentially overemphasizing cognitive inefficiencies that will likely be short term. Instead, I will try to find out about performance patterns and daily functioning."
Interpret observations	"When I asked her to bring photographs to her next session, Dr. N. wrote a note to herself on one of approximately eight 'sticky notes' that were affixed to her wallet. She seems comfortable with note-taking, but I am guessing that her notes do little to supplant her memory as she likely does not find them when she needs them."

Occupational Therapy Problem List

- Misattributions and misperceptions regarding personal competence
- Inadequate use of external information-processing strategies
- Disruption of personal routines, especially surrounding bedtime

Synthesize results	"Dr. N. did not link distracters, such as headache and fatigue, to episodes of memory failure and absent-mindedness or understand the implications of a limited working memory. I noticed that Dr. N. started writing lots of notes to herself but did not store or refer to them in a systematic manner. She worked off a mental plan each day but could not set priorities among multiple tasks. I am concerned about so much sleep in the early evening followed by more active household tasks. It is no wonder she is having difficulty with sleep."

Initial Occupational Therapy Goal List

The anticipated length of treatment was four to six sessions.

Dr. N. will complete 90% of work tasks on time by independently employing compensatory strategies including maintaining an up-to-date list of pending and completed tasks, using a daily schedule, and working on more difficult tasks in the morning when she is less fatigued.

During the work week, Dr. N. will take a 10-minute rest break both midmorning and midafternoon, take a 30-minute break when arriving home from work, complete home management activities by 8 pm, and go to bed by 10 pm.

Develop intervention hypotheses	"There seem to be many contributions to Dr. N.'s problems right now, including the aftereffects of mild TBI, anxiety associated with misattributions related to the problems she is experiencing, and a rather limited repertoire of information-processing strategies. Interventions in occupational therapy will focus on helping her make correct attributions related to performance problems and broadening her repertoire of information-processing and compensatory organizational strategies."
Consider the evidence	"There has been no empirical study of habit training for patients with mild TBI, but I have used this approach with other patients and seen them benefit."
Select an intervention approach	"I will use an education-consultative approach, teaching her about information processing and helping her refine her information management strategies."
Consider what will occur in therapy, how often, and for how long	"I think that she will need a relatively short duration of occupational therapy. I recommend that she come to therapy once per week for a few weeks, which will allow her to try out the strategies that we discuss, and we can work together to refine them accordingly."

Intervention

Dr. N. participated in five treatment sessions over 3 months, attending weekly sessions for 3 weeks and two follow-up sessions over 6 weeks. As cognitive inefficiencies were reframed as partly consequences of a working memory overload related to stress and the distraction of physical symptoms, Dr. N. eagerly explored methods to decrease the demands on internal information processing. She purchased a day planner and, with input from the therapist, established daily and weekly planning routines. Daily and weekly plans helped her set priorities among tasks and allocate time for leisure. She experimented with establishing routines for certain aspects of her "typical" day, scheduling breaks and allocating tasks with low cognitive demands to periods when her energy tended to be low. She changed her afterwork routine to set the timer for a 20–30-minute nap followed by a 30-minute walk. She also established a bedtime wind-down routine that decreased the amount of time she needed to fall asleep.

Assess the patient's comprehension Understand what she is doing Compare actual to expected performance Know the person Appreciate the context	"Dr. N. had relatively mild or subtle impairments that changed her cognitive capacity. Similar to many bright individuals, Dr. N. had never thought about her own thinking strategies and did not have a broad repertoire of techniques that she could default to. Furthermore, in her attempts to understand changes resulting from her injury and their implications, Dr. N. failed to appreciate the cumulative effect that subtle impairments, stress, reliance on premorbid cognitive strategies, and distractions associated with pain exerted on her information processing. She was relieved to learn that she was not 'losing it' and quickly engaged in problem solving with me regarding possible changes in strategies and routines that would buoy her everyday performance. Her relatively brief involvement in treatment shows the benefit of holistic occupational therapy services in dramatically improving an individual's occupational functioning and quality of life."

Next Steps

Discharge from occupational therapy.

Anticipate present and future patient concerns Decide whether the patient should continue or discontinue therapy and/or return in the future	"I do not expect that Dr. N. will need further therapy and anticipate that her overall functioning will continue to improve. She is making correct attributions related to cognitive inefficiencies and knows how and when to use compensatory strategies to lighten her load."

Clinical Reasoning in Occupational Therapy Practice

Taking Multiple Factors into Account in Treatment Planning for Mild Traumatic Brain Injury

Many people with mild traumatic brain injury return to normal functioning within 1–3 months without direct clinical intervention. What factors may have contributed to Dr. N.'s more lengthy recovery and persistence of symptoms? How might those factors affect your provision of occupational therapy services for Dr. N?

Summary Review Questions

1. What are some treatment planning implications related to age of onset of TBI? Describe the relevance of the cause of injury, developmental stage, and possible comorbidities.

2. In what ways do occupational therapists use information regarding mechanisms of injury of each patient in the clinical reasoning process? For example, how is the clinical presentation of a diffuse brain injury different from that of a focal brain injury? How can the therapist obtain information about the mechanisms of injury for a given patient?

3. Describe specific ways a patient's preinjury characteristics and background may affect rehabilitation and outcome.

4. Summarize terms used to describe patients in altered states of consciousness and why distinctions between these states are important to the occupational therapist.

5. What are some of the frequently cited predictors of prognosis and rehabilitation outcome after TBI? What are the occupational therapy implications of these predictors in planning treatment for patients in terms of goals, length of treatment, and needs of the family?

6. Describe the adjustment and adaptation process of the patient with TBI as compared to that of the family.

Detail what support and education patients and family members need from occupational therapy during each phase of recovery and adaptation.

7. How might the treatment approach used to optimize cognitive capacities and abilities for an inpatient be different from the treatment approach used in postacute rehabilitation or if the patient returns for services years later?

8. Compare Montgomery's (1995) multifactor explanation for disability after mild TBI with your own explanation of disability after severe TBI.

Glossary

Agitation—Subtype of delirium that is unique to survivors of TBI in altered states of consciousness in which there are excesses in behavior that include some combination of aggression, disinhibition, restlessness, and confusion.

Hematoma—Masses of blood confined to an organ or space caused by a broken blood vessel (Scott & Dow, 1995).

Mild traumatic brain injury—Brief alteration of mental status, such as confusion or disorientation, loss of memory lasting 24 hours or less, loss of consciousness lasting 30 minutes or less, and/or acute seizure after an impact to or forceful movement of the head (National Center for Injury Prevention and Control, 2003).

Post-traumatic amnesia—Inability to remember day-to-day events after brain injury including those

immediately before the injury (termed retrograde amnesia) and events that occur after the injury. The time elapsed from injury to recovery of continuous memory is one indicator used to describe the severity of brain damage.

Traumatic axonal injury—Axonal damage including shearing of axon clusters with reactive swelling and disconnection of strained and damaged axons as well as occasional tearing of axons. Previously termed diffuse axonal injury (DAI). Results from acceleration or deceleration injuries (Povlishock & Katz, 2005).

Traumatic brain injury—Alteration in brain function, or other evidence of brain pathology, caused by an external force (Menon et al., 2010).

References

Abreu, B. C., Seale, G., Podlesack, J., & Hartley, L. (1996). Development of paths of postacute brain injury rehabilitation: Lessons learned. *American Journal of Occupational Therapy, 50,* 417–427.

Abreu, B. C., & Toglia, J. P. (1987). Cognitive rehabilitation: A model for occupational therapy. *American Journal of Occupational Therapy, 41,* 439–448.

American Congress of Rehabilitation Medicine. (1995). Recommendations for use of uniform nomenclature pertinent to patients with severe alterations in consciousness. *Archives of Physical Medicine and Rehabilitation, 76,* 205–209.

Annegers, J. F., Grabow, J. D., Kurland, L. T., & Laws, E. R. (1980). The incidence, causes, and secular trends of head trauma in Olmsted County, Minnesota, 1935–1974. *Neurology, 80,* 912–919.

Ansell, B. J. (1993). Slow-to-recover patients: Improvement to rehabilitation readiness. *Journal of Head Trauma Rehabilitation, 8,* 88–98.

Ansell, B. J., & Keenan, J. E. (1989). The Western Neuro Sensory Stimulation Profile: A tool for assessing slow-to-recover head-injured patients. *Archives of Physical Medicine and Rehabilitation, 70,* 104–108.

Ashman, T. A., Spielman, L. A., Hibbard, M. R., Silver, J. M., Chandna, T., & Gordon, W. A. (2004). Psychiatric challenges in the first 6 years after traumatic brain injury: Cross-sequential analyses of Axis I disorders. *Archives of Physical Medicine and Rehabilitation, 85,* S36–S42.

Baron, E. M., & Jallo, J. I. (2007). TBI: Pathology, pathophysiology, acute care and surgical management, critical care principles, and outcomes. In N. D. Zasler, D. I. Katz, & R. D. Zafonte (Eds.),

Brain injury medicine: Principles and practice (pp. 265–282). New York: Demos.

Bell, K. R., Hoffman, J. M., Temkin, N. R., Powell, J. M., Fraser, R. T., Esselman, P. C., Barber, J. K., & Dikmen, S. (2008). The effect of telephone counseling on reducing post-traumatic symptoms after mild traumatic brain injury. *Journal of Neurology, Neurosurgery, and Psychiatry, 79,* 1275–1281.

Benton, A. (1979). Behavioral consequences of closed head injury. In G. L. Odom (Ed.), *Central nervous system trauma research status report* (pp. 220–231). Bethesda, MD: National Institute of Neurological and Communicative Disorders and Stroke.

Boortz-Marx, R. (1985). Factors affecting intracranial pressure: A descriptive study. *Journal of Neurosurgical Nursing, 17,* 89–94.

Bouska, M. J., & Gallaway, M. (1991). Primary visual deficits in adults with brain damage: Management in occupational therapy. *Occupational Therapy Practice, 3,* 1–11.

Brain Trauma Foundation. (2007). Guidelines for prehospital management of traumatic brain injury (2nd edition). *Prehospital Emergency Care, 12,* S1–S52. Retrieved December 1, 2011 from http://www.braintrauma.org/pdf/protected/Prehospital_Guidelines_2nd_Edition.pdf.

Brandstater, M. E., Bontke, C. F., Cobble, N. D., & Horn, L. J. (1991). Rehabilitation in brain disorders: 4. Specific disorders. *Archives of Physical Medicine and Rehabilitation, 72,* S332–S340.

Brown, M., Dijkers, M. P. J. M., Gordon, W. A., Ashman, T., Charatz, H., & Cheng, Z. (2004). Participation Objective, Participation Subjective: A measure of participation combining outsider and insider perspectives. *Journal of Head Trauma Rehabilitation, 19,* 459–481.

Bryant, R. A., & Harvey, A. G. (1998). Relationship between acute stress disorder and posttraumatic stress disorder following mild traumatic brain injury. *American Journal of Psychiatry, 155,* 625–629.

Bryant, R. A., Moulds, M., Guthrie, R., & Nixon, R. D. V. (2003). Treating acute stress disorder following mild traumatic brain injury. *American Journal of Psychiatry, 160,* 585–587.

Carr, J. H., & Shepherd, R. B. (1980). *Physiotherapy in disorders of the brain.* London: Heinemann Medical.

Center for Outcome Measurement in Brain Injury. (2011). COMBI: Featured scales. Retrieved October 20, 2011 from http://www.tbims.org/combi/list.html.

Charness, A. L. (1986). *Stroke/head injury: A guide to functional outcomes in physical therapy management* (Rehabilitation Institute of Chicago Series). Rockville, MD: Aspen.

Chestnut, R. M., Carney, N., Maynard, H., Mann, N. C., Patterson, P., & Helfand, M. (1999). Summary report: Evidence for the effectiveness of rehabilitation for persons with traumatic brain injury. *Journal of Head Trauma Rehabilitation, 14,* 176–188.

Cicerone, K. D., Dahlberg, C., Kalmar, K., Langenbahn, D. M., Malec, J. F., Bergquist, T. F., Felicetti, T., Giacino, J. T., Harley, J. P., Harrington, D. E., Herzog, J., Kneipp, S., Laatsch, L., & Morse, P. A. (2000). Evidence-based cognitive rehabilitation: Recommendations for clinical practice. *Archives of Physical Medicine and Rehabilitation, 81,* 1596–1615.

Cicerone, K. D., Dahlberg, C., Malec, J. F., Langenbahn, D. M., Felicetti, T., Kneipp, S., Ellmo, W., Kalmar, K., Giacino, J. T., Harley, J. P., Laatsch, L., Morse, P. A., & Catanese, J. (2005). Evidence-based cognitive rehabilitation: Updated review of the literature from 1998 through 2002. *Archives of Physical Medicine and Rehabilitation, 86,* 1681–1692.

Cicerone, K. D., Langenbahn, D. M., Braden, C., Malec, J. F., Kalmar, K., Fraas, M., Felicetti, T., Laatsch, L., Harley, J. P., Bergquist, T., Azulay, J., Cantor, J., & Ashman, T. (2011). Evidence-based cognitive rehabilitation: Updated review of the literature from 2003 through 2008. *Archives of Physical Medicine and Rehabilitation, 92,* 519–530.

Citta-Pietrolungo, T. J., Alexander, M. A., & Steg, N. L. (1992). Early detection of heterotopic ossification in young patients with traumatic brain injury. *Archives of Physical Medicine and Rehabilitation, 73,* 258–262.

Corrigan, J. D. (1989). Development of a scale for assessment of agitation following traumatic brain injury. *Journal of Clinical and Experimental Neuropsychology, 11,* 261–277.

Corrigan, J. D. (1995). Substance abuse as a mediating factor in outcome from traumatic brain injury. *Archives of Physical Medicine and Rehabilitation, 76,* 302–309.

Defense and Veterans Brain Injury Center (2013). DoD worldwide numbers for TBI. http://www.dvbic.org/dod-worldwide-numbers-tbi. Retrieved June 18, 2013.

DeKruijk, J. R., Twijnstra, A., & Leffers, P. (2001). Diagnostic criteria and differential diagnosis of mild traumatic brain injury. *Brain Injury, 15,* 99–106.

DePalma, R. G., Burris, D. G., Champion, H. R., & Hodgson, M. J. (2005). Blast injuries. *New England Journal of Medicine, 352,* 1335–1342

Dikmen, S. S., Machamer, J. E., Powell, J. M., & Temkin, N. R. (2003). Outcome 3 to 5 years after moderate to severe traumatic brain injury. *Archives of Physical Medicine and Rehabilitation, 84,* 1449–1457.

Dikmen, S., Machamer, J., & Temkin, N. (2001). Mild head injury: Facts and artifacts. *Journal of Clinical and Experimental Neuropsychology, 23,* 729–738.

Dikmen, S., Reitan, R. M., & Temkin, N. R. (1983). Neuropsychological recovery in head injury. *Archives of Neurology, 40,* 333–338.

DiPasquale, M. C., & Whyte, J. (1996). Use of quantitative data in treatment planning for minimally conscious patients. *Journal of Head Trauma Rehabilitation, 11,* 9–17.

Duff, D. (2001). Review article: Altered states of consciousness, theories of recovery, and assessment following a severe traumatic brain injury. *Axon, 23,* 18–23.

Eames, P., Haffey, W. J., & Cope, D. N. (1990). Treatment of behavioral disorders. In M. Rosenthal, E. R. Griffith, M. R. Bond, & J. D. Miller (Eds.), *Rehabilitation of the adult and child with traumatic brain injury* (pp. 410–432). Philadelphia: F. A. Davis.

Faul, M., Xu, L., Wahl, M. M., & Coronado, V. G. (2010). *Traumatic brain injury in the United States: Emergency department visits, hospitalizations and deaths 2002–2006.* Atlanta: Centers for Disease Control and Prevention, National Center for Injury Prevention and Control. Retrieved December 1, 2011 from http://www.cdc.gov/traumaticbraininjury/pdf/blue_book.pdf.

Giacino, J. T., Ashwal, S., Childs, N., Cranford, R., Jennett, B., Katz, D. I., Kelly, J. P., Rosenberg, J. H., Whyte, J., Zafonte, R. D., & Zasler, N. D. (2002). The minimally conscious state: Definition and diagnostic criteria. *Neurology, 58,* 349–353.

Giacino, J. T., & Kalmar, K. (1997). The vegetative and minimally conscious states: A comparison of clinical features and functional outcome. *Journal of Head Trauma Rehabilitation, 12,* 36–51.

Giacino, J. T., Zasler, N. D., Katz, D. I., Kelly, J. P., Rosenberg, J. H., & Filley, C. M. (1997). Development of practice guidelines for assessment and management of the vegetative and minimally conscious states. *Journal of Head Trauma Rehabilitation, 12,* 79–89.

Giles, G. M., & Clark-Wilson, J. (1993). *Brain injury rehabilitation: A neurofunctional approach.* San Diego: Singular.

Giles, G. M., Ridley, J. E., Dill, A., & Frye, S. (1997). A consecutive series of adults with brain injury treated with a washing and dressing retraining program. *American Journal of Occupational Therapy, 51,* 256–266.

Golisz, K. (2009). *Occupational therapy practice guidelines for adults with traumatic brain injury.* Bethesda, MD: AOTA Press.

Greenberg, D. A., Aminoff, M. J., & Simon, R. P. (1993). *Clinical neurology* (2nd ed.). East Norwalk, CT: Appleton & Lange.

Groswasser, Z., & Stern, M. J. (1998). A psychodynamic model of behavior after central nervous system damage. *Journal of Head Trauma Rehabilitation, 13,* 69–79.

Hagen, C. (1998). *Rancho levels of cognitive functioning: The revised levels* (3rd ed.). Downey, CA: Rancho Los Amigos Medical Center.

Hagen, C., Malkmus, D., & Durham, P. (1979). *Levels of cognitive functioning, rehabilitation of the brain-injured adult: Comprehensive physical management.* Downey, CA: Professional Staff Association of Rancho Los Amigos Hospital.

Hanks, R. A., Temkin, N., Machamer, J., & Dikmen, S. S. (1999). Emotional and behavioral adjustment after traumatic brain injury. *Archives of Physical Medicine and Rehabilitation, 80,* 991–997.

Hartl, R., & Ghajar, J. (2005). Neurosurgical interventions. In J. M. Silver, T. W. McAllister, & S. C. Yudofsky (Eds.), *Textbook of traumatic brain injury* (pp. 51–58). Washington, DC: American Psychiatric Publishing.

Healey, C., Osler, T. M., Rogers, F. R., Healey, M. A., Glance, L. G., Kilgo, P. D., Shackford, S. R., & Meredith, J. W. (2003). Improving the Glasgow Coma Scale score: Motor score alone is a better predictor. *Journal of Trauma, 54,* 671–680.

Heinemann, A. W., Saghal, V., Cichowski, K., Ginsburg, K., Tuel, S. M., & Betts, H. B. (1990). Functional outcome following traumatic brain injury rehabilitation. *Journal of Neurological Rehabilitation, 4,* 27–37.

Helman, D. L., Sherner, J. H., Fitzpatrick, T. M., Callender, M. E., & Shorr, A. F. (2003). Effect of standardized orders and provider education on head-of-bed positioning in mechanically ventilated patients. *Critical Care Medicine, 31,* 2285–2290.

Hibbard, M. R., Ashman, R. A., Spielman, L. A., Chun, D., Charatz, H. J., & Seton, M. (2004). Relationship between depression and psychosocial functioning after traumatic brain injury. *Archives of Physical Medicine and Rehabilitation, 85,* S43–S53.

Hirschberg, R., & Giacino, J. T. (2011). The vegetative and minimally conscious states: Diagnosis, prognosis and treatment. *Neurologic Clinics, 29,* 773–786.

Hoge, C. W., McGurk, D., Thomas, J. L., Cox, A. L., Engel, C. C., & Castro, C. A. (2008). Mild traumatic brain injury in U.S. soldiers returning from Iraq. *New England Journal of Medicine, 358,* 453–463.

Holden, M. K. (2005). Virtual environments for motor rehabilitation: A review. *CyberPsychology and Behavior, 8,* 187–211.

Holland, D., & Shigaki, C. L. (1998). Educating families and caretakers of traumatically brain injured patients in the new health care environment: A three phase model and bibliography. *Brain Injury, 12,* 993–1009.

Institute of Medicine. (2009). *Gulf War and health. Volume 7: Long-term consequences of traumatc brain injury.* Washington, DC: National Academies Press.

Institute of Medicine. (2011). *Cognitive rehabilitation therapy for traumatic brain injury: Evaluating the evidence.* Washington, DC: National Academies Press.

Ivanhoe, C. B., & Bontke, C. F. (1996). Movement disorders after traumatic brain injury. In L. J. Horn & N. D. Zasler (Eds.), *Medical rehabilitation of traumatic brain injury* (pp. 395–410). Philadelphia: Hanley & Belfus.

Jennett, B., Snoek, J., Bond, M. R., & Brooks, N. (1981). Disability after severe head injury: Observations on the use of the Glasgow Outcome Scale. *Journal of Neurology, Neurosurgery, and Psychiatry, 44,* 285–293.

Jennett, B., & Teasdale, G. (1981). *Management of head injuries.* Philadelphia: F. A. Davis.

Jones, R., Giddens, H., & Croft, D. (1983). Assessment and training of brain-damaged drivers. *American Journal of Occupational Therapy, 37,* 754–760.

Kalmar, K., & Giacino, J. T. (2005). The JFK Coma Recovery Scale—Revised. *Neuropsychological Rehabilitation, 15,* 454–460.

Katz, D. I. (1992). Neuropathology and neurobehavioral recovery from closed head injury. *Journal of Head Trauma Rehabilitation, 1,* 1–15.

Kelly, M. P., Johnson, C. T., Knoller, N., Drubach, D. A., & Winslow, M. M. (1997). Substance abuse, traumatic brain injury and neuropsychological outcome. *Brain Injury, 11,* 391–402.

Kessles, R. P. C., & de Haan, E. H. F. (2003). Implicit learning in memory rehabilitation: A meta-analysis on errorless learning and vanishing cues methods. *Journal of Clinical and Experimental Neuropsychology, 25,* 805–814.

Kim, E. (2002). Agitation, aggression, and disinhibition syndromes after traumatic brain injury. *NeuroRehabilitation, 17,* 297–310.

Langlois, J. A., Rutland-Brown, W., & Thomas, K. E. (2004). *Traumatic brain injury in the United States: Emergency department visits, hospitalization, and deaths.* Atlanta, GA: Centers for Disease Control and Prevention, National Center for Injury Prevention and Control.

Law, M., Baptiste, S., McColl, M. A., Carswell, A., Polatajko, H., & Pollock, N. (1994). *Canadian occupational performance measure.* Toronto, Canada: Canadian Association of Occupational Therapists.

Leathem, J. M., Murphy, L. J., & Flett, R. A. (1998). Self- and informant-ratings on the Patient Competency Rating Scale in patients with traumatic brain injury. *Journal of Clinical and Experimental Neuropsychology, 20,* 694–705.

Leech, R. W., & Shuman, R. M. (1982). *Neuropathology: A summary for students.* New York: Harper & Row.

Levin, H. S., Goldstein, F. C., & MacKenzie, E. J. (1997). Depression as a secondary condition following mild and moderate traumatic brain injury. *Seminars in Clinical Neuropsychology. 2,* 207–215.

Levin, H. S., High, W. M., Goethe, K. E., Sisson, R. A., Overall, J. E., Rhoades, H. M., Eisenberg, H. M., Kalisky, Z., & Gary, H. E. (1987). The Neurobehavioral Rating Scale: Assessment of the behavioral sequelae of head injury by the clinician. *Journal of Neurology, Neurosurgery, and Psychiatry, 50,* 183–193.

Lillehei, K. O., & Hoff, J. T. (1985). Advances in the management of closed head injury. *Annals of Emergency Medicine, 14,* 789–795.

Lippert-Grüner, M., & Terhaag, D., (2000). Multimodal early onset stimulation in rehabilitation after brain injury. *Brain Injury, 14,* 585–594.

Lippert-Grüner, M., Wedekind, C., & Klug, N. (2003). Outcome of prolonged coma following severe traumatic brain injury. *Brain Injury, 17,* 49–54.

Machamer, J., Temkin, N., & Dikmen, S. (2002). Significant other burden and factors related to it in traumatic brain injury. *Journal of Clinical and Experimental Neuropsychology, 24,* 420–433.

Malec, J. F., & Basford, J. S. (1996). Postacute brain injury rehabilitation. *Archives of Physical Medicine and Rehabilitation, 77,* 198–207.

Malec, J. F., Moessner, A. M., Kragness, M., & Lezak, M. D. (2000). Refining a measure of brain injury sequelae to predict postacute rehabilitation outcome: Rating scale analysis of the Mayo-Portland Adaptability Inventory. *Journal of Head Trauma Rehabilitation, 15,* 670–682.

Malec, J. F., & Thompson, J. M. (1994). Relationship of the Mayo-Portland Adaptability Inventory to functional outcome and cognitive performance measures. *Journal of Head Trauma Rehabilitation, 9,* 1–15.

Marion, D. W. (1996). Pathophysiology and initial neurosurgical care: Future directions. In L. J. Horn & N. D. Zasler (Eds.), *Medical rehabilitation of traumatic brain injury* (pp. 29–52). Philadelphia: Hanley & Belfus.

Mass, A. I., Harrison-Felix, C. L., Menon, D., Adelson, P. D., Balkin, T., Bullock, R., Engel, D. C., Gordon, W., Orman, J. L., Lew, H. L., Robertson, C., Temkin, N., Valadka, A., Verfaellie, M., Wainwright, M., Wright, D. W., & Schwab, K. (2010). Common data elements for traumatic brain injury: Recommendations from the interagency working group on demographics and clinical assessment. *Archives of Physical Medicine and Rehabilitation, 91,* 1641–1649.

Menon, K. D., Schwab, K., Wright, D. W, & Mass, A. I. on behalf of the Demographics and Clinical Assessment Working Group of the International and Interagency Initiative toward Common Data Elements for Research on Traumatic Brain Injury and Psychological Health. (2010). Position statement: Definition of traumatic brain injury. *Archives of Physical Medicine and Rehabilitation, 91,* 1637–1640.

Mitchell, P. H. (1986). Intracranial hypertension: Influence of nursing care activities. *Nursing Clinics of North America, 21,* 563–576.

Montgomery, G. K. (1995). A multi-factor account of disability after brain injury: Implications for neuropsychological counseling. *Brain Injury, 9,* 453–469.

Mortenson, P. A., & Eng, J. J. (2003). The use of casts in the management of joint mobility and hypertonia following brain injury in adults: A systematic review. *Physical Therapy, 83,* 648–658.

Muir, C. A., Rosenthal, M., & Diehl, L. N. (1990). Methods of family intervention. In M. Rosenthal, E. R. Griffith, M. R. Bond, & J. D. Miller (Eds.), *Rehabilitation of the adult and child with traumatic brain injury* (2nd ed., pp. 433–448). Philadelphia: F. A. Davis.

Multi-Society Task Force on PVS. (1994). Medical aspects of the persistent vegetative state: First of two parts. *New England Journal of Medicine, 330,* 1499–1508.

Mysiw, W. J., Fugate, L. P., & Clinchot, D. M. (1996). Assessment, early rehabilitation intervention, and tertiary prevention. In L. J. Horn & N. D. Zasler (Eds.), *Medical rehabilitation of traumatic brain injury* (pp. 53–76). Philadelphia: Hanley & Belfus.

Nakase-Richardson, R., Sherer, T., Seel, R. T., Hart, T., Hanks, R., Arango-Lasprilla, J. C., Yablon, S. A., Sander, A. M., Barnett, S. D., Walker, W. C., & Hammond, F. (2011). Utility of post-traumatic amnesia in predicting 1-year productivity following traumatic brain injury: Comparison of the Russell and Mississippi PTA classification intervals. *Journal of Neurology, Neurosurgery, and Psychiatry, 82,* 494–499.

National Center for Injury Prevention and Control. (2003). *Report to Congress on mild traumatic brain injury in the United States: Steps to prevent a serious public health problem.* Atlanta, GA: Centers for Disease Control and Prevention.

Neistadt, M. E. (1992). The Rabideau Kitchen Evaluation–Revised: An assessment of meal preparation skill. *Occupational Therapy Journal of Research, 12,* 242–253.

Neistadt, M. E. (1994a). A meal preparation treatment protocol for adults with brain injury. *American Journal of Occupational Therapy, 48,* 431–438.

Neistadt, M. E. (1994b). Perceptual retraining for adults with diffuse brain injury. *American Journal of Occupational Therapy, 48,* 225–233.

Nelson, D. L., & Lenhart, D. A. (1996). Resumption of outpatient occupational therapy for a young woman five years after traumatic brain injury. *American Journal of Occupational Therapy, 50,* 223–228.

O'Neill, J., Hibbard, M. R., Brown, M., Jaffe, M., Sliwinski, M., Vandergroot, D., & Weiss, M. J. (1998). Quality of life and community integration after traumatic brain injury. *Journal of Head Injury Rehabilitation, 13,* 68–79.

Pagulayan, K., Temkin, N. R., Machamer, J., & Dikmen, S. S. (2006). A longitudinal study of health-related quality of life after traumatic brain injury. *Archives of Physical Medicine and Rehabilitation, 87,* 611–618.

Palmer, M., & Wyness, M. A. (1988). Positioning and handling: Important considerations in the care of the severely head-injured patient. *Journal of Neuroscience Nursing, 20,* 42–50.

Phipps, E. J., DiPasquale, M., Blitz, C. L., & Whyte, J. (1997). Interpreting responsiveness in persons with severe traumatic brain injury: Beliefs in families and quantitative evaluations. *Journal of Head Trauma Rehabilitation, 12,* 52–69.

Povlishock, J. T., & Katz, D. I. (2005). Update of neuropathology and neurological recovery after traumatic brain injury. *Journal of Head Trauma Rehabilitation, 20,* 76–94.

Powell, J. M., Ferraro, J. V., Dikmen, S. S., Temkin, N. R., & Bell, K. R. (2008). Accuracy of mild traumatic brain injury diagnosis. *Archives of Physical Medicine and Rehabilitation, 89,* 1550–1555.

Powell, J. M., Temkin, N. R., Machamer, J. M., & Dikmen, S. S. (2007). Gaining insight into patients' perspectives on participation in home management activities following traumatic brain injury. *American Journal of Occupational Therapy, 61,* 269–279.

Prigatano, G. P. (1992). Personality disturbances associated with traumatic brain injury. *Journal of Consulting and Clinical Psychology, 60,* 360–368.

Rain, K. (2000). Survivor's voice. *TBI Challenge!, 4,* 6.

Rappaport, M., Hall, K. M., Hopkins, K., Belleza, & Cope, N. A. (1982). Disability Rating Scale for severe head trauma: Coma to community. *Archives of Physical Medicine and Rehabilitation, 63,* 118–123.

Rinehart, M. A. (1990). Strategies for improving motor performance. In M. Rosenthal, E. R. Griffith, M. R. Bond, & J. D. Miller (Eds.), *Rehabilitation of the adult and child with traumatic brain injury* (2nd ed., pp. 331–350). Philadelphia: F. A. Davis.

Rosenthal, M., & Bond, M. R. (1990). Behavioral and psychiatric sequelae. In M. Rosenthal, E. R. Griffith, M. R. Bond, & J. D. Miller (Eds.), *Rehabilitation of the adult and child with traumatic brain injury* (pp. 179–192). Philadelphia: F.A. Davis.

Ruff, R. M., Camenzuli, L., & Mueller, J. (1996). Miserable minority: Emotional factors that influence the outcome of mild traumatic brain injury. *Brain Injury, 10,* 551–565.

Sandel, M. E., Bell, K. R., & Michaud, L. J. (1998). Brain injury rehabilitation: 1. Traumatic brain injury: Prevention, pathophysiology, and outcome prediction. *Archives of Physical Medicine and Rehabilitation, 79,* S-3–S-9.

Schaffer, L., Kranzler, L. I., & Siqueira, E. B. (1985). Aspects of evaluation and treatment of head injury. *Neurology Clinics, 3,* 259–273.

Scherzer, B. P. (1986). Rehabilitation following severe head trauma: Results of a three-year program. *Archives of Physical Medicine and Rehabilitation, 67,* 366–374.

Scott, A. D., & Dow, P. W. (1995). Traumatic brain injury. In C. A. Trombly (Ed.), *Occupational therapy for physical dysfunction* (4th ed., pp. 705–733). Baltimore: Williams & Wilkins.

Sherer, M., Madison, C. F., & Hannay, H. J. (2000). A review of outcome after moderate to severe closed head injury with an introduction to life care planning. *Journal of Head Trauma Rehabilitation, 15,* 767–782.

Smith, D. H., Meaney, D. F., & Shull, W. H. (2003). Diffuse axonal injury in head trauma. *Journal of Head Trauma Rehabilitation, 18,* 307–316.

Sohlberg, M. M., McLaughlin, K. A., Todis, B., Larsen, J., & Glang, A. (2001). What does it take to collaborate with families affected by brain injury: A preliminary model. *Journal of Head Trauma Rehabilitation, 16,* 498–511.

Sparadeo, F. R., & Gill, D. (1989). Focus on clinical research: Effects of prior alcohol use on head injury recovery. *Journal of Head Trauma Rehabilitation, 4,* 75–82.

Stoeckmann, T. (2001). Casting for the person with spasticity. *Topics in Stroke Rehabilitation, 8,* 27–35.

Suter, P. (2004). Rehabilitation and management of visual dysfunction following traumatic brain injury. In M. J. Ashley (Ed.), *Traumatic brain injury: Rehabilitative treatment and case management* (2nd ed., pp. 209–249). Boca Raton, FL: CRC Press.

Taber, K. H., Warden, D. L., & Hurley, R. A. (2006). Blast-related traumatic brain injury: What is known? *Journal of Neuropsychiatry & Clinical Neurosciences, 18,* 141–145.

Teasdale, G., & Jennett, B. (1974). Assessment of coma and impaired consciousness: A practical scale. *Lancet, 2,* 81–84.

Thorton, M., Marshall, S., McComas, J., Finestone, H., McCormick, A., & Sveistrup, H. (2005). Benefits of activity and virtual reality based balance exercise programmes for adults with traumatic brain injury: Perceptions of participants and their caregivers. *Brain Injury, 19,* 989–1000.

Toglia, J. P. (1989). Approaches to cognitive assessment of the brain-injured adult. *Occupational Therapy Practice, 1,* 36–55.

Trexler, L. E., & Zappala, G. (1988). Neuropathological determinants of acquired attention disorders in traumatic brain injury. *Brain and Cognition, 8,* 291–302.

Trombly, C. A., Radomski, M. V., & Davis, E. S. (1998). Achievement of self-identified goals by adults with traumatic brain injury: Phase I. *American Journal of Occupational Therapy, 52,* 810–818.

Trombly, C. A., Radomski, M. V., Trexel, C., & Burnett-Smith, S. E. (2002). Occupational therapy and achievement of self-identified goals by adults with acquired brain injury: Phase II. *American Journal of Occupational Therapy, 56,* 489–498.

Vanderploeg, R. D., Schwab, K., Walker, W. C. Fraser, J. A., Sigford, B. J., Date, E. S., Scott, S. G., Curtiss, G., Salazar A. M., & Warden, D. L. for the Defense and Veterans Brain Injury Study Center Group. (2008). Rehabilitation of traumatic brain injury in active duty military personnel and veterans: Defense and Veterans Brain Injury Center randomized controlled trial of two rehabilitation approaches. *Archives of Physical Medicine and Rehabilitation, 89,* 2227–2238.

Warren, M. (1993). A hierarchical model for evaluation and treatment of visual perceptual dysfunction in adult acquired brain injury: Part 1. *American Journal of Occupational Therapy, 47,* 42–54.

Whyte, J., & DiPasquale, M. C. (1995). Assessment of vision and visual attention in minimally responsive brain injured patients. *Archives of Physical Medicine and Rehabilitation, 76,* 804–810.

Whyte, J., Hart, T., Bode, R. K., & Malec, J. F. (2003). The Moss Attention Rating Scale for traumatic brain injury: Initial psychometric assessment. *Archives of Physical Medicine and Rehabilitation, 84,* 268–276.

Williams, T. A. (1995). Low vision rehabilitation for a patient with a traumatic brain injury. *American Journal of Occupational Therapy, 49,* 923–926.

Wilson, J. T., Pettigrew, L. E., & Teasdale, G. M. (1998). Structured interviews for the Glasgow Outcome Scale and the extended Glasgow Outcome Scale: Guidelines for their use. *Journal of Neurotrauma, 15,* 573–585.

Wise, E. K., Mathews-Dalton, C., Dikmen, S., Temkin, N., Machamer, J. Bell, K., & Powell, J. M. (2010). Impact of traumatic brain injury on participation in leisure activities. *Archives of Physical Medicine and Rehabilitation, 91,* 1357–1362.

Ylvisaker, M., Jacobs, H. E., & Feeney, T. (2003). Positive supports for people who experience behavioral and cognitive disability after brain injury. *Journal of Head Trauma Rehabilitation, 18,* 7–32.

Yuen, H. K. (1997). Positive talk training in an adult with traumatic brain injury. *American Journal of Occupational Therapy, 51,* 780–783.

Acknowledgments

Thanks to Jenny Owens, OTD, OTR/L, for contributing the section on combat-related TBI and to Mechthild Rast, PhD, OTR/L, for her assistance with the section on positioning.

35

Neurodegenerative Diseases

Susan J. Forwell, Lucinda Hugos, Lois F. Copperman, and Setareh Ghahari

Learning Objectives

After studying this chapter, the reader will be able to do the following:

1. Describe four neurodegenerative diseases, including their courses and their symptoms.
2. Select appropriate standardized occupational therapy assessment and evaluation tools for clients with neurodegenerative diseases based on individual clients' characteristics and requirements.
3. Determine appropriate interventions for clients with neurode-generative disease based on their individual characteristics, requirements, the occupational therapy evaluation, and research evidence to maintain independent function at the highest possible level.

Neurodegenerative diseases are generally chronic, potentially progressive, and frequently require coping with disability and the threat of future loss of function. The underlying pathologies of four neurodegenerative diseases are described in this chapter and are shown to have mechanisms that attack the peripheral nervous system and central nervous system (CNS), resulting in impairments and limitations that affect all aspects of life. Although not curable, research and medical advances, including rehabilitation interventions, have led to treatments that allow people to live longer, more productive lives.

This chapter begins with an overview of occupational therapy for persons with neurodegenerative diseases. Broad considerations related to evaluation, goal setting, and intervention are reviewed, followed by detailed discussions of multiple sclerosis (MS), Parkinson's disease (PD), amyotrophic lateral sclerosis (ALS), and Guillain-Barré syndrome (GBS).

OCCUPATIONAL THERAPY FOR NEURODEGENERATIVE DISEASES

The unique contribution of occupational therapy for persons with neurodegenerative diseases is the consistent focus on participation in occupations and activities that are important and valued in their lives. There is no script, because the nature, type, intensity, and context of these occupations are as individual as each person with a neurodegenerative disease. By listening to each client coupled with professional expertise in occupation, however, occupational therapists provide a repertoire of systematic processes and diverse solutions.

Occupational therapy may frequently begin at diagnosis and continue throughout the continuum of comprehensive care; it may take place in inpatient acute care, inpatient rehabilitation, outpatient, in-home, or long-term care settings. Inpatient acute treatment usually follows a relapse or deterioration in the disease and/or a crisis and is short and limited to stabilizing symptoms with medical interventions. Inpatient rehabilitation may last one to several weeks, with daily therapy sessions to deal with changed symptoms. Outpatient therapy is usually weekly, with 45–60-minute individual sessions to maximize independence in the home, minimize the effects of symptoms on daily activities, and identify and obtain needed equipment. Occupational therapy in long-term care facilities may be similar to inpatient rehabilitation for people adjusting to changing symptoms to ensure maintenance of function or developing palliative care plans for patients. Occupational therapists attend to their own coping and maintain objectivity, especially when treating clients whose disease course portends increasing disability or death.

Occupational Therapy Evaluation

The occupational therapy evaluation begins with an interview to gather information about the client's valued roles and occupations, relevant history of his or her neurodegenerative disease, previous and current strategies used to manage daily life, and the nature of present concerns or problems. This interview must be sensitive to the client's changing function and fear of the unknown and also should attempt to illuminate areas that may not naturally arise such as fatigue, depression, sexual function, and cognitive concerns that impact the person's occupations and social network. With this information, the therapist selects assessments and measurement tools that will provide in-depth information on occupational areas of concern. For persons with neurodegenerative disease, the content of these measures may be limited to a few or cover a broad spectrum of occupational performance areas (such as activities of daily living [ADL], instrumental activities of daily living [IADL], work, recreation, and spiritual occupations) and/or symptoms (such as spasticity, weakness, and memory difficulties).

Occupational Therapy Intervention Process

The unplanned and profound impact of neurodegenerative disease frequently makes realistic goal setting and intervention complex and requires sensitivity, flexibility, and astute negotiation skills on the part of the occupational therapist. The therapist frequently helps the client modify behaviors and assumptions of a lifetime while assisting the person and significant others to move toward realistic new goals. Given the progressive nature of many neurodegenerative diseases, regular reassessment and reordering of goals and priorities may be necessary as intervention proceeds.

Because of the complexity of disability present with neurodegenerative disease, intervening in one area may affect several other symptoms or problems. Fatigue, for instance, may be related to pain and weakness. Interventions must be individually appropriate and may involve significant others, especially as the disease progresses. The following is an overview of ways occupational therapy optimizes performance in key roles for persons with neurodegenerative diseases.

Self-Maintenance Roles

In ADL and IADL, the occupational therapist assists the client to maintain independence in priority activities, use specialized equipment, and participate using energy-conserving methods such as

- assisting in setting priorities
- education in areas such as how the disease process affects motor or cognitive changes
- recommendation of environmental modifications at home to promote safety and independence
- range of motion (ROM) and strength exercises to facilitate occupations like bathing
- behavior modification such as use of energy and time management techniques
- use of smart phone and electronic tablet technology for grocery lists and to provide reminders
- balancing independence with assistance from others

Self-Advancement Roles

The onset of neurodegenerative diseases may affect employment in or outside of the home. Many individuals can and should continue to work rather than pursue disability benefits by seeking advice from an occupational therapist. Continued employment is beneficial for financial independence, access to diverse health care choices, maintaining one's social network, and supporting a productive identity and self-esteem. Therapists critically review job expectations and suggest modifications to the environment, behavioral changes, equipment, resources, and recommendations to the individual or the employer.

Self-Enhancement Roles

Maintaining leisure pursuits as well as involvement in community, neighborhood, and family activities may be a high priority for individuals with neurodegenerative diseases but are often the first roles or occupations to be abandoned.

Modifying activities, creative transportation solutions, and use of web-based interfaces enable the individual to continue to be involved in meaningful occupations.

The tasks associated with self-maintenance, self-advancement, and self-enhancement roles are supported by new and emerging mainstream technology including smart phones, electronic tablets, and environmental controls. For persons with neurodegenerative diseases, many of these advances have erased differences in participation, minimized the need for or altered the way adapted equipment and environmental modifications are implemented, and facilitated access to previously unavailable information and personal connections. (Refer to Chapter 18 for an in-depth discussion on technology.) With technology, however, there are a number of challenges particularly related to the vast amount of information. Occupational therapists assist clients by providing credible websites that can address questions. Examples of trustworthy sites for both occupational therapists and clients are found in Resources 35-1.

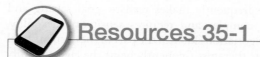 Resources 35-1

Neurodegenerative Diseases

Amyotrophic Lateral Sclerosis

ALS Association
www.alsa.org
Phone: 800-782-4747

Muscular Dystrophy Association, ALS Division
www.mda.org
Phone: 800-572-1717

Guillain-Barré Syndrome

Guillain-Barré Syndrome Foundation International
www.gbs-cidp.org

Guidelines for Physical and Occupational Therapy
www.gbs-cidp.org/wp-content/uploads/2012/01
/PTOTGuidelines.pdf
Phone: 866-224-3301

Guillain-Barré Syndrome Support Group
www.gbs.org.uk
Phone: 44-01529-469910

Multiple Sclerosis

National Multiple Sclerosis Society (NMSS)
www.nmss.org
Phone: 800-344-4867

Multiple Sclerosis Association of America (MSAA)
www.msassociation.org
Phone: 800-532-7667

Consortium of Multiple Sclerosis Centers (CMSC)
www.mscare.org
Phone: 201-487-1050

Parkinson's Disease

Parkinson Society Canada
www.parkinson.ca
Phone: 800-565-3000

American Parkinson Disease Association, Inc.
www.apdaparkinson.org
Phone: 800-223-2732

National Parkinson Foundation
www.parkinson.org
Phone: 800-327-4545; 800-473-4636 [helpline]

Michael J. Fox Foundation for Parkinson's Research
www.michaeljfox.org
Phone: 800-708-7644

Miscellaneous

National Organization of Rare Disorders (NORD)
www.rarediseases.org
Phone: 203-744-0100 or 800-999-6673 [voicemail]

Paralyzed Veterans of America (PVA)
www.pva.org
Phone: 800-424-8200

National Institute of Neurological Disorders and Stroke –
Clearinghouse on Disability Information
http://www.ninds.nih.gov/find_people/government_
agencies/volorg103.htm
http://www.ninds.nih.gov/
Phone: 202-245-7307 or 202-205-5637 (TTD)

Members and Roles of Rehabilitation Team

Depending on the type and severity of functional limitations, involvement of the rehabilitation team may vary but is essential in maintaining the highest level of function and quality of life (Martin & Wieler, 2003). When cognitive problems interfere with everyday occupations, psychologists, speech therapists, and occupational therapists are often consulted (Brown & Kraft, 2005). Depending on the setting, neuropsychologists may conduct in-depth cognitive assessments, and all three professionals may make recommendations and engage in intervention to augment or compensate for deficits in cognitive ability. Speech therapists may be involved when dysarthria or expressive communication is labored. In the presence of dysphagia, an occupational therapist, speech therapist, and/or dietician commonly form the intervention team. Social workers assist when there is a shift in financial or care needs and may help make applications to appropriate programs and counsel individuals and significant others to better cope with role change and demands. Physical changes as a result of weakness, spasticity, sensory problems, pain, and decreased endurance and ROM necessitate the services of physical therapy and occupational therapy to enhance mobility, upper extremity function, and overall conditioning to reduce falls and maintain participation. Occupational therapy services are used when individuals are having difficulty caring for themselves or their environment or engaging in work and/or familiar leisure occupations.

SPECIFIC NEURODEGENERATIVE DISEASES

The following sections focus on four neurodegenerative diseases: MS, PD, ALS, and GBS. The first section on MS provides detailed insights into the clinical reasoning for occupational therapy evaluation and treatment that may be applicable across conditions. For example, a client with ALS who has fatigue may benefit from the energy-conservation techniques described in the MS section. As such, issues occurring across neurodegenerative diseases are not elaborated upon in subsequent sections. Each neurological disorder, however, has its own underlying pathology, peculiarities, and prognosis. Understanding these issues helps the therapist develop appropriate intervention plans.

Multiple Sclerosis

MS is the most commonly diagnosed neurological disease that can cause disability in young adults. An estimated 400,000 people in the United States have MS (National Multiple Sclerosis Society [NMSS], 2012), and worldwide that number is 2.5 million (Multiple Sclerosis Trust, 2012). MS causes severe disability in some people, but many continue to lead active, productive lives and are not severely disabled (Rodriguez et al., 1994).

The precise cause of MS remains unknown. The present theory is that an environmental trigger or an infectious agent initiates the autoimmune response in people with genetic susceptibility (Trapp et al., 1998). The *multiple* in multiple sclerosis refers to both time and location of MS lesions and relapses. The *sclerosis* refers to the hardened or sclerotic plaques that are the scar tissue resulting from autoimmune attacks on the CNS (axons and myelin covering).

Axonal transection is considered as significant as demyelination in MS damage (McGavern et al., 2000). At least temporarily, demyelinated axons may remyelinate and provide conduction of nerve impulses. Transected axons are permanently destroyed and lose all potential for conduction. There is also evidence that disease activity continues even during periods that are clinically quiet or when no change in symptoms is apparent (Trapp et al., 1998). Inflammation occurs with demyelination and axonal damage, which may explain the rapid improvement often seen in treatment of relapses with corticosteroid anti-inflammatory agents.

Diagnosing Multiple Sclerosis

Individuals are typically diagnosed with MS between the ages of 15 and 50 years, although children are increasingly being diagnosed (Krupp & Macallister, 2005). Peak age of onset is at age 20–30 years. Women are two to three times as likely to have MS. Caucasians of northern European descent have the greatest risk of developing MS, whereas groups like the Norwegian Lapps, Inuit, and New Zealand Maoris who live in similar latitudes have no incidence of MS (NMSS, 2012).

The diagnosis of MS has evolved in the last 30 years owing to research and introduction of and advances in magnetic resonance imaging (MRI). The criteria, updated in 2010 and known as the Revised McDonald Criteria, are based on the combination of findings in the medical history, neurological examination, MRI results, and analysis of cerebrospinal fluid (Polman et al., 2011). Additional tests including visual evoked potential and blood tests may be used to corroborate evidence for the MS diagnosis or to rule out other possible diseases. Signs of MS include weakness, hyperreflexia, positive Babinski sign, dysmetria, nystagmus, and impaired vibratory or position sensation. The Expanded Disability Status Scale (Kurtzke, 1983) and the MS Functional Composite (MSFC) (Fischer et al., 2001) are the most commonly used impairment rating instruments in both clinical and research settings.

The Course of Multiple Sclerosis

The course of MS is typically categorized into four types: relapsing-remitting, secondary progressive, primary progressive, and progressive-relapsing. The relapsing-remitting course, the most common at the time of diagnosis, produces clearly defined relapses of acute worsening of neurological function followed by partial or complete improvement and then stable periods of remission between attacks (Trapp et al., 1998). People with secondary progressive MS start with a relapsing-remitting course of up to 10–15 years. The secondary progressive course is typically diagnosed when there is continued neurological deterioration. People with primary progressive MS have continuously declining neurological function from onset (Lublin & Reingold, 1996). The progressive-relapsing course is much less common and characterized by continued disease progression with superimposed relapses. Clinically isolated syndrome or the first neurological episode that may result in a MS diagnosis is important to identify so that treatments to minimize disease progression can be provided.

Medical Developments Changing Health Care for Multiple Sclerosis

There have been a number of developments in our understanding of MS and the ways to assess and treat problems. The most significant clinical medical advances that have consumed enormous research efforts and impacted clinical practice are the advent of disease modifying therapies (DMTs). There are five self-injectable immune-modulating medications approved for use in the United States (NMSS, 2012): interferon beta-1a (Avonex), interferon beta-1b (Betaseron), interferon beta-1b (Extavia), glatiramer acetate (Copaxone), and interferon beta-1a (Rebif). These drugs have been shown to reduce the number of lesions evidenced on MRI and the frequency and severity of relapses, although a recent study suggests that the beta interferons do not impact long-term disability (Shirani et al., 2012). Natalizumab (Tysabri), a monthly injectable, is administered by qualified practitioners and is approved for relapsing-remitting MS. Mitoxantrone (Novantrone), an immunosuppressant rather than an immunomodulator, is rarely used because of significant side effects. Fingolimod (Gilenya) is the only DMT that is taken orally and is generally used when the response to injectable DMTs has diminished. Another class of medications, neurofunctional modifiers, targets underlying pathophysiology and MS symptoms (Panitch & Applebee, 2012). Of these drugs, dalfampridine has been shown to improve walking ability in people with any type of MS (Goodman et al., 2009).

Clients may want to discuss their medications with therapists, asking their opinion about the efficacy of medications. This is true particularly for DMTs because they are designed not to reverse disability but to slow disease progression. The therapist's responsibility is to understand and explain the importance of taking medications because the benefits may further contribute to maintaining employment and participating in high-priority occupations for a longer period.

The client may also want to discuss the proposed presence of chronic cerebrospinal venous insufficiency (CCSVI), a narrowing of veins in the neck and chest resulting in reduced blood drainage from the brain to the spinal cord (Food and Drug Administration [FDA], 2012), which some suggest is a cause or contributing factor in MS (Zamboni & Carinci, 2011). Despite an international research effort, to date, there remains little to no evidence to support a significant relationship between CCSVI and MS (FDA, 2012; Mayer et al., 2011). The scientific community and health care providers, however, are at odds with the public and persons with MS as social media often portray positive if not miraculous messages about its treatment (Ghahari & Forwell, 2012). The resulting tension has played out in doctors' offices and MS clinics, such that there is an increased distrust, and patients are reluctant to discuss their thoughts or questions about CCSVI.

With conditions such as MS that are not curable and have a progressive course, unproven remedies may emerge periodically. The difference today, compared to past remedies, is the presence of the Internet that enables diverse ideas, including unproven remedies, to capture widespread attention. Occupational therapists must keep abreast of emerging remedies and trends and the research associated with them. Then while communicating the evidence in a balanced way, it is important to listen, to be sensitive to clients' situations, to provide honest, compassionate, accurate responses to their questions, and not to extinguish hope.

Potential Social, Emotional, and Economic Consequences

A disease that strikes young adults has substantial economic, social, and emotional costs that influence all aspects of life. Between the ages of 20 and 40 years, people typically are entering the labor market, establishing themselves in careers, meeting life partners, and forming families. MS, with its common symptoms of fatigue, weakness, difficulties with prolonged standing or walking, cognitive problems, and depression, can impede productivity at work and home and social engagement.

A body of research is developing that may influence family planning. The relapse rate in MS significantly declines during pregnancy, increases in the first 3 months following childbirth, and thereafter returns to prepregnancy levels (Vukusic et al., 2004). It is also known that the incidence of MS is increased between monozygotic twins and from mother to daughter (Sadovnick et al., 1993). Therapists must be aware of this research to assist clients seeking information and refer as appropriate.

Planning for the future is a precarious undertaking given the unknown disease progression in MS. This uncertainty may explain an estimated lifetime prevalence of 50% for depression (Sá, 2007) and 35% for anxiety (Korostil & Feinstein, 2007). Research suggests gaining control over the everyday management of MS is important for a satisfying life (Thorne, Paterson, & Russell, 2003).

Employment studies conducted prior to the development of DMTs showed that more than 70% of individuals with MS were out of the labor force 10–15 years after initial diagnosis (Kalb, 1996). Employment disability legislation such as the Americans with Disabilities Act, however, has resulted in opportunities for people to maintain productive paid employment for longer periods. It has been shown that persons with MS who leave the labor market are likely to have greater social isolation, psychological distress, and great burden of disease, as well as lower incomes and more limited access to health insurance than if they remain employed (Hakim et al., 2000). Maintaining employment has been shown to have high health-related quality of life (Buchanan, Haung, & Kaufman, 2012).

Symptoms Typically Addressed in Occupational Therapy

Occupational therapy intervention may reduce the impact of MS symptoms including weakness, sensory changes, balance disturbance, visual changes, bowel and bladder disturbance, cognitive changes, dysphagia, dizziness or vertigo, pain, ataxic gait, tremor, sexual dysfunction, depression, spasticity, and fatigue. A few of these are described here to exemplify therapy services.

Fatigue. Fatigue is the most common and pervasive MS symptom and a primary reason for referral to occupational therapy. It affects 60%–80% of people with MS and is a significant contributor to unemployment and overall disability (Julian et al., 2008). Fatigue in MS augments other MS symptoms, varies from slight to severe with worsening typically in the afternoon, and may be related to increased ambient and core body temperature (Leavitt et al., 2012).

Therapists must be aware of both the types of and factors contributing to fatigue in MS (see Definition 35-1) (Forwell et al., 2008; Stewart, Tran, & Bowling, 2007). Numerous screening measures for fatigue in MS include the Fatigue Severity Scale (Krupp et al., 1989), the Modified Fatigue Impact Scale (Fisk et al., 1994), and the Rochester Fatigue Diary (Schwid et al., 2002). The Comprehensive Fatigue Assessment Battery for MS (CFAB-MS) (Dawes, McCloy, & Forwell, 2010) was developed to identify factors contributing to MS fatigue and to guide clinicians' treatment decisions. Interventions are then directed at mitigating these factors as well as managing the primary MS fatigue.

Weakness. Weakness may occur in all parts of the body, resulting in referral to therapy. Weakness that increases after repeated muscle contractions or fatigue of the same muscle(s) is known as "nerve fiber fatigue." The cause is unknown but likely related to the conduction impairment in demyelinated nerves. An example is increased dorsiflexion weakness resulting in foot-drop after walking which may

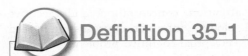

Definition 35-1

Types of Fatigue in Multiple Sclerosis

Primary multiple sclerosis (MS) fatigue—Fatigue caused by MS disease process, the cause of which is poorly understood.

Secondary MS fatigue—Fatigue resulting from untreated MS problem(s) such as walking difficulties.

Physical fatigue—Fatigue experienced in the limbs, torso, head, and neck such that the body is tired.

Cognitive fatigue—Fatigue that affects one's thinking, planning, memory, word-finding, and decision-making processes such that the brain feels exhausted.

Local or focal fatigue—Motor fatigue caused by inefficient nerve conduction to a selected area of the body.

Generalized fatigue—An entire body experience; a complete exhaustion that is physical and cognitive.

Normal fatigue—Fatigue experienced by humans after excessive energy output or several hours of being awake (a normal day) that benefits from rest or sleep.

Factors Shown to Contribute to Fatigue in Multiple Sclerosis

- Other medical issues such as anemia, arthritis, cardiac problems, respiratory inefficiency, infection, and thyroid problems
- Sleep problems, often related to muscle spasms, depression, or urinary problems
- Depression
- Stress
- Anxiety
- Pain
- Deconditioning
- Side effects to medications
- Nutrition or caloric intake
- Ambulation difficulties

increase stumbling, especially on uneven surfaces. Coupled with decreased balanced and gait impairment, the risk of falls is increased by 58% (Cattaneo et al., 2002). After resting, conduction and muscle contraction are improved.

Cognition. Up to 65% of people with MS have cognitive problems that vary considerably in severity (Patti, 2009) and that appear related to loss of brain volume, particularly grey matter (Hasan et al., 2011). It is estimated that 5%–10% of those with MS have cognitive problems that interfere with participation in everyday occupations (NMSS, 2012). Cognitive problems are seen at all stages of the disease and are significant in leading to unemployment in MS (Johnson, Bamer, & Fraser, 2009).

Common cognitive problems for people with MS include memory (acquiring and retaining new information);

word finding; attention, concentration, and executive function; and slowed information-processing speed (NMSS, 2012). Perceptual-cognitive problems may also occur such as visual-spatial impairments that might result in a tendency to get lost or a history of motor vehicle accidents. Cognitive issues in MS do not correlate with physical disability but are influenced by depression, stress, anxiety, and fatigue (Bol et al., 2010) and vary during the day, increasing in the afternoon or when sustained mental concentration is required (Krupp & Lekins, 2000). Both individuals and their families may be unaware that cognitive problems such as reduced insight and inflexible thinking are related to the disease and should not be mistaken for personality or psychological issues.

Many areas of cognition remain intact such that screens such as the Mini-Mental State Exam lack sensitivity to detect such problems (Beatty & Goodkin, 1990). Consequently, it is necessary to complete a lengthy neuropsychological evaluation. Fortunately, however, a 90-minute, six-test neuropsychological assessment battery was designed specifically for MS called the Minimal Assessment of Cognitive Function in MS (MACFIMS) (Benedict et al., 2002). In addition, three screening tools, the MS Neuropsychological Screening Questionnaire (Benedict et al., 2004), the Paced Auditory Serial Addition Test, and the Symbol Digit Modalities Test (SDMT) are quick to administer and have been found to be sensitive in MS (Foley et al., 2012). Of these, the oral version of the SDMT is considered a better screen because it has good test–retest reliability and is a predictor of unemployment. By identifying cognitive impairments, individualized compensation strategies can be recommended to reduce their impact on everyday life.

Pain. Pain is estimated to occur in 40%–60% of people with MS, with 48% reporting chronic pain (NMSS, 2012). Pain negatively impacts quality of life and independence (Douglas, Wollin, & Windsor, 2009) and is not related to age, length of time with MS, or degree of disability, although twice as many women report having pain than men. Pain in MS can be localized as in trigeminal neuralgia, Lhermitte's sign (a stabbing, electric shock along the spine when neck forward flexes), or pain as a result of spasticity (Solaro et al., 2004). Pain directly caused by the neurological lesions is considered primary to MS and is treated with medications. Pain secondary to MS is often due to posture, gait, and positioning problems and can be relieved by therapy and proper mobility equipment.

Spasticity. Spasticity in MS is usually greater in the lower extremities and may be source of pain, interrupted sleep, and activity limitations. Up to 30% of patients eliminate or modify activities because of spasticity (Rizzo et al., 2004). Factors that may precipitate or augment spasticity include infections, distended bladder, stress, or disease progression (Schapiro, 2011).

Tremor and Ataxia. Intention tremor is the most common tremor seen in MS and is one of the most difficult problems to manage (NMSS, 2012). As an activity progresses and the extremity approaches the target (a point when the greatest precision is required), the tremor is at its worse. Intention tremor occurs in the upper extremities but may also manifest in the lower extremities, torso, and neck. A comprehensive occupational therapy assessment was developed, the Multidimensional Assessment of Tremor (MAT), which measures both the severity and functional impact of intention tremor (Daudrich, Hurl, & Forwell, 2010).

Ataxia presents in the trunk and lower extremities where postural responses tend to occur before upper extremity movements. The functional challenges of ataxia are further magnified because of the multiple joints involved in the ataxic movement.

Dysphagia. Research on swallowing problems in MS that did not use videofluoroscopy (VF) suggested that 34%–43% of the individuals studied experienced dysphagia, although only half of these patients reported swallowing difficulties (Calcagno et al., 2002; Thomas & Wiles, 1999). When VF was used, however, swallowing abnormalities were identified that were not detected on non-VF swallow assessment (Weiser et al., 2002). These studies suggest that severity of disease and cerebellar or brainstem involvement are risk factors for dysphagia. Occupational therapists should routinely screen for choking, aspiration, and swallowing difficulties, for which additional information can be found in Chapter 43.

Adjusting to Multiple Sclerosis

Although only a small percentage of people with MS are severely disabled, the diagnosis can be devastating. The need to adjust to changing symptoms and impairments and the fear of and uncertainty about the disease process affect self-esteem, relationships, sexuality, physical activities, vocational goals, and recreational interests. From questions about pregnancy to cognitive changes influencing competence or safety, MS affects every role and relationship. The variability of the disease and the hidden nature of many symptoms, such as cognitive changes and fatigue, often make it difficult and uncomfortable to explain to friends, coworkers, and family members.

Each person's reaction to MS events varies and has implications for adjustment. Research has shown that emotion-focused coping techniques were used more often by those experiencing a MS relapse, whereas problem solving and using one's social network were used when in remission (Pakenham, 1999). This is supported by evidence that emotional involvement was a marginal indicator of new MS lesions as shown on MRI (Mohr et al., 2002). It has also been demonstrated that a greater use of problem-solving strategies appears to be an indicator of better psychological adjustment (Warren, Warren, & Cockerill, 1991).

For example, fewer lesions were found in persons who participated in a stress management program as compared to when the program was discontinued (Mohr et al., 2012).

Initially, people may be preoccupied with their diagnosis because it represents a major change that may challenge assumptions about the future. As time passes, particularly if individuals with MS return to full function, they frequently ignore the diagnosis and pay little attention to MS issues. As long as the inattention does not result in adverse decisions, this may be a healthy attitude. The therapist helps clients process the implications of changes and identifies modifications to minimize their effects. Information about new symptoms may be all a person needs to make a successful adjustment.

Occupational Therapy Evaluation

During the evaluation process of a person with MS, there are unique features that must be understood and incorporated from the individual's history with MS and from life experience. Occupational therapy assessment begins with an interview about the person's goals for therapy and a brief history of symptoms and treatment since diagnosis. This gives the therapist an understanding of the disease course and the person's past coping style. Throughout the interview, the therapist listens for hints of cognitive difficulties, being mindful that there may be further significant hidden impairments. Brief questions regarding dizziness, thinking problems, motivation or interest in doing things, numbness and tingling, manual dexterity, prolonged walking and standing, employment, home physical and social environment, leisure interests, bladder problems, ADL, IADL, energy, sleeping pattern, muscle cramping, pain, fine-motor activities, falling and balance problems, and vision can provide clues to the specific assessments that are likely to be relevant. If cognitive problems are present, a family member or significant other should be encouraged to attend the evaluation with the client's consent.

Analysis of Occupational Performance: Tools and Methods.
The initial interview gives the therapist an indication of the evaluation tools and methods to use including

- Canadian Occupational Performance Measure (COPM) (Law et al., 2005; Lexell, Iwarrson, & Lexell, 2006)
- Modified Fatigue Impact Scale to screen for fatigue severity (Fisk et al., 1994)
- 6-Minute Walk Test to assess endurance and fatigue (Pankoff et al., 2000)
- Multiple Sclerosis Walking Scale to assess mobility concerns (Hobart et al., 2003)
- Sleep history questionnaire or diary (Paralyzed Veterans of America [PVA], 1998)
- Home assessment
- Beck Depression Inventory-Fast Screen to assess depression (Benedict et al., 2003)
- MS Neuropsychological Screening Questionnaire to screen cognition (Benedict et al., 2004)

- Mobility section of the Functional Independence Measure (FIM™) to assess gait or bed mobility
- ADL, IADL, and dysphagia assessments
- Nine-Hole Peg Test or Purdue Pegboard to assess dexterity (see Chapter 37)
- Semmes-Weinstein Monofilaments to test sensation (see Chapter 9)
- Manual muscle testing (MMT), ROM testing, and grip strength (dynamometry) (see Chapter 7)
- Vestibular evaluation

There are also composite evaluations with a series of assessments that provide a more detailed or diverse estimation of an individual's ability. Examples are the MACFIMS (Benedict et al., 2002) for cognition; the MAT for intention tremor (Daudrich, Hurl, & Forwell, 2010); the MSFC (Fischer et al., 2001) for disability status; the CFAB-MS for fatigue (Dawes, McCloy, & Forwell, 2010); and the Brain Injury Visual Assessment Battery for Adults (biVABA) for vision (Warren, 1999).

Administering such measures requires the therapist to accurately interpret findings in the context of the client's situation and the complex interrelationship between functional challenges and symptoms. For example, therapists must differentiate among various types of fatigue by considering the results of several assessments. A high score on a depression index may indicate that depression is contributing to fatigue, whereas slow times on the 6-Minute Walk Test may also suggest a nerve fiber or motor fatigue component. Information from a sleep questionnaire may indicate that disturbed sleep caused by urinary frequency is a factor in daytime fatigue. It is common for persons with MS to have several sources of fatigue (Forwell et al., 2008), requiring intervention from multiple health care professionals.

Occupational Therapy Intervention Process

Clients' priorities and interests are the cornerstone of goal setting and treatment planning, necessitating a collaborative process to achieve realistic and satisfying outcomes. Frequently, both the person with MS and the referring provider mistakenly believe they have to live with problems as a result of MS that, in fact, are treatable through therapy. The intervention plan must then take into account the unique issues of individuals with MS. For example, Finlayson (2004) suggests that, for older adults with MS, the therapist must ensure they feel a sense of control over their future, work with families affected by the MS, and advocate for enhanced community support options. In addition, treatment that focuses on isolated symptoms is unlikely to be effective, and thus working with and coordinating intervention of the health care team is often indicated. Evidence Table 35-1 presents the best evidence for occupational therapy intervention for MS. Special considerations for activity strategies, equipment and environmental modifications, exercise programs, symptom management, and employment issues are discussed below.

Evidence Table 35-1 | Best Evidence for Occupational Therapy Practice Regarding Intervention Related to Multiple Sclerosis (MS)

Intervention	Description of Intervention Tested	Participants	Dosage	Type of Best Evidence and Level of Evidence	Benefit	Statistical Probability and Effect Size of Outcome	Reference
Efficacy and effectiveness of an energy–conservation course on fatigue, quality of life (QOL), and self-efficacy for persons with multiple sclerosis (MS)	Community-based energy conservation course including but not limited to importance of rest, effective communication, proper body mechanics, and modification of environments	One hundred sixty-nine persons with MS: 140 women, 29 men; mean age = 48 years	Energy conservation course for 2 hours per week for 6 weeks	Randomized control trial with a crossover design. Level: IA1a	The energy-conservation course significantly reduced the impact of the fatigue, improved vitality, and increased self-efficacy for performing conservation strategies.	Results were established at $p < 0.05$. Using Cohen's d for repeated measures, moderate to large effect sizes were shown for the fatigue subscales of cognition (0.52–0.57), physical (0.74–0.90), and social (0.69–0.77) as well as for three of eight subscales on the Short form-36 including role-physical (0.52–0.63), vitality (0.99–1.14), and mental health (0.53–0.60).	Mathiowetz et al. (2005)
Nintendo Wii Fit and its effect on physical activity behavior	Exercise program three times per week that included yoga, balance, strength, and aerobic training using Wii Fit in each session. Participants were telephoned to monitor adverse events and to encourage increase in the duration and frequency of using Wii Fit for the first 7 weeks.	Thirty participants: 23 women, 7 men; with relapsing-remitting MS; living within 40 miles of the University of Illinois, 18–60 years old, and able to walk 25 feet with or without a cane. Excluded if doing 2.5+ hours of activity per week, low vision, lower extremity amputation, pregnant, severe fatigue or depression, or cardiopulmonary disease	Wii Fit exercise program for 14 weeks, 3 days per week	One-group repeated measures design with 5-week baseline control period and 2-week Wii set-up and training followed by 14-week intervention. Level: IIIB3b	Balance and strength were significantly improved at week 7 but at week 14, physical activity levels declined relative to week 7, and the difference was no longer significant compared with the control period.	Results were determined using multivariate analysis of variance and showed physical activity improved at 14 weeks ($p = .001$; $ES = 0.65$) though declined at 21 weeks; self-efficacy progressively improved to 21 weeks ($p = 0.025$); and no difference in QOL or level of fatigue.	Plow & Finlayson (2011)
Using personal digital assistants (PDAs) as assistive technology for people with MS with cognitive impairment	Training to use a PDA as an organizer (i.e., calendar, alarm, contact list and "to do" list) and transferring data from computer to PDA)	Twenty people with MS: 16 women, 4 men; living in the community; having cognitive limitations; describing cognition as one of their major problems and having vision, hearing, and dexterity sufficient to use a PDA	After an 8-week baseline (no intervention) period, home visits for PDA training were completed over 3 weeks: two for 60 minutes, two for 90 minutes. Then 8 weeks of PDA usage.	One group pre and post treatment repeated measures; testing at weeks 1, 10, 12 and 21. Level: IIIB3b	Functional performance increased significantly with PDA use, which was maintained at 8-week follow-up.	Repeated-measures analysis of variance showed significant results on the COPM ($F = 96.02$, $p < 0.001$, for performance; $F = 104.92$, $p < 0.001$, for satisfaction). There was significant improvement during treatment, with a large effect size ($p < 0.001$, $r = 0.79$). The posttreatment scores remained higher than pretreatment.	Gentry (2008)

Activity Strategies and Energy Conservation. Based on the comprehensive assessment, the fatigue intervention begins with the occupational therapist providing explanations of each relevant underlying type and factor of fatigue impacting the individual (Definition 35-1). The client then completes a detailed activity diary that can be done on well-selected apps and makes a list of goals and priorities (PVA, 1998). The therapist and client use the diary to systematically analyze daily work, home, and leisure activities and understand rest–activity ratios. Identifying activity and environmental modifications, equipment, and technology to address fatigue issues then follows. Energy conservation strategies and exercise routines will also be incorporated to help the individual perform valued occupations and activities through optimal energy management techniques. Refer to the Definition 35-2 for examples of energy management strategies designed to enable persons with MS to use their limited energy on useful, meaningful activities and to exercise choice and control in everyday occupations.

Research has demonstrated the effectiveness of a face-to-face occupational therapy–led group intervention (Packer, Brink, & Sauriol, 1995) in energy conservation strategies for MS (Mathiowetz et al., 2005). A teleconference format (Finlayson & Holberg, 2007) and an online version of this energy conservation program (Ghahari, Packer, & Passmore, 2010) have also been shown to be effective. Further, there is a 6-week group video program called *Fatigue: Take Control!* that has been tested with positive outcomes (Hugos et al., 2010). In addition to these programs, occupational therapists should collaborate with physical therapists who treat fatigue through obtaining gait equipment, recommending appropriate aerobic exercise routines, and educating on the difference between energy expenditure during functional activities and exercise to increase endurance. With any of these interventions, written recommendations and summaries should be provided. Clients then return to occupational therapy for follow-up in 2–3 months, or sooner if changes in symptoms present or there are difficulties implementing strategies.

Equipment, Behavioral, and Environmental Modifications. Equipment, environmental, and behavioral modifications help persons with MS compensate for weakness, spasticity, tremor, fatigue, ataxia, and cognitive problems. Many standard pieces of adaptive equipment are helpful, (for example, scooters, electric wheelchairs, bath benches, shower chairs, and bed poles) in limiting fatigue and mitigating functional limitations related to weakness and spasticity. Because of fatigue, self-propelling manual wheelchairs are not indicated. As noted earlier, mainstream technology such as computers, motion sensors, and smart devices that have audio options reduce the impact of many MS symptoms. When appropriate, the therapist identifies consumer technology and adaptive equipment and facilitates equipment trials.

Behavioral changes, such as moving an exercise program from lunch to after work and incorporating a lunchtime

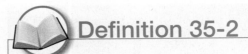

Definition 35-2

Energy Conservation

To save, conserve, or reduce consumption or expenditure of energy. An individual's conservation of energy and optimization of endurance during participation in occupations refers to efficiently using available energy while decreasing unnecessary expenditure. Examples of strategies used to conserve personal energy reservoir include employing a "brains rather than brawn" approach such as:

- Use high, low, and smart technology appropriately.
  - Use smart devices and helpful apps to save steps, such as voice options to replace touch typing.
  - Decrease prolonged standing and walking by modifying tasks to be done sitting.
  - Maintain a cooler body temperature by using, for example, an air conditioner, cooling wraps fitted comfortably at wrist or on neck or a cooling vest when active (Fig. 35-1).
  - Reduce the energy required to walk by using an ankle–foot orthosis, cane, or walker.
  - Obtain seating systems for trunk support in wheelchairs.
  - For work, use a fitted ergonomic chair with armrests, correct height, and back support.
- Plan approaches to occupation and daily schedule.
  - Do important activities in the morning.
  - Break large time-consuming activities into smaller tasks and do one task at a time.
- Problem solve using a step-by-step approach.
  - Use techniques to maintain cooler body temperature, for example layer clothing, have warm versus hot showers, and avoid electric blankets or down comforters when sleeping.
- Delegate necessary highly energy-consuming occupations.
- Manage environmental controls and modifications.
  - Adjust heights of work surfaces to avoid strain.
  - Avoids stairs in daily activities.
- Simplify or eliminate tasks.
  - Avoid multitasking.
  - Have tools required for the task readily available in arm's reach.
- Educate others about your energy limits.
  - Teach others about increased body temperature and effects on reduced function and energy.
  - Work with others to accomplish a task, sharing the energy expenditure.
- Punctuate activities with rest.
  - Alternate activity with intervals of rest, such as walking, sitting, and then walking.

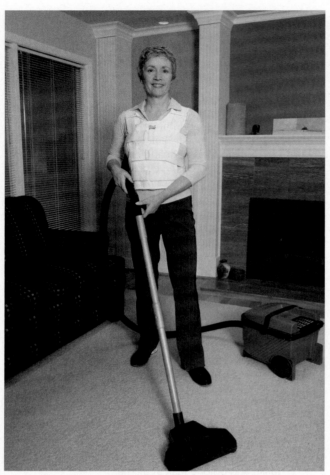

Figure 35-1 Woman in cooling vest vacuuming. Sensitivity to heat when participating in chosen occupation(s) can be mitigated by wearing cooling garments, such as cooling vests (as above) or cooling wraps comfortably worn on the neck or around the wrists.

nap, frequently improve an individual's ability to perform productively. Another example is using the elevator at work (rather than climbing stairs for exercise) to maximize energy for employment and engaging in exercise at another time. Environmental modifications may help in areas as diverse as maintaining independence in ADL to ensuring continued employment and involvement in the community. Home and/or work visits may be necessary to identify environmental modifications. The combination of the right equipment, behavior changes, and environmental modifications depend on the individual's needs, resources, and personal preferences. Scheduled follow-ups are recommended to determine the need for new or further modifications as changes occur.

Exercise Programs. Occupational therapists teach clients to monitor the effects of any MS exercise program on both fatigue and their ability to perform high-priority activities. Two MS symptoms, fatigue and spasticity, often decrease with regular exercise. A structured aerobic program has been shown to reduce fatigue and increase endurance (Kileff, 2005), and spasticity may be managed with a stretching program and rhythmic exercises such as walking or cycling. Therapists can be instrumental in assisting the client to integrate exercise into weekly routines so that exercise does not reduce ability to perform other activities.

An aerobic home program will vary based on several considerations. An employed individual may select a home stationary biking program for 20 minutes three or four times a week instead of a water exercise program at the closest cool water pool. Stretching exercises emphasize fewer repetitions and longer hold. Strengthening programs do not reverse neurological weakness resulting from MS, but they can reduce deconditioning as a result of weakness. A realistic exercise program performed regularly is more desirable than an ideal program that is never followed. Good illustrations and written instructions should accompany every home program.

Spasticity Interventions. The appropriate intervention for spasticity depends on the severity and the extent to which it interferes with function and impacts quality of life (Rizzo et al., 2004). In addition to stretching exercises, adapted dressing techniques may prove helpful, such as using a stool to maintain hip flexion to decrease extensor spasm and/or using dressing sticks to compensate for inability to reach the feet. A standing home program may also be employed, using a standing frame for 30–60 minutes per day. Other interventions include resting splints and posture and positioning techniques, such as bringing the hips into 90° or more of flexion to decrease extensor tone in the lower extremities (PVA, 2003).

Therapists should be familiar with the standard medications for spasticity, such as baclofen and tizanidine, and their side effect of drowsiness that may increase fatigue (PVA, 2003). Botox® (onabotulinumtoxin), a neurotoxin, results in relaxation of the targeted muscle and can last up to 3 months (Hyman et al., 2000). The intrathecal baclofen pump has been shown to reduce pain and improve function and quality of life for people with MS with moderate to severe spasticity (Erwin et al., 2011). Should a baclofen pump be indicated, the therapist may be involved in assessment prior to pump implantation and reevaluation following implantation.

Cognitive Compensation. Occupational therapy intervention for clients with cognitive problems focuses on compensation for deficits and inefficiencies in order to manage everyday life. Treating fatigue often improves self-reported cognitive performance (Diamond et al., 2008). Caution should be exercised in disclosing cognitive issues to employers, with careful consideration given to each circumstance. Education of clients and families about cognition is often beneficial. Awareness that these problems are due to MS and not personality eases stress and optimizes receptivity to modifications.

Interventions that include group therapy, stress management, personal digital assistants, electronic memory aids, and cognitive-behavioral therapy have been shown to have positive effects on cognitive function in MS (Brown & Kraft, 2005; Gentry, 2008; Johnson et al., 2009). Examples of cognitive techniques, strategies, and modifications include

- scheduling work responsibilities and cognitively demanding tasks to reduce the influence of the cognitive problems; for example, planning to do these in the morning or after breaks
- maintaining a paper, smart phone, or electronic diary as a memory aid and to help identify the timing of cognitive and fatigue problems as well as the environment in which these problems occur
- changing the environment to reduce distractions and interruptions and promote organization
- using problem-solving strategies for decision making rather than emotion-focused strategies
- supporting involvement of social network to assist with problem solving
- using step-by-step written home and/or work directions
- doing one activity at a time and avoiding multitasking
- incorporating assistive technology to improve function in high-order IADL, such as money management and bill payment, family schedules, and transportation options
- increasing time allotted for an activity and reducing the number of activities planned or undertaken
- delegating difficult tasks to others
- using repetition in the learning process
- assessing driving safety and recommending appropriate testing and interventions

Pain Intervention. For pain related to weakness or spasticity, interventions such as posture training, ergonomic seating, stretching, supportive splinting, and focal heat modalities on muscle trigger points may be effective. An ergonomic workstation (such as ergonomic chair with armrests, headsets, and mouse and keyboard trays) tailored to the individual can be beneficial. Exercise and mobility equipment to correct gait problems may also assist to minimize pain.

Tremor and Ataxia Intervention. The hallmarks of occupational therapy intervention for tremor and ataxia are proximal stabilization or support, modified approach to occupations, and adapted equipment and orthoses. Proximal stabilization includes supporting the trunk and larger joints of the upper and lower extremities are. For example, at mealtime, position the client's torso against the table with arms resting on the table (Gillen, 2000). Because the position is sitting, the lower extremities are supported, the trunk is stabilized by leaning against the table, and the shoulders and elbows are supported. A modified approach may be the use of hand-over-hand guidance for writing or dialing a cell phone. If one hand is unaffected by tremor, consider retraining the unaffected hand as tolerated. Orthoses might include a cervical collar to reduce the travel of the head and neck or wrist splints to minimize travel

and number of joints in motion. Weights on the wrist, for example, may also serve to dampen tremor (NMSS, 2012) but may contribute to fatigue. Peripheral cooling of the forearm has been shown to reduce tremor amplitude and frequency and increase functional capacity for up to 30 minutes (Feys et al., 2005). An occupational therapy intervention program, the Step-wise Approach to the Treatment of Intention Tremor (Hawes, Billups, & Forwell, 2010), developed specifically for MS was pilot tested and has shown some promising results.

Employment Modifications. The problems described in the preceding sections may affect the job performance of persons with MS. Modifications to maintain employment, productivity, and satisfaction may include

- changing the times at which tasks are performed
- limiting prolonged walking, standing, and travel by using conference calls, Internet, and apps
- using appropriate gait equipment and powered mobility devices
- changing to an office that is convenient to frequent activities
- modifying work hours
- working completely or partly at home
- arranging a space to rest periodically

Perspective in Intervention

Although referral to occupational therapy services can occur across the MS continuum, often it is those with relatively severe disability that are typically referred for therapy. Unfortunately, by that time, a tremendous window of opportunity has passed for interventions such as improving ambulation skills (and thereby reducing or delaying need for wheeled mobility aids), attending to fatigue and energy management and on-the-job modifications to support continued employment, and advancing self-management skills for living everyday with MS. It is essential that therapists educate physicians and other referral sources about the needs and benefits for early intervention for persons with MS.

It must also be recognized that people with MS, as well as those with other chronic conditions, play an integral role in the self-management of their conditions (Bodenheimer et al., 2002). Individuals with MS understand their needs and unique circumstances and can provide information that is complementary to the health professionals' knowledge. Research shows that those who participate in self-management programs have a higher quality of life and make better use of health professionals' time (Barlow, Turner, & Wright, 2000). There is also evidence that people with MS with poorly developed self-management skills feel less control and more uncertainty, have increased feelings of depression and hopelessness, and experience poor psychological adjustment (Bishop, Frain, & Tschopp, 2008). Self-management decisions for persons with MS involves taking control through planned strategies and routines and balancing the health care providers' expectations and advice against the practicality in their lives (Thorne, Paterson, & Russell 2003). It is for this reason that self-management is an important part of health care and critical for those living with MS everyday.

Parkinson's Disease

PD is a progressive, variable condition. It is most common in later adult years, with the mean age of onset of 55–60 years. The incidence of PD is 1%, or 1,000 per 100,000 persons in people older than 60 years of age (de Lau & Breteler, 2006). PD is gradual at onset, and symptoms may take years to develop (Baker & Graham, 2004). PD is defined by the three cardinal signs of tremor, rigidity, and bradykinesia. Postural instability is often added to this list (Conley & Kirchner, 1999). Tremor, often the first complaint, is a resting tremor that increases with stress and may present as pill-rolling (Gelb, Oliver, & Gilman, 1999). Rigidity tends to occur at more advanced stages of PD (Gelb, Oliver, & Gilman, 1999). Bradykinesia causes a lack of facial expression, or "mask face," and affects walking, involvement in activities, and eye blink (Conley & Kirchner, 1999). Postural instability begins with reduced arm swing, head and trunk leaning forward, and shorter strides that progress to a shuffling gait. Lack of postural reflexes results in falls and akinesia or episodes of motoric "freezing" that impede spontaneous initiation of walking, turning, and crossing thresholds (Hass et al., 2005; Ward & Robertson, 2004).

Other symptoms of PD, particularly in the middle to later stages, include swallowing changes, soft speech, festinating gait, autonomic deficits, constipation, fatigue, sleep disturbances, psychiatric complications (particularly depression and anxiety), and dementia (Shulman et al., 2002; Verbaan et al., 2007). When festinating gait is coupled with motoric "freezing" of gait, 37% report an increased occurrence of falls (Giladi et al., 2001). Swallowing problems can occur at any point in the course of PD and are not related to disease severity. These include difficulties with delayed swallow reflex, and abnormal tongue control that result in residues of food materials being left in the mouth (Plowman-Prine et al., 2009).

Dementia occurs in 15%–20% of persons with PD and tends to be among those who are older at diagnosis, have a history of PD, and experience depression (Aarsland et al., 1996). The cognitive functions most affected are motor planning, abstract reasoning, concentration, organizing, and sequencing (Ward & Robertson, 2004). It has been shown that persons with PD rely on external cues, feedback, and repetition when learning new tasks (Ward & Robertson, 2004).

The cause of PD is thought to stem from both hereditary and environmental factors. Hereditary factors have been linked to a chromosome 4 mutation in 5%–10% of cases, although the contribution of this mutation to PD is uncertain (Conley & Kirchner, 1999). Environmental factors implicated in PD include exposure to well water and pesticides and living on a farm (Marder et al., 1998).

The pathogenesis is related to loss of dopaminergic neurons of the substantia nigra that provide input to the corpus striatum and, in part, modulate the thalamus and its connections to the motor cortex (Ward & Robertson, 2004). Biochemical anomalies in the basal ganglia are also present (Conley & Kirchner, 1999). Medications to compensate for dopamine loss are effective for a limited period followed by "wearing off," particularly in later stages, and may result in difficult "on/off" fluctuations (Varanese et al., 2010). It is essential that occupational therapy intervention account for these fluctuations.

Diagnosing Parkinson's Disease

In autopsy studies, PD has been shown to be misdiagnosed in 25% of cases (Calne, 1995). In part, the difficulty is a result of the challenges associated with developing and subsequent lack of definitive preclinical biological markers (Wu, Le, & Jankovic, 2011). At present, diagnosis is based on clinical evidence using clinical diagnostic criteria specifically related to the cardinal signs of tremor, rigidity, bradykinesia, and postural stability (Jankovic, 2008).

The Course of Parkinson's Disease

PD has been described as having either five stages (Hoehn & Yahr, 1967) or three stages (Bradley, 1996) (Definition 35-3). These stages are broadly described by the presence of symptoms, functional implications, and response to medications.

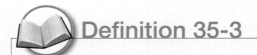

Definition 35-3

Stages of Parkinson's Disease

Stages as Defined by Hoehn and Yahr (1967)

Stage 1: Unilateral symptoms, no or minimal functional implications, usually a resting tremor.

Stage 2: Midline or bilateral symptom involvement, no balance difficulty, mild problems with trunk mobility and postural reflexes.

Stage 3: Postural instability, mild to moderate functional disability.

Stage 4: Postural instability increasing, though able to walk; functional disability increases, interfering with activities of daily living (ADL); decreased manipulation and dexterity.

Stage 5: Confined to wheelchair or bed.

Stages as Defined by Bradley (1996)

Early: Not disabling; monosymptomatic; responds well to medication; may remain at this level for years.

Nonfluctuating: Some disability; levodopa added to medication regimen; 80% of function is restored.

Fluctuating: Function limited; side effects to levodopa; difficult-to-control symptoms, postural instability, and gait disturbance become debilitating.

Potential Emotional, Social, and Economic Consequences

In the initial stages of PD, the degree of physical disability is minimal. The emotional burden and social consequences, however, can be marked. Resting tremor, rarely resulting in motor disability, is a frequent source of psychological distress, with many individuals reporting feeling embarrassed or self-conscious (Uitti, 1998). In later stages, tremor and rigidity were highly correlated with distress and reduced quality of life (Peto, Jenkinson, & Fitzpatrick, 1995). Other predictors of poor quality of life are depression, cognitive decline, social isolation, sleep disorders, mobility issues, fatigue, confusion, urinary incontinence, unpredictable on/off fluctuations, pain, and increasing dependence (Rahman et al., 2008). Major depression was found in 45% of those with PD, suggesting that early identification and intervention are crucial (Karlson et al., 1999).

The social consequences of PD are striking. In early stages, for example, handwriting may be shaky and micrographic, reducing legibility (Gillen, 2000). In intermediate and later stages, the voice softens and becomes monotone. Reduced facial expression and minimal hand gesturing contribute to reduced communication and negative messaging (Tickle-Degnen, 2006). The person with PD may have waning interest in social and previously enjoyed leisure activities. PD challenges relationships and roles in families. Both the individual and family members, typically a spouse or adult child, may have feelings of guilt, despair, and anger as caregiving increases (Baker & Graham, 2004).

Economic implications of PD are frequently related to medications, wheeled mobility, accessibility modifications, self-care and safety equipment, and in-home support. If employed, increasing limitations may require employment modifications, early retirement, and application for disability benefits that are usually accompanied by loss of income (Schrag & Banks, 2006). People with PD stop working 5–6 years earlier than the normal population (Dick et al., 2007). The caregiver is likely elderly and may require assistance and respite, which has further financial implications, and if required, long-term care placement is costly.

Occupational Therapy Evaluation

In the early stages of PD, occupational therapy is rarely indicated unless there are functional limitations or psychological issues. At this stage, it is recommended that interests and roles be maintained within and outside of the home, including employment, social activities, and driving (Baker & Graham, 2004). Occupational therapy is most often required in the intermediate and later stages of the disease (Hoehn & Yahr, 1967; stages 3–5). Evaluation should include a brief history and, in the intermediate stages, should identify occupational performance problems related to reduced mobility, safety issues, swallowing, fine-motor incoordination, slowed movements, cogwheel

rigidity, and depressed affect. A standardized quality of life measure, the Parkinson Disease Questionnaire–39, may be a useful screening tool. Its 39 items are clustered into eight domains relevant to occupational therapy: mobility, ADL, emotional well-being, stigma, social support, cognition, communication, and bodily discomfort (Peto, Jenkinson, & Fitzpatrick, 1995). The therapist should also note occupations that have been eliminated (Gillen, 2000). Examples of impairments and limitations in activities that may be included in evaluation are

- fine-motor activities at home, at work, and in the community (writing, eating, shaving, and fastening)
- safe mobility, such as walking, stair climbing, driving, and moving from sit to stand
- fatigue that affects most activities
- work evaluation at early stages of PD to reduce the risk of unemployment or early retirement
- bradykinesia, postural instability, and rigidity that limit participation in self-care, household tasks, and grocery shopping, etc.
- swallowing or other mealtime problems that prolong eating and reduce intake
- cognitive problems that affect activities associated with usual roles
- sexual activity limitations related to bradykinesia, fatigue, depression, and psychosocial issues
- sleep disturbances
- voice changes

Occupational Therapy Intervention Process

When setting goals with the client with PD and significant others, the therapist must balance activity energy demands with motivation and frustration as well as caregiver time in the context of the dependence-interdependence-independence continuum (Gillen, 2000). Participation of others in this process is crucial to the viability of interventions, which vary based on priorities and resources, stage of the disease, and occupational difficulties identified through the evaluation. Many of the interventions described in Procedures for Practice 35-1 may be incorporated at home and in other relevant environments. Numerous studies report an overall effectiveness of both occupational therapy and other rehabilitation interventions for PD (Dixon et al., 2007; Rao, 2010). A meta-analysis showed that 10 of the 15 studies reviewed demonstrated a positive effect for occupational therapy intervention and showed that 63% of those with PD who received therapy improved as compared to 37% who did not receive therapy (Murphy & Tickle-Degnen, 2001). A recent randomized control trial showed the efficacy of a self-management rehabilitation program for persons with PD (Tickle-Degnen et al., 2010). Other studies have tested the Lee Silverman Voice Treatment (LSVT) and Rehab-SelfCue-Speech programs.

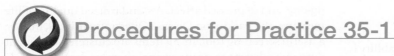

Procedures for Practice 35-1

Occupational Therapy for Parkinson's Disease

Interventions Related to Decreasing Isolation and Communication Problems

- Educate about timing activities to synchronize with maximum medication effectiveness.
- Modify leisure activities to encourage participation and decrease isolation.
- Provide information on support and advocacy groups.
- Educate caregivers about modifying communication and activities to support engagement
- Participate in programs such the LSVT and LSVT®BIG.
- Implement writing modifications, including using an enlarged felt-tip pen and writing when rested.
- Use communication aids, including smart devices such as electronic tablets (mobile phone may be too small), large-key telephones, and electronic aids to daily living (EADL)
- Provide home exercise program to maintain facial movement and expression for socializing.

Interventions Related to Safety

- Instruct in sit-to-stand and bed mobility using the Rehab SelfCue-Speech program.
- Instruct to manage motoric "freezing" while walking, includes avoiding crowds, narrow spaces, and room corners; reducing distractions and not carrying items while walking; reducing clutter in pathway; focusing when changing directions; using a rhythmic beat or counting to maintain momentum.
- Recommend equipment to increase independence such as a raised toilet seat and grab bars.
- Prescribe walking aids (walker for festinating gait).

- Recommend, if required, a wheelchair having a proper seating system, cushion, and adjusted foot/leg rests and armrests that is appropriate for transporting within the community.
- Recommend good, uniform lighting, particularly in narrow spaces and at doorways.
- Provide home exercises to maintain mobility, coordination, posture, and tolerance.
- Perform home assessment and recommend modifications that might include alterations to the bathroom (e.g., nonskid surfaces, bath bench/chair) and flooring (e.g., eliminating throw rugs), horizontal strips on the floor where "freezing" episodes occur, and reducing furniture congestion (Gillen, 2000).

Interventions to Maintain Independence and Participation

- Modify eating routine to include small portions, reduced distractions, schedule frequent meals that allow adequate time, and provide adapted equipment such as nonslip surfaces for plates and built-up handles.
- Recommend use of adult absorbent underwear to reduce embarrassment should a bathroom be difficult to access.
- Recommend that sexual activity be engaged in following rest and urination and when medications are most effective.
- Instruct on energy effectiveness strategies in home, leisure, and work activities.
- Reduce or eliminate the need for fine-motor control, such as clothing with minimal or no fasteners.
- Reduce the impact of perceptual problems by using visual cues and rhythmic music in a nondistracting environment; speak slowly using simple instruction.
- Perform a home assessment.

The LSVT is a 4-day-per-week, 4-week program designed to teach and habituate compensatory speech and voice strategies to facilitate a louder, clearer speech that is often run by occupational and/or physical therapists. The LSVT program is beneficial for motivated PD patients to improve vocal loudness, swallowing, speech, gestures used for communication, and facial expression (Sapir et al., 2007). A revision of the Lee Silverman program, known as LSVT®BIG, is used to promote high-amplitude movements in PD patients (Ebersbach et al., 2010). During this program, the participants are encouraged to think BIG. The quick, dramatic, explosive movements are aimed at mitigating the effects of bradykinesia.

The RehabSelfCue-Speech program was designed for people with PD who are in the mild to moderate stages (stage 3 on the Hoehn and Yahr scale) (Maitra, 2009; Maitra & Dasgupta, 2005). It is based on motor control principles and sensory feedback to target bradykinesia and uses self-cueing to initiate movement-related actions. In order to

practice of RehabSelfCue-Speech, the therapist helps the client choose tasks to perform and then selects action words to read aloud during the activity to facilitate the performance. The client practices using these cues during several sessions, with the goal of transferring these techniques to home activities. Here is an example: to get up from a chair, the action words can be SWAY, then RISE. These words are then used each time the client would like to stand up from a chair or from other surfaces. Evidence Table 35-2 presents the best evidence for occupational therapy intervention for PD.

Amyotrophic Lateral Sclerosis

ALS, popularly known as Lou Gehrig's disease, is a late-onset most often fatal neurodegenerative disease of upper motor neurons (UMN) and lower motor neurons (LMN). The incidence of ALS is 2 per 100,000 people, and it occurs more often in men (Amyotrophic Lateral Sclerosis

Evidence Table 35-2	Best Evidence for Occupational Therapy Practice Regarding Intervention Related to Parkinson's Disease					
Intervention	Description of Intervention Tested	Participants	Dosage	Type of Best Evidence and Level of Evidence	Benefit	Statistical Probability and Effect Size of Outcome	Reference
Interdisciplinary self-management rehabilitation program for persons with Parkinson's disease (PD)	Eighteen hours of group sessions include exercises for flexibility, strength, and speech; activities of daily living (ADL) and gait training and discussion about cognitive strategies, communication, stress management, and fall prevention.	One hundred nineteen persons with PD: 30 women, 90 men; mean age = 66 years	Participants were randomly assigned to one of these three groups: 1. No hours of rehab 2. Eighteen hours of clinic group rehab with 9 hours of social sessions 3. Twenty-seven hours of rehab (18 in group and 9 in-home or community individual sessions for skill transfer)	Randomized control trial. Level of evidence: IB2a	The two groups receiving rehab improved in health-related quality of life (HRQOL) as measured by the Parkinson's Disease Questionnaire-39 (PDQ-39) with relevant gains in communication and mobility. There was no difference between intervention groups for HRQOL.	Using repeated measures analysis of covariance (ANCOVA) the intervention effect post treatment and at follow-up was $F = 3.98$, $p = .02$, moderate effect size ($\eta = .26$). A significant response ($p = .03$) was shown for the HRQOL domains of communication (2-month follow-up) and mobility (6-month follow-up).	Tickle-Degnen et al. (2010)
LSVT®BIG, which is derived from the Lee Silverman Voice Treatment	The program focuses on intensive exercising of high-amplitude movements.	Fifty-eight people with PD at Hoehn & Yahr stages I–III; 36 women, 22 men	Participants were randomly assigned to one of three groups: 1. One-to-one training in (LSVT®BIG) 2. Group training of Nordic Walking (WALK) 3. Nonsupervised exercises (HOME)	Randomized control trial. Level: IC2b	Improvement to: 1. Unified Parkinson's Disease Rating Scale (UPDRS) motor score 2. Timed up-and-go (TUG) score 3. Timed 10-meter walk No differences for quality of life between groups.	Using analysis of covariance (ANCOVA) between group comparison, the LSVT®BIG program showed significant improvement on UPDRS ($F = 11.9$, $p = .001$) and TUG ($F = 3.64$, $p = .033$) while 10-meter walk ($F = 2.97$, $p = .059$) approached significant benefit.	Ebersbach et al. (2010)
Inpatient rehabilitation program for persons with PD	Rehabilitation included movement strategies and exercise offered by physical therapists and occupational therapists.	Twenty-eight persons with PD; mean age = 68 years hospitalized and at Hoehn & Yahr stage II or III, able to walk 10 meters, three times without assistance	A maximum of 16 sessions of up to 45 minutes per session over a 2-week inpatient period; number of sessions ranged from 5 to 16. Participants were randomized to the strategy group or the exercise group.	Randomized control trial. Level: IC1a	The movement-strategy group showed improvements on the UPDRS, 10-meter walk, 2-minute walk, balance, and quality of life as compared to the exercise group.	Significant improvement in QOL at discharge ($t = 3.65$, $p = .003$) and 3-month follow-up ($t = 3.65$, $p = .003$) and for the 2-minute walk at discharge ($t = -5.54$, $p = .000$) and follow-up ($t = 5.27$, $p = .000$). The UPDRS ($t = 3.16$, $p = .008$), the 10-meter walk ($t = 3.66$, $p = .003$) and balance ($t = 3.74$, $p = .002$) improved at discharge though not retained at 3 months.	Morris, Iansek, & Kirkwood (2009)

Association [ALSA], 2012). There is no test other than a clinical examination, so a selection of diagnostic tests is used in a careful, multistep system of exclusion of other diagnoses (ALSA, 2012). The cause remains unknown, and initial symptoms vary widely.

The average age at onset is 58 years, although adults as young as 20 have been diagnosed. Age at onset and the pattern of symptom development is useful for determining an individual's prognosis, with a younger onset of UMN origin having a somewhat better prognosis. It has also been shown that baseline scores on the Short Form-36 (SF-36) are significant predictors of health status over time (Norquist et al., 2003). Generally, the prognosis for individual patients is best left to neurologists with expertise in ALS.

In ALS, early manifestations indicating UMN or LMN disease vary with the site of the initial disease onset. UMN damage results in general weakness, spasticity, and hyperreflexia. LMN involvement results in weakness or muscle atrophy of the extremities, cervical extensor weakness, fasciculations, muscle cramps, and loss of reflexes. Early bulbar involvement affecting speech, swallowing, and breathing and/or advanced age at time of diagnosis tend to indicate a more progressive course of the disease (Mitsumoto, Chad, & Pioro, 1998). Speech impairment is common as the disease progresses (Ball, Beukelman, & Pattee, 2004), as are UMN and LMN symptoms. Cognition is rarely affected, and vision, bowel and bladder control, and sensation are spared.

No known cure or effective pharmacological treatment is available for ALS, although riluzole (Rilutek), an antiglutamate agent, shown to alter the course of the disease, is the only FDA–approved medication for the treatment of ALS. There are several other medications being investigated, as well as research in the use of stem cell therapy, offer hope to those with ALS (ALSA, 2012). Medications can also assist in the management of symptoms such as spasticity, anxiety, insomnia, and excessive saliva but do not affect the progression of the disease. Assisted ventilation, tracheotomies, and gastrostomies ease problems with eating and breathing (Mitsumoto, Chad, & Pioro, 1998). Because of the disease progression, numerous symptoms, and potential interventions, a multidisciplinary team improves the quality of life for those with ALS (Van den Berg et al., 2005).

The Course of Amyotrophic Lateral Sclerosis

Six stages of ALS are recognized and described according to clinical features (Table 35-1). The median duration of life after diagnosis ranges from 23 to 52 months, although a significant proportion survive 5 years or more (ALSA, 2012; Mitsumoto, Chad, & Pioro, 1998). Weakness of the arm, leg, or involvement of the bulbar area is a common initial symptom (Mitsumoto, Chad, & Pioro, 1998). Atrophy may begin in the hands, with wasting of the thenar and hypothenar eminences, as well as in the shoulder muscles. Finger extension is usually affected earlier than grip strength because of dorsal and palmar interossei wasting. Falling and problems with walking and bed mobility are common due to of lower extremity weakness.

Table 35-1 **Rehabilitation of Patients with Amyotrophic Lateral Sclerosis at Various Stages**

Stage	Clinical Features	Activities to Maintain Motor Function	Equipment
I	Ambulatory, no problems with ADL, mild weakness	Normal activities, moderate exercise in unaffected muscles, active ROM, and strength exercise	None
II	Ambulatory, moderate weakness in certain muscles, increased fatigue	Modification in living; modest exercise; active, assisted ROM exercise	Assistive devices, use of hands-free devices, electronic tablet
III	Ambulatory, severe weakness in certain muscles, increased difficulty with ADL; marked fatigue	Adaptations to continue active life; active, assisted, passive ROM exercise; joint pain management	Smart technology, adaptive devices, home equipment and environmental controls
IV	Wheelchair confined, almost independent, severe weakness in legs	Passive ROM exercise, modest strength exercise in uninvolved muscles	Smart technology, adaptive devices, home equipment, environmental controls, wheelchair
V	Wheelchair confined, dependent, marked leg and arm weakness	Passive ROM exercise, pain management, decubitus ulcer prevention	Smart technology, adaptive devices, home equipment, environmental controls, wheelchair
VI	Bedridden, unable to perform ADL, maximal assistance required	Passive ROM exercise, pain management, prevention of decubitus ulcers and venous thrombosis	Smart technology, adaptive devices and home equipment to assist caregiver(s), environmental controls, wheelchair

ADL, activities of daily living; ROM, range of motion.
From Mitsumoto, H., Chad, D., & Pioro, E. (1998). *Amyotrophic lateral sclerosis. Contemporary neurology series.* Philadelphia: Davis; Sinaki, M. (1980). Rehabilitation. In D. W. Mulder (Ed.), *The diagnosis and treatment of amyotrophic lateral sclerosis* (pp. 169–193). Boston: Houghton Mifflin.

Three forms of ALS have been described including sporadic, familial, and Guamanian (ALSA, 2012). The most common, sporadic, occurs in 90%–95% of those with ALS, whereas familial presents 5%–10% of the time and appears to have a genetic link occurring more than once in a family (ALSA, 2012). When a high ALS incidence appeared in Guam in the 1950s, the third form emerged.

Potential Emotional, Social, and Economic Consequences

ALS is a devastating disease for individuals and their families. Its relatively fast progression, coupled with early loss of upper extremity function and possibly speech and swallowing, means that the disease quickly affects ability to perform ADL and IADL and maintain employment and quality of life. It has been shown that those with ALS, as compared to normal controls, have more depression, external locus of control, and feelings of hopelessness (McDonald et al., 1994) and that this is not related to physical function or sociodemographic factors (Plahuta et al., 2002).

People with ALS and their families have little time to make psychological adjustment to the diagnosis and its implications before having to deal with their loved one's increasing disability. The acceptance of the ALS diagnosis by family members may affect willingness to be involved in planning, incorporating changes necessary to maximize the independence of the person with ALS, and making informed choices for intervention (Ball, Beukelman, & Pattee, 2004).

People frequently withdraw from work soon after diagnosis and may have to confront economic problems and health insurance issues. Because the age group most commonly affected is employed and actively involved in family and community activities, the abrupt change is devastating.

Occupational Therapy Evaluation

Assessments for clients with ALS should be based on clearly defined levels of function (see Table 35-1) and the individual's needs and priorities. Early interventions should target the individual's symptoms as they affect their occupations. As ALS progresses, interventions focus on individual function, as well as physical and social environment. This is supported by Neudert, Wasner, and Borasio (2004), who showed that the quality of life of a person with ALS with a supportive family and social network remains stable over time despite reduced health status.

To assist with the evaluation process, the ALS Functional Rating Scale (Mitsumoto, Chad, & Pioro, 1998) can be used. To determine ongoing functional ability, ADL and IADL assessments should be included in all evaluations. Functional limitations may be due to reduced upper extremity ability, and thus the Purdue Pegboard, 9-hole peg test or other timed upper extremity function tests and standard ROM and MMT are useful. Fatigue is shown to affect physical quality of life (Lou et al., 2003)

and can be assessed with the Multidimensional Fatigue Inventory or other screening measures described earlier in this chapter. As communication and swallowing decline (Higo, Tayama, & Nito, 2004), assessment and intervention is required to ensure that nutritional needs and social participation are maintained. Because of disease progression, reevaluation at each visit is required.

Occupational Therapy Intervention Process

The progressive nature of ALS necessitates that rehabilitation be compensatory, focusing on adapting to disability and preventing secondary complications. Goals center on keeping the person active and independent for as long as possible. Examples of occupational therapy goals in the early stages include

- optimizing strength and ROM using home exercise programs (Drory et al., 2001)
- maintaining function in ADL and IADL through use of assistive or adaptive devices
- decreasing fatigue in the neck and extremities through use of splints and orthotics
- managing pain and energy using joint protection and work simplification techniques

As function declines, mobility and self-care become increasingly difficult. Home evaluations and in-home therapy are important, and intervention focuses on enabling the caregiver to assist the client safely and effectively. The therapist helps the caregiver–client team to

- optimize safety and positioning, perform safe transfers, and maintain skin integrity
- enable communication using augmentative communication equipment (Ball, Beukelman, & Pattee, 2004)
- assess and manage dysphagia (Higo, Tayama, & Nito, 2004)
- optimize social participation
- identify and obtain equipment, such as a hospital bed, to allow continued mobility and comfort
- modify the environmental to enhance participation, safety and comfort

Throughout the stages of the disease, the occupational therapist must be sensitive to the client, family, and caregiver as physical demands, financial concerns, and transformation of the home into a hospital-like setting produce enormous stress and strain (Mitsumoto, Chad, & Pioro, 1998). Open discussions and close collaboration with clients, caregivers, and the ALS team help to address the client's changing needs.

Intervention Implementation. When treating clients with ALS, therapists must be aware of the client's level of gadget tolerance, financial resources, and social and cultural context. The special considerations for exercise, equipment, assistive technology, and dysphasia management for persons with ALS are reviewed below.

Exercise. Active and passive ROM, strengthening, endurance, stretching, and home breathing programs are appropriate at various stages of the disease and are effective for minimizing secondary complications (Mitsumoto, Chad, & Pioro, 1998). Attention to overexertion, potential secondary problems, muscle spasms, and careful monitoring of fatigue are important to a successful exercise program. A client may initially be able to perform an independent home stretching program, but as the disease progresses and the program becomes too fatiguing or difficult, the caregiver may become involved.

Equipment and Assistive Technology. The therapist will provide information and assist with accessing assistive technology and adaptive equipment that may help the client achieve optimal level of independence at the various stages of ALS (see Table 35-1). Assistive equipment such as a neck collar or universal cuff may be helpful. Because independent walking becomes difficult in a rapidly progressing disease such as ALS, ordering the wheelchair may need to be expedited. Mobility equipment, depending on level of function, may include a foot-drop splint, cane, and/or walker. A study showed that 57% of those with moderate disability used a mobility device in addition to a wheelchair (Trail et al., 2001). Together, a home assessment and client-caregiver consultation inform wheelchair selection. For specific features and details related to wheelchair selection refer to Chapter 17.

Mainstream technology and environmental controls are extremely useful as the disease progresses. This technology, for example, includes lighting and call alert systems, motion sensors, door (un)locking systems, and remote control for TV and radio. Use of smart devices with audio options (something that can be adjusted if the voice is weak) to replace the need for touch typing is helpful to conserve energy and to maintain communication. (see Chapter 18.)

Dysphasia. Swallowing difficulties may be present at any stage of ALS, particularly when bulbar involvement is apparent. Interventions may include, but are not limited to, reducing distractions during mealtime (limit conversation and other activities), altering food consistency (i.e., thicken liquids), teaching manual techniques to swallow, and ensuring adequate time for meals. Early introduction of an alternate route of nutrition may be indicated if nutrition and maintaining weight become issues.

Guillain-Barré Syndrome

GBS or acute inflammatory demyelinating polyneuropathy results in axonal demyelination of peripheral nerves (Meythaler, DeVivo, & Braswell, 1997). Characteristics include a quickly progressing, symmetrical ascending paralysis starting with the feet; pain in the legs; absence of deep tendon reflexes; mild sensory loss in glove-and-stocking distributions; cranial nerve dysfunction with possible facial palsy and swallowing problems; an autonomic nervous system response of postural hypertension and tachycardia; respiratory muscle paralysis; and pain, fatigue, and urinary dysfunction (Gregory, Gregory, & Podd, 2005). Cognition, however, remains intact (Guillian-Barré Syndrome–Chronic Inflammatory Demyelinating Polyneuropathy Foundation International [GBS-CIDP], 2012). Symptoms vary from so mild that medical attention is unlikely to severe disease that may cause death in 1%–10% of cases (Khan, 2004).

The cause of GBS is unclear. Its distribution is worldwide, with an incidence of 1.3–2 per 100,000 (GBS-CIDP, 2012). GBS is 1.5 times more common in men and occurs in adults 20–24 years and 70–74 years (van Doorn, Ruts, & Jacob, 2008). No hereditary susceptibility or vaccinations cause GBS (Hughes & Rees, 1997). Enteritis, however, precedes GBS in 41% of cases, as may respiratory infections and HIV or AIDS (Carroll, McDonnell, & Barnes, 2003; Jiang et al., 1997).

Diagnosing GBS

Diagnosis of GBS entails a history of symptoms and a physical and neurological examination that includes nerve conduction tests and cerebral spinal fluid analysis (GBS-CIDP, 2012). The medical interventions for GBS attempt to lessen the severity but do not cure the disease such that upon initial diagnosis, patients are admitted to hospital to monitor breathing and other functions until the GBS has stabilized (GBS-CIDP, 2012). Treatments include intravenous immunoglobulin, plasma exchange (otherwise known as plasmapheresis), and steroids (van Doorn, Ruts, & Jacob, 2008).

The Course of Guillain-Barré Syndrome

GBS has three phases. In more than 95% of people with GBS, the onset, or acute inflammatory phase, manifests as weakness in at least two limbs that progresses and reaches its maximum in 2–4 weeks accompanied by increasing symptoms (van Doorn, Ruts, & Jacob, 2008). Mechanical ventilation is required for 20%–30% of individuals (Dematteis, 1996). This is followed by the plateau phase of no significant change, which lasts for a few days or weeks, when the greatest disability is present. The third phase is progressive recovery, when remyelination and axonal regeneration occur and may last for up to 2 years, although the average length is 12 weeks (van Doorn, Ruts, & Jacob, 2008). Recovery starts at the head and neck and proceeds distally (Karavatas, 2005) and extent varies; approximately 50% of patients have complete return of function, and another 35% experience some residual weakness that may not resolve. The remaining 15% experience more significant permanent disability (Khan et al., 2010). Fatigue is the most common residual problem for 93% of patients (Parry, 2000). Subtle cognitive deficits in executive functions, short-term memory, and decision making may occur (Gregory, Gregory, & Podd, 2005).

Potential Emotional, Social, and Economic Consequences

Emotional and psychological reactions are a response to the rapid onset of symptoms and the degree of disability. Shock, despair, fear, and anger may be consuming (Dematteis, 1996). As recovery progresses and improvement is slow, adjustment, impatience, and frustration associated with disability persist (GBS-CIDP, 2012). At follow-up, GBS was reported to impact confidence and ability to live independently, with 18% having depression and 22% having anxiety (Khan et al., 2010).

For young adults, the impact of GBS can have educational, employment, and economic implications. This age group is launching careers and may have only small savings. For those who develop GBS in later years, the economic effect may be less. For those returning to work after GBS, there may be a renewed value for work, a need to cope with losing and recovering a work identity, and dilemmas about work adaptations that require coping strategies. Lack of public awareness of GBS may be a barrier for returning to work (Royal, Reynolds, & Houlden, 2009).

Occupational Therapy Evaluation

Referral to occupational therapy is common when the course of GBS is moderate to severe. Approximately 40% of all GBS patients require rehabilitation services (Meythaler, DeVivo, & Braswell, 1997). Assessment at the onset of the plateau phase typically occurs in the intensive care unit, when the individual is undergoing extensive medical procedures and pain can be significant. Therapists should complete an interview to understand the client's feelings and fears (GBS-CIDP, 2012) and evaluate communication, control of the environment, comfort, and level of anxiety. A sensory assessment is essential because marked sensitivity is typical of acute GBS; the guiding principle is to ask prior to touching the client (GBS-CIDP, 2012). Therapists should also be aware of the 7-point GBS disability scale that primarily assesses ambulation and the need for a ventilator (Hughes et al., 1978).

During the recovery phase, therapists evaluate self-care, communication, leisure, as well as mobility, sensation, strength, ROM and, as appropriate, reintegration into the workplace. Patients with GBS should not be pushed to fatigue, because recovery will be prolonged and fatigue may slow the rehabilitation process (GBS-CIDP, 2012). During this phase, occupational therapy services can be provided in an inpatient rehabilitation facility, through an outpatient program, and/or at home or work (Karavatas, 2005).

Occupational Therapy Intervention Process

Because the natural course of GBS is improvement, patients and caregivers tend to be optimistic about recovery.

The long-term goal is full recovery, so that the individual performs at the same level as prior to the onset of GBS with or without modification. Goals should focus on achieving optimal function at each level of recovery within tolerated pain levels (GBS-CIDP, 2012).

During the acute phase, the patient may be actively involved in directing care rather than physically involved, providing the opportunity for educating the patient and others about maintaining comfort in bed, protecting against bed sores, and future therapy (GBS-CIDP, 2012). Modifications during the acute and plateau phase should be considered temporary and may include

- communication tools, such as sign or picture board or voice-activated devices, if appropriate
- access to the nurse call button, TV, and lights by remote control, as appropriate
- use of hands-free telephone
- modification of lying and sitting positions for optimal function and comfort
- positioning trunk, head, and upper extremities for stability and comfort
- introducing strategies to reduce anxiety

Recovery-phase interventions are initially completed with few repetitions, punctuated with rest. The number and complexity of tasks should be increased gradually (GBS-CIDP, 2012). Examples of interventions include

- providing activities and dynamic splints to maintain ROM, particularly of wrists, fingers, and ankle (hinged drop-foot orthosis)
- instructing both caregiver and client in safe mobility and independent transfers
- providing a sensory stimulation or desensitization program, as appropriate
- training in modified self-care techniques and adapting other daily activities
- using smart devices to facilitate communication and conserve energy
- modifying and encouraging reengagement in routine activities, as appropriate
- adapting equipment for in home, leisure, and work activities
- instructing in energy conservation and fatigue management strategies
- modifying employment roles, tasks, and environment, as indicated
- recommending a fine-motor program to enhance strength, coordination, and sensation
- completing a home assessment and modifications, as appropriate, to facilitate return to home

The GBS-CIDP Foundation International provides guidelines for occupational and physical therapy assessment and treatment of GBS (Resources 35-1) and is an excellent resource about the services available.

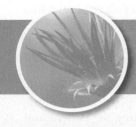

case example

Mrs. K: Continuing to Work with Multiple Sclerosis

Occupational Therapy Process	Clinical Reasoning Process	
	Objectives	Examples of Therapist's Internal Dialogue
Patient Information	Understand the patient's diagnosis and context of services	"This is not a new diagnosis for Ms. K., although it is her first interaction with OT because she may not have needed services in the past."
Ms. K., a 37-year-old woman diagnosed with relapsing-remitting multiple sclerosis (MS) 2 years prior to her first visit to occupational therapy (OT), had recently submitted her resignation to her employer of 15 years. Upset by having to quit her administrative job, she reported the following problems: (1) severe fatigue, which had increased in the past year and resulted in her inability to do her household tasks, perform her activities of daily living (ADL), and work without becoming exhausted; (2) increased lower extremity weakness, with decreased ability to perform tasks requiring prolonged walking or standing; (3) a feeling of heaviness and stiffness in upper and lower extremities; (4) decreased manual dexterity; (5) frequent falling; (6) daily headaches; (7) dizziness; (8) bladder problems; (9) vision problems; (10) disturbed sleep; and (11) attention and memory problems. Her adaptive equipment at the time of her initial therapy visit included a manual wheelchair and a quad cane. She had quit driving. Her husband was very supportive and had recently stopped adoption proceedings because of her MS. She was taking bladder medication and a disease-modifying therapy (DMT).	Know the person	"I will want to get to know how long Ms. K. has experienced her current problems and how she has tried to address them before her resignation from work. It appears that she has made some rather significant decisions about her future. In my experience, some patients respond to the relapse of MS symptoms by fearing the worst, not really understanding MS and all the potential treatment options. Getting a sense of 'where she is at' will be my priority."
Reason for Referral to Occupational Therapy	Appreciate the context	"Ms. K. is not working and is having difficulty at home. Because her husband is supportive, he will likely help to make any changes I suggest in therapy. She is probably using inadequate fatigue management strategies."
Referral was broad, indicating a need to improve overall function due to fatigue. Upon specific discussion with the health care team and Ms. K and her husband, the objective of the occupational therapy referral was to improve function at home and to re-evaluate employment and transportation options.	Develop provisional hypotheses	
Assessment Process and Results	Consider evaluation approach and methods	"I think I will start with an interview using the COPM to get to know Ms. K., her past coping strategies, and her primary concerns. Depending on that information and what I already know from the client information, I will use some specific assessments such as the Modified Fatigue Impact Scale, Modified Ashworth Scale, and the Functional Independence Measure (FIM™)."
The OT evaluation revealed the following: decreased strength in the lower extremities and her dominant upper extremity; increased tone in the lower extremities; decreased sensation and manual dexterity in the dominant upper extremity; severe dizziness with head movement; head, neck, and shoulder trigger points; and marked fatigue. Ms. K., determined not to give in to the disease, had made no adaptations to reduce energy expenditure in daily activities. She was scheduled to have a neuropsychological assessment to identify her current cognitive function and problem areas. Her equipment was self-selected and inappropriate for her problems. She was not taking medications to manage spasticity or fatigue. Her seating at home and work was not supportive. Ms. K. purposefully climbs the stairs in the morning and had a desk distant from the bathroom to get exercise, as she had no exercise program.	Interpret observations	"I'm thinking that fatigue underlies most of her occupational performance problems and that weakness and spasticity are adding to this. It also seems that her current equipment and environmental setup are not helping her. I am also very concerned about what (I think) is a premature resignation from her work and withdrawal from driving."
Occupational Therapy Problem List	Synthesize results	"Her occupational performance problems are due to inadequate information and modifications related to fatigue, inappropriate equipment, poor ergonomic layout, and lack of exercise routine."
The problems encountered by the patient include 1. use of inappropriate equipment 2. minimal use of fatigue management strategies 3. resigned from work without knowledge of options 4. is not involved in a home exercise program 5. has stopped driving without investigating options		

Occupational Therapy Goal List

In collaboration with Ms. K., the goals established were to

- obtain appropriate power mobility equipment
- incorporate at least six energy-saving strategies in her day
- withdraw resignation notice from employer
- make changes in work area by obtaining a headset and ergonomic chair and move her desk closer to the bathroom
- submit a request to her employer for automatic door openers on bathroom
- apply to vocational rehabilitation and work with therapist and vendor to install hand controls for driving
- educate Ms. K. in head, neck, and shoulder exercises

Develop intervention hypotheses	"I will sequence the intervention by focusing on what is most important to Ms. K. I hypothesize that education on energy effectiveness strategies will improve success in performing daily tasks and that assessment and alteration of the work environment and appropriate equipment will facilitate return to work. I will advocate the use of hand controls to return Ms. K. to driving."
Select an intervention approach	"I think the compensatory and educational approach will be most useful."
Consider what will occur in therapy, how often, and for how long	"I recommend one outpatient treatment session per week for 6 weeks. We will work with the physical therapist, who will attend to pain, gait, and exercise interventions."

Intervention

The occupational therapy intervention included (1) instruction in and adoption of energy-conservation techniques at home, at work, and in community (Hugos et al., 2010; Mathiowetz et al., 2005); (2) identifying and obtaining powered mobility equipment; (3) decreasing headaches with head, neck, and shoulder stretching; (4) identifying and obtaining equipment to decrease energy consumption and impact of cognitive issues at home and work (Mathiowetz et al., 2005; PVA, 1998); (5) obtaining ergonomic seating and workstation to decrease pain and energy consumption; (6) facilitating the use of hand controls to drive; (7) continuing full- or part-time employment; and (8) instruction in vestibular and strengthening home exercise program.

Assess the patient's comprehension	"Ms. K. was motivated to participate in therapy because of the potential to return to work. From my experience, I realize the success of therapy depends on her ability (and husband's) to incorporate techniques, access and use equipment, and implement ergonomic changes into her life."
Understand what she is doing	"When discussing fatigue, Ms. K. realized she was fighting the fatigue rather than managing it. At first, it was tough to incorporate suggestions like taking rests, but Ms. K. began to reduce long walks in favor of a short home exercise program."
Know the person	"Although she did not want a lot of equipment, Ms. K. was interested in getting appropriate items if it meant she could continue to do her usual activities."
Appreciate the context	"Because both her husband and employer were supportive, modifications at home and work could be accommodated."

Next Steps

Following the therapy evaluation, Ms. K. withdrew her job resignation and began making modifications in her work. She was also planning to resume driving with the appropriate hand control modifications.

Anticipate present and future concerns	"I will follow-up with Ms. K. when she has returned to work to assist with concerns related to the ergonomic changes and to help problem solve difficult job situations. It is important that she has a positive return-to-work experience without reservations."
Decide whether the patient should continue therapy and/or return in the future	"I will then follow up at the annual visit or earlier if changes in her function occur."

 Clinical Reasoning in Occupational Therapy Practice

One-Month Follow-Up: Successes and Continuing Issues

Ms. K. has met her goals for energy conservation and feels more confident that she can manage her fatigue. She was also able to withdraw her job resignation. However, she developed right foot drop, which affected her balance when fatigued. What kinds of work and mobility adaptations might the occupational therapist recommend to optimize her energy and functioning?

Summary Review Questions

1. What are the various courses of MS?
2. What symptoms of MS may require occupational therapy intervention?
3. What are the primary modifications that a therapist might recommend for a woman with severe MS fatigue who is working full time and has two young children?
4. How can an occupational therapist help a person with neurodegenerative disease stay employed?
5. What environmental modifications may be necessary in PD?
6. List the primary modifications you might recommend during a home safety visit for a person with a neurodegenerative disease.
7. Why is it important to include the significant others when developing interventions?
8. Plan an outpatient therapy session to treat a person with PD who has akinesia, bradykinesia, and rigidity and who is falling regularly.

Glossary

Akinesia—Impaired ability to initiate voluntary and spontaneous motor responses, such as the interruption of performance in movement when attention is distracted (e.g., freezing in Parkinson's disease).

Axonal transection—Separation of an axon from its postsynaptic neuron, permanently interrupting action potential propagation.

Bradykinesia—Slowness or poverty of body movement.

Cogwheel rigidity—Series of catches in the resistance during passive motion.

Demyelination—Myelin that covers nerve fibers is lost or damaged, resulting in an absence or impairment of nerve conduction typically manifesting in disability and limitations to function.

Fasciculations—Rapid, flickering twitching movements of a part of a muscle occurring irregularly in time and location.

Festinating gait—Marked by very small rapid steps which occurs in persons with Parkinson's disease when the posture of the head and trunk involuntarily lean forward ahead of the feet, moving the center of gravity (COG) forward. Rather than taking a large step to correct the imbalance, one takes several hurried small steps, increasing gait velocity, which results in running or "chasing" one's COG, which remains in front of the feet.

Intention tremor—A tremor that occurs during visually guided, goal-directed movement that is worse (meaning it has an increased tremor amplitude) as the proximity to the target nears and when increased precision is demanded. The functional repercussions, particularly for fine-motor skills, can be devastating.

Myelin—Lipid-rich insulating material covering nerve fibers that speeds conduction of impulses.

Rigidity—Hypertonicity of agonist and antagonist muscles that offers a consistent, uniform resistance to passive movement.

References

Aarsland, D., Tandberg, E., Larsen, J. P., & Cummings, J. L. (1996). Frequency of dementia in Parkinson disease. *Archive of Neurology, 53,* 538–542.

Amyotrophic Lateral Sclerosis Association. (2012). What is ALS? Retrieved March 31, 2012 from http://www.alsa.org/about-als.

Baker, M. G., & Graham, L. (2004). The journey: Parkinson's disease. *British Medical Journal, 329,* 611–614.

Ball, L. J., Beukelman, D. R., & Pattee, G. L. (2004). Acceptance of augmentative and alternative communication technology by persons with amyotrophic lateral sclerosis. *Augmentative and Alternative Communication, 20,* 113–122.

Barlow, J. H., Turner, A. P., & Wright, C. C. (2000). A randomized controlled study of the Arthritis Self-Management Programme in the UK. *Health Education Research, 15,* 665–680.

Beatty, W. W., & Goodkin, D. E. (1990). Screening for cognitive impairment in multiple sclerosis: An evaluation of the Mini-Mental State Examination. *Archives Neurology, 47,* 297–301.

Benedict, R. H., Cox, D., Thompson, L. L., Foley, F., Weinstock-Guttman, B., & Munschauer, F. (2004). Reliable screening for neuropsychological impairment in multiple sclerosis. *Multiple Sclerosis, 10,* 675–678.

Benedict, R. H., Fischer, J. S., Archibald, C. J., Arnett, C. A., Beatty, W. W., Bobholz, J., Chelune, G. J., Fisk, J. D., Langdon, D. W., Caruos, L., Foley, F., LaRocca, N. G., Vowels, L., Weinstein, A., DeLuca, J., Rao, S. M., & Munschauer, F. (2002). Minimal neuropsychological assessment of multiple sclerosis patient: A consensus approach. *Clinical Neuropsychology, 16,* 381–397.

Benedict, R. H. B., Fishman, I., McClellan, M. M., Bakshi, R., & Weinstock-Guttman, B. (2003). Validity of the Beck Depression Inventory-Fast Screen in multiple sclerosis. *Multiple Sclerosis, 9,* 393–396.

Bishop, M., Frain, M., & Tschopp, M. (2008). Self-management, perceived control, subjective quality of life in multiple sclerosis: an exploratory study. *Rehabilitation Counselling Bulletin, 52,* 45–56.

Bodenheimer, T., Lorig, K., Holman, H., & Grumbach, K. (2002). Patient self-management of chronic disease in primary care. *Journal of American Medical Association, 288,* 2469–2475.

Bol, Y., Duits, A. A., Hupperts, R. M. M., Verlinden, I., & Verhey, F. R. J. (2010). The impact of fatigue on cognitive functioning in patients with multiple sclerosis. *Clinical Rehabilitation, 24,* 854–862.

Bradley, W. E. (1996). *Neurology in clinical practice* (2nd ed.). Boston: Butterworth-Heinemann.

Brown, T. R., & Kraft, G. H. (2005). Exercise and rehabilitation for individuals with multiple sclerosis. *Physical Medicine and Rehabilitation Clinics of North America, 16,* 513–555.

Buchanan, R. J., Haung, C., & Kaufman, M. (2012). Health-related quality of life among young adults with multiple sclerosis. *International Journal of MS Care, 12,* 190–199.

Calcagno, P., Ruoppolo, G., Grasso, M. G., De Vincentiis, M., & Paolucci, S. (2002). Dysphagia in multiple sclerosis: Prevalence and prognostic factors. *Acta Neurological Scandinavia, 105,* 40–43.

Calne, D. B. (1995). Diagnosis and treatment of Parkinson's disease. *Hospital Practice, 30,* 83–86, 89.

Carroll, A., McDonnell, G., & Barnes, M. (2003). A review of the management of Guillian-Barré syndrome in a regional neurological rehabilitation unit. *International Journal of Rehabilitation Research, 26,* 297–302.

Cattaneo, D., De Nuzzo, C., Fascia, T., Macalli, M., Pisoni, I., & Cardini, R. (2002). Risks of falls in subjects with multiple sclerosis. *Archives of Physical Medicine and Rehabilitation, 83,* 864–867.

Conley, C. C., & Kirchner, J. T. (1999). Parkinson's disease: The shaking palsy. *Post Graduate Medicine, 109,* 39–52.

Daudrich, B., Hurl, D., & Forwell, S. J. (2010). Multidimensional assessment of tremor in multiple sclerosis: A useful instrument. *International Journal of MS Care, 12,* 23–32.

Dawes, L., McCloy, K., & Forwell, S. J. (2010). Development of a comprehensive fatigue assessment battery for multiple sclerosis. The Consortium of Multiple Sclerosis Centers 24th Annual Meeting, San Antonio, TX. Retrieved from June 2–5, 2010. http://annualmeeting.mscare.org/images/pdf/2010/S30.pdf.

de Lau, L. M. L., & Breteler, M. M. L. (2006). Epidemiology of Parkinson's disease. *Lancet Neurology, 5,* 525–535

Dematteis, J. A. (1996). Guillain-Barré syndrome: A team approach to diagnosis and treatment. *American Family Physician, 54,* 197–200.

Diamond, B. J., Johnson, S. K., Kaufman, M., & Graves, L. (2008). Relationships between information processing, depression, fatigue and cognition in multiple sclerosis. *Archives of Clinical Neuropsychology, 23,* 189–199.

Dick, S., Semple, S., Dick, F., & Seaton, A. (2007). Occupational titles as risk factors for Parkinson's disease. *Occupational Medicine-Oxford, 57,* 50–56.

Dixon, L., Duncan, D., Johnson, P., Kirkby, L., O'Connell, H., Taylor, H., & Deane, K. H. O. (2007). Occupational therapy for patients with Parkinson's disease. *Cochrane Database of Systematic Reviews (Online), 3.*

Douglas, C., Wollin, J. A., & Windsor, C. (2009). The impact of pain on the quality of life of people with multiple sclerosis: A community survey. *International Journal of MS Care, 11,* 127–136.

Drory, V. E., Gotsman, E., Reznick, J. G., Mosek, A., & Korczyn, A. D. (2001). The value of muscle exercise in patients with amyotrophic lateral sclerosis. *Journal of Neurological Sciences, 191,* 133–137.

Ebersbach, G., Ebersbach, A., Edler, D., Kaufhold, O., Kusch, M., Kupsch, A., & Wissel, J. (2010). Comparing exercise in Parkinson's disease: The Berlin BIG Study. *Movement Disorders, 25,* 1902–1908.

Erwin, A.,Gudesblatt, M.,Bethoux, F., Bennett, S.E., Koelbel, S., Plunkett, R., Sadiq, S., Stevenson, V. L., Thomas, A. M., Tornatore, C., Zaffaroni, M., & Hughes. M. (2011). Interthecal baclofen in multiple sclerosis: Too little, too late? *Multiple Sclerosis, 17,* 705–713.

Feys, P., Helsen, W. F., Liu, X., Nuttin, B., Lavrysen, A., Swinnen, S. P., & Ketelaer, P. (2005). Interaction between eye and hand movements in multiple sclerosis patients with intention tremor. *Movement Disorders, 20,* 705–713.

Finlayson, M. (2004). Concerns about the future among older adults with multiple sclerosis. *American Journal of Occupational Therapy, 58,* 54–63.

Finlayson, M., & Holberg, C. (2007). Evaluation of a teleconference-delivered energy conservation education program for people with multiple sclerosis. *Canadian Journal of Occupational Therapy, 74,* 337–347.

Fischer, J. S., Jak, A. J., Kniker, J. E., Rudick, R. A., & Cutter, G. (2001). *Multiple Sclerosis Functional Composite (MSFC): Administration and scoring manual.* New York: National Multiple Sclerosis Society.

Fisk, J., Pontefract, A., Ritvo, P. G., Archibald, C. J., & Murray, J. T. (1994). The impact of fatigue on patients with multiple sclerosis. *Canadian Journal of Neurological Sciences, 21,* 9–14.

Food and Drug Administration. (2012). FDA safety communication: Chronic cerebrospinal venous insufficiency treatment in multiple sclerosis patients. Retrieved May 20, 2012 from http://www.fda.gov/MedicalDevices/Safety/AlertsandNotices.

Foley, F. W., Benedict, R. H. B., Gromisch, E. S., & Deluca, J. (2012). The need for screening, assessment, and treatment for cognitive dysfunction in multiple sclerosis. *International Journal of MS Care, 14,* 58–64.

Forwell, S. J., Brunham, S., Tremlett, H., Morrison, W., & Oger, J. (2008). Differentiating primary and non-primary fatigue in MS. *International Journal on MS Care, 10,* 14–20.

Gelb, D. J., Oliver, E., & Gilman, S. (1999). Diagnostic criteria for Parkinson disease. *Archive of Neurology, 56,* 33–39.

Gentry, T. (2008). PDAs as cognitive aids for people with multiple sclerosis. *American Journal Occupational Therapy, 62,* 18–27.

Ghahari, S., & Forwell, S. J. (2012). CCSVI: The message in social media. Annual conference of the Consortium of MS Centers, San Diego, CA. Retrieved from May 30–June 2, 2012. http://annualmeeting.mscare.org/index.php?option=com_content &view=article&id=174&Itemid=105.

Ghahari, S., Packer, T. L., & Passmore, A. E. (2010). Effectiveness of an online fatigue self-management program for people with chronic neurological conditions: A randomized controlled trial. *Clinical Rehabilitation, 24,* 727–744.

Giladi, N., Shabtai, H., Rozenberg, E., & Shabtai, E. (2001). Gait festination in Parkinson's disease. *Parkinsonism and Related Disorders, 7,* 135–138.

Gillen, G. (2000). Improving activities of daily living performance in an adult with ataxia. *American Journal of Occupational Therapy, 54,* 89–96.

Goodman, A. D., Brown, T. R., Krupp, L. B., Schapiro, R. T., Schwid, S. R., Cohen, R., Marinucci, L. N., Blight, A. R., & the Fampridine MS-F203 Investigators. (2009). Sustained-release oral fampridine in multiple sclerosis: A randomised, double-blind, controlled trial. *Lancet, 373,* 732–738.

Gregory, M. A., Gregory, R. J., & Podd, J. V. (2005). Understanding Guillain-Barré syndrome and central nervous system involvement. *Rehabilitation Nursing, 30,* 207–212.

Guillian-Barré Syndrome–Chronic Inflammatory Demyelinating Polyneuropathy Foundation International. (2012). All about GBS. Retrieved March 31, 2012 from http://www.gbs-cidp.org/home/gbs/all-about-gbs.

Hakim, E. A., Bakheit, A. M., Bryant, T. N., Roberts, M. W., McIntosh-Michaelis, S. A., Spackman, A. J., Martin, J. P., & McLellan, D. L. (2000). The social impact of multiple sclerosis: A study of 305 patients and their relatives. *Disability and Rehabilitation, 22,* 288–293.

Hasan, K. M., Walimuni, I. S., Abid, H., Frye, R. E., Ewing-Cobbs, L., Wolinsky, J. S., & Narayana, P. A. (2011). Multimodal quantitative magnetic resonance imaging of thalamic development and aging across the human lifespan: Implications to neurodegeneration in multiple sclerosis. *Journal of Neuroscience, 31,* 16826–16832.

Hass, E. J., Waddell, D. E., Fleming, R. P., Juncos, J. L., & Gregor, R. J. (2005). Gait initiation and dynamic balance control in Parkinson's disease. *Archives of Physical Medicine and Rehabilitation, 86,* 2172–2176.

Hawes, F., Billups, C., & Forwell, S. J. (2010). Interventions for upper limb intention tremor in multiple sclerosis: A feasibility study. *International Journal of MS Care, 12,* 122–132.

Higo, R., Tayama, N., & Nito, T. (2004). Longitudinal analysis of progression of dysphagia in amyotrophic lateral sclerosis. *Auris Nasus Larynx, 31,* 247–254.

Hobart, J. C., Riazi, A., Lamping, D. L., Fitzpatrick, R., & Thompson, A. J. (2003). Measuring the impact of MS on walking ability: The 12-item MS walking scale (MSWS-12). *Neurology, 60,* 31–36.

Hoehn, M. M., & Yahr, M. D. (1967). Parkinsonism: Onset, progression and mortality. *Neurology, 17,* 427–442.

Hughes, R. A. C., & Rees, J. (1997). Clinical and epidemiologic features of Guillain-Barré syndrome. *Journal of Infectious Diseases, 176(Suppl. 2),* S92–S98.

Hughes, R. A., Newsom-Davis, J. M., Perkin, G. D., & Pierce, J. M. (1978). Controlled trial prednisolone in acute polyneuropathy. *Lancet, 2,* 750–753.

Hugos, C. L., Copperman, L. F., Fuller, B. E., Yadav, V., Lovera, J., & Bourdette, D. N. (2010). Clinical trial of a formal group fatigue program in multiple sclerosis. *Multiple Sclerosis, 16,* 724–732.

Hyman, N., Barnes, M., Bhakta, B., Cozens, A., Bakheit, M., Kreczy-Kleedorfer, B., Poewe, W., Wissel, J., Bain, P., Glickman, S., Sayer, A., Richardson, A., & Dott, C. (2000). Botulinum toxin (Dysportt) treatment of hip adductor spasticity in multiple sclerosis: A prospective, randomised, double blind, placebo controlled, dose ranging study. *Journal of Neurology Neurosurgery Psychiatry, 68,* 707–712.

Jankovic, J. (2008). Parkinson's disease: Clinical features and diagnosis. *Journal of Neurology Neurosurgery Psychiatry, 79,* 368–376.

Johnson, K. L., Bamer, A. M., & Fraser, R. T. (2009). Disease and demographic characteristics associated with unemployment among working-age adults with multiple sclerosis. *International Journal on MS Care, 11,* 137–143.

Johnson, K. L., Bamer, A. M., Yorkston, K. M., & Amtmann, D. (2009). Use of cognitive aids and other assistive technology by individuals with multiple sclerosis. *Disability Rehabilitation Assistive Technology, 4,* 1–8.

Julian, L. J., Vella, L., Vollmer, T., Hadjimichael, O., & Mohr, D. C. (2008). Employment in multiple sclerosis: Exiting and re-entering the work force. *Journal of Neurology, 255,* 1354–1360.

Kalb, R. C. (1996). *Multiple sclerosis: The questions you have–The answers you need.* New York: Demos.

Karavatas, S. G. (2005). The role of neurodevelopmental sequencing in the physical therapy management of a geriatric patient with Guillain-Barré syndrome. *Topics in Geriatric Rehabilitation, 21,* 133–135.

Karlson, K. H., Larsen, J. P., Tandberg, E., & Maeland, J. G. (1999). Influences of clinical and demographic variables in quality of life in patients with Parkinson's disease. *Journal of Neurology, Neuropsychiatry and Psychiatry, 66,* 431–435.

Khan, F. (2004). Rehabilitation in Guillain-Barré syndrome. *Australian Family Physician, 33,* 1013–1017.

Khan, F., Pallant, J. F., Ng, L., & Bhasker, A. (2010). Factors associated with long-term functional outcomes and psychological sequelae in Guillain-Barré syndrome. *Journal of Neurology, 257,* 2024–2031.

Kileff, J. (2005). A pilot study of the effect of aerobic exercise on people with moderate disability multiple sclerosis. *Clinical Rehabilitation, 19,* 165–169.

Korostil, M., & Feinstein, A. (2007). Anxiety disorders and their clinical correlates in multiple sclerosis patients. *Multiple Sclerosis, 13,* 67–72.

Krupp, L., LaRocca, N., Muir-Nash, J., & Steinberg, A.D. (1989). The fatigue severity scale: Application to patients with multiple sclerosis and systemic lupus erythematosus. *Archives of Neurology, 46,* 1121–23.

Krupp, L. B., & Lekins, L. E. (2000). Fatigue and declines in cognitive functioning in multiple sclerosis. *Neurology, 55,* 934–939.

Krupp, L. B., & Macallister, W. S. (2005). Treatment of pediatric multiple sclerosis. *Current Treatment Options in Neurology, 7,* 191–199.

Kurtzke, J. F. (1983). Rating neurologic impairment in multiple sclerosis: An Expanded Disability Status Scale (EDSS). *Neurology, 33,* 1444–1452.

Law, M., Baptiste, S., Carswell, A., McColl, M. A., Polatajko, H., & Pollock, N. (2005). *COPM: Canadian Occupational Performance Measure.* Ottawa, Canada: Canadian Association of Occupational Therapists.

Leavitt, V. M., Sumowski, J. F., Chiaravalloti, N., & DeLuca, J. (2012). Warmer outdoor temperature is associated with worse cognitive status in multiple sclerosis. *Neurology, 78,* 964–968.

Lexell, E. M., Iwarrson, S., & Lexell, J. (2006). The complexity of daily occupations in multiple sclerosis. *Scandinavian Journal of Occupational Therapy, 13,* 241–248.

Lou, J.-S., Reeves, A., Benice, T., & Sexton, G. (2003). Fatigue and depression are associated with poor quality of life in amyotrophic lateral sclerosis. *Neurology, 60,* 122–123.

Lublin, F. D., & Reingold, S. C. (1996). Defining the clinical course of multiple sclerosis: Results of an international survey. *Neurology, 46,* 907–911.

Maitra, K. K. (2009). Strategies for Curing with Self-Speech in People Living with Parkinson's Disease. In I. Sodenback (Ed.), *International Handbook of Occupational Therapy Interventions,* 317–324. New York: Springer.

Maitra, K. K., & Dasgupta, A. K. (2005). Incoordination of a sequential motor in Parkinson's disease. *Occupational Therapy International, 12,* 218–233.

Marder, K., Logroscino, G., Alfaro, B., Mejia, H., Halim, A., Louis, E., Cote, L., & Mayeux, R. (1998). Environmental risk factors for Parkinson's disease in an urban multiethnic community. *Neurology, 50,* 279–281.

Martin, W. R., & Wieler, M. (2003). Treatment of Parkinson's disease. *Canadian Journal of Neurological Science, 30(Suppl. 1),* S27–S33.

Mathiowetz, V., Finlayson, M. L., Matuska, K. M., Chen, H. Y., & Luo, P. (2005). Randomized controlled trial of an energy conservation course for persons with multiple sclerosis. *Multiple Sclerosis, 11,* 592–601.

Mayer, C. A., Pfeilschifter, W., Lorenz, M. W., Nedelmann, M., Bechmann, I., Steinmetz, H., & Ziemann, U. (2011). The perfect crime? CCSVI not leaving a trace in MS. *Journal of Neurology Neurosurgery Psychiatry, 82,* 436–440.

McDonald, E. R., Wiedenfeld, S. A., Hiller, A., Carpenter, C. L., & Walter, R. A. (1994). Survival in amyotrophic lateral sclerosis: The role of psychological factors. *Archives of Neurology, 51,* 17–23.

McGavern, D. B., Murray, P. D., Rivera-Quinones, C., Schmelzer, J. D., Low, P. A., & Rodrigues, M. (2000). Axonal loss results in spinal cord atrophy, electrophysiological abnormalities and neurological deficits following demyelination in a chronic inflammatory model of multiple sclerosis. *Brain, 123,* 519–531.

Meythaler, J. M., DeVivo, M. J., & Braswell, W. C. (1997). Rehabilitation outcomes of patients who have developed Guillain-Barré syndrome. *American Journal of Physical Medicine and Rehabilitation, 76,* 411–419.

Mitsumoto, H., Chad, D., & Pioro, E. (1998). *Amyotrophic lateral sclerosis.* Contemporary neurology series. Philadelphia: Davis.

Mohr, D. C., Goodkin, D. E., Nelson, S., Cox, D., & Weiner, M. (2002). Moderating effects of coping on the relationship between stress and the development of the new brain lesions in multiple sclerosis. *Psychosomatic Medicine, 64,* 803–809.

Mohr, D. C., Lovers, J., Brown, T., Cohen, B., Neylan, T., Henry, R., Siddique, J., Jin, L., Daikh, D., & Pelletier, D. (2012). A randomized trial of stress management for the prevention of new brain lesions in MS. *Neurology, 79,* 412–419.

Morris, M. E., Iansek, R., & Kirkwood, B. (2009). A randomized controlled trial of movement strategies compared with exercise for people with Parkinson's disease. *Movement Disorders, 24,* 64–71.

Multiple Sclerosis Trust. (2012). Prevalence and incidence of multiple sclerosis. Retrieved July 15, 2012 from http://www.mstrust.org.uk/atoz/prevalence_incidence.jsp.

Murphy, S., & Tickle-Degnen, L. (2001). The effectiveness of occupational therapy-related treatments for persons with Parkinson's disease: A meta-analytic review. *The American Journal of Occupational Therapy, 55,* 385–392.

National Multiple Sclerosis Society. (2012). About MS. Retrieved March 10, 2012 from http://www.nationalmssociety.org.

Neudert, C., Wasner, M., & Borasio, G. D. (2004). Individual quality of life is not correlated with health-related quality of life or physical function in patients with amyotrophic lateral sclerosis. *Journal of Palliative Medicine, 7,* 551–557.

Norquist, J. M., Jenkinson, C., Fitzpatrick, R., Swash, M., & the ALS-HPS Steering Group. (2003). Factors which predict physical and mental health status in patients with amyotrophic lateral sclerosis over time. *ALS and Other Motor Neuron Disorders, 4,* 112–117.

Packer, T. L., Brink, N., & Sauriol, A. (1995). *Managing Fatigue: A six week course for energy conservation.* Tucson, AZ: Therapy Skill Builders.

Pakenham, K. I. (1999). Adjustment to multiple sclerosis: Application of stress and coping model. *Health Psychology, 18,* 383–392.

Panitch, H., & Applebee, A. (2011). Treatment of walking impairment in multiple sclerosis: An unmet need for a disease-specific disability. *Expert Opinion on Pharmacotherapy, 12*(10), 1511–1521.

Pankoff, B., Overend, T., Lucy, D., & White, K. (2000). Validity and responsiveness of the 6 minute walk test for people with fibromyalgia. *Journal of Rheumatology, 27,* 2666–2670.

Paralyzed Veterans of America: Multiple Sclerosis Council for Clinical Practice Guidelines. (1998). *Fatigue and multiple sclerosis: Clinical Practice Guidelines.* Washington, DC: Paralyzed Veterans of America.

Paralyzed Veterans of America: Multiple Sclerosis Council for Clinical Practice Guidelines. (2003). *Spasticity management in multiple sclerosis: Clinical practice guidelines.* Washington, DC: Paralyzed Veterans of America.

Parry, G. J. (2000). Residual effects following Guillain-Barré. Retrieved from http://www.angelfire.com/home/gbs/residual.html.

Patti, F. (2009). Cognitive impairment in multiple sclerosis. *Multiple Sclerosis, 15,* 2–8.

Peto, V., Jenkinson, C., & Fitzpatrick, R. (1995). The development of validation of a short measure of functioning and well being for individuals with Parkinson's disease. *Quality of Life Research, 4,* 241–248.

Plahuta, J. M., McCulloch, B. J., Kasarskis, E. J., Ross, M. A., Walter, R. A., & McDonald, E. R. (2002). Amyotrophic lateral sclerosis and hopelessness: Psychosocial factors. *Social Science and Medicine, 55,* 2131–2140.

Plowman-Prine, E. K., Sapienza, C. M., Okun, M. S., Pollock, S. L., Jacobson, C., Wu, S. S., & Rosenbek, J. C. (2009). The relationship between quality of life and swallowing in Parkinson's disease. *Movement Disorders, 24,* 1352–1358.

Plow, M., & Finlayson, M. (2011). Potential benefits of Nintendo Wii Fit among people with multiple sclerosis. *International Journal of MS Care, 13,* 21–30.

Polman, C. H., Reingold, S. C., Banwell, B., Clanet, M., Cohen, J. A., Filippi, M., Fujihara, K., Havrdova, E., Hutchinson, M., Kappos, L., Lublin, F. D., Montalban, X., O'Connor, P., Sandberg-Wollheim, M., Thompson, A. J., Waubant, E., Weinshenker, B., & Wolinsky, J. S. (2011). Diagnostic criteria for multiple sclerosis: 2010 revisions to the McDonald criteria. *Annals of Neurology, 69*(2), 292–302.

Rahman, S., Griffin, H. J., Quinn, N. P., & Jahanshahi, M. (2008). Quality of life in Parkinson's disease: The relative importance of the symptoms. *Movement Disorders, 23,* 1428–1434.

Rao, A. K. (2010). Enabling functional independence in Parkinson's disease: Update on occupational therapy intervention. *Movement Disorders, 25,* S146–S151.

Rizzo, M. A., Hadjimichael, O. C., Preiningerova, J., & Vollmer, T. L. (2004). Prevalence and treatment of spasticity reported by multiple sclerosis patients. *Multiple Sclerosis, 10,* 589–595.

Rodriguez, M., Siva, A., Ward, J., Stolp-Smith, K., O'Brien, P., & Kurland, L. (1994). Impairment, disability, and handicap in multiple sclerosis: A population-based study in Olmsted County, Minnesota. *Neurology, 44,* 28–33.

Royal, E., Reynolds, F. A., & Houlden, H. (2009). What are the experiences of adults returning to work following recovery from Guillain-Barré syndrome? An interpretative phenomenological analysis. *Disability and Rehabilitation, 31,* 1817–1827.

Sá, M. J. (2007). Psychological aspects of multiple sclerosis. *Clinical Neurology and Neurosurgery, 110,* 868–877.

Sadovnick, A. D., Armstrong, H., Rice, G. P., Bulman, D., Hashimoto, L., Paty, D. W., Hashimoto, S. A., Warren, S., Hader, W., Murray T. J., Seland, T. P., Metz, L., Bell, R., Duquette, P., Gray, T., Nelson, R., Weinshenkar, B., Brunt, D., & Ebers, G. C (1993). A population-based study of multiple sclerosis in twins: update. *Annals of Neurology, 33,* 281–285.

Sapir, S., Spielman, J., Ramig, L., Story, B., & Fox, C. (2007). Effects of intensive voice treatment (LSVT®) on vowel articulation in dysarthric individuals with idiopathic Parkinson's disease: Acoustic and perceptual findings. *Journal of Speech Language and Hearing Research, 50,* 899–912.

Schapiro, R. T. (2011). Team approach to complex symptomatic management in multiple sclerosis. *International Journal of MS Care, 13,* 12–19.

Schrag, A., & Banks, P. (2006). Time of loss of employment in Parkinson's disease. *Movement Disorders, 21,* 1839–1843.

Schwid, S. R., Covington, M., Segal, B. M., & Goodman, A. D. (2002). Fatigue in multiple sclerosis: Current understanding and future directions. *Journal of Rehabilitation Research and Development, 39,* 211–224.

Shirani, A., Zhao, Y., Karim, M., Evans, C., Kingwell, E., van der Kop, M. L., Oger, J., Gustafson, P., Petkau, J., & Tremlett, H. (2012). Association between use of interferon beta and progression of disability in patients with relapsing-remitting multiple sclerosis. *Journal of the American Medical Association, 308,* 247–256.

Shulman, L. M., Taback, R. L., Rabinstein, A. A., & Weiner, W. J. (2002). Non-recognition of depression and other non-motor symptoms in Parkinson's disease. *Parkinsonism & Related Disorders, 8,* 193–197.

Sinaki, M. (1980). Rehabilitation. In D. W. Mulder (Ed.), *The diagnosis and treatment of amyotrophic lateral sclerosis* (pp. 169–193). Boston: Houghton Mifflin.

Solaro, C., Brichetto, G., Amato, M. P., Cocco, E., Colombo, B., D'Aleo, G., Gasperini, C., Ghezzi, A., Martinelle, V., Milanese, C., Patti, F., Trojano, M., Verdun, E., Mancardi, G. L., & the PaIMS Study Group. (2004). The prevalence of pain in multiple sclerosis: A multicenter cross-sectional study. *Neurology, 63,* 919–921.

Stewart, T. M., Tran, Z. V., & Bowling, A. (2007). Factors related to fatigue in multiple sclerosis. *International Journal of MS Care, 9,* 29–34.

Thomas, F. J., & Wiles, C. M. (1999). Dysphagia and nutritional status in multiple sclerosis. *Journal of Neurology, 246,* 677–682.

Thorne, S., Paterson, B., & Russell, C. (2003). The structure of everyday self-care decision making in chronic illness. *Qualitative Health Research, 13,* 1337–1352.

Tickle-Degnen, L. (2006, March). Wilma West Lectureship. USC Occupational Science Symposium, University of Southern California, Los Angeles, CA.

Tickle-Degnen, L., Ellis, T., Saint-Hilaire, M. H., Thomas, C. A., & Wagenaar, R. C. (2010). Self-management rehabilitation and health-related quality of life in Parkinson's disease: A randomized controlled trial. *Movement Disorders, 25,* 194–204.

Trail, M., Nelson, N., Van, J. N., Appel, S. A., & Lai, E. C. (2001). Wheelchair use by patients with amyotrophic lateral sclerosis: A survey of user characteristics and selection preferences. *Archives of Physical Medicine and Rehabilitation, 82,* 98–102.

Trapp, B. D., Peterson, J., Ransohoff, R. M., Rudick, R., Mork, S., & Bo, L. (1998). Axonal transection in the lesions of multiple sclerosis. *New England Journal of Medicine, 338,* 278–285.

Uitti, R. J. (1998). Tremor: How to determine if the patient has Parkinson's disease. *Geriatrics, 53,* 30–36.

Van den Berg, J. P., Kalmijn, S., Lindeman, E., Veldink, J. H., de Visser, M., Van er Graaff, M. M., Wokk, J. H. J., & Van der Berg, L. H. (2005). Multidisciplinary ALS care improves quality of life in patients with ALS. *Neurology, 65,* 1264–1267.

van Doorn, P. A., Ruts, L., & Jacobs, B. C. (2008). Clinical features, pathogenesis, and treatment of Guillain-Barré syndrome. *Lancet Neurology, 7,* 939–950.

Varanese, S., Birnbaum, Z., Rossi, R., & Di Rocco, A. (2010). Treatment of advanced Parkinson's disease. *Parkinson's disease.* Published online February 7, 2011. doi: 10.4061/2010/480260.

Verbaan, D., Marninus, J., Visser, M., van Rooden, S. M., Stigglebout, A. M., & van Hilten, J. J. (2007). Patient-reported autonomic symptoms in Parkinson disease. *Neurology, 69,* 333–341.

Vukusic, S., Hutchinson, M., Hours, M., Moreau, T., Cortinovis-Tourniaire, P., Adeleine, P., Confavreux, C., & the Pregnancy in Multiple Sclerosis Group. (2004). Pregnancy and multiple sclerosis (the PRIMS Study): Clinical predictors of post-partum relapse. *Brain, 127,* 1353–1360.

Ward, C. D., & Robertson, D. (2004). Rehabilitation in Parkinson's disease. *Reviews in Clinical Gerontology, 13,* 223–239.

Warren, M. (1999). biVABA (Brain Injury Visual Assessment Battery for Adults). visABILITIES Rehab Services Inc. Retrieved June 18, 2013 from www.visabilities.com/bivaba.

Warren, S., Warren, K. G., & Cockerill, R. (1991). Emotional stress and coping in multiple sclerosis exacerbations. *Journal of Psychosomatic Research, 35,* 37–47.

Weiser, W., Wetzel, S. G., Kappos, L., Hoshi, M. M., Witte, U., Radue, E. W., & Steinbrich, W. (2002). Swallowing abnormalities in multiple sclerosis: Correlation between videofluoroscopy and subjective symptoms. *European Radiology, 12,* 789–792.

Wu, Y., Le, W., & Jankovic, J. (2011). Preclinical biomarkers of Parkinson disease. *Archives of Neurology, 68,* 22–30.

Zamboni, P., & Carinci, F. (2011). Face, brain, and veins: A new perspective for multiple sclerosis onset. *Journal of Craniofacial Surgery, 22,* 376.

Orthopaedic Conditions

Colleen Maher

Learning Objectives

After studying this chapter, the reader will be able to do the following:

1. Identify the role of the occupational therapist in assessing and planning treatment for persons with occupational dysfunction secondary to injuries or diseases affecting the musculoskeletal system.
2. Select appropriate assessments and plan treatment according to the stages of recovery following a musculoskeletal injury or disease of the upper extremity.
3. Describe how to accomplish daily life tasks without causing adverse sequelae following fracture or surgery to the hip.
4. State the principles of body mechanics and describe how to apply them to activities and tasks of daily life.
5. Describe the phases of fracture management of the upper extremity and how to optimize occupational functioning at each stage.

Orthopaedic conditions include injuries, diseases, and deformities of bones, joints, and their related soft tissue structures: muscles, tendons, ligaments, and nerves. These conditions can be caused by traumatic events, such as motor vehicle, recreational, or work-related accidents; by cumulative trauma; by obesity; or by congenital anomaly. Furthermore, musculoskeletal conditions are most common in the elderly population, and it is projected that by the year 2030, the number of adults age 65 years and older will double. This rapidly expanding elderly population is most at risk for developing musculoskeletal injuries and conditions that will result in long-term chronic pain (American Academy of Orthopaedic Surgeons, 2008).

This chapter provides an overview of the occupational therapy assessments and treatment interventions used with adult clients who have orthopaedic or musculoskeletal conditions. Specifically, it reviews upper extremity and hip fractures and their sequelae, hip surgery for trauma and disease, shoulder injuries and their effects on function, and pain with a focus on low back pain.

PURPOSE AND ROLE OF OCCUPATIONAL THERAPY IN ORTHOPAEDICS

The aim of occupational therapy in orthopaedic rehabilitation is to help the client achieve maximal function of body and limb to restore occupational functioning. In the acute stage of recovery, the therapist's role is to help relieve pain, decrease swelling and inflammation, assist in wound care, maintain joint or limb alignment, and restore function at the injury site. The therapist teaches the client to safely perform tasks and activities while protecting the injury site for healing. As healing progresses to clinical union and then to consolidation, the occupational therapist retrains the client in activities of daily living (ADL) and other occupational tasks.

For individuals who have a chronic joint disease, such as osteoarthritis, or cumulative trauma, such as low back pain, the occupational therapist's role depends on the stage of recovery and the directives of the treatment team. The occupational therapist may directly help relieve pain, realign structures, or reduce the stress on soft tissue, or the occupational therapist may work closely with the physical therapist to relate the functional program to treatment offered in physical therapy. As the acute episode of pain decreases, the occupational therapist focuses on an individually tailored education program to help the client physically and psychologically make the required lifestyle changes to reach and sustain optimal occupational functioning.

OCCUPATIONAL THERAPY EVALUATION IN ORTHOPAEDICS

Evaluation is an ongoing process that is carefully coordinated with the stage of recovery. The therapist selects assessments that will provide sufficient information to plan and to direct treatment but will not threaten the injured or inflamed structure during healing. The therapist chooses assessments that correspond to the level of bone healing, the chosen method of reduction and stabilization, and the plan for movement during healing or the acute inflammatory episode. The therapist assesses participation in life roles including areas of occupations, performance skills and performance patterns, as well as impairments of capacities and abilities.

Participation in Life Roles

Although resumption of life roles may not be possible at the start of the aftercare program, life roles regulate the choices made during treatment planning and serve as the end point for treatment planning. In addition to noting the activities and tasks that can and cannot be accomplished, using the assessment tools described in Chapter 7, the therapist observes whether the client is magnifying the injury or appears to be adopting a sick role.

Impairments of Abilities and Capacities

Physical impairments are directly measured by various assessment instruments. See Chapter 7 for assessment of pain, edema, range of motion (ROM), sensation, strength, and endurance. The surgeon's protocol may stipulate no movement or no force at or near the fracture site, or it may require controlled range of motion beginning immediately or within the first 3–4 weeks after stabilization (Fig. 36-1). If the surgeon's protocol requires complete rest of the injured bone or joint, ROM measurements are deferred until movement is permissible. If the client is on a specific program, such as controlled ROM, the therapist measures the joint, adhering to the precautionary boundaries, and does not allow the client to exceed the limits of the surgeon's prescription. The adjacent joints are measured, and a treatment program is designed for any adjacent joint that demonstrates less than normal function. Detailed strength testing with applied resistance is deferred until there is bony consolidation or the acute inflammation has calmed. Because of the force required, grip and pinch testing are usually deferred for 2–4 weeks following cast removal in forearm fractures. *Safety Message: Assessing strength after a fracture should only be performed when ordered by the orthopaedist.* The occupational therapist not only focuses on direct measurement of the injured and adjacent anatomical regions but also closely observes the client's total body response in terms of postural changes, pain responses, and psychological reactions.

OCCUPATIONAL THERAPY TREATMENT IN ORTHOPAEDICS

The most important treatment goal is the restoration of occupational functioning. To achieve this, the client needs to be directed from the start of recovery to move and to use

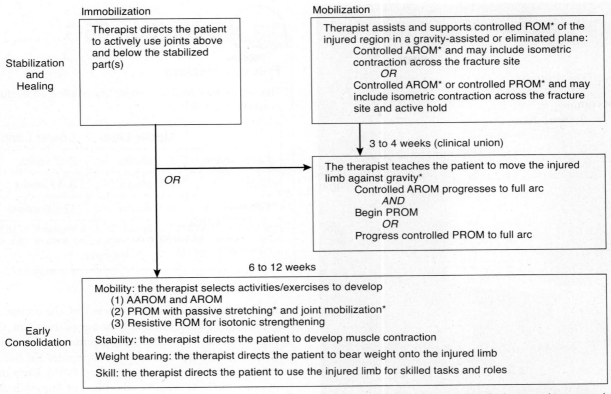

Figure 36-1 Guidelines for therapeutic intervention during fracture healing and consolidation. AAROM, active assisted range of motion; AROM, active range of motion; PROM, passive range of motion; ROM, range of motion.

all joints that are not affected by the injury or the disease. For patients who have an upper limb fracture or a short-term inflammation, the therapist may recommend temporary use of the uninjured hand alone to perform some ADL, assisted by adaptations such as pump bottles for toothpaste and shampoo, a button hook, or a rocker knife. Other ADL may require the temporary assistance of another person so as not to disturb the healing region. When the client is medically ready, the occupational therapist, through careful activity analysis, ascertains how the client can safely resume tasks that correspond with the achieved recovery status to reintegrate the injured or inflamed limb into activity safely. Attention is directed toward redeveloping the function of the injured limb to resume its capacity in mobility, stability, weight bearing, and ultimately skilled activity (see Fig. 36-1). When a condition is chronic, such as status post total hip replacement or low back pain, the therapist recommends alternative methods, adaptive equipment, or environmental modification for safe task completion.

Acute Trauma: Fractures

As long as orthopaedic surgeons have been treating fractures, there has been a controversy between the "movers" and the "resters." The surgeons prescribing rest as

a fracture treatment keep their clients immobilized in traction, plaster, or fiberglass for long periods after stabilization. For many surgeons, however, the goal in fracture treatment is to mobilize the injured structures as quickly as is compatible with healing and return the client to work and leisure activities (Salter, 1999).

The goal of fracture treatment is to achieve a precise and effective stabilization for optimal recovery and resolution of function. Closed fractures that are relatively undisplaced and stable may be managed by protection alone, without reduction or immobilization. Fractures that are undisplaced but unstable do not need reduction but do require positioning and immobilization by external fixation methods such as a sling, cast, or a fracture brace. Open reduction internal fixation surgically reduces open fractures and those closed fractures that are unstable, and where the bone fragments cannot be approximated accurately by closed manual reduction alone. The bone fragments are brought into a closer anatomical alignment during surgical reduction and are stabilized by insertion of an internal fixation device, such as a nail, pin, screw, rod, or compression plate or by an external fixator (McKinnis, 2010; Shin, 2011). Surgical repair also can include prosthetic devices that are implanted to restore joint motion.

Fracture healing, when the part is immobilized by a cast, splint, or fracture brace (Fig. 36-2), is accomplished

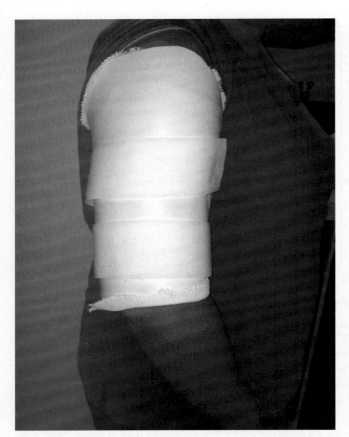

Figure 36-2 Thermoplastic humeral fracture brace to support the length of the humerus during healing.

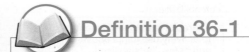

Definition 36-1

Fracture Healing

The estimate of healing time for uncomplicated fractures in adults is as follows:

	Upper Limb	Lower Limb
Callus visible	2–3 weeks	2–3 weeks
Union	4–6 weeks	8–12 weeks
Consolidation	6–8 weeks	12–16 weeks

Adapted from Solomon, L., Warwick, D. J., & Nayagam, S. (2005). *Apley's concise system of orthopaedics and fracture* (3rd ed.). London: Hodder Armold.

through the formation of immature woven bone or external callus. The woven bone then consolidates and remodels so that the fracture is repaired with lamellar bone (Smith et al., 2006). When internal fixation provides complete bone immobilization, external callus does not form, and direct healing occurs. When external callus forms first, more healing time is required. Fracture healing has a general timetable that is confirmed routinely by physical exam and x-rays to reveal the healing status before advancing the rehabilitation program (Definition 36-1). There are three phases of fracture healing: the inflammation phase (which involves up to10% of healing time), the reparative or fibroplastic phase (which accounts for up to 40% of total healing time), and the remodeling phase (which can account for up to 70% of healing time). Restoring bone to its optimal function is evident when consolidation or complete fracture repair has occurred—when there is fibrous union, the fracture site is no longer tender and painful, there is no radiologic evidence of the fracture line repair visible, and there is no movement when the fractured bone is manipulated (McKinnis, 2010).

Rehabilitation begins as soon as the cast is in place or within a day or two after reduction. The timing, amount, and kind of activity depend on the place and kind of fracture, the

method of fracture reduction selected by the orthopaedic surgeon, and, in some instances, the age of the client. Clinical experience has shown that early specific use of the injured limb during healing diminishes or eliminates the need for treatment after immobilization (Salter, 1999). Early movement prevents the unwanted side effects of immobilization: stiff joints, disuse atrophy, and muscle weakness.

Evaluation Process in Aftercare for Fractures

The evaluation is carefully designed and adjusted to the stage of recovery and the kind of fracture. This chapter presents the specialized focus for each fracture by the stage of recovery: immobilization and early mobilization or early consolidation.

Immobilization or Early Mobilization (0–6 Weeks). The therapist identifies the tasks and activities for which the client needs to learn an adaptation or obtain assistance during the temporary period of restricted movement so that the fracture site remains undisturbed. Measurements of ROM and circumference for swelling are conducted on adjacent joints. Assessment of ROM of the injured joints depends on the type of protection and stabilization used and the orthopaedic surgeon's protocol for aftercare, as discussed earlier. Clients with secure internal fixation of bone fragments may begin gentle ROM of the involved joints before the consolidation phase. This usually occurs at 1–2 weeks postoperatively under the close supervision of the surgeon.

Early Consolidation (6–8 Weeks). The therapist determines whether, and to what extent, the client can safely reintegrate the injured limb into purposeful and occupation-based tasks. The therapist continually assesses the client's ability to use the injured limb for functional tasks to correspond with clinical progress. The therapist initially measures active range of motion (AROM) of the involved joints with the exception of shoulder fractures, which are measured for active assisted/passive range of motion (AA/PROM). Edema and sensibility should be assessed. A 10-cm visual analog scale should be used to assess the client's pain level. Grip and pinch measurements are not taken until the surgeon orders strengthening. Observe the patient for signs of infection: redness, heat, swelling, pain, loss of function, or changes in circulation. To do so, look at the limb's skin color: purple, dusky, or white coloration indicates alterations in circulation, as does a skin surface that is too warm or too cold to the touch. Immediately report abnormal findings to the surgeon.

Treatment Process in Aftercare for Fractures

Intervention strategies for addressing orthopaedic injuries are based on the stage of recovery and the orthopaedic treatment protocol. The therapist selects and applies intervention strategies that are consistent with the orthopaedic surgeon's immobilization or mobilization plan, the restrictions or precautions, and goals.

Immobilization or Early Mobilization. Early mobilization treatment programs have specific and focused protocols indicating the timing, type, and quantity of desired movement (see Fig. 36-1). Advancement of the therapeutic program is determined for each client based on the stability of the fracture and radiographic signs of fracture healing (McKinnis, 2010). The cautiously controlled movement usually begins in a gravity-assisted or gravity-eliminated plane. The movement may be AAROM- or AROM-restricted to midrange and gradually upgraded to full ROM. Under careful guidance and manual handling, isometric contraction of the muscles whose bellies extend across the fracture site is encouraged to facilitate circulation and bone healing. Some protocols require controlled PROM, often followed by an active hold pattern. That is, the therapist passively moves the injured part through the prescribed arc, and then the client isometrically holds the achieved position briefly.

The therapist may have to fit the client with a sling, shoulder immobilizer, splint, or fracture brace during healing either to add protective support or to begin early controlled movement. To add to a client's comfort during stabilization in an external fixator, the therapist may recommend and fabricate a supportive static splint. Thermoplastic splinting alone is often used to achieve relative immobilization for fractures of the metacarpals and phalanges (see Chapters 15 and 37). Following the initial treatment of closed reduction of fractures in the shaft of long bones, such as humeral shaft fractures, the surgeon may prescribe a functional fracture brace as popularized by Sarmiento and shown in Figure 36-2 (Colditz, 2011). The lightweight thermoplastic fracture brace allows for motion above and below the fracture site and minimizes

the detrimental effects of prolonged immobilization. The patient is closely monitored for circulation, biomechanical alignment, and desired (controlled) movement. The therapist adjusts the shell to facilitate comfort, to respond to changes such as a reduction of limb volume, and to adjust the amount of movement the splint permits.

Early Consolidation. Therapy usually begins with focused, active use of the limb. Active therapy consists of activities and tasks to remediate the use of the muscles in the injured region. The therapist directs the client in a graduated program to resolve the presenting impairments and to reintegrate the limb into normal and customary use for functional tasks and role performance. If secondary changes are noted in the adjacent body parts or if there is a change in body posture, therapy is also directed to resolving those impairments.

Should edema persist even with elevation and active muscle contraction, additional methods, such as compression gloves or sleeves and gentle lymph massage, are used. To ameliorate stiffness and pain, the therapist may introduce modalities such as paraffin, fluidotherapy, or heat packs before or with exercise or activity (see Chapter 19). If stiffness prevails and the fracture is stable, joint mobilization and passive stretching are performed to facilitate the arthrokinetic accessory movements to increase the passive movement potential. These interventions should be approved by the surgeon before incorporating them into the treatment plan. Dynamic splinting, static progressive splinting, or the use of continuous passive motion (CPM) may also increase passive mobility over time. Adherent or hypertrophic scar formation after open reduction or soft tissue repair can also limit movement, increase pain, and alter sensation. To prevent this, the therapist teaches the patient deep pressure tissue massage and applies continuous pressure to the scar with a scar pad to facilitate scar remodeling (see Chapter 40).

FRACTURES

The care of fractures challenges both the surgeon and the occupational therapist to help the client ultimately reincorporate the injured limb into occupational performance. To initiate the care of a client who sustained a fracture, the therapist must understand the anatomy and biomechanics of the extremity and select intervention strategies that are consistent with the physiological process of fracture repair.

Shoulder Fractures

The shoulder complex is composed of the glenohumeral joint, scapulothoracic joint, sternoclavicular joint, and acromioclavicular joint. The shoulder complex provides a wide range of movements for hand placement but also provides the important functions of stabilization for hand use, lifting and pushing, reaching, and weight bearing (Greene & Roberts, 2005). The shoulder is considered the most challenging portion of the body to rehabilitate. After traumatic, degenerative, or surgical shoulder lesions, the therapy goals are delicately balanced to relieve pain, to restore movement and muscle strength, and to allow for callus formation and the approximation of the bony fragments in the injured region.

Immobilization of the shoulder results in stiffness and pain; therefore, nonoperative and postoperative therapy programs call for a specific regimen of PROM, AAROM, or AROM within a controlled, guarded range. Shoulder fractures are closely monitored by radiographs as initial controlled PROM and AAROM begin. There is controversy with regard to PROM. Some argue that passive motion is contraindicated, particularly in the elderly (Goldstein, 1999). Others say that passive movement is safe if the provided range corresponds to the surgeon's prescribed limitations. The therapist must also remember that PROM differs from passive stretching. PROM is movement of the limb by an external force to its available end range or prescribed end range. Passive stretching is movement of the limb by an external force to its available end range and then applying overpressure. *Safety Message: Passive stretching is contraindicated in the early stages of fracture healing.* Emphasis is on the patient resuming nonresistive functional activities and using the injured limb as soon as movement is allowed.

Because immobilization quickly results in stiffness, shoulder motion begins as soon as the acute pain diminishes in stable shoulder fractures. Therapy can begin as early as 7–10 days postinjury and includes pendulum exercises and sling immobilization (McKinnis, 2010). Exercises may progress to gentle P/AAROM (beginning with scapular elevation and external rotation. In 2–8 weeks, the client can begin AROM and light self-care activities. At 8 weeks, the sling is usually discarded, and the client can begin strengthening (Hodgson, 2006).

Unstable shoulder fractures usually require surgical intervention for fixation. The protocols are based on the classification of fracture, the type of surgical procedure, and the age and activity level of the client, and they often follow the guidelines as originally described by Neer (1990). Some postoperative protocols start with early mobilization programs, whereas others have a period of immobilization. Agorastides et al. (2007) found no difference in function in a study between those who received early mobilization immediately versus those who started mobilization 3 weeks postsurgical fixation. When approved by the surgeon, the sequence of exercise begins with Codman's pendulum exercises (Fig. 36-3). Codman's exercises are performed with the patient bending over so that the injured upper limb is perpendicular to the floor. In this gravity-assisted plane, the patient does clockwise and counterclockwise circular movements and flexion, extension, abduction, and adduction.

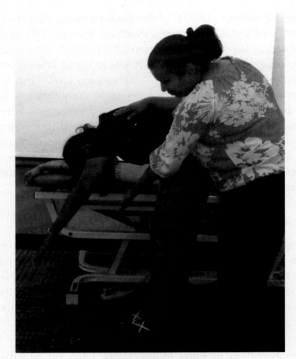

Figure 36-3 Codman's exercise (Pendulum exercise).

Safety Message: Codman's exercises may be contraindicated if the upper extremity is edematous. Also, during the first 6–8 weeks, progressive shoulder exercises for flexion and internal and external rotation are started, as are isometric exercises, a stimulant for fracture healing and callus formation; wall climbing; nonresistive therapeutic activities; and light ADL. PROM only begins when clinical union is evident and when there is no fear of disrupting the fracture.

Humeral head fractures that are unstable and significantly displaced are often surgically treated with humeral head replacement, known as hemiarthroplasty. A total shoulder arthroplasty is considered for clients with severe arthritis in combination with a proximal humerus fracture (Keenan & Mehta, 2006). A new surgical approach is the reverse total shoulder replacement. This approach is used when there is significant damage to the rotator cuff or severe arthritis of the glenohumeral joint. The major limitation of this surgery is impaired shoulder rotation (Gallinet et al., 2009; Garrigues et al., 2012).

Therapy for total shoulder arthroplasty varies with the design of the prosthesis and the surgical procedure. The rehabilitation program begins within the first 1–2 days after surgery. The exercises should not cause any pain. The key to a satisfactory functional result is early achievement of shoulder elevation and external rotation in the plane of the scapula.

Codman's pendulum exercises, passive shoulder elevation done lying supine with the opposite hand assisting the affected limb, and use of an exercise wand to perform passive external rotation are introduced during the first 2–3 days after surgery (Tan et al., 2011). The client is instructed to perform the exercises 4–6 times daily. Because the subscapularis tendon may be incised during surgery and the integrity of the rotator cuff may be disrupted, some surgeons introduce external rotation slowly in the first 4 weeks; others incorporate passive external rotation on the second postoperative day. The preferred position for passive external rotation exercise is with the humerus adducted. During this phase, the patient is instructed to begin nonresistive everyday activities, such as brushing teeth and self-feeding, while keeping the shoulder adducted to the side.

At 6 weeks postoperative, the client is instructed to add passive internal rotation, extension, and horizontal adduction. The client can progress to isometric strengthening and Thera-band® exercises for internal and external rotation. If the subscapularis was detached during surgery, the surgeon may restrict strengthening of this muscle at this time. At 8–12 weeks, Thera-band® exercises, free weights, and purposeful activities that emphasize shoulder elevation and rotational movements are initiated. At 12 weeks, the client is instructed in sports and work activities. Weight bearing on the injured arm is not allowed for at least 6 months (Neer, 1990; Tan et al., 2011).

Management of humeral shaft or humeral neck fractures is divided into three phases. Phase I includes positioning, Codman's pendulum exercises, and passive assistive exercises that are performed several times a day to prevent stiffness. Fractures of the humeral shaft and humeral neck both respond well to early passive movement and positioning. The occupational therapist may make a fracture brace conforming to the length of the humerus to provide the initial support after a humeral shaft fracture (see Fig. 36-2). *Safety Message: The therapist must be careful to flare and roll the edges of the shell to prevent compromise to circulation and nerve impingement while allowing available movement.* In the case of humeral shaft fracture, there is a risk of radial nerve damage because of the location of the injury relative to the course of the radial nerve. Radial nerve injury is characterized by the inability to extend the elbow, wrist, and digits. Other complications that are not uncommon with humeral shaft fractures are delayed union and nonunion. These complications may occur as a result of an injury to the nutrient artery located at midshaft when the humerus is fractured (McKinnis, 2010). A bone stimulator may be used to facilitate bone healing.

For phase II, the therapist encourages active assisted concentric and eccentric exercises, progressing to AROM and lightly resistive exercises. These patterns often begin with the client supine and progress to seated, in which the weight of the extremity is first supported by the therapist. Phase III addresses both stretching and strengthening. As healing permits, the client can combine shoulder forward flexion with abduction with or without external rotation

(Basti et al., 1994). Use of the injured extremity in occupation-as-end is encouraged.

Elbow Fractures

Elbow motion gives the individual the capacity to position the hand in space close to or far from the body for fine motor activities and to function as a stabilizer for strength activities (Davila, 2011). These movements are accomplished by two degrees of freedom: flexion and extension at the ulnohumeral and radiohumeral joints and pronation and supination at the proximal radioulnar joint. Intercondylar and supracondylar fractures (the extension type) are the most common of the distal humerus fractures that impact elbow function. These fractures are associated with complications that include malunion and peripheral nerve injury and have a risk of Volkmann's ischemia, a compartment syndrome of the forearm (McKinnis, 2010). Ischemia, considered an urgent medical matter, can be caused by edema within a fascia-surrounded compartment or by acute elbow flexion that compresses an artery against bone. Signs of ischemia include pale, bluish skin color; absence of forearm radial pulse; and decreased hand sensation accompanied by severe pain. *Safety Message: Report these signs immediately.* Immediate action is important because the peripheral nerves can withstand only 2–4 hours of ischemia, although they do have some potential to regenerate. The muscle can withstand up to 6 hours of ischemia, but it cannot regenerate (McKinnis, 2010; Salter, 1999). Prolonged occlusion allows for the progression to a contracture as the necrotic muscle becomes dense, shortened, fibrous scar tissue.

The nondisplaced or minimally displaced supracondylar fracture may be treated with closed reduction and immobilization in a removable cast or thermoplastic splint. After 1–2 weeks, the splint is removed daily for gentle AROM in a hinge splint (Beredjiklian, 2011). The splint is discharged after 6 weeks, and clients are encouraged to use their extremity for light ADL.

Complex elbow fractures, which include displaced supracondylar fractures and intercondylar fractures, are most often treated with open reduction and well-secured fixation. Active motion begins 2–3 days after surgery. The elbow fracture is splinted in 90° of flexion rather than extension because flexion has a greater functional importance. The splint is removed by the therapist to begin gentle A/AAROM. ROM of elbow flexion and extension is best performed in a supine position with the shoulder flexed to 90°. Gravity will assist with flexion, and the therapist will assist the client with extension. If the client also injured the collateral ligaments, restrictions on forearm rotation during elbow flexion and extension may be prescribed by the orthopaedic surgeon. Forearm ROM is performed in a seated position with the elbow flexed at 90° (Davila, 2011). Gentle PROM and light isotonic exercises are usually initiated between

6 and 8 weeks. Clients are encouraged to use their extremity for light self-care activities. At 8 weeks, there is an increased emphasis on restoring full ROM and increasing strength. In the elderly, elbow fractures are often treated with a sling alone, and active movement begins early to prevent stiffness and pain. A functional arc of motion for daily activities can be regained, but full ROM is not always achieved.

Radial head fractures can be treated with closed reduction or, depending on the severity, may require radial head excision. Radial head fractures seldom require more than a sling for immobilization. Active pronation and supination exercises are encouraged early. Emphasis should be placed on regaining active supination. Full supination is more difficult and painful than pronation (Davila, 2011). Supination and pronation exercises should be performed seated or standing, with the shoulder adducted to the side and elbow flexed to 90°. Exercises should be performed six times daily, with a minimum of two sets of 10 repetitions. Exercises should be pain free. CPM, dynamic supination splint, and static progressive splinting can be used to further encourage forearm rotation (see Chapter 37 for wrist and hand fractures).

ROTATOR CUFF PATHOLOGIES

The shoulder complex is the foundation of all upper extremity movements. The rotator cuff musculature plays an integral part in the function and control of the shoulder complex. The supraspinatus performs humeral elevation, the infraspinatus and teres minor perform external rotation, and the subscapularis performs internal rotation. Besides the actions they produce, the rotator cuff musculature functions as a force couple to control the head of the humerus on the glenoid fossa. Its anatomical location at the subacromial space, between the coracoacromial arch and the head of the humerus, makes the rotator cuff extremely vulnerable to compression. Charles Neer (1990) described a hooked acromion (type 3) as a possible cause of impingement syndrome that could progress to a tear. The supraspinatus also has an area of hypovascularity known as the critical zone. This zone is where the supraspinatus tendon inserts on the greater tuberosity of the humerus. Because of its anatomical location and area of hypovascularity, the tendon of the supraspinatus is the most commonly impinged rotator cuff tendon. Patients with rotator cuff pathology are often faced with the inability to perform the most personal self-care tasks. Activities such as toileting, hair care, and hooking a bra are all dependent on a normally functioning rotator cuff.

Shoulder Impingement Syndrome

Shoulder impingement syndrome is a compression of the structures found in the subacromial space. Structures found in the subacromial space (superior to inferior) include the subacromial bursa, supraspinatus, joint capsule, and long head of the biceps. Shoulder impingement syndrome is most commonly caused by a hooked acromion and or repetitive or sustained elevation of the shoulder above 90°. If shoulder impingement syndrome goes untreated, it can result in a rotator cuff tear. Neer (1990) developed a classification system to better understand the progression of shoulder impingement syndrome. Stage I is described as edema, inflammation, and hemorrhage. In this stage, the bursa and/or the tendons become irritated and inflamed. The symptoms can be reversed with occupational therapy intervention. The focus should be on activity modification. In stage II, the bursa and tendons become thick and fibrotic. At this stage, a person can be treated conservatively; however, recovery may take longer. In stage III, a person may present with bone spurs and partial- or full-thickness tears. A small tear is less than 1 cm, a medium tear is 1–3 cm, a large tear is 3–5 cm, and a massive tear is greater than 5 cm (Post, Silver, & Singh, 1983).

Rotator Cuff Tendonitis and Bicipital Tendonitis

A person may have rotator cuff tendonitis and or bicipital tendonitis but not shoulder impingement syndrome. The chief complaint of tendonitis is pain during humeral movement above 90°. In most cases, the client is independent with ADL; however, the patient will experience pain while performing these tasks. Common causes are repetitive overhead use, curved or hooked acromion, weakness of shoulder or scapula musculature, and capsular tightness. Tendonitis can be treated conservatively with pain modalities, activity modification, strengthening exercises, and occupation-based activities.

Bursitis

Shoulder bursitis is inflammation of the subacromial bursa. Subacromial bursitis can be differentiated from rotator cuff tendonitis if the patient has pain during passive shoulder elevation and is pain free during AROM and muscle testing of the rotator cuff. It is rarely a major source of pain and usually coexists with shoulder impingement syndrome (McMahon & Kaplan, 2006). See the section on shoulder impingement for causes.

Calcific Tendonitis

Calcific tendonitis results from calcium deposits laid down at the insertion of the tendon on the bone. In the shoulder, calcific tendonitis most commonly occurs in the supraspinatus and infraspinatus tendons. The cause is unknown. This type of tendonitis usually heals on its own by spontaneous reabsorption. Reabsorption of the calcium can take several months. During this time, the person may experience significant pain. Physical agent modalities, pain-free ROM, and activity modification are used to address the pain.

Rotator Cuff Tear

Tears of the rotator cuff can be of partial or full thickness. See the section on shoulder impingement syndrome for description of size of tear. Causes include trauma, progression of impingement syndrome, and degenerative changes of the tendon and aging. Patients with rotator cuff tears will present with difficulty performing activities above shoulder level and will often compensate by hiking the shoulder using the upper trapezius muscle. Rotational movements, such as reaching the small of the back to tuck a shirt in or remove a wallet from a back pocket, can also be limited. Rotator cuff tears can significantly limit a person's occupational functioning. Rotator cuff tears are diagnosed using magnetic resonance imaging (MRI) and magnetic resonance arthrography (MRA) (Toyoda et al., 2005). Some partial tears can be treated conservatively with activity modification and strengthening of scapula and rotator cuff muscles. Surgical options for those patients who do not benefit from conservative treatment include arthroscopic, mini-open, and open repairs. Postoperative therapy focuses on regaining full ROM, scapula and rotator cuff strengthening, practicing ADL, and other meaningful tasks.

Evaluation of the Nonsurgical Patient

The evaluation should begin with an occupational profile and a thorough history. Discuss the mechanism of injury. Was it a sudden onset or gradual onset? If it was a gradual onset, try to determine what activity or sustained posture led to the rotator cuff problem. Also discuss the client's level of pain (scale of 0–10). Is the pain localized or referred? What activities or occupations cause pain? Can the patient sleep on the involved side? The therapist should also observe the patient's posture and symmetry of the scapula at rest and during upward rotation. The physical assessments can then begin with asking the client to perform various functional movements such as reaching the small of the back, reaching the opposite axilla, and touching the top of the head. See Chapter 7 for assessment of AROM and PROM and manual muscle testing of the shoulder. Active cervical ROM and sensory testing the C4 to T1 dermatomes (see Chapter 9) should be performed to eliminate the possibility of cervical involvement. Palpation of the rotator cuff tendons will assess tenderness and swelling. Special tests should be administered to determine all the involved structures. Special tests for rotator cuff pathology include the Neer impingement sign, Hawkins test, empty can test, drop arm test, and biceps Speed's test (Procedures for Practice 36-1).

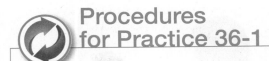

Procedures for Practice 36-1

Special Tests for Rotator Cuff Injuries

1. **Neer impingement sign:** Forced forward flexion with the shoulder internally rotated. If the patient expresses pain, the sign is positive, indicating compression and/or inflammation of the supraspinatus and/or long head of the biceps (Fig. 36-4).
2. **Hawkins test:** Shoulder and elbow are flexed to 90° followed by forced internal rotation. If the patient expresses pain (Fig. 36-5), the test is positive, indicating compression and/or inflammation of the supraspinatus and long head of the biceps.
3. **Empty can test:** Shoulder elevation to 45° and internal rotation (thumb facing down). Therapist applies resistance to abduction (downward force) (Fig. 36-6). Positive sign is weakness or pain. This test indicates a tear of the supraspinatus tendon. Repeat the same test at 90°. If pain is only experienced at 90° position, suspect bursitis.
4. **Drop arm test:** Patient's arm is positioned in 90° of abduction. The patient slowly lowers his or her arm to the side. The test is positive if the patient drops the arm to the side, indicating a supraspinatus tear (Fig. 36-7).
5. **Biceps Speed's test:** Shoulder flexed to 90°, forearm supinated, and elbow extended. Resistance is applied to flexion (downward force using a long lever arm). Positive sign is pain over bicipital groove (Fig. 36-8).

ADL should be assessed by observing the patient using the involved extremity during activities that are within low range (waist level), mid range (shoulder level), and high range (above shoulder level). The therapist should note any compensating or expressions of pain while performing the activities. There are also numerous standardized

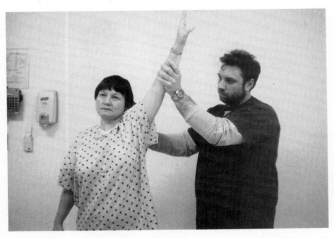

Figure 36-4 Neer impingement sign.

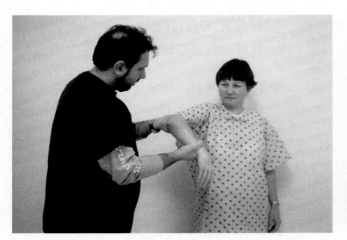

Figure 36-5 Hawkins test.

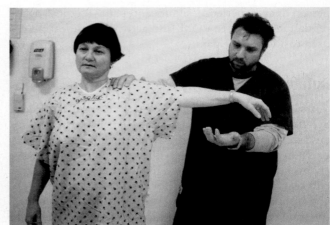

Figure 36-7 Drop arm test.

functional assessments specific to the shoulder, some of which should be included in the evaluation. Examples of standardized functional assessments that address World Health Organization International Classification of Functioning, Disability and Health (ICF) components: impairments, activity limitation, and participation restriction include the Disabilities of Arm, Shoulder and Hand (DASH), American Shoulder and Elbow Surgeons Self Report, Shoulder Disability Questionnaire, Shoulder Pain and Disability Index, and the Penn Shoulder Score (Dixon et al., 2008; Drummond et al., 2007; Hudak, Amadio, & Bombardier, 1996; McClure & Michener, 2003; Roy, MacDermid, & Woodhouse, 2009).

Evaluation of the Postsurgical Patient

The evaluation for the postsurgical patient will be guided by the surgeon. The decision to begin therapy and how to progress the client is based on many factors that include size and location of the tear, tissue quality, and surgical

approach (Ghodadra et al., 2009). Request for occupational therapy services can begin as early as 24 hours after surgery. Assessments of pain, PROM, and activity adaptation are the usual orders postoperatively. Depending on the type of repair, AROM can be assessed at 4–6 weeks, and strengthening can be tested at 8 weeks.

Treatment of the Nonsurgical Patient

Conservative treatment should begin with educating the patient on activity modification. The patient should be instructed to avoid above shoulder level activities until pain subsides. Sleeping postures should also be addressed. The patient should avoid sleeping with the arm above shoulder level or in an adducted and internally rotated position. Combined adduction and internal rotation for a long period of time can further compromise the blood supply of the supraspinatus tendon. Exercise should focus on pain-free ROM. Begin with PROM. As pain decreases, progress to AROM. Strengthening should include

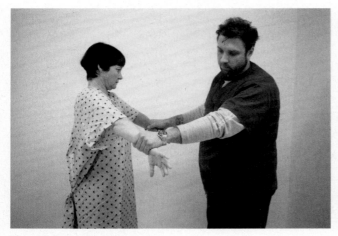

Figure 36-6 Empty can test.

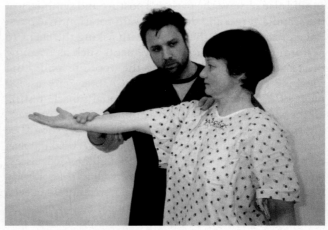

Figure 36-8 Biceps Speed's test.

isometric and isotonic exercises for the rotator cuff and scapula musculature. Also improve ROM and strength through functional activities such as dressing (Fig. 36-9, A–C). Investigate what occupations are most important to the patient and have him or her bring in the necessary equipment such as a golf club or tennis racquet. The long-term goal is to return the patient to unrestricted, pain-free occupational functioning.

Treatment of the Postsurgical Patient

Initiation of treatment following a rotator cuff repair will be based on the size of the tear, type of surgical repair, and tissue quality. After surgery, the client is placed in an abduction pillow brace. Following repair of a small or medium tear, the patient will begin with PROM/AAROM for the next 4–6 weeks. The movements emphasized should include pain-free Codman's pendulum exercises, passive shoulder elevation, and internal/external rotation in the slightly abducted position in the scapular plane. An ice pack should be used before, during, and after exercise to decrease pain and swelling. The client should be instructed to perform these exercises at home using the uninvolved arm to supply the power. Internal and external rotation is performed with the client supine and the shoulder slightly abducted to 30° (in the scapular plane) and elbow flexed to 90°. A cane or stick is held in both hands, whereas the uninvolved arm supplies the power to move the involved extremity toward the stomach (internal rotation) and away from the stomach (external rotation). Depending on the tension of the repair, the surgeon may set ROM limits. *Safety Message: Overhead pulleys are only used if requested by the surgeon because repetitive shoulder elevation may irritate the repair.* During this time, the patient should be instructed in one-handed techniques to perform ADL. The involved shoulder should not be used for any activity at this time, unless indicated by the surgeon. In between exercise sessions, the shoulder is protected in the abduction pillow brace. At 4–6 weeks, the client progresses to AROM. Begin in gravity-lessened positions and progress to against-gravity movements. Shoulder extension and internal rotation to the small of the back are added at 6–8 weeks. Encourage the patient to achieve functional ROM. Engage the patient in light ADL. Avoid compensatory movements such as hiking the scapula or lateral bending of the trunk. When performing against-gravity ADL, progress from waist level to above shoulder level activities. Strengthening can be initiated at 6 weeks to prepare the patient for functional activities. Initially, the strengthening program begins with isometric exercises for the rotator cuff and scapula stabilization exercises. Eight weeks after surgery, the patient progresses to isotonic exercises using Thera-band® and free weights. All strengthening should be performed below 90° and be pain free. Initially, exercises using free weights should begin supine to lessen gravity and prevent compensating. Then eventually increase to against-gravity strengthening remaining below 90° (Boissonnault et al., 2007; Butler, 2007; Ghodadra et al., 2009). Later, light ADL above shoulder level can be emphasized (if there is no hiking of the scapula), including cooking and folding laundry.

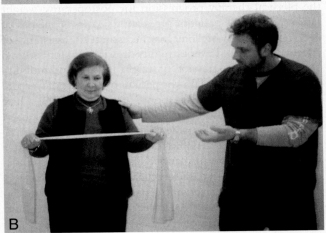

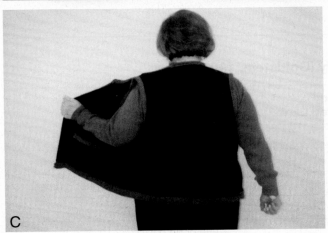

Figure 36-9 Progression of strengthening program. **A.** Isometric resistance to external rotation. **B.** Isotonic resistance to external rotation. **C.** Functional activity that incorporates external rotation.

At 12 weeks, the patient can begin resistive occupation-based tasks. Again, the long-term goal is to return the patient to normal pain-free occupational functioning.

Following repairs of large and massive tears of the rotator cuff, the client is immobilized in an abduction brace (O'Brien, Leggin, & Williams, 2011). ROM begins with pendulum exercises only. ROM restrictions vary depending on the surgeon's protocol. Some clients begin PROM within the first week, and others begin 6 weeks following surgery. The preparatory (exercise and ice) and purposeful activities are the same as for a small and medium tear, but the time frame of when they start are delayed. Time frames are determined by the surgeon. The treatment protocols given here are only guidelines; communication with the surgeon should be ongoing throughout the patient's rehabilitation.

HIP FRACTURES

Intertrochanteric hip fractures and femoral neck fractures are the most common fractures in adults older than 50 years of age (Altizer, 2005; Lareau & Sawyer, 2010). These fractures occur in bone that is markedly weakened by osteoporosis (Salter, 1999). Many of these patients have comorbidities, including congestive heart failure, coronary artery disease, hypertension, chronic obstructive pulmonary disease, or diabetes, that affect the duration and potential of the rehabilitation program (Altizer, 2005).

Hip fractures can be treated with closed reduction, which includes bed rest, traction, or early mobilization. The large majority of hip fractures are treated with open reduction with internal fixation using pins, nails, screws and plate, or rods (Keenan & Waters, 2003; Lareau & Sawyer, 2010). Hemiarthroplasty is the treatment for some fractures of the neck and head of the femur. Hemiarthroplasty is a partial joint replacement in which the femoral head

and neck are replaced by a prosthesis composed of ceramic with a titanium stem component. After excision of the femoral head, the stem of the prosthesis is inserted distally into the medullary canal of the femur so that its head articulates with the normal acetabulum (Lareau & Sawyer, 2010). If destructive changes have taken place in both the femur and the acetabulum, a total hip arthroplasty (THA) is necessary (Keenan & Waters, 2003).

Occupational Therapy Following a Hip Fracture and Surgery

The restrictions for weight bearing and hip movement on the operated leg are directly related to the severity and location of the fracture, the surgical approach, the ability of the fixation device or prosthesis to withstand stress, the integrity of the bone, the weight of the patient, and the patient's cognitive status (Goldstein, 1999). The physical therapist teaches the patient to use a walker or crutches, depending on percentage of body weight allowed on the operated limb (Definition 36-2). The occupational therapist teaches the patient to complete ADL safely, corresponding to the medical orders and the physical therapy progression for postoperative weight bearing. For some patients, preexisting factors or the risk of dislodging the new hip joint may necessitate the assistance of another person for lower extremity dressing and for bathing.

The rate of progression of weight bearing and mobility is individually tailored for the patient by the rate of fracture healing and the patient's response (Goldstein, 1999). Close communication among the members of the rehabilitation team is imperative to provide the patient with the best quality of care and consistency in learning how to function after surgery. Essential to the planned discharge following a hospital stay of less than a week, which is common for most, is the therapist's evaluation of the patient's ability to perform basic and instrumental ADL safely and independently and

 ## Definition 36-2

Progression of Weight Bearing after Hip Surgery (Goldstein, 1999)

Weight-Bearing Status	Percentage of Body Weight on Operated Limb	Ambulatory Device
Non–weight bearing	0	Walker (standard or rolling) or crutches
Touchdown weight bearing	10–15	Walker (standard or rolling) or crutches
Partial weight bearing	30	Walker (standard or rolling) or crutches
50% weight bearing	50	Cane
Full weight bearing	75–100	Cane or no device

From Goldstein, T. S. (1999). Geriatric orthopaedics: Rehabilitative management of common problems (2nd ed.). Gaithersburg, MD: Aspen.

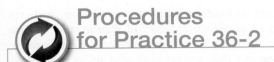

Procedures for Practice 36-2

Adaptations for Activities of Daily Living after Hip Replacement Surgery

Problem	Adaptation
Bathe feet	Long-handled bath sponge
Get in and out of tub	Nonskid bath mat; grab bar; tub bench
Don, doff shoes	Extended-handled shoehorn (medial side for posterior surgical approach and lateral for the anterior approach); elastic laces
Don, doff socks	Sock aide
Don pants	Reacher or dressing stick
Transfer to and from toilet, tub, and bed	Raised toilet seat, increased height of chair and bed
Sit in and rise from a chair	Wedge cushion with thick end of the wedge at the back of the chair
Open and close cabinets	Relocate frequently used items to eliminate the need to bend; use a reacher

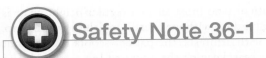

Safety Note 36-1

Movement Restrictions after Hip Surgery

- No hip flexion beyond 90°, including movement of the trunk over the thighs
- No hip rotation (avoid internal rotation for posterolateral approach and external rotation for anterolateral approach)
- No crossing the operated leg over the unoperated leg
- No adduction of the operated leg

the need for adapted equipment and/or assistance of others (Bargar, Bauer, & Borner, 1998; Sandell, 2008).

It is best to teach the patient who is restricted to non–weight bearing or touchdown weight bearing to sit to perform ADL to conserve energy and increase safety. Once the patient can do partial weight bearing, he or she can safely stand while grooming. For at least 6 weeks, and for some patients longer, movement is restricted. Because these restrictions preclude bending over or bringing the foot closer to the hands, adaptations (Procedures for Practice 36-2) are required to resolve problems in bathing, dressing, functional mobility, and home management.

Safety Message: The patient must be reminded that the operated hip is not to be flexed actively or passively or the leg adducted beyond the midline (Safety Note 36-1). Long-handled dressing and grooming devices are provided, and the therapist teaches the patient to bathe and dress the operated side using these devices to avoid bending over (flexion) or crossing the operated leg (adduction). For bathing, if permitted, some patients shower standing and require a grab assist bar and nonskid bath mat in the tub area for safety. Others prefer to sit to conserve energy or feel secure, and they require a bath bench. The bath bench must be high enough so the hip does not flex more than 80°–90°. These patients also require a nonskid bath mat and grab assist rail. Procedures for Practice 36-3 describes the procedure to get into and out of a bathtub after hip surgery.

To reduce hip flexion during sitting and rising, the patient is instructed to use a raised toilet seat, bed, and chair. Bed and chair heights are raised by putting wooden blocks under the legs. To increase mattress and chair cushion firmness to prevent passive hip flexion, plywood is inserted between the mattress and box spring or between the chair cushion and its frame. The patient is encouraged to sit in a reclined position enhanced by a wedge cushion or a small rolled pillow or towel at the junction of the chair's seat and back, as originally described by McKee (1975).

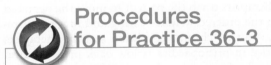

Procedures for Practice 36-3

Transferring into and out of a Bathtub after Hip Surgery

To get into the bathtub:

1. Stand with feet parallel to the tub with the operated leg next to the bathtub.
2. Shift body weight to unoperated leg.
3. Hold onto a grab assist rail for support.
4. Position the operated leg into hip extension and knee flexion; then abduct the hip to allow the leg to go over the edge of the bathtub.
5. Extend the knee on the operated side once the leg is over the tub edge.
6. Place the foot on the nonskid bath mat inside the tub.
7. When balance is secure, transfer the body weight to the operated leg.
8. Lift the unoperated leg over the edge of the tub and place the foot on the bath mat.

To get out of the bathtub:

1. Position self so feet are parallel to the side of the tub and the operated leg leads (goes out of the tub first).
2. Use the same procedure as for getting into the tub.

The patient who must sit in a regular-height chair is taught to stand up without overflexing the operated hip. In a chair with armrests, the patient scoots to the front edge of the seat, keeping the operated hip extended, and uses the armrests to push straight up without bending the trunk forward. In a chair without armrests, the patient moves to the side of the chair so that the operated thigh is over the edge with the foot placed at the midline of the chair. This places the operated hip in extension, puts the foot close to the center of gravity, and enables the person to gain momentum to stand without excessive hip flexion. With this technique, the unoperated hip, knee, and ankle are in position for weight bearing.

By 6 weeks, almost all patients walk with a cane, and some walk unassisted; most can return to driving a car, swimming, and work (Goldstein, 1999). Physical restrictions against bending to put on shoes or socks, sleeping on the operated side, and using a regular-height toilet seat are often lifted 8–12 weeks after surgery.

CHRONIC CONDITIONS

Some orthopaedic conditions are chronic. One is progressive hip pain from degenerative disease. When that pain interferes with activities and tasks of daily life despite medication, rest, reduction in lower extremity loading by the use of a cane, walker, or crutches, and physical therapy, hip surgery is indicated (Salter, 1999). After hip replacement surgery, therapists teach the patient to move the operated leg within the ordered weight-bearing and movement restrictions. Another chronic condition seen by therapists who practice in orthopaedics is low back pain. Medical costs for low back pain range between $20 and $50 billion annually (Hu et al., 2006). This section discusses occupational therapy both after hip replacement surgery and to relieve low back pain to enable occupational performance.

Occupational Therapy after Elective Hip Surgery Resulting from Disease

A number of surgical procedures are used for reduction of hip pain. They include osteotomy; arthrodesis, or hip fusion; hip resurfacing; and partial or total hip arthroplasty. To select the procedure, the orthopaedic surgeon considers not only the patient's age and physical status but also his or her occupational requirements and lifestyle.

Osteotomy is a procedure to correct the alignment of the femur to relieve weight bearing on the hip joint. When the osteotomy is done, compression plates stabilize the bone, and the patient can begin early postoperative mobilization with passive movement. Only partial weight bearing on the operated leg using crutches is allowed for 6 months, until the bone is healed. Osteotomies are not the treatment of choice for treating hip pain as a result of arthritis (Namba, Skinner, & Gupta, 2006).

Hip joint arthrodesis fuses the acetabulum with the femoral head at about 25°–30° of flexion and in neutral abduction and rotation. Arthrodesis is considered for patients younger than age 60 years who are in good physical condition and who have only one painful hip. It is not as common as other hip surgeries. A candidate for arthrodesis is a person who is not a candidate for a prosthetic hip implant because of heavy physical demands at work or recreational pursuits that are beyond the tolerances of an implant. This is also considered a salvage procedure for those whose prosthetic hip implant has failed. The patient is mobilized a week after the hip fusion and is allowed gradual weight bearing up to full weight in 2 months. Some patients do use a cane for a long time after surgery. The patient requires long-handled devices to assist with reaching the feet during bathing and dressing because of early postoperative flexion restrictions. In 6 months, when complete healing is established, the patient may be able to put on a sock and shoe when seated by flexing the knee to the side of the chair and reaching behind, using touch without visual guidance. The arthrodesis does leave the patient with a residual disability, but the hip is strong, stable, and pain free, and the patient has adequate endurance for everyday activities including work.

A THA surgically replaces the entire hip joint destroyed by disease or trauma. The main benefit of hip replacement is to resolve arthritic pain. Joint replacement surgery can also restore the length of the limb and its alignment, which has the potential to improve ROM and function (Drake, Ace, & Maale, 2002). This surgery replaces the arthritic acetabular cup with a titanium cup and polyethylene plastic liner. The femoral head is replaced with a femoral head implant made of ceramic and a titanium stem component.

The surgical approach to perform the THA varies among surgeons. The most common is the posterolateral approach (Youm, Maurer, & Stuchin, 2005). With this approach, there is no disruption to the gluteus medius and minimus muscles, and therefore, hip abduction is not compromised. The risk of the posterolateral approach is posterior dislocation. To avoid dislocation, immediately following surgery the patient is placed in an abduction pillow. Some surgeons also opt to place the ipsilateral knee in a knee immobilizer to further decrease the risk of dislocation. The patient is instructed to avoid hip flexion beyond 90°, adduction, and internal rotation. The second most common approach is the anterolateral approach (Youm, Maurer, & Stuchin, 2005). Although this approach decreases the risk for posterior dislocation and does not require an abduction pillow, the surgery requires division of the gluteus medius and minimus muscles and could disrupt the superior gluteal nerve, which leads to hip abductor weakness (Bertin & Rottinger, 2004). This weakness can result in a limp. The patient is instructed to avoid flexion beyond 90°, adduction, and internal and external rotation greater than 45° (Peak et al., 2005).

Another decision the surgeon must make when performing a THA is what type of implant fixation he or she will use. The choices are cemented, cementless, or hybrid prostheses (Namba, Skinner, & Gupta, 2006). The cemented total replacement usually requires 4–6 weeks of weight bearing to tolerance (WBTT) using a standard or rolling walker, and then the patient progresses to a straight cane. The cementless prosthesis, which depends on ingrowth of porous bone for stability, requires 6–12 weeks of partial weight bearing before a cane is used. Some surgeons may initially order non–weight bearing. In the case of the hybrid prosthesis, in which the femoral portion is cemented and the acetabulum is uncemented, 4–6 weeks of partial weight bearing precedes introduction of a cane (Youm, Maurer, & Stuchin, 2005).

Preoperative education should be the first phase of occupational therapy for the patient receiving a THA. Hip precautions, demonstration of long-handled equipment, and medically necessary durable medical equipment should be presented. Preoperative education has been linked to reducing anxiety (Spalding, 2003). The first 2 months after THA is critical for protection and function of the new hip joint. The postsurgical program is designed to allow for healing of the trochanter and soft tissues and for development of a capsule around the joint for future stability. *Safety Message: Until soft tissue is healed, hip flexion beyond 90°, hip adduction, and hip rotation (internal rotation for posterolateral approach and external rotation for anterolateral approach) are avoided.* The extremes of these movements during the first 2 months can dislocate the prosthesis. If dislocation occurs, the hip must be treated with closed reduction or be surgically realigned. The patient may be placed in a hip spica cast or knee immobilizer, delaying rehabilitation (Best, 2005). To protect the prosthesis, the occupational therapist instructs the patient in adaptive procedures and in methods to modify the environment to allow for safe performance of ADL and homemaking (Definition 36-2). The techniques used to help the patient following a THA parallel those described earlier: hip flexion and adduction are discouraged, limit hip rotation, and weight-bearing guidelines are carefully adhered to. Rehabilitation starts as early as 2 days after surgery.

For the client status post posterolateral approach, a foam abduction wedge is used with the patient lying down or sitting to encourage hip abduction. Once the patient achieves 55° of hip flexion in physical therapy, the patient can sit reclined on a raised chair using a rolled pillow or wedge cushion between the seat and the back of the chair and a foam abduction wedge between the legs. The patient learns to transfer from supine to standing without flexing the operated hip beyond 90° by keeping the knees apart (hips abducted) and sliding out of a raised bed to take weight on the unoperated leg. Some patients use an overhead trapeze bar to assist this transfer. The patient also needs to practice transferring from a variety of surfaces such as high chair (Fig. 36-10, A–C), tub bench, raised toilet seat, and a car seat.

The patient with a cemented or hybrid total hip prosthesis usually begins partial weight bearing with a walker

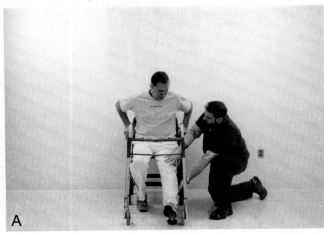

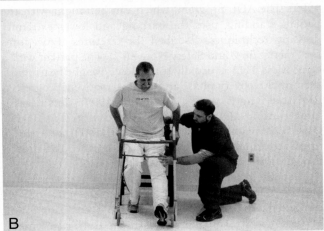

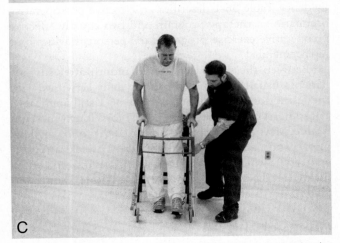

Figure 36-10 Sit-to-stand transfer for a patient with non–weight-bearing status post total hip arthroplasty (THA). **A.** Extends knee and pushes off arms of chair. **B.** Avoids flexing hip past 90° while pushing off. **C.** Maintains non–weight-bearing status when standing.

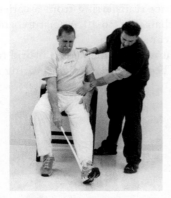

Figure 36-11 Removing shoe status post total hip arthroplasty (THA). Approach medial aspect of shoe with long-handled shoe horn to prevent internal rotation if surgery used a posterolateral approach.

or crutches immediately after surgery. In some instances, these patients can withstand full weight bearing within the first 3 days; however, many orthopaedic surgeons wait 3 weeks before ordering full weight bearing (Goldstein, 1999). The ADL program, which can be taught with the patient standing, uses the bathing and lower extremity dressing techniques described for fractures (Procedures for Practice 36-2 and Safety Note 36-1). The patient with a cementless THA is usually touchdown weight bearing for the initial recovery phase and is conservatively progressed to partial weight bearing (Goldstein, 1999). This necessitates learning ADL from the seated position (Fig. 36-11). Once 50% weight bearing is ordered, the ADL program is upgraded to allow for standing with a cane. The cane is used until the Trendelenburg gait disappears.

Usually, after a THA, patients do not receive outpatient therapy following inpatient rehabilitation, although many may receive home care occupational and physical therapy for safety assessment and/or treatment. Evidence Table 36-1 describes an effective postoperative occupational therapy program and two equally effective preoperative exercise programs for persons having joint replacement.

Between the second and third month after surgery, patients usually resume all routine daily activities, with the restrictions listed in Safety Note 36-1 still applicable. For some, this restriction may persist for a long time, even for life. Mayo Clinic has recommended the following low-impact sport activities permissible at >12 weeks after surgery: golf, swimming, cycling, bowling, sailing, and scuba diving (Healy, Iorio, & Lemos, 2001). Tennis, skiing, and jogging are discouraged.

Low Back Pain

Pain is defined as "An unpleasant sensory and emotional experience associated with actual or potential tissue damage, or described in terms of such damage" (International Association for the Study of Pain, 2012). Acute pain is proportional to the physical findings. It is often an indication that the patient has traumatized or damaged tissue. Physical and psychological responses to acute pain may include muscle guarding, anxiety, and increased pain behaviors (Healy, Iorio, & Lemos, 2001). Chronic pain is described as pain that extends beyond 3 months postinjury (International Association for the Study of Pain, 2012). Patients with chronic pain often become preoccupied with their symptoms, experience sleep deprivation, and have difficulties performing their ADL (Cieza et al., 2004).

Low back pain has been reported at one time or another by approximately 80% of the adult population (Hu et al., 2006; World Health Organization, 2003). Postural stress and disc degeneration are the most common causes of low back pain (Cohen, Argoff, & Carragee, 2008). Examples of postural stressors include poor sleeping and sitting postures, lifting or reaching with a rounded back, and prolonged standing or sitting (McKenzie, 2005). Other causes of back pain include spinal stenosis, vertebral fracture, tumor, infection, spondylolisthesis, and arthritis. Most episodes of low back pain are self-limiting; 90% of patients return to work within 6 weeks. However, 1% of patients have chronic pain and are out of work for more than 6 months (Hu et al., 2006).

The primary goal in medically managed back care is to prevent the patient from developing chronic pain that leads to occupational dysfunction. If pain is not alleviated, the objective findings of assessments done over time may have little or no association to a nociceptive stimulus. Chronic low back pain has become increasingly associated with psychological distress disorders and nonphysiological behaviors such as malingering or symptom magnification (in which one exaggerates the symptoms) and disease conviction or factitious disorder (convince self and others that the disease exists) (Manchikanti et al., 2003). This situation can be very difficult to treat and often requires a multidisciplinary approach.

The primary focus when treating patients with acute or chronic low back pain is to return them to work and to resumption of their daily activities as quickly as possible. All efforts should be made to prevent the development of chronic pain syndrome by adopting practices used in sports medicine treatment to calm the pain and relax the muscles. Bed rest is replaced with early application of physical therapy, a flexibility program, and active involvement in a graduated program of occupation-as-end. Studies have shown that exercise can significantly reduce sick leave in patients with low back pain (Kool et al., 2004). Because physical therapy helps the patient develop dynamic control of the lumbar spine through flexibility training, stretching, and ROM exercises, the occupational therapist directs the patient in performance of activities in a neutral lumbosacral position (the midpoint of available range between anterior and posterior pelvic tilt). The occupational

Evidence Table 36-1 — Best Evidence for Occupational Therapy Practice Regarding Hip Fracture

Intervention	Description of Intervention Tested	Participants	Dosage	Type of Best Evidence and Level of Evidence	Benefit	Statistical Probability and Effect Size of Outcome	Reference
Early postoperative individualized occupational therapy	Occupational therapy individual group: individual daily activities of daily living (ADL) and instrumental activities of daily living (IADL) training, including the use of technical aids plus one home visit. Control group: conventional care	One hundred patients aged ≥65 years having undergone surgery for hip fracture. All lived independently, and none used walking or technical aids prior to hospitalization (randomized to group). Ninety completed the study (10% attrition)	After the third to fourth postoperative day, the occupational therapy group received 45–60 minutes of individualized training (including technical aids) each weekday morning for 3–33 days. The control group received conventional care from the nursing staff for 3–23 days. All patients received instruction in walking with mobility aids.	Randomized controlled trial Level: IB1b	Yes. Occupational therapy sped up the ability of patients to perform ADLs, enhancing probability of discharge home. At discharge, the occupational therapy group had significantly better ability to dress, to toilet, personal hygiene, to take care of and to bathe independently compared with the control group. No other factors (e.g., age, sex, type of fracture, etc.) explained the outcome. After 2 months, all patients had regained independence.	Klein-Bell ADL Scale subtests: Dressing: $F_{(2,91)} = 79.0$, $p = 0.0001$, $r = 0.79.$[a] Toileting: $F_{(2,90)} = 5.97$, $p = 0.02$, $r = 0.34.$ Bathing/hygiene: $F_{(2,91)} = 17$, $p = 0.0001$, $r = 0.52.$ Mobility: $F_{(2,91)} = 2.20$, $p = 0.1$, $r = 0.21.$ Fifty-two percent of the occupational therapy group (only group evaluated) needed technical aids and adaptation of their homes. Preventative changes (remove loose rugs, etc.), were needed in 90% of the homes.	Hagsten, Svensson, & Gardulf (2004)
Preoperative land-based or pool-based exercise program	Each program included an education session, exercise classes (in pool or on land), a home exercise program, and an occupational therapy home assessment. The pool-based program included the benefits of buoyancy, hydrostatic pressure, and thermotherapy.	Patients (mean age = 70.3 years) waiting for total hip or knee replacement. Eighty-two subjects who (stratified by hip or knee replacement) were randomized to group: land n = 40; pool n = 42. 51 of the participants were females, and all but 8 were categorized as obese.	Both programs were conducted for 6 weeks and met two times per week. Each session lasted 1 hour.	Randomized controlled trial Level IB2b	Yes. Reduced pain and improved function was noted in both groups although there was no significant postintervention differences between land-based and pool-based programs. Participants in the pool-based program reported significantly ($p = 0.019$) less pain immediately following exercise.	The results indicated no significant difference for the main effect of group for the WOMAC[b] function ($F = 0.112$; $p = 0.739$) or the WOMAC pain ($F = 0.257$; $p = 0.614$) subscales. There were significant main effects for time (baseline to 7 weeks) of both function (land: $p = 0.000$; pool: $p = .016$) and pain (land: $p = 0.000$; pool: $p = 0.011$) measures. Baseline to week 15 assessment showed improvement in both groups for WOMAC function (land: $p = 0.012$; pool: $p = 0.045$), but only the land group for pain (land: $p = 0.015$; pool: $p = 0.431$).	Gill, McBarney, & Schutz (2009)

[a] r value was calculated from data reported, using a formula for F with $df_{numerator} > 1$. Effect size (r) is considered large if ≥0.50, medium if ≥0.30, and small if ≥0.10.

[b] The Western Ontario and McMaster Universities Arthritis Index (WOMAC).

therapist teaches the patient to understand, manage, and protect the low back by using proper body mechanics and alternative techniques to perform activities at home and at work (Sanders, 2004). As endurance training progresses in physical therapy, the occupational therapist upgrades the type and quantity of ADL and work-related task challenges. When return to usual and customary activities is imminent, the treatment addresses safety and prevention of recurrence.

Teaching patients about their back and body mechanics has been part of rehabilitation for many years. The multidisciplinary team usually consists of a physician, a physical therapist, an occupational therapist, and, in some instances, a social worker or psychologist. The philosophy is that education in anatomy, spine function, and proper body mechanics for daily living and leisure activities will help patients with low back pain take responsibility for long-term management of their back. Patients have reported that engagement in daily activities and being able to participate in social interactions is more of an indication of quality of life than the presence or absence of pain (Hush et al., 2009). The multidisciplinary approach to treating patients with low back pain can significantly reduce pain and improve occupational functioning (Guzman et al., 2001) (see Evidence Table 36-2).

Evaluation of the Patient with Low Back Pain

In the initial interview, the therapist asks about the pain history and pain reaction during activity. Patients are asked to describe their pain in relation to location, intensity (using a 0–10 pain scale), quality (the pain is sharp, throbbing, burning, etc.), and duration. Completion of an occupational profile will provide the therapist with information on what occupations are most meaningful to the client and how the client balances those activities throughout the day. In regard to the client's low back pain, additional questions may be needed to determine the person's extent of accommodation and methods for task completion. Observation of actual or simulated performance of tasks may be indicated to reveal the patient's functional limitations and decision-making process.

Treatment of the Patient with Low Back Pain

The occupational therapist facilitates the patient's active participation in tasks and activities by teaching body mechanics and how to perform activities safely. Based on research, effective therapies that may be included in the occupational therapy program include preparatory interventions such as hot packs, transcutaneous electrical nerve stimulation (TENS), stretching exercises, relaxation techniques for stress reduction, biofeedback for muscle control, and group educational sessions (Snodgrass, 2011). Body mechanics are taught relative to static and dynamic postures and transition patterns

(e.g., sit to stand, stand to stoop). The occupational therapist demonstrates body mechanics with commonly performed tasks to show the patient how to apply the principles to everyday tasks. The emphasis is on both cognitive and motor learning to develop the patient's understanding and ability to self-regulate motor activity safely. Therapeutic activity, including games, crafts, ADL, and work tasks, are selected for practice. Through feedback, the therapist guides the patient's performance during the activities and encourages development of self-regulation.

Body Mechanics

Good body mechanics entails practices to reduce the load or stresses on the spine in various positions or when moving objects. Compression and twisting of the spine are avoided, as are attempts to exert force in positions that poorly support the spine (Procedures for Practice 36-4). Suggestions for application of principles of body mechanics in various postures are as follows:

- While standing, for example to cook or wash dishes in the kitchen or to brush teeth at the bathroom sink, the patient places one foot on the shelf under the sink or on a low stool to achieve posterior pelvic tilt. This technique is used whenever prolonged standing is a requirement.
- To sit, the patient lowers the body by flexing the knees and hips without bending the spine. To do so, the patient places the hands on the chair's armrest, both to guide the descent and to provide support through the transition. A raised seat is recommended because it requires less muscle power, which reduces pain and stress on the back. A slightly reclined sitting posture is preferred for prolonged sitting. When seated to work at a table, the patient avoids bending over the work by moving the chair close to the work and raising or inclining the work surface as needed.
- When lying in bed, the ideal posture to decrease pressure on the spine is supine with the knees flexed. A pillow should be placed under the knees to maintain the flexed posture. Log roll to come to a seated position. For patients who sleep on their side, a pillow should be place between their legs with the knees slightly flexed.
- For tasks that ordinarily require excessive reaching and bending of the spine, such as sweeping, vacuuming, or raking, the patient is taught to move the body close to the task, that is, to walk with the broom or rake rather than reaching with it. For lifting objects from the floor, the choice of position depends on the size and weight of the object. To pick up a lightweight object, such as a newspaper, the patient faces the newspaper and lowers both knees in a semisquat (or a ballet position of plié) toward the floor while keeping the back straight and maintaining posterior pelvic tilt. When lifting a large or heavy object or a small child, the patient adds more central support by lowering one knee to the floor

Evidence Table 36-2   Best Evidence for Occupational Therapy Practice Regarding Pain Management

Intervention	Description of Intervention Tested	Participants	Dosage	Type of Best Evidence and Level of Evidence	Benefit	Statistical Probability and Effect Size of Outcome	Reference
Multidisciplinary pain management program	The program included physical, psychological, activity-based, and social interaction–based training and education. The team consisted of occupational therapist, psychologist, physician, physiotherapist, and social worker. Group-oriented program (eight to nine patients per group) but with individually tailored treatment for each patient.	One hundred eighty-eight patients with pain diagnoses (fibromyalgia, low back, whiplash, and myalgia). Males: 42; females: 146. Mean age = 41 years. Mean pain duration was 7.6 years for females and 5.8 years for males.	5–7 hours each session, once a week for 5 weeks	One-group, repeated-measures design Level: IIIA2a	Yes. There was significant improvement in occupational performance and performance satisfaction as measured by the Canadian Occupational Performance Measure (COPM); 30%–37% of patients increased two or more points on the COPM; 44%–56% increased more than one point in performance and satisfaction.	$p < 0.001$; insufficient data to allow calculation of the effect sizes	Persson, Rivano-Fischer, & Eklund (2004)

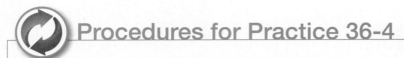

Procedures for Practice 36-4

Principles of Body Mechanics (Fig. 36-12, A–C)

The patient is taught to do the following:

- Incorporate a pelvic tilt during static sitting or standing to unload the facet joints, aid in pelvic awareness, and decrease muscular tension in the low back.
- Position the body close to and facing the task. This aids in balance by getting the objects as close to the center of gravity as possible. Objects held away from the body require increased force of all muscles to lift or hold them. Getting closer also helps to avoid twisting or bending the spine.
- Avoid twisting. Twisting causes stress on the ligaments and small muscles of the spine. Instead, turn the body by stepping with both legs to face the activity.
- Use the hip flexors and extensors to lower and raise the body. These are large muscles with leverage and power to handle heavy loads. The joints and muscles of the spine are much smaller, with less leverage and power.

- Avoid prolonged repetitive activity or static positions. Take microbreaks and walk briefly or stretch every hour.
- Balance activity with rest to facilitate endurance and safety. Incorporate rest periods into the course of a particular activity or alternate between two work patterns that challenge different muscle groups.
- Use a wide base of support. Stability while lifting is increased when the feet are at least hip distance apart. One foot slightly in front of the other provides additional support.
- Keep the back in proper alignment, ear over shoulder, shoulder over hips, and hips over knees and feet to maintain the natural curves of the back. Practice in front of a mirror.
- Test a load before lifting to decide whether the lift should be modified. Describe how to modify the lift: get help, split the load into more than one lift, or put the object on wheels.
- Stay physically fit. Strong muscles and flexible joints are the best defense against injury or recurrence of an injury.

(half-kneeling) so that the body is close to and facing the object. The goal is to bring and keep the weighted mass as close to the body's center of gravity as possible. A small child is encouraged to climb up into the lap. Once the object or child is grasped securely, the knee on the floor helps push the body up, and then both legs extend to lift the weight. The patient should be

instructed to lift to an intermediate height, such as a chair, if possible, rest briefly, and then lift to carry.
- The patient is taught to carry light, well-balanced loads of laundry, groceries, and parcels close to the body. Infants are best transported in a front or back baby carrier or a stroller. Through practice sessions, the patient learns his or her safe load tolerances over given distances and time.

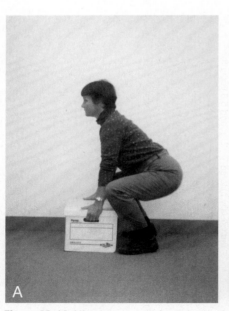 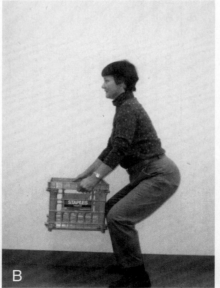 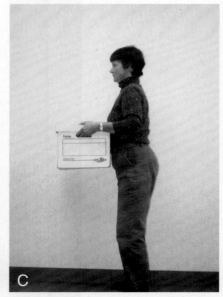

Figure 36-12 Lift using proper body mechanics. **A.** Move close to object being lifted. **B.** Lift with legs and maintain lumbar curve. **C.** Maintain lumbar curve throughout lifting activity.

It is important that practice employ common items, such as half a gallon of milk, which weighs 4 pounds, or a gallon of bottled water, which weighs 8 pounds.

Complementary and Alternative Medicine for Treating Pain

Complementary and alternative medicines (CAMs) are becoming more accepted as we attempt to move beyond our traditional forms of therapy toward more holistic approaches to addressing pain. Yoga is commonly used to treat arthritis, low back pain, and upper extremity conditions. Yoga combines alignment of posture, stretching, proper breathing, and relaxation. Several studies have shown yoga to be effective in treating pain; however, these studies did not address adverse effects that might occur as a result of using Yoga (Posadzski et al., 2011). Mindfulness meditation combines deep relaxation, meditation, and gentle exercise as an approach to manage pain and stress. Preliminary research on mindfulness meditation has shown promising results in the area of improved pain,

improved sleep, and improved quality of life (Morone et al., 2008). Participating in a 30-minute mindfulness meditation program 4–5 days a week has been shown to improve pain levels of clients diagnosed with chronic low back pain (Morone, Greco, & Weiner, 2008). Tai Chi is another complementary therapy that has been used by occupational therapists. The primary features of Tai Chi are slow sequential movements with a straight spine, proper abdominal breathing and different styles of pushing hands. Research on Tai Chi has found improved pain levels during ADL for clients diagnosed with fibromyalgia, osteoarthritis, and rheumatoid arthritis. Tai Chi is especially effective with improving lower extremity balance, strength and pain (Field, 2011). Therapists using CAMs in occupational therapy should demonstrate competency and be aware of licensure laws in regard to their use (American Occupational Therapy Association, 2011). Occupational therapists who are not specialized should consider referring their clients to other trained professionals to receive therapies such as acupuncture, Ayurveda, energy healing, and massage therapy.

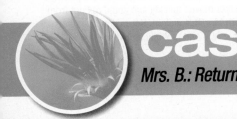

case example

Mrs. B.: Returning to Homemaking and Volunteer Roles after Total Hip Replacement

Occupational Therapy Process	Clinical Reasoning Process	
	Objectives	Examples of Therapist's Internal Dialogue
Patient Information	Understand the patient's diagnosis or condition	"Most patients who are status post cemented total hip replacement (s/p THR) can begin weight bearing as tolerated, and so I am hopeful that Mrs. B. will be given the same weight-bearing orders. The surgeon performed the total hip replacement using a posterior lateral approach, so precautions must be taken to avoid dislocation."
Mrs. B. is a 72-year-old married female who fell on ice 3 days ago when she walked from her house to her car. She was admitted to the hospital on the same day with a diagnosis of a right intertrochanteric hip fracture. Because of the severity of the hip fracture, Mrs. B. required surgical intervention the same day. She received a cemented total hip replacement. Mrs. B. anticipates returning home to be with her husband and eventually resuming her homemaking and volunteer roles.	Understand postsurgical precautions	
	Know the person	"Mrs. B. has a history of osteoarthritis in both hips; however, she has been able to manage the pain with Advil®."
	Know the environment that she will be discharged to	"Mrs. B. obviously values her home life and being active in the community."

Reason for Referral to Occupational Therapy

Mrs. B. was referred to occupational therapy for the duration of her acute-care postoperative hospital stay, approximately 3 days, to learn how to move safely while adhering to hip precautions, to practice transferring, and to begin to resume personal activities of daily living (ADL). She was also referred to physical therapy.

Appreciate the context	"Mrs. B. will have to follow the hospital's total hip replacement critical pathway, which allows a 3-day stay. I am glad she was referred to physical therapy, as we will be able to coordinate our services as well as cotreat during some of our sessions. I anticipate at the end of her 3-day stay that Mrs. B. will have improved occupational functioning by understanding hip precautions and practicing with long-handled equipment. The cotreatments with physical therapy will help to improve her confidence and ability to transfer."
Develop provisional hypotheses	

Assessment Process and Results

- The evaluation began with an occupational profile. Mrs. B. reports that she lives with her husband in a one-story ranch-style home. There are four steps to enter her home. The bathroom has a combined tub and shower. She reports her husband is retired and very supportive. She enjoys cooking for her husband and children.
- Bed mobility and transfers were assessed. Mrs. B. required minimal assistance for bed mobility and contact guard (CG) with verbal cues for tub and toilet transfer (using standard walker).
- Self-care: Dressing: hip precautions were reviewed, and use of long-handled adaptive equipment was demonstrated prior to the assessment. Mrs. B. was independent with upper body dressing but required moderate assistance for lower body dressing. Mrs. B. required constant verbal cueing on hip precautions during dressing assessment. Bathing: Mrs. B. is independent (I) in sponge bathing (bedside) her upper body but requires moderate assistance bathing her lower body (with aid of long-handled sponge).
- Upper extremity ROM: AROM is within functional limits (WFLs) throughout both upper extremities.
- Manual Muscle Test (MMT): 4 out of 5 muscle strength throughout both upper extremities.
- Pain (scale 0–10): Mrs. B. reported a 7 out of 10 for her right hip. Mrs. B. reports her pain is constant and interferes with her sleep and any movements she has been requested to do by nursing.

Consider evaluation approach and methods	"Because of the orthopaedic nature of Mrs. B.'s injuries, an approach that focused on her impaired performance skills and patterns was used to assess her impaired abilities and capabilities."
Interpret observations	"Pain was reported throughout the entire evaluation, which I was concerned might interfere with her progress. I contacted the patient's surgeon, and pain medications will be increased and administered to coordinate with occupational and physical therapy treatment sessions. ROM and muscle strength of both upper extremities were assessed to determine their ability to assist with transfers. I spoke with the physical therapist, and we agreed to start her with a standard walker because she has a history of falls. Although many clients use rolling walkers s/p THR, a rolling walker moves quickly and could roll out from underneath Mrs. B.'s weight. Her major limitations are with her ADL and mobility activities."

Occupational Therapy Problem List

- Pain that interferes with sleep and movement
- Impaired ADL status
- Unsafe transfers and mobility because of total hip replacement (THR)
- THR restrictions

Synthesize results	"Mrs. B. has the typical problems one faces following a THR."

Occupational Therapy Goal List

1. Mrs. B. will have a pain level of 3 out of 10 during all self-care activities.
2. Mrs. B. will be able to transfer to and from a chair, bed, tub bench, and toilet while adhering to the hip precautions.
3. Mrs. B. will demonstrate how to use long-handled equipment to independently perform functional tasks in the kitchen, bedroom, and bathroom while adhering to hip precautions.

Develop intervention hypotheses	"I feel Mrs. B. will have improved occupational performance by learning total hip replacement precautions. The structured daily therapy will also build her confidence for performing mobility and transfer tasks."
Select an intervention approach	"The OT intervention will use a combined compensatory/adaptation approach and restore/remediate approach."
Consider what will occur in therapy, how often, and for how long	"Following the critical pathway, Mrs. B. will have three individualized treatments from OT during her inpatient stay. An additional three cotreatments with physical therapy will be added to address mobility and transfers."

Intervention

Mrs. B. participated in six treatments over a 3-day inpatient stay. Her pain medication was coordinated with OT visits. Both the occupational therapist and physical therapist taught Mrs. B. postures and movements that would be safe for her operated hip during transfers, sitting, standing, lying in bed, and bending and reaching during ADL and instrumental activities of daily living (IADL). Transfers were performed using a standard walker. She practiced with long-handled equipment while adhering to hip precautions. Tasks or components of tasks that she could not complete satisfactorily were identified. Mr. B. attended all of the occupational therapy sessions with his wife, and he agreed to assist his wife with those activities identified as being difficult for Mrs. B. The therapist taught Mrs. B. energy conservation techniques to be used during ADL and IADL. Mrs. B. was given a written and illustrated brochure concerning restrictions related to ADL. The therapist determined that Mrs. B.'s husband, with the assistance of a home health aide, could provide the necessary care for ADL and IADL that she could not manage because of hip precautions. Therefore, the recommendation was to discharge her home rather than to a skilled nursing facility.

Next Steps

- Discharge to home with assistance of home health aide.
- Recommend home care occupational therapy.

Compare actual to expected performance	"Mrs. B. made significant improvement in her occupational performance with intensive therapy that used a team approach and family support."
Anticipate present and future patient concerns	"Mrs. B. is a highly motivated individual who will benefit from home care OT to further maximize her occupational performance. She understands the importance of her home program as well as continuing with structured supervised OT. I feel confident that, in 6 months, Mrs. B. will be successfully participating in those occupational roles that she identified as valuable in her life (wife, homemaker, and volunteer)."
Decide whether the patient should continue or discontinue therapy and/or return in the future	

Clinical Reasoning in Occupational Therapy Practice

Selecting Treatments for In-Home Therapy

Following Mrs. B.'s discharge to home, she is followed up with home care services. Based on her occupational profile, taken while she was an inpatient, knowledge of Mrs. B.'s surgical history, recovery history, and therapy experience and progress while hospitalized, what interventions might you select to enable pursuit of valued occupations and to assure adherence to hip surgery precautions if you were Mrs. B.'s in-home therapist?

Comprehension of Precautions

During the second occupational therapy session, you discuss her success in using the long-handled equipment issued to her in the hospital. Mrs. B. tells you that she is having her husband help until she is able to "bend over to dress herself without pain." How would you proceed with further treatment?

Summary Review Questions

1. What are the unwanted side effects of immobilization of any fracture?
2. How would you direct your patient to prevent adverse side effects of prolonged immobilization?
3. What is a major treatment goal for any patient with an upper extremity fracture?
4. Why is passive motion not used in the treatment of fractures of the elbow?
5. What are the guiding principles for advancing a patient in the aftercare therapy program following orthopaedic surgery?
6. What is clinical union, and why is it significant in terms of the therapy program?
7. Why are isometric contractions across the fracture site encouraged?
8. What type of activity modifications would you recommend to a client who is diagnosed with rotator cuff tendonitis?
9. Describe the type of preparatory interventions that can be performed at 6, 8, and 12 weeks post–rotator cuff repair surgery.
10. Describe the type of occupation-based activities that can be performed at 6, 8, and 12 weeks post–rotator cuff repair surgery.
11. What is the occupational therapist's role for the patient who underwent hip replacement surgery after a fractured hip?
12. After a hip fracture or total hip joint arthroplasty, the therapist directs the patient to perform occupational performance tasks safely. What specific tasks may threaten the integrity of the surgical procedure? Why?
13. List precautions that must be taught to a patient with a total hip arthroplasty (posterolateral and anterolateral approaches).
14. Describe how lower extremity dressing should be taught to a patient with low back pain, using all applicable body mechanics principles. Do the same for the tasks of sweeping the floor and working at a computer.

Glossary

Abduction pillow brace—A sling or brace that positions the shoulder in 30°–45° of abduction to protect the repaired supraspinatus.

Clinical union—Evidence of bony callus on radiographic examination, although the fracture line is still apparent (Salter, 1999).

Codman's pendulum exercises—Exercises prescribed for most shoulder surgeries in early recovery. The standing or sitting client bends over at the hips so that the trunk is parallel to the floor. The arm assumes a position away from the body and perpendicular to the floor, either with or without a sling. In this gravity-assisted position, the client moves the arm passively or actively, depending on the surgical protocol, forward into humeral flexion and backward into humeral extension; across and away from the body for shoulder abduction and adduction; and then in a circle for circumduction (Salter, 1999).

Controlled range of motion—Active or passive movement within a predetermined safe arc. Often, the allowed movement begins in the middle of the range and is gradually upgraded toward the full arc as healing occurs. A splint can be used to set the boundaries or block unwanted movement.

Deep pressure tissue massage—Firm manual pressure applied to the skin for about 5 seconds to blanch the underlying scar. This massage is initiated once sutures are removed. On a closed wound, lanolin or vitamin E can be used. Massage begins at the perimeter and gradually works toward and then over the surgical scar site.

Factitious disorder—A dysfunctional condition, one in which the person acts out an illness that they do not have.

Scapular plane—Scapular plane refers to the midpoint between shoulder flexion and abduction. The majority of functional activities occur in this plane.

Shoulder immobilizer—Used if strict immobilization is required. Adjustable elastic band that fits around the waist with two straps that position and secure the arm in a slightly abducted and internally rotated position.

Thera-band®—Exercise bands that come in various levels of resistance (denoted by eight different colors ranging from extra thin [tan] to maximum [gold]) used to improve strength. The most commonly used bands are red (2.7 pounds of force at 100% elongation), green (3.1 pounds), and blue (4.5 pounds).

Trendelenburg gait—Gait pattern that results from a weakened gluteus medius muscle. The client lurches toward the injured side to place the center of gravity over the hip. It is characterized by dropping of the pelvis on the unaffected side at heel strike of the affected foot.

Volkmann's ischemia—Increased compartment pressure in one anatomic area of the extremity as a result of a fracture or crush injury. In the upper extremity, it is most common in the forearm. Increased pressure results in closure of the small vessels. The client will experience severe pain, especially with passive stretching. Pressure greater than 30 mm Hg is considered a surgical emergency in which a fasciotomy would be performed (Bednar & Light, 2006).

Wall climbing, finger walking, palm gliding—Exercise to develop shoulder flexion. The client faces the wall, places the injured shoulder's hand on the wall, and either finger walks or glides the palm toward the ceiling and then the floor. For shoulder and scapular abduction, the client turns slightly away from the wall and abducts the shoulder in the plane of the scapula by placing the fingers or palm on the wall for finger walking or palm gliding. Commercially available finger climbers can be mounted on the wall or used on a tabletop with set increments for the finger walk; some climbers can be adjusted to different angles to allow for varying degrees of movement.

References

Agorastides, I., Sinopidis, C., El Meligy, M., Yin, Q., Brownson, P., & Frostick, S. P. (2007). Early versus late mobilization after hemiarthroplasty for proximal humerus fractures. *Journal of Shoulder and Elbow Surgery, 16,* S33–S38

Altizer, L. (2005). Hip fractures. *Orthopaedic Nursing, 24,* 283–292.

American Academy of Orthopaedic Surgeons. (2008). *The burden of musculoskeletal diseases in the United States: Prevalence, societal and economic cost.* Rosemont, IL: United States Bone and Joint Decade.

American Occupational Therapy Association. (2011). Complementary and alternative medicine [Position Paper]. *American Journal of Occupational Therapy, 65(Suppl.),* S26–S31.

Bargar, W. L., Bauer, A., & Borner, M. (1998). Primary and revision total hip replacement using the Robodoc system. *Clinical Orthopaedics and Related Research, 354,* 82–91.

Basti, J. J., Dionysian, E., Sherman, P. W., & Bigliani, L. U. (1994). Management of proximal humeral fractures. *Journal of Hand Therapy, 7,* 111–121.

Bednar, M. S., & Light, T. R. (2006). Hand surgery. In H. B. Skinner (Ed.), *Current diagnosis and treatment in orthopedics* (4th ed., pp. 568–569). New York: Lange Medical Books/McGraw-Hill.

Beredjiklian, P. K. (2011). Management of fractures and dislocations of the elbow. In T. M. Skirven, A. L. Osterman, J. M. Fedorczyk, & P. C. Amadio (Eds.), *Rehabilitation of the hand and upper extremity* (6th ed., pp. 1049–1060). Philadelphia: Elsevier Mosby.

Bertin, K. C., & Rottinger, H. (2004). Anterolateral mini-incision replacement surgery: A modified Watson-Jones approach. *Clinical Orthopedic Related Research, 429,* 248–255.

Best, J. T. (2005). Revision total hip and total knee arthroplasty. *Orthopaedic Nursing, 24,* 174–179.

Boissonnault, W. G., Badke, M. B., Wooden, M. J., Ekedahl, S., & Fly, K. (2007). Patient outcomes following rehabilitation for rotator cuff repair surgery: The impact of selected medical conditions. *Journal of Orthopaedic and Sports Physical Therapy, 37,* 312–319.

Butler, M. (2007). Common shoulder diagnoses. In C. Cooper (Ed.), *Fundamentals of hand therapy: Clinical reasoning and treatment guidelines for common diagnoses of the upper extremity* (pp. 150–182). St. Louis: Mosby Elsevier.

Cieza, A., Stucki, G., Weigl, M., Kullmann, L., Stoll, T., Kamen, L., Kostanjsek, N., & Walsh, N. (2004). ICF core sets for chronic widespread pain. *Journal of Rehabilitation Medicine, 44,* 63–68.

Cohen, S. P., Argoff, C. E., & Carragee, E. J. (2008). Management of low back pain. *British Medical Journal, 337,* a2718.

Colditz, J. C. (2011). Functional fracture bracing. In T. M. Skirven, A. L. Osterman, J. M. Fedorczyk, & P. C. Amadio (Eds.), *Rehabilitation of the hand and upper extremity* (6th ed., pp. 1061–1074). Philadelphia: Elsevier Mosby.

Davila, S. A. (2011). Therapist's management of fractures and dislocations of the elbow. In T. M. Skirven, A. L. Osterman, J. M. Fedorczyk, & P. C. Amadio (Eds.), *Rehabilitation of the hand and upper extremity* (6th ed., pp. 1061–1074). Philadelphia: Elsevier Mosby.

Dixon, D., Johnston, M., McQueen, M., & Court-Brown, C. (2008). The Disabilities of the Arm, Shoulder and Hand Questionnaire (DASH) can measure the impairment, activity limitations and participation restriction constructs from the International Classification of Functioning, Disability and Health (ICF). *BMC Musculoskeletal Disorders, 20,* 114–119.

Drake, C., Ace, M., & Maale, G. E. (2002). Revision total hip arthroplasty. *AORN Journal, 76,* 414–428.

Drummond, A. S., Sampaio, R. F., Mancini, M. C., Kirkwood, R. N., & Stamm, T. A. (2007). Linking the disabilities of arm, shoulder, and hand to the international classification of functioning, disability, and health. *Journal of Hand Therapy, 20,* 336–344

Field, T. (2011). Tai Chi research review. *Complementary Therapies in Clinical Practice, 17,* 141–146

Gallinet, D., Clappaz, P., Garbuio, P., Tropet, Y., & Obert, L. (2009). Three or four part complex proximal humerus fractures: Hemiarthroplasty versus reverse prosthesis: A comparative study of 40 cases. *Orthopaedic & Traumatology: Surgery and Research, 95,* 48–55.

Garrigues, G. E., Johnston, P. S., Pepe, M. D., Tucker, B. S., Ramsey, M. L., & Austin, L. S. (2012). Hemiarthroplasty versus reverse total shoulder arthroplasty for acute proximal humerus fractures in elderly patients. *Orthopedics, 35,* e703–e708.

Ghodadra, N. S., Provencher, M. T., Verma, N. N., Wilk, K. E., & Romeo, A. A. (2009). Open, mini-open, and all arthropscopic rotator cuff repair surgery: Indicators and implications for rehabilitation. *Journal of Orthopaedic & Sports Physical Therapy, 39,* 81–89.

Gill, S. D., McBarney, H., & Schutz, D. (2009). Land-based versus pool-based exercise for people awaiting joint replacement surgery of the hip or knee: Results of a randomized controlled trial. *Archives of Physical Medicine and Rehabilitation, 90,* 388–394.

Goldstein, T. S. (1999). *Geriatric orthopaedics: Rehabilitative management of common problems* (2nd ed.). Gaithersburg, MD: Aspen.

Greene, D. P., & Roberts, S. L. (2005). *Kinesiology: Movement in the context of activity* (2nd ed.). St. Louis: Mosby/Elsevier.

Guzman, J., Esmail, R., Karjalainen, K., Malmivaara, A., Irvin, E., & Bombardier, C. (2001). Multidisciplinary rehabilitation for chronic low back pain: Systematic review. *Journal of British Medicine, 322,* 1511–1516.

Hagsten, B., Svensson, O., & Gardulf, A. (2004). Early individualized postoperative occupational therapy training in 100 patients improves ADL after hip fracture: A randomized trial. *Acta Orthopedica Scandinavica, 75*, 177–183.

Healy, W. L., Iorio, R., & Lemos, M. (2001). Athletic activity after joint replacement. *American Journal of Sports Medicine, 29*, 377–388.

Hodgson, S. (2006). Proximal humerus fracture rehabilitation. *Clinical Orthopaedic & Related Research, 442*, 131–138.

Hu, S. S., Tribus, C. B., Tay, B. K., & Bhatia, N. N. (2006). Disorders, diseases, and injuries of the spine. In H. B. Skinner (Ed.), *Current diagnosis and treatment in orthopedics* (4th ed., pp. 221–297). New York: Lange Medical Books/McGraw-Hill.

Hudak, P. L., Amadio, P. C., & Bombardier, C. (1996). Development of an upper extremity outcome measure: The DASH (disabilities of the arm shoulder and hand). *American Journal of Industrial Medicine, 29*, 602–608.

Hush, J. M., Refshauge, K., Sullivan, G., De Souza, L., Maher, C. G., & McAuley, J. H. (2009). Recovery: What does this mean to patients with low back pain? *Arthritis & Rheumatism, 61*, 124–131.

International Association for the Study of Pain. (2012). IASP pain terminology. Retrieved September 8, 2012 from http://www.iasp-pain.org/content/NavigationMenu/GeneralResourceLinks/PainDefinitions/default.htm.

Keenan, M. E., & Mehta, S. (2006). Rehabilitation. In H. B. Skinner (Ed.), *Current diagnosis and treatment in orthopedics* (4th ed., pp. 671–728). New York: Lange Medical Books/McGraw-Hill.

Keenan, M. E., & Waters, R. L. (2003). Rehabilitation. In H. B. Skinner (Ed.). Current diagnosis and treatment in orthopedics (3rd ed., pp. 689–693). New York: Lange Medical Books/McGraw-Hill.

Kool, J., Bie, R. D., Oesch, P., Knusel, O., Brandt, P. V. D., & Bachmann, S. (2004). Exercise reduces sick leave in patients with non-acute non-specific low back pain: A meta analysis. *Journal of Rehabilitation Medicine, 36*, 49–62.,

Lareau, C., & Sawyer, G. (2010). Hip fracture surgical treatment and rehabilitation. *Medicine & Health/Rhode Island, 93*, 108–111.

Manchikanti, L., Fellows, B., Singh, V., & Pampati, V. (2003). Correlates of non-physiological behavior in patients with chronic low back pain. *Pain Physician, 6*, 159–166.

McClure, P., & Michener, L. (2003). Measures of adult shoulder function. *Arthritis & Rheumatism, 49*, 50–58.

McKee, J. I. (1975). Foam wedges aid sitting posture of patients with total hip replacement. *Physical Therapy, 55*, 767.

McKenzie, R. (2005). *Treat your own back* (7th ed.). New Zealand: Spinal Publication.

McKinnis, L. N. (2010). *Fundamentals of musculoskeletal imaging.* Philadelphia: F.A. Davis Company.

McMahon, P. J., & Kaplan, L. D. (2006). Sports medicine. In H. B. Skinner (Ed.), *Current diagnosis and treatment in orthopedics* (4th ed., pp. 163–220). New York: Lange Medical Books/McGraw-Hill.

Morone, N. E., Greco, C. M., & Weiner, D. K. (2008). Mindfulness meditation for the treatment of chronic low back pain in older adults: A randomized controlled pilot study. *Journal of the International Association for the Study of Pain, 134*, 310–319.

Morone, N. E., Lynch, C. S., Greco, C. M., Tindle, H. A., & Weiner, D. K. (2008). "I felt like a new person": The effect of mindfulness meditation on older adults with chronic pain: Qualitative narrative analysis of diary entries. *Journal of Pain, 9*, 841–848.

Namba, R. S., Skinner, H. B., & Gupta, R. (2006). Adult reconstructive surgery. In H. B. Skinner (Ed.), *Current diagnosis and treatment in orthopedics* (4th ed., pp. 381–423). New York: Lange Medical Books/McGraw-Hill.

Neer, C. S., II. (1990). *Shoulder reconstruction.* Philadelphia: Saunders.

O'Brien, M. J., Leggin, B. G., & Williams, G. R. (2011). Rotator cuff tendinopathies and tears: Surgery and therapy. In T. Skirven, A. L. Osterman, J. Fedorczyk, & P. C. Amadio (Eds.), *Rehabilitation of the hand and upper extremity* (6th ed., pp. 1157–1173). Philadelphia: Mosby Elsevier Inc.

Peak, L. E., Parvizi, J., Ciminiello, M., Purtill, J. J., Sharkey, P. F., Hozack, W. J., & Rotman, R. H. (2005). The role of patient restrictions in reducing the prevalence of early dislocation following hip arthroplasty: A randomized prospective study. *Journal of Bone and Joint Surgery, 87-A*, 247–253.

Persson, E., Rivano-Fischer, M., & Eklund, M. (2004). Evaluation of changes in occupational performance among patients in a pain management program. *Journal of Rehabilitation Medicine, 36*, 85–91.

Posadzski, P., Ernst, E., Terry, R., & Lee, M. S., (2011). Is yoga effective for pain? A systematic review of randomized clinical trials. *Complementary Therapies in Medicine, 19*, 281–287.

Post, M., Silver, R., & Singh, M. (1983). Rotator cuff tear: Diagnosis and treatment. *Clinical Orthopedic, 173*, 78.

Roy, J.-S., MacDermid, J. C., & Woodhouse, L. J. (2009). Measuring shoulder function: A systematic review of four questionnaires. *Arthritis Care & Research, 61*, 623–631.

Salter, R. B. (1999). *Textbook of disorders and injuries of the musculoskeletal system* (3rd ed.). Baltimore: Williams & Wilkins.

Sandell, C. (2008). A multidisciplinary assessment and intervention for patients awaiting total hip replacement to improve their quality of life. *Journal of Orthopaedic Nursing, 12*, 26–53.

Sanders, M. J. (2004). Ergonomics of child care. In M. J. Sanders (Ed.), *Ergonomics and the management of musculoskeletal disorders* (2nd ed., pp. 410–417). St. Louis: Butterworth & Heinemann.

Shin, E. K. (2011). Fractures: General principles of surgical management. In T. M. Skirven, A. L. Osterman, J. M. Fedorczyk, & P. C. Amadio (Eds.), *Rehabilitation of the hand and upper extremity* (6th ed., pp. 351–360). Philadelphia: Elsevier Mosby.

Smith, W. R., Agudelo, J. F., Parekh, A., & Shank, J. R. (2006). Musculoskeletal trauma. In H. B. Skinner (Ed.), *Current diagnosis and treatment in orthopedics* (4th ed., pp. 138–264). New York: Lange Medical Books/McGraw-Hill.

Snodgrass, J. (2011). Effective occupational therapy interventions in the rehabilitation of individuals with work related low back injuries and illnesses: A systematic review. *American Journal of Occupational Therapy, 65*, 37–43.

Solomon, L., Warwick, D. J., & Nayagam, S. (2005). *Apley's concise system of orthopaedics and fracture* (3rd ed.). London: Hodder Armold.

Spalding, N. J. (2003). Reducing anxiety by pre-operative education: Make the future familiar. *Occupational Therapy International, 11*, 278–293.

Tan, V., Leggin, B. G., Kelley, M. J., & Williams, G. (2011). Surgical and postoperative management of the shoulder arthritis. In T. M. Skirven, A. L. Osterman, J. M. Fedorczyk, & P. C. Amadio (Eds.), *Rehabilitation of the hand and upper extremity* (6th ed., pp. 351–360). Philadelphia: Elsevier Mosby.

Toyoda, H., Ito, Y., Tomo, H., Nakao, Y., Koike, T., & Takaoka, K. (2005). Evaluation of rotator cuff tears with magnetic resonance arthrography. *Clinical Orthopaedics and Related Research, 439*, 109–115.

World Health Organization. (2003). *WHO Technical Report Series: The burden of musculoskeletal conditions at the start of the new millennium.* Geneva, Switzerland: World Health Organization.

Youm, T., Maurer, S. G., & Stuchin, S. A. (2005). Postoperative management after total hip and knee arthroplasty. *Journal of Arthroplasty, 20*, 322–324.

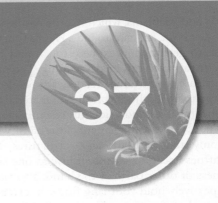

37

Hand Impairments

Cynthia Cooper

Learning Objectives

After studying this chapter, the reader will be able to do the following:

1. State principles and general precautions of hand therapy evaluation and intervention.
2. Select splinting (orthotic) positions that minimize, prevent, or correct hand deformity.
3. Describe clinical features of common hand impairments.
4. Recognize and foster favorable tissue responses to hand therapy interventions.
5. Promote pain-free occupational functioning of persons with hand impairment.

Hand problems, which may be cosmetic or functional or both, are hard to hide. Hands function exquisitely to gesture and express, touch and care, dress and feed. Impairment can be devastating. The purposes of this chapter are to introduce readers to the elements of hand therapy, to highlight the breadth of material that hand therapy encompasses, and to identify resources for further study.

The complex arrangement of the hand, with its intimate anatomy and multiarticulate structures, is unforgiving of stiffness, scar, or edema. Injury at one site can lead to stiffness of other parts of the hand. To test this for yourself, passively hold your ring finger in extension and then try to make a fist. This example, called the quadriga effect, demonstrates the interconnectedness of digits, whereby limited movement of one digit may cause restricted motion in uninjured digits (Giambini et al., 2010). For this and other reasons, hand therapists must look at more than the isolated site of injury and must continually reexamine the patient's performance in the areas of occupation.

Hand therapy originated during World War II. Devastating upper extremity injuries of that era and of subsequent wars prompted a team approach to medical care. Today, members of the rehabilitation team in hand therapy can include physicians and physician assistants, nurses, occupational therapists and occupational therapy assistants, physical therapists and physical therapy assistants, and aides or technicians. Workers' compensation representatives or case managers representing payers may also be involved.

Certified hand therapists are occupational therapists or physical therapists with advanced clinical skills who have passed the examination for certification in hand therapy. A minimum of 5 years of clinical experience and other criteria are prerequisites to taking the examination. It is advisable to establish a strong generalist background in occupational therapy before specializing in hand therapy.

Hand therapy differs from other occupational therapy specializations, such as pediatrics or gerontology, because it merges occupational therapy and physical therapy, and it has its own professional organizations. Although most hand therapists are occupational therapists, actual clinical practice may often look more like physical therapy than occupational therapy. Occupational therapy hand therapists should embrace an occupational therapy identity by grounding intervention in core concepts of our profession. To this end, hand therapists should not become so focused on specific anatomical structures that they overlook the person attached to the hand. They should treat the hand and should also address performance skills and performance patterns of the occupational human whose hand it is.

PSYCHOSOCIAL FACTORS AFFECTING THERAPEUTIC OUTCOMES

Why do some people with minor hand injuries wind up with large disabilities and others with devastating injuries have only small disabilities? Adaptive responses to hand impairment are influenced by body image as well as individual functional needs and contextual elements. The personal or symbolic meaning of the hand, self-esteem, family and friend support systems, and coping strategies all influence outcome. Whenever possible, encourage patients to participate in their care. Introduce yourself, maintain eye contact, listen well, use nonmedical terminology and instructional diagrams, and encourage some amiable conversation as appropriate (Vranceanu, Cooper, & Ring, 2009). It can be helpful to touch patients' hands supportively and to make positive remarks (see Chapter 14).

Motivation is the most important variable favorably influencing recovery. Realistic expectations and appropriate communication that emphasizes participatory decision making and education are also important (Moorhead & Cooper, 2007). Psychological symptoms related to hand trauma resolve best when intervention occurs early.

HAND THERAPY CONCEPTS

The following concepts are keys to clinical reasoning for all diagnoses of hand impairment. Intervention should not be determined by diagnosis per se. Rather, hand therapy relies on an understanding of anatomy and physiology, wound healing, biomechanics, tissue tolerances, psychosocial issues, and probable outcomes. Given the infinite variations among people, no two intervention plans should be the same.

Tissue Healing

Tissue heals in phases as follows: inflammation, fibroplasia, and maturation or remodeling. The inflammation phase lasts several days. It includes vasoconstriction followed by vasodilation, with white blood cell migration to promote phagocytic removal of foreign bodies and dead tissue. Depending on the diagnosis, immobilization to provide rest is often advised during the inflammation phase (Fess et al., 2005).

The fibroplasia phase starts at approximately day 4 and continues for 2–6 weeks. In this phase, fibroblasts synthesize scar tissue. The wound's tensile strength increases gradually with the increase in collagen fibers. At this time, active range of motion (AROM) and orthotics may be appropriate to protect healing tissues and promote balance in the hand (Fess et al., 2005).

The maturation, or remodeling, phase may last for years, but tissue is usually more responsive early rather than late in this period. The remodeling phase reflects the changing architecture and improved organization of collagen fibers and the associated increased tensile strength. Gentle resistive activity may be appropriate during maturation, but it may also generate inflammatory responses, which should be avoided. Gentle application of corrective dynamic or static orthoses may also be appropriate (Fess et al., 2005). Tolerance of tissues to controlled stress requires monitoring throughout all phases of intervention. As tissue continues to heal, the wound contracts, and the scar shrinks. Collagen continues to remodel, as it is constantly doing in uninjured tissue.

Antideformity Positioning

Upper extremity injury and disuse are associated with predictable deforming hand positions. Edema, which typically accompanies injury, creates tension on extrinsic extensor structures. This leads to a zigzag collapse with a resulting deformity position of flexed wrist, hyperextended metaphalangeals (MPs), flexed proximal interphalangeals (PIPs) and distal interphalangeals (DIPs), and adducted thumb (Pettengill, 2011).

Hand joints are anatomically destined to stiffen in predictable positions. Specifically, the MP joint is prone to stiffen in extension. This is because the protruding or cam shape of the metacarpal head causes the collateral ligament to be slack in MP extension and taut in MP flexion. Conversely, the interphalangeal (IP) joints are prone to become stiff in flexion because of shortening of the volar plate and collateral ligaments (Hahn et al., 2010).

When prolonged or constant immobilization is necessary and range of motion (ROM) is at risk, it is usually best to splint the patient's hand in the antideformity position, also called the intrinsic-plus position (Fig. 37-1). This position places the wrist in neutral or extension, the MPs in flexion, the IPs in extension, and the thumb in abduction and opposition. The antideformity position allows the collateral ligaments at the MP joints and the volar plate at the IP joints to maintain their length, which counteracts the forces that promote zigzag collapse. Certain diagnoses, such as flexor or extensor tendon repair,

are not compatible with antideformity positioning. The physician can assist in this determination.

The Myth of No Pain, No Gain

Regarding tissue tolerances, the myth of "no pain, no gain" must be dispelled in hand therapy. A better mindset would be no pain, more gain. Well-intentioned therapists and overzealous family members of patients have too often caused irreversible damage by applying passive range-of-motion (PROM) forces beyond the tissues' tolerances. Pain induced by therapy can also cause complex regional pain syndrome (CRPS), which is discussed later.

People with upper extremity problems often arrive at therapy prepared for painful intervention. Some patients do not tell the therapist when intervention hurts. It is essential to educate patients about this. In addition, watch the patient's body language and face for signs of pain. Wincing and withdrawing the upper extremity are obvious signals. Proximal guarding is another revealing response. Change the intervention accordingly, and if necessary, try a hands-off approach wherein the therapist coaches and instructs while the patient self-treats.

Passive Range of Motion Can Be Injurious

PROM can be injurious to the delicate tissues of the hand. Specifically, PROM can disturb healing tissues and incite further inflammatory reactions, resulting in increased scar production. PROM can damage articular structures and can even trigger CRPS. A tissue's timeline for remodeling is maximized by noninflaming intervention and is cut short by intervention that is inflaming or provoking. For all of these reasons, if PROM is clinically appropriate, be sure it is done gently and in a pain-free manner. Low-load, long-duration splinting is a safer and more effective method for remodeling tissue and increasing PROM (Fess et al., 2005).

The potential for harm may be compounded if PROM is performed following external application of heat. External application of heat, such as a hot pack, is a popular way to prepare tissues for stretching. Unfortunately, the clinical concerns of externally applied heat have received less attention than they deserve. Heat increases edema, which acts like glue. Heat may degrade collagen and contribute to microscopic tears (Chen et al., 2011). Heat may also incur a rebound effect, with stiffening following its use. *Safety Message: Do not use heat on patients who have edema or sensory loss or whose limb appears inflamed.* Overall, it is safer to use aerobic exercise to warm up the tissues of people with hand impairments. If external application of heat is used, elevate the upper extremity, be gentle with exercise, and promote active movement in conjunction with the heat. Continue to monitor for immediate and subsequent signs of inflammation.

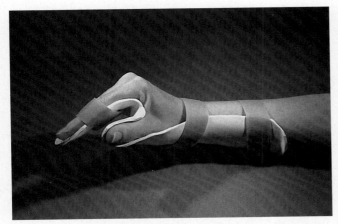

Figure 37-1 Antideformity or intrinsic-plus position: wrist in neutral or extension, MPs in flexion, IPs in extension, and thumb in abduction and opposition.

Isolated Exercise, Purposeful Activity, and Therapeutic Occupation

Technically, it is necessary to treat hand impairments with a structure-specific approach to isolate and care for the discrete components that are involved. It may seem easiest to accomplish this type of exacting intervention in the form of isolated exercise. Traditional valuing of the appearance of highly technical clinical environments, medical model indoctrination, busy schedules, and financial or material constraints may contribute to the perpetuation of hand therapy identifying itself within an environment that looks like an exercise gymnasium.

Although some hand therapists do incorporate purposeful activity into intervention, more support is needed for an alternative approach to hand therapy that leads with concepts of therapeutic occupation. One way to achieve this is to integrate patient-directed goals and activities of daily living (ADL) into hand therapy intervention planning and implementation. Whenever possible, encourage upper extremity use in ordinary daily activities as appropriate to the diagnosis. Explore the capabilities in the clinic, and then teach patients to do activities at home. For example, folding socks and underwear can be upgraded to folding heavy towels and jeans, which require greater strength and endurance.

Occupation elicits adaptive responses that do not occur with exercise alone. Compared to isolated exercise, purposeful activity or occupation promotes more coordination and better movement quality (Omar, Hegazy, & Mokashi, 2012). An example of isolated hand therapy exercise to increase grip strength is gross grasp with therapy putty or exercise grippers. An example of purposeful activity to increase strength would be putting away groceries, starting with light items and progressing to heavier objects.

Occupation-as-means instills occupational therapy's heritage in what might otherwise be a less function-oriented context (Trombly, 2011). The examples cited earlier become therapeutic occupation with the use of activity that is meaningful to the particular person to accomplish the therapeutic goal. If the patient enjoys baking, then rolling dough with a rolling pin would be a therapeutic occupation to promote grip function.

EVALUATION

History

History taking as part of the occupational profile offers an excellent opportunity to establish therapeutic rapport. Review medical reports, including radiographs, when possible; learn hand dominance, age, occupation, and avocational interests (Seftchick et al., 2011). Assess deficits in the areas of occupation by asking what the patient cannot do that he or she wants to do, needs to do, or is expected to do. Also discuss the case with the physician.

For trauma, learn the date of injury, dates of any surgery, where and how injury occurred, mechanism of injury, posture of the hand when it was injured, and any previous intervention. For nontraumatic problems, learn the date of onset, whether the symptoms are worsening, sequence of onset of symptoms, functional effects, and what worsens and/or lessens the symptoms (Seftchick et al., 2011).

Pain

Pain may be acute or chronic. Acute pain has a sudden and recent onset, usually has a limited course with an identifiable cause, and can last a few minutes to 6 months. Acute pain serves a physiological purpose, signaling the need to protect tissue from further damage. Chronic pain lasts months or years longer than expected and may not serve a physiological purpose. Myofascial pain, which may be chronic or acute, stems from local irritation in fascia, muscle, tendon, or ligament. It has specific reproducible pain patterns and associated autonomic symptoms. Evaluation of pain may include a graphic representation of pain, in which the patient marks painful areas on a drawing of the human body; analog pain rating scales (see Chapter 5); joint or muscle palpation to identify areas of local pain or qualitative changes in soft tissue; and trigger point sensitivity (Klein, 2007a).

Physical Examination

It is helpful to observe the positioning and use of the patient's upper extremity in the waiting area before the meeting. On examination, look at the entire unclothed upper extremity for posture, guarding and gesturing, atrophy, and edema (Klein, 2007a). Because distal symptoms are often caused by proximal problems, it is important to perform a cervical screening, which is a proximal screening assessment of the neck and shoulder, to identify additional areas requiring intervention (Butler, 2007).

Wounds

Safety Message: Always follow universal precautions (see Chapter 44). Evaluate wound size in terms of length, width, and depth. Wound drainage (exudate) is bloody (sanguinous), serous (clear or yellow), purulent (pus), or deep or dark red (hematoma). Wound odor is absent or foul (Klein, 2007a).

The three-color concept (red, yellow, or black) dictates wound care. Wounds can be one of or a combination of these three colors. A red wound is healing, uninfected, and composed of revascularization and granulation tissue. A yellow wound has an exudate that requires cleansing and debridement. A black wound is necrotic and requires debridement. The goal of wound care is to convert yellow and black wounds to red wounds (von der Heyde & Evans, 2011).

Scar Assessment

Observe scar location, length, width, and height. Hypertrophic scars stay confined to the area of the original wound and usually resolve within a year. Keloids proliferate outside the area of the original wound and do not usually become smaller or less pigmented with time. Note any scar tethering or adherence of skin and tendon causing restricted movement. Any wound or scar crossing a joint may form a contracture, which restricts passive motion. An immature scar has a red or purplish color imparted by its vascularity. It blanches to touch. A mature scar is flatter and softer. It has a neutral color and does not blanch to touch (Klein, 2007a).

Vascular Assessment

Cyanosis, erythema, pallor, gangrene, or grayish color indicates vascular compromise. To test digital capillary refill, apply pressure to the fingernail or distal pad of the involved digit. Color should return within 2 seconds of release of pressure. Compare the refill time to that of uninvolved digits (Klein, 2007a).

Edema

Circumferential measurement is quick to perform and provides a good alternative when it is not possible to use a volumeter (Klein, 2007a). Be consistent with measuring tape placement and tension. Volumetric measurement is contraindicated for open wounds, percutaneous pinning such as Kirschner wires, plaster casts, or vasomotor instability (see Chapter 7 for volumetric and circumferential measurement procedures).

Range of Motion

In hand therapy, both AROM and PROM should be evaluated and compared to the uninjured extremity (see Chapter 7). Facilities usually have their own guidelines for measuring ROM. As expected, consistency of retesting is important.

Total active motion (TAM) or total passive motion (TPM) measures the sum of composite digital flexion and extension. This measurement is used in some studies. Normal TAM and TPM are 270° (Fess, 2002/2011) (see Procedures for Practice 37-1).

Grip and Pinch

When properly calibrated, the Jamar dynamometer is one of the best instruments to assess grip strength because of its reliability, face validity, and accuracy (see Chapter 7). Hand therapy authorities recommend comparing scores with those of the contralateral extremity rather than using

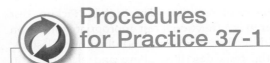

Procedures for Practice 37-1

Total Active Motion (TAM) and Total Passive Motion (TPM)

- Add the measurements for flexion of the MP, PIP, and DIP joints.
- Subtract the combined deficits in extension for those joints.
  For example, if the digital AROM is MP: 10–50, PIP: 20–70, DIP: 0–40, the total active motion (TAM) would be 160 (flexion total) minus 30 (extension deficits total) = 130 TAM.

norms (Fess, 2002/2011). Goals for grip and pinch strength depend on occupational factors and dominance. There may be approximately 10%–15% difference in strength between dominant and nondominant hands, with dominant hands usually being stronger. It is routine to measure three pinch patterns: lateral, three-jaw chuck, and tip. As with grip, compare pinch scores with those of the contralateral extremity.

No linear relationship exists between improvement in grip and pinch strength and improvement in function. Rice, Leonard, and Carter (1998) noted that even debilitated, deformed hands could be surprisingly functional. These authors found only weak relationships between grip and pinch strength and the forces required to open six containers used commonly in the home. Thus, grip and pinch testing are not substitutes for ADL assessment with contextual relevance (Liepert, 2010). To promote occupational functioning of people with hand impairments, it is far better to have intervention and goals reflect personally meaningful ADL than grip or pinch strength measures.

Manual Muscle Testing

Manual muscle testing is particularly useful for monitoring progress following peripheral nerve lesions (see Chapter 7). Facilities usually have their preferred method of grading, which may be numerical or descriptive.

Sensibility

Inspect the patient's hand for dryness, moistness, and calluses (see Chapter 9). Blisters may be an alert to injurious hand use because of sensory loss. "Wear marks" illustrate where and how the hand is used and which parts of the hand avoid use, indicating sensory impairment (Callahan, 2011).

The Semmes-Weinstein Monofilament Test and the Two-Point Discrimination (2PD) test are most commonly used in hand therapy. The Semmes-Weinstein Monofilament Test assesses pressure threshold, and the 2PD assesses density of receptors. The Moberg Pickup Test (see Chapter 9) is a functional test appropriate for use on patients with median or median and ulnar nerve lesions. Although the tests described above and elaborated in Chapter 9 are very useful clinically, there is no one tool that evaluates the hand's actual functional sensibility (Moberg, 1991).

Dexterity and Hand Function

No one evaluation covers all features of hand function (Yancosek & Howell, 2009). Standard terminology regarding hand function is lacking, and there is limited evidence that the assessment of hand function indicates the patient's actual performance in ADL. Thus, hand function tests should not substitute for assessments of ADL or other areas of occupation. Hand function tests, however, can be helpful measures of improvement of performance skills.

For dexterity tests to be reliable, therapists must administer them using the standard procedures from the original articles or test manuals, and they must decide whether a specific test is valid for the intended use. The tests described in this section all require further validation.

Box and Block Test

The Box and Block Test measures gross manual dexterity. It was developed to test people with severe problems affecting coordination (Fig. 37-2). The subject transfers 1-inch blocks from one side of the box to the other. The score

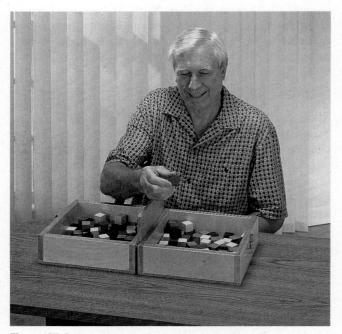

Figure 37-2 Box and Block Test of manual dexterity. (Photo used with permission from Patterson Medical, Bolingbrook, IL.)

is the number of blocks transferred in 1 minute for each hand. Procedures for Practice 37-2 presents procedures for administration of the test (Mathiowetz et al., 1985).

Test–retest reliability and interrater reliability of the Box and Block Test is high, with an intraclass correlation coefficient of 0.99 (Yancosek & Howell, 2009) and demonstrated validity (Faria-Fortini et al., 2011; Higgins et al., 2006). One systematic review concluded that this test provided "robust" data and was recommended for clinical use (Connell & Tyson, 2012). Norms for persons aged 20–75 years and older appear in Table 37-1.

Purdue Pegboard Test

The Purdue Pegboard Test of finger dexterity (Tiffin, 1968) assesses picking up, manipulating, and placing little pegs into holes with speed and accuracy. It tests finger or fine motor dexterity (Amirjani et al., 2011). It has a wooden board with two rows of tiny holes plus reservoirs for holding pins, collars, and washers. The four subtests are performed with the subject seated. To begin, there is a brief practice. The subtests for preferred, nonpreferred, and both hands require the patient to place the pins in the holes as quickly as possible, with the score being the number of pins placed in 30 seconds. The subtest for assembly requires the patient to insert a pin and then put a washer, collar, and another washer on the pin, with the score being the number of pieces assembled in 1 minute. The Purdue Pegboard Test manual provides normative data using percentile tables for adults and different categories of jobs and for children 5–15 years of age by age and sex.

One-trial administration of the Purdue Pegboard Test produced good test–retest reliability of 0.60–0.76 in healthy subjects and 0.85–0.9 in patients (de la Llave-Rincon et al., 2011). Three-trial administration produced excellent reliabilities (>0.80) (Buddenberg & Davis, 2000). Among subjects with multiple sclerosis, test–retest reliability coefficients were excellent, with no significant practice effects ($r = 0.85$–0.96) (Gallus & Mathiowetz, 2003).

Nine-Hole Peg Test

The Nine-Hole Peg Test measures finger dexterity among patients of all ages. Test administration is brief, involving the time it takes to place nine pegs in holes in a 5-inch square board and then remove them. The Nine-Hole Peg Test was found to have high test–retest reliability coefficients (0.95 for right hands and 0.92 for left hands) (Wang et al., 2011). High interrater reliability has been reported (Higgins et al., 2006).

The Purdue Pegboard Test is preferred to the Nine-Hole Peg Test in the measurement of finger dexterity. Of the two, the Purdue Pegboard Test has good test–retest reliability; it is time limited; it is for both unilateral and bilateral assessment; and its normative data reflect a broader age range (Gallus & Mathiowetz, 2003).

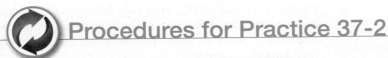

Procedures for Practice 37-2

Administration Procedures for the Box and Block Test (Mathiowetz et al., 1985)

- Place the test box lengthwise along the edge of a standard-height table (Fig. 37-2).
- The 150 cubes are in the compartment of the test box to the dominant side of the patient.
- Sit facing the patient to monitor the blocks being transported.
- Give these instructions: "*I want to see how quickly you can pick up one block at a time with your right [left] hand [the therapist points to the dominant hand]. Carry the block to the other side of the box and drop it. Make sure your fingertips cross the partition. Watch me while I show you how.*"
- Transport three cubes over the partition in the same direction the patient is to move them. After the demonstration, say, "*If you pick up two blocks at a time, they will count as one. If you drop one on the floor or table after you have carried it across, it will still be counted, so do not waste time picking it up. If you toss the blocks without your fingertips crossing the partition, they will not be counted. Before you start, you will have a chance to practice for 15 seconds. Do you have any questions? Place your hands on the sides of the box. When it is time to start, I will say 'Ready' and then 'Go.'*"

- Start the stopwatch at the word *go*. After 15 seconds, say "*Stop.*"
- If the patient makes mistakes during the practice period, correct them before beginning the actual testing.
- On completion of the practice period, return the transported cubes to the compartment.
- Mix the cubes to ensure random distribution, and then say, "*This will be the actual test. The instructions are the same. Work as quickly as you can. Ready; go. [After 1 minute:] Stop.*"
- Count the blocks transported across the partition. This is the patient's score for the dominant hand.
- If the patient transports two or more blocks at the same time, subtract the number of extra blocks from the total.
- After counting, return the blocks to the original compartment and mix randomly.
- Turn the test around so that the blocks are on the nondominant side.
- Administer the test to the nondominant hand using the same procedures as for the dominant hand, including the 15-second practice.

From Mathiowetz, V., Volland, G., Kashman, N், & Weber, K. (1985). Adult norms for the box and block test of manual dexterity. *American Journal of Occupational Therapy, 39*, 386–391.

Table 37-1   **Average Performance of 628 Normal Subjects on the Box and Block Test[a]**

Age (Years)	Males Mean	SD	Females Mean	SD	Age (Years)	Males Mean	SD	Females Mean	SD
20–24					50–54				
Right hand	88.2	8.8	88.0	8.3	Right hand	79.0	9.7	77.7	10.7
Left hand	86.4	8.5	83.4	7.9	Left hand	77.0	9.2	74.3	9.9
25–29					55–59				
Right hand	85.0	7.5	86.0	7.4	Right hand	75.2	11.9	74.7	8.9
Left hand	84.1	7.1	80.9	6.4	Left hand	73.8	10.5	73.6	7.8
30–34					60–64				
Right hand	81.9	9.0	85.2	7.4	Right hand	71.3	8.8	76.1	6.9
Left hand	81.3	8.1	80.2	5.6	Left hand	70.5	8.1	73.6	6.4
35–39					65–69				
Right hand	81.9	9.5	84.8	6.1	Right hand	68.4	7.1	72.0	6.2
Left hand	79.8	9.7	83.5	6.1	Left hand	67.4	7.8	71.3	7.7
40–44					70–74				
Right hand	83.0	8.1	81.1	8.2	Right hand	66.3	9.2	68.6	7.0
Left hand	80.0	8.8	79.7	8.8	Left hand	64.3	9.8	68.3	7.0
45–49					75+				
Right hand	76.9	9.2	82.1	7.5	Right hand	63.0	7.1	65.0	7.1
Left hand	75.8	7.8	78.3	7.6	Left hand	61.3	8.4	63.6	7.4

[a]The values indicate the number of cubes transferred in 1 minute (Mathiowetz et al., 1985).

TEMPA

TEMPA is an acronym from the French for Upper Extremity Performance Test for the Elderly. It consists of nine tasks, five bilateral and four unilateral, reflecting daily activity (Desrosiers et al., 1993). Each task is measured by the three subscores of speed, functional rating, and task analysis. The nine tasks are to pick up and move a jar, open a jar and take a spoonful of coffee, pour water from a pitcher into a glass, unlock a lock, take the top off a pillbox, write on an envelope and affix a postage stamp, put a scarf around one's neck, shuffle and deal cards, use coins, and pick up and move small objects. Instructions are in the manual. The test takes about 15–20 minutes for an unimpaired elderly subject and about 30–40 minutes for an impaired elderly subject. Advantages of the TEMPA are clinical use, especially with hand patients older than 60 years of age; provision of both quantitative and qualitative data; simulation of ADL; test applicability; test availability; and acceptability to patients (Rallon & Chen, 2008). Normative data for young adults has been determined (Nedelec et al., 2011).

TEMPA norms were established on adults 60 years of age or older ($n = 360$) by 10-year age groups and by gender. Interrater reliability of the TEMPA ranged from 0.96 to 1.00. Test–retest reliability was excellent (Rallon & Chen, 2008). Concurrent validity with the Action Research Arm test was 0.90–0.95, and with the Box and Block Test, it was 0.73–0.78 (Desrosiers et al., 1994).

CLINICAL REASONING AND INTERVENTION

Questions to Ask

Close communication with the patient's physician is always advisable. Choosing which questions to ask depends on the diagnosis and structures involved. General categories of questions may include the physician's expectations for functional recovery; tendon status, such as fraying or vascular compromise; whether the patient is medically cleared for AROM only or AROM and/or PROM; and whether the patient is medically cleared for low-load, long-duration dynamic splinting.

Activities of Daily Living and Occupational Role Implications

The functional use of the upper extremity and the patient's ability to perform in the areas of occupation are what really matter. Hand therapists must be careful not to become so focused on the technical aspects of the patient's injury that they overlook the patient's function, personal goals, and life needs. In some circumstances, it may actually be better for patients to accept a stiff finger and get on with life using compensatory techniques than to interrupt the flow of their lives for

therapy (Merritt, 1998). This may be true if gains are exceedingly slow, if function is not dramatically compromised, or if there are other priorities, such as ill family members, for example.

Goal Setting

Express hand therapy goals or projected outcomes in terms that reflect the patient's occupational functioning. Ultimately, the number of degrees achieved in ROM is less important than whether the patient can open a door, get dressed, or return to work. One way to integrate concrete and functional outcomes is to measure the movement needed to accomplish an appropriate patient-specific functional task and incorporate that measurement into the stated goal. For example, if a patient wants to be able to splash water on his or her face but lacks forearm supination to do so, have the patient perform the activity with the opposite upper extremity. Measure the supination needed to perform the task. In this instance, the goal could be stated as "sufficient forearm supination (60°) for ability to wash the face."

Quality of Movement

Poor quality of movement (called dyscoordinate cocontraction) may result from cocontraction of antagonist muscles. The cause may be habit, fear of pain, guarding, or excessive effort. Poor quality of movement looks awkward and unpleasant. It is important to identify dyscoordinate cocontraction early and to work on retraining a smooth, comfortable, effective quality of motion. Pain-free occupation is the best way to promote good quality of motion. Oscillations are rhythmic therapeutic movements that may be helpful, but they must be pain free. Imagery, such as pretending to move the extremity through water or gelatin, may also help (Cooper, 2007). Biofeedback may aid in muscle reeducation as well.

What Structures Are Restricted, and Does Passive Range of Motion Exceed Active Range of Motion?

Hand therapists strive to be structure specific in identifying and treating upper extremity limitations. It is not adequate to identify a general problem, such as decreased ROM. Rather, it is important to understand and treat the specific structures causing the restriction. Limited PROM may be due to pericapsular structures, such as adhered or shortened ligaments, or actual joint limitations, such as mechanical block or adhesions. PROM that exceeds AROM may be due to disruption of the musculotendinous unit, adhesions restricting excursion of the tendon, or weakness. When PROM exceeds AROM, promote active movement and function of the restricted structures with differential tendon gliding exercises, blocking exercises, place-and-hold exercises, and functional orthoses (discussed later). When PROM equals AROM, discern whether the restriction is joint or musculotendinous or both (see section on Joint versus Musculotendinous Tightness), and promote both passive and active flexibility.

Joint versus Musculotendinous Tightness

With joint tightness, the PROM of the particular joint *does not change* with repositioning of the joints proximal and/or distal to it. With musculotendinous tightness, the PROM of the particular joint *does vary* with repositioning of joints crossed by that multiarticulate structure (Colditz, 2011). Treat joint tightness with dynamic splinting, static progressive splinting, or serial casting, followed by AROM. Treat musculotendinous tightness the same as extrinsic tightness (discussed later).

Lag versus Contracture

A lag is a limitation of active motion in a joint that has passive motion available. A joint contracture is a passive limitation of the joint. A patient with a PIP extensor lag cannot actively extend the PIP joint even though passive extension is available. A patient with a PIP joint flexion contracture lacks passive extension of that joint.

Treat lags by facilitating motion of the restricted structure with scar management, blocking exercises in mechanically advantageous positions, place-and-hold exercises, static splinting to promote normal length of the involved structure, and functional splints. Treat contractures the same as for joint tightness (discussed later).

An advantageous position to test or treat extensor lag at the PIP level is to maintain MP flexion while trying to extend actively at the PIP. An advantageous position to test or treat extensor lag at the DIP level is to maintain MP and PIP flexion while trying to extend actively at the DIP. This is contraindicated if the diagnosis is acute mallet finger (see section on Extensor Tendon Injury).

Intrinsic versus Extrinsic Tightness

Compare the PROM of digital PIP and DIP flexion with the MP joint flexed and again with the MP joint extended. With extrinsic tightness, there is less PIP and DIP passive flexion with the MP joint flexed. With intrinsic tightness, there is less PIP and DIP passive flexion with the MP joint extended (Colditz, 2011).

Treat intrinsic tightness with functional splinting with MPs hyperextended and IPs free. In other words, promote IP flexion with MPs hyperextended. Treat extrinsic extensor tightness with MPs flexed and IPs free, and promote composite digital flexion. Use blocking exercises with an advantageous proximal position (discussed later). Try dynamic or static progressive splinting.

Tightness of Extrinsic Extensors or Extrinsic Flexors

With extrinsic extensor tightness, there is less passive composite digital flexion available with the wrist in flexion than with the wrist in extension. In contrast, with extrinsic flexor tightness, there is less passive composite digital extension available with the wrist in extension than with the wrist in flexion (Colditz, 2011). Treat extrinsic flexor or extensor tightness with place-and-hold exercises, static splinting comfortably at end range (especially useful at night), dynamic or static progressive splinting during the day, and functional splinting.

BASIC INTERVENTIONS

Edema Control

Elevation, active exercise, and compression have been the mainstays of edema control. Treatment of upper extremity edema has also historically included retrograde massage, string wrapping, compression garments, and modalities such as an intermittent pressure pump.

Research has challenged hand therapists to reexamine the anatomical and physiological bases of our treatment of edema. This inquiry has resulted in a new approach to the treatment of upper extremity edema, called manual edema mobilization (Artzberger, 2007), a technique for stimulating the lymphatic system to remove the excess large plasma proteins that cause sustained edema leading to fibrotic tissue and stiffness. This hands-on technique, which must be learned in workshops that last 2 days or longer, can lead to dramatic and effective results (Knygsand-Roenhoej & Maribo, 2011; Priganc & Ito, 2008). The approach used in manual edema mobilization is very different from and, in some ways, opposite to traditional retrograde massage techniques. Furthermore, manual edema mobilization raises questions about whether retrograde massage is sometimes more damaging than helpful. Manual edema mobilization is a wonderful example of the groundbreaking changes in hand therapy, based on scholarly questioning and research, that keep the profession interesting.

Scar Management

Compression (e.g., Isotoner™ gloves, Tubigrip™, or Coban™ wrap) and desensitization are traditionally used to promote scar softening and maturation. Silicone gel applied over the scar helps promote scar maturation, presumably through neutral warmth. Other inserted materials such as padding, otoform, or elastomer can also be used. Application of micropore tape over incision scars is gaining popularity. It has been shown to be very effective and is much more affordable than the other options (von der Heyde & Evans, 2011).

There are three ways of making a fist:

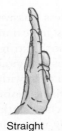 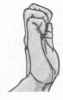

Straight   Hook fist   Straight fist   Full fist

Figure 37-3 Differential flexor tendon gliding exercises. The four positions: straight, hook, straight fist, and full fist. (Adapted with permission from Skirven, T. M., Osterman, A. L., Fedorczyk, J. M., & Amadio, P. C. [Eds.]. [2011]. *Rehabilitation of the hand and upper extremity* [6th ed.]. Philadelphia: Mosby.)

Although friction massage has typically been advocated for scar softening, legitimate questions have been raised as to whether this more aggressive technique may in fact cause inflammation, resulting in deposition of even more scar tissue. Manual edema mobilization may be a more effective alternative. Research is needed in this area.

Differential Digital Tendon Gliding Exercises

Tendon gliding exercises maximize total gliding and differential gliding of digital flexor tendons at the wrist (Fig. 37-3) (Bardak et al., 2009). Because tendon gliding exercises promote digital and joint motions, they are a mainstay of most home exercise programs.

Blocking Exercises

Various blocking tools and orthotics are available commercially or can be made easily with scraps of splinting materials (Fig. 37-4). Digital cylinders blocking the IPs help to isolate and exercise MP flexion and extension. A blocking splint with the MPs extended promotes intrinsic stretch as well as IP flexion. A blocking splint with the MPs flexed promotes extrinsic extensor stretch and recovery of composite fisting [flexion at all finger joints of the hand simultaneously]. A PIP cylindrical block encourages DIP isolated flexion and flexor digitorum profundus

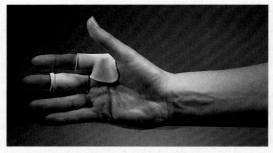

Figure 37-4 Blocking splints. MP splint blocks MP motion, promoting PIP and DIP motion. Digital splint blocks PIP motion, promoting MP, and/or DIP motion.

(FDP) excursion at the DIP. A DIP cap facilitates PIP flexion and flexor tendon excursion at the PIP.

Instruct patients who do blocking exercises to exercise comfortably into the end range to remodel the tissue. Teach them to do the exercises frequently and slowly, holding at the comfortable end range for 3–5 seconds.

Place-and-Hold Exercises

Place-and-hold exercises are effective for achieving increased ROM when PROM exceeds AROM. To perform them, use comfortable PROM to position the hand (e.g., composite fisting). Then release the assisting hand while the patient tries to sustain the position in a pain-free way. Place-and-hold exercises can be effective in combination with blocking exercises.

Mirror Box

Growing interest in neuroplasticity has provided fascinating additions to the traditional repertoire of hand therapists. The use of a mirror box (also called mirror visual feedback or mirror training) is based on research on neural responses to intentional visual confusion, with stimulation of neurons called mirror neurons. Mirror training is used for pain, sensory, and motor problems and can be used in conjunction with laterality and graded imagery interventions. It has been used with clients who have had a cerebral vascular accident (CVA) and is being used more recently with clients with peripheral and orthopedic problems of the upper extremities (Lamont, Chin, & Kogan, 2011; Rosén & Lundborg, 2005, 2011) (see Fig. 37-5).

End Feel and Splinting

If there is a soft end feel (a favorable spongy quality at end range indicative of potential to remodel), it is reasonable to try low-load, long-duration dynamic splinting for a medically cleared patient. Dynamic splint forces must be prolonged and gentle for tissue to remodel. Forceful splinting is contraindicated because it causes pain and injury, hence inflammation and scarring (Fess et al., 2005). Follow dynamic orthotic use with activity that challenges and incorporates the limited motion. For a firmer or hard end feel (an unyielding quality at end range), try increasing the time in the orthosis and decreasing the force. If there is a hard end feel, dynamic splinting may not be effective, and serial casting or static progressive splinting may be more useful.

Splints (Orthotics)

Terminology related to splinting has changed. It is now recommended to use the term "orthotics," especially in regard to occupational therapy documentation and billing. These two terms are used interchangeably in this chapter. Functional splints (or orthotics) can be used in ordinary

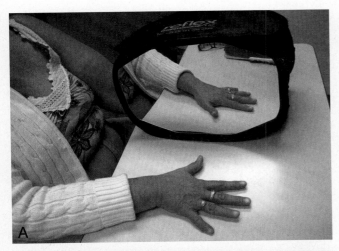

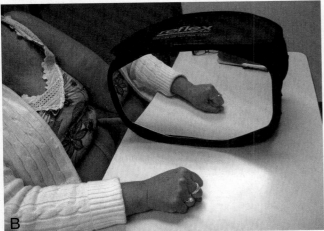

Figure 37-5   Mirror box. **A.** Hand open. **B.** Hand fisted.

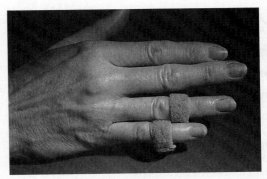

Figure 37-6   Offset buddy straps. Interdigital strap accommodates different phalangeal lengths of adjacent digits. Used to allow one digit to assist the next in achieving motion and for protection.

COMMON DIAGNOSES

Hand therapists 15 years ago treated more hand trauma than cumulative trauma, and surgical cases constituted most of the caseload. Nowadays, many hand therapists see a substantially greater number of patients with a soft tissue diagnosis, such as tendinitis or cumulative trauma disorders (see Resources 37-1 for informational products).

Stiff Hand

Any upper extremity injury can result in the serious and sometimes irreversible problem of a stiff hand. Even an injury in the proximal upper extremity can cause serious stiffening of the digits. The stiff hand is what hand therapists try to prevent. Edema is the main culprit in the series of events leading to a stiff hand. Edema is a natural response to trauma, occurring in the inflammatory phase. The challenge for hand therapy is to strike a balance between rest and movement. Too much rest may increase the edema. Too much movement may increase the inflammation. The right amount of rest in an appropriate position reduces inflammation and promotes healing. Proximal motion plus well-tolerated hand and wrist exercise and functional use, particularly while elevated, help to reduce edema and restore motion.

Encourage the patient to achieve gentle full arcs of available motion with functional use or exercise instead of performing quick or incomplete arcs of motion that are less effective. Make exercises relevant to occupational functioning or at least goal oriented whenever possible (e.g., grasping and releasing items). If the patient's hand is painful or more swollen after use or exercise, it is imperative to decrease temporarily the amount of exercise being performed (Colditz, 2011).

Avoid aggressive PROM. It is okay to coax tissues to lengthen within their available comfortable range, but always respect the feeling of tissue resistance, and do not exceed it. Gentle passive motion, if indicated, should be accompanied by joint traction to promote gliding of the joint surfaces. Sustained holding of a position is much

daily activity to promote mobility of restricted structures. For example, if the index finger PIP joint lacks flexion and the MP joint moves normally, try a hand-based index finger MP blocking splint, used off and on throughout the day. When the splint is in use, the patient achieves PIP flexion exercise while performing normal grasping activities.

Buddy straps allow one digit to assist a neighboring digit to achieve greater motion. The offset buddy strap (Fig. 37-6) accommodates different phalangeal lengths of adjacent digits (Jensen & Rayan, 1996). Buddy straps are also useful to retrain keyboard users who habitually maintain the small finger MP in hyperextension or repetitively hyperabduct the small finger when keyboarding.

A dorsal MP flexion blocking orthosis promotes composite flexion incorporating MP flexion and is particularly helpful when there is extrinsic extensor tightness. If the patient has difficulty incorporating MP flexion into composite fisting and instead extends the MPs while flexing the IPs, a dorsal hood maintaining MP flexion promotes recovery of composite fist incorporating MP flexion (see Chapters 15 and 16 for further splinting guidelines.)

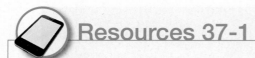

Resources 37-1

Websites

American Society for Surgery of the Hand

Phone: 847-384-8300
http://www.assh.org/Public/HandConditions/Pages/
CarpalTunnelSyndrome.aspx
http://www.assh.org/Public/HandConditions/Pages/
CubitalTunnelSyndrome.aspx
http://www.assh.org/Public/HandConditions/Pages/
deQuervainsTendonitis.aspx
http://www.assh.org/Public/HandConditions/Pages/
TriggerFinger.aspx
http://www.assh.org/Public/HandConditions/Pages/
DupuytrensDisease.aspx
http://www.assh.org/Public/HandConditions/Pages/
GanglionCysts.aspx

Arthritis Foundation

Phone: 800-283-7800
http://www.arthritistoday.org/daily-living/index.php
http://www.arthritistoday.org/fitness/stretching-and-
flexibility/index.php
http://www.arthritistoday.org/fitness/yoga-and-tai-chi/index.
php

Books

Minnesota Hand Rehabilitation, Inc.

Phone: 651-646-4263
Reiner, M. (2004). *The illustrated hand*. St. Paul: Minnesota
Hand Rehabilitation.

CD ROM

Primal Pictures Ltd.

Phone: 44-207-637-10100
McGroutier, D. A., & Colditz, J. (1998). *Interactive hand
therapy*. London: Primal Pictures.

Tests

Physiopro

805 rue Longpre
Sherbrooke, Quebec J1G 5B8, Canada
TEMPA

Videos

(Be aware that resources on youtube may not be clinically
accurate)
http://www.youtube.com/watch?v=65mjCLGrGTE—Hand
and wrist examination.
http://www.youtube.com/
watch?v=jUaWhNji9a8&feature=related—Examination of
the hand.
http://www.youtube.com/
watch?v=vTcgJuwoPis&feature=related—Wrist pain
causes and treatment.

---

more effective than fast jerky stretches, which frequently add to the inflammation.

During the acute inflammatory stage, static splinting is usually most appropriate. After the inflammation has subsided and while the joint displays a soft end feel, dynamic splinting is productive. Inflamed tissue is not as flexible as uninflamed tissue (Glasgow et al., 2011). Watch closely for signs of inflammation and return to static splinting as indicated. Later, if there is a hard end feel, serial static or static progressive splinting will most likely be needed (Glasgow, Tooth, & Fleming, 2010). Many patients with hand impairments complain of morning stiffness. Night splinting, which can be very helpful for this problem, also corrects tissue tightness that limits daytime use of the hand.

Tendinitis/Tendinosis

The pain associated with tendinitis/tendinosis can be severe and can seriously impact performance in all areas of occupation. Symptoms include pain with AROM, with resistance, and with passive stretch of the involved structures. Tendons are made up of connective tissues that are not well vascularized. Tendinitis has been treated historically as if it is an inflammatory phenomenon. More recent histological evidence has shown that the pathology of tendinitis includes alterations in tissue with disorganized and degenerated collagen and atypical vascular granulation tissue. These findings are described as angiofibroblastic hyperplasia or angiofibroblastic tendinosis. It is now believed that the patients who are diagnosed with tendinitis actually have tendinosis. Because the pathology is not primarily inflammatory, treatment approaches now emphasize interventions that restore nourishment to collagen (Ashe, McCauley, & Khan, 2004). The question of use of modalities with this diagnosis remains intriguing. Most authorities report that modalities are effective in reducing pain, normalizing the vascular status of the involved tissue, and quieting inflammation if it exists.

Debate is ongoing over the cause of musculoskeletal problems; whether such problems are work related remains controversial (Seror & Seror, 2012). Tendons are vulnerable because they are relatively avascular. Cell damage may become chronic (Barr, 2006). Biomechanical deficits include muscular weakness, inflexibility, and scar tissue. Early treatment of an acute traumatic case typically has a better prognosis than after the injury has become chronic.

Evaluation

An overaggressive evaluation that provokes pain can set the treatment timetable back significantly and undermine the trust of and rapport with the patient. Start the evaluation with a cervical screening to look for proximal causes of distal symptoms. Compare both extremities. Assess for pain that may be local or diffuse, swelling, sensory changes, and loss of function. Tendinitis typically is accompanied by pain with AROM, with resistance, and with passive stretch of the involved structures. Compare subjective and objective findings, but remember that symptoms are often elusive and may occur dynamically or intermittently. Patients who seem angry or hostile may understandably be depressed over their loss of function.

It is essential to identify the activity causing the pain. Occupational therapists possess unique skills for ergonomic-related analysis of occupational performance and activity modification. It is best to observe the actual activity. If this is not possible, simulate the activity. Ergonomic risk factors for tendinitis include forceful, rapid, repetitive movements. A movement is considered repetitive if it is performed more than once every 30 seconds or for more than half the total work time. Additional risk factors include a history of soft-tissue problems, pressure and shear forces, stress and muscle tension, and hypermobility.

Intervention

Treat the acute phase with ice, compression, elevation of the involved structures, and rest if needed to manage pain. Anti-inflammatory physical agent modalities may be useful at this time (see Chapter 19), but remember that tendinitis/tendinosis is no longer thought to be primarily inflammatory. Splinting is individualized to the patient's and physician's preferences. Orthotic intervention may be most beneficial and least problematic at night. There are also clinical compromises associated with disuse from immobilization. Soft supports may be very helpful. In weighing the advantages and disadvantages of orthotic use, consult closely with the referring physician, try to avoid pain, and monitor the clinical responses. Active pain-free motion is the best way to begin revascularizing the involved tissues.

After the inflammation subsides, upgrade intervention to restore normal function through gradual mobilization balanced with rest. Most importantly, pain must be avoided. Instruct in tendon gliding exercises in a pain-free range

appropriate to the particular structures involved. Progress from isometric exercises with gentle contractions of involved structures to isotonic exercises (Cooper & Martin, 2007). Gradually introduce low-load, high-repetition strengthening in short arcs of motion. Then increase the arc of motion and modify proximal positions to be more challenging if appropriate for work simulation. Instruct in gentle flexibility exercises in a pain-free range. It is often difficult for patients to learn to perform slow and pain-free passive stretch. Aerobic exercises and proximal conditioning are essential.

Prevent reinjury through education (Cooper & Martin, 2007). Simulation and biofeedback (see Chapter 19) can promote biomechanically efficient upper extremity use. Teach the patient to avoid reaching and gripping with an extended elbow or a flexed or deviated wrist. First, solve the easily recognizable issues, such as obviously poor posture or trunk twisting with reaching and lifting. Instruct in pacing to avoid fatigue that leads to reinflammation. Unsupported upper extremity use is taxing, as are nonsymmetrical upper extremity use, nonfrontal trunk or upper extremity alignment, and unilateral upper extremity work. Many people with distal symptoms recover well by focusing intervention on posture, conditioning, and proximal strengthening. Using handheld tools with ergonomic design can be helpful. Even a small ergonomic adjustment, such as learning to lift bilaterally with proper body mechanics or making use of a telephone headset instead of laterally flexing the neck and elevating the shoulder to hold the receiver, can often lead to dramatic improvement.

Lateral Epicondylitis or Tennis Elbow

Lateral epicondylitis involves the extrinsic extensors at their origin. The extensor carpi radialis brevis is most commonly involved. Pain is at the lateral epicondyle and extensor wad (the proximal portion of the extensor muscles). This diagnosis is differentiated clinically from radial tunnel syndrome, in which tenderness occurs more distally over the radial tuberosity. Test for radial tunnel syndrome with the middle finger test (positive if there is pain secondary to resisting the middle finger proximal phalanx while the patient maintains elbow extension, neutral wrist, and MP extension) or by percussing distally to proximally over the superficial radial nerve. This percussion test is positive if it elicits paresthesia (Fedorczyk, 2011).

Exercises should include proximal conditioning and scapular stabilizing. Instruct the client to use built-up handles. If using an orthosis, support the wrist in extension, especially at night. Splinted wrist position recommendations range from neutral to about 30°. Also try a counterforce strap, which is a strap placed over the extensor wad to prevent full muscle contraction and to reduce the load on the tendon during the day with activity. *Safety Message: Avoid applying the counterforce strap too tightly, because this can cause radial tunnel syndrome.*

Medial Epicondylitis, or Golfer's Elbow

Medial epicondylitis involves the extrinsic flexors at their origin. The flexor carpi radialis (FCR) is most commonly involved. Pain is at the medial epicondyle and flexor wad (the proximal portion of the flexor muscles) and worsens with resisted flexion and pronation. Exercise should promote proximal conditioning. Avoid activity that requires force at end ranges. Provide built-up handles. If using an orthosis, maintain the wrist in neutral, and try a counterforce strap over the flexor wad.

De Quervain's Tenosynovitis

De Quervain's tenosynovitis is tendinitis involving the abductor pollicis longus (APL) and extensor pollicis brevis (EPB) tendons at the first dorsal compartment. It is the most common upper extremity tenosynovitis. Finkelstein's test is positive if there is exquisite pain with passive wrist ulnar deviation while flexing the thumb (Fig. 37-7). This diagnosis occurs frequently among golfers, knitters, and racquet sports players. Thumb posture in sustained hyperabduction at the computer space bar may also be provoking. Differential diagnosis is for carpometacarpal (CMC) arthritis, scaphoid fracture, intersection syndrome, and FCR tendinitis (Crop & Bunt, 2011).

Teach patients to avoid wrist deviation, especially in conjunction with pinching. Provide built-up handles. If splinting, use a forearm-based thumb spica, leaving the IP free. Watch for irritation from the radial splint edge along the first dorsal compartment.

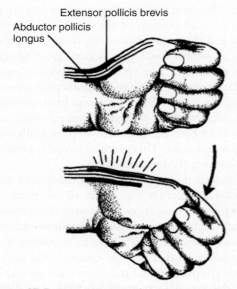

Extensor pollicis brevis

Abductor pollicis longus

Figure 37-7 Finkelstein's test for de Quervain's disease. (Adapted with permission from Rayan, G., & Akelman, E. [2011]. *The hand: Anatomy, examination, and diagnosis.* Philadelphia: Lippincott Williams & Wilkins.)

Intersection Syndrome

Intersection syndrome presents as pain, swelling, and crepitus of the APL and EPB muscle bellies approximately 4 cm proximal to the wrist, where they intersect with the wrist extensor tendons (extensor carpi radialis brevis and extensor carpi radialis longus). This diagnosis is associated with repetitive wrist motion and occurs in weight lifters, rowers, and canoers. Differential diagnosis is for de Quervain's disease, but both diagnoses can occur concomitantly. Teach patients to avoid painful or resisted wrist extension and forceful grip. Orthotic selection is the same as for de Quervain's disease (Mellick & Mellick, 2012).

Extensor Pollicis Longus Tendinopathy

Also called drummer boy palsy, tendinitis of the extensor pollicis longus (EPL) reveals pain and swelling at Lister's tubercle (a dorsal prominence at the distal radius around which the EPL passes). It is less common than other forms of tendinitis, but if left untreated, it can lead to tendon rupture. EPL tendinitis is associated with activities requiring repetitive use of the thumb and wrist, as seen in drummers. Rupture of the EPL may occur in persons with rheumatoid arthritis (RA) or Colles' fracture (Kardashian et al., 2011).

Help patients to identify and eliminate provocative activities. Enlarge the girth of utensils. The orthotic choice is a forearm-based thumb spica that includes the IP.

Extensor Carpi Ulnaris Tendinopathy

Tenosynovitis of the extensor carpi ulnaris (ECU) occurs fairly frequently. It causes pain and swelling distal to the ulnar head and is associated with repetitive ulnar deviation motions. Subluxation of the ECU tendon elicits a painful snap with forearm supination and wrist ulnar deviation. Differential diagnosis includes instability of the distal radioulnar joint and ulnocarpal abutment or tears of the triangular fibrocartilage complex. Teach patients to avoid ulnar deviation with activities. Orthotic intervention consists of a forearm-based ulnar gutter or a wrist cock-up splint.

Flexor Carpi Radialis Tendinopathy

With tendinitis of the FCR, pain is over the FCR tendon just proximal to the wrist flexor creases. Differential diagnosis is for a volar ganglion or arthritis of the scaphotrapeziotrapezoid joint. Orthotic intervention consists of a wrist cock-up in neutral or a position of comfort.

Flexor Carpi Ulnaris Tendinopathy

Flexor carpi ulnaris (FCU) tendinitis is more common than FCR tendinitis. It causes pain along the volar–ulnar side of the wrist. Inflammation occurs where the FCU inserts at the pisiform. Differential diagnosis is pisiform fracture and pisotriquetral arthritis (Verdon, 1996) or triangular fibrocartilage complex injury. Teach patients to avoid wrist flexion with ulnar deviation. Orthotic intervention consists of a forearm-based ulnar gutter. For comfort, pad the ulnar head if it is prominent, so the splint does not rub or irritate it.

Flexor Tenosynovitis, or Trigger Finger

Trigger finger is also called stenosing tenosynovitis of the digital flexor. The usual cause is stenosis at the A-1 pulley, which is part of the fibro-osseous tunnel that prevents bow-stringing of the digital flexors (Taras, Martyak, & Steelman, 2011). Tenderness is over the A-1 pulley of the digital flexor (Fig. 37-8) along with pain with resisted grip and painful catching or locking of the finger in composite flexion (Lee, Biafora, & Zelouf, 2011).

The origin of this impairment can be inflammatory or not. It has been strongly associated with diabetes and RA. Medical management often consists of a mixture of steroid and local anesthetic injected into the flexor sheath. The injection may be repeated a few times. Therapy consists of splinting the MP in neutral to prevent composite digital flexion (preventing triggering), while promoting tendon gliding, and place-and-hold fisting that avoids triggering. Built-up handles, padded gloves, and pacing strategies are helpful. Instruct the patient to avoid triggering, as this reinflames the tissue (Valdes, 2012). If symptoms persist, the surgeon may surgically release the A-1 pulley.

Nerve Injury

When injury or disease occurs to a neural structure in the upper extremity, there is a high likelihood that multiple areas of neural pathology will develop. This phenomenon is known as the double or multiple crush syndrome (Novak & Mackinnon, 2005). Remembering this concept lessens the possibility of missing relevant clinical findings.

The various mechanisms of nerve injury include acute or chronic compression, stretch ischemia, electrical shock, radiation, injection, and laceration (Smith, 2011). Compression and laceration, impairments that are commonly seen by hand therapists, are described next.

Nerve Compression

Median Nerve Compression at the Wrist, or Carpal Tunnel Syndrome. Carpal tunnel syndrome is the most common upper extremity nerve entrapment. It results from compression of the median nerve at the wrist. The carpal bones form the floor of the carpal tunnel. The transverse carpal ligament, also called the flexor retinaculum, forms the roof of the tunnel and acts as a pulley for the flexor tendons during gripping (Amadio, 2011). Inside the carpal canal are nine flexor tendons (four FDP, four flexor digitorum superficialis [FDS], and the flexor pollicis longus) and the median nerve, which is most superficial (Fig. 37-9).

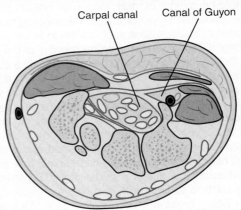

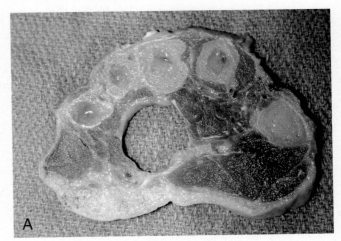

Figure 37-9 **A, B.** Carpal tunnel cross-section. (Adapted with permission from Rayan, G., & Akelman, E. [2011]. *The hand: Anatomy, examination, and diagnosis.* Philadelphia: Lippincott Williams & Wilkins.)

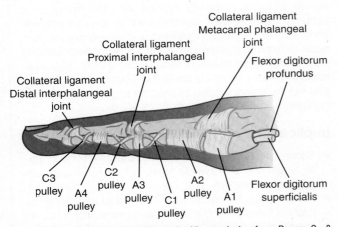

Figure 37-8 Pulley system. (Adapted with permission from Rayan, G., & Akelman, E. [2011]. *The hand: Anatomy, examination, and diagnosis.* Philadelphia: Lippincott Williams & Wilkins.)

Swelling or thickening of the tendons can lead to pressure on the nerve, resulting in sensory symptoms in the distribution of the median nerve (van Doesburg et al., 2012).

Typical complaints include hand numbness, particularly at night or when driving a car, along with pain and paresthesia in the distribution of the median nerve (thumb through radial ring finger pads), and clumsiness or weakness (Zhang et al., 2011) (see Research Note 37-1). Associated diagnoses include RA, Colles' fracture, diabetes, deconditioning, obesity, and thyroid disease. Transient carpal tunnel syndrome is fairly common in pregnancy. Carpal tunnel syndrome may be associated with repetitive use or flexor tenosynovitis caused by increased friction between the tendons and nerve. For these people, focus intervention on resolving the tendinitis.

Evaluation. Perform a cervical screening, and evaluate posture, ROM, grip and pinch, and a manual muscle test looking for independent excursion of FDP and FDS. Also do Tinel's, Phalen's, Semmes-Weinstein Monofilament, and two-point discrimination tests. Tapping at the volar wrist elicits Tinel's sign, which is a sensation of tingling or electric shock if the median nerve is compromised. Phalen's test provokes sensory symptoms in the median nerve distribution if positive, created by maintaining the wrist in flexion for 60 seconds. Phalen's test should be done with extended elbows to avoid confusing these findings with a positive elbow flexion test (see section on cubital tunnel syndrome). Advanced cases of carpal tunnel syndrome reveal thenar atrophy of the abductor pollicis brevis, which can be functionally debilitating (Seftchick et al., 2011).

Intervention. Conservative medical management may include steroid injection (Amadio, 2011). Conservative therapy for carpal tunnel syndrome includes night splinting with the wrist in neutral because this position minimizes pressure in the carpal tunnel, exercises for median nerve gliding at the wrist (Fig. 37-10), differential flexor tendon gliding exercises (Fig. 37-3), aerobic exercise, proximal conditioning, ergonomic modification, and postural training (Schmid et al., 2012). Teach patients to avoid extremes of forearm rotation or of wrist motions and to avoid sustained pinch or forceful grip. Provide padded gloves and built-up handles. Thick padded automobile steering wheel covers are helpful.

Surgical intervention consists of decompression of the carpal tunnel by division of the transverse carpal ligament (Amadio, 2011). Carpal tunnel release is one of the 10 most

Research Note 37-1

Zhang, W., Johnston, J. A., Ross, M. A., Smith, A. A., Coakley, B. J., Gleason, E. A., Dueck, A. C., & Santello, M. (2011). Effects of carpal tunnel syndrome on adaptation of multi-digit forces to object weight for whole-hand manipulation. *PLoS ONE, 6,* e27715. doi: 10.1371/journal.pone.0027715. Retrieved May 14, 2012 from www.plosone.org.

Abstract

The delicate tuning of digit forces to object properties can be disrupted by a number of neurological and musculoskeletal diseases. One such condition is carpal tunnel syndrome (CTS), a compression neuropathy of the median nerve that causes sensory and motor deficits in a subset of digits in the hands. Whereas the effects of CTS on median nerve physiology are well understood, the extent to which it affects whole-hand manipulation remains to be addressed. CTS affects only the lateral three and a half digits, which raises the question of how the central nervous system integrates sensory feedback from affected and unaffected digits to plan and execute whole-hand object manipulation. We addressed this question by asking CTS patients and healthy controls to grasp, lift, and hold a grip device (445, 545, or 745 g) for several consecutive trials. We found that CTS patients were able to successfully adapt grip force to object weight. However, multidigit force coordination in patients was characterized by lower discrimination of force modulation to lighter object weights, higher across-trial digit force variability, the consistent use of excessively large digit forces across consecutive trials, and a lower ability to minimize net moments on the object. Importantly, the mechanical requirement of attaining equilibrium of forces and torques caused CTS patients to exert excessive forces at both CTS-affected digits and digits with intact sensorimotor capabilities. These findings suggest that CTS-induced deficits in tactile sensitivity interfere with the formation of accurate sensorimotor memories of previous manipulations. Consequently, CTS patients use compensatory strategies to maximize grasp stability at the expense of exerting consistently larger multidigit forces than controls. These behavioral deficits might be particularly detrimental for tasks that require fine regulation of fingertip forces for manipulating light or fragile objects.

Implications for Practice

- Clients with CTS have sensory loss that affects hand dexterity and use of the whole hand, not just the fingers with sensory impairment.
- Hand therapy for clients with CTS should address occupational tasks that incorporate use of the whole hand, not just those digits with sensory innervation of the median nerve.

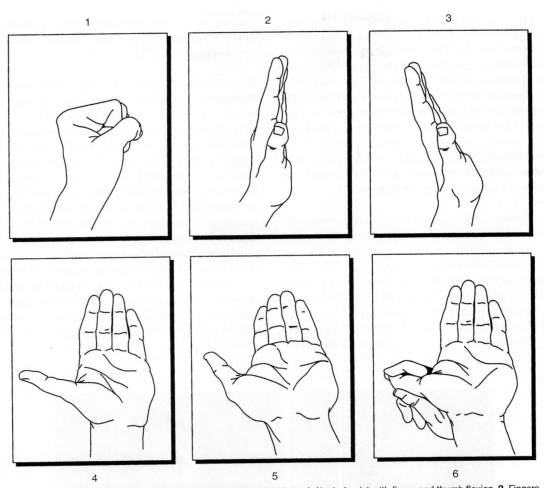

Figure 37-10 Median nerve gliding exercises at the wrist. Positions: **1.** Neutral wrist with finger and thumb flexion. **2.** Fingers and thumb extended. **3.** Wrist and fingers extended with thumb in neutral. **4.** Thumb extended. **5.** Forearm supinated. **6.** Thumb gently stretched into extension. (Adapted with permission from Cooper, C. [2007]. *Fundamentals of hand therapy*. St. Louis: Mosby.)

frequent surgeries performed in the United States. Postoperative therapy, when necessary, consists of edema control, scar management, desensitization as needed, nerve and tendon gliding exercises (Evans, 2011a), and eventual strengthening. Many therapists postpone strengthening exercises until at least 6 weeks following carpal tunnel release to avoid inflammation. Patients with new and mild symptoms tend to recover best.

Ulnar Nerve Compression at the Elbow, or Cubital Tunnel Syndrome. Cubital tunnel syndrome is the second most common upper extremity nerve entrapment and is the most commonly compressed site of the ulnar nerve, at its location between the medial epicondyle and the olecranon (Oskay et al., 2010). Typical complaints include proximal and medial forearm pain that is aching or sharp; decreased sensation of the dorsal and palmar surfaces of the small finger and the ulnar half of the ring finger; and weakness of interossei, adductor pollicis (AP),

FCU, and FDP of the ring and small fingers. Clawing may be more evident if the FDP is not involved because the long flexors are unopposed. Wartenberg's sign, the inability to adduct the small finger, and Froment's sign, in which effort at lateral pinch elicits thumb IP flexion because of weakness of the AP, may be seen. Grip and pinch strength are decreased, and patients complain of dropping things. Symptoms are worse when the elbow is flexed repeatedly or is kept in flexion because this position dramatically reduces the volume of the cubital tunnel (Porretto-Loehrke & Soika, 2011). Understandably, symptoms may increase at night if the person sleeps with the elbow flexed.

Cubital tunnel syndrome may result from trauma, such as a blow to the elbow or fracture or dislocation of the supracondylar or medial epicondylar area, or it may be due to chronic mild pressure on the elbow. Associated diagnoses include osteoarthritis (OA), RA, diabetes, and Hansen's disease.

Evaluation. Tapping over the cubital tunnel elicits a positive Tinel's sign. However, Tinel's sign may also be positive in 20% of normal people. The elbow flexion test is positive if passively flexing the elbow and holding it flexed for 60 seconds produces sensory symptoms. Keep the wrist neutral while performing the elbow flexion test so as not to confound the findings with Phalen's test. Look for digital clawing and for muscle atrophy in the first web space, hypothenar eminence, and medial forearm. Perform grip and pinch testing and manual muscle testing as appropriate, and test sensation. Goldman et al. (2009) provide an excellent review of ulnar neuropathy assessment.

Intervention. Conservative therapy for cubital tunnel syndrome includes edema control; splinting or padding the elbow; and positioning guidelines to avoid leaning on the elbow, to avoid elbow-flexed postures, and to avoid elbow-intensive activity. An elbow orthosis helps prevent sleeping with the elbow flexed. Types of orthotics include elbow pads or soft splints, pillows, and anterior or posterior thermoplastic orthoses. The splinted elbow position for sleeping is usually about 30° of flexion. Additional therapy includes proximal conditioning, postural and ergonomic training, and ulnar nerve gliding exercises (Porretto-Loehrke & Soika, 2011) (Fig. 37-11).

Radial Nerve Compression, or Posterior Interosseous Nerve Syndrome. Posterior interosseous nerve syndrome is purely motor. It presents two clinical pictures. In one, paralysis affects all muscles innervated by the posterior interosseous nerve, with inability to extend the MP joints of thumb, index, long, ring, or small fingers. Wrist extension occurs only radially because of paralysis of extensor digitorum and ECU. In the other presentation of this syndrome, the person cannot extend the MP joint of one or more digits. Paralysis may spread to other digits if it is not treated on a timely basis (Duff & Estilow, 2011).

A common site of entrapment of the posterior interosseous nerve is at the supinator muscle, where it pierces the two heads of this muscle. Other causes include soft tissue tumors, RA with synovial proliferation, and radial head fractures or dislocations. Therapy focuses on maintaining PROM and orthotic selection to prevent deformity and promote function.

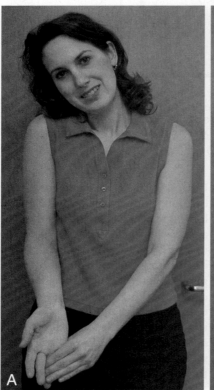
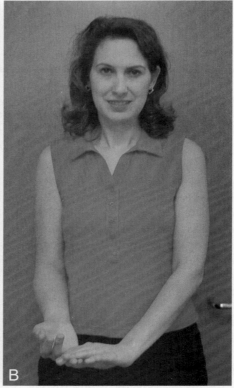

Figure 37-11 Neural mobilization for cubital tunnel syndrome in highly irritable stage. **A.** Ipsilateral scapular elevation and cervical side-bending while the wrist, ring, and small fingers are extended with the forearm remaining supinated and the elbow extended. **B.** Return the scapula and cervical spine to neutral as the patient brings the wrist, ring, and small fingers into slight flexion. Perform this in a slow and in rhythmic manner. (Adapted with permission from Skirven, T. M., Osterman, A. L., Fedorczyk, J. M., & Amadio, P. C. [Eds.]. [2011]. *Rehabilitation of the hand and upper extremity* [6th ed.]. Philadelphia: Mosby.)

Nerve Laceration

Nerve lacerations are categorized as complete or partial. Stretching and contusion injuries can occur along with the laceration. Nerve reconstruction is termed primary if within 48 hours, early secondary if within 6 weeks, and late secondary after 3 months. The advantages associated with primary repair are that nerve stump retraction is limited, and electrical stimulation can be used to identify distal fascicles [nerve bundles] (Smith, 2011).

A neuroma, a disorganized mass of nerve fibers, can follow nerve injury. Significant nerve pain is elicited by tapping over the neuroma, with hypersensitivity limiting functional use of the hand. Desensitization techniques are helpful, along with padding over the painful area to promote functional use.

Following nerve injury, therapy promotes functional performance in the areas of occupation with ADL training and adaptive equipment and assists in prevention of deformity with orthotics and appropriate PROM. Hand therapy provides valuable education to patients about their diagnosis and general recovery sequence and teaches protective guidelines to compensate for sensory loss. Hand therapy monitors changes in sensory and motor function and helps prevent joint contractures and imbalance by reevaluating ROM, sensation, and muscle status. Orthotic modifications are based on clinical changes over time.

Low Median Nerve Lesion. Median nerve laceration at the wrist results in low median nerve palsy, with denervation of the opponens pollicis and abductor pollicis brevis of the thumb and of the lumbricals to the index and long fingers. Clawing of the index and long fingers does not usually occur because the interossei remain ulnarly innervated. Loss of sensation of the radial side of the hand is present. With the absence of thumb abduction and opposition, the thumb rests in adduction, where it may become contracted (Fig. 37-12). Fabricate a hand-based thumb abduction orthosis to maintain balance, to substitute for lost thumb opposition, and to prevent overstretching of denervated muscles (Moscony, 2007a).

Median nerve laceration creates serious functional loss of manipulation and sensibility of the thumb, index, and long fingers. Motor recovery usually occurs before sensory recovery. Be sure to teach compensatory strategies to avoid reinjury while sensibility is impaired. Instruct the patient to perform PROM to maintain joint mobility. Fabricate orthotics to sustain thumb abduction and digital MP flexion with IP extension to promote functional hand use and to counteract the deforming forces of the injury.

High Median Nerve Lesion. Injury near or at the elbow is called a high median nerve injury. Along with the motor loss identified earlier, there is denervation of FDP to index and long fingers, FDS to all digits, pronator teres, and

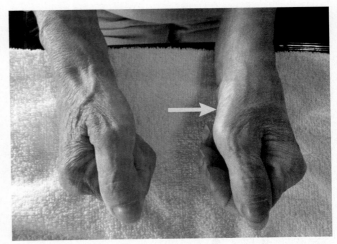

Figure 37-12 Thenar wasting (atrophy of thumb muscles) caused by median nerve problem.

pronator quadratus. The median nerve is considered the most important sensory nerve, and its loss severely compromises hand function. In therapy, prepare patients for probable tendon transfers by preventing deformity with orthotics and by maintaining PROM of pronation, of digital MPs in flexion, of digital IPs in extension, and of thumb CMC abduction. Visual cues, adaptive devices, and modified handles may help compensate for the functional loss.

Low Ulnar Nerve Lesion. Laceration of the ulnar nerve at the wrist level is called a low ulnar lesion. This injury results in loss of most of the hand intrinsics. Denervation of the abductor digiti minimi, flexor digiti minimi, and opponens digiti minimi results in flattening of the hand with loss of the ulnar transverse metacarpal arch; denervation of thumb AP and deep head of flexor pollicis brevis results in loss of thumb adduction and MP support; denervation of dorsal and volar interossei results in loss of digital abduction or adduction; and denervation of lumbricals to the ring and small fingers results in extrinsic imbalance. The ring and small fingers present a claw deformity, a position of MP hyperextension and PIP flexion associated with muscle imbalance in ulnar-innervated structures (Fig. 37-13). Fine manipulation skills are compromised. Sensory loss involves the ulnar digits.

Orthotic intervention for ulnar nerve palsy aims to prevent overstretching of the denervated ring and small finger intrinsics. An MP blocking orthosis that maintains slight MP flexion and prevents MP extension is recommended (Moscony, 2007a) (see Chapter 15). Teach patients to compensate for sensory loss and to maintain passive range of the MPs in flexion and the IPs in extension. It is very important to prevent PIP flexion contractures. Built-up handles in conjunction with the MP blocking orthosis may be helpful.

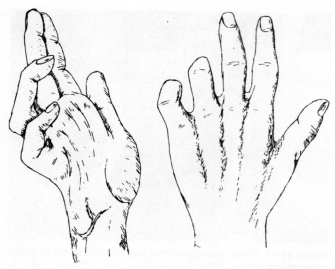

Figure 37-13 Clawing of digits seen with ulnar nerve problems. (From Snell, R. S. [2003]. *Clinical anatomy* [7th ed.]. Baltimore: Lippincott Williams & Wilkins.)

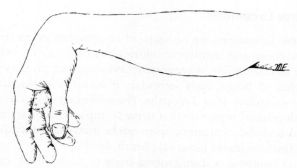

Figure 37-14 Wrist drop caused by radial nerve problem. (From Snell, R. S. [2003]. *Clinical anatomy* [7th ed.]. Baltimore: Lippincott Williams & Wilkins.)

High Ulnar Nerve Lesion. A high ulnar nerve lesion is often identified with trauma at or proximal to the elbow. There is involvement of the muscles listed earlier and denervation of FDP of ring and small fingers and of FCU. Ring and small finger clawing is less apparent with the high lesion but becomes noticeable as the FDP are reinnervated and are unopposed by the still-absent intrinsics. Orthotic intervention and treatment are the same as for a low ulnar nerve lesion. If the FDP is absent, teach the patient to maintain full PROM of the IPs of the ring and small fingers to prevent contractures (Colditz, 2011).

Low Radial Nerve Lesion. Low radial nerve injury of the deep motor branch is called posterior interosseous palsy. Presentations vary (see section on Radial Nerve Compression), but brachioradialis and extensor carpi radialis longus function is usually present. Efforts to extend the wrist yield strong radial deviation. MP extension is affected. Sensation on the dorsal radial hand is affected (Wu, Hsu, & Wang, 2010). Therapy is similar to that described for radial nerve compression, with emphasis on maintaining PROM for wrist, thumb, and digital extension and orthotics to promote tenodesis for functional pinch, grip, and release.

High Radial Nerve Lesion. A high radial nerve injury is seen commonly with humeral fractures because this nerve spirals around the humerus. Wrist and digital extensors are absent (Fig. 37-14). Sensory loss occurs on the dorsal–radial hand, which interferes less with function than does sensory loss on the palmar hand. Triceps function remains, but the supinator and all wrist and finger extensors lose function. Tenodesis is lost (Tuncel, Turan, & Kostakoglu, 2011).

Splinting restores tenodesis and may be useful for the many months during the wait for reinnervation, which occurs at approximately 1 inch per month. Various static and dynamic orthoses are available; the dynamic orthotics are most useful functionally. Many patients make good use of both types of orthoses. Compliance tends to be good because of the functional value of these orthoses. It is important to maintain joint suppleness while awaiting reinnervation or reconstructive surgery.

Fractures

Distal Radius Fracture

Distal radius fractures are among the most common upper extremity fractures (Medoff, 2011). Hand therapists frequently treat patients with this diagnosis. Distal radius fractures should not be confused with fractures of the carpal bones. The main complication associated with distal radius fracture is traumatic arthritis caused by poor articular congruency. Decreased wrist ROM, decreased grip strength, alteration of the carpal alignment, and instability may ensue. Other complications include tendon rupture, compression of the median or ulnar nerve, and complex regional pain syndrome (CRPS) (Michlovitz & Festa, 2011).

Therapy during Immobilization. Appropriate early therapy intervention can make a huge difference in the patient's overall functional recovery. If digits are allowed to become swollen and stiff, the long-term functional results can be devastating. These fractures are common among older people with osteoporosis and balance problems. Temporary loss of independence following fracture can trigger an irreversible downward spiral in their occupational functioning.

Typical medical management of Colles' fracture is cast immobilization, usually above elbow with the elbow in 90° of flexion to prevent forearm rotation during the first 3 weeks. When the patient is put in a short arm cast and the elbow is freed, begin elbow AROM for flexion and extension, but avoid resisted elbow motion so as not to stress the fracture healing. Do not perform elbow PROM without medical clearance, and be very gentle. Biceps tightness commonly follows elbow immobilization.

Certain fractures require some form of fixation. Some physicians delay the referral of patients to therapy, but postponing the initiation of therapy can result in significant problems with edema and decreased ROM. It is a good idea to communicate with referring physicians and encourage routine early therapy referral for this diagnosis.

While the patient has percutaneous pins, provide pin site care as the physician prescribes using sterile technique and universal precautions. Teach the patient digital ROM and tendon gliding exercises, and instruct in precautions related to cast wearing. It is critical to monitor for cast tightness because a tight cast can cause CRPS. Call the physician if the cast is too tight. Discourage the use of slings because they promote unnecessary proximal stiffness, guarded posture, and disuse.

Insidious onset of shoulder restrictions is problematic and best avoided. Physicians most assuredly appreciate therapists' input regarding early signs of this problem. To prevent a frozen shoulder, proximal ROM is a high treatment priority (Michlovitz & Festa, 2011). Instruct in shoulder flexion, abduction, internal rotation, and external rotation. Perform as thorough a physical assessment as tolerated and as cast constraints permit. This may have to be done in phases. Early identification of guarding, excessive pain, or autonomic signs can alert the team to the possibility of CRPS.

Following distal radius fracture, the recovery of function depends on restoration of motion and strength and on maximizing the length-tension relationship of the digital flexors and extensors (Moscony, 2007b). Edema can contribute to decreased ROM at uncasted areas. Patients are often surprised that uninjured and uncasted areas can stiffen.

The goals of early therapy during immobilization are to normalize edema and to achieve as nearly normal AROM of uncasted areas as possible. During this period, intrinsic tightness, extrinsic tightness, and digital joint tightness may occur. The chance of tendon adherence is increased following open reduction and its accompanying incisional scar. Various blocking splints may be used with functional activity and exercise to resolve joint or musculotendinous tightness (Fig. 37-4). Differential tendon gliding exercises are extremely important. Frequent exercise throughout the day is better than a few long sessions. It is generally advised to perform exercises every hour or two, perhaps 5–10 repetitions each, maintaining the end position comfortably for 3–5 seconds. Incorporate exercises into occupation, including ADL, as much as possible (Moscony, 2007b).

If extrinsic musculotendinous tightness persists, it may be appropriate to add night static progressive splinting or low-load, long-duration dynamic splinting in conjunction with exercise to normalize extrinsic length. Consult the physician before making this determination.

Therapy after Immobilization Stage. When fracture immobilization is discontinued, physicians often recommend a custom-fabricated volar wrist orthosis. This is protective and can be corrective to help restore functional wrist motion (usually extension). This temporary support is particularly helpful if the patient maintains habitual wrist flexion because this "doggy paw" posture leads to development of the undesirable deformity position of MP extension, PIP flexion, and thumb adduction and extension discussed earlier.

At this stage of therapy, there is usually measurable limitation in ROM, with patients reporting awkwardness and decreased function (Bruder et al., 2011). Consult the physician for medical clearance and guidelines for forearm and wrist ROM. *Safety Message: Do not initiate PROM of the wrist without medical clearance because this may be injurious.* Teach the patient to wean off the protective orthosis according to the physician's guidelines, which are individualized. Edema control continues to be the highest priority until it is resolved. AROM and ADL can help correct the edema.

At any time, but especially in this early stage, overzealous therapy is harmful. Patients and families who think they should be aggressive in their home programs need education and reinforcement to avoid overdoing it. Use written material and illustrations to teach them how to observe tissue responses and monitor inflammation. Temperature elevation or redness over the joints of digits may indicate that intervention is eliciting an inflammatory reaction and should be adjusted accordingly (Michlovitz & Festa, 2011).

It is extremely important to retrain the wrist extensors to function independently of the extensor digitorum. Have the patient practice wrist extension with available composite digital flexion, being especially sure the MPs are flexed. Then have the patient flex the wrist with digits relaxed but extended to isolate the wrist flexors. Because substitution patterns are hard to overcome, early training of biomechanically efficient movement is best. Progressive grasp-and-release activities reinforce this tenodesis training. It is also important to retrain the extensor digitorum to function independently of the intrinsics. Have the patient extend the MPs with the IPs slightly flexed to isolate the extensor digitorum.

Gradually upgrade therapy with increasingly challenging motions, combined motions, and activities aiming to restore joint suppleness and musculotendinous lengths. Dexterity activities, such as cat's cradle, and games, such as pick-up sticks, promote spontaneous functional movements.

Sorting drawers and folding small items of clothing are good home activities. Initiate graded functional strengthening with medical clearance, usually after good motion has been achieved. Again, it is easy to be too aggressive with these patients. Upgrade carefully, monitor patient and tissue responses, and adjust the intervention accordingly.

Scaphoid Fracture

Some 60% of carpal fractures affect the scaphoid (also called the navicular) bone, making scaphoid fractures the most common of all carpal fractures. The mechanism of injury is usually a fall on the outstretched hand (called FOOSH) with wrist radial deviation. Associated ligamentous injury may also be present. Tenderness in the anatomical snuffbox, a depression at the base of the thumb between the EPL and EPB tendons, where snuff used to be placed, is a classic finding. Scaphoid fracture may be difficult to confirm radiographically initially and may not become apparent until 3 weeks following injury because of resorption at the fracture site. Once fracture is confirmed, the thumb is usually included in the cast, with the IP joint free (Doornberg et al., 2011; Geissler et al., 2012).

Proximal scaphoid fractures may be at risk for developing avascular necrosis because of the pattern of vascular supply. Casting time may be long for this reason. Hand therapy principles are the same as for distal radius fracture (Dell, Dell, & Griggs, 2011).

Nonarticular Hand Fracture

Fracture occurs more often in the hand than any other area, and more than 50% of hand fractures occur at work. Motor vehicle accidents, household injuries, and recreational accidents also account for many of these injuries (Feehan, 2011).

Distal Phalanx Fracture. Distal phalanx digital fractures typically result from a crushing injury and occur most often in the thumb and middle finger. Tuft fractures occur at the distal tip. They are extremely painful, in part because there is often a subungual (i.e., beneath the nail) hematoma (Moscony, 2007b). Following a distal phalanx fracture, hypersensitivity, pain, and decreased ROM of the DIP joint may occur. Monitor closely for signs of DIP extensor lag or the inability to extend the DIP joint actively despite full available passive extension.

Middle Phalanx Fracture. At the middle phalanx, fractures angulate according to their relation to the FDS insertion. Medical management and early positioning guidelines vary among caregivers. Following middle phalanx fractures, decreased PIP and DIP ROM are common problems. Fractures at this site may require long immobilization time for healing, with resulting stiffness. When the patient is medically cleared for therapy, isolated FDS

exercises are very important. Here, too, PIP joint flexion contractures are serious complications that can occur in as little as 2 weeks of immobilization in flexion. Consult with the physician for therapy guidelines based on fracture stability and healing (Moscony, 2007b).

Proximal Phalanx Fracture. At the proximal phalanx, fractures tend to angulate with a palmar apex. This deforming force is due to the action of the intrinsic muscles on the proximal fragment. With proximal phalanx fractures, a hand-based orthosis in intrinsic-plus (antideformity) position is useful at night. A digit-based extension orthosis provides support and protection in the day except during exercise. Again, the physician provides therapy guidelines based on fracture stability and healing. PIP joint flexion contractures are the most likely and most difficult complication. Watch for these, and catch them early. Better yet, avoid them with appropriate orthotics and structure-specific exercise. PIP extensor lag and flexor tendon adherence at the fracture site are other serious problems (Moscony, 2007b).

Metacarpal Fracture. Unless there is associated trauma, metacarpal fractures at the base are frequently stable. Metacarpal fractures at the shaft may be transverse, oblique, or spiral. Metacarpal fractures at the neck are common, occurring most often in the small finger. They may result in muscle imbalance between the intrinsics and extrinsics (Moscony, 2007b).

With metacarpal fractures, dorsal hand edema is a frequent complication that can contribute to MP joint dorsal capsular tightness. If there is associated soft tissue injury, intrinsic contracture or extensor digitorum adherence may occur. Appropriate early therapy and preventive edema control are important (Feehan, 2011).

Unstable fractures require fixation to achieve stability and allow early ROM (Soong, Got, & Katarincic, 2010). Kirschner wires, a common form of fixation used for hand fractures, may be used alone or in conjunction with additional fixation. Other forms of internal fixation include tension band wires, lag screws, plates, and mini external fixators (Belsky & Leibman, 2011). Functional recovery relates to anatomical restoration. To maximize functional outcomes, the ideal situation allows for early motion. Preventing stiffness of uninvolved digits is a high priority that can itself be challenging. Prolonged immobilization is associated with edema and pain. Persistent edema results in joint and tendon scar and adhesions, atrophy, and osteoporosis.

Collateral Ligament Injury

Proximal Interphalangeal Joint Sprain

PIP joint sprains often result from sports involving balls. Their severity, which may be underappreciated, is described as grade I through grade III. In grade I, the ligament

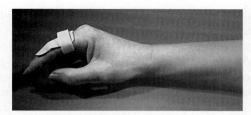

Figure 37-15 Dorsal PIP extension–blocking splint. Protective digit-based splint maintains slight PIP flexion. Used to prevent full extension to protect volar plate injury.

remains intact, but there is diffuse individual fiber disruption. In grade II, there is complete disruption of one of the joint capsule's major retaining ligaments. In grade III, there is complete disruption of one collateral ligament in addition to injury to dorsal and/or volar capsular structures. Pain, decreased ROM, and risk of flexion contracture are the most common problems associated with grades I and II injuries. Joint instability may occur with grade III injuries (Little & Jacoby, 2011).

Therapy focuses on edema control, joint protection, and ROM. Buddy straps are helpful to protect or to promote movement. They may be offset to improve fit (Fig. 37-6). Orthotic intervention is both protective and corrective. A dorsal extension blocking orthosis is often ordered early on for volar plate injuries associated with dorsal PIP joint dislocation (Fig. 37-15). Persistent thickening about the joint commonly occurs, interfering with recovery of ROM.

Skier's Thumb

Disruption of the ulnar collateral ligament of the thumb MP joint occurs with acute radial deviation. This diagnosis, which may entail avulsion of bone fragment at the ligamentous insertion, is often seen among people who fall while skiing (Ritting, Baldwin, & Rodner, 2010). Injury to the radial collateral ligament of the thumb MP occurs only one-tenth as often (Tang, 2011). Following surgical repair, the wrist and thumb are casted. When therapy begins, IP ROM is the priority because full MP flexion may not be achieved, especially among older patients. Avoid resistive exercise until medically cleared. Then begin with lateral pinch but avoid tip pinch until further medical clearance, which may not be for 12 weeks, because tip pinch is strenuous on the injured structures. Use a hand-based spica orthosis for protection. Scar hypersensitivity caused by the underlying radial sensory nerve is common.

Flexor Tendon Injury

Surgical repair of flexor tendon injury is a complex undertaking performed by specialists in the field. Like the surgery, hand therapy for these patients is a complicated and specialized area. Therapy can be time consuming,

and it entails substantial education of the patient, with subtle but significant changes in splinting and exercise at every session to promote function while protecting fragile repaired structures. Multiple structures are often involved, and there are many precautions and contraindications that vary according to the details of the patient's surgery and the surgeon's specifications and preferences. It is essential to maintain close communication with the patient's surgeon. A therapist experienced in the treatment of these patients should closely supervise their care.

Five anatomical zones describe flexor tendon injury to the index, long, ring, and small digits (Fig. 37-16). Zone I is from the insertion of the FDS to the insertion of the FDP. Zone II is the area where the FDS and FDP both lie within the flexor sheath, from the A-1 pulley to the FDS insertion. This region has memorably been dubbed "no man's land" to reflect the technical challenge and historically poor prognosis for repair in this area (Taras, Martyak, & Steelman, 2011). Zone III describes the area from the distal edge of the carpal tunnel to the A-1 pulley of the flexor sheath, including the lumbrical muscles. Zone IV is where the flexor tendons lie under the transverse

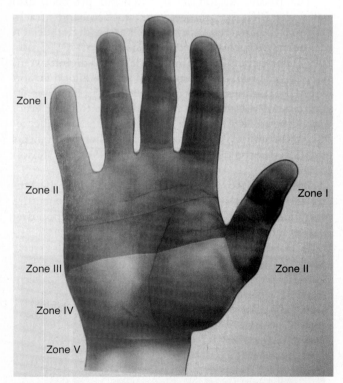

Figure 37-16 The five zones of the hand based on flexor tendon anatomy. Zone I contains flexor digitorum profundus tendon; zone II is the tendon sheath containing flexor digitorum superficialis and flexor digitorum profundus tendons; zone III is the lumbrical muscle zone; zone IV is the carpal tunnel region; and zone V is the forearm area. (From Rayan, G. M., & Akelman, E. [2012]. *The hand: Anatomy, examination, and diagnosis* [Kindle Locations 704–707]. Philadelphia: Lippincott [Wolters Kluwer Health]. Kindle Edition. Used with permission.)

carpal ligament in the carpal tunnel. Injuries in this zone may include the median and ulnar nerves. Zone V is the area from the forearm flexor musculotendinous junction to the border of the transverse carpal ligament (Taras, Martyak, & Steelman, 2011).

Physicians usually indicate specific postoperative positioning guidelines to protect repaired structures following flexor tendon repair. The goals are twofold and contradictory: to minimize adhesion formation and to prevent gap or attenuation of the repaired tendon (Korstanje et al., 2010, 2012). These dual goals highlight the complexity of therapy associated with this diagnosis. Various protocols exist for controlled mobilization, using a dorsal orthosis with the wrist in 10°–30° of flexion, MP joints in 40°–60° of flexion, and IP joints ideally in full extension (unless there has also been a digital nerve repair). The involved IP joints may have to be in some flexion if a digital nerve has been repaired. The Duran protocol entails passive digital flexion and extension within the protective orthosis to achieve 3–5 mm of differential digital tendon excursion (Lalonde & Kozin, 2011). With this protocol, gentle active motion begins with medical clearance about 4 weeks after surgery.

The passive flexion–active extension protocol, also called the Kleinert protocol, uses rubber band attachments to the fingernails to provide passive digital flexion within the protective dorsal orthosis (Fig. 37-17) (Groth, 2005). The patient performs gentle active digital extension, and the rubber band provides passive digital flexion within the confines of the protective orthosis. Exercises are gradually increased to 10 repetitions comfortably every waking hour. At night, the digits may be strapped carefully and comfortably to the dorsal hood of the orthosis to counteract the tendency to develop PIP or DIP flexion contractures.

The Chow protocol uses a combination of the Duran and Kleinert techniques. With advances in suture techniques, flexor tendons protocols are incorporating

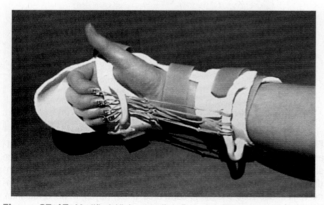

Figure 37-17 Modified Kleinert splint. Dorsal splint maintains the wrist in 30° of flexion, MPs in 70° of flexion, and IPs in extension. Rubber band attachments provide passive digital flexion.

early active motion in patients who are good candidates (Chesney et al., 2011; Griffin et al., 2012).

When the physician gives medical clearance to discontinue the dorsal protective orthosis, begin a graded program to promote functional movement. Edema control and scar management remain high clinical priorities. Assess closely and determine tissue-specific limitations that guide the therapy program. Tendon gliding exercises and place-and-hold exercises are typical early techniques. Corrective splinting is useful, along with ADL, graded activity, and upgraded exercise as appropriate.

Staged Flexor Tendon Reconstruction

Staged flexor tendon reconstruction is a complex two-part procedure. It is highly advisable to have an experienced hand therapist supervise the treatment. Staged flexor tendon surgery is chosen when there is significant scarring of the tendon yet potential for eventual function. It may be used in cases of flexor tendon rupture or when primary repair is not possible, such as with a complex injury involving bone and multiple tissues. In the first stage, a tendon implant replaces the scarred tendon, capsular contractures are released, and pulleys are reconstructed. The implant, which may be active or passive, stimulates formation of a new biological sheath. In the second stage, after about 3 months, a tendon graft replaces the implant (Diao & Chee, 2011).

Extensor Tendon Injury

Therapy of extensor tendon injuries is complicated and requires supervision by experienced hand therapists. Various protocols are available for immobilization, controlled passive motion, or active short arc of motion following extensor tendon repair (Klein, 2007b).

Seven zones describe the digital extensors for the index, long, ring, and small fingers, and five zones describe the thumb extensors (Fig. 37-18). Injury in zones I and II leads to a mallet deformity, which follows disruption of the terminal extensor tendon and manifests itself as DIP extensor lag (Fig. 37-19). Depending on the nature of the problem, in nonoperative cases, therapy may include continuous splinting of the DIP in extension for 6–8 weeks as determined by the physician while the tendon heals (Anderson, 2011). It is essential to maintain normal PIP ROM during immobilization at the DIP. When initiating ROM of the DIP after the terminal tendon has healed, watch closely for recurrence of DIP extensor lag and resume splinting as needed to recover DIP extension. Some physicians recommend continuation of night splinting when DIP AROM is begun.

Extensor injuries in zones III and IV lead to a boutonniere deformity, an imbalanced digital position of PIP flexion and DIP hyperextension (Fig. 37-20). The deformity is

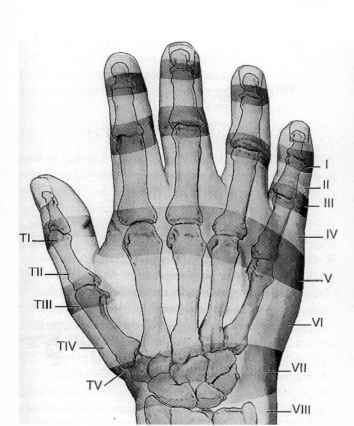

Figure 37-18 The seven zones of the hand based on extensor tendon anatomy. The odd zones I, III, V, and VII belong to distal interphalangeal, proximal interphalangeal, metacarpophalangeal, and wrist joints, respectively. The even zones II, IV, and VI belong to phalanx 2, phalanx 1, and metacarpal. (From Rayan, G. M., & Akelman, E. [2012]. *The hand: Anatomy, examination, and diagnosis* [Kindle Locations 742–744]. Philadelphia: Lippincott [Wolters Kluwer Health]. Kindle Edition. Used with permission.)

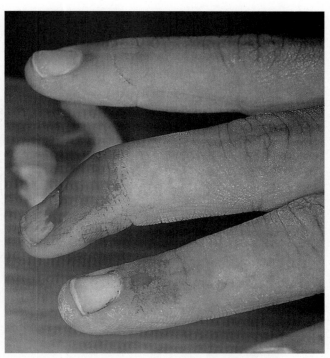

Figure 37-19 Mallet finger. (From Anderson, M. K., Parr, G. P., & Hall, S. J. [2009]. *Foundations of athletic training: Prevention, assessment and management* [4th ed.]. Philadelphia: Lippincott Williams & Wilkins. Used with permission).

Tenolysis

Tenolysis is a surgical procedure to release tendon adhesions that restrict movement. Physicians do not usually perform this procedure until injured tissues have matured and PROM is maximized, as demonstrated by a plateau in progress during therapy. Therapy following tenolysis may begin as early as a few hours after surgery. The first few days following surgery are considered crucial. The physician's referral should include information on the integrity

due to volar displacement of the lateral bands secondary to involvement of the central slip (Williams & Terrono, 2011). In nonoperative cases, splint the PIP in full extension for 6 weeks, and promote DIP active and passive flexion to prevent stiffness of the oblique retinacular ligament. In operative cases, follow the physician's guidelines, which may vary in timing and technique of mobilization and splinting. When the patient is medically cleared to begin PIP active exercises, watch closely for PIP extensor lag, and modify therapy and splinting accordingly.

Injury in zones V and VI may be treated by immobilization or by controlled early motion (Evans, 2011b) (see Evidence Table 37-1). Specific positioning and motion guidelines vary from surgeon to surgeon and are modified according to each patient's tissue responses. Multiple complex orthotics may be needed to achieve a program that balances rest and motion appropriately.

Injury in zone VII is likely to result in restrictions because of development of adhesions. Communicate closely with the surgeon for specific positioning and motion guidelines.

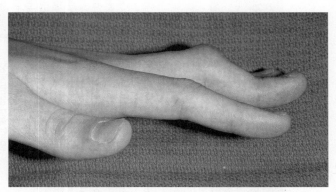

Figure 37-20 Boutonniere deformity. (From Anderson, M. K., Parr, G. P., & Hall, S. J. [2009]. *Foundations of athletic training: Prevention, assessment and management* [4th ed.]. Philadelphia: Lippincott Williams & Wilkins. Used with permission).

Evidence Table 37-1 | Best Evidence for Occupational Therapy Practice Regarding Treatment of Hand Impairments

Intervention	Description of Intervention Tested	Participants	Dosage	Type of Best Evidence and Level of Evidence	Benefit	Statistical Probability and Effect Size of Outcome	Reference
Postoperative treatment protocols for zones V and VI extensor tendon lacerations of the hand	Immobilization (IM): complete immobilization of wrist at 40°–45°, metacarpophalangeal (MCP) and IPs at 0° for 3 weeks in a splint. Early passive motion (EPM): dorsal dynamic splint and controlled passive motion. Early active motion (EAM): palmar blocking splint and active motion	Twenty-seven patients from three sites, within 5 days post surgery for zones V and VI extensor tendon lacerations; randomized to 3 groups (n = 9 per group); mean age = 30.4 years 33% attrition at 6 weeks: 5 (IM); 4 (EPM); 0 (EAM). Defaulters claimed recovery had occurred and no further treatment was necessary.	IM: Splint was discontinued at 6 weeks, with gradual increase of resistive activity and return to heavy manual labor by the end of 12 weeks. EPM: Passive extension exercises 20 times per hour in the splint and active MP flexion. Passive wrist tenodesis and IP joint motion supervised by therapist. Splint discontinued at 5 weeks, with graded mobilization. Remainder of the protocol same as IM group. EAM: Active motion exercises performed 10 times per hour as allowed by palmar blocking splint extended to the IP joint. At 3 weeks, splint adjusted to allow 70° MCP flexion, and active hook fists were initiated for extensor digitorum glides. At week 5, same as EPM protocol.	Randomized controlled trial (RCT). Level: IC2a	Yes. EAM appears beneficial.	Outcome measured at 3, 6, and 12 weeks. All patients showed steady improvement of total active motion (TAM) during the study period ($F_{2,46}$ = 75.6, $p < 0.001$). There was a significant ($p < 0.004$) difference among the groups in TAM over time, but the pairwise, post-hoc statistics were not reported. EAM group gained more active motion, had less extension lag, more self-reported improvement in function, and greater grip strength; however, none of these differences were significant. A type II error (no difference when one actually existed) could have occurred because of the small sample. Effect sizes for TAM calculated from reported means ± S.D. do indicate moderate strength of relationship between treatment and outcome (EAM versus EPM: r = 0.40; EAM versus IM: r = 0.48)[1]	Hall et al. (2010)

| Intensive lumbrical splint/stretch combination and less intensive lumbrical splint/stretch combinations | Lumbrical splints with wrist in 0° of extension and MCP joints free in 0°–10° of flexion. Prefabricated cock-up splints with wrist in 0° of extension and MCP joints free. Lumbrical stretching and massage. General stretches for composite wrist/hand flexion and extension. LspLst: lumbrical splint/lumbrical stretch group (intensive lumbrical intervention). LspGst: lumbrical splint/general stretch group. GspLst: general splint/lumbrical stretch group. GspGst: general splint/general stretch group. | One hundred twenty-four volunteers with mild to moderate carpal tunnel syndrome (CTS) randomized to 4 groups: lumbrical splint/lumbrical stretch (LspLst) n = 31; lumbrical splint/general stretch (LspGst) n = 34; general splint/lumbrical stretch (GspLst) n = 34; general splint/general stretch (GspGst) n = 28. One hundred three subjects remained at 4 weeks (17% attrition rate). Ninety-five subjects remained at 12 weeks; attrition rate 23% from baseline. Eighty-nine subjects remained at 24 weeks; attrition rate 29% from baseline. | Randomized clinical trial Level: IA2b | Four-week regimen. Subjects wore splints at night and performed exercises 10 times per session, six sessions per day, 7-second hold for each stretch. | At 4 weeks, all splint/ stretch combinations were equally effective as measured by the DASH (Disabilities of the Arm, Shoulder, and Hand) and Carpal Tunnel Questionnaire. At 12 weeks, LspGst and GspLst groups demonstrated continued improvement, and the other two groups did not. At 24 weeks, only the GspLst group improved in function to a clinically important degree. From baseline (chi square analysis significant at $\alpha = .05$) By 24 weeks, 25.5% of subjects chose to undergo surgery; no significant difference between groups. | At 4 weeks, 66% of subjects achieved clinically important improvement in symptoms, but only 34% achieved clinically important improvement in function. At 12 weeks, 68% of subjects achieved clinically important improvement in function. At 24 weeks, a significantly greater percentage of subjects in the GspLst group achieved a clinically important improvement in function. Conclusion: a cock-up splint combined with stretches targeting the lumbricales is a more effective long term treatment for functional gains than splinting or stretching alone or other tested combinations for people with mild to moderate CTS. | Baker et al. (2012) |

significant p ≤ .001

(continued)

Evidence Table 37-1 | Best Evidence for Occupational Therapy Practice Regarding Treatment of Hand Impairments (continued)

			Dosage			
Conservative interventions for osteoarthritis (OA) of the hand to relieve pain, prevent joint deformity, and/or to increase function	Splinting, joint protection instruction with provision of adapted devices, local application of heat (paraffin or hot pack), exercises, and home exercise program	Systematic review of 21 RCT and cohort studies published between 1986 and 2009 that met the following criteria: (1) patients had OA of hands; (2) treatment of OA was conservative. Ten studies were of high quality, 10 were of moderate quality, and 1 was poor quality.	NA	Systematic review Level: I	Conclusion: (1) High to moderate evidence to support carpometacarpal (CMC) orthotics to lessen pain and increase function; (2) moderate evidence to support hand exercise, low-level heat, and CMC orthotics to increase grip strength; (3) moderate evidence to support hand exercises, joint protection education and provision of adapted equipment, use of CMC orthotics to increase hand function; (4) moderate evidence to support hand exercises to increase range of motion (ROM) (5) moderate evidence to support hand exercises, joint protection education and provision of adapted equipment, low level heat to decrease pain; and (6) weak evidence for paraffin to decrease pain and increase ROM and function Moderate evidence that low level laser therapy is no better than placebo to increase function or decrease pain or stiffness	No statistics or effect sizes reported	Valdes & Marik (2010)

[1] Cohen, J. (1992). A power primer. *Psychological Bulletin, 112*, 155–159; Rosenthal, R., & Rosnow, R. L. (1991). *Essentials of behavioral research: Methods and data analysis* (2nd ed.). New York: McGraw-Hill, Inc.

of the tendon and expected ROM goals based on intra-operative findings (Culp, Feldscher, & Rodriguez, 2011). First priorities are edema control and ROM; observe and respect the tolerances of these fragile tissues.

Complex Regional Pain Syndrome

Any upper extremity injury, whether as minor as a paper cut or as major as a complex crush injury, has the potential to result in devastating reflex sympathetic dystrophy (RSD), renamed complex regional pain syndrome (CRPS) by the International Association for the Study of Pain. CRPS type I follows a noxious event. Pain that is not limited to the territory of a single peripheral nerve occurs spontaneously and is disproportionate to the inciting noxious event. Edema is present, with abnormality of skin color or abnormal sudomotor activity in the painful area since the onset. The diagnosis of CRPS is excluded by other existing conditions that may cause the pain and dysfunction (van de Meent et al., 2011).

CRPS type II is the same as type I except that it develops after a nerve injury, whereas type I does not involve a nerve injury. CRPS type III refers to a group not otherwise specified and includes patients who do not fulfill the criteria for types I or II (Veizi, Chelimsky, & Janata, 2012) .

Pain that is disproportionate to the injury is the hallmark of CRPS. Constant attention to the patient's pain level and autonomic responses can lead to early medical management, if not prevention, of this challenging problem. The earlier this problem is diagnosed, the more successfully it may resolve (Walsh, 2011).

The four cardinal symptoms and signs of CRPS are pain, swelling, stiffness, and discoloration. Secondary symptoms and signs include osseous demineralization, sudomotor changes (sweating), temperature changes, trophic changes, vasomotor instability, palmar fasciitis (thickening of palmar fascia), and pilomotor activity (goose pimples or hair standing on end).

Elegant animal studies have shown that self-protection through immobilization, intended to avoid pain, is itself a risk factor for the diagnosis of CRPS. People with CRPS must learn to use the extremity in ways that are pain free and biomechanically efficient. Normalizing sensory input also helps interrupt the vicious cycle of pain and stiffness (Goebel, 2011).

Therapy for Complex Regional Pain Syndrome

The most important therapy guideline is no PROM or painful intervention. The first thing is to control the pain. This includes management through medications, sympathetic blocks such as stellate ganglion blocks, and modalities such as TENS as appropriate. Close communication with medical experts specializing in pain management is ideal (Veizi, Chelimsky, & Janata, 2012).

Provide vasomotor challenge through stress loading (described later), temperature biofeedback, and posture changes during activity. It also helps to reset the sensory thresholds through contrast baths, vibration, and desensitization (see Chapter 22). Water aerobics and functional activities are excellent ways to provide active movement incorporating reciprocal motion. Use stress loading routinely with patients who are at risk for CRPS. Stress loading is proposed to change sympathetic efferent activity. Although the physiological mechanisms of stress loading are not known (Carlson & Watson, 1988), it is popular among hand therapists for treating active CRPS, not the sequelae (Veizi, Chelimsky, & Janata, 2012).

The two components of stress loading are "scrubbing the floor" (performed literally on all fours if possible), in brief sessions, three times per day initially, and carrying a weighted briefcase, done with the extremity in extension. The weight should be light and tolerable. Be sure it is not too heavy. Scrubbing and carrying achieve compressive loading and distraction of the upper extremity. If actual scrubbing cannot be tolerated, substitute comfortable weight-bearing exercises.

The frequency and duration of scrub and carry are upgraded as tolerated. If wrist ROM limitations or injury precautions do not allow the patient to assume the scrub position, positions may be adapted to accomplish comfortable weight bearing (see online Chapter A). Also instruct the patient to perform frequent pain-free proximal AROM bilaterally.

Avoid PROM or other therapy until the pain and swelling begin to subside, and then monitor responses closely. Incorporate traditional hand therapy, including orthotics and other nonaggravating modalities, with edema control, joint ROM, differential tendon gliding, restoration of musculotendinous lengths, strengthening, desensitization, physical agents including transcutaneous electrical nerve stimulation (TENS) and ultrasound as appropriate, and functional activity within tolerance. Manual edema mobilization is effective with this diagnosis.

Perhaps with CRPS more than other diagnoses, patient-directed therapy is essential. It is better to perform gentle, pain-free active exercises frequently for short periods than fewer and longer sessions. Light massage and active exercise help to interrupt the pain cycle. Make the exercise program bilateral and include reciprocal upper extremity motions. Allow the progress to be as slow as necessary to prevent worsening of symptoms. This diagnosis can be overwhelming and discouraging. Provide the patient with appropriate encouragement and reassurances that progress can be made over time.

CRPS typifies the difficult clinical problems that hand therapists are trying to avert or avoid. Intervention programs that are progressing well can be suddenly and unexpectedly derailed by this disorder. For this reason, it is advisable to approach all hand therapy patients supportively and with a very careful eye, regardless of their diagnosis. Early identification of CRPS is a key to resolving it.

Osteoarthritis

Idiopathic OA is the most common type of OA. In the upper extremity, it often affects the DIP and PIP joints. Osteophytes at the DIP are called Heberden's nodes, and osteophytes at the PIP are called Bouchard's nodes (Beasley, 2012). For painful DIP nodes, small cylindrical splints or a light Coban™ wrap may promote function while decreasing pain (Biese, 2007).

Hand therapy for OA focuses on alleviating symptoms through education in principles of joint protection, protective and supportive splinting, and provision of adaptive devices for ADL (Hochberg et al., 2012) (see Evidence Table 37-1). For OA of the thumb CMC, a hand-based thumb spica orthosis (Fig. 37-21) is often extremely helpful (Beasley, 2011). Some therapists prefer to use a forearm-based spica orthosis, particularly when there is pantrapezial involvement rather than just CMC joint involvement.

Thumb CMC arthroplasty is a common postoperative diagnosis seen by hand therapists. Surgical techniques and timelines for therapy vary among physicians. Patients are often sent to therapy a few weeks after surgery for fabrication of a static forearm-based thumb spica orthosis with the IP free. The physician indicates appropriate guidelines for AROM according to the particular surgical procedures performed. Postoperative therapy goals are to promote pain-free stability and function. ADL modification and joint protection remain a priority.

Rheumatoid Arthritis

Unlike OA, RA is a systemic disease that primarily affects the synovium. Its debilitating and crippling effects can be severely disabling. RA presents as inflammation of synovial membranes of joints and of tendon sheaths, with redness, swelling, pain, and heat in the areas of involvement (Alter, Feldon, & Terrono, 2011).

Digital involvement at the DIP is less common than at the PIP. If DIP involvement does occur, a mallet finger may result. Involvement at the PIP may result in swan-neck or boutonniere deformities (see the section on extensor tendons for clinical management of mallet and boutonniere deformities). A swan-neck deformity presents as MP flexion, PIP hyperextension, and DIP flexion (Fig. 37-22). Fabricate a digital dorsal splint in slight PIP flexion to minimize deforming forces and enhance FDS function. At the level of the MP joints, deformity usually manifests as MP ulnar drift and palmar subluxation. Thumb deformities include boutonniere (primary thumb MP involvement) and swan-neck (primary CMC involvement) deformities. The thumb may also demonstrate stiff, unstable, and painful joints at the levels of the IP, MP, or CMC. RA often affects the wrist (Beasley, 2012). This is significant because the wrist is anatomically critical to proper hand function. Wrist involvement is compounded by concomitant hand deformity. Synovitis at the wrist can lead to flexor or extensor tendon ruptures (Alter, Feldon, & Terrono, 2011).

In evaluating patients with RA, observe deformities and abnormal posture, any atrophy, and skin condition. Identify crepitus of joint or tendon, palpable nodules, tendon integrity, and joint stability. Ask about morning stiffness, fatigue, and pain. The appearance of the deformity (cosmesis) is also relevant (Beasley, 2011).

The goals of upper extremity orthotics for RA include reducing inflammation, supporting weak tissues, and minimizing deforming forces. Orthotic intervention also provides functional assistance. Orthotics are used especially in the acute stage, when inflamed structures are at risk for further damage. Forearm-based resting orthoses may support the wrist and entire hand, the wrist and MPs, or only the wrist.

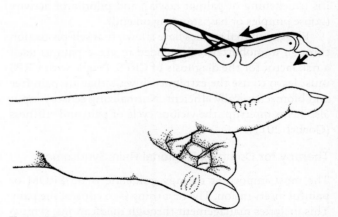

Figure 37-22 Swan-neck deformity: hyperextension of the PIP joint and dorsal migration of the lateral bands. (From Rayan, G. M., & Akelman, E. [2012]. *The hand: Anatomy, examination, and diagnosis* [Kindle Locations 2124–2127]. Philadelphia: Lippincott [Wolters Kluwer Health]. Kindle Edition. Used with permission.)

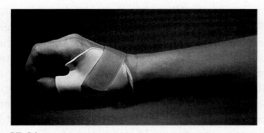

Figure 37-21 Hand-based thumb spica splint. Used to provide pain relief and promote functional pinch.

Determine orthotic design according to the pathomechanics of the disease. Involved MP joints are at risk for volar subluxation. Therefore, splint the wrist in neutral or slight extension, the MP joints in available extension, and the PIP joints in slight flexion (Biese, 2007). Radial deviation of the wrist encourages ulnar drift of the digits at the MP joints because of the zigzag deformity. An orthosis to correct MP ulnar drift often improves the biomechanics of hand use. Talk with the patient to identify individual preferences and needs in terms of ADL and joint protection. Adapt the straps and practice with patients to be sure they can open and close them. For some people who require bilateral orthotics, it may be easier to use one at a time on alternate nights.

CONCLUSION

Wilson (1998) stated, "The hand is not merely a metaphor or an icon for humanness, but often the real-life focal point—the lever or the launching pad—of a successful and genuinely fulfilling life" (p. 14). Occupational therapy can be the launching pad for people with hand impairments to reestablish fulfilling lives.

Client-Focused Activity Analysis Case Example
Client-Focused Activity Analysis: Task of Blow-Drying Hair Independently for Improved Upper Extremity Strength and Function

Patient Information

Mrs. V. is a 59-year-old right dominant female who sustained a left distal humerus fracture and underwent a delayed open reduction internal fixation with plating. Occupational therapy (OT) assessment identified limitations in range of motion (ROM) and strength limiting ability to use the left upper extremity (UE) in self-care including grooming activities. Mrs. V. had worked as a hair stylist in the past and was very concerned about being able to groom herself independently. The therapist decided to incorporate a grooming task into the intervention plan to help Mrs. V. achieve the following goal: *Mrs. V will use her left UE to blow-dry her hair for 10 minutes with pain rating of less than 2 out of 10 and thereby improve her strength and function.*

Task Analysis Process		Intervention Planning	Clinical Transactions: Preparation for and Interactions at the Occupational Therapy Session	Clinical Reasoning: Example of Therapist's Internal Dialogue
S E L E C T I O N	Specify the primary goal that performing this task is intended to advance	Independent grooming	The therapist selected a setup that included a mirror as a venue for grooming activities.	"The therapeutic aim of this task is to improve upper extremity strength and function in unsupported overhead activity. Mrs. V. has told me how important it is for her to become independent in her grooming activities."
	Specify the primary abilities and capacities that the task is intended to challenge: • ROM • Strength • Motor behavior • Praxis • Sensation • Vision-visual perception • Cognition	ROM Strength	The therapist positioned a blow-dryer on the counter in front of the mirror and asked Mrs. V. to use her left UE to lift it into position for blow-drying. She timed the interval that Mrs. V. was able to hold the blow-dryer in position before fatiguing.	"Even reaching for and lifting the blow-dryer is good for ROM and strengthening."

(continued)

A N A L Y S I S	Evaluate the therapeutic value of activity based on these characteristics: 1. Inherently evoke desired response 2. Be gradable to progress the patient to higher function 3. Be within patient's capabilities 4. Be meaningful 5. Be repetitive	Use of strengthening and flexibility task that relates to Mrs. V.'s personal goal of improved grooming using left UE.	Weight and position of the blow-dryer can be adjusted to increase difficulty reaching and holding it in position.	"Mrs. V. will get practice with this task because she wants to perform grooming activities every morning."
G R A D A T I O N & A D A P T A T I O N	Specify task parameters to calibrate difficulty level of the task: • Method of instruction • Nature and level of cueing • Objects and their properties (materials, equipment) • Environmental demands • Social demands • Sequence and timing • Required actions and performance skills • Required body functions • Required body structures • Context or environment	Lighter versus heavier blow-dryer; smaller versus larger blow-dryer; varying handle sizes of blow-dryer; positioned lower and then higher; activity performed over increasingly longer periods of time before taking a rest.	The therapist monitored Mrs. V.'s responses and tolerance and modified the physical demands of the task accordingly.	"Mrs. V. is so eager to blow-dry her hair independently that she might overlook her fatigue level. I will help provide opportunities to pace this task so she can do it successfully without pain afterward."

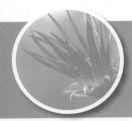

case example

Miss L.: Recovery of Upper Extremity Function and Independent Self-Care, Homemaking, and Job Duties Post Distal Radius Fracture

Occupational Therapy Process	Clinical Reasoning Process	
	Objectives	Examples of Therapist's Internal Dialogue
Patient Information Miss L. is a 49-year-old athletic computer software manager with dominant right hand. She is single and lives alone. Miss L. fell on an outstretched hand while on vacation out of state, sustaining a comminuted displaced right distal radius fracture. She was initially treated with closed reduction and a long-arm cast. Ten days later, after returning home, she underwent open reduction internal fixation of the right distal radius with a volar plate. Family members came to stay with her to assist with self-care and activities of daily living (ADL) needs. At the time of her injury, she was looking forward to a kayaking vacation.	Understand the patient's diagnosis or condition Know the person	"Miss L. sustained a significant injury to her dominant upper extremity (UE) requiring fixation and bone grafting. The immobilization time prior to surgery could potentially lead to significant stiffness of multiple structures." "Miss L. is an independent and active woman who hopes to go on a kayaking trip in a few months. She is not used to depending on others for self-care or other assistance. She likes living alone, driving her sports car, and going on business trips, but right now these aspects of her life are disrupted."
Reason for Referral to Occupational Therapy Miss L. was referred to outpatient hand therapy the day after surgery to maximize her functional abilities while her dominant hand was immobilized and to promote wound and fracture healing, edema control, and mobility of nonimmobilized structures.	Appreciate the context	"Miss L.'s family is with her initially to help her function while she relies on her nondominant UE for use. Although she prefers living alone, it is good that she has some help initially. Her desire to perform her occupational roles will help her recover more quickly."
Assessment Process and Results Miss L. had severe pain (9 out of 10), significant edema, and increased autonomic signs including vasomotor instability and guarded positioning of the right UE. She had extremely limited range of motion (ROM) of the digits of her right hand and was also hesitant to actively move her shoulder or elbow.	Develop provisional hypotheses Consider evaluation approach and methods Interpret observations	"I do not want to impose pain with my evaluation, so I will measure only active range of motion (AROM) in a gentle fashion. I will provide encouragement and explain how autonomic responses can be normalized with pain-free motion, elevation, and edema control." "Miss L. is at risk for complex regional pain syndrome (CRPS) and for significant stiffness of joints and tendons. Managing the edema is a high priority in order to normalize all tissue responses."
Occupational Therapy Problem List • Disruption of independent living and job performance • Interruption of frequent job-related travel • Inability to sleep or to perform self-care or home activities because of pain, edema, and decreased ROM • Risk of developing CRPS with degradation of functional and clinical status as evidenced by increased autonomic signs	Synthesize results	"Miss L. has multiple severe problems that could lead to permanent stiffness and loss of function. Despite this, she is a highly motivated successful professional, and she is eager to recover."

Occupational Therapy Goal List

1. Normalize autonomic signs and ameliorate pain interfering with function and sleep
2. Promote spontaneous pain-free use of the right upper extremity in daily activity
3. Achieve independent self-care and homemaking and resume job-related travel and engagement in athletic activity

Develop intervention hypotheses	"I believe that a gradual and gentle upgrade of exercises to promote healing and recover flexibility will be far more effective than overstressing her delicate healing tissues."
Select an intervention approach	"Occupational therapy will focus on promoting healing and restoring normal joint motions and musculotendinous lengths in order to recover UE function."
Consider what will occur in therapy, how often, and for how long	"Miss L. will need upgrades to her home program weekly. Splints will need to be revised, as well as exercises and instructions/practice in using her right UE for self-care and nonresistive home tasks."
Assess the patient's comprehension	"I can tell that Miss L. understands her instructions because she demonstrates her activities well. She is exploring what new abilities she has with her right hand and is trying to use it as much as possible in a pain-free way. She demonstrates accurate placement of her splints and describes effective choices in using them. Her follow-through at home is exactly as I hoped it would be. And she understands when to rest her hand so that she does not develop new signs of swelling or pain."
Understand what she is doing	
Compare actual to expected performance	

Intervention

Miss L. began a home program of education about the expected clinical course and recovery; edema control; and shoulder, elbow, and digital ROM in pain-free ranges. Emphasis was on shoulder active exercise and upper extremity elevation. A week after surgery, Miss L.'s autonomic signs were resolving. Her digits remained edematous, and AROM was still limited throughout the upper extremity except for her shoulder, which was functional. Gentle wrist AROM was initiated.

At 2 weeks after surgery, digital AROM and passive range of motion (PROM) were slowly improving but still limited. Miss L.'s home program was upgraded to include edema control, functional grip and release activities, blocking exercises with thermoplastic supports, place-and-hold exercises, night composite digital extension static splinting, and day dynamic digital composite extension splinting. She was encouraged to use her injured arm in light self-care and in light household activity as well as desk work in order to reestablish use of the arm in her occupations. Differential digital flexor tendon gliding was restricted by adherence at the volar distal forearm incisional site, which was still healing. She had extrinsic extensor tightness, extrinsic flexor tightness, and intrinsic tightness. Fortunately, Miss L. was not developing PIP flexion contractures. She had been relying on her nondominant left hand for handwriting and all self-care. She returned to work soon after surgery and was once again traveling frequently on business.

At 3 weeks after surgery, when incision sites were healed, manual edema mobilization began, and all functional activities, splints, and exercises were upgraded in a pain-free fashion. Paper tape was applied to incision sites at night for scar management. Miss L. continued to make slow but measurable progress. Her physician reported good radiographic alignment.

At 6 weeks after surgery, Miss L.'s fixator was removed. Her physician reported good reduction and stability of the distal radioulnar joint. She was severely limited in forearm pronation and supination and in wrist AROM and PROM. She was instructed in pain-free forearm and wrist AROM. A thermoplastic volar wrist splint was fabricated for support and to correct limited wrist extension. Miss L. began to resume use of her right upper extremity for handwriting intermittently and for home activities as tolerated. Although she was very compliant with her home program, her progress was slow. She had become quite adept at using her left hand for dexterity tasks.

At 10 weeks after surgery, Miss L. began to demonstrate dramatic gains in suppleness (Fig. 37-23, A & B). She was significantly improved in digital edema and in all ROM. Elbow extension was normal. Forearm supination and pronation were better, with AROM being equal to PROM. Isolated wrist extension was improved. Digital composite fisting and flexor digitorum profundus (FDP) and flexor digitorum superficialis (FDS) differential tendon gliding were nearly normal, and tightness of the extrinsic flexors was almost fully resolved. Miss L. was using her right hand for all handwriting and grooming and for driving her sports car. She was eager to begin simulating kayaking, because she had kept her plans for a kayaking vacation. Miss L. said that her dynamic splints and night static composite extension splints were helpful to her, so these were modified and upgraded. Strengthening exercises were gradually and cautiously upgraded as well.

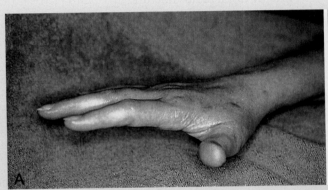 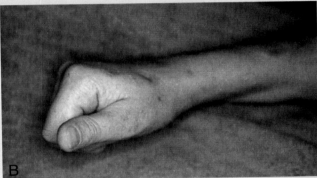

Figure 37-23 Case example at 10 weeks postsurgery. **A.** active digital extension; **B.** active digital flexion.

Next Steps

Discharge from occupational therapy with home activities and splints.

Anticipate present and future patient concerns

Decide whether the patient should continue or discontinue therapy and/or return in the future

"Miss L. was able to go on her kayaking trip and enjoyed it. She still exercises and knows that it is important not to overdo it. She has learned how to keep her tissues flexible and has gained good strength as well."

 Clinical Reasoning in Hand Therapy Practice

Effects of Promoting Occupational Engagement on Upper Extremity Function

Miss L. initially had to rely on her uninjured arm for one-handed self-care and was not able to picture herself resuming enjoyable activities such as kayaking. What recommendations should be made to her regarding her home program to incorporate occupation-based treatment as soon as possible? What clinical activities would be helpful to encourage more functional use of the arm?

Summary Review Questions

1. Why should painful treatment be avoided? What signs are indicative of overaggressive intervention?
2. Name the phases of tissue healing and approximate timelines.
3. Define joint versus musculotendinous tightness, intrinsic versus extrinsic tightness, and tightness of extrinsic extensors versus extrinsic flexors.
4. Describe the antideformity position of the wrist and hand and explain why it is used.
5. What function is lost with a low radial nerve injury? What kind of orthotic intervention (splinting) is appropriate, and why?
6. What distribution of sensation is usually impaired with carpal tunnel syndrome? What musculature might be atrophied in an advanced case? What night orthotic (splint) position is best for carpal tunnel syndrome, and why?
7. Describe CRPS and discuss intervention priorities for this diagnosis.
8. What symptoms are associated with a trigger finger?
9. Name four self-care or home activities that are safe and therapeutic for a person in a short arm cast with a healing distal radius fracture.

Glossary

Antideformity position (intrinsic-plus position)— Position of digital MP flexion and IP extension that maintains the length of the collateral ligaments and volar plate.

Buddy straps— Straps between an injured and an adjacent digit to protect or to promote movement.

Carpal tunnel syndrome— Nerve entrapment involving compression of the median nerve at the wrist causing sensory symptoms typically involving the thumb, index, and long finger and radial half of the ring finger.

Cervical screening— Proximal screening assessment of neck and shoulder to identify causes of or contributors to distal symptoms.

Claw deformity— Position of MP hyperextension and PIP flexion associated with muscle imbalance in ulnar-innervated structures.

Complex regional pain syndrome (CRPS)— Previously called reflex sympathetic dystrophy. CRPS is characterized by pain that is disproportionate to the injury, along with swelling, stiffness, and discoloration. Sudomotor (sweating) changes are often seen.

Contracture— Lack of passive motion caused by tissue shortening.

Counterforce strap— Support or strap used over flexor or extensor muscle wads to support muscles and prevent maximum muscle contraction, decreasing load on the tendon. Often used to reduce symptoms of lateral or medial epicondylitis.

Cubital tunnel syndrome— Nerve entrapment involving compression of the ulnar nerve at the elbow between the medial epicondyle and olecranon. Sensory symptoms affect the small finger and ulnar half of the ring finger.

Motor symptoms affect the FCU, FDP of the ring and small fingers, AP, and interossei.

De Quervain's tenosynovitis— Inflammation of the APL and EPB tendons at the first dorsal compartment.

Extensor lag— Inability to extend a joint actively while passively being able to.

Hard end feel— Unyielding quality of joint motion at end range when moved passively; indicates an established joint restriction.

Kirschner wires— Fixation devices used alone or in conjunction with other forms of fixation to treat unstable fractures of the hand. Kirschner wires are wires or pins that are driven through the skin, into the bone. They may protrude outside the skin, or they may be buried below the skin surface. If they protrude, the physician may request pin site care to prevent infection.

Neuroma— Disorganized mass of nerve fibers that can occur following nerve injury. Significant nerve pain with associated hypersensitivity is elicited by tapping over the neuroma.

Oscillations— Rhythmic movements that may be helpful to reduce guarding and pain.

Place-and-hold exercises— Passive motion used gently to achieve a position, with the patient then actively sustaining or holding that position.

Soft end feel— Spongy quality of joint motion at end range when moved passively; indicates favorable potential for tissue remodeling.

Tenolysis— Surgical procedure to release tendon adhesions that restrict movement.

References

Alter, S., Feldon, P., & Terrono, A. L. (2011). Pathomechanics of deformities in the arthritic hand and wrist. In T. M. Skirven, A. L. Osterman, J. M. Fedorczyk, & P. C. Amadio (Eds.), *Rehabilitation of the hand and upper extremity* (6th ed., pp. 1321–1329). Philadelphia: Mosby.

Amadio, P. C. (2011). Carpal tunnel syndrome: Surgeon's management. In T. M. Skirven, A. L. Osterman, J. M. Fedorczyk, & P. C. Amadio (Eds.), *Rehabilitation of the hand and upper extremity* (6th ed., pp. 657–665). Philadelphia: Mosby.

Amirjani, N., Ashworth, N. L., Olson, J. L., Morhart, M., & Chan, K. M. (2011). Validity and reliability of the Purdue Pegboard Test in carpal tunnel syndrome. *Muscle & Nerve, 43,* 171–177.

Anderson, D. (2011). Mallet finger. *Australian Family Physician, 40,* 47–48.

Artzberger, S. (2007). Edema reduction techniques: A biologic rationale for selection. In C. Cooper (Ed.), *Fundamentals of hand therapy: Clinical reasoning and treatment guidelines for common diagnoses of the upper extremity* (pp. 36–52). St. Louis: Mosby.

Ashe, M. C., McCauley, T., & Khan, K. M. (2004). Tendinopathies in the upper extremity: A paradigm shift. *Journal of Hand Therapy, 17,* 329–334.

Baker, N. A., Moehling, K. K., Rubinstein, E. N., Wollstein, R., Gustafson, N. P., & Baratz, M. (2012). The comparative effectiveness of combined lumbrical muscle splints and stretches on symptoms and function in carpal tunnel syndrome. *Archives of Physical Medicine and Rehabilitation, 93,* 1–10.

Bardak, A. N., Alp, M., Erhan, B., Paker, N., Kaya, B., & Onal, A. E. (2009). Evaluation of the clinical efficacy of conservative treatment in the management of carpal tunnel syndrome. *Advances in Therapy, 26,* 107–116.

Barr, A. E. (2006). Tissue pathophysiology, neuroplasticity and motor behavioural changes in painful repetitive motion injuries. *Manual Therapy, 11,* 173–174.

Beasley, J. (2011). Therapist's examination and conservative management of arthritis of the upper extremity. In T. M. Skirven, A. L. Osterman, J. M. Fedorczyk, & P. C. Amadio (Eds.), *Rehabilitation of the hand and upper extremity* (6th ed., pp. 1330–1343). Philadelphia: Mosby.

Beasley, J. (2012). Osteoarthritis and rheumatoid arthritis: Conservative therapeutic management. *Journal of Hand Therapy, 25,* 163–172.

Belsky, M. R., & Leibman, M. (2011). Extra-articular hand fractures: Part I. Surgeon's management—A practical approach. In T. M. Skirven, A. L. Osterman, J. M. Fedorczyk, & P. C. Amadio (Eds.), *Rehabilitation of the hand and upper extremity* (6th ed., pp. 377–385). Philadelphia: Mosby.

Biese, J. (2007). Arthritis. In C. Cooper (Ed.), *Fundamentals of hand therapy: Clinical reasoning and treatment guidelines for common diagnoses of the upper extremity* (pp. 348–375). St. Louis: Mosby.

Bruder, A., Taylor, N. F., Dodd, K. J., & Shields, N. (2011). Exercise reduces impairment and improves activity in people after some upper limb fractures: A systematic review. *Journal of Physiotherapy, 57,* 71–82.

Buddenberg, L. A., & Davis, C. (2000). Test-retest reliability of the Purdue Pegboard Test. *American Journal of Occupational Therapy, 54,* 555–558.

Butler, M. W. (2007). Common shoulder diagnoses. In C. Cooper (Ed.), *Fundamentals of hand therapy: Clinical reasoning and treatment guidelines for common diagnoses of the upper extremity* (pp. 151–182). St. Louis: Mosby.

Callahan, A. D. (2011). Sensibility assessment for nerve lesions-in-continuity and nerve lacerations. In T. M. Skirven, A. L. Osterman, J. M. Fedorczyk, & P. C. Amadio (Eds.), *Rehabilitation of the hand and upper extremity* (6th ed.). Philadelphia: Mosby.

Carlson, L. K., & Watson, H. K. (1988). Treatment of reflex sympathetic dystrophy using the stress-loading program. *Journal of Hand Therapy, 1,* 149–154.

Chen, J.-J., Jin, P.-S., Zhao, S., Cen, Y., Liu, Y., Xu, X.-W., Duan, W.Q., & Wang, H. S. (2011). Effect of heat shock protein 47 on collagen synthesis of keloid in vivo. *ANZ Journal of Surgery, 81,* 425–430.

Chesney, A., Chauhan, A., Kattan, A., Farrokhyar, F., & Thoma, A. (2011). Systematic review of flexor tendon rehabilitation protocols in zone II of the hand. *Plastic and Reconstructive Surgery, 127,* 1583–1592.

Colditz, J. C. (2011). Therapist's management of the stiff hand. In T. M. Skirven, A. L. Osterman, J. M. Fedorczyk, & P. C. Amadio (Eds.), *Rehabilitation of the hand and upper extremity* (6th ed., pp. 894–921). Philadelphia: Mosby.

Connell, L. A., & Tyson, S. F. (2012). Clinical reality of measuring upper-limb ability in neurologic conditions: A systematic review. *Archives of Physical Medicine and Rehabilitation, 93,* 221–228.

Cooper, C. (2007). Fundamentals of clinical reasoning: Hand therapy concepts and treatment techniques. In C. Cooper (Ed.), *Fundamentals of hand therapy: Clinical reasoning and treatment guidelines for common diagnoses of the upper extremity* (pp. 3–21). St. Louis: Mosby.

Cooper, C., & Martin, H. A. (2007). Common forms of tendinitis /tendinosis. In C. Cooper (Ed.), *Fundamentals of hand therapy: Clinical reasoning and treatment guidelines for common diagnoses of the upper extremity* (pp. 286–300). St. Louis: Mosby.

Crop, J. A., & Bunt, C. W. (2011). "Doctor, my thumb hurts." *The Journal of Family Practice, 60,* 329–332.

Culp, R. W., Feldscher, S. B., & Rodriguez, S. (2011). Flexor and extensor tenolysis: Surgeon's and therapist's management. In T. M. Skirven, A. L. Osterman, J. M. Fedorczyk, & P. C. Amadio (Eds.), *Rehabilitation of the hand and upper extremity* (6th ed., pp. 555–568). Philadelphia: Mosby.

de la Llave-Rincon, A. I., Fernandez-de-las-Penas, C., Perez-de-Heredia-Torres, M., Martinez-Perez, A., Valenza, M. C., & Pareja, J. A. (2011). Bilateral deficits in fine motor control and pinch grip force are not associated with electrodiagnostic findings in women with carpal tunnel syndrome. *American Journal of Physical Medicine and Rehabilitation, 90,* 443–451.

Dell, P. C., Dell, R. B., & Griggs, R. (2011). Management of carpal fractures and dislocations. In T. M. Skirven, A. L. Osterman, J. M. Fedorczyk, & P. C. Amadio (Eds.), *Rehabilitation of the hand and upper extremity* (6th ed., pp. 988–1001). Philadelphia: Mosby.

Desrosiers, J., Hebert, R., Dutil, E., & Bravo, G. (1993). Development and reliability of an upper extremity function test for the elderly: The TEMPA. *Canadian Journal of Occupational Therapy, 60,* 9–16.

Desrosiers, J., Hebert, R., Dutil, E., Bravo, G., & Mercier, L. (1994). Validity of the TEMPA: A measurement instrument for upper extremity performance. *Occupational Therapy Journal of Research, 14,* 267–281.

Diao, E., & Chee, N. (2011). Staged/delayed tendon reconstruction. In T. M. Skirven, A. L. Osterman, J. M. Fedorczyk, & P. C. Amadio (Eds.), *Rehabilitation of the hand and upper extremity* (6th ed., pp. 479–486). Philadelphia: Mosby.

Doornberg, J. N., Buijze, G. A., Ham, J., Ring, D., Bhandari, M., & Poolman, R. W. (2011). Nonoperative treatment for acute scaphoid fractures: A systematic review and meta-analysis of randomized controlled trials. *Journal of Trauma, 71,* 1073–1081.

Duff, S. V., & Estilow, T. (2011). Therapist's management of peripheral nerve injury. In T. M. Skirven, A. L. Osterman, J. M. Fedorczyk, & P. C. Amadio (Eds.), *Rehabilitation of the hand and upper extremity* (6th ed., pp. 619–633). Philadelphia: Mosby.

Evans, R. B. (2011a). Therapist's management of carpal tunnel syndrome: A practical approach. In T. M. Skirven, A. L. Osterman, J. M. Fedorczyk, & P. C. Amadio (Eds.), *Rehabilitation of the hand and upper extremity* (6th ed., pp. 666–677). Philadelphia: Mosby.

Evans, R. B. (2011b). Clinical management of extensor tendon injuries: The therapist's perspective. In T. M. Skirven, A. L. Osterman, J. M. Fedorczyk, & P. C. Amadio (Eds.), *Rehabilitation of the hand and upper extremity* (6th ed., pp. 521–554). Philadelphia: Mosby.

Faria-Fortini, I., Michaelsen, S. M., Cassiano, J. G., & Teixeira-Salmela, L. F. (2011). Upper extremity function in stroke subjects: Relationships between the international classification of functioning, disability, and health domains. *Journal of Hand Therapy, 24,* 257–265.

Fedorczyk, J. M. (2011). Elbow tendinopathies: Clinical presentation and therapist's management of tennis elbow. In T. M. Skirven, A. L. Osterman, J. M. Fedorczyk, & P. C. Amadio (Eds.), *Rehabilitation of the hand and upper extremity* (6th ed., pp. 1098–1108). Philadelphia: Mosby.

Feehan, L. M. (2011). Extra-articular hand fractures: Part II. Therapist's management. In T. M. Skirven, A. L. Osterman, J. M. Fedorczyk, & P. C. Amadio (Eds.), *Rehabilitation of the hand and upper extremity* (6th ed., pp. 386–401). Philadelphia: Mosby.

Fess, E. E. (2002/2011). Documentation: Essential elements of an upper extremity assessment battery. In E. J. Mackin, A. D. Callahan, T. M. Skirven, L. H. Schneider, & A. L. Osterman (Eds.), *Rehabilitation of the hand and upper extremity* (5th ed., pp. 263–284). St. Louis: Mosby. Archived online in T. M. Skirven, A. L. Osterman, J. M. Fedorczyk, & P. C. Amadio (Eds.), *Rehabilitation of the hand and upper extremity* (6th ed.). Philadelphia: Mosby.

Fess, E. E., Gettle, K. S., Philips, C. A., & Janson, J. R. (2005). *Hand and upper extremity splinting: Principles and methods* (3rd ed.). St. Louis: Mosby.

Gallus, J., & Mathiowetz, V. (2003). Test-retest reliability of the Purdue Pegboard for persons with multiple sclerosis. *American Journal of Occupational Therapy, 57,* 108–111.

Geissler, W. B., Adams, J. E., Bindra, R. R., Lanzinger, W. D., & Slutsky, D. J. (2012). Scaphoid fractures: What's hot, what's not. *Journal of Bone and Joint Surgery, 94,* 169–181.

Giambini, H., Ikeda, J., Amadio, P. C., An, K. N., & Zhao, C. (2010). The quadriga effect revisited: Designing a "safety incision" to prevent tendon repair rupture and gap formation in a canine model in vitro. *Journal of Orthopedic Research, 28,* 1482–1489.

Glasgow, C., Tooth, L. R., & Fleming, J. (2010). Mobilizing the stiff hand: Combining theory and evidence to improve clinical outcomes. *Journal of Hand Therapy, 23,* 392–401.

Glasgow, C., Tooth, L. R., Fleming, J., & Peters, S. (2011). Dynamic splinting for the stiff hand after trauma: Predictors of contracture resolution. *Journal of Hand Therapy, 24,* 195–206.

Goebel, A. (2011). Complex regional pain syndrome in adults. *Rheumatology, 50,* 1739–1750.

Goldman, S. B., Brininger, T. L., Schrader, J. W., & Koceja, D. M. (2009). A review of clinical tests and signs for the assessment of ulnar neuropathy. *Journal of Hand Therapy, 22,* 209–220.

Griffin, M., Hindocha, S., Jordan, D., Saleh, M., & Khan, W. (2012). An overview of the management of flexor tendon injuries. *Open Orthopedics Journal, 6,* 28–35.

Groth, G. N. (2005). Current practice patterns of flexor tendon rehabilitation. *Journal of Hand Therapy, 18,* 169–174.

Hahn, S. B., Kang, H. J., Kang, E. S., & Choi, Y. R. (2010). Correction of long standing proximal interphalangeal flexion contractures with cross finger flaps and vigorous postoperative exercises. *Yonsei Medical Journal, 51,* 574–578.

Hall, B., Lee, H., Page, R., Rosenwax, L., & Lee, A. H. (2010). Research scholars initiative: Comparing three postoperative treatment protocols for extensor tendon repair in zones V and VI of the hand. *American Journal of Occupational Therapy, 64,* 682–688.

Higgins, J., Salbach, N. M., Wood-Dauphinee, S., Richards, C. L., Cote, R., & Mayo, N. E. (2006). The effect of a task-oriented intervention on arm function in people with stroke: A randomized controlled trial. *Clinical Rehabilitation, 20,* 296–310.

Hochberg, M. C., Altman, R. D., April, K. T., Benkhalti, M., Guyatt, G., McGowan, J., Towheed, T., Welch, V., Wells, G., & Tugwell, P. (2012). American College of Rheumatology 2012 recommendations for the use of nonpharmacologic and pharmacologic therapies in osteoarthritis of the hand, hip, and knee. *Arthritis Care and Research, 64,* 465–474.

Jensen, C., & Rayan, G. (1996). Buddy strapping of mismatched fingers: The offset buddy strap. *Journal of Hand Surgery, 21,* 317–318.

Kardashian, G., Vara, A. D., Miller, S. J., Miki, R. A., & Jose, J. (2011). Stenosing synovitis of the extensor pollicis longus tendon. *Journal of Hand Surgery, 36A,* 1035–1038.

Klein, L. J. (2007a). Evaluation of the hand and upper extremity. In C. Cooper (Ed.), *Fundamentals of hand therapy: Clinical reasoning and treatment guidelines for common diagnoses of the upper extremity* (pp. 73–97). St. Louis: Mosby.

Klein, L. J. (2007b). Tendon injury. In C. Cooper (Ed.), *Fundamentals of hand therapy: Clinical reasoning and treatment guidelines for common diagnoses of the upper extremity* (pp. 320–347). St. Louis: Mosby.

Knygsand-Roenhoej, K., & Maribo, T. (2011). A randomized clinical controlled study comparing the effect of modified manual edema mobilization treatment with traditional edema technique in patients with a fracture of the distal radius. *Journal of Hand Therapy, 24,* 184–194.

Korstanje, J.-W. H., Schreuders, T. R., van der Sijde, J., Hovius, S. E. R., Bosch, J. G., & Selles, R. W. (2010). Ultrasonographic assessment of long finger tendon excursion in zone V during passive and active tendon gliding exercises. *Journal of Hand Surgery, 35A,* 559–565.

Korstanje, J.-W. H., Soeters, J. N. M., Schreuders, T. R., Amadio, P. C., Hovius, S. E. R., Stam, H. J., & Selles, R. W. (2012). Ultrasonographic assessment of flexor tendon mobilization: Effect of different protocols on tendon excursion. *Journal of Bone and Joint Surgery, 94,* 394–402.

Lalonde, D. H., & Kozin, S. (2011). Tendon disorders of the hand. *Plastic and Reconstructive Surgery, 128,* 1e. Retrieved May 14, 2012 from www.PRSJournal.com.

Lamont, K., Chin, M., & Kogan, M. (2011). Mirror box therapy-seeing is believing. *Explore, 7,* 369–372.

Lee, M. P., Biafora, S. J., & Zelouf, D. S. (2011). Management of hand and wrist tendinopathies. In T. M. Skirven, A. L. Osterman, J. M. Fedorczyk, & P. C. Amadio (Eds.), *Rehabilitation of the hand and upper extremity* (6th ed., pp. 569–588). Philadelphia: Mosby.

Liepert, J. (2010). Evidence-based therapies for upper extremity dysfunction. *Current Opinion in Neurology, 23,* 678–682.

Little, K. J., & Jacoby, S. M. (2011). Intra-articular hand fractures and joint injuries: Part I. Surgeon's management. In T. M. Skirven, A. L. Osterman, J. M. Fedorczyk, & P. C. Amadio (Eds.), *Rehabilitation of the hand and upper extremity* (6th ed., pp. 402–416). Philadelphia: Mosby, Inc.

Mathiowetz, V., Volland, G., Kashman, N., & Weber, K. (1985). Adult norms for the box and block test of manual dexterity. *American Journal of Occupational Therapy, 39,* 386–391.

Medoff, R. J. (2011). Distal radius fractures: Classification and management. In T. M. Skirven, A. L. Osterman, J. M. Fedorczyk, & P. C. Amadio (Eds.), *Rehabilitation of the hand and upper extremity* (6th ed., pp. 941–948). Philadelphia: Mosby.

Mellick, G. A., & Mellick, L. B. (2012). Bilateral intersection syndrome. *Journal of the American Osteopathic Association, 112,* 98.

Merritt, W. H. (1998). Written on behalf of the stiff finger. *Journal of Hand Therapy, 11,* 74–79.

Michlovitz, S., & Festa, L. (2011). Therapist's management of distal radius fractures. In T. M. Skirven, A. L. Osterman, J. M. Fedorczyk, & P. C. Amadio (Eds.), *Rehabilitation of the hand and upper extremity* (6th ed., pp. 949–962). Philadelphia: Mosby.

Moberg, E. (1991). The unsolved problem: How to test the functional value of hand sensibility. *Journal of Hand Therapy, 4,* 105–110.

Moorhead, J. F., & Cooper, C. (2007). Clients with functional somatic syndromes or challenging behavior. In C. Cooper (Ed.), *Fundamentals of hand therapy: Clinical reasoning and treatment guidelines for common diagnoses of the upper extremity* (pp. 117–125). St. Louis: Mosby.

Moscony, A. M. B. (2007a). Common peripheral nerve problems. In C. Cooper (Ed.), *Fundamentals of hand therapy: Clinical reasoning and treatment guidelines for common diagnoses of the upper extremity* (pp. 201–250). St. Louis: Mosby.

Moscony, A. M. B. (2007b). Common wrist and hand fractures. In C. Cooper (Ed.), *Fundamentals of hand therapy: Clinical reasoning and treatment guidelines for common diagnoses of the upper extremity* (pp. 251–285). St. Louis: Mosby.

Nedelec, B., Dion, K., Correa, J. A., & Desrosiers, J. (2011). Upper extremity performance test for the elderly (TEMPA): Normative data for young adults. *Journal of Hand Therapy, 24,* 31–43.

Novak, C. B., & Mackinnon, S. E. (2005). Evaluation of nerve injury and nerve compression in the upper quadrant. *Journal of Hand Therapy, 18,* 230–240.

Omar, M. T. A., Hegazy, F. A., & Mokashi, S. P. (2012). Influences of purposeful activity versus rote exercise on improving pain and hand function in pediatric burn. *Burns, 38,* 261–268.

Oskay, D., Meric, A., Kirdi, N., Firat, T., Ayhan, D., & Leblebiciogly, G. (2010). Neurodynamic mobilization in the conservative treatment of cubital tunnel syndrome: Long-term follow-up of 7 cases. *Journal of Manipulative and Physiological Therapeutics, 33,* 156–163.

Pettengill, K. S. (2011). Therapist's management of the complex injury. In T. M. Skirven, A. L. Osterman, J. M. Fedorczyk, & P. C. Amadio (Eds.), *Rehabilitation of the hand and upper extremity* (6th ed., pp. 1238–1251). Philadelphia: Mosby.

Porretto-Loehrke, A., & Soika, E. (2011). Therapist's management of other nerve compressions about the elbow and wrist. In T. M. Skirven, A. L. Osterman, J. M. Fedorczyk, & P. C. Amadio (Eds.), *Rehabilitation of the hand and upper extremity* (6th ed., pp. 695–709). Philadelphia: Mosby.

Priganc, V. W., & Ito, M. A. (2008). Changes in edema, pain, or range of motion following manual edema mobilization: A single-case design study. *Journal of Hand Therapy, 21,* 326–335.

Rallon, C. R., & Chen, C. C. (2008). Relationship between performance-based and self-reported assessment of hand function. *American Journal of Occupational Therapy, 62,* 574–579.

Rice, M. S., Leonard, C., & Carter, M. (1998). Grip strengths and required forces in accessing everyday containers in a normal population. *American Journal of Occupational Therapy, 52,* 621–626.

Ritting, A. W., Baldwin, P. C., & Rodner, C. M. (2010). Ulnar collateral ligament injury of the thumb metacarpophalangeal joint. *Clinical Journal of Sport Medicine, 20,* 106–112.

Rosén, B., & Lundborg, G. (2005). Training with a mirror in rehabilitation of the hand. *Scandinavian Journal of Plastic and Reconstructive Surgeryand Hand Surgery, 39,* 104–108.

Rosén, B., & Lundborg, G. (2011). Sensory reeducation. In T. M. Skirven, A. L. Osterman, J. M. Fedorczyk, & P. C. Amadio (Eds.), *Rehabilitation of the hand and upper extremity* (6th ed., pp. 634–645). Philadelphia: Mosby.

Schmid, A. B., Elliott, J. M., Strudwick, M. W., Little, M., & Coppieters, M. W. (2012). Effect of splinting and exercise on intraneural edema of the median nerve in carpal tunnel syndrome: An MRI study to reveal therapeutic mechanisms. *Journal of Orthopedic Research.* Retrieved May 14, 2012 from wileyonlinelibrary.com.

Seftchick, J. L., De Tullio, L. M., Fedorczyk, J. M., & Aulicino, P. L. (2011). Clinical examination of the hand. In T. M. Skirven, A. L. Osterman, J. M. Fedorczyk, & P. C. Amadio (Eds.), *Rehabilitation of the hand and upper extremity* (6th ed., pp. 55–71). Philadelphia: Mosby.

Seror, P., & Seror, R. (2012). Hand workload, computer use and risk of severe median nerve lesions at the wrist. *Rheumatology, 51,* 362–367.

Smith, K. L. (2011). Nerve response to injury and repair. In T. M. Skirven, A. L. Osterman, J. M. Fedorczyk, & P. C. Amadio (Eds.), *Rehabilitation of the hand and upper extremity* (6th ed., pp. 601–610). Philadelphia: Mosby.

Soong, M., Got, C., & Katarincic, J. (2010). Ring and little finger metacarpal fractures: Mechanisms, locations, and radiographic parameters. *Journal of Hand Surgery, 35A,* 1256–1259.

Tang, P. (2011). Collateral ligament injuries of the thumb metacarpophalangeal joint. *Journal of the American Academy of Orthopedic Surgeons, 19,* 287–296.

Taras, J. S., Martyak, G. G., & Steelman, P. J. (2011). Primary care of flexor tendon injuries. In T. M. Skirven, A. L. Osterman, J. M. Fedorczyk, & P. C. Amadio (Eds.), *Rehabilitation of the hand and upper extremity* (6th ed., pp. 445–456). St. Louis: Philadelphia.

Tiffin, J. (1968). *Purdue Pegboard: Examiner manual.* Chicago: Science Research Associates.

Trombly, C. A. (2011). Occupation: Purposefulness and meaningfulness as therapeutic mechanisms. In R. Padilla & Y. Griffiths (Eds.), *A professional legacy: The Eleanor Clarke Slagle lectures in occupational therapy 1955–2010* (3rd ed.). Bethesda, MD: AOTA Press.

Tuncel, U., Turan, A., & Kostakoglu, N. (2011). Acute closed radial nerve injury. *Asian Journal of Neurosurgery, 6,* 106–109.

Valdes, K. (2012). A retrospective review to determine the long-term efficacy of orthotic devices for trigger finger. *Journal of Hand Therapy, 23,* 334–351.

Valdes, K., & Marik, T. (2010). A systematic review of conservative interventions for osteoarthritis of the hand. *Journal of Hand Therapy, 25,* 89–96.

van de Meent, H., Oerlemans, M., Bruggeman, A., Klomp, F., van Dongen, R., Oostendorp, R., & Frolke, J. P. (2011). Safety of "pain exposure" physical therapy in patients with complex regional pain syndrome type 1. *Pain, 152,* 1431–1438.

van Doesburg, M. H. M., Henderson, J., Yoshii, Y., van der Molen, A. B. M., Cha, S. S., An, K. N., & Amadio, P. C. (2012). Median nerve deformation in differential finger motions: Ultrasonographic comparison of carpal tunnel syndrome patients and healthy controls. *Journal of Orthopedic Research, 30,* 643–648.

Veizi, I. E., Chelimsky, T. C., & Janata, J. W. (2012). Chronic regional pain syndrome: What specialized rehabilitation services do patients require? *Current Pain and Headache Reports, 16,* 139–146.

Verdon, M. E. (1996). Overuse syndromes of the hand and wrist. *Primary Care, 23,* 305–319.

von der Heyde, R. L., & Evans, R. B. (2011). Wound classification and management. In T. M. Skirven, A. L. Osterman, J. M. Fedorczyk, & P. C. Amadio (Eds.), *Rehabilitation of the hand and upper extremity* (6th ed., pp. 219–232). Philadelphia: Mosby.

Vranceanu, A.-M., Cooper, C., & Ring, D. (2009). Integrating patient values into evidence-based practice: Effective communication for shared decision-making. *Hand Clinics, 25,* 83–96.

Walsh, M. T. (2011). Therapist's management of complex regional pain syndrome. In T. M. Skirven, A. L. Osterman, J. M. Fedorczyk, & P. C. Amadio (Eds.), *Rehabilitation of the hand and upper extremity* (6th ed., pp. 1479–1492). Philadelphia: Mosby.

Wang, Y.-C., Magasi, S. R., Bohannon, R. W., Reuben, D. B., McCreath, H. E., Bubela, D. J., Gershon, R. C., & Rymer, W. Z. (2011). Assessing dexterity function: A comparison of two alternatives for the NIH toolbox. *Journal of Hand Therapy, 24,* 313–321.

Williams, K., & Terrono, A. L. (2011). Treatment of boutonniere finger deformity in rheumatoid arthritis. *Journal of Hand Surgery, 36A,* 1388–1393.

Wilson, F. R. (1998). *The hand: How its use shapes the brain, language, and human culture.* New York: Pantheon Books.

Wu, Y.-Y., Hsu, W.-C., & Wang, H.-C. (2010). Posterior interosseous nerve palsy as a complication of friction massage in tennis elbow. *American Journal of Physical Medicine and Rehabilitation, 89,* 668–671.

Yancosek, A. E., & Howell, D. (2009). A narrative review of dexterity assessments. *Journal of Hand Therapy, 22,* 258–270.

Zhang, W., Johnston, J. A., Ross, M. A., Smith, A. A., Coakley, B. J., Gleason, E. A., Dueck, A. C., & Santello, M. (2011). Effects of carpal tunnel syndrome on adaptation of multi-digit forces to object weight for whole-hand manipulation. *PLoS ONE, 6,* e27715. Retrieved May 14, 2012 from www.plosone.org.

Acknowledgments

Heartfelt thanks to John L. Evarts, BS, for the photography and for his valuable ideas, contribution to content, and ongoing technical and emotional support. I also thank Cecelia M. Skotak, OTR, CHT; and Virgil Mathiowetz, PhD, OTR, for their input to a previous version of this chapter.

38

Spinal Cord Injury

Michal S. Atkins

Learning Objectives

After studying this chapter, the reader will be able to do the following:

1. Define key terms and concepts central to spinal cord injury and its care.
2. Value the physical, psychosocial, and occupational challenges associated with spinal cord injury.
3. Describe the tests and procedures appropriate for occupational therapy assessment.
4. List the roles and priorities of the occupational therapist in each of the treatment phases.
5. Recognize functional expectations of patients with various levels of injury.

spinal cord injury (SCI) is a devastating event that disrupts every facet of life. Diminished physical capacities, inability to get around and carry out daily routines, and feelings of confusion and despair are coupled with fears about gainful employment and questions about the ability to return home. The occupational therapist may share this burden. With such devastating losses, where does the therapist begin? How do we help patients rebuild a sense of efficacy and self-esteem? How do we set priorities for our treatment interventions?

This chapter provides beginning answers to these questions. First, it introduces epidemiological data, definitions, and classifications of SCI. Next, it discusses the course after injury, followed by information about occupational therapy evaluations, interventions, and a case study. Research data, resources, and suggested readings are listed to assist the therapist in exploring SCI beyond the material outlined in this chapter.

EPIDEMIOLOGY

SCI is relatively rare, afflicting approximately 12,000 people a year in the United States. The number of people with SCI alive today in the United States is estimated to be in the range of 236,000 to 327,000 (National Spinal Cord Injury Statistical Center [NSCISC], 2012). The NSCISC, a federally funded organization established in 1973, collects SCI epidemiological data in the United States. The causes of SCI as tracked by NSCISC since 2005 are as follows. Approximately 39.2% of SCIs are caused by motor vehicle accidents, 28.3% by falls, 14.6% by violence (mostly gunshot wounds), and 8.2% by sports injuries. Other causes, such as nontraumatic SCI, account for the remaining 9.7% (NSCISC, 2012). Nontraumatic SCI is caused by spinal stenosis, tumors, ischemia, infection, and congenital diseases (van den Berg et al., 2010). In large metropolitan areas in the United States, violence, specifically gun violence, accounts for a greater percentage of SCIs (Nobunaga, Go, & Karunas, 1999). In other countries, violence accounts for only a small fraction of injuries. Most SCIs occur in males with a ratio of four injured males per females in the United States (NSCISC, 2012).

The following demographic data paints a picture of those with SCI. Globally, as in the United States, the etiology and age distribution of injury has changed over the past decade with the average age of injury rising (to be further discussed later). SCI occurs mostly in adolescents and young adults (ages 15–29 years of age) and in elderly people aged 65 years and older, and the most common causes of traumatic SCI are vehicular accidents and falls, respectively (van den Berg et al., 2010). In the United States, 66% of those injured are Caucasian, and there is a greater representation of minority groups than in the general population: 26.8% of those injured are African Americans, 8.3% Hispanics, 2% Asian, and 2.9% for all other non-Caucasian ethnic groups (NSCISC, 2010).

Close to half of persons in the National Institute on Disability and Rehabilitation Research SCI Model System of Care have completed high school, and 57.1% were employed at onset (NSCISC, 2010, 2012). Generally, the level of education of injured individuals is somewhat lower and the unemployment rate is somewhat higher than in the general population. At injury, 51.95% of individuals are single, and the likelihood of getting married postinjury is somewhat lower than the general population.

The clinical implications of the SCI epidemiological data have great relevance to the work of occupational therapists. Therapists must appreciate that the patients' ethnic, gender, socioeconomic, and educational backgrounds may differ from their own (see Chapter 3). For example: What language would be best to communicate in? What is the best learning style of the person? What kind of written materials should be given to a patient with little education? Additionally, given that most therapists are females and most patients are males, sexual, bowel, and bladder management issues must be addressed with great sensitivity, and therapists must become comfortable with their role in these matters.

COURSE AFTER SPINAL CORD INJURY

SCI causes a disruption in the motor and sensory pathways at the site of the lesion (Fig. 38-1). Because the nerve roots are segmental, a thorough evaluation of motor and sensory function can identify the level of lesion (Fig. 38-2). For example, if the spinal cord is completely severed at the level of the 6th cervical nerve root, motor and sensory information below that level no longer can travel to and from the brain. This results in paralysis of muscular activity and absence of sensation below the level of injury.

Immediately after the injury, a period of spinal shock occurs, characterized by areflexia at and below the level of injury. Spinal shock may last hours, days, or weeks. As soon as spinal shock subsides, reflexes below the level of injury return and become hyperactive. At the level of injury, areflexia may remain as the reflex arc is interrupted.

Neurological Classification of Spinal Cord Injury

To understand the typical course of recovery from SCI, occupational therapists must be familiar with commonly used terms that describe SCI impairment and know how levels of impairment relate to prognosis.

| Evidence Table 38-1 | Comparing Interventions and Their Outcomes | | | | | |

Intervention	Description of Intervention Tested	Participants	Dosage	Type of Best Evidence and Level of Evidence	Benefit	Statistical Probability	Reference
Intervention to improve voluntary hand function in individuals with incomplete C4–C7 spinal cord injury	Comparison of two treatment groups: conventional occupational therapy and functional electrical stimulation (FES) therapy	Twenty-two individuals with incomplete C4–C7 tetraplegia; single site	Dose defined as 60 min per day, 5 days per week (for 8 weeks). Conventional occupational therapy group: two units of conventional occupational therapy. FES group: one unit of conventional occupational therapy and one unit of FES.	Randomized controlled trial; small groups (10 and 12); no control who did not receive treatment Level: IB	Group that received FES and conventional occupational therapy showed greater improvement than group that had 2 hours of conventional occupational therapy.	FIM™ $p = 0.015$; Spinal Cord Independence Measure upper extremity subscale <0.0001; Hand test Toronto Rehabilitation Institute Hand Function Test: 10 objects = 0.054; Rectangular blocks = 0.124; able to hold wooden bar $p = 0.065$	Kapadia et al. (2011)
Intervention to improve self-efficacy, ability to set/achieve goals, and perceived independent-living status	Occupational therapists and other health care providers conducted health promotional seminars, group discussions, physical and recreational activities.	SCI = 16 MS = 12	Ten full day sessions: twice a month for 5 months	One group, quasiexperimental repeated-measures; nonrandomized Level: IIIC	Yes. Self-efficacy and ability to formulate and achieve goals in the areas of independent-living skills improved for intervention participants.	Statistically significant difference in the change in self-efficacy scores $p = 0.007$; $d = 0.925$ (large effect size)	Block et al. (2010)

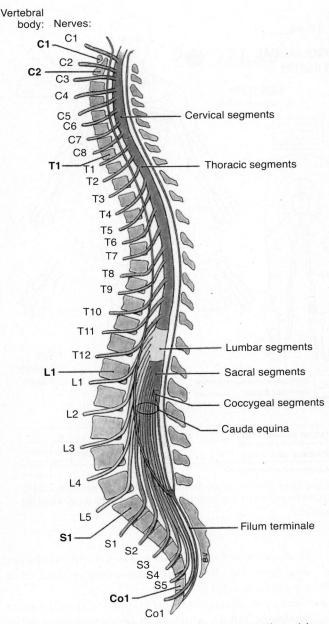

Vertebral
body: Nerves:

C1 — C1

C2 — C2
        C3
        C4
        C5
        C6
        C7
        C8

T1 — T1
        T2
        T3
        T4
        T5
        T6
        T7
        T8
        T9

        T10
        T11
        T12

L1 — L1
        L2
        L3
        L4
        L5

S1 — S1
        S2
        S3
        S4
        S5

Co1 — Co1
        Co1

Cervical segments

Thoracic segments

Lumbar segments

Sacral segments

Coccygeal segments

Cauda equina

Filum terminale

Figure 38-1 Spinal cord and spinal nerves in relation to the vertebrae. (From Agur, A. M. R. [1991]. *Grant's atlas of anatomy* [9th ed.]. Baltimore: Williams & Wilkins.)

Definitions

Tetraplegia results in functional impairment in the arms, trunk, legs, and pelvic organs. The term tetraplegia, which has replaced quadriplegia, is defined as impairment in motor and/or sensory function in the cervical segments of the spinal cord (American Spinal Injury Association [ASIA], 2011). It is caused by damage to neural elements within the vertebral canal, and the term is not used to describe injuries to peripheral nerves. Paraplegia refers to motor and sensory impairment at the thoracic, lumbar, or sacral segments of the cord. Likewise,

it refers only to damage to the neural elements inside the vertebral canal. Paraplegia results in sparing of arm function and, depending on the level of the lesion, impairment in the trunk, legs, and pelvic organs. The terms paraparesis and tetraparesis, which were used in the past to describe incomplete injuries, should no longer be used (ASIA, 2011).

The neurological level is diagnosed by the physician according to the motor and sensory level. The motor level is determined by testing 10 key muscles on each side of the body, and the sensory level is determined by testing sensation of 28 key points on each side of the body (Fig. 38-2). The *neurological level of injury* (NLI) is the lowest segment of the spinal cord at which key muscles grade 3 or above out of 5 on manual muscle testing (MMT), and sensation is intact for this level's dermatome. Also, the level above must have normal strength and sensation. For example, a person is diagnosed as having C6 tetraplegia when radial wrist extensors test 3 out of 5 and sensation is intact for the C6 dermatome. Furthermore, all motor and sensory status above the C6 level is intact. Skeletal level refers to the level of greatest vertebral damage (ASIA, 2011).

Functional level, a term used by occupational and physical therapists, refers to the lowest segment at which strength of important muscles (key and non-key muscles by ASIA terms) is graded 3+ or above out of 5 on MMT and sensation is intact. These muscles significantly change functional outcomes (Zigler et al., 2011). The ASIA muscle list for the physician's motor examination (Fig. 38-2) includes only some of the muscles considered important to determine a functional level.

Two other terms commonly used with people with spinal injuries are complete and incomplete injuries (Definition 38-1). Complete injury consists of the absence of sensory and motor function in the lowest sacral segments (S4–S5) (ASIA, 2011). Consider the patient in the Case Example who has a C6 complete injury (also called AIS A). He does not have either sensation or motor have either sensation or motor function in S4-S5 but does have some muscle and sensory function above that level. The term incomplete injury should be used only when there is partial preservation of sensory and/or motor function below the neurological level and must include the sacral segments (ASIA, 2011). The physician tests innervation at the lowest sacral segment, including anal sensation and sphincter contraction. The degree of impairment of people with complete and incomplete injuries has been classified to ensure international diagnostic consistency. This impairment scale is called the American Spinal Injury Association Impairment Scale (or AIS) (see Definition 38-1).

The term *zone of partial preservation* is used for patients with complete injuries only who have partial innervation in dermatomes below the neurological level (ASIA, 2011). A patient may have a C5 AIS A neurological level and the radial wrist extensors innervated by C6 are functional. This patient's zone of partial preservation is C6.

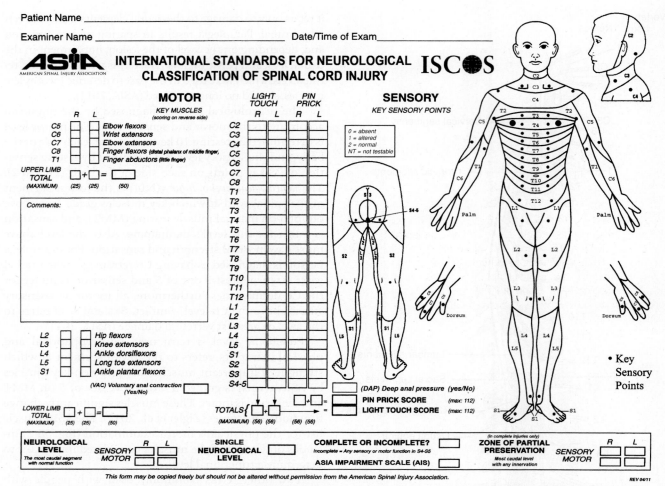

Figure 38-2 International standards for neurological classification of spinal cord injury. (Courtesy of the American Spinal Injury Association. [2011]. *International standards for neurological classification of spinal injury.* Atlanta, GA: American Spinal Injury Association. This form may be copied freely but should not be altered without permission from the American Spinal Injury Association.)

Some specific cord lesions cause a common pattern of clinical findings.

- Central cord syndrome, the most common syndrome, is an incomplete injury, often caused by falls; it results in greater weakness in the upper limbs than in the lower limbs. This injury occurs mostly to older people and is often associated with cervical stenosis (ASIA, 2011).
- Brown-Sequard syndrome is an incomplete injury with damage to half of the cord causing ipsilateral proprioceptive and motor loss and contralateral loss of pain and temperature sensation. This syndrome is rarely seen in its pure form (ASIA, 2011).
- Anterior cord syndrome is a rare syndrome associated with absent blood supply to the cord causing the loss of motor control, pain, and temperature sensation below the injury. Proprioception and light touch are preserved (ASIA, 2011).
- Cauda equina syndrome is a lower motor neuron injury to the lumbosacral nerve roots within the spinal canal.

It results in areflexic bladder and bowel and paralysis or weakness of the lower limbs (depending on the level of injury) (ASIA, 2011).

- Conus medullaris syndrome is similar to cauda equina syndrome but in addition to lesions to the lumbar nerve roots, the cord is also damaged, resulting in a mixed physical picture with some preservation of reflex activity. The bladder, bowel, and lower limbs are affected (ASIA, 2011).

Prognosis

Not surprisingly, recovery is very much on the minds of patients, families, and staff. Neural recovery during rehabilitation is common and can result in significant improvement in function. In patients with complete injuries, muscles in the zone of partial preservation strengthen, which may result in significant functional change. This is true especially if a key muscle, such as extensor carpi radialis, strengthens enough to enable the person to

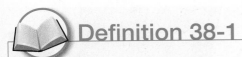

Definition 38-1

ASIA Impairment Scale (AIS)

AIS A = Complete. No sensory or motor function is preserved in the sacral segments S4–S5.

AIS B = Sensory Incomplete. Sensory but not motor function is preserved below the neurological level and includes the sacral segments S4–S5 (light touch, pin prick at S4–S5 or deep anal pressure [DAP]), AND no motor function is preserved more than three levels below the motor level on either side of the body.

AIS C = Motor Incomplete. Motor function is preserved below the neurological level**, and more than half of key muscles below the single neurological level of injury (NLI) have a muscle grade of <3 (Grades 0–2).

AIS D = Incomplete. Motor function is preserved below the neurological level**, and *at least half* (half or more) of key muscles below the NLI have a muscle grade of ≥3.

AIS E = Normal. If sensation and motor function as tested with the International Standards for Neurological Classification of Spinal Cord Injury are graded as normal in all segments, and the patient had prior deficits, then the AIS grade is E. Someone without an initial SCI does not receive an AIS grade.

Note: To receive a grade of C or D, a person must have sensory or motor function in the sacral segments S4–S5. In addition, the individual must have either (1) voluntary anal sphincter contraction or (2) sparing of motor function more than three levels below the motor level.

**For an individual to receive a grade of C or D (i.e., motor incomplete status), they must have either (1) voluntary anal sphincter contraction or (2) sacral sensory sparing with sparing of motor function more than three levels below the motor level for that side of the body. The Standards at this time allows even non-key muscle function more than three levels below the motor level to be used in determining motor incomplete status (AIS B versus C).

Note: When assessing the extent of motor sparing below the level for distinguishing between AIS B and C, the **motor level** on each side is used, whereas to differentiate between AIS C and D (based on proportion of key muscle functions with strength grade 3 or greater) the **single neurological level** is used.

---

extend the wrist and hold objects. Patients with incomplete injury have a better prognosis, and their spontaneous recovery is less predictable in its pattern and outcome than patients with complete injury (Fawcett et al., 2007).

Immediately after the injury, all reflexes cease to function. When spinal shock resolves, patients have an excellent chance to regain motor and sensory function. As time after injury increases, however, the recovery rate declines. Most motor and sensory spontaneous return in both complete and incomplete injuries occurs in the first 3 months post onset. The rate of recovery declines but persists for up to 18 months or longer (Fawcett et al., 2007). Following encouraging discoveries of adult brain plasticity in the recovery after stroke, some new encouraging brain studies point to similar developments in SCI. These studies point to new formation of neural links associated with prolonged repetitive motion of affected limbs (Hoffman & Field-Fote, 2009). They open a window for future physical improvements over time and are yet to be fully investigated.

Because patients and significant others hope for complete recovery, it is important that the therapist maintain hope while planning a realistic course of treatment. Research data can assist the clinician in predicting recovery and outcomes. The therapist should be sensitive and cautious about sharing this information with patients when they are most vulnerable.

Long-term survival of people with SCI has improved dramatically over the past 50 years and is only slightly less than the general population (Fawcett et al., 2007). The major causes of death are respiratory complications and infections (NSCISC, 2010).

As the search for cure continues, many drug therapies have been introduced to decrease the initial damage to the cord and restore function. Some of the research strategies to heal the spinal cord have included studying nerve protection, nerve regeneration, bridging, and cell replacement (Maddox, 2007).

Some of the most common questions that patients often ask are "Will I walk again?" or "When will I be able to walk?" In many cases, the patient may repeat such questions to different clinicians in an attempt to make sense of their condition, to find a glimpse of hope in their new dire situation and to adjust to their new body. It takes time to learn to answer such questions in a truthful, supportive yet hopeful way. The new therapist may find help in answering such questions through discussion with the rest of the team.

Impairments and Their Therapeutic Implications

Paralysis is the most common result of SCI. This injury is accompanied by a variety of frequent complications.

The therapist must be aware of these impairments to provide a safe therapeutic environment and educate patients in understanding how to live a safe and healthy life.

Respiration

Many patients with SCI have compromised breathing. This is true especially for individuals with cervical injuries. Respiratory complications, specifically pneumonia, have been identified as the leading cause of death in the first year of life after SCI (NSCISC, 2010). In lesions above C4, damage to the phrenic nerve results in partial or complete paralysis of the diaphragm. These patients require mechanical ventilation (Fig. 38-3) (Consortium for Spinal Cord Medicine, 2005b). Lower cervical and thoracic spine injuries can result in paralysis of other breathing muscles, such as the intercostals, abdominals, or latissimus dorsi (Kendall et al., 2005). Thus, patients with such injuries also have impaired respiration.

Use of proper techniques and infection control standards are important for respiratory care. Under the direction of the physician, the physical and respiratory therapists and the health care team work to achieve adequate bronchial hygiene and to facilitate good breathing at rest and during activities. Good communication with the team allows the occupational therapist to support breathing goals.

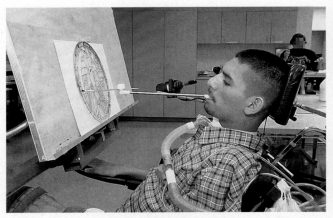

Figure 38-3 A person with C2 complete tetraplegia, ventilator dependent, using a mouthstick. Notice the plastic hose attached to a tracheostomy tube in the neck. A portable ventilator enables the person to be mobile.

Autonomic Dysreflexia

Autonomic dysreflexia, a sudden dangerous increase in blood pressure, is a possibly life-threatening complication associated with lesions at the T6 level or above (Safety Note 38-1). It is brought on by an unopposed sympathetic response to noxious stimuli. Some of the more common causes of autonomic dysreflexia are distended bladder,

Safety Note 38-1

Safety Concerns for Patients with Spinal Cord Injury

Autonomic Dysreflexia

Individuals with injuries at the T6 level or above may develop dangerously high blood pressure in response to a noxious stimulus. This condition is brought about by unopposed hyperactivity of the autonomic nervous system. If not promptly treated, autonomic dysreflexia may result in a stroke or sudden death. An increase of 20 mm Hg or more in systolic blood pressure is a sign that must be attended to. A pounding headache is the most common symptom. Other signs and symptoms include heavy sweating, flushed skin, goose bumps, blurry vision, a stuffy nose, anxiety, difficulty breathing, and chest tightness (Consortium for Spinal Cord Medicine, 1997).
Take the following steps:

1. Ask the person to stop any ongoing activity, as it may further increase blood pressure.
2. Check blood pressure. If high:
3. Have the person sit up with head elevated to avoid excessive blood pressure to the brain.
4. Loosen clothing, abdominal binder, and any other constrictive devices.
5. Check the urinary catheter for kinks or folds and straighten any.

6. Continue to monitor blood pressure and seek medical assistance, which may include bladder irrigation, manual fecal evacuation, and medications.

Orthostatic or Postural Hypotension

In contrast to autonomic dysreflexia, in orthostatic hypotension, blood pressure drops to dangerously low levels in response to assuming an upright position. If it is not treated immediately, the person may lose consciousness. Symptoms of orthostatic hypotension include light-headedness, pallor, and visual changes. To resolve the problem:

1. Check blood pressure.
2. If the person is in bed, lower the head of the bed.
3. If the person is in a wheelchair, lift his or her legs and observe for signs of relief. If symptoms persist, recline the wheelchair to place the head at or below the level of the heart.
4. If symptoms persist, put the patient to bed.
5. Continue to monitor blood pressure and seek medical assistance. Do not leave the patient unattended until a nurse or a physician is present.

Principles for treatment of autonomic dysreflexia are derived from Consortium for Spinal Cord Medicine (1997). Principles for treatment of postural hypotension are derived from Alverzo et al. (2009).

urinary tract or other infection, bladder or kidney stones, fecal impaction, pressure ulcers, ingrown toenails, invasive procedures such as urinary catheterization or enema, and pain. The main symptoms are hypertension and a pounding headache (Consortium for Spinal Cord Medicine, 1997).

Orthostatic Hypotension or Postural Hypotension

Orthostatic hypotension is a sudden drop in blood pressure occurring when a person assumes an upright position (Safety Note 38-1). Most common in patients with lesions at the T6 level and above, it is caused by impaired autonomic regulation. A decrease occurs in the returning blood supply to the heart, commonly because of blood pooling in the lower extremities. Orthostatic hypotension is aggravated by a prolonged stay in bed. When the patient attempts to sit up, the blood rushes down to the legs. The patient may complain of light-headedness or dizziness and may faint on moving from reclined to upright. The therapist must use caution when sitting the patient up by having the patient move slowly and in stages and letting the blood pressure adjust to the change. Elevating the head of the bed, using a tilt table, or using a reclining wheelchair can accomplish this. To control this problem further, patients benefit from wearing abdominal binders and elastic stockings (Alverzo et al., 2009).

Pressure Ulcers and the Maintenance of Skin Integrity

Individuals with SCI are in perpetual danger of developing pressure ulcers (Jackson et al., 2010). Most patients do not have the sensory feedback that periodically cues them to shift position in their bed or wheelchair. The constant pressure caused by maintaining a static position without shifting weight can lead to skin breakdown. All individuals with SCI must adhere to a weight-shifting pressure-relief schedule. Generally, in the wheelchair, people that have strong upper limbs perform pressure relief by leaning forward or side to side. Individuals that cannot perform these skills must rely on a powered wheelchair that tilts back (either a tilt-in-space wheelchair or one that reclines).

Although most pressure-relief efforts are aimed at the buttocks, many other parts of the body are vulnerable. All insensate areas must be inspected daily. For high tetraplegic patients, these areas may also include the spine of the scapula and the back of the head.

The pressure-relief program is successful only if individuals with SCI incorporate this practice in their daily routines following hospitalization (Jackson et al., 2010). They must become responsible for carrying out pressure-relief procedures themselves or for asking assistance in doing so. This may sound easy, but data suggest that most people with SCI develop at least one pressure ulcer during their lifetime. This underscores the challenge of living life fully while having to stay vigilant, perform routine thorough skin inspections, shift weight routinely, maintain equipment in

good repair, and make minute-by-minute choices about activity levels and durations (Fogelberg et al., 2009). Recent research suggests that intervals of 2 minutes of pressure relief every hour while seated in the wheelchair is required for tissue oxygen perfusion, rather than 1 minute as previously thought (Makhsous et al., 2007). While in bed, people with SCI must change position every 2 hours.

Any client interaction must be viewed as an opportunity for a "teachable moment" (Wolfe, Potter, & Sequeira, 2004). Educational materials, such as the Consortium for Spinal Cord Medicine Clinical Practice Guidelines, *Consumer Guides—Pressure Ulcers: What You Should Know* (2002) and www.PressureUlcerPrevention.com, a user-friendly website for consumers and therapists, are helpful supplements for reinforcing the program. However, education is not enough to prevent ulcers.

Examples of occupational therapy roles in pressure ulcer prevention include

- training in motor skills, such as checking the skin in bed and in the wheelchair
- establishing routines, such as inspecting and wiping any wetness in vulnerable areas
- assessing environmental and contextual factors, such as helping select high-protein, healthy foods when going to the market (Clark et al., 2006; Jackson et al., 2010)
- recommending appropriate equipment such as seating systems, cushions, and padded shower chairs
- assisting in creating a typical day that allows for rest periods and other preventive measures

Bowel and Bladder Function and Management

Bowel and bladder function is controlled in the S2–S5 spinal segments. Therefore, all persons with complete lesions at and above the S2–S5 levels lose their ability to void and defecate voluntarily. With the presence of intact reflex activity but with a lack of cortical voluntary control, patients void and defecate reflexively. Incomplete injuries and disruption at the S2–S5 levels, as seen in conus medullaris and cauda equina, may present with a mixed sensory and/or motor picture. For example, a person may feel the urge but may lack the ability to void and defecate voluntarily. The goal of a sound bowel and bladder program is to allow the person to develop an elimination routine that supports health, reduces potential complications, and allows the freedom to engage in life roles without disruption (Consortium for Spinal Cord Medicine, 1998, 2006).

Following a thorough medical examination that includes studies of the structure and function of the digestive and urinary tracts, a physician establishes a safe elimination program. Most programs involve behavioral and pharmacological interventions (Consortium for Spinal Cord Medicine, 1998, 2006). Surgery is also an option that is typically offered years postinjury to further ease elimination and reduce problems.

Nurses are the primary trainers of bowel and bladder routines, and occupational therapists have a vital role in supporting the acquisition of these new skills and habits. A typical bowel program for a person with paraplegia includes taking oral medications to allow for optimal feces consistency and establishing a daily routine of transferring to the toilet, managing clothing, inserting a suppository, and, after waiting for some time, inserting a finger to the anus (called digital stimulation), which causes reflexive defecation. The occupational therapist may assist in facilitating skill acquisition in a person with poor vision and/or cognitive deficits. A magnifying mirror and a lamp may be placed on the floor to help the person see the process, which helps to further break down the activity to better reinforce each step. Persons with low tetraplegia have added challenges in becoming independent in bowel care. They may achieve independence or assist in managing their bowel care only after much practice. To compensate for poor trunk control, individuals perform the bowel program on a commode; to compensate for finger paralysis, they require a tool called a dill stick to stimulate the anal reflex to defecate (Fig. 38-4); and to compensate

for lack of sensation in the anus and/or parts of the hand, they require a mirror. For safe task performance, occupational therapists may practice commode mobility and dill stick insertion, focusing on effective visual compensation. When patients become skillful at bowel evacuation practices, they decrease the risk of complications. Most individuals, after discharge, opt to carry out their bowel program in the morning every other day and can complete the procedure within 45 minutes (Kirshblum et al., 1998).

As with the bowel program, the goal of the bladder program is to achieve a simple routine with minimal risk of complications. Recurring urinary tract infection is a frequent complication and the most frequent cause of rehospitalization after SCI (Cardenas et al., 2004). To avoid complications, patients must empty their bladder routinely.

An indwelling catheter, which is a catheter that stays in the urethra and is changed only periodically, is commonly inserted soon after the person is admitted to the acute care hospital (Consortium for Spinal Cord Medicine, 2008). Although some patients continue to use an indwelling catheter, an effort is made to find other ways to empty the bladder to reduce the chance of urinary tract infections (Consortium for Spinal Cord Medicine, 2006).

Some common bladder practices include use of either intermittent catheterization (IC) or reflex voiding. IC involves the manual insertion of a catheter into the bladder (Fig. 38-5) at fixed intervals of approximately 4–6 hours. Reflex voiding refers to spontaneous urination when the bladder is full. This voiding method requires that males use a condom catheter and a leg bag and that females use a diaper (Consortium for Spinal Cord Medicine, 2006). As with the bowel program, the bladder programs of persons with tetraplegia need more intervention, and the occupational therapist must become thoroughly familiar with individual techniques. Interventions may include finding

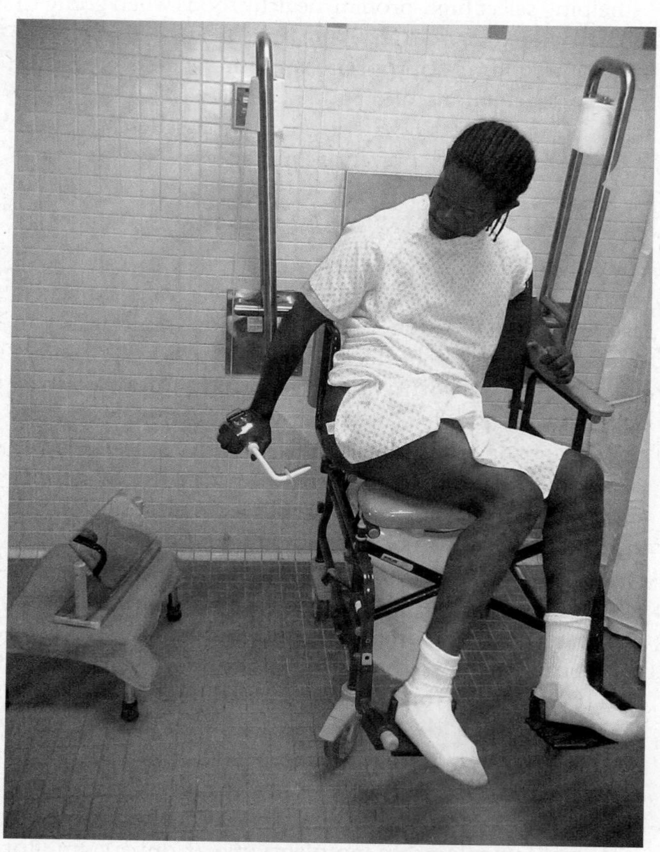

Figure 38-4 A simulation of a bowel program for a person with low-level tetraplegia (AIS A). The person is hooking his left arm under the handle for stability. He is using a dill stick to stimulate reflexic evacuation and a mirror to compensate for his lack of sensation in the anal area.

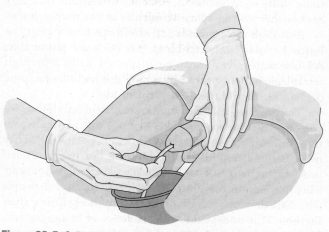

Figure 38-5 Catheterization: Inserting a catheter into the bladder and waiting for urine to flow.

a way to keep down the pants when performing IC in the wheelchair and training with a tool that helps insert the catheter into the urethra. Urinary management is more challenging to females than to males. Women have a shorter urethra and the opening is between the folds of the labia, so it is much harder for women to insert a catheter. In addition, women often need to wear diapers because their shorter urethra is more prone to leakage, and there are currently no acceptable female external collection devices that can keep the skin dry.

To best meet the person's environmental and contextual demands, the occupational therapist must think and practice beyond the hospital or clinic when helping patients rehearse and refine bowel and bladder routines. As patients rebuild new routines and habits, the therapist helps identify and embed these new functional skills in real-life scenarios such as emptying a full leg bag at a party, changing clothes when an accident happens in a mall, and performing IC while attending school.

Sexual Function

The need for emotional and physical intimacy does not diminish after SCI, and questions about intimacy, sexuality, fertility, and reproduction must be answered by a team of sensitive and knowledgeable professionals. SCI affects both sexual intercourse and reproduction, both of which are determined by the level of injury and its completeness. Most male patients with complete injuries are unable to have psychogenic (voluntary) erections and ejaculations. They can, however, have reflex erections that may be controlled by stimulation, such as pulling the pubic hairs or using a vibrator. Although most cannot feel orgasms, many describe developing new erogenous zones, such as around the neck and face (Consortium for Spinal Cord Medicine, 2010). Patients with complete injuries at S2–S5 lose bowel, bladder, and genital reflexes and have a complete loss of erection. As with physical performance, male fertility is decreased after SCI. Advances in technology, however, provide ways for male patients to sustain an erection and improve the chances of fathering children (Consortium for Spinal Cord Medicine, 2010).

Although sexual and reproductive functioning is less affected in women, sex, fertility, and menopause are still issues of concern. Some consequences related to these issues are dysreflexia and bladder incontinence during intercourse and complications of pregnancy and delivery (Consortium for Spinal Cord Medicine, 2010).

For both men and women, other psychological, social, and physical issues add to the difficulty in resuming satisfying sexual roles. Problems with mobility, dependency, and societal role expectations are some of the issues the person with SCI must face. Individual counseling, often by a psychologist, takes place after a thorough evaluation by

a physician. Some areas addressed are sexual satisfaction, sexual function, fertility, and desirability. Patients learn that, despite their injury, they can continue to be desirable and have an active sex life (Consortium for Spinal Cord Medicine, 2010).

Optimally, experienced clinicians who are a part of an interdisciplinary team specializing in sexual functioning facilitate candid discussion about the topic. In this context, the role of the occupational therapist is to address varied individual needs. The therapist may become involved in helping people groom themselves to improve their appearance and to feel more attractive, help create a cozy environment that allows for intimacy, or find equipment to either compensate for lack of hand function or to help position the person for optimal, safe physical contact. In discussing sexual issues, the therapist must be particularly sensitive to the needs of the individual. To learn more about sexuality and reproductive health, *Sexuality and Reproductive Health in Adults with Spinal Cord Injury: A Clinical Practice Guideline for Health-Care Professionals* is an excellent comprehensive resource (see Resources 38-1) (Consortium for Spinal Cord Medicine, 2010).

Temperature Regulation

Many people with SCI cannot regulate body temperature, which can lead to hypothermia or heat stroke (Alverzo et al., 2009). Because of decreased sensation, patients may become severely sunburned or frostbitten. Education in the importance of neutral temperatures and the prevention of skin exposure to sun and severe temperatures is an important part of the occupational therapy program (Hill, 1986).

Pain

Acute and chronic pain (duration of more than half a year) are common after SCI. Studies vary greatly in estimating the prevalence of chronic pain, with the reported range of pain being 26%–96% regardless of completeness and level of injury (Dijkers, Bryce, & Zanca, 2009). Considering the violent nature of most injuries and the courses of illnesses that affect the spinal cord, it is not surprising that most patients have pain at onset and that pain persists for a long time. The Bryce-Ragnarsson Pain Taxonomy and the International Association for the Study of Pain task force on SCI pain created taxonomies and algorithms to help diagnose and treat the patient with pain (Bryce & Ragnarsson, 2000; Siddall, Yezierski, & Loeser, 2000). These algorithms simplify somewhat the complex nature of pain and SCI. These algorithms share some concepts in classifying pain according to location either being above, below, or at the level of injury and sharing two other major pain taxonomies: nociceptive and neuropathic. Nociceptive pain is caused by a normal reaction to a noxious stimulus like inflammation, or tissue tear. Examples of

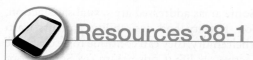

Resources 38-1

Organizations

Paralyzed Veterans of America (PVA)

www.pva.org
This organization offers many resources for consumers and for clinicians.

Consortium for Spinal Cord Medicine
Publications of clinical practice guidelines available to clinicians and consumers (see reference list for individual guidelines). Guides for people with SCI. Booklets cover topics such as bladder management, autonomic dysreflexia, and bowel management.

Hammond, M. C., & Burns, S. C. (2000). *Yes, you can! A guide to self-care for persons with spinal cord injury* (3rd ed.). Washington, DC: Paralyzed Veterans of America.

PVA Magazines
PN
Sports 'n Spokes

National Spinal Cord Injury Association (NSCIA)

www.spinalcord.org

American Spinal Cord Injury Association (ASIA)

www.asia-spinalinjury.org
Provides educational materials to physicians and other health care professionals.

The Spinal Cord Injury Statistical Center (NSCISC) and the Spinal Cord Injury Information Network

www.spinalcord.uab.edu
Includes detailed reports and data from the U.S. Model System Network. Targets mostly clinicians and researchers.

Christopher & Dana Reeve Foundation

www.christopherreeve.org
Target audience: Consumers.

The Spinal Cord Injury Rehabilitation Evidence (SCIRE)

www.scireproject.com
Provides evidence based syntheses and recommendations for best practice in SCI rehabilitation interventions. Some topics are upper limb, spasticity, cost and depression.

SCI ACTION Canada

http://pvamag.com/sns/magazine/issue/ (for sports n spokes magazine)
Online physical activity guidelines for adults with spinal cord injury.

Paralinks

www.paralinks.net

For a list of more organizations:

See www.sci-info-pages.com/spinal-cord-organizations.html

Other Publications

New Mobility

www.newmobility.com

---

nociceptive pains are local soft tissue pains above the level of injury associated with the injury or pain common in the shoulder of the person with tetraplegia because of muscle imbalance and overuse of weak muscles. Neuropathic pain originates in the nervous system and may be caused by different mechanisms such as misdirected neural sprouting after the injury. Neuropathic pain is hard to treat. Individuals with gunshot wounds often have severe shooting and burning neuropathic pains below the level of their injury.

Because most people with SCI experience pain, often in more than one location and throughout their life, the occupational therapist has many tools that help reduce pain levels and manage and cope with pain, including the following:

- Listen to the person, watch for signs of pain (such as facial expressions), and communicate clearly about the pain. The experience of pain is subjective and must be honored for what it is.
- Modify plans to help relieve the pain prior to activities. For example, instruct the patient to take pain medication half an hour prior to your session.
- Consider the contributing factors to pain such as feeling sad, being tired, or sitting too long and adjust your interventions accordingly.
- Be aware that people with complete injury (AIS A) with no sacral sensory and motor sparing may experience pain below their injury level, and this pain has to be taken seriously because it may signal medical problems such as bowel obstruction or skin breakdown.
- Facilitate positive and meaningful experiences that teach the power of diversion and meaningful occupations in reducing, managing, and coping with pain. For example, the patient may resist going shopping because of pain but after doing so report having enjoyed the outing and feeling less pain.
- Educate and practice routines to prevent long-term complications such as chronic shoulder pain caused by pushing a manual wheelchair. Guidelines for such programs are available from the PVA Clinical Practice Guideline: *Preservation of upper limb function following spinal cord injury* (Consortium for Spinal Cord Medicine, 2005a) and from a strengthening program derived from a 2011 study: *Strengthening and optimal movements for shoulders* (STOMPS) (Mulroy et al., 2011).

Fatigue

Physiological, psychological, and environmental factors all contribute to patients' fatigue. Persistent pain, antispasmodic medications, and prolonged bed rest are physical factors that can make the patient feel tired or sleepy. These factors are often compounded by restless nights interrupted by hospital routines, such as repositioning patients in bed and waking them for checking vital signs and administering medications. Occupational therapists must be aware of these constraints and observe and listen to the patient. They must find the optimal waking hours for activities and report nighttime sleep disturbances, any changes of behavior that medication may cause, and other factors.

Spasticity and Spasms

An injury to the spinal cord often results in an increase in transmission within the synaptic stretch reflex. This results in spasticity. Spasticity develops into clonic or tonic spasms triggered by sensory stimuli such as sudden touch, infection, or other irritation. Management of spasticity is important in maximizing a patient's functional independence. Severe spasticity may hinder function. For example, the hypertonicity of the hip and knee adductors can make donning pants difficult. The most common way to decrease spasticity is to use a muscle relaxant, such as baclofen or diazepam. An intrathecal pump, motor point, or nerve blocks may be used in severe cases (Botte, Peace, & Pacelli, 2011). Spasticity can lead to contractures and so routine positioning in bed (Fig. 38-6) and in the wheelchair and range-of-motion exercise are essential; patient and family must participate in these measures for continuity of care (see Chapter 20).

Deep Vein Thrombosis

Deep vein thrombosis is the formation of a blood clot, most often in a lower extremity or the abdomen or pelvic area. A clot may develop further and dislodge from the venous wall, forming an embolus. This condition poses a threat to the patient because the embolus may travel and occlude pulmonary circulation (Consortium for Spinal Cord Medicine, 1999). The therapist helps prevent this condition by observing any asymmetry in the lower extremities in color, size, and/or temperature. When deep vein thrombosis is identified, the patient must have complete bed rest and anticoagulants to prevent embolus (Consortium for Spinal Cord Medicine, 1999). This is a good time to inform the patient and family about the symptoms, prevention, and care of deep vein thrombosis.

Heterotopic Ossification

Heterotopic ossification, which is pathological bone formation in joints, has been recorded in 15%–53% of SCI patients (van Kuijk, Geurts, & van Kuppevelt, 2002). It is a condition in which connective tissue calcifies around the joint. Heterotopic ossification usually appears 1–4 months after injury.

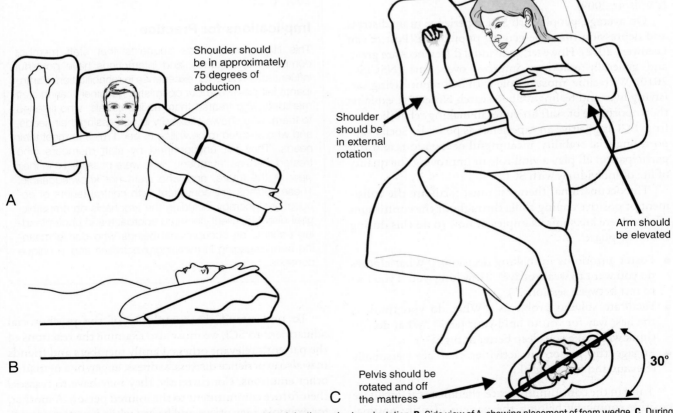

Figure 38-6 Positioning in bed. **A.** Alternate the arm in shoulder abduction and external rotation. **B.** Side view of A, showing placement of foam wedge. **C.** During side-lying, keep the upper back flat on the bed to protect the weighted shoulder. (Printed with permission from Rancho Los Amigos National Rehabilitation Center, Downey, CA.)

The symptoms are a warm, swollen extremity; fever; and/or range-of-motion limitations. Most often seen in the hip and shoulder joints, heterotopic ossification can result in joint contractures. Positioning in bed and in the wheelchair (see Fig. 38-6) and daily range of motion prevent or control heterotopic ossification. Because the first indication of heterotopic ossification most typically is range-of-motion limitation, the occupational therapist must use each range-of-motion session to monitor joint ranges, especially in patients with spastic muscles (Garland, 1991).

Psychosocial Adaptation

SCI, independent of its severity, is an emotionally traumatic event. During the first days after injury and often during acute rehabilitation, paralysis, multiple medical problems, and the need to rely on others for basic functions is overwhelming. Patients may experience a myriad of feelings such as confusion, anxiety, loss, hope, grief, depression, and helplessness. Family and significant others may also experience similar emotions (Consortium for Spinal Cord Medicine, 2008). Despite the paucity of evidence-based data specific to SCI, stage-based models have been prevalent in past decades. Fortunately, they have been replaced with a more open and fluid understanding of an individualized coping process (Magasi, Heinemann, & Wilson, 2009).

On average, people with SCI experience more distress and depression than the general population (Post & van Leeuwen, 2012). However, individual differences are great, and generally emotions improve over time (NSCISC, 2010). With time, most people with SCI report living satisfying lives and feeling well. Research Note 38-1 explains the importance of staff attitudes in making rehabilitation from SCI as positive an experience as possible. Social support, financial stability, meaningful occupations and full participation all play a vital role in improving the quality of life of individuals with SCI.

The occupational therapist must facilitate the enlistment of positive coping skills throughout the continuum of care. Here are some examples of how to do this during the acute phase.

- Foster autonomy in making decisions ("What clothes do you want to wear today?" "How long would you like to rest between sessions?").
- Facilitate solving problems ("What do you think is the best way for you to hold your pen?" "What do you think will make you sleep better at night?")
- Engage the person in activities that are personally relevant and meaningful.

Later in the continuum of care, therapists can facilitate positive coping by helping the patient identify optimal transportation, reduce environmental barriers, and facilitate the return to gainful employment.

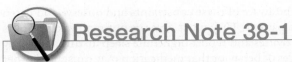

Research Note 38-1

Hammell, K. W. (2007). Experience of rehabilitation following spinal cord injury: A meta-synthesis of qualitative findings. *Spinal Cord, 45,* 260–274.

Abstract

In this comprehensive literature synthesis, the author reviewed qualitative articles that describe the subjective experience of rehabilitation following SCI. The author conducted a thematic comparison and found seven concepts that were identified as key factors in shaping the rehabilitation experience. These are: "(1) the importance of specific staff qualities; (2) the need for a vision of future life possibilities; (3) the importance of peers; (4) the relevance of program content; (5) the institutional context of rehabilitation; (6) the importance of reconnecting the past to the future; (7) the importance of meeting the needs of the real world" (Hammell, 2007, p. 260). In conclusion, the author states: "If rehabilitation services are to be evidence-based, relevant, and effective in meeting the needs of people with SCI, they must be informed by the perspectives of people with SCI. The findings of this review suggest that the most important dimension of rehabilitation for people with SCI is the caliber and vision of the rehabilitation staff" (Hammell, 2007, p. 260).

Implications for Practice

This literature synthesis suggests that staff member competence, attitudes, and interactions have powerful influences on patients' experience in rehabilitation. Participants felt positive about optimistic, genuinely caring staff members who treated them as individuals, who listened to them, who showed flexibility in addressing their needs, and who seemed to be willing to bend rules to meet their needs. They felt unsupported by staff members who treated them as "numbers," who were pessimistic in their view of the future, and who were not knowledgeable. These findings are consistent with central tenets of occupational therapy including the emphasis on empathic, goal-directed, client-centered approach and understanding patients as occupational beings who derive meaning from engaging in meaningful activities and in unique contexts.

To understand the complexity of the psychosocial adjustment to SCI, we must also examine the reactions of the patient's relevant others. Family members and friends may also experience distress, sadness, anger, or a myriad of other emotions. Concurrently, they may have to reassess their future commitment to the injured person. A mother, for example, may grieve and be sad while having to decide whether to take her fully dependent son home after a turbulent adolescence.

We must also examine our own emotional reactions and the influence of these emotions on the patient and therapeutic process. For example, sometimes upon interviewing a newly injured person, I become especially sad as I strongly identify with something in the patient's life narrative (e.g., the struggles of a mother with two young children). I am reminded of my projection, as the patient may be more accepting and positive. As occupational therapists, we contribute to psychosocial adaptation after SCI by incorporating the following considerations into evaluation and treatment:

- Set aside all preconceived biases about who the patient is and how he or she should feel or behave. Instead, concentrate on learning to know patients' factors, their unique life contexts, and their individual reactions to their trauma or illness.
- Provide psychological support. At times when the patient is overwhelmed with sadness, it is okay just to be present and available to the person. It is okay to stop an activity, find a quiet environment, possibly outside, and listen, affirm, and educate.
- Select activities with a just-right challenge. After weeks of being dependent, patients find hope by being able to feed themselves or use their cell phone independently.
- When providing information, do not overwhelm the person with too much detail. Find the opportunity for a "teachable moment" for a particular "chunk" of information, and be sensitive of patients' signs to help you determine how to proceed and when to stop (Potter et al., 2004; Wolfe, Potter, & Sequeira, 2004).
- Accept patients' emotional states without judging them (Hammell, 1995). Lack of evidence of depression or anger does not necessarily mean that individuals are coping poorly with their injury. They may be using ways of coping that are not the textbook ones. Remember that there is no requirement to mourn to learn to accept and live with the injury (Magasi, Heinemann, & Wilson, 2009). Consult with the team physician and mental health providers if the person expresses suicidal ideations (Magasi, Heinemann, & Wilson, 2009).
- Create opportunities for peer education and support. Peers with SCI are often very effective in reaching patients and helping them feel less isolated and more optimistic. Individuals with similar levels of injury can truly understand the pain that comes with SCI and may help the therapeutic process.

ASSESSMENT: GETTING TO KNOW THE PATIENT

Prior to the assessment, the occupational therapist checks the medical chart for medical clearance to begin the evaluation. The patient often has other trauma, such as lacerations of internal organs, closed head injury, and fractures. Special care is taken to review records and communicate with the physician to ensure the safety of the patient. The initial evaluation is often difficult, because the newly injured patient may be sedated, in pain, and/or confused. Furthermore, this assessment may be interrupted by numerous medical procedures and may be restricted by medical and spinal precautions. Therefore, the occupational therapist must be flexible in choosing an appropriate evaluation time, in gathering bits of information in interrupted sessions, and in choosing the right tool for the moment when the patient is available. In essence, the evaluation process should not be limited to set scheduled intervals, and the therapist must view each encounter with the patient as part of an ongoing evaluation. Information should be also collected from relevant others and other team members. Thus, at the end of the assessment period, the therapist assembles all fragments of information into a full, initial evaluation (American Occupational Therapy Association, 2008). Treatment begins while the evaluation is in progress. This prevents further complications, such as range-of-motion limitations and edema. The therapist may also address patients' immediate needs, for example making them more comfortable in bed, which further establishes rapport and trust.

A positive trend toward an initial interdisciplinary team evaluation in which a few members of the team (physician, nurse, social worker, case manager, occupational therapist, and physical therapist) evaluate the patient together allows for organized information gathering with no redundancy. Next, the occupational therapist completes more detailed assessments with the patient alone.

Occupational Profile

The goals of the initial evaluation include beginning to establish rapport and trust, teaching patients about their potential, and learning about who they are and what is important to them. From the first encounter, the therapist also begins to educate the patient and to plan discharge. This is true especially today, when hospital stays have been cut to a bare minimum. In the acute phase and shortly after the injury, patients may be quite limited in their knowledge of the nature of their injury, prognosis for recovery, and potential for function. It is important not to overwhelm the patient with more than can be absorbed at that moment. The therapist must always leave room for hope without deceiving the patient.

To gather deeper understanding of patients' roles, activities, and the meaning behind the activities, use open-ended questions. Charting a typical day's schedule prior to injury allows for creative questioning and enables the therapist to sketch a person's habits, routines, and other activities.

The Canadian Occupational Performance Measure (COPM) is an excellent tool for working with the SCI population. It focuses on finding out patients' occupational goals and their priorities (Donnelly et al., 2004) (see Chapters 3 and 4). If patients are not psychologically ready to formulate goals that are important to discharge, first goals may be directed toward attaining more control over their immediate environment.

Evaluation of Performance Skills

Spinal stability must be established prior to any physical contact with the patient. The occupational therapist must clarify with the primary physician how much movement and load are allowed without jeopardizing spinal integrity.

The physical evaluation includes upper extremity range of motion, strength, muscle tone, and sensation (see Chapters 7 and 9). The therapist also observes the patient's endurance, trunk balance, fatigability, and pain. The Manual Muscle Test is most widely used to measure strength. This test is useful in determining the functional level of the person. The appearance of the upper extremities can reveal signs of Complex Regional Pain Syndrome, which is a chronic limb disease marked by severe pain, swelling, and skin changes. Such findings are vital for prevention of further deformity by immediately initiating an aggressive treatment regimen.

Hand and Wrist of the Patient with Tetraplegia

Evaluation of the hands and wrists is both physical and functional. Following the administration of the Manual Muscle Test and range-of-motion and tone assessments, most therapists observe hand use while the person is performing activities such as eating and picking up coins or pieces of a game (see Fig. 38-9 A–C). Standardized hand function tests, specific or nonspecific for people with tetraplegia, are typically not performed during acute rehabilitation. Some such tests are the Sollerman Hand Function Test (Sollerman & Ejeskar, 1995) and the Jebsen Test of Hand Function (Jebsen et al., 1969). Most tetraplegia hand tests have been specifically developed to assess hand function before and after hand reconstruction and hand neuroprosthesis surgeries (e.g., the Motor Capacities Scale [Fattal, 2004] and the Grasp and Release Test [Wuolle et al., 1994]) (van Tuijl, Janssen-Potten, & Seelen, 2002). Hand muscle function and pinch and grip strength are measured by dynamometers (van Tuijl, Janssen-Potten, & Seelen, 2002). To measure weak pinch and grip, more sensitive instruments than the standard dynamometer and pinch meter are used. Finally, by asking the person to list functions they want and need to perform with their hands and then examining their performance in these areas, the thera-

pist can concentrate on those functional components most relevant to the person.

Evaluation of Performance in Areas of Occupation

Selection of appropriate functional evaluations is determined by level of injury and stage of recovery. Occupational therapists rely on observations and standardized and nonstandardized assessments to evaluate activities of daily living (ADL) and instrumental activities of daily living (IADL), leisure, school, vocational interests, and aptitudes (see Chapter 4).

Activities of Daily Living and Instrumental Activities of Daily Living

Often, full ADL evaluation is postponed because of medical and spinal restrictions, and predictions regarding length of stay and functional outcomes are rendered without complete data. The Spinal Cord Independence Measure III (Catz et al., 2007) is a new SCI-specific instrument that is widely accepted in the United States (Anderson et al., 2011). It measures ADL, respiration, sphincter management, and mobility. Using a simple one-sheet scoring sheet, clinical staff scores performance while the patient engages in routine activities. The Quadriplegia Index of Function (Gersham et al., 1986) is a tetraplegia-specific instrument that is less widely used. A non–SCI-specific measure that is widely used in the United States is the Functional Independence Measure (FIM™) (see Chapter 4).

Leisure and Sports

Finding relevant and meaningful leisure activities is of great importance for improving quality of life (see Chapter 29). Leisure assessments may include the COPM and interest inventories. Because SCI typically occurs to young men, it is not surprising that sports are meaningful to many patients and become a big part of their lives. Assessing the potential for engaging in sports following the injury may include activities such as an outing to a game and/or being introduced to a wheelchair sports program. Most able-bodied sports are available to people with paraplegia and low tetraplegia. To enhance performance and safety, specialized equipment is available, such as a racing wheelchair or a specialized handle to compensate for a weak hand grip (Rice et al., 2009). With less physical capacities, finding meaningful recreational activities for people with high cervical injuries is challenging. Evolving high-tech solutions such as voice-activated computers allow people with high tetraplegia to find and access community resources and to engage in activities such as social networking and gaming.

School and Vocation

A full vocational evaluation is rarely performed during acute rehabilitation because patients are focused on more immediate challenges. Many have lost the physical ability to engage in prior occupations. Vocational exploration begins with defining patients' abilities and interests. Observation of factors such as hand function and work habits contribute information for the prevocational team and department of vocational rehabilitation.

Home and Community

The home visit is an invaluable assessment tool for the person with SCI, and the earlier it is performed, the better. This visit allows the therapist to assess home accessibility and safety and to evaluate the capacity of patients and their families to problem solve (Atkins, 1989).

Assessing transportation issues is important, because persons with SCI must often find new ways to get around. This evaluation may involve taking a bus for the first time or referring the patient to special driving services for the disabled (see Chapters 10, 26, and 31).

SETTING GOALS: ORDERING PRIORITIES FOR MEANINGFUL AND RELEVANT ACTIVITIES

Setting treatment goals in the acute phase may seem overwhelmingly difficult for both patient and therapist. Complications hinder progress, and patients are often confused, fearful, and uncertain about their impairments and abilities. Answers to the following questions help patient and therapist set priorities, establish short-term goals, and start treatment while evaluation is still in progress:

- What must be done to prevent further deformities and complications?
- What activity is important for the patient to engage in right now?
- What skills must patients and caregivers have for a safe return home?

The development of short-term goals stems from the therapist's ability to perform an activity analysis. Short-term goals may address functional performance areas and tasks, underlying problems, or activity demands. For example, a person with C4 tetraplegia who wants to use a mouthstick for word processing on a computer must first tolerate sitting upright in the wheelchair for significant periods. Increasing tolerance for sitting upright is an appropriate short-term goal for achieving the independence of mouthstick computer use.

Functional Expectations

Data collected from disability outcome measures inform the clinician of performance capacities of individuals with a similar clinical picture. This knowledge assists in formulating realistic goals and in selecting optimal activities that the person can perform successfully. These data also help the therapist predict how much help a person may need following discharge from rehabilitation.

Expected functional outcome charts (see Appendix 38-1) predict the degree of functional independence for a particular level of injury. One such chart was published in a 1999 document, *Outcomes Following Traumatic Spinal Cord Injury: Clinical Practice Guidelines for Health Care Professionals* (Consortium for Spinal Cord Medicine, 1999).

When studying this chart, consider the following (see Appendix 38-1):

- Expected functional outcome charts represent functional performance outcomes of individuals with complete (AIS A) injuries. As stated previously, when patients have complete injuries (AIS A), the muscle paralysis is more symmetrical, and the prognosis is somewhat more predictable, making it easier to set goals.
- The data were collected 1 year after injury and thus represent the functional level after people completed their inpatient rehabilitation stays.
- Patients with incomplete injuries (not represented in this chart; mostly individuals with AIS C and D) present greater challenges in goal formulation. With AIS C and D, muscle return is unpredictable and not symmetrical, making recovery and outcomes more individual and harder to predict.
- Expected functional outcome charts do not address many of the tasks, activities, and occupations that individuals would like to engage in. For example, they do not inform us about functions such as writing or driving a car.

Age-Specific Considerations

Although every patient has unique considerations in treatment planning, this chapter highlights the unique needs of adolescents and older adults with SCI.

Adolescence and Young Adulthood

The adolescent with SCI must deal with complex normal developmental factors coupled with new impairments and disabilities (Smith et al., 1996). Psychological adaptation to the injury may be especially difficult for adolescents, because the injury comes in the midst of development of adult self-image, identity, and independence. The therapist is challenged to maintain a delicate balance between the sometimes competing needs to support patients and families and to encourage the young person to be self-reliant. Warning the family about avoiding overindulgence can lead to more engaged and assertive participation by the patient (Smith et al., 1996). At times, when the adolescent exhibits brooding or defiant behaviors that are harmful to progress, a strict behavioral program becomes necessary to draw the adolescent into positive participation (Massagli & Jaffe, 1990). Along with establishing independence, primary goals for the adolescent must include the following.

- Reentering the student role—Goals may include meeting with school personnel and visiting the school with the patient (Massagli & Jaffe, 1990; Wilkins, 2011).
- Sexual roles—Adolescents must be assured that individuals with SCI can remain sexually active (Massagli & Jaffe, 1990).
- Driver role—Initial evaluation and referral may be carried out in the acute rehabilitation phase and may be continued in the transition and adaptation phases. Driving, if possible, may provide the adolescent with a valuable sense of empowerment, independence, and increased motivation.
- At times, it is hard to remember that adolescents are minors and that all fundamental decisions must be made with parental participation and consent. The parents must be supported and must be part of the team, helping the patient make appropriate choices. Parents must also participate in educational sessions to ensure consistency in treatment, for example, with pressure relief.

The Older Adult

With rising longevity and greater participation of older adults, the number of people age 60 years and older with SCI is rising worldwide. The etiology of SCI of older adults is mostly falls and nontraumatic SCI such as tumors, vertebral degeneration, and vascular problems. In this population, etiology is often less clear because several medical conditions can cause spinal trauma (van den Berg et al., 2010). Falls, the number one cause of injury for this population, result in lesions at the cervical level, often causing central cord syndrome.

Having SCI and being elderly may be considered a dual diagnosis. The physiological process of aging can make rehabilitation from SCI particularly difficult, and older patients tend to have more medical complications (Scivoletto et al., 2003). The geriatric patient may require downgrading of expected functional outcomes, given physical and/or cognitive limitations. Some important factors are decreases in muscle strength, endurance, energy, and physical fitness; joint degeneration; bone decalcification; skin integrity; cognition; vision; and emotional changes. Older patients may require more assistance in ADL, and

hence, the focus of rehabilitation may be helping them identify resources in the community, teaching them to effectively direct their care, and involving family members in therapy (Scivoletto et al., 2003).

INTERVENTION

The occupational therapist treats individuals with SCI at various settings and at various times. Throughout this treatment continuum of acute care, acute rehabilitation, transition, and adaptation, most treatment principles remain the same. The focus of care changes, however, as the patient's internal processes (such as the psychological adjustment to the injury) and external environments change.

Acute Recovery: Focus on Support and Prevention

Immediately after injury, most patients are admitted to an intensive care unit, where the focus is on preservation of life and stabilizing fluids, electrolytes, cardiopulmonary and other vital functions. The patient is immobilized in traction and waiting to hear whether surgery is required to stabilize the spine. For prevention of pressure ulcers, the patient is put in a rotating bed (Consortium for Spinal Cord Medicine, 2008). In the intensive care unit, medical and surgical procedures take precedence over therapy. The therapist must be flexible, often seeing the patient for brief periods throughout the day. One or two 15-minute sessions per day are often helpful to the patient, who may be in pain, fatigue easily, and become confused or overwhelmed by this fast-paced environment of electronic devices and medical procedures. The occupational therapist's initial contact should be within the first few days after admission and when medically cleared by a physician. Treatment begins as the initial evaluation is in progress, allowing the therapist to begin to gain a full picture of the patient (Hammell, 1995). In addition to ongoing patient and family support and education, the focus of therapy in the acute recovery phase includes the following:

1. Providing some environmental controls to help the patient get some control of their immediate environment such as nurse call button or bed controls.
2. With individuals with tetraplegia, maintaining normal upper limb joint range of motion and preventing edema and deformities (Consortium for Spinal Cord Medicine, 2008).

To prevent range-of-motion limitations, therapists use positioning techniques and assist with range-of-motion exercises. In bed, most persons with tetraplegia tend to lie with their arms adducted close to their body, internally rotated, and with elbows flexed (Consortium for Spinal Cord Medicine, 2005a). Therefore, movement in joints particularly susceptible to contractures must be monitored daily. Important movements include scapular rotation, shoulder scaption (the functional motion between abduction and flexion), shoulder external rotation, elbow extension, and forearm pronation. Hands are fitted with resting hand splints. Upper limbs are placed in either some abduction or external rotation (see Fig. 38-6, A & B). Alternating arms between these positions puts all vulnerable joints in stretch. It is important to note, however, that although the goal is to preserve range of motion, one must consider the comfort of patients to allow them a good night's sleep.

Range of motion to the hand of the patient with tetraplegia is performed in a special way to facilitate tenodesis grasp: passive opening of the fingers when the wrist is flexed and closing of the fingers when the wrist is extended (Fig. 38-7, A & B) (Wilson et al., 1984). The patient, family, and others are taught how to perform range-of-motion exercises to the arm and to facilitate tenodesis. Again, range-of-motion exercises must be augmented with proper positioning in bed and in the wheelchair.

During the acute phase and when medically cleared, the occupational therapist may also evaluate the person's ability to swallow, sit upright, and begin evaluating and training in appropriate ADL (Consortium for Spinal Cord Medicine, 2008).

Acute Rehabilitation: Focus on Support, Education, Acquiring Performance Skills and Meaningful Activities

In the United States in the 1970s, the mean length of stay in acute SCI rehabilitation was 144.8 days. By the late 1990s, mean length of stay had decreased to 97 days and is now less than 37 days (NSCISC, 2010). To a lesser extent, this trend of shortening rehabilitation length of stays has been also occurring worldwide. With such short stays, individuals are discharged way before their physical condition plateaus. Because rehabilitation institutions are the major venues for delivering intensive therapy, this trend has been difficult for patients and clinicians alike, who must make tough decisions about what is most important to accomplish during inpatient stay. The growing availability of ambulatory services have helped ease the sense of urgency somewhat, allowing patients and therapists to focus their attention on the present and near future while in rehabilitation.

During acute rehabilitation, occupational therapy continues to focus on providing education and support to patients and helping them begin to explore meaningful activities that restore a sense of efficacy and self-esteem. Treatments must always be structured with these overriding goals in mind. This chapter offers basic information. For specific detailed interventions, consult the reference and suggested reading lists.

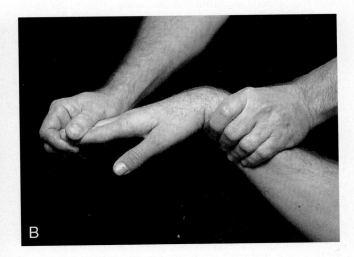

Figure 38-7 Ranging to facilitate tenodesis grasp. **A.** When the wrist is extended, the fingers are flexed. **B.** When the wrist is flexed, the fingers are extended.

Educating Patients and Family

Each encounter with patients and families must be viewed as an educational opportunity. The style, quantity, and direction of each session must be carefully considered (Hammell, 1995; Wolfe et al., 2004). While patients are learning to put on a shoe, for example, the therapist may ask if they have checked skin integrity and, by so doing, draw attention to the importance of skin inspection. This discussion may also inform the patient about preferable shoe styles and sizes, pedal edema, and deep vein thrombosis. These "teachable moments" arise often and help embed details of newly learned skills and routines (Wolfe et al., 2004). Nurses, the only team members who see the patient throughout the day, are pivotal in enforcing a daily routine. The therapist must communicate with them daily to ensure a coherent and consistent program.

Education is often enhanced by learning and problem solving with a peer or in a group (Hammell, 1995; Wolfe, 2004). Group learning is widely used in SCI centers, to inform and invite group dialogue on topics such as home modifications, accessibility rights, attendant management, assertiveness, travel, and driving. Experiential group activities, such as going to a restaurant, are recommended for building emotional and social alliances with peers while learning from each other's successes and failures. Educational materials and videos are available through groups such as the Paralyzed Veterans of America and the Spinal Cord Injury Association (Resources 38-1). Participation in self-initiated learning, such as surfing the Internet, empowers the patient. On the Internet, many SCI consumer websites offer tips, personal stories, and chat rooms, which can provide a lively forum for communication, self-expression, and information. Family education must result in competence in range of motion, positioning, pressure relief, assistance in ADL, and use of equipment. Home and weekend passes provide an excellent opportunity to develop and refine skills.

Self-Efficacy and Self-Management Skills

Patients' medical and psychological status, as well as being in a hospital environment, invite passivity and submission to hospital routines and to professional staff recommendations of care. The therapist and the rest of the health care team must encourage patients in taking an active role in managing their care, in evaluating behaviors, and in self-reflection about failures and successes (Lorig, 2003; Radomski, 2000). In addition, our challenge as therapists is to recruit, educate, and empower our patients to be problem solvers. By so doing, we encourage active participation, generalization of information, and the transfer of learning to the post-discharge environment (Radomski, 1998; Wolfe et al., 2004). When planning an outing, for example, ask the group to prepare a list of items to be checked to ensure a safe, successful outing.

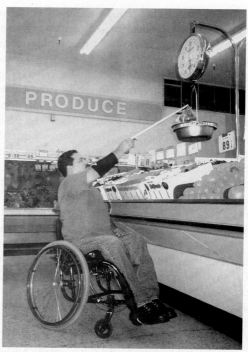

Figure 38-8 A person with paraplegia using a reacher to retrieve hard-to-reach items on a shopping outing.

Upon return to the hospital, encourage discussion of the outing to reflect on ways future outings can be improved (Fig. 38-8). Practical issues such as restaurant accessibility to wheelchairs and self-catheterization in public bathrooms may arise. This discussion is also a good time to reflect on performance accomplishments during the outing and to share failures and success experiences in a supportive environment.

Balancing Self-Maintenance Skills and Meaningful Activities

In acute rehabilitation, most patients are relearning skills that they mastered in childhood, such as eating and dressing independently. This training is an important part of our job. For many patients, however, this training is frustrating, time consuming, tiring, and a constant reminder of their impairments and disabilities. The therapist has the difficult task of helping the patient see when relearning skills is valuable and when the skill should be accomplished by a caregiver, either for now or permanently. The ultimate goal of rehabilitation is no longer viewed as the attainment of maximal functional independence. Rather, it is the attainment of optimal desired functional independence. Functional expectations charts (see Appendix 38-1 at the end of this chapter) help us understand the range of expectations for a given level of injury considering only the motor and sensory status of the patient. These charts do not answer such questions as these: Why should the patient dress for half an hour when his wife can dress him in 5 minutes? Will it still take that long after adequate training? What will the patient do when his wife is away? Such discussions encourage patients and families to explore the range and consequences of their choices. The novice therapist will find books such as *Spinal Cord Injury: A Guide to Functional Outcomes in Occupational Therapy* (Hill, 1986) and *Physical Management for the Quadriplegic Patient* (Ford & Duckworth, 1987) especially valuable because they contain photographs that demonstrate various skills, their sequencing, and the use of assistive devices (both books are out of print but can be found in libraries and as used books for purchase on the Internet).

Choosing Equipment

Initially, when pain, spinal precautions, and orthoses, such as a body jacket, may stand in the way of accomplishing goals, assistive devices may be handy facilitators. When obstacles diminish, some equipment, such as a dressing stick, can be eliminated. Only essential equipment should be sent home with the patient, because much of it is costly, and it may further complicate the person's life. Also, a universal device should be favored over multiple assistive devices.

Most persons with SCI require lifetime use of wheelchairs for their mobility. Choosing the optimal wheelchair requires great expertise and has important implications for ease of mobility, accessibility, and participation (see Chapter 17). The therapist and the patient must consider many factors in weighing the advantages and disadvantages of specific chairs (Consortium for Spinal Cord Medicine, 2005a). For example, if a young adult with a functional level of C6 is returning to college following a rehabilitation stay and would like to use an attractive manual wheelchair to look and feel less disabled, questions about the layout of campus, the terrain, and distances between classes must first be answered prior to recommending the optimal wheelchair. The person's endurance, posture, and transportation are factors that must all be weighed in selecting either a manual wheelchair or a power wheelchair.

Patients and families should be involved also in the purchase of any other major equipment, such as commode, other bathroom equipment, or a bed.

The Patient with High Tetraplegia: C1 to C4

Patients with complete C1–C3 require an external breathing device because their diaphragm is either paralyzed or only partially innervated (C3). Most persons with C4 tetraplegia require assistance with ventilation during acute care, but as the diaphragm strengthens, they are able to breathe independently. The most common device for assisted breathing is the ventilator, a pneumatic electric machine that forces room air into the lungs. Expiration is passive. This device is attached via plastic tubes directly to a hole in the trachea (see Fig. 38-3).

People with complete high tetraplegia are paralyzed from the neck down. These patients require a highly specialized team to stabilize them medically and to prevent further complications, such as respiratory infections and pressure sores. The occupational therapist who works with this population must be comfortable with nursing procedures. These tasks include suctioning (removing secretions from the trachea), manually ventilating the patient with a manual resuscitator (Ambu-bag), and proficiently managing a ventilator (Consortium for Spinal Cord Medicine, 2005b). The rehabilitation team must also be well coordinated, providing the patient and family with care while preparing them for discharge. Patients with high lesions have a myriad of issues to deal with in many domains of their life. It may be surprising to realize that, despite seemingly insurmountable obstacles to success, many patients with such lesions live healthy and meaningful lives (Whiteneck et al., 1989).

Some additional roles the therapist may have in treating persons with high cervical injury include teaching them to direct their own care; helping them select specialized and sophisticated equipment (see Chapter 18) for life support, mobility, and ADL; and training them in the use of mouthsticks, which are rigid long rods held in the mouth that allow the patient to perform activities such as turning pages, drawing, typing, painting, and playing board games (see Fig. 38-3) (Atkins, Clark, & Waters, 2010; Hammell, 1995).

The Patient with Lower Cervical Injuries: C5 to C8

As in the acute recovery phase, physical intervention includes positioning in bed and in the wheelchair (see Fig. 38-6), splinting the upper extremities, daily upper extremity range of motion, and strengthening. Strengthening, an important goal in this phase, can be performed by using weights, pulley systems, tabletop skateboards, suspension slings, mobile arm supports (discussed later), and modalities such as biofeedback neuromuscular electrical stimulation and robotics (Hill, 1986; Hoffman & Field-Fote, 2009) (see Chapters 19, 20, and 22).

New evidence of neuroplasticity once thought unattainable in the adult brain shows some promise for upper extremity recovery. Emerging research demonstrates that mass repetitive upper extremity task practice with sensory stimulation can bring about greater brain excitability in the corresponding brain sites and some improvement in function (Hoffman & Field-Fote, 2009). A growing number of rehabilitation centers offer intense repetitive upper extremity training with the aid of robotic arms and/or video games to enhance repetitive motion with the hope of increasing function.

To enhance function and engage in a variety of activities, the therapist works closely with the patient, exploring wrist and hand compensatory techniques and finding devices to compensate for hand paralysis (Curtin, 1999) (see Fig. 38-9, A–E).

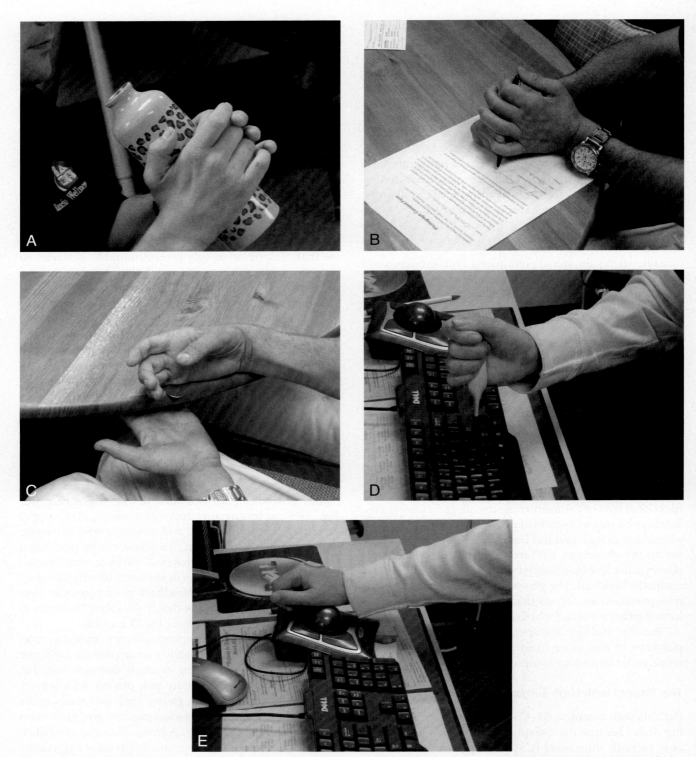

Figure 38-9 Hand compensatory techniques. **A.** Pressing one hand against the other to lift a bottle. **B.** Pressing one hand against the other to write. **C.** Dragging the coin to the edge of the table in order to pick it up. **D.** Using devices to compensate for lack of ability to point and isolate finger movements. **E.** Using a track ball instead of a mouse.

Patients with C5 Tetraplegia. Initially, the deltoids and biceps, key muscles for this level of injury, are weak, so upper limbs require support to function. The mobile arm support, also called a ball-bearing feeder, is a mechanical device attached to the wheelchair. (See Chapter 15 for further discussion of this device.) This shoulder and elbow support carries the weight of the arm (Wilson et al., 1984). The mobile arm support can assist the patient in driving the wheelchair, feeding, hygiene and grooming, and carrying out tabletop activities, such as writing and cooking (Atkins et al., 2008). If and when the strength of the deltoids and biceps is 3+/5 or greater and endurance is good, patients can engage in activities without mobile arm supports (Zigler et al., 2011).

Patients with C5 complete tetraplegia need a way to grasp and hold objects, because their wrists and hands are paralyzed. First, the wrist must be stabilized with a splint or orthosis. Next, a device is attached to the hand to enable the person to perform activities. The universal cuff is a simple, inexpensive utensil holder is worn around the palm (Fig. 38-10). Other U- or C-shaped clamps can be attached to objects such as telephone receiver or a shaver. Some splints, devices, and orthoses accommodate the wrist and the hand as a unit. To maximize functional gain with any device, the patient must have adequate time and repeated training sessions.

Most patients with C5 tetraplegia can master tabletop activities. They lack trunk control and muscles below the shoulder, however, so they are mostly dependent in dressing and bathing (see Appendix 38-1) (Consortium for Spinal Cord Medicine, 1999). With adequate emotional and financial resources, persons with C5 tetraplegia engage in meaningful, productive activities. Case in point: Mr. L. is a financial consultant who lives on his own and has part-time caregivers. He lives a busy life full of business trips and leisure activities with friends. He attributes his success to much planning and good organizational skills.

Patients with C6 and C7 Tetraplegia. Patients with C6 and C7 tetraplegia may attain significantly higher levels of independence than those with C5 injury. The addition of radial wrist extensors allows patients to close their fingers with a tenodesis grasp. This is a critical functional enhancement because, with it, light objects may be picked up, held, and manipulated. The wrist-driven wrist–hand orthosis (also called the flexor hinge splint or tenodesis splint) is a metal device that transfers power from the extended wrist to the radial fingers, allowing a stronger pinch (Fig. 38-11) (Atkins et al., 2010; Consortium for Spinal Cord Medicine, 1999).

More fully innervated proximal scapular and shoulder muscles, such as the rotator cuff, deltoids, and biceps, allow for an increase in upper limb strength and endurance. Patients can also roll in bed, and their arms can cross the midline more forcefully, with the addition of the clavicular pectoralis muscle. The ability to use the triceps, the

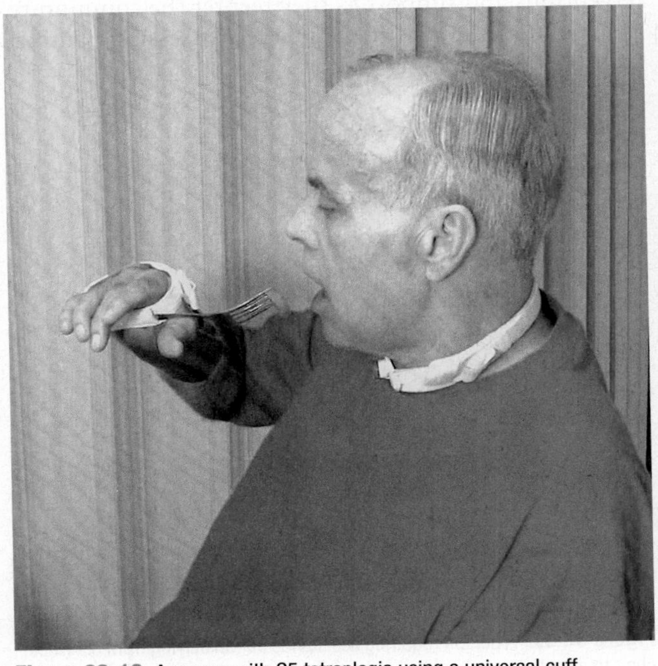

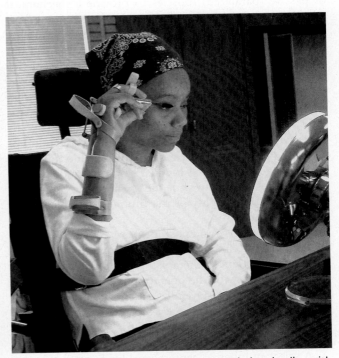

Figure 38-10 A person with C5 tetraplegia using a universal cuff.

Figure 38-11 A woman with C6 complete tetraplegia using the wrist-driven wrist–hand orthosis to apply makeup. This device enables the person to hold on to objects tightly despite finger paralysis.

key muscle for C7 tetraplegia, allows the patient to reach for objects above head level, such as items on a store shelf; transfer with greater ease; and push a manual wheelchair.

Patients with C8 Tetraplegia. Hand function is significantly improved with the addition of extrinsic finger muscles and thumb flexors. Hand dexterity and strength are limited by the absence of intrinsic finger and thumb muscles. A person with complete C8 tetraplegia grasps objects with the metacarpophalangeal joints in extension and the proximal interphalangeal and distal interphalangeal joints in flexion. This is called a claw hand or intrinsic minus hand (Zigler et al., 2011).

Surgical Options for the Upper Extremities. Restoring hand function is the top priority of many individuals with tetraplegia (Moberg, 1978; Snoek et al., 2004). To improve hand function, persons with C5, C6, C7, or C8 injuries may have surgical options. These options do not provide for a normal hand but aim to restore pinch, grasp, and reach. Tendon transfer surgeries are recommended only after full spontaneous motor and sensory recovery has occurred and no earlier than a year after injury because most of these procedures permanently alter the musculoskeletal structures (Waters et al., 1996).

Upper limb reconstructive surgeries, although not frequently performed, are available for increasing motion and function of the upper extremities. These surgeries may shorten or change the direction of pull of tendons of passive (paralyzed) muscles to provide a mechanical advantage to the thumb or fingers. Other common procedures may entail tendon transfers of functioning muscles. Typically, a proximal functional muscle with strength of 4 out of 5 or above is attached to a tendon of a distal paralyzed muscle. Following the surgery, the patient learns to contract a proximal muscle to move a distal joint (Waters et al., 1996). An example of a hand tendon transfer surgery is the brachioradialis to flexor pollicis longus. This surgery restores lateral pinch by attaching the tendon of a strong (4 out of 5 muscle or above) brachioradialis to a paralyzed flexor pollicis longus. To pinch an object, the patient flexes the elbow while the forearm is in pronation. To improve the stability of the thumb, the interphalangeal joint is fused.

The preoperative and postoperative evaluation, education, wound care, and muscle reeducation must be carried out by an experienced therapist. Additionally, consistent communication with the operating physician is vital for favorable outcomes. Overall, patients who have gone through reconstructive surgeries perceive their surgeries positively and as improving their function and appearance (Jaspers Focks-Feenstra et al., 2011).

A select number of centers worldwide offer complex procedures for achieving hand function. One such system is the second generation neuroprosthesis, a permanently

implanted electrical stimulation device, which allows the person with C5–C6 injury to open and close the hand by moving the opposite shoulder. This electrical device is composed of 12 electrodes implanted into various muscles, electrode leads, transmitter, and a shoulder sensor. An external controller box attached to the wheelchair controls the device remotely with no connecting wires. Often, the neuroprosthesis surgery is either combined with or follows other hand surgeries that allow for optimal use of the device (Kilgore, 2008).

The Patient with Paraplegia

Most people with complete or incomplete paraplegia become independent in self-maintenance, self-enhancement, and self-advancement roles, although they require assistance with heavy housekeeping and physically demanding vocational pursuits (Consortium for Spinal Cord Medicine, 1999). Paraplegics with injuries at T10 and below may attain skills more easily and rapidly than patients with higher injuries (Fig. 38-12). Good trunk control enables a person with low paraplegia to bend down and from side to side without fear of falling forward. Skills performed while upright (e.g., bowel management, lower body dressing, undressing, and bathing) require the patient with a higher injury to secure the trunk by supporting the body with one arm while performing the activity with the other to prevent falls (Zigler et al., 2011).

Typically, patients with paraplegia have fewer medical complications than those with tetraplegia, and self-maintenance skills are learned quickly. Patients with paraplegia are discharged quickly from acute rehabilitation settings and may benefit greatly from more interventions and support as they reenter the community. These interventions often include reassessing routines

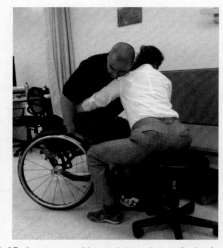

Figure 38-12 A person requiring assistance in transferring from his wheelchair to a mat.

such as re-examining self-care skills, facilitating return to school, and exploring work and leisure interests, skills, and opportunities.

The Ambulatory Patient: Incomplete Paraplegia and Tetraplegia

Typically, when we think of spinal cord injuries, we picture a person using a wheelchair, yet many individuals with incomplete SCI are able to walk (Fig. 38-13). Walking potential is mostly determined by the level and completeness of the injury (Consortium for Spinal Cord Medicine, 1999). Other factors may include body weight, age, upper extremity involvement, and pain. Ambulation, a primary goal for most patients, carries with it some unique challenges to the patient and occupational therapist.

For expedient and relevant treatment planning, the occupational therapist must clearly understand ambulation goals soon after admission. Early discussion with the physical therapist helps clarify goals and enables the occupational therapist to outline a treatment course that takes walking into consideration. Answers to the following questions guide treatment planning:

1. Will upper extremity aids be needed to assist in walking (e.g., a forearm trough walker)? If so, how will the patient carry objects if both hands are occupied?
2. What lower extremity braces are needed? Will the patient require assistance in donning and doffing the braces?
3. Is the goal to walk short distances only? Will the patient need a wheelchair for mobility in the community?
4. What can be done for fall prevention: Better lighting, the removal of area rugs and extension cords?

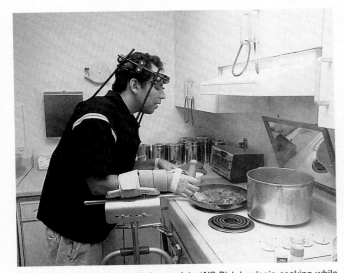

Figure 38-13 A person with incomplete (AIS D) tetraplegia cooking while using an arm trough walker. The 8- to 10-pound Halo vest interferes with balance and limits vision.

Not surprisingly, ambulatory patients with tetraplegia pose the greatest challenge with their often weak upper extremities. In the wheelchair, equipment such as lapboards, armrests, and mobile arm supports support weak arms and allow for function. When upper limb proximal muscles are weak, hand function becomes difficult or impossible, because the patient lacks a mechanism for bringing the hand to the mouth or face. Various devices are available that enable the person to both lift and support the arm. A solution for supporting the arm depends on the pattern of upper extremity muscle strength (e.g., a table versus a chair-mounted mobile arm support). Frequently, however, these devices are less than optimal.

Concomitant Brain Injury and Cognitive Deficits

Much attention is given to the visible paralysis of the injured patient, whereas less visible traumatic brain injury may be overlooked and unattended to. If we think about the velocity of the body at the time of impact in injuries caused by motor vehicle accidents and falls, it becomes apparent that head injuries are common. The percentage of patients who suffer concomitant injuries to the brain and spinal cord may be as high as 40%–50% (Davidoff, Roth, & Richards, 1992). These injuries may be diffuse or focal and mild or severe. Because Chapter 34 is solely devoted to traumatic brain injury, the discussion here is limited to elements that are unique to the dual diagnosis.

The occupational therapist must be vigilant for clues of brain injury in the first encounters with the patient. A period of unconsciousness and post-traumatic amnesia raises a red flag (Consortium for Spinal Cord Medicine, 2008). Therapists should ask patients directly whether they have trouble remembering events or sense any changes in their thinking. Patients may lack insight, however. Often, the family is an excellent source of information because they usually know the premorbid cognitive status of the patient. The evaluation of the patient is made more challenging with factors such as fatigue, medication side effects, pain, depression, sleep deprivation, and sensory deprivation (Davidoff, Roth, & Richards, 1992). A formal screening can determine whether a detailed neuropsychological assessment is indicated. It is common in many hospitals to request such consultations automatically if the patient had a period of unconsciousness or post-traumatic amnesia.

Cognitive deficits in the SCI population may not be limited to those incurred as a result of the injury. Factors such as previous head injuries, learning disabilities, and a history of alcohol and drug abuse are often present, and they affect the patient's cognitive functioning (Davidoff, Roth, & Richards, 1992). Although the effects of a mild brain injury associated with SCI may diminish over time, the prognosis for recovering from a preexisting cognitive deficit is poor (Davidoff, Roth, & Richards, 1992).

Transitions: Restoring Roles at Home and in the Community

With the short length of acute rehabilitation hospitalization stays, the health care team and occupational therapists are challenged to transition quickly from a protective role to a "launching" role, exposing the person to the real world and promoting autonomy and self-efficacy. This may include offering patients an increased number of activity choices, having them assess their own competence in performing a skill, requiring them to prepare for the activity on their own (call in preparation for an outing or search the internet, for example). After completing activities, having feedback sessions to celebrate successes and reflect on failures further helps to facilitate self-efficacy and a feeling of autonomy.

If therapists conclude that the rehabilitation program is too short for achieving optimal outcomes, they must be prepared to articulate and document the need for longer hospitalization. This is especially true if the short stay may jeopardize the safety of the patient. The therapist may also be called upon to find resources that allow the patient to continue to receive care and engage in occupations following discharge.

If geographically possible, many patients benefit from outpatient occupational therapy services. In a prospective U.S. study on the amount of therapy given after discharge from acute rehabilitation care within a year postinjury, Whiteneck et al. (2011) found that 52% of the total therapy time (inpatient and outpatient) was delivered in an outpatient setting. There was, however, a great variability between centers, and 8% of patients received no outpatient care because of such factors as location, and lack of reimbursement (Whiteneck et al., 2011). Not surprising, this study also found that the highest number of hours of occupational therapy, both inpatient and outpatient, was spent with patients with tetraplegia.

Most patients continue to gain strength during the first year after their injury, allowing them to become more independent. In outpatient clinics, the occupational therapist continues to facilitate performance skills and performance patterns and explore meaningful occupations in greater depth. Outpatient programs teach clients to use newly acquired voluntary movements and offer them additional ADL training. As clients gain strength and endurance and improve their balance, they reassess and reprioritize their goals. For example, a person with tetraplegia who once could not carry out a bowel program but who now exhibits normal strength in manual muscle testing of the triceps and latissimus dorsi and exhibits improved body handling skills can begin bowel training.

To ensure good fit and function, training in the use of orthoses and devices often begins during the last days of hospitalization and continues during outpatient visits.

Outpatient evaluation and training in the use of other equipment is beneficial because the patient and family can use the equipment at home and provide ongoing feedback about its fit and use.

The outpatient occupational therapist should begin and/or continue working on goals and skills that move the patient toward greater community integration (e.g., driving and vocational evaluation and training). The outpatient education of family members and attendants must continue to assure continuity and progress.

With the help of the social worker, liaison nurse, or case manager, the therapist can minimize barriers to receiving therapy after discharge. A frequent barrier is a lack of transportation. If patients cannot leave home, an agency such as the Visiting Nurses Association may provide occupational therapy services at home for a limited time.

Other transitional services, such as support groups and transitional living centers, must be identified. Independent living centers are federally funded programs designed to promote reintegration. They are located in most large cities in the United States and provide resources and access to financial, vocational, rehabilitative, and community-based programs (Forchheimer & Tate, 2004).

To further ease clients' transition from hospital to home, models are continuing to emerge and evolve and reflect third-party payers' growing awareness of the benefits of less costly alternatives to hospitalization, preventing complications, enhancing health and quality of life, and supporting the goal of full participation. Examples of such models include the following:

- Clients living for days to months in a transitional residence with family members and/or attendants. Clients and their families are encouraged to seek health care providers' help only when they cannot solve problems independently. Such residential programs are often located in close proximity to acute rehabilitation centers.
- Following discharge, clients sometimes receive the assistance of a federal or state transitional services team, which may include a case manager, an occupational therapist, a physical therapist, a vocational counselor, and others. They may assist in finding accessible housing, implementing home modifications, and finding financial benefits.

Adaptation: Focus on Facilitation toward Full Participation, Improved Quality of Life, and Wellness

The path from being a dependent patient to becoming a person with a sense of efficacy and self-esteem is long and individual. Occupational therapists are increasingly involved in helping individuals with SCIs to be aware of their special health risks, how to prevent secondary conditions, engage in productive, meaningful activities, and sustain a good quality of life. Some newly emerging programs were created to meet these challenges:

- Lifestyle Redesign® is a program that encourages participants to select health promoting personalized goals and to work toward their achievement and maintenance (Mandel et al., 1999). The therapist helps the individual identify risks and health-promoting behaviors and build routines to sustain healthy behaviors. For example, if a young adult loves to play wheelchair basketball for hours at a time and forgets his pressure reliefs, both the therapist and the person work together to identify the problem, find alternative solutions, test them, and incorporate them into the game and other daily activities.

- Telehealth, an all-encompassing term for electronic technologies that promote and maintain health, is becoming more prevalent and opens new avenues for interventions (Carson, 2012). It offers an ongoing communication with consumers through technologies such as two-way computer monitors, texting, and phone calls, thereby assisting individuals in developing skills, forming new routines and habits, and problem solving together with occupational therapists. This is especially important in rural communities and in areas with harsh winters that make it difficult for clients to get to a hospital (Carson, 2012). During telehealth sessions, the client may ask the therapist to look at a wheelchair or cushion that suddenly does not feel the same.

- Wellness programs are offered by an increasing number of rehabilitation hospitals, independent living centers, nonprofit organizations, and other agencies. They typically offer wellness classes, supervised adapted exercise programs, community recreation programs such as sailing and skiing, adaptive driving programs, computer access programs, and counseling services.

- Patient self-management programs, which provide group support and patient education for prevention of secondary conditions and facilitation of healthy living habits, with peers and clinicians acting as facilitators. These models of health care are offered to address the challenge of providing care throughout the life span in an environment of minimal resources (Dames et al., 2009).

Living Fully and Growing Older

Long-term survival rates of patients with SCI have improved dramatically in recent decades. Along with the decline of normal aging, some unique problems arise in this population. Multiple secondary health conditions and rehospitalizations are common with people with SCI. Clinicians must address these conditions throughout the individual's life span (Krause & Saunders, 2011). Conditions most linked to decreased life expectancy are pressure ulcers, amputations, infections, and clinical depression. Not

surprisingly, rehospitalizations, multiple health problems, and pain have also been linked to reduced reported subjective well-being. Other common body changes include decreased bone density with susceptibility to fractures, and renal and bowel problems. Other concerns and risk factors include impaired cardiovascular fitness, because of the inability to walk and limitations in engaging in aerobic exercises, as well as the early development of diabetes. As a result of a more sedentary life, many also become overweight, which makes engaging in self-care and other activities more challenging. To address obesity, occupational therapists and other clinicians are involved in creating and testing programs that facilitate adherence to a healthy lifestyle, focusing on routine exercise and nutrition, by offering supportive environments with education classes, exercise regimens, and mechanisms to encourage the maintenance of healthy routines (Radomski et al., 2011).

Often, to achieve better health, the occupational therapist must ask the person to make difficult choices. Having to make functional adjustments, modify routines and habits, and reduce intensity and occupational engagement is difficult for most people but especially for individuals with SCI who have over many years learned to live with their disability. Therefore, the need to modify daily occupations to meet declining physical capacities or to add exercise to the daily routine must be addressed with great respect and sensitivity. The occupational therapist and client must work together to optimize daily occupations with dialogue, practice, and problem solving. Often, this involves performing detailed activity analyses to better understand and modify routines and habits. An aging client once independent in all self-maintenance skills may need help in the morning to conserve energy for work. A grandmother who wants to interact with her toddler grandson may have to teach him to climb onto her lap rather than picking him up.

For many people with SCI, pain contributes to limited activity, lack of participation, and depression. Available treatments include prescription and nonprescription medications, physical agent modalities, medical procedures such as nerve blocks, and psychotherapy (Widerstrom-Noga, 2009). The occupational therapist's contribution to pain management includes a thorough evaluation and a myriad of possible interventions. Although treatment goals are often directed toward reducing impairments, our main contribution is in changing habits and roles and in facilitating engagement in meaningful activities with full participation. This approach is especially valuable because most persons continue to live with some pain throughout their lives and new pains arise with aging.

The World Health Organization's development of the International Classification of Functioning, Disability and Health (ICF) (World Health Organization, 2001) reflects a growing global recognition of the importance of people with disabilities living healthy, productive lives; engaging in social, vocational, and avocational pursuits; and feeling well. This model parallels occupational therapy values and beliefs. Occupational therapists around the world are at the forefront of creating innovative programs and challenging old models in order to create greater opportunities for people with SCI. Although some laws (e.g., the Americans with Disabilities Act) aim to encourage individuals with SCI to participate fully in all societal roles, many barriers continue to hinder full participation. The unemployment rate of individuals with SCI is significantly higher than in the general population, and income is lower (Lidal et al., 2009).

As all of health care moves toward preventative care and healthy living, occupational therapy has a great opportunity to continue developing, shaping, and implementing new programs to better serve people with SCI. To fill this role, we must continue to seek work in group homes and governmental agencies and to engage in shaping public policy (Baum, 2000; Hammell, 2004).

As occupational therapists, we have the opportunity and obligation to educate consumers, the public, and policy makers with the goal of enabling people with SCI to live full, meaningful lives by facilitating full participation in their desired life roles.

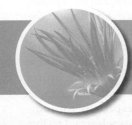

case example

Able: Optimizing Occupational Performance after Spinal Cord Injury

Occupational Therapy Process	Clinical Reasoning Process	
	Objectives	**Examples of Therapist's Internal Dialogue**
Patient Information Able is a 19-year-old man with C6 AIS A (complete) tetraplegia resulting from an ocean diving accident 3 months ago. Able is a sophomore at a community college. He came to the United States from Samoa to attend college on a football scholarship. Able is single and lives with fellow students in a rented house near campus. He has a large and supportive family in Samoa. After his injury, Able's mother, aunt, and two of his sisters came to be with him for a month. Able is fluent in English. He was hoping to stay in California and resume his studies. He did not have a discharge destination. Following his injury, Able was sent to a trauma center, where he underwent posterior fusion surgery to stabilize C4–C7 vertebrae and was placed in a Philadelphia collar, a rigid collar that limits neck motion. Following surgery, Able was prescribed spine restrictions in order to protect the surgical site. Precautions allowed Able to perform shoulder bilateral/symmetrical activities with minimal resistance (no greater than 3+/5) and unilateral, active-only activities with no resistance.	Understand the patient's diagnosis or condition	"If Able has a functional level of C6, he may be able to achieve independence in many areas. Unfortunately, because he has an AIS A (complete) injury, his muscle and sensory return will most likely be only in the zone of partial preservation (ZPP)."
During the postoperative hospital stay, Able was on a rotating bed to prevent pressure sores. The occupational therapist performed daily upper limb range-of-motion exercises. She established a shoulder-positioning program and fitted Able with prefabricated resting hand splints. In conversations with the patient and his family, the therapist began to explain the process of rehabilitation. The occupational therapist documented that the family was engaged and supportive and that the patient appeared passive and quiet. Able was transferred to a rehabilitation center 3 weeks post injury.	Know the person	"Able is passive and quiet and seems quite depressed. Knowing that the best predictor of future behaviors and disposition is premorbid personality and behaviors, I am very hopeful that he soon will feel better, as he sees his renewed abilities. It is excellent that he has such a supportive, loving family; however, later in the course of rehabilitation, we will request that they limit their visits somewhat, in order to enable Able to see that he can manage without them, to allow him to become more active in his rehabilitation, and to encourage him to begin directing his own care. Prompt identification of discharge destination and potential caregivers is crucial for goal setting. Therefore, the social worker must address these important issues as soon as possible."

Reason for Referral to Occupational Therapy

Able was referred to occupational therapy to address limitation in performance skills and patterns.

Appreciate the context	"Able's past accomplishments and tough school/sports schedule required him to be disciplined and structure his time efficiently. I think this will help him in the acute rehabilitation setting, a place that requires hard work. More importantly, his past level of engagement is an indicator that he will be able to continue a life full of participation in meaningful occupations."

Assessment Process and Results

Occupational profile: Interviews included establishing rapport; in-depth interviews about Able's typical day, interests, routines, habits and roles; and administering of the Canadian Occupational Performance Measure. Initially, because of Able's withdrawn mood, the therapist secured Able's permission and interviewed his family about his life and about family goals.

Findings: Able was clear about wanting to stay in California and resume his studies. His family was going to go back to Samoa in a few weeks. He and his family described his busy schedule. Football occupied most of his nonstudy time. For fun, he "hung out" with his roommates, some of whom were also from Samoa. Information from the social worker indicated no clear discharge destination and no knowledge of who will assist Able with his care.

Physical evaluation: Physical evaluation included measuring bilateral upper extremities (BUE) passive range of motion, tone, sensation (pain, light touch, proprioception, and object identification), and Manual Muscle Test (MMT). Observations of reach and hand use included activities such as picking up a coin or a tissue and pushing a button.

Results of MMT:
Scapulae and shoulder muscles: 3+ or above/5 throughout.
Elbows: 4/5 flexion; 0/5 extension.
Forearms: 4/5 supination; 2/5 pronation.
Wrist: Radial wrist extensors: Right 3+/5; left 3/5; bilateral ulnar wrist extension and flexion 0/5
Fingers and thumbs: 0/5
Sensory level: C2–C6 dermatomes intact; impaired C7 and absent below (see Fig. 38-2).
Tone throughout both upper limbs: Within normal limits.
Hand use: Drags objects to edge of table; picks up objects with the two hands

Summary of upper limb findings: Right hand dominant. Symmetry in strength with right arm slightly stronger than left. Shoulder strength 3+/5 and above. Deficits in reaching away from body and in pronation. Fair tenodesis action bilaterally; beginning effective hand compensatory techniques for picking up and manipulating objects.

Activities of daily living (ADL): Able was given a universal cuff in the acute hospital, and he is able to feed himself with a spoon and a fork and to brush his teeth. He needs assistance with setup for these activities (Functional Independent Measure-5). He is dependent with all other self-maintenance skills.

Consider evaluation approach and methods	"Two casual contacts were made, establishing rapport with Able and his family and meeting Able's immediate needs. These included making Able more comfortable in bed and assessing his ability to press key pads (nurse call light, phone use, and bed and TV controls). The installation of key pads allowed Able to stay alone in his room for short periods of time and increased his autonomy."
Interpret observations	"I hope that Able's roommates and friends will help and support him when his family is no longer here. When he indicates that he wants his friends around, we will encourage them to visit and be involved in his therapy."
	"Able had a large repertoire of occupations prior to his injury, and his self-efficacy is strong. He has excellent potential for resuming his studies. I need to further explore his engagement with football and, as he gains skills and feels more self-confident and competent, explore with him the range of options for engaging in sports. For example, either being a spectator and/or acquainting him to wheelchair sports."
	"Initial spinal precautions limit full resistive exercises to neck, scapulae, and shoulders and allow only for minimal-resistance, symmetrical exercises. This will be achieved with routine activities such as washing the face. A full strengthening program can be carried out to elbows and wrists. The left wrist will also benefit from neuromuscular electrical stimulation (NMES) to radial wrist extensors."
	"Able is beginning to compensate for his finger paralysis. He has learned to drag objects to the edge of a table and to hold objects with two hands to compensate for weak grip. Further education and experiential training will help him with other compensatory techniques such as weaving objects through his fingers."

Occupational Therapy Problem List

- Decreased performance skills: moderate depression, lack of engagement with the rehabilitation team, excessive dependency on family.
- Decreased performance skills: upper limbs weakness, sensory deficit, decreased endurance and control.
- Limitations in all performance patterns including ADL, instrumental activities of daily living (IADL), education, work, leisure, and social participation.
- Decreased knowledge of spinal cord injury (SCI) management, resources, and of directing own care.

| Synthesize results | "The problem list is overwhelming because Able's disability is devastating, affecting physical capacities and all his occupational roles. I have to remind myself that tackling this long list will sort itself out daily, as we reassess Able's engagement in the program, his progress, and his evolving list of priorities." |

Occupational Therapy Goal List (In the Acute Rehabilitation Facility)

Initially, Able had difficulty coming up with goals, as he appeared overwhelmed with his paralysis and was not able to determine what he would be able to physically do. With the help of his therapist, the team, and his family, his short-term goals included strengthening his arms, feeding, brushing his teeth, shaving, upper body dressing, writing, and using the phone and the computer.

Other goals included:

- Learn routine SCI precautions for skin care, pressure relief, bowel and bladder care, and autonomic nervous system functioning.
- Learn to direct own care.
- Learn SCI resources in the community.
- Select and trial a cushion and wheelchair.

"Able views his primary role as an athlete. It is not surprising that exercising the arms is his first goal. This activity has the potential of transforming Able's attitude toward therapy, becoming more engaged in the process. Strengthening his weak muscles will improve his sense of control and feelings of renewed hope. Feeding, brushing teeth, writing, and using the computer are skills that will be easy for Able to develop. Able will have a harder time dressing, especially his lower body. The reality of the amount of energy and time it takes to complete this task right now may help Able sort out his priorities as to what a caregiver will do for him and what he will do himself."

| Select an intervention approach | "The occupational therapy intervention approach will focus on compensatory techniques." |

| Consider what will occur in therapy, how often, and for how long | "I must remember that the interventions in acute care are only the beginning of a long process of rehabilitation toward participation. His acute rehabilitation stay provides intense therapy for only a few weeks: 3–5 hours of combined OT and PT per day, 6 days a week for 4–5 weeks. |

Intervention in the acute rehabilitation facility

First 3 weeks:

- Upper limbs passive and active exercises (nonresistive shoulder exercises because of spinal precautions).
- Wrist strengthening program through exercises, activities, and NMES.
- ADL training including feeding, brushing teeth, and grooming using a universal cuff.
- Exploration and training in writing, computer skills, and telephone use with adaptive equipment.
- Hand use in routine activities, such as compensatory techniques in swiping a card, handling money, and opening pill bottles.
- Individual, short educational sessions focused on specific interventions, such as how to use the hand and how to best maximize hand function.
- Trialing different power wheelchairs.

| Compare actual to expected performance | "Able's premorbid self-discipline and high level of occupational engagement were, indeed, reliable predictors of his ability to engage in therapy despite his depression. In the first few weeks, he talked little, and although not fully engaged, he went along with the program as if 'going through the motions' of therapy. As he gained some independence, he became more animated. He enjoyed working with the computer because he realized that going back to school would be possible. It was wonderful to get to know Able as his warm and engaging personality began to emerge when his depression lifted. He began initiating ideas, |

| Know the person | solved problems easily, and seemed interested in newly introduced equipment. He also became more outgoing and started socializing with other patients. Able's family needed to return to Samoa close to his discharge from acute rehabilitation. The shift from family to friends' support happened naturally as all his acquaintances understood his need for support." |

Weeks 4 and 5:

- Spinal precautions were lifted, allowing Able to move his neck and shoulders freely and engage in a full strengthening program. Evaluation for the use of right wrist-driven wrist–hand orthosis with clinic trial equipment. Ordering, checking fit, and beginning training in use of orthotics. Training in upper body dressing and beginning of lower body dressing.
- Expanded on student role activities such as using a computer and an iPad and handling books and papers.
- Education: Individual and group. Group experiential training in topics such as taking public transportation, assertiveness training, and directing care. Individual: Daily self range-of-motion exercises.
- Training in hand use with and without the orthosis through activities with peers (for example, board games).
- Ordering of a wrist-driven wrist–hand orthosis.
- Ordering of cushion and permanent wheelchair.

Predischarge goals:

- Prepare Able to live in a transitional living center (TLC).
- Train a caregiver in assisting Able with his care.
- Engage Able in directing his care.

Predischarge interventions:

Visiting a transitional living center and meeting the staff.

Postscript:

Able was accepted to a TLC. This facility offered continued rehabilitation services at reduced intensity and cost. The strong support of his friends helped his transition. He resided in the facility for 8 months, sharing a room with a roommate. He received assistance from a caregiver twice a day. With the help of the TLC team and his occupational therapist, he established a daily routine that enabled him to continue learning new skills, managing his care, and exploring his return to school. His caregiver came in the morning for 3 hours assisting Able in getting out of bed, bathing, dressing, and setting up his breakfast. In the evening, the caregiver came again for 3 hours to help Able manage his dinner, bowel program, undressing, and getting into bed.

During the day, Able received TLC services. His occupational therapy program included individual and group therapy sessions, engaging in activities such as learning to use his new wrist-driven wrist–hand orthosis and learning to empty his bladder independently by carrying out self-intermittent catheterization. Other activities included attending Able's college football team's game, touring his college to assure full wheelchair accessibility, and meeting with the disabled students counselor.

Throughout his TLC stay, Able established new habits. As previously predicted, he worked hard, became more independent, and directed his caregiver effectively. Before leaving the TLC, Able explored community resources to support a healthy lifestyle. He found accessible transportation and a venue for routine exercise. After leaving the TLC, Able rented an apartment with a roommate he met at the TLC and resumed college.

Appreciate the context	"Because Able decided to stay in California with no family around, team meetings involved finding alternatives for further care because all felt that Able would not be ready to live alone postdischarge. Able liked the idea of an interim discharge to a transitional living facility (TLC). This would enable him to acquire more skills and to attain greater self-efficacy prior to returning to school and to independent living."
Assess outcomes	
Prepare for discharge from acute rehabilitation	"Being admitted to the TLC requires hiring a caregiver because Able requires assistance in ADLs. He must learn to direct his own care effectively, to supervise the activities of a caregiver, and to be vigilant about new daily routines such as daily skin inspection and bowel and bladder care."

Clinical Reasoning in Occupational Therapy

Helping the Client Hire a Caregiver

Able is hiring his first caregiver. A. What activities will the caregiver need to perform? B. What important precautions does the caregiver need to exercise? C. As Able's therapist how would you facilitate the caregiver's learning?

Summary Review Questions

1. List three key epidemiological factors of the SCI population and describe how these factors influence evaluation and treatment.
2. List three precautions the therapist must consider in planning for an outing with a patient with C5 injury.
3. What is a tenodesis grasp? Why is it important, and how can the occupational therapist facilitate it?
4. List five parts of the initial occupational therapy evaluation of a patient with SCI.
5. Describe a typical feeding setup for a person with C5 tetraplegia.
6. What are the functional expectations for the patient with a C7 injury?
7. You read in the medical chart that a patient lost consciousness at the time of injury. How do you modify your evaluation? Describe how concomitant brain injury may alter your treatment goals and interventions.
8. What are the roles of the occupational therapist in the transition phase?

Glossary

Dermatome—"The area of skin innervated by the sensory axons within each segmental nerve (root)" (ASIA, 2011, p. 7).

Complete injury—"Absence of sensory and motor function in the lowest sacral segments (S4–S5) (i.e., no 'sacral sparing')" (ASIA, 2011 p. 10).

Functional level—Lowest segment at which strength of important muscles is graded 3+ or above out of 5 on MMT and sensation is intact.

Incomplete injury—"Preservation of any sensory and/or motor function below the neurological level that includes the lowest sacral segments S4–S5 (i.e., presence of 'sacral sparing')" (ASIA, 2011, p. 9).

Paraplegia—Loss or impairment in motor and/or sensory function in the thoracic, lumbar, or sacral segments of the cord resulting in impairment in the trunk, legs, and pelvic organs and sparing of the arms (ASIA, 2011).

Skeletal level—Level of greatest vertebral damage.

Tenodesis grasp—Passive opening of the fingers when the wrist is flexed and closing of the fingers when the wrist is extended (Wilson et al., 1984).

Tetraplegia (in the past called quadriplegia)—Loss or impairment in motor and/or sensory function in the cervical segments of the spinal cord resulting in functional impairment in the arms, trunk, legs, and pelvic organs (ASIA, 2011).

Appendix 38-1
Expected Functional Outcomes*

EXPECTED FUNCTIONAL OUTCOMES TABLES

Outcome-based practice guidelines can provide estimates of the effect of rehabilitation on functional status or activity restrictions. In the expected functional outcomes charts that follow, the Consortium for Spinal Cord Medicine has put forth its best description, based on outcome studies and expert consensus, of outcomes of people with motor complete spinal cord injury (SCI) 1 year after injury. These outcome guidelines are presented with the full recognition that outcomes are not fully under the influence or control of health care providers. Differences in patient characteristics; the course of medical events; psychological, social, and environmental supports; and cognitive abilities have strong influences on outcomes.

These outcome-based guidelines can be used to establish goals, provide information for quality improvement, and compare performance across facilities with similar populations. When used appropriately, outcome-based practice guidelines provide a benchmark for comparing programs and services while improving both the processes and outcomes of care that have an enduring impact on long-term functioning in the community. Disability outcome measures are generally focused on the degree to which a person can independently complete an important function or activities of daily living (ADL). This definition of disability is consistent with the World Health Organization model of disablement in which disability is measured at the level of the person interacting with the environment during daily routines. In the completion of daily tasks, adaptive equipment becomes a crucial adjunct to the independence of the person with SCI.

The following charts present expectations of functional performance of SCI at 1 year postinjury for each of eight levels of injury (C1–C3, C4, C5, C6, C7–C8, T1–T9, T10–L1, and L2–S5). The outcomes reflect a level of independence that can be expected of a person with motor complete SCI, given optimal circumstances.

The categories presented reflect expected functional outcomes in the areas of mobility, ADL, instrumental ADL, and communication skills. The guidelines are based on consensus of clinical experts, available literature on functional outcomes, and data compiled from the Uniform Data System and the National Spinal Cord Injury Statistical Center (NSCISC). Within the functional outcomes for people with SCI listed in the tables that follow, the panel has identified a series of essential daily functions and activities, expected levels of functioning, and the equipment and attendant care likely to be needed to support the predicted level of independence at 1 year postinjury. These outcome areas include the following:

- **Respiratory, bowel, and bladder function.** The neurological effects of spinal injury may result in deficits in the ability of the individual to perform basic bodily functions. Respiratory function includes the ability to breathe with or without mechanical assistance and to adequately clear secretions. Bowel and bladder function includes the ability to manage elimination, maintain perineal hygiene, and adjust clothing before and after elimination. Adapted or facilitated methods of managing these bodily functions may be required to attain expected functional outcomes.

- **Bed mobility, bed/wheelchair transfers, wheelchair propulsion, and positioning/pressure relief.** The neurological effects of SCI may result in deficits in the ability of the individual to perform the activities required for mobility, locomotion, and safety. Adapted or facilitated methods of managing these activities may be required to attain expected functional outcomes.

- **Standing and ambulation.** SCI may result in deficits in the ability to stand for exercise or psychological benefit or to ambulate for functional activities. Adapted or facilitated methods of management may be required to attain expected functional outcomes in standing and ambulation.

- **Eating, grooming, dressing, and bathing.** The neurological effects of SCI may result in deficits in the ability of the individual to perform these ADL. Adapted or facilitated methods of managing these ADL may be required to attain expected functional outcomes.

- **Communication (keyboard use, handwriting, and telephone use).** The neurological effects of SCI may result in deficits in the ability of the individual to communicate. Adapted or facilitated methods of communication may be required to attain expected functional outcomes.

- **Transportation (driving, attendant-operated vehicle, and public transportation).** Transportation activities are critical for individuals with SCI to become maximally independent in the community. Adaptations may be required to facilitate the individual in meeting the expected functional outcomes.

---

* Reprinted with permission from the Paralyzed Veterans of America (PVA). Consortium for Spinal Cord Medicine. (1999). *Outcome following traumatic spinal cord injury: Clinical practice guidelines for health care professionals.* Washington, DC: Paralyzed Veterans of America.

- **Homemaking (meal planning and preparation and home management).** Adapted or facilitated methods of managing homemaking skills may be required to attain expected functional outcomes. Individuals with complete SCI at any level will require some level of assistance with homemaking activities. The hours of assistance with homemaking activities are presented in the tables.
- **Assistance required.** The Expected Functional Outcomes charts include the number of hours that may be required from a caregiver to assist with personal care and homemaking activities in the house. Personal care includes hands-on delivery of all aspects of self-care and mobility, as well as safety interventions. Homemaking assistance is also included in the recommendation for hours of assistance and includes activities previously presented. The number of hours presented in both the panel recommendations and the self-reported Craig Handicap Assessment and Reporting Technique (CHART) (Whiteneck et al., 1992) data is representative of skilled and unskilled and paid and unpaid hours of assistance. The 24-hour-a-day requirement noted for the C1–C3 and C4 levels includes the expected need for unpaid attendant care to provide safety monitoring.

Adequate assistance is required to ensure that the individual with SCI can achieve the outcomes set forth in the expected functional outcomes charts. The hours of assistance recommended by the panel do not reflect changes in assistance required over time as reported by long-term survivors of SCI (Gerhart et al., 1993), and they also do not take into account the wide range of individual variables mentioned throughout this document that may affect the number of hours assistance required. The Functional Independence Measure (FIM™) estimates are widely variable in several categories. One does not know whether the representative individuals with SCI in the individual categories attained the expected functional outcomes for their specific level of injury or whether there were mitigating circumstances such as age, obesity, or concomitant injuries that would account for variability in assistance reported. An individualized assessment of needs is required in all cases.

- **Equipment requirements.** Minimum recommendations for durable medical equipment and adaptive devices are identified in each of the functional categories. The most commonly used equipment is listed, with the understanding that variations exist among SCI rehabilitation programs and that use of such equipment may be necessary to achieve the identified functional outcomes. Additional equipment and devices that are not critical for the majority of

individuals at a specific level of injury may be required for some individuals. The equipment descriptions are generic to provide for variances in program philosophy and financial resources. Rapid changes and advances in equipment and technology will be made and therefore must be considered.

Health care professionals should keep in mind that the recommendations set forth in Appendix 38-1 are not intended to be prescriptive, but rather to serve as guidelines. The importance of individual functional assessment of people with SCI prior to making equipment recommendations cannot be overemphasized. All durable medical equipment and adaptive devices must be thoroughly assessed and tested to determine medical necessity to prevent medical complications (e.g., postural deviations, skin breakdown, or pain) and to foster optimal functional performance. Electronic aids to daily living (EADL), the new name for environmental control units, and telephone modifications may be needed for safety and maximal independence, and each person must be individually evaluated for the need for this equipment. Disposable medical product recommendations are not included in this document.

- **FIM™.** Evidence for the specific levels of independence provided in Appendix 38-1 relies both on expert consensus and data from the FIM™ in large-scale, prospective, and longitudinal research conducted by NSCISC. FIM™ is the most widely used disability measure in rehabilitation medicine. Although it may not incorporate all of the characteristics of disability in individuals recovering from SCI, it captures many basic disability areas. FIM™ consists of 13 motor and 5 cognitive items that are individually scored from 1 to 7. A score of 1 indicates complete dependence, and a score of 7 indicates complete independence. The sum of the 13 FIM™ motor score items can range from 13, indicating complete dependence for all items, to 91, indicating complete independence for all items. FIM™ is a measure usually completed by health care professionals. Different observers, including the patient, family members, and caregivers, can contribute information to the ratings. Each of these reporters may represent a different type of potential bias. It should also be noted that, although the sample sizes of FIM™ data for certain neurological level groups are quite small, the consistency of the data adds confidence to the interpretation. Other pertinent data regarding functional independence must be factored into outcome analyses, including medical information, patient factors, social participation, quality of life, and environmental factors and supports.

In Appendix 38-1, FIM™ data, when available, are reported in three areas. First, the expected FIM™ outcomes are documented based on expert clinical consensus. The second number reported is the median FIM™ score, as compiled by NSCISC. The interquartile range for NSCISC FIM™ data is the third set of numbers. In total, the FIM™ data represent 1-year postinjury FIM™ assessment of 405 survivors with complete SCI. The sample size for FIM™ and assistance data is provided for each level of injury. Different outcome expectations should clearly apply to different patient subgroups and populations.

Some populations are likely to be significantly older than the referenced one. Functional abilities may be limited by advancing age (Penrod, Hedge, & Ditunno, 1990; Yarkony et al., 1988).

- **Home modifications.** To provide the best opportunity for individuals with SCI to achieve the identified functional outcomes, a safe and architecturally accessible environment is necessary. An accessible environment must take into consideration, but not be limited to, entrance and egress, mobility in the home, and adequate setup to perform personal care and homemaking tasks.

Appendix 38-1 | Expected Functional Outcomes

Level C1-3

Functionally relevant muscles innervated: Sternocleidomastoid; cervical paraspinal; neck accessories
Movement possible: Neck flexion, extension, rotation
Patterns of weakness: Total paralysis of trunk, upper extremities, lower extremities; dependent on ventilator

FIM™/Assistance Data: Exp = expected FIM™ score; **Med** = NSCISC median; **IR** = NSCISC interquartile range
NSCISC Sample Size: FIM™ = 15; Assist = 12

	Expected Functional Outcomes	Equipment	FIM™/Assistance Data		
			Exp	Med	IR
Respiratory	• Ventilator dependent • Inability to clear secretions	• Two ventilators (bedside, portable) • Suction equipment or other suction management device • Generator or battery backup			
Bowel	Total assist	Padded reclining shower-commode chair (if roll-in shower available)	1	1	1
Bladder	Total assist		1	1	1
Bed mobility	Total assist	Full electric hospital bed with Trendelenburg feature and side rails			
Bed, wheelchair transfers	Total assist	• Transfer board • Power or mechanical lift with sling	1	1	1
Pressure relief, positioning	Total assist; may be independent with equipment	• Power recline and/or tilt wheelchair • Wheelchair pressure-relief cushion • Postural support and head control devices as indicated independent with equipment • Hand splints may be indicated • Specialty bed or pressure-relief mattress may be indicated			
Eating	Total assist		1	1	1
Dressing	Total assist		1	1	1
Grooming	Total assist		1	1	1

(continued)

Appendix 38-1   Expected Functional Outcomes *(continued)*

Level C1-3

	Expected Functional Outcomes	Equipment	FIM™/Assistance Data		
			Exp	Med	IR
Bathing	Total assist	• Handheld shower • Shampoo tray • Padded reclining shower-commode chair (if roll-in shower available)	1	1	1
Wheelchair propulsion	Manual: Total assist Power: Independent with equipment	• Power recline and/or tilt wheelchair with head, chin, or breath control and manual recliner • Vent tray	6	1	1–6
Standing, ambulation	Standing: Total assist Ambulation: Not indicated				
Communication	Total assist to independent, depending on workstation setup and equipment availability	• Mouth stick, high-tech computer access, environmental control unit • Adaptive devices everywhere as indicated			
Transportation	Total assist	Attendant-operated van (e.g., lift, tie-downs) or accessible public transportation			
Homemaking	Total assist				
Assist required	• 24-hour attendant care to include homemaking • Able to instruct in all aspects of care		24*	24*	12–24*

*Hours per day

Level C4

Functionally relevant muscles innervated: Upper trapezius; diaphragm; cervical paraspinal muscles
Movement possible: Neck flexion, extension, rotation; scapular elevation; inspiration
Patterns of weakness: Paralysis of trunk, upper extremities, lower extremities; inability to cough, endurance and respiratory reserve low secondary to paralysis of intercostals

FIM™/Assistance Data: Exp = expected FIM™ score; **Med** = NSCISC median; **IR** = NSCISC interquartile range
NSCISC Sample Size: FIM™ = 28; Assist = 12

	Expected Functional Outcomes	Equipment	FIM™/Assistance Data		
			Exp	Med	IR
Respiratory	May be able to breathe without a ventilator	If not ventilator free, see C1–C3 for equipment requirements			
Bowel	Total assist	Reclining shower-commode chair (if roll-in shower available)	1	1	1
Bladder	Total assist		1	1	1
Bed mobility	Total assist	Full electric hospital bed with Trendelenburg feature and side rails			
Bed, wheelchair transfers	Total assist	• Transfer board • Power or mechanical lift with sling	1	1	1

Appendix 38-1 Expected Functional Outcomes *(continued)*

Level C4

	Expected Functional Outcomes	Equipment	FIM™/Assistance Data		
			Exp	Med	IR
Pressure relief, positioning	Total assist; may be independent with equipment	• Power recline and/or tilt wheelchair • Wheelchair pressure-relief cushion • Postural support and head control devices as indicated • Hand splints may be indicated • Specialty bed or pressure-relief mattress may be indicated			
Eating	Total assist		1	1	1
Dressing	Total assist		1	1	1
Grooming	Total assist		1	1	1
Bathing	Total assist	• Shampoo tray • Handheld shower • Padded reclining shower-commode chair (if roll-in shower available)	1	1	1
Wheelchair propulsion	Power: Independent Manual: Total assist	• Power recline and/or tilt wheelchair with head, chin, or breath control and manual recliner • Vent tray	6	1	1–6
Standing, ambulation	Standing: Total assist Ambulation: Not usually indicated	• Tilt table • Hydraulic standing table			
Communication	Total assist to independent, depending on workstation setup and equipment availability	Mouth stick, high-tech computer access, environmental control unit			
Transportation	Total assist	Attendant-operated van (e.g., lift, tie-downs) or accessible public transportation			
Homemaking	Total assist				
Assist required	• 24-hour care to include homemaking • Able to instruct in all aspects of care		24*	24*	16–24*

*Hours per day.

(continued)

Appendix 38-1 | **Expected Functional Outcomes** *(continued)*

Level C5

Functionally relevant muscles innervated: Deltoid, biceps, brachialis, brachioradialis, rhomboids, serratus anterior (partially innervated)
Movement possible: Shoulder flexion, abduction, and extension; elbow flexion and supination; scapular adduction and abduction
Patterns of weakness: Absence of elbow extension, pronation, all wrist and hand movement; total paralysis of trunk and lower extremities

FIM™/Assistance Data: Exp = expected FIM™ score; **Med** = NSCISC median; **IR** = NSCISC interquartile range
NSCISC Sample Size: FIM™ = 41; Assist = 35

	Expected Functional Outcomes	Equipment	FIM™/Assistance Data		
			Exp	Med	IR
Respiratory	Low endurance and vital capacity secondary to paralysis of intercostals; may require assist to clear secretions				
Bowel	Total assist	Padded shower, commode chair, or padded transfer tub bench with commode cutout	1	1	1
Bladder	Total assist	Adaptive devices may be indicated (electric leg bag emptier)	1	1	1
Bed mobility	Some assist	• Full electric hospital bed with Trendelenburg feature with patient's control • Side rails			
Bed, wheelchair transfers	Total assist	• Transfer board • Power or mechanical lift	1	1	1
Pressure relief, positioning	Independent with equipment	• Power recline and/or tilt wheelchair • Wheelchair pressure-relief cushion • Hand splints • Specialty bed or pressure-relief mattress may be indicated • Postural support devices			
Eating	Total assist for setup, then independent eating with equipment	• Long opponens splint • Adaptive devices as indicated	5	5	25–55
Dressing	Lower extremity: Total assist Upper extremity: Some assist	• Long opponens splint • Adaptive devices as indicated	1	1	1–4
Grooming	Some to total assist	• Long opponens splints • Adaptive devices as indicated	1–3	1	1–5
Bathing	Total assist	• Padded tub transfer bench or shower-commode chair • Handheld shower	1	1	1–3
Wheelchair propulsion	Power: Independent Manual: Independent to some assist indoors on uncarpeted, level surface; some to total outdoors	Power: Power recline and/or tilt with arm drive control frame with hand rim modifications assist Manual: Lightweight rigid or folding	6	6	5–6

Appendix 38-1 Expected Functional Outcomes (continued)

Level C5

	Expected Functional Outcomes	Equipment	FIM™/Assistance Data		
			Exp	Med	IR
Standing ambulation	Total assist	Hydraulic standing frame			
Communication	Independent to some assist after setup with equipment	• Long opponens splint • Adaptive devices as needed for page turning, writing, button pushing			
Transportation	Independent with highly specialized equipment; some assist with accessible public transportation; total assist for attendant-operated vehicle	Highly specialized modified van with lift			
Homemaking	Total assist				
Assist required	• Personal care: 10 hours per day • Home care: 6 hours per day • Able to instruct in all aspects of care		16*	23*	10–24*

*Hours per day.

Level C6

Functionally relevant muscles innervated: Clavicular pectoralis; supinator; extensor carpi radialis longus and brevis; serratus anterior; latissimusdorsi
Movement possible: Scapular protraction; some horizontal adduction, forearm supination, radial wrist extension
Patterns of weakness: Absence of wrist flexion, elbow extension, hand movement; total paralysis of trunk and lower extremities

FIM™/Assistance Data: Exp = expected FIM™ score; **Med** = NSCISC median; **IR** = NSCISC interquartile range
NSCISC Sample Size: FIM™ = 43; Assist = 35

	Expected Functional Outcomes	Equipment	FIM™/Assistance Data		
			Exp	Med	IR
Respiratory	Low endurance and vital capacity secondary to paralysis of intercostals; may require assist to clear secretions				
Bowel	Some to total assist	• Padded tub bench with commode cutout or padded shower-commode chair • Other adaptive devices as indicated	1–2	1	1
Bladder	Some to total assist with equipment; may be independent with leg bag emptying	Adaptive devices as indicated	1–2	1	1
Bed mobility	Some assist	• Full electric hospital bed • Side rails • Full to king standard bed may be indicated			

(continued)

Appendix 38-1 Expected Functional Outcomes *(continued)*

Level C6

	Expected Functional Outcomes	Equipment	FIM™/Assistance Data		
			Exp	Med	IR
Bed, wheelchair transfers	Level: Some assist to independent Uneven: Some to total assist	• Transfer board • Mechanical lift	3	1	1–3
Pressure relief, positioning	Independent with equipment and/or adapted techniques	• Power recline wheelchair • Wheelchair pressure-relief cushion • Postural support devices • Pressure-relief mattress or overlay may be indicated			
Eating	Independent with or without equipment except cutting, which is total assist	Adaptive devices as indicated (e.g., U-cuff, tenodesis splint, adapted utensils, plate guard)	5–6	5	4–6
Dressing	Independent upper extremity; some to total assist for lower extremities	Adaptive devices as indicated (e.g., button hook; loops on zippers, pants, socks; Velcro® on shoes)	1–3	2	1–5
Grooming	Some assist to independent with equipment	Adaptive devices as indicated (e.g., U-cuff, adapted handles)	3–6	4	2–6
Bathing	Upper body: Independent Lower body: Some to total assist	• Padded tub transfer bench or shower-commode chair • Adaptive devices as needed • Handheld shower	1–3	1	1–3
Wheelchair propulsion, standing, ambulation	Power: Independent with standard arm drive on all surfaces Manual: Independent indoors; some to total assist outdoors Standing: Total assist Ambulation: Not indicated	Manual: Lightweight rigid or folding frame with modified rims Power: May require power recline or standard upright power wheelchair Hydraulic standing frame	6	6	4–6
Communication	Independent with or without equipment	Adaptive devices as indicated (e.g., tenodesis splint; writing splint for keyboard use, button pushing, page turning, object manipulation)			
Transportation	Independent driving from wheelchair	• Modified van with lift • Sensitized hand controls • Tie-downs			
Homemaking	Some assist with light meal preparation; total assist for all other homemaking	Adaptive devices as indicated			
Assist required	• Personal care: 6 hours per day • Home care: 4 hours per day		10*	17*	8–24*

*Hours per day.

Appendix 38-1	**Expected Functional Outcomes** *(continued)*

Level C7–C8

Functionally relevant muscles innervated: Latissimusdorsi; sternal pectoralis; triceps; pronator quadratus; extensor carpi ulnaris; flexor carpi radialis; flexor digitorum profundus and superficialis; extensor communis; pronator/flexor/extensor/abductor pollicis; lumbricals (partially innervated)

Movement possible: Elbow extension; ulnar/wrist extension; wrist flexion; finger flexion and extension; thumb flexion/extension/abduction

Patterns of weakness: Paralysis of trunk and lower extremities; limited grasp release and dexterity secondary to partial paralysis intrinsic muscles of the hand

FIM™/Assistance Data: Exp = expected FIM™ score; **Med** = NSCISC median; **IR** = NSCISC interquartile range

NSCISC Sample Size: FIM™ = 38; Assist = 35

	Expected Functional Outcomes	Equipment	FIM™/Assistance Data		
			Exp	Med	IR
Respiratory	Low endurance and vital capacity secondary to paralysis of intercostals; may require assist to clear secretions				
Bowel	Some to total assist	• Padded tub bench with commode cutout or shower-commode chair • Adaptive devices as needed	1–4	1	1–4
Bladder	Independent to some assist	Adaptive devices as indicated	2–6	3	1–6
Bed mobility	Independent to some assist	Full electric hospital bed or full to king standard bed			
Bed, wheelchair transfers	Level: Independent Uneven: Independent to some assist	With or without transfer board	3–7	4	2–6
Pressure relief, positioning	Independent	• Wheelchair pressure-relief cushion • Postural support devices as indicated • Pressure-relief mattress or overlay may be indicated			
Eating	Independent	Adaptive devices as indicated	6–7	6	5–7
Dressing	Independent upper extremities; independent to some assist lower extremities	Adaptive devices as indicated	4–7	6	4–7
Grooming	Independent	Adaptive devices as indicated	6–7	6	4–7
Bathing	Upper body: Independent Lower extremity: Some assist to independent	• Padded transfer tub bench or shower-commode chair • Handheld shower • Adaptive devices as needed	3–6	4	2–6
Wheelchair propulsion	Manual: Independent all indoor surfaces and level outdoor terrain; some assist with uneven terrain	Manual: Rigid or folding; lightweight or folding wheelchair with modified rims	6	6	6
Standing, ambulation	Standing: Independent to some assist Ambulation: Not indicated	Hydraulic or standard standing frame			

(continued)

Appendix 38-1 | Expected Functional Outcomes *(continued)*

Level C7–C8

	Expected Functional Outcomes	Equipment	FIM™/Assistance Data		
			Exp	Med	IR
Communication	Independent	Adaptive devices as indicated			
Transportation	Independent car if independent with transfer, wheelchair loading and unloading; independent driving modified van from captain's seat	• Modified vehicle • Transfer board			
Homemaking	Independent light meal preparation and homemaking; some to total assist for complex meal prep and heavy housecleaning	Adaptive devices as indicated			
Assist required	• Personal care: 6 hours per day • Home care: 2 hours per day		8*	12*	2–24*

*Hours per day.

Level T1–T9

Functionally relevant muscles innervated: Intrinsics of the hand including thumbs; internal and external intercostals; erector spinae; lumbricals; flexor/extensor/abductor pollicis
Movement possible: Upper extremities fully intact; limited upper trunk stability; endurance increased secondary to innervation of intercostals
Patterns of weakness: Lower trunk paralysis; total paralysis lower extremities

FIM™/Assistance Data: Exp = expected FIM™ score; **Med** = NSCISC median; **IR** = NSCISC interquartile range
NSCISC Sample Size: FIM™ = 144; Assist = 122

	Expected Functional Outcomes	Equipment	FIM™/Assistance Data		
			Exp	Med	IR
Respiratory	Compromised vital capacity and endurance				
Bowel	Independent	Elevated padded toilet seat or padded tub bench with commode cutout	6–7	6	4–6
Bladder	Independent		6	6	5–6
Bed mobility	Independent	Full to king standard bed			
Bed, wheelchair transfers	Independent	May or may not require transfer board	6–7	6	6–7
Pressure relief, positioning	Independent	• Wheelchair pressure-relief cushion • Postural support devices as indicated • Pressure-relief mattress or overlay may be indicated			
Eating	Independent		7	7	7
Dressing	Independent		7	7	7

Appendix 38-1   Expected Functional Outcomes *(continued)*

Level T1–T9

	Expected Functional Outcomes	Equipment	FIM™/Assistance Data		
			Exp	Med	IR
Grooming	Independent		7	7	7
Bathing	Independent	• Padded tub transfer bench or shower-commode chair • Handheld shower	6–7	6	5–7
Wheelchair propulsion	Independent	Manual rigid or folding lightweight wheelchair	6	6	6
Standing, ambulation	Standing: Independent Ambulation: Typically not functional	Standing frame			
Communication	Independent				
Transportation	Independent in car, including loading and unloading wheelchair	Hand controls			
Homemaking	Independent with complex meal prep and light housecleaning; total to some assist with heavy housekeeping				
Assist required	Homemaking: 3 hours per day		2*	3*	0–15*

*Hours per day.

Level T10–L1

Functionally relevant muscles innervated: Fully intact intercostals; external obliques; rectus abdominis
Movement possible: Good trunk stability
Patterns of weakness: Paralysis of lower extremities

FIM™/Assistance Data: Exp = expected FIM™ score; **Med**= NSCISC median; **IR** = NSCISC interquartile range
NSCISC Sample Size: FIM™ = 71; Assist = 57

	Expected Functional Outcomes	Equipment	FIM™/Assistance Data		
			Exp	Med	IR
Respiratory	Intact respiratory function				
Bowel	Independent	Padded standard or raised padded toilet seat	6–7	6	6
Bladder	Independent		6	6	6
Bed mobility	Independent	Full to king standard bed	7	7	6–7
Bed, wheelchair transfers	Independent				
Pressure relief, positioning	Independent	• Wheelchair pressure-relief cushion • Postural support devices as indicated • Pressure-relief mattress or overlay may be indicated			

(continued)

Appendix 38-1 Expected Functional Outcomes *(continued)*

Level T10–L1

	Expected Functional Outcomes	Equipment	FIM™/Assistance Data		
			Exp	Med	IR
Eating	Independent		7	7	7
Dressing	Independent		7	7	7
Grooming	Independent		7	7	7
Bathing	Independent	• Padded transfer tub bench • Handheld shower	6–7	6	6–7
Wheelchair propulsion	Independent all indoor and outdoor surfaces	Manual rigid or folding lightweight wheelchair	6	6	6
Standing, ambulation	Standing: Independent Ambulation: Functional, some assist to independent	• Standing frame • Forearm crutches or walker • Knee, ankle, foot orthosis (KAFO)			
Communication	Independent				
Transportation	Independent in car, including loading and unloading wheelchair	Hand controls			
Homemaking	Independent with complex meal prep and light housecleaning some assist with heavy; housekeeping				
Assist required	Homemaking: 2 hours per day		2*	2*	0–8*

*Hours per day.

Level L2–S5

Functionally relevant muscles innervated: Fully intact abdominals and all other trunk muscles; depending on level, some degree of hip flexors, extensors, abductors, adductors; knee flexors, extensors; ankle dorsiflexors, plantar flexors.
Movement possible: Good trunk stability; partial to full control lower extremities.
Patterns of weakness: Partial paralysis lower extremities, hips, knees, ankle, foot

FIM™/Assistance Data: Exp = expected FIM™ score; **Med** = NSCISC median; **IR** = NSCISC interquartile range
NSCISC Sample Size: FIM™ = 20; Assist = 16

	Expected Functional Outcomes	Equipment	FIM™/Assistance Data		
			Exp	Med	IR
Respiratory	Intact function				
Bowel	Independent	Padded toilet seat	6–7	6	6–7
Bladder	Independent		6	6	6–7
Bed mobility	Independent				
Bed/wheelchair transfers	Independent	Full to king standard bed	7	7	7
Pressure relief/positioning	Independent	• Wheelchair pressure-relief cushion • Postural support device as indicated			

Appendix 38-1   Expected Functional Outcomes *(continued)*

Level L2–S5

	Expected Functional Outcomes	Equipment	FIM™/Assistance Data		
			Exp	Med	IR
Eating	Independent		7	7	7
Dressing	Independent		7	7	7
Grooming	Independent		7	7	7
Bathing	Independent	• Padded tub bench • Handheld shower	7	7	6–7
Wheelchair propulsion	Independent on all indoor and outdoor surfaces	Manual rigid or folding lightweight wheelchair	6	6	6
Standing/ambulation	Standing: Independent Ambulation: Functional, independent to some assist	• Standing frame • Knee-ankle-foot orthosis or ankle-foot orthosis • Forearm crutches or cane as indicated			
Communication	Independent				
Transportation	Independent in car, including loading and unloading wheelchair	Hand controls			
Homemaking	Independent complex cooking and light housekeeping; some assist with heavy housekeeping				
Assist required	Homemaking: 0–1 hour per day		0–1*	0*	0–2*

*Hours per day.

References

Alverzo, J. P., Rosenberg, J. H., Sorensen, C. A., & Shultz DeLeon, S. (2009). Nursing care and education for patients with spinal cord injury. In S. A. Sisto, E. Druin, & M. Macht Sliwinski (Eds.), *Spinal cord injuries: Management and rehabilitation* (pp. 37–68). St. Louis: Mosby.

American Occupational Therapy Association. (2008). Occupational therapy practice framework: Domain and process (2nd ed.). *American Journal of Occupational Therapy, 62,* 625–700.

American Spinal Injury Association. (2011). *International standards for neurological classification of spinal injury*. Atlanta, GA: American Spinal Injury Association.

Anderson, K. D., Acuff, M. E., Arp, B. G., Backus, D., Chun, S., Fisher, K., Fjerstad, J. E., Graves, D. E., Greenwald, K., Groah, S. L., Harkema, S. J., Horton, J. A., Huang, M.-N., Jennings, M., Kelley, K. S., Kessler, S. M., Kirshblum, S., Koltenuk, S., Linke, M., Ljungberg, I., Nagy, J., Nicolini, L., Roach, M. J., Salles, S., Scelza, W. M., Read, M. S., Reeves, R. K., Scott, M. D., Tansey, K. E., Theis, J. L., Tolfo, Whitney, M., Williams, C. D., Winter, C. M., & Zanca, J. M. (2011). United States (US) multi-center study to assess the validity and reliability of the Spinal Cord Independence Measure (SCIM III) *Spinal Cord, 49,* 880–885.

Atkins, M. S. (1989). *A descriptive study: The occupational therapy pre-discharge home visit program for spinal cord injured adults* (Unpublished master's thesis). University of Southern California, Los Angeles, CA.

Atkins, M. S., Baumgarten, J. M., Yasuda, Y. L., Adkins, R., Waters, R. L., Leung, P., & Requejo, P. (2008). Mobile arm supports: evidence-based benefits and criteria for use. *Journal of Spinal Cord Medicine, 31,* 388–393.

Atkins, M. S., Clark, D., & Waters, R. (2010). Upper limb orthoses. In V. W. Lin (Ed.), *Spinal cord medicine: Principles and practice* (2nd ed., pp. 663–674). New York: Demos.

Baum, C. (2000). Occupation-based practice: Reinventing ourselves for the new millennium. *OT Practice, 1,* 12–15.

Block, P., Vanner, E. A., Keys, C. B., Rimmer, J. H., & Skeels, S. E. (2010). Project Shake-It-Up: Using health promotion, capacity building and a disability studies framework to increase self-efficacy. *Disability and Rehabilitation, 32,* 741–754.

Botte, M. J., Peace, W. J., & Pacelli, L. L. (2011). Complications of the musculoskeletal system following spinal cord injury. In J. E. Zigler, F. J. Eismont, S. R. Garfin, & A. R. Vaccaro (Eds.), *Spine trauma* (2nd ed.). Rosemont, IL: American Academy of Orthopaedic Surgeons.

Bryce, T. N., & Ragnarsson, K. T. (2000). Pain after spinal cord injury. *Physical Medicine & Rehabilitation Clinics of North America, 11,* 157–168.

Cardenas, D. D., Hoffman, J. M., Kirshblum, S., & McKinley, W. (2004). Etiology and incidence of rehospitalization after traumatic spinal cord injury: A multicenter analysis. *Archives of Physical Medicine and Rehabilitation, 85,* 1757–1763.

Carson, J. (2012). Telehealth opportunities in occupational therapy through the affordable care act. *American Journal of Occupational Therapy, 66,* 131–136.

Catz, A., Itzkovich, M., Tesio, L., Biering-Sorensen, F., Weeks, C., Laramee, M. T., Craven, B. C., Tonack, M., Hitzig, S. L., Glaser, E., Zeilig, G., Aito, S., Scivoletto, G., Mecci, M., Chadwick, R. J., El Masry, W. S., Osman, A., Glass, C. A., Silva, P., Soni, B. M., Gardner, B. P., Savic, G., Bergstrom, E. M., Bluvshtein, V., & Ronen, J. (2007). A multicenter international study of the Spinal Cord Independent Measure, Version III: Rasch psychometric validation. *Spinal Cord, 45,* 275–291

Clark, F. A., Jackson, J. M., Scott, M. D., Carlson, M. E., Atkins, M. S., Uhles-Tanaka, D., & Rubayi, S. (2006). Data-based models of how pressure ulcers develop in daily-living contexts of adults with spinal cord injury. *Archives of Physical Medicine & Rehabilitation, 87,* 1516–1525.

Consortium for Spinal Cord Medicine. (1997). *Acute management of autonomic dysreflexia: Adults with spinal cord injury presenting to health care facilities.* Washington, DC: Paralyzed Veterans of America.

Consortium for Spinal Cord Medicine. (1998). *Neurogenic bowel management in adults with spinal cord injury: Clinical practice guidelines.* Washington, DC: Paralyzed Veterans of America.

Consortium for Spinal Cord Medicine. (1999). *Outcome following traumatic spinal cord injury: Clinical practice guidelines for health care professionals.* Washington, DC: Paralyzed Veterans of America.

Consortium for Spinal Cord Medicine. (2005a). *Preservation of upper limb function following spinal cord injury: A clinical practice guidelines for health-care professionals.* Washington, DC: Paralyzed Veterans of America.

Consortium for Spinal Cord Medicine. (2005b). *Respiratory management following spinal cord injury: A clinical practice guideline for health-care professionals.* Washington, DC: Paralyzed Veterans of America.

Consortium for Spinal Cord Medicine. (2006). *Bladder management for adults with spinal cord injury: A clinical practice guideline for health-care professionals.* Washington, DC: Paralyzed Veterans of America.

Consortium for Spinal Cord Medicine. (2008). *Early acute management in adults with spinal cord injury: A clinical practice guideline for health-care professionals.* Washington, DC: Paralyzed Veterans of America.

Consortium for Spinal Cord Medicine. (2010). *Sexuality and reproductive health in adults with spinal cord injury.* Washington, DC: Paralyzed Veterans of America. www.pva.org

Curtin, M. (1999). An analysis of tetraplegic hand grips. *British Journal of Occupational Therapy, 62,* 444–450.

Dames, T. M., Jackson, G. L., Powers, B. J., Bosworth, H. B., Cheng, E., Anderson, E. J., Guihan, M., LaVela, S., Rajan, S., & Plue, L. (2009). Implementing evidence-based patient self-management programs in the Veterans Health Administration: Perspectives on delivery system design considerations. *Journal of General Internal Medicine, 25,* 68–71

Davidoff, G. N., Roth, E. J., & Richards, J. S. (1992). Cognitive deficits in spinal cord injury: Epidemiology and outcome. *Archives of Physical Medicine and Rehabilitation, 73,* 275–284.

Dijkers, M. Bryce, T., & Zanca, J. (2009). Prevalence of chronic pain after spinal cord injury: A systematic review. *Journal of Rehabilitation Research and Development.* 46:13–30

Donnelly, C., Eng, J. J., Hall, J., Alford, L., Giachino, R., Norton, K., & Kerr, D. S. (2004). Client-centered assessment and the identification of meaningful treatment goals for individuals with spinal cord injury. *Spinal Cord, 42,* 302–307.

Fattal, C. (2004). Motor capacities of upper limbs in tetraplegics: A new scale for the assessment of the results of functional surgery on upper limbs. *Spinal Cord, 42,* 80–90.

Fawcett, J. W., Curt, A., Steeves, J. D., Coleman, W. P., Tuszynski, M. H., Lammertse, D., Bartlett, P. F., Blight, A. R., Dietz, V., Ditunno, J., Dobkin, B. H., Havton, L. A., Ellaway, P. H., Fehlings, M. G., Privat, A., Grossman, R., Guest, J. D., Kleitman, N., Nakamura, M., Gaviria, M., & Short, D. (2007). Guidelines for the conduct of clinical trials for spinal cord injury as developed by the ICCP panel: Spontaneous recovery after spinal cord injury and statistical power needed for therapeutic clinical trials. *Spinal Cord, 45,* 190–205.

Fogelberg, D., Atkins, M., Blanche, E., Carlson, M., & Clark, F. (2009). Decisions and dilemmas in everyday life: Daily use by individuals with spinal cord injury and the impact on pressure ulcer risk. *Topics in Spinal Cord Injury Rehabilitation, 15,* 16–32

Forchheimer, M., & Tate, D. G. (2004). Enhancing community re-integration following spinal cord injury. *NeuroRehabilitation, 19,* 103–113.

Ford, J. R., & Duckworth, B. (1987). *Physical management for the quadriplegic patient* (2nd ed.). Philadelphia: Davis.

Garland, D. E. (1991). A clinical perspective on common forms of acquired heterotopic ossification. *Clinical Orthopaedics and Related Research, 242,* 169–176.

Gerhart, K. A., Bergstorm, E., Charlifue, S., Mentor, R. R., & Whiteneck, G. G. (1993). Long-term spinal cord injury: Functional changes over time. *Archives of Physical Medicine and Rehabilitation, 74,* 1030–1034.

Gersham, G. E., Labi, M. I., Dittmar, S. S., Hicks, J. T., Joyce, S. Z., & Phillips Stehlik, M. A. (1986). The Quadriplegia Index of Function

(QIF): Sensitivity and reliability demonstrated in a study of thirty quadriplegic patients. *Paraplegia, 24,* 38–44.

Hammell, K. W. (1995). *Spinal cord injury rehabilitation.* Suffolk, UK: Chapman & Hall.

Hammell, K. W. (2004). Exploring quality of life following high spinal cord injury: A review and critiques. *Spinal Cord, 42,* 491–502.

Hammell, K. W. (2007). Experience of rehabilitation following spinal cord injury: A meta-synthesis of qualitative findings. *Spinal Cord, 45,* 260–274.

Hill, J. (1986). *Spinal cord injury: A guide to functional outcomes in occupational therapy.* Rockville, MD: Aspen.

Hoffman, L. R., & Field-Fote, E. C. (2009). Upper extremity training for individuals with cervical spinal cord injury: Functional recovery and neuroplasticity. In E. C. Field-Fote (Ed.), *Spinal cord rehabilitation* (pp. 259–290). Philadelphia: F. A. Davis.

Jackson, J., Carlson, M., Rubayi, S., Scott, M. D., Atkins, M., Blanche, E., Saunders-Newton, C., Mielke, S., Wolfe, M. K., & Clark, F. (2010). Qualitative study of principles pertaining to lifestyle and pressure ulcer risk in adults with spinal cord injury. *Disability and Rehabilitation, 32,* 567–578.

Jaspers Focks-Feenstra, J. H., Snoek, G. J., Bongers-Janssen, H. M., & Nene, A. V. (2011). Long-term patient satisfaction after reconstructive upper extremity surgery to improve arm-hand function in tetraplegia. *Spinal Cord, 49,* 903–908.

Jebsen, R., Taylor, N., Trieschmann, R., Trotter, M., & Howard, L. (1969). An objective and standardized test of hand function. *Archives of Physical Medicine and Rehabilitation, 50,* 311–319.

Kapadia, N. M., Zivanovic, V., Furlan, J., Craven, B. C., McGillivray, C., & Popovic, M. R. (2011). Functional electric stimulation therapy for grasping in traumatic incomplete spinal cord injury: Randomized control trial. *Artificial Organs, 35,* 212–216.

Kendall, F. P., McCreary, E. K., Provance, P. G., Rodgers, M. M., & Romani, W. A. (2005). *Muscles: Testing and function, posture and pain* (5th ed.). Baltimore, MD: Lippincott Williams & Wilkins.

Kilgore, K. L., Hoyen, H. A., Bryden, A. M., Hart, R. L., Keith, M. W., & Peckham, H. (2008). An implanted upper-extremity neuroprosthesis using myoelectric control. *Journal of Hand Surgery, 33,* 539–550.

Kirshblum, S. C., Gulati, M., O'Conner, K. C., & Voorman, S. J. (1998). Bowel care practices in chronic spinal cord injury patients. *Archives of Physical Medicine and Rehabilitation, 79,* 20–23.

Krause, J. S., & Saunders, L. L. (2011). Health, secondary conditions, and life expectancy after spinal cord injury. *Physical Medicine and Rehabilitation, 92,* 1770–1775.

Lidal, I. B., Hjeltnes, N., Roislien, J., Stanghelle, J. K., & Biering-Sorensen, F. (2009). Employment of persons with spinal cord lesions injured more than 20 years ago. *Disability and Rehabilitation, 31,* 2174–2184.

Lorig, K. L. (2003). Self-management education, more than a nice extra. *Medical Care, 41,* 699–701.

Maddox, S. (2007). *Paralysis resource guide.* Short Hills, NJ: Christopher & Dana Reeve Foundation.

Magasi, S., Heinemann, A. W., & S. Wilson (2009). Psychological aspects of living with SCI: Emotional health, quality of life and participation. In E. C. Field-Fote (Ed.), *Spinal cord rehabilitation* (pp. 211–228). Philadelphia: F. A. Davis.

Makhsous, M., Priebe, M., Bankard, B. S., Rowles, D., Zeigler, M., Chen, D., & Lin, F. (2007). Measuring tissue perfusion during pressure relief maneuvers: Insights into preventing pressure ulcers. *Journal of Spinal Cord Medicine, 30,* 497–507

Mandel, D. R., Jackson, J. M., Zemke, R., Nelson, L., & Clark, F. A. (1999). *Lifestyle redesign: Implementing the Well Elderly Program.* Bethesda, MD: American Occupational Therapy Association.

Massagli, T. L., & Jaffe, K. M. (1990). Pediatric spinal cord injury: Treatment and outcome. *Pediatrician, 17,* 244–254.

Moberg, E. (1978). *The upper limb in tetraplegia.* Stuttgart: Thieme.

Mulroy, S. J., Thompson, L., Kemp, B., Hatchett, P. P., Newsam, C. J., Lupold, D. G., Haubert, L. L., Eberly, V., Ge, T. T., Azen, S. P.,

Winstein, C. J., & Gordon, J. (2011). Strengthening and optimal movements for painful shoulders (STOMPS) in chronic spinal cord injury: A randomized controlled trial. *Physical Therapy, 91,* 305–324.

National Spinal Cord Injury Statistical Center. (2010). *Annual report for the model spinal cord injury care systems.* Birmingham: University of Alabama.

National Spinal Cord Injury Statistical Center. (2012). *Spinal cord injury: Facts and figures at a glance.* Birmingham: University of Alabama.

Nobunaga, A. I., Go, B. K., & Karunas, R. B. (1999). Recent demographic and injury trends in people served by the Model Spinal Cord Injury Systems. *Archives of Physical Medicine and Rehabilitation, 80,* 1372–1382.

Penrod, L. E., Hedge, S. K., & Ditunno, J. F., Jr. (1990). Age effect on prognosis for functional recovery in acute traumatic central cord syndrome (CCS). *Archives of Physical Medicine and Rehabilitation, 71,* 963–968.

Post, M. W., & van Leeuwen, C. M. (2012). Psychosocial issues is spinal cord injury: A review. *Spinal Cord, 50,* 382–389.

Potter, P. J., Wolfe, D. L., Burkell, J. A., & Hayes, K. C. (2004). Challenges in educating individuals with SCI to reduce secondary conditions. *Topics in Spinal Cord Injury Rehabilitation, 10,* 30–40.

Radomski, M. V. (1998). Problem-solving deficits: Using a multidimensional definition to select a treatment approach. *Physical Disabilities Special Interest Section Quarterly, 21,* 1. Bethesda, MD: American Occupational Therapy Association.

Radomski, M. V. (2000). Self-efficacy: Improving occupational therapy outcomes by helping patients say "I can." *Physical Disabilities Special Interest Section Quarterly, 23,* 1–3. Bethesda, MD: American Occupational Therapy Association.

Radomski, M. V., Finkelstein, M., Hagel, S., Masemer, S., Theis, J., & Thompson, M. (2011). A pilot wellness and weight management program for individuals with spinal cord injury: Participants' goals and outcomes. *Topics in Spinal Cord Injury and Rehabilitation, 17,* 59–69

Rice, I., Cooper, R. A., Cooper, R., Kelleher, A., & Boyles, A. (2009). Sports and recreation for people with spinal cord injuries. In S. A. Sisto, E. Druin, & M. M. Sliwinski (Eds.), *Spinal cord injury: Management and rehabilitation* (pp. 455–477). St. Louis: Mosby

Scivoletto, G., Morganti, B., Ditunno, P., Ditunno, J. F., & Molinari, M. (2003). Effects on age spinal cord lesion patients' rehabilitation. *Spinal Cord, 41,* 457–464.

Siddall, P. J., Yezierski, R. P., & Loeser, J. D. (2000). Pain following spinal cord injury: Clinical features, prevalence and taxonomy. *IASP News-letter, 3,* 3–7.

Smith, Q. W., Frieden, L., Nelson, M. R., & Tilbor, A. G. (1996). Transition to adulthood for young people with spinal cord injury. In R. R. Benz & M. J. Mulcahey (Eds.), *The child with a spinal cord injury* (pp. 601–612). Rosemont, IL: American Academy of Orthopedic Surgeons.

Snoek, G. J., Ijzerman, M. J., Hermens, H. J., Maxwell, D., & Biering-Sorensen, F. (2004). Survey of the needs of patients with spinal cord injury: Impact and priority for improvement in hand function in tetraplegics. *Spinal Cord, 42,* 526–532.

Sollerman, C., & Ejeskar, A. (1995). Sollerman Hand Function Test: A standardized method and its use in tetraplegia patients. *Scandinavian Journal of Plastic Reconstructive Surgery and Hand Surgery, 29,* 167–176.

van den Berg, M. E. L., Castellote, J. M., Mahillo-Fernandez, I., & de Pedro-Cuesta, J. (2010). Incidence of spinal cord injury worldwide: A systematic review. *Neuroepidemiology, 34,* 184–192.

van Kuijk, A. A., Geurts A. C., & van Kuppevelt, H. J. (2002). Neurologic heterotropic ossification in spinal cord injury. *Spinal Cord, 40,* 313–326.

van Tuijl, J. H., Janssen-Potten, Y. J. M., & Seelen, H. A. M. (2002). Evaluation of upper extremity motor function tests in tetraplegics. *Spinal Cord, 40,* 51–64.

Waters, R. L., Sie, I. H., Gellman, H., & Tognella, M. (1996). Functional hand surgery following tetraplegia. *Archives of Physical Medicine and Rehabilitation, 77,* 86–94.

Whiteneck, G. G., Gassaway, J., Dijkers, M. P., Lammertse, D. P., Hammond, F., Heinemann, A. W., Backus, D., Charlifue, S., Ballard, P. H., & Zanca, J. M. (2011). Impatient and postdischarge rehabilitation services provided in the first year after spinal cord injury: Findings from the SCIRehab study. *Archives of Physical Medicine and Rehabilitation, 92,* 361–368.

Whiteneck, G. G., Lammertse, D. P., Manley, S., & Mentor, R. (Eds.). (1989). *The management of high quadriplegia.* New York: Demos.

Widerstrom-Noga, E. (2009). Pain after spinal cord injury: Etiology and management. In E. C. Field-Fote (Ed.), *Spinal cord injury rehabilitation* (pp. 427–444). Philadelphia: Davis.

Wilkins, J. (2011). *Reentry programs for out-of-school youth with disabilities: Characteristics of reentry programs.* Clemson, SC: National Dropout Prevention Center for Students with Disabilities, Clemson University.

Wilson, D. J., McKenzie, M. W., Barber, L. M., & Watson, K. L. (1984). *Spinal cord injury: A treatment guide for occupational therapists* (2nd ed.). Thorofare, NJ: Slack.

Wolfe, D. L., Potter, P. J., & Sequeira, K. A. J. (2004). Overcoming challenges: The role of rehabilitation in educating individuals with SCI to reduce secondary conditions. *Topics in Spinal Cord Injury Rehabilitation, 10,* 41–50.

World Health Organization. (2001). *International classification of functioning, disability and health.* Geneva, Switzerland: World Health Organization.

Wuolle, K. S., Van Doren, C. L., Thrope, G. B., Keith, M. W., & Peckham, P. H. (1994). Development of a quantitative hand grasp and release test for people with tetraplegia using a hand neuroprosthesis. *Journal of Hand Surgery, 9,* 209–218.

Yarkony, G. M., Roth, E. J., Heinemann, A. W., & Lovell, L. L. (1988). Spinal cord injury rehabilitation outcomes: The impact of age. *Journal of Clinical Epidemiology, 41,* 173–177.

Zigler, J. E., Resnik, C., Carroll, L., Ramirez, A., Atkins, M. S., & Thompson, L. (2011). In J. E. Zigler, F. J. Eismont, S. R. Garfin, & A. R. Vaccaro (Eds.), *Spine trauma* (2nd ed., pp. 651–699). Rosemont, IL: American Academy of Orthopaedic Surgeons.

Suggested Reading

American Spinal Injury Association. (2011). *International standards for neurological classification of spinal injury patients* (Rev. ed.). Chicago: American Spinal Injury Association.

Ford, J. R., & Duckworth, B. (1987). *Physical management for the quadriplegic patient* (2nd ed.). Philadelphia: Davis. (Out of print but can be found in libraries and can be purchased used, on the Internet)

Hammell, K. W. (1995). *Spinal cord injury rehabilitation.* London: Chapman & Hall.

Hill, J. (1986). *Spinal cord injury: A guide to functional outcomes in occupational therapy.* Rockville, MD: Aspen. (Out of print but can found in libraries and can be purchased used on the Internet)

Magasi, S., Heinemann, A. W., & S. Wilson (2009). Psychological aspects of living with SCI: Emotional health, quality of life and participation. In E. Field-Fote (Ed.), *Spinal cord rehabilitation.* Philadelphia: F. A. Davis.

Sisto, S. A., Druin, E., & Sliwinski, M. M. (Eds) (2009). *Spinal cord injury: Management and rehabilitation.* St. Louis: Mosby

Whiteneck, G., Charlifue, S., Gerhart, K., Overholser, J., & Richardson, G. Quantifying handicap: a new measure of long-term rehabilitation outcomes. (1992). *Archives of Physical Medicine and Rehabilitation, 73,* 519–526.

Personal Accounts of People Living with SCI

Hockenberry, J. (1995). *Moving violations: War zones, wheelchairs, and declarations of independence.* New York: New York. Hyperion, ISBN 9780786881623. This author's favorite book about the experience of living with SCI: Funny, well written, and educational.

Reeve, C. (1998). *Still me.* New York: Ballantine. Christopher Reeve's moving account.

Acknowledgement

I thank the patients and staff at Rancho Los Amigos National Rehabilitation Center, who have inspired and taught me so much over the years. I also thank my parents, Miriam and Zeev Schmidt of Hod-Hasharon, Israel, who taught me the love and joy of learning and engaging in meaningful occupations. Last, I thank my husband Richard Atkins and the photographer, the late Paul Weinreich.

Rheumatoid Arthritis, Osteoarthritis, and Fibromyalgia

Alison Hammond

Learning Objectives

After studying this chapter, the reader will be able to do the following:

1. Describe key features of rheumatoid arthritis, osteoarthritis, and fibromyalgia.
2. Identify clinical sequelae that interfere with meeting occupational performance goals.
3. Select assessments to optimize occupational performance for clients with rheumatoid arthritis, osteoarthritis, and fibromyalgia.
4. Describe interventions to enable clients to continue, resume, and/or adopt new occupational performance goals.
5. Describe methods of helping clients understand and adopt self-management methods during occupational performance.

Many people with rheumatoid arthritis (RA), osteoarthritis (OA), and fibromyalgia (FM) find performing everyday activities painful, tiring, and frustrating, affecting their well-being. Occupational therapy aims to

- improve clients' ability to perform daily occupations (i.e., activities and valued life roles in work, the home, in leisure, and socially)
- reduce pain and fatigue
- prevent losses of function
- improve or maintain psychological status
- help people self-manage their condition and successfully adapt to disruptions in lifestyle
- achieve occupational balance.

Those with participation restrictions have poorer psychological outcomes, which is linked with poorer physical outcomes. Maintaining or increasing participation is the goal of therapy (American Occupational Therapy Association [AOTA], 2008). Treatment enables behavioral change by using self-management approaches such as ergonomics (joint protection techniques), fatigue management, orthoses (if applicable), stress management, and increasing physical activity. Occupational therapists see clients with RA, OA, or FM mainly as outpatients or community patients.

RHEUMATOID ARTHRITIS

RA is an autoimmune, chronic inflammatory disease affecting joints. Symptoms are symmetrical, polyarticular pain and swelling; early morning stiffness; malaise; and fatigue. It also affects the eyes, skin, lungs, heart, gastrointestinal system, kidneys, nervous system, and blood. There is no cure, but earlier diagnosis and start of medication help prevent or slow effects.

RA affects about 1.5 million people in the United States (Helmick et al., 2008). Prevalence is 0.5%–1.0%. Peak onset is at age 40–70 years. Some 60% are of working age when diagnosed (Symmons et al., 2002). Usually, onset is slow, with hands and feet affected first. Onset is rapid for 20%: waking up one morning with multiple painful, stiff and swollen joints, and they may be admitted via the Emergency Department.

Etiology and Pathophysiology

Genetic, hormonal, environmental, and lifestyle factors contribute to developing RA. Joint damage can occur within months of symptom onset. Changes include the following:

- Synovitis, i.e., thickening of the synovial membrane with increased synovial fluid (swelling). The pressure resulting stretches nociceptors in surrounding tissues, causing pain.

- Protein-degrading enzymes released from inflammatory cells. Inflammatory tissue (pannus) invades bone and cartilage at the joint margins. Chondral and subchondral erosions develop.
- Continued, prolonged joint swelling stretches and weakens ligaments and capsules, disrupting joint stability.
- Muscle mass is lost (cachexia) as inflammatory processes affect muscles and the metabolism.
- Inflammatory proteins (e.g., tumor necrosing factor alpha) are released, causing marked fatigue.
- Abnormal movement occurs in joints with weakened ligaments and disrupted structures. Joint deformity may occur.

Joint Involvement and Natural History

The upper limb joints affected are the wrists (85% of people with RA), metacarpophalangeal (MCP) joints (80%), elbows (70%), proximal interphalangeal (PIP) joints (65%), and shoulders (60%). In the lower limb, knees (80%), ankles (70%), metatarsophalangeal (MTP) joints (70%), and hips (30%) are affected. Additionally, the cervical spine (35%) and temporomandibular joint (25%) can be affected (Arthur & Hill, 2006).

The natural history of RA varies considerably. Three disease courses have been identified:

1. Monocyclic: About 20% have one episode ending within 2–5 years of initial diagnosis and not reoccurring. Early diagnosis and/or aggressive treatment with disease-modifying antirheumatic drugs (DMARDs) can help achieve this.
2. Polycyclic: About 75% experience fluctuating disease activity over the course of the condition. RA can last many years.
3. Progressive: In 5% RA continues to rapidly increase in severity and is unremitting (Centers for Disease Control and Prevention [CDC], 2012).

Management of Rheumatoid Arthritis

Medical management aims to suppress inflammation rapidly to prevent or limit joint damage, thereby limiting pain and fatigue. The earlier the person starts DMARDs, the better the outcome. Methotrexate is the drug of choice. Combination therapy (e.g., methotrexate, and/or leflunomide, sulphasalazine, or hydroxychloroquine) is recommended in moderate to severe disease (Singh et al., 2012) and has better outcomes than monotherapy, with no difference in drug tolerability or toxicity (National Institute for Health and Clinical Excellence [NICE], 2009). If DMARDs are ineffective, or there are poor prognostic indicators, biologic drugs are considered (e.g., etanercept, infliximab, or adalimumab) (Singh et al., 2012). In the last

5 years, increasingly early, aggressive use of combination DMARD therapy and biologics have improved outcomes of those newly diagnosed.

Multidisciplinary team (MDT) management, self-management, and condition education are essential. Ergonomic education, exercise, and fatigue management are key components. From an early stage, some 60% have hand and activities of daily living (ADL) problems, and 28%–40% stop work within 5 years of diagnosis (NICE, 2009). Once unemployed, they are unlikely to return to work (Verstappen et al., 2004). This suggests that two-thirds could benefit from OT for hand and activities of daily living (ADL) difficulties, and at least a third could benefit from work rehabilitation (NICE, 2009). Clinical guidelines for the management of RA (including nonpharmacological management) have been produced in Europe (Combe et al., 2007) and the United Kingdom (NICE, 2009).

OSTEOARTHRITIS

OA is the most common form of arthritis and one of the leading causes of pain and disability worldwide. OA is a clinical syndrome of joint pain linked with degenerative joint changes. OA affects 27 million adults in the United States (CDC, 2012). Symptoms are joint pain, initially on activity, which reduces with rest. Over time, pain becomes persistent and disturbs sleep. Pain arises from stretching of nociceptors in the joint capsule caused by focal synovitis, from increased vascular pressure in subchondral bone, and from spasm of surrounding muscle. Stiffness occurs after sleep or prolonged inactivity (called the gel phenomenon). This usually lasts 5–30 minutes and reduces with movement. There is no cure.

Etiology and Pathophysiology

There are multiple risk factors:

- Genetic (heritability accounts for 40%–60% of hand, knee, and hip OA)
- Constitutional factors (more common in women, with age, and with higher body weight)
- Biomechanical factors (e.g., joint injury, greater occupational or leisure use of a joint, reduced muscle strength, joint laxity, or misalignment)

Any synovial joint can develop OA, but structural changes do not always cause symptoms. OA is a metabolically active, dynamic process involving all joint tissues (cartilage, bone, synovium, capsule, ligaments, and muscle). Pathophysiological changes include fibrillation, loss of articular cartilage, and remodelling of adjacent bone with new bone formation (osteophytes). Focal synovial membrane inflammation can occur because of irritation from osteophytes and other joint changes. These changes suggest OA is a repair process, which

is initially effective, resulting in a structurally altered but symptom-free joint. However, continued damage or ineffective repair means symptomatic OA results (NICE, 2008).

Joint Involvement and Natural History

The prevalence of symptomatic OA is:

- hand OA: 8% of people older than 60 years of age
- knee OA: 12% of people older than 60 years of age and 16% older than 45 years of age
- hip OA: 4.4% of people older than 55 years of age (CDC, 2012)

OA may affect one joint or be multifocal. It usually develops gradually. It is often accepted as part of getting older and as inevitably getting worse. However, different types of OA have different prognoses. People with interphalangeal (IP) joint OA (Heberden's and Bouchard's nodes) no longer have symptoms after a few years, although joint changes remain that can affect function. Thumb base OA frequently continues causing pain and disability. After 5 years of knee OA, about a third have improved, a third are the same, and a third have gotten worse. Why this is so is unclear, although obesity may be an important factor in worsening disease. Hip OA tends to have the worst outcome, with a significant number needing hip replacements after 1–5 years (NICE, 2008).

Management of Osteoarthritis

Core interventions are self-management and condition education, including local muscle strengthening exercise and aerobic exercise to improve fitness, weight-loss advice (if necessary), and ergonomics education. Acetaminophen and topical nonsteroidal anti-inflammatory drugs (NSAIDs, e.g., ibuprofen gel) are recommended for pain relief. If necessary, oral NSAIDs may be prescribed. Capsaicin cream or intra-articular injections may be used if problems continue (NICE, 2008).

Amongst those seeking medical care, 82% reported difficulties with ADL (74% with hand OA and 83% with knee and multifocal OA). Problems include shopping (57% of participants), housework (43%), and dressing (21%) compared to 12%, 21%, and 13%, respectively, of age-matched controls (Fautrel et al., 2005). One in five with OA have to give up work or retire early because of their condition, and four out of five are in constant pain (Arthritis Care, 2004). This suggests that many could benefit from OT. Clinical guidelines for the MDT management of OA have been produced in the United States (Hochberg et al., 2012) and of knee OA (Jordan et al., 2003), hip OA (Zhang et al., 2005), and hand OA (Zhang, Doherty, & Leeb, 2007) in Europe (NICE, 2008).

FIBROMYALGIA

FM is neurogenic in origin and considered a disorder of the stress system following prolonged physical and/or mental overburdening. It is part of a spectrum of such disorders, including chronic fatigue syndrome. People experience chronic widespread pain, sleep disturbance, fatigue, and psychological distress. Other symptoms can include morning stiffness; tingling or numbness in hands and feet; headaches, including migraines; irritable bowel syndrome; and problems with thinking and memory (sometimes called "fibro fog"). It affects about 5 million adults in the United States. Prevalence is 2%–5%, and 80% are women (Arnold, Clauw, & McCarberg, 2011; CDC, 2012). FM seems to be underdiagnosed in men. Peak age of onset is 40–55 years, but it can occur at any age.

The American College of Rheumatology diagnostic criteria are pain lasting more than 3 months and of unknown origin, with a widespread pain index score of >9 out of 19 possible pain locations and symptom severity score of >9 out of 13 (including fatigue, cognitive, and somatic symptoms) (Wolfe et al., 2010). There can be long delays to diagnosis (average 5 years), resulting in poor management. Some health care professionals still do not consider FM to be a "real" condition, which causes distress and confusion to clients (Ablin et al., 2011).

Etiology and Pathophysiology

The cause of FM is likely to be multifactorial. Triggers include early life stressful events, physical trauma, catastrophic events, infections, and peripheral joint conditions (e.g., RA or OA). Predisposing factors may include a tendency to overexert physically and/or mentally. There can be familial associations, indicating that hereditary and social factors also play a role. Physical or psychological stresses can disrupt the hypothalamic-pituitary-adrenal pathway (i.e., the stress response mechanism in the brain) altering neuroendocrine functions. Functional magnetic resonance imaging shows FM is also associated with abnormal pain processing in the central nervous system. There is central sensitization of pain perception, with allodynia and hyperalgaesia, resulting in altered levels of neurotransmitters in pain pathways including increased substance P (increasing pain perception), reduced endorphins (increasing pain perception and reducing mood), and reduced serotonin (reducing sleep, mood, and cognition and altering circadian rhythms).

If C-size peripheral nerve fibers are repeatedly exposed to painful stimuli, there is progressively greater stimulation in the dorsal horn receptors in the spinal cord. This is known as "wind up" (pain is increasingly perceived at higher intensity over time). Substance P released in the dorsal horn cells can diffuse to synaptic connections in nearby myotomes, thus "spreading" pain perception to other uninjured sites. Pain wind up helps explain why some people with RA and OA go on to develop secondary FM. Appropriate use of pain medication is therefore important. Negative thoughts (fears, anxiety, depression, and poor self-efficacy) can also increase pain perception (Ablin et al., 2011).

Natural History

Community-based studies suggest that symptoms are relatively stable and quality of life improves as people with FM learn to cope with their condition. However, longitudinal studies of those referred to secondary care [rehabilitation] indicate that symptoms progress over a long period, remission is rare, and many are high users of health care services (Sallinen et al., 2009) (see Research Note 39-1).

Management of Fibromyalgia

Providing a diagnosis as soon as possible with a clear explanation about FM effects, the importance of self-management, and taking the person seriously are central to successful management. Three drugs are licensed for use in FM: pregabalin reduces the release of noradrenalin and substance P, improving pain, sleep, and fatigue; and milnacipran and duloxetine are dual reuptake inhibitors of serotonin and norepinephrine, improving pain, physical function, and fatigue. The side effects are generally mild. Tramadol also improves pain and physical function and is well tolerated.

Team management should provide multimodal therapy, because this is more effective than single therapies, and should include medication; exercise (moderate-intensity aerobic exercise including large body movements at least two or three times a week for at least 6 weeks; this can be water or land based, e.g., walking, Tai Chi); progressive strength training; cognitive-behavioral therapy (CBT); self-management education using CBT approaches such as stress, pain, and fatigue (sleep and pacing) management; relaxation; and ergonomics (Glombiewski et al., 2010; Hauser et al., 2009).

In a national community-based survey, 90% of women with FM reported difficulties in heavy household tasks and strenuous activities; 60% in light household tasks, carrying, climbing stairs, and walking over half a mile; and 25% in self-care (Jones et al., 2008). Work disability rates vary between 23% and 66% (Henriksson, Liedberg, & Gerdle, 2005). This suggests that many with FM can benefit from OT. Guidelines for the MDT management of FM have been produced by EULAR (Carville et al., 2007).

HAND INVOLVEMENT IN RHEUMATOID ARTHRITIS, OSTEOARTHRITIS, AND FIBROMYALGIA

Hand function is commonly affected in RA, OA, and FM. Therefore, understanding how the hands are affected helps appreciate the rationale behind interventions

Research Note 39-1

Sallinen, M., Kukkurainen, M. L., Peltokallio, L., & Mikkelsson, M. (2009). Women's narratives on experience of work ability and functioning in fibromyalgia. *Musculoskeletal Care, 8,* 18–26.

Abstract

Little is known about the long-term effects of fibromyalgia (FM) in everyday life or on work ability. A narrative interview study explored the experiences of work ability and functioning of 20 women with a long history of FM. Four types of experience were identified: confusion, coping with fluctuating symptoms, being "in between," and being over the edge of exhaustion. Severe pain and fatigue symptoms, combined with a demanding life situation and ageing, led to substantial decreases in work ability and functioning. Vocational rehabilitation or adjustments to work tasks were rarely seen or started too late to be effective. Exploring the women's life stories revealed perceived causes and consequences of FM related to work ability and disability. Such insights can be used in developing effective interventions to support work ability and avoid premature retirement in people with FM.

Implications for Practice

- Understanding the impact of FM from the client's perspective is essential. Qualitative studies provide valuable insights into how symptoms affect occupational performance. They help in understanding the barriers people may face from health care and social security systems in getting support and the possible negative attitudes of employers.
- Loss of work can lead to depression and anxiety in FM, making symptoms worse.
- In the occupational therapy process, the impact of FM on work must be assessed, and vocational rehabilitation must be provided. Ergonomic and fatigue management education are essential.
- Once unemployed, people with FM see a return to work as unrealistic. Early vocational rehabilitation to prevent work disability is essential.

used, such as ergonomics, exercise, and orthoses, and in explaining these to clients.

The Hand and Rheumatoid Arthritis

In women with early RA (<2 years), average losses are 20° of wrist extension, 30° wrist flexion, 15° MCP flexion, and 60% of normal power and pinch grip strength (Hammond et al., 2000). A third develop hand deformities (Eberhardt et al., 1990). There have been no recent studies of hand deformity development. The effect of earlier aggressive DMARD therapy may mean these losses now occur less. Deformities develop because of a combination of persistent synovitis, disrupted joint structures that alter joint mechanics, and both normal and abnormal forces over joints that arise from normal hand use (Adams et al., 2008). For example, power grip requires MCP ulnar deviation, especially in the fourth and fifth fingers, promoting ulnar deviation at weakened MCP joints. During lifting, external pressures in a volar or longitudinal direction increase strain on weakened wrist ligaments. Strong pinch grips increase intrinsic muscle pull, promoting imbalance at the IP joints (see Fig. 39-1).

Wrist Joint Changes

The ulnar side of the wrist is an early inflammation site. The triangular fibrocartilage is disrupted, allowing the proximal carpal row to rotate ulnarward. The distal row compensates by sliding radially, resulting in a gradually radially deviating wrist. Persistent synovitis promotes laxity of the wrist ligaments. Radioulnar ligament laxity allows rotation of the radius and ulna, with the ulnar styloid becoming more prominent. Extensor carpi ulnaris then displaces volarly, passing beneath the wrist joint axis, exerting a flexor pull. This, combined with wrist ligament laxity, and the natural volar incline of the distal radius, increases risk of wrist volar subluxation. Radial deviation at the wrist disrupts biomechanics of the extensor and flexor tendons, causing these to exert an ulnar pull at the MCP joints.

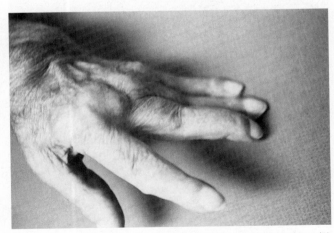

Figure 39-1 The hand and rheumatoid arthritis: synovitis at the wrist, metacarpophalangeal (MCP) and interphalangeal (IP) joints; swan-neck deformity in the third, fourth, and fifth fingers.

Metacarpophalangeal Joint Changes

Persistent synovitis weakens MCP collateral ligaments, volar plates, and dorsal hoods, leading to joint instability. The finger extensors can slip volarly and ulnarly, increasingly acting as weak flexors. Normal MCP joint features further contribute to ulnar deviation once joint structure is disrupted. These include (1) the flexor tendons normally approach the index and middle fingers from an ulnar direction exerting a significant ulnar torque, (2) the metacarpal head anatomically predisposes to tendons slipping ulnarward, and (3) the ulnar interossei exert a stronger pull than the radial ones.

Interphalangeal Joint Changes

Persistent synovitis can also disrupt positioning of the extensor tendon central slip and lateral bands at the PIP joints, allowing a Boutonniere deformity to develop. MCP joint inflammation can also cause protective spasms in the interossei, causing MCP flexion during finger extension (the intrinsic plus position), which further contributes to Boutonniere and swan-neck deformity development. Similar changes can result in Z deformity of the thumb.

The Hand and Osteoarthritis

The repair process in hand OA can lead to osteophyte formation at joint margins and focal synovitis in affected joints. Hand OA most commonly affects the DIP joints and carpometacarpal (CMC) joint. Bony enlargement and persistent synovitis can cause joint ligament laxity. Combined with forces exerted on the hands during daily use, deformities can result. At the PIP joints, bony enlargements are known as Bouchard's nodes, and at the

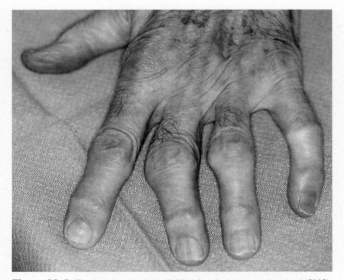

Figure 39-2 The hand and osteoarthritis: showing carpometacarpal (CMC); Bouchard's nodes (proximal interphalangeal [PIP] joint) and Heberden's nodes (distal interphalangeal [DIP] joint).

distal interphalangeal (DIP) joints, they are known as Heberden's nodes (Fig. 39-2). Mallet finger deformity results at the DIP joint if the distal extensor digitorum communis tendon attachment is disrupted by bony enlargement. The classic thumb deformity of squaring at the CMC joint, with Z deformity of the thumb, results from CMC joint adduction, MCP joint hyperextension, and IP joint flexion. Muscle wasting is noticeable in the thenar eminence, and finger, thumb, and wrist movement reduces (Bland, Melvin, & Hasson, 2000). People with combined finger and CMC OA have worse function. In women with hand OA, grip strength is only 57% of normal (Kjeken et al., 2005).

The Hand in Fibromyalgia

Hand function problems can be common in FM. They are due to hand pain, muscle weakness, and stiffness, resulting in poor grip. In women with moderate FM, hand grip strength was 19.3 kg of grip force, and in women with severe FM, hand grip strength was 16.9 kg compared to healthy women (29.5 kg) (Aparicio et al., 2011). There are no synovial or bony changes occurring in FM, and deformities do not develop.

ASSESSMENT AND EVALUATION

Assessment identifies clients' treatment priorities, their degree of motivation to use self-management approaches, and how their condition affects them. Treatment effectiveness can be evaluated if standardized, reliable, valid measures are used.

Initial Interview

Obtain information about the client's medical history and current medication from his or her medical records. For new clients, start with a brief explanation of OT because many, particularly in an early disease stage, may not be aware of the services occupational therapists provide. Explain that the initial assessment aims to identify key goals for therapy based on his or her needs. The interview includes

- a relevant past medical history, including comorbidities
- current medication information. For RA, knowing how long the person has been taking his or her DMARD or biologic drugs is helpful because, if started recently, functional gains may be expected. Ask about pain medication, when and how regularly, and note the client's attitude toward taking it.
- social history: whether they live alone or with others; type of house

The initial interview also focuses on occupational performance: ADL (personal and instrumental); rest and sleep; work (paid or volunteer); education (formal or informal); leisure, social, and community activities

(AOTA, 2008). For example, the Canadian Occupational Performance Measure (COPM) is a semistructured interview that focuses on activity limitations and participation. It takes 20–40 minutes to complete (Law et al., 2005). At the end, the person identifies the five most important problems he or she is experiencing in self-care, work, or leisure and rates each for importance, performance, and satisfaction with performance.

As problems are reported, explore why they are occurring: Is it due to pain? Fatigue? Stiffness? Physical limitations (e.g., in movement, strength, endurance)? Environmental factors (e.g., barriers, lack of equipment)? Psychological factors such as poor concentration, low mood, or lack of confidence (self-efficacy)? Performing specific activities because of fears of increasing pain and/or fatigue? Or a lack of information about alternatives?

Ask how clients spend a typical weekday and a typical weekend day. How much time do they spend in activity and in rest? Do they take regular rest breaks or keep pushing themselves even though fatigued? Have leisure activities become a rarity? How are they coping with competing demands of work and home life? What are they satisfied and dissatisfied about in their daily lives? How confident are they about managing difficulties they are experiencing? How much do they understand about why they are experiencing problems, about their condition, and what they could do themselves to make a difference? During the interview, gauge their mood, observe their body language, and listen carefully to their intonation and choice of words. This will help judge how ready and willing the person is to learn about self-management approaches, find solutions, and make changes.

Objective and subjective assessments are selected according to priority issues identified. Subjective assessments include patient-reported outcome measures. Interview may be more appropriate for some issues (e.g., intimate relations). An extensive review of rheumatology measures for body functions, activity limitations, participation, and personal factors was published by the ACR (2011). Some measures are described below and in Assessment Table 39-1.

Body Functions and Activity Limitations

Using self-reported questionnaires saves time and facilitates comprehensive evaluation.

The Evaluation of Daily Activity Questionnaire

The Evaluation of Daily Activity Questionnaire (EDAQ) is a detailed assessment (Nordenskiold, Grimby, & Dahlin-Ivanoff, 1998) now translated into English, updated with input from people with RA, OA, and FM, psychometrically tested in RA (Hammond et al., 2011, 2012) and being tested in OA, FM, and five other musculoskeletal conditions. Explain that the EDAQ helps clients identify their

own problems and priorities, enabling collaboratively finding solutions. The client completes it in his or her own time at home. There are three sections to this evaluation: body functions, activity limitations, and use of assistive devices.

Observation of ADL is more appropriate with those unable to self-report activity limitations because of severe comorbid cognitive problems and those post surgery as changing circumstances mean the client may not know his limitations. Interview is often more appropriate for those with low mood.

Activity Diaries

A diary of how the client spends a typical weekday and a typical weekend day, with each day divided into half-hour periods, helps identify occupational balance. Several designs exist. For example, the person can write his main activity each half hour, indicate on a scale of 0–10 the level of pain and fatigue experienced, and whether he took a rest.

Other Activity Limitation Patient-Reported Outcome Measures

- The Arthritis Impact Measurement Scale 2 (Meenan et al., 1992) is useful as an outcome measure, although lacking detail for treatment planning (10–20 minutes).
- The Health Assessment Questionnaire (HAQ) (Pincus et al., 1983). Scores are worsened if assistive devices are used, making it unsuitable as an outcome measure in OT. However, it is widely used in rheumatology clinics and useful for screening for OT (5 minutes).
- The Fibromyalgia Impact Questionnaire Revised (Bennett et al., 2009) specifically targets the issues affected in FM (5–10 minutes).

Mobility and Hand and Upper Limb Function

Overall movement can be assessed, if necessary, using the gait arms legs spine (GALS), a reliable, valid musculoskeletal screening examination (Plant et al., 1993) that takes 5–10 minutes to administer. There is a video posted online (http://www.youtube.com/watch?v=9jTZ03CbZm0) that shows the exam being conducted.

Hand and Upper Limb Assessment. In RA, a tender and swollen joint count can be conducted for hand splint assessment or to monitor progress over time. An online video (http://www.youtube.com/watch?v=RnvsbD6NKoc) shows this assessment performed as part of the Disease Activity Score 28 (Prevoo et al., 1995). Swelling in any condition can also be assessed using volumetry. In RA and OA, recording hand appearance, e.g., presence of joint swelling, pain, and deformity, on a hand chart is particularly useful, as is digital photography. Range of movement and appearance can be observed using the upper limb part of the GALS or using standard goniometric methods.

Assessment Table 39-1 — Summary of Assessments of Occupational Performance Related to Practice for Rheumatoid Arthritis, Osteoarthritis, or Fibromyalgia

Instrument and Reference	Description	Time to Administer	Validity	Reliability	Sensitivity	Strengths and Weaknesses
Evaluation of Daily Activity Questionnaire (EDAQ) (Hammond et al., 2011; 2012; Nordenskiöld, Grimby, & Dahlin-Ivanoff, 1998)	Self-assessment of daily activity ability Ordinal (4-point) scale: 138 items in 14 domains; scores range from 0 to 24 or 56 depending on number of domain items	30–60 minutes	Correlations with HAQ r_s = 0.72–0.89; SF36 Physical function = −0.57 to −0.86	Internal consistency r_s = 0.89–0.97 Test-retest r_s = 0.54–0.87	Minimal detectable difference = 1.60–4.61	Strengths: Patient generated; very detailed; free Weaknesses: Length not acceptable to all
Workplace Activity Limitations Scale (WALS) (Gignac, 2005) http://www.acreu.ca/research/measures.html	Self-assessment of ability at work Ordinal (4-point) scale: scores range from 0 to 48; 12 items	5 minutes	Correlations with other work measures: RA Work Instability Scale, r = 0.77; Work Limitations Questionnaire, r = 0.61	Internal consistency determined by inter-item correlation coefficient = 0.81–0.86 Test-retest reliability not established Interrater reliability not established	Standardized Response Mean = −0.79–0.50	Strengths: Data have been collected in rheumatoid arthritis (RA) and osteoarthritis (OA) to date; free Weaknesses: Items based on literature review and did not include patients in scale development; psychometrics incomplete; not yet used as an end point in clinical trials
Michigan Hand Outcomes Questionnaire (Chung et al., 1998; Waljee et al., 2010) http://sitemaker.umich.edu/mhq	Self-assessment of hand function, appearance, pain and satisfaction Ordinal (5-point Likert) scale: 37 items in six subscales (overall hand function, activities of daily living (ADL), pain, work, aesthetics, and satisfaction with hand function. Scores converted to a 0 (worst) to 100 (best) scale.	30 minutes	In RA: correlations with Arthritis Impact Measurement Scales 2 (AIMS2) subscales r = 0.2–0.77, with highest for function, ADL, work, pain and AIMS2 physical function In OA: correlations with Cochin Hand Scale (r_s = 0.82) and hand strength (r_s = 0.5–0.65)	Internal consistency; intra-class correlation coefficient (ICC) = 0.75–0.94 in RA Test-retest ICC = 0.95 (RA) and 0.85 (OA)	Minimal Clinically Important Difference (MCID); pain subscale = 3; function = 11 and ADL = 13	Strengths: Good psychometric qualities in arthritis; includes appearance and satisfaction; useful postsurgery; free Weaknesses: Longer completion time
Measure of Activity Performance of the Hand (MAP-HAND) (Paulsen et al., 2010)	Self-assessment of hand function Ordinal (4-point) scale: 18 items of hand function; scores range from 18 (best) to 72 (worst)	3 minutes	Correlations with AIMS2 in RA: hand and finger function, r = 0.78; arm scale, r = 0.66; pain, r = 0.65 Unidimensional	Person Separation reliability index = 0.93. Test-retest ICC = 0.94	Not established	Strengths: Patient-generated items; quick; free Weaknesses: Needs testing in other conditions

Grip strength can be assessed using the Jamar® dynamometer, although this is less accurate for weak grip. Pinch strength can be measured with a B&L® pinch gauge, which is also reliable. Normative data are published for grip and pinch measured using the Jamar® and B&L® gauges (Crosby & Wehbe, 1994).

Reliable, valid hand assessments include the Grip Ability Test, which takes 5 minutes to complete and score and consists of pouring water from a jug, placing a paper clip on an envelope, and pulling Tubigrip® over the hand and forearm (Dellhag & Bjelle,1995); and the Sequential Occupational Dexterity Assessment (SODA) (Van Lankveld et al., 1996), which takes 15–20 minutes, if a more detailed assessment is required. Two self-report hand function measures are reviewed in the Assessment Table 39-1.

Participation

Measures of work and involvement in other valued roles are important in the rehabilitation of persons with arthritis or FM.

The Work Environment Survey–Rheumatic Conditions. A detailed semistructured interview, taking about 45 minutes, identifies problems experienced by working people, such as getting ready for and going to and from work, workplace access, completing job activities (physical, mental, and time demands), relationships with people at work, environmental factors, company policies, and work-life balance (Allaire & Keysor, 2009).

The Ergonomic Assessment Tool for Arthritis. The Ergonomic Assessment Tool for Arthritis (EATA) includes describing tasks, equipment used, a diary of typical activities at work during one day, work postures, work demands, and work station layout. It helps guide observation and recording during a work site visit and job analysis or can be conducted as an interview and/or client self-report (Backman, Village, & Lacaille, 2008).

For those who are unemployed, the Worker Role Interview identifies clients' perceptions of abilities and limitations, expectations of success, and enjoyment of and commitment to work (Braveman et al., 2005). An observational and functional assessment of work ability, the Functional Capacity Evaluation (FCE) describes the person's ability to perform work activities. FCE is an umbrella term, and there are several evaluation systems available: the WorkHab, Isernhagen Work Systems, and Matheson systems are examples (Gouttebarge et al., 2004).

Other Work Assessments. The RA-Work Instability Scale (Gilworth, Chamberlain, & Harvey, 2003) is a screening tool taking 5 minutes to administer. It has cut points identifying risk levels of work instability: <10 = low; 10–17 = moderate; and >17 = high risk, predictive of future work disability. People scoring 10 or more are recommended to receive

work rehabilitation. The Workplace Activity Limitations Scale evaluates the degree of difficulties experienced during work tasks (Gignac, 2005). (See Assessment Table 39-1).

Valued Life Activities Scale

The Valued Life Activities Scale is a brief measure of participation (33 items) that also includes some self-care items. Activities include leisure and social activities, work, travel, caring, household tasks, and gardening (Katz et al., 2009).

Educational and Psychological Assessments

Self-management education needs can be assessed using the Educational Needs Assessment Tool (Ndosi et al., 2011), which has 39 items and takes 5–10 minutes to administer. In RA, self-efficacy to use self-management approaches can be evaluated using the RA Self Efficacy Scale (RASE) (Hewlett et al., 2001). Other psychological measures are reviewed in the ACR (2011) outcome measures review.

INTERVENTIONS

Interventions are summarized in Procedures for Practice 39-1. Choice is guided by the priority occupational performance problems identified in assessment, the client's adjustment to the disease process, and his or her psychological status and self-management education needs. Occupational performance can be affected by limited

- knowledge of the condition and its progress
- knowledge and skills to adopt ergonomic approaches during occupational performance to reduce pain, fatigue, and joint strain
- energy to manage a full day of activity and ability to balance rest and activity
- range of movement and deformity
- muscle strength and endurance
- self-efficacy to use self-management approaches and to redesign lifestyle

Comprehensive OT programs sustain improvements in function (Helewa & Goldsmith, 1991; Steultjens et al., 2004) and increase self-management in early RA (Hammond, Young, & Kidao, 2004). Typically, key interventions are ergonomic approaches and fatigue management, self-management education, psychosocial support and cognitive-behavioral approaches to improve coping and reduce stress, hand and upper limb exercise, and orthoses.

Ergonomic Approaches

Ergonomic approaches include

- altering movement patterns and use of proper joint and body mechanics

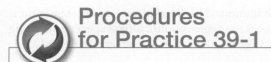

Procedures for Practice 39-1

Comprehensive List of Occupational Therapy Interventions in Rheumatology

- Activities of daily living (ADL) rehabilitation
- Work rehabilitation: including on-site work assessments, ergonomics; work assistive devices; employer liaison; work environment adaptation; functional capacity evaluation; work hardening
- Avocational rehabilitation: voluntary work, adult education and leisure opportunities; modifying leisure activities
- Stress and pain management
- Relaxation training
- Communication and assertiveness training
- Counseling (may also include cognitive-behavioral therapy if the therapist has post graduate training)
- Family/carer liaison and support
- Advice on social security benefits and community resources
- Exercise for health and well-being (e.g., Tai Chi, yoga, swimming, walking, low impact dance programs)
- Self-management education (individual and group work) using cognitive-behavioral approaches
- Activity/role planning; goal clarification and setting
- Ergonomic education (joint protection); fatigue management.
- Assistive devices and adaptive equipment
- Orthoses (e.g., resting and working hand splints; elbow and neck orthoses)
- Hand and upper limb therapy and exercises
- Therapeutic activities
- Home assessment, recommendations for environmental and housing adaptations
- Mobility aids prescription (including wheelchair/powered aids); driving/transport advice
- Foot care advice and simple orthoses (e.g., metatarsal pads, arch supports, insoles)

From Hammond, A. (2004). What is the role of the occupational therapist? *Best Practice and Research in Clinical Rheumatology, 18,* 491–505; NICE, 2009.

- restructuring activities, work simplification, and altering the environment
- using ergonomic equipment and assistive technology
- activity pacing, planning, prioritizing, and problem solving to modify activities and routines (discussed in the Fatigue Management section)

Ergonomic approaches are also termed joint protection and energy conservation techniques. Joint protection was first developed in practice relating to RA and is now applied in practice with other rheumatic conditions causing joint or soft tissue pain and swelling (Cordery & Rocchi, 1998). Some conditions, such as FM and soft tissue rheumatisms,

do not affect joints, so "ergonomics" is a more relevant term. How to provide self-management education to help people use ergonomic approaches enough in daily life to be effective is discussed at the end of this section.

Aims of Ergonomics

In inflammatory and degenerative rheumatic conditions (e.g., RA and OA), the aims of the ergonomics approach are to

- reduce pain during activity, and at rest, resulting from pressure on nociceptive endings in joint capsules, caused by inflammation and/or mechanical forces on joints
- reduce forces on joints: internal (i.e., from muscular compressive forces, e.g., during strong grip) or external (i.e., forces applied to joints whilst carrying or pulling/pushing objects)
- reduce secondary inflammation and subsequent strain on soft tissues resulting from excess (i.e., beyond tolerability) force on already inflamed and/or disrupted joints
- reduce loading on articular cartilage and subchondral bone
- help preserve joint integrity and reduce risk of development and/or progression of deformities

Additionally, in RA, OA, and FM, the aims of the ergonomic approach are to

- reduce pain resulting from overuse (i.e., beyond tolerability) of deconditioned muscles
- reduce fatigue, by reducing effort required for activity performance
- improve or maintain function

Ergonomics must be combined with exercise in order to maintain or improve muscle strength and endurance. Additionally, in RA and OA, exercise increases joint stability and improves the shock-absorbing capabilities of joints.

Evidence for Effectiveness of Ergonomics

Ergonomics is effective in RA and hand OA in reducing pain and improving function. However, effective teaching techniques must be used to help people make sufficient changes to gain benefits. (See the Self-Management Education section later for how to do this.) A number of randomized controlled trials (RCTs) of ergonomic education (joint protection) have shown education using cognitive-behavioral and/or self-efficacy–enhancing approaches is significantly more effective than traditional education. At 1 year, those receiving group behavioral education had significantly better use of joint protection, functional ability, reduced hand pain, general pain, and early morning stiffness than those receiving traditional education (Hammond & Freeman, 2001). Benefits continued for 4 years, and the behavioral group had fewer hand deformities (Hammond & Freeman, 2004) (see Evidence Table 39-1). An individual program, based on similar approaches, demonstrated at 3 months significant improvements in use of ergonomics and in

Evidence Table 39-1		Best Evidence for Occupational Therapy Practice Regarding Rheumatic Diseases					
Intervention	Description of Intervention Tested	Participants	Dosage	Type of Best Evidence and Level of Evidence	Benefit	Statistical probability and effect size of outcome	Reference
Ergonomics (i.e., joint protection [JP])	Standard arthritis education program versus a JP program using educational, behavioral, motor learning, and self-efficacy–enhancing strategies	$n = 65$ (JP); $n = 62$ (standard) programs; RA: mean age: 50 years; 30 men, 97 women	JP: 4×2-hour weekly meetings JP training. Standard: $4 \times 2h$ weekly meetings (2.5 hours typical JP education + 5.5 hours re RA, exercise, pain management, foot care).	Randomized controlled trial Level: IA2a	Yes. At 4 years posttreatment, the JP group continued to have better joint protection adherence and activities of daily living (ADL) scores.	JP group significantly more improvement in ADL: $p = 0.04$, effect size, $r = 0.15$; and behavioral assessment: $p = 0.001$, $r = 0.27$ as compared to the control (standard) group	Hammond and Freeman (2004)
Work rehabilitation	Vocational rehabilitation (VR) and comprehensive occupational therapy versus usual care	VR/OT = 16; usual care = 16. RA: mean age = 50 years; 2 men, 28 women; all employed, but at risk for work disability.	VR/OT = 6–8 OT sessions: work rehab, splinting, education, ADL advice, ergonomics, work visit (and usual care). Usual care = medication and clinic visits	Randomized controlled trial Level: IB2a	Yes. At 6 months, there was significant reduction in work instability and improved functional ability and pain.	6 months: VR/OT group: Work instability $p = 0.04$, $r = 0.31$; COPM performance $p = 0.001$, $r = 0.55$; COPM satisfaction $p = 0.001$, $r = 0.55$; VAS (visual analog scale) pain $p = 0.007$, $r = 0.43$. These are medium to large effects.	Macedo et al. (2009)

self-efficacy (Niedermann et al., 2011). Furst et al. (1987) demonstrated that behavioral education was more effective than traditional in increasing the amount of daily activity people with RA were able to do. In hand OA, at 6-month follow-up, a hand joint protection intervention (based on the Looking After Your Joints Programme of Hammond & Freeman [2001]) led to significant improvements in hand pain, hand disability, global improvement, and self-efficacy (Dziedzic et al., 2011).

Ergonomic Methods

Hand ergonomics in RA includes changing movement patterns to limit strong grips, twisting movements, and sustained grips to reduce MCP forces; to limit lifting heavy objects and sustained wrist radial positioning to reduce wrist volar and radial forces; and to limit tight, prolonged key, tripod, and pinch grips to reduce volar and ulnar forces on the MCP, IP, and CMC joints. Approaches are similar in OA, although there is no need to emphasize reducing ulnar forces on the second through fifth MCPs, because these are not affected. The rapid hand function decline often seen in early RA and hand OA suggests that effective ergonomic education should be provided early to improve and maintain function or prevent problems. There is no need to "protect joints" in FM, because these are not affected, but ergonomic approaches help reduce forces on the hand that cause pain and help to compensate for weak grip.

Ergonomic Principles

Altering Movement Patterns and Use of Proper Joint and Body Mechanics. In hand activities, two hands can be used, and the load can be spread over the palmar surface (e.g., see Figs. 39-3 and 39-4). Movement patterns can be changed by, for example, turning a jar lid using the thumb, index, ring fingers, and thumb web space. The fingers are kept in correct anatomic alignment, and ulnar forces are avoided (Fig. 39-5).

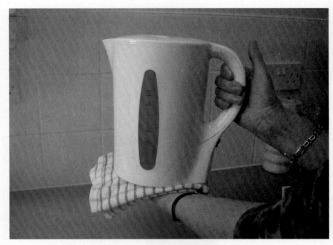

Figure 39-4 Distribute load: using two hands to carry a kettle.

Objects should be kept closer to the body when lifting and carrying, and/or a stronger larger joint can be used. For example, avoid carrying a shopping bag using a hook grip in the hand. Instead use a bag with longer handles and put it over the shoulder (Fig. 39-6), or use a rucksack. Avoid prolonged sitting and standing. Change position regularly. For people with knee and foot pain, a perch stool reduces standing when preparing food or ironing. Work surfaces are within the reach envelope of the arms. Maintain efficient postures when working, e.g., avoid sitting with the head poking forward whilst working at a desk or reading. Book stands, writing slopes, and document holders help. Keep the back straight using supportive seating such as ergonomic office chairs and higher back, supportive sofas. Poor posture and positioning increases muscle fatigue and pain because greater energy is

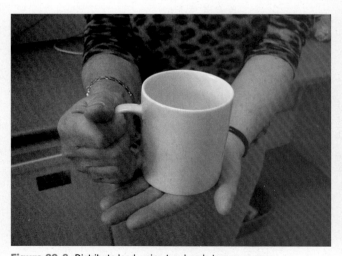

Figure 39-3 Distribute load: using two hands to carry a mug.

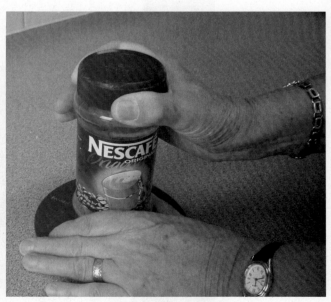

Figure 39-5 Altering movement patterns: opening a jar.

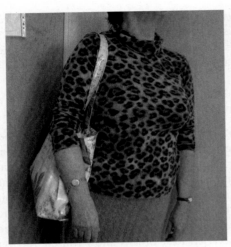

Figure 39-6 Using a stronger, larger joint: carrying a bag.

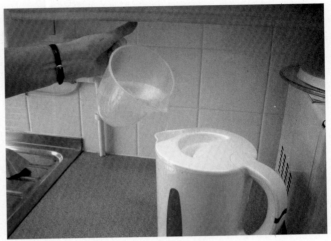

Figure 39-7 Altering working methods: using a light jug to fill a kettle.

used to maintain biomechanically inefficient postures (see Procedures for Practice 39-2).

Restructuring Activities, Work Simplification, and Altering the Environment. Can an activity be done differently? For example, rather than taking a kettle to the tap, holding it whilst it fills and carrying it back across the kitchen, fill it with a lightweight jug instead (Fig. 39-8). Could shopping be done via the Internet to save driving, walking, and carrying bags? Reorder the sequence of tasks within activities to increase efficiency. Eliminate unnecessary tasks: Do all those items need to be ironed? Keep frequently used equipment within the reach envelope. Reorganize work areas to streamline work processes. Make work areas uncluttered. Locate equipment to promote correct joint positioning, e.g., keyboards. Raise or lower work surfaces to maintain good posture. Ensure storage is efficient, e.g., use stepped shelves in cupboards and sliding racks so jars, cans, and boxes are easily reached.

Using Ergonomic Equipment and Assistive Technology. Reduce the effort required by using ergonomic equipment or products with universal design, i.e., designed to be easy for all to use. There are many kitchen and household products available in stores and via the Internet (Figs. 39-7 and 39-9).

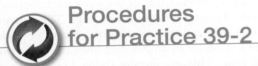

Procedures
for Practice 39-2

Ergonomic (Joint Protection) Principles

- Respect pain
- Distribute load over several joints
- Reduce the force and effort required in activities
- Use correct patterns of movement
- Use good body positioning, posture and moving and handling techniques
- Use the strongest, largest joint available for the job
- Avoid staying in one position for too long
- Use ergonomic equipment, assistive devices, and labor-saving gadgets
- Pace activities: balance rest and activity, alternate heavy and light tasks, take microbreaks
- Use work simplification: plan, prioritise, and problem solve
- Modify the environment and equipment location to be ergonomically efficient
- Maintain muscle strength and range of movement

Modified from Cordery, J., & Rocchi, M. (1998). Joint protection and fatigue management. In J. Melvin & G. Jensen (Eds.), *Rheumatologic rehabilitation series: Assessment and management* (Vol. 1, pp. 279–321). Bethesda, MD: American Occupational Therapy Association; Hammond, A. (2010). Joint protection. In K. Dziedzic & A. Hammond (Eds.), *Rheumatology: Evidence based practice for physiotherapists and occupational therapists* (pp. 137–150). Edinburgh: Churchill Livingstone.

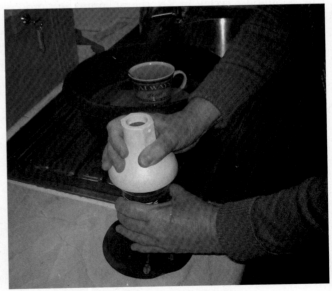

Figure 39-8 Using an ergonomic device: a jar opener.

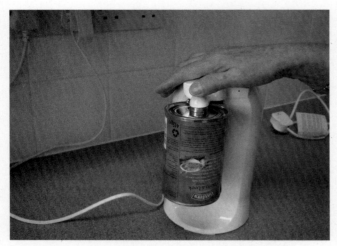

FIGURE 39-9 Using an ergonomic device: an electric can opener.

For example, avoid lifting by using wheels: put shopping in a folding hand cart, easily kept in the boot of the car when not in use. Encourage people to consider features of good design when selecting products (see Procedures for Practice 39-3). For example, to avoid bending and kneeling, sit on a garden kneeler/stool when weeding. Wear cushioned, shock-absorbing insoles in shoes to reduce pressure on foot and knee joints when walking and standing. At work, use voice-activated software to reduce keyboarding and a wireless telephone headset or hands-free mobile instead of a handset.

Fatigue Management

Fatigue occurs in all three conditions. Causes can be physical: pain, increased physical demands because of altered joint biomechanics, deconditioning because of insufficient physical activity, and/or overdoing activities (the boom-bust cycle). In RA, the inflammatory process contributes to fatigue and also causes anemia and muscle cachexia. Psychosocial factors, e.g., depression, anxiety, helplessness, stress, poor self-efficacy, and poor social support (e.g., lack of understanding from family and friends),

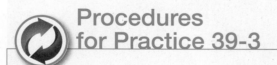

Procedures for Practice 39-3

Selecting Ergonomic Products

- Lightweight, durable, compact
- Larger, nonslip handles
- Comfortable to hold and easy to maneuver
- Attractive and acceptable to the user
- Simple to operate; multipurpose (if appropriate)
- Reduces stress to all joints needed to operate the device
- Affordable

and work pressures contribute to fatigue. A variety of strategies help reduce fatigue, including ergonomic approaches at home and work, activity pacing, exercise, and stress management.

Activity Pacing, Planning, Prioritizing, and Problem Solving

Pacing. Many find taking a rest break difficult because it can be seen as "giving in." Rest "recharges the batteries," allowing people to keep going for longer. Rest recommendations include taking microbreaks for 30 seconds every 5–10 minutes or so, stretching and relaxing joints and muscles being most used, or taking a rest break for up to 5 minutes every 30–60 minutes. Frequency depends on fatigue severity. Rest breaks allow muscle recovery time. Help develop habits by using computer screen prompts or a kitchen timer or mobile phone alarm (or set to vibrate) to remind the person to take the rest break.

Planning. Balance activities to alternate between light, medium, and heavy tasks during the day and week. A "boom-bust" cycle is common, with people doing too much on good days and suffering the consequences for the next few. Breaking this habit requires attitudinal change. Many fear the consequences of failing to meet responsibilities. Activity diaries help people see boom-bust patterns. Use a diary with a line for each day of the week, each divided into 24 hours, showing 7 days on one page. The person completes this over a week, coloring the hours of high activity in red, medium in amber, and low in green, with rest colored blue. This graphically shows how they are overdoing activity and why they are fatigued.

Sleep Hygiene. A sleep diary helps identify why sleep is problematic. Solutions depend on problems and can include having a more supportive mattress and pillow (e.g., memory foam); establishing a regular bedtime and relaxing evening routine (e.g., listening to a relaxation recording, warm bath, or hot milky drink); avoiding stimulants (coffee, tea, alcohol, nicotine, and caffeinated soft drinks) several hours before bedtime; reducing stimuli in the bedroom (e.g., no TV or computer use), black-out curtains; and muted colors. Fatigue can also be aided by reducing stress and increasing physical activity (see later sections). At 6-month follow-up, an RCT of a multimodal fatigue management program in moderate to severe RA showed significant reductions in fatigue (Hewlett et al., 2011).

Self-Management Education: Applying Theory to Practice

Self-management education is problem focused and practical and emphasizes clients' ability to develop problem-solving skills and generate action plans. It includes educational, behavioral, and cognitive approaches to influence health knowledge, attitudes, beliefs, and behaviors and to promote independence, maintain, or adjust life roles and address the psychological impact of disease (Iversen, Hammond, & Betteridge, 2010). Making changes to lifestyle is not easy. How it is applied in an ergonomics (i.e., joint protection, fatigue management, and hand exercise) program (the Looking After Your Joints Programme) is discussed below (Hammond & Freeman, 2001, 2004). Techniques can be applied to teach any self-management strategy.

The Transtheoretical Model

Identify the person's readiness to change and the benefits and barriers, both practical and psychological, to the person using ergonomics. People cycle through five stages of change when modifying health behaviors (Prochaska, DiClemente, & Norcross, 1992), with lapses at any stage possible. The stages are the following:

- Precontemplation: not knowing why or how to change or not wanting to.
- Contemplation: weighing the pros and cons of change.
- Preparation: starting to plan for change. Small steps are being taken, but they could easily remain "wishful thinking."
- Action: making changes and establishing new routines.
- Maintenance: keeping up the health behavior(s) for over 6 months.

To help identify a client's stage of change regarding pain management, during the initial assessment, ask

- "What do you do now to help manage your pain?"
- "Does pain and fatigue affect you doing activities you need and want to do in life?"

What does the response indicate? For example, "I take the tablets and keep on working through the pain" suggests the person is not self-managing effectively (precontemplation). Probe further to identify whether the person does not know what to do (limited knowledge), knows but lacks confidence to try other actions (poor self-efficacy), knows but does not believe anything else works (limited perceived benefit), or is angry/upset or denying the need to change (limited attitudinal change). This guides your choice of what to do next.

Precontemplation and Contemplation. If the person is not yet ready to make changes, cognitive and affective strategies are more important to use. Either (as relevant) provide small amounts of information incrementally about how, why, and what to do (increasing knowledge, perceived benefit, and self-efficacy) or discuss the person's attitudes toward having the condition and use counselling or motivational interviewing (attitudinal change) as relevant. See also Chapter 13 concerning motivational interviewing. Encourage using self-evaluation and self-monitoring. Explore what activities and roles are important to the person: How are these affected by arthritis, what difficulties result (e.g., pain, fatigue, stiffness, or frustration)? How is the person's pain and fatigue at the end of the day or when doing activities he or she must do (e.g., work)? How will they be in a year or 5 years if things go on as they are or get worse? If resistance is encountered, roll with it (Mason & Butler, 2010). Encourage further self-reflection. This helps the person weigh up the pros and cons of change. Facing up to the negative consequences he or she fears for the future may prompt change. A technique then used in motivational interviewing is to ask

- How important is it for you to reduce these symptoms and continue these activities, on a scale of 0–10?
- How confident do you feel about making changes on a scale of 0–10?
- How ready are you to make changes on a scale of 0–10?

Zero means that the activity is not at all important or the person is not confident or ready. Ten means that the activity is extremely important or that the person is confident and ready (Mason & Butler, 2010). If the person's score is less than 7 for any of these questions, he or she is less likely to see the need for or be willing to change. If this is the case, explore what she thinks might increase these beliefs and her confidence in and readiness to use ergonomics; discuss that ergonomics and fatigue management are proven effective and the benefits gained, that is, reduced pain and fatigue, having more energy and ability to do what he or she needs and wants to in life (playing with the kids, working, running the home, and social activities), staying independent, reducing frustration, better physical and psychological well-being. Let the person discuss his or her concerns, which are commonly about negative self-image, embarrassment, not wanting to use assistive devices, wanting to remain as he or she is, not wanting to take the time to change, or concerns that using ergonomics makes tasks slower and more difficult.

Market ergonomics effectively. It can be perceived as excessive rest and giving up activity. Emphasize that it is adapting activities and movements to reduce strain or force on joints and soft tissues, just as in industry. Ergonomic practices do not mean stopping doing activities and appearing different, they mean change. Focus first on using altered working methods, planning, pacing, and restructuring activities (rather than assistive devices and splints). Such methods are less obvious, and many with arthritis strive not to appear different.

Change is a choice. The person may have good reasons for not using ergonomic approaches. There may be other priorities such as managing new medication, work, child care, increased exercise, or counseling. Ensure there are regular opportunities for people to be rereferred for education.

Preparation and Action. Identify the knowledge and skills the person has, emphasize that he or she has already started problem solving and will extend the amount and frequency of change to further reduce strain and pain. Teach some ergonomic skills specific to individual patient's priorities (e.g., in cooking). Teach self-monitoring: observing one's own behavior and how pain and fatigue are less when practicing an ergonomic method. This helps the person self-evaluate to determine whether change helps. Do not promote overly ambitious goals too soon. Engage family and friends in planning ergonomic changes, buying gadgets to help as presents, and reading advice leaflets to help support the client to change.

Once the person has started practicing techniques at home and work, use a coaching and educational-behavioral approach to teach ergonomic principles and their application across different activities. Motor learning approaches, with sufficient supervised practice and feedback, help psychomotor skill development. Teach

- task analysis: to help identify actions and activities to change
- problem solving: applying joint protection principles to generate new solutions, help overcome barriers, and prevent lapses
- goal setting: to regularly set and review action plans and identify internal rewards for meeting these

Workbooks, diaries, and action plans help recall of information and recording of activities, ergonomic behaviors practiced, and intentions to change. Increase and support self-efficacy by collaboratively developing a home program with the client to practice regularly.

Maintenance

Follow-up support can include telephone calls a few weeks or months later to check progress, booster sessions, and review of progress at rheumatology annual review appointments. Help clients be aware of how to cope with lapses.

Integrating Social Cognitive Theory

Increasing self-efficacy is key in teaching ergonomics. In the preparation, action, and maintenance phases, important strategies are the following (Bandura, 1977):

- Mastery experience: i.e., performing tasks successfully. Major barriers to change are altering automatic movement patterns and habitual daily routines. Provide sufficient practice of skills, with feedback, starting with simpler to more complex skills. Plan together how routines can change to accommodate extra practice and pacing.
- Vicarious experience (role modeling): watching others like ourselves successfully perform actions enhances our beliefs that we can also succeed.
- Verbal persuasion, i.e., encourage the person to try. Although widely used by health professionals,

supervised practice time and modeling are more effective. Persuasion is an adjunct.
- Reinterpretation of physiological signals, i.e., help people perceive differences in disease symptoms and increased symptoms (e.g., aches, fatigue, and joint swelling) from overdoing activities. Explain that symptoms from overdoing can be controlled through ergonomics and fatigue management.

Teaching in groups is very effective to enable modeling, problem solving, peer support, and ideas exchange, as well as being more efficient. Treating six patients in a 10-hour program takes less time than seeing each for 2 hours. Individuals get much more teaching time, which is significantly more likely to enable change.

Cognitive-Behavioral Approaches and Goal Setting

Change is the person's responsibility, but it is the therapist's responsibility to help him or her weigh the pros and cons of change and then provide effective interventions once the person decides to change. In preparation and action, goal setting and action plans support self-management. First, help clients identify long-term goals to aid motivation, for example, to be able to stay at work. Explain how ergonomics helps achieve this. Practicing with a therapist aids correct skill development, but continued home practice is essential for habit development. Help the person set a weekly action plan, including relevant short-term goals the person believes lead toward longer term goals. Short-term goals should state what, how much, when, how often, and the time frame. Plans must be achievable. Ask how confident the person is about achieving, on a scale of 0–10, each goal and the whole plan. If the answer is less than 7 for any or all, recommend the person review the plan to make it achievable. Failure reduces self-efficacy. Better to progress slowly and successfully. At the end of each session, help the person set an action plan until the next session. At the beginning of the next session, discuss progress toward meeting goals. If goals were not met, help problem solve about barriers.

Educational Approaches in Joint Protection

In the preparation and action phases, effective education techniques improve understanding and recall. Audiovisual aids are best kept simple. An A3 easel presenter portfolio (a table top presentation tool; e.g., see http://www.phillipsdirect.co.uk/a2-easel-presenter-portfolio-p-130.html), with preprinted sheets is cheap, informal, quick to set up, and very unlikely to go wrong. Group comments can be added to spare sheets. Help people remember by

- Using advance organizers: Before they come, send a booklet about ergonomics that they can read (e.g., the Arthritis Foundation's "Managing Your Pain" pages 15–17) (See Resources 39-1).

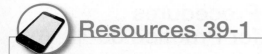

Resources 39-1

Patient and Professional Education

Arthritis Foundation

www.arthritis.org
Patient education brochures on conditions and self-management available for free download. Online store sells books with practical tips, e.g., "Good Living with . . ." Series (includes RA, OA, and FM). Branches in every state run exercise programs (e.g., *Tai Chi for Arthritis*, *Walk for Ease*, *People with Arthritis Can Exercise*, aquatic exercise) and organize arthritis self-management courses.

Arthritis Society of Canada

www.arthritis.ca
Includes sections about conditions and *Tips for Living Well*

American College of Rheumatology: Arthritis Health Professionals in Rheumatology

http://www.rheumatology.org
The clinical support section of the website includes standards of practice for rheumatology, bibliography of clinical guidelines and health assessments, and practice guidelines and patient resources. The education section includes access to some free educational materials.

American Occupational Therapy Association

www.aota.org
Patient education: *Tips for Living Life to the Fullest: Living with Arthritis* (2012).

Tai Chi for Arthritis

http://www.taichiforarthritis.com/ and http://www.youtube.com/watch?v=SvN8oawFlXl

Self-help book

Lorig, K., & Fries, J. F. (2006). *The arthritis help book*. Cambridge, MA: De Capo Press.

- Simplification: Give a few key messages each session. Explain technical terms when necessary (e.g., inflammation). Use nontechnical words (e.g., bend rather than flex). Keep explanations short.
- Explicit categorization: Structure information to "tell them what you are going to tell them, tell them, and tell them what you told them." Summarize before and after each topic, and at the beginning and end of the session.
- Repetition: Ensure that key facts are repeated by paraphrasing. Ask the person to repeat back or paraphrase what he learned. Repetition is an important part of education for both facts and skills.

Psychomotor Skills Teaching Applied to Ergonomics

Ensure there is sufficient space, without obstacles. Check that your client(s) can see clearly. Move furniture, equipment, or people if need be. Have all the equipment you need to hand; be familiar with its use. Put anything not immediately required aside to avoid visual distraction. Explain why the skill is performed, its relevance to the client, objectives of the session, and how they will be participating. Teach skills using four steps:

1. Confidently demonstrate the whole skill at normal speed *without* commentary, providing a clear image of what is to be learnt, without distraction.
2. Demonstrate *with* commentary: break it down step-by-step. Use clear, *short* instructions. Too much information distracts.
3. Demonstrate whilst asking the person to tell you step-by-step what to do. Start/continue each step as a prompt if need be.
4. The person demonstrates the skill with commentary. Errors need correcting, but allow a few seconds for self-correction first. If not, provide prompts to identify errors. Tell the answer if the client is unsure.

This gives plenty of opportunity to watch and hear about new actions before doing it themselves. In a group, the last two stages can be shared amongst members (working in pairs or threes), each trying the skill in turn. Developing psychomotor skills helps clients successfully perform ergonomic actions correctly and integrate them into daily life. Repetition helps this. Simply knowing what to do and why does not necessarily lead to behavior change.

Teach skills gradually over three to four treatment sessions. Start with blocked practice of one part of an activity (i.e., repeating individual tasks such as opening a jar). Use self-monitoring. In RA and OA, highlight the hand limitations they already have (reduced grip strength, range of movement, any early deformities). Explain how deformities occur in RA and OA, e.g., forces on joints contributing to ulnar deviation in RA. Between sessions, ask them to self-monitor: watch movements during common activities (e.g., making a meal, at work) as they normally do them. What forces occur? Is there aching, pain, or fatigue? Ask them to reflect and compare with ergonomic approaches they are learning. Could these help? In the second session, discuss their experience doing this. Often "the penny drops"; the clients begin to see the connection between ergonomic approaches and a reduction in pain and fatigue. Progress to whole practice, i.e., sequences of activities such as making a hot drink and snack meal, requiring more ergonomic methods to be integrated. OT facilities may mean practice is limited to cooking and household activities, but if possible, also try this process with work and leisure activities. Encourage the client to apply ergonomics in these in his or her action plan.

Physical Activity and Exercise

Ergonomic approaches are not used in isolation. Many with RA, OA, and FM have occupational performance problems because of reduced range of movement, muscle strength, and endurance. Exercise and physical activity are essential. Whilst tailored exercise programs are provided by physiotherapists, occupational therapists should explain the benefits of physical activity—how it reduces pain, improves fitness, and increases energy levels as muscle strength and aerobic capacity increase, and in RA and OA, how it helps protect joints as stronger muscles compensate for weakened ligaments. The occupational therapist helps clients to integrate physical activity into daily routines.

Occupational therapists should be able to confidently teach home exercise maintenance programs for range of movement, strength, and aerobic exercises, such as are described in widely available patient information booklets. Exercise programs should be recommended, such as the Arthritis Foundation's Walk with Ease program and the Tai Chi for Arthritis program (see Resources 39-1). People need advice tailoring exercise and activity to suit their changing ability and how to gradually progress, rather than overdoing it. People with FM especially should not do too much too soon, because sensitization means that incidence of delayed onset muscle soreness is high and can contribute to fear of exercising. Aerobic exercise programs are safe and effective in RA, OA, and FM. Those more physically active have less pain and fatigue, better function, and well-being (Busch et al., 2011; NICE, 2008, 2009). Refer to physical therapy for specialist advice.

Hand Exercises

Several trials demonstrate that exercise is effective in improving grip and pinch strength and hand function and reducing pain in RA. Two studies used intensive exercise (i.e., 10 repetitions, at least 15 minutes per day of resisted exercise using soft dough or therapeutic putty,

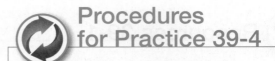

Procedures
for Practice 39-4

A Home Hand Exercise Program

Find a comfortable position: support the arm to avoid shoulder aching. Warm up by moving the joints a little first and/or soaking in warm water for a few minutes. Exercise 3 days the first week, increasing repetitions and number of days over 2–4 weeks, to 10 repetitions most/every day.

Range of Movement

- Wrist extension/flexion
- Wrist pronation/supination
- Tendon gliding exercise
- Radial finger walk

Muscle Strength and Dexterity Exercise

Use a good handful of Play-doh® or therapeutic putty. Five minutes initially, gradually increasing to 10–15 minutes.

- Gently knead and squeeze
- Push fingers into dough and push out straight
- Pinch off dough with each finger/thumb in turn
- Roll into a sausage (two hands)
- Form a "ring doughnut" from the sausage. Put the fingers/thumbs in the hole; stretch out.
- Use an elastic band over fingers and thumb and stretch.
- Grip a 0.5-L (16.9-fl oz) drink bottle (with a "waist" filled with water or sand). Support the forearm. Lift bottle up and down slowly, first with palm facing down 10 times, and then with the palm facing up 10 times.

plus range of movement exercise). No adverse effects were reported (Brorsson et al., 2009; Ronningen & Kjeken, 2008). In hand OA, exercises can improve grip by up to 25% and reduce pain (Valdes & Marik, 2010). However, exercise must be sustained, otherwise the benefits are lost. A simple home program is described in Procedures for Practice 39-4 (see also Fig. 39-10). These exercises should be taught effectively, using the strategies discussed above to promote behavioral change. Exercise diaries and goal setting help people sustain exercising. Opportunities to remind people to restart, if they lapse, are essential.

Hand Orthoses

Splinting is used to

- reduce local inflammation
- reduce soft tissue and joint pain

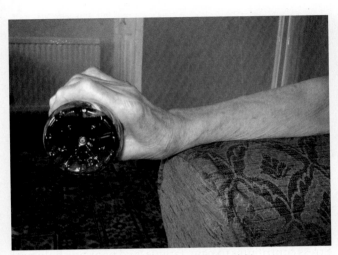

FIGURE 39-10 Wrist exercise with a homemade weight.

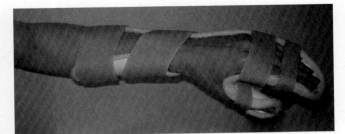

FIGURE 39-11 A resting splint.

- correctly position joints and improve joint stability
- improve hand function

Adherence to splint wear is variable and affected by belief in efficacy and quality of fit. People may believe splints cause muscle weakness and/or stiffness and therefore fear relying on them. An RCT demonstrated adherence with splint wear is significantly improved by how the therapist explains the splint's purpose, wear regimen, and whether he or she conducts a positive interaction with the client (Feinberg & Brandt, 1992). Hand exercises should be taught when providing splints, recommending the person does these most days.

Static Resting Splints

In RA, resting splints reduce localized pain and inflammation by providing support in an anatomically correct position at rest. They can be worn at night and/or during daytime rest periods. Trials give conflicting results. Adams et al. (2008) conducted an RCT, with 12-month follow-up, in early RA ($n = 116$). There were no significant differences in strength, hand function, or ulnar deviation progression as a result of using resting splints. However, by study end, adherence had reduced considerably. In contrast, Silva et al. (2008a), in an RCT with 3-month follow-up of 50 persons with established RA, identified significant improvements in pain, hand function, and grip and pinch strength. Adherence was good throughout the study. This suggests careful attention is needed to willingness to wear the splint and adherence. These splints are effective in established RA, but in early RA, acceptability may be less, or there may be only a short-term need until drug therapy reduces pain (Fig. 39-11).

Compression Gloves

Compression gloves can be prescribed for nocturnal pain in RA, OA, and FM and to reduce pain during daytime activities, because they are easily worn in activity. Several small RCTs indicate that gloves reduce pain and stiffness in established RA (McKnight & Kwoh, 1992; Oosterveld & Rasker, 1990). People with hand OA and FM also report reduced pain during night and day wear and improved function with day wear. There are no trials evaluating gloves in OA and FM.

Wrist Orthoses

Wrist orthoses are widely used in RA, and many designs are available. A close fit, not impeding MCP and thumb movement, is needed. They can be worn for nighttime pain relief if the person has wrist but not MCP or IP pain. Their main aim is to reduce torque during heavy tasks involving the wrist and to stabilize the wrist in a functionally effective position (i.e., 10°–15° of extension). RCTs show that wrist orthoses are effective in reducing hand pain (Kjeken, Moller, & Kvien, 1995; Veehof et al., 2008) but not improving grip strength or hand function. Their benefit is largely when being worn, and clients regularly report they are helpful for heavier activities, such as ironing, gardening, housework, and at work (Fig. 39-12).

Metacarpophalangeal Splints

MCP splints either are small palm-based splints or may also have a wrist and forearm component. They aim to

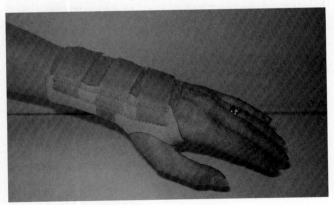

FIGURE 39-12 A wrist splint.

reduce medial force on the MCPs and maintain fingers in correct alignment. There is no evidence that they help prevent deformities because no trials have been conducted. One small study demonstrated that they maintained alignment and that function was easier in people with established RA with MCP deformities (Rennie, 1996).

Finger Splints

Swan-neck splints apply three-point pressure around the PIP joint to prevent PIP joint hyperextension and subsequent PIP flexion. They can be made or bought in thermoplastics or made in silver. The latter are more popular and adherence is better (Adams, 2010). Trials have demonstrated that they improve dexterity and hand function, although not pain or grip strength (van der Giesen et al., 2009; Zijlstra, Heijnsdijk-Rouwenhorst, & Rasker, 2004).

Thumb Splints

In RA and OA, thumb splints aim to reduce pain and improve function and grip. They may be a short, hand-based splint immobilizing the CMC joint only or a longer hand/forearm splint if pain extends to the wrist. A systematic review concluded that CMC joint splints for OA reduce pain and improve function and may help clients postpone or avoid surgery. Many prefer a short flexible splint to longer, more rigid versions (Valdes & Marik, 2010). A trial in RA identified that CMC splints significantly reduced pain (Silva et al., 2008b) (Fig. 39-13).

Effects of Combined Ergonomic and Exercise Interventions

Several RCTs evaluated combined interventions in RA. At 8-month follow-up, a 12-hour program of ergonomics, exercise, cognitive pain management, and relaxation, with monthly telephone follow-up, led to significant

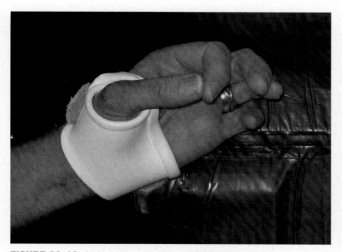

FIGURE 39-13 A short carpometacarpal (CMC) splint.

improvements in pain, functional ability, and physical status (Masiero et al., 2007). At 1-year follow-up, the Lifestyle Management for Arthritis Programme (LMAP) (including ergonomics, exercise, and fatigue, pain, and stress management) led to significantly improved pain, functional and physical ability, self-efficacy, and psychological status compared to a group receiving standard arthritis education (Hammond, Bryan, & Hardy, 2008). In hand OA, at 1-year follow-up, a combined program of joint protection, hand exercises, and splinting led to significant improvements in pain, stiffness, and daily activities (Boustedt, Nordenskiold, & Lundgren, 2009).

Stress Management

Stress contributes to pain, fatigue, and poor psychological status. Managing stress is a key component for FM management especially and is often best addressed first. Explain the link between stress, pain, and fatigue and how stress can lower neurochemical levels, such as serotonin and noradrenaline, which help control sleep cycles and energy levels. In FM, these are already lowered, and stress makes the situation worse. Stress management methods help increase neurochemical levels. Effective stress reduction approaches include mindfulness therapy, relaxation, and CBT, combined with condition education (Glombiewski et al., 2010). Multimodal therapy is more effective. Undertaking additional training in such techniques can make a valuable contribution to OT, especially in FM.

Vocational Rehabilitation

Vocational rehabilitation (VR) can include

- job modifications or "accommodations" such as ergonomic changes (restructuring work tasks, assistive technology and adaptations, work station/place redesign, and splints)
- psychosocial and informational strategies (increasing confidence to ask for job modifications, work rights, statutory [imposed by law] VR service availability, and coping strategies)
- liaising with employers (about job and hours flexibility and better understanding of the condition), occupational health, and statutory services

Two OT studies in RA have demonstrated positive effects. An RCT with working people with RA ($n = 32$) randomized participants to both comprehensive occupational therapy and VR (work assessment, job modifications, help with daily living problems, ergonomic advice, splinting, and group education: provided over six to eight sessions) or a waiting list control group. At 6 months, self-perceived ability to manage self-care, work, and leisure, work instability, work satisfaction, and pain significantly improved (Macedo et al., 2009) (see Evidence Table 39-1). A Canadian proof of principle study with people with RA ($n = 19$) evaluated a five-session group VR and self-management program plus an occupational therapy visit using the EATA to identify problems (Backman, Village, & Lacaille, 2008). At 1 year, 80% reported increased confidence in requesting job accommodations, 74% had requested at least one, and 71% of requests were implemented (Lacaille et al., 2008).

An RCT of a job-retention program with people with arthritis (RA, knee OA, systemic lupus erythematosus, or ankylosing spondylitis) led to significant reductions in job loss in the intervention group compared to the control group. The intervention group received two 1.5-hour individual VR sessions including a structured interview (the Work Experience Survey–Rheumatic Conditions [WES-RC]). Barriers were prioritized, potential solutions were discussed, and action plans were developed. Information on employment rights and guidance on disclosing arthritis to employers and asking for job accommodations were given (Allaire, Li, & La Valley, 2003). The intervention was provided by VR counsellors, but occupational therapists could provide a similar intervention.

CLINICAL OUTCOMES

The interventions described assist clients in adapting their lifestyle to improve self-management and occupational balance. Changing habits and routines is not easy. On average, adherence rates are about 50% for many interventions. Providing patient education about the condition, motivational interviewing, and counselling to help people prepare for change, followed by effective self-management education, takes time. But without doing so, we are wasting time if people do not follow the advice given. Delivering interventions effectively is a priority.

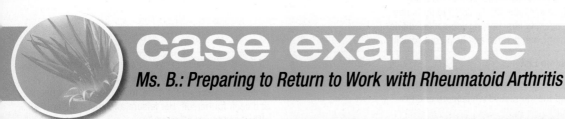

case example
Ms. B.: Preparing to Return to Work with Rheumatoid Arthritis

Occupational Therapy Assessment Process	Objectives	Clinical Reasoning Process
		Examples of Therapist's Internal Dialogue
Patient Information Ms. B. is 45 years old and has a 3-year history of rheumatoid arthritis (RA). She is stable on disease-modifying antirheumatic drugs (DMARDs). At her last 6-monthly rheumatology appointment, she complained of increasing right wrist, metacarpophalangeal (MCP), and shoulder pain (she is right handed) and pain in her feet. She is a full-time fourth-grade schoolteacher, and her work is affected, although she has not taken time off work. She lives in a first floor, one-bedroom apartment.	Understand the patient's diagnosis or condition	"Ms. B. has mild inflammatory RA affecting hands, feet, and shoulder. Her work problems might be walking around school because of foot pain, using a personal computer (PC), marking books because of hand pain, writing on the whiteboard because of her arm problems, and interacting with schoolkids because of fatigue."
	Know the person	"She enjoys teaching, wants to continue working, and is keen to help herself. A good candidate for self-management education and work rehabilitation."
Reason for Referral to Occupational Therapy Ms. B. was referred by her rheumatologist for assessment of hand function, help with work problems, and self-management education. Ms. B. wants to keep working full time.	Appreciate the context	"How much is she affected by fatigue? Does she have energy for leisure and social life?"
	Develop provisional hypotheses	"She is likely to do well as she is motivated to keep working, enjoys her job, and is keen to learn."

Assessment Process and Results

Ms. B.'s priority is work. She was assessed using the Work Environment Survey—Rheumatic Conditions (WES-RC) and an activity diary. Every day, she regularly uses an interactive whiteboard and PC, moves round the classroom helping small groups of children and bends to do so. She drives to work and has a full briefcase to carry to the car. She buys lunch at the school cafe. Work takes all her time and energy. She buys ready meals (although likes cooking) and has let her housework go. She does not like this but has supportive friends who help out. She spends weekends recovering, and the pain reduces, but she is often still tired. Her sleep is disturbed by hand pain at night. Her pain and fatigue is much less during school vacations. The pain, fatigue, and having given up some leisure activities gets her down at times, but teaching helps keep her positive.

Physical examination of Ms. B.'s hands, wrist, shoulder and feet (using the gait arms legs spine [GALS]) and tender and swollen joint count showed a mild inflammatory process and no deformity. Bilateral grip strength was 19 kg (norm is 28 kg). On a Visual Analog Scale (VAS) for pain and for fatigue, Ms. B. scored 7 out of 10 for both after workday.

Ms. B. took the Evaluation of Daily Activity Questionnaire (EDAQ) home to complete (see Assessment Table 39-1). She had problems including, e.g., cooking (viz., opening jars, peeling vegetables, lifting pans), cleaning (viz., vacuuming), handicrafts, and going out socially.

Consider evaluation approach and methods	"Her joint swelling wasn't too bad, but poor grip strength, pain, and fatigue scores helped me understand why things are difficult. The activity diary showed which activities are painful, she doesn't rest much in the day, sleeps poorly, and doesn't do a lot at weekends. The WES-RC and EDAQ identified activities she has difficulty with."
Interpret observations	"Her joint pain and inflammation seem aggravated by resisted activities, regular shoulder elevation using the whiteboard, and regular standing. Overuse is a likely cause as at weekends and vacations she has less pain and fatigue. Her mood is likely to improve if her job is made easier, and she can do more things in the home and during her leisure time."

Occupational Therapy Problem List

1. Right wrist, MCP, shoulder, and foot pain worsen during the work day, especially using the interactive whiteboard and PC and standing a lot.
2. Difficulty with home maintenance.
3. Difficulty preparing meals.
4. Limited leisure activities.
5. Poor sleep because of nocturnal hand pain.

Synthesize results	"If Ms. B. continues to overdo activity and push through pain at work, it may get more difficult for her to continue working full time, look after her apartment, and cook for herself. Her leisure and social life are already seriously affected."

Occupational Therapy Goal List

1. Use ergonomic approaches to reduce wrist, MCP, shoulder, and foot pain during work, home, and meal preparation activities.
2. Use fatigue management (activity pacing) to reduce fatigue.
3. Wear right wrist orthosis during heavier activities and compression glove at night to reduce pain.
4. Perform hand exercises daily to improve grip strength and endurance.

Develop intervention hypotheses	"It can be difficult using ergonomic principles. Focusing specifically on her goals and helping her problem solve should help her cope in new situations as they arise. Educating Ms. B. about the positive effects of hand exercises and orthoses will help her understand why these help."
Consider the evidence	"She wants to keep teaching, so she is more likely to want to learn about making work and daily activities easier. She seems trapped in a cycle of fatigue, pain, and overwork and needs help tackling problems step by step, to increase her self-efficacy to manage RA. She is doing some things to help herself (**preparation** stage of change)."
Select an intervention approach	"I think I will use ergonomic and self-management education using cognitive-behavioral and self-efficacy enhancing approaches to facilitate change."
Consider what will occur in therapy, how often, and for how long	"Ms. B. will be seen in occupational therapy (OT) as an outpatient for five 1-hour sessions over 5 weeks. The sessions will focus on ergonomic teaching, problem solving, self-management, and provision of orthoses and hand exercises."

Intervention

1. Identify which activities are most important to Ms. B. to accomplish each day at work, home, and in the community. Identify long-term goals and set priorities together; teach how to action plan short-term goals.
2. Provide ergonomic education emphasizing self-analysis of activity, problem solving and practicing alternative methods to reduce joint stress. Practice each session.
3. Explore alternative equipment to operate the interactive whiteboard to reduce shoulder movement (e.g., light pens); alternative mouse and keyboard designs, use of voice-activated software to reduce keyboarding time.
4. Explore adapted equipment for carrying heavy briefcase: e.g., wheeled briefcase, folding hand cart. Discuss use of online assessment with kids to reduce marking and getting books home.
5. Explore using a stool with wheels around classroom to scoot between tables and save standing/bending.
6. Discuss fatigue management: pacing activities, microbreaks. Discuss goals to practice and how to fit into routines.
7. Review meal preparation activities; teach ergonomic methods; and review equipment available in shops to reduce wrist and MCP stress, e.g., easy jar and can openers, Good Grip® knives.
8. Review driving: padded steering wheel, hand and arm positioning.
9. Identify and fit appropriate right wrist splint, fit right compression glove. Explain wearing time of orthoses and purpose. Train in appropriate donning, doffing, and general care.
10. Teach intensive hand exercise program (range of movement and strength): practice and grade up weekly.
11. Review adapative equipment to help with handicrafts.

Assess the patient's comprehension	"We easily identified long- and short-term goals, and she is used to the concept of action planning. Finding ergonomic approaches makes sense to her."
Understand what she is doing	"Ms. B. is finding it hard to break habits during classroom activities; wonders how the kids will respond."
Compare actual to expected performance	"Using ergonomic methods and equipment, wearing glove at night and wrist splint at home (but not work), and finding pacing hard at school, pain and fatigue scores were reduced to 4 out of 10 at the end of the day. Exercise was well tolerated, and grip increased to 23 kg."
Know the person	"Ms. B. is well motivated and has made a number of changes. She is willing to continue to change."
Appreciate the context	"Pacing is difficult in school; I recommend she adds some 'quiet time' work-alone activities to most lessons (5 minutes), e.g., doing online tests that automatically score. She can take microbreaks while the children are completing these activities."

Next Steps

Discuss continuing to set weekly action plans. Schedule review appointment in 6 weeks to evaluate effect of changes at work and home, and give opportunity to raise problems not solved herself. Discuss how managing with pacing at school and attitude to splint wearing. Telephone after further 4 weeks to discuss progress. Then discharge and recommend that she contact occupational therapy via rheumatology if she needs help in future.

Anticipate present and future patient concerns	"Possible continuing problems are pacing and accepting wearing the wrist splint at school. I will encourage Ms. B. to focus on how pacing will help her keep going for longer and be able to do more for the kids in the long run."
Analyze patient's comprehension	"Ms. B. understands all of the concepts well but still struggles to accept pacing because she always puts the children's needs first."
Decide whether he or she should continue or discontinue therapy and/or return in the future	"A review appointment in 6 weeks will encourage her to keep setting action plans and review progress. The final follow-up call will be to check whether changes have been embedded into routines."

 Clinical Reasoning in Occupational Therapy Practice

Activity Analysis: Cooking

Ms. B. does very little cooking, mostly relying on ready meals and eating at the school cafeteria. The therapist taught ergonomic approaches during cooking skills but also wants Ms. B. to be able to apply ergonomic principles to finding solutions for herself in the future. How can she teach problem-solving skills? What tasks are involved in the activity of making a simple meal (soup and cheese on toast)? How can each task be made easier using ergonomic principles?

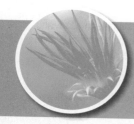

case example

Mrs. S.: Activities of Daily Living and Instrumental Activities of Daily Living with Osteoarthritis

Occupational Therapy Process	Clinical Reasoning Process	
	Objectives	**Examples of Therapist's Internal Dialogue**

Patient Information

Mrs. S. is 65 years old and lives with her husband in their own home. They owned and operated a small café for 25 years until they had to retire 5 years ago because the café site was redeveloped. Mrs. S. has bilateral knee pain and now can only walk short distances until she has to sit or lie down. She has pain in the right carpometacarpal (CMC) joint, especially when cooking, doing housework, and gardening (all of which she used to enjoy), but her husband now helps a lot. She has been having difficulty using the bath and toilet. She does not go out much. They have no children.

Understand the patient's diagnosis or condition

"Her medical records identify x-ray changes of joint narrowing in both knees, right CMC joint, and Heberden's nodes, with a diagnosis of osteoarthritis (OA). She is overweight (14 stones [196 pounds]), which will make her knee pain worse."

Know the person

"Mrs. S. used to be a sociable, busy person in the café. She now feels her arthritis has taken over and has given up many activities she enjoyed."

Reason for Referral to Occupational Therapy

Mrs. S. was referred by her family doctor because of her difficulties in personal care, home activities, and gardening.

Appreciate the context

"Her doctor thinks her pain is worse than expected considering the x-ray changes. He thinks psychosocial factors are contributing. He has advised about weight loss and exercise, but Mrs. S. does neither."

Develop provisional hypotheses

"Her pain is being made worse by low mood (from being forced to retire, pain, and helplessness), being overweight (putting extra stress on knee joints), deconditioning, lack of physical activity and use of ergonomic approaches, and poor occupational balance."

Assessment Process and Results

Mrs. S. was tearful during the initial interview. The Canadian Occupational Performance Measure (COPM) was used. (She did not have the concentration to do a self-report questionnaire). She identified her five most important activities as using the bathroom (bath and toilet), cooking, gardening, walking more, and getting out socially. She rated her performance between 2 and 4. She felt that there was little she could do to control pain and that she is relying too much on her husband (who has heart problems) because he helps lift her out of the bath, cooks, and does the housework.

On a Visual Analog Scale for knee pain, her scores after walking short distances are 8 out of 10; her hand pain was 8 out of 10; her QuickDASH (Quick Disabilities Arm Shoulder Hand) hand function score was 70.5 out of 100 (see Chapter 9); right pinch strength (B&L® pinch gauge) was 1.5 (norm is 4.5 kg).

Consider evaluation approach and methods

"Mrs. S.'s low mood is the priority. She wants to do more but feels helpless. With help, she could identify goals. Her concern about overburdening her husband (who has health problems) is a motivator for change."

Interpret observations

"She doesn't know where to start without making the pain worse. She fears exercise and believes doing more will make her joints worse.

"Many physical problems are due to poor grip and pinch strength and thumb/hand pain and reduced lower limb strength and endurance."

Occupational Therapy Problem List

1. Difficulties in activities of daily living (ADL) (toilet and bathing) because of knee pain, reduced mobility, and poor grip.
2. Difficulty with cooking because of poor grip and standing tolerance.
3. Difficulty with gardening: poor grip and standing tolerance, difficulty bending and kneeling, lack of stamina.
4. Reduced mobility: deconditioned and fearful of consequences of physical activity.
5. Limited social activities: because of low mood and poor mobility (was a very social person before retirement).
6. Lack of knowledge of self-management approaches: pain management, ergonomics, and physical activity.

Synthesize results

"If Mrs. S. continues as she is, her psychological and physical problems will get worse, her husband will have increasing difficulties, and he could have a heart attack."

Occupational Therapy Goal List

1. Use ergonomic approaches and adaptive equipment during personal care (toilet, bath), cooking, gardening and any other valued activities.
2. Increase occupational balance: engaging in more social, leisure, and community activities.
3. Perform hand exercises most days to increase hand muscle strength.
4. Increase physical activity to increase upper and lower limb muscle strength and endurance.
5. Wear a right CMC splint to reduce pain during activity.

Develop intervention hypotheses	"Mrs. S. is stuck in a cycle of pain, fear about making it worse, and unhappiness because of not doing activities she enjoys. We'll have to take things step by step, in valued activity–related goals, and explore new activities. I will help her see change is possible."
	"She was forced to retire, she never planned her retirement, and OA got in the way of doing so. Her low mood is due to poor occupational balance, social isolation, fear, and pain."
Select an intervention approach	"I will use motivational interviewing to enhance change and educate about condition/self-management. As Mrs. S. moves to preparation/action, I will start ergonomic and self-management education using cognitive-behavioral and self-efficacy enhancing approaches."
Consider what will occur in therapy, how often, and for how long	"Mrs. S. will be seen in occupational therapy as an outpatient for five 1-hour sessions over 8 weeks, plus a home visit after the first session."

Intervention

Session 1:

1. Motivational interviewing: explore pros and cons of changing/not changing. ("I am confident I can move her to preparation as her concern about husband's health is already beginning to overtake her own fears.")
2. Explain about OA and self-management, i.e., exercise and physical activity will not damage joints; can manage pain through ergonomic and other approaches.
3. Assess for toilet and bath aids; practice techniques.
4. Practice some ergonomic approaches in making a hot drink.
5. Home visit: fit bathroom aids and practice; do a kitchen and gardening assessment; discuss with Mrs. S. and husband how he can help Mrs. S. make changes; explore social, leisure, and physical activities they might both be interested in.

Sessions 2–5:

6. Practice ergonomic approaches and use of ergonomic equipment during kitchen activities (e.g., jar openers, Good Grip® knife and vegetable peeler, perch stool) and gardening activities (easy kneeler; long handled tools). Provide booklets with ideas on making house and garden activities easier.
7. Discuss activity pacing and help set weekly goals to gradually increase activity duration (household, gardening, and leisure activities).
8. Educate about importance of physical activity in reducing pain and improving muscle strength. Introduce to a walking program (loan pedometer to monitor activity). Introduce to Tai Chi (practice warm-up twice for 10 minutes). Set weekly goals to increase physical activity and locate a Tai Chi class to join.
9. Teach intensive hand exercise program (range of movement and strength; progress gradually)
10. Identify and fit appropriate CMC splint: explain wearing time and purpose. Train in donning, doffing, and splint care. Include splint use when practicing activities.

Assess the patient's comprehension	"Mrs. S. was surprised her pain was not made worse when trying ergonomic approaches and hand exercises and that the thumb splint made a difference."
Understand what she is doing	"She is doing more now; looks forward to Tai Chi (husband goes too) and chatting to class in the leisure center café after. She says it 'Feels like the old times.' Two class members used to go to their café!"
Compare actual to expected performance	"Hand and mobility pain scores improved to 4 out of 10, QuickDASH to 30.8, and pinch strength to 2.5 kg. Average daily steps increased from 2,000 to 4,500."
Know the person	"She is keen to learn more methods and is getting more confident. She is now looking for social groups they can join."
Appreciate the context	"Her husband is very supportive and keen to do things with his wife (e.g., Tai Chi). He read the booklets and is making changes to make things easier at home. He loves that Mrs. S. is more like her old self again."

Next Steps

Discuss with Mrs. and Mr. S. about setting weekly action plans to help continue making changes. Schedule a telephone review in 4 weeks to discuss progress, plans for future, and joining social group(s). Refer to physical therapy for knee exercises. Then discharge and recommend that they contact occupational therapy via family doctor if they need help in the future.

Anticipate present and future patient concerns	"Mrs. S. could lapse if her knee pain got worse or her mood lowers again (e.g., if husband's health got worse). Developing a social network will help provide support in future as they have no family."
Analyze patient's comprehension	"Her apprehension initially meant needing to start slowly and ensure she was 'on board.'" But once she decided to change, she gained confidence with my and her husband's support."
Decide whether he or she should continue or discontinue therapy and/ or return in the future	"A review call will give Mrs. and Mr. S. a goal to look forward to; they have been keen every week to tell me about progress. I am confident they will continue after discharge."

Summary Review Questions

1. List the primary differences between RA and OA.
2. Describe joint problems that can lead to diminished occupational performance for people with RA and OA
3. Besides joint problems, what other issues affect occupational performance for people with RA?
4. What are the major symptoms of FM that lead to diminished occupational performance?
5. What assessments can be used to evaluate occupational performance for people with RA, OA, and FM?
6. Describe ergonomic approaches in RA to prevent or restore occupational performance.
7. Describe a home hand exercise program suitable for people with RA or hand OA.
8. Name three resources for people with RA, OA, and FM to find alternate methods and assistive devices to improve occupational performance.
9. How does splinting help people with RA and OA improve occupational performance?
10. Describe strategies the OT can use to help people increase self-management.

Glossary

Allodynia—Pain in response to a normally nonpainful stimulus.

Bouchard's nodes—Hard, bony outgrowths at the PIP joints caused by OA.

Boutonniere deformity—Flexion of the PIP joint and hyperextension at the DIP joint.

Chronic fatigue syndrome—A condition characterized by persistent fatigue (lasting more than 6 months) not caused by ongoing exertion nor relieved by rest or known to be caused by other medical conditions. There can be multiple causes.

Disease-modifying antirheumatic drugs (DMARDs)—Drugs that affect the immune response or suppress the disease process (e.g., methotrexate).

Energy conservation techniques—Breaking up physically active periods with rest periods, resulting in increased amount of physical activity (Cordery & Rocchi, 1998).

Fibrillation—The initial degenerative changes in OA, marked by softening of the articular cartilage and development of vertical clefts between groups of cartilage cells.

Heberden's nodes—Hard, bony outgrowths at the DIP joints caused by OA.

Hyperalgaesia—Increased response to painful stimuli.

Joint protection techniques—The application of ergonomic principles in daily activities, work, and leisure to reduce internal and external stress on joints and soft tissues.

Mallet finger deformity—Deformity resulting from damage to the extensor tendon at the DIP joint.

Patient-reported outcome measures—Self-reported measures facilitating insight into the way patients perceive their health and the impact that treatments or adjustments to lifestyle have on their abilities and/or quality of life.

Stress system—The complex interplay between the nervous system and stress hormones. The hormonal system is known as the hypothalamic-pituitary-adrenal axis, a feedback loop by which signals from the brain trigger the release of hormones needed to respond to stress.

Swan-neck deformity—Hyperextension of the PIP joint and flexion at the DIP joint.

Synovitis—Inflammation of the synovial membrane (which lines synovial joint capsules, the function of which is to produce synovial fluid, which lubricates joints).

Volumetry—A water displacement measure of hand volume, conducted by inserting the hand to a specified depth in a measuring cylinder containing a specified amount of water.

Z deformity of the thumb—hyperextension of the interphalangeal joint and flexion of the MCP joint of the thumb.

References

Ablin, J. N., Buskila, D., Van Houdenhove B, Luyten, P., Atzeni, F., Sarzi-Puttini, P. (2011). Is fibromyalgia a discrete entity? *Autoimmunity Reviews, 11*(8),585-588.

Adams, J. (2010). Orthotics of the hand. In K. D. Dziedzic & A. Hammond (Eds.), *Rheumatology: Evidence based practice for physiotherapists and occupational therapists* (pp. 163-170). Edinburgh: Churchill Livingstone.

Adams, J., Burridge, J., Mullee, M., Hammond, A., & Cooper, C. (2008). The clinical effectiveness of static resting splints in early rheumatoid arthritis: A randomized controlled trial. *Rheumatology, 45,*1548-1553.

Allaire, S., & Keysor, J. J. (2009). Development of a structured interview tool to help patients identify and solve rheumatic condition-related work barriers. *Arthritis Care and Research, 61,* 988–995.

Allaire, S. H., Li, W., & La Valley, M. P. (2003). Reduction of job loss in persons with rheumatic diseases receiving vocational rehabilitation: A randomised controlled trial. *Arthritis & Rheumatism, 48,* 3212–3218.

American College of Rheumatology. (2011). Patient outcomes in rheumatology, 2011: A review of measures. *Arthritis Care and Research, 63 (Suppl.),* S1–S490.

American Occupational Therapy Association. (2008). Occupational therapy practice framework: Domain & process (2nd ed.). *American Journal of Occupational Therapy, 62,* 625–683.

Aparicio, V. A., Ortega F. B., Heredia J. M., Carbonnell-Baeza, A., Sjostrom, M., & Delgado-Fernandez, M. (2011). Hand grip strength test as a complementary tool in the assessment of fibromyalgia severity in women. *Archives of Physical Medicine and Rehabilitation, 92*(1),83-88.

Arnold, L. M., Clauw, D. J., & McCarberg, B. H. (2011). Improving the recognition and diagnosis of fibromyalgia. *Mayo Clinic Proceedings, 86,* 457–464.

Arthritis Care. (2004). OA Nation. London: Arthritis Care. Retrieved April 1, 2012 from http://www.arthritiscare.org.uk/@3235/Forhealthprofessionals/OANation.

Arthur, V., & Hill, J. (2006). The musculoskeletal system and the rheumatic diseases. In J. Hill (Ed.), *Rheumatology nursing: A creative approach* (2nd ed., pp. 25–92). Chichester, UK: John Wiley and Sons Ltd.

Backman, C., Village, J., & Lacaille, D. (2008). The Ergonomic Assessment Tool for Arthritis: Development and pilot testing. *Arthritis Care and Research, 59,* 1495–1503. Retrieved April 1, 2012 from http://ergotool.arthritisresearch.ca/.

Bandura, A. (1977). Self-efficacy: Towards a unifying theory of behavior change. *Psychology Reviews, 84,* 191–215.

Bennett, R. M., Friend, R., Jones, K. D., Ward, R., Han, B. K., & Ross, R. L. (2009). The Revised Fibromyalgia Impact Questionnaire (FIQR): Validation and psychometric properties. *Arthritis Research and Therapy, 11,* R120.

Bland, J. H., Melvin, J. L., & Hasson, S. (2000). Osteoarthritis. In J. L. Melvin, & K. M. Ferrell (Eds.), *Adult rheumatic diseases: Rheumatologic rehabilitation series* (Vol. 2, pp. 94–99). Bethesda, MD: American Occupational Therapy Association.

Boustedt, C., Nordenskiold, U., & Lundgren, N. A. (2009). Effects of a hand-joint protection programme with an addition of splinting and exercise: One year follow-up. *Clinical Rheumatology, 28,* 793–799.

Braveman, B., Robson, M., Velozo, C., Kielhofner, G., Fisher, G., Forsyth, K, & Kerschbaum, J. (2005). *The Worker Role Interview 10.1 Manual.* Chicago: University of Chicago Model of Human Occupation Clearing House. Retrieved April 1, 2012 from http://www.uic.edu/depts/moho/assess/wri.html

Brorsson, S., Hilliges, M., Sollerman, C., & Nilsdotter, A. (2009). Six-week hand exercise programme improves strength and hand function in patients with rheumatoid arthritis. *Disability and Rehabilitation, 41,* 338–342.

Busch, A. J., Webber, S. C., Brachaniec, M., Bidonde, J., Bello-Haas, V. D., Danyliw, A. D., Overend, T. J., Richards, R. S., Sawant, A., & Schachter, C. L. (2011). Exercise therapy for fibromyalgia. *Current Pain & Headache Reports, 15,* 358–367.

Carville, S. F., Arendt-Nielsen, S., Bliddal, H., Blotman, F., Branco, J. C., Buskila, D., Da Silva, J. A., Danneskiold-Samsoe, B., Dincer, F., Henriksson, C., Henriksson, K. G., Kosek, E., Longley, K., Mc Carthy, G. M., Perrot, S., Puszczewicz, M., Sarzi-Puttini, P., Silman, A., Spath, M., & Choy, E. H. (2007). EULAR evidence based recommendations for the management of fibromyalgia syndrome. *Annals of the Rheumatic Diseases, 67,* 536–541.

Centers for Disease Control and Prevention. (2012). Arthritis-related statistics. Retrieved April 1, 2012 from http://www.cdc.gov/arthritis/data_statistics/arthritis_related_stats.htm.

Chung, K. C., Pillsbury, M. S., Walters, M. R., & Hayward, R. A. (1998). Reliability and validity testing of the Michigan Hand Outcomes Questionnaire. *Journal of Hand Surgery, 23A,* 575–587.

Combe, B., Landewé, R., Lukas, C., Bolosiu, H. D., Breedveld, F., Dougados, M., Emery, P., Ferraccioli, G., Hazes, J. M., Klareskog, L., Machold, K., Martin-Mola, E., Nielsen, H., Silman, A., Smolen, J., & Yazici, H. (2007). EULAR recommendations for the management of early arthritis: Report of a task force of the European Standing Committee for International Clinical Studies Including Therapeutics (ESCISIT). *Annals of the Rheumatic Diseases, 66,* 34–45.

Cordery, J., & Rocchi, M. (1998). Joint protection and fatigue management. In J. Melvin & G. Jensen (Eds.), *Rheumatologic rehabilitation series: Assessment and management* (Vol. 1, pp. 279–321). Bethesda, MD: American Occupational Therapy Association.

Crosby, C. A., & Wehbe, M. A. (1994). Hand strength: Normative values. *Journal of Hand Surgery, 19,* 665–670.

Dellhag, B., & Bjelle, A. (1995). A grip ability test for use in rheumatology practice. *Journal of Rheumatology, 41,* 138–163.

Dziedzic, K., Hill, S., Nicholls, E., Hammond, A., Handy, J., Thomas, E., & Hay, E. (2011). Self-management, joint protection and hand exercises in hand osteoarthritis: A multicentred randomised controlled trial in the community. *Annals of the Rheumatic Diseases, 70 (Suppl. 3),* 746.

Eberhardt, K. B., Rydgren, L. C., Pettersson, H., & Wollheim, F. A. (1990). Early rheumatoid arthritis: Onset, course and outcome over two years. *Rheumatology International, 10,* 135–142.

Fautrel, B., Hilliquin, B., Rozenberg, S., Allaert, F. A., Coste, P., Leclerc, A., & Rossignol, M. (2005). Impact of osteoarthritis: A nationwide survey of 10,000 patients consulting for OA. *Joint Bone Spine, 72,* 235–240.

Feinberg, J., & Brandt, K. D. (1992). Effect of the arthritis health professional on compliance with use of resting hand splints by patients with rheumatoid arthritis. *Arthritis Care and Research, 5,* 17–23.

Furst, G., Gerber, L. H., Smith, C. C., Fisher, S., & Shulman, B. (1987). A program for improving energy conservation behaviours in adults with rheumatoid arthritis. *American Journal of Occupational Therapy, 41,* 102–111.

Gignac, M. A. (2005). Arthritis and employment: An examination of behavioural coping efforts to manage workplace activity limitations. *Arthritis and Rheumatism,* [now called *Arthritis Care and Research*] *53,* 328–336.

Gilworth, G., Chamberlain, M. A., & Harvey, A. (2003). Development of a work instability scale for rheumatoid arthritis. *Arthritis Care and Research, 49,* 349–353.

Glombiewski, J. A., Sawyer, A. T., Guterman, J., Koenig, K., Rief, W., & Hofmann, S. G. (2010). Psychological treatments for fibromyalgia: A meta-analysis. *Pain, 151,* 280–295.

Gouttebarge, V., Wind, H., Kuijer, P. F. M., Sluiter, J. K., & Frings-Dresen, M. H. (2004). Reliability and validity of Functional Capacity Evaluation methods: A systematic review with reference to Blankenship system, Ergos work simulator, Ergo-Kit and Isernhagen work system. *International Archives of Occupational and Environmental Health, 77,* 527–537

Hammond, A. (2004). What is the role of the occupational therapist? *Best Practice and Research in Clinical Rheumatology, 18,* 491–505.

Hammond, A. (2010). Joint protection. In K. Dziedzic & A. Hammond (Eds.), *Rheumatology: Evidence based practice for physiotherapists and occupational therapists* (pp. 137–150). Edinburgh: Churchill Livingstone.

Hammond, A., Bryan, J., & Hardy, A. (2008). Effects of a modular behavioural arthritis education programme: A pragmatic parallel group randomized controlled trial. *Rheumatology, 47,* 1712–1718.

Hammond, A., & Freeman, K. (2001). One year outcomes of a randomised controlled trial of an educational-behavioural joint protection programme for people with rheumatoid arthritis. *Rheumatology, 40,* 1044–1051.

Hammond, A., & Freeman, K. (2004). The long-term outcomes of a randomised controlled trial of an educational-behavioural joint protection programme for people with rheumatoid arthritis. *Clinical Rehabilitation, 18,* 520–528.

Hammond, A., Kidao, R., & Young, A. (2000). Hand impairment and function in early rheumatoid arthritis. *Arthritis and Rheumatism, 43 (Suppl. 9),* S285.

Hammond, A., Tennant, A., Tyson, S., Nordenskiold, U., & Gill, R. (2011). Development of the United Kingdom Evaluation of Daily Activities Questionnaire in Rheumatoid Arthritis using Rasch Analysis. *Arthritis & Rheumatism, 63(Suppl. 10),* S1000.

Hammond, A., Tyson, S., Tennant, A., Nordenskiold, U., & Greenhill, Y. (2012). Development of the United Kingdom Evaluation of Daily Activity Questionnaire in rheumatoid arthritis: Psychometric testing. *Annals of the Rheumatic Diseases, 71(Suppl. 3),* 753.

Hammond, A., Young, A., & Kidao, R. (2004). A randomised controlled trial of occupational therapy for people with early rheumatoid arthritis. *Annals of the Rheumatic Diseases, 63,* 23–30.

Hauser, W., Bernardy, K., Arnold, B., Offenbacher, M., & Schiltenwolf, M. (2009). Efficacy of multicomponent treatment in fibromyalgia syndrome: A meta-analysis of randomized controlled clinical trials. *Arthritis Care and Research, 61,* 216–224.

Helewa, A., & Goldsmith, C. H. (1991). Effects of occupational therapy home service on patients with rheumatoid arthritis. *Lancet, 337,* 1453–1457.

Helmick, C. G., Felson, D. T., Lawrence, R. C., Gabriel, S., Hirsch, R., Kwoh, C. K., Liang, M. H., Kremers, H. M., Mayes, M.D., Merkel, P. A., Pillemer, S. R., Reveille, J. D., & Stone, J. H. (2008). Estimates of the prevalence of arthritis and other rheumatic conditions in the United States: Part I. *Arthritis & Rheumatism, 58,* 15–25.

Henriksson, C., Liedberg, G., & Gerdle, B. (2005). Women with fibromyalgia: Work and rehabilitation. *Disability and Rehabilitation, 27,* 685–695.

Hewlett, S., Ambler, N., Almeida, C., Cliss, A., Hammond, A., Kitchen, K., Knops, B., Pope, D., Spears, M., Swinkels, A., & Pollock, J. (2011). Self-management of fatigue in rheumatoid arthritis: A randomised controlled trial of group cognitive-behavioural therapy. *Annals of the Rheumatic Diseases, 70,* 1060–1067.

Hewlett, S., Cockshott, Z., Kirwan, J., Barrett, J., Stamp, J., & Haslock, I. (2001). Development and validation of a self-efficacy scale for use in British patients with rheumatoid arthritis (RASE). *Rheumatology, 40,* 1221–1230.

Hochberg, M. C., Altman, R. D., April, K. T., Benkhalti, M., Guyatt, G., McGowan, J., Towheed, T., Welch, V., Wells, G., & Tugwell, P. (2012). American College of Rheumatology 2012 recommendations for the use of nonpharmacological and pharmacological therapies in osteoarthritis of the hand, hip and knee. *Arthritis Care and Research, 64,* 465–474.

Iversen, M., Hammond, A., & Betteridge, N. (2010). Self-management of rheumatic diseases: State of the art and future directions. *Annals of the Rheumatic Diseases, 69,* 955–963.

Jones, J., Rutledge, D. N., Jones, K. D., Matallana, L., & Rooks, D. S. (2008). Self-assessed physical function levels of women with fibromyalgia: A national survey. *Women's Health Issues, 18,* 406–412.

Jordan, K. M., Arden, N. K., Doherty, M., Bannwarth, B., Bijlsma, J. W., Dieppe, P., Gunther, K., Hauselmann, H., Herrero-Beaumont, G., Kaklamanis, P., Lohmander, S., Leeb, B., Lequesne, M., Mazieres, B., Martin-Mola, E., Pavelka, K., Pendleton, A., Punzi, L., Serni, U., Swoboda, B., Verbruggen, G., Zimmerman-Gorska, I., & Dougados, M. (2003). EULAR recommendations 2003: An evidence based approach to the management of knee osteoarthritis: Report of a Task Force of the Standing Committee for International Clinical Studies Including Therapeutic Trials (ESCISIT). *Annals of the Rheumatic Diseases, 62,* 1145–1155.

Katz, P., Morris, A., Gregorich, S., Yazdany, J., Eisner, M., Yelin, E., & Blanc, P. (2009). Valued life activity disability played a significant role in self-rated health among adults with chronic health conditions. *Journal of Clinical Epidemiology, 62,* 158–166.

Kjeken, I., Dagfinrud, H., Slatkowsky-Christensen, B., Mowinckel, P., Uhlig, T., Kvien, T. K., & Finset, A. (2005). Activity limitations and participation restrictions in women with hand osteoarthritis: Patients' descriptions and associations between dimensions of functioning. *Annals of the Rheumatic Diseases, 64,* 1633–1638.

Kjeken, I., Moller, C., & Kvien, T. (1995). Use of commercially produced elastic wrist orthoses in chronic arthritis. *Arthritis Care and Research, 8,* 108–113.

Lacaille, D., White, M. A., Rogers, P. A., Backman, C. L., Gignac, M. A., & Esdaile, J. M. (2008). A proof-of-concept study of the "Employment and Arthritis: Making It Work" program. *Arthritis Care and Research, 59,* 1647–1655.

Law, M., Baptiste, S. Carswell, A., McColl, M. A., Polatajko, H., & Pollock, N. (2005). *The Canadian occupational performance measure* (4th ed.). Ottawa, Canada: Canadian Association of Occupational Therapists.

Macedo, A., Oakley, S. P., Panayi, G. S., & Kirkham, B. W. (2009). Functional and work outcomes improve in patients with rheumatoid arthritis who receive targeted, comprehensive occupational therapy. *Arthritis Care and Research, 61,* 1522–1530.

Masiero, S., Boniolo, A., Wassermann, L., Machiedo, H., Volante, D., & Punzi, L. (2007). Effects of an educational-behavioural joint protection programme on people with moderate to severe rheumatoid arthritis: A randomised controlled trial. *Clinical Rheumatology, 26,* 2043–2050.

Mason, P., & Butler, C. C. (2010). *Health behaviour change: A guide for practitioners* (2nd ed.). Edinburgh: Churchill Livingstone.

McKnight, P. T., & Kwoh, C. K. (1992). Randomised controlled trial of compression gloves in rheumatoid arthritis. *Arthritis Care and Research, 5,* 223–227.

Meenan, R. F., Mason, J. H., Anderson, J. J., Guccione, A. A., & Kazis, L. E. (1992). AIMS2. The content and properties of a revised and expanded arthritis impact measurement scales health status questionnaire. *Arthritis and Rheumatism, 35*, 1–10.

National Institute for Health and Clinical Excellence. (2008). *Osteoarthritis: National clinical guideline for care and management in adults.* London, UK: Royal College of Physicians.

National Institute for Health and Clinical Excellence. (2009). *Rheumatoid arthritis: National clinical guideline for the management and treatment in adults.* London, UK: Royal College of Physicians.

Ndosi, M., Tennant, A., Bergsten, U., Kukkurainen, M. L., Machado, P., de la Torre-Aboki, J., Vlieland, T. P., Zangi, H. A., & Hill, J. (2011). Cross-cultural validation of the Educational Needs Assessment Tool in RA in 7 European countries. *BMC Musculoskeletal Disorders, 12*, 110. Retrieved August 17, 2012 from http://www.biomedcentral.com/1471-2474/12/110.

Niedermann, K., de Bie, R. A., Kubli, R., Ciurea, A., Steurer-Stey, C., Villiger, P. M., & Buchi, S. (2011). Effectiveness of individual resource-oriented joint protection education in people with rheumatoid arthritis. A randomized controlled trial. *Patient Education & Counseling, 82*, 42–48.

Nordenskiold, U., Grimby, G., & Dahlin-Ivanoff, S. (1998). Questionnaire to evaluate the effects of assistive devices and altered working methods in women with rheumatoid arthritis. *Clinical Rheumatology, 17*, 6–16.

Oosterveld, F. G. J., & Rasker, J. J. (1990). The effect of pressure gradient and thermolactyl control gloves in arthritis patients with swollen hands. *British Journal of Rheumatology, 29*, 197–200.

Paulsen, T., Grotle, M., Garratt, A., & Kjeken, I. (2010). Development and psychometric testing of the patient-reported Measure of Activity Performance of the Hand (MAP-HAND) in rheumatoid arthritis. *Journal of Rehabilitation Medicine, 42*, 636–644.

Pincus, T., Sumney, J. A., Soraci, S. A., Wallston, K. A., & Hummon, N. P. (1983). Assessment of patient satisfaction in activities of daily living using a modified Stanford health assessment questionnaire. *Arthritis and Rheumatism, 26*, 1346–1353.

Plant, M. J., Linton, S., Dodd, E., Jones, P. W., & Dawes, P. T. (1993). The GALS locomotor screen and disability. *Annals of the Rheumatic Diseases, 52*, 886–890.

Prevoo, M., Van't Hof, M., Kuper, H., van Leeuwen, M. A., van de Putte, L. B., & van Riel, P. L. (1995). Modified disease activity scores that include twenty-eight joint counts. Development and validation in a prospective longitudinal study of patients with rheumatoid arthritis. *Arthritis & Rheumatism, 38*, 44–48.

Prochaska, J. O., DiClemente, C. C., & Norcross, J. C. (1992). In search of how people change. Applications to addictive behaviours. *American Psychologist, 47*, 1102–1114.

Rennie, H. (1996). Evaluation of the effectiveness of a metacarpophalangeal ulnar deviation orthosis. *Journal of Hand Therapy, 9*, 371–377.

Ronningen, A., & Kjeken, I. (2008). Effect of an intensive hand exercise programme in patients with rheumatoid arthritis. *Scandinavian Journal of Occupational Therapy, 15*, 173–183 .

Sallinen, M., Kukkurainen, M. L., Peltokallio, L., & Mikkelsson, M. (2009). Women's narratives on experience of work ability and functioning in fibromyalgia. *Musculoskeletal Care, 8*, 18–26.

Silva, A. C., Jones, A., Silva, P. G., & Natour, J. (2008). Effectiveness of a night-time hand positioning splint in rheumatoid arthritis: A randomised controlled trial. *Journal of Rehabilitation Medicine, 40*, 749–754.

Silva, P. G., Lombardi, I., Breitschwerdt, C., Poli Araujo, P. M., & Natour, J. (2008). Functional thumb orthosis for type I and II boutonniere deformity on the dominant hand in patients with rheumatoid arthritis: A randomized controlled study. *Clinical Rehabilitation, 22*, 684–689.

Singh, J. A., Furst, D. E., Bharat, A., Curtis, J. R., Kavanaugh, A. F., Kremer, J. M., Moreland, L. W., O'Dell, J., Winthrop, K. L., Beukelman, T., Bridges, S. L., Jr., Chatham, W. W., Paulus, H. E., Suarez-Almazor, M., Bombardier, C., Dougados, M., Khanna, D., King, C. M., Leong, A. L., Matteson, E. L., Schousboe, J. T., Moynihan, E., Kolba, K. S., Jain, A., Volkmann, E. R., Agrawal, H., Bae, S., Mudano, A. S., Patkar, N. M., & Saag, K. G. (2012). 2012 update of the American College of Rheumatology 2008 recommendations for the use of non-biologic and biologic disease modifying antirheumatic drugs in rheumatoid arthritis. *Arthritis Care and Research, 64*, 625–639.

Steultjens, E. M. J., Dekker, J., Bouter, L. M., van Schaardenburg, D., van Kuyk, M. A., & van den Ende, C. H. (2004). Occupational therapy for rheumatoid arthritis. *Cochrane Database of Systematic Reviews, 1*, CD003114.

Symmons, D., Turner, G., Webb, R., Asten, P., Barrett, E., Lunt, M., Scott, D., & Silman, A. (2002). The prevalence of rheumatoid arthritis in the United Kingdom: New estimates for a new century. *Rheumatology, 41*(7), 793–800.

Valdes, K., & Marik, T. (2010). A systematic review of conservative interventions for osteoarthritis of the hand. *Journal of Hand Therapy, 23*, 334–351.

van der Giesen, F. J., van Lankveld, W. J., Kremers-Selten, C., Peeters, A. J., Stern, E. B., Le Cessie, S., Nelissen, R. G., & Vliet Vlieland, T. P. (2009). Effectiveness of two finger splints for swan neck deformity in patients with rheumatoid arthritis: A randomized, crossover trial. *Arthritis Care and Research, 61*, 1025–1031.

Van Lankveld, W., van't Pad Bosch, P., Bakker, J., Terwindt, S., Franssen, M., & van Riel, P. (1996). Sequential occupational dexterity assessment (SODA): A new test to measure hand disability. *Journal of Hand Therapy, 9*, 27–32.

Veehof, M. M., Taal, E., Heijnsdijk-Rouwenhorst, L. M., & van de Laar, M. A. (2008). Efficacy of wrist working splints in patients with rheumatoid arthritis: A randomized controlled study. *Arthritis Care and Research, 59*, 1698–1704.

Verstappen, S. M. M., Boonen, A., Bijlsma, J. W. J., Buskens, E., Verkleij, H., Schenk, Y., van Albada-Kuipers, G. A., Hofman, D. M., & Jacobson, J. W. (2004). Working status among Dutch patients with rheumatoid arthritis: Work disability and working conditions. *Rheumatology, 44*, 202–206.

Waljee, J. F., Chung, K. C., Kim, H. M., Burns, P. B., Burke, F. D., Wilgis, E. F., & Fox, D. A. (2010). Validity and responsiveness of the Michigan Hand Questionnaire in patients with rheumatoid arthritis: A multicentre, international study. *Arthritis Care and Research, 62*, 1569–1577.

Wolfe, F., Clauw, D. J., Fitzcharles, M. A., Goldenberg, D. L., Katz, R. S., Mease, P., Russell, A. S., Russell, I. J., Winfield, J. B., & Yunus, M. B. (2010). The American College of Rheumatology preliminary diagnostic criteria for fibromyalgia and measure of symptom severity. *Arthritis Care and Research, 62*, 600–610.

Zhang, W., Doherty, M., Arden, N., Bannwarth, B., Bijlsma, J., Gunther, K. P., Hauselmann, H. J., Herrero-Beaumont, G., Jordan, K., Kaklamanis, P., Leeb, B., Lequesne, M., Lohmander, S., Mazieres, B., Martin-Mola, E., Pavelka, K., Pendelton, A., Punzi, L., Swoboda, B., Varatojo, R., Verbruggen, G., Zimmermann-Gorska, I., & Dougados, M. (2005). EULAR evidence based recommendations for the management of hip osteoarthritis: Report of a task force of the EULAR Standing Committee for International Clinical Studies Including Therapeutics (ESCISIT). *Annals of the Rheumatic Diseases, 64*, 669–681.

Zhang, W., Doherty, M., Arden, N., Bannwarth, B., Bijlsma, J., Gunther, K. P., Hauselmann, H. J., Herrero-Beaumont, G., Jordan, K., Kaklamanis, P., Leeb, B., Lequesne, M., Lohmander, S., Mazieres, B., Martin-Mola, E., Pavelka, K., Pendelton, A., Punzi, L., Swoboda, B., Varatojo, R., Verbruggen, G., Zimmermann-Gorska, I., & Dougados, M. (2007). EULAR evidence based recommendations for the management of hand osteoarthritis: Report of a Task Force of the EULAR Standing Committee for International Clinical Studies Including Therapeutics (ESCISIT). *Annals of the Rheumatic Diseases, 66*, 377–388.

Zijlstra, T., Heijnsdijk-Rouwenhorst, L., & Rasker, J. J. (2004). Silver ring splints improve dexterity in patients with rheumatoid arthritis. *Arthritis Care and Research, 51*, 947–951.

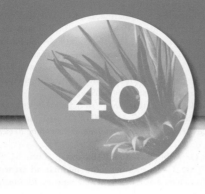

40

Burn Injuries

Monica A. Pessina and Amy C. Orroth

Learning Objectives

After studying this chapter, the reader will be able to do the following:

1. Describe differences between superficial, superficial partial-thickness, deep partial-thickness, and full-thickness burn injuries.
2. Explain the rationale for splinting and positioning programs for patients with burn injuries.
3. Outline occupational therapy treatment techniques for each phase of burn recovery.
4. Give examples of using activity as a modality in the acute and rehabilitation phases of burn recovery.
5. Describe potential complications and treatment strategies for hand burns.
6. Discuss the effects of a burn injury on a patient's psychosocial functioning.

Approximately 450,000 burn injuries that required medical treatment occurred in the United States in 2011, resulting in 3,000 fire- and burn-related deaths (American Burn Association [ABA], 2011). Thermal damage to the skin can be caused by fire, contact with a hot object or hot liquid (scald burn), radiation, chemicals, or electricity. According to statistics from 2001 to 2010, the majority of burns in adults occur in males (70%); the most common cause of burns is fire/flame (44%); and most burns occur in the home, followed by injuries in the workplace (ABA, 2011). These data also show that hot food and liquid spills are the most common source of burns to children. Approximately one-half of patients with burn injuries are admitted to regional burn centers designated by the American Burn Association; the remainder are treated at local or regional hospitals (ABA, 2011). Therefore, every occupational therapist should understand the principles of care and rehabilitation of patients with burn injuries. Treatment of these injuries requires a comprehensive approach by a qualified burn treatment team, including a skilled occupational therapist. This chapter explores the unique role of occupational therapy in treatment of burn patients, from the initial injury to the patient's return to independent function. Topics include various phases of burn rehabilitation, scar management, psychosocial issues, and reconstructive surgery. We hope to convey the unique and rewarding aspects of working with patients with burn injuries.

BURN CLASSIFICATION

In the past, burn depth was classified as first, second, or third degree. Today, the preferred classification system more accurately describes the level of cellular injury. The terms in use are superficial, superficial partial-thickness, deep partial-thickness, and full-thickness. Burns typically have mixed depths, which necessitates that the burn team carefully assess the appearance and progress of each area of the wound site. Disruption of any portion of the skin has the potential to interfere with its normal functions, which include temperature regulation, excretion, sensation, vitamin D synthesis, and acting as a barrier against infection and dehydration (Falkel, 1994). Occupational therapists may treat patients with all levels of thermal injury. It is important to differentiate among the classifications to plan appropriate intervention.

Superficial Burns

Superficial burns damage cells only in the epidermis (Malick & Carr, 1982; Staley, Richard, & Falkel, 1994) (Fig. 40-1). These injuries are painful and red. With a well-nourished and intact epithelial bed at the base of the hair follicles, these injuries heal spontaneously within approximately 7 days and leave no permanent scar (Malick & Carr, 1982).

Superficial Partial-Thickness Burns

Superficial partial-thickness burns damage cells in the epidermis and the upper level of the dermis (Malick & Carr, 1982; Staley, Richard, & Falkel, 1994). The most common sign of a superficial partial-thickness burn is intact blisters over the injured area (Staley, Richard, & Falkel, 1994). Hair follicles remain intact, because these are found in the deeper layers of the dermis. In addition, these injuries are painful because of the irritation of the nerve endings in the dermal layer. Superficial partial-thickness burns heal spontaneously within 7–21 days and leave minimal or no scarring (Staley, Richard, & Falkel, 1994).

Deep Partial-Thickness Burns

Deep partial-thickness burns cause cell injury in the epidermis and severe damage to the dermal layer (Malick & Carr, 1982; Staley, Richard, & Falkel, 1994). These injuries appear blotchy, with areas of whitish color interspersed throughout the wound, which is the result of damage to the blood vessels in the dermal layer (Malick & Carr, 1982). The injury site is painful. Pressure sensation is intact, but light-touch sensation is diminished because of the relative locations of receptors for these modalities (Staley, Richard, & Falkel, 1994). Spontaneous healing of deep partial-thickness burns is sluggish (3–5 weeks) because vascularity in the dermal layer is impaired. Therefore, the risk of significant scarring is increased (Staley, Richard, & Falkel, 1994). For this reason, deep partial-thickness burns are often grafted to expedite healing and minimize scarring.

Full-Thickness Injury Burns

In a full-thickness injury, both the epidermis and the dermal layer are destroyed (Malick & Carr, 1982; Staley, Richard, & Falkel, 1994). These wounds appear white or waxy because of the underlying adipose tissue and are inherently insensate because of the complete destruction of the dermal nerve endings (Malick & Carr, 1982). Full-thickness burns require surgical intervention, such as skin grafting (Malick & Carr, 1982; Staley, Richard, & Falkel, 1994), because there are no dermal elements to support the regrowth of epithelial tissue. Some burns, such as electrical burns, may damage structures below the dermis, including subcutaneous fat, muscle, or bone.

RULE OF NINES

The rule of nines is a commonly used technique to determine burn size in adults (Fig. 40-2). For example, if an adult received a burn that included the anterior and posterior surfaces of his right arm (9%), his anterior head and neck (4.5%), and his anterior chest (18%), then his total body surface area (TBSA) affected would be 31.5%. To determine the TBSA of a burn injury in children and infants, a modification of this technique, the Lund-Browder chart, is used. In addition, in

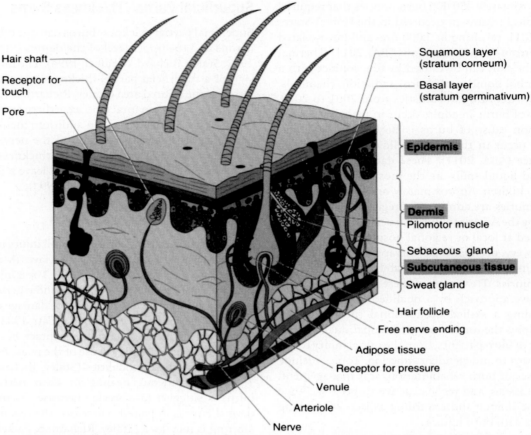

Figure 40-1 Cross section of the skin. (From Willis, M. C. [1996]. *Medical terminology: The language of health care.* Baltimore: Williams & Wilkins.)

both children and adults, it is a widely used estimate that the palmar surface of one's hand is approximately 1% TBSA. The burn percentage TBSA is used for the following:

- Calculating nutritional and fluid requirements
- Determining level of acuity to establish the level of medical treatment needed (i.e., admission to an intensive care unit)
- Classifying patients for use of standardized protocols

PHASES OF BURN MANAGEMENT AND REHABILITATION

Identifying specific phases of burn management helps to describe the role of occupational therapy for patients with burn injuries. These include the emergent, acute, and rehabilitation phases. Each of the phases, along with accompanying occupational therapy considerations, are described.

Emergent Phase

The emergent phase of a burn injury is considered to be from initial injury to approximately 72 hours after the burn (Grigsby deLinde & Miles, 1995).

Medical Management

During the emergent phase, the medical team attempts to stabilize the patient. This may include fluid resuscitation, establishment of adequate tissue perfusion by means of mechanical ventilation, and achievement of cardiopulmonary stability. Associated injuries, such as fractures, are also evaluated and treated during this time.

Inhalation Injury. An important consideration in the emergent phase is the possibility of an inhalation injury. Damage to the upper airway from inhaling either smoke or noxious gases results in an inhalation injury. This damages the respiratory epithelium and can impair gas exchange. Inhalation injuries can significantly increase mortality rate (Cioffi & Rue, 1991). Singed eyebrows, soot around the nares, and facial edema are indications of an inhalation injury (Cioffi & Rue, 1991). Diagnosis is confirmed by analysis of arterial blood gases, chest radiographs, and bronchoscopy. In addition, edema can quickly develop in the airway and constrict breathing. Therefore, patients with significant burn injuries are usually intubated (placed on mechanical ventilation) to maintain an open airway until the risk of airway closure caused by edema has diminished.

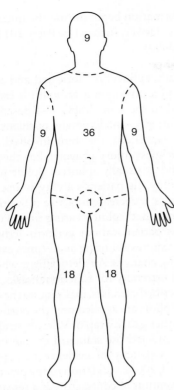

Figure 40-2 Rules of nines. (Reprinted with permission from Malik, M. H., & Carr, J. A. [1982]. *Manual on management of the burn patient.* Pittsburgh: Harmarville Rehabilitation Center.)

Escharotomy and Fasciotomy. Circulation can be compromised when burn injuries encircle a body segment. This is due to the inelasticity of the eschar (burned tissue) combined with increased internal pressure within fascial compartments. Local increase in pressure in the extremities compresses blood vessels and reduces blood flow (Sheridan et al., 1995). Symptoms of increased compartmental pressure include paresthesias, coldness, and decreased or absent pulses in the extremities. In the trunk, inelastic eschar can act as a corset, limiting lung expansion and preventing adequate respiration. In both cases, surgical intervention (escharotomy and/or fasciotomy) is required to relieve the pressure and prevent tissue death. An escharotomy is a surgical incision through the eschar, whereas a fasciotomy is a deeper incision extending through the fascia. Unless exposed tendon is present, the escharotomy region can be mobilized during therapy (Grigsby deLinde & Miles, 1995).

Dressings. After the initial burn assessment, the nursing staff applies dressings. The functions of dressings include protecting the wound against infection, maintaining contact between the topical agent and the wound, superficially debriding the wound, and providing comfort for the patient (Grigsby deLinde & Miles, 1995). Debriding is the

removal of devitalized tissue from the wound site. Types of topical agents vary widely, although most are wide-spectrum antimicrobials. Examples include mafenide acetate (Sulfamylon), silver sulfadiazine (Silvadene), and 0.5% silver nitrate solution (Duncan & Driscoll, 1991). As a rule, the nursing staff changes the dressings; however, by periodically participating in dressing removal and application, the occupational therapist makes opportunities to view the healing wounds. This allows the therapist to monitor healing and adjust the therapy program accordingly.

Infection Control. One of the functions of the skin is to act as a barrier against infection (Falkel, 1994). Therefore, a patient with a burn injury is susceptible to infection. It is essential that all staff, family, and visitors adhere to infection control procedures. This includes frequent hand washing, use of gloves when necessary, and avoiding cross-contamination through instruments and equipment (Procedures for Practice 40-1).

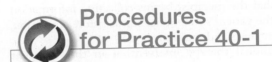

Procedures for Practice 40-1

Hand Hygiene

Proper hand hygiene, either by use of traditional hand washing with soap and water or the use of hand disinfectants, is essential in the reduction of infections for you and your clients. A study by Kampf and Löffler (2009) noted that nosocomial infection rates can be reduced as much as 40% by proper hand hygiene. A nosocomial infection is a hospital-acquired infection.

When to Perform Proper Hand Hygiene

- Before and after all patient contact
- After removing gloves used to perform a task involving contact with blood, body fluids, or infectious material
- After handling possibly infectious devices or equipment
- Before and after preparing and eating food

General Procedure for Hand Washing

- Dispense paper towel
- Push up long sleeves
- Wet hands and wrists
- Apply antiseptic solution or soap
- Use friction to clean between fingers, under nails, and palms and backs of hands; effective scrubbing lasts at least 20–30 seconds
- Rinse hands and towel dry
- Turn off faucet using paper towel
- Dispose of paper towel in appropriate trash barrel
- Waterless hand cleaner can be used if hand washing facilities are available

Contracture Formation

Patients with burn injuries are at significant risk for contractures. Wound contracture, a normal physiological response to an open wound (Greenhalgh & Staley, 1994; Jordan, Daher, & Wasil, 2000) combined with prolonged immobilization, creates an opportunity for permanent soft tissue contracture. Contractures tend to occur in predictable patterns, usually flexed, shortened positions (e.g., elbow flexion, shoulder adduction, or knee flexion) and can considerably limit the patient's ability to perform activities of daily living (ADL). For example, decreased elbow extension may limit the patient's ability to dress.

Occupational Therapy during the Emergent Phase

During the emergent phase, the occupational therapist performs a screen of the patient's needs. A full evaluation is deferred until after the emergent phase, when the patient is more medically stable. During the screen, the therapist notes the distribution of the burn and which joints are involved. This allows the occupational therapist to establish an appropriate splinting and positioning program. It is also during this time that the therapist begins collecting information regarding the patient's functional status before admission, including interests and social supports.

Occupational therapy intervention in the emergent phase focuses on the prevention of early contracture formation through the use of splints and positioning programs. It is ideal to initiate occupational therapy intervention as early as 24–48 hours after burn, because collagen synthesis and contracture formation begin during the initial response to thermal injury (Dewey, Richard, & Parry 2011; Jordan, Daher, & Wasil, 2000).

Splinting. Ideally, splints are fabricated and applied in the initial visit, and a positioning program is established and communicated to the team. Table 40-1 describes common contracture patterns, antideformity positions, and appropriate splints. Generally, any joint involved in a superficial partial-thickness injury or worse has the potential for contracture and is usually splinted. Splint wearing times are determined by the patient's ability to use the involved extremity. That is, a decrease in active movement indicates the need for increased splint wearing time. For example, a heavily sedated patient cannot perform active movement and therefore requires splinting at all times except for therapy and dressing changes. An alert patient who can use his or her affected extremity for functional tasks, such as self-feeding or prescribed exercises, may require the use of splints only at night. Splints are applied over the burn dressing and secured with either gauze wrap or Velcro® straps. Although splinting is considered the standard of care in burn treatment, there is a paucity of evidence to support its use (Richard & Ward, 2005). Validation of the practice of splinting for the prevention of contracture is a research area that may be addressed by occupational therapists in the future.

Positioning. Antideformity positioning, which is used as an adjunct to splinting for prevention of contractures, can be initiated in the first visit. For example, if a patient is

Table 40-1 Anticontracture Positioning by Location of Burn

Location of Burn	Contracture Tendency	Anticontracture Positioning and/or Typical Splint
Anterior neck	Neck flexion	Remove pillows; use half-mattress to extend the neck; neck extension splint or collar
Axilla	Adduction	120° abduction with slight external rotation; axilla splint or positioning wedges; watch for signs of brachial plexus strain
Anterior elbow	Flexion	Elbow extension splint in 5°–10° flexion
Dorsal wrist	Wrist extension	Wrist support in neutral
Volar wrist	Wrist flexion	Wrist cock-up splint in 5°–10° extension
Hand dorsal	Claw hand deformity	Functional hand splint with MP joints 70°–90°, IP joints fully extended, first web open, thumb in opposition (safe position; see Chapter 37)
Hand volar	Palmar contracture Cupping of hand	Palm extension splint MPs in slight hyperextension
Hip-anterior	Hip flexion	Prone positioning; weights on thigh in supine; knee immobilizers
Knee	Knee flexion	Knee extension positioning and/or splints; prevent external rotation, which may cause peroneal nerve compression
Foot	Foot drop	Ankle at 90° with foot board or splint; watch for signs of heel ulcer

Reprinted with permission from Pessina, M. A., & Ellis, S. M. (1997). Rehabilitation. *Nursing Clinics of North America, 32,*367.

unable to be fitted with a custom wrist extension splint, supporting the hand on a rolled pillow can, at least temporarily, maintain appropriate joint position. Elevating the upper extremities can also help to minimize upper extremity edema. Elevation can be done with foam wedges, pillows, or specialized arm troughs attached to the bed. A risk of upper extremity elevation is the potential for brachial plexus strain. Symptoms of brachial plexus strain include tingling, numbness, and cold fingers.

Acute Phase

The acute phase begins after the emergent phase and continues until the wound is closed, either by spontaneous healing or skin grafts (Grigsby deLinde & Miles, 1995). The acute phase can last several days to several months, depending on the extent of the burn and the amount of grafting required. For example, a patient with a 10% TBSA may have an acute phase of 1 week, during which the patient is mobile and undergoes one excision and grafting procedure. However, a patient with a 70% TBSA burn may be in the acute phase for several weeks, during which the patient is in an intensive care unit and undergoes many grafting procedures to close the wounds.

Support and Psychosocial Adjustment in the Acute Phase

All patients with burn injuries, regardless of age, exhibit some of the same psychological responses, including withdrawal, denial, fear of death, regression, anxiety, depression, and grief (Wright, 1984). In addition, various factors can influence a burn patient's psychological status. These include emotional trauma arising from the hospital stay, the length of the hospital stay, adjustment to physical changes, adjustment to others' reactions, and location and depth of the burn injury (Baker et al., 1996; LeDoux et al., 1996). The psychosocial challenges of burn patients vary as the patient moves through each stage of physical recovery (Weichman & Patterson, 2004). Patients in the acute stage deal with issues of depression and anxiety and may begin to exhibit signs of both acute and post-traumatic stress disorder. Also at this time, any preinjury psychopathology may become more apparent (Weichman & Patterson, 2004).

LeDoux et al. (1996) state that the burn team can foster healthy coping strategies while working with the burn patient by using these techniques:

1. Identify strengths that each patient can emphasize, reminding him or her of the strength already involved in surviving a painful and frightening experience.
2. Validate sadness and fear.
3. Assist patient to achieve goals; this helps to show hope for the future.
4. Instill a belief that the patient can succeed.

Team Communication

Communication with all members of the team, including the patient and the patient's family and/or support system, throughout hospitalization is essential. During this acute phase, collaboration between the occupational therapist and the burn team is essential for several reasons, including the following (Pessina & Ellis, 1997):

1. Alerting the team to developing contractures and response to therapeutic intervention.
2. Planning for perioperative splinting.
3. Clarifying range-of-motion orders based on graft integrity.
4. Teaching the team about environmental modifications or communication systems.
5. Advocating on the patient's behalf regarding eventual outpatient needs.

Medical Management

Skin grafting, which occurs primarily in the acute phase, is required when the dermal bed is sufficiently destroyed to prevent or significantly impair spontaneous regrowth of the epithelial tissue (Grigsby deLinde & Miles, 1995). If reepithelialization of the burn site has not occurred within 14 days of the injury or is not expected, grafting would be considered (Kagan & Warden, 1994). Skin grafting is generally performed for all full-thickness burns and for large, deep partial-thickness burns. Skin grafting entails both excision of necrotic (dead) tissue and the placement of skin or a skin substitute over the wound bed.

Types of Grafts. A variety of grafting procedures are available to the burn team. According to the size of the burn and the medical stability of the patient, the team may opt to use one or more of the graft types described next.

Autografts. Skin harvested from an unburned area of the patient is an autograft. Split-thickness autografts, the most frequently used, are taken at the level of the mid-dermis (Institute for Healthcare Quality [IHQ], 1997; Staley, Richard, & Falkel, 1994). Donor sites are ideally selected for the best match of color and texture to the affected area. As donor sites produce mild scarring, their location, when possible, is in an inconspicuous site, such as the upper thigh. The harvested skin can be left as a solid sheet (sheet graft) or perforated to increase surface area (meshed graft) (Staley, Richard, & Falkel, 1994). Meshing allows the surface area of the harvested skin to cover up to four times the original area. Both sheet and meshed grafts have advantages and disadvantages. A sheet graft has the best cosmetic outcome and is thus preferred for the face and hands (Hazani, Whitney, & Wilhelmani, 2012). Infection and the development of hematoma under a sheet graft, however, can cause complete graft loss and require regrafting. A meshed graft, although less cosmetically appealing (the meshed pattern is retained permanently), covers large areas when the donor site is limited. In addition, meshed grafts allow drainage of blood and exudate, which prevents hematomas and improves graft adherence (Hazani, Whitney, & Wilhelmani, 2012).

Temporary Grafts. In cases of extensive burn injuries, where there is not sufficient donor skin to cover all of the affected area with autograft, the burn team may opt to use temporary grafts until the donor site has healed sufficiently for reharvesting. These temporary dressings are either biologic, such as allografts or xenografts (from cadaver and bovine skin, respectively) or synthetic, such as Biobrane® composed of nylon and silastic. These dressings aid in wound management by decreasing infection, stimulating healing and preparing the wound bed for autograft skin, decreasing pain, and protecting exposed tendons, nerves, and blood vessels (Halim, Khoo, & Mohd Yussof, 2010).

Occupational Therapy during the Acute Phase

During the acute phase, the occupational therapist performs a detailed initial evaluation. This includes a thorough chart review to determine the history of the wound and associated injuries. Previous medical history is also important. Associated diagnoses that may limit occupational performance, such as psychiatric illness, diabetes, or lung disease, are to be noted and accounted for during occupational therapy treatment planning. Areas specifically assessed by the occupational therapist during the initial evaluation include client factors (e.g., mental functions, cognitive skills, communication and social skills, sensory functions, neuromusculoskeletal and movement-related functions, joint mobility/stability, and muscle strength/tone/endurance) and ADL and instrumental activities of daily living.

Evaluation can consist of observation during task performance and interviews with patient and family. The potential for permanent scarring and disfigurement may cause significant anxiety and limit the patient's ability to participate in rehabilitation. Thus, early assessment of the patient's support systems allows the therapist to identify resources that may aid in early patient motivation and goal setting.

Because of the acute medical nature of many burn injuries, occupational therapy intervention in the acute phase focuses on capacities and abilities such as range of motion and strength. These are addressed through continued splinting, positioning, exercise, and functional activity. Whenever possible, activities in treatment should reflect each patient's interests. For example, using sports analogies to encourage performance in active range of motion may benefit one patient, while using images of nature and music may benefit another. Other potential treatment activities include environmental modifications, pain remediation, environmental adaptation, and patient and family education. In the acute phase, the individual's ability to participate in treatment related to self-care and functional retraining is often limited by complex medical issues. These areas are addressed in detail during the rehabilitation phase.

Splinting and Positioning. During the acute phase, the splinting and positioning programs established in the emergent phase are continually monitored and adjusted. Splinting schedules are adjusted according to the individual's ability to participate in an exercise and positioning program. For example, if a patient consistently uses an affected elbow for self-feeding and ADL during the day, decreasing the wearing time for the elbow splint to nights and rest periods is appropriate. Conversely, a patient who cannot follow through with an exercise and positioning program because of impaired alertness or poor motivation should wear a splint continuously except for dressing changes and therapeutic activity. It is imperative to check all splints often to ensure proper fit and function (Dewey, Richard, & Parry, 2011). In addition, teaching the nursing staff proper fit and application of splints can decrease the potential for complications (Pessina & Ellis, 1997).

Exercise and Activity. In the acute phase, splinting and positioning are used in combination with exercise and activity (Schneider et al., 2012). Exercise is especially important to control edema and prevent muscle atrophy, tendon adherence, joint stiffness, and capsular shortening (Dewey, Richard, & Parry 2011; Harden & Luster, 1991). Exercise types include passive range of motion, active range of motion, active assistive range of motion, and functional activity. If the patient cannot participate in active exercise or activity because of poor medical status or impaired level of alertness, passive range of motion is indicated. Active exercise is encouraged whenever possible, however (Burke Evans et al., 1996; Wright, 1984), and it is the role of the therapist to guide the patient toward function. Within a single treatment session, a patient may participate in all of these forms of exercise. In fact, functional activities may be used to improve active range of motion. For example, ring toss games are entertaining and easily adapted by changing height and distance to meet upper extremity range of motion goals. Exercise and activity programs are performed up to five times daily (Wright, 1984). Contraindications to exercise include exposed tendons, recent autografts (approximately 5–10 days), acute medical complications, and fractures (Dewey, Richard, & Parry, 2011; Grigsby deLinde & Miles, 1995; Staley, Richard, & Falkel, 1994). In addition, periodic inspection of the wound by the occupational therapist is essential to determine status of wound healing and skin integrity as related to tolerance of the exercise program.

Perioperative Care. The 5–10 days after a skin graft procedure is the perioperative period. A patient with a large burn injury may make many trips to the operating room for skin grafting. Each surgical procedure begins a new perioperative stage. For example, a patient needing grafting on the trunk, arms, and legs may make three trips to the operating room, with each successive area requiring proper perioperative care. The role of the occupational therapist in the perioperative period is to fabricate custom splints to immobilize the newly grafted areas in antideformity positions. Ideally, splints are fabricated immediately prior to or during surgery and applied at the conclusion of the surgery. These splints usually stay in place, along with the primary dressing, for 5–10 days (Dewey, Richard, & Parry, 2011; Grigsby deLinde & Miles, 1995). During this time, range-of-motion exercises are contraindicated to allow for graft adherence. After the primary dressing is removed, the burn team assesses the graft adherence, and a determination is made regarding the appropriateness of resuming exercise.

Pain Management. The occupational therapist must address pain issues that arise during treatment. Many patients in intensive care cannot verbalize a subjective response to manipulation, such as during dressing changes or exercise. In these cases, the therapist monitors objective responses to pain, such as blood pressure, heart rate, and respiratory rate, and adjusts the treatment accordingly. If necessary, the time of the treatment may be changed to allow pain medication to be administered. Decreased repetitions and increased rest breaks during exercise sessions may also be appropriate. Other techniques used to manage pain throughout recovery include distraction strategies, relaxation techniques, and preparatory information (informing/preparing the client regarding procedures to be performed) (Connor-Ballard, 2009). Activity context and emotional state can also affect perception of pain (Dubner & Ren, 1999). Recently, the effectiveness of virtual reality distraction for reducing pain associated with burn injuries has been reported (Hoffman et al., 2011).

Environmental Adaptation. Beginning in the acute phase and throughout recovery, the occupational therapist provides modified call buttons and bed controls, voice-activated telephone systems, and modified utensils (Fig. 40-3) and self-care items. These modifications, combined with patient, staff, and family education, can increase a patient's sense of control and independence. The development of environmental modifications is limited only by the patient's motivation and the therapist's creativity.

Patient and Family Teaching The occupational therapist provides members of the patient's support system with guidance regarding ways to interact with and support the patient during recovery. They may be encouraged to make tape recordings and posters or to bring in favorite music or

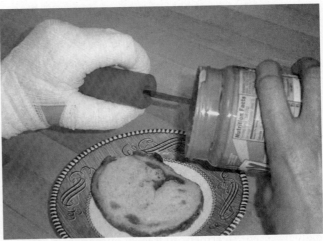

Figure 40-3 Modified utensils can increase independence in the acute phase.

foods. They may need to learn new ways to touch or comfort their loved one. In addition, the family and friends provide a source of information regarding the patient's vocational and avocational roles and available community resources if the patient cannot communicate this information. An educated family and/or support system can be an important asset for ensuring follow-through of exercise and splinting programs and for encouraging participation in functional activities (Duran-Coleman, 1991).

Discharge Planning

Because hospital stays are generally short, discharge planning begins as soon as possible after admission (Fletchall & Hickerson, 1995; Rivers & Jordan, 1998). Many patients in the acute phase are discharged directly home or leave a burn center for continued care on a rehabilitation unit. Elements to consider during discharge planning are the availability of community resources for outpatient or follow-up care, support systems available to the patient, and physical demands of the home environment. When patients who have sustained major burns cannot return to the hospital where they received acute care, it is important for the inpatient occupational therapist to establish a relationship with a therapist in the patient's community to ensure continuity of care throughout the rehabilitation phase. In accordance with the knowledge and experience of the community therapist, the discharging therapist provides appropriate literature and written, photographic, and/or videotaped descriptions of the rehabilitation program. This establishes a communication channel for the community therapist so questions and concerns can be addressed in a timely manner. Whenever possible, all authorization from third-party payers should be established prior to discharge (Fletchall & Hickerson, 1995) to avoid delays in the initiation of outpatient therapy. If a patient cannot be discharged directly to home, transfer to an inpatient rehabilitation facility is appropriate; again, early communication with the receiving therapist is necessary to ensure continuity of care. Regardless of the discharge setting, well-briefed patients are best able to advocate for appropriate care.

Rehabilitation Phase

The rehabilitation phase follows the acute phase and continues until scar maturation (Rivers & Jordan, 1998). Scar maturation can take 6 months to 2 years (Rivers & Jordan, 1998; Staley, Richard, & Falkel, 1994). It is considered complete when the scar becomes pale and the rate of collagen synthesis stabilizes (Grigsby deLinde & Miles, 1995). The level of direct involvement of the occupational therapist during this extended time is varied. It may range from daily inpatient treatment to weekly outpatient treatment to annual clinic visits.

Occupational Therapy during the Rehabilitation Phase

During the rehabilitation phase, the occupational therapist continues to assess capacities and abilities such as range of motion and strength. In addition, functional assessments specific to self-care and homemaking are valuable in guiding treatment planning and preparing for discharge. The overall goal of occupational therapy intervention during this phase is to facilitate the patient's return to his or her previous level of occupational performance. Patients are encouraged to take increasing responsibility for their care, including helping to establish meaningful goals. In addition to range of motion and strength, occupational therapy also focuses on activity tolerance, sensation, coordination, scar management, and self-care and home management skills.

Range of Motion. In the rehabilitation stage, the patient continues to benefit from daily stretching routines established in the acute phase of care. In the early part of this phase, the rate of collagen synthesis is increased (Staley, Richard, & Falkel, 1994), requiring the patient to stretch frequently throughout the day. As the scar matures and collagen synthesis slows, frequency of stretching should be reduced. At all times, skin integrity must be monitored during stretching to prevent tearing. Massage using a non–water-based cream should precede stretching to help prevent dry skin from rupturing (Rivers & Jordan, 1998). An appropriate stretch consists of bringing the tissue to the point of blanching, or becoming pale, and holding it in that position for several seconds. The patient should report tension but not pain. Overzealous stretching can result in tissue tears and edema, which increase joint stiffness. Stretching is initially performed by the occupational therapist. With training, however, the patient and/or caregiver can also complete stretching routines.

Strength. Resistive exercise and graded functional activities can improve strength. Patients may be taught an independent exercise program with resistive rubber ribbon or tubing, such as Theraband®, to increase proximal upper body strength. Functional activities can also be graded to increase strength. For example, patients may gain strength as they perform self-care activities with increasing demands, as when progressing from sitting to standing for hygiene activities.

Activity Tolerance. A key feature of rehabilitation is mobilizing the patient as much as possible, thereby increasing his or her activity tolerance. For an inpatient, this includes increased time spent out of bed and trips to the gym and off the nursing unit. Activity time can be increased by 15 minutes every 2 days, if there is no evidence of fatigue. Fatigue can be monitored by patient self-report and clinician observation. For an outpatient, this may mean resuming leisure activities and going on community outings.

Sensation. Newly healed skin and grafted skin may be hypersensitive, which can significantly limit functional performance. Hypersensitivity can be addressed effectively by systematic desensitization. This can be achieved by asking the patient to manipulate objects with varying textures in the environment. Initially, the patient practices holding soft textures, such as cotton balls or lambswool, and then progresses to manipulating objects with rougher textures, such as Velcro® or burlap. A formal system such as the Downey desensitization program (Barber, 1990) can be used (see Chapter 22).

Coordination. Coordination can be impaired by a variety of factors, including limited range of motion, strength, or sensation. Coordination can be improved through the use of selected progressive tasks designed to challenge the patient's skills. For example, a patient may be asked first to take lids off large jars and then smaller containers (Fig. 40-4).

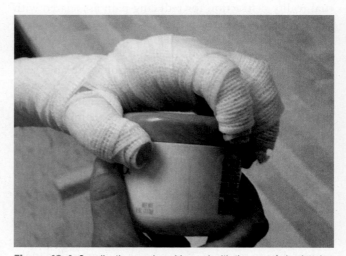

Figure 40-4 Coordination can be addressed with the use of simulated or actual functional tasks.

The patient may also trace large letters or patterns before attempting fine motor writing tasks such as working a crossword puzzle from the newspaper.

Scar Management. Scar tissue formation is a natural response to wound healing (Grisby deLinde & Miles, 1995). It begins in the emergent phase and may take up to 2 years to mature (Jordan, Daher, & Wasil, 2000). A hypertrophic scar is an aberration of the normal healing process and presents as a red, raised, and inelastic scar (Dewey, Richard, & Parry, 2011) (Fig. 40-5). A hypertrophic scar contains an increased number of fibroblasts as compared to normal skin, and the collagen fibers are arranged in a nodular as opposed to parallel fashion (Abston, 1987). The cause is thought to be a disruption in the balance between collagen synthesis and lysis (Grigsby deLinde & Miles, 1995). The tendency for hypertrophic scarring is unique to each individual. In general, patients with large amounts of pigment in the skin and young patients are most prone to hypertrophic scarring. Hypertrophic scarring is also inversely related to the depth of the initial burn wound (Staley, Richard, & Falkel, 1994). In addition to being cosmetically unappealing, hypertrophic scars can limit functional skills by restricting joint range of motion.

Occupational Therapy Assessment of Scars. The Burn Scar Index (Vancouver Scar Scale) is the most widely used standardized scar assessment tool and is used to rate the pliability, vascularity, height, and pigmentation of scars (Sullivan et al., 1990). Used periodically, the Burn Scar Index can help guide the occupational therapist in determining

effective scar management and evaluating the stage of scar maturation. Other assessments include the Patient and Observer Scar Assessment Scale (Draaijers et al., 2004) and the Matching Assessment of Scars and Photographs (Masters, McMahon, & Svens, 2005).

Occupational Therapy Intervention for Scar Management. The occupational therapist attempts to prevent or limit the development of hypertrophic scars. Treatment methods include a combination of techniques, including massage, pressure therapy, and the use of specialized inserts.

Massage. Massage may be useful in reducing scar contracture (Roh, Seo, & Jang, 2010; Staley, Richard, & Falkel, 1994). Scar massage is initiated when it is determined that the injured area can withstand slight friction. In addition, scar massage maintains suppleness, often at risk as normal sweat and oil gland function is disrupted. Scar massage also aids in desensitization. Scar massage is performed several times daily with deep pressure (enough to blanch the scar temporarily) in either a circular pattern or perpendicular to the long axis of the scar. Lotion is used during massage to reduce friction. Perfume-free lotions are preferred to decrease potential irritation to newly healed skin. Initially, scar massage is the responsibility of the occupational therapist so that skin integrity and tolerance can be monitored. Once an established routine has been developed, the therapist teaches the patient and/or caregivers to assume responsibility for daily scar massage.

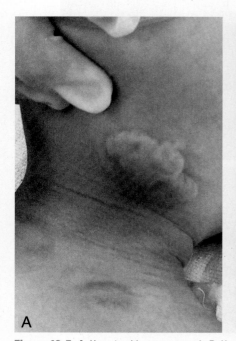 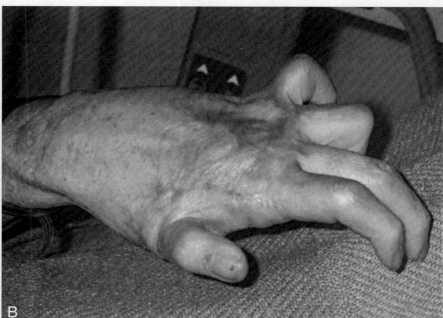

Figure 40-5 **A.** Hypertrophic scars on neck. **B.** Hypertrophic scars on hand. The hypertrophic scar on the dorsum of the hand causes claw hand deformity.

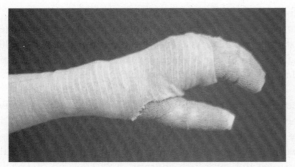

Figure 40-6 Gentle pressure is applied using Coban™ and Tubigrip™.

Pressure Dressings and Garments. Pressure dressings and garments are another form of scar management that has been advocated in the literature (Chang et al., 1995; Li-Tsang, Zheng, & Lau, 2010; Ward, 1991). The flattened, smooth, supple appearance of the scar after application of pressure has been reported clinically, but objective support has been inconclusive (Bloemen et al., 2009; Grigsby deLinde & Miles, 1995). The occupational therapist initiates

the application of gentle pressure via Tubigrip™, elastic bandage wraps, Coban™, or Isotoner® gloves (Fig. 40-6). Initially, pressure dressings are applied for 2-hour intervals. Wearing time is gradually increased by 2-hour increments until 24-hour wear is tolerated. Tolerance is determined by lack of blisters or open areas. At this point, increased pressure using customized products such as Jobst® or Bioconcepts™ garments is indicated (Fig. 40-7). Staley, Richard, and Falkel (1994) suggest that the application of 25 mm Hg of pressure is ideal to aid in collagen organization, which ultimately helps decrease scar tissue formation. Custom garments cause notable shearing during application and removal and thus should be used only when the skin is healed sufficiently to withstand these forces. Wearing of custom garments continues until the scar is inactive, or mature, as described earlier. The therapist's role is to initiate the ordering of custom garments and oversee their use. Most providers of custom garments send trained personnel to measure the patient for custom fitting. For facial burns, the patient may use a transparent facial orthosis secured by elastic straps to provide even pressure distribution. These orthoses are usually fabricated by a specially trained orthotist at the request of the therapist.

Inserts are often used in conjunction with pressure garments. They may be constructed from products such as Otoform®, or closed cell foam (Fig. 40-8, A & B). Their purpose is to increase pressure in concave areas, such as the web spaces and the sternoclavicular depression. Silicone inserts have also been demonstrated to be effective in improving some characteristics of hypertrophic scars

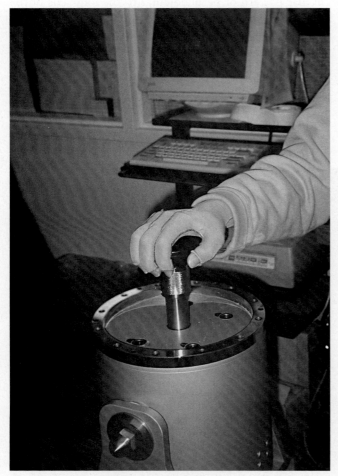

Figure 40-7 Custom pressure garments can be worn while performing simulated functional activity.

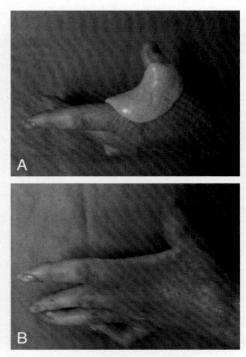

Figure 40-8 **A.** Use of Otoform® insert. **B.** Without insert.

(Ahn, Monafo, & Mustoe, 1989), although the mechanism of action remains to be determined. The design of a scar management program is determined by the available resources, careful clinical observation, and the patient's ability to comply with the program (Evans & McAuliffe, 1995). Periodic outpatient visits to occupational therapy or an established burn clinic throughout the rehabilitation phase allow for monitoring and adjustments of the scar management program.

Self-Care and Home Management Skills. If neuromuscular limitations impede the patient's performance of functional tasks, the therapist may provide adaptive equipment, such as built-up handles for impaired grasp or long-handled utensils for decreased elbow flexion. Teaching adaptive techniques, such as performing certain activities using two hands for extra support, may also improve function.

Patient and Family Teaching. Patients and their family members should understand the rationale for each of the splints and techniques used in their care. They participate in the development of goals, so that they are invested in achieving them. Skin care is an important element in discharge teaching. Patients practice monitoring their skin for breakdown and caring for their skin, including the daily use of a moisturizer. They learn to use a sunscreen with an SPF of at least 15 (reapplied frequently) if they anticipate exposure to the sun (Staley, Richard, & Falkel, 1994). In addition, patients should have a basic understanding of wound healing and tissue response to exercise and scar management techniques.

Support and Psychosocial Adjustment during the Rehabilitation Phase. Although the patient and family typically focus on survival immediately after injury, many other issues arise during rehabilitation. According to Weichman and Patterson (2004), patients in the rehabilitation phase face challenges in three areas: physical (such as decreases in function), social (such as body image and changing roles), and psychological (such as anxiety and depression). The increase in activity in the rehabilitation phase not only assists physical rehabilitation but also assists patients to discover how their injury affects their daily lives. Emotional reactions to the realization of loss may produce a wide range of behaviors, such as crying or expression of anger. In addition, guilt or embarrassment regarding the injury may lead the patient to withdraw. Patients may also have responses related to post-traumatic stress disorder, such as flashbacks.

One of the most difficult challenges for the burn therapist is caring for patients as they grieve for a functional limitation or alteration in body image (Pessina & Ellis, 1997). The occupational therapist supports the patient by encouraging questions and verbalization of feelings about the burn injury (Pessina & Ellis, 1997). The occupational therapist also chooses treatment activities to restore confidence and self-esteem. Group activities provide opportunities for socialization and sharing of concerns in a safe environment (Summers, 1991). Given the extensive contact with the patient throughout all phases of recovery, the occupational therapist is in a unique position to identify and address psychosocial issues, but collaboration with other specialists on the burn team (e.g., nursing staff, family members, social workers, and psychologists) is essential.

Potential Complications

In addition to the potential for soft tissue contractures and loss of joint range of motion, other complications may occur in any phase of burn recovery.

Pruritus

Pruritus (persistent itching) is a common complication (IHQ, 1997; Staley, Richard, & Falkel, 1994), presumably caused by nerve regeneration. It usually resolves within 2 years of the initial injury (Poh-Fitzpatrick, 1992). The use of compression garments, skin moisturizers, cold packs, and medications such as antihistamines may alleviate itching (IHQ, 1997).

Microstomia

Patients with facial burns in the area of the mouth are at risk for oral commissure contracture (microstomia) (Rivers & Jordan, 1998), which is tightening of the musculature around the lip area that limits mouth opening. In extreme cases, urgent surgical revision is required. This risk is exaggerated if the patient has undergone prolonged periods without eating or speaking because of intubation or respiratory compromise. In addition to daily scar massage, the therapist can teach the patient facial stretching exercises, such as yawning or grinning widely and pursing lips together. The exercises can be combined with the wearing of a microstomia splint to stretch the oral commissure. The splint may be worn as tolerated, usually starting with 10 minutes and gradually increasing to 60 minutes twice a day. These devices can be purchased or constructed by the occupational therapist. The cognitive level of the patient is an extremely important factor in use of a microstomia device because of the risk of an unexpected airway emergency. For example, a heavily sedated or confused patient may attempt to swallow the device.

Heterotopic Ossification

Heterotopic ossification, or myositis ossificans, is the development of new bone in tissues that normally do not ossify. It occurs in up to 13% of patients with major burns

(Dutcher & Johnson, 1994). The most common location in the burn-injured population is the elbow, although the shoulder, knee, and hip can also be affected (Dutcher & Johnson, 1994). Heterotopic ossification causes pain, swelling, and rapid loss of range of motion. The therapist must be aware of the symptoms and alert the team so treatment options, including medications and surgery, can be discussed. *Safety Message: Aggressive range-of-motion exercise is contraindicated.*

Heat Intolerance

Heat intolerance is caused by loss of sweating, because split-thickness skin grafts do not contain sweat glands (Grigsby deLinde & Miles, 1995; Rivers & Jordan, 1998). To compensate for this, patients may sweat excessively in remaining unburned areas. Patients in extremely hot climates may require additional air conditioners in the home to maintain comfort (Rivers & Jordan, 1998). The lack of sweat glands also makes healed grafts susceptible to extreme dryness (Grigsby deLinde & Miles, 1995; Staley, Richard, & Falkel, 1994), and patients are encouraged to use moisturizing cream often throughout the day.

RECONSTRUCTIVE SURGERY

An important element in burn recovery is the planning and execution of reconstructive procedures. Despite diligent efforts by the burn team and patient, contractures may develop. Reconstructive surgery can be useful in correcting these deformities. Surgery is typically performed once the scar tissue is mature; however, it may be necessary to perform reconstructive surgery before scar maturation if a severe functional deficit is present (Robson et al., 1992). For example, an axillary contracture, which limits abduction to 80°, may significantly interfere with dressing and hygiene. A surgical procedure, a Z-plasty, can be performed to elongate soft tissue (Robson et al., 1992; Staley, Richard, & Falkel, 1994). A skin graft to cover the deficit may be necessary once the contracture is released.

Occupational Therapy Related to Reconstructive Procedures

When results of functional assessment suggest that the patient's progress toward his or her self-management goals has ceased because of a contracture, the occupational therapist communicates to the burn team the possible need for surgical release of the contracture.

Postoperatively, the occupational therapist provides a custom splint to immobilize and protect the graft in its new lengthened position. After approximately 10–14 days, the therapist initiates an exercise program beginning with gentle active range of motion and progressing to more aggressive exercise and activity as skin integrity tolerates.

Pressure therapy over the newly grafted area minimizes scarring. This includes the use of a pressure garment and an insert fabricated to match the contours of the new graft.

RETURN TO WORK

Returning to work before final scar maturation preserves function and improves the patient's self-concept (Rivers & Jordan, 1998). During the initial evaluation in the acute phase, the occupational therapist gathers information regarding the work history of the patient and specific job demands the patient previously encountered daily. With this information, the occupational therapist can guide treatment activities to prepare for return to the previous level of functioning. For example, if the patient was employed as a mechanic prior to injury, tool use should be incorporated into treatment activities as soon as possible. Patients may require job retraining if the extent of the injury renders the original job demands now unrealistic. In this case, the occupational therapist works with the patient and employer to explore appropriate job modifications.

Return-to-work parameters are ideally based on the percentage of body surface area affected, whether the job requires the use of the affected body part, and the depth of the burn (IHQ, 1997). Fletchall and Hickerson (1995) investigated the effectiveness of a daily 6-hour outpatient program beginning immediately after discharge. Patients in this program, with burns to the upper extremity and hands averaging less than 25% of TBSA, returned to work in an average of 8 weeks; patients in a similar population who participated in traditional outpatient therapy returned in an average of 19 weeks. In addition, the experimental program was shown to reduce the overall costs to the health care payer (Fletchall & Hickerson, 1995). Assignment of a case manager early during the inpatient phase also facilitated the progression from rehabilitation to return to work (Fletchall & Hickerson, 1995).

In addition to physical limitations, burn survivors may encounter psychosocial barriers to returning to the work. These include nightmares, flashback, concern regarding appearance and depression. Patients exhibiting these symptoms may benefit from psychological intervention that, when started early in their recovery, may enable them to return to work sooner (Esselman et al., 2007).

SPECIAL CONSIDERATIONS FOR HAND BURNS

Hand burns resulting in significant functional limitations occur quite frequently. The high rate of injury to the hand is because individuals use their hands to protect themselves or to extinguish the fire (Tanigawa, O'Donnell,

& Graham, 1974). Dorsal hand burns occur more frequently than palmar injuries (Tanigawa, O'Donnell, & Graham, 1974). As previously noted, significant edema usually occurs in response to thermal injury. This pulls the hand into a position of deformity (Sheridan et al., 1995) characterized by thumb adduction, digital metacarpal hyperextension, interphalangeal joint flexion, and flattening of the palmar arches (Wright-Howell, 1989). If this position is maintained, the result is joint contracture and severe functional limitation.

Evaluation of Hand Burns

A comprehensive hand evaluation includes determination of whether range-of-motion limitations are due to joint stiffness, intrinsic muscle tightness, extrinsic muscle tightness, or inelasticity of skin. Other factors that limit hand flexibility and decrease range of motion include pain, bulky dressings, exposed tendons, and the presence of eschar, which is inelastic. Once the clinician determines the cause of range-of-motion limitations, an effective treatment plan can be devised.

Treatment of Hand Burns

The occupational therapist must provide appropriate splinting and exercise programs to prevent contracture and expedite functional use of the burned hand. The appropriate splinting position of the hand is described in Table 40-1. In this position, the collateral ligaments of the metacarpophalangeal (MP), proximal interphalangeal (PIP), and distal interphalangeal joints are positioned at length, preventing ligamentous contracture so that maximum digital range of motion is preserved.

Two distinct options exist for thumb position. Radial abduction maintains the first web space at maximum length. We prefer palmar abduction, however, because this is a position of function. Hand burns are typically dorsal. When present, a deep palmar burn can lead to palmar contracture. In this case, a volar hand extension splint is appropriate. When using this position, however, careful monitoring of MP flexion is critical to prevent shortening of the collateral ligaments. Unfortunately, evidence is lacking regarding specific splint positions and schedules. According to Richard and Ward (2005), "Controversy about splinting in burn care is not based on the rationale for and success of splinting, but exists because of the paucity of validation of its use" (p. 392). A list of splinting options for the conditions previously discussed follows (see Chapter 16 for splint illustrations):

- Dynamic PIP extension splint such as LMB™, or banana splints for PIP stiffness: start 10 minutes three times a day, increase wearing time as tolerated, not to exceed 60 minutes at a time.

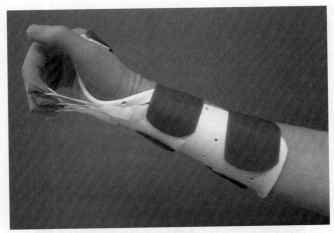

Figure 40-9 Dynamic flexion splint and pressure glove combination.

- Dynamic flexion splint in which the MPs are blocked in full extension while the IPs are passively flexed (for intrinsic muscle tightness): start 10 minutes three times a day, increase wearing time as tolerated, not to exceed 60 minutes at a time.
- Forearm-based dynamic flexion splint that offers composite MP-IP flexion (Fig. 40-9) (for extrinsic extensor tightness or inelastic skin that limits composite flexion): start 10 minutes three times a day, increasing as tolerated but not to exceed 40 minutes.
- Volar forearm-based static extension splint (for extrinsic flexor tightness): wear at night.
- Forearm-based dynamic extension splint (for extrinsic flexor tightness): wear periodically during the day, starting with 10 minutes three times per day and progressing to 45 minutes as tolerated.

Often, individuals do not present with a single limitation; rather, a combination of factors limits the individual's range of motion. The clinician must determine which factor is the primary source of dysfunction and treat accordingly. Appropriate splints are always used in conjunction with exercises, functional activities, and scar management techniques. Splints should never be used to the extent that they limit or prevent performance of ADL.

Potential Complications of Hand Burns

Normal hand anatomy can be characterized by a balance of levers and pulleys that work harmoniously to achieve motion. Damage to this balanced network results in significant functional limitations.

Extensor Tendon Injury

Extensor tendon injury is often associated with dorsal hand burns because they lie superficially on the dorsal

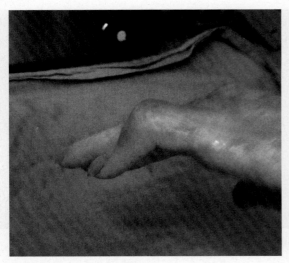

Figure 40-10 Boutonniere deformity.

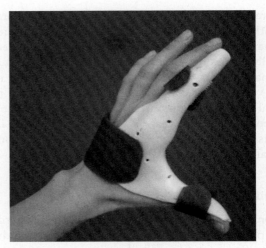

Figure 40-11 C-splint in radial abduction.

aspect of the hand. Limitations can be due to direct thermal injury or tendon ischemia (Wright-Howell, 1989). Because of the close proximity of structures, the formation of scar tissue can greatly limit tendon excursion and create imbalance. This can result in contracture development. Boutonniere (Fig. 40-10) and swan-neck deformities are the result of extensor tendon damage (Evans & McAuliffe, 1995; Rosenthal, 1995; Wright-Howell, 1989).

Web Space Contractures

Web space contractures can be due to overgrafting of the web spaces, muscle shortening (contracture of the adductor pollicis brevis resulting in a first web space contracture), joint stiffness, or skin graft contracture in a normal response to tissue healing. Splints, scar management, and exercise are effective treatment modalities. First web space contractures (between the thumb and index finger) respond well to a web space C-splint (Fig. 40-11) that is lined with Otoform®, a silicon gel sheet. This is usually worn at night for 6–8 hours. During the day, the individual performs stretching, massage, and functional activities that encourage full range of motion of the affected area. For example, an individual with a first web space contracture is asked to pick up containers or game pieces of various sizes, using palmar abduction to promote full abduction of the thumb. A dynamic splint with an insert that exerts pressure over the second, third, and fourth web spaces can be appropriate for digital web space contractures. Another option is the addition of web space inserts under a Jobst® or Isotoner® glove.

OUTCOME STUDIES

Long-term outcomes and quality of life after major burn injuries are of significant concern to those working in the field of burn rehabilitation. A research tool that has

been established to address this issue is the Burn Specific Health Scale (BSHS) (Blalock, Bunker, & DeVellis, 1994). This scale is a 31-item instrument that includes items in seven categories: simple functional abilities, work, body image, interpersonal relationships, affect, heat sensitivity, and treatment programs.

Kildal and colleagues (2004) performed an outcome study using a brief version of the Burn Specific Health Scale (BSHS-B) and the Coping with Burns Questionnaire to determine the relationship between coping strategies, burn injury characteristics, social and economic status, and long-term functional outcome. Data were collected from 161 adult survivors of burn injury. The authors concluded that, for most patients, extensive use of avoidant coping and low use of emotional support were related to the lowest long-term functional outcomes. This suggests that early attempts should be made to guide patients toward the most effective coping strategies.

Another study investigated hand function after acute hand burns (Sheridan et al., 1995). The study examined 659 patients with a total of 1,047 hand burns. It was reported that normal function was resumed in 97% of patients with superficial injuries and 81% of patients with deep dermal or full-thickness injuries. Of the patients with severe injuries, which included tendon damage or joint capsule or bone involvement, only 9% had normal function, whereas 90% were able to compensate for this and independently perform ADL (Sheridan et al., 1995).

Another study published by Sheridan et al. in 2000 investigated the long-term outcome of children surviving major burn injuries (>70% TBSA) using a validated quality-of-life scale administered an average of 14 years postinjury. The authors reported that most children had a satisfying quality of life. The majority of the subjects (72%) were either full-time students or gainfully employed. Statistical analysis revealed that key factors such as early return to pre-burn activities and comprehensive burn care that included experienced multidisciplinary aftercare played an important role in recovery (Sheridan et al., 2000). The authors are careful to note that "Children who survive massive burns will have major cosmetic and functional impairments that can never be completely corrected" (Sheridan et al., 2000, p. 73).

When outcomes were assessed in adult survivors of severe burn injuries, the results were similar (Druery et al., 2005). Using an abbreviated form of the BSHS to assess function and quality of life in adults surviving burns >40% TBSA, it was determined that the majority of these burn survivors developed functional independence and a good quality of life (Druery et al., 2005).

Although evidence is growing that patients who sustain burn injuries can expect generally positive outcomes, little evidence is available to guide the occupational therapy clinician in choosing specific treatment approaches and modalities. The lack of evidence in this field prevents a formal assessment of evidence related to occupational therapy practice. It highlights the need of occupational therapists to participate in outcome-based research related to the treatment of patients with burn injuries. As specialists in the evaluation and treatment of function, occupational therapists have a responsibility to continue to enhance the knowledge base in this area (see Resources 40-1). Evidence Table 40-1 shows evidence of benefits of occupational therapy for patients with burns.

FUTURE DIRECTIONS

Exciting progress has occurred in regards to reconstruction techniques for the burn patient. Recent advances include hand and face transplants. To date, 18 successful face transplants have occurred worldwide (Singhal, Pribaz & Pomahac, 2011), and patients have undergone unilateral and bilateral hand transplants as well. In both cases, clients must undergo a rigorous evaluation process to determine appropriateness. Rejection is a constant concern

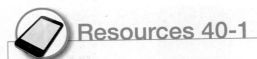

Resources 40-1

Burns

American Burn Association (ABA)

311 S. Wacker Drive, Suite 4150
Chicago, IL 60606
Phone: 312-642-9260
Fax: 312-642-9130
http://www.ameriburn.org

Phoenix Society for Burn Survivors Inc.

1835 R. W. Berends Dr., SW
Grand Rapids, MI 49519-4955
Phone: 800-888-2876 or 616-458-2773
E-mail: info@phoenix-society.org

Journal of Burn Care & Research

Official journal for the American Burn Association
Published by Lippincott Williams & Wilkins
http://journals.lww.com/burncareresearch

with these individuals, because current protocols require that transplant recipients must stay on a lifelong immunosuppressive medications to prevent transplant rejection. These medications can have significant side effects including increased risk of cancer and organ toxicity. The major goals of face and hand transplants include functional and sensory improvements; however, the potential impact they have on an individual's life satisfaction, body image, and social interaction cannot be overlooked. As occupational therapists, focused on functioning in daily activities, we can assist these patients through the use of splinting, exercise, and environmental adaptations to maximize functional independence.

Evidence Table 40-1	Best Evidence for Occupational Therapy Practice Regarding Burns

Intervention	Description of Intervention Tested	Participants	Dosage	Type of Best Evidence and Level of Evidence	Benefit	Statistical Probability and Effect Size of Outcome	Reference
Effects of pressure therapy (PG), silicone gel sheeting (SGS), and combined therapies (CTG) on hypertrophic scar	Four groups (PG, SGS, CTG, and control group); blinded assessment of hypertrophic scar at five time intervals: pretreatment; at 2, 4, and 6 months during treatment; and 1 month after treatment using various validated instruments	One hundred four patients mean age 21.8 ± 18.7 years (scar size of <16 cm²) with baseline Vancouver Scar grade of >5	Application of garment and/or silicone 24 hours per day (except bathing or 15 minutes of daily massage)	Randomized, double blind, prospective controlled clinical trial Level IB1a	CTG most effective for improving thickness of scar after 2 months. CTG and PG both resulted in improved thickness after 6 months, with CTG showing greatest change. SGS most effective in relieving pain and pruritus.	Using two-way repeated analysis of variance, all noted significant effects, p values ≤ 0.001	Li-Tsang, Zheng, & Lau (2010)
Inpatient burn rehabilitation	Standard of care rehabilitation program. Tested range of motion (ROM) of shoulder, elbow, hip, and knee Hand function assessed via Jebsen Hand Function test Balance assessed using Berg balance scale	Eleven inpatients in regional burn hospital All subjects >18 years of age	All subjects received physical & occupational therapy for 3 hours daily five times per week	Prospective one-group, pre- post-test pilot study Level IIIC3c	Demonstrated improvement in ROM by 64% as well as improvement in hand function and balance in response to rehabilitation intervention	Significant improvements in ROM, hand function, and balance from admission to discharge (p < 0.05).	Schneider et al. (2012)

case example
Mrs. J.: Burn Rehabilitation

Occupational Therapy Intervention Process	Clinical Reasoning Process	
	Objectives	**Examples of Therapist's Internal Dialogue**
Patient Information Mrs. J. is a 42-year-old woman who sustained a 45% total body surface area (TBSA) burn as a result of a house fire. She presented to the emergency department with superficial and superficial partial-thickness burns to her face and neck and deep partial- and full-thickness burns to both upper extremities and hands (dorsal aspect only), chest, and proximal aspect of her bilateral lower extremities. She also sustained an inhalation injury and was intubated and sedated. She was admitted to the intensive care unit. No significant medical history was reported. Split-thickness skin grafts (STSGs) were performed to her chest and upper thighs 3 days after admission. STSGs were performed to her arms and hands 10 days after admission. After skin grafting was complete, Mrs. J. was extubated and moved to a private room. She was on a regular diet and could walk independently. She was noted to be withdrawn and was concerned regarding her ability to care for her 3-year-old daughter. Her husband and sister were present and supportive throughout her hospitalization.	Understand the patient's diagnosis or condition Know the person	"STSGs have the potential for contracture, which means we will have to work hard to ensure full return of her upper extremity function. In addition, STSGs may result in some scarring, which means a scar management program will need to begin as soon as possible." "From the pictures her family has brought in, it seems she took great pride in caring for her daughter—doing her hair, getting her dressed, etc. I can work with her to create goals related to care for her daughter that will be motivating for her and will reassure her that she will, in fact, be able to resume care for her child. Also, it appears that Mrs. J. has good family support. I wonder how available her husband and sister will be now that Ms. J. is beginning rehabilitation. It seems that often, after the acute crisis is over, many family members need to return to their jobs, at least to some extent."
Reason for Referral to Occupational Therapy Mrs. J. was referred to occupational therapy (OT) during the acute phase to prevent contractures that might result in deficits in occupational functioning, to provide patient and family education, and to address psychosocial sequelae related to the burn injury.	Appreciate the context Develop provisional hypotheses	"I am going to suggest regular team meetings to discuss goals and monitor Mrs. J.'s progress. It will be important for the team to recognize if she is becoming more withdrawn or depressed. I will also need to know what services will be available as she prepares for discharge. I anticipate that occupational therapy intervention can help in many aspects of recovery, from restoring performance skills, such as range of motion (ROM), to returning to important life roles such as caring for her family."
Assessment Process and Results The following assessment was performed on transition to the rehabilitation phase: Assessment of wound healing: Immature scar noted on bilateral forearms and dorsum of both hands Assessment of cognitive/social status: Awake and alert for several short periods throughout the day; also noted to appear withdrawn, not seeking social interaction Biomechanical assessment: ROM and strength: Decreased elbow flexion, decreased grasp (metacarpophalangeal [MP] flexion limited) and decreased upper extremity strength bilaterally Role and interest assessment: Ability to care for daughter is of primary importance Functional assessment: Observed having difficulty using utensils and difficulty using nurse call button and observed to fatigue easily	Consider evaluation approach and methods Interpret observations	"Mrs. J. receives many services throughout the day and has limited activity tolerance. In my experience, observational methods are the most efficient way to gather assessment information during this phase of burn recovery." "Mrs. J.'s limited ROM is not unexpected at this stage of recovery. Fortunately, these patients usually respond well to occupational therapy treatment. In addition to working to remediate her biomechanical limitations, I would like to try to quickly improve her independence in activities by issuing some adaptive equipment. This may help her feel more in control and less dependent."
Occupational Therapy Problem List • Unable to feed or dress independently because of impaired strength and ROM in both upper extremities • Impaired ability to care for her daughter • Withdrawn behavior • Activity tolerance limited to 5 minutes	Synthesize results	"Biomechanical limitations are affecting her ability to perform tasks independently. Before the fire, Mrs. J. was so competent and in control of her activities that I'm sure her current functional status is contributing to feelings of dependence and poor self-esteem."

Occupational Therapy Goal List

- Mrs. J. will use splinting, positioning, exercise, and activity to prevent loss of ROM in her upper extremities.
- Mrs. J. will be able to perform 10 repetitions of active assistive ROM of bilateral upper extremities.
- Mrs. J. will improve ability to grasp utensils by increasing flexion in her right MP joints from 40° to 75°.
- Mrs. J. will eat 90% of her meal independently, using adaptive equipment as needed.
- Ms. J. will be able to comb her daughter's hair for 5 minutes while sitting independently.
- Mrs. J. will cope with anxiety and withdrawal by attainment of goals and through increased knowledge of the burn recovery process.

Develop intervention hypotheses	"I believe that through the use of carefully selected activities, Mrs. J. will regain basic skills, as well as quickly gain confidence in her ability to perform tasks that are important to her."
	"Splinting is not fully evaluated in the literature, yet it is the standard of care. So I will carefully evaluate and document the effects of my splinting program and modify my intervention accordingly."
Select an intervention approach	"The most limiting factors in her task performance are her biomechanical limitations. Therefore, I need to address these as a priority. However, I will accomplish biomechanical goals by using activities that also address psychosocial needs."
Consider what will occur in therapy, how often, and for how long	"In my experience, occupational therapy treatment six times a week is appropriate for the remainder of Mrs. J.'s acute hospitalization (2–3 weeks). Initially, she may be frustrated and discouraged. However, I expect that, with the proper motivation, she will quickly regain function. This means that her goals will need to be continually reviewed and adjusted appropriately. I really want her to know that she is part of setting the goals for treatment, so she can take pride in her achievements in therapy."

Intervention

OT occurred six times a week. Bilateral elbow and hand splints were fabricated. Adaptive equipment, such as modified call button and built-up utensils, were provided. The therapist encouraged the family to bring in recordings of get-well messages that Mrs. J. could listen to with headphones. Mrs. J. was taken to the OT gym as much as possible, and private time with her daughter was added to her daily schedule.

Understand what she is doing Know the person Appreciate the context	"Mrs. J. is slowly beginning to ask me and the other team members appropriate questions regarding her treatment. She is demonstrating beginning awareness of the course of recovery and expected outcomes from this type of injury. She is smiling more and appears more open as she realizes that she will be able to resume activities that are meaningful to her. Her family is responding well to her new brightness. This is a nice cycle that is further motivation for Mrs. J."

Next Steps

As the scars matured, Mrs. J. was provided with both verbal and written instructions regarding scar management and skin care. As discharge neared, a local therapist was contacted to follow Mrs. J. three times a week.

Anticipate present and future patient concerns	"As Mrs. J. transitions to home, she may be initially fearful of being home again, but we will plan close follow-up to quickly address any new issues that arise. Also, as she becomes more competent in her daily activities, her focus may shift to concerns about her appearance. She will likely have many questions in the next few months. I believe that the more she knows about the scar maturation process and scar management treatments, the more empowered she will feel. A burn garment will be needed, and I will order it prior to discharge, so trials can begin under the supervision of an experienced therapist."
	"I will need to be sure that I have opened the lines of communication with her local therapist who may also have questions about types of treatment, appropriate goals, and so on."
Decide whether the patient should continue or discontinue therapy and/or return in the future	"In addition to local follow-up, I would like to see Mrs. J. in the burn clinic in 1 month to assess outpatient care and provide additional recommendations as needed."

Clinical Reasoning in Occupational Therapy Practice

Poor Functional Grasp

In therapy, Mrs. J. has been making steady gains in range of motion of her wrist and digits, and her grasp strength has improved as well. However, she has difficulty performing functional tasks such as holding a utensil for eating or buttoning her shirt. Her hand grafts are well healed with no remaining open areas, and her available range of motion for these tasks seems sufficient. What methods might the therapist use to determine what is limiting functional performance?

Summary Review Questions

1. In your own words, what is the primary goal of burn care?
2. How is the role of the occupational therapist unique to the burn team?
3. Describe key differences between superficial, superficial partial-thickness, deep partial-thickness, and full-thickness burns.
4. What splinting and positioning program would you establish for a patient who is intubated in the intensive care unit with deep partial-thickness burns to the axilla, elbow, and wrist?
5. How would your approach differ with the same patient awake and alert?
6. Describe the correct positioning for a deep dorsal hand burn and explain the anatomical justification behind your answer.
7. What factors would you consider when designing a scar management program for your patient?
8. As the occupational therapist on the burn unit, how would you help to address the psychosocial issues of your patients?
9. List five complications you might encounter as your patient recovers from a significant burn injury.
10. What might you, as an occupational therapist, find difficult about treating a patient with a burn injury? How would you address these issues?

Glossary

Antideformity positions—Positions opposite to common patterns of deformity used to prevent contractures.

Blanching—Applying sufficient pressure to interrupt blood flow temporarily: an assessment of capillary flow rate.

Debriding—Removing eschar and loose or necrotic tissue to prevent infection and promote healing.

Deep partial-thickness burn—Thermal injury that destroys cells from the epidermis to the deep dermal layer.

Dermis—Layer of skin below the epidermis that contains blood vessels, nerve endings, hair follicles, and sweat and oil glands; supports the regrowth of new epithelial tissue.

Epidermis—Most superficial layer of the skin; acts as a barrier. It is continually sloughed and replaced.

Eschar—Burned tissue.

Full-thickness burn—Thermal injury in which the epidermis and dermis are destroyed.

Superficial burn—Thermal injury that involves only cells in the epidermis.

Superficial partial-thickness burn—Thermal injury in which the epidermis and upper portion of the dermal layer are destroyed.

Wound contracture—Part of normal healing in which myofibroblasts in the wound bed contract to minimize the skin defect.

Z-plasty—Surgical procedure in which a Z-shaped incision is made and tissue is transposed to increase tissue length.

References

Abston, S. (1987). Scar reaction after thermal injury and prevention of scars and contractures. In J. A. Boswick Jr. (Ed.), *The art and science of burn care* (pp. 359–371). Rockville, MD: Aspen.

Ahn, S. T., Monafo, W. W., & Mustoe, T. A. (1989). Topical silicone gel: A new treatment for hypertrophic scars. *Surgery, 106,*781–787.

American Burn Association National Burn Repository. (2011). Version 7.0.

Baker, R. A., Jones, S., Sanders, C., Sadinski, C., Martin-Duffy, K., Berchin, H., & Valentine, S. (1996). Degree of burn, location of burn, and length of hospital stay as predictors of psychosocial status and physical functioning. *Journal of Burn Care and Rehabilitation, 17,* 327–333.

Barber, L. M. (1990). Desensitization of the traumatized hand. In J. M. Hunter, E. J. Mackin, & A. D. Callahan (Eds.), *Rehabilitation of the hand* (p. 721). St. Louis: Mosby.

Blalock, S. J., Bunker, B. J., & DeVellis, R. F. (1994). Measuring health status among survivors of burn injury: Revisions of the Burn Specific Health Scale. *Journal of Trauma, 36,* 508–515.

Bloemen, M. C., van der Veer, W. M., Ulrich, M. M., van Zuijlen, P. P., Niessen, F. B., & Middelkoop, E. (2009). Prevention and curative management of hypertrophic scar formation. *Burns, 35,* 463–475.

Burke Evans, E., Alvarado, M. I., Ott, S., McElroy, K., & Irwin, C. (1996). Prevention and treatment of deformity in burned patients. In D. N. Herndon (Ed.), *Total burn care* (pp. 443–454). Philadelphia: Saunders.

Chang, P., Laubenthal, K. N., Lewis, R. W., Rosenquist, M. D., Lindley-Smith, P., & Kealy, G. P. (1995). Prospective, randomized study of the efficacy of pressure garment therapy in patients with burns. *Journal of Burn Care and Rehabilitation, 16,* 473–475.

Cioffi, W. G., & Rue, L. W. (1991). Diagnosis and treatment of inhalation injuries. *Critical Care Nursing Clinics of North America, 3,* 191–198.

Connor-Ballard, P. A. (2009). Understanding and managing burn pain: Part 2. *American Journal of Nursing, 109,*54–62.

Dewey, W. S., Richard, R. L., & Parry, I. S. (2011). Positioning, splinting, and contracture management. *Physical Medicine and Rehabilitation Clinics of North America, 22,* 229–247.

Draaijers, L. J., Tempelman, F. R., Botman, Y. A., Tuinebreijer, W. E., Middelkoop, E., Kreis, R. W., & van Zuijlen, P. P. (2004). The patient and observer scar assessment scale: A reliable and feasible tool for scar evaluation. *Plastic and Reconstructive Surgery, 113,* 1960–1965.

Druery, M., La, H., Brown, T., & Muller, M. (2005). Long term functional outcomes and quality of life following severe burn injury. *Burns, 31,* 692–695.

Dubner, R., & Ren, K. (1999). Endogenous mechanisms of sensory modulation. *Pain, 82 (Suppl. 1),* S45–S53.

Duncan, D. J., & Driscoll, D. M. (1991). Burn wound management. *Critical Care Nursing Clinics of North America, 3,* 199–220.

Duran-Coleman, L. A. (1991). Rehabilitation of the burn survivor. *Progress Report: A Rehabilitation Journal, 3,* 1–8.

Dutcher, K., & Johnson, C. (1994). Neuromuscular and musculoskeletal complication. In R. L. Richard & M. J. Staley (Eds.), *Burn care and rehabilitation: Principles and practice* (pp. 576–602). Philadelphia: Davis.

Esselman, P. C., Askay, S. W., Carrougher, G. J., Lezotte, D. C., Holavanahalli, R. K., Magyar-Russell, G., Fauerbach, J. A., & Engrav, L. H. (2007). Barriers to return to work after burn injuries. *Archives of Physical Medicine and Rehabilitation, 88 (Suppl. 2),* S50–S56.

Evans, R. B., & McAuliffe, J. A. (1995). Wound classification and management. In J. M. Hunter, E. J. Mackin, & A. D. Callahan (Eds.), *Rehabilitation of the hand: Surgery and therapy* (pp. 217–235). St. Louis: Mosby Year Book.

Falkel, J. E. (1994). Anatomy and physiology of the skin. In R. L. Richard & M. J. Staley (Eds.), *Burn care and rehabilitation: Principles and practice* (pp. 10–18). Philadelphia: Davis.

Fletchall, S., & Hickerson, W. L. (1995). Quality burn rehabilitation: Cost-effective approach. *Journal of Burn Care and Rehabilitation, 16,* 539–542.

Greenhalgh, D. G., & Staley, M. J. (1994). Burn wound healing. In R. L. Richard & M. J. Staley (Eds.), *Burn care and rehabilitation: Principles and practice* (pp. 70–102). Philadelphia: Davis.

Grigsby de Linde, L., & Miles, W. K. (1995). Remodeling of scar tissue in the burned hand. In J. M. Hunter, E. J. Mackin, & A. D. Callahan (Eds.), *Rehabilitation of the hand: Surgery and therapy* (pp. 1265–1303). St. Louis: Mosby Year Book.

Harden, N. G., & Luster, S. H. (1991). Rehabilitation considerations in the care of the acute burn patient. *Critical Care Nursing Clinics of North America, 3,* 245–253.

Halim, A. S., Khoo, T. L., & Mohd Yussof, S. J. (2010). Biologic and synthetic skin substitutes: An overview. *Indian Journal Plast Surgery, 43 (Suppl.),* S23–S28.

Hazani, R., Whitney, R., & Wilhelmi, B. J. (2012). Optimizing aesthetic results in skin grafting. *The American Surgeon, 78,* 151–154.

Hoffman, H. G., Chambers, G. T., Meyer, W. J., Arceneaux, L. L., Russell, W. J., Seibel, E. J., Richards, T. L., Sharar, S. R., & Patterson, D. R. (2011). Virtual reality as an adjunctive non-pharmacologic analgesic for acute burn pain during medical procedures. *Annals of Behavioral Medicine, 41,* 183–191.

Institute for Healthcare Quality. (1997). *Quality first position paper: Burns.* Minneapolis: Author.

Jordan, R. B., Daher, J., & Wasil, K. (2000). Splints and scar management for acute and reconstructive burn care. *Clinics of Plastic Surgery, 27,* 71–85.

Kagan, R. J., & Warden, G. D. (1994). Management of the burn wound. *Clinical Dermatology, 12,* 47–56.

Kampf, G., & Löffler, H. (2009). Hand disinfection in hospitals: Benefits and risks. *Journal der Deutschen Dermatologischen Gesellschaft, 8,* 978–983.

Kildal, M., Willebrand, M., Andersson, G., Gerdin, B., & Ekselius, L. (2004). Coping strategies, injury characteristics and long term outcome after burn injury. *Injury, 36,* 511–518.

LeDoux, J. M., Meyer, W. J., Blakeney, P., & Herndon, D. (1996). Positive self-regard as a coping mechanism for pediatric burn survivors. *Journal of Burn Care and Rehabilitation, 17,* 472–476.

Li-Tsang, C. W., Zheng, Y. P., & Lau, J. C. (2010). A randomized clinical trial to study the effect of silicone gel dressing and pressure therapy on post-traumatic hypertropic scars. *Journal of Burn Care and Research, 31,* 448–457.

Malick, M. H., & Carr, J. A. (1982). *Manual on management of the burn patient.* Pittsburgh: Harmarville Rehabilitation Center.

Masters, M., McMahon, M., & Svens, B. (2005) Reliability testing of a new scar assessment tool, Matching Assessment of Scars and Photographs (MAPS). *Journal of Burn Care and Rehabilitation, 26,* 273–284.

Pessina, M. A., & Ellis, S. M. (1997). Rehabilitation. *Nursing Clinics of North America, 32,* 365–374.

Poh-Fitzpatrick, M. B. (1992). Skin care of the healed burn patient. *Clinical Plastic Surgery, 19,* 745–751.

Richard, R., & Ward, R. S. (2005). Splinting strategies and controversies. *Journal of Burn Care and Rehabilitation, 26,* 392–396.

Rivers, E. A., & Jordan, C. L. (1998). Skin system dysfunction: Burns. In M. J. Neistadt & E. B. Crepeau (Eds.), *Willard and Spackman's occupational therapy* (9th ed., pp. 741–755). Philadelphia: Lippincott.

Robson, M. C., Barnett, R. A., Leitch, I. O., & Hayward, P. G. (1992). Prevention and treatment of postburn scars and contracture. *World Journal of Surgery, 16,* 87–96.

Roh, Y. S, Seo, C. H., & Jang, K. U. (2010). Effects of a skin rehabilitation nursing program on skin status, depression, and burn-specific health in burn survivors. *Rehabilitation Nursing, 35,* 65–69.

Rosenthal, E. A. (1995). The extensor tendons: Anatomy and management. In J. M. Hunter, E. J. Mackin, & A. D. Callahan (Eds.), *Rehabilitation of the hand: Surgery and therapy* (pp. 519–564). St. Louis: Mosby.

Schneider, J. C., Qu, H. D., Lowry, J., Walker, J., Vitale, E., & Zona, M. (2012). Efficacy of in-patient burn rehabilitation: Prospective pilot study examining range of motion, hand function, and balance. *Burns, 38,* 164–171.

Sheridan, R. L., Hinson, M. I., Liang, M. H., Nackel, A. F., Schoenfeld, D. A., Ryan, C. M., Mulligan, J. L., & Tompkins, R. G. (2000). Long-term outcome of children surviving massive burns. *Journal of the American Medical Association, 283,* 69–73.

Sheridan, R. L., Hurley, J., Smith, M. A., Ryan, C. M., Bondoc, C. C., Quinby, W. C., Tompkins, R. G., & Burke, J. F. (1995). The acutely burned hand: Management and outcome based a ten-year experience with 1047 acute hand burns. *Journal of Trauma, 38,* 406–411.

Singhal, D., Pribaz, J. J., & Pomahac, B. (2012). The Brigham and Women's Hospital face transplant program: A look back. *Plastic and Reconstructive Surgery, 129,* 81e–88e.

Staley, M. J., Richard, R. L., & Falkel, J. E. (1994). Burns. In S. B. O'Sullivan & T. J. Schmitz (Eds.), *Physical rehabilitation: Assessment and treatment* (pp. 509–532). Philadelphia: Davis.

Sullivan, T., Smith, J., Kermode, J., McIver, E., & Courtemanche, D. J. (1990). Rating the burn scar. *Journal of Burn Care and Rehabilitation, 3,* 256–260.

Summers, T. M. (1991). Psychosocial support of the burned patient. *Critical Care Nursing Clinics of North America, 3,* 237–244.

Tanigawa, M. C., O'Donnell, O. K., & Graham, P. L. (1974). The burned hand: A physical therapy protocol. *Physical Therapy, 54,* 953–958.

Ward, R. S. (1991). Pressure therapy for the control of hypertrophic scar formation after burn injury: A history and review. *Journal of Burn Care and Rehabilitation, 12,* 257–262.

Weichman, S. A., & Patterson, D. R. (2004) Psychosocial aspects of burn injuries. *BMJ, 329,* 391–393.

Wright, P. C. (1984). Fundamentals of acute burn care and physical therapy management. *Physical Therapy, 64,* 1217–1231.

Wright-Howell, J. (1989). Management of the acutely burned hand for the non-specialized clinician. *Physical Therapy, 69,* 1077–1089.

Acknowledgments

We thank the patients, physicians, and staff of the Sumner Redstone Burn Unit at Massachusetts General Hospital and the staff of the occupational therapy and hand therapy departments.

41

Amputations and Prosthetics

Sarah Mitsch, Lisa Smurr Walters, and Kathleen Yancosek

Learning Objectives

After studying this chapter, the reader will be able to do the following:

1. Design treatment programs for preprosthetic and prosthetic management of upper limb amputations.
2. Discuss upper limb amputation levels and respective prosthetic systems and components.
3. Discuss treatment program considerations for persons with lower limb amputations.
4. Describe the psychological implications of amputation and the therapeutic management.
5. Discuss challenges of treating individuals with multiple limb loss.

Amputation can result from several causes including trauma, vascular disease, tumors, infection, or congenital limb deficiencies that present as missing or partially developed limbs. This chapter addresses adults with acquired amputation, that is, amputations that occurred after birth.

INCIDENCE, LEVELS, AND CLASSIFICATION OF AMPUTATION

There are nearly two million people living with limb loss in the United States (Ziegler-Graham et al., 2008). Annually, more than 185,000 persons in the United States have amputations, with the ratio of arm to leg amputations estimated to be 1:3 (Goodney et al., 2009). Some 57% of upper limb amputations are transradial, that is, below the elbow through the radius and ulna. Trauma rather than disease is the primary cause (close to 75%) of upper limb amputations in adults, with injury occurring primarily to males aged 15–45 years in work-related accidents (Esquenazi, 2004). Upper limb amputations can also result from other causes, such as gunshot wounds and electrical burns. Disease is the primary reason for lower limb amputations, with peripheral vascular disease and diabetes being the most common causes in people older than 60 years of age (Dillingham, Pezzin, & MacKenzie, 2004). An increasing prevalence of diabetes as well as continued overseas combat military operations is causing an overall increase in amputation rates (Darnall, 2009; Johannesson et al., 2009; Rayman et al., 2004). As of January 2012, over 1,400 military service members have sustained limb loss as a result of the wars in Iraq and Afghanistan, with over 200 service members sustaining an upper extremity amputation (Harvey, Loomis, et al., 2012).

When amputation is necessary, the surgeon's aim is to preserve as much limb length as possible and still retain healthy skin, soft tissue, blood supply, sensation, muscles, bones, and joints (Smith, Michael, & Bowker, 2004). A residual limb that is pain free and functional is the final surgical goal.

The levels of upper extremity amputation are illustrated in Figure 41-1. The term forequarter describes an amputation of the arm, scapula, and clavicle. The term transhumeral describes an amputation through the humerus; transradial describes an amputation through the radius and ulna. The level of amputation may affect the use of a prosthesis. The higher the upper extremity amputation, the more difficult it will be to use a prosthesis because fewer joints and muscles are available to control the prosthesis. Furthermore, the weight of the prosthesis is greater, and more complex systems are needed for active control. Therefore, for a variety of reasons, a patient may choose not to be a full-time prosthetic user in his or her daily activities (Biddiss & Chau, 2007).

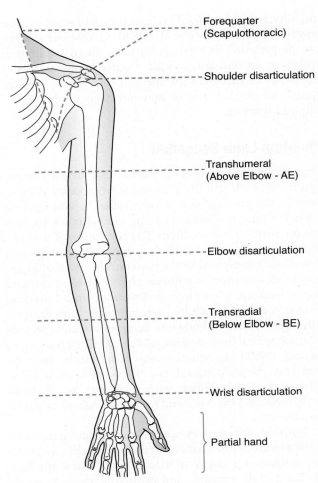

Figure 41-1 Levels of amputations.

REHABILITATION: A TEAM APPROACH

The members of the professional team are the physician, prosthetist, occupational therapist, physical therapist, and the patient. The social worker, psychologist, and vocational counselor should be consulted as needed. Patients are always active, equal members of the team and must be given the opportunity to explain their needs, preferences, and goals. The occupational therapist is essential to the rehabilitation process, because he or she works so closely with patients after their amputation.

PREPROSTHETIC THERAPY

The preprosthetic therapy program occurs from the postsurgical period until the patient receives a temporary (test) or permanent prosthesis. This is a preparatory time for both physical and emotional healing.

Postoperative Care

Postoperative care, required immediately after surgery, addresses wound care, maintenance of skin integrity, joint mobility, reduction of edema, prevention of scarring, and control of pain (Smurr et al., 2008). Outpatient therapy can be provided in a rehabilitation unit, rehabilitation center, or an outpatient clinic. Future inpatient admissions may be necessary for infections, revisions, or other complications that may or may not delay prosthetic fitting and training.

Phantom Limb Sensation

Therapists must reassure the patient that after an amputation, he or she will likely continue to experience sensations in the missing limb. This is called "phantom limb sensation" and is common among individuals with limb loss (Eichenberger et al., 2008). The perception of the presence of the amputated limb is a universal phenomenon that is remarkably real to the patient. The cause of phantom limb sensation is still not clearly understood, and research into it is continuing. Phantom limb sensation is most common in adults with traumatic amputations, although it has been known to occur in aplasics (persons with congenital limb absence) (Price, 2006). According to Melzack (1989), the neural system exists within the brain even when the body input is cut off by amputation. These perceptions are strongest with amputations of upper extremities, and the hand and fingers are felt more vividly than the arm.

With time, the patient may feel that the distal portions of the phantom limb have moved closer to the site of the amputation; this is called "telescoping." Phantom limb sensation often remains, and ordinarily, the patient accepts it. The patient may view it as an annoyance if the sensation is mild burning or tingling or may find it useful, as when learning myoelectric control for externally powered prostheses. Open discussion and ongoing patient education regarding this common phenomenon are imperative.

Phantom Limb Pain

Phantom limb pain is even less clearly understood, and its causation and management remain controversial; again, research continues (Hompland, 2004). This pain can be felt as extremely intense burning or cramping sensations or shooting pain in the residual limb and is most common in traumatic amputations. At least 90% of individuals with limb loss experience phantom limb pain (Chan et al., 2007). Central nervous system changes and peripheral nervous system damage are thought to be causes of phantom limb pain (Flor, Nikolajsen, & Jensen, 2006), whereas psychological factors have been identified as triggers to phantom limb pain (Desmond & MacLachlan, 2006).

Often, pain increases with stress. The therapist is advised to avoid emphasizing pain when possible. Treatments for those with severe pain include analgesics and surgery, such as nerve blocks and neurectomies. In the

rehabilitation setting, limb percussion (See Chapter 22), ultrasound, and transcutaneous electrical nerve stimulation (TENS) have been used (Smurr et al., 2008). Acupuncture, psychotherapy, hypnotherapy, and relaxation techniques have also been used. No one approach, however, has proven to be clearly successful. Using both a team approach and a patient-centered approach to find the best pain relief methods for the patient and to integrate them into the overall treatment plan is recommended.

Mirror therapy is another available treatment option to explore for treating phantom limb pain. Over 15 years ago, Ramachandran and Rogers-Ramachandran (1996) published a key article on the novel use of a mirror for the treatment of phantom limb pain. Albeit a small case report, 60% of their subjects had an improvement in phantom limb pain with the use of mirror therapy. In 2007, Chan et al., published the first randomized, sham-controlled trial on the use of mirror therapy versus imagery therapy for phantom limb pain in lower extremity amputees. The results were impressive: 100% of those performing mirror therapy experienced improvement in phantom limb pain, whereas 89% of those who switched to mirror therapy from the two sham-controlled conditions also experienced improvement.

The use of mirror therapy is now widely accepted as standard therapy for limb amputation (Weeks, Anderson-Barnes, & Tsao, 2010). The process of mirror therapy involves the use of a mirror placed at midline and against the patient's chest or groin depending on the level of amputation that is being addressed. The residual limb is placed behind the mirror and the intact limb is placed in front of the mirror, so that the patient observes the reflection of the intact limb in the mirror. The mirror should be placed close enough to the body to obstruct view of the residual limb as shown in Figure 41-2. The patient is then

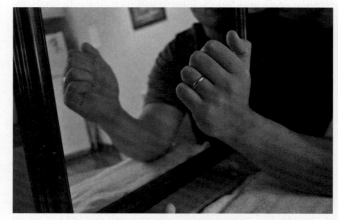

Figure 41-2 A patient with a transhumeral amputation performing mirror box therapy. Position the mirror at the patient's midline with the residual limb behind the mirror. Instruct him to continuously look at the reflection of the intact limb while performing mirror box therapy.

directed to focus on the reflection of the intact limb in the mirror during the process. He or she is instructed to place the intact limb in the position that the residual limb feels as though it is in. As tolerated, the patient should slowly move the intact limb and attempt to move the phantom limb through motions that do not elicit pain in the phantom or residual limb. The patient is encouraged to perform movements that he or she is capable of doing with the phantom limb and at a speed that requires attention but does not create a challenge. Typically, the therapist will observe movement in the residual limb when the patient feels able to move the phantom limb. It is recommended that mirror therapy be conducted in a quiet environment to reduce distractions.

Oftentimes, patients beginning mirror therapy will fatigue easily, so it is not uncommon for the patient to initially only tolerate 8–12 minutes. Patients should be encouraged to work up to 15–20-minute sessions daily over a 4-week period as part of their home program. Encourage patients to perform mirror therapy daily and as needed when phantom limb pain is disruptive to daily activity, including sleep. Daily use of a visual analogue scale and tracking of the number and duration of phantom pain episodes are recommended to determine whether mirror therapy is beneficial.

Psychological Aspects of Limb Loss

Upper limb loss results in a change in the ability to grip, feel, and manipulate objects; physically engage in social interaction; and communicate through gestures. This loss can profoundly influence the person's body scheme, self-esteem, and sense of efficacy (Desmond, 2007). Limb loss affects not only physical function but also the patient's competence and satisfaction in life roles: self-maintenance, family, and home; self-enhancement, such as engaging in leisure and community activities; and self-advancement as a worker or student (see Chapter 1) (Murray, 2005). Reactions to amputation are as complex as the unique nature of each human, and an individual's personality and belief system may influence how he or she responds to limb loss. Often, an early response is shock and disbelief; furthermore, when both upper extremities are amputated, a feeling of helplessness is common. In a review of the literature relating to psychosocial adjustment to amputation, Horgan and MacLachlan (2004) found that depression rates in amputees are higher than general population rates for up to 2 years postamputation. Anxiety rates were also higher but seemed to readjust to comparable general population rates after 1 year. Sometimes the patient may project negative feelings onto the therapist, family members, and friends. What can the occupational therapist do? The therapist should encourage open discussion, develop a relationship based on trust and respect, and work with the other treatment team members to facilitate the patient's psychological adjustment and reintegration into previous roles.

- Give the patient information. Explain the therapy process and establish realistic goals and outcomes. This can clarify the patient's expectations and reduce fear and anxiety. The therapist can prepare the patient during the preprosthetic phase by showing various prostheses that are appropriate to the amputation level and discussing prosthetic components. The therapist must listen to the patient and understand his or her life roles and future goals. A collaborative relationship between therapist and patient fosters a sense of trust and control for the patient.
- Introduce the patient to a peer visitor who has a similar amputation to facilitate discussion on stages of recovery, the rehabilitation process, and problem-solving strategies. Recommend that the patient attend local amputee support groups and research appropriate available Internet resources.
- Provide the patient with reference material; topics can include information on coping and adjusting to the amputation, information on prosthetic options, tips on how to manage one's activities of daily living (ADL) independently, and a list of organizations as resources (Resources 41-1).
- Communicate with (and, when necessary, refer the patient to) the psychologist, spiritual counselor, and other team members throughout the psychosocial adjustment periods of survival, recovery, and reintegration after limb loss described by Van Dorsten (2004).

Preprosthetic Program Guidelines

Occupational therapy (OT) during the preprosthetic period for the upper extremity includes providing emotional support, ensuring maximal limb shrinkage and shaping, desensitizing the residual limb, maintaining range of motion and strength, facilitating independence in ADL, and change of dominance.

Provide Emotional Support

Establish an ongoing supportive, trusting relationship with the patient and family to facilitate open discussion (see Chapter 14). Collaborate with the team regarding the patient's needs and refer the patient for additional services if needed.

Instruct in Limb Hygiene and Expedite Wound Healing

- Instruct the patient to wash the limb daily with mild soap and dry it thoroughly (after clearance from the surgeon to get the residual limb wet).
- Provide basic wound care such as wound cleansing or debridement.
- Use creams to massage at the scar line to decrease scar adhesions.

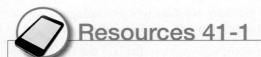

Resources 41-1

Publications for Consumers and Professionals

Challenge Magazine

Disabled Sports USA

451 Hungerford Drive, Suite 100
Rockville, MD 20850
Phone: 301-217-0960
www.dsusa.org

First Step and *Inmotion*

Amputee Coalition of America

900 E. Hill Avenue, Suite 205
Knoxville TN, 37915-2566
Phone: 888-267-5669
TTY: 865-525-4512
www.amputee-coalition.org

Handwriting for heroes: Learn to write with your non-dominant hand in 6 weeks

Phone: 888-761-6268
www.handwritingforheroes.com

One-Handed in a Two-Handed World

3rd ed, revised September 2007
Prince-Gallison Press
P.O. Box 23, Hanover Station
Boston, MA 02113
Phone: 617-367-5815
http://www.princegallison.com/

Organizations

American Amputee Foundation

P.O. Box 94227
North Little Rock, AK 72190
Phone: 501-835-9290
www.americanamputee.org

Amputee Coalition

900 E. Hill Avenue, Suite 205
Knoxville, TN 37915-2566
Phone: 888-267-5669
TTY: 865-525-4512
www.amputee-coalition.org

Challenged Athletes Foundation

9591 Waples Street
San Diego, CA 92121
Phone: 858-866-0959
www.challengedathletes.org

Disabled Sports USA

451 Hungerford Drive Suite 100
Rockville, MD 20850
Phone: 301-217-0960
www.dsusa.org

National Amputation Foundation

40 Church Street
Malvern, NY 11565
Phone: 516-887-3600
www.nationalamputation.org

Websites on Topics Related to Limb Loss

Amputee Information Network Arm Amp

www.arm-amp.com/
www.activeamp.org

DARPA: Defense Advanced Research Projects Agency

3701 North Fairfax Drive
Arlington, VA 22203-1714
Phone: 703-526-6630
www.darpa.mil

Manufacturers and Distributors

Hosmer

561 Division Street
Campbell, CA 95008
Phone: 800-827-0070
www.hosmer.com
Manufactures primarily BP components.

LTI: Liberating Technologies, Inc.

325 Hopping Brooke Road, Suite A
Holliston, MA 01746
Phone: 508-893-6363
www.Libertytechnology.com
Manufactures electronic elbows, control systems, hands, and gloves.

Motion Control, Inc.

115 N Wright Brothers Drive
Salt Lake City, UT 84116
Phone: 888-696-2767
www.utaharm.com/
Manufactures multiple electric elbows and terminal devices.

(continued)

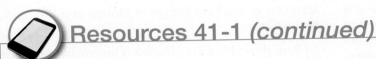

Resources 41-1 *(continued)*

Ottobock

14630 28th Avenue N .
Minneapolis, MN 55447
Phone: 800-328-4058
www.ottobock.com
Manufactures electronic hands and hooks; wrist, elbow, and other electronic systems; and BP components.

Single-Handed Solutions, LLC

http://singlehandedsolutions.blogspot.com/

Latour Anchor

E-mail: LatourAnchor@gmail.com
Cutaneous Anchor Technology for body-powered prostheses.

Touch Bionics

3455 Mill Run Drive
Hilliard, OH 43026
Phone: 855-MY-ILIMB (855-694-5462)
www.touchbionics.com
Manufacturer of iLimb and Prodigits.

TRS, Inc. (Therapeutic Recreation Systems)

3090 Sterling Circle, Studio A
Boulder, CO 80301-2338
Phone: 800-279-1865
www.oandp.com/products/trs/
Manufactures VC terminal devices and adaptations for sports and other recreational activities.

Maximize Limb Shrinkage and Limb Shaping

The goal is to shrink and shape the residual limb so that it is tapered at the distal end; this allows for optimal prosthetic fit. The following interventions can be used to achieve this goal.

- Elastic bandage. The patient is taught to wrap the limb in a figure-of-eight pattern and is expected to do so independently unless physical or cognitive limitations prevent it. In this case, a family member, friend, or caregiver is instructed in the process. The residual limb must be wrapped in a figure-of-eight diagonal configuration, with the most pressure applied at the end of the limb. *Safety Message: The limb must never be wrapped in a circular manner, as this causes a tourniquet effect and restricts circulation.* The bandage must conform firmly to the limb and be wrapped in a distal to proximal direction (Fig. 41-3). The wrap should

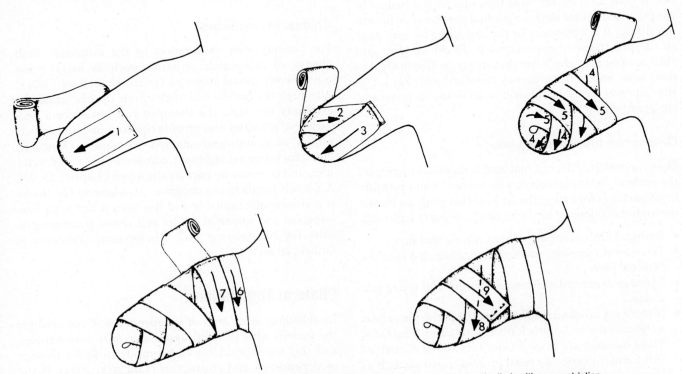

Figure 41-3 Wrapping technique for transhumeral amputation. Repeat diagonal turns as necessary to cover the limb with no constriction.

be worn continuously and reapplied immediately if it loosens. *Safety Message: The patient is advised to remove the bandage two to three times daily to examine the skin for any redness or excessive pressure.* A clean bandage should be applied at least every 2 days. Bandages can be washed with mild soap and laid flat to dry but not squeezed or machine dried.

- Elastic shrinker. Another option is an elasticized sock or shrinker. If the shrinker loosens, a smaller shrinker size will be needed. Shrinkers should be worn when not wearing the prosthesis and while sleeping in order to maintain residual limb shaping and size.
- Early postoperative prosthesis. The early postoperative prosthesis is strongly recommended for bilateral upper extremity amputations (Uellendahl, 2004) to reduce dependency for self-care activities. This temporary prosthesis may facilitate acceptance and use of the permanent prosthesis. Studies support the premise that early fitting and prosthetic training ensure acceptance of the prosthesis and its use (Fletchall, 2005; Lake & Dodson, 2006). If an early postoperative prosthesis is chosen by the team as an intervention, it is imperative that there is daily communication among the patient, occupational therapist, and prosthetist in order to maintain proper fit and use, including necessary, often daily, adjustments to improve function.

Prosthesis Wear Schedule

Early in this phase, it is important to begin patient and family education on the wear time and wear schedule of the prosthesis. Wear time is a gradual process after the initial fitting. It is important in the beginning to limit wear of the prosthesis to approximately 15–30 minutes and then remove it to check for skin integrity. Gradually, the daily wear time will increase as tolerance and skin integrity improves. The schedule will be set by the therapist and the prosthetist.

Desensitize the Residual Limb

Desensitization of the residual limb is necessary to prepare the patient's residual limb to tolerate touch and pressure in preparation for fitting the socket. This goal can be met through the following interventions (see also Chapter 22).

- Residual limb wrapping or wearing of a shrinker.
- Percussion (tapping, rubbing, and vibration) over the residual limb.
- Massage to prevent or release adhesions and soften scar tissue.
- If there are no contraindications, the patient may bear weight on the end of the limb against various surfaces. These surfaces are graded from very resilient, such as soft foam, to variously resistant and textured, such as layers of felt, a bucket of rice, and a mound of clay.

Maintain or Increase Range of Motion and Strength of the Limb

A physical conditioning program is instituted to increase or maintain the range of motion of all joints proximal to the amputation. Increasing muscle strength of the residual limb and shoulder area are also important to address. Include the contralateral side if limitations are noted. For patients with high-level amputations, a shift of weight and center of gravity can occur. Core strengthening will promote postural control, balance, and endurance and prevent asymmetry. Mobilization of the limb also increases circulation and reduces edema. This conditioning regimen should be practiced at home. Encourage the patient with unilateral limb loss to incorporate the residual limb into bilateral tasks during daily activities. Patient education on the risks of overuse of the contralateral limb should be discussed, especially if the patient elects to do all tasks one-handed. Those risks include biomechanical overuse syndromes, learned nonuse of the amputated side, and reduction of the cortical representation of the amputated part.

Facilitate Independence in Activities of Daily Living

It is important that the patient develop skills to be proficient with and without a prosthesis in his or her ADLs. A patient may only have one prosthesis; therefore, there may be times when the patient does not have the prosthesis and will still have to complete daily tasks without it.

Change of Dominance

For persons with amputation of the dominant limb, change of dominance activities, such as handwriting, must receive special attention (Yancosek & Howell, 2011). Although the patient will instinctively use the remaining extremity for ADL, the therapist can introduce a wide variety of activities and provide tips for one-handed techniques or recommend adaptive equipment (Yancosek, 2008) for home management, communication, desk activities, and community participation (see Chapters 25–27). A 6-week handwriting program, *Handwriting For Heroes*, is commercially available and has been tested with non-impaired and impaired adults and shows promising results for handwriting skill development (Yancosek & Gulick, 2008).

Bilateral Amputation

Establishing some level of independence is essential for the patient with bilateral upper extremity amputations, and this must be addressed promptly to lessen feelings of dependency and frustration (Yancosek, 2011). If the patient has enough length in one of the residual limbs, immediately provide the patient with a universal cuff, which is useful for holding a utensil or toothbrush; this is a temporary substitute for grasp. Inserting a small pencil into the universal cuff with eraser end downward can be used to operate cell phones, telephones, and allow for text messaging. For patients with smartphones, a stylus with thermoplastic, silicon, elastic, or neoprene tip can be fabricated to be mounted around the residual limb; however, the stylus must have direct contact with the skin to receive the natural electric charge from the skin in order to effectively operate the smart phone.

Early fitting with a temporary prosthesis on at least one limb is by far the best approach. Adapted devices may be needed to assist the patient in performing basic self-maintenance tasks, such as eating, toileting, grooming, and dressing (Davidson, 2002). For patients with high-level amputation, specifically designed prostheses may be helpful for accomplishment of critical tasks, for example eating (Hung & Wu, 2005). Use of the feet should be encouraged if at all possible, and other modifications of performance can be suggested, such as use of the chin, knees, and teeth (Edelstein, 2004). The therapist and patient can analyze tasks and solve problems together. Typically, the longer residual limb will be chosen as the dominant extremity.

CHOOSING THE PROSTHESIS

As a member of the team, the occupational therapist contributes to the recommendation for the upper limb prosthesis. The therapist has come to know the patient in some depth during the preprosthetic program and can contribute information regarding the patient's social and cultural contexts (Procedures for Practice 41-1).

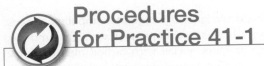

Procedures for Practice 41-1

Choosing the Prosthesis

Consider these factors:

- Residual limb: length, range of motion, skin integrity, strength
- Preference for cosmesis and function
- Hand dominance
- Prior level of function and activity levels
- Activities at work, home, school, community and recreational interests
- Patient goals, motivation, and attitude
- Financial coverage: health care insurance, ability to pay privately, and alternative funding sources
- Cognitive abilities to learn to use various components

The occupational therapist and prosthetist educate the patient about upper extremity prosthetic systems appropriate to the level of amputation. A candid discussion needs to occur between the patient, therapist, and the prosthetist about the different types of prostheses and terminal devices (TDs) and the advantages and disadvantages of each system. This discussion assists the patient in establishing realistic expectations of the prosthesis and its function.

Prosthetic Systems

The most common upper extremity prosthetic options currently available are body-powered (BP), externally powered, hybrid, activity-specific, and passive prostheses. A BP system uses motions from the body, proximal to the amputation, to operate a TD. Tension is produced from the contralateral limb, and the scapulohumeral motions are transferred to a TD through a cable. An externally powered system uses power external to the body for operation. These devices are more commonly known as myoelectric systems. Myoelectric systems require electrical signals produced from muscle contractions to operate powered elbow and electric TDs. A hybrid system is a combination of a BP and externally powered components. This type of system often includes a BP elbow and a myoelectrical TD. This system is often an option for patients with elbow disarticulation or transhumeral amputations. An activity-specific prosthesis is designed for a specific function or activity. A passive prosthesis is another option. It is endoskeletal, contoured to the shape of the arm and covered with resilient foam. It is often lightweight, contains an internal pylon shaft, and is designed with the physical characteristics of the natural arm and hand. There is no functional component to a passive prosthesis. These prostheses are available to replace any part of a limb, from a single digit to a whole arm (Leow, Pho, & Pereira, 2001). Each option has specific socket designs for each level of amputation, as well as harnessing and suspension options, and available TDs

Socket Designs

Transradial Amputation. The residual limb is encased in the socket of the prosthesis with total contact. A standard forearm socket encases the full length of the residual forearm but can be modified to allow for more active pronation and supination if the patient has a long residual limb as well as for more elbow flexion and extension. The supracondylar socket (modified Muenster) is a frequent choice for the short transradial limb; the proximal brim grips the humeral lateral and medial epicondyles and the posterior olecranon (Fig. 41-4). Additionally, the

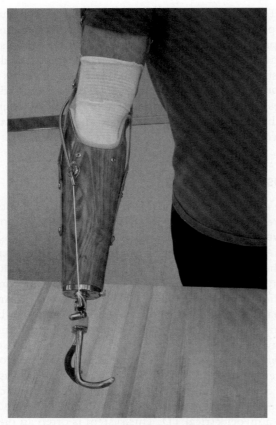

Figure 41-4 Body-powered transradial prosthesis with a modified Muenster socket and a standard voluntary opening hook.

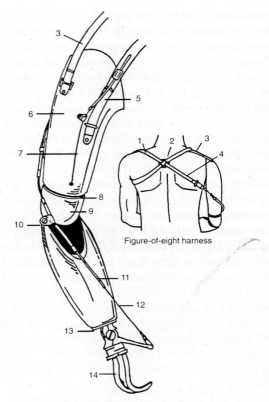

Figure 41-6 Standard transhumeral prosthesis. 1, axilla loop; 2, Northwestern University (NU) ring; 3, lateral support strap; 4, control attachment strap; 5, elastic anterior support strap; 6, socket; 7, elbow lock cable; 8, turntable; 9, internal elbow lock unit; 10, lift loop; 11, housing; 12, cable; 13, wrist unit; and 14, TD. (Illustration by Gregory Celikyol.)

supracondylar design is widely used for the myoelectric prostheses because it is self-suspending and thus requires no harnessing (Fig. 41-5).

Transhumeral Amputation. The conventional socket edge is generally just near or above the acromion, depending

on residual limb length. If rotational stability is of concern there are other variations to socket design that the prosthetist may consider. An example of a transhumeral BP prosthesis is shown in Figure 41-6.

Shoulder Disarticulation and Forequarter Amputation. Most socket designs at this level consist of a plastic laminated shoulder cap or frame socket with carbon fiber reinforcements. Another choice is an endoskeletal passive arm that is lightweight and contains an internal pylon shaft.

Harness and Other Control System Options

The harness serves two purposes: (1) to suspend, or hold, the prosthesis firmly on the residual limb and (2) to allow for force (through body motions) to be transmitted to the control cable on a BP or hybrid system. Several types of harnesses are available to include figure-of-eight, figure-of-nine, and chest strap. A new alternative option to harnessing for a BP prosthesis is the cutaneous anchor technology available through Single-Handed Solutions (Resource 41-1). This kit system uses movement from the same side of the body as the residual limb to activate the

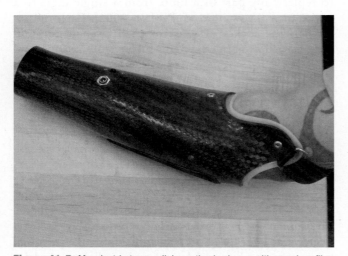

Figure 41-5 Myoelectric transradial prosthesis shown with a carbon fiber socket and without a terminal device.

prosthesis, thus eliminating the need for body motion from the contralateral side through a harness.

Wrist Units. The wrist rotation unit provides a means to attach the TD to the forearm. It also provides an important function: the TD can be rotated to positions of supination, pronation, or midposition before engaging in an activity. This is termed prepositioning and is an important substitute movement for reduced or absent active forearm rotation. Common types of wrist units include the constant friction wrist unit and quick change units.

Wrist flexion units provide the user with the ability to manually flex at the wrist often at neutral, 30° of flexion, or 50° of flexion. Wrist flexion units are indispensable for the person with bilateral amputations because of their usefulness in reaching the midline for toileting, dressing, and eating.

Elbow Units

Two kinds of elbow units are available for the BP transhumeral prosthesis: (1) an internal elbow locking unit for a standard or short transhumeral amputation and (2) an external elbow locking unit for a long transhumeral or elbow disarticulation amputation. Manual elbow components are also available with a locking mechanism. For a shoulder disarticulation prosthesis, the elbow lock can be activated using a chin nudge lever, a manual elbow lock mechanism, or through myoelectric control.

For an above-elbow externally powered prosthesis, the elbow is controlled by electromechanical switches or by myoelectric control. There are numerous types currently available. Depending on the company's design specifics, some elbows can be matched with certain available externally powered wrist and hand components and TDs. Each unit will have a charging mechanism such as an internal or external battery. Battery life can vary between products and manufactures.

Body-Powered Terminal Device Prehensors

TD prehensors for a BP prosthesis can be classified as operating by a voluntary opening (VO) mechanism or voluntary closing (VC) mechanism. The fingers of a VO device remain closed by springs for a mechanical hand or by rubber bands for a hook. The force of pinch on the hook can be increased by adding rubber bands, approximately 1 pound for each band, or by adjusting the spring mechanism for the hands. In a VC mechanism, the amount of pinch force is decreased or increased by the amount of tension the patient applies on the cable to close the TD. Patients should be made aware of the advantages of a hook over a hand, including precision grasp for small items; a minimally obstructed view, making it easier to visualize the object for grasp or release; and light weight.

The choice of a hand TD would be made by a person who values cosmesis over function.

Voluntary Opening Terminal Devices. The VO hook is widely used and can vary in size. Hooks are made of aluminum, titanium, or stainless steel; some have rubber-lined fingers. The lining provides a firm grip and prevents slippage. Many available hooks can withstand the rigors of heavy mechanical activity and are able to facilitate holding tools in activities. The VO mechanical hands operate similarly to the VO hooks except that, in the hand, the thumb and first two fingers open when the cable is pulled. These fingers oppose in a three-point prehension pattern.

Voluntary Closing Terminal Devices. A VC TD has strong variable prehension and is controlled by the amount of force the individual can exert. It is possible that a grasp of more than 30 pounds can be attained. This TD may be appealing for individuals who are active in sports, heavy physical work, or recreational activities. A VC mechanical hand has a thumb that can be manually adjusted and locked in two positions to achieve a 1.5- or 3-inch opening.

Electrically Powered Terminal Device Prehensors

The electrically powered prehensors are heavier (approximately 1 pound) but provide stronger pinch force (approximately 20–40 pounds) than the BP TDs. Examples of these are shown in Figure 41-7. These devices are activated through myoelectric or switch control. The two speed systems are (1) digital control (constant speed), in which muscle contractions cause opening and closing at a given speed; and (2) proportional control (variable speed), in which the speed and pinch force increase in proportion to the intensity of muscle contraction.

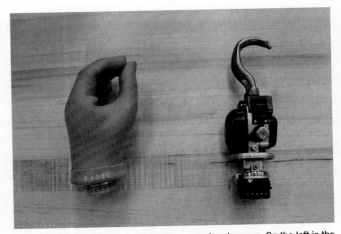

Figure 41-7 Examples of externally powered prehensors. On the left is the Ottobock System Electric Hand (Otto Bock, Minneapolis, MN) with a cosmetic cover. On the right is the Electric Terminal Device by Motion Control, Inc. (Salt Lake City, UT).

Electric Hands. The Sensorhand Speed by Ottobock has a motor in the hand mechanism that drives the thumb and first two fingers as a unit to provide palmar (three-point) prehension. The hand automatically increases force on an object if it detects slippage by a sensor in the thumb. There are multiple other electric hand devices being developed, tested, marketed, and manufactured. The ultimate goal of these types of devices is to have individual articulating digits to include an opposable thumb and multiple grips, pinch, and grasp patterns available that allow users to better master everyday tasks.

Electric Hooks. The Ottobock electric Greifer TD is only available in one size, and its two "fingers" move symmetrically in opposition to one another for precision pinch, whereas a more proximal, expanded contact area provides for a cylindrical grasp (Figure 41-8). This device may be chosen when the activity requires prehension force up to 40 pounds.

Myoelectric Control and Terminal Devices. There are numerous myoelectrically controlled TDs available, and each has advantages and disadvantages, but it is often up to the user to decide which TD he or she finds most useful and functional. It is beyond the scope of this chapter to elaborate on all available types of myoelectic TDs because technology quickly advances, and control schemes vary based on TD function and user preference. It is important that the therapist consult the patient's prosthetist to understand the capabilities and control mechanisms of the specific TD the user has received in order to effectively train the patient to operate the myoelectric TD.

Myoelectric Site Testing and Training. Muscle site testing is necessary for patients choosing a myoelectric prosthesis. This testing results in choosing the optimal location for

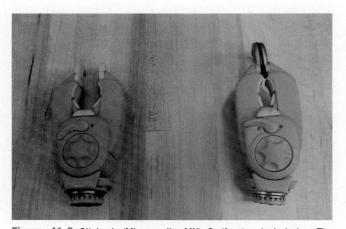

Figure 41-8 Ottobock (Minneapolis, MN) Greifer terminal device. The Greifer on the left has the interchangeable standard hooks and is in open position. The Greifer on the right has interchangeable extended hooks and is in the closed position.

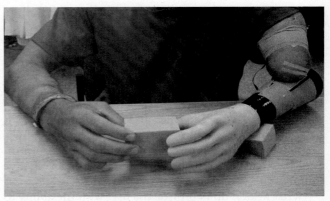

Figure 41-9 Myoelectric site training during the preprosthetic training phase at midline. The electrodes are placed on the patient's biceps and triceps myosites. The electrode leads are connected to a universal carbon fiber demonstration socket with an Ottobock System Electric Hand (Minneapolis, MN) with a standard hand shell covering the terminal device. Use of the demonstration socket allows the patient to experience what it is like to control an actual myoelectric terminal device. This patient is practicing grasp and release with a foam block; use of this type of object is often for practicing proportional control during grasping.

the control site or sites. The goal is to find a site where the patient can hold a steady contraction for at least 1–2 seconds and relax for that time. Ordinarily, the agonist and antagonist are chosen, such as wrist extensors and flexors for transradial amputation and biceps and triceps for transhumeral amputation. It is possible to use only one muscle to control two functions: a strong contraction controls one function, and a weaker contraction controls another; relaxation turns the system off; however, this system is difficult to learn and use without error. There is a wide variety of alternative control setups that can be programmed by the prosthetist.

During muscle site testing and training, skin electrodes are strapped to the residual limb or encased in a test socket. A myotester such as Myolab II by Motion Control, Inc. (Salt Lake City, UT) or Myoboy® by Ottobock, a biofeedback computer program (see Chapter 19), or an electronic demonstration hand is used to provide feedback (Fig. 41-9). Once the optimal electrode placement for control of the prosthesis is determined, the user practices with the feedback device to operate the electronic motor on command. See Chapter 13 for teaching and learning principles and practices.

Cosmetic Gloves

Prosthetic hands will have some type of rubberized covering or gloves. These gloves are available in a variety of colors and sizes to cover mechanical, electric, and passive hands. The glove needs to be replaced when damaged.

A stock production glove is one type of covering available. The skin color choices are made from a selection of sample swatches to match skin tones. These polyvinyl

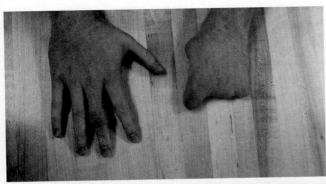

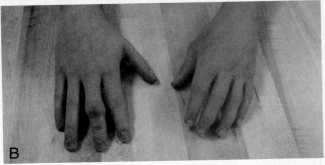

Figure 41-10 A. An individual with a left partial hand amputation. **B.** The same individual with a left-hand custom-sculpted and painted silicone glove. This custom glove is designed to resemble the intact hand.

chloride (PVC) gloves are the least expensive but are susceptible to staining from contact with such items as newsprint, clothing dyes, and ballpoint ink. The glove can deteriorate with extreme temperature and when exposed to sunlight.

A silicone covering is more expensive than PVC. A wider range of color choices is available, and details, such as veins, are painted on the glove to render a more realistic covering. These silicone gloves can withstand extremes of temperature and do not stain as easily as those made of PVC.

A custom-sculpted and painted silicone glove, also called an anatomical cover, truly attempts to replicate the individual's remaining hand (Fig. 41-10, A & B). To make the glove, the remaining hand is cast in silicone, which duplicates its contours in great detail. It is then reversed. A cosmetic restorationist adds to the realistic appearance of the hand by painting the glove and adding veins and other features. This glove is more costly than the stock production gloves.

Bilateral Upper Extremity Prostheses Considerations

Individuals with bilateral upper extremity amputations present unique challenges when selecting the prosthetic systems. Many factors influence this selection and frequently a combination of systems is selected: for example, a system that includes a BP prosthesis with

a hook as one system and a myoelectric system with an electric hand as the other system. There is no ideal setup for all individuals with bilateral upper extremity amputations. It is recommended to listen to the patient and his or her needs and goals and also consult with other team members for other perspectives. In the end, the patient will select the system best for him or her (Fig. 41-11, A & B).

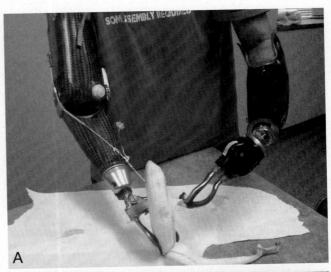

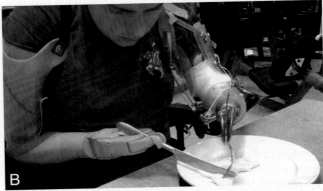

Figure 41-11 A. A patient with bilateral upper extremity amputations using final prosthetic sockets. This picture demonstrates this individual using his prostheses to peel a banana. This activity requires a high level of proportional control to hold the banana without crushing it as well as a high level of skill to control the prosthesis and terminal device while peeling the banana. This individual has a through-elbow amputation on his right and is wearing a body-powered prosthesis with the N-Abler V Series Body-powered Five Function Wrist by Texas Assistive Devices, LLC (Brazoria, TX). On his left, he has a transradial amputation and is wearing a myoelectric prosthesis with an ETD by Motion Control, Inc. (Salt Lake City, UT) with a flexion wrist component. **B.** Bilateral upper extremity prosthetic test socket system. This patient has a myoelectric test socket on the left with a Dynamic Arm and Griefer from Otto Bock (Minneapolis, MN). The test socket is made of a clear heavy thermoplastic and is used until the individual's limb volume has stabilized. On the right, the individual has a body-powered test socket with the N-Abler V Series Body-powered Five Function Wrist by Texas Assistive Devices, LLC (Brazoria, TX).

The Final Choice: A Discussion

"In the upper extremity, the prosthesis meets its greatest challenge. Here the lost function can only be imitated. . . . We must fit the prosthesis not only to the patient's limb but to his whole personality" (Kessler, 1947, p. 5).

Comfort and function have long been accepted as important factors in the acceptance and use of the prosthesis by the patient. Studies have attempted to reveal additional predictor variables of prosthetic use. In one study of 107 upper limb amputees, 56% wore a prosthesis for approximately 11 hours per day for an average of 24 days per month; this study identified longer length of the residual limb, the absence of phantom limb pain, and married status as variables associated with use of a prosthesis (Raichle et al., 2009). Military service members from current conflicts have higher than previously recorded acceptance and use rates that may be a result of improved comfort and function of prostheses (Gailey et al., 2010; McFarland et al., 2010; Reiber et al., 2010). The patient's desire for a prosthesis is strongest after surgery and may wane as time passes, particularly for those with unilateral amputations, because compensatory one-handed techniques are typically quickly mastered. The patient with bilateral upper extremity amputations needs to function and therefore is likely to accept and use one or both prostheses in order to achieve some level of independence. Therapists may also be involved in evaluating the patient's satisfaction with the prosthesis using standardized measurement tools as well as measuring performance while using a prosthesis (Resnik & Borgia, 2011).

What defines a success? The definition is unique to the individual. When the prosthesis is viewed as necessary or meaningful for any activity, such as leisure activities, or for cosmesis, it has added to the quality of life and thus can be seen as successful. A patient with a unilateral amputation may use the prosthesis for particular activities, such as for sports, and these interests can change with time. The end goal is for self-selection of the type of prosthesis for activities and tasks that facilitate the highest level of independence and competency in life roles that are meaningful to the patient. However, this does not always assume prosthetic use in all daily activities. It is the team's responsibility to present all the options to the patient.

Although prosthetic use is the goal, another important discussion topic is the risk for development of a musculoskeletal overuse syndrome in the neck/upper back, the shoulders, and the remaining limb (Ostlie et al., 2011).

PROSTHETIC TRAINING PROGRAM

Initial Stage of Prosthetic Training

The initial stage of treatment can generally be covered in one or two therapy sessions. Procedures for Practice 41-2 has treatment guidelines for this stage.

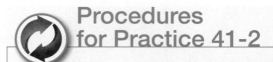

Procedures for Practice 41-2

Treatment Guidelines for Initial Stage of Prosthetic Training

- Evaluate to determine roles, tasks, and activity needs and preferences.
- Evaluate the prosthesis.
- Explain program goals to the patient.
- Describe the functions of each component; give the patient an illustration of the prosthesis with components labeled.
- Teach the patient to don and doff the prosthesis.
- Discuss the wearing schedule with the patient.
- Teach limb hygiene care.
- Teach care of the prosthesis.
- Begin controls training using the terminal device.

Evaluation of the Prosthesis

The therapist evaluates the prosthesis before training begins. The evaluation is to determine (1) compliance with the prescription, (2) comfort of fit of the socket and harness, (3) satisfactory operation of all components, and (4) appearance (features) of the prosthesis and its parts. If the patient is fitted with a myoelectrically controlled prosthesis, it is important that the therapist have a good understanding of the prosthetic control setup in order to direct prosthetic controls training. Control setup refers to how the patient switches between modes (i.e., elbow control, wrist control, and hand open and close). The therapist should contact the prosthetist if there are any questions about the prosthesis setup.

First Therapy Session

Generally, patients with unilateral amputations attend therapy on an outpatient schedule several days a week; therefore, the first visit is important. The initial goal is to minimize negative experiences in order to facilitate future acceptance and use of the prosthesis. In addition to evaluation of the prosthesis, the following must also be covered during the first visit: (1) donning and removing the prosthesis, (2) wearing schedule, and (3) hygienic care of the residual limb if the patient did not receive preprosthetic care in the clinic.

Donning and Removing the Prosthesis. Donning and doffing of the full prosthetic system as independently as possible is critical to prosthetic use. The full prosthetic system includes (1) residual limb sock, (2) prosthetic donning liner, (3) alcohol-based lubricant gels, or powder, (4) prosthetic socket, and (5) harnessing as appropriate (Smurr et al., 2008).

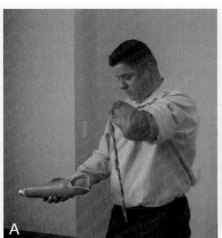
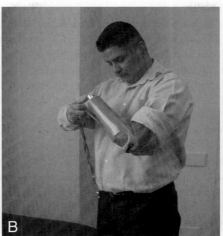
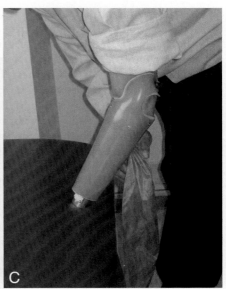

Figure 41-12 Transradial myoelectric prosthetic donning method with pull sock. This method can also be used to don transhumeral level myoelectric prosthesis. **A.** Don the pull sock over the residual limb. **B.** Pull the laynard of the pull sock through the socket opening. **C.** Pull the pull sock completely through to ensure good skin contact.

There are a number of different methods for donning and doffing the BP prosthesis, but the two most common methods are (1) the coat method and (2) the pull-over method. To use the coat method, the residual limb is inserted into the socket, which is held in place with the intact hand, with the harness and axilla loop dangling behind the back. The intact arm reaches behind and slips into the axilla loop; a forward shrug of the shoulders positions the prosthesis in place. For the pullover method, the patient places the prosthesis in front of him or her, and the intact arm is placed through the axilla loop while the residual limb is placed into the socket. Both limbs are raised to lift the prosthesis and harness over the head as the harness falls into place. Initially, the prosthesis can be placed on a bed or dresser to support it as the patient slips into the prosthesis. When donning a myoelectric prosthesis, the patient may use a pull sock on the residual limb that helps to guide the residual limb into the socket and is pulled through an opening in the socket and allows for good skin and socket interface (Fig. 41-12, A–C). To allow for the highest level of independence of donning and removing the prosthesis, the patient, therapist, and prosthetist may need to collaborate to determine the simplest or most ideal method.

Wearing Time. The patient must increase wearing time gradually to develop tolerance to the socket and harness or type of suspension. The initial wearing time may be two to three 15–30-minute sessions spread out over the course of a day. Each time the prosthesis is removed, the residual limb must be examined for excessive redness or irritation and must not be reapplied until any redness subsides. *Safety Message: Redness that does not disappear after approximately 20 minutes should be reported to the prosthetist for adjustment of the prosthesis.* Otherwise, prosthetic wearing time can be increased in 30-minute increments until the prosthesis can be worn all day. The importance of gradually increasing the wearing time cannot be overemphasized, particularly for patients with decreased sensation and scar tissue (Smurr et al., 2008).

Limb Hygiene. The residual limb is enclosed in a rigid socket where excessive perspiration can macerate the skin. Therefore it is important to instruct the patient to inspect the residual limb each time the prosthesis is removed to look for any skin changes or areas of irritation and to wash the residual limb daily with mild soap and lukewarm water and pat dry. If the patient experiences excessive sweating with the wear of the prosthesis, it is recommended the patient and therapist discuss this with the prosthetist. This discussion may identify any socket modifications or socks, liners, or special antiperspirant formulas that may be worn with the prosthesis without compromising the fit and suspension and without interfering with myosite electrodes. Alternative strapping methods for suspension may also be examined.

Operational Prosthetic Knowledge: Componentry and Maintenance

Componentry Knowledge. With all prostheses, the patient must obtain and demonstrate knowledge of prosthesis componentry terminology and a general understanding of proper prosthetic maintenance. The prosthestist will provide education on the componentry and maintenance, and the therapist should reinforce this education during therapy. Basic common terminologies include but is not limited to (1) socket and harness design; (2) component identification, operation, and care; (3) types of TDs; (4) type of control system used; and (5) basic prosthesis mechanics. The goal is for the patient to be able to articulate problems to the prosthetist and therapist using correct terminology if the prosthesis malfunctions.

Care of Prosthesis. Mild soap and warm water are recommended for daily cleaning of the interior of the socket to remove any residues of powders, lubricants, and perspiration. It can also be wiped with rubbing alcohol every several weeks. The patient must be cautioned about agents that may stain or damage gloves. If using hand sanitizer, caution against using those with an added fragrance. The hook is rugged, but care must be taken during work in areas where there is excessive dirt, grease, or water. The patient must be especially careful with powered components and know which components must avoid contact with water or which are water resistant. Other special concerns are care of the batteries, methods of charging the batteries, and operation of the on/off switch.

Regardless of the type of prosthesis, basic prosthetic maintenance procedures that the patient is expected to become proficient with include (1) socket daily maintenance (i.e., daily cleaning and socket inspection), (2) routine battery charging procedures appropriate for the prosthesis, (3) component maintenance (i.e., routine cleaning and lubrication), (4) harness adjustment, and (5) rubber band replacement and cable system changes for BP prosthesis (Smurr et al., 2008). The therapist is responsible for ensuring the patient is appropriately trained and achieves maximal independence in all of the above procedures and can complete each task proficiently within his or her everyday environment.

Intermediate Stage of Prosthetic Training

The therapy program for the prosthesis is addressed in two phases: (1) prosthetic controls training and (2) prosthetic functional use training. Please refer to Figures 41-13 and 41-14 for schematic overview of controls training for BP and myoelectric prostheses by level of amputation.

Prosthetic Controls Training

Therapy for BP controls training begins with teaching the operation of each control, beginning with the TD. The therapist guides the patient to practice repetitive activation of each component. Transradial prostheses have a single control system that activates the TD

by cable pull. Patients are instructed to activate the TD (Fig. 41-15) through humeral flexion and scapular abduction (protraction). Transhumeral prostheses have a dual control system for the TD and elbow. The motions required to lock and unlock the elbow are a combination of scapular depression, and humeral extension and abduction (Fig. 41-16). Chest expansion can also be useful for patients with higher level amputations or with nerve involvement or other injuries impacting the residual limb; however, harnessing may need to be adjusted to capture this motion (Atkins & Edelstein, 2006). TD activation is achieved in the same manner as with the transradial controls except that the elbow must be locked. The patient with a transhumeral prosthesis may also have to learn to use the turntable to rotate the arm medially and laterally. For very short transhumeral amputations, the prosthetist may fit the patient with a shoulder joint as well, so the user should be trained how to position the shoulder to better accommodate specific activities.

Currently, myoelectric prostheses are frequent choices for prosthetic systems. Ideally, the patient has already received muscle site controls training during the preprosthetic period. When a myoelectric tester is used (a biofeedback unit can also be used), the goals are to isolate muscle contractions and increase muscle strength (see Chapter 20). Figure 41-17 depicts a two-state transradial system whereby two separate muscle groups are used to operate the TD. The intent is to choose muscles that physiologically closely correspond to the outcome motion and also produce strong electrical signals when contracted. It is also essential that the contractions can be isolated from one another. Cocontraction may be used to switch between functions (i.e., wrist rotation and TD control). Wrist extensors and flexors are commonly chosen to achieve opening and closing of the TD. For transhumeral amputations, the common choices are the biceps and triceps. For higher level amputations, as in shoulder disarticulation or forequarter amputations, the choices for control may be pectoralis or infraspinatus.

The therapy program begins with evaluation of the prosthesis, with special emphasis on the control system. Additional factors to be addressed with externally powered prostheses include the following:

- Are the electrodes aligned along the direction of the muscle fiber and placed over the site offering the best muscle control potential?
- Is there good contact between the electrodes and the skin? An imprint should be visible on the skin when the prosthesis is removed but should not be deep enough to cause irritation.
- Can the patient open and close the hand in various planes?
- If there is an internal battery, can the patient manage the battery charging strategy?

Controls Training for Body-Powered Prosthesis by Level of Amputation

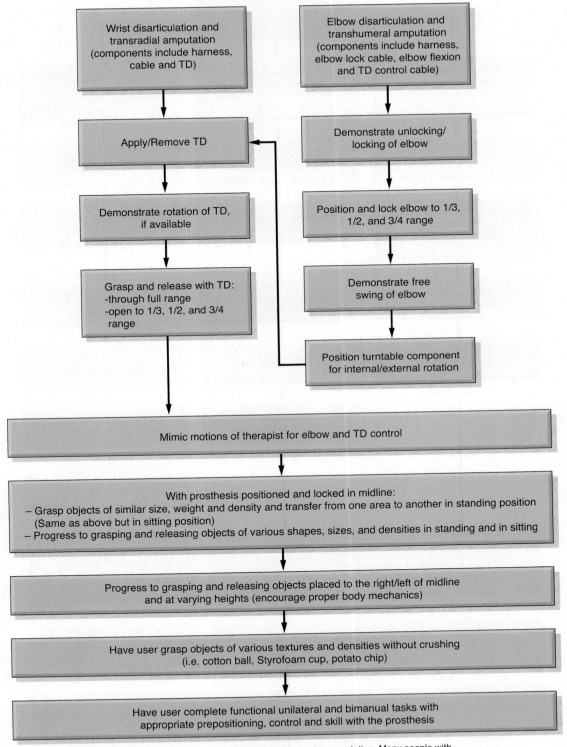

Wrist disarticulation and transradial amputation (components include harness, cable and TD)

Elbow disarticulation and transhumeral amputation (components include harness, elbow lock cable, elbow flexion and TD control cable)

Apply/Remove TD

Demonstrate unlocking/ locking of elbow

Demonstrate rotation of TD, if available

Position and lock elbow to 1/3, 1/2, and 3/4 range

Grasp and release with TD:
-through full range
-open to 1/3, 1/2, and 3/4 range

Demonstrate free swing of elbow

Position turntable component for internal/external rotation

Mimic motions of therapist for elbow and TD control

With prosthesis positioned and locked in midline:
– Grasp objects of similar size, weight and density and transfer from one area to another in standing position
  (Same as above but in sitting position)
– Progress to grasping and releasing objects of various shapes, sizes, and densities in standing and in sitting

Progress to grasping and releasing objects placed to the right/left of midline and at varying heights (encourage proper body mechanics)

Have user grasp objects of various textures and densities without crushing (i.e. cotton ball, Styrofoam cup, potato chip)

Have user complete functional unilateral and bimanual tasks with appropriate prepositioning, control and skill with the prosthesis

*Note: This diagram does not include shoulder disarticulation or forequarter amputation. Many people with these levels of amputation are unable to generate necessary motions to produce excursion through the harness and cables to operate a body-powered system, therefore they are rarely seen clinically.

Figure 41-13 Controls training for body-powered prosthesis by level of amputation. TD, terminal device.

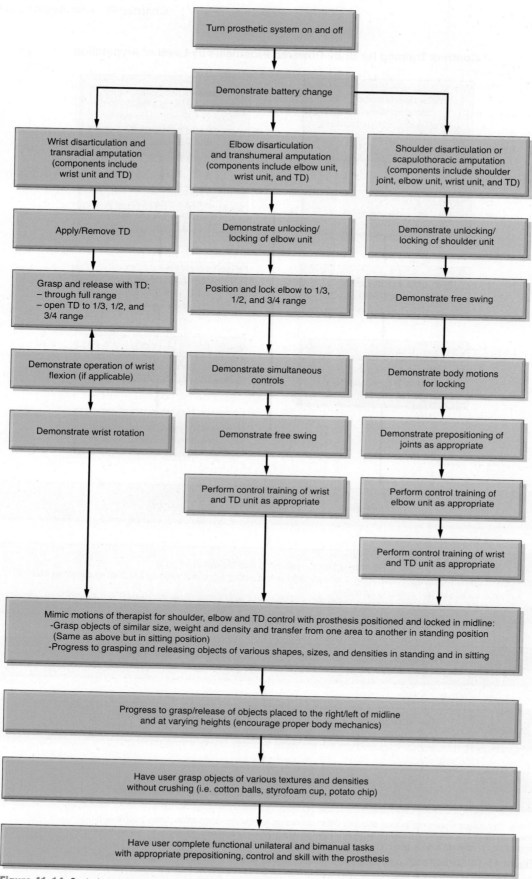

Figure 41-14 Controls training for myoelectric prosthesis by level of amputation. TD, terminal device.

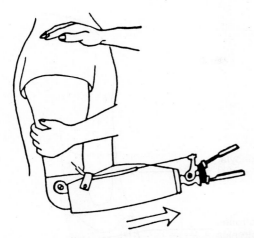

Figure 41-15 Teaching activation of voluntary opening (VO) terminal device (TD). With elbow locked, the therapist guides the patient's upper arm forward to open TD. (Illustration by Gregory Celikyol.)

- If there is an external battery, can the patient remove and replace the battery with ease?

The therapist should consult with the prosthetist for guidance with any concerns with system setup and operation.

Practice in control drills requires instructing and coaching the patient in patterns of reach, grasp, and release of objects that vary in weight, size, texture, and

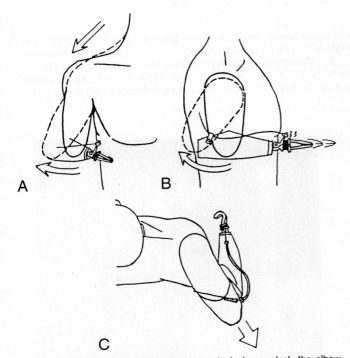

Figure 41-16 Motions (*arrows*) necessary to lock or unlock the elbow of a transhumeral prosthesis. **A.** Abduction with depression. **B.** Extension. **C.** Combined movement pattern of extension, depression, and abduction. (Illustration by Gregory Celikyol.)

configuration. Ordinarily, the sequence is from large, hard objects to smaller, softer, and more fragile ones. These assortments are subject to the therapist's ingenuity and the patient's interests. Initially, objects are placed on a tabletop for prehension practice; they are then transported to various locations in the room. The therapist instructs the patient to determine the most natural and efficient position for the TD before grasping an item and to rotate it in the wrist unit. This is called prepositioning the TD.

Eventually, the therapist instructs the patient to perform motion patterns in different planes away from midline through the functional envelope, such as overhead, at tabletop, and at floor level. The functional envelope refers to the area of space in which the patient can operate the upper limb prosthesis. Overhead use is the most difficult because of the harnessing system; overhead use is particularly difficult, sometimes impossible, for individuals with high amputations. The person with bilateral amputations may have a harness system that is bilaterally attached; therefore, the patient must practice relaxing the musculature on the contralateral side while using one prosthesis.

Prosthetic Functional Use Training

Spontaneous, automatic skillful prosthetic use is a goal for functional use training, particularly with bimanual tasks. Another is completion of activities within a reasonable length of time while using minimal extraneous movement and energy expenditure. Figures 41-18 to 41-25 show functional tasks. The therapist encourages patients to analyze and see similarities among situations and reminds them of relevant principles. This prepares the patient to respond with a sense of control in unpredictable situations.

A person with a unilateral amputation can be expected to use the prosthesis primarily for sustained holding or for stabilization. Table 41-1 suggests how some activities can be accomplished; Yancosek (2011) offers additional task suggestions. A key component to successful training is deliberate practice using the prosthesis for realistic, functional tasks. A landmark study by Lake in 1997 that has never been replicated revealed that individuals who received prosthetic training surpassed those who did not in efficiency of use, skill, and spontaneity.

Several factors affect the degree of independence of the person with bilateral amputations, the major one being the level of amputations. Some adaptations may be necessary for those with high-level bilateral amputations. These adaptations may range from a simple buttonhook or dressing frame—a stand in which coat hooks are inserted to hold clothing—to high-tech solutions, such as electronic aids for daily living and computers controlled

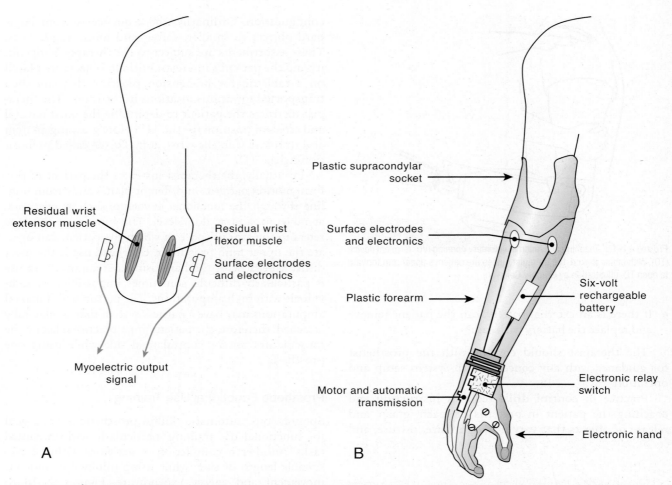

A

B

Figure 41-17 Myoelectric prosthesis, a two-state system in which two separate muscle groups operate the terminal device. **A.** 1, The muscle contracts and creates an electrical signal that can be measured in microvolts (1 millionth of a volt). 2, The EMG signal is detected by the surface electrode. 3, The EMG signal is processed by the electronics and transmitted to the electronic relay in the hand. **B.** 1, When the electronic relay receives an EMG signal from the wrist flexors, the circuit is complete, and the electricity from the battery runs the motor to close the hand. 2, When the relay receives an EMG signal from the wrist extensors, the motor runs in the opposite direction to open the hand. (Illustration courtesy of Jack Hodgins, CPO, Kessler Institute for Rehabilitation, West Orange, NJ.)

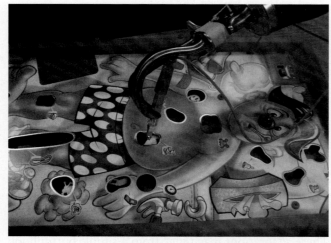

Figure 41-18 An individual using a body-powered prosthesis to play a tabletop game. Using the prosthesis as the primary mover during the game requires a high level of prosthetic control and skill. This type of activity would be appropriate during advanced prosthetic training.

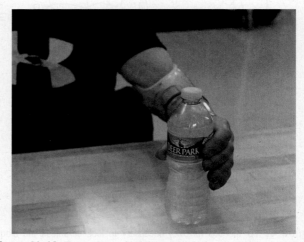

Figure 41-19 The practice of holding a bottle of water with a myoelectric prosthesis and electric hand is an excellent functional activity to learn proportional control and build individual confidence in the prosthesis.

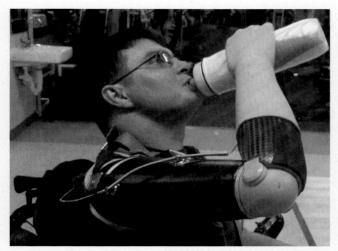

Figure 41-20 Individual with final hybrid prosthesis drinking from a water bottle. This demonstrates prosthetic integration into activity.

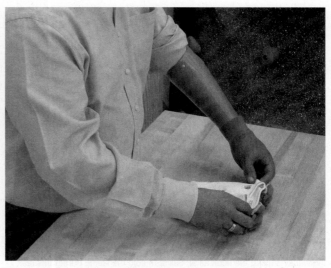

Figure 41-22 Practicing folding laundry with a myoelectric prosthesis with electric hand to learn to integrate the device during bimanual tasks.

by breath, voice, or mouthstick. The therapist is advised to encourage foot use when patients show potential and are agile. Persons who have developed this ability at an early age have a high degree of independence. Feet have the advantage of having sensibility, which serves well in all activities and surpasses prosthetic use.

Final Stage of Prosthetic Training: Instrumental Activities of Daily Living

In the final stage, prosthetic functional use skills are further developed, and daily living activities that are more demanding are introduced. Discharge planning should include exploration of vocational and recreational interests, driving, the use of public transportation, community reintegration, and adaptive sports. Visits to the community, home, school, and work are strongly advised. This brings the patient and therapist into the actual environment, away from simulated, static settings of a clinic. Patients may be encouraged to attend an amputee peer support group. These groups vary in their goals, but most provide a forum wherein people can interact and share experiences. Many groups provide ongoing educational programs on new prosthetic developments or on sports and recreational activities. See Resources 41-1 for organizations that may have local chapters.

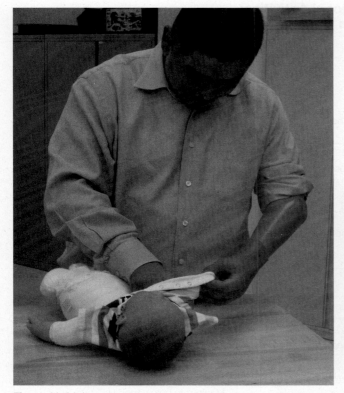

Figure 41-21 Practicing bimanual tasks with a myoelectric prosthesis and electric hand. This individual changing a diaper and dressing a doll using his prosthesis as an assist.

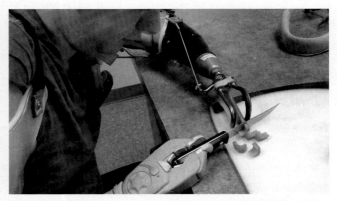

Figure 41-23 Cutting vegetables using a body-powered prosthesis and a myoelectric prosthesis. It is important for the a patient with bilateral upper extremity amputations to learn how to hold a knife in the terminal device for functional activities such as cutting.

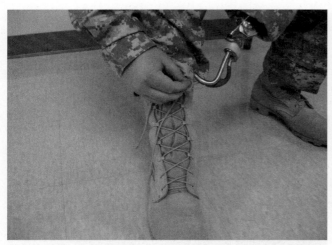

Figure 41-24 Tying military boots with a body-powered prosthesis. The individual is using the hook as an assist to hold the lacing during this task.

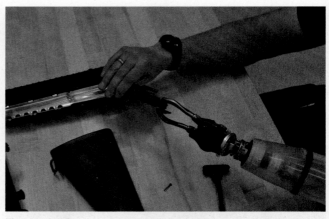

Figure 41-25 Assembling a mock weapon using a myoelectric prosthesis with a wrist rotator and wrist flexion component. This is a meaningful and purposeful activity for service members.

Sports and Recreation

Increasing numbers of individuals with amputations are pursuing recreational and sporting activities, and as a result, several customized prosthetic sockets and components are available for sports and recreational activities. Figures 41-26 to 41-29 show activity-specific sockets and

activity-specific TDs used to facilitate participation in sports activities. The Internet is a good source of information for this and related topics.

Driving

Driving is of considerable importance in today's society. Many patients are eager to return to driving following

Table 41-1	Suggested Approaches for Functional Activities: Unilateral Upper Limb Amputation	
Task	**Prosthesis**	**Sound Limb**
Eating		
Cut food	Hold fork	Cut with knife
Butter bread	Stabilize bread	Spread toward body
Fill glass from faucet	Hold glass	Turn knob or lever
Carry tray	TD in midposition to hold	Hold in midposition
Peel fruit	Stabilize with TD	Peel
Dressing		
Don and doff shirt or blouse	Don: prosthesis in sleeve first; doff: remove sound arm first	Don: sound arm last; doff: remove prosthesis last
Put clothing on hanger	Hold hanger	Place clothing on hanger
Buckle belt	Stabilize belt	Push belt through buckle
Tie bow	Stabilize lace	Manipulate and make loops
Button cuff on sound side	Use buttonhook (or sew on button using elastic thread)	Hold cuff in place with fingertips while using buttonhook
Use zipper	Hold fabric with TD	Pull zipper
Desk skills		
Write	Stabilize paper	Write
Insert letter in envelope	Hold, stabilize envelope at end	Insert letter and seal
Use phone, dial, take notes	Hold receiver: TD or with chin and shoulder	Dial and write
Draw line with ruler; use paper clip	Stabilize ruler; hold paper	Draw line; apply clip
General skills		
Take bill from wallet	Hold wallet or stabilize on table	Manipulate wallet and remove bill
Wrap and unwrap package	Stabilize box and paper	Manipulate box, paper; tie
Thread needle	Hold needle	Thread needle

TD, terminal device.

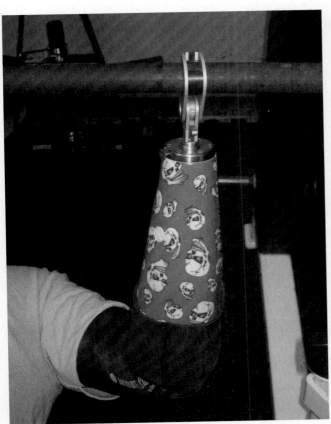

Figure 41-26 Activity-specific prosthesis for weightlifting. This particular terminal device for weightlifting is from Texas Assistive Devices, LLC (Brazoria, TX).

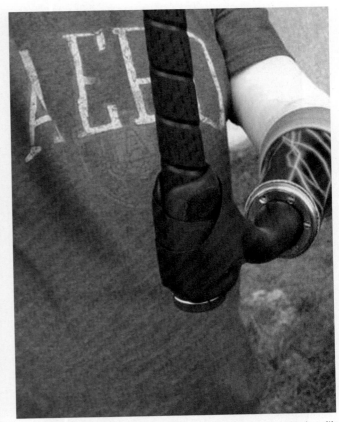

Figure 41-28 Commercially available activity-specific prosthesis with baseball bat attachment terminal device.

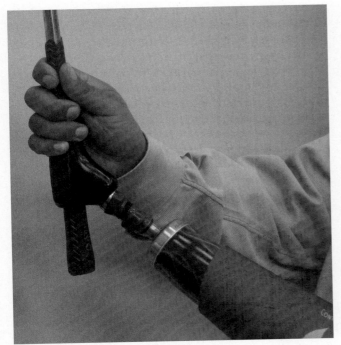

Figure 41-27 Commercially available activity-specific prosthesis with golfing attachment terminal device.

either an upper and/or lower limb amputation. Safe and independent driving involves a complex interaction of multiple systems to include one's physical, visual, cognitive, and behavioral abilities. When appropriate, the therapist makes the referral for a comprehensive driving assessment. The driving rehabilitation specialist will do a thorough chart review, patient interview, and clinical assessment, which may include a behind the wheel evaluation. The driving rehabilitation specialist will make recommendations for any needed adaptive equipment or vehicle modifications. For example, a spinner knob or driving ring may be recommended for patients with a unilateral upper extremity amputation. Installation of a left-foot accelerator bar and pedal may be necessary for a person with a right lower extremity amputation. Hand controls can be installed for patients with bilateral leg amputations (see Chapter 26). There are companies available that may be consulted to do van conversions for patients who require multiple adaptations. Patients are encouraged to contact their state licensing agency or department of motor vehicles to determine whether there are any limitations or driving restrictions for those individuals with amputations.

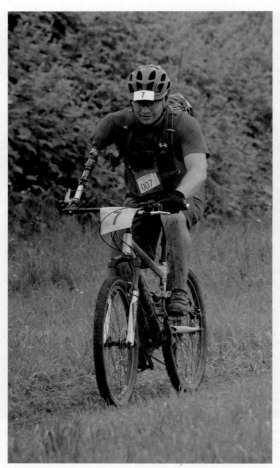

Figure 41-29 An individual with a short transhumeral amputation mountain biking wearing a custom activity-specific prosthesis. (Courtesy of Disabled Sports USA, Rockville, MD.)

OUTCOME ASSESSMENTS

A special interest group of rehabilitation professionals called the Upper Limb Prosthetic Outcome Measures (ULPOM) group was formed to address the need for validated outcome measures for amputees (Hill et al., 2009). These specific instruments are needed because traditional dexterity assessments (e.g., Box and Blocks, 9-Hole Pegtest, and Purdue Pegboard) do not provide meaningful data for patients with amputation using a prosthesis for fine motor movements. Anecdotally, occupational therapists may use these traditional assessments to assess changes in performance pre- and postprosthetic training (Fig. 41-30); however, they are inadequate for determining true outcomes of the effectiveness of prosthetic interventions. Clinicians who frequently treat patients with upper limb amputations are interested in compiling normative data on this specialized patient population and developing the evidence base for intervention selection; therefore, they need more valid measuring instruments. Although more work is needed in

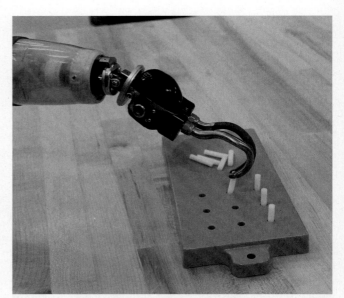

Figure 41-30 An individual with a transradial amputation completing the 9-Hole Peg Test using a test socket with wrist rotation and flexion wrist components as well as the Motion Control ETD by Motion Control, Inc. (Salt Lake City, UT).

the area of outcome assessments for patients with upper limb amputation, there are five assessments worthy of consideration and use. Assessment Table 41-1 provides information on these assessments.

DISCHARGE PLANNING

At discharge, the team will educate the patient and the family on the process of follow-up with the clinic if occupational therapy is needed for future therapy, questions, or any other issues that may arise. The patient may continue an ongoing relationship with the prosthetist and return for modifications or if a new prosthesis is needed. As patients return to their occupational roles and lives, their needs may change, and in the future they may want to explore different prosthetic options and TDs for different activities. When new devices are received, more therapy and training in occupational therapy may be needed.

PARTIAL HAND AMPUTATIONS

As with any amputation, the surgeon performing a partial hand amputation attempts to preserve length with intact sensibility. At this level, retaining residual digits with adequate skin coverage and some degree of mobility and sensation is far superior to any prosthesis and is the goal. The principles of preprosthetic therapy (discussed earlier) apply to this level of amputation as well. Devices available for persons with partial hand amputations can be described as cosmetic, passive functional, or active functional prostheses.

Assessment Table 41-1	Summary of Outcome Assessments for Prosthetic Use by Upper Extremity Amputees				
Instrument and Reference	Description	Time to Administer	Validity	Reliability	Sensitivity	Strengths and Weaknesses
Trinity Amputation and Prosthesis Experience Scales-Revised (TAPES-R) (Gallagher & MacLachlan, 2000)	A self-report instrument that consists of three scales (psychosocial adjustment, activity restriction, and satisfaction with the prosthesis), each one containing three subscales (Gallagher et al., 2010). Higher scores indicate greater levels of the factor measured.	Not reported	Face validity in that subscales resembled what they intended to measure (Gallagher & MacLachlan, 2000). Construct validity as compared to the World Health Organization Quality of Life Questionnaire ($r \geq 0.618$), the Impact of Event Scale ($r \geq 0.26$), and the Trait Meta Mood Scale ($r \geq 0.337$) (Gallagher & MacLachlan, 2000).	All scales showed good internal consistency. Chronbach's $\alpha \geq$ 0.89 (Gallagher et al., 2010), as did the subscales: prosthesis satisfaction: $\alpha = 0.94$, activity restriction: $\alpha = 0.72-0.94$, psychosocial adjustment: $\alpha = 0.788-0.907$ (Desmond & MacLachlan, 2005). Interrater and test-retest reliability not reported.	Not reported	Strengths: The patient can complete on his own and mail the results back. Available free from http://www. psychoprosthetics.ie/ tapes-r.html Weaknesses: The psychometrics are incomplete.
Assessment of Capacity for Myoelectric Control (ACMC) (Hermansson et al., 2005; Hermansson, Bodin, Eliasson, 2006)	The ACMC is administered and scored on clinical observations of the myoelectric prosthesis user (Hermansson et al., 2005). It measures the ability to use a myoelectrically controlled prosthesis for bimanual tasks on 30 items in four different areas: gripping, holding, releasing, and coordinating between hands. Each person's performance is rated on a 4-point capability scale: 0 = not capable, 3 = spontaneously capable.	Not reported	Validated for ages 2–57 years. Determined to have internal scale validity by Rasch analysis (Hermansson et al., 2005).	Intrarater reliability was excellent ($\kappa = 0.81$) in the experienced raters; interrater reliability was fair ($\kappa = 0.60$) in the experienced raters (Hermansson, Bodin, Eliasson, 2006).	Not reported	Strengths: Patient performs a functional task of choice & Rasch analysis determines patient's score in relation to difficulty of task (Wright, 2009). Intra-rater reliability is also a strength. Weaknesses: Administering this assessment requires substantial training and clinical experience. The scores must be entered into the ACMC database and converted to interval-level linear measures, using the Rasch measurement analysis in the ACMC website (http://acmc.se/).

(continued)

Assessment Table 41-1		Summary of Outcome Assessments for Prosthetic Use by Upper Extremity Amputees *(continued)*				

Instrument and Reference	Description	Validity	Time to Administer	Reliability	Sensitivity	Strengths and Weaknesses
Orthotics and Prosthetics User Survey (OPUS) (Heinemann, Bode, & O'Reilly, 2003)	A paper and pencil measure of upper extremity and lower extremity functional status, health-related quality of life, and client satisfaction with prosthesis/orthosis and services.	Rasch analysis determined the survey possesses good internal consistency and construct validity (Burger et al., 2008; Heinemann, Gershon, & Fisher, 2006). Content validity based on input from patients, orthotists, prosthetists, physical therapists, occupational therapists and physiatrists.	Not reported	Not reported	Not reported	Strengths: Modules exist for upper and lower extremity function. The instrument is copyrighted to maintain integrity but is available free of charge from Dr. Heinemann (a-heinemann@ northwestern.edu) Weaknesses: No psychometric data available, including intra-rater reliability.
The Southampton Hand Assessment Procedure (SHAP) (Light, Chappell, & Kyberd, 2002)	Assesses the use of an upper limb prosthesis with 8 object manipulation and 14 ADL tasks. A functionality profile and an index of function are generated.	Content validity established by expert peer review.	20–30 minutes	Test-retest reliability and interrater reliability were established using analysis of variance and 95% confidence intervals.	Not reported	Strengths: One-hour training Available from http:// www.shap.ecs.soton. ac.uk/index.php Weaknesses: A kit must be purchased or an evaluator hired. Psychometric data were not provided.
Activities Measure for Upper Limb Amputees (AM-ULA) (Resnik et al., 2013) Copies of the measure are available free of charge. Contact: Linda.Resnik@va.gov	The AM-ULA is an 18-item observational measure of activity performance for adults with upper limb amputation that considers task completion, speed, movement quality, skillfulness of prosthetic use, and independence in its rating system. Items are graded on a scale of 0–4 with 0 = unable, 1 = poor, 2 = fair, 3 = good, and 4 = excellent. A summary score is obtained. The potential scores range from 0 to 40.	Content: Occupational and physical therapists with expertise in rehabilitation of adults with upper limb amputation identified and refined content, scoring elements and criteria. Convergent: The AM-ULA was moderately correlated with most dexterity tests and with self-reported function. Known Group Validity: Subjects with more distal levels of limb loss had better scores than those with more proximal levels ($p < 0.01$).	30–45 minutes. More time may be needed for persons with more proximal level amputations.	Test-retest reliability: One study reported ICCs of 0.88–0.91. Interrater reliability: One study reported ICCs of 0.84–0.89 Internal consistency: Cronbach's α values were 0.89–0.91. (Resnik et al., 2013)	Sensitivity to change has not been reported to date. Minimum detectable change (MDC) 90 was 3.7 points MDC 95 was 4.4 points	Strengths: The AM-ULA is appropriate for users of all types of upper limb prosthetic devices and addresses the need for a validated performance-based measure of activity for adults with upper limb amputation.

ICC, intraclass correlation; ADL, activities of daily living.

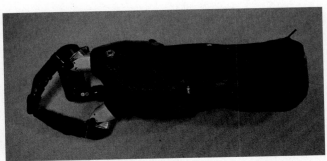

Figure 41-31 An example of a final prosthesis for an individual with a partial hand amputation using ProDigits™ by Touch Bionics, Inc. (Hilliard, OH).

Some patients with a partial hand amputation may want a prosthesis that closely replicates the look of the hand and provides dexterity as well. Although cosmetic hand coverings are truly artistic endeavors, once they fit over the residual hand, tactile sensation is lost, which limits function. The passive functional prosthesis may be a highly specialized device that is task specific, or it may be a simple post to provide opposition. ProDigits™ (Touch Bionics, Hillard, OH) provide myoelectic control for partial hand amputations, specifically those with transmetacarpal level amputations (Fig. 41-31). Each ProDigit™ by Touch Bionics, Inc. (Hilliard, OH) is a self-contained finger that is individually powered through remote electrodes called force-sensitive resistors, more commonly known as FSRs. The prosthetist determines which setup will work best for the patient. Ultimately, these devices provide fine motor pinch, touch, grasp, and pointing that the patient had previously lost as a result of amputation (Harvey, Potter et al., 2012).

MANAGEMENT OF LOWER LIMB AMPUTATIONS

As previously mentioned, the primary reason for lower extremity amputations is disease. Patients may have a primary diagnosis of diabetes or vascular disease with secondary complicating factors that affect therapy, such as sensory deficits, kidney disease, cardiovascular disease, chronic infection, respiratory disease, and arthritis. Other factors influencing function and safe performance of ADL are impaired vision and memory deficits. The therapeutic program for patients with lower limb amputations requires collaboration between the physical therapist and occupational therapist. This may occur in the acute care setting immediately following amputation, in an outpatient clinic, or in the patient's home.

Both therapists will perform an evaluation of the patient. The physical therapist is responsible for limb wrapping, core and lower limb strengthening exercises, range of motion, preprosthetic, prosthetic, and gait training. Initial patient treatment sessions by both disciplines

may focus on ADL to include patient and family education on wound care, limb wrapping, bed mobility, transfers, and basic wheelchair propulsion and management skills. Safety is a major concern with lower limb amputations, particularly for patients with other comorbidities. Patient and family are educated on safety precautions with specific activities such as transfers. Treatment sessions may include safe transfers from the wheelchair to the bed, toilet, furniture, and car. Early patient education on desensitization of the residual limb is also addressed.

The occupational therapist may also include other self-maintenance skills, such as kitchen tasks, housecleaning and bed making during the treatment sessions. Home and community visits with the patient may be indicated. During standing activities and ambulation, special attention is paid to balance, posture, and equal weight bearing through both lower extremities. This may be challenging for certain individuals and the therapist should use visual or verbal cues if necessary. The physical therapist or the occupational therapist will teach fall recovery to the patient and the family because safety after amputations is always important.

The occupational therapist may recommend home modifications and equipment to the patient and family. Equipment often includes a transfer tub bench or shower chair for use while showering and bathing and safety arm rails around the toilet. These rails provide a means of arm support that assists with lowering to the toilet and coming to the standing position safely.

The primary surgical or medical team will clear the patient to start wearing a shrinker on his or her lower residual limb prior to receiving the first prosthesis. The patient needs to be educated on the proper shrinker donning techniques and care of the shrinkers and liners. The shrinkers should have no wrinkles, and seams should not be over bony areas or the scar. The patient must inspect the skin on the residual limb everyday to check for any changes in skin integrity before and after shrinker, liner, or prosthetic wear. If the patient has difficulty inspecting the residual limb, a long-handled mirror may be used to assist.

The physical therapist will assess and recommend the lower extremity prosthetic wearing schedule, the amount of assistance required, and assistive devices needed, as well as readiness for any standing or ambulation activities. A patient needs to be able to don and doff the lower extremity prosthesis independently. If unable, a family member needs to be educated and able to demonstrate the proper technique in donning and doffing the prosthesis. The occupational therapist continues to address ADL with the patient both with and without the prosthesis. The occupational therapist works with the patient to identify how to incorporate the prosthesis into daily activities while assessing energy, effort, balance, transfer, and mobility skills. Energy conservation methods should be included in the program. It is important to recognize that energy expenditures are affected by limb amputation and prosthetic ambulation. The percentage increase in energy costs of prosthetic ambulation is 9%–28% for unilateral transtibial, 40%–60% for a unilateral transfemoral, 41%–100% bilateral transtibial, and 280% for bilateral transfemoral amputations (Shah, 2010).

MULTIPLE LIMB LOSS

Individuals with multiple limb loss present a unique set of challenges for the rehabilitation and prosthetic teams. With the U.S. military "surge" in 2010, there was a two-fold increase in the number of service members evacuated from the theater of operations who had sustained triple and quadruple limb amputations (Anderson et al., 2012). This created a need for additional rehabilitation expertise in treating individuals with multiple limb amputations. Early focus is on basic ADL such as eating, bathing, toileting, and transfer techniques along with core strengthening and residual limb preprosthetic exercises. Early application of a prosthesis for at least one limb fosters adaptation and learning. It is highly recommended to have a team meeting with all team members, including the patient and family, regarding initial focus of rehabilitation, achievable goals, and progression of prosthetic training for both upper and lower extremity amputations (Harvey et al., 2012a).

The rehabilitation team and patient must discuss initial mobility options such as ambulating with or without wearing a upper limb prosthesis (Yancosek, Schnall, & Baum, 2008), use of an electric wheelchair versus a manual wheelchair for mobility, and the direct effects mobility choices have on areas such as home modifications and vehicle selection. As the patient progresses and is fitted with various prosthetic systems, it is imperative for the entire team to have open communication in how specific therapies are progressing to achieve the patient's goals and obtain higher levels of independence in both ADL and instrumental activities of daily living (IADL). General considerations that will influence rehabilitation for this subset of the amputee population include (1) increased body temperature secondary to reduced body surface area; (2) increased risk of joint contractures, weight gain, deconditioning, and bone resorption as a result of immobility; (3) unique pain management needs given architectural changes to the musculoskeletal system; (4) psychosocial issues, such as the importance of body image acceptance and return to work; and (5) likely ongoing medical risks, such as cardiovascular disease, metabolic dysfunction, musculoskeletal pain, and arthritis (Davidson, 2002; Naschitz & Lenger, 2008; Ostlie et al., 2011).

The therapeutic program must be structured to meet the patient's needs. As the patient masters the basics of prosthetic control systems and practices their use in

activities, with the therapist's guidance as a facilitator, the patient chooses tasks that he or she values. The approach of analyzing tasks and problem solving on how best to use this tool, the prosthesis, regardless of its complexity, serves the patient well throughout life.

EMERGING TRENDS IN PROSTHETICS

Research and development activities increase during times of armed conflict, as is currently the case with military operations. As a result, attention is focused on the increase in numbers of amputations in a young, previously healthy population, whose members will hopefully live long, productive lives using prosthetic devices.

Recent improvements in lower extremity prosthetic devices related to materials include improved suspension sleeves and gel interfaces that directly contact the skin. The use of carbon fiber, urethane, and titanium combined with improved mechanical and microprocessor components has advanced the state of the art for lower extremity prosthetics (Harvey et al., 2012b). Innovations such as the iWalk BiOM (Bedford, MA) allow plantar flexion in a lower limb extremity prosthesis by way of on-board sensors relaying information to actuators during gait.

The next area of promise is in using pattern recognition to allow for a more natural (instinctive) control of the prosthesis. The C-leg from Ottobock (Minneapolis, MN) has a microprocessor (computerized) knee and has stumble recovery capability that improves static and dynamic balance in response to perturbation. Ottobock has also developed new computerized leg prostheses, the Ottobock X2 (microprocessor knee), and the Genium™ Bionic Prosthetic System, which offer features for more athletic wearers who wish to ambulate backward or on uneven terrain, carry weighted loads, or run without stopping to change settings. To address the frequent problem of low back pain common to lower extremity amputees, the Ossur Power knee (Aliso, Viejo, CA) produces knee extension and limits the physiological and mechanical work for the amputee. Regeneration and purposeful directing of biomechanical energy within a prosthesis shows promise for improved control options for individuals with lower limb amputations (Au, Berniker, & Herr, 2008; Ha, Varol, & Goldfarb, 2011; Hitt et al., 2010).

Developments in upper limb prosthetics include the capability to perform (limited) isolated digit motions and some natural actions such as "reflexive responses" triggered by sensors in the prosthetic hand that detect slip and automatically adjust grip, thereby reducing the mental load required of the user to visually monitor grasp. Although no commercial electric shoulder is currently available, LTI has developed an electric lock actuator to lock the manually positioned shoulder. Wrist flexion and rotation units are available on both BP as well as electric TDs. Motion Control (Salt Lake City, UT) has a mechanical flexion/rotation component to incorporate with the electric TD.

Current Research Topics

The surgical approach called osseointegration requires the implantation of a titanium peg fixed to the bone to which a prosthesis can be attached. This approach reportedly has been successful for lower limb amputations and has further potential for upper limb prosthetics. If successful in higher level upper limb amputations, the need for suspension is eliminated because it provides a stable fixation for prosthetic attachment. It has the added advantage of enhanced proprioceptive feedback from the artificial limb. This has been a treatment option in Sweden since 1980 (Hagberg & Branemark, 2009), but the practice is still under investigation in the United States (Shelton et al., 2011) and is not currently approved by the Food and Drug Administration.

Targeted muscle-reinnervation (TMR) is a surgical technique to increase the number of myoelectric control sites available in a higher level amputation. After limb loss, the brachial plexus and peripheral nerves may remain intact in the residual limb. This procedure takes advantage of expendable regions of remaining muscle by denervating and reinnervating sections of tissue. When successful, this can result in myoelectric sites that correlate physiologically with prosthetic functions: the radial nerve innervates musculature that contracts when the subject attempts to extend the elbow; the distal radial nerve reinnervated area contracts to open the hand; the median nerve area contracts to close the hand (Kuiken et al., 2009). Additionally, while undergoing TMR, targeted sensory reinnervation can be undertaken to allow some sensory nerves from the amputated limb to be directed to chest skin (Kuiken et al., 2007). This results in perceived touch of the missing limb at nearly normal ranges and can be used for sensory feedback within a prosthesis. Early indications suggest that sensory reinnervation may be tapped to enhance control of multiple functions in the artificial arm (Kuiken et al., 2004). There is an existing OT protocol for amputees who have undergone TMR that should be used when working with these specific patients (Stubblefield et al., 2009).

Currently, surface EMG (electromyography) will only allow up to four channels of control in the forearm, but 18 extrinsic muscles supply the hand and wrist. Development is proceeding on implantable myoelectric sensors (IMES) small enough to be injected, with the hope of extending myoelectric control to multiple degrees of freedom in the hand simultaneously (Weir et al., 2003).

The Defense Advanced Research Project Agency (DARPA) Revolutionizing Prosthetics program has set its mission "to create a fully functional (motor and sensory) upper limb that responds to direct neural control, within this decade" (DARPA, 2012). DARPA has teamed with DEKA Integrated Solutions Corporation (Manchester, NH) and Johns Hopkins Applied Physics Laboratory (APL) (Laurel, MD) to meet its mission. This partnership has resulted in advances in socket design, electronics, componentry, signal processing, and implantable devices that can produce arm control for those with limb loss or other neurologic conditions affecting upper extremity function.

As of the time of this publication, the DEKA Arm System is still in the research and development phase and is not commercially available. The intent of the DEKA Arm System is to provide a device with capabilities far exceeding those in available prostheses. It includes a flexible socket design for improved comfort, up to 18° of freedom, 10 of the degrees powered, depending on level of amputation, multiple hand and pinch grips, and versatile control inputs (Resnik, 2010). The expectation is that this device will offer greater function, improved comfort, control scheme design flexibility, and more intuitive control for the user.

The goal of the DARPA APL arm project was to determine whether it was possible to operate a prosthetic arm by direct brain control. In September 2011, the first human volunteer was able to move a DARPA-funded arm through mind control. This accomplishment sets the stage for clinical trials to begin over the next several years. Future advances in engineering, medicine, and prosthetics promise technical improvements in the fit and function of prosthetics.

Vascularized composite allotransplantation (VCA) is an emerging field that has presented the option of hand transplantation to potentially replace and restore tissue, function, and nearly normal aesthetics after limb loss. According to the American Society of Transplantation (2011), "VCA refers to the transplantation of multiple tissues such as muscle, bone, nerve and skin, as a functional unit (e.g., a hand, or face) from a deceased donor to a recipient with a severe injury." As of July 1, 2011, 46 patients worldwide had received 66 hand transplants (American Society of Transplantation, 2011).

Currently, most hand transplantations occur as part of approved clinical trials, and thus an extensive medical, surgical, and psychological screening process determines eligibility. The procedure and rehabilitation is costly and complex (Lanzetta, Dubernard, & Petruzzo, 2007). There are inherent risks associated with hand transplantation such as immunosuppressive therapies and possible rejection of the transplant. However, the transplanted hand may not only restore the natural cosmetics of the physical hand but may also provide psychological recovery to the individual's sense of wholeness and normalcy after limb loss. The functional results of VCA are by no means immediate and require dedicated time for intensive rehabilitation (Dubernard et al., 2003; Lee et al., 2011). There still exists considerable controversy over the risk-to-benefit ratio of undergoing hand transplantation (Schneeberger, Ninkovic, & Margreiter, 2008), and the therapist working with a patient with an amputation does well to study this topic because it may be of interest to the patient who may seek guidance in considering all his or her options. After treating five patients with eight transplanted hands, the occupational therapists at the University of Pittsburgh Medical Center outlined a rehabilitation protocol to assist other therapists facing such challenging patients (Pace & Macguire, 2011).

CONCLUSION

Rehabilitation of an individual with an amputation requires a holistic approach that addresses the psychosocial adjustment to limb loss as well as the physical recovery (Hannah, 2011). This approach includes working with the patient to achieve tolerance to wearing and efficiency in using a pros-

thesis to facilitate participation in activities and occupations. The therapist needs to understand the technology available to this population, which means communicating with the prosthetist and other team members to make decisions about prosthetic selection. Rehabilitation progresses across time to accommodate the phases of adjustment, acceptance, healing, recovery, and ultimate mastery of skills needed to achieve higher levels of function and independence. The field of prosthetics is rapidly developing and necessitates therapists to stay abreast of emerging technologies; however, keystone principles of occupation-based, patient-centered rehabilitation remain the foundation for a successful rehabilitation experience. The occupational therapist operating from a biopsychosocial perspective is poised to help an individual that has an amputation adjust, adapt, and facilitate success (Borrell-Carrio, Suchman, & Epstein, 2004).

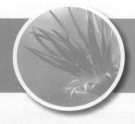

case example
Z.M.: A Military Service Member with Multiple Limb Amputations

| **Occupational Therapy Process** | **Clinical Reasoning Process** | |
	Objectives	**Examples of Therapist's Internal Dialogue**
Patient Information Z.M. is a 25-year-old active duty right-hand–dominant married male injured while deployed to Afghanistan. Z.M. is an infantryman with 5 years of service. This was his second deployment. He was on foot patrol with his unit and stepped on an improvised explosive device. As a result, he sustained bilateral transtibial and right transradial amputations. He was treated and then transferred to a U.S. military treatment facility. Z.M. spent 2.5 months as an inpatient before his discharge to an outpatient facility. He currently resides in on-campus apartment housing with his wife of 3 years and their 1-year-old son. As an inpatient, he received daily occupational therapy and physical therapy for preprosthetic training for both his upper and lower extremity amputations. He was discharged from inpatient rehabilitation with a tub transfer bench, a rental power wheelchair, and a rental manual wheelchair. The power chair allows him increased independence and mobility from where he is living to the hospital and in the hospital. If he is traveling by vehicle, the manual chair can be stored in the vehicle, and he will be pushed by his family once they arrive at their destination.	Understand the patient's diagnosis or condition	"Z.M. is an individual with three amputated limbs. He lost his dominant hand. I have several individuals on my caseload currently with similar injuries. One of my other patients was in Z.M.'s unit and injured 2 months prior to him."
	Know the person	"Z.M. has a strong military background. He excelled on both of his deployments and was respected by his peers and unit. He had planned to make the military a career, serve 20 years, and then retire. Although he has a positive attitude, I know there may be stress in his family related to their understanding of his injuries and the impact the injuries may have on his future. With these types of injuries, there are changes initially in occupational roles. His wife is caring for both him and their son and attending all his medical appointments with him. They do have strong family support."
Reason for Referral to Occupational Therapy Z.M. will transition to outpatient OT for continued amputee care, preprosthetic training, prosthetic training, wheelchair mobility, community reintegration, adaptive sports, and driving.	Appreciate the context	"I will be Z.M.'s occupational therapist for the duration of his rehab here. I have worked with his physical therapist and his prosthetist with multiple prior patients, and we all have a good multidisciplinary approach. I think Z.M. has the potential to do very well and be both an upper extremity and lower extremity prosthetic user in his daily activities. He should be fitted soon with all of his initial sockets."

Assessment Process and Results

During his initial outpatient appointment, the goals and expectations of the patient and his family were determined. Z.M.'s activities of daily living (ADL) status was evaluated, including the current level of assistance needed to complete tasks (e.g., donning and doffing upper and lower extremity shrinkers) and his primary means for mobility and transfers. Also evaluated was the extent of education he and his family has received about the amputee care program. During the evaluation, he reported that his pain usually is 3 out of 10 and is usually in his legs. He does report having phantom pain at night.

| Consider evaluation approach and methods | "I need to understand and observe Z.M.'s functional levels now before he gets his prostheses in order to develop my treatment plan. I am sure there will be tasks that Z.M. will find easier to complete with his upper extremity prosthesis, and I need to work with Z.M. to identify which tasks and in what sequence he performs these tasks." |

"Z.M. arrived in the clinic in his power wheelchair. His wife accompanied him. They stated that he still needs assistance with bathroom transfers and all ADL areas. He states he is compliant with shrinker wear and is very excited for his fitting for his upper and lower extremity prostheses this week."

Occupational Therapy Problem List

1. ADL dependent.
2. Need to change upper extremity dominance.
3. Active range of motion (ROM) deficit of right elbow, bilateral knees.
4. Passive ROM deficit of right elbow.
5. At risk for contractures of right elbow and bilateral knees.
6. At risk for falls.
7. Weakness of abdominal muscles and back muscles.
8. Activity tolerance limited to decreased conditioning.
9. Unable to ambulate.
10. Unable to independently transfer from wheelchair to toilet, bed, bath, or chair.
11. Unable to perform tasks one handed.

Synthesize results

"Like many of my patients with multiple limb loss, Z.M. has many areas that need to be addressed, which may be overwhelming at times both for Z.M. and for me as a therapist. I need to engage Z.M. during each therapy session about his functional levels and review what he is working on outside of therapy."

Occupational Therapy Goal List

Long-term goal: Z.M. will be independent in ADL and instrumental activities of daily living (IADL) with and without his prostheses and be a community ambulator with least restrictive assistive device in 12 months. Initial short-term goals:

1. Z.M. will be able to be moderately independent in his ADL.
2. Z.M. will be able to independently don and doff his shrinkers, liners, and sockets.
3. After completing his wear schedule, Z.M. will be able to wear his upper extremity prosthesis for 6–8 hours and use it for functional activities.
4. Z.M. will complete the *Handwriting for Heroes* change of dominance program.
5. Z.M. will attend two community reintegration events each month (e.g., attend lunch and a movie with community reintegration group).
6. Z.M. will attend his unit's redeployment ceremony in 4 months and will stand to welcome his unit back from deployment.

Develop intervention hypotheses

"Z.M. appears to be learning how to control his upper extremity prosthesis quickly. I can use principles of learning with practice of functional activities to improve his independence in activities of daily living tasks."

Select an intervention approach

"I selected controls training tasks in the clinic that allowed Z.M. to master control of his body-powered and myoelectric prostheses for grasping, holding, releasing, and reaching for various objects. I increased the difficulty when appropriate and added bilateral tasks. Finally, I simulated daily living tasks in the clinic as well as instructed Z.M. to use his prosthesis at home in activities."

Consider what will occur in therapy, how often, and for how long

"Z. M. will attend both occupational and physical therapy daily Monday through Friday for at least an hour in each for approximately the next year. He will also have multiple appointments with both his upper and lower extremity prosthetists for casting, fitting, and adjustments of his sockets. I have the ability to discuss any problems or issues with the multidisciplinary team weekly at our outpatient meeting for all of our patients. Encouraging participation in community reintegration both with his peers and his family early is important. Attending the redeployment ceremony is an important military tradition and will be beneficial psychologically for Z. M., his family, and his unit."

Intervention

Z.M. is expected to be compliant with his daily therapy appointments. His military job while here is to heal and progress to higher levels of function and independence. His daily OT sessions may vary day to day in the activities, tasks, and focus. Once fitted with his initial upper extremity preparatory prosthesis, focus will be on increasing prosthesis wearing time, donning, doffing, and controls training with various terminal devices. These activities may be performed while sitting in his wheelchair or while standing as he progresses in his wearing schedule for his legs. Mirror therapy will be used to decrease pain.

Next Steps

1. Continue to assess and improve ADL and transfer status.
2. Facilitate community reintegration and adaptive sports participation.
3. Begin vocational exploration.
4. Discuss driving and vehicle options and refer for evaluation.
5. Arrange for him to discuss the pros and cons of returning to military duty versus military retirement with military unit, his therapists, and his family.
6. Identify needed future home adaptations.
7. Provide patient and family education concerning advances in prosthetic components.

Know the person Appreciate the context	"Z.M. performed well during his preprosthetic training as an inpatient and continued as an outpatient. He is able to demonstrate isolated control of his forearm flexors and extensors and understands how these movements will eventually help him control his myoelectric prosthesis. Z.M. is highly motivated in therapy and has good family support."
Anticipate present and future patient concerns Decide whether he or she should continue or discontinue therapy and/ or return in the future	"Z.M. has the potential and motivation to do very well and be able to become very independent in his ADL and IADL. He wants to return to his previous level of function and be able to participate in leisure activities that he enjoyed previously such as fishing, running, and skiing. As he progresses and improves in function, it is very important that all members of the treatment team, including Z.M., are communicating well and identifying any issues that may arise. Z.M. has verbalized an intention to remain in the service after rehabilitation; however, he also states that he will continue to evaluate his functional levels and his ability to perform his military duties with his prostheses. He also values the future needs of his family in this important decision."

 # Clinical Reasoning in Occupational Therapy Practice

Prosthesis Training

Z.M. demonstrated effective use of his body-powered and myoelectric prostheses but verbalizes that he is challenged by current child care tasks that he would like to be able to do with his son, such as changing diapers, dressing, and preparing food and bottles. How can the therapist incorporate these concerns into the treatment program?

Summary Review Questions

1. Why is a shrinker used on the residual limb?
2. What are the most common causes of acquired upper and lower limb amputations?
3. What are the types of upper extremity prosthetic systems?
4. Which body movements are required for a patient using a body-powered prosthesis?
5. How does myoelectric control work?
6. What is the purpose of controls training and use training?
7. What are tasks a therapist might start with for functional (use) training with a prosthesis?
8. Why might an individual reject a prosthesis?
9. What is the role of the occupational therapist in the rehabilitation of the patient with lower extremity amputations?
10. What is TMR? How does this improve control of a prosthesis?
11. What are the challenges of treating a patient with multiple limb loss?

Glossary

Acquired amputation—Surgical amputation after birth as a result of trauma or disease.

Actuators—Motorized mechanisms or signals that activate a device or system.

Body-powered (BP) prosthesis—Person's own effort through body motion is used to apply tension on the control cable to activate the TD and/or the elbow unit.

Externally powered or myoelectric prosthesis—Electric or other motor that provides impetus to move the prosthesis or terminal device.

Functional envelope—The area of space in which the patient can operate an upper extremity prosthesis.

Hybrid prosthesis—Combines BP and myoelectric-powered control to operate the system; only available for prostheses for transhumeral amputations or elbow disarticulation amputations.

Myoelectric prosthesis—Has electrodes embedded in the prosthetic socket that pick up electromyographic signals that activate prosthetic components to open, close, or move.

Preprosthetic therapy program—Period from the postsurgical procedure until a test-socket (temporary prosthesis) or the permanent prosthesis is received.

Terminal device (TD)—Prosthetic hook, hand, or other prehensile device that is inserted into the wrist unit of the prosthesis.

Transfemoral amputation—Amputation across the axis of the femur; previously called above knee (AK).

Transhumeral amputation—Amputation across the axis of the humerus; previously called above elbow (AE).

Transradial amputation—Amputation across the axis of the radius and ulna; labeled by the larger of two adjacent bones; previously called below elbow (BE).

Transtibial amputation—Amputation across the axis of the fibula and tibia; labeled according to the larger of two adjacent bones; previously called below knee (BK).

Visual analogue scale—A straight line 10-centimeter scale with 0 centimeters meaning no pain and 10 centimeters meaning the worst pain imaginable; the patient marks a point along the scale that matches the amount of pain.

Voluntary closing (VC) mechanism—TD that remains open until tension is applied to the control cable for grasp.

Voluntary opening (VO) mechanism—TD that remains closed until tension is applied to the control cable to open it.

References

American Society of Transplantation. (2011). Vascularized composite allotransplantation (VCA) research: emerging field. Retrieved March 10, 2012, from http://www.a-s-t.org/public-policy/vascularized-composite-allotransplantation-vca-research.

Anderson, R. C., Fleming, M., Forsberg, J. A., Gordon, W. T., Nanos, G. P., III, Charlton, M. T., & Ficke, J. R. (2012). Dismounted complex blast injury. *Journal of Surgical Orthopedica Advances, 21,* 2–7.

Atkins, D. J., & Edelstein, J. E. (2006). Training patients with upper-limb amputations. In K. Carroll & J. E. Edelstein (Eds.), *Prosthetics and patient management. A comprehensive clinical approach* (pp. 167–177). New York: Slack, Inc.

Au, S., Berniker, M., & Herr, H. (2008). Powered ankle-foot prosthesis to assist level-ground and stair-descent gaits. *Neural Networks, 21,* 654–666.

Biddiss, E. A., & Chau, T. T. (2007). Upper limb prosthesis use and abandonment: A survey of the last 25 years. *Prosthetics and Orthotics International, 31,* 236–257.

Borrell-Carrio, F., Suchman, A. L., & Epstein, R. M. (2004). The biopsychosocial model 25 years later: Principles, practice, and scientific inquiry. *Annals of Family Medicine, 2,* 576–582.

Burger, H., Fanchignoni, F., Heinemann, A. W., Kotnik, S., & Giordano, A. (2008). Validation of the orthotics and prosthetics user survey upper extremity functional status module in people with unilateral upper limb amputation. *Journal of Rehabilitation Medicine, 40,* 393–399.

Chan, B. L., Witt, R., Charrow, A. P., Magee, A., Howard, R., Pasquina, P. F., Heilman, K. M., & Tsao, J. W. (2007). Mirror therapy for phantom limb pain. *New England Journal of Medicine, 357,* 2206–2207.

Darnall, B. D. (2009). Self-delivered home-based mirror therapy for lower limb phantom pain. *American Journal of Physical Medicine & Rehabilitation, 88,* 78–81.

Davidson, J. H. (2002). Management of the multiple limb amputee. *Disability and Rehabilitation, 24,* 688–699.

Defense Advanced Research Project Agency. (2012). DARPA website. Retrieved March 1, 2012 from www.darpa.mil.

Desmond, D. M. (2007). Coping, affective distress, and psychosocial adjustment among people with traumatic upper limb amputations. *Journal of Psychosomatic Research, 62,* 15–21.

Desmond, D. M., & MacLachlan, M. (2005). Factor structure of the Trinity Amputation and Prosthesis Experience Scales (TAPES) with individuals with acquired upper limb amputations. *American Journal of Physical Medicine and Rehabilitation, 84,* 506–513.

Desmond, D. M., & MacLachlan, M. (2006). Affective distress and amputation-related pain among older men with long-term, traumatic limb amputations. *Journal of Pain and Symptom Management, 31,* 362–368.

Dillingham, T., Pezzin, L., & MacKenzie, E. J. (2004). Limb amputation and limb deficiencies: Epidemiology and recent trends in the United States. *Disability and Rehabilitation, 26,* 831–836.

Dubernard, J. M., Petruzzo, P., Lanzetta, M., Parmentier, H., Martin, X., Dawahra, M., Hakim, N. S., & Owen, E. (2003). Functional results of the first human double-hand transplantation. *Annals of Surgery, 238,* 128–136.

Edelstein, J. E. (2004). Rehabilitation without prostheses. In D. G. Smith & J. H. Bowker (Eds.), *Atlas of amputations and limb deficiencies: Surgical, prosthetic and rehabilitation principles* (pp. 745–755). Rosemont, IL: American Academy of Orthopedic Surgeons.

Eichenberger, U., Neff, F., Sveticic, G., Björgo, S., Petersen-Felix, S., Arendt-Nielsen, L., & Curatolo, M. (2008). Chronic phantom limb pain: The effects of calcitonin, ketamine, and their combination on pain and sensory thresholds. *Anesthesia & Analgesia, 106,* 1265–1273.

Esquenazi, A. (2004). Amputation rehabilitation and prosthetic restoration. From surgery to community reintegration. *Disability and Rehabilitation, 26,* 831–836.

Fletchall, S. (2005). Returning upper-extremity amputees to work. *O&P Edge, 4,* 28–33.

Flor, H., Nikolajsen, L., & Jensen, T. S. (2006). Phantom limb pain: A case of maladaptive CNS plasticity? *Nature Reviews Neuroscience, 7,* 873–881.

Gailey, R., McFarland, L. V., Cooper, R. A., Czerniecki, J., Gambel, J. M., Hubbard, S., Maynard, C., Smith, D. G., Raya, M., & Reiber, G. E. (2010). Unilateral lower-limb loss: Prosthetic device use and functional outcomes in servicemembers from Vietnam war and OIF/OEF conflicts. *Journal of Rehabilitation Research & Development, 47*(4), 317–331.

Gallagher, P., Franchignoni, F., Giordano, A., & MacLachlan, M. (2010). Trinity amputation and prosthesis experience scales (TAPES): A psychometric assessment using classical test theory and Rasch analysis. *American Journal of Physical Medicine and Rehabilitation, 89,* 487–496.

Gallagher, P., & MacLachlan, M. (2000). Development and psychometric evaluation of the Trinity Amputation and Prosthesis Experience Scales (TAPES). *Rehabilitation Psychology, 45,* 130–154.

Goodney, P. P., Beck, A. W., Nagle, J., Welch, H. G., & Zwolak, R. M. (2009). National trends in lower extremity bypass surgery, endovascular interventions, and major amputations. *Journal of Vascular Surgery, 50,* 54–60.

Ha, K. H., Varol, H. A., & Goldfarb, M. (2011). Volitional control of a prosthetic knee using surface electromyography. *IEEE Transactions on Biomedical Engineering, 58,* 144–151.

Hagberg, K., & Branemark, R. (2009). One hundred patients treated with osseointegrated transfemoral amputation prostheses rehabilitation perspective. *Journal of Rehabilitation Research & Development, 46,* 331–344.

Hannah, S. D. (2011). Psychosocial issues after a traumatic hand injury: Facilitating adjustment. *Journal of Hand Therapy, 24,* 95–103.

Harvey, Z. T., Loomis, G. A., Mitsch, S., Murphy, I. C., Griffin, S. C., Potter, B. K., & Pasquina, P. (2012). Advanced rehabilitation techniques for the multi-limb amputee. *Journal of Surgical Orthopedica Advances, 21*(1), 50–57.

Harvey, Z. T., Potter, B. K., Vandersea, J., & Wolf, E. (2012). Prosthetic advances. *Journal of Surgical Orthopedica Advances, 21*(1), 58–64.

Heinemann, A. W., Bode, R. K., & O'Reilly, C. (2003). Development and measurement properties of the Orthotics and Prosthetics Users' Survey (OPUS): A comprehensive set of clinical outcome instruments. *Prosthetics and Orthotics International, 27,* 191–206.

Heinemann, A. W., Gershon, R., & Fisher, W. P. (2006). Development and application of the orthotics and prosthetics user survey: Applications and opportunities for health care quality improvement. *Journal of Prosthetics and Orthotics, 18,* 80–84.

Hermansson, L. M., Bodin, L., & Eliasson, A. C. (2006). Intra- and inter-rater reliability of the assessment of capacity for myoelectric control. *Journal of Rehabilitation Medicine, 38,* 118–123.

Hermansson, L. M., Fisher, A. G., Bernspång, B., & Eliasson, A. C. (2005). Assessment of capacity for myoelectric control: A new Rasch-built measure of prosthetic hand control. *Journal of Rehabilitation Medicine, 37,* 166–171.

Hill, W., Kyberd, P., Norling-Hermansson, L., Hubbard, S., Stavdahl, O., & Swanson, S. (2009). Upper Limb Prosthetic Outcome Measures (ULPOM): A working group and their findings. *Journal of Prosthetics & Orthotics, 21,* P69–P82.

Hitt, J. K., Sugar, T. G., Holgate, M., & Bellman, R. (2010). An active foot-ankle prosthesis with biomechanical energy regeneration. *Journal of Medical Devices, 4,* 011003.

Hompland, S. (2004). Pain management for upper extremity amputation. In D. J. Atkins & R. H. Meier III (Eds.), *Functional restoration of adults and children with upper extremity amputation* (pp. 89–105). New York: Demos Medical Publishing.

Horgan, O., & MacLachlan, M. (2004). Psychosocial adjustment to lower-limb amputation: A review. *Disability and Rehabilitation, 26,* 837–850.

Hung, J. W., & Wu, Y. H. (2005). Fitting a bilateral transhumeral amputee with untensil prostheses and their functional assessment 10 years later: A case report. *Archives of Physical Medicine & Rehabilitation, 86,* 2211–2213.

Johannesson, A., Larsson, G. U., Ramstrand, N., Turkiewicz, A., Wiréhn, A. B., & Atroshi, I. (2009). Incidence of lower-limb amputation in the diabetic and nondiabetic general population. *Diabetes Care, 32,* 275–280.

Kessler, H. H. (1947). *Cineplasty.* Springfield, IL: Charles C. Thomas.

Kuiken, T. A., Dumanian, G. A., Lipschutz, R. D., Miller, L. A., & Stubblefield, K. A. (2004). The use of targeted muscle reinnervation for improved myoelectric prosthesis control in a bilateral shoulder disarticulation amputee. *Prosthetics and Orthotics International, 28,* 245–253.

Kuiken, T. A., Li, G., Lock, B. A., Lipschutz, R. D., Miller, L. A., Stubblefield, K. A., & Englehardt, K. B. (2009). Targeted muscle reinnervation for real-time myoelectric control of multifunction artificial arms. *Journal of the American Medical Association, 301*(6), 619–628.

Kuiken, T. A., Marasco, P. D., Lock, B. A., Harden, R. N., & Dewald, J. P. A. (2007). Redirection of cutaneous sensation from the hand to the chest skin of human amputees with targeted reinnervation. *Proceedings of the National Academy of Sciences, 104,* 20061–20066.

Lake, C. (1997). Effects of prosthetic training on upper-extremity prosthesis use. *Journal of Prosthetics & Orthotics, 9*(1), 3–9.

Lake, C., & Dodson, R. (2006). Progressive upper limb prosthetics. *Physical Medicine and Rehabilitation Clinics of North America, 17,* 49–72.

Lanzetta, M., Dubernard, J. M., & Petruzzo, P. (2007). *Hand transplantation.* New York: Springer.

Lee, J., Garcia, A. M., Lee, W. P. A., & Munin, M. C. (2011). Inpatient rehabilitation challenges in a quadrimembral amputee after bilateral hand transplantation. *American Journal of Physical Medicine & Rehabilitation, 90,* 688–693.

Leow, M. E., Pho, R. W., & Pereira, B. P. (2001). Esthetic prostheses in minor and major upper limb amputations. *Hand Clinics, 17,* 489–497.

Light, C. M., Chappell, P. H., & Kyberd, P. J. (2002). Establishing a standardized clinical assessment tool of pathologic and prosthetic hand function: Normative data, reliability and validity. *Archives of Physical Medicine and Rehabilitation, 83,* 776–783.

McFarland, L. V., Hubbard-Winkler, S. L., Heinemann, A. W., Jones, M., & Esquenazi, A. (2010). Unilateral upper-limb loss: Satisfaction and prosthetic-device use in veterans and servicemembers from Vietnam and OIF/OEF conflicts. *Journal of Rehabilitation Research and Development, 47,* 299–316.

Melzack, R. (1989). Phantom limbs, the self and the brain. *Journal of Canadian Psychology, 30,* 1–16.

Murray, C. D. (2005). The social meanings of prosthesis use. *Journal of Health Psychology, 10,* 425–441.

Naschitz, J. E., & Lenger, R. (2008). Why traumatic leg amputees are at increased risk for cardiovascular disease. *Quarterly Journal of Medicine, 101,* 251–259.

Ostlie, K., Franklin, R. J., Skjeldal, O. H., Skrondal, A., & Magnus, P. (2011). Musculoskeletal pain and overuse syndromes in adult acquired major upper-limb amputees. *Archives of Physical Medicine & Rehabilitation, 92,* 1967–1973.

Pace, M., & Macguire, K. (2011). Hand and upper extremity transplantation: A rehabilitation process. *OT Practice, 16*(8), 17–22.

Price, E. H. (2006). A critical review of congenital phantom limb cases and a developmental theory for the basis of body image. *Consciousness and Cognition, 15,* 310–322.

Raichle, K. A., Hanley, M. A., Ivan Molton, I., Kadel, N. J., Campbell, K., Phelps, E., Ehde, D., & Smith, D. G. (2009). Prosthesis use in persons with lower- and upper-limb amputation. *Journal of Rehabilitation Research & Development, 45,* 961–973.

Ramachandran, V. S., & Rogers-Ramachandran, D. (1996). Synaesthesia in phantom limbs induced with mirrors. *Proceedings of Biological Science, 263,* 377–386.

Rayman, G., Krishnan, T. M. S., Baker, N. R., Wareham, A. M., & Rayman, A. (2004). Are we underestimating diabetes-related lower-extremity amputation rates? *Diabetes Care, 27,* 1892–1896.

Reiber, G. E., McFarland, L. V., Hubbard, S., Maynard, C., Blough, D. K., Gambel, J. M., & Smith, D. G. (2010). Service members and veterans with major traumatic limb loss from Vietnam war and OIF/OEF conflicts: Survey methods, participants, and summary findings. *Journal of Rehabilitation Research & Development, 47,* 275–298.

Resnik, L. (2010). Guest Editorial: Research Update: VA study to optimize DEKA Arm. *Journal of Rehabilitation Research & Development, 47,* ix–x.

Resnik, L., Adams, L., Borgia, M., Delikat, J., Disla, R., Ebner, C., & Smurr Walters, L. (2013). Development and evaluation of the activities measure for upper limb amputees (AM-ULA). *Archives of Physical Medicine and Rehabilitation, 94*(3), 488–494.

Resnik, L., & Borgia, M. (2011). Reliability of outcome measures for people with lower-limb amputations: Distinguishing true change from statistical error. *Physical Therapy, 91,* 555–565.

Schneeberger, S., Ninkovic, M., & Margreiter, R. (2008). Hand transplantation: The Innsbruck experience. In C. W. Hewitt & W. P. A. Lee (Eds.), *Transplantation of composite tissue allografts* (pp. 234–250). New York: Springer.

Shah, S. K. (2010). Cardiac rehabilitation. In W. R. Frontera, B. M. Gans, N. E. Walsh, & L. R. Robinson (Eds.), *DeLisa's physical medicine & rehabilitation: Principles and practice* (5th ed.). Philadelphia: Lippincott Williams & Wilkins.

Shelton, T. J., Beck, J. P., Bloebaum, R. D., & Bachus, K. N. (2011). Percutaneous osseointegrated prostheses for amputees: Limb compensation in a 12-month bovine model. *Journal of Biomechanics, 44,* 2601–2606.

Smith, D. G., Michael, J. W., & Bowker, J. H. (2004). *Atlas of amputations and limb deficiencies: Surgical, prosthetic, and rehabilitation principles* (3rd ed.). Rosemont, IL: American Academy of Orthopaedic Surgeons.

Smurr, L. M., Gulick, K., Yancosek, K., & Ganz, O. (2008). Managing the upper extremity amputee: A protocol for success. *Journal of Hand Therapy, 21,* 160–175.

Stubblefield, K. A., Miller, L. A., Lipschutz, R. D., & Kuiken, T. A. (2009). Occupational therapy protocol for amputees with targeted muscle reinnervation. *Journal of Rehabilitation Research & Development, 46,* 481–488.

Uellendahl, J. E. (2004). Bilateral upper limb prostheses. In D. G. Smith, J. W. Michael, & J. H. Bowker (Eds.), *Atlas of amputations and limb deficiencies: Surgical, prosthetic and rehabilitation principles* (pp. 311–325). Rosemont, IL: American Academy of Orthopaedic Surgeons.

Van Dorsten, B. (2004). Common emotional concerns following limb loss. In D. J. Atkins & R. H. Meier III (Eds.), *Functional restoration of adults and children with upper extremity amputation* (pp. 73–78). New York: Demos Medical Publishing.

Weeks, S. R., Anderson-Barnes, V. C., & Tsao, J. W. (2010). Phantom limb pain: Theories and therapies. *Neurologist, 16,* 277–286.

Weir, R. F., Troyk, P. R., DeMichele, G., & Kuiken, T. (2003). *Implantable myoelectric sensors (IMES) for upper-extremity prosthesis control-preliminary work.* Paper presented at the 25th Annual International Conference of the IEEE EMBS, Cancun, Mexico, September 17–21, 2003.

Wright, V. (2009). Prosthetic outcome measures for use with upper limb amputees: A systematic review of the peer-reviewed literature, 1970–2009. *Journal of Prosthetics and Orthotics, 21*(4s), 3–63.

Yancosek, K. (2008). One-handed backpacks. *inMotion, Nov/Dec,* 33–34.

Yancosek, K. E. (2011). Amputations and prosthetics In T. Skirvin, L. Osterman, J. Fedorczyk, & P. Amadio (Eds.), *Rehabilitation of the hand* (Vol. 2, 6th ed.). Philadelphia: Mosby, Inc.

Yancosek, K. E., & Gulick, K. (2008). *Handwriting for heroes.* Ann Arbor, MI: Loving Healing Press.

Yancosek, K. E., & Howell, D. (2011). Systematic review of interventions to improve or augment handwriting ability in adult clients. *Occupational Therapy Journal of Research, 31,* 55–63.

Yancosek, K. E., Schnall, B. L., & Baum, B. S. (2008). Impact of upper-limb prosthesis on gait: A case study. *Journal of Prosthetics and Orthotics, 20,* 163–166.

Ziegler-Graham, K., MacKenzie, E. J., Ephraim, P. L., Travison, T. G., & Brookmeyer, R. (2008). Estimating the prevalence of limb loss in the United States: 2005 to 2050. *Archives of Physical Medicine and Rehabilitation, 89,* 422–429.

ACKNOWLEDGMENT

The authors wish to acknowledge the work of the authors of this chapter for previous editions: Kathy Stubblefield and Anne Armstrong (6th edition), and Felice Gadaleta Celikyol (4th and 5th editions). The authors thank Dr. Catherine Trombly Latham for her work on the assessment table.

The information and use of product names in this chapter does not reflect the official policy, position, or endorsement of the Department of the Army, Department of Defense, Department of Veterans Affairs, or the U. S. Government.

42

Cardiac and Pulmonary Diseases

Nancy Huntley

Learning Objectives

After studying this chapter, the reader will be able to do the following:

1. Recognize the signs and symptoms of exercise/activity intolerance.
2. Identify the common cardiac diagnoses and their treatment in occupational therapy.
3. Understand various cardiac and pulmonary diagnostic studies and how these tests assist with treatment planning in occupational therapy.
4. Know the controllable risk factors for heart disease and ways to ameliorate their effect.
5. Be able to instruct patients with pulmonary disease in breathing techniques.
6. Know resources for further guidelines in cardiac and pulmonary rehabilitation.

INCIDENCE OF CARDIAC AND PULMONARY DISEASE

Between 1998 and 2008, the mortality rate from cardiovascular disease (CVD) decreased by 30.6% (American Heart Association [AHA], 2012). However, CVD remains the leading cause of mortality, causing one out of every three deaths in the United States (AHA, 2012). According to Summary Health Statistics for U.S. Adults 2010, 12% of Americans have been told by a health professional that they have heart disease, and 6% have been told they have coronary heart disease. There is a positive correlation between advancing age and increased incidence of heart disease (Schiller et al., 2010).

Pulmonary disease is also a significant cause of death in the United States. Chronic obstructive pulmonary disease (COPD) is the third leading killer of Americans (American Lung Association, 2012). Lung disease is not only a killer; it is also chronic and significantly alters the lives of those who have it. Of people with COPD, 50% say that the disease limits their ability to work, and 70% say it limits their ability to do normal daily exertion (American Lung Association, 2008).

Even though a clinician is not working in either cardiac or pulmonary rehabilitation, the diagnosis of cardiac or pulmonary disease in a patient's medical history has implications for the occupational therapist's treatment plan. For instance, a patient may carry the primary diagnosis of a recent stroke. If that stroke occurred shortly after coronary artery bypass surgery, certain precautions should be taken to protect the patient's sternum. When the patient has a history of heart disease, the therapist should also routinely measure heart rate and blood pressure both at rest and with activity to determine his or her cardiovascular response to rehabilitation. The occupational therapist must therefore be aware of these disease processes and know how they will influence treatment.

HEART DISEASE

Heart disease may be due to a blockage of the coronary arteries, diseases of the heart muscle, or structural anomalies of the heart. A myocardial infarction (MI), or heart attack, is death of the heart muscle caused by lack of blood flow caused by an obstruction of a coronary artery by thrombosed plaque or spasm. The patient's clinical history, along with several diagnostic tests, is considered when diagnosing a heart attack. The patient may first have an onset of symptoms known as acute coronary syndrome (ACS), which indicates acute myocardial ischemia and encompasses unstable angina, non-ST elevation myocardial infarctions (non-STEMIs) and ST elevation myocardial infarctions (STEMIs) (Kim, Kini, & Fuster, 2008). The patient may first have symptoms such as chest pain or pressure, which may radiate to the teeth, jaw, ear, arm, or midback. These symptoms may be accompanied by diaphoresis, shortness of breath (SOB), nausea, vomiting, and/or fatigue. The patient may present with one or more of these symptoms, and the severity and intensity varies from person to person. (Not everyone who has these symptoms will have a heart attack, but it helps to triage them to the appropriate treatment.) An electrocardiogram (EKG) will show where the damage to the heart muscle occurred. Meanwhile, blood tests for certain structural proteins and cardiac enzymes will confirm a heart attack and give an idea of the amount of damage done to the heart muscle.

If a person realizes he or she is having a heart attack, it is important to seek treatment immediately. It has been demonstrated in numerous multicenter trials that aggressive treatment with angiographic revascularization and antiplatelet drugs produces better results (Kim, Kini, & Fuster, 2008). The greatest benefit, especially with large heart attacks, is when treatment is initiated within the first 60–90 minutes after symptom onset (Antman, 2008). The sooner the patient receives treatment, the more heart muscle can be saved.

The left ventricle is the main pump of the heart. It pumps the blood from the heart to the rest of the body. Because the left ventricle does more work, it has a higher oxygen requirement than the rest of the heart. It is usually the first area of the heart to suffer from any coronary artery perfusion deficiency.

Types of Myocardial Infarction

In evaluating an MI, an EKG is an important adjunct in determining the location of the MI and the severity of the infarction (see Fig. 42-1). An MI that involves all three layers of the heart muscle is called transmural, and

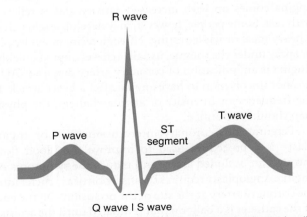

Figure 42-1 Basic EKG. (Google Images, 2012.) P wave reflects when the atria contract, the R wave reflects the ventricular contraction, and the T wave represents when the heart is repolarizing. If the ST segment is elevated, it is significant for myocardial injury. If the ST segment is depressed, there is myocardial ischemia. If there is a Q wave one-third the depth of the R wave, the patient has had a previous myocardial infarction.

it usually produces ST elevation on the EKG. It is referred to as an ST elevation MI, or STEMI. Most of these MIs will later produce a Q wave over EKG leads affected by the MI (Antman & Braunwald, 2008). A Q wave is an identifying characteristic showing where damage occurred. In STEMIs, the size of the infarct is important. If the STEMI is large or if the STEMI is small to moderate in a person with previous STEMIs, the prognosis is poor (Antman, 2008). An anterior STEMI is considered the most serious because of the large amount of muscle mass lost and decrease in the effectiveness of ventricular pumping action (Meyers, 2005). (See Definition 42-1 for a review of common diagnostic procedures.)

When the thrombus in the coronary artery is incomplete, less damage is done, and it is called a non-ST elevation MI or a non-STEMI. The majority of these MIs do not develop a Q wave. These MIs are called non-STEMIs or non–Q wave MIs (Antman & Braunwald, 2008). Although the immediate prognosis is better in patients with a non-STEMI, their future risk is often higher for death or further cardiac events because of a history of previous heart events, comorbidities or because of the extent of their underlying heart disease (Cannon & Braunwald, 2008).

Blockage in the left main or left anterior descending artery of the heart will cause damage to the front of the left ventricle and is called an anterior MI. When the right coronary artery is involved, the back and bottom of the left ventricle are damaged; this is called an inferior MI. The circumflex artery feeds the lateral wall of the heart, and blockage in this artery results in a lateral MI (Fig. 42-2).

Angina pectoris is heart pain caused by a temporary inadequate supply of blood to the heart muscle. Angina might be described as pain, aching tightness, or pressure. It is usually diffuse and located in the midchest, but it may radiate to the midback, teeth, ear, jaw, or arm. Typically, angina comes on with increased activity and is relieved with rest. Some people, however, may develop angina after a heavy meal or while resting. Nitroglycerin, taken by pill or spray under the tongue, usually relieves angina quickly. Angina is an indication of coronary artery disease (CAD); it is not uncommon to have angina after a heart attack. If the frequency or intensity of angina changes, the physician should be notified.

Percutaneous coronary intervention (PCI) or angioplasty is a procedure used to improve the blood flow through an occluded artery and reduce the symptoms of angina. Angioplasty requires the insertion of a catheter into the coronary artery at the site of the occlusion. On the end of the catheter is a balloon that is inflated until the arterial walls, at the point of the occlusion, are pushed out to allow more blood flow through the area. When just angioplasty is done on a blood vessel, the restenosis rate is high. Of patients with angioplasty, 30%–50% will experience restenosis within the first year (Shaffer, 2008). Currently, a stent,

which resembles a spring in a ballpoint pen, is usually used with the balloon. The stent lies over the balloon, and when the balloon is inflated, the stent opens and imbeds itself in the artery wall, forming a structure to keep the artery open. Stents without drugs are called bare metal stents. Stents with drugs coating them are called drug-eluting stents. When a bare metal stent is used, the success of the procedure increases to about 70%–80% (Popma, Baim, & Resnic, 2008). When a drug-eluting stent is used, the restenosis rate drops to less than 5% (Baim, 2010). Getting a patient who is having an MI quickly to the catheterization lab for an angioplasty/stent to the involved artery is now considered the standard of care. For each 30 minutes of delay in having a PCI after the onset of symptoms, there is an 8% increase in 1-year mortality (Antman, 2008).

For those patients whose lesions are too calcified to insert the angioplasty catheter, another procedure is available. It is called atherectomy. In atherectomy, the catheter inserted into the coronary artery has a rotating blade that cuts out the plaque. As it cuts the plaque, suction pulls the plaque through a tube and out of the body. Arthrectomy is usually followed with stent placement (Barsness & Murphy, 2007).

Open Heart Surgery

Open heart surgery is a procedure that usually involves a sternotomy that allows the surgeon to work on the heart. There are several types of open heart surgery.

Coronary artery bypass graft (CABG) is the replacement of occluded coronary arteries with artery or vein grafts. The patient is first put on a heart lung machine so that the heart can be stopped while the surgeon works and oxygenated blood will continue to be pumped through the body. The harvested grafts are then attached to the aorta and reconnected below the occlusion in the coronary artery. Sometimes the mammary artery, which comes directly off the aorta, is dissected from its original destination and used as a graft. Another arterial graft is the radial artery. Arteries are preferred as grafts, because they stay patent longer than vein grafts. Vein grafts are harvested from the legs.

Valve replacement and/or repair may be necessitated by destruction of a heart valve caused by disease or congenital malformation. If the surgeon is unable to repair the valve, it is replaced with a prosthetic or tissue valve. Prosthetic valves are very durable and last a lifetime. If a prosthetic valve is used, patients will have to take thrombolytics for the rest of their lives. The thrombolytics will prevent blood from clotting as it goes through the valve. A tissue or biothesis valve is from humans or pigs. These valves do not require the patient to be on thrombolytic therapy. Bioprosthetic valves last at least 15 years for 94% of the patients with an aortic valve and for 78% of

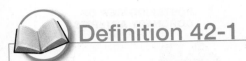

Definition 42-1

Common Diagnostic Studies for Heart Disease

Blood Tests

Blood tests are usually drawn on patients with symptoms of a probable heart attack. The cells of the heart contain isoenzymes and structural proteins, which are specific to that organ. Death of the heart's cells causes those isoenzymes and structural proteins to be released into the bloodstream where an increase in their levels can be measured. CPK MB is an isoenzyme that shows up in the blood within 6 hours after a heart attack and peaks in 24 hours (Davis, 2008). Troponin I and troponin T are two structural proteins whose levels rise with heart damage. Troponin I is the preferred structural protein to examine because of its specificity and sensitivity for myocardial ischemia (Blue Verrier & Hargrove Deelstra, 2010). Troponin levels start rising after 3–6 hours and stay elevated for up to 14 days, allowing detection of a myocardial infarction (MI) in patients who wait to seek treatment (Davis, 2008).

Natriuretic peptides BNP and pro-BNP are neurohormones made in the left ventricle, whose values increase in the bloodstream with ventricular wall stress. BNP is a strong diagnostic tool in CHF and a predictor of clinical outcomes in CHF, unstable angina, and non-STEMIs (Cannon & Braunwald, 2008).

Stress Echocardiogram

A stress echocardiogram is an exercise test usually conducted on a treadmill. Before starting the test, an ultrasound recording is taken of the function of the heart at rest. The patient is then exercised to his or her maximum capacity. After exercising, another ultrasound recording of the heart is done to show how the heart responds to work. It will show whether the heart muscle and valves work normally under pressure or if some parts respond suboptimally. It is also possible to measure how much blood the heart ejects with each beat. This number is the ejection fraction (EF).

A normal EF is >60%. A person is mildly impaired with an EF of 50%–59%. A person with an EF of 40%–50% has moderate impairment. An EF below 40% is considered significant impairment. The lower the EF, the higher the risk the patient has for further events and complications. In most cardiac conditions, the EF is a strong predictor of outcome and is helpful in determining treatment (Connolly & Oh, 2012). The EF does not always accurately reflect an individual patient's ability to work, but the EF is helpful as a starting point for making appropriate exercise and activity recommendations and precautions.

Stress echocardiography is approximately 85% accurate in predicting CVD depending on the cohort of the study (ACSM, 2010a). When a stress test is given without the echo, the accuracy is reduced to 75% in predicting heart disease, but patient's maximum exercise capacity and maximum heart rate with exercise are known.

Nuclear Stress Test

A nuclear stress test is conducted with a 12-lead electrocardiogram (EKG) as patients exercise to their maximum capacity on a treadmill. During this test, the patient is injected with a radioactive isotope when the patient feels only able to exercise for one more minute. The patient is then placed under a special instrument called a scintillation camera, which can detect the presence of the radioactive isotope in the heart muscle. This isotope has special properties, which allows it to be readily picked up by healthy myocardium cells, more slowly by cells with poor perfusion, and not at all by infarcted myocardium. Those areas with restricted blood flow may eventually "fill in" with the radioactive isotope, and these areas are said to have a reversible defect. Areas that do not "fill in" are infarcted, and the deficit is permanent (Nishimura et al., 2010). Because this process may take several hours, the nuclear test usually involves an initial scan, with another scan administered 2–3 hours later.

Transesophogeal Echocardiography

A transesophageal echocardiography (TEE) involves intubating the esophagus with a TEE ultrasound probe to visualize the cardiac structures such as the condition of the valves, both native and prosthetic; tumors; atrial septal defects; and congenital anomalies (Scordo, 2008).

Magnetic Resonance Imaging

Magnetic resonance imaging (MRI) is a noninvasive technique that uses radio waves, magnets, and computers to create pictures of the heart. It provides diagnostic information about the blood vessels, tissue, size of MI, the condition of valves, and neoplasms (Soine & Crawley, 2010). Often, contrast dyes are used with it.

Computed Tomography

In computed tomography (CT), the patient is surrounded by a 360° gantry of x-ray tubes, which gives excellent pictures of the coronary arteries and veins, valves, and patency of stents and picks up tumors and congenital abnormalities (Soine & Cawley, 2010). It is often used to assess coronary artery disease (CAD) in the symptomatic patient. When used for diagnosis of CAD, it has a 95% sensitivity, 60%–85% positive predictive value, and a 99% negative predictive value (Vora, 2011). There is radiation exposure with CT, and contrast dyes may be used with it.

Coronary Angiography

Coronary angiography is currently the most definitive test in the diagnosis of CAD. A catheter is inserted into a blood vessel in the groin and threaded back into the heart, and a radiopaque dye is injected through it into the coronary blood vessels. The extent of the obstruction in any coronary blood vessel can be visualized. A blockage must be greater than 70%–75% of the lumen to be considered significant. A lesion greater than 50% in the left main artery is considered equivalent to two-vessel disease. The length of coronary artery lesion(s) is also taken into consideration. In addition, heart valve function, ventricular wall motion abnormalities, and some heart defects can be detected (Paganda & Paganda, 2011).

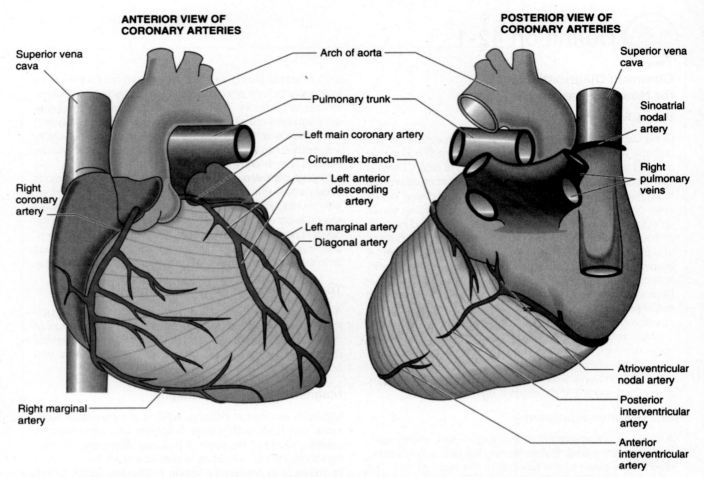

ANTERIOR VIEW OF CORONARY ARTERIES

Superior vena cava
Arch of aorta
Pulmonary trunk
Left main coronary artery
Circumflex branch
Right coronary artery
Left anterior descending artery
Left marginal artery
Diagonal artery
Right marginal artery

POSTERIOR VIEW OF CORONARY ARTERIES

Superior vena cava
Sinoatrial nodal artery
Right pulmonary veins
Atrioventricular nodal artery
Posterior interventricular artery
Anterior interventricular artery

Figure 42-2 Coronary arteries. Location of damage to the heart depends on which coronary arteries are blocked. (From Willis, M. C. [1996]. *Medical terminology: The language of health care.* Baltimore: Williams & Wilkins.)

the patients with a mitral valve, before they need to be replaced (Acar & Theodore, 2010).

Differently invasive bypasses or valve surgery are new techniques in which the bypass or valve replacement operations are done through small incisions (minimally invasive bypass) or are performed on a beating heart. In both cases, the patient is not put on a heart lung machine used during a standard bypass operation (Sabek, Bansilal, & Lyle, 2008). Minimally invasive surgery is done through several small incisions made between the ribs. In bypass surgery done on a beating heart, the patient has a sternotomy, but special instruments stop the heart from beating for a few seconds so the surgeon can sew the new bypass graft to the native coronary artery. In both types of differently invasive surgeries, the recovery time is much less than usual. However, the skill level to do both these operations is high, and they are generally done only when the arteries in the front of the heart are being bypassed or on the aortic valve.

Atrial septal defects are the most common type of congenital defect (Marelli, 2011). About 30% of people with

atrial septal defect will develop symptoms in the third decade of life, but 75% will have symptoms by their 50s (Moons et al., 2008). When the heart has been attempting to compensate for a defect for a long time, it may become enlarged, and the patient may complain of fatigue and SOB. The current standard of practice is to repair these heart defects before the patient has significant symptoms or sustains myocardial damage.

Other Heart Diagnoses and Procedures

Congestive heart failure (CHF) describes the inability of the heart to function as an effective pump. The heart muscle becomes stretched beyond its ability to contract efficiently, resulting in the collection of fluid in the lungs or the extremities. In Western civilization, 60%–65% of cases of CHF are caused by CAD (Francis, Wilson Tang, & Walsh, 2012). CHF may also result from a number of other disease processes such as hypertension, incompetent valves, and cardiomyopathy (CM). Patients with CHF experience SOB and fatigue and may have an increase in weight and

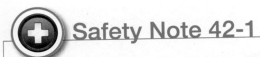

Safety Note 42-1

Signs and Symptoms of Congestive Heart Failure

- Sudden gain in weight
- Inability to sleep lying down flat
- Persistent dry hacking cough, often with white frothy sputum
- Shortness of breath with normal activity
- Swelling in ankles or feet or legs
- Fatigue with activity
- Lack of appetite
- Difficulty focusing one's attention

From Mayo Clinic. (2010). Heart failure: Symptoms. Retrieved March 20, 2012 from www.mayoclinic/health/heart-failure/.

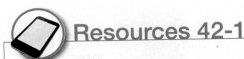

Resources 42-1

Two organizations dominate the administration and policies of cardiac rehabilitation. One is the American Association of Cardiovascular and Pulmonary Rehabilitation (AACVPR), which published the book *Guidelines for Cardiac Rehabilitation and Secondary Prevention Programs*. Government agencies and third-party payers use this publication to determine appropriate cardiac rehabilitation policies and procedures. The second is the American College of Sports Medicine, which has multiple publications of use for those working in cardiac rehabilitation. Both organizations offer continuing education courses in cardiac rehabilitation. Together these two organizations shape the practice of cardiac rehabilitation.

AACVPR

401 North Michigan Avenue, Suite 2200
Chicago, IL 60611
Phone: 312-321-5146
www.aacvpr.org

ACSM National Center

401 West Michigan Street
Indianapolis, IN 46202-3233
Phone: 317-637-9200
www.acsm.org

a dry hacking cough. Often, they complain of coughing or being SOB in a recumbent position (see Safety Note 42-1 for signs and symptoms). The B-type natriuretic peptide (BNP) is a lab test routinely drawn to differentiate CHF from other causes of SOB (Hollenberg & Parrillo, 2010). The number of medication treatment options for patients with CHF has increased significantly, yet the mortality rate for CHF is high. Of those with CHF, 50% will die within 5 years (AHA, 2012).

CM refers to diseases of cardiac muscle. The three main types of CM are dilated, hypertrophic, and restrictive (Wynne & Braunwald, 2010). According to the American Heart Association Heart and Stroke Update (2012), dilated CM is the most common type of cardiomyopathy. Many diseases can cause dilated CM, but symptoms are an enlarged heart with decreased pumping capacity that usually results in CHF (Mestroni et al., 2012). Depending on the cohort of the study, 10%–50% of those people presenting to the hospital with CHF died within the first year (Hare, 2008). Approximately one-fourth of patients with dilated CM, for unknown reasons, improve or stabilize over time (Wynne & Braunwald, 2010). However, the most reliable predictor of a poor outcome is the decreased pumping function of the left ventricle as expressed by a low ventricular ejection fraction (EF) (Mestroni et al., 2012).

CARDIAC REHABILITATION

Cardiac rehabilitation usually involves a multidisciplinary team. Doctors, nurses, occupational and physical therapists, exercise physiologists, dieticians, chaplains, psychologists, and social workers may all play a part in the patient's recovery. Doctors, dieticians, chaplains, psychologists, and social workers perform their conventional roles in treating the cardiac patient. None of the other allied health professionals, however, are trained specifically to work in cardiac rehabilitation, and all need additional training. Geographical tradition and availability of staff seem to determine what role each allied health professional plays. Members of each discipline use their own special skills in dealing with patients with heart disease, but their job expectations and responsibilities may essentially be the same. (See Resources 42-1 for information on organizations that develop policies and certifications in cardiac rehabilitation and Evidence Table 42-1 for the best evidence for cardiac rehabilitation.)

Occupational therapists are invaluable when treating the patient with heart disease. Therapists are able to evaluate and analyze the patient's activities of daily living (ADL). The therapist can then assist patients in modifying activities, if necessary, so that they can resume those activities they previously enjoyed. The occupational therapist's expertise in the rehabilitative process and knowledge of comorbid diseases is extremely important when evaluating and adapting treatment for the individual needs of the patient. Patients who have undergone lifestyle changes and experienced life-threatening diseases also benefit from occupational therapy intervention to help with psychosocial adjustment to their new situation.

Evidence Table 42-1 | Best Evidence for Cardiac Rehabilitation

Intervention	Description of Intervention Tested	Participants	Dosage	Type of Best Evidence and Level of Evidence	Benefit	Statistical Probability and Effect Size of Outcome	Reference
Phase II cardiac rehabilitation (CR)	Two groups of women with syndrome X. One group was assigned to symptom monitoring and the other group attended a phase II CR program and symptom monitoring program.	Sixty-four women, 57.3 ± 8.6 years, who had chest pain and normal coronary arteries (syndrome X)	The cardiac rehab group received 8 weeks of exercise and symptom monitoring. The other group monitored symptoms for 8 weeks.	Randomized controlled trial. Level: 1B2a	Those who received CR showed improvements in exercise tolerance, quality of life, psychological morbidity, symptom severity, and cardiovascular risk. These improvements were not found in the symptom monitoring group.	Statistically significant differences between CR and symptom monitoring groups in terms of decreased symptom severity ($p = 0.009$, $r = 0.17$), hospital anxiety ($p = 0.008$, $r = 0.21$), depression ($p = 0.004$, $r = 0.24$), SF-36 physical functioning ($p = 0.006$, $r = 0.20$), and pain ($p = 0.028$, $r = 0.18$) and increased exercise tolerance on shuttle walk test ($p < 0.001$, $r = 0.32$).	Asbury et al. (2008)
Any form of supervised or unsupervised structured exercise program compared to a control group	Inpatient, outpatient, or community-based setting exercise program	6,111 patients	Varied from study to study. The minimum was 2 weeks with a minimum follow-up of 12 weeks	Systematic review and meta-analysis of 34 randomized, controlled trials Level: I	Yes, patients in exercise-based cardiac rehab programs had a lower rate of reinfarction, cardiac, and all-cause mortality.	Reduction in all-cause mortality (odds ratio [OR]) = 0.74; 95% confidence interval [CI] = 0.58–0.95) Reduction in cardiac mortality (OR = 0.64); lower risk of reinfarction (OR = 0.53); 95% CI = 0.38–0.76	Lawler, Filion, & Eisenberg (2011)

| Any form of supervised or unsupervised structured exercise program (compared with usual care) | Inpatient, outpatient, or community- or home-based setting exercise program either with or without psychosocial and educational interventions | 8,940 patients | Varied from study to study. Median intervention time was 3 months. | Meta-analysis of 48 trials Level: I | Yes, significant reduction in all-cause mortality and total cardiac mortality, a significant reduction in total cholesterol and triglycerides and systolic blood pressure, and lower self-reports of smoking | Reduction in all-cause mortality (OR = 0.80; 95% CI = 0.68–0.93) Reduction in cardiac mortality (OR = 0.74; 95% CI = 0.61–0.96) Reduction in total cholesterol level (weighted mean difference = –0.37 mmol/L; 95% CI = –0.63 to –0.11 mmol/L) Reduction in total triglyceride level (weighted mean difference = –0.23 mmol/L; 95% CI = –0.39 to –0.07 mmol/L) Reduction in systolic blood pressure (weighted mean difference = –3.2 mm Hg; 95% CI = –5.4 to –0.9 mm Hg) Reduction in smoking (OR = 0.64; 95% CI = 0.50–0.83). | Taylor et al. (2004) |

Risk Factors for Heart Disease

One of the main goals of all phases of cardiac rehabilitation is primary and secondary prevention of heart disease. Primary prevention refers to efforts to prevent the development of heart disease. Primary prevention efforts are usually limited to health fairs and lecture series because health insurance currently does not cover its cost. Those costs are borne either by a sponsor (i.e., a hospital) or by charging admission. Therefore, most of the therapist's efforts are directed toward secondary prevention. Secondary prevention pertains to efforts designed to stop or slow the progression of heart disease. Improving an individual's risk factor profile is the method used by therapists for secondary prevention of heart disease.

Ten risk factors increase one's likelihood of developing CAD. The three risk factors that are not controllable are age, family history, and gender. With advancing age, an individual is at greater risk for heart disease. A family history of a first-degree relative, such as father, mother, brother, or sister, developing heart disease before age 55 years for males and before age 65 years for females increases one's risk (Johns Hopkins Health Alert, 2010). If one's father has premature heart disease, a man's risk doubles and a woman's increases by 70% (AHA, 2012). The risk of developing heart disease for both men and women doubles when another sibling has the disease (AHA, 2012). Men are more likely to develop heart disease 10–15 years earlier than women, but as women approach menopause, they lose the protective effect of estrogen, and their risk of heart disease increases (Stewart, 2008). Although heart disease is commonly considered a male problem, it is an equal opportunity killer. It remains the number one cause of death for both men and women (AHA, 2012).

Controllable Risk Factors

The risk factors that one can control are smoking, hyperlipidemia, hypertension, sedentary lifestyle, obesity, diabetes, and psychological stress.

Smoking is a major modifiable risk factor that contributes to heart disease in multiple ways. The incidence of heart disease is two to four times higher in people who smoke than in nonsmokers (Sohn et al., 2010). Smoking damages the endothelial lining of the coronary arteries, making them more susceptible to plaque formation. Nicotine causes vasoconstriction of the arteries and increases heart rate. Smoking makes the heart more susceptible to lethal ventricular arrhythmias and predisposes it to coronary artery spasm (Ridker & Libby, 2008). Carbon monoxide in cigarette smoke binds with the hemoglobin faster than oxygen, resulting in less oxygen being distributed to the tissues. Nicotine alters the metabolism of fats, increasing the levels of atherogenic low-density lipoprotein (LDL) cholesterol and decreasing the levels of the heart-protective high-density lipoprotein (HDL) cholesterol. Smoking also causes the blood to coagulate more quickly and promotes thrombus formation (Ridker & Libby, 2008). Even those who are regularly exposed to secondhand smoke at work or home have a 25% increase in their risk of CVD (AHA, 2012). However, if a person quits smoking after their first MI, the benefits accrue quickly. Within a year, their risk for heart disease drops by 50%. Their risk continues to decline over time, so that after 15 years of smoking abstinence, their risk of coronary heart disease is equal to someone who has never smoked (Sohn et al., 2010).

Hyperlipidemia or a high lipid level is a major risk factor among Americans. It has been determined that a total cholesterol level below 200 mg/dL is desirable. LDL or "bad" cholesterol is acceptable below 130 mg/dL for those without risk factors for heart disease. LDL should be below 100 for those at risk of heart disease, and LDL should be below 70 for those with known CAD. HDL or "good" cholesterol of less than 40 mg/dL for men and 50 mg/dL for women significantly increases the risk of heart disease. Triglycerides should be under 150 mg/dL to be considered normal (Mayo Clinic, 2012). Cholesterol levels may be lowered through a low-fat diet, regular aerobic exercise, and weight loss. If these options are unsuccessful, the physician will put a patient on a lipid-lowering drug. Others are put on lipid lowering drugs because they inherit an inability to metabolize lipids normally. They have very high lipid levels in their blood because they manufacture high levels of their own cholesterol. According to multiple trials on lipid-lowering drugs, these medications decrease the risk of heart disease by lowering blood cholesterol (Blaha et al., 2012).

The American Heart Association Heart and Stroke Update (2012) classifies blood pressures greater than 140/90 at rest as being hypertensive. Hypertension causes damage to the arterial walls and causes increased myocardial oxygen consumption because of the need for the heart to do more work against high pressures (Medline Plus, 2012). People with hypertension have a two- to fourfold higher risk of heart disease and heart failure than normotensive individuals (Dennison, Miller, & Cunningham, 2010). Other than taking medication, individuals can improve their blood pressure by weight loss, eating a low fat diet, reducing sodium intake, eating lots of fruits and vegetables, regular aerobic exercise, moderation in alcohol intake, and controlling other risk factors for CAD (Blaha et al., 2012).

Sedentary lifestyle is a risk factor for heart disease. The relative risk of a sedentary lifestyle for heart disease is comparable to the risk associated with smoking, hypercholesterolemia, and high blood pressure (Sohn et al., 2010). Regular physical exercise assists with weight control, lowers blood pressure, and improves the lipid profile and glucose tolerance (Ridker & Libby, 2008). The Centers for Disease Control and Prevention (CDC) and the American College of Sports Medicine (ACSM) recommend that adults get 30 minutes or more of moderate physical activity on most and preferably all days of the week (CDC, 2008). Results of a meta-analysis of multiple studies suggested that patients who undergo cardiac rehabilitation exercise training after an MI have 25% reduction in cardiovascular and all-cause mortality (Clinical Knowledge Summaries, 2007). Because of the effect of exercise on the heart, circulatory system, and other risk factors, aerobic exercise is an effective weapon against heart disease.

In the United States, 68% of adults are overweight or obese (AHA, 2012). Obesity is now the second leading preventable cause of death (Burke et al., 2010). Obesity is closely related to and influences negatively a number of risk factors for heart disease such as hypertension, diabetes, hyperlipidemia, and physical activity. The distribution of body fat is important in disease promotion. Central or abdominal obesity is linked to increased risk of CAD (Warzeski et al., 2008). The loss of even 5%–10% of one's weight, however, can have a positive influence on risk factors such as hypertension, lipid levels, and sleep apnea (Warzeski et al., 2008).

Diabetes has long been recognized as a risk factor for heart disease. The incidence of type II diabetes has doubled in the past 30 years and parallels the increase in obesity (AHA, 2012). Women who have diabetes lose the protective effect of their hormones against heart disease, and their risk of CAD is significantly higher than that of nondiabetic women (Sweeney, 2010). Compared to people who do not have diabetes, people with diabetes have two to four times the death rate from heart disease (AHA, 2012). Keeping blood sugar levels in good control through medication, diet, and exercise reduces macro- and microvascular disease in patients with type I and type II diabetes and thus reduces the risk of heart disease (Cade, 2008).

Stress is also considered to be a risk factor for heart disease, but its effect is difficult to quantify. Several studies have shown that depression, low social support, and stress increase one's risk for CAD and other adverse life events (O'Connell-Edwards, York, & Blumenthal, 2008). Chronic stress negatively affects the cardiovascular system by increasing the heart rate, blood pressure, blood lipid levels, and blood clotting. Managing chronic stressors with relaxation techniques or through behavioral change is helpful in eliminating or minimizing the effect of stress on the body.

As part of secondary prevention, the therapist must direct considerable energy toward educating the patient regarding the significance of these risk factors and methods of ameliorating them. Education may take place in one-on-one sessions, such as with the patient while doing a home program, or with groups of patients before, during, or after exercise.

Inpatient Cardiac Rehabilitation or Phase I

The goals of inpatient cardiac rehabilitation are to prevent muscle loss from bed rest, monitor and assess the patient's ability to function, instruct the patient in appropriate home activities, educate the patient about individual risk factors, and teach methods to lessen these risks.

Therapists treat each patient at least once a day and usually twice daily as soon as the patient's medical status has stabilized, often within the first 24–48 hours after admission. Hospital stays for coronary events have declined significantly in the past 10 years. The average stays are 1 day for the uncomplicated non-STEMI, 2–3 days for STEMIs, and 3–7 days for open heart surgery.

The occupational therapist working in cardiac rehabilitation initiates therapy on a one-on-one basis so that the therapist can interview the patient regarding lifestyle and assess the patient's cardiovascular response to exercise. During exercise, physical measurements of heart rate, blood pressure, EKG response, and symptoms are noted. Occupational therapists working in cardiac rehabilitation need to take an EKG reading course. See Procedures for Practice 42-1 for instructions regarding blood pressure measurement and pulse taking.

Although programs vary in the type of exercise done, many begin with mild calisthenics for 2-minute bouts followed by a 1-minute rest for people post bypass or those with CHF. Initially, the total time of the calisthenics added together is 4–8 minutes, depending on the patient's tolerance. As the patient progresses, the amount of time the patient may spend doing calisthenics typically increases to 8–10 minutes. Hall walking, treadmill, and/or stairs are added to those with surgery and CHF as soon as they can tolerate it. With patients who have had non-STEMIs, STEMIs, or percutaneous transluminal coronary revascularization (PTCR)/stents, the therapist usually starts with hall walking or treadmill and may add stair climbing. Other modalities, such as NuStep® and bicycle ergometer, may be added to all of the diagnoses as tolerated (Fig. 42-3). Regardless of the modality used, each is started gradually (treadmill walking at 0.8–2.5 mph or less for about 3–15 minutes) with progression based on the patient's tolerance and diagnosis. It is important for the therapist to assess the patient's heart rate, blood pressure, EKG, and symptoms to establish the patient's tolerance for exercise (see Safety Note 42-2).

Home Programs

Each patient is given a home program before discharge from the hospital. The type of program given is individualized to the patient and his or her particular diagnosis. The general components of a home program are activity and exercise guidelines, work simplification, pacing, temperature precautions, social activity, sexuality, signs and symptoms of exercise intolerance, and/or a discussion of risk factors. Depending on the diagnosis, certain aspects

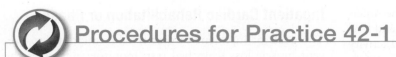

Procedures for Practice 42-1

Measuring Blood Pressure and Pulse

Measuring Blood Pressure

1. Wrap blood pressure cuff 1 to 1.5 inches above the antecubital space.
2. The cuff should be wrapped smoothly and firmly around the arm.
3. The bladder of the cuff should cover 80% of the arm circumference.
4. Palpate the brachial pulse on the medial aspect of the arm.
5. Place the stethoscope over the pulse.
6. Close the valve on the inflation ball.
7. Inflate the cuff 20 mm Hg greater than the point where you hear the pulse obliterated.
8. Slowly open the valve on the inflation ball so the mercury or arrow drops at the rate of 2–3 mm per second.
9. The first sound heard is the systolic pressure; make a note of that number.
10. Continue to listen until the pulse starts to muffle and finally disappears.
11. The point at which the pulse disappears is the diastolic pressure; make a note of that number.
12. Be sure to listen for 30 mm Hg longer to make sure you heard the exact last pulsation.
13. Completely deflate the cuff and remove from the patient (Berman & Snyder, 2012).

To be considered normal, blood pressure must be under 140/90 at rest. Systolic blood pressure should rise with exercise. Diastolic blood pressure should stay the same or drop slightly. With exercise, diastolic blood pressure should not increase more than 10 mm Hg compared with resting. The blood pressure response of patients with a history of high blood pressure is likely to be exaggerated with exercise.

Pulse Taking

1. Locate indentation on lateral side of wrist about 0.5 inch proximal to the wrist crease.
2. Palpate the radial artery with the index and middle finger.
3. Count the number of pulsations for 10 seconds.
4. Multiply that number by six to determine the number of beats per minute.
5. Notice if the pulse is regular or irregular.
6. Also note any "skipped" or early beats.

A normal heart rate (HR) range at rest is between 60 and 100 beats per minute (bpm). Someone who is very fit, such as a runner, may have a heart rate in the 40s or 50s. After open heart surgery, a patient often has a heart rate in the low 100s. It is not uncommon for patients who have valve repair or replacement to develop a rapid heart rhythm called atrial fibrillation. This rhythm is usually controlled with medication or by cardioversion. *Safety Message: If the patient's HR is uncontrolled and is 120 bpm or higher at rest, exercise is contraindicated.*

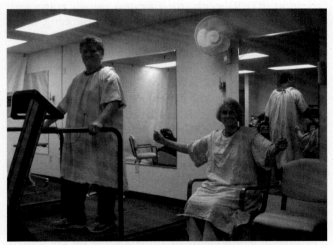

Figure 42-3 Patients exercising in inpatient cardiac rehabilitation to maintain muscle tone and endurance. The exercises also allow the therapist to evaluate the patients' cardiovascular response to light-to-moderate activity while they recuperate from significant myocardial infarction, congestive heart failure, or open heart surgery.

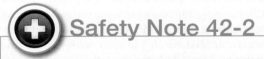

Safety Note 42-2

Signs and Symptoms of Exercise Intolerance

- Chest pain or pain referred to the teeth, jaw, ear, or arm
- Excessive fatigue
- Shortness of breath
- Light-headedness or dizziness
- Nausea or vomiting
- Unusual weight gain of 3–5 pounds in a 1–3-day period

If a Patient Needs to Take Nitroglycerin

A patient with chest pain or angina, who has a prescription for nitroglycerin, should try a nitroglycerin pill under the tongue. If the chest pain has not disappeared within 3–5 minutes, another nitroglycerin pill should be tried, and 911 (or the within-hospital emergency number) should be called. The patient may take a third nitro pill after another 5 minutes if he or she needs it. The doctor should be notified when the patient first has angina or if there are changes in the frequency or intensity of episodes of angina. Notify the physician if other symptoms of exercise intolerance persist after resting.

of the home program are emphasized or minimized. The information should be pertinent to the patient's lifestyle, including favorite activities, work, and/or hobbies with suggestions for resuming these activities.

Open Heart Surgery Home Program Patients who have had open heart surgery are given directions that are more specific. They are in pain and under the influence of analgesics, which may affect retention of information. They are told specifically what to do and what to avoid. They are also given information on stretches and mild exercises to assist in incisional pain management. In these patients, the sternum has been broken, and it must be treated like any other broken bone. Surgical patients are to avoid lifting, pushing, or pulling greater than 10 pounds for 6–12 weeks. Therapists should make recommendations for alternative ways of doing activities to avoid one-sided pulling. For example, when pulling open a heavy door, it is desirable to use two hands, or when picking up a heavy coffeepot, put one hand covered with an oven mitt on the bottom of the pot and the other hand on the handle. Patients who complain of feeling sternal shifting or clicking are told to try to avoid the activity that causes it and to stop any upper extremity (UE) exercises. Usually, the clicking goes away with just a little care. Be aware that individual surgeons have their own views regarding the exact length of time to avoid lifting and the amount of arm activity they will allow. Walking schedules that increase gradually, such as 1 minute per day for those very deconditioned or 2–5 minutes a day for those with small MIs, are issued. Patients are also given information regarding the possible emotional and physical responses they may expect during the healing process, such as easy fatigability or depression. Patients are encouraged to express their affection and intimacy. After open heart surgery, it is generally suggested that patients wait 6–8 weeks before resuming sexual intercourse (Levine et al., 2012). When patients initially resume sexual intercourse, they may wish to try positions that avoid strain on the sternum, such as side-lying or sitting in a chair facing each other.

Congestive Heart Failure Home Program Patients with CHF and/or CM often have limited endurance. Their home program puts heavy emphasis on pacing and work simplification. It also includes a mild exercise program. Information regarding their diagnosis is given to help these patients understand that overexertion could put them back into heart failure. Signs and symptoms of CHF are included to alert the patient to signs of worsening medical status (see Safety Note 42-1).

Myocardial Infarction Home Program The home program of a patient who has had an STEMI will tend to highlight how to evaluate activity/exercise and determine the correct energy expenditure during the patient's recovery.

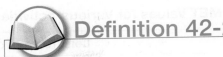

Definition 42-2

METs

METs, or metabolic equivalents, are a unit of measure used to describe the amount of oxygen the body needs for a given activity. One MET is equal to oxygen consumption at rest or 3.5 ml of oxygen per kilogram of body weight per minute (ACSM, 2010b). Extensive oxygen consumption tests have been done on a number of activities, and a small sampling of activities is included in Table 42-1. These values are still approximate because they do not take into account environmental factors or skill. The more the body moves and has to work against resistance, the higher the MET level.

Healing of the heart muscle takes about two to four weeks depending on the amount of damage sustained. Patients are usually asked to restrict their activities to the 2–4-MET range during this time (Definition 42-2 and Table 42-1). Pacing and work simplification may also be explained. This is especially important when the patient has had a significant amount of heart damage. A walking or biking exercise schedule is issued. Depression and sexuality are discussed because certain cardiac medications can play a significant role in mood as well as sexual function and desire. Patients should be told that, if there is a change in sexual ability or desire after their cardiac event, they should talk to their doctor to explore the role of any new medications in those changes. The AHA suggests that post-MI patients who can tolerate activities between 3 and 5 METs without symptoms, are ready to resume sexual intercourse (Levine et al., 2012).

Angioplasty Home Program Patients admitted for ACS and who have revascularization PCI are usually seen for home instruction. The goal of this home program is to teach risk factor recognition and patient awareness of ways to modify these risks. An aerobic exercise program positively affects most risk factors for heart disease. Therefore, a variety of ways to exercise are discussed, with the goal of finding one or several modes of aerobic exercise that might interest the patient. For example, if the patient chooses walking, options such as mall walking, treadmill and video walking programs, and outdoor walking are explored. Patients are given instruction in how to start an exercise program and taught how to assess their physical response to exercise using the Borg Rating of Perceived Exertion (RPE) Scale (ACSM, 2010a) and heart rate monitoring, if appropriate. Again, the therapist reviews signs and symptoms of exercise intolerance. Stress reduction techniques may be covered, and other resources for stress reduction are given. If the patient is a smoker, his or her willingness to quit is

Table 42-1 **MET Values for Various Activities**

Home	Leisure and Vocational	Exercise and Sports
1.0–2.5 METs		
Sweeping floors	Power boating	Walking at slow pace
Dusting	Fishing from boat	Playing catch with a baseball or football
Straightening up	Pumping gas	Horseback riding, walking
Serving food	Typing, computer	
Table setting	Sitting for light office work	
Knitting and crocheting	Card playing, sitting	
Putting away groceries	Board games	
Making bed	Playing piano or organ	
Standing quietly in line	Driving tractor	
Mowing lawn with a riding mower	Sewing with a machine	
Sexual activity (general, moderate effort)	Driving an auto or truck	
Dressing and undressing	Sitting to study, read, or write	
Sleeping	Casino gambling–standing	
Watching TV		
Dish washing		
Bathing–sitting		
Changing light bulbs		
Hairstyling–standing		
2.6–4.0 METs		
Child care bathing and grooming	Pitching horseshoes	Very light stationary biking
Walk, run, and play with children (moderate)	Home auto repair	Weight lifting of light-to-moderate effort
General house cleaning	Planting seedlings and shrubs	Stretching, yoga
Walking downstairs	Playing the drums	Golf using a cart
Sweeping garage or sidewalk	Home wiring or plumbing	Snowmobiling
Raking lawn	Feeding small farm animals	Walking at moderate speed
Walking and carrying load of 15 pounds	Standing doing light-to-moderate effort	Water aerobics
	Bartending–standing	Walking pushing a wheelchair
	Walking and picking up yard	Bicycling (<10 mph)
	Sailing	Activity videos moderate effort (i.e., Wii Fit™ aerobics and weight training)
	Motorcycle riding	Curves™ exercise for women
>4.0–6.0 METs		
Major house cleaning, such as washing windows, vigorous effort	Laying carpet or tile	General calisthenics, moderate effort
Moving furniture	Slow wood chopping	Shooting hoops
Scrubbing floors on hands and knees	Farming, feeding cattle	Softball, fast or slow pitch
Cleaning gutters	Carpentry on outside of house	Low-impact or dance aerobics
Painting the outside of house	Carpentry, refinishing surfaces	Dodgeball or hopscotch
Painting and wallpapering inside of house	Hunting–general	Bicycling (10–11.9 mph)
Weeding or cultivating	Road building, carrying heavy loads	Walk/jog (with jogging part less than 10 minutes)
Walking carrying a 15-pound load	Roofing	Elliptical, moderate effort
	Golf, carrying clubs	
6.0–10 METs		
Carrying groceries upstairs	Farming, bailing hay	High-impact aerobics
Moving household items in boxes	Concrete masonry	Running 10–12 minutes/mile
Shoveling more than 16 pounds per minute (heavy)	Moving heavy objects such as furniture	Basketball game
Walking or standing with objects weighing 50–74 pounds	Firefighter carrying hoses	Jump roping
		Race walking
		Swimming laps at a moderate pace
		Bicycling at moderate pace (>12 mph)

From Ainsworth, B. W., Haskell, W. L., Herrmann, S. D., Meches, N., Bassett, D. R., Jr., Tudor-Locke, C., Greer, J. L., Vezina, J., Whitt-Glover, M. C., & Leon, A. S. (2011). Compendium of physical activities: A second update of codes and met levels. *Medicine & Science in Sports & Exercise, 43*, 1575–1581; Ainsworth, B. W., Haskel, W. L., Leon, A., Jacobs, D., Jr., Montoye, H., Sallis, J., & Paffenbarger, R. (1998). Compendium of physical activities: Classification of energy costs of human physical activities. In J. Roitman (Ed.), *ACSM's resource manual for exercise testing and prescription* (pp. 656–667). Baltimore, MD: Williams & Wilkins.

assessed. If the patient is in the planning or action phase of quitting, information regarding the effects of nicotine on the body is given, as well as assistance in planning how to beat the urge to smoke and resources for support groups. All information is written so that the patient may refer to it later.

Patients with PCI, MI, CABG, or valve replacement or repair are all referred to outpatient cardiac rehabilitation to continue skilled monitoring of exercise and risk factor education and modification. Patients who have CHF are not covered by Medicare for outpatient cardiac rehabilitation.

Discharge Planning

Discharge planning begins early because of shortened hospital stays. The cardiac occupational therapist provides information regarding the level of physical function the patient tolerates at discharge. The therapist also makes recommendations for further therapies and gives input regarding the possible need for home health or extended care facility.

Outpatient Cardiac Rehabilitation or Phase II

Outpatient cardiac rehabilitation is a multifaceted program of EKG-monitored exercise and education for secondary prevention of heart disease. Outpatient cardiac rehabilitation is designed to

1. Continue medical surveillance and assessment of an individual's cardiovascular response to exercise
2. Limit the physiological and psychological effects of heart disease
3. Instruct on risk factors for heart disease and how to reduce their impact
4. Maximize psychosocial and vocational status.

Patients are usually started in outpatient cardiac rehabilitation 1–2 weeks after discharge from the hospital. The program runs 3 days a week for 8–12 weeks. Often, the therapist must take a careful history to determine risk stratification based on the patient's EF, hospital course, heart rate and blood pressure response, symptoms, and/or possible EKG changes with exercise. Risk stratification refers to determination of the patient's risk for further cardiac events based on the past medical history.

After assessing the patient's risk stratification, the therapist will need to determine the appropriate exercise intensity using one of the following means. The therapist could determine 50%–85% of the patient's maximum age-adjusted heart rate (MAHR) (see Procedures for Practice 42-2 regarding how to calculate MAHR). If, however, the patient is on a beta blocker medication, such as Toprol or Metoprolol, his or her heart rate response will be blunted, making the heart rate calculation inaccurate. Using the Borg RPE Scale is an additional way to measure the patient's tolerance of

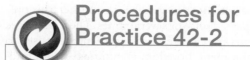

Procedures for Practice 42-2

Determining the Maximum Age-Adjusted Heart Rate

1. Take the number 220.
2. Subtract the patient's age.
3. The difference is that patient's maximum age-adjusted heart rate (MAHR).
4. To establish his or her exercise heart range, multiply the MAHR by 50%–85% to obtain the heart rate for exercise.

For example, a 50-year-old patient's MAHR would be 170 (220 − 50). To determine the exercise heart rate, multiply 170 by 0.50 and 0.85. The 50-year-old patient's exercise heart rate range is 85–149 bpm.

exercise. The patient is usually asked to rate the intensity of the exercise on the Borg RPE Scale. Initially, the patient should try to keep the score between 11 and 13; later in the rehabilitation program, a score between 12 and 15 may be appropriate (ACSM, 2010a). The patient's cardiovascular response and/or symptoms all assist in formulating the exercise prescription.

The exercise goal varies per individual depending on the function of his or her heart and physical condition. Usually, those with good heart function and physical condition achieve between 5 and 6 METs. The patient's previous vocational and leisure interests, however, must also be considered in determining the patient's exercise goal.

The elderly, those who are sedentary, or those who have low functional capacity can still benefit by increasing their maximum MET level. For example, a patient with MI and CHF may have a functional capacity of 2.5 METs after a hospitalization. If they can increase their MET level to 3.5–4 METs, they have significantly increased the number of activities or tasks they can do.

The two primary methods of achieving exercise goals are continuous and discontinuous exercise. For some, continuous exercise works well. For others, short bouts of exercise on various pieces of equipment followed by a short rest of 1–2 minutes are preferable.

The first goal is to increase the total duration of continuous exercise to at least 20–40 minutes. Later, intensity is gradually increased. The advantages of continuous exercise are that less equipment and space are needed and the exercise more closely mimics what the patient will be doing at home. The disadvantages are that only certain muscle groups are targeted on one piece of equipment and the patient is exposed to just one form of aerobic exercise.

In discontinuous exercise, the patient stays on one piece of equipment for one-half or one-third of the allotted exercise time. After finishing the time on one piece of equipment, the patient then switches to another; this process may be repeated once or several times. The advantages of discontinuous exercise are that the patient is exposed to a variety of equipment, boredom is minimized, and multiple muscle groups are used. The disadvantages are that discontinuous exercise takes a lot of space and equipment, it is sometimes hard to coordinate patients shifting equipment at the same time, and it does not reflect what the patient will be doing for aerobic exercise at home. With both methods of conditioning, however, the patients can achieve the same MET levels over time.

In outpatient cardiac rehabilitation, a variety of exercise equipment may be used. Treadmills, bicycle ergometers, recumbent bikes, rowing machines, arm ergometers, and so on are used, depending on the patient's preference and to accommodate any existing orthopedic problem the patient may have. Weight training is usually started 1–2 weeks postevent if weights below 10 pounds are used. For instance, a patient post bypass might start with 1–3-pounds weights, whereas a patient post–non-STEMI might start at 5-pound weights and gradually progress upward. If the program starts with heavier weights such as 50% of one repetition maximum, the ACSM recommends waiting at least 5 weeks post-MI or bypass. Patients post percutaneous transluminal coronary revascularization (PTCR) may start 2–3 weeks postprocedure (ACSM, 2010). Prior to weight training, patients must meet certain criteria regarding their exercise capacity, blood pressure (BP) control, and heart rhythm (ACSM, 2010).

Risk factor modification is a key focus of outpatient cardiac rehabilitation. Therapists help patients identify their own risk factors and choose which risk factors they would like to try to modify or eliminate. Risk factor education occurs in a variety of ways. Some centers have specific times on various days where health professionals will lecture on a particular topic. Other hospitals have short education sessions before, during, or after exercise sessions. The goal of these educational sessions is to give patients the information they need to modify their risk factors.

Psychosocial issues must be evaluated with the patient who has heart disease. Depression post-MI is linked to negative outcomes (Madan & Sivarajan Froelicher, 2010). Many centers use standardized questionnaires to determine depression or anxiety such as the Beck Depression Inventory or the Center for Epidemiological Studies Depression Scale (ACSM, 2010b). The results of testing will indicate whether the patient needs referral to a chaplain, social worker, or psychologist based on their circumstance or preference.

Community-Based Phase III Cardiac Rehabilitation

Phase III is a community-based cardiac rehabilitation with larger groups of patients and fewer staff members per participant. Phase III programs are often located in community centers, school gyms, or YMCAs. Such programs may follow outpatient or phase II cardiac rehabilitation. Patients may skip phase II, however, and go directly to phase III if they are low risk and have been active in the past. Only a small percentage of patients go to phase III after phase II because it is generally not covered by insurance. Because reimbursement is difficult, it also means that these programs run on a very low budget and usually are lucky to break even.

A physician must refer a participant to a phase III program. Sometimes a stress test is required, or the physician establishes heart rate guidelines. Trained personnel monitor BP response and assist patients with monitoring their heart rate. EKG monitoring is typically limited to once per month. Goal setting for risk management continues, as does the education component, although the education may be more informal. Participants also enjoy the support and encouragement of others who have a common goal of reducing their incidence of heart disease.

CHRONIC OBSTRUCTIVE PULMONARY DISEASE

COPD is a combination of emphysema and bronchitis (American Lung Association, 2010). Emphysema is the progressive and irreversible destruction of the alveoli walls (American Lung Association, 2008). The walls of the alveoli have elastic fibers, and when these are destroyed, the lung loses some of its elasticity, resulting in air trapping. This air trapping reduces the ability of the lung to shrink during exhalation; the lung then inhales less air with the next breath (American Lung Association, 2010). Chronic bronchitis is defined as excessive sputum production and cough of at least 3 months in duration occurring 2 years in a row. This inflammation also causes the bronchial tubes to increase their production of mucus. The result of these processes is that the patient experiences sudden SOB and may wheeze or cough (Davis, 2012). Patients with COPD have characteristics of all these diseases (see Definition 42-3 for a description of pulmonary function tests). COPD is a chronic and progressive condition (American Lung Association, 2010). Medications and good health habits can lessen the symptoms and maximize function.

The feeling of breathlessness, called dyspnea, is a key feature of COPD. Damage to the lung results in a flattening of the diaphragm caused by hyperinflation. This flattening takes away the ability of the diaphragm to act effectively in assisting with expansion of the lungs during inspiration (Hill & Schmitt, 2010). To compensate for the lack of inspiratory pressure, patients with COPD tend to use their shoulder girdle muscles to expand their lungs, making it difficult to use those muscles in unsupported UE activities (Celli, 2009a).

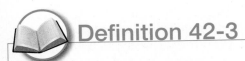

Definition 42-3

Pulmonary Function Tests

- Patients are asked to exhale forcefully as much air as possible into a spirometer. The amount of air exhaled in 1 second is called the forced expiratory volume (FEV1). Age-related norms for the FEV1 are available (Celli, 2009b).
- Arterial blood gases are drawn to determine the lungs' ability to oxygenate blood, remove CO_2, and maintain the body's acid–base status (Tiep & Carter, 2009). It is helpful to draw blood gases before and after exercise to see how well oxygenation is maintained during activity.
- A pulse oximeter is a noninvasive test to determine the amount of oxygen in the blood. A probe is wrapped around a fingertip. A light shines through the finger, and the amount of light reaching the other side indicates the amount of oxygen in the blood. Hemoglobin is red, and the more hemoglobin in the blood, the less light is able to penetrate the fingertip (Tiep & Carter, 2009). The oximeter can occasionally give false readings. If the patient is anemic, wears nail polish, or has poor circulation, the pulse oximetry may be inaccurate. Often, the oximetry machine will also determine the patient's pulse. If the palpated pulse and the oximetry machine pulse match, it is likely that the oxygen saturation (O_2 Sat) will be accurate.

Dyspnea, fatigue, cough, and sputum production are part of the disease process. The effort of breathing takes so much energy that often COPD patients find themselves without enough energy to do their daily tasks, including ADL and vocational and leisure endeavors. They are unable to increase their ventilation enough to meet physiological demands. Because of the unpleasant sensation of SOB, patients reduce their physical activities, resulting in muscle weakness and the inability to use oxygen efficiently (Celli, 2009a).

Eating is an activity that is made difficult by lack of air. Maintaining adequate nutrition is a problem for many patients with COPD, and nutrition problems are independent predictors of mortality (American Association of Cardiovascular and Pulmonary Rehabilitation [AACVPR], 2011). Some patients lose weight because of the excessive energy costs of their breathing efforts. Others use steroids to reduce lung inflammation, resulting in weight gain, that contributes to additional problems (AACVPR). Weight gain exacerbates the problem of not having enough oxygen to metabolize food, and extra weight requires more oxygen to do any activity, including eating.

In a large study of over 7,400 people, individuals with COPD had a rate of depression slightly higher at 23.1% compared to those without COPD whose depression rate was 16.8% (Schneider et al., 2010). As with any chronic disease process, the changes in lifestyle, the struggle to accomplish normal daily activities, the fear of extreme SOB, and feelings of hopelessness all contribute to the depression that many patients with COPD feel.

PULMONARY REHABILITATION

The AACVPR sets standards of practice for pulmonary rehabilitation, which are used by insurers and the Joint Commission of Hospital Organizations. The AACVPR (2011) has published a book called *Guidelines for Pulmonary Rehabilitation Programs* to guide practice. It has also instituted a certification for pulmonary rehabilitation programs (see Resources 42-1). A team of health professionals, including doctors, respiratory therapists, dieticians, pharmacists, and occupational and physical therapists, is ideally involved in the pulmonary rehabilitation program. As with other diagnostic categories, the roles may overlap in reinforcing behaviors to enhance function.

Occupational therapy goals in pulmonary rehabilitation are patient centered and patient driven and may include

1. ADL evaluation and training to increase functional endurance
2. Instruction and training in appropriate breathing techniques with ADL
3. Evaluation and strengthening of the UE
4. Instruction in work simplification and energy conservation
5. Evaluation of the need for adaptive equipment
6. Assistance in adapting leisure activities
7. Education in stress management and relaxation techniques.

Evidence Table 42-2 lists the best evidence for occupational therapy practice regarding pulmonary rehabilitation.

Activities of Daily Living Evaluation and Training

Patients with COPD are often limited in their ability to perform their ADL because of dyspnea. It is common to have significant muscle wasting from disuse. The therapist should note the patient's breathing pattern during the ADL evaluation. Often, patients with COPD hold their breath, breathe shallowly and fast, or elevate their shoulders as they breathe. The amount of oxygen in the blood or oxygen saturation (O_2 Sat) with activity should also be measured by pulse oximetry (Procedures for Practice 42-3). If the O_2 Sat falls below 90% as the patient performs ADL, the use of oxygen with activity should be considered. If the patient does not have home oxygen, the physician should be informed of the patient's low O_2 Sat. Currently, the O_2 Sat must be below 88% to qualify for reimbursement for home oxygen from Medicare or other supplemental insurances (Crouch, 2009). As part of the

Evidence Table 42-2	Best Evidence for Occupational Therapy Practice Regarding Pulmonary Rehabilitation

Intervention	Description of Intervention Tested	Participants	Dosage	Type of Best Evidence and Level of Evidence	Benefit	Statistical Probability and Effect Size of Outcome	Reference
Eight studies evaluated a cognitive-behavioral– or psychotherapeutically based intervention, and one evaluated a taped progressive muscle relaxation.	Studies that had detailed psychologically based interventions for treatment of anxiety associated with chronic obstructive pulmonary disease (COPD)	Five hundred twenty-three patients with confirmed COPD. Four studies had patients with moderate-to-severe COPD, one had mild-to-moderate COPD, and others did not classify severity.	Varied from study to study in number of sessions and duration of each session	Systematic review and meta-analysis of nine studies Level: I	Yes. Meta-analysis found a small but significant reduction for anxiety, but only when compared within the intervention group, but not compared to control.	Significant decrease in pre- and postanxiety scores from eight studies ($n = 222$, CI = -0.419 to -0.141, $p = 00004$).	Baraniak & Sheffield (2011)
Compare effectiveness of short-term pulmonary rehabilitation with brief advice	Rehabilitation group: Patients came to hospital. Sessions included exercise and education. Brief advice group: Individuals were given instruction and advice on exercise along with a printed handout. They were asked to keep a record of their exercise.	One hundred three patients with severe COPD were randomly assigned to group program or advice program. Fifty-four were in the group program, and 48 were in the advice program.	Those in rehabilitation group were seen twice per week for 6 weeks. Advice patients received 1 hour of individual advice and education.	Randomized controlled trial Level: 1A2a Trial did not have blinded therapists or participants; difference in amount of intervention time.	Yes, the rehabilitation group increased the shuttle walking distance compared to the advice group.	Statistically significant differences between group rehabilitation program and brief advice groups at 3 months in terms of shuttle walking distance (34.1 m; 3.0–65.3 confidence interval; $p < .05$).	White et al. (2002)

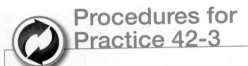

Procedures for Practice 42-3

Breathing Techniques

Patients are instructed to practice these techniques while sitting in a relaxed position. After they become proficient using these breathing methods at rest, patients should try using them while doing pleasant activities such as reading or watching television. Finally, patients should try using one of these techniques while doing a task that is difficult, such as stair climbing (Coppola & Wood, 2009).

Pursed Lip Breathing

- Breathe in through your nose.
- With lips pursed, exhale air slowly.
- Try to take twice as much time to exhale as it did to inhale.

Active expiration is the contraction of the abdominal muscles during exhalation.

According to the AACVPR *Guidelines for Pulmonary Rehabilitation* (2011), abdominal or diaphramatic breathing is no longer used because of lack of evidence of efficacy. Instead active expiration is recommended.

---

functional assessment, measurements of heart rate and blood pressure should also be taken.

Breathing Techniques

It is important that the patient practice use of breathing techniques with ADL. After becoming familiar with pursed lip breathing and active expiration, the patient should attempt to use these breathing techniques while performing tasks that previously caused them to be breathless. The pulse oximeter helps to reinforce the improvement in the O$_2$ Sat with use of a breathing technique. Timing the breath with work is also helpful. For example, the patient should breathe out while pushing the vacuum cleaner, and breathe in while pulling the vacuum cleaner. Exhaling with the exertion of lifting is less taxing not only on the lungs but also on the cardiovascular system because it prevents the Valsalva maneuver (see Procedures for Practice 42-3 for breathing techniques).

Upper Extremity Function

UE muscle strength must be evaluated. Pulmonary patients are often on steroids, have systemic inflammation, are older and hypoxic, and therefore often have muscle weakness (American Association of Cardiac and Pulmonary Rehabilitation, 2011). Patients with COPD

commonly use the accessory muscles of the shoulder girdle to help them breathe, which makes it difficult for them to use these muscles in unsupported upper extremity activity (Celli, 2009a). UE strengthening has been found to improve the quality of life by increasing the capacity to work and reducing the oxygen requirement of UE activity. Use of free weights, Theraband®, an arm ergometer, and other upper body strengthening techniques are all helpful in increasing upper body strength. Additional improvement in functional status is seen when leg training is added (Celli).

Work Simplification and Energy Conservation

Because their work capacity is significantly reduced, patients with COPD will benefit from instruction in work simplification and energy conservation. Bathing is a particularly strenuous activity because the hot humid air makes breathing difficult. Therapists encourage patients to use the ventilation fan or leave the door open while bathing to keep the humidity level down. Recommending the use of a chair in the shower and using a thick terry robe after showering instead of toweling off are two suggestions that are helpful in reducing energy expenditure. Unsupported UE activity is very fatiguing for patients with COPD. It is important to teach these patients to support their arms during UE activities such as hair combing or shaving. Sometimes, a machine like an electric toothbrush can be of assistance. Scheduling of activities that require more energy expenditure for the time following the use of a bronchodilator will also allow patients to accomplish more (AACVPR, 2011).

Not all patients with COPD will need adaptive equipment. As the disease progresses in severity, however, some adaptive equipment is useful (Fig. 42-4). Because bending

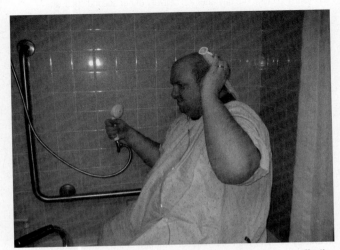

Figure 42-4 Using adaptive aids for self-care activities can be an effective way to conserve energy and maintain independence for those with cardiac or respiratory conditions.

over to tie shoes or put on pants may cause significant SOB, elastic shoe laces, a long-handled shoehorn, or a reacher to assist with putting on slacks may be helpful.

Promoting Self-Enhancement Roles

People with COPD tend to feel isolated. Just completing daily necessities takes so much energy that little, if any, is left for leisure activities. Many patients fear becoming very SOB in front of others or are embarrassed using oxygen. The occupational therapist can help the patient evaluate previously enjoyed activities and see whether those activities can be adapted to fit the current health status. Providing patients with information regarding programs or activities available in their community is also helpful. Sometimes, involving a helper or companion may make an activity more feasible.

Stress Management

The feeling of being unable to get enough air is truly frightening. Patients with COPD often experience a sense of panic with breathlessness. Teaching patients methods to cope with extreme SOB can lessen their fear. Leaning forward and resting their arms on the table releases the diaphragm and makes breathing easier. Using pursed lip and/or active expiration helps to slow the pace of breathing so that the patient is not breathing shallowly and rapidly. A stress management technique such as visualization may help patients calm themselves by mentally transporting them out of the stressful situation. It is important that the patient practice these options prior to actually needing them. Having a well-practiced plan of action for the panic associated with breathlessness will give patients confidence in their ability to control the situation.

Heart disease and pulmonary disease, as the first and third leading causes of death, respectively, pose a major health problem. As either a primary or a secondary diagnosis, both heart disease and COPD require specialized attention in planning occupational therapy intervention. If a patient has a history of heart disease or COPD, the occupational therapy practitioner must assess the patient's cardiovascular response to activity or exercise. Precautions for the patient's cardiac or pulmonary problem must be incorporated into the treatment program.

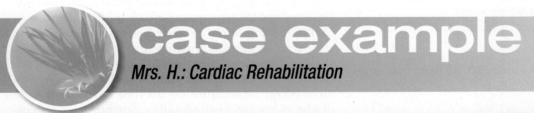

case example
Mrs. H.: Cardiac Rehabilitation

		Clinical Reasoning Process
Occupational Therapy Process	**Objectives**	**Examples of Therapist's Internal Dialogue**
Patient Information	Understand the patient's diagnosis or condition	"Cardiomyopathy after pregnancy is rare. If she improves within the 6 months after diagnosis, she will probably be able to lead a normal life."
Mrs. H. is a married, 32-year-old full-time health worker and mother of a 3-year-old child. The day after the delivery of her second child, she suddenly developed a migraine headache. Her condition deteriorated quickly. She became very SOB and needed a rebreather mask with 10 L of oxygen to maintain her O_2 saturation. Her heart rate was 135–140 bpm. The next day, she was diagnosed as having an anterior wall myocardial infarction (MI). Several days later, her pulmonary edema had resolved, and she had a coronary angiogram. The angiogram showed normal coronary arteries and an ejection fraction (EF) of 25%–30%. She was subsequently diagnosed with a cardiomyopathy.	Know the person	"Mrs. H. will be a busy lady, working and taking care of two children younger than 3 years old. She works in the health care system and has some knowledge of health issues. Mrs. H. is used to a full-time income and taking care of herself, her home, and family. It must be stressful to have to rely on others to take care of something she normally did herself."
Initially, she was referred to inpatient cardiac rehab for general conditioning and instructions for appropriate activities at home. She had very limited endurance. She had a 10-pound lifting restriction, which, with a newborn, made her dependent on family and friends.		
She was seen by home health occupational therapy for several weeks. She was given exercises to increase her endurance and instructed in energy conservation techniques. Although she became somewhat stronger, she was still dependent on volunteers around the clock to do the majority of household tasks and take care of the children. This caused her a great deal of stress. Her therapist instructed her in stress management techniques and practiced them with Mrs. H.		

Reason for Referral to Cardiac Occupational Therapy Phase II

Mrs. H. was referred to outpatient cardiac rehabilitation for physical conditioning and education.

| Appreciate the context | "I will talk with the husband to get his view of how things are going at home and get a feel for how supportive he is to Mrs. H. I will also need to consider whether Mrs. H. is getting secondary gain from all the attention." |

Assessment Process and Results

Mrs. H. arrived in outpatient cardiac rehabilitation via wheelchair because she felt she was too weak to walk from the car and exercise. She was now doing her own self-care but still relied on volunteers for most of her household chores and caring for her children. She admitted she was stressed by her diagnosis, the number of volunteers in her home, and financial worries. She reported that she slept excessively and was exhausted with exercise. She also reported that she had a history of depression and complained of being somewhat depressed. She was able to walk slowly on the treadmill at 2.0 mph for 20 minutes with normal cardiovascular response. A recent echocardiogram revealed her EF to now be up to 50%.

| Consider evaluation approach and methods | "Initially, Mrs. H. is allowed to demonstrate what she can comfortably do physically. After 20 minutes of walking, she still is tolerating the exercise well." |

| Interpret observations | "Mrs. H. does not seem to correlate her ability to easily walk 20 minutes at a strolling pace as indicative of her ability to do many household chores, such as dishwashing, folding clothes, making beds, etc. I will continue to assess Mrs. H. to see if she may need referral for psychiatric help for possible depression." |

Occupational Therapy Problem List

- Low physical capacity for work less than 3 METs.
- Inability to engage in previous work and leisure pursuits because of decreased endurance.
- Possible depression over feelings of dependency and concern over cardiac diagnosis.
- Dependence on volunteers for most instrumental activities of daily living (IADL).

| Synthesize results | "Mrs. H. seems to be overwhelmed with her diagnosis and has not assimilated that her heart function has now improved to near normal. With an exercise program to increase her physical capacity, she should be able to return to her job and all her IADLs. Stress management technique training will assist her to cope with difficulties caused by illness." |

Occupational Therapy Goal List

- Learn to monitor physical response to exercise and activity through use of Borg RPE Scale and pulse monitoring.
- Gradually increase capacity for work through aerobic exercise and strengthening exercises (2–5 METs).
- Gradually resume household and leisure pursuits (1.5–5 METs).
- Learn to pace household activities.
- Learn stress management techniques to cope with difficulties caused by illness.
- Instruct patient in risk factors for heart disease.
- Identify patient's personal risk factors and ways to ameliorate their effects.
- Start a regular home aerobic exercise program.

| Select an intervention approach | "As Mrs. H. increases her endurance, we can gradually shift her back to some of her household responsibilities of the same energy or MET level. In the meantime, learning stress techniques will help her handle her current situation. Education about her current health problem will help her understand that she is truly getting better."

"Cardiac rehabilitation will concentrate on an aerobic exercise and strengthening program. Brief educational sessions will be conducted as she exercises or after the exercise session." |

| Consider what will occur in therapy, how often, and for how long | "Mrs. H. is highly motivated to improve, but conditioning takes time. I will see her three times a week for 6 weeks. During that time, I will help her understand the connection between workload on treadmill or exercise cycle and home activities. Together we can develop a plan on how she will start resuming household tasks. I will also instruct her in a home exercise program to assist in improving her conditioning. After exercising, we will practice some stress management techniques." |

Intervention

As she regained physical strength through exercise, Mrs. H. could start resuming more of her usual activities and reduce her dependence on volunteers. Instructing Mrs. H. in how to assess her own physical response to exercise and activity gave her confidence that she was in control. Because Mrs. H. had difficulty with pacing, the therapist had her keep a diary of her daily routine. Later, they reviewed it, and the occupational therapist reviewed work simplification techniques and methods of pacing. The therapist also assigned her tasks within her current aerobic capacity to assist her in resuming her home responsibilities. Mrs. H. was also instructed in stress management techniques to help her deal with the stresses of her illness. Because of her previous history of depression, the therapist reviewed information about the relationship of depression and fatigue. The occupational therapist explored with Mrs. H. the possibility of seeking professional help and/or medication to deal with her depression. Additionally, Mrs. H. was instructed in the risk factors for heart disease. Her individual risk factors were identified, and information was provided on how to ameliorate their effects. As part of her risk factor reduction, Mrs. H. initiated a walking program.

Assess the patient's comprehension

Know the person

Appreciate the context

"Mrs. H. was a quick learner. As she fully understood that her heart function was near normal, she really started to gain confidence that her life could return to normal. However, she needed some concrete direction to translate what she was learning into action. Adding the additional home exercise program helped to increase her capacity more quickly, but depression was holding her back from making a complete recovery. Even with her health care background, she did not realize the effect of depression on her physically. With more information about depression, she was more willing to seek professional help."

Next Steps

Discharge from outpatient cardiac rehabilitation.

Decide whether the patient should continue or discontinue therapy and/ or return in the future

"Mrs. H. was making significant strides in returning to her previous activity level. She seemed to benefit significantly from activity modification, education, and information on heart disease. She had initiated a home walking program, and she planned to return to work within a month."

 Clinical Reasoning in Occupational Therapy Practice

Implications of a Diagnosis

When treating Mrs. H., what signs or symptoms would cause you to discontinue treatment and/or call the doctor?

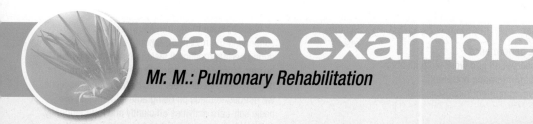

case example
Mr. M.: Pulmonary Rehabilitation

Occupational Therapy Process	Clinical Reasoning Process	
	Objectives	Examples of Therapist's Internal Dialogue

Patient Information

Mr. M. is an 85-year-old male with a medical history of congestive heart failure (CHF), chronic obstructive pulmonary disease (COPD), and diabetes. He also has a history of coronary artery disease and has had a myocardial infarction in the past. He has been on home oxygen but reports he was not always using it despite it being prescribed. He lives alone in an apartment building with an elevator. Prior to this hospitalization, he had recently begun receiving home visits from a nurse and was getting food from Meals on Wheels™. Up until this point, he has been independent with dressing, toileting, bathing, laundry, and finances. He is ambulating without an assistive device but owns a front-wheeled walker and a wheelchair. He also stated that he owns a shower chair and has a handheld shower head but has not needed to use the shower chair for bathing. He does not drive and is provided with transportation by various family members. He is currently on 6 L of oxygen and is receiving steroids and inhalers to improve breathing. He states that he has had "a little" education for COPD/CHF management in the past.

His goal was to return to his apartment after discharge from the hospital, to which he was admitted for increased shortness of breath (SOB). He was open to receiving more assistance from family or outside agencies if necessary.

Objectives: Understand the patient's diagnosis or condition

Know the person

Internal Dialogue: "Mr. M. has been on 6 L of oxygen chronically at home and has other medical conditions that indicate to me that he likely has poor endurance and may have had some difficulty managing activities of daily living (ADL) at home."

"The lack of Mr. M.'s use of energy conservation techniques and his prescription for oxygen during daily activities suggests that he would benefit from education in these areas. His daughter reports some forgetfulness in the patient, and therefore, I need to keep in mind that he may need to have education repeated and in written form, as well as hands-on practice and demonstration, for the most success in learning new information."

Reason for Referral to Occupational Therapy

Mr. M. was admitted to the hospital because of increased shortness of breath. He was referred to occupational therapy for an evaluation and further treatment to improve efficiency with functional activities. Because Mr. M. lives alone, it is especially important that he be as independent as possible to allow him to reach his goal of returning to his apartment.

Objectives: Appreciate the context

Develop provisional hypotheses

Internal Dialogue: "I believe that Mr. M. will benefit from the combination of education and adaptive equipment use, as well as exercise to improve his activity tolerance at home. I am hoping that as Mr. M. gets more competent and confident with using breathing techniques, he will be more inspired to combine them with adaptive equipment use to improve his efficiency. I am glad that he has a supportive family that is working to keep Mr. M. as independent as possible."

Assessment Process and Results

Mr. M.'s assessment took place in his hospital room. He was on 6 L of oxygen via nasal cannula. He appeared to be comfortable at rest, but following activity, his oxygen saturations decreased to 85%. He was able to complete pursed lip breathing with cues, and his saturations increased to 93% after 90 seconds of rest and pursed lip breathing. His upper body strength and range of motion were within functional limits. He was able to demonstrate ability to physically complete grooming, dressing, and toileting independently but was limited by decreased endurance and rapid shortness of breath. He frequently had to stop what he was doing to rest and, for that reason, took extra time or chose not to complete some tasks. He was able to complete basic transfers and ambulate in his room with standby assistance and no assistive device. A basic cognitive screen indicated that Mr. M.'s cognition was intact. His daughter did report that he has been more forgetful lately.

Objectives: Consider evaluation approach and methods

Internal Dialogue: "My focus was primarily on Mr. M.'s functional status and assessing his level of fatigue during functional tasks. I did spend some time observing him completing activities of daily living (ADL) as well as interviewing him about his perceived level of fatigue and level of difficulty completing tasks. I monitored his oxygen saturations throughout our treatment sessions and observed his levels of dyspnea."

"We discussed what ADL were a priority for him versus less important tasks, and we were able to narrow our focus and set specific goals."

Occupational Therapy Problem List

- Limited endurance affecting ADL performance
- Limited education of energy conservation and work simplification techniques and pursed lip and diaphragmatic breathing
- Decreased awareness of adaptive equipment resources and oxygen use
- Mild memory impairment

Occupational Therapy Goal List

(anticipated length of treatment: four or five sessions)
- Patient will be able to verbalize and demonstrate understanding of pursed lip breathing and active exhalation during functional activities by discharge.
- Patient will verbalize or demonstrate understanding of two or three work simplification and energy conservation techniques during self-care activities, community activities, and laundry and other homemaking tasks by discharge.
- Patient will complete tub transfer independently using adaptive equipment to increase activity tolerance by discharge.
- Patient will have all recommended adaptive equipment or resources for pursuing purchase of equipment by discharge.
- Patient will be independent with a 10–15-minute upper extremity exercise program while using pursed lip breathing to improve overall endurance and ability to tolerate ADL.

Intervention

Mr. M.'s treatment plan consisted of education for specific breathing techniques (pursed lip and active exhalation). He was instructed on how to incorporate these breathing techniques into his daily routine. He was then provided with more education in energy conservation and work simplification to allow him to be more efficient. Discussion about adaptive equipment needs took place, and recommendations were made. He was instructed in an upper extremity exercise program to increase endurance, and he was provided with a handout to encourage him to continue with the exercises after he was discharged. Mr. M. was provided with written instruction for all education because of memory impairments. Repetition and hands-on training were also provided whenever possible.

Providing education was key to allow Mr. M. to understand how to manage his COPD symptoms better. He was better able to manage his shortness of breath and fatigue during activities by using pursed lip breathing combined with work simplification and energy conservation techniques. Discussion about the benefits of adaptive equipment use and incorporation into Mr. M.'s daily routine has allowed him to complete more tasks independently and with less fatigue. He was in agreement with using a shower chair, handheld showerhead, and long-handled bath sponge to ease the burden that bathing once had been. Mr. M. elected to purchase a long-handled bath sponge from the hospital before discharge, and he already had a shower chair and handheld showerhead at his apartment. He was encouraged to use his oxygen for all activities, including showering, to maintain a desirable oxygen saturation level for his safety. By participating in a daily exercise program, Mr. M.'s endurance improved, which allowed him to complete his ADL with much less shortness of breath and fewer rest breaks. Mr. M. was seen for six sessions by occupational therapy. He met all of his established goals and was discharged back to his apartment

Synthesize results	"It was apparent to me that Mr. M. was not conserving the maximum amount of his energy during certain functional tasks. Occasionally when he was fatigued, he would not complete grooming or hygiene tasks at all. I feel that, because he lives alone, we needed to focus on being able to complete his basic self-care activities efficiently and independently. At this point, he was not able to complete all self-care activities because of fatigue and shortness of breath."
Develop intervention hypotheses	"I plan on providing Mr. M. with instruction on breathing techniques, energy conservation, adaptive equipment recommendations, and resources. This education will provide him with improved activity tolerance and give him a greater sense of independence. I believe that it is important to provide him with the opportunity to prioritize the importance of completing certain tasks and allowing him to participate in the goal-setting process."
Select an intervention approach	"My intervention will primarily focus on an adaptive approach with a focus on patient education."
Consider what will occur in therapy, how often, and for how long	"Mr. M. will likely only be hospitalized for 5–6 days, and therefore, we will need to strive to meet our goals in that time frame. I will focus mostly on completing functional tasks while providing education throughout the sessions. Written materials will also be provided, as well as family education when possible."
Assess the patient's comprehension	"I could see the initial frustration that Mr. M. had when he was not fully able to complete tasks because of dyspnea. He was hesitant to try pursed lip breathing initially because he thought it was 'too confusing' and that he would 'forget how to do it.' However, with repetition and encouragement, he was able to quickly learn the technique and feel the benefits. Once we started to incorporate the use of adaptive equipment (such as a shower chair, handheld showerhead, and long-handled bath sponge), Mr. M. was appearing more positive and confident in his abilities. He really was a rewarding patient to work with because he dramatically improved with simple modifications to his routine."
Understand what he is doing	

Next Steps

Discharge to his apartment with recommendation of home occupational therapy evaluation and to resume Meals-on-Wheels™ as was established previously.

| Anticipate present and future patient concerns | "I am recommending a home occupational therapy evaluation to reinforce the use of adaptive equipment and oxygen in Mr. M.'s home setting. I feel that Mr. M. was able to fully appreciate the benefits of using pursed lip breathing and oxygen to extend his endurance. He was comfortable with |
| Decide whether the patient should continue or discontinue therapy and/ or return in the future | the idea of using adaptive equipment and work simplification techniques incorporated into his everyday routine. He is confident in his abilities to complete his daily activities and to return to his apartment independently. His family is comfortable with his abilities to care for himself, and they feel he has the resources he needs to be successful." |

Clinical Reasoning in Occupational Therapy Practice

Implications of a Diagnosis

How could you show Mr. M. that using pursed lip breathing is effective in keeping the oxygen level in his blood at the proper levels? What would be an appropriate percentage of O_2 in the blood for someone with moderate-to-severe COPD?

Summary Review Questions

1. A person is admitted to the hospital with an acute STEMI. He is given thrombolytics to reverse clot formation in his coronary arteries, but the thrombolytics cause a cerebral bleed. In evaluating and treating for stroke-related deficits, what physiological parameters should the therapist take to measure the workload on the patient's heart? What factors might increase these parameters?

2. What cardiac symptoms might a patient who has a previous heart history exhibit if he or she were not tolerating the treatment you prescribed for the patient's current shoulder injury?

3. What symptoms would a person going into CHF exacerbation exhibit?

4. In reviewing a patient's medical record after hip replacement surgery, what cardiac diagnoses might influence your treatment? What cardiac diagnostic tests might provide information to help you make decisions about the severity of his or her heart disease?

5. Describe in detail the differences between a home program for a patient with a STEMI, a CABG, and an angioplasty. How would you customize the program for the individual?

6. Describe the different ways of conditioning an outpatient in cardiac rehabilitation. What are the advantages and disadvantages of each method?

7. List the risk factors for heart disease. What methods might an occupational therapist use to decrease a patient's risk for CAD?

8. Describe pursed lip breathing and active exhalation. How would you teach it to a patient with COPD?

9. If you were the only occupational therapist in a small rural hospital, where could you find information pertaining to the treatment of the patient with cardiac or pulmonary disease?

10. Develop a treatment plan for a patient with COPD, who is having problems with SOB while doing her ADLs.

Glossary

Acute coronary syndrome (ACS)—A term that includes unstable angina and myocardial infarction (MI), both non-ST elevation MI (non-STEMIs) and ST elevation MIs (STEMIs). This designation is used to triage and manage patients with symptoms of myocardial ischemia (Kim, Kine, & Fuster, 2008).

Angina pectoris—A temporary lack of blood flow to the myocardium, which causes the sensation of chest pain, fullness, tightness, or pressure. The pain or discomfort from angina can be referred to the teeth, jaw, back, ear, or arm. Angina is relieved with nitroglycerin or rest.

Atherogenic—Causing the development of plaque in an artery.

Atrial fibrillation—A rapid firing of cells in the atria of the heart with irregular response of the ventricles causing a fast irregular heart rhythm. With uncontrolled atrial fibrillation, the patient often feels short of breath and fatigued.

Cardioversion—Electrical shock delivered to the heart to stop a serious dysrhythmia, with the hope that the heart will restart in a normal sinus rhythm.

Diaphoresis—A cold clammy sweat that comes on suddenly.

Oxygen saturation (O$_2$ Sat)—Measurement of the amount of oxygen carried by the hemoglobin in the blood. A normal O$_2$ Sat is greater than 95%.

Sternotomy—A procedure used in open heart surgery where the sternum is split in half to allow the surgeon access to the chest cavity. After surgery, the sternum is wired together.

References

Acar, C., & Theodore, P. (2010). Surgery for valvular heart disease. In M. Crawford, J. DiMarco, W. Paulus (Eds.), *Cardiology* (pp. 1345–1355). Philadelphia: Mosby Elsevier.

Ainsworth, B. W., Haskell, W. L., Herrmann, S. D., Meches, N., Bassett, D. R., Jr., Tudor-Locke, C., Greer, J. L., Vezina, J., Whitt-Glover, M. C., & Leon, A. S. (2011). Compendium of physical activities: A second update of codes and met levels. *Medicine & Science in Sports & Exercise, 43,* 1575–1581.

Ainsworth, B. W., Haskel, W. L., Leon, A., Jacobs, D., Jr., Montoye, H., Sallis, J., & Paffenbarger, R. (1998). Compendium of physical activities: Classification of energy costs of human physical activities. In J. Roitman (Ed.), *ACSM's resource manual for exercise testing and prescription* (pp. 656–667). Baltimore, MD: Williams & Wilkins.

American Association of Cardiovascular and Pulmonary Rehabilitation. (2011). *Guidelines for pulmonary rehabilitation* (4th ed.). Champagne: Human Kinetics.

American College of Sports Medicine. (2010a). Exercise prescription for patients with cardiac disease. In W. R. Thompson, N. F. Gordon, & L. Pescatello (Eds.), *ACSM's guidelines for exercise testing and prescription* (8th ed., pp. 207–224). Philadelphia: Wolters Kluwer.

American College of Sports Medicine. (2010b). In J. K. Ehrman, A. Dejong, B. Sanderson, D. Swain, A. Swank, & C. Womack (Eds.), *ACSM's resource manual for guidelines for exercise testing and prescription.* Philadelphia: Wolters Kluwer.

American Heart Association. (2012). *Heart disease and stroke statistics—2012 update: A report from the American Heart Association. Circulation, 125,* (pp. e2–220). DOI: 10.1161/CIR.ObO13e31823aco46m.

American Lung Association. (2008). Lung disease data: Chronic obstructive lung disease. In *Epidemiology & statistics* (pp. 41–47). Retrieved January 11, 2012 from www.lungusa.org.

American Lung Association. (2010). Chronic obstructive lung disease. In *State of lung disease in diverse communities 2010* (pp. 35–36). Washington, DC: American Lung Association.

American Lung Association. (2012). Lung diseases: COPD. Retrieved January 11, 2012 from www.lungusa.org.

Antman, E. (2008). ST-elevation myocardial infarction management. In P. Libby, R. Bonow, D. Mann, D. Zipes, & E. Braunwald (Eds.), *Braunwald's heart disease* (pp. 1233–1299). Philadelphia: Sanders Elsevier.

Antman, E., & Braunwald, E. (2008). ST-elevation myocardial infarction: Pathology, pathophysiology & clinical features. In P. Libby, R. Bonow, D. Mann, D. Zipes, & E. Braunwald (Eds.), *Braunwald's heart disease* (pp. 1207–1232). Philadelphia: Sanders Elsevier.

Asbury, E. A., Grant, A., Evans, L., Barbir, M., & Collins, P. (2008). Cardiac rehabilitation for the treatment of women with chest pain and normal coronary arteries. *Menopause, 5,* 454–460.

Baim, D. (2010). Percutaneous coronary intervention. In J. Loscalzo (Ed.), *Harrison's cardiovascular medicine* (pp. 414–421). New York: McGraw Hill.

Baraniak, A., & Sheffield, D. (2011). The efficacy of psychologically based interventions to improve anxiety, depression and quality of life in COPD: A systematic review and meta-analysis. *Patient Education and Counseling, 83,* 29–36.

Barsness, G., & Murphy, J. (2007). Principles of interventional cardiology. In J. Murphy & M. Lloyd (Eds.), *Mayo clinic cardiology* (pp. 1369–1379). Rochester: Mayo Clinic Publishing.

Berman, A., & Snyder, S. (2012). *Fundamentals of nursing* (9th ed.). Boston: Pearson.

Blaha, M., Ketlogetswe, I., Ndumele, D., Gluckman, T., & Blumenthal, R. (2012). Preventative strategies for heart disease. In V. Fuster, R. Walsh, & R. Harrington (Eds.), *Hurst's the heart* (13th ed.). Retrieved March 31, 2012 from http://www.accessmedicine.com/content.aspx?aID=7817557.

Blue Verrier, J. M., & Hargrove Deelstra, M. (2010). Acute coronary syndromes. In S. L. Woods, E. S. Sivarajan Froelicher, S. Adams Motzer, & E. J. Bridges (Eds.), *Cardiac nursing* (pp. 511–536). Philadelphia: Lippincott Williams & Wilkins.

Burke, L. E., Tuite, P. K., & Warziski Turk, M. (2010). Obesity: An overview of assessment and treatment. In S. L. Woods, E. S. Sivarajan Froelicher, S. Adams Moser, & E. J. Bridges (Eds.), *Cardiac nursing* (pp. 861–875). Philadelphia: Lippincott Williams & Wilkins.

Cade, W. T. (2008). Diabetes related microvascular and macrovascular disease in the physical therapy setting. *Physical Therapy, 88,* 1322–1335.

Cannon, C., & Braunwald, B. (2008). Unstable angina & non-ST-elevation myocardial infarctions. In P. Libby, R. Bonow, D. Mann, D. Zipes, & E. Braunwald (Eds.), *Braunwald's heart disease* (pp. 1183, 1319–1351). Philadelphia: Sanders Elsevier.

Cannon, C. P., & Braunwald, E. (2012). Unstable angina & Non-ST elevation MI. In R. Bonow , D. Mann, D. Sipes & P. Libby (Eds.), *Braunwald's heart disease* (9th ed., pp. 1178–1209). Philadelphia: Sanders Elsevier.

Celli, B. R. (2009a). Exercise in the rehabilitation of patients with respiratory disease. In J. E. Hodgkins, B. R. Celli, & G. L. Connors (Eds.), *Pulmonary rehabilitation: Guidelines to success* (4th ed., pp. 129–141). St. Louis: Mosby Elsevier.

Celli, B. R. (2009b). Pathophysiology of chronic obstructive pulmonary disease. In J. E. Hodgkins, B. R. Celli, & G. L. Connors (Eds.), *Pulmonary rehabilitation: Guidelines to success* (4th ed., pp. 18–38). St. Louis: Mosby Elsevier.

Centers for Disease Control and Prevention. (2008). Activity guidelines for adults. Retrieved January 31, 2012 from www.cdc.gov/physicalactivity /everyone.

Clinical Knowledge Summaries. (2007). Myocardial secondary prevention evidence: Evidence for exercise comprehensive rehabilitation following myocardial infarction. Retrieved January 31, 2012 from http://cks.nice.org.uk/mi-secondary-prevention#!supportingevidence1:6.

Connolly, H. M., & Oh, H. J. (2012). Echocardiography, evaluation of systolic and diastolic dysfunction. In R. Bonow, D. C. Mann, D. Sipes, & P. Libby (Eds.), *Braunwald's heart disease* (pp. 200–269). Philadelphia: Saunders and Elsevier.

Coppola, S., & Wood, W. (2009). Occupational therapy to promote functions and health related quality of life. In J. Hodgkin, B. R. Celli, & G. L. Connors (Eds.), *Pulmonary rehabilitation: Guidelines to success* (p. 199). St. Louis: Mosby Elsevier.

Crouch, R. (2009). Physical and respiratory therapy for the medical and surgical patient. In J. Hodgkins, B. R. Celli, & G. L. Connors (Eds.), *Pulmonary rehabilitation: Guidelines to success* (p. 170). St. Louis: Mosby Elsevier.

Davis, D. P. (2012). *What are the symptoms of chronic bronchitis?* Retrieved February 9, 2012 from www.medicinenet.com.

Davis, L. (2008). Care of patients with acute coronary syndrome: Unstable angina and non-ST-segment elevation myocardial infarction. In D. Moser, & B. Reigel (Eds.), *Cardiac nursing* (pp. 789–810). St. Louis: Saunders Elsevier.

Dennison, C. R., Miller, N. H., & Cunningham, S. G. (2010). Hypertension. In S. L. Woods, E. S. Sivarajan Froelicher, S. Adams Moser, & E. J. Bridges (Eds.), *Cardiac nursing* (pp. 799–822). Philadelphia: Lippincott Williams & Wilkins.

Francis, G., Wilson Tang, W., & Walsh, R. (2012). Pathophysiology of heart failure: Conclusion. In W. Furster, R. Walsh, & R. Harrington (Eds.), *Hurst's the heart* (13th ed.). Retrieved March 31, 2012 from http://www.accessmedicine.com/content.aspx?aiD=7809772.

Google. (2012). Google images: EKG. Retrieved February 1, 2012 from www.google.com.

Hare, J. (2008). The dilated, restrictive and infiltrative cardiomyopathies. In P. Libby, R. Bonnow, D. Mann, D. Zipes, & E. Braunwald (Eds.), *Braunwald's heart disease* (pp. 1739–1762). Philadelphia: Sanders Elsevier.

Hill, N. S., & Schmitt, G. A. (2010). Acute ventilatory failure: Acute ventilatory failure due to airway obstruction. In R. J. Mason, V. C. Broaddus, T. R. Martin, T. E. King, Jr., D. E. Schraufnagel, J. E. Murray, & J. Nadel (Eds.), *Murray and Nadels textbook of respiratory medicine* (5th ed., pp. 2146–2154). Philadelphia: Saunders Elsevier.

Hollenberg, S., & Parrillo, J. (2010). Acute heart failure and shock. In M. Crawford, J. Dimarco, & W. Paulus (Eds.), *Cardiology* (pp. 951–967). Philadelphia: Mosby Elsevier.

Johns Hopkins Health Alert. (2010). The importance of family history in heart disease. Retrieved January 28, 2012 from www.johnshopkinshealthalerts.com.

Kim, M., Kinin, A., & Fuster, V. (2012). Definitions of acute coronary syndromes: Non-ST-segment elevation myocardial infarctions. In V. Fuster, R. Walsh, & R. Harrington (Eds.), *Hurst's the heart* (13th ed.). Retrieved March 31, 2013 from http://www.accessmedicine.com/content.aspx?aiD=7819488.

Lawler, P. R., Filion, K. B., & Eisenberg, M. J. (2011). Efficacy of exercise-based cardiac rehabilitation post myocardial infarction: A systematic review and meta-analysis of randomized controlled trials. *American Heart Journal, 162,* 571–584.

Levine, G. N., Steinke, E. E., Bakaeen, F. G., Bozkurt, B., Cheitlin, M. D., Conti, J. B., Foster, E., Jaarsma, T., Kloner, R. A., Lange, R. A., Lindau S. T., Maron, B. J., Moser, D. K., Ohman, E. M., Seftel, A. D., & Stewart, W. J. (2012). Sexual activity and cardiovascular disease: A scientific statement from the American Heart Association. *Circulation, 125,* 1058–172.

Madan, S. K., & Sivarajan Froelicher, E. S. (2010). Psychosocial risk factors: Assessment and management interventions. In S. L. Woods, E. S. Sivarajan Froelicher, S. Adams Motser, & E. J. Bridges (Eds.), *Cardiac nursing* (pp. 769–782). Philadelphia: Lippincott Williams & Wilkins.

Marelli, A. J. (2011). Congenital heart disease in adults. In L. Goldman & A. I. Schafer (Eds.), *Cecil Goldman's medicine* (24th ed., pp. 397–409). Philadelphia: Elsevier Saunders.

Mayo Clinic. (2010). Heart failure symptoms. Retrieved March 20, 2013 from http://www.mayoclinic.com/health/heart-failure/DS00061/DSECTION=symptoms.

Mayo Clinic. (2012). *High cholesterol.* Retrieved January 10, 2012 from www.mayoclinic.com/health/cholesterol-levels/CL00001.

Medline Plus. (2012). Hypertensive heart disease. Retrieved February 1, 2012 from http://www.nlm.nih.gov/medlineplus/ency/article/000163.htm.

Mestroni, L., Gilbert, E., Lowes, B., & Bristow, M. (2012). Dilated cardiomyopathies. In V. Fuster, R. Walsh, & R. Harrington (Eds.), *Hurst's the heart* (13th ed.). Retrieved March 31, 2012 from http://www.accessmedicine.com/content.aspx?aiD7811432.

Meyers, J. (2005). Exercise and activity. In S. Woods, E. Froelicher, S. Motser, & E. Bridges (Eds.), *Cardiac nursing* (pp. 842–860, 916–936). Philadelphia: Lippincott Williams & Wilkins.

Moons, P., Cannobbio, M., Nickolaus, M., & Verstappen, A. (2008). Care of adults with congenital heart disease. In D. Moser & B. Riegel (Eds.), *Cardiac nursing* (pp. 1085–1109). St. Louis: Saunders Elsevier.

Nishimura, R. A., Gibbons, R. D. J., Glockner, J. F., & Tajik, A. J. (2010). Noninvasive cardiac imaging: Echocardiography, nuclear cardiology, and MRI, CT imaging. In J. Loscalzo (Ed.), *Harrison's cardiovascular medicine* (pp. 99–111). New York: McGraw Hill Medical.

O'Connell-Edwards, C. F., York, E., & Blumenthal, J. A. (2008). Psychosocial risk factors and coronary disease. In J. L. Durstine, G. E. Moore, M. J. LaMonte, & B. A. Franklin (Eds.), *Pollock's textbook of cardiovascular disease and rehabilitation* (pp. 235–245). Champagne, IL: Human Kinetics.

Paganda, K. D., & Paganda, T. J. (2011). Cardiac catherization. In *Mosby's diagnostic & laboratory test reference* (pp. 225–231). St. Louis: Elsevier Mosby.

Popma, J. J., Baim, D. S., & Resnic, F. S. (2008). Percutaneous coronary and valvular intervention. In P. Libby, R. O. Bonow, D. L. Mann, & D. P. Zipes (Eds.), *Braunwald's heart disease* (pp. 1419–1449). Philadelphia: Saunders Elsevier.

Ridker, P., & Libby, P. (2008). Risk factors for atherothrombic disease. In P. Libby, R. Bonow, D. Mann, D. Zipes, & E. Braunwald (Eds.), *Braunwald's heart disease* (pp. 1003–1029). Philadelphia: Saunders Elsevier.

Sabek, J., III, Bansilal, S., & Lyle, B. (2012). Coronary bypass surgery: Current operative strategies & risks. In V. Fuster, R. Walsh, & R. Harrington (Eds.), *Hurst's the heart* (13th ed.). Retrieved March 31, 2012 from http://www.accessmedicine.com/content.aspx?aiD=7822960.

Schiller, J., Lucas, J., Ward, B., Peregay, J. (2010). Summary health statistics for U.S. adults: National Health Survey, 2010. In *Vital & Health Statistics* (Series 10, No. 52, p. 16). Retrieved January 23, 2012 from http://www.cdc.gov/nchs/data/series/sr_10/sr10_252.

Schneider, C., Jick, S., Bothner, U., & Meier, C. (2010). COPD and the risk of depression. *Chest, 137,* 341–347.

Scordo, K. A. (2008). Nurse's role in exercise testing and non invasive imaging. In D. Moser & B. Riegel (Eds.), *Cardiac nursing* (pp. 350–374) St. Louis: Saunders Elsevier.

Shaffer, R. (2008). Care of patients undergoing fibrolytic therapy and percutaneous intervention. In D. Moser & B. Reger (Eds.), *Cardiac nursing* (pp. 823–851). St. Louis: Saunders Elsevier.

Sohn, M., Hawk, M., Martin, K., & Sivarajan Froelicher, S. S. (2010). Smoking cessation and relapse prevention. In S. L. Woods, E. S. Sivarajan Froelicher, S. Adams Motser, & E. J. Bridges (Eds.), *Cardiac nursing* (6th ed., pp. 783–798). Philadelphia: Lippincott Williams & Wilkins.

Soine, L. A., & Crawley, P. J. (2010). Nuclear, magnetic resonance and computed tomography. In S. L. Woods, E. S. Sivarajan Froelicher, S. Adams Motzer, & E. J. Bridges (Eds.), *Cardiac nursing* (6th ed., pp. 291–299). Philadelphia: Lippincott Williams & Wilkins.

Stewart, S. (2008). Epidemiology of coronary artery disease. In D. Moser, B. Riegal (Eds.), *Cardiac nursing* (pp. 9–30). St. Louis: Saunders Elsevier.

Sweeney, M. (2010). Therapeutic approaches to the diabetic patient. In M. Crawford, J. Demarco, & W. Paulus (Eds.), *Cardiology* (pp. 59–77). Philadelphia: Mosby Elsevier.

Taylor, R., Brown, A., Ebrahim, S., Jolliffe, J., Moorani, H., Rees, K., Skidmore, B., Stone, J., Thompson, D., & Oldridge, N. (2004). Exercised-based rehabilitation for patients with coronary heart disease: Systematic review and meta-analysis of randomized controlled trials. *American Journal of Medicine, 116,* 682–692.

Tiep, B. L., & Carter, R. (2009). Therapeutic oxygen. In J. E. Hodgkins, B. R. Celli, & G. L. Connors (Eds.), *Pulmonary rehabilitation: Guidelines to success* (4th ed., pp. 115–128). St. Louis: Mosby Elsevier.

Vora, T. (2011). Cardiovascular diagnostic testing. Lecture at Matters of the Heart Women's Health Conference, February 18, 2011.

Warzeski, M., Choo, J., Novak, J., & Burke, L. (2008). Obesity. In D. Moser & B. Reigel (Eds.), *Cardiac nursing* (pp. 446–462). St. Louis: Saunders Elsevier.

White, R. J., Rudkin, S. T., Harrison, S. T., Day, K. L., & Harve, I. M. (2002). Pulmonary rehabilitation compared with brief advice given for severe chronic obstructive pulmonary disease. *Journal of Cardiopulmonary Rehabilitation, 22,* 338–344.

Willis, M. C. (1996). *Medical terminology: The language of health care.* Baltimore: Williams & Wilkins.

Wynne, J., & Braunwald, E. (2010). Cardiomyopathy and myocarditis. In J. Loscalzo (Ed.), *Harrison's cardiovascular medicine* (pp. 241–253). New York: McGraw Hill.

Acknowledgment

Thanks to Stacey Larson, MA, OTR/L, staff therapist from Detroit Lakes, Minnesota, for submitting the case study on COPD.

43

Dysphagia

Wendy Avery

Learning Objectives

After studying this chapter, the reader will be able to do the following:

1. Discuss normal swallowing.
2. Identify types of dysphagia and their presentation.
3. Describe how to perform a clinical dysphagia assessment.
4. Employ basic compensatory and rehabilitative strategies to treat dysphagia.
5. Describe instrumental evaluation procedures for dysphagia.

D ysphagia, or difficulty with any stage of swallowing, interferes with functional independence for many recipients of occupational therapy services in many settings. Safe swallowing is a critical and life-supporting activity of daily living that is addressed by occupational therapists in many environments, including acute care and psychiatric hospitals, acute and subacute rehabilitation centers, outpatient clinics, nursing homes, home health settings, and schools. Dysphagia is prevalent in adult diagnostic groups often seen by occupational therapists, including in 81% of clients with acute stroke (Warnecke et al., 2008), 50% of those with Parkinson's disease (Crary & Groher, 2003), and 55% of the elderly presenting with pneumonia (Cabre et al., 2010).

Occupational therapists assist clients with dysphagia in rehabilitation of abilities that affect swallowing, including self-feeding, cognition, perception, sensory and motor skills, postural control, and in rehabilitation of or compensation for an altered swallowing mechanism. Clients with acute, chronic, congenital, and acquired dysphagias may all benefit from intervention. In some settings, experienced occupational therapists serve as the primary swallowing therapist (American Occupational Therapy Association [AOTA], 2011); in other settings, speech and language pathologists serve as the primary swallowing therapist. Even when occupational therapists are not the primary dysphagia therapist, their contribution to swallowing rehabilitation is significant, and an understanding of the anatomy and physiology of the swallowing mechanism is most useful. Dysphagia care may be provided by a multidisciplinary dysphagia team, often including the occupational therapist, attending or primary care physician, nurse, respiratory therapist, speech language pathologist, and specialty physicians including the radiologist. The patient as a self-advocate and consumer is also a member, as are caregivers.

This chapter introduces the entry-level skills required for the evaluation and treatment of dysphagia in adults. Independent intervention with the dysphagic patient requires advanced knowledge and skills on the part of the occupational therapy clinician. AOTA (2007) delineates entry-level and advanced-level skills in dysphagia care for occupational therapists and occupational therapy assistants. It should be noted that dysphagia care is an advanced practice area for occupational therapists (AOTA, 2007). The contents of this chapter are not a substitute for formal education and training in dysphagia care. Further information about dysphagia can be acquired by seeking advanced learning opportunities, researching new developments, attending workshops and conferences, and receiving mentoring.

NORMAL SWALLOWING

Deglutition is a complex process involving both volitional and nonvolitional behaviors. The cranial nerves

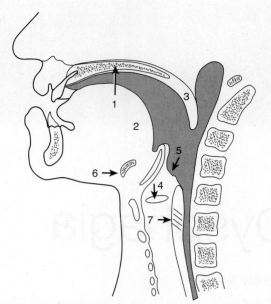

Figure 43-1 The oral, pharyngeal, and esophageal structures involved in swallowing. 1. The hard palate. 2. The base of the tongue. 3. The soft palate and uvula. 4. The vocal cords. 5. The laryngeal vestibule. 6. The hyoid bone. 7. The upper esophageal sphincter. (Adapted with permission from Groher, M. E. [1997]. *Dysphagia: Diagnosis and management* [3rd ed.]. Boston: Butterworth-Heinemann.)

execute the sensory and motor processes that constitute swallowing. Cortically mediated factors, including appetite, attitude, attention span, appreciation of food, and body position influence swallowing and must be considered in evaluation and treatment. Oral, pharyngeal, and esophageal structures involved in swallowing are shown in Figure 43-1.

The stages of swallowing include the preoral, oral preparatory, oral, pharyngeal, and esophageal stages (Definition 43-1). The preoral, oral preparatory, and oral stages are voluntary. The length of the oral preparatory stage varies with the type of bolus (Mendell & Logemann, 2007) and age (Logemann et al., 2002). Oral transit time, the length of time to accomplish the oral stage, is normally 1–1.5 seconds (Mendell & Logemann, 2007). The pharyngeal stage is involuntary, although volitional movements can alter it. Normal pharyngeal transit time is 1 second (Mendell & Logemann, 2007). Although the patient's position may affect the esophageal stage because of the effects of gravity, this stage is involuntary.

IMPAIRED SWALLOWING

Many disease processes and trauma cause dysphagia, including those that affect the central nervous system, peripheral nervous system, motor end plate, muscles, and other anatomical structures. Dysphagia can lead to

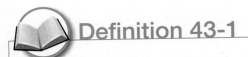

Definition 43-1

The Stages of Swallowing

Preoral Stage

The food is visually and olfactorily appreciated. This stimulates salivation, and there are preparatory movements of the mouth to ready the oral cavity to receive and mobilize the food or liquid. Spontaneous upper extremity movements occur as the person reaches for and grasps the utensil, cup, or finger food and brings it to the mouth.

Oral Preparatory Stage

The food is received and contained by the mouth. It is then formed into a bolus of food and mixed with saliva. Pureed or liquid boluses require little mastication and may briefly be held centrally in the mouth by the tongue and cheek musculature. If solid, the food may need to be bitten off to be contained in the mouth. The bolus is chewed in a rotary motion by the molars and is moved between the left and right molars. The buccal muscles contract to prevent food from pocketing between the cheeks and the teeth. Once masticated or formed, the bolus is brought to the center of the tongue.

Oral Stage

As the cheek and tongue muscles retain the bolus centrally in the mouth, the tongue squeezes it against the hard palate, moving it posteriorly to the level of the faucial arches.

Pharyngeal Stage

The soft palate elevates to close off the nasopharynx. The larynx and hyoid elevate and protract, minimizing the size of the laryngeal vestibule (its opening) as the epiglottis tips to cover the vestibule. Breathing stops (termed "swallowing apnea"), which reduces the possibility of aspiration or laryngeal penetration of food or liquid. The vocal cords close. Simultaneously, the pharyngeal constrictor muscles sequentially contract to propel the bolus through the pharynx. The elevation of the larynx causes the upper esophageal sphincter (UES) to relax, allowing the bolus to pass through it.

Esophageal Stage

The UES returns to its normal tonic state, and the bolus is transported through the esophagus via esophageal peristalsis and gravity. The lower esophageal sphincter relaxes, allowing the bolus to pass through into the stomach.

---

dehydration (Leibovitz et al., 2007), malnutrition (Foley et al., 2009), pressure ulcers (Westergren et al., 2001), and pulmonary complications caused by aspiration. These complications include aspiration pneumonia (Eisenstadt, 2010), airway obstruction (Eckberg & Feinberg, 1992), and death (Eisenstadt, 2010). The limited ability to participate in social and cultural activities because of chronic dysphagia can profoundly affect an individual.

Types of Dysphagia

Dysphagia occurs in three types: paralytic, pseudobulbar, and mechanical. Paralytic dysphagia results from lower motor neuron involvement that causes weakness and sensory impairment of oral and pharyngeal structures, including weakness or absence of the swallowing reflex. Pseudobulbar dysphagia results from upper motor neuron involvement, causing hypotonicity or hypertonicity of oral and pharyngeal structures and a slow or poorly coordinated swallowing reflex. Mechanical dysphagia is caused by loss of oral, pharyngeal, or esophageal structures; weakness; and/or sensory deficits caused by trauma or surgery. Pulmonary complications may complicate the presentation. Debility, lack of appetite, and poor overall nutritional status can affect a client's stamina and ability to participate in

dysphagia and overall rehabilitation (Safety Note 43-1 and Definition 43-2).

DYSPHAGIA ASSESSMENT

A dysphagia assessment involves two components, a clinical assessment and an instrumental evaluation.

Clinical Assessment

Clinical assessment of dysphagia must be thorough, with examination of all areas relevant to swallowing. It is best done using a reliable and valid tool (Latella & Meriano, 2010). A reliable and valid tool allows for accurate assessment and reassessment by different test administrators and ensures that each test item provides accurate assessment of performance components. The Dysphagia Evaluation Protocol (1997) is an example of a standardized assessment developed by occupational therapists. Figure 43-3 illustrates the use of a chartable form to document evaluation results.

History, Nutrition, and Respiratory Considerations

The clinician reviews the patient's medical and surgical history, with special attention to any diagnoses and procedures that are relevant to dysphagia. The patient

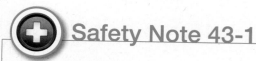

Safety Note 43-1

Pulmonary Concerns

Respiratory problems may contribute to dysphagia and vice versa because the respiratory and swallowing mechanisms share anatomy and physiology.

Secretion Management

The patient's airway must be clear of excessive secretions. Intermittent suctioning through the nose or tracheostomy may be needed to clear the airway. The swallowing therapist should work closely with nursing and respiratory staff to assess whether airway protection and the ability to maintain oxygenation are adequate. Personnel should be available to suction the airway as necessary.

Tracheostomy

A tracheostomy tube reroutes breathing through a stoma in the neck. Tracheostomy tubes may be temporary or permanent and are used to keep the airway open (Fig. 43-2). Tracheostomies provide easy access for suctioning or ventilator use but can cause or exacerbate dysphagia. They cause reduced smell and taste sensation because the patient is not breathing through the nose. Tracheostomy reduces the ability to clear the upper airway if laryngeal penetration occurs. It increases the risk of aspiration caused by pooling in the pharynx, delays trigger of the swallow reflex, decreases duration of vocal cord closure, and reduces laryngeal movement. An inflated tracheostomy cuff further reduces laryngeal elevation and increases the risk of silent aspiration (Ding & Logemann, 2005). An "open" tracheostomy, in which the tube is not covered or "capped," eliminates the subglottic pressure, reducing the force of the swallow response (Gross, Mahlmann, & Grayhack, 2003).

Mechanical Ventilators

Ventilators are machines that assist patients to breathe if they cannot do so on their own. Positive pressure ventilators may be used temporarily, to assist a patient through an acute illness, or chronically, for a patient with a long-term respiratory challenge. Positive pressure ventilators deliver breaths to patients through a tube in the nose or mouth or through a tracheostomy. Patients who use a ventilator to breathe via a tracheostomy may be able to eat by mouth.

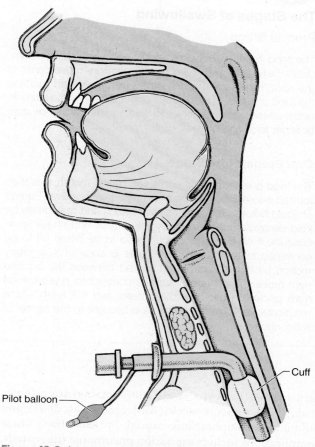

Figure 43-2 A tracheostomy tube. Tubes come in different sizes and may come with or without the cuff as pictured. The pilot balloon is used to inflate the cuff with a syringe and indicates relative inflation of the cuff. The inflated cuff prevents food or secretions from falling further into the airway.

Breathing ceases during the swallow. A well-coordinated swallow is needed to interpose the swallow between inhalation and exhalation. Patients who have had mechanical ventilation for more than a week have been shown to have multiple swallowing deficits once the ventilator is removed (Macht et al., 2011). Patients who are ventilator dependent via tracheostomy are prone to aspiration during eating (Macht et al., 2011).

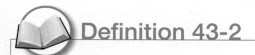

Definition 43-2

Clinical Dysphagia Presentation for Various Diagnostic Groups

This is not an exhaustive list of diagnoses prone to dysphagia; however, it includes those most often encountered.

Alzheimer's Disease: Pseudobulbar Dysphagia

- Decreased attention span and apraxia for swallowing and self-feeding may be seen.
- Oral and pharyngeal responses slow and a need for physical and verbal cues to self-feed are needed.
- Difficulty with self-feeding is common, and challenges with initiating the meal may be present (Edahiro et al., 2012).
- Agitation and behavioral challenges can hamper the eating process (Edahiro et al., 2012).
- Clients prefer sweet-flavored and pureed foods.
- Clients are prone to aspiration (van der Maarel-Wierink et al., 2011) and more difficulty with self feeding (Edahiro et al., 2012) in later stages of the disease.

Brain Injury: Pseudobulbar, Paralytic Dysphagia

- Type and severity of dysphagia in brain injury depends on the cause of the injury and location and size of brain lesions.
- Behavioral and cognitive problems affect self-feeding and swallowing.
- Abnormal pathological reflexes can affect oral and pharyngeal control.
- Increased or reduced muscle tone may cause decreased mouth opening, decreased lip closure, drooling, decreased tongue control, and pocketing of the bolus in the cheek (Logemann, Pepe, & Mackay, 1994; Mackay, Morgan, & Bernstein, 1999).
- Delayed pharyngeal swallow trigger, nasal regurgitation, decreased base of tongue movement, and decreased laryngeal elevation with resulting pharyngeal residue may be seen (Logemann, Pepe, & Mackay, 1994).
- Overall mealtime may be slow (Mackay, Morgan, & Bernstein, 1999).

Cerebrovascular Accident: Pseudobulbar and Paralytic

- Pharyngeal and laryngeal sensory deficits may occur in right and left hemispheric as well as subcortical strokes (Aviv et al., 1996).
- Symptoms vary with lesion location and size.
- Patients with right hemispheric stroke (pseudobulbar dysphagia) display mild oral transit delays and some delay in pharyngeal trigger and laryngeal elevation. The pharyngeal stage lasts longer, and there may be penetration of the larynx and aspiration (Robbins et al., 1993). There may be neglect or denial of swallowing problems,

and sensory loss can slow motor responses to bolus presence.

- Patients with left hemispheric stroke (pseudobulbar dysphagia) display delays in initiating the oral stage and in triggering the pharyngeal stage. The pharyngeal stage takes longer (Robbins et al., 1993). There may be apraxia for eating and swallowing.
- Patients with subcortical stroke (paralytic dysphagia) demonstrate mild oral transit delays and a delay in triggering the swallow. There is general weakness of pharyngeal swallow, as seen in reduced laryngeal elevation, reduced tongue base retraction, and unilateral pharyngeal weakness (Horner et al., 1991; Robbins et al., 1993). There may also be reduced upper esophageal sphincter (UES) opening (Horner et al., 1991).

Developmental/Intellectual Disabilities: Pseudobulbar, Paralytic Dysphagia

- Cerebral palsy (CP) and mental retardation, together or in isolation, may present deficits of bolus formation and transit, delayed swallow reflex, pharyngeal dysmotility, esophageal disease, and aspiration (Sullivan, 2008).
- Abnormal oral reflexes and oral hyposensitivity or hypersensitivity may be observed.
- Poor postural, head, neck, and limb control can affect swallowing.
- Behaviors such as eating too quickly and putting too much food in the mouth can affect efficiency and safety of swallowing (Samuels & Chadwick, 2006)

Head and Neck Cancer: Mechanical Dysphagia

- Swallowing problems with head and neck cancer vary with tumor type, size, and location.
- Bolus control and containment problems result from surgery to the lip (Nguyen et al., 2008).
- Resection of tumor from the floor of the mouth causes difficulty with bolus control, reduced laryngeal elevation, and its accompanying reduction in UES opening (Hara et al., 2003).
- Glossectomy, or removal of some or all of the tongue, causes difficult or absent bolus mobilization; a resection of the tongue base limits the elevation needed to initiate the pharyngeal swallow (Lazarus, 2006).
- Unilateral laryngeal cancer may require a vertical laryngectomy or hemilaryngectomy; this may cause reduced vocal cord closure, reduced posterior tongue movement, and reduced UES opening (McConnel & O'Connor, 1994).
- Supraglottic laryngectomy reduces glottic closure, laryngeal elevation, and opening of the UES (McConnel & O'Connor, 1994).

(continued)

Definition 43-2 *(continued)*

- Extensive cancer of the larynx necessitates a total laryngectomy, which separates the foodway and airway tracts and creates a permanent anatomical tracheostomy. Although aspiration is no longer a threat, there is reduced movement through the pharynx, remaining laryngeal tissue, and esophagus (Maclean, Cotton & Perry, 2009).
- Adjunctive radiation therapy causes edema in areas adjacent to the radiation field, fibrosis, and reduced salivary flow, causing dry mouth or xerostomia.
- Radiation therapy combined with chemotherapy without surgery can reduce tongue base movement, laryngeal elevation, and pharyngeal range of motion and speed (Lazarus et al., 1996).
- Radiation therapy combined with surgery can cause longer oral transit time, increased pharyngeal residue, and reduced UES opening (Pauloski, 2008).

Multiple Sclerosis: Pseudobulbar, Paralytic Dysphagia

- Dysphagia symptoms vary with location of plaques in the central and peripheral nervous systems. Dysphagia worsens with disease progression (Poorjavad et al., 2010).
- Weakness of the oral structures and the neck muscles may be seen (Poorjavad et al., 2010).

- Delayed pharyngeal swallow and weakness of pharyngeal contractions may be seen (Poorjavad et al., 2010).

Neoplasms of the Brain: Pseudobulbar, Paralytic Dysphagia

- Dysphagia may be due either to a tumor or to metastasis in the brain or to medical or surgical interventions.
- Symptoms vary with the location and extent of the client's neoplasm and interventions, and symptoms may be similar to those found in clients with stroke (Wesling et al., 2003).

Parkinson's Disease: Pseudobulbar Dysphagia

- Impulsiveness and poor judgment can affect swallowing.
- Jaw rigidity, abnormal head and neck posture, impaired coordination of tongue movements and mastication. Mastication and orofacial motions are affected (Bakke et al., 2011) along with tongue control (van Lieshout, Steele, & Lang, 2011). Alterations in the pharyngeal aspect of the swallow occur (Noyce et al., 2012) including pharyngeal residue and delayed pharyngeal elevation. Abnormal head, neck, and trunk posture along with difficulty coordinating upper extremity movements for self-feeding are seen.
- Feeding and swallowing may be too slow and laborious to allow sufficient nutritional intake.
- Orofacial fatigue may make eating and swallowing more difficult as a meal progresses (Solomon, 2006).

and caregiver also provide information about any history of swallowing disorders. Specific signs and symptoms and modifications in behaviors relevant to mealtime are noted, as are changes in food intake and weight loss. The current nutritional sources are recorded, including the length of time the patient has been NPO, or not eating by mouth, if applicable. The therapist also documents any cultural and religious dietary preferences and practices. Information regarding respiratory status is gathered from the hospital chart and staff, including the presence of a tracheostomy and/or mechanical ventilation, and the level of independence with secretion management.

Assessment of Cognitive, Perceptual, and Physical Abilities

Important cognitive and perceptual considerations include the level of alertness and arousal, orientation, ability to attend to a feeding session or meal, ability to follow multistep commands, and any visual deficits or unilateral neglect. The clinician notes the patient's

insight into his or her dysphagia and observes head, neck, trunk, and limb control and endurance for being out of bed at mealtimes. The ability to self-position and self-feed and need for or use of adaptive eating equipment are assessed.

Assessment of Oral and Pharyngeal Abilities

Once direct physical assessment begins, the clinician must observe universal precautions to prevent exposure to pathogens for both the clinician and the patient (Safety Note 43-2). Then the occupational therapist assesses oral and pharyngeal control including tone, range of motion, strength, and sensation of the lips, tongue, jaw, and cheeks and any abnormal oral reflexes. To assess pharyngeal control, the therapist observes soft palate movement, gag reflex, vocal quality, and volitional cough. A stethoscope may be used to listen for pooling of fluid above the level of the vocal cords, as pooled liquids resonate during breathing. The therapist rates the patient's hunger and level of enthusiasm for a snack or meal.

DYSPHAGIA
Evaluation Protocol

RECORD FORM

Client name: Doe, John   DOB: 1/1/40   Age: 73   Date: 1/1/13
Physician: Dr. Smith   Location: bedside   Type of service: Neuro
Type of eval: ☑ Initial ☐ Re-eval   Assistive or postural devices used: wheelchair.
Diagnosis: (L)CVA, (R) hemi   Date of onset: 12/29/12   Reason for referral: dysphagia
Last oral feeding: breakfast   Clinician/Title: Wendy Avery, MS OTR/L

HISTORY AND OBSERVATIONS

Feeding History

Normal preexisting function?   ☑ No   ☐ Yes
  When did change occur? Describe change.
coughing c̄ all textures p̄ CVA
Has consistency of food changed?   ☐ No   ☑ Yes
  When, and how did client compensate? MD
ordered thick puree
Has food intake changed?   ☐ No   ☑ Yes
  When, and how? poor oral intake
Weight loss?   ☑ No   ☐ Yes
  Number of lbs: _____   When? _____
  Other changes: _____
_____

Nutritional Status

Nutritional Route:
  ☐ NPO   ☑ PO
Alternative feeding method used:
  ☐ NGT   ☐ PEG   ☐ TPN   ☑ Other: IV for
                                   fluids
Current diet:
  ☐ Regular   ☑ Other: thick puree
Special dietary requirements:
  ☐ No concentrated sweets   ☐ Low salt   ☐ Kosher
  ☐ Other: None

Respiratory Status

Auscultation of pooling?   ☑ No   ☐ Yes
Suctioning required?   ☑ No   ☐ Yes
  Frequency: _____   Route: _____
Tracheostomy?   ☑ No   ☐ Yes
  Type: ☐ Cuffed   ☐ Cuffless
          ☐ Fenestrated   Size: _____
  Position of cuff:
  ☐ Fully inflated   ☐ Partially inflated   ☐ Deflated
Comments: _____
_____

Ventilator?   ☑ No   ☐ Yes   ☐ Cannot be removed
  Weaning parameters: _____

Receiving chest physical therapy?   ☑ No   ☐ Yes
  Type of treatment: _____
Comments: _____
_____

General Status

Alertness:
  ☑ No deficit   ☐ Partial deficit   ☐ Moderate/Severe deficit
Follows directions:
  ☑ verbal   ☐ gesture
  ☑ 3-step   ☐ 2-step   ☐ 1-step   ☐ Unable
If client responds to fewer than 3-step directions, note reason
for difficulty: _____
_____

*If the client has difficulty with two- or three-step directions,
see Alternative Administration Protocol section of the manual
for information about continuing the evaluation.*

Recognizes swallowing problems:
  ☑ Good insight   ☐ Partial insight   ☐ No insight

*Record the appropriate rating of this item after observing
client's performance during the Feeding Trial portion of
the evaluation.*

Perceptual/Cognitive observations:
  ☑ No deficit   ☐ Partial deficit   ☐ Severe deficit
Comments: _____

Physical Status

Assistance needed to attain and maintain position:
  ☑ Independent   ☐ Minimal/Moderate assistance
  ☐ Maximal assistance
Comments: _____
_____

Head and neck control
  Range of motion: ☐ Normal   ☑ Impaired
  Manual muscle testing: ☐ Normal   ☑ Impaired
  ☐ Nonfunctional for eating

*If head and neck control is nonfunctional for eating, stop the
evaluation and refer to the Manual for additional information.*

Upper-extremity control
  for self-feeding: ☐ Normal   ☑ Impaired
                      ☐ Nonfunctional

Record rating for upper-extremity control during the feeding trial.

Comments: ↓ tone (R) neck, needs cues
to keep head erect, decreased
(R) U/e tone for utensil manipulation

1

IMPRESSIONS

Summary

This 73 y o gentleman is s/p CVA c̄ Ⓡ hemi and aphasia. He shows reduced oral tone and control of Ⓡ tongue and cheek. He manages soft, formed boluses c̄ extra time for oral manipulation and a slowed swallow response. No pooling or coughing was noted after swallowing. There were no clinical signs of aspiration or laryngeal penetration.

Functional Level (Physical and verbal assistance needed for positioning, hand-to-mouth movements, and swallowing):

Pt was able to self-feed c̄ hand-over-hand guiding to use utensil but was able to use cup Ⓘ with both hands. He needed verbal cues to prepare his tray to eat and supervision to transfer to wheelchair to eat.

Intermittent supervision at meals and snacks and assistance to self-feed c̄ right hand is recommended.

Recommendations/Plan:

- ☐ NPO (No food by mouth)
- ☐ Nutrition consultation:
- ☑ Videofluoroscopy TO assess safety with fluids
- ☐ Prefeeding program
- ☑ Special positioning, Adaptive equipment: Seated in chair to eat
- ☐ Mealtime supervision ☐ Constant ☐ Intermittent ☐ Set-up
- ☑ Diet recommendation: Thick puree, trial thick fluids
- ☑ Other: short-term goals
  1. Trial of honey thick fluids
  2. Tolerate soft chewables without s/s of aspiration
  3. Ⓘ techniques to maintain lip closure + prevent food pocketing
  4. Ⓘ vocal cord adduction exercises
  5. Modified Ⓘ self-feeding c̄ adaptive equipment

0761644121
Printed in the U.S.A.
1 2 3 4 5 6 7 8 9 10 11 12 A B C D E

Figure 43-3 *(continued)*

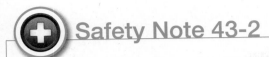

Safety Note 43-2

Precautions for the Therapist and Patient

The swallowing therapist stays close to the patient during eating and is exposed to oral secretions and respirations. Likewise, the patient is exposed to pathogens on the therapist's clothing and hands and in the therapist's respiratory tract. Universal (also called "standard") precautions should be used. The use of gloves is mandatory anytime the therapist touches the face or inside the oral cavity.

Dysphagia patients are prone to difficulty with airway obstruction and aspiration during eating. For the safety of the patient, the swallowing therapist should be trained in suctioning of the airway, the Heimlich maneuver, and cardiopulmonary resuscitation.

Signs and Symptoms of Potential or Actual Aspiration

Although laryngeal penetration or aspiration may be silent, occurring without overt warning signs and symptoms, the following indicate that it may occur or be occurring. If observed during a dysphagia evaluation, these signs or symptoms can indicate that a feeding trial should not be initiated or should be discontinued. Specific items of concern are as follows (Avery-Smith, Rosen, & Dellarosa, 1997):

1. The patient cannot remain awake for the clinical evaluation.
2. The oral and/or pharyngeal sensation and motion assessment reveal poor ability to manipulate and contain the bolus.
3. The bolus remains in the mouth, and the patient cannot initiate or complete the oral preparatory stage within a reasonable time.
4. There is excessive coughing or choking before, during, or after swallowing.
5. There is no swallow response once the oral stage is completed.
6. There is a change in voice quality, often wet, or no voice after swallowing.
7. Severe pooling or wetness is heard on auscultation or by the naked ear; secretions are poorly managed.
8. Silent aspiration is suggested by a change in the patient's color and/or respiratory rate, increased congestion on auscultation of the chest, and/or a reduction in oxygen level in the blood as recorded by pulse oximetry.

The Feeding Trial

Interventions that maximize performance can be initiated before the feeding trial begins (Procedures for Practice 43-1). The safest food textures are chosen for the trial. Easy-to-manage foods and thick fluids are attempted first, especially if the patient has been NPO and/or has a diagnosis or clinical picture that suggests a high risk of aspiration. During the oral stage, the clinician observes bolus containment, formation, propulsion, and mastication. During the pharyngeal stage, the clinician assesses laryngeal elevation, voice quality after swallow, repetitive swallows, and cough reflex. The therapist should observe for signs and symptoms of laryngeal penetration or aspiration, especially during the first feeding trial (Safety Note 43-2). The evaluation concludes with a summary, recommendations, and a plan (Latella & Meriano, 2010).

Specific techniques are helpful during the feeding trial. Auscultation (listening) to the swallow with a stethoscope held lateral to the larynx (Fig. 43-5) can reveal the efficiency and safety of the oral and pharyngeal stages (Borr, Hielscher-Fastabend, & Lücking, 2007). Gentle palpation of the neck (Fig. 43-6) during the swallow reveals symmetry, strength, and speed of oral pharyngeal movement and may be done simultaneously with auscultation. Use of a pulse oximeter, a noninvasive monitoring device that measures the patient's oxygen saturation in the bloodstream, may be effective in assessing whether aspiration or respiratory difficulties are occurring (Salvador et al., 2009). Normal oxygen saturation in the bloodstream falls in between 93% and 98%; a level below 92% after swallowing suggests aspiration. If the patient can self-feed, palpation and auscultation may be done simultaneously. If the patient needs help to self-feed, auscultation and guiding with hand-to-mouth efforts may be done simultaneously.

Recommendations and Plan

Once the clinical evaluation is complete, recommendations and a plan are formulated. As seen in Figure 43-4, recommendations may include whether eating by mouth is advisable, whether an instrumental evaluation is advised, whether a nutritional consultation with a dietitian is needed, recommended diet type, mealtime positioning and supervision, adaptive equipment, and type and amount of assistance. Evaluation of the patient is ongoing, and with additional information from clinical observations, instrumental evaluations, and input from

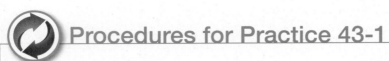

Procedures for Practice 43-1

Preparation for Eating

Prior to the feeding trial portion of an evaluation and snacks or meals, measures must be taken to optimize the patient's swallowing performance. Because these strategies do not involve ingestion of food, they are indirect therapy techniques.

- Provide a quiet environment to encourage concentration.
- Position the patient upright in a chair to minimize the risk of aspiration. The feet should be supported, and the arms should be free for self-feeding. Patients with pseudobulbar dysphagia may need special attention to positioning before eating and special positioning devices; they may need assistance to maintain head and neck alignment and facilitation to stimulate oral and pharyngeal motions prior to and during eating (Fig. 43-4).
- Complete oral hygiene activities before the trial because this stimulates sensation and range of motion in oral structures.
- Present a simplified visual array of food and utensils for the patient with visual neglect and/or other visual deficits. Anchors, colorful cues to call attention to the side of the plate, are helpful for patients with neglect.
- Present appetizing, culture-specific foods, utensils, and tableware.
- Provide adaptive equipment and/or use hand-over-hand guidance to facilitate self-feeding.
- Provide simple explanations and one-step verbal directions if necessary.
- If the patient eats too quickly or is confused by multiple food choices, present one food at a time.
- Use small-bowled utensils and verbal or manual assistance to load just a teaspoon-sized bolus. Pinch the straw to limit the amount of liquid consumed or use a covered cup with a small opening.

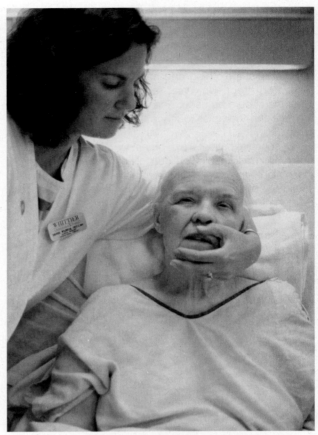

Figure 43-4 Using the half-nelson position to assist with head and neck control. The therapist can also assist with jaw, cheek, and lip control at the same time.

other dysphagia team members, the treatment plan and goals change.

Instrumental Evaluation

Clinical assessment goes hand in hand with instrumental evaluation, which uses imaging and diagnostic studies to provide critical information about the unseen parts of the oral, pharyngeal, and esophageal stages of swallowing. Various types of instrumental evaluations for dysphagia are discussed in Definition 43-3. These evaluations are usually performed by physicians, often together with the occupational therapist. Aspiration of food or fluid may be silent (Leder, Suiter, & Green, 2011). Imaging studies, such as videofluoroscopy, and fiberoptic endoscopic evaluation of

swallowing (FEES) are needed to identify aspiration, but they may not identify aspiration in all instances, because client skills can vary, and the testing situation in the radiology suite may not reliably approximate an actual eating situation. However, these studies do provide important information about the quality of the swallow and the efficacy of compensatory therapy techniques used during swallowing.

DYSPHAGIA INTERVENTION

Remedial and Compensatory Goals

One consideration in treatment is remedial versus compensatory goals. Remedial, also referred to as "rehabilitative" treatment, focuses on restoring a normal level of

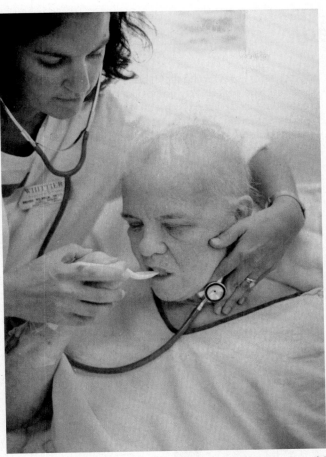

Figure 43-5 Auscultation of the swallow using a stethoscope. The therapist may be able to facilitate head position and guide self-feeding while listening to the sounds of the swallow.

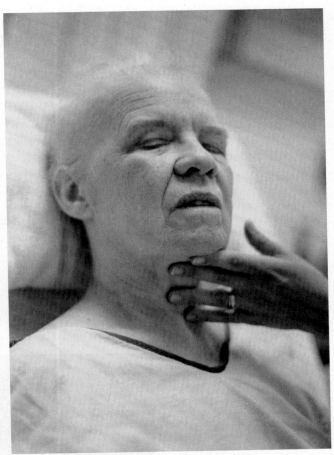

Figure 43-6 Palpation of the neck during swallowing. The first finger is under the chin, the second finger is at the base of the tongue, the third finger is over the thyroid cartilage, and the fourth finger is at the base of the throat. A very light touch should be used so as not to inhibit motion.

 Definition 43-3

Instrumental Evaluation of Swallowing

Instrumental evaluation uses technology, including the following.

Electromyography

Electrodes are placed either into the muscle via a small needle or on the skin over a muscle to record contractions of the muscle. Surface electrodes have been used to assess aspects of oral bolus management in neurological dysphagia patients and pharyngeal, laryngeal, and esophageal activity (Stepp, 2012).

Fiberoptic Endoscopic Evaluation of Swallowing

A fiberoptic laryngoscope, a narrow flexible tube with a small camera on its tip, is introduced through the nose into the nasopharynx, where structures including the palate, pharynx, and larynx are viewed for assessment of anatomy and movement. Food is administered in different consistencies to observe posterior oral and pharyngeal function and airway protection during eating.

Manometry

A catheter with transducers to measure pressure is introduced into the esophagus. The force, timing, and sequence of the esophageal contractions are measured.

Scintigraphy

A radioactive isotope is mixed with food. As the bolus is swallowed, a gamma camera tracks the radioactive particles. This test measures the speed of bolus transit and can accurately measure the amount of bolus that is aspirated.

(continued)

Definition 43-3 *(continued)*

Ultrasonography

An ultrasound transducer held under the chin produces images of oral and pharyngeal stages of swallow, revealing the mobility of structures and boluses swallowed.

Videofluoroscopy

The patient is seated between a movable camera and a fluorescent screen. Radiographic images of oral, pharyngeal, and esophageal structures are delivered to a screen from the camera as barium or barium-impregnated fluids and foods are swallowed. The images are recorded on videotape or DVD. Figure 43-7 illustrates a videofluoroscopic image of the oral, pharyngeal, and upper esophageal structures. Swallowing pathology and the effectiveness of compensatory swallowing techniques and positions can be observed. The patient may be positioned in a lateral and/or anteroposterior position to view structure and function from both perspectives. Videofluoroscopies are often repeated to assess progress. A swallowing therapist is usually present to ensure that the test reproduces compensatory maneuvers and food textures being used and to ensure that it mimics real eating as accurately as possible. In some instances, the swallowing therapist may perform the videofluoroscopy. Therapists assisting with or performing videofluoroscopies must be expert swallowing clinicians; they must be fully trained in use of the equipment and procedures used in videofluoroscopy. Videofluoroscopy of swallowing may also be known as "modified barium swallow" or "MBS."

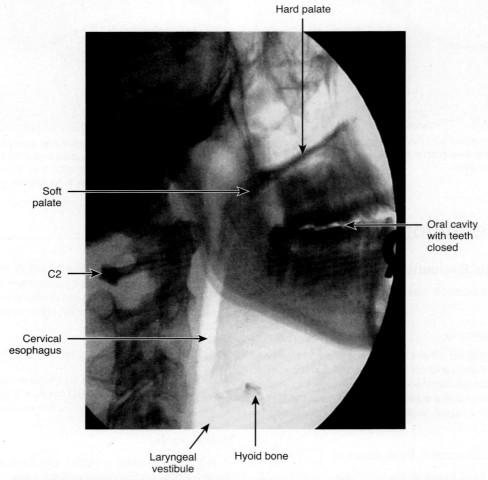

Figure 43-7 A videofluoroscopic image of the oral, pharyngeal, and esophageal structures. (Videoprint image courtesy of Bette Pomerleau, MS, SLP, and Ray Autiello, LPN, RT, of Universal Mobile Services, Haverhill, MA.)

swallowing function. Potential for partial or full recovery is anticipated when goals are strictly remedial. This approach may be used with an acute stroke patient for whom complete or near complete recovery is anticipated. Compensatory treatment circumvents impairments with the use of alternative strategies and techniques. These techniques are used when full recovery is not anticipated, for example, for a patient with advancing Parkinson's disease. Compensatory techniques may also be used to enable a safe, functional swallow prior to recovery of normal swallowing, for example, with a patient with an acute pneumonia for whom full recovery is anticipated. Table 43-1 discusses compensatory and remedial interventions for specific swallowing deficits. Compensatory swallowing maneuvers and their indications are discussed in Procedures for Practice 43-2, and instrumental interventions are explained in Definition 43-4. Goals may be remedial and then change to compensatory once a plateau in function is reached.

Indirect and Direct Therapy

Another consideration is the type of therapeutic techniques used. Indirect therapy addresses the prerequisite abilities or the capacity to swallow without ingestion of food or liquid. Patients who are at high risk for aspiration often begin with indirect therapy only. Indirect therapy can include range of motion, strengthening, and coordination exercises for weak or hypotonic oral and pharyngeal musculature; strengthening of pharyngeal and laryngeal structures; techniques to reduce or stimulate sensitivity of oral musculature; and techniques to improve the pharyngeal swallowing response. Indirect therapy also involves increasing the patient's level of arousal to implement treatment, and manipulating the environment to optimize behaviors that affect swallowing (see Procedures for Practice 43-1).

Direct therapy rehabilitates prerequisite abilities or the capacity to swallow during therapeutic snacks or meals. This involves exercises and/or the use of compensatory swallowing maneuvers that include ingestion of food. Indirect therapy may continue once direct therapy has begun. An individualized treatment plan usually includes a selection of direct and indirect techniques. The complexity of interventions depends on the ability of the patient and/or caregiver to process complex information. Treatment techniques may be evaluated by videofluoroscopy or fiberoptic endoscopy to assess their efficacy, especially in the pharyngeal stage, where the effects of techniques are unseen. Although not discussed in depth here, optimizing self-feeding skills is an important goal to address together with swallowing goals. Although not yet proven in the literature, the sensory inputs and motor patterns used for self-feeding are probably related to those used in the partly voluntary swallow, and facilitating both skills enhances each.

Progression of Diet with Swallowing Therapy

As indirect therapy begins, some patients may receive all nutrition, hydration, and medication via a nonoral source, such as intravenous or gastrostomy tube feedings. As the patient recovers the ability to swallow without laryngeal penetration or aspiration, direct therapy with the therapist present begins during snacks and progresses to meals. As improvement continues and the patient learns compensatory techniques, he or she may progress to eating under the supervision of nursing personnel and trained significant others and then progress to eating independently. Calorie counts are initiated by the dietitian to assess the adequacy of oral intake. Once food intake improves and calories are consistently sufficient, nonoral feeding sources may be used only for hydration and/or medication. Finally, as the patient improves and fluids and medications are safely ingested by mouth, the use of nonoral feeding sources can be discontinued. Diet textures are upgraded as skills develop. Depending on the diagnosis and potential for recovery, patients may level off at any point in the described progression (Procedures for Practice 43-2).

Dysphagia Diets

Dysphagia diets are designed to provide stepwise gradation of food and fluid textures that are matched to the patient's improving oral and pharyngeal skills. A diet of mechanical soft foods (foods that have been chopped or ground) that form a moist, cohesive bolus and thickened fluids may reduce the incidence of aspiration compared with pureed foods and thin fluids (Groher et al., 2006). Specific textures and flavors can stimulate optimal oral and pharyngeal motion; for example, sour flavors may stimulate swallowing responses (Pelletier & Lawless, 2003). Patients may have strong preferences; those with dementias may prefer sweet flavors and reject foods that require chewing. Dysphagia diets for most patients follow this general progression:

1. Thick purees, such as pudding and applesauce
2. Very soft moist chewables, such as soft cooked vegetables, fruits, and soft pastas
3. Drier chewables, such as cookies and breads
4. Foods requiring biting, firmer chewables such as meats, and mixed textures like cereals and milk or pills and water.

The progression of fluids advances thus:

1. No fluids at all
2. Honey-thick fluids
3. Nectar-thick fluids
4. Thin, flavored fluids
5. Water

Table 43-1 **Compensatory and Remedial Interventions for Specific Problems**

Patient Problem	Compensatory Intervention	Remedial Intervention
Swallowing apraxia		Provide a natural mealtime setting; enhance self-feeding skills to facilitate oral skills; provide a variety of boluses to stimulate oral movements
Weakness of cheeks, lips	Provide soft solids and thick fluids for easy oral manipulation; place food at back and stronger side of mouth; tilt head toward stronger side; massage cheek to prevent pocketing; hold lips closed; inspect mouth after meals to check for residue	Use tapping, vibration, and quick stretch to stimulate movement (refer to Web Chapter C for further information on these interventions); provide range-of-motion and stretching exercises progressing to resistive sucking and blowing exercises
Abnormal oral reflexes	Avoid stimuli that provoke rooting, bite, tongue thrust, sucking, or hyperactive gag reflexes; elicit movements antagonistic to undesirable reflex (for example, encourage mouth opening to weaken bite reflex); seat patient with body well supported to minimize proximal extensor tone, which can provoke abnormal distal movements and reflexes	
Facial, intraoral hypersensitivity		Provide systematic desensitization to face and intraoral area; if sensory defensiveness affects whole body, a program of graded sensory stimulation to body should precede stimulation to oral area, followed by careful introduction of food; use systematic desensitization with guided imagery to reduce muscle tone and anxiety regarding eating and mouth
Oral hyposensitivity	Place bolus on more sensitive areas of mouth; use warmer or colder bolus and flavorful food to stimulate sensation (Logemann et al, 1998); use heavy or viscous boluses	Sensory diet providing heightened tactile and proprioceptive input to intraoral structures may stimulate sensation and movement before and during a meal or snack
Reduced lingual control	Introduce diet requiring little oral manipulation, including soft solids and thick fluids; use posterior and/or lateral placement of food on stronger side; inspect mouth for residue after meals	Introduce active and passive tongue range-of-motion exercises, activities; provide quick stretch to tongue with tongue depressor or gloved fingers; provide articulation and tongue strengthening exercises (Robbins et al., 2005)
Slow oral transit time	Use cold boluses to hasten oral transit time (take care in case they melt into a difficult-to-manage liquid) sour boluses, such as those infused with lemon juice, can speed oral manipulation	
Delayed swallow	Use a sour bolus to reduce swallow delay (Logemann et al., 1998); try chin tuck to enhance airway protection; increase bolus volume and viscosity to reduce pharyngeal delay time (Bisch et al., 1994)	Try thermal-tactile stimulation: stroke anterior faucial arches with iced laryngeal mirror (Fig. 43-8) which hastens initiation and overall speed of swallow immediately after application (Rosenbek et al., 1996)
Reduced laryngeal elevation	Use Mendelsohn maneuver to prolong elevation of the larynx or chin tuck to elevate larynx; use supraglottic or super-supraglottic swallow to clear or minimize any material in airway	Use "Shaker" exercises (a program of capital flexion exercises) to strengthen suprahyoid musculature and prolong opening of the upper esophageal sphincter (UES) (Shaker et al., 2002)
Reduced laryngeal closure	Use supraglottic or super-supraglottic swallow to enhance airway protection (Logemann et al., 1998) or chin tuck to elevate and close off larynx	Introduce vocal cord adduction exercises (Logemann et al., 1998)
Tracheostomy	Occlusion of tracheostomy tube minimizes aspiration and improves swallow biomechanics (Logemann, Pauloski, & Colangelo, 1998); use of one-way speaking valve can decrease frequency of aspiration (Dettelbach et al., 1995); chin tuck may be useful	

The swallowing therapist typically has to try several interventions, preferably with the assistance of videofluoroscopy, to assess which techniques work most effectively. Clinicians should work under the guidance of an experienced therapist when using a technique that is new to them.

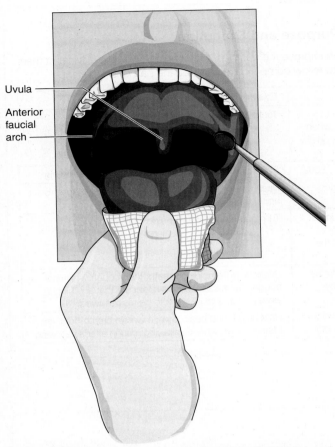

Uvula

Anterior
faucial
arch

Figure 43-8 Thermal-tactile stimulation of swallow. An iced laryngeal mirror is used to stroke the faucial arches to elicit or improve strength of the swallowing reflex.

Fluids are easily thickened with commercial thickeners, which can be mixed with hot or cold beverages. Unthickened or "free" water is sometimes provided to dysphagia clients on the assumption that consuming small amounts of water creates little risk of pneumonia and can improve hydration (Carlaw et al., 2011). However, occupational therapists always comply with the patient-specific swallowing program, providing liquids only as designated. Because bacterial pathogens in the mouth may be aspirated into the lungs, meticulous oral hygiene before and after meals is needed with any oral intake to reduce the risk of pneumonia (Yamaya et al., 2001). It is important that all caregivers know and understand an individual patient's diet so that no foods or fluids are provided that are not allowed.

Patient and Caregiver Training

Although the occupational therapist alone may carry out treatment, the plan for intervention also includes education of the patient, nursing staff, and caregivers. The patient and family should understand the cause of and prognosis for the patient's dysphagia and the importance of strategies to be carried out at home. It may be helpful to have the patient view the videofluoroscopy or fiberoptic endoscopy to fully comprehend his or her condition and the benefits of compensatory techniques. Mealtime positioning, adaptive equipment, and the type and amount of assistance must be taught to caregivers. Meal preparation practice and community outings can reinforce diet modifications, enhance patient and family education in various settings, and motivate the patient.

EFFECTIVENESS OF DYSPHAGIA INTERVENTION

Numerous studies cite the effectiveness of dysphagia intervention in both acute and chronic populations. More recent research is focusing on efficacy in the form of systematic reviews. One systematic review revealed that dysphagia interventions in acute stroke reduced incidence of aspiration pneumonia (Foley et al., 2008). Another demonstrated that compensatory swallowing and head positioning maneuvers can be effective in neurological populations (Ashford et al., 2009). Evidence Table 43-1 lists evidence for the benefits of occupational therapy interventions for dysphagia.

Studies have also evaluated the efficacy of specific intervention techniques in diagnostic cohorts. For instance, Logemann et al. (2008) concluded that providing honey-thick fluids was the most effective technique in eliminating aspiration in a population with Parkinson's disease and dementia. Other examples of proven therapeutic techniques to manage dysphagia are presented earlier in the chapter.

Although much research focuses on how well interventions eliminate aspiration from a clinical perspective, other studies evaluate how dysphagia interventions can improve the patient's quality of life. The SWAL-QOL and the SWAL-CARE tools assess quality of life and quality of care/patient satisfaction, respectively (McHorney et al., 2002). Since the publication of these and similar assessments and their publication in other languages, studies have been introduced to assess quality of life and care of patients with dysphagia around the world.

As the emphasis on evidence-based medicine and rehabilitation advances, clinicians must keep abreast of new knowledge. Useful resources on dysphagia care for both beginning- and advanced-level swallowing therapists are noted under Resources 43-1. The author encourages the reader to explore further learning and expertise in dysphagia care. In many facilities, problem-oriented rehabilitation team goals are supplanting discipline-specific goals to target improvement of specific abilities that pose barriers to discharge, creating a need for occupational therapists versed in dysphagia management. Early discharge from acute care and rehabilitation hospitals and minimized staffing in health care facilities create situations in which competence in dysphagia intervention has become a mandatory skill for occupational therapy practitioners. Occupational therapists, with their background in the many abilities and capacities that influence eating and swallowing, make logical primary swallowing therapists.

Compensatory Swallowing Maneuvers: Their Purpose and Execution

The following techniques are ways to use volitional movement to improve the quality of the pharyngeal swallow. Most of them are complex and require a good attention span and the ability to follow complex directions on the part of the patient.

Maneuver	Purpose	Execution
Chin tuck	Moves base of tongue back; narrows opening to larynx, protecting airway; helps protect airway when larynx is low and swallow is delayed; improves quality of the swallow (Ertekin et al., 2001)	Tuck chin down toward chest while swallowing
Effortful	Helps to elevate base of tongue (Lazarus et al., 2002)	Squeeze hard with throat muscles while swallowing
Mendelsohn maneuver	Prolongs opening of upper esophageal sphincter (UES) when larynx is low (Lazarus et al., 2002)	Push tongue into roof of mouth; try to keep Adam's apple up while swallowing
Neck rotation	Closes weaker side of pharynx; uses stronger intact musculature in cases of unilateral weakness of pharynx and/or vocal folds; improves quality of the swallow (Ertekin et al., 2001)	Turn head to the weaker side while swallowing
Supraglottic swallow	Compensates for weak vocal cord closure, reduces penetration of food into larynx during swallow by closing vocal cords (Lazarus et al., 2002)	Swallow while holding breath; then cough. Volitional cough after swallow helps to ensure that anything in airway returns to pharynx to be reswallowed.
Super-supraglottic swallow	Reduces penetration of food into larynx during swallow by narrowing opening to airway (Lazarus et al., 2002)	Hold breath and bear down; maintain breath-hold, keep bearing down while swallowing; cough after swallowing

Definition 43-4

Instrumental Intervention

Surface electromyography provides patients with improved awareness of swallowing function, providing for better swallowing. This intervention has been shown to be useful in populations with stroke (Crary et al., 2004; Freed et al., 2001). One example of this is VitalStim Therapy®, which uses a specially designed electrical stimulation unit with surface electrodes placed on the neck (Fig. 43-9).

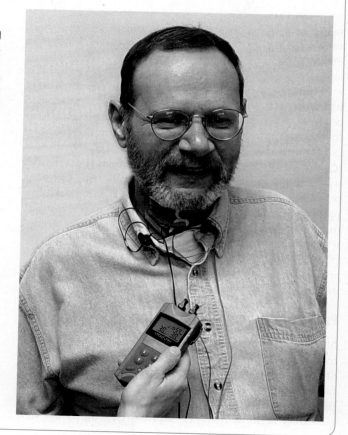

Figure 43-9 VitalStim, a specially developed neuromuscular stimulation unit that facilitates contraction of the muscles used in swallowing, in place on a dysphagic patient's neck. (©2005 Encore Medical, L.P. VitalStim is a registered trademark of VitalStim, LLC.)

| Evidence Table 43-1 | | Best Evidence for Dysphagia Interventions Used in Occupational Therapy | | | | |

Intervention	Description of Intervention Tested	Participants	Dosage	Type of Best Evidence and Level of Evidence	Benefit	Statistical Probability and Effect Size of Outcome	Reference
Remedial	Effect of thermal-tactile stimulation as assessed pre- and poststimulation by videofluoroscopy	Thirteen patients with Parkinson's disease and dysphagia	Thermal tactile stimulation applied to faucial pillars in pharynx	Pre-post non-experimental design Level III C1a	Yes. Median pharyngeal transit time for swallowing both fluid and paste textures was improved. Oral transit time was unaffected with both textures.	Pharyngeal transit time for fluids: $p = 0.004$; for paste $p = 0.01$	Regan, Walshe, & Tobin (2010)
Compensatory	Comparison of three interventions for aspiration in patients with dementia and/or Parkinson's disease: chin down posture, nectar-thickened liquids, and honey-thickened liquids	Seven hundred eleven patients who aspirated on thin liquids assessed with videofluoroscopy	1. Chin-down posture 2. Nectar-thickened liquids 3. Honey-thickened liquids	Randomized controlled study Level IA1a	Yes. Honey-thickened fluids were more effective than nectar-thickened fluids to eliminate aspiration, and both were more effective than chin-down position with thin fluids.	1. Chin down versus nectar thickened $p < 0.001$ 2. Chin down versus honey thickened $p < 0.0001$ 3. Nectar thickened versus honey thickened $p < 0.0001$	Logemann et al. (2010)

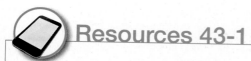

Resources 43-1

Dysphagia-Related Resources

American Dietetic Association

Offers National Dysphagia Diet:
Standardization for Optimal Care
Phone: 800-877-1600
http://www.eatright.org

Dysphagia Resource Center

www.dysphagia.com
This website provides information and links on anatomy
and physiology pertinent to dysphagia, organizations, print
materials, case studies, research information, and funding.
Information for clinicians and lay persons.

Dysphagia Evaluation Protocol

Pearson Assessment
Phone: 800-627-7271
http://www.pearsonassessment.com
Assessment of dysphagia in adults developed by
occupational therapists and tested for reliability and validity.
Chartable record form and easy-to-use flip book format.

Dysphagia Research Society

Houston, TX
www.dysphagiaresearch.org

Dysphagia

Official journal of the Dysphagia Research Society
Springer-Verlag
Phone: 713-965-0566
http://www.springer.de/
Peer-reviewed journal devoted to publication of scholarly
articles about dysphagia. Abstracts and subscription
information available online. Subscription information
available by telephone.

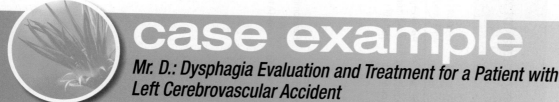

case example

Mr. D.: Dysphagia Evaluation and Treatment for a Patient with Left Cerebrovascular Accident

Occupational Therapy Process	Clinical Reasoning Process	
	Objective	Examples of Therapist's Internal Dialogue
Patient Information Mr. D. is an 73-year-old man with a left hemispheric cerebrovascular accident (CVA). He was admitted to an acute-care hospital with aphasia and right upper extremity weakness, with a prior history of hypertension, transient ischemic attacks (TIAs) with aphasia, and chronic heart failure.	Understand the patient's diagnosis or condition	"According to my experience and the literature, patients with dysphagia caused by an acute single stroke eventually swallow safely without compensatory techniques. However, Mr. D. has had prior TIAs (possible permanent damage), which may limit his swallowing recovery. I expect that his symptoms will resolve, at least in part. He does have some control of his lips, cheek, and tongue, but reduced competence of his airway protection skills indicate that oral feeding should proceed cautiously."
	Know the person	"Although he is frail, Mr. D. is enthusiastic about advancing his diet and participates fully in his dysphagia intervention, and I believe that he will take responsibility for following through with his rehabilitation program. He enjoys meals at home and assists with meal preparation. He has a supportive spouse who will help to carry over mealtime recommendations and exercise programs. Because he is ambulatory, I believe that follow-up dysphagia therapy will occur on an outpatient basis."

Reason for Referral to Occupational Therapy

Mr. D. was referred to occupational therapy for dysphagia intervention, as well as to improve his upper extremity skills including self-feeding. The medical staff wants to be sure that he does not need alternative nutritional routes (nasogastric feedings or intravenous) to nourish and hydrate himself while in the hospital and wants assurance that he is not at risk for aspiration. The doctors also want to assure that he can maintain his nutritional requirements so that he can safely be discharged home.

Assessment Process and Results

A dysphagia evaluation was done using the Dysphagia Evaluation Protocol (see Resources 43-1). The evaluation (Fig. 43-3) revealed that Mr. D. had hypotonicity and reduced control of his lips, cheek, and tongue on the right side. Decreased airway protection skills were evidenced by his inability to phonate because of vocal cord weakness, inability to cough volitionally, and reduced laryngeal elevation during swallowing. He was not aphasic. Mr. D. was able to swallow foods from the beginning level dysphagia diet, including foods with soft, moist textures, such as pudding and applesauce, with mild food spillage out of the mouth because of poor lip control, delayed formation and propulsion of the bolus, and delayed initiation of the swallow. He had difficulty grasping utensils and cups because of hypotonicity of his dominant right hand.

Occupational Therapy Problem List

1. Hypotonicity of oral, pharyngeal, and laryngeal structures, resulting in
   • delay in and reduced coordination of bolus control both in the mouth and in propelling the bolus posteriorly to initiate the swallow
   • delayed initiation of the swallow
2. Reduced upper extremity control, making use of his dominant arm to self-feed awkward

Occupational Therapy Goal List

(5 daily treatments prior to discharge)
1. Mr. D. will tolerate a more advanced dysphagia diet, adding soft chewables such as cooked fruit and soft pasta.
2. Mr. D. will tolerate these textures without clinical signs of aspiration (see Safety Note 43-2).
3. Mr. D. will be independent in vocal cord adduction exercises.
4. Mr. D. will support the right side of his lower lip and massage the right cheek during the oral preparatory stage to prevent food spillage and pocketing in his right cheek.
5. Mr. D. will feed himself with his right hand with built-up utensils and an adapted cup while weight bearing on his right elbow.

Appreciate the context	"Mr. D. is being seen as a hospital inpatient. Although eating and mealtime in this setting is very different from being home, because of natural recovery, his level of function may improve quickly, and I should be alert to update goals on a daily basis. I'll be working together with the dietician to care for Mr. D.; she will monitor that he is eating and drinking enough and initiate any changes in diet that I recommend."
Develop the provisional hypotheses	"Because Mr. D.'s muscle tone is low, I may be working with him to reinforce muscle activity for both muscles involved in swallowing and his upper extremity muscles involved in self-feeding."
Consider evaluation approach and methods	"I have chosen a standardized evaluation of dysphagia skills that also examines self-feeding and includes all components of swallowing that I need to assess."
Interpret observations	"Given the evaluation results and observation over the course of several meals, Mr. D. should be able to nourish and hydrate himself with supplementary (not by mouth) nutrition or hydration."
Synthesize results	"Reduced muscle tone is evidenced with both his swallowing and self-feeding."
Develop intervention hypotheses	"I believe that focusing occupational therapy within a functional mealtime context can efficiently address both swallowing and self-feeding."
Select an intervention approach	"Because Mr. D.'s stroke is acute and has great potential for improvement, the initial approach will be remedial, although a compensatory dysphagia modification will be used to reduce any possible risk of aspiration or laryngeal penetration at meal or snack time."
Consider what will occur in therapy, how often, and for how long	"Because Mr. D. has had an acute stroke, the intervention plan should be intensive; exercises should be done once or twice daily, and mealtime techniques be employed each time he eats, for both safety and to facilitate improvement."

Intervention

Mr. D. was seen daily for occupational therapy during a week as a hospital inpatient. Constant supervision at mealtime was accomplished, and all meals and snacks took place with him seated upright in the chair. Occupational therapy intervention addressed exercises and positioning to enhance tone and control of oral motor skills, laryngeal exercises to strengthen his vocal cords and improve laryngeal elevation, and facilitation of tone and movement in his hypotonic right upper extremity to improve self-feeding skills. Mr. D. and his caregiver were educated and given handouts on the nature of his dysphagia, exercises, and mealtime procedures and precautions.

Next Steps

Mr. D. was discharged from the hospital to home in the company of his wife. He and his wife were taught to thicken fluids with commercial thickeners at home. As his vocal cord strength returned, his volitional cough became stronger, and he gradually became able to speak in a loud whisper; laryngeal strengthening exercises continued. Mr. D. was able to discontinue use of external lip control strategies as oral motor control returned. He continued use of built-up utensils and weight bearing at the elbow while self-feeding. He continued with outpatient occupational therapy for 4 more weeks. During that time, the following long-term goals were accomplished:

1. Mr. D. will tolerate a regular diet consisting of a variety of solid and liquid textures, dry cut-up chewable solids, and thin liquids without signs or symptoms of aspiration.
2. Mr. D. will eat independently with his right upper extremity without use of adaptive equipment and without compensatory movements.

Assess the patient's comprehension Understand what he is doing Compare actual to expected performance Know the person	"Mr. D., with the help of his wife, was able to understand all instructions and followed through with the treatment plan. He was anxious to progress to his normal diet and eating habits. He understood that the supervision at mealtime and exercises would help him to improve and prevent complications such as aspiration. He demonstrated improvements daily, and although his appetite initially was limited, he showed definite improvement through the week in terms of his intake. His progress was on target with what I expected, given that he developed no further medical complications. Happily, he achieved his short-term goals within a week."
Anticipate present and future patient concerns Decide whether the patient should continue or discontinue therapy and/or return in the future	"I know that Mr. D. will likely be anxious to resume a normal diet and enjoy a normal range of food textures. I anticipate that he will also be concerned about being able to eat in a restaurant or with friends without his 'elbow on the table' weight-bearing strategy to improve his upper extremity control. For this reason and because of continued expected improvement, I'll continue to see him as an outpatient until the remedial long-term goals are accomplished. Once he has regained 'normal' function, I'll discharge him."

Clinical Reasoning in Occupational Therapy Practice

Determining Treatment Approach Based on Past Response to Therapy

Mr. D., the patient encountered in the case study, successfully completed six outpatient dysphagia therapy visits with his occupational therapist. He was able to achieve a normal swallow as shown by a follow-up modified barium swallow (MBS), and eat with his right hand. A month later, Mr. D. was rehospitalized with an acute episode of chronic heart failure, pneumonia, and recurrence of his right-sided weakness. During his intensive care stay, his swallowing was reevaluated, and his evaluation results were similar to those on his prior admission. However, he did not demonstrate progress, and experienced low levels of aspiration and hypotonicity on the right side of his face and oral structures, making bolus containment and mobilization difficult, and a continued delay of his swallow. How would your treatment approach be different with this second course of intervention?

Summary Review Questions

1. What are the stages of swallowing, and what events occur during each stage? Which stage or stages are most amenable to therapeutic intervention, and why?
2. What is aspiration, and what are its warning signs and symptoms?
3. Outline the three types of dysphagia; compare the specific dysphagia symptoms of selected diagnoses with the typical manifestations of the appropriate category: paralytic, pseudobulbar, and mechanical dysphagia.
4. Which components of a thorough dysphagia evaluation are most accurately completed with a patient who can follow multistep commands? How would you alter bedside evaluation for patients with various cognitive and perceptual deficits?
5. What are the instrumental evaluations for dysphagia, and how does the information that each provides assist in dysphagia rehabilitation?
6. What recommendations should a dysphagia evaluation provide?
7. Define compensatory and remedial and direct and indirect dysphagia treatments and provide examples of each for specific diagnoses.

Glossary

Aspiration—Entrance of food or secretions into the larynx below the level of the vocal cords.

Bolus—Food or liquid in the mouth.

Deglutition—The act of swallowing.

Direct therapy—Therapeutic techniques involving ingestion of food or liquids.

Dysphagia—Difficulty with any stage of swallowing.

Eating—Ingestion of food and liquid, including the preoral, oral preparatory, oral, pharyngeal, and esophageal stages.

Feeding—Taking or giving nourishment.

Fiberoptic endoscopic evaluation of swallowing (FEES)—Direct visualization of the swallow using a small illuminated camera at the end of a flexible tube (endoscope), which is introduced into the pharynx through the nose

Indirect therapy—Therapy addressing the prerequisite capacities associated with swallowing without ingestion of food or liquid.

Instrumental evaluation—Use of technology to assess aspects of swallowing.

Laryngeal penetration—Entrance of food or secretions into the larynx above the level of the vocal cords.

NPO (nil per os)—Latin for "nothing by mouth": no food or medication to be administered orally.

Swallowing—Ingestion of nourishment, beginning with introduction of food into the mouth and ending with reception of food into the stomach; includes the preoral, oral preparatory, oral, pharyngeal, and esophageal stages.

Videofluoroscopy—Moving radiographic images of swallowing structure and physiology, also known as "modified barium swallow study," recorded on videotape or DVD.

References

American Occupational Therapy Association. (2007). Specialized knowledge and skills for feeding, eating and swallowing in occupational therapy practice. *American Journal of Occupational Therapy, 61,* 686–700.

American Occupational Therapy Association. (2011). Fact sheet: Occupational therapy, a vital role in dysphagia care. Retrieved from www.aota.org/Practitioners/Resources/Docs/FactSheets/38514.

Ashford, J., McCabe, D., Wheeler-Hegland, K., Frymark, T., Mullen, R., Musson, N., Schooling, T., & Smith Hammond, C. (2009). Evidence-based systematic review: Oropharyngeal dysphagia behavioral treatments. Part III. Impact of dysphagia treatments on populations with neurological disorders. *Journal of Rehabilitation Research and Development, 46,* 195–204.

Avery-Smith, W., Rosen, A. B., & Dellarosa, D. (1997). *Dysphagia evaluation protocol.* San Antonio, TX: Harcourt Assessment.

Aviv, J. E., Martin, J. H., Sacco, R. L., Zagar, D., Diamond, B., Keen, M. S., & Blitzer, A. B. (1996). Supraglottic and pharyngeal sensory abnormalities in stroke patients with dysphagia. *Annals of Otology, Rhinology and Laryngology, 105,* 92–97.

Bakke, M., Larsen, S. L., Lautrup, C., & Karlsborg, M. (2011). Orofacial function and oral health in patients with Parkinson's disease. *European Journal of Oral Science, 19,* 27–32.

Bisch, E. M., Logemann, J. A., Rademaker, A. A. W., Kahrials, P. J., & Lazarus, C. L. (1994). Pharyngeal effects of bolus volume, viscosity, and temperature in patients with dysphagia resulting from neurologic impairment and in normal subjects. *Journal of Speech and Hearing Research, 37,* 10541–1059.

Borr, C., Hielscher-Fastabend, M., & Lücking, A. (2007). Reliability and validity of cervical auscultation. *Dysphagia, 22,* 225–234.

Cabre, M., Serra-Prat, M., Palomera, E., Almirall, J., Pallares, R., & Clavé, P. (2010). Prevalence and prognostic implications of dysphagia in elderly patients with pneumonia. *Age and Ageing, 39,* 39–45.

Carlaw, C., Finlayson, H., Beggs, K., Visser, T., Marcoux, C., Coney, D., & Steele, C. M. (2011). Outcomes of a pilot water protocol project in a rehabilitation setting. *Dysphagia, 27,* 297–306. Retrieved August 15, 2013 from http://www.springerlink.com/content/3r563v645028rj73/.

Crary, M. A., Carnaby Mann, G. D., Groher, M. E., & Helseth, E. (2004). Functional benefits of dysphagia therapy using adjunctive sEMG biofeedback. *Dysphagia, 19,* 160–164.

Crary, M. A., & Groher, M. E. (2003). *Introduction to adult swallowing disorders.* St. Louis: Butterworth-Heinemann.

Dettelbach, M. A., Gross, R. D., Mahlman, J., & Eibling, D. E. (1995). Effect of the Passy-Muir valve on aspiration in patients with tracheostomy. *Head and Neck, 17,* 297–302.

Ding, R., & Logemann, J. A. (2005). Swallow physiology in patients with trach cuff inflated or deflated: A retrospective study. *Head Neck, 27,* 809–813.

Eckberg, O., & Feinberg, M. (1992). Clinical and demographic data in 75 patients with near-fatal choking episodes. *Dysphagia, 7,* 205–208.

Edahiro, A., Hirano, H., Yamada, R., Chiba, Y., Watanabe, Y., Tonogi, M., & Yamane, G. Y. (2012). Factors affecting independence in eating among elderly with Alzheimer's disease. *Geriatrics & Gerontology International, 12,* 481–490.

Eisenstadt, S. E. (2010). Dysphagia and aspiration pneumonia in older adults. *Journal of the American Academy of Nurse Practitioners, 22,* 17–22.

Ertekin, C., Keskin, A., Kiylioglu, N., Kirali, Y., On, A. Y., Tarlaci, S., & Aydogdu, I. (2001). The effect of head and neck positions on oropharyngeal swallowing: A clinical and electrophysiologic study. *Archives of Physical Medicine and Rehabilitation, 82,* 1255–1260.

Foley, N. C., Martin, R. E., Salter, K. L., & Teasell, R. W. (2009). A review of the relationship between dysphagia and malnutrition following stroke. *Journal of Rehabilitation Medicine, 41,* 707–713.

Foley, N., Teasell, R., Salter, K., Kruger, E., & Martino, R. (2008). Dysphagia treatment post stroke: A systematic review of randomized controlled trials. *Age and Ageing, 37,* 258–264.

Freed, M. L., Freed, L., Chatburn, R. L., & Christian, M. (2001). Electrical stimulation for swallowing disorders caused by stroke. *Respiratory Care, 46,* 466–474.

Groher, M. E., Crary, M. A., Carnaby Mann, G., Vickers, Z., & Aguilar, C. (2006). The impact of rheologically controlled materials on the identification of airway compromise on the clinical and videofluoroscopic swallowing examinations. *Dysphagia, 21,* 218–225.

Gross, R. D., Mahlmann, J., & Grayhack, J. P. (2003). Physiologic effects of open and closed tracheostomy tubes on the pharyngeal swallow. *Annals of Otology, Rhinology, and Laryngology, 112,* 143–152.

Hara, I., Gellrich, N. C., Duker, J., Schon, R., Nilius, M. Fakler, O., Schmelzeisen, R., Ozeki, S., & Honda, T. (2003). Evaluation of swallowing function after intraoral soft tissue reconstruction with microvascular free flaps. *International Journal of Oral and Maxillofacial Surgery, 32,* 593–599.

Horner, J., Buoyer, F. G., Alberts, M. J., & Helms, M. J. (1991). Dysphagia following brainstem stroke. *Archives of Neurology, 48,* 1170–1173.

Latella, D., & Meriano, C. (2010). *Clinical evaluation of dysphagia in dysphagia care and related feeding concerns for adults* (2nd ed., pp. 83–120). Bethesda, MD: AOTA Press.

Lazarus, C. (2006). Tongue strength and exercise in healthy individuals and in head and neck cancer patients. *Seminars in Speech and Language Pathology, 27,* 260–267.

Lazarus, C. L., Logemann, J. A., Pauloski, B. R., Colangelo, L. A., Kahrilas, P. J., Mittal, B. B., & Pierce, M. (1996). Swallowing disorders in head and neck cancer patients treated with radiotherapy and adjuvant chemotherapy. *Laryngoscope, 106,* 1157–1166.

Lazarus, C., Logemann, J. A., Song, C. W., Rademaker, A.W., & Kahrilas, P. J. (2002). Effects of voluntary maneuvers on tongue base function for swallowing. *Folia Phoniatrica et Logopaedica, 54,* 171–176.

Leder, S. B., Suiter, D.M., & Green, B. G. (2011). Silent aspiration risk is volume-dependent. *Dysphagia, 26,* 304–309.

Leibovitz, A., Baumoehl, Y., Lubart, E., Yaina, A., Platinovitz, N., & Segal, R. (2007). Dehydration among long-term care elderly patients with oropharyngeal dysphagia. *Gerontology, 53,* 179–183.

Logemann, J. A., Gensler, G., Robbins, J. A., Brandt, D., Hind, J., Kosek, S., Dikeman, K., Kazandjian, M., Gramigna, G. D., Lundy, D., McGarvey-Toler, S., & Miller Gardner, P. J. (2008). A randomized study of three interventions for aspiration of thin liquids in patients with dementia or Parkinson's disease. *Journal of Speech, Language, and Hearing Research, 51,* 173–183.

Logemann, J. A., Gensler, G., Robbins, J. A., Lindblad, A., Brandt, D., Hind, J., Kosek, S., Dikeman, K., Kazandjian, M., Gramigna, G. D., Lundy, D., & McGarvey-Toler, S, & Gardner, P. J. M. (2010). A randomized study of three interventions for aspiration of thin liquids in patients with dementia or Parkinson's disease. *Journal of Speech Language Hearing Research, 51,* 173–183.

Logemann, J. A., Pauloski, B. R., & Colangelo, L. (1998). Light digital occlusion of the tracheostomy tube: A pilot study of effects on aspiration and biomechanics of the swallow. *Head and Neck, 20,* 52–57.

Logemann, J. A., Pauloski, B. R., Rademaker, A. W., & Kahrilas, P. J. (2002). Oropharyngeal swallow in younger and older women: Videofluoroscopic analysis. *Journal of Speech, Language, and Hearing Research, 45,* 34–44.

Logemann, J. A., Pepe, J., & Mackay, L. E. (1994). Disorders of nutrition and swallowing: Intervention strategies in the trauma center. *Journal of Head Trauma Rehabilitation, 9,* 43–56.

Macht, M., Wimbish, T., Clark, B. J., Benson, A. B., Burnham, E. L., Williams, A., & Moss, M. (2011). Postextubation dysphagia is persistent and associated with poor outcomes in survivors of critical illness. *Critical Care, 15,* 231–236.

Mackay, L. E., Morgan, A. S., & Bernstein, B. A. (1999). Swallowing disorders in severe brain injury: Risk factors affecting return to oral intake. *Archives of Physical Medicine and Rehabilitation, 80,* 365–371.

Maclean, J., Cotton, S., & Perry, A. (2009). Post-laryngectomy: It's hard to swallow: An Australian study of prevalence and self-reports of swallowing function after a total laryngectomy. *Dysphagia, 24,* 172–179.

McConnel, F. M. S., & O'Connor, A. (1994). Dysphagia secondary to head and neck cancer surgery. *Acta Oto-Rhino-Laryngologica Belgica, 48,* 165–170.

McHorney, C. A., Robbins, J., Lomax, K., Rosenbek, J. C., Chignell, K., Kramer, A. W., & Bricker, D. E. (2002). The SWAL-QOL and SWAL-CARE outcomes tool for oropharyngeal dysphagia in adults: III. Documentation of reliability and validity. *Dysphagia, 17,* 97–114.

Mendell, D. A., & Logemann, J. A. (2007). Temporal sequence of swallow events during the oropharyngeal swallow. *Journal of Speech Language and Hearing Research, 50,* 1256–1271.

Nguyen, N. P., Vos, P., Moltz, C. C. Frank, C., Millar, C., Smith, H. J., Dutta, S., Alfieri A., Lee, H., Martinez, T., Karlsson, U., Nguyen, L. M., Sallah, S. (2008). Analysis of the factors influencing dysphagia severity upon diagnosis of head and neck cancer. *British Journal of Radiology, 81,* 706–710.

Noyce, A. J., Silveira-Moriyama, L., Gilpin, P., Ling, H., Howard, R., & Lees, A. J. (2012). Severe dysphagia as a presentation of Parkinson's disease. *Movement Disorders, 27,* 457–458.

Pauloski, B. R. (2008). Rehabilitation of dysphagia following head and neck cancer. *Physical Medicine & Rehabilitation Clinics of North America, 19,* 889–928.

Pelletier, C. A., & Lawless, H. T. (2003). Effect of citric acid and citric acid-sucrose mixtures on swallowing in neurogenic oropharyngeal dysphagia. *Dysphagia, 18,* 231–241.

Poorjavad, M., Derakhshandeh, F., Etemadifar, M., Soleymani, B., Minagar, A., & Maghi, A. H. (2010). Oropharyngeal dysphagia in multiple sclerosis. *Multiple Sclerosis, 16,* 362–365.

Regan, J., Walshe, M., & Tobin, W. O. (2010). Immediate effects of thermal-tactile stimulation on timing of swallow in idiopathic Parkinson's disease. *Dysphagia, 25*, 207–215.

Robbins, J., Gangnon, R. E., Theis, S. M., Kays, S. A., Hewitt, A. L., & Hind, J. A. (2005). The effects of lingual exercise on swallowing in older adults. *Journal of the American Geriatrics Society, 53*, 1483–1489.

Robbins, J. A., Levine, R.L., Maser, A., Rosenbek, J.C., Kempster, G.L. (1993). Swallowing after unilateral cerebral stroke, Archives of Physical Medicine and Rehabilitation, 74, 1295-1300.

Rosenbek, J. C., Roecher, E. B., Wood, J. L., & Robbins, J. (1996). Thermal application reduces the duration of stage transition in dysphagia after stroke. *Dysphagia, 11*, 225–233.

Salvador, R., Watson, T. J., Herbella, F., Dubecz, A., Polomsky, M., Jones, C. E., Raymond, D. R., & Peters, J. H. (2009). Association of gastroesophageal reflux and O_2 desaturation: A novel study of simultaneous 24-h MII-pH and continuous pulse oximetry. *Journal of Gastrointestinal Surgery, 13*, 854–861.

Samuels, R., & Chadwick, D. D. (2006). Predictors of asphyxiation risk in adults with intellectual disabilities and dysphagia. *Journal of Intellectual Disability Research, 50*, 522–527.

Shaker, R., Easterling, C., Kern, M., Nitschke, T., Massey, B., Daniels, S., Grande, B., Kazandjian, M., & Dikeman, K. (2002). Rehabilitation of swallowing by exercise in tube-fed patients with pharyngeal dysphagia secondary to abnormal UES opening. *Gastroenterology, 122*, 1314–1321.

Solomon, N. P. (2006). What is orofacial fatigue and how does it affect function for swallowing and speech? *Seminars in Speech and Language, 27*, 268–282.

Stepp, C. E. (2012). Surface electromyography for speech and swallowing systems: Measurement, analysis, and interpretation. *Journal of Speech Language Hearing Research, 55*, 1232–1246.

Sullivan, P. B. (2008). Gastrointestinal disorders in children with neurodevelopmental disabilities. *Developmental Disabilities Research Review, 14*, 128–136.

Van der Maarel-Wierink, C. D., Vanobberben, J. N., Bronkhorst, E. M., Schols, J. M., & de Baat, C. (2011). Risk factors for aspiration pneumonia in frail older people: A systematic literature review. *Journal of the American Medical Directors Association, 12*, 344–354.

van Lieshout, P. H., Steele, C. M., & Lang, A. E. (2011). Tongue control for swallowing in Parkinson's disease: Effects of age, rate, and stimulus consistency. *Movement Disorders, 26*, 1725–1729.

Warnecke, T., Teisman, I., Maimann, W., Olenber, S., Zimmersman, J., Kramer, C., et al. (2008). Assessment of aspiration risk in acute ischaemic stroke: Evaluation of the simple swallowing provocation test. *Journal of Neurology, Neurosurgergy, & Psychiatry, 79*, 312–314.

Wesling, M., Brady, S., Jensen, M., Nickell, M., Starkus, D., & Escobar, N. (2003). Dysphagia outcomes in patients with brain tumors undergoing inpatient rehabilitation. *Dysphagia, 18*, 203–210.

Westergren, A., Karlsson, S., Andersson, P., Ohlsson, O., & Hallberg, I. R. (2001). Eating difficulties, need for assisted eating, nutritional status and pressure ulcers in patient admitted for stroke rehabilitation. *Journal of Clinical Nursing, 10*, 257–269.

Yamaya, M., Yanai, M., Ohrui, T., Arai, H., & Sasaki, H. (2001). Interventions to prevent pneumonia among older adults. *Journal of the American Geriatric Society, 49*, 85–90.

Acknowledgments

I thank Denise Jules, OTR, for her assistance with photographs used in this chapter. Thanks also to Bette Pomerleau, MS, SLP, and Ray Autiello, LPN, RT, formerly of Universal Mobile Services in Haverhill, Massachusetts, for their assistance with the videofluoroscopic image reproduced in this chapter.

44

Human Immunodeficiency Virus

Karin J. Opacich

Learning Objectives

After studying this chapter, the reader will be able to do the following:

1. Convey the social and epidemiological history of HIV/AIDS in the United States, focusing on the populations most prevalently infected.
2. Summarize the natural history of HIV and its concomitant social trajectory.
3. Extrapolate the effect of HIV/AIDS at points along the disease trajectory on the occupations of people within different populations.
4. Select tools and assessment strategies to ascertain the specific occupational needs of individuals living with HIV/AIDS.
5. Describe interventions to preserve, restore, and adapt meaningful occupations of individuals living with HIV/AIDS.

ince the symptoms associated with human immunodeficiency virus (HIV) were first described in 1981 (Gottlieb et al., 1981; Masur et al., 1981; Siegal et al., 1981), over a million cases have been recorded in the United States alone. Acquired immunodeficiency syndrome (AIDS) was officially defined in 1993 and periodically updated (Centers for Disease Control and Prevention [CDC], 1993), and surveillance systems for both HIV and AIDS have been established and revised by the Centers for Disease Control and Prevention (CDC, 1999; Nakashima & Fleming, 2003). HIV/AIDS is regarded as a global pandemic because it has dramatically affected nations and populations throughout the world. Initially thought to be a fatal diagnosis, life expectancies have increased because of advances in medical management. HIV/AIDS is now considered a chronic disease. Although the science associated with HIV/AIDS has rapidly compounded, arresting the disease still depends largely on individual compliance with prevention strategies. Biological and physical aspects of HIV/AIDS have been systematically studied and documented, but the more variable social trajectory is shaped by the sociopolitical context in which individuals experience the disease. Consequently, quality of life after diagnosis is highly contingent on resources, support, and access to relevant treatment. Among the services that can impact the lives of people with HIV/AIDS, occupational therapy can be valuable.

EPIDEMIOLOGICAL HISTORY

Epidemiologists have now established that HIV and AIDS are the result of human exposure to a chimpanzee virus in Africa that mutated perhaps as early as the 1920s. It is conjectured that this mutant viral strain has spread in modern times because of increased slaughter and consumption of primate meat, widespread prostitution, and use of contaminated needles. After reexamination of stored specimens, it appears that HIV entered the United States sometime in the 1970s (Armstrong, Calabrese, & Taege, 2005; Vahlne, 2009). In the ensuing years, an increasing incidence of rare cancers and opportunistic infections precipitated curiosity among health scientists (Fan, Connor, & Villareal, 2004).

THE GLOBAL PICTURE

According to the World Health Organization (WHO), 34 million people were living with HIV/AIDS by 2010 (WHO & UNAIDS, 2011), a figure revised downward from earlier estimates. Of those living with HIV/AIDS in 2010, 3.4 million were women and children. In the 2011 joint report of global progress, *Global HIV/AIDS Response* (WHO, 2011), between 2.4 and 2.9 million people were newly infected with HIV in 2010. Estimates of the extent of the global HIV/AIDS pandemic are complicated by differences in surveillance methodology. Although new measurement techniques have added to a more nuanced understanding of the pandemic, these changes have made comparisons over time especially difficult (Brookmeyer, 2010). Nevertheless, it does appear that annual AIDS-related deaths peaked at around 2.2 million in 2005 as compared to 1.8 million world deaths in 2010. The decline in deaths has been attributed to increased access to antiretroviral therapy particularly in sub-Saharan Africa (WHO, 2011).

It is now understood that populations and subgroups most affected by HIV/AIDS vary greatly by country. Epidemiological histories are similarly unique. The most common routes of transmission continue to be unprotected sex and injection drug use, but behavior varies from population to population. These variations have in part been attributed to prevailing social, economic, and political influences and conditions. The *Global HIV/AIDS Response* report cites six indicators that have contributed to improvements in the overall world outlook. First and foremost is the decline in new infections. Although many people in middle and lower income brackets remain untested and unaware of their HIV status, access to testing and counseling has increased, especially for pregnant women. By 2011, reportedly 22,400 health facilities were able to provide access to antiretroviral therapy, reducing the number of deaths and new infections. Highly effective pharmaceutical interventions have continued to diminish maternal–child infection, and children infected with HIV have increased access to drug therapies (WHO, 2011).

Although there has been irrefutable progress in managing and arresting the progression of HIV/AIDS globally, the three United Nations Millennium Goals (United Nations, 2012) associated with HIV/AIDS and tailored to each participating country remain unmet by middle- and low-income countries, most notably sub-Saharan Africa, where the epidemic is largest and where adult women are infected 1.4 times more often than men. New infections are on the rise in the Middle East and North Africa. Europe and Central Asia have achieved goals related to reduction of infant and child mortality but still struggle with containing both HIV and tuberculosis as a coexisting opportunistic infection (Pontali et al., 2011). A consortium of global agencies reiterates the ongoing need for collaboration and continuing investment in science and health infrastructure (Stuckler, Basu, & McKee, 2010).

HIV/AIDS in the United States

Unlike the epidemiological history in Africa, HIV/AIDS in the United States first manifested among gay men. In the early years of the epidemic in the United States, those considered most at risk for infection were gay men, people requiring blood products, and users of injected drugs (Fan, Connor, & Villareal, 2004). Women and children initially represented a very small proportion of those infected.

Although predicted transmission has been contained, men who have sex with men of all races still comprise the largest cohort of people with HIV/AIDS in the United States (CDC, 2012b). Data accumulated through 2009 show that women now represent nearly 25% of all people with HIV/AIDS and 23% of the new cases in the United States. Black women are infected at 15 times the rate of white women and more than 3 times the rate of Latinas. Incidence among children rose until studies in the late 1990s demonstrated that drug therapies administered during the perinatal period could reduce transmission from mother to child. HIV infection among infants has been diminished, with only 13 new cases reported in children younger than age 13 years in 2009 (CDC, 2011). According to the CDC, nearly 619,400 people have died in the United States during the epidemic. The best line of defense remains to be prevention, and there are still approximately 50,000 people in the United States newly infected with HIV each year.

THE DISEASE MECHANISM

HIV is a retrovirus that results in a gradual deterioration of the immune system. Once the virus enters the human body, it overwhelms the CD4+ T cells that usually defend the body against viruses. HIV uses the cell machinery to convert its own RNA into a form that can be recognized and replicated using the DNA of the host, a process called transcription. Once emitted into the cytoplasm of the cell, this reconfigured virus translates itself prolifically, producing new copies and long chains of viral proteins that mature into new infectious particles that are emitted into other cells (National Institute of Allergy and Infectious Diseases [NIAID], 2009, 2012). The most efficient vehicle for transmission is blood and contact with delicate mucosal tissue susceptible to cuts and tears. Studies have shown that HIV is not spread through casual contact with saliva, sweat, tears, urine, or feces. HIV status is confirmed by blood tests such as enzyme-linked immunosorbent assay (ELISA), which detects exposure to the HIV virus via the presence of antibodies, or Western blot, which targets the presence of the virus itself. Home screening kits are now available as well. Despite the availability of laboratory tests, initial diagnosis is sometimes not made until a person is hospitalized for pneumonia, persistent diarrhea, or other AIDS-related illness.

Although it is rare for health care providers to contract HIV through patient contact or even accidental needlesticks (NIAID, 2012), precautions (Safety Note 44-1) are advised, particularly if the provider is handling blood and blood products. Surgeons performing extraordinarily bloody procedures (e.g., orthopedists) are at greatest risk. Special care should be taken to avoid exposing HIV-positive persons to infectious agents because their compromised immunity makes them more vulnerable to serious infections.

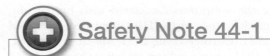

Safety Note 44-1

Standard Precautions

You must routinely use standard precautions to protect yourself from exposure to blood or body fluids from all patients, regardless of their diagnosis. Standard precautions consist of the use of protective barriers to prevent contamination of the skin, clothing, and mucous membranes (eyes, ears, and nose). Hepatitis B virus, hepatitis C virus, and HIV are communicated through blood-borne pathogens. Modes of transmission include sexual contact involving the sharing of body fluid, needlestick, contact with blood through mucous membranes or broken skin, childbirth, receiving blood or blood products, and organ transplantation. Proper use of protective barriers prevents exposure. Protect yourself by always following these recommendations:

- Wear and change gloves.
- Do not wash or decontaminate disposable (single-use) gloves.
- Wear a fluid- or moisture-resistant gown, apron, or lab coat when you anticipate contact with bodily fluids.
- Wear surgical cap and/or hood and shoe covers and/or boots when gross contamination is likely.
- Wear mask and eye protection with side shields and face shield when there is potential for splash, spray, or splattering of body fluids to the eyes, nose, or mouth.
- Wash your hands before and after contacting patients.
- Use a pocket mask or other ventilation guard device when doing cardiopulmonary resuscitation (CPR).

Needlestick or puncture is the most common mechanism for transmission for occupational therapists. To minimize risk, follow these precautions used by medical personnel:

- Use caution when handling all sharp objects.
- Do not bend, break, or manipulate items by hand.
- Place disposable sharp objects in a puncture-resistant container immediately after use.
- Do not recap or remove needles from syringe by hand unless no alternative exists.
- Use a device instead of your hand to pick up or remove contaminated needles or other sharp objects.
- Place reusable sharp objects in containers that are puncture resistant, leak proof on sides and bottom, and labeled.
- Use a mechanical device to clean up broken glassware.
- Promptly report all exposures to your supervisor and health care authorities.

SYMPTOMS

Within 2–4 weeks of initial exposure, most, although not all, people infected with HIV experience flulike symptoms, such as fever, headache, fatigue, and enlarged lymph nodes. Until the body's immune system is depleted of resources to combat the virus, the infected person may not experience further symptoms. Symptoms reported before progression to full-blown AIDS include lack of energy, weight loss, fevers and sweats, yeast infections, skin rashes, pelvic inflammatory disease unresponsive to treatment, and short-term memory loss. In many people, progression to AIDS takes 10–12 years, although approximately 10% of those who are HIV positive will progress to AIDS within 2–3 years of infection (NIAID, 2009, 2012). According to the prevailing CDC (1993) definition, HIV-infected people with fewer than 200 CD4 + T cells per cubic millimeter of blood and manifesting at least one Category C opportunistic illness are considered to have AIDS. As the disease progresses and opportunistic illnesses accrue, people with HIV often experience cognitive, motor, and behavioral manifestations including memory impairment, poor concentration, incoordination, weakness, irritability, and depression. More severe neurological deterioration may occur, especially with high viral loads (NIAID, 2009, 2012).

MEDICAL INTERVENTIONS AND ADVANCES

Clearly, the best treatment for HIV is prevention. Prevention strategies entail raising public awareness, providing education, and promoting individual behaviors that avoid risk or minimize harm. Prevention strategies can have a dramatic effect as illustrated by the reduction in the rates of new infection among gay men in Thailand where safe-sex campaigns have been successful (Curran, 2003). Bailey et al. (2007) established that male circumcision is effective in reducing HIV transmission in sub-Saharan Africa, where heterosexual infection is highest. Scientists continue to focus on developing effective barriers to the virus and vaccinations that would protect people from sexual transmission (Armstrong, Calabrese, & Taege, 2005).

For those already infected with HIV, advances in pharmaceutical interventions have made notable effect upon survival and extended years of quality life. It is no longer unusual for people to experience 15 or more years of quality life from the time of diagnosis. The use of zidovudine during pregnancy (CDC, 1994) is among the most successful advances; it dramatically reduces transmission of the virus to infants born to HIV-positive mothers to a rate of about 1% (NIAID, 2009, 2012). Even though they may test positively for antibodies to HIV at birth, only a very small number of newborns now go on to develop the disease. Because women tend to underestimate their risk and because prenatal transmission to infants can be prevented, in 2001, the CDC recommended that all pregnant women be routinely tested for HIV.

For seropositive adults, three categories of drugs have evolved and are currently used to treat HIV. Reverse transcriptase inhibitors interrupt the viral cycle early in its proliferation, and protease inhibitors interrupt it later. The third class of drugs, fusion inhibitors, interferes with viral reproduction by blocking the cell membrane, preventing permeation of HIV. Combination therapies, called highly active antiretroviral therapy or HAART, are aimed at curtailing HIV at multiple points along its reproductive cycle. For those who tolerate and respond to HAART, the drugs can retard the progression of HIV and even restore some immune functions for those with AIDS (NIAID, 2009, 2012). Long-term use of HAART does seem to be associated with detrimental side effects including fat redistribution, insulin resistance, poor lipid profiles, and increased risk of myocardial infarction (Armstrong, Calabrese, & Taege, 2005; NIAID, 2009, 2012).

PROGNOSIS AND MITIGATING FACTORS

Numerous strains of HIV have been identified, and the virus tends to customize itself within the individual. Some people seem to be more resistant to rapid translation than others. Viral load and strength of the particular HIV strain also seem to be associated with the rate of progression of the disease. Concurrent diseases or poor health status before infection can increase vulnerability and complicate medical interventions. Early detection of infections and adherence to medication regimens can prevent or slow the virus from usurping the entire immune system. Unfortunately, not everyone has access to testing, and not everyone responds positively to the drugs. For many people infected with HIV, sociopolitical circumstances erect barriers to health.

The Sociopolitical Context of HIV/AIDS

HIV infection is most frequently attributed to unprotected sexual intercourse and behaviors that are generally not socially acceptable, such as illegal intravenous drug use and commercial sex. Globally, HIV manifested initially in the heterosexual population, and infections rates are highest among women who have sex with men. Based on 2012 data, sub-Saharan Africa represents 68% of global HIV infections, and 59% of those infected are women (WHO, 2012). Impoverished individuals in poor countries with few resources are more vulnerable to the spread of HIV. History demonstrates that people tend to underestimate their risk of exposure, and HIV infections are now permeating the mainstream heterosexual population in the United States. People with HIV often report being stigmatized or marginalized, and the potential for discrimination is very real. In the United States, HIV is still most prevalent among men who have sex with men. Minorities, especially poor women of color, are disproportionately infected and vulnerable to exclusion, stigmatization, and discrimination (Dean et al., 2005; Duffy, 2005). The distribution of HIV represents one among many disconcerting health disparities globally and in the United States.

Gay Men

Although discrimination against gay men has long been an issue, the gay community has some attributes that yielded some positive preventive responses. Higher levels of education, access to resources, and community mobilization allowed the gay community to promote education and prevention strategies (Curran, 2003; Fan, Connor, & Villareal, 2004). Concerns about confidentiality and employer discrimination may deter access to appropriate health care. To be effective, occupational therapists providing treatment to gay and bisexual men must be culturally sensitive. Non-traditional life partners and families are likely to be involved in care, and the occupational therapist should be aware that the gay community has established many agencies, programs, and support networks that can enhance quality of life for people living with HIV/AIDS.

Women with HIV/AIDS

Poor women of color are disproportionately represented among those with HIV infection. According to the 2010 population data, African Americans and Hispanics together constitute approximately 30% of the total population but bear a disproportionate disease burden. For all U.S. HIV cases, 39.7% represent black women, and 11.8% represent Latina women in stark contrast to 2.6% among white women (CDC, 2011, 2012b, 2013; U.S. Census Bureau, 2010). Similar to their international counterparts, the women are generally socioeconomically disadvantaged and often disempowered. Their stories often reveal family violence, disrupted education, dependency on exploitive men, and engagement in high-risk behaviors such as drug and alcohol use and commercial sex (Gielen et al., 2007). General health literacy is poor, and health status even before infection may have been compromised. Therapists need to be particularly sensitive to the context in which these women live to avoid unreasonable expectations of them and exposure to increased harm from unempathic people. To attend to their own health, these women may need housing and transportation assistance, child care, and partner or family counseling.

People Who Abuse Drugs and Alcohol

For people who have been actively using drugs and/or alcohol, sobriety is critical to improving health. HIV infection often leads to an epiphany that provides a powerful incentive for getting clean and sober (Opacich, 2004). Because chemical dependency is a complex biopsychosocial phenomenon, it is important to collaborate closely with expert colleagues and to encourage participation in programs designed to support sobriety.

Effect on Scientific and Health Resources

Despite the tremendous social and economic effect of HIV/AIDS on nations worldwide, resources are still inadequate to meet needs. Over the years, programs have emerged that attend to the social complexities as well as the medical needs of people with HIV/AIDS. Many of these programs rely on grants and resources from international, state, federal, and private agencies. Treating HIV/AIDS successfully requires an array of health and human services and a culturally competent workforce to deliver those services. Labor statistics reveal shortages in many of those disciplines.

Using an accounting tool developed by UNAIDS (the Joint United Nations Programme on HIV/AIDS), data were collected from 28 countries to determine what proportion of total health care spending went to prevention and treatment of HIV/AIDS in sub-Saharan Africa where the infection rates are highest. The authors concluded that 19.4% of total health spending, reflecting billions of dollars, went to HIV prevention and treatment and translated to $9.34 to $118 spent per capita (Amico, Aran, & Avila, 2010). In the United States, the 2012 presidential budget request included $28.4 billion, a 34% increase over the 2007 budget request, for domestic and global HIV/AIDS-related activities, which represents less than 1% of the total federal budget. Of that total request, 53% ($14.9 billion) was allocated for treatment and 4% ($1 million) for prevention (Kaiser Family Foundation, 2011). In the United States, efforts toward the prevention of AIDS, along with other sexually transmitted diseases, have largely been funded by the CDC. According to CDC surveillance data from 2009, each new case of HIV is expected to accrue an average lifetime cost of $379,668 (in 2010 dollars) (CDC, 2012a). Savings from prevention efforts (cases averted) from 2001 to 2006 totaled $129.9 billion. The Ryan White Comprehensive AIDS Resources Emergency Act (CARE Act) (Government Accounting Office, 2005) provided over $2.3 billion in assistance including drug subsidies to individuals and families through state-administered programs in FY 2012 (Kaiser Family Foundation, 2013). However, poor health literacy, disempowerment, and stigmatization may still limit access to health resources.

CONTRIBUTION OF OCCUPATIONAL THERAPY IN THE TREATMENT OF HIV/AIDS

A growing body of professional literature attests to successful and potential occupational therapy contributions in addressing the needs of people with HIV/AIDS. Disease trends have stimulated research about the particular needs of women and the challenges people with HIV face in returning to work. To date, most of the literature has yielded program recommendations and educational strategies rather than evidence of effectiveness. Occupational therapy interventions for HIV/AIDS can be enhanced by the use of instruments that address underlying abilities and capacities that lead to competency in occupational performance and that measure outcomes of therapy.

Neurobiological Changes That Affect Occupation

At times, it can be difficult to distinguish symptoms associated with HIV/AIDS and those related to the treatment of the virus. Nevertheless, these symptoms can impact quality of life. For many years, the Whalen Symptom Index (Whalen et al., 1994) has been used to indicate how frequent and troublesome the symptoms are. Since the 1990s, over 30 indices designed to capture both the severity and the individual's experience of symptoms have emerged. These indices include the Revised Sign and Symptom Checklist for HIV (Holzemer et al., 2001), the HIV/AIDS Stress Scale (Pakenham & Rinaldis, 2002), the World Health Organization QOL HIV Instrument (Fang, O'Connell, & WHO HIV/AIDS Quality of Life Group, 2002), the Body Image Scale (Martinez et al., 2005), and the Assessment of Body Change and Diarrhea Scale (Guaraldi et al., 2006). Combined with other data, a symptom index informs the occupational therapist and other health providers so they may help the person with HIV to manage symptoms.

Based on the outcome of these assessments, occupational therapists can recommend lifestyle modifications and compensatory strategies to cope with symptoms. O'Brien et al. (2010) compiled a summary review of instruments used to describe disability as experienced by people with HIV that occupational therapy practitioners may find useful in their work. Another group led by Worthington et al. (2012) reviewed instruments and evidence specific to workforce participation, some of which are reflective of occupation.

Psychosocial Manifestations

Awareness of the social trajectory is equally important in the treatment of people with HIV/AIDS. As with any serious illness, initial diagnosis is usually followed by a grief response. Depression is common both initially and intermittently throughout the disease process. Education is vitally important at this time because many misperceive HIV as a certain and imminent death sentence. Some programs link newly diagnosed people with a peer outreach worker who can comfort and inform them about HIV and helpful resources. If connected to relevant services, the person with HIV is less likely to become socially isolated or marginalized. As the disease progresses, neurological changes may predispose the person with HIV to mood swings, prolonged depression, and cognitive impairment. Occupational therapists should be prepared to employ psychosocial strategies to combat the psychomotor retardation that often accompanies depression and

to facilitate participation in family and community life (see Chapter 30).

Fatigue and Its Effect on Occupation

Among the most vexing symptoms of HIV is fatigue. Fatigue in contrast to tiredness is pervasive and persistent, contributing to a kind of occupational inertia. Although fatigue is associated with numerous diseases and disorders, it can affect people with HIV even when they are healthy and stable. There have been many attempts to discern the causes of fatigue in HIV (Jong et al., 2010). Most often, conclusions point to depression and anxiety in the absence of medical explanations. Some studies suggest that pharmacotherapies, for example, zidovudine or HAART, may themselves be responsible for fatigue. Stressful life events such as unemployment seem to contribute, as do poor sleep and coexisting medical conditions. Whatever the source, fatigue can be disabling and must be considered when addressing occupations (Stout & Finlayson, 2011).

It is suggested that practitioners use an assessment tool to measure the extent of fatigue that the client is experiencing to determine the effect on meaningful engagement. One such tool is the seven-item version of the Fatigue Severity Scale (Lerdal et al., 2011). Another assessment, the Energy Conservation Strategies Survey (Mallik et al., 2005) has been found to be useful in measuring changes in behaviors surrounding fatigue. Any number of qualitative and/or quantitative assessments in the occupational therapist's repertoire can enhance insight into the lived experience of a person with HIV that can lead to strategies to support participation and meaningful engagement (See additional discussion in Chapter 3).

With a clear understanding of the client's fatigue, the occupational therapy practitioner can assist in selecting appropriate strategies. Work simplification and energy conservation are long-standing tools. Habit training and lifestyle counseling may also be useful. Just being HIV positive entails rigorous adherence to medication regimens and frequent health care appointments that may exacerbate fatigue, and practitioners can assist clients to establish schedules and routines to maximize their energy. Some findings suggest that physical exertion is important in reducing feelings of fatigue, and therapists can help clients to select and to plan physical activities that benefit them.

Framing Occupational Problems and Developing Interventions

HIV insinuates itself into the human body and into every aspect of daily life. Although the diagnosis of HIV is devastating to some people, it becomes the vehicle to a more meaningful and productive life to others. An individual's response to untoward events, including HIV infection, seems to depend on both internal and external resources and individual capacities. When establishing goals for occupational therapy treatment, it will help the therapist to think in terms of occupational role integrity, occupational competencies, and overall occupational coherence.

Because occupational functioning is the culmination of abilities and capacities that shape activities, tasks, and roles, multiple strategies may be needed to sort out occupational dysfunction. Although some problems in occupation may be directly attributable to AIDS-related illness, others may reflect contextual challenges or histories that prevented the development of occupational competency.

Integrity of Occupational Roles

In the initial interview, the occupational therapist working with a person with HIV/AIDS needs to develop a clear picture of the roles that characterize the person's life. Depending on the point along the disease trajectory at which the therapist encounters the recipient of services, evidence of role strain, role disruption, or role abandonment may be present. The therapist may find it useful to plot the person's role status on the Matrix of Occupational Status (Table 44-1) to establish a baseline for decision making and intervention.

Role Strain. The occupational therapist should ascertain whether the HIV-positive person is responsible for the care of others. If there are children, life partners, elderly adults, or even pets in the household, the person with HIV may be experiencing the strain of taking care of others given the added burden of managing HIV. In addition, others in the family, however that family is constituted, may also have HIV.

Most people sustain multiple roles, and life is an exercise of juggling priorities and meeting obligations. Some individuals are very tenacious about their roles, even when their health is compromised. Because those with HIV frequently experience fatigue, it is important to designate time for rest and restoration throughout the day. The occupational therapist can help the person with HIV to establish role priorities, reserving time and energy to attend to personal health needs. This may entail negotiating and relinquishing some responsibilities and tasks to others or arranging for support (e.g., homemaker services).

Role Disruption. When immune system failure results in illness, the person with HIV might be confined to bed or

Table 44-1　Matrix of Occupational Status for People with HIV/AIDS

Occupational Domain	Occupational Role	Discontinued	Disrupted	Adapted	No Change	Expanded
Work	Parent/caregiver Homemaker (IADL) Employee Entrepreneur Vocational trainee Student					
Play/leisure	Participant/observer Spectator Hobbyist Athlete					
Self-care	Personal care (ADL) IADL Health-related care Self-advocacy Intimacy/sexual expression Spiritual/devotional expression					
Description of occupational context	Neighborhood/ community Home environment Health care setting Social network Employment setting					

By writing brief narratives regarding specific occupational roles in the box(es) corresponding to the domain/role status, the therapist can develop an occupational profile that can be used to generate therapeutic goals and priorities.
ADL, activities of daily living; IADL, instrumental activities of daily living.

hospitalized for brief or extended periods of time. This is not an unusual pattern and should be anticipated. The occupational therapist can help to plan strategies for dealing with health emergencies. Such strategies may include identifying babysitters, notifying family members, enlisting help from neighbors, calling health care providers, and arranging sick leave. When the individual with HIV is ready to resume a former role after a period of illness, the occupational therapist can assess, modify, and design rehabilitative strategies consistent with the person's state of health and abilities.

Role Abandonment. Many stories elicited from people with HIV reveal role abandonment. For those whose lives were dominated by chemical dependency, development may have been arrested and efforts diverted to the procurement of drugs or alcohol. For others who are HIV positive, depression or shame may have interrupted life plans. For still others, the symptoms and sequelae of HIV itself may have prevented full participation. Whatever the case, if reasonable health can be restored, then the occupational therapist may be the primary facilitator of role resumption or role exploration.

Occupational Competencies

At the start of therapy, the occupational therapist should generate a list of occupational competencies or skills relative to the roles the client fulfills. For example, if remunerative employment is relevant, the occupational therapist can help to delineate the skills the client has or needs to acquire to resume or pursue work. Some people with HIV/AIDS who had been unable to work have been restored to a level of health through HAART that makes employment feasible again (Kielhofner et al., 2004a). The therapist might advocate on behalf of the client to accommodate special needs (e.g., flexible work schedules, longer rest periods, or accommodations for adaptive equipment). The occupational therapist may need to assist clients to develop strategies to compensate for low vision or for poor coordination.

If the HIV-positive person is a homemaker, establishing routines to accomplish cleaning, shopping, laundry, and so on will be important. Safety in the kitchen, especially when handling sharp utensils, will prevent exposure of others to HIV-positive blood. If the person is living with family members or friends, the occupational therapist can help the individual to negotiate household responsibilities, rest and privacy needs, and accurate understanding of HIV/AIDS and healthy behaviors. Work simplification and energy conservation principles may be useful for coping with changes in strength, endurance, and sequencing tasks and activities. It is important to acknowledge that many people living with HIV/AIDS are impoverished and may be living in poor housing and unsafe environments, which

pose additional challenges. For some, the social assistance surrounding HIV care may present new housing opportunities; the occupational therapist can guide the person through the establishment of a household, from obtaining utilities to paying bills to preparing meals.

Occupational Coherence

Occupational coherence speaks to the complementarity of roles, routines, habits, and behaviors that contribute to a life that, in totality, makes sense (Opacich, 2004). Coherence is a notion introduced by Antonovsky (1987), a sociologist, and later expanded by Nyamathi (1993). Coherence was first applied to occupations by Christiansen (1999) and Christiansen, Little, and Backman (1998) as an indicator for outcomes in the face of threats to health. Research on women with HIV/AIDS illustrated the construct by contrasting the lives of women living amidst chaos and uncertainty with those whose lives were more coherent (Opacich, 2004). If a person is ill with HIV, actively chemically dependent, and homeless, one would not describe that person as leading an occupationally coherent life. If that same person became sober, adhered to medical recommendations for arresting HIV, procured safe housing, and resumed remunerative employment, life would appear to be occupationally coherent and built on meaningful doing. The ultimate goal of occupational therapy with people with HIV might well be the achievement of occupational coherence.

Assessment

Occupational therapists use both qualitative and quantitative assessments to determine the occupational needs of persons with HIV/AIDS.

Qualitative Assessment Strategies

Each theoretical model of occupation is associated with instruments and strategies for framing occupation. An array of qualitative tools reflecting the naturalistic paradigm can be useful to reveal the nature of experience, in this case how an individual experiences HIV. Among these strategies, semistructured interviews can elicit narrative reflecting occupations. One of the published narrative tools, the *Occupational Performance History Interview II*, is reflective of the Model of Human Occupation (Kielhofner et al., 2004b). This particular template is used to probe how a given illness, condition, or untoward event shaped or altered the person's occupations. These narrative data can be analyzed by a number of ways and used to generate plans and strategies for reconstructing occupation. Based on the same model, two other instruments, the *Occupational Self-Assessment* (Baron et al., 2006) and the *Worker Role Interview* (Braveman et al., 2005) may be useful.

Quantitative Assessment Strategies

Quantitative strategies are useful when the phenomenon in question is well defined and the query is focused. An example of a quantitative criterion-referenced tool useful for people with AIDS is the *Assessment of Motor and Process Skills* (Fisher, 2012). This tool enables the therapist to observe the person with HIV engaging in familiar tasks, to quantify and compare the person's occupational performance, and to recommend strategies and levels of support necessary for safe living. The therapist might consider incorporating quality-of-life measures that reflect occupations and inform decision making (Robinson, 2004). Another developing occupational therapy tool for measuring the effects of neurocognitive impairment on task performance is the *PRPS (Perceive, Recall, and Perform System of task analysis)* (Ranka & Chapparo, 2010).

Intervention: Preserving, Restoring, and Adapting Meaningful Doing

The Occupational Functioning Model organizes roles and the definition of self into self-maintenance, self-advancement, and self-enhancement (see Chapter 1). Occupational therapy may address any or all of these aspects with the person with HIV/AIDS, depending on the occupational status of that person both before and after HIV infection. As previously noted, some cohorts of people with HIV have led marginal lives that are likely to have stymied their occupational potential.

Preservation

In the early stages of HIV infection, it is important that the individual resume or establish routines, habits, and behaviors that preserve healthfulness. Along with established roles, the newly diagnosed person must now incorporate medication regimens and attend appointments for regular lab tests and check-ups. For those whose lifestyles involved drug use or commercial sex, HIV treatment also entails intensive redirection, psychotherapy, and peer support. If pharmaceutical interventions or the virus itself results in symptoms, the person with HIV can face additional challenges in work, parenting, self-care, or other occupational pursuits. Whether the patient is a child or an adult, preserving and adapting occupational roles is critically important for both physical and mental health. For people whose lifestyles entailed maladaptive behaviors, occupational therapy may well require

role exploration that may have been derailed in childhood or adolescence or abandoned in adulthood. Strategies may include parenting classes, practicing independent living skills (e.g., laundry), and job training/retraining.

Restoration

As the disease progresses, it is common for people to experience periods of ill health and disruption of normal routines. Those with HIV/AIDS are immunocompromised and are therefore susceptible to illness and opportunistic infections. Improvement in health can occur when symptoms are addressed and HIV medication regimens bolster the immune system. Similar to cardiac rehabilitation, occupational therapy can be useful while the person is reconditioning and the illness is abating. During these times, therapy may entail work simplification or rebuilding endurance. Roles, routines, and habits related to work, self-care, and leisure may need to be negotiated and adjusted. When symptoms persist or abilities are permanently altered, the occupational therapist and the HIV-positive client should focus on adaptation.

Adaptation

As the immune system is overwhelmed, the person with HIV/AIDS is likely to lose abilities. Sensory deficits, weakness, incoordination, compromised memory, and other sequelae can compromise occupational roles and independent living. During this stage of illness, occupational therapy can facilitate adaptations that enable the person with HIV/AIDS to participate in daily life as fully as possible. This may entail environmental adjustments, adaptive strategies or assistive devices, personal assistance, or changes in living situation (see Chapters 18, 25, 27, and 28).

EVIDENCE OF EFFECTIVENESS OF OCCUPATIONAL THERAPY FOR PERSONS WITH HIV/AIDS

The literature pertaining to occupational therapy in HIV/AIDS is largely phenomenological. It reflects the experience of people with HIV/AIDS and informs the development of programs and services. A number of those studies have been mentioned in this chapter. Very few studies have been designed to examine particular interventions or to quantitatively measure effectiveness of occupational therapy interventions (see Evidence Table 44-1).

Evidence Table 44-1 | Best Evidence for Occupational Therapy Practice Regarding HIV/AIDS

Intervention	Description of Intervention Tested	Participants	Dosage	Type of Best Evidence and Level of Evidence	Benefit	Statistical Probability and Effect Size of Outcome	Reference
Four-phase vocational program: (1) 8 weeks of self-assessment and preparation for work, (2) effort to reacquire productive roles through experiences, (3) support successful employment, and (4) support sustained employment	Model of Human Occupation (MOHO)–based program customized to individual needs to explore, develop skills, and seek employment	Convenience sample of 129 men and women with HIV/AIDS (106 males, 21 females, and 2 transgendered persons; mean age = 41 years); 30% attrition rate (39 of 129 participants)	Phase 1: 8 weeks, group session one time a week plus individual sessions; length of subsequent phases varied by individual.	Qualitative research Participatory action research to examine and improve the program as it unfolded Level: N	Yes, 50 participants achieved employment, 2 returned to school, and 8 participated in volunteer or internship programs from 6 to 24 months after the program. Persons with a history of mental illness were more likely to benefit.	Ninety participants completed program; 67% of those achieved successful outcome (achieved employment, returned to school, or started volunteering); effect size not reported.	Kielhofner et al. (2004b)
A program designed to increase productive participation; implemented in supported living environments	Experimental treatment based on MOHO and the Social Model of Disability: Enabling Self-Determination (ESD) aimed at achieving productive participation (employment, school or training, volunteering), consisted of group sessions focused on empowerment and the employment process, use of peer mentors; individual meetings with therapists on request. Control: standard care: education related to employment and productivity, written materials on community resources, option of individual meetings with therapists.	Sixty-five recruited; 38 (31 men; 7 women) received ESD and 27 (21 men; 6 women) received control treatment. Seventy percent African American. No significant differences between groups before or after attrition; 29.3% attrition	Both conditions overseen by occupational therapists. ESD: 2-hour initial evaluation session that focused the participant, eight 1-hour weekly group sessions, optional individual sessions for client-driven consultation, peer mentoring. Control: 1-hour peer week for 8 weeks group sessions, monthly presentations on employment & productivity for 9 months, written materials, optional meetings with therapist. Evaluation at 3, 6, and 9 months.	Nonrandomized two-group design Level: IIC2a	Yes. The ESD group achieved higher levels of participation than the control group at each interval of the study.	Intention-to-treat analysis indicated significantly more ESD participants were engaged productively: 3 months: $\chi^2_{(df=1)} = 6.08$ ($p = 0.015$), odds ratio (OR) = 3.89; 6 months: $\chi^2_{(df=1)} = 8.88$ ($p = 0.004$), OR = 5.44; 9 months: $\chi^2_{(df=1)} = 5.75$ ($p = 0.018$), OR = 3.96. The ORs indicate large effects for the ESD program, with those participants twice as likely to be productively engaged at all three time points.	Kielhofner et al. (2008)

(continued)

Evidence Table 44-1 | Best Evidence for Occupational Therapy Practice Regarding HIV/AIDS (continued)

Intervention	Description of Intervention Tested	Participants	Dosage	Type of Best Evidence and Level of Evidence	Benefit	Statistical Probability and Effect Size of Outcome	Reference
A 2-year pilot program to improve balancing health, work, and daily life that combined job skills training with chronic disease self-management	The job skills training program entailed daily participation to which six biweekly sessions were added to address disease self-management, vocational health, performance, and quality of life.	Six groups of adults (n = 53) participated in the program over a 2-year period, 28 females and 25 males diagnosed with HIV 4+ years. Forty-two participants contacted 3–5 months postintervention. Twenty-one percent lost to follow-up.	For 6–7 weeks, 6 hours per day. Six 1.5-hour self-management focused sessions were integrated into an existing job skills training program to facilitate transition to work. Topics included balancing work and daily life, energy conservation, and nutrition.	Nonrandomized groups (6) received the same intervention over a 2-year period with pre- and postexamination of up to 42 individuals on key outcomes as measured by 11 scales, including the Canadian Occupational Performance Measure. Level: IIIB2b	Yes. Fifty-two percent of retained participants were working successfully, with another 41% actively seeking employment.	Outcome was determined using paired t tests and effect sizes. Three of the 11 scales indicated moderate to large effect sizes upon follow-up: perceived ability to balance health, work, and daily life ($r = 0.46$); health management and work ($r = 0.61$); and perceived ability to work ($r = 0.72$). However, only perceived ability to work showed significant ($p = 0.00$) improvement after treatment, which indicates that the outcome is probably not due to chance.	Bedell (2008)

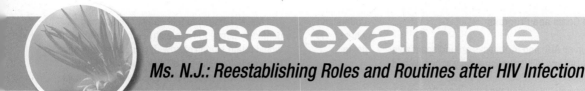

case example

Ms. N.J.: Reestablishing Roles and Routines after HIV Infection

Occupational Therapy Intervention Process	Clinical Reasoning Process	
	Objectives	Examples of Therapist's Internal Dialogue

Patient Information

Ms. N.J., a 49-year-old African American female with AIDS, participated in an outpatient occupational therapy assessment. The following problems were identified: (1) insufficient endurance for some activities of daily living (ADL) and instrumental activities of daily living (IADL), (2) mild memory impairment and confusion that interferes with self-care, (3) ambiguity of roles and routines, (4) intermittent loss of balance impacting environmental mobility, and (5) paresthesias that affect the execution of fine motor tasks.

The assessment process in general, including ascertaining personal background information, is described in Chapters 3–9.

Appreciate the context — "Ms. N.J.'s poor endurance is a direct result of her extended hospitalization and convalescence, during which she was bedridden and tube fed. Since her recovery, she has abandoned former dysfunctional pursuits, leaving her to redefine her roles, habits, and routines. Her remaining symptoms are natural sequelae of HIV/AIDS and/or drug interventions."

Select an intervention approach — "The first order of therapy will be to identify critical ADL and IADL that support recovery, such as adherence to medication regimens, establishing intermittent rest periods, and planning for proper nutrition. Given the reported sensory and cognitive issues, precautions and compensatory strategies need to be implemented to assure the patient's safety. Finally and probably most importantly, the patient needs to be supported in her role exploration and resumption for maximal participation in family and community life."

Reflect on competence — "Do I have adequate understanding of the relevant epidemiology, neurobiology, pharmacology, and psychodynamics? Am I sufficiently culturally competent, and can I be effective with this patient? I will need to collect tools and strategies for role exploration and practice any specific administration protocols."

Recommendations

The occupational therapist recommended home-based care two times a week initially for 4 weeks and one time a week for the next 2 months. In collaboration with Ms. N.J., goals for treatment were established as follows: (1) Ms. N.J. will identify which ADL and IADL tasks are indispensable to her management of HIV and will establish a daily schedule and record system for these, (2) Ms. N.J. will learn and implement home safety strategies relying on cue cards posted where most needed, and (3) Ms. N.J. will explore two roles or interests that will lead to safe and productive use of time.

Consider what will occur in therapy, how often, and for how long

Ascertain the patient's endorsement of plan

"Since the initiation of the highly active antiretroviral therapy (HAART) protocol, Ms. N.J. has been slowly regaining her health and is more hopeful than she has been in years. She describes herself as having died and been reborn to a different life, and she says that she is actually grateful for HIV. She sees herself as having some special purpose. Because she once had many occupational competencies, she seems eager and able to reach her goals. Ms. N.J. is currently residing with her daughter and young grandchildren; they have agreed to support her in these goals and to be present for at least one in-home occupational therapy session each week."

Summary of Short-Term Goals and Progress

1. Ms. N.J. will identify which ADL and IADL tasks are indispensable to her management of HIV and will establish a daily schedule and a record system for these.

    Ms. N.J. and her therapist identified the following ADL and IADL tasks as indispensable: 15 minutes of morning meditation, showering once a day, preparing her own breakfast and lunch, eating her evening meal with the family, taking her medications at 6-hour intervals, and taking a nap for 1 hour in the afternoon. Ms. N.J. developed a schedule for herself that she kept next to her bed and checked off after completing each task. At each occupational therapy session, the therapist reviewed these with Ms. N.J. and addressed any problems.

2. Ms. N.J. will learn and implement home safety strategies relying on cue cards posted where most needed.

    Ms. N.J. and her therapist practiced safe methods of handling sharp objects in the kitchen and posted pictures of her using these procedures under the cabinets. With the assistance of the therapist, the family installed grab bars in the bathroom. The therapist also instructed Ms. N.J. in the use of a walker for those days when her balance felt precarious. Ms. N.J. also generated a list of emergency numbers that she programmed into her cell phone. The family also established a call system to check on her well-being.

3. Ms. N.J. will explore two roles or interests that will lead to safe and productive use of time.

    Through interviews with the therapist, Ms. N.J. will tell stories of things that she did in the past that she found enjoyable and fulfilling. Responding to the *Occupational Performance History Interview*, Ms. N.J. related that she loved to sing, and she began attending choir practice one evening a week and singing in the church choir on Sundays. She also decided that she would like to try working in her daughter's grocery store, and she began doing this for 2 hours two times a week in the early afternoon.

Next Steps

Revised short-term goals (1 month):

- Ms. N.J. will identify one household task for which she will take responsibility on a daily basis.
- Ms. N.J. will continue to adhere to established safety strategies and will report to the therapist any problems or other situations that seem to pose a threat to safety.
- Ms. N.J. will increase her hours at the grocery store to a maximum of 3 hours daily depending on the state of her health.

Understand what she is doing

"As Ms. N.J. began to feel better, she seemed genuinely happy to have a structure to her life. She would relate stories of how dysfunctional she had become before she got so sick. Even on the days when she was very tired or experienced a setback, she expressed gratitude for being here to help raise her grandchildren."

Assess the patient's comprehension

Know the person

"Ms. N.J. felt that she did not need the safety procedures most of the time, but she began to accept that it was better to be cautious than to have an unnecessary accident. Even her family members would remind her to do things 'like in the pictures.' Ms. N.J. took the walker with her when she left the house because it just made her feel a little safer if she got dizzy."

Appreciate the context

"Ms. N.J. really enjoyed singing in church, and joining the choir gave her the opportunity to make some new friends who were very supportive. Working in her daughter's grocery store was tiring at first, but Ms. N.J. felt like she was able to help out and even began to repair the strained relationship with her eldest child. Even though she shares a room with her grandchildren in her youngest daughter's apartment, she seems very happy to be there."

Anticipate present and future patient concerns

Analyze patient's comprehension

"Ms. N.J. seems much healthier in a short period of time. She is enthusiastic about the church choir, and a few of the ladies have even begun to visit her at home. She is acutely aware of how important it is for her to eat well, rest, and take her medication. She has a frank and wonderful rapport with her physician, and she trusts her advice. Ms. N.J. has a tendency to do a little too much, and she needs to be reminded to add things into her schedule gradually. Despite everything that has happened to her, she is not at all bitter and seems to have accepted her diagnosis and its implications in her life."

Clinical Reasoning in Occupational Therapy Practice

A Transition Plan for Returning to Work after a Period of Illness

You are assessing a new client today in an ambulatory clinic setting associated with a hospital that specializes in HIV/AIDS care. According to your phone intake, C.H. is a 32-year-old gay man who has been HIV positive for 6 years. C.H. was a meeting and event planner for an upscale hotel, and he really enjoyed the work. Although he was quite ill last year, his new highly active antiretroviral therapy (HAART) protocol has been very successful, and he would like to transition back to work. Having been a highly valued employee, he has been on leave of absence for the last year, but his employer does not know that he has HIV. His job entails attention to details, management of staff, coordination with vendors, and long hours. What will you need to further assess or explore with him to make a transition plan?

Summary Review Questions

1. How does the epidemiology of HIV differ in the United States compared with other countries?
2. By what mechanisms does HIV overwhelm the immune system?
3. What are the routes of transmission for HIV?
4. What are the precautions that an occupational therapist should observe when working with persons with HIV/AIDS or other blood-borne diseases?
5. Which populations are most vulnerable to HIV/AIDS and why?
6. What information is yielded from particular qualitative strategies and quantitative measures that is useful for developing interventions for people with HIV/AIDS?
7. How are occupational roles affected by HIV/AIDS?
8. How does the illness trajectory impact occupational therapy interventions?

Glossary

Disease trajectory—The expected biological and physiological manifestations of disease over time.

Global pandemic—An epidemic that affects many countries similarly.

HAART—An acronym for highly active antiretroviral therapy; combinations of pharmaceutical interventions configured to act on HIV at different points of reproduction of the virus.

Health disparities—Unintended differences in health status or health outcomes; seemingly associated with race/ethnicity, socioeconomic status, education, and access to health care.

Naturalistic paradigm—Research methodology that focuses on the lived experience, people in their natural environments; generally yields qualitative data, rather than quantitative data, from which themes or meanings are extracted.

Occupational coherence—Fluidity and complementarity of occupations that make outcomes predictable.

Occupational competencies—Skills and abilities associated with effective execution of occupations and occupational roles.

Occupational role integrity—Clusters of skills and abilities that support the tasks and activities associated with a given role; intactness of an occupational role.

Opportunistic illness—Infections and diseases that manifest because the normal protective responses of the immune system have been disabled.

Retrovirus—A virus that replicates itself using the mechanisms of host cells to convert RNA to DNA.

Social trajectory—The evolving social and behavioral responses that emerge as a disease progresses.

References

Amico, P., Aran, C., & Avila, C. (2010). HIV spending as a share of total health expenditure: An analysis of regional variation in a multi-country study. *PLoS One, 5,* e12997.

Antonovsky, A. (1987). *Unraveling the mystery of health: How people manage stress and stay well.* San Francisco: Jossey-Bass.

Armstrong, W., Calabrese, L., & Taege, A. J. (2005). HIV update 2005: Origins, issues, prospects, and complications. *Cleveland Clinic Journal of Medicine, 72,* 73–78.

Bailey, R. C., Moses, S., Parker, C. B., Agot, K., Maclean, I., Krieger, J. N., Williams, C. F. M., Campbell, R. T., & Ndinya-Achola, J. O. (2007). Male circumcision for HIV prevention in young men in Kisumu, Kenya: A randomised controlled trial. *Lancet, 369,* 643–656.

Baron, K., Kielhofner, G., Iyenger, A., Goldhammer, V., & Wolenski, J. (2006). *The Occupational Self-Assessment (OSA) (Version 2.2).* Chicago: Model of Human Occupation Clearinghouse, Department of Occupational Therapy, College of Applied Health Sciences, University of Illinois at Chicago.

Bedell, G. (2008). Balancing health, work, and daily life: Design and evaluation of a pilot intervention for persons with HIV/AIDS. *Work, 31,* 131–144.

Braveman, B., Robson, M., Velozo, C., Kielhofner, G., Fisher, G., Forsyth, K., & Kerschbaum, J. (2005). *Worker Role Interview (WRI) (Version 10.0).* Chicago: Model of Human Occupation Clearinghouse, Department of Occupational Therapy, College of Applied Health Sciences, University of Illinois at Chicago.

Brookmeyer, R. (2010). Measuring the HIV/AIDS Epidemic: Approaches and challenges. *Epidemiological Review, 32,* 26–37.

Centers for Disease Control and Prevention. (1993). *Revised classification system for HIV infection and expanded surveillance case definition for AIDS among adolescents and adults.* Washington, DC: U.S. Government Printing Office.

Centers for Disease Control and Prevention. (1994). Recommendations of the U.S. Public Health Service Task Force on the use of zidovudine to reduce perinatal transmission of human immunodeficiency virus. *Morbidity and Mortality Weekly Report, 43,* RR-11.

Centers for Disease Control and Prevention. (1999). *CDC guidelines for national human immunodeficiency virus case surveillance, including monitoring for human immunodeficiency virus infection and acquired immunodeficiency syndrome.* Washington, DC: U.S. Government Printing Office.

Centers for Disease Control and Prevention. (2001). *Revised recommendations for HIV screening of pregnant women.* Washington, DC: U.S. Government Printing Office.

Centers for Disease Control and Prevention. (2011). Diagnoses of HIV infection and AIDS in the United States and Dependent Areas, 2009, HIV Surveillance Report, Volume 21. Retrieved June 25, 2012 from http://www.cdc.gov/hiv/surveillance/resources/reports/2009 report/index.htm.

Centers for Disease Control and Prevention. (2013). Division of HIV/AIDS Prevention: Fact sheet–HIV/AIDS among women. Retrieved July 18, 2013 from http://www.cdc.gov/hiv/risk/gender/women/index.html.

Centers for Disease Control and Prevention. (2012a). HIV cost-effectiveness. Retrieved April 10, 2012 from www.cdc.gov/hiv/topics/preventionprograms/ce/index.htm#Overview.

Centers for Disease Control and Prevention. (2012b). HIV in the United States: At a glance. National Center for HIV/AIDS, Viral Hepatitis, STD, and TB Prevention, Division of AIDS Prevention. Retrieved April 5, 2012 from www.cdc.gov/hiv/resources/factsheets/us.htm.

Christiansen, C. H. (1999). Defining lives: Occupation as identity: An essay on competence, coherence, and the creation of meaning. *American Journal of Occupational Therapy, 53,* 547–558.

Christiansen, C. H., Little, B. R., & Backman, C. (1998). Personal projects: A useful approach to the study of occupation. *American Journal of Occupational Therapy, 52,* 439–446.

Curran, J. W. (2003). Reflections on AIDS, 1981–2031. *American Journal of Preventive Medicine, 24,* 281–284.

Dean, H., Steele, C., Satcher, A., & Nakashima, A. (2005). HIV/AIDS among minority races and ethnicities in the United States, 1999–2003. *Journal of the National Medical Association, 97(Suppl.),* 5S–12S.

Duffy, L. (2005). Suffering, shame, and silence: The stigma of HIV/AIDS. *Journal of the Association of Nurses in AIDS Care, 16,* 13–20.

Fan, H. Y., Connor, R. F., & Villareal, L. P. (2004). *AIDS science and society* (4th ed.). Sudbury, MA: Jones and Bartlett.

Fang, C. T., O'Connell, K., & the World Health Organization's Quality of Life Instrument HIV Group. (2002). Initial steps to developing the World Health Organization's Quality of Life Instrument (WHO-QOL) module of international assessment in HIV/AIDS. *AIDS Care, 15,* 347–357.

Fisher, A. G. (2012). *Assessment of motor and process skills* (7th ed.). Fort Collins, CO: Three Star Press.

Gielen, A. C., Ghandour, R. T., Burke, J. G., Mahoney, P., McDonnell, K. A., & O'Campo, P. (2007). HIV/AIDS and intimate partner violence: Intersecting women's health issues in the United States. *Trauma Violence Abuse, 8,* 178–198.

Gottlieb, M. S., Schroff, R., Schanker, H. M., Weisman, J. D., Fan, P. T., Wolf, R. A., & Saxon, A. (1981). *Pneumocystis carinii* pneumonia and mucosal candidiasis in previously healthy homosexual men: Evidence of a new acquired cellular immunodeficiency. *New England Journal of Medicine, 305,* 1425–1431.

Government Accounting Office. (2005). *Ryan White CARE Act: Factors that impact HIV and AIDS funding and client coverage* (GAO-05-841T). Washington, DC: U.S. Government Accounting Office.

Guaraldi, G., Orlando, G., Murri, R., Vandelli, M., De Paola, M., Beghetto, B., Nardini G., Ciaffi, S., Vichi, F., & Wu, A. W. (2006). Quality of life and body image in the assessment of psychological impact of lipodystrophy: Validation of the Italian version of Assessment of Body Change and Distress Questionnaire. *Quality of Life Research, 15(1),* 173–178.

Holzemer, W. L., Hudson, A., Kirksey, K. M., Hamilton, M. J., & Bakken, S. (2001). The revised Sign and Symptom Check-List for HIV (SSC-HIVrev). *Journal of the Association of Nurses in AIDS Care, 12,* 60–70.

Jong, E., Oudhoff, L., Epskamp, C., Wagener, M. N., van Duijn, M., Fischer, S., & van Gorp, E. C. M. (2010). Predictors and treatment strategies of HIV-related fatigue in the combined antiretroviral therapy era. *AIDS, 24,* 1387–1405.

Kaiser Family Foundation. (2013). U.S. Federal Funding for HIV/AIDS: The President's FY2014 Budget Request. Retrieved July 19, 2013 from http://www.kff.org/search/?s=US+federal+funding+for+HIV/AIDS.

Kielhofner, G., Braveman, B., Finlayson, M., Paul-Ward, A., Goldbaum, L., & Goldstein, K. (2004). Outcomes of a vocational program for persons with AIDS. *American Journal of Occupational Therapy, 58,* 64–72.

Kielhofner, G., Braveman, B., Fogg, L., & Levin, M. (2008). A controlled study of services to enhance productive participation among people with HIV/AIDS. *American Journal of Occupational Therapy, 61,* 36–45.

Kielhofner, G., Mallinson, T., Crawford, C., Nowak, M., Rigby, M., Henry, A., & Walens, D. (2004). *The user's manual for the Occupational Performance History Interview (Version 2.1) OPHI-II.* Chicago: Model of Human Occupation Clearinghouse, Department of Occupational Therapy, College of Applied Health Sciences, University of Illinois at Chicago.

Lerdal, A., Kottorp, A., Gay, C., Aouizerat, B. D., Portillo, C. J., & Lee, K. A. (2011). A 7-item version of the fatigue severity scale has better psychometric properties among HIV-infected adults: An application of a Rasch model. *Quality of Life Research, 20,* 1447–1456.

Mallik, P., Finlayson, M., Mathiowetz, V., & Fogg, L. (2005). Psychometric evaluation of the Energy Conservation Strategies Survey. *Clinical Rehabilitation, 19,* 538–543.

Martinez, S. M., Kemper, C. A., Diamond, C., Wagner, G., & California Collaborative Treatment Group. (2005). Body image in patients with HIV/AIDS: Assessment of a new psychometric measure and its medical correlates. *AIDS Patient Care and STDs, 19,* 150–156.

Masur, H., Michelis, M. A., Greene, J. B., Onorato, I., Stoue, R. A., Holzman, R. S., Wormser, G., Brettman, L., Lange, M., Murray, H. W., & Cunningham-Rundles, S. (1981). An outbreak of community-acquired *Pneumocystis carinii* pneumonia: Initial manifestation of cellular immune dysfunction. *New England Journal of Medicine, 305,* 1431–1438.

Nakashima, A. K., & Fleming, P. L. (2003). HIV/AIDS surveillance in the United States, 1981–2001. *Journal of Acquired Immune Deficiency Syndrome, 32 (Suppl. 1),* S68–S85.

National Institute of Allergy and Infectious Diseases. (2009). *HIV infection and AIDS: An overview.* Retrieved June 25, 2012 from http://www.niaid.nih.gov/topics/HIVAIDS/Understanding/howHIVCausesAIDS/Pages/howhiv.aspx.

National Institute of Allergy and Infectious Diseases. (2012). *How HIV causes AIDS.* Retrieved June 25, 2012 from http://www.niaid.nih.gov/topics/hivaids/understanding/howhivcausesaids/Pages/cause.aspx.

Nyamathi, A. M. (1993). Sense of coherence in minority women at risk for HIV infection. *Public Health Nursing, 10,* 151–158.

O'Brien, K., Bayoumi, A., Strike, C., Young, N., King, K., & Davis, A. (2010). How do existing HIV-specific instruments measure up? Evaluating the ability of instruments to describe disability experienced by adults living with HIV. *Health and Quality of Life Outcomes, 8,* 88. doi:10.1186/1477-7525-8-88. Retrieved June 25, 2012 from http://www.hqlo.com/content/8/1/88.

Opacich, K. J. (2004). Reconstructing occupation after HIV infection: Lessons from women's experiences. *International Journal of Therapy and Rehabilitation, 11,* 516–524.

Pakenham, K. I., & Rinaldis, M. (2002). Development of the HIV/AIDS Stress Scale. *Psychology & Health, 17,* 203–219.

Pontali, E., Pasticci, M. B., Matteelli, A., Baldelli, F., & Migliori, G. B. (2011). Tuberculosis and HIV Co-infection: Do we have a surveillance system in Europe? *European Respiratory Journal, 38,* 1258–1260.

Ranka, J. L., & Chapparo, C. J. (2010). Assessment of productivity performance in men with HIV associated neurocognitive disorder (HAND). *Work, 36,* 193–206.

Robinson, F. (2004). Measurement of quality of life in HIV disease. *Journal of the Association of Nurses in AIDS Care, 15(Suppl.),* 14S–19S.

Siegal, F. P., Lopez, C., Hammer, G. S., Brown, A. E., Kornfeld, S. J., Gold, J., Hassett, J., Hirschman, S. Z., Cunningham-Rundles, C., Adelsberg, B. R., Parham, D. M., Siegal, M., Cunningham-Rundles, S., & Armstrong, D. (1981). Severe acquired immunodeficiency in male homosexuals, manifested by chronic perianal ulcerative herpes simplex lesions. *New England Journal of Medicine, 305,* 1439–1444.

Stout, K., & Finlayson, M. (2011). Fatigue management in chronic illness. *OT Practice, 16*(1), 17–19. www.aota.org.

Stuckler, D., Basu, S., & McKee, M. (2010). Drivers of inequality in millennium development goal progress: A statistical analysis. *PLoS Medicine, 7,* e1000241. DOI:10.1371/journal.pmed.1000241.

United Nations. (2012). *United Nations Millennial Development Goals.* Retrieved April 9, 2012 from http://www.un.org/millenniumgoals/.

U.S. Census Bureau. (2010). *American Fact Finder.* Retrieved April 5, 2012 from http://factfinder2.census.gov/faces/nav/jsf/pages/index.xhtml.

Vahlne, A. (2009). A historical reflection on the discovery of human retroviruses. *Retrovirology, 6,* 40ff. doi: 10-1186/1742-4690-6-40. Retrieved June 27, 2012 from http://www.retrovirology.com/content/6/1/40.

Whalen, C., Antani, M., Carey, J., & Landefeld, C. (1994). An index of symptoms for infection with human immunodeficiency virus: Reliability and validity. *Journal of Clinical Epidemiology, 47,* 537–546.

World Health Organization & UNAIDS. (2011). *Global HIV/AIDS Response–epidemic and health sector progress towards universal access–Progress report 2011.* Geneva: World Health Organization.

World Health Organization. (2012). Global Health Observatory: HIV/AIDS. Retrieved June 25, 2012 from http://www.who.int/gho/hiv/en/index.html.

Worthington, C., O'Brien, K., Zack, E., McKee, E. & Oliver, B. (2012). Enhancing labour force participation for people with HIV: A multi-perspective summary of the research evidence. *AIDS and Behavior, 16,* 231–243.

45

Cancer

Mary Vining Radomski, Mattie Anheluk, Kim Grabe, Shayne E. Hopkins, and Joette Zola

Learning Objectives

After studying this chapter, the reader will be able to do the following:

1. Describe general information regarding cancer incidence, cancer categories, and cancer care.
2. Appreciate the contribution of occupational therapy to cancer rehabilitation, survivorship, and palliative care.
3. Identify occupational therapy–specific assessment and intervention approaches with this population.
4. Address the psychosocial and communication needs of those affected by cancer.
5. Advocate for the provision of occupational therapy services for persons with cancer.

CANCER: BACKGROUND

The term "cancer" refers to a group of diseases that are characterized by growth of abnormal cells. Cells become abnormal because of a change in the cell's deoxyribonucleic acid (DNA) or genetic material. Abnormal DNA can be inherited; however, most changes occur during cell reproduction or as a result of exposure to something in the environment, and typically, the cause of cancer for a given individual cannot be determined. Unlike normal damaged cells, cancer cells do not die when damaged. They continue to reproduce and form new abnormal cells that are capable of invading normal tissue (National Cancer Institute, 2012c).

Cancer Classification

Oncologists and pathologists classify cancer in a number of ways. Doing so enables them to specify a diagnosis, plan treatment, consider patient eligibility for clinical trials, and determine a prognosis. One way cancers are classified is by the type of tissue from which the cancer originates (histological type). Histological classification includes six major categories: carcinoma, sarcoma, myeloma, leukemia, lymphoma, and mixed types (National Cancer Institute, n.d.[a]) (see Table 45-1). Carcinomas are the most common form of cancer and account for 80%–90% of all cases (National Cancer Institute, n.d.[a]). Cancer is also classified by the location in the body where the cancer first developed (primary site). Characterizing the spread of cancer is also used to classify the disease. Sometimes cancer cells get into the bloodstream or lymph vessels, travel to other parts of the body, and form new tumors; this is called metastasis. Cancers that have metastasized to different areas of the body are named for the location where it started (e.g., breast cancer with metastasis to the bones).

In addition to cell type and body location, cancers are often classified by grade and stage. Tumors are graded in terms of degree of differentiation, that is, the degree to which the cell resembles the source tissue (Hutson, 2004). Grading varies based on the type of cancer, but in general, the more abnormal the cell appears, the higher the grade, and conversely, the lower the grade, the better the prognosis (National Cancer Institute, n.d.[b]). Staging is the process of determining the severity of a person's cancer based on the degree to which a cancer has spread (National Cancer Institute, 2010a) (see Definition 45-1). Common elements in most staging systems consider the site of the primary tumor, tumor size and number, spread into lymph nodes, cell type and grade, and presence or absence of metastasis (National Cancer Institute, 2010a). The TNM staging system is the most common method and includes identification of tumor size (T), lymph node involvement (N), and the presence of metastasis, or distant spread of the cancer (M) (National Cancer Institute, 2010a). Staging helps physicians select the type of treatment that will be most appropriate for the patient, and it contributes to the estimate of prognosis.

Types of Cancer

As discussed earlier, cancers are labeled based on the location of the body in which the cancer starts. In this chapter, five types of cancer are described that reflect diagnostic groups often seen by occupational therapists in acute hospitals and rehabilitation settings (Table 45-2). Readers are referred to the Resources 45-1 for more websites and texts that offer additional information on an array of other cancer types and interventions.

Lung Cancer

The two major types of lung cancer are small-cell lung cancers, derived from neuroendocrine cells, and non–small-cell lung cancers, which arise from the epithelial types of tissues that line the lungs (American Cancer Society, 2012c). Cigarette smoking is the leading cause of lung cancer. Secondhand smoke, asbestos, radiation, air pollution, and exposure to toxic heavy metals have also been determined to increase lifetime risk of cancer.

Lung cancer is the deadliest form of cancer for both men and women (American Cancer Society, 2012b). Lung cancers tend to be diagnosed at later stages, when the cancer has metastasized to other sites and when other symptoms, such as weight loss, fatigue, pain, or osteoarthropathy (arthritis-like bone and joint pain), have become more prevalent and affect the individual's daily routines. Treatment of these cancers may entail surgery, chemotherapy, and/or radiation, which is determined by the type and stage of cancer and the goals of treatment (i.e., curative or palliative). People with lung cancer tend to be referred to occupational therapy to address quality-of-life issues related to maximizing performance in light of steady decline. However, new roles may be emerging for rehabilitation practitioners as

Table 45-1	Classification of Cancer Based on Tissue of Origination
Category	**Origination**
Carcinoma	Skin or lining of the internal organs
Sarcoma	Bone, cartilage, fat, muscle, blood vessels, or other connective or supportive tissue
Myeloma	Plasma cells of bone marrow
Leukemia	Blood-forming tissue such as the bone marrow
Lymphoma	Glands or nodes of the lymphatic system
Central nervous system	Tissues of the brain and spinal cord

From National Cancer Institute. (n.d.[a]). Surveillance, epidemiology and end result (SEER) training modules: Cancer classification. Retrieved September 20, 2012 from http://training.seer.cancer.gov/disease/categories/classification.html.

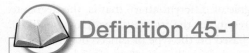

Definition 45-1

Grading and Staging Systems

In order to plan assessment and intervention, occupational therapists must understand terminology used in the medical record to characterize a patient's disease. Although criteria for stages vary based on type of cancer, for many cancers, TNM combinations correspond to one of five stages (National Cancer Institute, 2010a) as exemplified below.

Classification	TNM Interpretation	Stage (0–IV)
T1, N0, M0 breast cancer	T1: primary breast tumor is less than 2 cm across N0: no lymph node involvement M0: has not spread to distant parts of the body	Stage I
T3, N1, M1 breast cancer	T3: tumor more than 50 mm (2 inches) across N1: spread to nearby lymph nodes M1: cancer found in another part of the body	Stage IV

Staging Using the TNM System

T	Tumor size	T(X): tumor cannot be evaluated T(0): no evidence of primary tumor T(is): cancer in situ-abnormal cells that have not spread to surrounding tissue T(1–4): the greater the number, the larger and more invasive the tumor
N	Extent of spread to the lymph nodes	N(X): lymph nodes cannot be evaluated N(0): no lymph node involvement N(1–3): the greater the number, the greater the lymph node involvement
M	Presence of metastasis	M(X): metastasis cannot be evaluated M(0): no known distant metastasis M(1): distant metastasis is present

Stages of Cancer (0–IV)

Stage	Definition
0	Carcinoma in situ for most cancers. A very early stage in which cancer is present only in the layer of cells in which it began and has not spread. Note: not all cancers have a stage 0.
I	Cancer that is the next least advanced; patients often have good prognosis.
II–III	Cancer involving more extensive disease as indicated by greater tumor size and/or spread of the cancer to nearby lymph nodes and/or organs.
IV	Cancer that has spread to other organs.

From American Cancer Society. (2012e). Staging. Retrieved November 12, 2012 from http://www.cancer.org/treatment/understandingyour diagnosis/staging; National Comprehensive Cancer Network. (n.d.). Cancer staging guide. Retrieved November 12, 2012 from http://www.nccn.com/ understanding-cancer-cancer-staging.html.

Table 45-2	Problems Relevant to Occupational Functioning for Five Types of Cancer by Location

Location	Problems That May Interfere with Occupational Functioning
Breast cancer	Weakness, fatigue, body-image issues, pain, lymphedema, limited range of motion (ROM), brachial plexus injury, cognitive inefficiencies
Lung cancer	Fatigue, dyspnea, weakness, limited ROM, limited endurance
Brain cancer	Cognitive problems, impaired balance, decreased sensation, dysphasia, hemiparesis, impaired coordination, personality changes
Head and neck cancer	Limited cervical ROM, shoulder dysfunction, loss of scapular stability, difficulty swallowing, speech problems
Sarcoma	Possible amputation or issues associated with limb salvage, body-image issues

From Smith-Gabai, H. (Ed.). (2011). *Oncology*. Bethesda, MD: AOTA Press.

evidence suggests possible benefits of inpatient rehabilitation that addresses pulmonary function and exercise capacity (Spruit et al., 2006).

Breast Cancer

Breast cancer is the most common cancer among women and the second leading cause of death for women (Centers for Disease Control and Prevention, 2012), with over 250,000 Americans diagnosed each year (American Cancer Society, 2012a). Breast cancer death rates have been steadily declining since the 1990s because of progress with early detection, improved treatment, and possibly reduced incidence (American Cancer Society, 2012a). Risk factors for breast cancer include age, heredity, physical inactivity, weight gain, use of hormone replacement therapy, and race. African American women have the highest breast cancer death rates of all racial and ethnic groups, possibly because they often have cancers that grow faster and are harder to treat and may not have access to preventive and medical care (Centers for Disease Control and Prevention, 2012). Inherited gene mutations account for approximately 5%–10% of all breast cancer cases (American Cancer Society, 2012a). Individuals with a strong family history of breast cancer are often encouraged to seek genetic counseling to determine lifetime risk and whether preventive measures should be considered.

As with other types of cancer, treatment for breast cancer may contribute to decrements in occupational functioning. Treatment for breast cancer typically involves surgery to remove the tumor. Options include breast-conserving procedures (e.g., lumpectomy) or mastectomy (simple mastectomy in which the entire breast is removed,

modified radical mastectomy that also involves removal of axillary lymph nodes, or radical mastectomy in which pectoral muscles under the breast are removed as well) and sometimes reconstructive surgery (American Cancer Society, 2012f). Surgery may contribute to decreased shoulder range of motion (ROM). If axillary lymph nodes are removed, the patient is at risk for lymphedema, arm swelling caused by disruption in the lymphatic drainage system. Lymphedema causes the arm to become painful, swollen, and tight and may interfere with extremity use, performance of daily activities, and clothing options.

Some breast cancer survivors (and those with other types of cancer) report cognitive declines after chemotherapy, a condition that they call "chemobrain" or "brain fog." This may contribute to short-term occupational dysfunction for some and more permanent problems for others (Wefel & Schagen, 2012). The cause of this cognitive dysfunction is not clear, but some attribute the problem to chemotherapy-related neurobiological changes in the brain (Wefel & Schagen, 2012). Fatigue and pain, which often accompany cancer treatment, contribute to cognitive difficulties in and of themselves (Kahol et al., 2008; Seminowicz & Davis, 2007). Common cognitive deficits include attention, memory, processing speed, executive dysfunction, verbal ability, and visuospatial abilities (Biglia et al., 2012; Jim et al., 2012; Wefel & Schagen, 2012).

Brain Cancer

Each year, more than 22,000 adults in the United States are informed they have a brain tumor (National Cancer Institute, 2012a). Pathologists determine whether brain tumors are benign or malignant. Benign tumors do not contain cancer cells and usually do not grow back once removed. Malignant tumors contain cancer cells and are often considered more serious and life threatening. Tumors that originate in the brain are considered primary tumors, whereas those that result from cancers that have spread from other locations in the body are referred to as metastatic brain tumors (National Cancer Institute, 2012a). Metastatic brain tumors outnumber primary brain tumors by 10 to 1, occurring in 20%–40% of cancer patients (National Cancer Institute, 2012c). The most common types of primary brain tumors in adults are astrocytoma (which begin in glial cells called astrocytes), meningioma (which arise from the meninges), and oligodendroglioma (involving the protective covering of nerves) (National Cancer Institute, 2009). Glioblastoma multiforme, a type of astrocytoma, is the most common primary malignant brain tumor and the deadliest (Chandana et al., 2008).

Brain tumors of all kinds are capable of causing functional deficits, depending on their size and location on the brain (Smith-Gabai, 2011). Common deficits for which rehabilitation services are needed include impaired cognition, weakness, visual-perceptual deficits, sensory loss, and bowel–bladder dysfunction (Mukand et al., 2001).

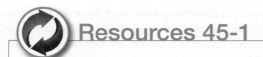

Resources 45-1

Resources for Cancer Rehabilitation

Recommended books

Cooper, J. (Ed.). (1997). *Occupational therapy in oncology and palliative care*. London: Whurr Publishers Ltd. Treatment suggestions across the continuum of cancer care.

Lenhard, R. E., Osteen, R. T., & Gansler, T. (2001). The American Cancer Society's clinical oncology. Atlanta: American Cancer Society. Medical overview of various cancers, medical treatment, and symptom management.

Silver, J. K. (2006). After cancer treatment, heal faster, better, stronger. Baltimore: John Hopkins Press. Practical guide to help cancer patients that offers a step-by-step plan for physical healing.

Websites for additional information

American Cancer Society
www.cancer.org
Dedicated to helping persons who face cancer. Supports research, patient services, early detection, treatment, and education.

breastcancer.org
www.breastcancer.org
Nonprofit organization that provides information on breast cancer.

Cancer Net
www.cancer.net.
Patient information from the American Society of Clinical Oncology. Includes cancer types, treatments, survivorship, advocacy, resources, podcasts, and news.

Livestrong Foundation
http://www.livestrong.org/
The Livestrong Foundation (formerly the Lance Armstrong Foundation) unites, inspires, and empowers people affected by cancer.

Leukemia and Lymphoma Society
www.lls.org
The Leukemia & Lymphoma Society helps patients with blood cancers live better, longer lives.

National Cancer Institute
www.cancer.gov
Accurate, up-to-date, comprehensive cancer information from the U.S. government's principal agency for cancer research.

http://www.cancer.gov/clinicaltrials
Information from the National Cancer Institute on how to find cancer clinical trials, what clinical trials are, recent research, and resources for researchers.

National Coalition for Cancer Survivorship (NCCS)
www.canceradvocacy.org
Get help dealing with cancer, order cancer resources for your patients, and find out what NCCS is doing to advocate for quality cancer care for all people.

National Comprehensive Cancer Network
www.nccn.org
An alliance of 21 of the world's leading cancer centers, this is an authoritative source of comprehensive cancer care.

National Lymphedema Network
www.lymphnet.org
Internationally recognized nonprofit organization that provides education and guidance to lymphedema patients, professionals, and the public.

Survivorship Training and Rehab (STAR Program®)
http://www.oncrehab.com/
Provides certification for cancer rehabilitation programs and clinicians.

Susan G. Komen Breast Cancer Foundation
www.komen.org
Funds research grants, support education, screening, and treatment projects in communities around the world.

The Wellness Community
www.cancersupportcommunity.org
Nonprofit organization that provides professional programs and support groups.

These individuals may also need rehabilitation intervention to address fatigue, sleep issues, and role resumption (Vargo, 2011).

Head and Neck Cancers

Head and neck cancers begin in squamous cells that line the oral cavity, nasal cavities, thyroid gland, and pharynx (National Cancer Institute, 2012b); they are further categorized based on the specific area in which they begin.

Men are two times more likely to be diagnosed with head and neck cancers than women (American Cancer Society, 2012b). Most head and neck cancers are caused by tobacco and excessive alcohol use (National Cancer Institute, 2012b). While the general incidence rate of head and neck cancer has been declining, incidence of oropharynx cancer has been increasing over the last few years because of a rise in the human papillomavirus (HPV) (National Cancer Institute, 2012b). Symptoms of these cancers are often overlooked because they initially do not appear dangerous.

Treatment for head and neck cancers (which almost always involves surgery) may cause disfiguration, pain, and weakness and interfere with communication and swallowing (Goldstein, Genden, & Morrison, 2008). Furthermore, sometimes patients with head and neck cancer experience anxiety and guilt regarding the cause of cancer and implications for their loved ones (Goldstein, Genden, & Morrison, 2008).

Sarcoma

As a collection of diseases, sarcomas include both soft tissue sarcomas and primary bone tumors (American Cancer Society, n.d.). Soft tissue sarcomas include tumors that develop from fat, muscle, nerve, fibrous tissues surrounding joints, blood vessels, and deep skin tissues. Primary bone tumors arise from both bone and cartilage. Most sarcomas are found in the arms and legs, but they can arise in any part of the body (American Cancer Society, n.d.). Soft tumor sarcomas have no identified etiological factor, although some genetic conditions and previous treatment for cancer have been identified as predisposing factors (Yasko et al., 2001).

Surgery is the primary treatment for sarcoma, and in some cases of bone sarcoma, the affected limb has to be amputated. People who have either primary bone tumors or soft tissue sarcomas typically require the services of rehabilitation professionals during the course of treatment, particularly in the postoperative period. The needs and concerns of individuals with sarcoma may vary widely depending on the nature of the tumor and its location but may include peripheral neuropathy, fatigue, lymphedema, and inability to perform daily tasks and valued roles because of surgery to remove the tumor. Tumor growth may also impair circulatory function, resulting in edema, and can compress nerves and invade muscle or joint structures, causing pain or altered sensory perception and limiting ROM.

PHASES OF THE CANCER JOURNEY: IMPLICATIONS FOR OCCUPATIONAL THERAPY

Patients and providers often use metaphors to describe a person's experience with cancer (Harrington, 2012; Penson et al., 2004). Metaphors contribute to communication by using familiar experiences to represent unfamiliar medical concepts (Harrington, 2012); clinicians are advised to follow the patient's lead in this realm. The military metaphor, that of the fight against cancer, resonates with many patients and providers. However, many providers avoid this analogy because poor response to treatment may infer "failure" and the suggestion that the patient did not fight hard enough (Penson et al., 2004). Many patients and providers prefer to discuss the cancer journey, which emphasizes the illness experience as part of a larger narrative and supports each patient's path as unique (Harrington, 2012).

We now employ the journey metaphor to discuss phases of the cancer experience to provide context for occupational therapy assessment and intervention.

Diagnosis

At first you just can't believe it, surely they've got the wrong chart, surely this isn't mine. It can't be true. Then I hoped that the cancer was not very advanced. Hope keeps moving along. . . . (Penson et al., 2007, p. 1106)

Most people are shocked by a cancer diagnosis (Leigh, 2006; Penson et al., 2007). They must adjust their identity from one of health to that of illness; rapidly gather information to make decisions regarding the course of treatment; and alter plans, activities, and roles to accommodate. This potentially traumatic experience may be accompanied by clusters of stress-related symptoms ("I can't sleep" or "I can't stop thinking about it") and/or emotional avoidance and withdrawal ("I don't want to talk about it") (Penson et al., 2004).

Medical Treatment

Following my diagnosis, I underwent nine months of treatment—surgery, chemotherapy, radiotherapy, and brachytherapy. I felt as if I had a new full-time job on my hands, a project which took up all my time. It was structured around appointments and moved through defined stages to a clear end goal. (Ennis-O'Connor, n.d.)

Medical therapies for cancer typically involve surgical removal of the tumor, chemotherapy, and/or radiation. All of these interventions have potential consequences and side effects that may interfere with the patient's daily functioning (see Table 45-3). Surgery and medical treatment may impact patients' ability to perform activities of daily living (ADL), instrumental activities of daily living (IADL), and life roles, including driving and work (Campbell et al., 2012; Hoving, Broekhuizen, & Frings-Dresen, 2009; Yuen et al., 2007). In addition to the nature and extent of the patient's cancer, the ability to work during treatment is influenced by opportunities to work flexibly around appointments (and availability of paid time off), support of coworkers, and ability to manage fatigue (Pryce, Munir, & Haslam, 2007).

Cancer rehabilitation may begin after surgery and continue concurrent with chemotherapy and/or radiation and into the survivorship phase. These services are provided in acute medical settings, in inpatient rehabilitation units, or as outpatient services. In addition to occupational therapists, the cancer rehabilitation team includes physiatry, oncology nursing, psychosocial services, nutritional support services, pharmacy, pastoral care, physical therapy, speech language pathology, and comprehensive multidisciplinary lymphedema services (Committee on Cancer Survivorship: Improving Care and Quality of Life, 2006) (see Fig. 45-1). Patients may also be referred to

Table 45-3 **Types of Cancer Treatment and Possible Effects on Occupational Performance**

Type of Cancer Treatment	Description	Side Effects or Secondary Effects That May Interfere with Functioning
Surgery	Used to diagnose, treat, and prevent cancer	• Complications from surgery: blood transfusions, damage to internal organs, reaction to anesthesia • Pain (most common side effect) • Infection from wound site • Lymphedema
Chemotherapy	Medicines or drugs that are used to treat cancer; can be used to contain or slow tumor growth or kill cancer cells	• Fever and chills • Nausea and vomiting • Hair loss • Fatigue • Sores in the mouth or throat • Constipation or diarrhea • Itching or rash • Muscle or joint pain • Memory changes
Radiation	The use of high-energy particles or wavelengths to kill the cancerous cells and shrink tumors	• Fatigue • Skin irritation at radiation site • Fever/chills

From American Cancer Society. (2012d). Questions people ask about cancer. Retrieved November 25, 2012 from http://www.cancer.org/cancer/cancerbasics/questions-people-ask-about-cancer.

exercise and fitness programs during chemotherapy and/or radiation. There is evidence that moderate to vigorous exercise interventions are associated with reduced anxiety, depression, fatigue, and sleep disturbances and improved physical functioning (Mishra et al., 2012).

Survivorship

It was only when treatment ended and that structure fell apart, that the full impact of what had happened hit me. I felt cut adrift. There is an expectation that when you walk out of hospital on that final day of treatment, your cancer story has ended, but the reality is that in many ways your story is only just beginning. (Ennis-O'Connor, n.d.)

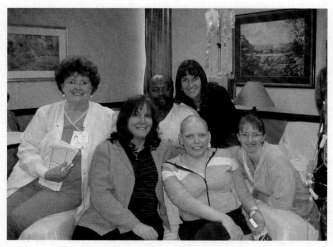

Figure 45-1 A patient with leukemia and her rehabilitation team.

When primary medical treatment concludes, the patient transitions from patienthood into survivorship (Thorne & Stajduhar, 2012). To the surprise of some patients and providers, the emotional relief associated with completing medical care may be accompanied by a sense of disequilibrium, fear of recurrence, and challenge in reorienting their lives (Thorne & Stajduhar, 2012). With the completion of their formal medical treatment, cancer survivors must figure out how to manage long-term health consequences of cancer treatments and lingering problems with physical functioning, fatigue, and cognition. Although increasing numbers of people are surviving cancer, more cancer survivors report poor mental and physical health-related quality of life than adults without cancer ($p < 0.0001$) (Weaver et al., 2012). Many survivors demonstrate resilience and even personal growth from their cancer experience, but others may experience psychological distress; young survivors are particularly at risk (Costanzo, Ryff, & Singer, 2009). In addition, cancer survivors may face roadblocks in returning to "normal" life. For example, cancer survivors have a higher risk of unemployment than healthy controls (Tamminga et al., 2010).

To address these concerns, the Institute of Medicine recommended the development of Survivorship Care Plans to summarize information about cancer type, treatments received and their potential consequences, timing and content of medical follow-up, recommendations regarding preventive and wellness practices, information about employment, and resources regarding psychosocial services in the community (Committee on Cancer Survivorship: Improving Care and Quality of Life, 2006).

However, the extent to which this recommendation has been implemented is unclear.

Palliative Care

> . . . I want to live as usual but it's not possible. . . . I can't cook. . . . I can't go for a walk. . . . (Appelin & Berterö, 2004, p. 68; comments from a recipient of palliative care regarding fatigue)

Although most people who are diagnosed with cancer experience either a full recovery or live many years with cancer as a chronic condition (American Cancer Society, 2012d), some experience steady and significant decline from their disease. Many of those patients and their families choose to receive palliative care, an approach that aims to improve quality of life by addressing the emotional, physical, practical, and spiritual aspect of cancer for patients and their family who are facing life-threatening illness (National Cancer Institute, 2010b). An interdisciplinary team, including occupational therapists, provides relief from symptoms such as pain, fatigue, insomnia; addresses fear and depression; and assists in coordinating services that pertain to legal, financial, and employment concerns. Palliative care is available from the time of diagnosis through cancer treatment and beyond, including the transition to end-of-life care (National Cancer Institute, 2010b). During this phase of the cancer journey, occupational performance may continue to be limited by the disease process or medical treatment as described earlier (pain, fatigue, cognitive changes, strength and ROM, and home and community access and mobility). Intervention may emphasize supporting caregivers and making environmental changes as means of optimizing patient performance.

OCCUPATIONAL THERAPY ACROSS THE PHASES OF THE CANCER JOURNEY

Individuals with cancer have complex needs and priorities that can change, sometimes rapidly, depending on severity of illness, response to treatment, stage of cancer, and stage of treatment. The diversity of cancers and treatment regimens makes it challenging to establish definitive guidelines for practice. It is essential to continually reevaluate the patient's performance, adaptation, and plan of care, staying attuned to his or her goals and priorities. Therapy goals and activities must be relevant and understandable to the patient and family as the spector of a potentially life-threatening illness brings their priorities into focus.

It is fitting that this is the final chapter in this textbook because occupational therapy for persons with cancer draws on most if not all of the book's contents. Assessment, for example, may involve evaluating the patient's upper extremity strength, ROM, or swelling (Chapter 7); cognition (Chapter 6); performance of ADL or IADL roles (Chapter 4);

and/or environmental accessibility (Chapter 10). Similarly, intervention methods for patients with cancer will follow that which is described in the intervention sections of the book. Furthermore, patients with cancer may present much like those described in some of the diagnostic chapters, depending on the location of the tumor (and consequences of surgery). For example, individuals with spinal cord tumors may have issues that are similar to those with spinal cord injury (Chapter 38). Individuals with brain cancer may have sensory motor, visual, cognitive problems that resemble those of stroke (Chapter 33) or traumatic brain injury (Chapter 34). Therapists are advised to refer to Chapter 43 on dysphagia when treating patients with head and neck cancer and to Chapter 41 if caring for patients whose cancer has resulted in amputation.

In this section, we provide additional information about cancer-specific assessments and interventions, beginning with overarching considerations when serving this population.

Awareness of Psychosocial and Family Needs

Many people view their experience of cancer as life altering. Some use the diagnosis as a springboard for growth and development, regardless of outcome. Almost all the people that we have encountered in our practices have experienced psychosocial adjustment issues, and many of them note that intervention and support to help with the resolution of these issues is lacking among health care professionals. Occupational therapists are well equipped to address these issues throughout their involvement with a given patient and family.

Psychosocial Adjustment Issues

Effective patient–clinician communication is the foundation of any effort to address patients' psychosocial adjustment, and health care professionals who provide care for patients with cancer may benefit from communications skills training (Uitterhoeve et al., 2010). Communicating with individuals who have cancer is similar to communicating with those with other chronic conditions. There are, however, unique cancer-related factors that may affect communication. Experts suggest that "few other illnesses are both life-threatening and potentially curable; that care involves numerous clinicians and multiple treatment modalities (such as oral and intravenous medications, radiation, and surgery); that there is often a long period of uncertainty after treatment; and that the patient's health care team often changes over time" (Epstein & Street, 2007, p. 1). Epstein and Street (2007) developed a framework that describes the following six core functions of patient–clinician communication: nurturing healing relationships, sharing information, responding to emotions, managing uncertainty, making decisions, and facilitating patient self-management.

Occupational therapists contribute to psychosocial adjustment in many ways. As suggested above, it is essential that clinicians ask questions that begin the dialogue about adjustment and allow time during sessions to simply listen (also see Chapter 14 on Therapeutic Rapport). Clinicians may also encourage or recommend stress-relieving practices to patients and family, such as journaling, exercise, meditation, and yoga. Further, supporting leisure activities (both new and familiar) throughout the cancer journey may contribute to occupational engagement that is critical to socialization, health, and wellness.

Family Needs

Attending to the psychosocial needs of caregivers is also imperative for optimal occupational outcomes. Caregiver goals for the patient can at times differ from the patient's priorities, and it is critical that all areas be addressed. Caregivers may also need guidance in setting realistic expectations for functional recovery and training in strategies to promote patients' optimal participation in occupations.

Caregivers may be involved in supporting a person with cancer in many ways including eating, bathing, using the bathroom, medication management, shopping, cleaning, financial management, attending medical appointments, and coordinating care (American Cancer Society, 2012g). In addition to supporting their loved ones ADL/IADL, caregivers may have less time to care for their own needs. Amid these changes in their routines and roles, caregivers are often coping with the uncertainty and loss involved with their loved one's cancer diagnosis and occupational changes.

Occupational therapists help caregivers acquire the knowledge and skills required for supporting their loved ones with cancer. Clinicians support family members and caregivers by revisiting their need for information at various junctures in the illness trajectory (DuBenske et al., 2008). Therapists also incorporate caregiver skills training into their sessions and may refer caregivers to counseling, both of which have been demonstrated to decrease caregiver burden and improve coping and self-efficacy (Northouse et al., 2010). The rehabilitation team also collaborates with the patient to ensure that the informational and psychological needs of his or her young children are addressed as well.

Assessment

Occupational therapists establish rapport with a client by addressing immediate needs and by understanding who this person is, was, and wants to be through his or her narrative. The type of assessment chosen and the length of the evaluation process depend on the individual's medical and cognitive status. Information is obtained from significant others, team members, and chart review. The clinician needs to understand the client's medical history, previous responses to and side effects of treatments, prognosis,

and the current and potential impact of the disease and treatment on performance areas. In addition, precautions, such as immunosuppression, thrombocytopenia, isolation (to prevent exposure to vancomycin-resistant *Enterococcus, Clostridium difficile,* fungoides, etc.), and anemia should be noted, because these factors impact functioning and occupational therapy treatment (see Safety Note 45-1 for other precautions).

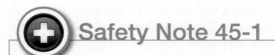

Safety Note 45-1

General Precautions in Treatment

If the patient is an inpatient:

- Before you enter a patient's room, read the chart and check with the patient's nurse to find out if any events or changes have occurred since your last visit.
- Monitor vital signs, because cancer treatments are capable of impacting cardiopulmonary and nervous system function.
- Practice universal precautions. You will protect the patient and prevent spread of infection to others.
- Be familiar with handling oncological emergencies and observe precautions as necessary. Categories of oncological emergencies include obstructive/compressive, hematological/immune, metabolic, those related to increased pressure or fluid accumulation, and pathological fractures (Garrett & Kirchner, 1995; Hockett, 2004; Tatu, 2005). Although some of these conditions/emergencies may not prevent you from working with individuals who have cancer, you should know how to respond should one occur.

Regarding the use of physical agent modalities:

- Follow all standard precautions regarding their use.
- Do NOT apply thermal or electrical modalities over areas of active or potential malignancies.
- Avoid areas with altered skin integrity (i.e., radiation sites, graft versus host disease, chemotherapy burns, etc.).
- Inappropriate use of modalities may exacerbate conditions, such as lymphedema.

Regarding the use of exercise:

- Consider the impairment or condition. Aggressive exercise may be contraindicated, as in the presence of spinal cord compression, lymphedema, or pathologic fracture.
- Manual muscle testing is contraindicated for patients with metastatic disease to the bones because it may lead to fracture.
- Verify use of stretching or resistive activity because of low platelet levels and risk of uncontrolled bleeding.
- When in doubt, consult with your clinical instructor or supervisor.

The Canadian Occupational Performance Measure (Law et al., 1998) and the Occupational Performance History Interview II (Kielhofner et al., 1998) are occupation-based assessments that facilitate identification of a client's sense of self-efficacy and self-esteem, as well as satisfaction with life roles in self-maintenance, self-advancement, and self-enhancement. Observing clients as they perform tasks and activities provides information about performance levels, abilities, and habits. Other assessments may be indicated to determine limiting factors and underlying reasons for diminished ability to meet activity demands.

Fatigue is the most common problem reported by individuals with cancer. The Brief Fatigue Inventory (Mendoza et al., 1999) provides a quick assessment of the severity of fatigue and its impact on daily function. Cleeland et al. (2000) also developed a global symptoms assessment, the M. D. Anderson Symptom Inventory, which measures the severity of many cancer-related symptoms and the degree to which they interfere with daily function. Either of these tools can be used routinely to monitor changes in the individual's status, side effects of treatment, and effectiveness of rehabilitation.

The Functional Assessment of Cancer Therapy (FACT) measures quality of life in persons undergoing cancer treatment (Cella et al., 1993). There are many versions of the original tool that are part of the FACIT measurement system, all of which are available for free online (FACIT.org, 2010). Several versions have been developed that are specific to different types of cancer (e.g., FACT-B for patients with breast cancer) and for various symptoms of cancer (e.g., FACT-Cog for patients with cognitive issues).

Occupational therapists have also recently developed cancer-specific measures. The Manual Ability Measure in Oncology-20 (MAM) is a self-report instrument composed of a list of commonly performed tasks requiring hand function (e.g., writing, clipping nails) that are rated using a four-point ordinal scale related to the patient's perceived level of difficulty (Hill & Chen, 2012). It may be particularly useful with patients who have had surgery for breast cancer or brain cancer. An earlier, 36-item version of the MAM was evaluated with patients who had hand dysfunction associated with neurological and musculoskeletal conditions (Chen & Bode, 2010). The MAM-36 demonstrated acceptable unidimensionality and psychometric properties. The Valued Activity Inventory for Adults with Cancer (VAI-AC) is a self-report instrument that measures activity limitations in tasks valued by individual patients undergoing chemotherapy (Lyons et al., 2012). Patients rate the importance and difficulty levels of various everyday tasks. The VAI-AC demonstrated moderate test–retest reliability, and evaluation of construct validity demonstrated that there was logical association with other related measures (Lyons et al., 2012).

Intervention Planning: Goal Setting across the Continuum of Care

The goal of therapy is to enable clients to optimize their quality of life by engaging in meaningful occupations and to facilitate living regardless of life expectancy. Many of the goals that are meaningful to the client who has cancer are the same as those encountered with persons who have other diagnoses. With cancer, however, distinct moderating variables may affect realistic goal setting. People with cancer experience rapid changes in medical and functional status across the continuum of care. It is sometimes difficult for the person and the therapist to determine how permanent these changes might be. The severity of the disease and the individual's expectations regarding function and recovery may be incongruous. The occupational therapist should continually monitor these changes and help the individual to modify valued goals and roles accordingly. At the same time, the therapist must walk a fine line to avoid dispelling hope.

The role of the occupational therapist varies according to the point at which he or she enters the patient's course of treatment. Duration of treatment depends on acuity of the condition and severity of the disease, along with the patient's wishes. Regardless, the treatment plan should be individualized and address the performance skills required to function at that point in the continuum of care. The patient's long-term goals should guide him or her toward resuming activities such as work, driving, leisure, social interaction, play, and education. Most patients are able to resume normal activities with few, if any, long-term restrictions.

The occupational therapy intervention plan will also be shaped by the composition of the broader medical and/or cancer rehabilitation team. All team members are advised to practice self-care strategies to optimize their own professional quality of life so that they may best serve their patients (Procedures for Practice 45-1).

Intervention

Occupational therapists rely on their general knowledge and expertise related to intervention for patients with physical dysfunction in treating patients with cancer. This section highlights areas of intervention that exemplify cancer-specific interventions that are within occupational therapists' scope of practice.

Arm Function

Occupational therapists address the consequences of cancer-related surgery on arm function, using exercise and activity to improve ROM, strength, and coordination (Campbell, Pergolotti, & Blaskowitz, 2009; Penfold, 1996). Occupational therapists with specialized training

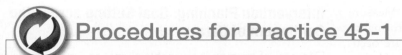

Procedures for Practice 45-1

Maintaining Compassion Satisfaction and Preventing Compassion Fatigue

Professional quality of life is an important concept in health care today and its significance is gaining increased interest among researchers, health care administrators, and health care professionals. Compassion satisfaction is the positive feature of professional quality of life and involves the desirable effects of helping others (Stamm, 2010). Facilitating engagement in clients' occupations and roles at various stages and points of cancer recovery offers many opportunities for rewarding experiences that can lead to high compassion satisfaction (Prochnau, Liu, & Boman, 2003). The results of a qualitative study of occupational therapists working in palliative care suggested that clinicians derive high levels of satisfaction from their work and see it as a source of personal growth, in part because of rewarding relationships with patients and families (Prochnau, Liu, & Boman, 2003).

Occupational therapists are among health care professionals who are also at risk for compassion fatigue, which derives from the negative aspects involved in professional caregiving. The Professional Quality of Life Scale (ProQOL) is a measure often used to explore the positive and negative aspects of professional quality of life. The ProQOL is a free measure available on the internet to be used for research, to monitor the professional quality of life among workers in an

organization, and to monitor one's own status for personal use (Stamm, 2010).

It is important for occupational therapists to monitor and prevent compassion fatigue and to nurture a sense of compassion satisfaction. This can be accomplished through habitual use of prevention and self-care strategies. Costa (2005) recommends the following self-care skills for occupational therapy practitioners:

- Maintain your relationships with coworkers, family members, and friends.
- Practice healthy boundaries with your personal and work-related relationships.
- Develop self-awareness of activities that nurture and exhaust your energy.
- Seek life balance.
- Practice effective time management.
- Practice positive self-talk.
- Focus on your physical health.
- Learn from experiences when a client reminds you of a source of conflict.
- Make time for self-reflection of your values and strengths.
- Seek a mentor.
- Participate in educational and professional opportunities.
- Set measurable and timely goals surrounding your personal, professional, and work life.

---

in lymphedema management use techniques such as manual lymph drainage, wrapping, and garment fitting to treat lymphedema (Longpré, 2012). An occupational therapy program for women with cancer-related lymphedema that incorporated exercise and education was found to result in improvements in upper extremity swelling, arm flexibility, and mood (McClure et al., 2010) (see Evidence Table 45-1 for further discussion).

Fatigue

Occupational therapists often provide instruction in energy conservation and stress management techniques to patients with cancer who are experiencing fatigue (Longpré, 2012; Penfold, 1996; Vockins, 2004). A recent evidence review of 27 studies of psychosocial interventions to address cancer-related fatigue (including instruction in energy conservation, relaxation, and stress management) suggests that these interventions are effective in reducing fatigue, especially those programs that are specific to fatigue as compared to more general psychosocial interventions (Goedendorp et al., 2009). There is also increasing evidence to support the benefits of moderate-intensity exercise in modulating cancer-related fatigue and improving overall function (Anderson et al., 2012;

Brown et al., 2011), another important consideration in occupational therapy intervention for fatigue.

Cognition

Occupational therapists address problems with memory, concentration, and problem solving that may occur as a result of brain surgery (Campbell, Pergolotti, & Blaskowitz, 2009) or associated with patients' self-described "chemobrain." Many people with cancer, including those with breast cancer, experience mild cognitive impairment after chemotherapy in the areas of attention, learning, executive function, and information processing speed (Joly et al., 2011; Wefel et al., 2010). For some, these problems persist well past their completion of and recovery from chemotherapy (Wefel et al., 2004). Although there appears to be a linkage between chemotherapy and deficits on neuropsychological testing, the etiology and linkage to emotional factors and fatigue remain unclear (Poppelreuter et al., 2004). Cancer survivors who experience chemobrain indicate that it impacts their life economically, emotionally, and interpersonally (Boykoff, Moieni, & Subramanian, 2009). Despite the prevalence of this issue and its potential to disrupt everyday functioning, no specific interventions have been specified or recommended based on

Evidence Table 45-1	Best Evidence for Occupational Therapy Intervention for Cancer					
Intervention	Description of Intervention Tested	Participants	Dosage	Type of Best Evidence and Level of Evidence	Benefit	Statistical Probability	Reference
Breast Cancer Recovery Program (BCRP) for lymphedema	BCRP consisted of education regarding lymphedema management and instruction in relaxation techniques (deep diaphragmatic breathing, progressive muscle relaxation). Controls received usual medical care.	Women with stage I or II unilateral breast cancer-related lymphedema (BCRL) with ≥10% increased affected arm size compared with unaffected arm (16 in each group)	Ten biweekly, 1-hour sessions for 5 weeks	Randomized controlled trial Level IC3b	Those receiving BCRP demonstrated significant treatment effects (extracellular fluid, arm flexibility, range of motion [ROM], and mood) compared to controls.	Extracellular fluid in affected arm (measured via bioimpedance): $p = 0.049$, $r = 0.43$ Total shoulder active ROM: $p = 0.034$, $r = 0.50$ Mood as measured by Beck Depression Inventory: $p = 0.03$, $r = 0.41$ Quality of life as measured by SF-36: $p = 0.03$, $r = 0.52$ (general health)	McClure et al. (2010)
Exercise to address cancer-related fatigue (CRF)	Various exercise interventions (24 studies of aerobic exercise, 6 studies of resistance exercise, 11 studies of a combination, 6 with other types like yoga and Tai Chi).	3,254 participants with various types and stages of cancer	Average length of intervention was 11.5 weeks. Mean level of exercise was 3.5 days per week for an average of 48.5 minutes per session.	Meta-analysis involving 44 studies Level IA1a	Statistically significant improvements in CRF (all cancers)	$d = 0.31$ (95% confidence interval 0.22–0.40)	Brown et al. (2011)
Problem Solving Occupational Therapy (PST-OT)	PST to help subjects identify and analyze problematic activities and design compensatory approaches. Control group received usual care.	Rural patients with breast cancer (stages I–III) who were undergoing chemotherapy PST-OT ($n=15$), Control ($n = 16$)	Six weekly sessions via telephone	Feasibility study of PST-OT	Established feasibility of intervention	Ninety-seven percent of all planned sessions were completed; 92% of participants reported PST-OT to be helpful in overcoming performance restrictions; 81% study retention rate	Hegel et al. (2011)

scientific research (Joly et al., 2011). Occupational therapy intervention largely focuses on teaching patients to modify their approach or the environment to minimize cognitive load and implementing compensatory cognitive strategies (see Chapter 24), but there is little scientific literature at present to support this approach.

Intervention to Address Activity Limitations

Occupational therapists provide intervention to reduce activity limitations by providing ADL, IADL, and transfer training to persons with cancer (Campbell, Pergolotti, & Blaskowitz, 2009; Penfold, 1996; Vockins, 2004). This may involve providing equipment and optimizing access within the home, particularly for individuals receiving palliative care (Kealey & McIntyre, 2005; Keesing & Rosenwax, 2011). It is noteworthy that even though patients with cancer appear to have driving-related concerns (Yuen et al., 2007), this aspect of IADL intervention is not currently described in the literature.

Intervention to Address Role Resumption and Prevent Occupational Disengagement

Ultimately, all occupational therapy intervention for persons with cancer should contribute to role resumption and engagement in valued occupations. This emphasis is aligned with what many cancer survivors want and need, as underscored by a qualitative study of people participating in a hospice day program (Lyons et al., 2002). These individuals described the importance of remaining socially engaged, doing for themselves, and trying new things, even with life-threatening illness (Lyons et al., 2002). Unfortunately, in many cases, these participation-related needs go unmet (Taylor & Currow, 2003). In a survey of patients receiving cancer or palliative services over a 1-year period at a cancer center, over 30% reported that they had unmet needs—work, leisure, and driving needs were most frequently reported (Taylor & Currow, 2003). Of note, 19% of patients at this center were referred to occupational therapy, and 31% of that subgroup also reported unmet needs.

New programs such as Problem Solving and Occupational Therapy (PST-OT) demonstrate the potential contributions of occupational therapists in reducing participation restrictions (Hegel et al., 2011). PST-OT was a telephone-delivered 6-week, six-session intervention for women with breast cancer who were undergoing chemotherapy. Each session focused on a patient-established goal, using the person-environment-occupation model (Law et al., 1996) as the foundation for problem solving. Common patient-identified problems included maintaining aerobic exercise, IADL (housecleaning, shopping, and childcare), and work. Researchers found high levels of satisfaction and use of therapy-related action plans among participants (Hegel et al., 2011).

Finally, successful return to work is increasingly recognized as a problem for many cancer survivors (Pryce, Munir, & Haslam, 2007). A work-directed intervention that involves early contact with vocational specialists and development of a return-to-work plan is described in the literature (Tamminga et al., 2010), but no outcomes of this program have been reported as yet. Occupational therapists have the education and expertise to address this important aspect of functioning.

ADVOCACY

As more people continue to survive cancer (American Cancer Society, 2012b), cancer rehabilitation services, including that provided by occupational therapists, will be increasingly important in remediating disease and treatment-related sequelae and helping people return to personally valued roles and activities. There is evidence, however, to suggest that we could be doing more, because many cancer survivors report unmet rehabilitation needs (Taylor & Currow, 2003; Thorsen et al., 2011). As we better articulate the breadth of our potential contributions to cancer care and conduct research to provide evidence of the impact of our services, occupational therapists are well positioned to substantively contribute to the cancer rehabilitation field.

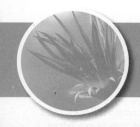

case example

Ms. S.: Evaluation and Treatment for a Patient with Breast Cancer

Occupational Therapy Process	Clinical Reasoning Process	
	Objectives	**Examples of Therapist's Internal Dialogue**

Patient Information

Medical

Ms. S. (Sarah) is a 32-year-old woman who was diagnosed with stage II breast cancer. She has a family history of breast cancer. She underwent bilateral mastectomy and is preparing for reconstructive surgery. She currently has expanders in place on her chest wall and hopes to complete the procedure in 6 weeks. She reports discomfort on both chest walls that is interfering with her sleep. She is currently receiving chemotherapy and has two of four cycles left to complete. She receives the medication on a 1 week on, 2 weeks off regimen.

Social

Sarah has been married for 12 years and has a 6-year-old daughter and 18-month-old son. Another son died from an undiagnosed heart condition when he was age 3 years. This occurred 6 months before her cancer diagnosis. Her sister lives in town, but the rest of her family is out of state. She reports that her husband is supportive but travels a lot with his job. She is primarily responsible for the household management tasks and care of her children. She is active in her church and teaches religion classes.

Vocational

Sarah works in human resources at a local hospital. She has always worked full time and hopes to return to her position as soon as she has medical clearance from her doctor. She has been off of work for 12 weeks and has used up her Family Medical Leave. She reports that her manager is supportive. She plans to return to work in 1 month. Sarah drove herself to the appointment and reports no community mobility concerns.

Understand the patient's diagnosis or condition

Know the person

"I would be so overwhelmed if I were her. She is used to being so healthy and able to manage so many life roles."

"I wonder how much effect the pain and lack of sleep are having on her function. I wonder how she is tolerating the chemotherapy. I wonder what coping strategies she is using."

"I need to contact her physical therapist. She has so many life demands and appointments. We need to see which one of us will address the positioning concerns related to her disrupted sleep as well as her walking program."

"She has had to manage so much loss this past year: her son, her health, and temporarily her role as a full time worker. I hope she is working with a counselor."

"She appears to be a type A personality. I cannot believe she is still volunteering and managing her home and children throughout her chemo treatments. It may be difficult for her to incorporate fatigue management strategies."

"I am concerned about her returning to work in 1 month. She will still be getting chemotherapy treatments and needs to finish up her reconstructive surgery. I wonder if that start date is a work requirement or if that is more of a personal requirement?"

"I need to make sure she is confident in her driving skills, especially when she is tired."

Reason for the Referral to Occupational Therapy

Sarah had an appointment with her physiatrist and reported concerns related to excessive fatigue, memory errors, and frustrating incidents in which she lost items and track of what she was doing. She is afraid this will affect her job performance. She has recently started to use the calendar on her cell phone, but it frustrates her because she never had to do so before. She is starting to make lists but usually forgets them at home.

She recently had diagnostic brain imaging and does not have any metastases.

Appreciate the context

"She is demonstrating the common symptoms of mild cognitive impairment related to cancer treatments. She sounds resistant to using strategies typical of someone who prided herself on good memory. I am going to need some quick wins to get her to embrace changes. I really need to listen to her story when I meet her and focus on the area she cares most about."

"I am so relieved that she does not have metastases to the brain. We can really focus on showing her ways she can regain some control with good strategy use."

She reports that she is managing all of her medical needs; she is caring for her children and resumed her volunteer teaching role last week. She has more difficulty completing all of her roles during chemotherapy weeks, but she is determined and has been able to get it all done. Despite feeling very tired, she is having difficulty sleeping because of her expanders. She does not want to take any sleep medications; she feels that the chemotherapy is too many toxins already. She told her doctor she is not sure she needs occupational therapy (OT) and is worried about her return-to-work schedule.

| Develop provisional hypotheses | "I will need to address fatigue management fairly quickly in her treatment. She seems like someone that has worked hard all her life and will need some tips and support to work smarter and take care of her own needs." |
| | "I think she will have a good outcome. I will likely need to see her weekly for 1 month and then have a follow up visit when she returns to work. I will talk with her about possibly postponing work until she has finished chemotherapy and then with a gradual increase in hours." |

Assessment Process and Results

FACT-Cog: score of 44.83 (top score is 131.78)
Higher scores indicate better quality of life.
Goals identified by the Canadian Occupational Performance Measure

1. Consistently effective parenting
2. Consistently effective household management
3. Effective/accurate worker
4. Consistent with care of self
5. Continue volunteer commitments to a lesser extent

Consider evaluation approach and methods	"I think it would be counterproductive to administer cognitive tests that highlight her cognitive inefficiencies. I am going to need to identify what roles she values, figure out what is frustrating her, and give her some tools to cope better."
Interpret observations	"Her score on the FACT-Cog indicates that she is experiencing stress related to her cognitive changes. She is really focused on what she is not doing well or accurately. I am really going to need her to be part of the strategy selection if she is going to accept the need to use these."
	"She really puts others first; I will need to make sure she talks with her counselor about the importance of taking care of herself first."
	"If I start with concepts to give her some control and strategies to help with parenting, I may get her to invest energy into the solutions."

Occupational Therapy Problem List

1. Disrupted sleep and ongoing fatigue
2. Difficulty with information management
3. Disrupted routines/habits
4. Difficulty with consistency of care of others
5. Decreased participation in community including volunteer work and vocational pursuits
6. Difficulty with time management within her activity tolerance capabilities

| Synthesize the results | "She is not consistently managing her own needs first, and this results in fatigue and inefficiencies that affect the quality of her life roles. She will continue to spiral down if I cannot get her to be aware of the effects of her choices." |
| | "I think I need to start by addressing the areas of her life that need to be managed for best function: sleep, nutrition, physical exercise, and stress reduction." |

Occupational Therapy Goal List

1. Patient will consistently employ bedtime routines for her children and herself evidenced by going to bed and getting up at the same time 5 out of 7 days, 4 out of 4 weeks.
2. Patient will independently and consistently use the calendar on her cell phone, including the alarm options, evidenced by no missed appointments.
3. Patient will effectively manage her fatigue throughout the day/week by prioritizing her tasks and initiating breaks with cues from the alarms on her cell phone.

| Develop intervention hypotheses | "I suspect that as Sarah gets a handle on her fatigue and puts in place some new cognitive strategies, she will realize improved cognitive function. If I can also give her a few strategies that help decrease her errors and/or frustration, she will likely start to develop her own strategies and need less occupational therapy." |
| Select an intervention approach | "I know she values taking care of her children and feels badly when she is too tired to engage with them. I think changing bedtime routines could be a quick win for everyone. I will suggest she focus on moving bedtime up by 45 minutes for the children and herself. I will help her think through the cues or changes she may need in her day to make this happen. I wonder if she would try using a timer. I will send one home if she is willing." |

4. Patient will spontaneously manage the distracters in her environment evidenced by accurately completing high-consequence tasks such as paying bills in a quiet environment with limited interruptions.	Consider what will occur in therapy, how often, and for how long	"I will start therapy one time per week for five sessions after initial assessment. She will likely need a 1 month follow-up as she returns to work."

Interventions

1. Education on importance of routines/habits
   a. Develop routines/checklists for different activities of daily living (ADL) tasks: getting ready for bed, leaving the house, daily planning
   b. Create a weekly activity template
2. Education on fatigue management strategies
   a. Develop/employ strategies that assist in effective use of her energy: pacing, planning, prioritizing, and taking breaks
   b. Pedometer use/walking program to increase her energy level
   c. Education on good nutrition
   d. Education on sleep hygiene, options for positioning to decrease discomfort from the expanders when sleeping
3. Education on information processing
   a. Develop/employ strategies related to calendar/alarm use on her cell phone
   b. Develop/employ use of strategies to manage information from meetings when she resumes her job; explore technology that could be useful
4. Education on time-management skills
   a. Develop/employ strategies to help her manage ADL roles
   b. Develop/employ strategies to manage home-management roles
   c. Develop/employ strategies to manage her vocational roles

Assess the patient's comprehension

Understand what she is doing

Compare actual to expected performance

Know the person

Appreciate the context

"I have to make sure she summarizes what she learned and what she will focus on the next week at the end of each session. She could easily get overwhelmed and do nothing. I do not want her to feel like she failed at treatment."

"I will issue a grid so she can check off if she used the strategy each day or not. I need to make sure she understands that she can change the strategy to meet her needs or decide not to use it if it is not helpful. Each week she comes back I will review the use of her strategies by looking at the grid, and she can decide if the strategies are ones she will continue to use or discard."

"I need to make sure that as she understands the concepts and her confidence is growing, I let her really find her strategies or solutions more independently."

"I need to make sure that the concepts and strategies do not add stress to her life but help decrease it as she uses her energy more wisely."

"I will use motivational interviewing techniques to help her come up with her own strategies or modifications."

Next Steps

1. Sarah has decided not to return to work until 2 weeks after she has finished her chemotherapy to ensure she has adequate activity tolerance. Occupational therapy can assist in crafting work accommodations.
2. Follow-up at 1 month to ensure that she is habitually employing her strategies and effectively managing her life roles.
3. She may need a few additional sessions once she has returned to work to develop any new strategies she may need to be successful at work.

Anticipate present and future patient concerns

Decide whether the patient should continue or discontinue therapy and/or return in the future

"She will very likely learn how to use her energy well enough to consistently care for her children and her home. I need to make sure that she understands that she may notice more cognitive difficulties when she first returns to work. The increased demands may lead to fatigue again. She will need to plan for that and either delegate more at home or return part time with a gradual increase in hours."

"I am going to schedule a follow-up session 1 week prior to return to work to assist her in thinking through the challenges and having some strategies she can use to minimize errors. At that session we can determine whether she needs an additional 1 month follow-up or whether she is ready for discharge."

 Clinical Reasoning in Occupational Therapy Practice

Building a Therapeutic Alliance

What can the therapist do to establish rapport and a therapeutic alliance with Sarah early on in their work together?

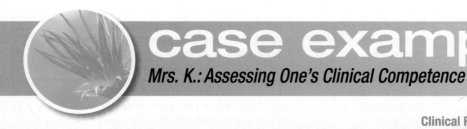

case example
Mrs. K.: Assessing One's Clinical Competence

Occupational Therapy Intervention Process	Clinical Reasoning Process	
	Objectives	**Examples of Therapist's Internal Dialogue**

Patient Information

Mrs. K. is a 50-year-old woman with a diagnosis of left postmastectomy lymphedema with multiple infections and fibrosis. Mrs. K. underwent mastectomy for left breast cancer 15 months ago and had 20 of her lymph nodes removed on the left side. She had chemotherapy and radiation therapy and now shows no evidence of disease. She recently saw her oncologist with complaints of left upper extremity swelling and aching heaviness in the arm and across her chest and back. She reported difficulty with fit of clothing on the left, which causes her increasing embarrassment at work. Her sleep is also disturbed because of left arm discomfort. She is referred to outpatient occupational therapy for evaluation and treatment of lymphedema, including manual lymph drainage, compressive bandaging, fitting of custom compressive garments, and instruction in home exercises and skin care.

Although the occupational therapist had previous experience treating cancer patients and instructing in self-care, home management, and work-simplification strategies, she had no specific or specialized training in the area of lymphedema management. Because this new area of practice interested her, she searched the Internet for information. She readily found information on lymphedema and its treatment (www.cancer.org) and guidelines for contacting a lymphedema treatment center, information about training programs, and names of clinicians with specialized training (www.lymphnet.org). She searched the National Library of Medicine (www.nlm.nih.gov) for abstracts of research regarding treatment of lymphedema.

Appreciate the context

"I wonder how much Mrs. K. knows about lymphedema and how to manage it. I wonder what kind of work she does along with other kinds of activities. Do any of these need to be modified in order to prevent recurrence of lymphedema once it is under control? Does Mrs. K. have a support system in place to which she can delegate tasks to prevent further exacerbation of the lymphedema?"

Develop intervention hypotheses

"It appears that Mrs. K. needs a specialized form of intervention."

Reflect on competence

"I am an occupational therapist working in a small physical disabilities setting at a suburban hospital in the Midwest. I have 5 years of experience, working in long-term care for 1 year and for 4 years in my present position. I typically work with both inpatients and outpatients, primarily with orthopedic or neurological problems. I am concerned that I do not have the expertise that is required to perform the manual lymph drainage or the fitting for a compression garment in this case."

Recommendations

Having some preliminary information, the occupational therapist used American Occupational Therapy Association Standards of Continuing Competence (American Occupational Therapy Association, n.d.) to assess her competence to treat Mrs. K. She concluded that she did not have the knowledge, critical reasoning, or performance skills necessary to assess and treat Mrs. K. She used information from her Internet search to provide Mrs. K. with suggestions to help minimize the impact of lymphedema in her daily life and to refer Mrs. K. to another facility with specially trained therapists. She also decided to pursue training herself to make these services available to patients at her hospital.

Summary Review Questions

1. Define two methods of classifying cancer and how an occupational therapist might use this information.
2. Describe common medical treatments for breast cancer.
3. List potential side effects of cancer treatments that may interfere with occupational performance.
4. Summarize clinician practices that may help prevent compassion fatigue. Propose the unique circumstances that make use of self-care strategies particularly important for occupational therapists involved in cancer care.
5. Explain why it is important to address the needs of caregivers for persons with cancer.
6. Discuss three strategies you could employ to meet the needs of caregivers.
7. Describe potential occupational needs a client with cancer may have throughout the cancer journey.
8. Summarize occupational therapy interventions for fatigue and cognition. How might those interventions be different for patients in medical treatment or survivorship phases as compared to those receiving palliative care?

Glossary

Compassion satisfaction—The positive feature of professional quality of life that involves the desirable effects of helping others (Stamm, 2010). Its opposite is compassion fatigue.

Lymphedema—A buildup of lymph fluid in the fatty tissues under the skin that causes swelling. It is often a sequela to surgery and/or radiation that involves one or more lymph nodes and remains a lifetime risk for cancer survivors (American Cancer Society, 2011).

Metastasis—The term to describe the situation in which cancer cells get into the bloodstream or lymph system, travel to other parts of the body, and form new tumors

Palliative care—An approach that aims to improve quality of life for patients who are facing life-threatening illness and for their families. It provides relief from pain and other distressing symptoms and provides support to help patients live as actively as possible as well as for coping and bereavement (World Health Organization, 2012).

Peripheral neuropathy—Numbness, tingling, and/or pain caused by nerve damage.

Survivorship—The phase of the cancer journey beginning as the patient completes medical treatment and continuing throughout his or her life.

References

American Cancer Society. (2011). Understanding Lymphedema. Retrieved November 17, 2012 from http://www.cancer.org/treatment/treatmentsandsideeffects/physicalsideeffects/lymphedema/index.

American Cancer Society. (2012a). Breast cancer. Retrieved November 14, 2012 from http://www.cancer.org/cancer/breastcancer/detailedguide/breast-cancer.

American Cancer Society. (2012b). Cancer Facts & Figures 2012. Retrieved November 23, 2012 from http://www.cancer.org/research/cancerfactsfigures/cancerfactsfigures/cancer-facts-figures-2012.

American Cancer Society. (2012c). Lung cancer. Retrieved November 25, 2012 from http://www.cancer.org/cancer/lungcancer/index.

American Cancer Society. (2012d). Questions people ask about cancer. Retrieved November 25, 2012 from http://www.cancer.org/cancer/cancerbasics/questions-people-ask-about-cancer.

American Cancer Society. (2012e). Staging. Retrieved November 12, 2012 from http://www.cancer.org/treatment/understandingyourdiagnosis/staging.

American Cancer Society. (2012f). Surgery for breast cancer. Retrieved November 13, 2012 from http://www.cancer.org/cancer/breastcancer/detailedguide/breast-cancer-treating-surgery.

American Cancer Society. (2012g). What you need to know as a cancer caregiver. Retrieved November 23, 2012 from http://www.cancer.org/treatment/caregivers/caregiving/whatyouneedtoknow/index.

American Cancer Society. (n.d.). Sarcoma—Adult soft tissue cancer. Retrieved November 11, 2012 from http://www.cancer.org/cancer/sarcoma-adultsofttissuecancer/index.

American Occupational Therapy Association. (n.d.). Occupational therapy practice areas in the 21st Century. Retrieved November 25, 2012 from http://www.aota.org/Practitioners/PracticeAreas.aspx.

Anderson, R. T., Kimmick, G. G., McCoy, T. P., Hopkins, J., Levine, E., Miller, G., Ribisl, P., & Mihalko, S. L. (2012). A randomized trial of exercise on well-being and function following breast cancer surgery: The RESTORE trial. *Journal of Cancer Survivorship, 6,* 172–181.

Appelin, G., & Berterö, C. (2004). Patients' experiences of palliative care in the home. *Cancer Nursing, 27,* 65–70.

Biglia, N., Bounous, V. E., Malabaila, A., Palmisano, D., Torta, D. M., D'Alonzo, M., Sismondi, P. P., & Torta, R. R. (2012). Objective and self-reported cognitive dysfunction in breast cancer women treated with chemotherapy: A prospective study. *European Journal of Cancer Care, 21,* 485–492.

Boykoff, N., Moieni, M., & Subramanian, S. K. (2009). Confronting chemobrain: An in-depth look at survivors' reports of impact on work, social networks, and health care response. *Journal of Cancer Survivorship, 3,* 223–232.

Brown, J. C., Huedo-Medina, T. B., Pescatello, L. S., Pescatello, S. M., Ferrer, R. A., & Johnson, B. T. (2011). Efficacy of exercise interventions in modulating cancer-related fatigue among adult cancer survivors: A meta-analysis. *Cancer Epidemiology, Biomarkers, & Prevention, 20,* 123–133.

Campbell, C. L., Pergolotti, M., & Blaskowitz, M. (2009). Occupational therapy utilization for individuals with brain cancer following a craniotomy: A descriptive study. *Rehabilitation Oncology, 27*, 9–13.

Campbell, K. L., Pusic, A. L., Zucker, D. S., McNeely, M. L., Binkley, J. M., Cheville, A. L., Harwood, K. J. (2012). A prospective model of care for breast cancer rehabilitation: Function. *Cancer, 118(Suppl.)*, 2300–2311.

Cella, D. F., Tulsky, D. S., Gray, G., Sarafian, B., Linn, E., Bonomi, A., Silberman, M., Yellen, S. B., Winicour, P., Brannon, J., Eckberg, K., Lloyd, S., Purl, S., Blendowski, C., Goodman, M., Barnicle, M., Stewart, I., McHale, M., Bonomi, P., Kaplan, E., Taylor, Samuel IV, Thomas, C. R. Jr., & Harris, J. (1993). The functional assessment of cancer therapy scale: Development and validation of the general measure. *Journal of Clinical Oncology, 11*, 570–579.

Centers for Disease Control and Prevention. (2012). Breast cancer disparities. Retrieved November 14, 2012 from http://www.cdc.gov/features/vitalsigns/breastcancer/.

Chandana, S. R., Movva, S., Arora, M., & Singh, T. (2008). Primary brain tumors in adults. *American Family Physician, 77*, 1423–1430.

Chen, C. C., & Bode, R. K. (2010). Psychometric validation of the Manual Ability Measure-36 (MAM-36) in patients with neurologic and musculoskeletal disorders. *Archives of Physical Medicine and Rehabilitation, 91*, 414–420.

Cleeland, C. S., Mendoza, T. R., Wang, X. S., Chou, C., Harle, M., Morrissey, M., & Engstrom, M. C. (2000). Assessing symptom distress in cancer: The M. D. Anderson symptom inventory. *Cancer, 89*, 1634–1646.

Committee on Cancer Survivorship: Improving Care and Quality of Life, National Cancer Policy Board (2006). *From Cancer Patient to Cancer Survivor: Lost in Transition.* Washington, DC: National Academies Press.

Costa, D. M. (2005). Compassion fatigue: Self-care skills for practitioners. *OT Practice, 10*, 13–20.

Costanzo, E. S., Ryff, C. D., & Singer, B. H. (2009). Psychosocial adjustment among cancer survivors: Findings from a national survey of health and well-being. *Health Psychology, 28*, 147–156.

DuBenske, L. L., Wen, K. Y., Gustafson, D. H., Guarnaccia, C. A., Cleary, J. F., Dinauer, S. K., & McTavish, F. M. (2008). Caregivers' differing needs across key experiences of the advanced cancer disease trajectory. *Palliative & Supportive Care, 6*, 265–272.

Ennis-O'Connor, M. (n.d.). Journeying beyond breast cancer. Retrieved November 22, 2012 from http://journeyingbeyondbreastcancer.com/about/.

Epstein, R. M., & Street, R. L. (2007). *Patient-centered communication in cancer care: Promoting healing and reducing suffering* (NIH Publication No. 07-6225). Bethesda, MD: National Cancer Institute.

FACIT.org. (2010). Questionnaires. Retrieved November 25, 2012 from http://www.facit.org/FACITOrg/Questionnaires.

Garrett, K., & Kirchner, S. (1995). Oncologic emergencies: The role of physical therapy and occupational therapy. *Rehabilitation in Oncology, 13*, 10–24.

Goedendorp, M. M., Gielissen, M. F., Verhagen, C. A., & Bleijenberg, G. (2009). Psychosocial interventions for reducing fatigue during cancer treatment in adults. *Cochrane Database of Systematic Reviews, (1)*, CD006953.

Goldstein, N. E., Genden, E., & Morrison, R. S. (2008). Palliative care for patients with head and neck cancer: "I would like a quick return to a normal lifestyle." *Journal of the American Medical Association, 299*, 1818–1825.

Harrington, K. J. (2012). The use of metaphor in discourse about cancer: A review of the literature. *Clinical Journal of Oncology Nursing, 16*, 408–412.

Hegel, M. T., Lyons, K. D., Hull, J. G., Kaufman, P., Urquhart, L., Li, Z., & Ahles, T. A. (2011). Feasibility study of a randomized controlled trial of a telephone-delivered problem-solving-occupational therapy intervention to reduce participation restrictions in rural breast cancer survivors undergoing chemotherapy. *Psychooncology, 20*, 1092–1101.

Hill, A. E., & Chen, C. (2012). The Manual Ability Measure in oncology: An occupation-based hand assessment. *OT Practice, 17*, CE-1–CE-7.

Hockett, K. (2004). Oncologic emergencies. In C. Varricchio, T. B. Ades, P. S. Hinds, & M. Pierce (Eds.), *A cancer source book for nurses* (8th ed., pp. 447–465). Atlanta: American Cancer Society.

Hoving, J. L., Broekhuizen, M. L., & Frings-Dresen, M. H. (2009). Return to work of breast cancer survivors: A systematic review of intervention studies. *BMC Cancer, 9*, 117.

Hutson, L. M. (Ed.). (2004). *Breast cancer* (8th ed.). Atlanta: American Cancer Society.

Jim, H. S., Phillips, K. M., Chait, S., Faul, L. A., Popa, M. A., Lee, Y. H., Hussin, M.G., Jacobsen, P. B., & Small, B. J. (2012). Meta-analysis of cognitive functioning in breast cancer survivors previously treated with standard-dose chemotherapy. *Journal of Clinical Oncology, 30*, 3578–3587.

Joly, F., Rigal, O., Noal, S., & Giffard, B. (2011). Cognitive dysfunction and cancer: Which consequences in terms of disease management? *Psychooncology, 20*, 1251–1258.

Kahol, K., Leyba, M. J., Deka, M., Deka, V., Mayes, S., Smith, M., Ferrara, J. J, & Panchanathan, S. (2008). Effect of fatigue on psychomotor and cognitive skills. *American Journal of Surgery, 195*, 195–204.

Kealey, P., & McIntyre, I. (2005). An evaluation of the domiciliary occupational therapy services in palliative cancer care in a community trust: A patient and carers perspective. *European Journal of Cancer Care, 14*, 232–243.

Keesing, S., & Rosenwax, L. (2011). Is occupation missing from occupational therapy in palliative care? *Australian Occupational Therapy Journal, 58*, 329–336.

Kielhofner, G., Mallinson, T., Crawford, C., Nowak, M., Rigby, M., Henry, A., & Walens, D. (1998). *A user's manual for the Occupational Performance History Interview* (Version 2.0). Chicago: University of Illinois at Chicago.

Law, M., Baptiste, S., Carswell, A., McColl, M. A., Polatajko, H., & Pollock, N. (1998). *Canadian occupational performance measure* (3rd ed.). Toronto, Canada: Canadian Association of Occupational Therapists.

Law, M., Cooper, B., Strong, S., Stewart, D., Rigby, P., & Letts, L. (1996). The person-environment-occupation model: A transactive approach to occupational performance. *Canadian Journal of Occupational Therapy, 63*, 9–23.

Leigh, S. (2006). Cancer survivorship: A first-person perspective. *American Journal of Nursing, 106(Suppl.)*, S12–S14.

Longpré, S. M. (2012). Breast cancer: A holistic perspective. *[AOTA] Physical Disabilities Special Interest Section Quarterly, 35*, 1–3.

Lyons, K. D., Hegel, M. T., Hull, J. G., Li, Z., Balan, S., & Bartels, S. (2012). Reliability and validity of the Valued Activity Inventory for Adults with Cancer (VAI-AC). *Occupational Therapy Journal of Research, 32*, 238–245.

Lyons, M., Orozovic, N., Davis, J., & Newman, J. (2002). Doing-being-becoming: Occupational experiences of persons with life-threatening illnesses. *American Journal of Occupational Therapy, 56*, 285–295.

McClure, M. K., McClure, R. J., Day, R., & Brufsky, A. M. (2010). Randomized controlled trial of the Breast Cancer Recovery Program for women with breast cancer-related lymphedema. *American Journal of Occupational Therapy, 64*, 59–72.

Mendoza, T., Wang, X. S., Cleeland, C. S., Morrissey, M., Johnson, B. A., Wendt, J. K., & Huber, S. L. (1999). The rapid assessment of fatigue severity in cancer patients: Use of the Brief Fatigue Inventory. *Cancer, 85*, 1186–1196.

Mishra, S. I., Scherer, R. W., Snyder, C., Geigle, P. M., Berlanstein, D. R., & Topaloglu, O. (2012). Exercise interventions on health-related quality of life for people with cancer during active treatment. *Cochrane Database of Systematic Reviews, (8)*, CD008465.

Mukand, J. A., Blackinton, D. D., Crincoli, M. G., Lee, J. J., & Santos, B. B. (2001). Incidence of neurologic deficits and rehabilitation of patients with brain tumors. *American Journal of Physical Medicine and Rehabilitation, 80*, 346–350.

National Cancer Institute. (2009). What you need to know about brain cancer: Types of primary brain tumors. Retrieved November 17, 2012 from http://www.cancer.gov/cancertopics/wyntk/brain/page3#c2.

National Cancer Institute. (2010a). Cancer staging. Retrieved November 10, 2012 from http://www.cancer.gov/cancertopics/factsheet/detection/staging.

National Cancer Institute. (2010b). Palliative care in cancer. Retrieved November 6, 2012 from http://www.cancer.gov/cancertopics/factsheet/Support/palliative-care.

National Cancer Institute. (2012a). General information about adult brain tumors. Retrieved November 14, 2012 from http://www.cancer.gov/cancertopics/pdq/treatment/adultbrain/HealthProfessional#Section_619.

National Cancer Institute. (2012b). Head and neck cancers. Retrieved November 17, 2012 from http://www.cancer.gov/cancertopics/factsheet/Sites-Types/head-and-neck.

National Cancer Institute. (2012c). What is cancer? Retrieved November 10, 2012 from http://www.cancer.gov/cancertopics/cancerlibrary/what-is-cancer.

National Cancer Institute. (n.d.[a]). Surveillance, epidemiology and end results (SEER) training modules: Cancer classification. Retrieved September 20, 2012 from http://training.seer.cancer.gov/disease/categories/classification.html.

National Cancer Institute. (n.d.[b]). Tumor grade. Retrieved November 11, 2012 from http://www.cancer.gov/cancertopics/factsheet/detection/tumor-grade.

National Comprehensive Cancer Network. (n.d.). Cancer staging guide. Retrieved November 12, 2012 from http://www.nccn.com/understanding-cancer/cancer-staging.html.

Northouse, L. L., Katapodi, M. C., Song, L., Zhang, L., & Mood, D. W. (2010). Interventions with family caregivers of cancer patients: Meta-analysis of randomized trials. *CA: A Cancer Journal for Clinicians, 60,* 317–339.

Penfold, S. L. (1996). The role of the occupational therapist in oncology. *Cancer Treatment Reviews, 22,* 75–81.

Penson, R. T., Gu, F., Harris, S., Thiel, M. M., Lawton, N., Fuller, A. F., Jr., & Lynch, T. J., Jr. (2007). Hope. *Oncologist, 12,* 1105–1113.

Penson, R. T., Schapira, L., Daniels, K. J., Chabner, B. A., & Lynch, T. J., Jr. (2004). Cancer as metaphor. *The Oncologist, 9,* 708–716.

Poppelreuter, M., Weis, J., Kulz, A. K., Tucha, O., Lange, K. W., & Bartsch, H. H. (2004). Cognitive dysfunction and subjective complaints of cancer patients. A cross-sectional study in a cancer rehabilitation centre. *European Journal of Cancer, 40,* 43–49.

Prochnau, C., Liu, L., & Boman, J. (2003). Personal-professional connections in palliative care occupational therapy. *American Journal of Occupational Therapy, 57,* 196–204.

Pryce, J., Munir, F., & Haslam, C. (2007). Cancer survivorship and work: Symptoms, supervisor response, co-worker disclosure and work adjustment. *Journal of Occupational Rehabilitation, 17,* 83–92.

Seminowicz, D. A., & Davis, K. D. (2007). Interactions of pain intensity and cognitive load: The brain stays on task. *Cerebral Cortex, 17,* 1412–1422.

Smith-Gabai, H. (Ed.). (2011). *Oncology.* Bethesda, MD: AOTA Press.

Spruit, M. A., Janssen, P. P., Willemsen, S. C. P., Hochstenbag, M. M. H., & Wouters, E. F. M. (2006). Exercise capacity before and after an 8-week multidisciplinary inpatient rehabilitation program in lung cancer patients: A pilot study. *Lung Cancer, 52,* 257–260.

Stamm, B. H. (2010). The Concise ProQOL Manual (2nd ed.). Retrieved June 13, 2013 from http://proqol.org/uploads/ProQOL_Concise_2ndEd_12-2010.pdf.

Tamminga, S. J., de Boer, A. G., Verbeek, J. H., Taskila, T., & Frings-Dresen, M. H. (2010). Enhancing return-to-work in cancer patients, development of an intervention and design of a randomised controlled trial. *BMC Cancer, 10,* 345.

Tatu, B. (2005). Physical therapy intervention with oncological emergencies. *Rehabilitation Oncology, 23,* 4–17.

Taylor, K., & Currow, D. (2003). A prospective study of patient identified unmet activity of daily living needs among cancer patients at a comprehensive cancer care centre. *Australian Occupational Therapy Journal, 50,* 79–85.

Thorne, S. E., & Stajduhar, K. I. (2012). Patient perceptions of communications on the threshold of cancer survivorship: Implications for provider responses. *Journal of Cancer Survivorship, 6,* 229–237.

Thorsen, L., Gjerset, G. M., Loge, J. H., Kiserud, C. E., Skovlund, E., Fløtten, T., & Fosså, S. D. (2011). Cancer patients' needs for rehabilitation services. *Acta Oncologica, 50,* 212–222.

Uitterhoevew, R. J., Bensing, J. M., Grol, R. P., Demulder, P. H. M., & Achterberg, T. V. (2010). The effects of communication skills training on patient outcomes in cancer care: A systematic review of the literature. *European Journal of Cancer Care, 19,* 442–457.

Vargo, M. (2011). Brain tumor rehabilitation. *American Journal of Physical Medicine & Rehabilitation, 90(Suppl. 1),* S50–S62.

Vockins, H. (2004). Occupational therapy intervention with patients with breast cancer: A survey. *European Journal of Cancer Care, 13,* 45–52.

Weaver, K. E., Forsythe, L. P., Reeve, B. B., Alfano, C. M., Rodriguez, J. L., Sabatino, S. A., Hawkins N. A., & Rowland, J. H. (2012). Mental and physical health-related quality of life among U.S. cancer survivors: Population estimates from the 2010 National Health Interview Survey. *Cancer Epidemiology, Biomarkers, & Prevention, 21,* 2108–2117.

Wefel, J. S., Lenzi, R., Theriault, R. L., Davis, R. N., & Meyers, C. A. (2004). The cognitive sequelae of standard-dose adjuvant chemotherapy in women with breast carcinoma: Results of a prospective, randomized, longitudinal trial. *Cancer, 100,* 2292–2299.

Wefel, J. S., Saleeba, A. K., Buzdar, A. U., & Meyers, C. A. (2010). Acute and late onset cognitive dysfunction associated with chemotherapy in women with breast cancer. *Cancer, 116,* 3348–3356.

Wefel, J. S., & Schagen, S. B. (2012). Chemotherapy-related cognitive dysfunction. *Current Neurology and Neuroscience Reports, 12,* 267–275.

World Health Organization. (2012). WHO definition of palliative care. Retrieved November 6, 2012 from http://www.who.int/cancer/palliative/definition/en/.

Yasko, A. W., Shreyaskumar, R. P., Pollack, A., & Pollock, R. E. (Eds.). (2001). *Sarcomas of soft tissue and bone.* Atlanta: American Cancer Society.

Yuen, H. K., Gillespie, M. B., Barkley, R. A., Day, T. A., Bandyopadhyay, D., & Sharma, A. K. (2007). Driving performance in patients with cancer in the head and neck region: A pilot study. *Archives of Otolaryngology: Head & Neck Surgery, 133,* 904–909.

Acknowledgements

We recognize the contributions of Margarette L. Shelton, Joanna B. Lipoma, and E. Stuart Oertli, the previous authors of this chapter.